W9-CBF-894

Schalm's
VETERINARY HEMATOLOGY

Schalm's
VETERINARY HEMATOLOGY

Nemi C. Jain, BVSc and AH, MVSc, PhD
Department of Clinical Pathology
School of Veterinary Medicine
University of California
Davis, California

FOURTH EDITION

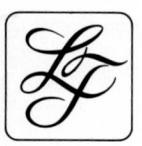 Lea & Febiger   *Philadelphia*   1986

Lea & Febiger
600 Washington Square
Philadelphia, PA   19106-4198
U.S.A.
(215) 922-1330

First Edition, 1961
Second Edition, 1965
   Reprinted, 1967, 1971
Third Edition, 1975
   Reprinted, 1977, 1979, 1981

Library of Congress Cataloging in Publication Data

Schalm, O. W. (Oscar William), 1909-
   Schalm's Veterinary hematology.

   Rev. ed. of: Veterinary hematology / O.W. Schalm,
N.C. Jain, E.J. Carroll. 3rd ed. c1975.
   Includes bibliographies and index.
   1. Veterinary hematology. I. Jain, Nemi C.
(Nemi Chand), 1936-   . II. Title. [DNLM:
1. Hematologic Diseases—veterinary. 2. Veterinary
hematology. SF 771 S298v]
SF769.5.S3   1985   636.089'615   84-27811
ISBN 0-8121-0942-2

PRINTED IN THE UNITED STATES OF AMERICA

Print number: 5   4   3   2   1

Dedicated to
my spiritual Sād-Guru,
Shri Sai Sham,
and
in memory of my beloved father,
Shri Mangilal Kishanlal Jain

Preface

Eleven years have passed since the publication of the third edition of *Veterinary Hematology*. Great expansion in the fields of veterinary and human hematology and immunology during this period necessitated an extensive revision and expansion of this book. The current edition is titled *Schalm's Veterinary Hematology*, honoring the immense contributions of the late Dr. Oscar W. Schalm to veterinary hematology and his establishing it as a vital discipline of veterinary medicine. Due to the untimely demise of Drs. Schalm and Carroll, the fourth edition has evolved primarily as a single-author text.

The text has been extensively reorganized, revised, and expanded. The use of color plates has been expanded from 20 to 25 plates containing 202 individual figures; some old plates have been replaced. The number of black and white illustrations has been increased from 230 to 286. Extensive use has been made of scanning and transmission electron photomicrographs to depict the ultra-structure of leukocytes, erythrocytes, and platelets.

Two new chapters have been added: Chapter 1, concerning examination of the blood and bone marrow in general, and Chapter 11, concerning avian hematology. The normal hematology of common domestic animals is presented separately for each species in Chapters 4 through 10. The information on platelets, normal erythrocytes, erythrocytes in disease, and leukocytes, which comprised one chapter each in the third edition, has been greatly expanded and is now presented in several individual chapters. Thus, Chapters 15 to 17 concern platelet production, struc-

ture, function, and abnormalities; Chapters 18 through 25, erythrocytes and their abnormalities, including anemias; and Chapters 26 through 31, various leukocytes and their abnormalities and responses to disease. The comparative cytochemistry of normal and leukemic human and animal leukocytes is presented separately in Chapter 33, in view of the increasing use of cytochemistry in the diagnosis of leukemia. Other chapters have been revised, updated, and expanded.

The book is aimed at undergraduate and graduate veterinary students, veterinary practitioners, veterinarians engaged in teaching and research, and other scientists interested in comparative hematology. The subject has been presented primarily from the point of view of its application to clinical veterinary medicine, yet provides some in-depth information about the fundamentals of hematology necessary to understand the pathophysiology of hematopoietic disorders. Up-to-date references have been incorporated wherever possible. Although an extensive literature search was made for all the chapters, it was impossible to cite all references. Selection of reference citations has not been an easy task, and I apologize for omission of a particular reference deemed important by the reader.

I am thankful to Dr. Joseph G. Zinkl for contributing the chapter on avian hematology and to Dr. Bernard F. Feldman for his contributions to the chapter on blood coagulation. The assistance of Dr. John W. Switzer in preparing the chapter on immunohematology and of Dr. Prem Handagama in preparing several photographs to illustrate cell morphology is acknowledged. The courtesy of various investigators and colleagues in supplying their published and unpublished photographs for inclusion in the book is highly appreciated. I express my sincere gratitude to Mrs. Constance S. Kono, for her painstaking efforts in overseeing the minute details necessary to publication of this book and my thanks to Rosanna Ullrich for skillfully word processing some challenging tables and parts of the manuscript and to Mrs. Carroll for typing some references. I am thankful to the staff of Lea & Febiger for preparing this fourth edition for publication.

Finally, my deepest gratitude is due to my entire family, without whose unceasing moral support this book would have not come to fruition. My lovely children Kamal, Madhu, and Anant gave their untiring help in searching the literature, typing and cross-checking references, and typing parts of the manuscript. Special thanks and indebtedness are due to my wife, Javitri, and my mother, Shrimati Manfulbai, for their understanding and perseverance in making the dream of publication of this book come true.

Davis, California   *Nemi C. Jain*

Contents

1. Examination of the Blood and Bone Marrow 1

2. Hematologic Techniques 20

3. Blood Volume and Water Balance ... 87

4. The Dog: Normal Hematology with Comments on Response to Disease .. 103

5. The Cat: Normal Hematology with Comments on Response to Disease .. 126

6. The Horse: Normal Hematology with Comments on Response to Disease .. 140

7. Cattle: Normal Hematology with Comments on Response to Disease 178

8. The Sheep: Normal Hematology with Comments on Response to Disease .. 208

9. The Goat: Normal Hematology with Comments on Response to Disease .. 225

10. The Pig: Normal Hematology with Comments on Response to Disease .. 240

11. Avian Hematology—Joseph G. Zinkl 256

12. Normal Values in Blood of Laboratory, Fur-Bearing, and Miscellaneous Zoo, Domestic, and Wild Animals 274

13. The Hematopoietic System 350

14. Coagulation and Its Disorders—B.F. Feldman, E.J. Carroll, N.C. Jain 388

15. Megakaryocytopoiesis and Platelet Production, Survival, and Distribution 431

16. The Platelets: Structural, Biochemical, and Functional Aspects 446

17. Qualitative and Quantitative Disorders of Platelets 466

18. Erythropoiesis and Its Regulation.... 487

19. Hemoglobin Synthesis and Destruction....................... 514

20. The Erythrocyte: Its Morphology, Metabolism, and Survival.............. 527

21. Clinical and Laboratory Evaluation of Anemias and Polycythemias 563

22. Blood Loss or Hemorrhagic Anemias 577

23. Hemolytic Anemias Associated with Some Infectious Agents............. 589

24. Hemolytic Anemias of Noninfectious Origin 627

25. Depression or Hypoproliferative Anemias 655

26. The Neutrophils 676

27. The Eosinophils.................... 731

28. The Basophil and the Mast Cell 756

29. The Monocytes and Macrophages ... 768

30. The Lymphocytes and Plasma Cells.. 790

31. Clinical Interpretation of Changes in Leukocyte Numbers and Morphology 821

32. The Leukemia Complex 838

33. Cytochemistry of Normal and Leukemic Leukocytes 909

34. The Plasma Proteins, Dysproteinemias, and Immune Deficiency Disorders 940

35. Immunohematology................ 990

36. Blood Pictures in Some Common Diseases of Domestic Animals.......... 1040

Appendix 1087

Index 1169

ix

1

Examination of the Blood and Bone Marrow

EXAMINATION OF THE PERIPHERAL BLOOD 1
Collection of Blood 1
Handling the Blood Sample 2
Developing a Hemogram 2
Leukocyte Morphology in Old Blood 5
Species Variation in Blood Morphology 5
Physiological Considerations in Interpretation of Blood Values 7
General Considerations regarding Normal Values in Blood 7

EXAMINATION OF THE BONE MARROW 11
Characteristics and Classification of Cells in Marrow Aspirates 12
Bone Marrow Evaluation 15
General Comments about Bone Marrow Cytology 15
The Myeloid:Erythroid Ratio 17
Bone Marrow Biopsy 18

EXAMINATION OF THE PERIPHERAL BLOOD

Blood is a fluid tissue that circulates through vascular channels carrying the necessities for life to all cells of the body, and it receives the waste products of metabolism for transport to the organs of excretion. Blood examination is performed for several reasons: as a screening procedure to assess general health; as an adjunct to patient evaluation or to diagnosis of a disease; to assess the body's ability to fight infection; and to evaluate the progress of certain disease states. A thorough history and physical examination are essential for meaningful interpretation of hematologic data and other laboratory tests concerning the subject under investigation.

Abnormal findings in a hemogram are most commonly nonspecific; that is, they can be associated with a variety of diseases or conditions provoking a similar response. Infrequently, however, they may be diagnostic, as when leukemic cells or hemoparasites are found in blood. A single hemogram may be adequate for general physical examination, but sequential hemograms must be developed to follow recovery from the disease state. A blood examination may also provide clues as to the necessity of bone marrow examination and other laboratory tests.

This chapter presents a general approach to examination of the peripheral blood and bone marrow in different animal species. Many of the topics discussed here are covered more fully in other chapters. General references in medical literature on examination of blood and bone marrow also provide additional information (Williams et al., 1983; Wintrobe et al., 1981).

Collection of Blood

Blood is readily drawn from large vessels, but several alternate sites have been found suitable for blood collection from various animal species (p. 25). Blood clots upon removal from the body; later the clot retracts releasing the serum commonly used in biochemical analysis. Hematologic examination requires blood in liquid form. For this purpose, blood is collected into a vial containing an appropriate anticoagulant (p. 23). EDTA, which prevents coagulation by complexing Ca^{++}, is the anticoagulant of choice for most hematologic and biochemical analyses. Blood collected with heparin, unless processed immediately, yields poor staining of blood cells. Sodium citrate is recommended for blood platelet studies. Blood should be drawn from the animal at rest and under conditions of least excitement to minimize physiologic variations in cell counts. Blood should be drawn gently. Vacutainers are best for collecting blood; they must be filled to capacity to yield the desired blood-to-anticoagulant ratio. When syringe and needles are used, the needle should be removed from the syringe before transferring blood to the vial containing the anticoagulant to prevent hemolysis. The blood and the anticoagulant should be mixed adequately by inverting the vial a dozen times. A clean venipuncture should be attempted to avoid formation of blood clots from contamination with tissue juice. A fasting blood sample is preferred to obviate processing problems associated with postprandial lipemia.

Handling the Blood Sample

Blood samples should be processed as soon as possible after collection. If a delay is anticipated, it should be refrigerated at 4°C. The blood sample should be mixed several times before a portion is removed for a test procedure. Automatic devices providing a continuous rocking or circular motion have been found satisfactory, but prolonged mixing should be avoided, particularly on a device with circular motion, to prevent mechanical trauma to various blood cells, especially erythrocytes. The steps involved in performing several routine blood tests are described in Chapter 2. The optimal time up to which the sample would be good for performing the desired tests must be kept in mind. In any event, blood films should be made immediately after blood collection, either directly from fresh blood or after anticoagulation. Blood films should be dried quickly and protected from dust and flies until stained. Blood films can be made on glass slides or coverslips. Automatic stainers are made to process only glass slides.

Developing a Hemogram

Essential hematologic techniques are described in detail in Chapter 2. The veterinarian would benefit most by establishing a set of tests for initial screening to be followed by a more detailed hematologic examination. The choice of tests will vary according to the purpose of the patient evaluation, and further laboratory investigation may be required. Initial screening should include at least one of the red blood cell (RBC) parameters, preferably packed cell volume (PCV) or hemoglobin determination, total plasma protein and fibrinogen concentrations, and total and differential leukocyte counts. A detailed hemogram or complete blood count (CBC), as performed at the Veterinary Medical Teaching Hospital at the University of California, Davis (VMTH-UCD) and our laboratories, includes determinations of RBC, Hb, PCV, MCV, MCHC, MCH, icterus index, total plasma protein concentration, fibrinogen, WBC, and a 200-cell differential leukocyte count. (Abbreviations are spelled out in the list below.) Reticulocyte counts are performed on all blood samples, except those from the horse, when PCV is below the minimum normal for the species. ESR is performed for canine and feline patients. Morphologic evaluation of the various blood cells is made from Wright-stained blood films, and abnormalities observed are described briefly following the guidelines outlined in Table 1–1. A subjective evaluation of platelet numbers—above, below, or within normal range for the species—is made from distribution on the stained blood film, and a platelet count is made when specifically requested by the clinician or thrombocytopenia is suspected.

To conserve space in tables of data presented in this and other chapters, particularly Chapters 4 through 10, the unit of measurement for each blood component is listed below.

Blood Entity	*Expressed in*
Erythrocytes (RBC)	Millions per μl of blood
RBC diameter	Micrometers (μm)
Hemoglobin (Hb)	Grams per deciliter (g/dl)
Packed cell volume (PCV)	Volume percent
Mean corpuscular volume (MCV)	Femtoliters (fl)
Mean corpuscular hemoglobin (MCH)	Picograms (pg)
Mean corpuscular hemoglobin concentration (MCHC)	Percent (%) of red cells
Erythrocyte sedimentation rate (ESR)	mm fall in 1 hour
Reticulocytes	Number per 100 red cells or percent

Nucleated erythrocytes (Nuc RBC)	Number per 100 leukocytes
Erythrocyte resistance to hypotonic saline (also called red cell fragility test)	Percent saline in solution producing initial and complete hemolysis
Leukocytes, total count (WBC)	Number per µl of blood
Leukocytes, differential count	Percent
Leukocytes, differential absolute count	Number per µl of blood
Bone marrow, differential cell count	Percent
Thrombocytes (platelets)	Number per µl of blood
Icterus index	Units of color as compared to standards prepared from potassium dichromate
Plasma protein, total	Grams per deciliter (g/dl)
Plasma fibrinogen	Grams per deciliter (g/dl) or milligrams per deciliter (mg/dl)

RBC and WBC counts in modern laboratories are performed using an electronic counter, e.g., the Coulter counter. *Platelet counts* are commonly performed by the hemocytometer method, using ordinary illumination or phase-contrast microscopy, but they can also be performed using an automatic counter designed for this purpose. Blood cell counts obtained by electronic particle counting machines are highly accurate and more reliable than those obtained with the hemocytometer method. Because of species variations in erythrocyte number and morphology, adjustments are necessary in dilution of blood and calibration of the cell-counting equipment. Indirect platelet counts, obtained from viewing a stained blood film for platelets and determining their distribution relative to leukocytes, are highly subjective and inaccurate; they should not be used as a substitute for direct platelet counts.

A *reticulocyte count* is performed by counting at least 1,000 erythrocytes in smears prepared from a mixture of a few drops of blood and an equal to double volume of reticulocyte stain containing new methylene blue (Chapter 2). The reticulocyte count is essential to assess response to anemia in various species, the horse being an exception. In the latter species, a reticulocyte count performed on a bone marrow sample yields similar information. A "corrected" blood reticulocyte count or "reticulocyte production index" is calculated for a more meaningful assessment of erythropoietic response to anemia (Chapter 18).

PCV should be determined by the microhematocrit method rather than by the Wintrobe method. Adequate centrifugal force and time are essential to minimize trapped plasma and obtain accurate PCV values. Even with the microhematocrit method, goat and sheep bloods require longer centrifugation times (10–20 minutes), while 5 minutes is sufficient for other species' blood. PCV values obtained from electronic counters may be erroneous because they are derived from calculations based on MCV, which varies widely among animal species; thus the instrument must be recalibrated each time a different species' blood sample is processed.

Gross examination of the hematocrit tube provides a rough evaluation of both compartments of the blood—the plasma and the formed elements. Centrifugation of blood separates it into three layers: the plasma at the top, the buffy coat in the middle, and the red blood cell mass at the bottom. Plasma color suggests the presence of hemolysis, lactescence, lipemia, and bilirubin. The *icterus index*, which is a measure of the amount of bilirubin in the blood, is determined by comparing plasma color with standards prepared from 1.0% potassium dichromate solution. The presence of hemolysis, lactescence, and lipemia interferes with estimation of the icterus index. The *buffy coat* is an off-white layer composed of platelets above and leukocytes below. Generally the platelet layer is whitish and should not be mistaken for the leukocyte layer, which is tinged reddish due to admixture of erythrocytes of low specific gravity, e.g., reticulocytes and leptocytes. The platelet layer is most noticeable and clearly distinguishable from the leukocyte layer in cat blood.

Hemoglobin determination is best performed by the cyanmethemoglobin method, which measures almost all types of circulating hemoglobin. The oxyhemoglobin method measures functional hemoglobin; hence it generally provides somewhat lower values than the

Table 1–1.   Outline for Examination of a Wright-Stained Blood Smear*

  I.   Platelets
      1. Distribution
      2. Estimated number
      3. Morphologic abnormalities, e.g., hypogranulation, basophilia, vacuolation, and megathrombocytes
  II.   Erythrocytes
      1. Size
         a. Anisocytosis
         b. Normocytic
         c. Macrocytic
         d. Microcytic
      2. Shape
         a. Poikilocytes
         b. Leptocytes
         c. Target cells
         d. Acanthocytes
         e. Spherocytes
         f. Schistocytes
         g. Other forms (for additional terminology see Chapter 20)
      3. Distribution
         a. Single
         b. Rouleau formation
         c. Agglutination
      4. Color
         a. Normochromic
         b. Hypochromic
         c. Polychromasia
      5. Abnormal structures
         a. Howell-Jolly bodies
         b. Heinz bodies
         c. Pappenheimer bodies
         d. Basophilic stippling
         e. Nucleated red cells
         f. Parasites
         g. Inclusion bodies, e.g., distemper inclusions
         h. Nuclear fragmentation and other structures
 III.   Leukocytes
      1. Estimated number
      2. Differential leukocyte count
      3. Morphologic abnormalities
         a. Toxic changes such as azurophilic granules, vacuolation, foaminess, basophilia, and Döhle bodies in
            neutrophils
         b. Nuclear degeneration
         c. Hypersegmentation of neutrophil nucleus
         d. Hyposegmentation of neutrophil nucleus (Pelger-Huët anomaly)
         e. Giant bizarre forms
         f. Other abnormal findings
      4. Cytoplasmic inclusions, e.g., *Ehrlichia* organisms, distemper inclusions, phagocytosed red cells and bac-
         teria, etc.
 IV.   Other findings
      1. A variety of cells including mast cells, plasma cells, macrophages, megakaryocytes, and tumor cells
      2. Hemoparasites, e.g., trypanosomes
      3. Microfilariae of heart worm

*Various subjective findings may be graded from slight to marked (e.g., slight polychromasia) or rare to many (e.g., many Heinz bodies).

cyanmethemoglobin method and has yielded significantly lower values in rare instances of methemoglobinemia in cats anesthetized with ketamine. Such is also the case in other instances of methemoglobinemias from oxidant drugs. Spectrophotomatic measurement of hemoglobin is erroneous when blood is lipemic or contains Heinz bodies in large numbers (Chapter 2). Sahli's hemoglobinometer method is less accurate because of variations due to sampling error and subjective evaluation of color.

Erythrocyte indexes, namely, *MCV*, *MCHC*, and *MCH* are a must for evaluation of an anemic patient and can be used as a guide to the accuracy of various erythrocyte parameters (RBC, Hb, and PCV). For evaluation of anemias, the indexes are more applicable to the dog, as to humans, but have limited application to the cat and cow and are of little practical use in other species. As a guide to the accuracy of erythrocyte parameters, these indexes are applicable to blood of all species. The accuracy of the erythrocyte indexes is as good as those of the parameters used in their derivation. Hence errors in RBC, PCV, and Hb will become compounded in these indexes. Erythrocytic indexes should be interpreted in conjunction with an assessment of erythrocyte morphology in Wright-stained blood films (see Table 1–1). For example, a sample with distinct dimorphic erythrocyte morphology may yield normal erythrocytic indexes, and slight changes in red cell size and hemoglobin may not be reflected in corresponding indexes.

Total plasma protein concentration can be estimated using a refractometer. Plasma present in a 75-mm-long hematocrit tube used for determination of PCV is usually sufficient for this purpose. Plasma can also be obtained after centrifugation of some blood in a Wintrobe hematocrit tube (15 minutes at 2,000 G). Hemolysis, lactescence, and lipemia interfere with proper refractometer reading, giving falsely higher values. Similarly, higher values have been obtained for samples having increased blood sugar and cholesterol levels. Postprandial lactescence and lipemia can be avoided if blood samples are collected before the animal is fed in the morning. *Fibrinogen* content of plasma can be readily estimated by the heat precipitation method and by using a refractometer. It is an important procedure in evaluating inflammatory response and disseminated intravascular coagulation (DIC). In cattle, fibrinogen determination is of considerable value in determination of internal inflammatory lesions.

The *erythrocyte sedimentation rate* is a nonspecific test suggestive of an organic abnormality. It is often performed on human blood and occasionally has been found useful in the dog and cat. The test is set up in a Wintrobe hematocrit tube and read at the end of 1 hour. The observed ESR value must be corrected for the PCV of the blood before it is interpreted. A procedure to conduct the test in a 75-mm capillary tube has also been described (Jain and Kono, 1975).

The *differential leukocyte count* should be performed on a minimum of 200 cells unless the blood sample has well below the normal number of leukocytes. A standard procedure should be followed to perform the differential count. Simultaneously, any abnormality in the morphologic appearance of various cell types should be recorded. Smears prepared on slides or coverslips can be used. Smears should be prepared to provide a monolayer of cells, and the staining method used should produce quality results with discernible cellular details. The need for optimal staining of blood and bone marrow films for satisfactory cytologic examination cannot be overemphasized. Precipitate and other staining artifacts should be avoided because they might be mistaken for certain blood cell features such as erythrocyte parasites or toxic changes in leukocytes. Platelets, particularly in equine blood, and basophils, particularly in canine and feline bloods, could be overlooked in poorly stained films. Erythrocyte morphology may appear defective in poorly fixed blood films.

Leukocyte Morphology in Old Blood

The leukocyte may degenerate in blood that is several hours old or that was exposed to high ambient temperature before the blood film was made. Degeneration occurs principally in the nucleus. The monocyte is one of the first leukocytes to be affected by aging; the nucleus splits into a number of fragments, producing a pattern suggestive of the radiating petals of a flower (Fig. 4–3). The neutrophil nucleus becomes hypersegmented, with many small, rounded lobes interconnected by filaments (Fig. 4–4); later, the individual lobes break away, becoming pyknotic blobs of chromatin. The lymphocyte nucleus tends to form one or more large, bud-like projections (Fig. 4–4). These changes are more common in oxalated blood than in blood anticoagulated with EDTA.

Species Variation in Blood Morphology

Wright stain or any other Romanowsky stain provides the best available means of morphologic evaluation of blood and bone marrow. Supravital staining as with new methylene blue may be performed to demonstrate certain cellular structures such as the reticulum of reticulocytes and Heinz bodies. Blood films must be examined under an oil immersion lens so that necessary details can be observed and leukocyte differential counts performed. Mechanical trauma to blood cells from smear making and contact of blood with the glass surface creates artifacts of morphology. For example, red cells may appear highly crenated and acquire teardrop form; lymphocytes may become deformed because of compression from red cells; granules of neutrophils, eosinophils, and, rarely, basophils may be found scattered from ruptured cells. These findings should not be confused with pathologic changes. For this reason, finding of abnormal red cell morphology in doubtful cases should be confirmed by examination of blood in wet mounts between plastic surfaces. The veterinarian, being knowledgeable about the patient under investigation, will benefit most by examining blood and bone marrow films himself rather than relying completely on results provided by the laboratory technician.

Mammalian platelets and erythrocytes are non-nucleated, whereas both are nucleated in birds, reptiles, and fish. Mammalian platelets appear as small, roundish or oblong structures with a cluster of reddish purple (azurophilic) granules in a pale blue matrix enclosed by a delicate membrane. Their morphology is generally similar in various animals. Slight variation in size is apparent, with an occasional platelet being about twice as large as an average platelet and rarely as big as the red blood cell. Equine platelets generally stain lightly, and some may appear elongated or filamentous (Fig. 16–2A). Platelet activation occurs upon slightest injury to their surface membrane, and so some platelet aggregation is common in blood films. Increased platelet clumping results in their irregular distribution and gives a false impression of thrombocytopenia.

Normal erythrocytes are biconcave discs with a light center and a small rim of hemoglobin. Slight variation in size (anisocytosis) is common among erythrocytes of various species, while variations in shape (poikilocytosis) may be artifactual (such as crenation) or a natural occurrence (sickle cells in the deer and fusiform and spindle-shaped red cells in Angora goats) or a pathologic abnormality (schistocytes). Pig erythrocytes have a marked tendency to crenate. Other artifacts include adherence of stain precipitate to the red cells or their margins, vacuolation, target cell formation, and flattening (loss of central pallor) along the periphery of the blood film. In a blood film, teardrop or oblong red cells produced as a result of mechanical pull during smear making are generally oriented in the same direction in contrast to pathologic ovalocytes or rod-shaped cells, which are distributed randomly; these artifacts are not seen in wet mounts of blood as indicated above. Elliptical red blood cells are characteristic of the family Camellidae (e.g., camels, llamas, and alpacas; see Chapter 12). Rouleau formation (roll of red blood cells like a pile of coins) is prominent in the horse, and some rouleaux are apparent in dog and cat blood. Increased rouleau formation in dog and cat blood is suggestive of increased total plasma protein concentration. Bovine erythrocytes normally do not form rouleaux. Red blood cell agglutination is certainly an abnormality and must be distinguished from rouleaux. Erythrocytes coated with IgM tend to aggregate and form macroscopic and/or microscopic clumps. Young polychromatic erythrocytes (reticulocytes) are normally found in small numbers in the human, dog, and cat, but not in the horse and cow. Howell-Jolly bodies are occasionally seen in small numbers in the erythrocytes of the cat and horse. Nucleated erythrocytes are usually absent in the peripheral blood, but an occasional one may be encountered in the dog and cat. They are found in the peripheral blood under a variety of circumstances (p. 569). Splenectomy or reduced splenic function is commonly associated with increased numbers of erythrocytes with Howell-Jolly bodies and nucleated red cells. Heinz bodies can occur naturally in the cat. Red blood cell inclusions such as basophilic stippling (aggregation of ribosomal material), Pappenheimer bodies (iron particles), and Cabot's rings (remnants of mitotic spindle) are abnormal findings.

Leukocyte morphology, except for some minor differences, is generally similar in various species. The neutrophil, eosinophil, and basophil are collectively referred to as granulocytes, and the neutrophil often as the polymorphonuclear leukocyte or segmenter. Similarly, the lymphocyte and monocyte are referred to as agranulocytes and also as the mononuclear leukocytes. Species differences occur not only with regard to the WBC count, but also in the proportion of the different leukocytes. For example, neutrophils predominate in the human, dog, and cat, while in the horse they slightly exceed lymphocytes and in ruminants and laboratory animals such as rats and mice neutrophils are outnumbered by lymphocytes. Nuclear segmentation in animal neutrophils is not as prominent as in human neutrophils. Cytoplasm presents fine, pinkish or pale granules. In some animals (e.g., the rabbit and guinea pig), the granules are conspicuous and reddish; the cells are then designated heterophils. The eosinophil and basophil usually have a less polymorphous nucleus than the neutrophil. Their cytoplasm contains large and distinctive granules—reddish orange in the eosinophil and purplish red in the basophil. Some animals have a characteristic eosinophil, e.g., the horse with large round granules and the cat with rod-shaped granules. Basophils are rare in normal blood and exhibit some species variations. Canine basophils have very few granules, and granules of feline basophils lack metachromasia and stain pale gray. An immature feline basophil may exhibit both darkly stained and lightly stained granules. The lymphocyte is the most prominent leukocyte in the cow, sheep, goat, mouse, and rat. The size, shape, and staining features of lymphocytes vary from blood to blood within a species. The most common form has a roundish nucleus and a small amount of light to deep blue cytoplasm. An occasional lymphocyte, especially in the cow, may contain some large azurophilic granules in the cytoplasm. Large lymphocytes are seen in the cow more often than in the dog and cat, and some of them may be difficult to distinguish from monocytes. The monocyte is generally the largest of the leukocytes in blood. Its nucleus tends to be ameboid; hence it assumes varied morphology. The cytoplasm stains grayish blue and may present some vacuoles and/or dust-like (azurophilic) granules. The presence of broken or degenerated cells in stained films is suggestive of mechanical damage during smear making or increased cellular fragility as in old blood or blood containing abnormal cells (leukemia). Some free nuclei may swell from hydration and present separated chromatin giving the appearance of "basket cells."

For details of normal and abnormal cellular morphology see Chapters 4 through 12 on hematology of various animal species.

Physiological Considerations in Interpretation of Blood Values

Some of the blood values are significantly influenced by age and to a lesser extent by sex and breed. Emotional disturbance, excitement, and strenuous exercise, which contract the spleen and force stored cells into the circulation, influence certain blood parameters, e.g., erythrocyte and platelet numbers. Neutrophil numbers increase owing to mobilization of cells from the marginal pool in microvasculature. Lymphocyte numbers, particularly in young animals, are similarly elevated by emotions and exercise because of increased input from the thoracic duct. Dehydration leads to loss of water from the plasma resulting in hemoconcentration and thus in increased erythrocyte parameters, total plasma protein concentration, and blood urea nitrogen.

General Considerations regarding Normal Values in Blood

The student will find it helpful to think of the normal blood standards as reflecting certain characteristics of the animal in question (Tables 1–2, 1–3, and 1–4).

Hemoglobin is a respiratory pigment, and its concentration in the blood, in health, is in proportion to the propensity of the animal for sustained muscular activity or ability to meet demands for sudden bursts of speed. The dog, horse, and human are representative of the more active types, and thus their hemoglobin needs and values are greater than those of the more lethargic animals, such as the cow, sheep, goat, and cat.

The size and number of erythrocytes vary among the animal species; the smaller the red cell the greater the number per unit volume of blood. The distribution of the hemoglobin

Table 1–2. Some Differential Characteristics in Blood Morphology of Domestic Animals

Animal	Rouleaux	Central Pallor	Mean Diameter (μm)	Reticulocytes in Peripheral Blood in Health (%)	Special Features (Erythrocytes)	Approximate Neutrophil: Lymphocyte Ratio	Special Features (Leukocytes)
Dog	+	+ +	7.0	± 1.0	Essentially uniform in size.	70:20	Basophils rare. Eosinophil granules do not fill cell; granules variable in size and stain lightly. Cytoplasm shows through and takes pale blue stain.
Cat	+ +	+	5.8	± 0.5	Crenation with few blunt processes. Slight anisocytosis. Eccentric Howell-Jolly body in 1% of cells.	60:30	Basophils rare. Eosinophil granules rod-like and stain dull grayish-orange. Majority of lymphocytes of small size. Few band neutrophils are normally present.
Cow	−	+	5.5	0	Anisocytosis is common. Giant forms may occur.	28:58	Eosinophil granules small, round, intensely stained, and fill cell. Azurophil granules of large size may occur in lymphocytes. Vacuoles common in monocytes.
Sheep	±	+	4.5	0	Regular in size and shape with small central pale spot.	30:60	Neutrophil nucleus usually multilobed. Eosinophil granules well-stained, ovoid and fill cell. Frequent large azurophil granules in lymphocytes. Monocyte nucleus amoeboid.
Horse	+ + +	±	5.7	0	Marked rouleaux, a consistent finding. Cells uniform in size. Occasional Howell-Jolly body. Immature RBC almost never found in peripheral blood.	cold-blooded, 55:35 hot-blooded, 50:45	Eosinophil very characteristic; granules very large and fill cell. Majority of lymphocytes are small. Monocytes usually have kidney-bean nucleus.
Pig	+ +	±	6.0	± 1.0	Crenation with sharp points is a characteristic feature. Slight anisocytosis. Occasional polychromatophilia.	35:50	Eosinophil granules ovoid, pale pink-orange, fill cell. Band neutrophils occur in health (ave. 1%). Lymphocytes vary from small to large.

Table 1–3. Ranges and Means for the Normal Differential Absolute Leukocyte Number per µl of Blood[a]

Animal	Total Leukocyte Count	Band Neutrophils	Mature Neutrophils	Lymphocytes	Monocytes	Eosinophils	Basophils
Dog	6,000–17,000 (11,500)	0–300 (70)	3,000–11,500 (7,000)	1,000–4,800 (2,800)	150–1,350 (750)	100–1,250 (550)	Rare
Cat	5,500–19,500 (12,500)	0–300 (100)	2,500–12,500 (7,500)	1,500–7,000 (4,000)	0–850 (350)	0–1,500 (650)	Rare
Cow	4,000–12,000 (8,000)	0–120 (20)	600–4,000 (2,000)	2,500–7,500 (4,500)	25–840 (400)	0–2,400 (700)	0–200 (50)
Sheep	4,000–12,000 (8,000)	Rare	700–6,000 (2,400)	2,000–9,000 (5,000)	0–750 (200)	0–1,000 (400)	0–300 (50)
Goat	4,000–13,000 (9,000)	Rare	1,200–7,200 (3,250)	2,000–9,000 (5,000)	0–550 (250)	50–650 (450)	0–120 (50)
Horse (hot-blooded)	5,500–12,500 (9,000)	0–100 (20)	2,700–6,700 (4,700)	1,500–5,500 (3,500)	0–800 (400)	0–925 (375)	0–170 (50)
Pig	11,000–22,000 (16,000)	0–800 (150)	3,200–10,000 (5,500)	4,500–13,000 (8,000)	250–2,000 (800)	50–2,000 (500)	0–400 (80)

[a]Ranges for dog, cat, cow, and horse represent two standard deviations from the mean, with slight modification with respect to minimum numbers of lymphocytes for the dog and cat. Ranges for sheep, goat, and pig represent estimates from raw data.

Table 1-4. Normal Ranges and Means for Blood Values in Domestic Animals[a]

Animal	RBC (×10⁶/μl)	Hb (g/dl)	PCV[b] (%)	MCV (fl)	MCHC (%)	WBC (×10³/μl)	Differential Leukocyte Count (%)					
							Neutrophils		Lympho-cytes	Mono-cytes	Eosino-phils	Basophils
							Band	Mature				
Dog	5.5–8.5 (6.8)	12–18 (15)	37–55 (45)	60–77 (70)	32–36 (34)	6.0–17.0 (11.5)	0–3 (0.8)	60–77 (70)	12–30 (20)	3–10 (5)	2–10 (4)	Rare
Cat	5.0–10.0 (7.5)	8–15 (12)	24–45 (37)	39–55 (45)	30–36 (33)	5.5–19.5 (12.5)	0–3 (0.5)	35–75 (59)	20–55 (32)	1–4 (3)	2–12 (5)	Rare
Cow	5.0–10.0 (7.0)	8–15 (11)	24–46 (35)	40–60 (52)	30–36 (33)	4.0–12.0 (8.0)	0–2 (0.5)	15–45 (28)	45–75 (58)	2–7 (4)	2–20 (9)	0–2 (0.5)
Sheep	8.0–16.0 (12.0)	8–16 (12)	24–50 (38)	23–48 (33)	31–38 (33)	4.0–12.0 (8.0)	Rare	10–50 (30)	40–75 (62)	0–6 (2.5)	0–10 (5)	0–3 (0.5)
Goat	8.0–18.0 (13.0)	8–14 (11)	19–38 (28)	15–30 (23)	35–42 (38)	4.0–13.0 (9.0)	Rare	30–48 (36)	50–70 (56)	0–4 (2.5)	1–8 (5)	0–1 (0.5)
Horse (hot-blooded)	6.5–12.5 (9.5)	11–19 (15)	32–52 (42)	34–58 (46)	31–37 (35)	5.5–12.5 (9.0)	0–2 (0.5)	30–65 (49)	25–70 (44)	1–7 (4)	0–11 (4)	0–3 (0.5)
Pig	5.0–8.0 (6.5)	10–16 (13)	32–50 (42)	50–68 (63)	30–34 (32)	11.0–22.0 (16.0)	0.4 (1)	28–47 (37)	39–62 (53)	2–10 (5)	1–11 (3)	0–2 (0.5)

[a]For influence of age on the total and differential leukocyte counts in the cow, see Tables 7–4 and 7–5; for the horse, see Table 6–6.
[b]PCV obtained at 14,000 G for 2 minutes for dog, cat, cow, sheep, and horse bloods and for 12 minutes for goat blood. Pig blood PCV based on Wintrobe method at 2,260 G for 30 minutes.

in a greater number of smaller units results in increasing the surface area of the erythrocytic mass, thereby enhancing the exchange of gases. Because of this feature, certain breeds of horses are best suited for use in racing and other active sports. The Arabian horse and all breeds that have stemmed from it, the "hot-blooded" horses, are unique in having erythrocytes that are smaller and present in greater number than in the so-called cold-blooded breeds.

The goat has the smallest red cell among the domestic animals and also the greatest number, and the sheep follows as a close second. The ancestors of the sheep and goat lived in the rarefied atmosphere of mountaintops. In this environment, efficient respiration was required, and this may in part explain why domestic sheep and goats have an arrangement for more efficient respiration than is needed for life under domestication.

The total leukocyte number and differential distribution in peripheral blood are influenced by the stress hormone secreted by the adrenal cortex. The dog and cat respond well to stress, as is reflected in significant changes in their leukocyte picture in disease. The cow, sheep, and goat respond less dramatically to the stress of disease insofar as their total and differential leukocyte counts are concerned. These latter animals tend to have lower total leukocyte counts in health and more lymphocytes than neutrophils.

Sedimentation of erythrocytes in plasma is dependent to a great extent on the tendency of the erythrocytes to form rouleaux. Rouleaux are especially prominent in drawn equine blood, of which rapid sedimentation is a normal characteristic feature. The red cells of the dog, cat, and pig are intermediate in tendency toward rouleau formation, so the influence of disease on the sedimentation rate can be best studied in these animals. The cow, sheep, and goat red cells show little or no rouleaux, and so erythrocyte sedimentation is minimal in these animals.

Turbidity or lactescence of blood plasma occurs principally in dog blood as a physiologic effect following a meal high in lipids (Plate II–4). This is called postprandial lipemia, because it occurs generally between 2 and 12 hours after a meal (Jasper and Jain, 1964). When blood is taken from dogs at random, cloudy plasmas are common and may interfere with some observations, e.g., icterus index, hemoglobin measurement, and plasma protein concentration. Lactescence can generally be prevented by taking blood 12 hours after the last meal.

Important general references on hematology of animals are Burnett, 1917, a summary of the literature to 1917 on the blood of the horse, cow, sheep, goat, dog, cat, pig, rabbit, and domestic fowl; Scarborough, 1931–1932, an extensive compilation of data appearing in the literature through 1926 and including the rabbit, guinea pig, rat, dog, cat, cow, sheep, goat, horse, monkey, and birds; Wirth, 1950, a German-language text on the hematology of domestic animals; Albritton, 1952, a manual on standard values in blood of humans, the domestic animals, and some of the lower vertebrates which was compiled with the help of several hundred contributors and reviewers; Altman, 1961, which presents data on humans and animals gathered from many sources and covering blood and body fluids; Schermer, 1954, a German-language text on the blood morphology of laboratory animals, and Schermer, 1967, an English-language text on the same subject; Lucas and Jamroz, 1961, a text on avian hematology; Andrew, 1965, a text on comparative hematology of vertebrates and nonvertebrates; Archer and Jeffcott, 1977, a text on comparative clinical hematology of the common domestic animals with chapters on hematology of humans, birds, primates, laboratory animals, and wild animals; Hawkey, 1975, a text on comparative mammalian hematology; and Mitruka and Rawnsley, 1977, a text on hematology and clinical chemistry of laboratory animals. Several atlases and laboratory manuals have also become available in recent years (Keller and Freudiger, 1983; Lewis and Rebar, 1979; Rich, 1974; Sanderson and Phillips, 1981; Schalm, 1980, 1984a, 1984b).

EXAMINATION OF THE BONE MARROW

Bone marrow examination provides information about hematopoietic status of the individual. It is a necessary adjunct to hematologic examination, but must not be performed indiscriminately. Various indications of marrow examination include: nonresponsive anemias, megaloblastic or microcytic anemias, persistent neutropenia, thrombocytopenia, drug toxicities, irradiation, lymphoproliferative disorders including multiple myeloma, myeloproliferative disorders, and infiltrative diseases. Marrow examination is unnecessary in regenerative anemias unless the response is inadequate. At present marrow examination is the principal means of evaluating response to anemia in the horse. Sometimes marrow examination may be rewarding in parasitic diseases such as leishmaniasis in that parasitized macrophages can be found in marrow aspirates and not in the peripheral blood. Blood examination provides clues as to the necessity of a bone marrow examination, and it is imperative that a blood sample always be collected along with the bone marrow specimen for

proper evaluation. The techniques of bone marrow aspiration and procedures for making and staining marrow films are described in Chapter 2. Iron staining of marrow smears provides information about iron stores and helps differentiate iron deficiency anemias from anemias of chronic inflammatory disease. Marrow smears can also be processed to demonstrate direct immunofluorescence of antibody-coated megakaryocytes in patients suspected of immune-mediated thrombocytopenia.

Characteristics and Classification of Cells in Marrow Aspirates

The terminology employed here conforms to the reports of the Committee for Clarification of the Nomenclature of Cells and Diseases of the Blood and Blood-Forming Organs 1948–1950. The following is a brief description of various morphologically recognizable bone marrow cells.

MATURATION OF THE ERYTHROCYTE

Rubriblast (proerythroblast, pronormoblast)	Round cell presenting a narrow rim of dark blue cytoplasm. The nucleus occupies most of the cell, is usually centrally located but may be eccentric. The chromatin is finely stippled and of reddish tinge. Nucleoli or nucleolar rings are present.	Plates IV–1, IV–3 (dog); Plate IV–5 (cat); Plates V–1, VI–4, VI–6 (horse)
Prorubricyte (basophilic or early erythroblast or normoblast)	Similar in appearance to the rubriblast, with the exception that the nuclear chromatin may have minimal condensation, and nucleoli or rings are absent.	Plate IV–2 (dog); Plate VI–5 (horse)
Basophilic Rubricyte (basophilic erythroblast or normoblast)	The cell is smaller than the prorubricyte. It retains the narrow rim of deep blue cytoplasm. The nuclear chromatin is condensed and separated by light streaks giving the so-called cartwheel appearance.	Plates V–1, VI–5 (horse); Plate IV–3 (dog); Plate V–2 (cat)
Polychromatophilic Rubricyte (early polychromatic erythroblast or normoblast)	Synthesis of hemoglobin is well under way, and this produces a change in color of the cytoplasm to light blue or gray. Condensation of nuclear chromatin has continued so that the appearance is one of dark blobs separated by light streaks.	Plates IV–1, IV–2, IV–3 (dog); Plates IV–5, V–2 (cat); Plates VI–2, VI–5, VI—6 (horse)
Normochromic (orthochromatic) Rubricyte	This stage is most commonly encountered in the cat and horse. The nucleus remains viable, while the cytoplasm stains similarly to the mature erythrocyte.	Plate VI–6 (horse)
Metarubricyte (late polychromatic erythroblast or normoblast)	This stage is depicted by the presence of a nonviable nucleus. The nucleus is solidly black or pyknotic. It may be fragmented, partially extruded, or partially autolyzed. The cytoplasm may be polychromatic or normochromic, depending on the extent of hemoglobin synthesis.	Plates V–1, VI–5; VI–6 (horse); Plates IV–5, V–2 (cat); Plates IV–2, XVII–3 (dog)

Reticulocyte	Non-nucleated erythrocyte that, when stained with new methylene blue, presents one or more granules or a diffuse network of fibrils. With Romanowsky stains, the reticulocyte is commonly polychromatophilic and infrequently may contain an eccentrically placed nuclear remnant called a Howell-Jolly body.	Plates IV–3, XVII–3 (dog); Plate IV–6 (cat)
Erythrocyte	Non-nucleated, definitive cell of the series.	

MATURATION OF THE GRANULOCYTES

Myeloblast	Large cell, round to irregular in shape, with finely stippled chromatin containing one or more nucleoli or nucleolar rings. The cytoplasm is blue (basophilic) but generally lighter in color than that of the rubriblast. There are no granules in the cytoplasm.	Plate V–3 (dog): Plates V–5, VI–1 (horse)
Promyelocyte (progranulocyte)	Similar in size to the myeloblast. The nuclear chromatin is finely stippled. Nucleolus or nucleolar ring is absent. The cytoplasm is basophilic and commonly presents reddish azurophilic granules. There are no specific granules.	Plates V–4, XII–3 (dog); Plate VI–2 (horse)
Myelocyte, neutrophilic	Smaller than the progranulocyte, with beginning condensation of the nuclear chromatin. The cytoplasm is light blue and contains few to numerous neutrophilic granules. These granules when properly stained are dust-like and faintly pink.	Plate V–6 (horse): Plate IV–4 (cat)
Myelocyte, eosinophilic	This cell is generally larger than the neutrophilic myelocyte. The cytoplasm is more basophilic, and the granules are distinctly reddish orange.	Plate V–5 (horse)
Myelocyte, basophilic	Not a very common cell in bone marrow preparations. In the cat, the granules are of two types: numerous small, round, and pinkish and fewer large, round, and black. In other animals, granules are metachromatic or black.	Plates V–2, XII–4 (cat); Plate VI–3 (horse)
Metamyelocyte, neutrophilic, eosinophilic, and basophilic	The nucleus is indented to assume a kidney-bean shape. This cell is no longer capable of division. The cytoplasm may retain a slight basophilia in the neutrophil, but the other two forms retain a bluish cytoplasm as characteristic of the mature cell of the series. The specific granules identify the cell as neutrophilic, eosinophilic, or basophilic.	Plate V–3 (dog); Plates V–5, V–6, VI–3 (horse)
Band neutrophil	The nucleus has parallel sides but twists to conform to the space within the cytoplasm. Horseshoe or S-forms are common. The nuclear membrane is smooth. Irregularity of the nuclear membrane or beginning indentation are features indicating that maturity has been attained, requiring classification as a segmenter and not a band form.	Plates V–6, VI–4, VII–8 (horse); Plate IV–4 (cat)
Segmenter neutrophil (polymorphonuclear leukocyte)	The nucleus may be monolobed, but the nuclear membrane is irregular (moth-eaten) or several lobes are separated by filaments. This cell is called a heterophil in some species.	Plate VII–1 (cow); Plate VII–8 (horse); Plate VII–9 (dog); Plate IX–4 (cat)
Eosinophil	Cytoplasm contains eosinophilic granules which vary in intensity of reddish color between species. Granules vary in size, shape, and number with the species of animal. The cytoplasm is light blue.	Plate VII–4 (cow; Plate VII–7 (horse); Plate XII–1 (dog); Plates VII–6, IX–1 (cat)
Basophil	Cytoplasm is basophilic with few to many metachromatic granules, depending on the species. Granules are round and pinkish in the cat, although some basophils may retain a few small, darker-staining granules.	Plate VII–5 (cow); Plate VII–6, XII–5 (cat); Plate VII–7 (horse); Plate XII–1 (dog)

MATURATION OF THE MEGAKARYOCYTE

Megakaryoblast	The first recognizable cell of this series is larger than other blast cells of bone marrow. It has 1 to 4 reddish nuclei with a distinct chromatin pattern. The cytoplasm is small in amount and takes a deep blue stain.	Plates III–1, III–3 (dog)
Promegakaryocyte	Maturation leads to multiplication of nuclei by mitotic division without division of the cytoplasm (endomitosis). Number of nuclei may be 8 or more. In the larger cells, the nuclei are commonly fused into a single irregular mass. The cytoplasm stains deep to moderate blue and is limited to a relatively narrow rim around the nuclear mass.	Plates III–2, III–4 (dog)
Megakaryocyte	The cytoplasm is pale blue and presents pinkish azurophilic granules. The cytoplasm is increased considerably over that of the promegakaryocyte. The formation of granules begins in the perinuclear zone and gradually extends to the periphery of the cell. Cell size is variable and depends on the number of nuclear divisions that had taken place before DNA synthesis was terminated by the beginning maturation of the cytoplasm. In films of aspirated bone marrow, some megakaryocytes may present pseudopod-like extensions and a nuclear mass without cytoplasm, or cytoplasm without a nucleus may be encountered.	Plates III–4, III–5 (dog)
Platelets (thrombocytes)	Individual platelets are cytoplasmic fragments of megakaryocytes. They vary in shape and size and contain reddish granules in a light blue field. In blood, they are often commonly clumped.	Plate IX–1 (cat)

OTHER CELLS

Osteoclast	Large cells, irregular in shape and presenting multiple oval nuclei distinctly separated in a pinkish granular cytoplasm. These cells are not to be confused with megakaryocytes.	Plate III–6 (dog)
Mitotic figures	These are not numerous in normal marrow. Cells in mitosis in the erythrocytic series are usually readily identifiable as belonging to that series. Otherwise, they are recorded as "other cells."	
Hematogones	Round, pyknotic free nuclei extruded from metarubricytes.	Plate IV–2 (dog)
Lymphocytes	Small lymphocytes may be encountered in aspirated bone marrow. In the cat, they may contribute 10% to 15% of the total nucleated cells.	Plate XV–8 (cat)
Monocytes	Cells morphologically typical of monocytes may occur in small numbers. Monocytes originate in the bone marrow from promonocytes.	Plates VIII–1 to VIII–9 (dog)
Macrophages	Phagocytic cells are present in bone marrow. They are best recognized as such when they contain phagocytosed iron particles, pyknotic nuclear material, or erythrocytes, and rarely an entire leukocyte.	Plate XI–1 (horse); Plates XV–6, XV–7 (cat)
Plasma cells	Cells of irregular shape but usually round with a large amount of light blue cytoplasm and round, eccentrically placed nucleus. The nucleus is similar in appearance to the rubricyte nucleus but with greater contrast between chromatin and parachromatin. There may be a pale area of cytoplasm near one side of the nucleus. An infrequently encountered plasma cell is filled with round structures called Russell bodies.	Plates XI–4, XI–5, X–12 (dog)

RE nuclei	Bone marrow aspirations contain pinkish-staining roundish structures presenting one or more blue nucleoli. These are classified as free nuclei of reticuloendothelial cells.	Plate XI–2 (dog)
Unclassified cells	Cells may be present in normal bone marrow that do not fit the description of any of the many stages of hematopoietic cells undergoing maturation.	
Degenerated cells	Cells presenting fragmented, pyknotic nuclei or irregularly roundish, pinkish structures without nucleoli or a net-like pinkish structure, commonly referred to as a basket cell, are degenerating cells. They are included in a bone marrow differential cell count.	Plate V–2 (cat); Plate XI–2 (dog)

Bone Marrow Evaluation

Ability to classify the various cells in the bone marrow smears comes only with practice. The beginner will learn more quickly to differentiate the many different maturation stages of hematopoietic cells by starting with the megakaryocytic series (Plate III). In bone marrow films on coverslips, the megakaryocytes are concentrated along the base or long straight border of the film. The low-power objective is used to detect these large cells, and then the high dry objective is used to study cellular detail. Next, the film should be scanned, using the high dry objective, to locate good areas of the film where cellularity is adequate and morphology is satisfactory for cell identification. An oil immersion lens is then used to study details of various bone marrow cells. In the learning process, the next step is to acquire skill in classifying cells within the erythrocytic maturation series. Here it is best to begin with the metarubricyte (Plates V–1, V–2) and proceed through the series, recognizing the salient characteristics of decreasing immaturity at each classified stage of cellular maturation (Plates IV, VI). Finally, the granulocytic series is studied using the same approach as applied to the erythrocytic series (Plates V, VI). Osteoclasts can be recognized at low magnification, and relative distribution of other cells such as mast cells, plasma cells, and lymphocytes can be determined under high dry magnification.

General Comments about Bone Marrow Cytology

The following general principles apply to the cytology of bone marrow.

1. Megakaryocytes increase in size by endomitosis. That is, the nucleus undergoes division, but the cell itself does not divide (Plate III–2). The promegakaryocyte is capable of nuclear division only if the cytoplasm remains basophilic and devoid of azurophilic granules. Once formation of granules is initiated, nuclear division ceases. Thus mature megakaryocytes may vary considerably in size and are recognized by the presence of azurophilic granules. Extrusion of megakaryocyte nuclei may occur during the process of making films of marrow aspirates. See Chapter 16 for details of megakaryocytopoiesis.

2. Cells of the erythrocytic and granulocytic series decrease in size with each successive stage of maturation. However, cells at the same stage of maturation also vary in size. Classification is based not on size but on cytoplasmic and nuclear characteristics.

3. The earliest blast cells contain nucleoli that stain light blue because of their content of RNA. After the first mitotic division, the nucleolus loses its blue color, but may persist as a ring-like structure (Plate V–3).

4. The cytoplasm is basophilic in the blast and pro cells and stains progressively less blue as maturation proceeds. The cytoplasm in immature cells of the erythroid series is highly basophilic compared to that in the granulocytic series.

5. Cytoplasmic granules are not present in blast cells. Azurophilic granules occur commonly in promyelocytes and are not apparent in the myelocytes that display

the specific granules. When a nucleolar ring and azurophilic granules are both present in the cell, the latter characteristic takes precedence in classifying the cell as a promyelocyte (Plate V–4).

6. Nuclear chromatin is diffuse and finely stippled in blast cells. Beginning condensation of chromatin takes place in pro cells and becomes more pronounced with each successive stage of the maturation series. The condensing, darker-staining basichromatin is separated by lighter-staining parachromatin. The nuclear chromatin stains darker in the erythrocytic series than in the granulocytic series because the former has a higher content of DNA. The nuclear chromatin pattern of the polychromatic rubricyte is somewhat suggestive of a cartwheel (Plate IV–1). In the granulocytic series, the clumped basichromatin finally becomes concentrated along the nuclear membrane, causing it to become "bumpy" in the mature neutrophil (Plate VII–8).

7. The nucleus and cytoplasm usually mature together. Asynchronous maturation is an indication of disease. Diseases that depress granulopoiesis may lead to skipped mitotic divisions, resulting in giant forms with bizarre nuclear patterns. Such forms are frequently seen in diseased cats (Plate XV–8). The occurrence in cells of the granulocytic series of double nuclei, bluish and foamy cytoplasm (Plates VIII–11, VIII–12, IX–3), isolated deep blue granular objects (Döhle bodies; Plates IX–2, XII–6), and scattered or uniformly distributed azurophilic granules ("toxic" granulation; Plates XI–12, XV–12) are all signs of aberrant or abnormal granulopoiesis in disease. Enzymatic abnormalities can also be detected in the granulocytic series because of asynchrony of cellular maturation during leukemic process.

8. The cells of the granulocytic series are more susceptible to rupture during preparation of the film than the cells of the erythrocytic series. Thus degenerated cells are usually granulocytic in origin. Nuclei containing several prominent blue nucleoli originate from rupture of marrow reticuloendothelial cells.

9. Mature lymphocytes are present in small numbers in aspirated marrow of common domestic animals. They are usually more numerous (10–15%) in bone marrow preparations of the cat than in other species. Dilution of marrow with blood will bring increased numbers of lymphocytes into the sample from those animals in which lymphocytes normally outnumber neutrophils in the blood, e.g., the cow. Marrow of small laboratory animals such as the mouse, guinea pig, and rat often contains a large number of lymphocytes.

10. Plasma cells are infrequent in normal bone marrow. They appear in increased numbers in the bone marrow in diseases involving continuous antigenic exposure (Plate XI–4) and in plasma cell myeloma. The plasma cell is distinguished from the polychromatic rubricyte on the basis of greater size, a lower nuclear:cytoplasmic ratio, and the hue of its basophilic cytoplasm. Plasma cells with one or more nucleoli may be encountered in marrows with intense plasma cell production.

11. The band neutrophil and the reticulocyte stages immediately precede the mature cell of the respective cell series. Both are classified as immature cells, and their occurrence in increased numbers in blood indicates intensification of their production in the bone marrow.

12. Deficiencies of vitamin B_{12} and folic acid lead to reduced replication of nucleoprotein and affect cells of both erythrocytic and granulocytic series. Maturation arrest occurs at the prorubricytic and basophilic rubricyte stages. This is accompanied by the occurrence of some large metamyelocytes in the bone marrow and some hypersegmented neutrophils in blood and bone marrow (Plate XI–7). Such cells tend to have larger than normal nuclei with stippled chromatin pattern (Plate XIX–1). Depressed DNA synthesis causes nuclear maturation to be out of step with hemoglobinization of the cytoplasm. When hemoglobin

synthesis reaches a certain level of concentration, the nucleus stops dividing, usually short of normal mitotic divisions, and the cell begins to mature. The extrusion of the nucleus from such cells results in formation of macrocytic erythrocytes characteristic of macrocytic anemia of vitamin B_{12} and folic acid deficiency. The abnormal precursor cells are called megaloblasts or megaloblastoid cells (Plate XIX–1). Somewhat similar cells occur in erythremic myelosis and erythroleukemia of the cat (Plates XV–4, XIX–2, XX–3). In iron deficiency, decreased hemoglobin synthesis leads to retention of a viable nucleus beyond the normal number of cell divisions. Some cell lines undergo additional mitosis, producing the microcytic erythrocytes typical of iron deficiency anemia (Plates XVII–1, XVII–2). See Chapter 25 for further details of mechanisms of anemia in these conditions.

The Myeloid:Erythroid Ratio

The myeloid:erythroid (M:E) ratio is obtained by dividing the number of nucleated cells of the erythrocytic series into the number of all cells of the granulocytic series. Thus it is also called the G:E ratio. Commonly 500 cells are differentiated and tallied on a bone marrow evaluation tally sheet (Fig. 1–1). All cells including degenerated cells are included in the 500-cell differentiation, but cells other than the erythroid and granulocytic series are excluded from calculation of the ratio. Some hematologists also exclude cells of the eosinophil and basophil series, and others prefer to exclude mature neutrophils (Wintrobe et al., 1981). Excluding eosinophils and basophils is inconsequential because bone marrow ordinarily contains very few of them, but excluding mature neutrophils significantly lowers the value. The normal ranges and means of M:E ratios for the various domestic animals are given in Table 1–5. Examples of bone marrow differential counts in selected canine diseases are prevented in Table 4–9.

An M:E ratio of 1.0:1.0 indicates that nucleated erythrocytes and granulocytes are present in equal numbers. When the ratio is less than 1.0, the usual inference is that eryth-rocyte production exceeds granulopoiesis, and when the ratio is greater than 1.0, granulopoiesis exceeds erythropoiesis. However, the former could also occur if granulopoiesis were suppressed, and the latter if erythropoiesis were diminished. Therefore, the M:E ratio cannot be interpreted properly without reference to the total and differential leukocyte counts and reticulocyte count in blood. When a significant neutrophilia exists in the blood, especially accompanied by a left shift (presence of excessive numbers of immature neutrophils in blood), intensified granulopoiesis is indicated. An M:E ratio greatly in excess of unity then would not necessarily reflect a depression of erythropoiesis. In this instance, the reduction in nucleated erythrocytes in the bone marrow differential count would be relative rather than absolute. In comparison, when the total leukocyte count is within the normal range for the species in question, the M:E ratio is a valuable tool to indicate intensification (decreased M:E ratio) or depression of erythropoiesis (increased M:E ratio). Reticulocytosis in blood or bone marrow indicates increased erythropoiesis, and in such cases, granulopoiesis must similarly be evaluated relative to the degree of erythropoiesis. In some cases, e.g., chronic inflammatory disease, both erythrocytic and granulocytic series may be simultaneously affected. Interpretation of the M:E ratio in such cases would require awareness of pathogenetic mechanisms involved in hematopoietic changes associated with such disease processes.

Developing an M:E ratio based on differentiation of maturation stages in each cell series is time-consuming and delays reports to clinicians. A satisfactory substitute is a narrative of impressions gained from examination of morphology and distribution of sequential developmental stages of various hematopoietic cell lines. Although smears of marrow aspirates are believed not to reflect true marrow cellularity, comments should also be made regarding impressions gained about general cellularity of smears, particularly after a search has been made for marrow spicules. The presence of megakaryocytes, plasma cells, mast cells, lymphocytes, mitotic cells, and cells foreign to the bone marrow

BONE MARROW EVALUATION TALLY SHEET

Case No._____ Animal_____ Date_____

Cell Type	Total	Cell Type	Total
Rubriblast		Myeloblast	
Prorubricyte		Progranulocyte	
RUBRICYTES Basophilic		MYELOCYTES Neutrophilic	
Polychromatic		Eosinophilic	
Normochromic		Basophilic	
Metarubricyte		METAMYELOCYTE Neutrophilic	
Mitotic		Eosinophilic	
TOTAL CELLS ERYTHROCYTIC =		Basophilic	
Hematogones*		BAND Neutrophilic	
Lymphocytes		Eosinophilic	
Plasma cells		Basophilic	
Monocytes		SEGMENTER Neutrophilic	
Mitotic cells		Eosinophilic	
Megakaryocytes		Basophilic	
Osteoclasts		SEGMENTER Neutrophilic	
Macrophages		Eosinophilic	
Unclassified cells		Basophilic	
Degenerated cells		TOTAL CELLS GRANULOCYTIC =	
*free metarubricyte nucleus		M:E ratio =	

Fig. 1–1.   Example of a bone marrow evaluation tally sheet.

Table 1–5.   Normal Myeloid:Erythroid Ratios of Some Animal Species

Species	Range	Mean
Dog	0.75–2.53	1.25
Cat	1.20–2.15	1.63
Horse	0.94–3.76	1.64
Cow	0.31–1.85	0.70
Sheep	0.77–1.68	1.09
Goat	—	0.69
Pig	—	1.77

should be specifically noted. A quick M:E ratio can be obtained by counting different developmental stages of each series as a group rather than in various subcategories as shown in Figure 1–1. If necessary, erythroid as well as myeloid cells may be classified under mitotic and maturative compartments and granulocytic cells also under storage com-partments to gain information regarding rel-ative distribution of cells in these functional pools. Such grouping may be desirable in cases of megaloblastic anemia, microcytic hy-pochromic anemia, and granulocytic leuke-mias.

For additional information on bone marrow cytology of various species, see appropriate sections in Chapters 4 through 12.

Bone Marrow Biopsy

In most cases, marrow aspirates are ade-quate to evaluate response to disease. How-ever, marrow biopsy may be desired in some situations, particularly when information re-garding marrow topography, gross cellular-ity, and relative distribution of various cells is needed (Burkhardt et al., 1982). Needle biopsy is preferred in situations such as when hypocellularity of marrow smears is suspected to have resulted from hypoplasia rather than hemodilution. Other indications of marrow biopsy include: repeated failure to obtain adequate marrow samples ("dry taps"), pancytopenias, lymphoproliferative disorders including myelomas, tumor metastasis, granulomatous diseases involving the bone marrow, and myelofibrosis. Marrow biopsies can be taken from the iliac crest using a Jamshidi needle in a manner similar to that described for marrow aspiration (see Chapter 2). A marrow aspirate must also be collected for simultaneous cytologic examination. When this is not possible, touch preparations of marrow tissue should be prepared although they are not as satisfactory as smears of marrow aspirate.

Paraffin-embedded bone marrow biopsy specimens are unreliable for assessment of various hematopoietic elements, especially the immature stages (Rowden et al., 1982). This major disadvantage stems from processing artifacts of tissue shrinkage. Newer techniques of embedding bone marrow in various plastics, particularly methacrylate and glycol methacrylate, provide superior means of evaluating 1–2 μm thin sections for overall cellularity and cell types with high resolution and minimum artifacts (Rowden et al., 1982). In addition, cytochemical and immunocytochemical staining techniques can be applied to such specimens (Beckstead et al., 1981). These techniques have not yet been applied in veterinary medicine.

REFERENCES

Albritton, E.C.: Standard Values in Blood. W.B. Saunders, Philadelphia, 1952.

Altman, P.L.: Blood and Other Body Fluids. Federation of American Societies for Experimental Biology, Washington, D.C., 1961.

Andrew, W.: Comparative Hematology. Grune & Stratton, New York, 1965.

Archer, R.K., and Jeffcott, L.B.: Comparative Clinical Haematology. Blackwell Scientific Publications, Oxford, 1977.

Beckstead, J.H., et al.: Enzyme Histochemistry and Im-munohistochemistry on Biopsy Specimens of Pathologic Human Bone Marrow. Blood, *57*:1088, 1981.

Burkhardt, R., et al.: Bone Biopsy in Haematologic Disorders. J. Clin. Pathol., *35*:257, 1982.

Burnett, S.H.: The Clinical Pathology of the Blood of Domesticated Animals. 2nd ed., Macmillan, New York, 1917.

Committee for Clarification of the Nomenclature of Cells and Diseases of the Blood and Blood-Forming Organs: First report, Amer. J. Clin. Path., *18*:443, 1948. Second report, ibid. *19*:56, 1949. Third, fourth, and fifth reports, ibid., *20*:562, 1950.

Hawkey, C.M.: Comparative Mammalian Haematology. William Heinemann Medical Books, London, 1975.

Jain, N.C., and Kono, C.S.: Erythrocyte Sedimentation Rate in the Dog and Cat: Comparison of Two Methods and Influence of Packed Cell Volume, Temperature and Storage of Blood. J. Small Anim. Pract., *16*:671, 1975.

Jasper, D.E., and Jain, N.C.: Postprandial Lipemia in Dogs. Calif. Vet., *18*:27 May–June, 1964.

Keller, P., and Freudiger, U.: Atlas zur Hämatologie von Hund und Katze. Verlag Paul Parey, Berlin, 1983.

Lewis, H.B., and Rebar, A.H.: Bone Marrow Evaluation in Veterinary Practice. Ralston Purina Co., St. Louis, 1979.

Lucas, A.M., and Jamroz, C.: Atlas of Avian Hematology. Agriculture Monograph 25, U.S. Dept. of Agriculture, Washington, D.C., 1961.

Mitruka, D.M., and Rawnsley, H.M.: Clinical Biochemical and Hematological Reference Values in Normal Experimental Animals. Masson, New York, 1977.

Rich, L.J.: The Morphology of Canine and Feline Blood Cells. Ralston Purina Co., St. Louis, 1974.

Rowden, G., et al.: Plastic Embedded Specimens for Evaluation of Bone Marrow. Topical Rev. Haemat., *2*:1, 1982.

Sanderson, J.H., and Phillips, C.E.: An Atlas of Laboratory Animal Hematology. Clarendon Press, Oxford, 1981.

Scarborough, R.A.: The Blood Picture of Normal Laboratory Animals: A Compilation of Published Data. Yale J. Biol. Med., *3*:64 (rabbit), 169 (guinea pig), 267 (rat), 272 (mouse), 1930–1931, and *4*:199 (monkey), 1931–1932.

Schalm, O.W.: Manual of Feline and Canine Hematology. Veterinary Practice Publishing Co., Santa Barbara, 1980.

Schalm, O.W.: Manual of Equine Hematology. Veterinary Practice Publishing Co., Santa Barbara, 1984a.

Schalm, O.W.: Manual of Bovine Hematology. Veterinary Practice Publishing Co., Santa Barbara, 1984b.

Schermer, S.: Die Blutmorphologie der Laboratoriumstiere. Barth, Leipzig, 1954.

Schermer, S.: The Blood Morphology of Laboratory Animals. 3rd ed., F.A. Davis, Philadelphia, 1967.

Williams, W.J., et al.: Hematology. 3rd ed., chaps. 2 and 3. McGraw-Hill, New York, 1983.

Wintrobe, M.M., et al.: Clinical Hematology. 8th ed., chaps. 2 and 3. Lea & Febiger, Philadelphia, 1981.

Wirth, D.: Grundlagen einer Klinischen Hämatologie der Haustiere. 2nd ed., Urban und Schwarzenberg, Vienna, 1950.

2

Hematologic Techniques

THE MICROSCOPE 21

CLEANING GLASSWARE 22
   Slides and Coverslips 22
   Hematology Pipettes 22
   Wintrobe Hematocrit Tubes 22
   Hemocytometers 23

**COLLECTING AND HANDLING BLOOD FOR
   LABORATORY STUDY 23**
   Anticoagulants 23
   Obtaining the Blood Sample 24
   Handling the Blood 28

THE BLOOD FILM 29
   Slide Method 29
   Coverslip Method 29

**STAINING BLOOD FILMS WITH
   ROMANOWSKY STAINS 31**
   Basic Principles 31
   Neutralization of Distilled Water 32
   Phosphate Buffer 32
   Wright Stain 32
   Giemsa Stain 33
   Wright-Leishman Stain 33
   Staining Procedure 34
   Quick Stains 34
   Causes and Correction of Poor Staining 34

**MICROSCOPIC EXAMINATION OF A
   STAINED BLOOD FILM 35**
   General Examination and Differential
     Count 35
   Number of Cells to Be Differentiated 36

**HEMATOCRIT OR PACKED CELL
   VOLUME 36**
   The Wintrobe Hematocrit 37
   The Microhematocrit 41

DETERMINATION OF HEMOGLOBIN 41
   Direct Matching 43
   Hematin Method 43
   Oxyhemoglobin Method 44
   Spectrophotometric Methods 44
   Hemoglobinometer 45

**COUNTING ERYTHROCYTES AND
   LEUKOCYTES IN THE
   HEMOCYTOMETER 45**
   Filling the Pipette 45
   The Counting Chamber 46
   Cell Count and Calculations 47
   Inherent Errors in the Blood Cell Count
     Obtained with the Hemocytometer 48
   Unopette Method for Blood Dilution and
     Cell Counting 48

THE ELECTRONIC CELL COUNTERS 48

**THE WINTROBE ERYTHROCYTE
   INDEXES 52**
   Mean Corpuscular Volume (MCV) 52
   Mean Corpuscular Hemoglobin (MCH) 52
   Mean Corpuscular Hemoglobin
     Concentration (MCHC) 52
   Errors in Erythrocyte Indexes 53

**ERYTHROCYTE SEDIMENTATION RATE
   (ESR) 53**
   Factors Influencing ESR and Changes in
     Disease 54

**ESTIMATION OF TOTAL PLASMA PROTEIN
   BY REFRACTOMETER 56**

**ESTIMATION OF PLASMA FIBRINOGEN BY
   REFRACTOMETER 58**

**BLOOD EXAMINATION BY WET-FILM
   METHOD 59**

**STAINING BLOOD FILMS WITH NEW
   METHYLENE BLUE 59**
   Comments on Structures Discernible in
     Blood Films 60
   Comments on Other Applications of New
     Methylene Blue Stain 62

SPECIAL STAINING PROCEDURES 62
Staining and Counting Reticulocytes 62
Demonstration of Basophilic Stippling 63
Permanent Stain for Heinz Bodies 63
Staining for Sideroleukocytes 63
Iron Stain 64
Cytochemical Stains 64

COUNTING EOSINOPHIL LEUKOCYTES 64

COUNTING PLATELETS 65
Indirect Method 65
Direct Method 65

COAGULATION TESTS 66

ASPIRATION OF BONE MARROW 66
Technique for the Dog 66
Technique for the Cat 67
Technique for the Cow and the Horse 67

**ESTIMATION OF TOTAL LEUKOCYTE
COUNT BY DNA VISCOSITY TEST 67**

**ERYTHROCYTE OSMOTIC FRAGILITY
TEST 69**

**CROSS-MATCHING BLOOD FOR
TRANSFUSION 71**
Cross-Matching Donor and Recipient Bloods
for Compatibility 71

Cross-Matching for Blood Transfusion in the
Horse 71

**DETECTION OF ANTIBODIES TO
ERYTHROCYTES 73**
Coombs Tests 73
Agglutination of Papain-Treated
Erythrocytes 75

**DETECTION OF ANTIPLATELET
ANTIBODIES 75**
Platelet Factor 3 (PF-3) Test 75
Direct Immunofluorescence of
Megakaryocytes 77

**DETECTION OF ANTINUCLEAR
ANTIBODIES 77**
Indirect Immunofluorescence Test 78
The Lupus Erythematosus (LE) Cell Test 78

**EXAMINATION OF CANINE BLOOD FOR
MICROFILARIAE 79**
Direct Blood Film 80
Stained Blood Film 80
Microcapillary Hematocrit Method 80
Whole Blood Concentration Method 81
Serum Methods 82
Periodicity in Peripheral Blood 82

The discipline of hematology has much to offer the field of clinical veterinary medicine. The veterinary practitioner should select a few techniques to serve as screening procedures on blood, the results of which, when combined with history and clinical examination, will offer valuable diagnostic information and will also indicate when additional and more specific procedures should be applied.

The routine use of the hematocrit in combination with the stained blood film will reveal unsuspected derangements. In many instances, of course, it will reveal that the blood is normal, and such knowledge is also valuable to the clinician. A specific diagnosis can seldom be made from laboratory findings alone, but laboratory results often provide clues that, together with the history and physical examination, make for a more critical diagnosis and provide for prognosis and proper treatment.

THE MICROSCOPE

A good microscope, properly cared for, will last a lifetime. When purchasing a microscope, one should give serious consideration to the quality of the lenses, the magnification, and the advantages of the binocular over the less expensive monocular.

Lenses are the most important components of the microscope. The *ocular* is the eyepiece lens, and the *objective* is the lens in contact with the specimen. The cost of the microscope is influenced by the type of lenses in the objectives. *Achromatic lenses* are suitable for low-power and high dry objectives. However, for oil immersion work, *apochromatic lenses* are desirable. Both planachromatic and planapochromatic lenses provide a flat field of view, but the latter are preferred for quality microphotography.

The *resolving power* of an objective refers to the ability of the lens to show distinctly separate elements only a short distance apart. The *numerical aperture* is a statement of the resolving power of the lens. The numerical aperture multiplied by 100,000 indicates the number of lines to the inch that can be resolved by the objective, e.g., NA 0.25 = 25,000 lines to the inch, or NA 1.25 = 125,000 lines to the inch.

Magnification of the specimen is determined by a combination of ocular and objective, e.g., 100× objective and 10× ocular provide a final magnification of 1,000×. The *depth of focus* refers to the sharpness with which all elements of the specimen can be seen. It is inversely proportional to both the numerical aperture and the magnification. Thus the depth of focus is reduced as NA and magnification are increased. For this reason, it is important not to employ a greater magnification than necessary. A microscope fitted with 10×, 25×, 40×, and 97× or 100× objective lenses (40× can be high dry or oil immersion; 97× and 100× are oil immersion) and 10× eyepiece lenses is ideally suited for cytologic examination of blood, bone marrow, and other body fluids and tissues.

The *oil immersion* objective requires a drop of special oil to be placed between the objective and the slide. The oil should not be left on the objective when the microscope is not in use. The oil is removed by wiping with special lens paper. It is not necessary to use xylol to remove oil at the end of each period of use of the microscope. The *ocular* lens may become coated with a grease-like film from the eyelashes. This film can be removed by fogging the lens with breath and wiping with lens paper. The *condenser lens* and *substage mirror* should be wiped with lens paper when oil contacts the former and dust appears on the latter.

Critical illumination is important in observing fine cellular details often required for cell identification. Modern microscopes generally have a built-in light source, but the substage condenser and iris diaphragm must be properly positioned and the light beam centered for proper illumination. Older microscopes fitted with a substage mirror to reflect light through the specimen should be similarly adjusted for correct illumination. There is a *plane* and a *concave* side to each mirror; the plane mirror should be used with microscopes equipped with a condenser. If the concave mirror is employed together with a condenser, the apex of the cone of light falls within the condenser, rather than at the level of the microscope slide, reducing the effectiveness of the light beam.

CLEANING GLASSWARE

Slides and Coverslips

The better grade of slides and coverslips are generally grease-free and suitable for use as they come from the original package. A camel's hair brush is helpful to remove the small amount of lint or dust that may be on the surface of the glass. Poor-grade slides and coverslips should be placed in isopropyl alcohol or ethanol and dried with a clean, soft cloth.

Hematology Pipettes

A water-pump aspirator is useful to draw distilled water through the pipette until it is clean, followed by enough acetone to dry it. When the pipettes are clean and dry, the glass bead in the bulb will move freely. Pipettes should be inspected frequently to see that scum is not adhering to the inside, especially in the capillary portions. If the pipette is not absolutely clean, fill with concentrated chlorine solution, and after several minutes, rinse with water and finally with acetone. In the event that this procedure should not clean the pipette, fill with the chlorine solution or dichromate cleaning solution* and after leaving it overnight, blow the acid out of the pipette by means of rubber tubing, and clean in the usual way.

Wintrobe Hematocrit Tubes

A stainless steel, U-shaped tube called the hematocrit tube cleaner is connected to a water suction pump by means of rubber tubing. The hematocrit tube is inverted on the U-tube and placed into a beaker of water (Fig. 2–1). When the suction is applied, the blood

---

*Commercial potassium dichromate, 60 g; tap water, 300 ml. Heat to dissolve, cool, and then add, slowly with continuous stirring, commercial sulfuric acid, 460 ml.

is withdrawn from the hematocrit tube, and water follows. After all the water has been sucked through the hematocrit tube, the suction is continued for a short time to draw air into the tube to dry it. Hematocrit tubes that are not clean following the suction method should be filled with dichromate cleaning solution and left overnight or longer. Disposable Wintrobe hematocrit tubes are also available.

Hemocytometers

Hemocytometers and coverslips should be rinsed with distilled water and dried with clean facial tissue or a soft clean cloth after each use. Polish with clean facial tissue before each use, since the counting chamber will not fill properly if not absolutely clean. Care must be taken not to scratch the chamber or coverslip.

COLLECTING AND HANDLING BLOOD FOR LABORATORY STUDY

A 5-ml volume of blood is adequate for routine blood study, but with cats and small dogs, it may be necessary to limit the volume to 2 ml. Use of a calibrated syringe is desirable to ensure the collection of an exact volume of blood to correspond with the amount of anticoagulant contained in the sample vial. Blood-collecting vacuum specimen tubes, e.g., Vacutainer (Becton-Dickinson) and Venoject (Kimble-Terumo) tubes, constitute an ideal system for bleeding small and large domestic animals. They are available with a wide variety of capacities and additives to meet the needs of both morphological and biochemical studies. It is necessary to permit blood to flow into the tube until all vacuum has been satisfied, or else the concentration of additive will exceed that desired for the purpose intended.

Anticoagulants

Anticoagulants in common use are ethylenediaminetetraacetate (EDTA: [ethylenedinitrilo]tetraacetic acid), heparin, and sodium citrate. Sodium and potassium oxalates are no longer in general use as anticoagulants. EDTA, sodium citrate, and oxalates prevent blood coagulation by complexing calcium ions required in the clotting mechanism.

Heparin prevents blood coagulation by complexing with antithrombin III and thereby potentiating the ability of antithrombin III to neutralize the action of thrombin and activated coagulation factors XII, XI, IX, and X.

EDTA is the preferred anticoagulant for blood morphology studies. It is available as disodium or dipotassium salt; the latter is preferable because it is more soluble. EDTA is commonly used at a concentration of 0.5–2.0 mg/ml of blood or as a 15% solution of K_2-EDTA at the rate of 0.01 ml/ml of blood. Excessive EDTA causes shrinkage of erythrocytes and seriously affects the validity of the packed cell volume (PCV) in the hematocrit test (Doyle, 1967; Penny et al., 1970); e.g., PCV of a feline blood sample may be reduced by 5–10%. Consequently, errors are also introduced in the calculations of mean corpuscular volume (MCV) and mean corpuscular hemoglobin concentration (MCHC). Hemoglobin estimation is not affected by an excess of EDTA. Vacutainers contain liquid EDTA to yield a final concentration of 1.5 mg/ml of blood. Blood should be drawn to completely fill the tube to avoid excessive concentration of the anticoagulant. Vacutainers with EDTA may not prevent clotting of blood having high calcium levels as from horses with kidney disease.

Blood anticoagulated with EDTA is suitable for thrombocyte counts and blood film preparation up to several hours. Refrigerated blood is suitable for PCV, hemoglobin, and cell counts up to 24 hours post collection. Blood anticoagulated with EDTA is suitable for determination of blood urea nitrogen, total plasma proteins, and plasma fibrinogen and for a preliminary test for blood glucose concentration by dipstick method.

EDTA in dry bulk form can be prepared inexpensively for anticoagulation of blood as follows: Transfer a quantity of EDTA powder to a mortar and grind to fineness. Transfer the powder to shell vials with a special spatula that delivers approximately 4.0 mg/vial for collection of 2–3 ml of blood or 10.0 mg/vial for 5 ml. To make the spatula, carve pits in the opposite ends of a wooden tongue depressor with a sharp scalpel blade to hold about 4.0 mg and 10.0 mg of powder, respectively. Dip the spatula into the powder, and then draw it across the edge of a second tongue depressor to fill the pit and remove excess powder (Fig. 2–2). Shell vials containing anticoagulant can be prepared rapidly by this method and should then be closed with rubber stoppers. When blood is added, tip the vial gently back and forth a dozen times to dissolve the anticoagulant.

Heparin (from the Greek *hepar*, "liver") is a natural anticoagulant occurring in various tissues and found abundantly in the liver. Excess heparin does not alter erythrocyte volume (Pennock and Jones, 1966), but it has a serious disadvantage in cell morphology studies (Schmidt et al., 1953). It interferes with staining of leukocytes, resulting in a hazy appearance of cells (Table 2–1). Heparin is commonly employed as a 1.0% solution (1,000 USP units/ml), at which concentration 0.1 ml is adequate to prevent coagulation of 5.0 ml of blood (0.2 mg or 20 units/ml of blood). This quantity of heparin will moisten the inside of a syringe employed to withdraw 5.0 ml of blood. Heparin appears to interfere with plasma fibrinogen determination, and it is not suitable for blood coagulation studies because it inhibits the action of thrombin and several other activated coagulation factors (p. 23).

Sodium citrate is used for anticoagulation at the rate of one part of 3.8% aqueous solution to nine parts of blood. This introduces a 10% dilution of the blood and is, therefore, not generally used for complete blood count (CBC). It is used, however, to collect blood for study of platelet morphology and functions. Sodium citrate forms a component of the various solutions used for collection of blood for transfusion purposes.

For transportation of bovine blood, a formalin-containing anticoagulant (Titriplex IV) was found to provide satisfactory leukocyte stability (Valli et al., 1980). Titriplex IV consisted of 22.5% dipotassium EDTA, 25 ml formalin (36% solution), 0.1 g acetylsalicylic acid, and 225 ml distilled water. It was used at the rate of 0.1 ml/ml of blood.

Obtaining the Blood Sample

Common sites and needle sizes for collection of blood from various species are given in Table 2–2. The use of a syringe or Vacutainer is governed by the size of the animal and quantity desired. In large animals, the

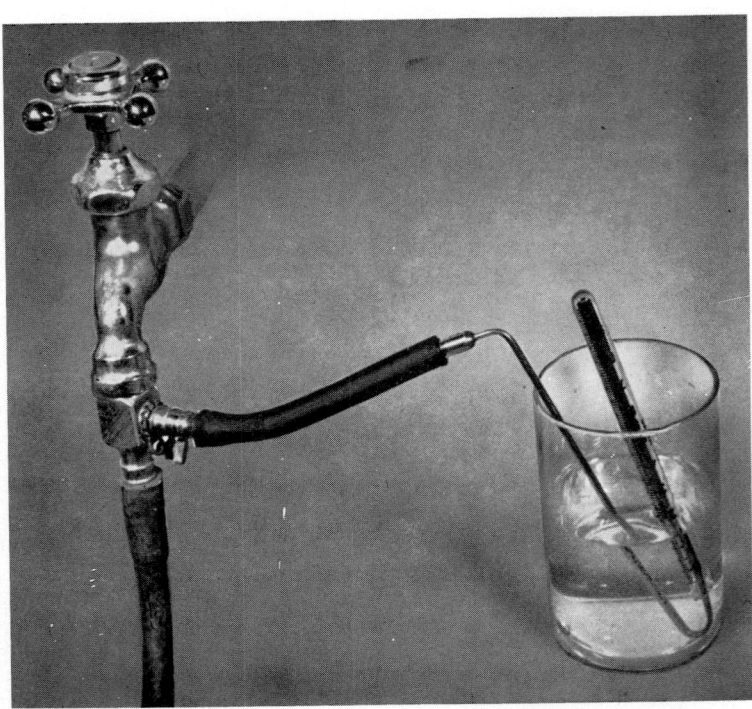

Fig. 2–1. A convenient method for cleaning the Wintrobe hematocrit tube by means of a water vacuum pump.

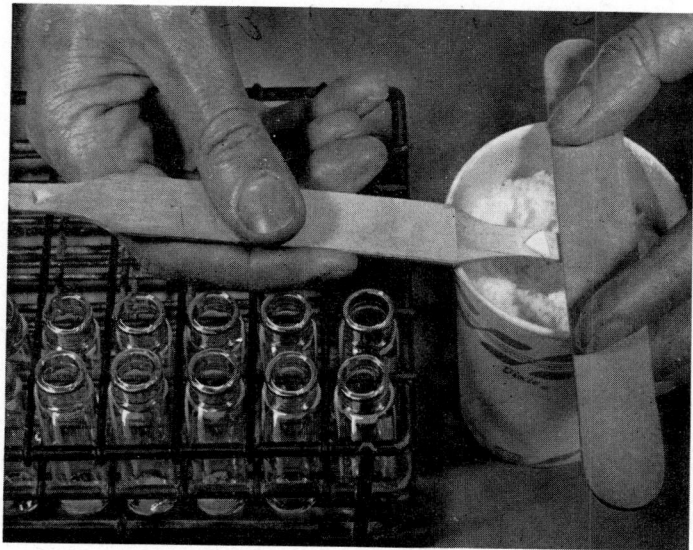

Fig. 2–2. Method for dispensing EDTA anticoagulant powder into vials. The pit in the end of the spatula containing the powder holds 10 mg of EDTA when filled level with the surface of the spatula. The pit in the opposite end of the spatula is for dispensing 4 mg of EDTA anticoagulant powder.

Table 2–1.   The Effects of Heparin and EDTA Anticoagulants on Leukocyte Morphology

Observation	Time Interval (hours)	Heparin (0.1 ml of 1.0%/ 5 ml of blood)	EDTA (10.0 mg/5 ml of blood)
Autolysis of cell nuclei	1	+ +[a]	—
	6	+ +	+
	24	+ +	+ +
Clarity of cell morphology	1	+[b]	+ + + +
	6	+	+ + +
	24	+	+ + +
Stainability	1	+ +	+ + + +
	6	+ +	+ + + +
	24	+ +	+ + + +
Quantity of platelets	1	+ +	+ + + +
	6	+	+ + + +
	24	+	+ + + +

Modified from Schmidt et al., 1953.
[a]Cells distorted and poorly preserved.
[b]Cells very hazy.

Table 2–2.   Sites and Needle Sizes Commonly Used for Collection of Blood from Various Animals

Animal	Site	Needle Size Gauge	Length (in.)
Horse	Jugular vein	16–19	1½–2
Cow	Jugular vein	16–19	1½–2
Sheep and goat	Jugular vein	18–20	1½–2
Pig	Anterior vena cava	20	1½–4
Dog	Cephalic, jugular, or saphenous vein	20–22	1½
Cat	Cephalic, jugular, or femoral vein	22–25	1
Rabbit	Heart	18	3
Small primates	Femoral artery	22–26	⅝–1
Rat and mouse	Orbital sinus	Micro blood-collecting tube	

needle of proper size is introduced percutaneously into the distended vein, and the blood is drawn into a syringe or collected directly into the Vacutainer tube. The Vacutainer system may also be used for sampling larger dogs, but a syringe is preferred for cats and smaller dogs to prevent collapse of vein from excessive vacuum. A syringe is employed for collecting blood when heart puncture is done as with the pig and small laboratory animals (rabbits and guinea pigs).

Venipuncture should be made with least tissue injury to avoid contamination with tissue juices having a procoagulant. Animals should be restrained with minimal physical force, and other precautions should be taken to obtain blood samples representative of the animal at rest. To prevent hemolysis from occurring, certain precautions must be taken. Hemolysis in a needle is directly related to flow velocity and conduit radius (Moss and Stauton, 1970). Needles of small gauge have decreased flow rate, which in turn decreases velocity, turbulence, and hemolysis. The needle and syringe must be dry to allow free flow of blood into the syringe with minimum use of suction or pumping action and to avoid rupture of some red cells by hypotonic moisture. Before the blood is transferred to the vial, the needle should be removed because forcing the blood through the needle under pressure may rupture red cells. Goat blood is very sensitive to hemolysis because of smaller red cell size. Goat blood undergoes some lysis in Vacutainers and also when heparin is used as the anticoagulant; EDTA in powder or liquid form is a satisfactory anticoagulant. Use of a syringe fitted with a 19- or 20-gauge, 1-inch needle is recommended.

The jugular vein is the most suitable site for blood collection for hematologic analyses in many animals. Blood samples may also be collected from the tail (coccygeal) vein of cattle as an alternate to the jugular vein (Sears et al., 1978). Cephalic and saphenous veins can be used in the dog and cephalic and femoral veins in the cat. It is also convenient with cats to puncture a marginal ear vein with a sharp scalpel blade and to draw blood directly into an anticoagulated capillary hematocrit tube and into pipettes for cell counts and hemoglobin estimation. Carle and Dewhirst

(1942) were the first to employ the anterior vena cava as a site for bleeding of swine (Fig. 2–3). Restraint, equipment, and special anatomic considerations for this method of bleeding have been described (Hoerlein et al., 1951). Other sites of blood sampling from the pig include auricular vascular system (Hultsch and Ellendorff, 1979), internal thoracic vein (Brown, 1979), and cardiac puncture (Calvert et al., 1977). Miniature pigs have been sampled from the ophthalmic venous sinus (Stier and Leucht, 1980) and femoral vein (Benjaminsen and Karlberg, 1979; Brown et al., 1978). Methods have been described for bleeding small animals such as mink and ferrets (Baker and Gorham, 1951), guinea pigs (Vallejo-Freire, 1951), mice (Kassel and Levitan, 1953), and small zoo animals (Wallach, 1970). See also Chapter 12. The carotid artery is a suitable site for sampling blood for pH and gas analysis.

Collecting blood from the rabbit, mouse, or rat by cardiac puncture may be followed by death of some of the animals unless the operator has acquired expertise in the method. A technique for collection of blood from the orbital sinus (Fig. 2–4) of the rat and mouse (Stone, 1954; Riley, 1960) is as follows:

The animal is held by the back of the neck and the loose skin of the head is tightened with the thumb and middle finger. With the aid of the index finger the eye is made to bulge slightly by further traction on the skin adjacent to the eye. The tip of the pipette* is placed at the lower or inner corner of the eye and gently but firmly slid alongside of the eyeball to the ophthalmic venous plexus which lines the back of the orbit. The venous capillaries rupture on contact with the tip of the pipette and the resulting hemorrhage fills the orbital cavity. A slight withdrawal of the pipette frees the tip so that the accumulated blood is immediately drawn into the tube by capillary action. [Riley, 1960]

The volume of blood collected is 0.2 ml from mice and up to 1.0 ml from rats. Bleeding usually stops immediately upon withdrawal of the pipette. The same mice have been bled repeatedly from both orbits for periods of several months without evidence of blindness or other serious damage. Anesthesia is generally not required.

---

*Micro-Blood Collecting Tubes, Scientific Products, Division of American Hospital Supply Corporation.

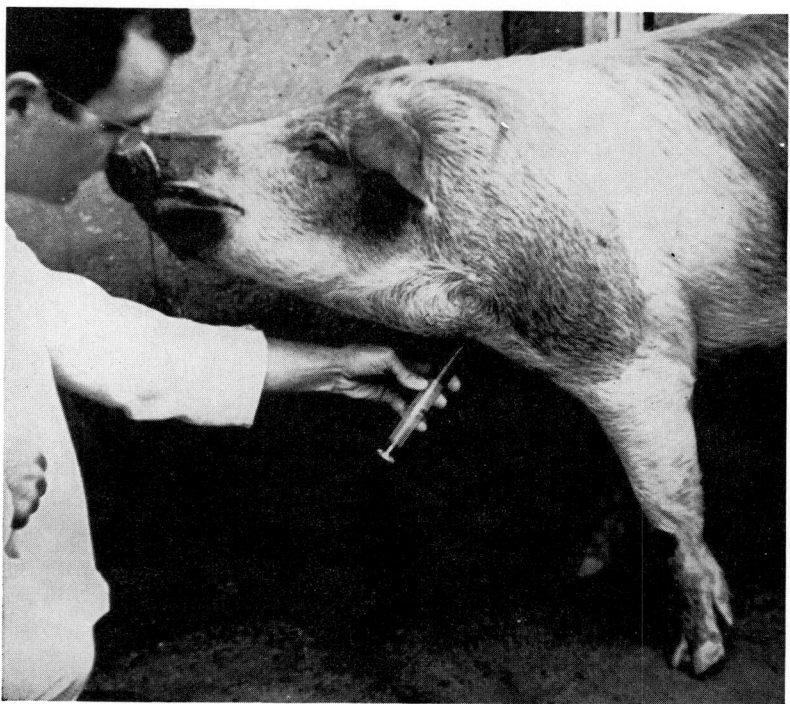

Fig. 2–3. Collecting blood from the anterior vena cava of a 200-pound pig. (From Carle and Dewhirst, 1942; courtesy of the *Journal of the American Veterinary Medical Association.*)

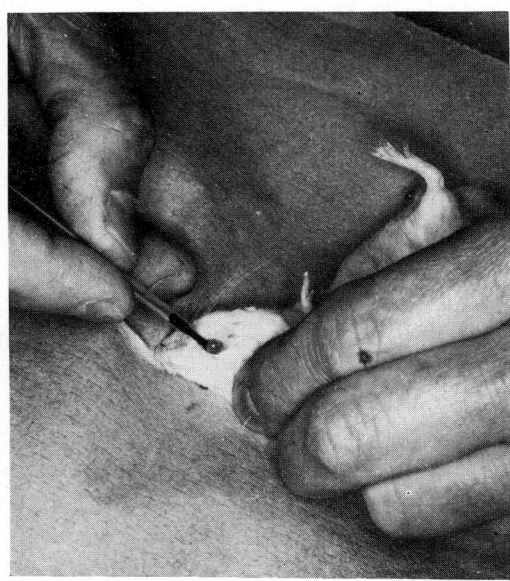

Fig. 2–4. Demonstration of the orbital bleeding technique on a mouse, using a micro blood-collecting tube.

A procedure for collection of blood from small nonhuman primates is as follows (Cooper, 1972): Good immobilization is absolutely essential. Two persons are generally required to position even the smallest primate infants. From the tiny 50-g bush baby *(Galago crassicaudatus)* and the 40-g tamarin *(Leontocebus* sp.) 0.2–0.4 ml of blood can be withdrawn with a 1-ml tuberculin syringe and a short 26-gauge needle. For all larger infants (100–400 g) and for a prosimian or monkey of any size or age from which 1.0 ml of blood or less is to be taken, a ⅝-inch, regular bevel 25-gauge needle is used. For all primates larger than 400 g, a 22-gauge needle and a 2.5-, 5.0- or 10.0-ml syringe is used. Syringes with plain tips and needles with clear plastic hubs should be used so that blood can be visualized immediately as it reaches the end of the needle tube.

Immobilize the primate on a tabletop with two animal holders on the side opposite the person collecting the blood. One holder pins the back and shoulders of the subject to the table with his right hand across the chest and arms while his left hand presses the left leg

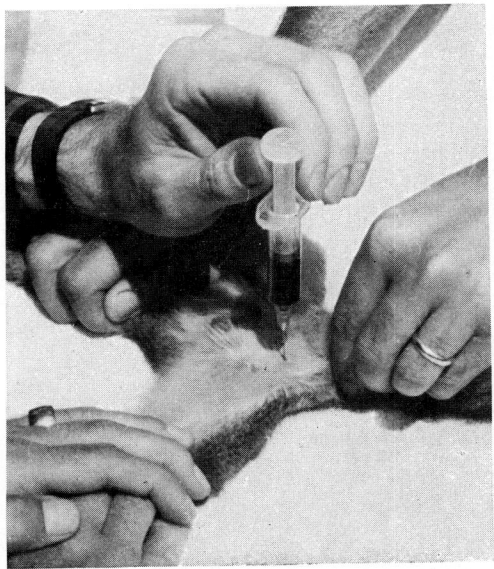

Fig. 2–5. Collection of blood from the femoral vein of a small nonhuman primate.

against the table in frog-leg fashion (Fig. 2–5). The other holder presses the right leg to the table, keeping one hand free for later use. It is important to press the legs as flat as anatomically possible without bringing the restraining hand beyond the distal portion of the femur and without stretching the skin or otherwise displacing tissue in the area of the femoral triangle. When thick hair is present, it should be clipped. Palpate the femoral artery as it emerges from beneath the inguinal ligament; in some species this closely coincides with the anterior edge of the pubis. Hold the syringe and needle in a straight, upright position with the needle bevel facing the flow of blood from the lower limb. Push the needle point through the skin 3 or 4 mm medial to the femoral arterial pulse, the actual distance depending on the size of the animal. Pass the needle completely through the femoral vein; it will actually hit the pubis near the femoral head in some species. Then withdraw the barrel slightly to produce negative pressure in the syringe. Withdraw the needle slowly until the needle tip re-enters the lumen of the vein and blood flows into the syringe. Gentle digital pressure for 30–60 seconds produces hemostasis. Animals may be bled repeatedly by this method at intervals of several days to a week for long periods of time without difficulty. It has been possible to draw safely from healthy primates a volume of blood equal to 0.5% of the total body weight, assuming 1.0 ml of blood to be equal to 1 g.

A comparison of peripheral blood from the ear and femoral venous blood of infant baboons revealed erythrocyte values to be higher in the former than in the latter (Berchelmann et al., 1973). The leukocyte counts in capillary blood from the ear were too variable for accuracy in estimation of cell numbers.

Handling the Blood

Immediately after withdrawal, blood must be thoroughly mixed with the anticoagulant to prevent clotting. The blood should always be mixed gently to avoid formation of air bubbles and hemolysis. Gentle mixing to avoid hemolysis is especially important with lipemic blood (Plate I–2) and goat blood.

When the blood is allowed to stand in the vial, separation of cells and plasma takes place. The rate of settling of cells varies with animal species and disease. Horse blood often separates within minutes; dog, cat, and pig blood may be rapid or slow in separation; cow, sheep, and goat blood seldom settles out. Because of the tendency of the cells to settle, it is necessary to mix the sample thoroughly each time a portion is removed for a test. In a laboratory where many blood samples are handled, it is convenient to use a device with gentle rocking motion or to employ a vertical turntable to which the vials are attached by clips for purposes of obtaining a uniform suspension of the blood cells in the plasma. All tests should be completed within a reasonable time. Blood can be kept at room temperature for an hour or two while various tests are performed. However, if blood examination is to be postponed for several hours or overnight, make blood films immediately, perform erythrocyte sedimentation rate (ESR), and then refrigerate the sample; leave blood films at room temperature. An icebox or cold-packs should be used to transport or dispatch blood samples to a distant laboratory.

In routine blood studies, a definite procedure should be followed to perform a CBC. The following sequence of tests is suggested:

1. Prepare the blood films and set them aside, protected from flies and moisture, until they can be stained.
2. Fill a microhematocrit tube for determination of PCV, and if ESR is to be performed, fill a Wintrobe hematocrit tube and set it vertically at room temperature.
3. Set up platelet and reticulocyte counts, if so desired.
4. Perform the erythrocyte and leukocyte counts.
5. Determine the hemoglobin concentration by cyanmethemoglobin method. With Coulter automatic hemoglobinometer, determine hemoglobin concentration from blood dilution used for the leukocyte count.
6. Record the ESR, PCV, buffy coat, and icterus index.
7. Determine total plasma protein and fibrinogen concentrations by means of a refractometer.
8. Stain and examine the blood films.

Additional tests such as erythrocyte osmotic fragility, Coombs test, etc., should be performed as time permits.

THE BLOOD FILM

The blood film should be made immediately from fresh blood and as soon as possible from anticoagulated blood, preferably within an hour of sampling. It may be prepared on a slide or a coverslip.

Slide Method

Place a clean slide on a level surface, and deposit a very small drop of thoroughly mixed blood near one end of the slide. The inexperienced person has a tendency to use too large a drop of blood. A round applicator stick can be used to transfer blood to the slide. Spread the blood in an even film with another slide. The spreading edge should be perfectly smooth (free of chipped spots), and the corners of the slide preferably should be cut off in order to make the spreading edge slightly less wide than the slide on which the film is to be made. Lay the spreader slide on the inner surface of the index finger or hold it

between the thumb and finger and draw it toward the drop of blood (Fig. 2–6); as it makes contact, the blood will spread along the edge of the spreader slide, which is then moved forward in a smooth glide. The angle at which the spreader slide is held determines the thickness of the blood film, i.e., the greater the angle, the thicker the film. Generally, about a 30° angle is satisfactory. Wave the slide in the air to hasten drying; slow drying leads to movement of water out of the erythrocytes resulting in *crenation*. Waving the film over a low gas flame will hasten drying and improve results. The criteria of a good slide blood film are:

1. It has a *smooth, even appearance, free from holes*. A wavy film is caused by a jerking movement when the blood is spread, and holes in the film are usually caused by grease or dirt on the surface of the slide. Clear streaks are the result of a chipped edge on the spreader slide.
2. *The film has long straight borders* that are about 2 mm from the edge of the slide.
3. *The erythrocytes are distributed in a single layer* over a greater portion of the film. Blood films with a monolayer of cells appear translucent and exhibit a rainbow spectrum when held against light. Thick films are difficult to study because of the lack of cellular details.

A modified method is to make blood and bone marrow films essentially similar to the coverslip method described below but using glass slides instead. In our experience, this method provides an even distribution of animal leukocytes comparable to the coverslip method and provides preparations suitable for staining employing an automatic stainer.

Coverslip Method

1. Use No. 1½, 22-mm-square coverslips. With a clean camel's hair brush, remove dust particles from the surfaces to receive the blood.
2. Holding a coverslip by two of its corners, place a very small drop of blood (1–2 mm in diameter) on its surface near the center with the applicator stick (Fig. 2–7).

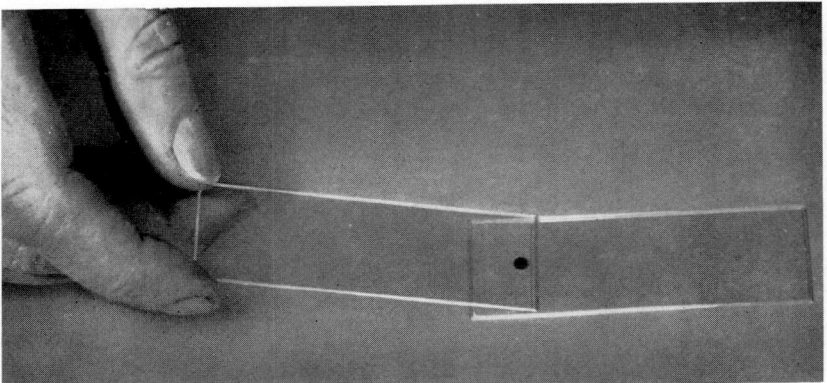

Fig. 2–6. Method for preparing a blood film on a slide. (1) The spreader slide is drawn toward the small drop of blood; (2) as soon as contact with the blood is made, the spreader is moved forward in a smooth glide.

3. Quickly drop another coverslip on the first in crosswise fashion. If the coverslip is clean and free of particles, the blood will spread quickly and evenly between the two surfaces (Fig. 2–8).

4. Just before spreading is complete and soon after rays have appeared along the edges (Fig. 2–10), separate the two coverslips by sliding (not lifting) them apart.

5. Immediately wave the films in the air, preferably over a low gas flame, to hasten drying.

An alternative method is to hold two coverslips simultaneously, separated between the thumb and index finger (Fig. 2–9A). Briefly brush the upper surface of the top coverslip and the lower surface of the bottom coverslip to remove dust particles. Place the small drop of blood near the center of the upper coverslip, and immediately move the lower coverslip into position with the other hand and drop it parallel upon the opposite one (Fig. 2–9B) so that it covers about three-quarters of its surface. Grasp the free corners of the projecting edge of the upper coverslip, and slide the two coverslips apart immediately after rays have appeared along the advancing edge of the spreading blood film (Fig. 2–10).

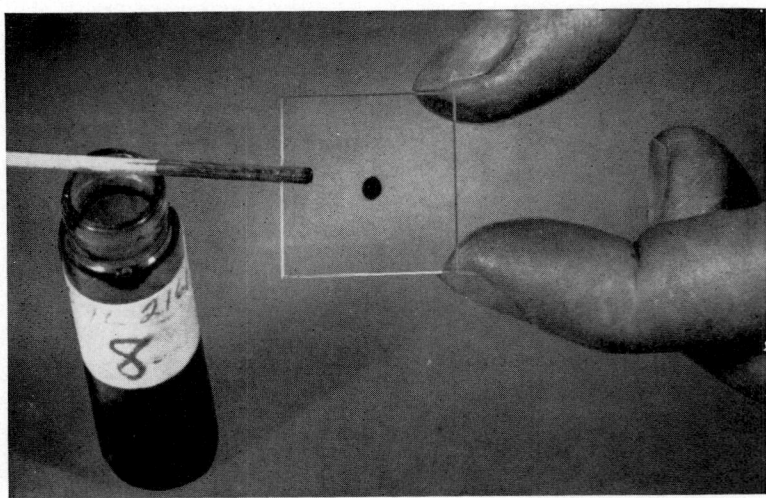

Fig. 2–7. An applicator stick is used to place a small quantity of blood on a glass coverslip in preparation for making a blood film.

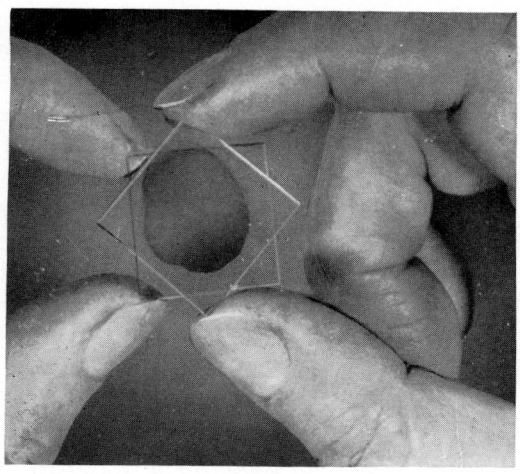

Fig. 2–8. In preparing blood films on coverslips, a second coverslip is dropped crosswise onto the coverslip containing the small drop of blood. The blood spreads quickly between the coverslips, and at the moment spreading is complete, the two coverslips are separated by sliding them apart.

STAINING BLOOD FILMS WITH ROMANOWSKY STAINS

Basic Principles

An understanding of the physicochemical principles involved in the differential staining of blood cells is a prerequisite to the satisfactory use of Wright or Giemsa stains. Romanowsky, in 1891, stimulated by Ehrlich's work on staining leukocytes with anionic and cationic dyes, combined eosin and methylene blue to stain blood. He realized that the differential staining effect obtained was not entirely due to the two stains and that additional dyes had formed. The present-day blood stains that employ eosin and methylene blue are commonly referred to as "modified Romanowsky stains." Recent developments in the chemistry and technology of these stains have been reviewed (Marshall, 1978).

Methylene blue readily oxidizes to form azure dyes called Azure A, B, and C. Methylene blue solution, upon standing or aging, forms the azure dyes and is then referred to as "polychrome methylene blue." Oxidation of methylene blue can be hastened by boiling in the presence of alkali. *Wright stain* is a mixture of methylene blue, polychromated with sodium bicarbonate and heat, and eosin. Eosin enters into chemical combination with the basic dyes present, and a compound insoluble in water precipitates. This precipitate is the Wright stain powder, which is soluble in absolute alcohol.

Giemsa stain consists of Azure II–eosin and Azure II in the ratio of 15:4. Azure I and II are trade names, and it is said that Azure B predominates in Azure I and that Azure II is a mixture of Azure I and methylene blue in equal parts.

The azures are basic dyes, and they are therefore attracted to the acidic nuclei,

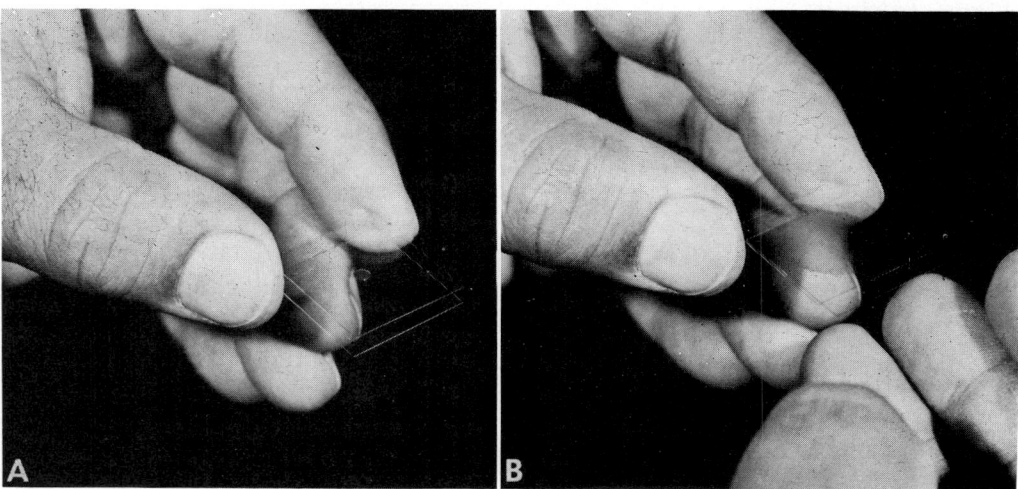

Fig. 2–9. A method for making coverslip blood films. *A,* Hold two coverslips between thumb and forefinger, separated as shown. *B,* As blood spreads between the two coverslips, watch for lines developing along the spreading edge (see Fig. 2–10), and slide the two glasses apart as soon as the lines appear to form.

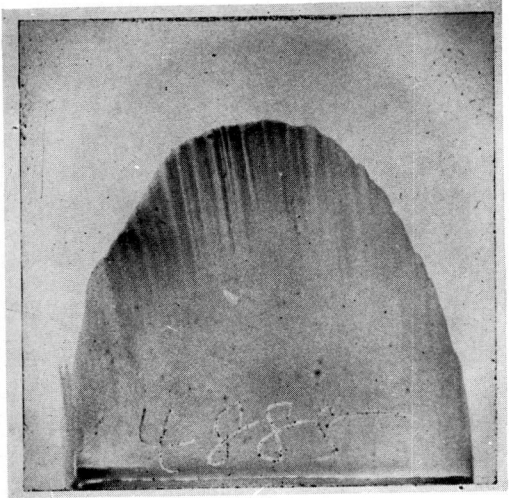

Fig. 2–10. A coverslip blood film prepared according to the procedure outlined in Figure 2–9 and text.

whereas eosin is an acid dye and is attracted to the alkaline cytoplasmic constituents. This combination of basic and acid dyes, in the form of chlorides for the basic dye and sodium or potassium salts for the acid dyes, is referred to as a "neutral stain" (Conn, 1969).

The neutral stains are soluble in absolute methyl or ethyl alcohol, but the alcoholic solutions tend to retain the dyes so that they are not adsorbed to the protoplasm of the cell. Thus it is necessary to force the dyes out of solution by the addition of water, which precipitates the stain. The water must be neutral or of proper pH to provide the best differential staining. Water that is too alkaline favors the methylene blue and azure stains, causing the cells to become too blue, whereas too acid a medium leads to overemphasis of the eosin stain, with little or no staining on the part of the nuclei of cells. Distilled water is usually too acid because of dissolved CO_2, and tap water may be too alkaline. A buffer solution is preferred for this step of staining (see below).

Blood and tissue cells treated with a mordant show a greater affinity for the stain. This is accomplished by fixing blood films with absolute methyl alcohol. The methyl alcohol should be neutral in reaction and free of acetone and acid. The same purity of methyl alcohol is required for use in dissolving the powdered stain in making the stock solution.

Wright stain is used in concentrated form, while Giemsa stain is employed as a diluted stain. Thus staining with Wright stain is accomplished more rapidly but may lead to more difficulty. Fixation of the blood film with Wright stain is accomplished directly by the alcoholic staining solution. With Giemsa stain, the blood film is fixed in absolute methyl alcohol before exposure to the diluted stain. Prior fixation of the blood film has been found to improve results with the Wright stain.

Neutralization of Distilled Water

Rinse a clean test tube in the water to be neutralized, and to 5 ml of the water add a few crystals of hematoxylin.

Neutral water—becomes pale lavender in 10 seconds.

Acid water—becomes yellow and remains yellow for more than 5 minutes.

Alkaline water—becomes reddish purple immediately or within 1 minute.

Neutral water may be prepared by adding 1% potassium carbonate, drop by drop, to acid water in quantity sufficient to neutralize it or by adding 1% HCl to alkaline water. The neutralized water should be prepared each day, and it should be kept in a polyethylene or Pyrex bottle with no rubber connections.

Phosphate Buffer

Phosphate buffer, pH 6.6–6.8, for use in lieu of neutral distilled water, is prepared as follows:

34 mM Na_2HPO_4: 2.41 g dissolved in 500 ml of distilled water

34 mM KH_2PO_4: 4.63 g dissolved in 500 ml of distilled water

Mix both solutions in proportion of one part Na_2HPO_4 solution to two parts KH_2PO_4 solution. If necessary, adjust pH by adding a few ml of the former solution when pH is below 6.6 or the latter solution when it is above 6.6.

Wright Stain

Wright stain ready for use is available commercially, or it can be prepared as follows:

Place 0.1 g of powder stain in a mortar. Add 60 ml of absolute methyl alcohol (free of acetone and acetic acid), a few milliliters at a time, while grinding the powdered stain. Continue grinding for about 5 minutes after all alcohol has been added. Transfer to a tightly stoppered brown bottle and store in the dark. Allow the stain to age 2–4 weeks, and filter it through paper before use. Aging may be hastened by storing at 37°C.

A modified formula (Reich, 1954) of Wright stain contains 300 mg of Wright stain and 30 mg of Giemsa stain ground in a mortar until dissolved in 100 ml of absolute methyl alcohol. It can be used after 24 hours. A stable Romanowsky stain has been developed recently by Marshall et al. (1978).

A procedure to stain an occasional blood film with Wright stain is as follows:

1. To conserve stain, mark off with a wax pencil the area of the film to be stained.
2. Place the slide on the staining rack, and with a medicine dropper add 4–10 drops of stain. Allow the concentrated stain to act for 1 minute. (Sufficient stain must be added so that the alcohol will not evaporate during the fixation period.)
3. Add an equal number of drops of buffer or neutral water, and mix thoroughly by blowing or by applying air with the medicine dropper. Continue mixing until a metallic film forms on the surface of the stain-buffer mixture.
4. Let the diluted stain act for 2–4 minutes (staining period). Each batch of stain has its own time requirements. When testing a new batch of stain, start with a 4-minute period and modify the time as necessary. With modified Wright formula, a staining time of 2–3 minutes has been satisfactory.
5. Float off the metallic film with neutral water. This is an important step. It is accomplished by quickly flooding water from a 50-ml beaker over the slide. *Excessive exposure to water will wash out the stain, while insufficient washing leaves stain precipitate.*

An alternate method is to fix the blood film in absolute methyl alcohol for 30 seconds and then stain with dilute Wright stain (four parts stock stain and six parts neutral distilled water or buffer).

When more than an occasional blood film is to be stained, it is convenient to have stock Wright stain and buffer in separate screw-capped coplin jars. The slide is first fixed in absolute methyl alcohol, then placed in the stain, transferred to the buffer, and finally rinsed briefly in tap water and stood on edge to air dry. A similar procedure can be used for blood films prepared on coverslips. In this case small coplin jars (Columbia staining dishes) with screw caps are used. Where staining load is heavy, jars with ground glass covers are best.

Giemsa Stain

Commercial Giemsa stock solution is used for staining slides or coverslips. The coplin jar, with screw cap, is preferable.

1. Place the blood film in absolute methyl alcohol for 3–5 minutes and air dry.
2. Fill a coplin jar with Giemsa stain prepared as follows: To each ml of neutral distilled water add one drop of stock Giemsa stain. The large coplin jar holds about 60 ml, and the small coplin jar 9 ml.
3. Place the blood film into the diluted stain for 30–45 minutes.
4. Wash the film with neutral distilled water for 30 seconds and drain dry.

Wright-Leishman Stain

The following is the method for staining coverslip blood and bone marrow films as employed in the Clinical Pathology Laboratory, School of Veterinary Medicine, University of California, Davis. Consistently good results are obtained by adhering strictly to all details given for preparation and use of the stain.

1. *Neutralization of Alcohol.* Neutralize 1 gallon of absolute methyl alcohol, anhydrous and acetone- and acid-free, by adding a very small amount of buffer salts (25 mg or the quantity retained on the tip of the small spatula). A slight excess of buffer salts does not matter because they are only slightly soluble in the alcohol. Prepare the dry buffer by mixing 6.20 g of Na_2HPO_4 with 3.22 g of KH_2PO_4. A crystal of hematoxylin added

to a small quantity (5 ml) of alcohol is acidic.

2. *Preparation of Solution I, Wright Stain.* Place 0.6 g of powdered Wright stain, 5.0 ml of glycerin, and 300 ml of neutralized absolute methyl alcohol into a 500-ml Pyrex flask containing approximately 20 glass beads. With extreme caution and constant agitation, gently heat the mixture until the solution reaches a temperature that is just below the boiling point. Permit the solution to cool a few minutes, and repeat the heating process three times. Tightly stopper the flask while the solution is still warm, and store in the dark to age a minimum of 2 weeks. When preparing a new batch of stain, use the same flask without discarding any residual stain or sediment. This procedure helps to fortify the staining solution.

3. *Preparation of Solution II, Leishman Stain.* Substitute 0.6 g of powdered Leishman stain in the above formula, and prepare the solution for use in the same manner.

4. *Wright-Leishman Stain.* Mix aged stains in a ratio of four parts solution I to one part solution II. Filter a small quantity into a plastic bottle, and transfer filtered stain to the coplin jar as needed.

Staining Procedure

Three Columbia jars with covers are used to hold neutralized absolute methyl alcohol, stain, and buffer solution. Fortify the buffer solution of pH 6.6 with stain by adding about 20 drops of stain to 7.0 ml of buffer in the Columbia jar and mixing with an applicator stick. Start with fresh alcohol, stain, and fortified buffer each day.

1. Immerse the blood film in the alcohol for a minimum of 5 minutes to fix the cells. Drain excess alcohol from the coverslip before transferring it to the stain. Change the alcohol after every four blood films have been fixed.

2. Place the blood film in the stain for 3 minutes. Replace the stain daily.

3. Transfer the blood film to the fortified buffer solution without draining off excess stain, and leave it in for 6 minutes.

Replace the buffer solution after every eight blood films.

4. Rinse briefly by dipping the film in neutral distilled water in two separate beakers. Be careful not to rinse excessively or the stain will be washed out.

5. Stand the coverslip on end to facilitate draining and drying.

6. Mount the coverslip, blood film down, on a clean slide with mounting medium such as Pro-Texx (distributed by Scientific Products).

7. Examine as usual.

If staining is light, stain another coverslip film giving longer time in freshly prepared fortified buffer. If the same film is to be restained, remove the mounting medium by briefly dipping the coverslip film in xylol, and then repeat steps 2 through 6 using freshly prepared fortified buffer.

Bone marrow smears can be stained similarly, with 4 minutes in stain (step 2) and 10 minutes in buffer (step 3). Examine the stained films unmounted (omit step 6) under high dry magnification and restain, if necessary, repeating steps 2 through 5.

Leukemic blood and bone marrow cells may stain poorly with the above procedure. In such instances, satisfactory staining can be obtained by additional staining in diluted Giemsa stain (1 drop/ml of the phosphate buffer) for 10 minutes.

Quick Stains

A number of quick stains are available commercially. With these, only a few minutes are required to obtain a stained preparation. Our experience is limited to Camco Quik (Scientific Products) and Harleco Diff Quick (Curtis Matheson Scientific, Inc.) stains. Both are Wright stain preparations. These stains can be recommended for use by the busy practitioner. Staining instructions are supplied by the manufacturer, but some modifications may be required to obtain desired differential staining of various blood and bone marrow cells.

Causes and Correction of Poor Staining

Delay in preparing smears introduces degenerative changes in leukocytes, and delayed fixing or staining may result in poor staining quality.

1. *Irregularity in staining intensity of various regions of the film:*
   (a) Failure to obtain thorough mixing of stain and buffer.
   (b) Variation in pH of the surface of the slide due to careless cleaning.
   (c) Water allowed to remain on parts of the film during drying. Always stand the slide or coverslip on end to hasten drying after washing.
2. *Washed-out appearance of the stain over entire film:*
   (a) Water was allowed to act too long in washing, or film was not drained dry quickly enough.
   (b) Insufficient staining time or failure to add a sufficient number of drops of buffer to the stain after the fixation period, when staining was conducted directly on the slide rather than in a jar.
3. *Nuclei stain faintly, but erythrocytes and granules of eosinophils have an intense eosin stain:*
   (a) Water or buffer used in staining or washing was acidic.
   (b) Surface of slide was acidic.
4. *Nuclei intensely blue, erythrocytes greenish or blue, cytoplasm of leukocytes not stained:*
   (a) Water or buffer used in staining or washing was alkaline.
   (b) Surface of slide was alkaline.
5. *Film covered with precipitate:*
   (a) Failure to float off the metallic scum from the slide or insufficient stain placed on the slide during the period of fixation so that the alcohol evaporated, leaving a precipitated stain.
   (b) Inadequate rinsing of slide or coverslip when stained in coplin jars.
6. *Overstaining:*
   Remove stain by dipping the film in 95% methyl alcohol, and restain, reducing the staining time.

MICROSCOPIC EXAMINATION OF A STAINED BLOOD FILM

General Examination and Differential Count

Initially, the blood film should be examined with low-power objective (25×) to locate areas that consist of well-spread blood cells in a monolayer and that are satisfactory for study. High dry magnification (40×) is used to gain an overall impression of (a) degree of variation in size and shape of erythrocytes, (b) existence of excessively high or low number of leukocytes, and (c) the occurrence and relative distribution of thrombocytes. The experienced technician may conduct the differential leukocyte count under high dry magnification, but the oil immersion lens is preferred. The latter objective is essential for studying cellular details and recognizing various abnormalities encountered in pathologic specimens, such as red cell parasites, azurophilic granules, toxic changes, and other leukocyte and red cell abnormalities. A pattern of examination of blood films should be developed for consistency. Blood platelets should be looked at first, then erythrocytes, then the leukocytes should be examined for various abnormalities, and finally the blood film should be checked for other abnormalities. Various features to be kept in mind during blood examination are given in Table 1–1. Freshly mounted coverslip blood films should be examined carefully under the oil immersion lens and the oil left unremoved because the mounting medium takes a few days to dry. Blood smears on slides must be covered with a coverslip or coated with a thin film of immersion oil before satisfactory inspection is possible at low or high dry magnification. To remove oil, wipe the slide with facial tissue or cheesecloth; avoid using xylene.

When blood is spread on a slide, there is a tendency for the neutrophils to flow to the edges of the film and the lymphocytes to remain mainly in the body of the smear, while the monocytes and eosinophils tend to distribute evenly. MacGregor et al. (1940) compared three methods for making the differential count in blood films on slides (Fig. 2–11). The straight edge method, which follows the edge of the film, gave consistently higher neutrophil and lower lymphocyte counts than those obtained by the cross-sectional method, which consists of going back and forth across the slide. These workers found the battlement method of counting to give values that compared favorably with the differential leukocyte count made by exami-

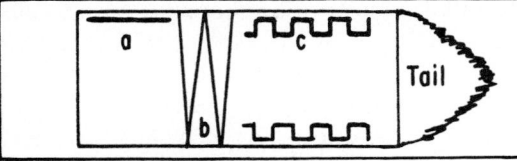

a = Straight-edge method
b = Cross-sectional method
c = Battlement method

Fig. 2–11. Three methods for selecting areas for the differential leukocyte count in blood films on slides. The battlement method *(c)* was reported to produce the most accurate result.

Table 2–3.   The 95% Confidence Limits for Differential Leukocyte Counts*

Percentage of Given Cell Type	100 Cells Counted	200 Cells Counted
0	0.0– 3.0	0.0– 1.5
1	0.5– 4.7	0.2– 3.1
2	0.4– 6.3	0.7– 4.6
3	0.8– 7.7	1.3– 5.9
4	1.4– 9.1	2.0– 7.2
5	2.0–10.5	2.7– 8.5
10	4.0–16.0	5.8–14.2
20	12.0–28.0	14.3–25.7
30	20.8–39.2	23.5–36.5
40	30.2–49.8	33.1–46.9
50	40.0–60.0	42.9–57.1
60	50.2–69.8	53.1–66.9
70	60.8–79.2	63.5–76.5
80	72.0–88.0	74.3–85.7
90	84.0–96.0	85.8–94.2

From Wintrobe et al., 1981.
*For percentages of 5 or less the limits were derived by assuming a Poisson rather than a binomial distribution.

nation of the entire blood film. In describing the battlement method, they stated: "It implies a count made of three horizontal edge fields followed by two fields toward the center (so as to give three vertical fields), followed by two fields in a horizontal and then two fields in the vertical direction to reach the edge again." This limits the counting of cells in an area of 1 mm of the edge of the blood film. In order to use the battlement method of counting, it is necessary to obtain films having reasonably long straight edges. They also stated that in blood films on coverslips the cells tend to gather toward the center, and, provided a large enough number of cells is counted in the central area, a good average figure is obtained. General experience is that the leukocytes are more evenly distributed in blood films prepared on coverslips.

Number of Cells to Be Differentiated

The differential leukocyte count determines the percentage distribution of the various leukocyte types in peripheral blood. The procedure is subject to considerable error because an extremely small portion of the total number of leukocytes is observed. The unavoidable error in differential count has been discussed (Barnett, 1933). It has been shown to vary as a result of chance distribution of cells. At least 400 cells must be counted before the results can be considered reliable, and even then the chance error may be as much as 7.5% of the total count. For total leukocyte counts of more than 20,000/μl of blood, it has been suggested that an additional 100 cells may be differentiated for each 10,000 increment in the total leukocyte count. The probable error and 95% confidence limits of a differential count

in relation to the number of cells counted have been determined (Table 2–3). The larger the number of cells counted and the greater the proportion of a particular cell, the greater the accuracy. Considering the time involved in performing a differential leukocyte count and compromising the accuracy, at least 200 leukocytes should be differentiated routinely, except when this is too time-consuming in instances of marked leukopenia. The results should be reported for each leukocyte type as percentage of total count and as absolute number per μl of blood. The latter is calculated by multiplying the total leukocyte count by the percentile fraction. For example, the absolute neutrophil number for a blood sample having a leukocyte count of 15,000/μl and 60% neutrophils would be 15,000 × 0.6 = 9,000/μl of blood. *Interpretation of the differential leukocyte count should be based not on the relative percentage distribution but on the absolute number*, which provides a more accurate assessment of the situation because each leukocyte behaves largely independently with regard to its production, distribution, functions, and response to disease.

HEMATOCRIT OR PACKED CELL VOLUME

The word "hematocrit" is derived from two Greek words *(haima, blood; krinein, to sepa-*

rate) meaning "to separate blood." Centrifugation separates the blood into three distinct compartments: *(a)* the erythrocyte mass at the bottom, called the packed cell volume or PCV; *(b)* a white to gray layer of leukocytes and thrombocytes occurring immediately above the red cell mass and called the buffy coat; and *(c)* the blood plasma (Plate I–1). By common usage the word hematocrit has become, though incorrectly, synonymous with PCV.

The Wintrobe Hematocrit

The Wintrobe hematocrit tube (Wintrobe, 1933) has a uniform 3-mm bore and is calibrated by a double 10-cm scale with millimeter divisions. The scale on the left is read from top to bottom, while the scale on the right is in reverse. The volume percent of each compartment of the blood, after adequate centrifugation, is determined by directly observing the height of each compartment in millimeters.

About 1 ml of blood is required to fill the Wintrobe hematocrit tube. The tube is filled by means of a special pipette with a long, narrow delivery tip. The tip of the pipette is inserted to the bottom of the hematocrit tube, and as blood is forced out by pressure on the rubber bulb, the pipette is slowly withdrawn. When the column of blood reaches the level of the 0 mark on the left-hand scale, the proper amount of blood has been deposited. While the tube is being filled, the tip of the pipette should remain just below the advancing level of blood in order to avoid the formation of bubbles. With practice, the hematocrit tube can be filled quickly and easily.

The purpose of centrifugation is to obtain maximum packing of the erythrocyte so that little or no plasma remains trapped between the cells (see p. 92). The centrifuge must produce sufficient relative centrifugal force (RCF) to accomplish this purpose. Maximum packing in human blood is obtained with a force of 2,260 G for 30 minutes (Wintrobe, 1967). Species variations with regard to red cell size and rouleau formation influence the required RCF and time of centrifugation necessary to produce complete packing. When the proper RCF is applied, satisfactory packing for routine study is accomplished in 30 minutes with dog and horse blood. With cattle and pig blood, a centrifugation time of 60 minutes is required (Bunce, 1954). With sheep and goat blood, an RCF much greater than 2,260 G is required for complete packing of the red blood cells. When packing is complete, the red cell column has a translucent appearance. This phenomenon is called Koeppe's criterion for complete packing. Koeppe's criterion is regularly apparent in the red cell column of the Drummond microcapillary hematocrit. It is generally not observed in the Wintrobe hematocrit tube with normal animal bloods, but may be seen in anemia in remission when PCV is low and the erythrocytes are large. Interconversion of the RCF and G force can be made from Figure 2–12.

The Packed Cell Volume

The column of packed erythrocytes (PCV) is measured in mm and expressed as a percentage of the total volume, or as a ratio (SI unit). Normally, a direct relationship exists between hemoglobin concentration and PCV. In all species having normal average MCHC of 33%, the ratio of PCV to hemoglobin concentration is 3:1. With such a relationship, it is possible to approximate the amount of hemoglobin from the PCV by dividing the latter by 3. The PCV is erroneously decreased in blood samples with excessive EDTA (see p. 23) or marked hemolysis, in which cases the relationship with hemoglobin becomes spurious.

Anemia exists when the PCV falls below the normal range for the species in question (Figs. 2–13*B* and 2–14*A*), and hemoconcentration may be present when the PCV exceeds the normal range. An anemic animal in a state of marked dehydration, however, may have a PCV within the normal range. Interpretation of the PCV must always be made in light of the water balance of the animal as determined by the physical examination and estimation of total plasma proteins.

The Buffy Coat

In blood from a normal animal, the buffy coat consists of a white to gray layer, 0.5–1.2 mm deep, occurring immediately above the packed erythrocytes (Fig. 2–14). A delicate black line is often observed at the point of contact of the buffy coat and erythrocytes.

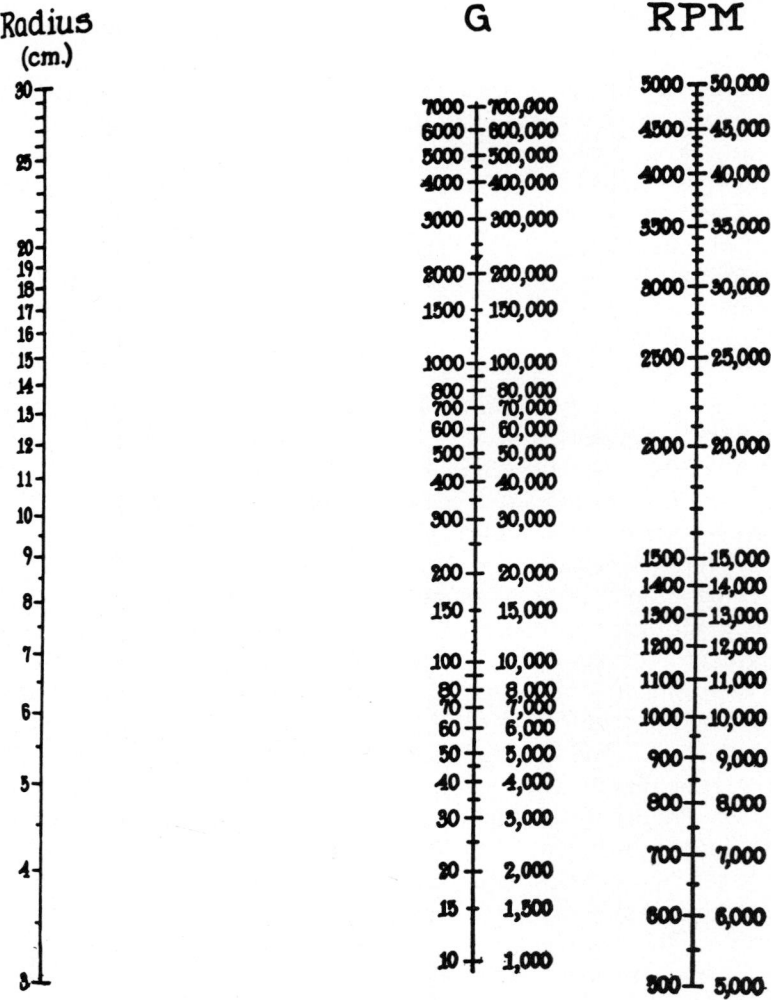

Fig. 2–12. A nomogram depicting the relationship of the radius of a centrifuge head and the relative centrifugal force (RCF) to gravity (G). (From Dole and Cotzias, 1951. By permission from Science, *113*:553, 1951. Copyright 1951 by the AAAS.)

This dark line is the result of action of the leukocyte upon the hemoglobin of the red cells, whereby the oxygen is removed and reduced hemoglobin is produced. The thrombocytes are arranged at the very top of the buffy coat, with the leukocytes below (Plates I–2, II–2). The platelet layer is whitish compared to the leukocyte layer and can be distinguished on close examination with a magnifying glass or 10× ocular lens, particularly in feline blood. In exceptional circumstances, the platelet layer may be so large from thrombocytosis that it could be mistaken for the leukocyte layer (Plate I–4).

A rough estimation of total leukocyte count can be made from height of the buffy coat (excluding the platelet layer). The estimate however, may vary considerably from actual count because of variations in size and relative packing of various leukocytes and intermixing in varying numbers of platelets at the top and young erythrocytes (reticulocytes) at the bottom. However, a rough estimate can be obtained by considering the first mm equal to 10,000 leukocytes and each additional mm, 20,000 leukocytes. For routine clinical application, a buffy coat of less than 0.5 mm would suggest leukopenia, while that above 1.5 mm would suggest a leukocytosis (Fig. 2–14A, Plate II–2).

In chronic diseases erythrogenesis is often affected, with the result that erythrocytes of

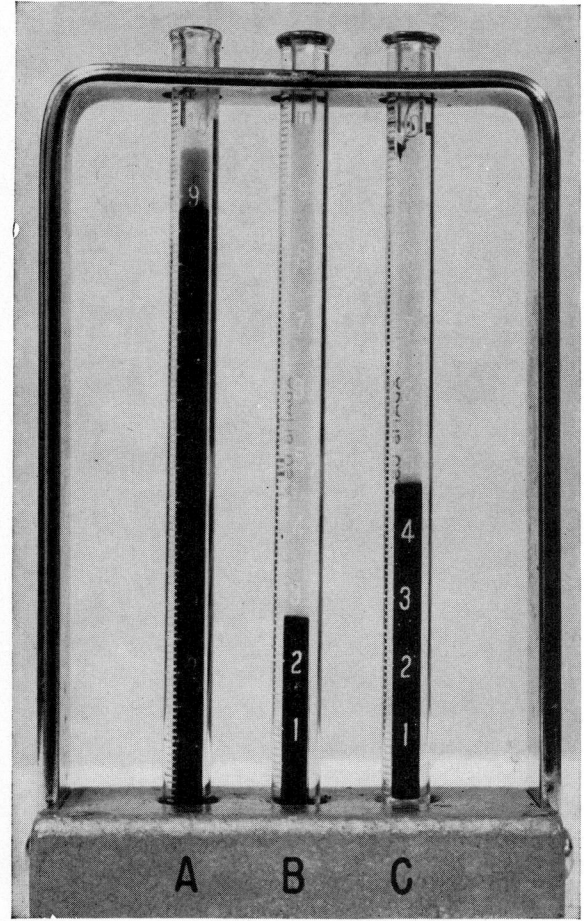

Fig. 2–13. A diphasic erythrocyte sedimentation rate in canine blood is shown in tube *A*. The same blood, after centrifugation for the hematocrit, is shown in *B*. For comparison with tube *B*, tube *C* contains a canine blood with the PCV within the normal range. The hazy plasma zone of tube *A* reflects the trailing-out of reticulocytes during the 1 hour required for the erythrocyte sedimentation test. The PCV in tube *B* reveals the presence of an anemia. Combining the results of *A* and *B* leads to the conclusion that anemia exists and the bone marrow is responding with release of reticulocytes to peripheral blood. However, the latter assumption should be verified by examination of a blood film stained with new methylene blue.

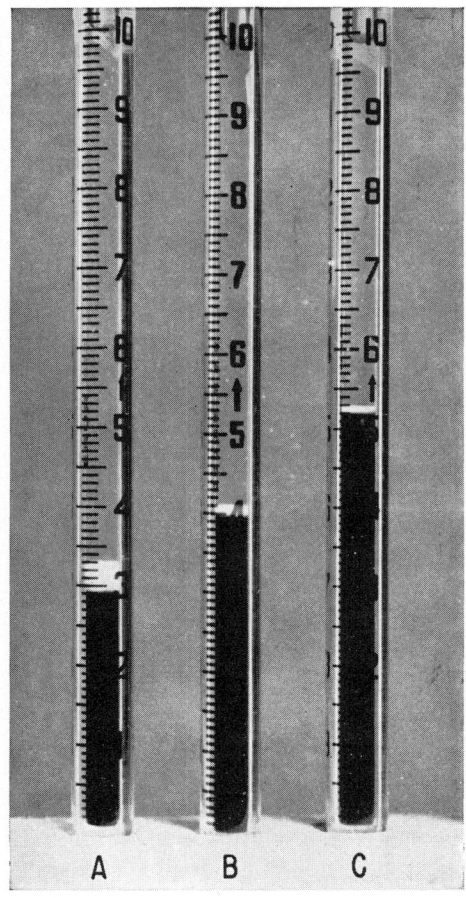

Fig. 2–14. Three canine bloods in the Wintrobe hematocrit tubes. In *A*, PCV is 29%, indicating anemia, and the buffy coat is 4 mm, indicating a marked leukocytosis. Tubes *B* and *C* are representative of the normal ranges for PCV and buffy coat (See also Plate I–1).

abnormal morphology are produced. Such erythrocytes, as well as reticulocytes, do not participate in the formation of rouleaux, and for this reason they tend to accumulate at the top of the erythrocyte column and may even be involved in the lower portions of the buffy coat, where they impart a red tinge (Plates I–1, II–2). Admixture of leukocytes and abnormal erythrocytes and/or reticulocytes in the buffy coat is enhanced when ESR is conducted before centrifugation for the hemato-

crit test. A red-tinged buffy coat indicates that erythrogenesis has been affected by the disease process. When many reticulocytes are present, they mix uniformly with the leukocytes during centrifugation, giving the appearance of the absence of a buffy coat. Examination of the buffy coat area by magnifying glass will demonstrate the intensely red buffy coat of admixed leukocytes and reticulocytes.

The Plasma Compartment and Icterus Index

The volume of plasma normally exceeds 50% of whole blood. Bilirubin, a product of hemoglobin catabolism, imparts a yellow color to the plasma. This yellow color increases in hemolytic anemia, in certain forms of hepatopathy, and in bile-duct obstruction.

The degree of yellow pigmentation of the plasma is referred to as the *icterus index*. The icterus index is determined by matching the plasma color in the hematocrit tube with standards prepared from potassium dichromate. The icterus index is recorded in units from 0 to 100 (Plates II–1, II–2).

Icterus index standards for 2, 5, 7.5, 10, 15, 25, 50, 75, and 100 units can be prepared with the proper dilution of potassium dichromate. One unit is defined as the color produced by one part $K_2Cr_2O_7$ in 10,000 parts distilled water. One gram of potassium dichromate in 100 ml of water equals 100 units of color. By dilution, the various unit standards indicated above are easily prepared. Disposable Wintrobe hematocrit tubes or 75 mm $\times$ 1 mm capillary hematocrit tubes are filled with solutions representing the various units of color and sealed. Color comparison must be made with standards filled in tubes of size (bore and thickness) identical to the hematocrit tubes containing plasma. Commercially available standards are designed to compare with Wintrobe hematocrit tubes.

In normal carnivorous animals such as the dog and cat, the yellow color is due entirely to bilirubin. In these animals, the icterus index is generally less than 5 units. A reading of 7.5 units in the dog or cat should be regarded with suspicion, and a reading of over 7.5 units is definitely abnormal. Thus color equal to 10 units of icterus is clinically significant in the dog and cat. In the cow and horse, the yellow pigments, carotenoids of plants and vegetables of diet impart additional color to the plasma and make the establishment of an upper limit for icterus index score rather unsatisfactory. In addition, the horse has a higher bilirubin concentration than other domestic species (Cornelius et al., 1960), and fasting for 48 hours causes a striking increase in plasma bilirubin (Ramsay, 1945). For these reasons, the icterus index score is not as useful in certain herbivores as in the carnivores. In general, the normal icterus index score in the cow is between 5 and 15 units and may be as high as 20 to 25 units when the animal is on green feed; a reading of 20 to 25 icterus units may also be seen in instances of acute disease with accompanying hemoconcentration. In the horse, icterus index scores of 7.5

to 20 units are common; the intensity of color due to bilirubin is in direct proportion to the magnitude of the PCV in the horse (see p. 160). It is important to take into consideration the type of feed and state of water balance of the animal when using the icterus index score in the cow and horse. Animals with yellow body fat, such as cattle, horses, and chickens, are the ones that will develop yellow plasma color from plant pigments. Sheep, pigs, goats, and water buffaloes do not show plasma color from plant pigments.

In hemolytic disease in which the erythrocytes are being destroyed by the mononuclear phagocyte (reticuloendothelial) system, bilirubin accumulates because the liver is unable to conjugate and excrete the bilirubin as rapidly as it is produced. Bilirubin also accumulates in blood during intrahepatic and extrahepatic bile duct obstruction. Under these conditions, the yellow color of the plasma increases. In certain diseases, intravascular hemolysis of erythrocytes may occur, with development of hemoglobinemia. In such cases, the plasma is red.

In the horse, the icterus index may reach 50 to 100 units without evidence of hemolytic disease. This occurs when food and water intake are significantly reduced in any illness, but especially in diseases involving the gastrointestinal tract (Appendix Case 65; Tables 6–16, 6–17).

A turbid plasma indicates lipemia or the presence of a fine emulsion of fatty substance. Examination of such blood in wet film will reveal myriads of tiny particles in brownian motion; these particles are called chylomicra. In the dry, unfixed blood film treated with new methylene blue stain, the chylomicra appear as small, spherical refractile bodies adhering to the surface of the erythrocytes (Fig. 2–25:2). When lipids are present in the plasma in large amount, the plasma may appear uniformly lactescent, or a white opaque layer of chylomicra may appear at the top of the plasma column (Plates II–3, II–4). The plasma in the latter instance is often red because of the presence of free hemoglobin. The hemoglobinemia indicates the presence of a lytic agent, most probably neutral fat and fatty acids (Freeman and Johnson, 1940; Loewy et al., 1943; Swank and Roth, 1954). The hemolysis in lipemic blood is produced after the blood is withdrawn from the animal and is enhanced by physical force, such as shaking the blood sample or forcing the blood from the syringe through the needle (Jasper and Jain, 1965). Care must be employed in handling lipemic blood to prevent hemolysis. The icterus index of hemolyzed, lactescent, or lipemic plasma is spurious because of interference with proper color comparison.

The plasma of the hematocrit is suitable for estimation of concentrations of total plasma protein and fibrinogen by the refractometer method described later in this chapter.

The Microhematocrit

The advantages of the microhematocrit over the Wintrobe method are several: (a) more accurate and reproducible PCV values are possible because there is less trapping of plasma; (b) much less time is required for the entire procedure; and (c) the amount of blood required is minimal. There are two disadvantages: (a) a special reader is required to determine the hematocrit value, and (b) because of the small size of the capillary tube, the erythrocyte sedimentation rate, the buffy coat value, and the icterus index score are not so easily observed and determined as with the Wintrobe method (Plate I–1).

The microhematocrit method makes use of a high-speed centrifuge that permits a corresponding reduction in the time required for complete packing of the erythrocytes. Time required to produce complete packing with human blood was shown to be 1 minute at 28,000 G; 2 minutes at 12,000 G; 4 minutes at 8,000 G; and 9 minutes at 4,000 G (Strumia et al., 1954).

Capillary tubes containing anticoagulant may be purchased for filling directly from a punctured vein; plain capillary tubes are available for use on anticoagulated blood. The Drummond microhematocrit centrifuge (Fig. 2–15), with a fixed speed of 16,000 rpm (approximately 14,000 G), employs capillary tubes measuring 32 mm × 0.8 mm. After they are filled with blood to two-thirds to three-fourths capacity by capillary traction, the outside is wiped off and the opposite end is carefully flame sealed. The sealed capillary is centrifuged for 2 minutes, and the PCV is de-

termined using a special reader. Buffy coat layer should be excluded from the red cell mass when the PCV is read.

Other types of microhematocrit centrifuges (Fig. 2–16) make use of somewhat larger capillary tubes, i.e., 75 mm × 1.0 mm. The blood is drawn into the tube by capillary traction to three-fourths its length. The tube is tipped to permit the blood to flow toward the free end to provide sufficient space to prevent outflow when the opposite end is sealed. The outside of the capillary is wiped free of blood, and the index finger is placed over the moist end to hold the column of blood in place as the opposite dry end is forced into the sealing material to form a tight plug. The capillary tube is placed in the centrifuge with the sealed end pointing outward. The blood is centrifuged for 5 minutes for most species, 10 minutes for the sheep, and 10–20 minutes for the goat. PCV is determined by a reader card or scale attached to the centrifuge head. The 75 mm × 1.0 mm capillary tube, when adequately filled, contains sufficient plasma for measurement of icterus index and total plasma proteins.

Although the microhematocrit method has replaced the Wintrobe method because of the speed and accuracy of its PCV value, the Wintrobe tube remains ideal for obtaining erythrocyte sedimentation rate, after which the tube can be centrifuged at 1,500–2,000 G for 10 minutes to clear the plasma of cells. Icterus index can then be determined, and plasma can be used to determine total plasma protein and fibrinogen concentrations by refractometer.

DETERMINATION OF HEMOGLOBIN

The hemoglobin molecule consists of protoporphyrin, native globin, and ferrous iron. It is a protein with a molecular weight of 64,458.

The iron content is 0.335%, or 3.35 mg/g of hemoglobin. The oxygen-carrying capacity is 1.36 cm³/g of hemoglobin. The most accurate methods for hemoglobin measurement are based on the chemical determination of iron content or oxygen-carrying capacity. These methods are too involved for practical clinical hemoglobinometry, and therefore a number

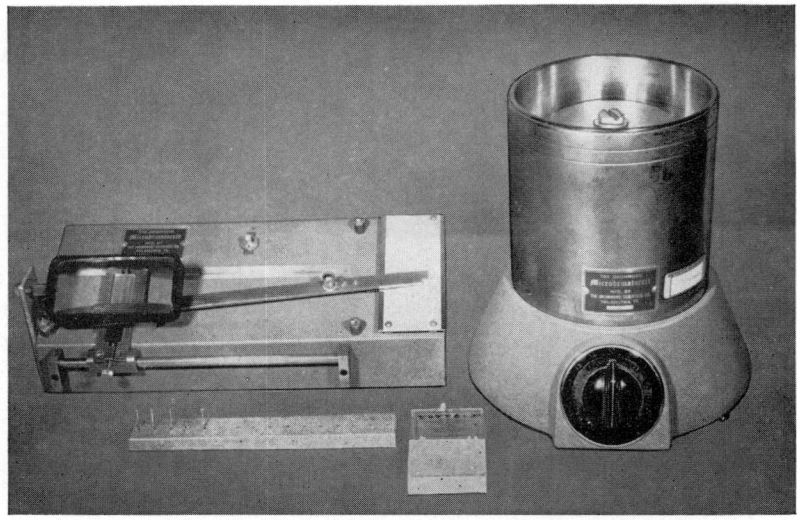

Fig. 2–15. Drummond microhematocrit high-speed centrifuge on the right and special reader on the left. In foreground is a box of capillary tubes and the metal block for holding the tubes.

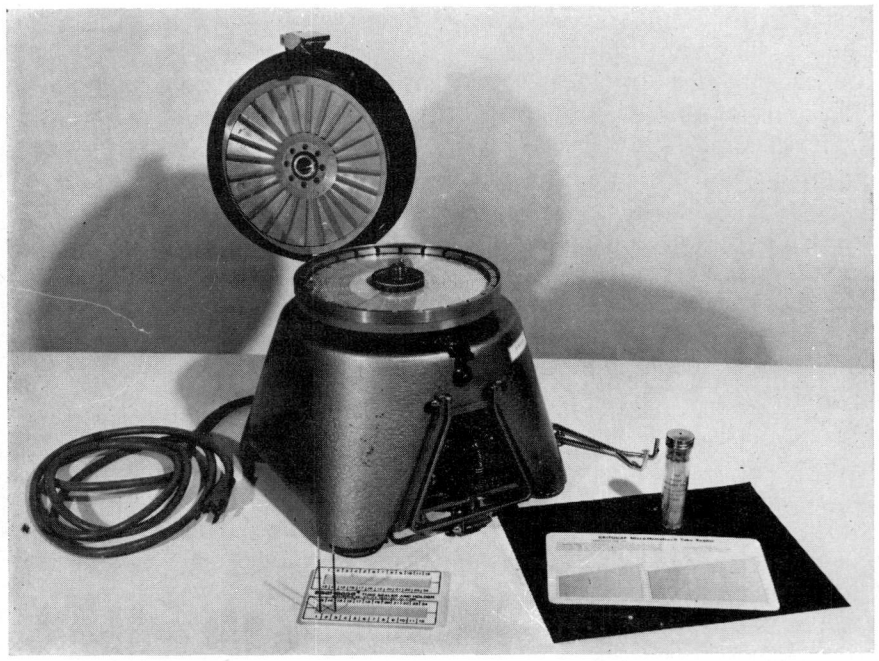

Fig. 2–16. An Adams Autocrit centrifuge along with a reader and other accessories needed for determining PCV.

of rapid procedures have been developed based on (a) direct matching of the red color with artificial standards; (b) converting the hemoglobin to acid hematin and matching the brown color with glass standards; (c) measuring oxyhemoglobin by its light absorption in the green portion of the spectrum; or (d) measuring light absorption of oxyhemoglobin, cyanmethemoglobin, or carboxyhemoglobin by means of the photoelectric colorimeter or spectrophotometer (Tables 2–4, 2–5). Special instruments have been developed to measure hemoglobin concentration of a hemolyzed specimen within seconds. To avoid confusion, hemoglobin concentration should be expressed in g/dl of blood rather than in percentage of a fixed standard value.

For a thorough review of the problems of measurement of hemoglobin, see the *Symposium on Clinical Hemoglobinometry* (Sunderman et al., 1953).

Direct Matching

Hemoglobin is red, and the depth of color it imparts to the blood is directly proportional to the concentration of iron. As early as 1900, Tallqvist proposed a method for evaluation of the quantity of hemoglobin in the blood by direct comparison of a drop of blood on blotting paper to lithographed color standards. In the same year, Dare described a hemoglobinometer in which undiluted blood is placed in a capillary space between two pieces of glass, and the color compared, through an eyepiece, with graded glass standards. The errors with these methods are said to range from 10% to 40%.

Hematin Method

Sahli introduced a method for hemoglobin determination that is used in various modifications, such as the Sahli-Adams, Sahli-Haden, Haden-Hausser, and Newcomer hemoglobinometers.

A measured quantity of blood is treated with 0.1 N HCl. The acid separates the globin from the hemoglobin molecule, producing acid hematin, which has a brown color. Maximum color develops only after 40 minutes have elapsed, after which the color begins to fade. The various hemoglobinometers employing the acid hematin method use brown glass standards adjusted to color intensity so that the result can be read within a stated time period, such as 1, 5, 10, or 30 minutes. It is important to make the final reading within the exact time period for which the instrument is adjusted to obtain greatest accuracy. By careful technique, the error in acid hematin method may be held to 5% to 10%.

The errors of the acid hematin method resulting from variation in content of protein and lipid in the plasma in disease may be overcome if the acid hematin is converted to

Table 2–4. Methods for Clinical Hemoglobinometry

Type of Method	Remarks
Colorimetric	
Direct matching	Artificial standards, not same color. Inaccurate.
Acid hematin	Erratic. Matching difficult with colored glass. Fading. Plasma constituents affect color.
Alkaline hematin	Less erratic than acid hematin but same difficulties.
Oxyhemoglobin	Simple, rapid. Fading. Does not measure hemoglobin derivatives.
Pyridine hemochromogens	Precise, rapid. Fairly good color. Unpleasant odor.
Carboxyhemoglobin	Rapid, precise. Stable color. Requires source of carbon monoxide.
Cyanmethemoglobin	Rapid, precise. Measures hemoglobin derivatives. Employs cyanide reagents.
Physical measurements	
Specific gravity	
Hematocrit readings	Indirect. Not entirely specific for hemoglobin.
Refractive index	
Gasometric	
Oxygen capacity	Precise. Requires special equipment. Time-consuming. May not measure all
Carbon monoxide capacity	hemoglobin derivatives present.
Chemical	
Iron concentration	Precise. Time-consuming. Method of choice for checking and calibration purposes. Assumes nonhemoglobin iron to be negligible.

From Sunderman et al., 1953; courtesy of *The American Journal of Clinical Pathology.*

Table 2–5.   Comparison of Results with Several Methods for Hemoglobin Determination on the Same Blood (g/dl of blood)

Blood	Leitz Photo-meter[a]	Coleman Jr. Spectro-photometer[a]	Haden-Hausser (electric)	Haden-Hausser (daylite)	Spencer Hb-meter	Sahli-Adams #1[b]	Sahli-Adams #2[b]
Cow #1	14.3	14.0	11.8	12.5	14.0	12.0	13.0
Cow #2	14.3	13.8	12.5	13.0	14.4	12.8	13.0
Cow #3	8.6	8.9	8.5	9.0	8.6	7.0	7.5
Cow #4	9.0	9.0	8.5	8.0	8.8	7.0	8.0
Cow #5	7.4	6.8	7.8	7.5	6.4	5.5	6.0
Dog #1	8.0	8.4	8.0	8.5	8.0	6.5	7.0
Dog #2	13.0	13.25	11.5	12.0	12.6	11.0	11.5
Dog #3	15.0	14.4	13.0	14.0	14.5	13.0	13.0
Ave. variation from Coleman reading	+0.2	0	−0.8	−0.5	−0.1	−1.65	−1.2

[a]Oxyhemoglobin method.
[b]Two separate Sahli-Adams hemoglobinometers.

alkaline hematin by the addition of sodium hydroxide (Wu, 1923). This suggestion has not been followed in methods commonly available.

Oxyhemoglobin Method

The Spencer hemoglobin meter (American Optical, 1010D) measures oxyhemoglobin by light absorption using a green filter. A drop of blood is placed in a shallow depression on a glass plate and laked by a hemolytic agent present on the tip of an applicator stick. The proper thickness of laked blood is obtained by placing a second piece of glass on top of the chamber and pressing the two glasses together. The glass chamber is inserted into the hemoglobinometer and the green color matched with the standard. The hemoglobinometer can be illuminated by flashlight batteries and is thus adaptable to field use.

Spectrophotometric Methods

Spectrophotometric procedures have been developed for measurement of hemoglobin in the form of oxyhemoglobin (Wong, 1928) and cyanmethemoglobin (Drabkin and Austin, 1935; van Kampen and Zijlstra, 1961, 1965). The cyanmethemoglobin method is one of the most accurate methods available. It has been internationally adapted as the reference method for hemoglobin determination. It entails conversion of all hemoglobin derivatives by ferricyanide to methemoglobin, which in turn is converted by cyanide ions to the stable red compound, cyanmethemoglobin. The latter is measured spectrophotometrically.

To prepare the cyanmethemoglobin reagent (Drabkin's solution), place 500 ml water in a 1-L volumetric flask and add 1 g sodium bicarbonate ($NaHCO_3$), 0.05 g potassium cyanide (KCN), and 0.02 g potassium ferricyanide ($K_3Fe(CN)_6$). Dissolve the contents and add water to make the total volume 1 L. The procedure for hemoglobin determination is as follows:

1. Carefully transfer 5 ml of Drabkin's solution to a clean, dry cuvette.
2. Measure 20 µl of blood by using Sahli's hemoglobin pipette and transfer it to the cuvette, rinsing the pipette several times therein. This gives a blood-to-reagent dilution of 1:251.
3. Mix well and allow 10 minutes for cyanmethemoglobin to form.
4. Read optical density in a spectrophotometer at 540 nm, using 5 ml of Drabkin's solution as the "blank."
5. Calculate hemoglobin concentration from the standard curve. A standard curve is prepared by making serial dilutions of a cyanmethemoglobin standard in Drabkin's solution, reading optical densities of various dilutions spectrophotometrically at 540 nm against the reagent "blank," and plotting on linear graph paper optical density versus hemoglobin in g/dl.

Alternatively, process a known hemoglobin standard simultaneously with the blood and calculate hemoglobin concentration as follows:

$$\text{Hemoglobin concentration (g/dl of blood)} = \frac{\text{Optical density of blood}}{\text{Optical density of standard}} \times \text{Hemoglobin concentration of standard}$$

Spuriously high hemoglobin values result with the spectrophotometric method if blood is lipemic or contains erythrocytes with large numbers of Heinz bodies. Chylomicra and Heinz bodies increase the optical density of the diluent containing the hemolyzed blood. Heinz bodies should be sedimented by centrifugation (1,000 G for 2 minutes) to obtain a valid optical density representative of the hemoglobin concentration in the diluted blood. A discrepancy in the MCHC and MCH values often provides clues to such an occurrence.

Hemoglobinometer

The Coulter hemoglobinometer (Coulter Electronics) provides a direct digital reading of hemoglobin concentration in a simple, one-step procedure. Blood is diluted 1:500 in Isoton II (Coulter Electronics), or dilution that has been prepared for total leukocyte count by the Coulter counter (described later in this chapter) is used. Three drops of Zapoglobin (Coulter Electronics) are added to lyse red cells and convert hemoglobin to cyanmethemoglobin. The contents are poured through the machine to read hemoglobin concentration in g/dl of blood. The machine is equipped with a flow-through cuvette to receive the sample and has automatic rinsing, reset, and self-blanking features.

A hemoglobinometer measuring oxyhemoglobin provides comparatively low values of total hemoglobin concentration because other hemoglobin types are not measured. This is especially true for patients with methemoglobinemia (certain dogs and cats). The discrepancy is detected when MCHC and MCH are calculated from such data.

COUNTING ERYTHROCYTES AND LEUKOCYTES IN THE HEMOCYTOMETER

It is advisable to select equipment claimed by the manufacturer to meet the specifications for accuracy of the National Bureau of Standards.

Filling the Pipette

The diluting pipette consists of a calibrated stem and a bulb or mixing chamber containing a glass bead to facilitate uniform dispersion of the cells in the diluting fluid. The stem is divided into 10 equal parts, totaling one unit. The volume of the bulb in the white-cell pipette is 10 units and in the red-cell pipette 100 units. Therefore, on the opposite side of the bulb, the number 11 appears on the white-cell pipette and the number 101 on the red-cell pipette. The volume of fluid required to fill a pipette to the upper mark does not represent a specific amount. The marks on each individual pipette, however, indicate comparable volumes for that pipette.

A rubber tube fitted with a mouthpiece is attached to the upper end of the pipette. By gentle suction, blood is drawn into the stem to the mark desired. In routine blood work for humans, the 0.5 mark is used for both leukocyte and erythrocyte counts. When the column of blood reaches the proper mark, the lips are parted slightly to stop the flow of blood into the stem. If blood is drawn beyond the desired mark, the excess may be removed by touching the tip of the pipette with tissue paper. The tip is wiped clean, and diluting fluid is drawn into the pipette to the 11 or 101 mark, depending on the pipette. As the diluting fluid enters, the pipette should be rolled back and forth to facilitate mixing. To avoid an error in dilution, the fluid should be stopped exactly at the upper mark.

The white-cell pipette gives a dilution of 1:20, and the red-cell pipette, a dilution of 1:200 when blood is drawn to the 0.5 mark and diluted (Fig. 2–17). Because all domestic animals normally have many more erythrocytes per μl of blood than humans, the use of blood to 0.5 mark allows too many cells in the hemocytometer chamber. Erythrocyte counts in normal animals may be obtained by drawing blood to the 0.3 mark of the red blood cell pipette. When anemia is known to exist, blood is drawn to the 0.5 mark. In extreme anemias, the white-cell pipette can be employed for erythrocyte count, and in blood

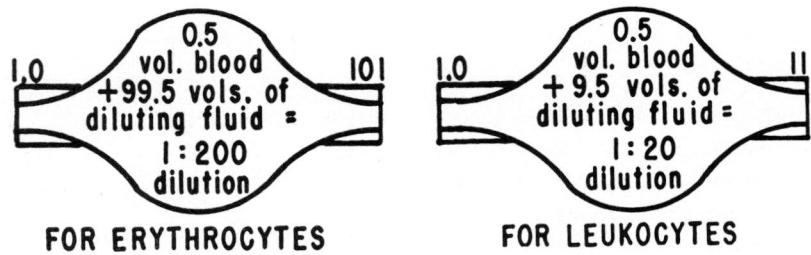

Fig. 2–17. In counting the red and white blood cells, the appropriate blood diluting pipette is employed and blood is drawn into the capillary portion to the 0.5 mark. The proper diluent is then drawn into the pipette, which moves the blood from the stem into the bulb of the pipette, where it becomes diluted as shown above.

having exceedingly high leukocyte numbers the red-cell pipette can be used.

The diluting fluid for the white-cell count consists of an acid to lyse the erythrocytes. Either 1% HCl or 2% acetic acid can be used. One ml of a 1% aqueous solution of gentian violet can be added to each 100 ml of leukocyte diluting fluid to distinguish it from the red-cell diluting fluid.

The diluting fluid for the red-cell count should be isotonic. Those in common use are:

Hayem's Solution

Mercuric chloride	0.5 g
Sodium sulfate	5.0 g
(or anhydrous, 2.2 g)	
Sodium chloride	1.0 g
Distilled water	200.0 ml

Gower's Solution

Sodium sulfate	12.5 g
Glacial acetic acid	33.3 ml
Distilled water	200.0 ml

Physiologic Solution

Sodium chloride	0.85 g
Distilled water q.s. to	100.0 ml

Hayem's solution may cause agglutination of erythrocytes in some bloods by action of the mercury salt on the plasma proteins. Agglutination is especially likely to occur with cow, sheep, and goat bloods. Gower's solution has the advantage of preventing agglutination in most bloods. If agglutination is a problem with certain animal bloods, physiologic saline may be used as the diluent. A disadvantage of Gower's solution is that a brownish deposit is left in the pipette with continued use. Hypochlorite cleaning solution (Clorox) drawn into the pipette generally removes the sediment. The brownish deposit can usually be prevented by rapid filling while actively rotating the pipette. A similar

precipitate may also form in the white-cell pipette when it is filled slowly.

The Counting Chamber

The counting chamber consists of a rectangular thick glass slide with two raised crossbars on which the coverslip rests. In the central area between the crossbars are two platforms, each of which is completely surrounded by a moat. The polished surface of each platform is 0.1 mm below the coverslip so that when the chamber is filled, the depth of fluid is 0.1 mm. Each platform presents a ruled area consisting of nine primary squares, each of which encompasses 1 square mm. Each of the four corner primary squares is subdivided into 16 secondary squares to facilitate the counting of leukocytes. The center primary square is used for the erythrocyte count and is divided into 25 secondary squares, each of which is further subdivided into 16 tertiary squares. The total number of tertiary squares in this central area is 400. The borders of the secondary squares of the red-cell-counting area are made up of two or three parallel lines to facilitate selection of erythrocytes to be included in the count. It is customary to count all erythrocytes in five of the secondary squares, using the four corners and the center square.

Before filling the chamber, shake the pipette for 2 minutes to bring about a uniform dispersion of the blood cells in the diluting fluid. Hold the pipette by placing the thumb over the tip and the index or middle finger over the opposite end. To shake the pipette, use a back-and-forth movement at right angles to its long axis. If it is shaken in the same direction as the long axis, cells may be forced from the mixing chamber into the stem, and an error may be introduced. Blow out and discard up to half the contents of the pipette to remove the cell-free fluid from the stem; touch the tip of the pipette to the edge of the platform of the counting chamber and allow the fluid to flow under the coverslip by capillary traction. The chamber should be filled by uniform movement of the fluid across the surface of the platform. The amount of fluid should be controlled so as to just fill the chamber without spilling into the moat. Fill one side of the chamber from the white-cell pipette and the other side from the red-cell pipette. Count the leukocytes first, thus permitting sufficient time for the erythrocytes to settle to the surface of the platform. Alternatively, both chambers may be filled from the same pipette to obtain a duplicate count for each cell type.

A definite system of counting must be followed to avoid missing cells or counting cells more than once (Fig. 2–18). The usual practice is to start at the upper left square and include in the count for each respective square all cells touching the lines forming the upper and left borders and ignore cells touching the bottom and right borderlines. Move across the top row of squares from left to right, and then drop down to the second row and proceed from right to left. Repeat this pattern until all squares have been covered as required for either the white-cell or red-cell count.

Cell Count and Calculations

The low-power objective (10×) is used for the white-cell count. At this power, the field is filled by the area of one primary square. It is customary to count the leukocytes in the four corner primary squares and multiply by a factor of 50 to obtain the number of cells in 1 μl of blood. The factor is derived as follows:

Area of each primary square	1 mm²
Depth of each primary square	$\frac{1}{10}$ mm
Fluid volume of each primary square	$\frac{1}{10}$ μl
Fluid volume in four primary squares	$\frac{4}{10}$ μl
Dilution factor	$\frac{1}{20}$
Amount of undiluted blood counted	$\frac{4}{10} \times \frac{1}{20} = \frac{1}{50}$ μl.

When nucleated erythrocytes (NuRBC) are present in blood, they are included in the total leukocyte count whether done by the hemocytometer method or electronic counter (described below). The observed leukocyte count thus requires an appropriate correction. The number of NuRBC encountered while making the differential count of 100 leukocytes in the stained blood film is noted separately and employed to correct the total leukocyte count as follows:

$$\frac{100}{100 + \text{number of NuRBC}} \times \text{WBC count}$$

$$= \text{corrected WBC count}$$

Expression of nucleated red cells as a part of the differential leukocyte count may be an easy and practical approach to correction of the leukocyte count (Weiser, 1981), but it introduces an error in relative values of the differential counts.

The high dry objective is employed in making the erythrocyte count. The number of cells in five secondary squares (80 tertiary squares) is determined and multiplied by 10,000. This is accomplished by adding four zeros to the

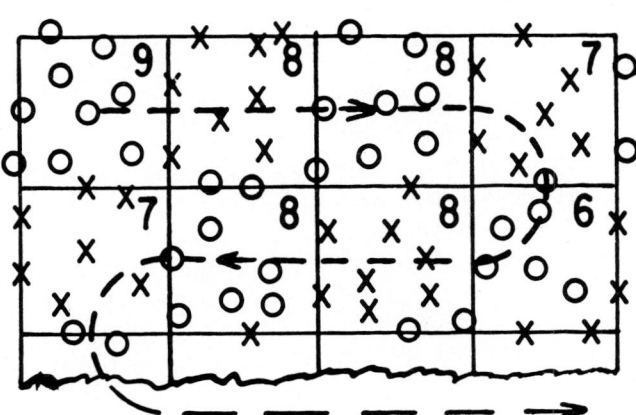

Fig. 2–18. The recommended pattern for counting blood cells in the hemocytometer chamber.

total number of cells counted. This represents the number of erythrocytes per μl of blood. The factor of 10,000 is derived as follows:

Area of each secondary square	$\frac{1}{5} \times \frac{1}{5} = \frac{1}{25}$ mm^2
Fluid volume of each secondary square	$\frac{1}{25} \times \frac{1}{10} = \frac{1}{250}$ μl
Fluid volume in five secondary squares	$\frac{1}{50}$ μl
Dilution factor	$\frac{1}{200}$
Amount of undiluted blood counted	$\frac{1}{50} \times \frac{1}{200} = \frac{1}{10,000}$ μl

When blood is drawn to the 0.3 rather than the 0.5 mark in the diluting pipette, the factor is recalculated or the erythrocyte number obtained in the hemocytometer is divided by 3 and the quotient multiplied by 5. Four zeros are then added to give the number of erythrocytes per μl of blood.

Inherent Errors in the Blood Cell Count Obtained with the Hemocytometer

Berkson et al. (1940) investigated the inherent error in the procedure. Errors arise for the following reasons:

1. The cell count of a large volume is estimated with a very small sample.
2. The random settling of cells in the counting area of the chamber, even in properly mixed samples, is subject to chance, referred to as the "error of the field."
3. Filling separate counting chambers leads to variations in count, called the "error of the chamber."
4. Filling of different pipettes leads to variations in count, called the "error of the pipette."

The total error inherent in the procedure for a mean count of 5 million erythrocytes/μl was found to be ± 7.8% at the level of 1 standard deviation and ± 16% at 2 standard deviations from the mean. Similarly, for a leukocyte count of 7,000, the total inherent error was found to be ± 21%. This error can be minimized when experienced technicians are performing the counts. The electronic cell counter, however, is the method of choice for greatest accuracy.

Unopette Method for Blood Dilution and Cell Counting

The Unopette (Becton Dickinson) system employs a premeasured volume of diluent in a thin-walled plastic reservoir. An exact volume of blood is drawn by capillary traction into a tube of uniform length and base and transferred into the reservoir (Fig. 2–19).

The Unopette system removes the error of sampling and dilution that may occur with the standard red- and white-cell pipettes. Unopettes are available for most routine hematologic tests and many biochemical determinations. Unopettes for counting both leukocytes and platelets, using the same diluent, are also available. Instructions supplied with specific Unopettes are to be followed for counting cells and calculating their number per μl of blood.

THE ELECTRONIC CELL COUNTERS

The Coulter Counter (Fig. 2–20) and other electronic particle counters were developed specifically for blood-cell enumeration and are based on the principle that cells are poor electrical conductors. A measured volume of diluted suspension of cells (in an electrically conductive medium) is drawn through a minute aperture between two electrodes (Fig. 2–21). Each cell passing through the aperture displaces an equal volume of the electrolyte solution and introduces resistance in the electric circuit. A voltage pulse proportional to the particle size is produced and visualized on an oscilloscope. The pulses resulting from all cells in the measured volume drawn through the electric field are counted electronically and displayed on the digital readout. Thus the Coulter Counter has the capability of determining both the number and size of the particles.

Blood is diluted with buffered isotonic NaCl solution (see formula below) for erythrocyte count. The erythrocyte count includes the leukocytes because both are registered as they pass through the aperture. Error due to the presence of leukocytes is generally less than 1%, but it could be greater in leukemic blood, especially if anemia is also present. Dog blood having leukocytosis of 50,000/μl would present a 1.0% error in an erythrocyte count of 5 million/μl of blood. Saponin is added to a cell suspension in buffered NaCl solution to lyse erythrocytes for making the leukocyte count. When Coulter reagents are used, blood

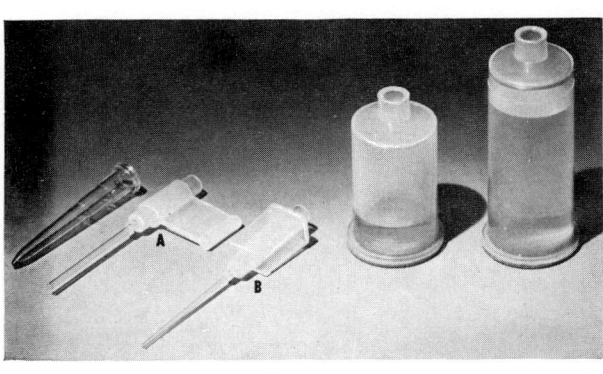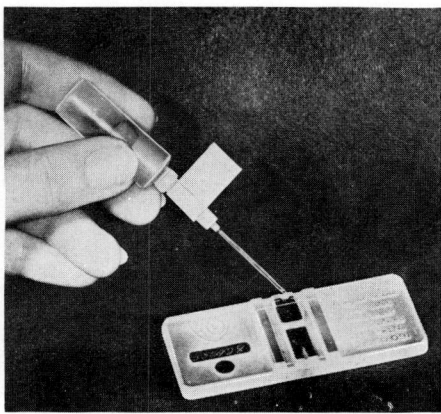

Fig. 2–19. *Left,* Unopette reservoirs with diluting fluid showing old-style *(A)* and new-style *(B)* capillary holders. (Courtesy of Becton Dickinson.) *Right,* Filling the hemocytometer chamber with diluted blood from the Unopette.

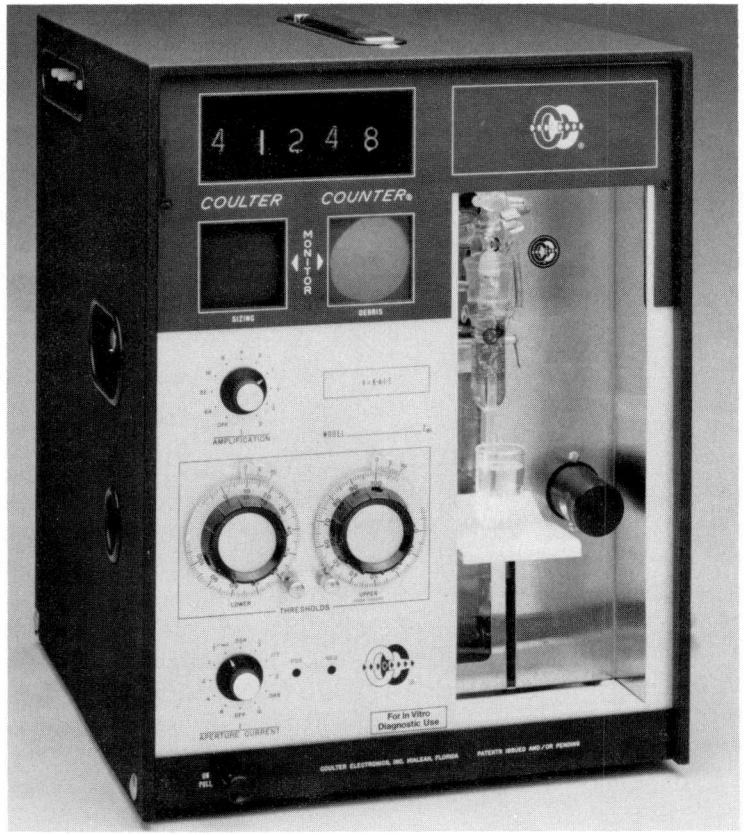

Fig. 2–20. The Coulter Counter, model ZBI. (Courtesy of Coulter Electronics Inc.)

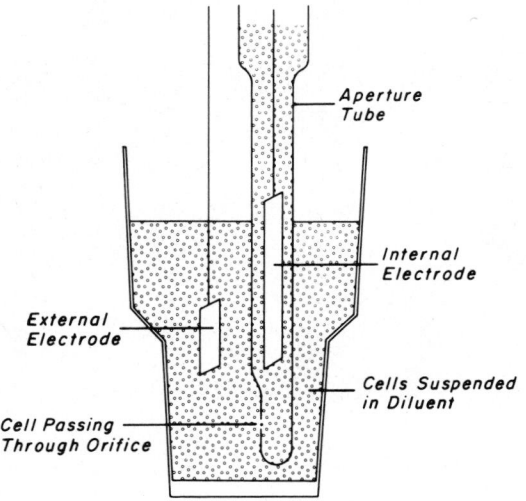

Fig. 2–21. Sample container for electronic cell counting.

is diluted in Isoton II, and Zapoglobin II is used to lyse red cells for making the leukocyte count. The instrument cannot distinguish between blood cells and particles of debris. Therefore the glassware and diluting fluids must be as free as possible of dust particles and extraneous material. The manufacturer (Coulter Electronics) states that "the accuracy of the measurement is not limited by the instrument but is simply a matter of the degree of care exercised in its use." A threshold dial is incorporated to permit selection of the minimal size of the cells to be counted. In this manner it is possible to exclude most debris and limit the background count. Since erythrocyte size is characteristic of each animal species, the instrument must be calibrated for the blood of each species under investigation.

The following threshold settings on Coulter Counter models F and F_N were found suitable for red cell and white cell counts on the blood of different animal species. A calibration factor, determined by mean cell threshold (Pruden and Winstead, 1964), of about 2.5 μl/threshold division was used with settings for sensitivity control of 1 for attenuation and 8 for aperture current. The diluent used is described on page 51.

Threshold Settings	Species
Red Cell Counts	
4	Goat
5	Sheep
7	Cat, cow, horse, mouse, pig, rat
10	Dog, donkey, guinea pig, human, monkey, rabbit

White Cell Counts	
22	Cow, goat, pig, sheep
25	Cat, dog, donkey, guinea pig, horse, human, monkey, mouse, rabbit, rat

Red-cell counts in an occasional blood sample required lowering of the threshold to 4 for the sheep and to 5 for the cow and horse. The calibration factor may increase slightly with use of the instrument. When Isoton II is used as the diluent, a threshold of 10 is generally used to count red and white cells of common domestic animals except the goat red cells, for which the threshold is kept at 4.

Coulter model ZBI is used at different settings. Red and white cells are counted at an amplification of ½ and aperture current of 1. A 100-μm aperture is used, and counts are made from a fluid volume of 500 μl. A threshold setting of 10 is used for both red- and white-cell counts of different species except for bovine and ovine white cells, which are counted at a threshold of 14 (otherwise counts obtained are too high), and the goat red cells, which are counted at a setting of 4. Platelet count is performed at the same amplification setting, but a 70-μl aperture tube is used, aperture current is set at ½, and fluid volume utilized is 100 μl.

With species for which the threshold settings are not established, the height of voltage pulses seen on the oscilloscope is observed; then the threshold is set to slightly less than half the major pulse height. Counts are done at a few threshold settings below that chosen to assure that no small cells are missed. If the count of the higher threshold is the same as the count of the lower threshold setting, the higher threshold setting is chosen for greater accuracy. In such instances, as well as with certain abnormal bloods, counts should also be done with the hemocytometer to assure reliability of the electronic cell counts.

The dilution of cells must be adequate to reduce the coincidence of two or more cells entering the aperture simultaneously. The instrument counts such occurrences as single cells, and thus the actual count is reduced. Coincidence is predictable or standard for a given cell concentration and aperture (Mattern et al., 1957), and therefore a correction table for coincidence is supplied by the manufacturer. Most blood samples are routinely diluted 1:50,000 for the erythrocyte count and 1:500 for the leukocyte count, using an automatic diluter. The ratio of blood to diluent for erythrocyte count may need to be varied in order to compensate for the wide range of red cell numbers characteristic of the various animal species (Weide et al., 1962; Wisecup and Crouch, 1963). Blood is preferably diluted to give counts below 80,000/0.5 ml of the diluent. Goat blood usually needs to be diluted two to three times, and sheep and horse bloods sometimes require twice the regular dilution.

The Coulter Counter method is more accurate and less time-consuming than the hemocytometer method for counting erythrocytes and leukocytes (Brecher et al., 1956; Richar and Breakell, 1959; Weide et al., 1962). Total error with the electronic count is less than 2% for the red cell count and 3% for the leukocyte count (Wintrobe et al., 1981).

The Coulter Counters are available in several models. The model F_N and the model ZBI (Fig. 2–20) are used to count erythrocytes and leukocytes and can be used to count platelets by replacing the 100-μm-aperture tube with a 70-μm tube and changing the metering section with a switch. A hemoglobin accessory, a hematocrit accessory, and MCV computer unit can be attached to the system to determine hemoglobin concentration, PCV, and MCV automatically. Model S, S-Senior, and S-Plus simultaneously perform RBC, WBC, Hb, and MCV determinations and then automatically calculate PCV, MCHC, and MCH. This is accomplished within 20 seconds, utilizing about 1 ml of blood, and data are automatically printed on a report form. As little as 40 μl of blood sample may be prediluted and used for analysis. Model S-Plus is also good for platelet counts. These instruments are calibrated to perform optimally for human blood and require appropriate adjustments for use on animal blood (Weiser, 1983). They are well suited for use in large hospitals and commercial laboratories. The Coulter Channelyzer provides volume distribution curves for the erythrocytes, leukocytes, and platelets. A technique for obtaining automatic equine differential leukocyte counts by analysis of volume distribution curves using the Coulter Channelyzer has been described (Allen, 1981).

Diluent and lysing solutions used for making RBC and WBC counts with the Coulter Counter are commercially available. They can also be prepared as follows:

Diluent

Stock Solutions:
  A. 1.5 *M* acetate buffer, pH 6.0:

Sodium acetate ($NaC_2H_3O_2\ 3H_2O$)	408.2 g
Thimerosal	0.2 g
Deionized water	2,000 ml

Mix well, correct pH to 6.0 with glacial acetic acid.
  B. 18.4% NaCl:

NaCl	368 g
Deionized water	2,000 ml

  C. Formalin (40% formaldehyde)

Filter solutions A, B, and C twice through a medium-porosity sintered glass filter.

Working Solution:

Deionized water	2,700 ml
Stock solution A	150 ml
Stock solution B	150 ml
Stock solution C	3 ml

Lysing Solution

Saponin (obtained from Coulter Electronics)	5 g
Working solution of the diluent (from above)	95 ml

Use 1 drop per 20 μl of blood in diluent.

Several cell-counting errors may be introduced by blood abnormalities:

1. In autoimmune hemolytic anemia, the osmotic fragility of erythrocytes may at times be so great that significant hemolysis may occur in 0.85% saline (Fig. 20–10). In such instances, the electronic erythrocyte count is lower than the actual count because highly fragile erythrocytes undergo lysis in the diluent. The low counts will give erroneously high MCV and MCH values (Table 24–3). Erythrocyte counts on such samples may be more accurately performed by the hemocytometer method.
2. Electronic erythrocyte counts are erroneously low on blood samples showing

marked agglutination of red cells. Similarly, small blood clots will introduce an error.

3. Oscilloscope observation is very important in detecting marked abnormalities in cell size or volume. Large numbers of microcytic erythrocytes or leptocytes may not be counted if the threshold is not lowered. If routine settings are used in these cases, the erythrocyte counts will be too low, and the MCV will be too high.

4. Leukergy (nonspecific clumping of leukocytes) and fragile leukocytes will give erroneously low electronic leukocyte counts. Some bovine leukocytes, namely, lymphocytes of leukemic and preleukemic cattle, may be lysed by saponin; therefore, it is advisable to check by hemocytometer all bovine leukocyte Coulter Counter counts that exceed 12,000/μl (Theilen, 1975). Examination of the blood film may be helpful in such cases. An 8% to 48% discrepancy was observed between hemocytometer and electronic leukocyte counts in bloods from neutrophilic dogs exhibiting varying degrees of left shift (Faulkner et al., 1982). Destruction of immature neutrophils in preparation of hemocytometer counting was found to be the major cause.

5. Abnormally large platelets or clumps of platelets, particularly in the cat, will be counted while RBC or WBC counts are being made by electronic counters. This introduces a significant error in the WBC count and also in the RBC count in severe anemia. For this reason, WBC counts on domestic cats are routinely performed in our laboratories by hemocytometer method, and RBC counts are similarly checked whenever discrepancies appear among various erythrocyte parameters.

6. Large numbers of nucleated red cells equal to or greater in size than the small lymphocyte will be counted, adding to the leukocyte count as with the hemocytometer count. The corrected WBC count is calculated from the formula given on p. 47.

THE WINTROBE ERYTHROCYTE INDEXES

The PCV, the erythrocyte count, and the hemoglobin concentration are the data required for calculation of these indexes (Wintrobe, 1929; 1932). The validity of the indexes is dependent on the accuracy of the data needed for their calculations. These indexes are useful in morphologic classification of anemia and to evaluate erythropoietic responses. See Chapter 21 for interpretations.

Mean Corpuscular Volume (MCV)

This index expresses in fl (femtoliter, 10^{-15}) the average volume of a population of erythrocytes. Given a PCV of 42% and an erythrocyte count of 6 million/μl, the MCV would be 70 fl from the following:

$$\frac{PCV \ (ml/dl \ or \ \%)}{RBC \ (million/\mu l)} \times 10$$

$$\text{Example: } \frac{42}{6} \times 10 = 70 \ \text{fl}$$

Red cell volume measurements are performed electronically in certain automated blood cell counters. The MCV value so obtained is used to calculate PCV automatically based on the above relationship.

Mean Corpuscular Hemoglobin (MCH)

This index expresses in picograms (10^{-12}) the weight of hemoglobin in an average erythrocyte of a population of cells.

$$\frac{Hb \ (g/dl)}{RBC \ (million/\mu l)} \times 10$$

$$\text{Example: } \frac{14}{6} \times 10 = 23.3 \ \text{pg}$$

Mean Corpuscular Hemoglobin Concentration (MCHC)

This index expresses the ratio of weight of the hemoglobin to the volume of the erythrocyte, and the unit is percentage or grams per deciliter of red cells.

$$\frac{Hb \ (g/dl)}{PCV \ (ml/dl \ or \ \%)} \times 100$$

$$\text{Example: } \frac{14}{42} \times 100 = 33.3\% \text{ or g/dl of red cells}$$

The student of hematology should know that the expression of MCHC in SI units as g/dl does not relate to a deciliter of blood, as other CBC parameters are expressed. Instead, it refers to a deciliter of red cells (i.e., if the red cells were so concentrated). Moreover, it implies that a certain amount of hemoglobin is present per deciliter of red cells, whereas by definition the term "mean corpuscular hemoglobin concentration" calls for a value indicative of the concentration of hemoglobin in an average red cell of a given population. Thus, the SI unit (g/dl) for MCHC is misleading compared to the conventional unit (percent), which is a better expression of its intended purpose.

In health, the MCHC normally ranges between 30% and 35% for domestic animals except for the family Camellidae in which it is over 40%. Hypochromic anemia is characterized by MCHC falling below 30%.

Errors in Erythrocyte Indexes

Mathematical derivation of erythrocytic indexes suggests that errors in RBC count would influence MCV and MCH; errors in hemoglobin level would influence MCH and MCHC; and errors in PCV value would influence MCV and MCHC. Inherent errors in the RBC count by the hemocytometer method, in the PCV determination by the Wintrobe method, and in the hemoglobin determination by Sahli's hemoglobinometer introduce wide variations in the erythrocyte indexes. Errors may arise in the RBC counts obtained by the electronic cell counter at improper threshold settings for the species or in the case of extremely anemic bloods because thrombocytes are included in the RBC counts. In such cases, both MCV and MCH are decreased. This has been noted with both dog and cat blood samples. Similarly, automatic calculation of MCV and PCV may be in error if the electronic cell counter is not properly calibrated for the species in question.

An excess of EDTA in a blood sample produces shrinkage of erythrocytes (see p. 23). The PCV is reduced, although erythrocyte count and hemoglobin concentration are not affected. This reduction in PCV results in a reduction in MCV and an increase in MCHC. Significant hemolysis leads to erroneously increased values for MCH and MCHC because the free hemoglobin in the plasma is mathematically incorporated in the remaining nonhemolyzed erythrocytes.

Spectrophotometric methods for determination of hemoglobin concentration lead to errors when the blood is lipemic or contains a large number of Heinz bodies. Both situations lead to increasing optical density of the diluent, which in turn causes erroneously high estimations of hemoglobin. When Heinz bodies are involved, a valid hemoglobin determination is possible after centrifugation of the blood-diluent mixture. It is important to remember this when handling feline blood samples because Heinz bodies are frequently encountered in cats even during nonanemic states. During methemoglobinemia, the oxyhemoglobin method underestimates the hemoglobin level, and consequently MCH and MCHC are reduced.

When the method for obtaining PCV fails to minimize trapped plasma in the erythrocyte column, MCV is increased and MCHC is decreased. This occurs with cow, sheep, and goat blood when PCV is obtained by the Wintrobe hematocrit method, and with goat and sheep blood centrifuged for a short period (5 minutes instead of 10–20 minutes) in a microhematocrit centrifuge.

ERYTHROCYTE SEDIMENTATION RATE (ESR)

In clinical hematology, the ESR is performed as an aid to diagnosis and evaluation of the disease process. The test is especially applicable to canine blood, but its usefulness is limited for blood of other domestic animals.

Several methods have been devised to perform the test, and micromethods have been developed for use on small blood samples (Lloyd, 1958; Miale, 1967). The ESR on animal bloods is generally measured by the Wintrobe method. It is conducted as follows: A Wintrobe hematocrit tube is filled to the zero mark and placed in a perfectly vertical position at room temperature, and the level to which the erythrocytes have fallen in exactly 1 hour is observed. ESR may also be conducted in a 75 × 1 mm microhematocrit tube (Jain and Kono, 1975). Several technical factors are known to affect the ESR; hence ESR values obtained by various methods should not be considered equivalent, although conclusions drawn may be similar. The ESR is influenced by the length and temperature of storage of blood (Jain and Kono, 1975). If the test cannot be conducted within the hour of sampling, the blood should be stored at 4°C and the test conducted within 6 hours. Sedimentation rate is directly influenced by ambient temperature, and so maintenance of a uniform laboratory temperature is advisable (Wartman, 1946).

Suspension stability or sedimentation of erythrocytes in blood is influenced by red cell and plasma characteristics. Such an influence is reflected in species differences seen in the ESR in health and changes in ESR during disease. Basically, red cells settle in plasma because of their greater density. The speed of settling is inversely proportional to the number of red cells in the sample. Since the red cell number or PCV varies widely in health and is affected by the state of water balance, it is important to compare the *observed ESR* of a given blood sample with the *anticipated ESR* for the PCV of that sample. Any difference between the observed and anticipated rate is called the *corrected ESR*. It is the corrected, not the observed, ESR that should be used to evaluate the influence of disease. Anticipated ESR values for various PCV levels have been developed for the dog (Table 2–6). These values apply to ESR determined only with the Wintrobe method. In general, these values have also been found useful to correct observed ESR values for domestic cats for which a separate correction table is currently not available.

Factors Influencing ESR and Changes in Disease

In addition to being affected by various technical factors, ESR is positively influenced by rouleau formation and plasma content of fibrinogen, α_2-globulins, and γ-globulins, while it is negatively influenced by reticulocytes, leptocytes, and plasma content of albumin (Gordon and Wardley, 1943; Gray and Mitchell, 1942). Among the domestic animals, the erythrocytes of ruminants show little or no natural tendency to form rouleaux. There-

Table 2–6. Relative Anticipated Erythrocyte Sedimentation Rate of Canine Blood in mm in 1 Hour for PCV value from 9 to 50

PCV	ESR	PCV	ESR	PCV	ESR
9	82	23	40	37	13
10	79	24	38	38	12
11	76	25	36	39	11
12	73	26	34	40	10
13	70	27	32	41	9
14	67	28	30	42	8
15	64	29	28	43	7
16	61	30	26	44	6
17	58	31	24	45	5
18	55	32	22	46	4
19	52	33	20	47	3
20	49	34	18	48	2
21	46	35	16	49	1
22	43	36	14	50	0

Examples: *(a)* PCV 43, observed ESR 45, anticipated ESR 7 (from the table: Corrected ESR 45 − 7 = +38.
(b) PCV 24, observed ESR 16, anticipated ESR 38 (from the table): Corrected ESR 16 − 38 = −22.

fore there is little or no ESR in health, and only a serious tissue alteration in disease will result in significant rouleau formation. This statement holds true especially for cattle, so that when significant rouleau formation is seen in blood films, such an occurrence should be interpreted as reflecting a grave disease process. The ESR is not ordinarily determined on the blood of cattle, sheep, and goats because of the insignificant settling of red cells within the usual period of 1 hour. However, considerable separation of erythrocytes and plasma may take place in the vial of blood left standing in a refrigerator overnight when severe disease, particularly inflammation, is present. On the other hand, the natural tendency of equine blood to form extreme rouleaux results in such rapid settling of erythrocytes as to make the test almost useless as a measure of the intensity of a morbid process. ESR is commonly performed on canine blood in the evaluation of a disease state. Additional knowledge is needed before ESR can be properly evaluated in feline and porcine bloods.

Reticulocytes and young erythrocytes do not readily participate in rouleau formation and therefore trail in the plasma producing a hazy reddish zone above the main mass of settling red cells. By the end of the hour, only the first few mm of plasma are usually clear, followed by the hazy reddish zone, which gradually merges with the main red cell mass (Fig. 2–13*A*, Plate I–2). The ESR in such cases is referred to as *diphasic*. Thus when reticulocytes are present in significant numbers in blood, the observed ESR is usually less than the anticipated value and may be diphasic. A diphasic negative corrected ESR also may develop when the blood contains a large number of thin erythrocytes, called leptocytes.

Since ESR is significantly influenced by the concentration of certain plasma proteins, a negative corrected value is a common occurrence in hypoproteinemia and a positive value in hyperproteinemia. Neonatal dogs have plasma protein levels of less than 6.0 g/dl (Table 4–1), and albumin is in excess of the globulin fraction. Furthermore, fibrinogen level is low in the normal pup. Thus negative corrected ESR values can be anticipated in young, growing dogs, even though PCV is often in the low normal range. On the other hand, occurrence of a positive corrected ESR in a neonate would indicate existence of an abnormality. Increase in ESR during pregnancy (Simms, 1940; Anderson and Gee, 1958) is probably related to physiologic hemodilution as well as reduced red-cell numbers.

Fibrinogen and α-globulin are commonly elevated in a variety of inflammatory or tissue-destroying diseases (Longworth et al., 1939). Although fibrinogen levels may be elevated significantly in disease, a significant positive corrected ESR is not always obtained. Reasons for this discrepancy remain unknown, but may involve interaction of various other plasma proteins including acute phase proteins. Hemoconcentration may adversely affect the ESR by increasing the influence of the albumin fraction. End stage kidney disease in the dog is commonly associated with rapid sedimentation of erythrocytes. It is noteworthy that plasma fibrinogen is commonly elevated in diseases of the kidney; furthermore, in glomerulonephritis the loss of albumin in the urine lowers the albumin content of the blood.

The anticipated ESR increases in proportion to the reduction in erythrocyte number. Thus it would be expected, a priori, that an elevated ESR would accompany anemia. This generally holds true when the anemia is normocytic normochromic (secondary anemia) and the plasma protein concentration is normal or increased. However, when the anemia is due to hemorrhage (blood loss), plasma proteins are lost along with erythrocytes. In addition, reticulocytes entering the peripheral blood during anemia in remission generally do not clump but remain dispersed in the plasma. Reticulocytosis and hypoproteinemia are associated with a lower than anticipated ESR. Under these circumstances, the corrected ESR is negative. Anemia, reticulocytosis, and hypoproteinemia represent a triad that is the hallmark of blood loss. When ESR is a positive corrected value in hemorrhage, one should look for a bleeding lesion such as leiomyoma of the gut.

The ESR is a nonspecific test that indicates the existence of an abnormal process in much the same way as elevations in body temperature or abnormal leukocyte counts. A positive corrected ESR indicates the presence of a morbid process. This procedure is useful in detecting occult disease and in following the progress of a chronic disease. In the dog, when PCV is $\geq 50\%$, any settling of red cells is significant and cause should be found. Small positive corrected ESR values, occurring at the extreme ends of the PCV range, are as significant as high corrected ESR values. For example, a 3+ ESR at PCV of 55% is as significant as a value of 27+ at PCV of 20%. Similarly, a negative ESR is as meaningful as a positive ESR. The sedimentation rate may be expected to vary from day to day because of the changing composition of the blood as it reflects the disease state. A declining rate suggests healing, an increasing rate suggests that the disease is uncontrolled, and a continuing abnormal rate indicates that recovery has not as yet taken place. The following comments apply specifically to the dog.

An elevated ESR is to be anticipated in:

(*a*) All acute generalized infections.

(*b*) Localized acute inflammatory diseases of the serous membranes such as the pleura, pericardium, and peritoneum.

(*c*) Chronic localized infections—the rate varies with the extent and tissue involved. In formation of an abscess, the rate is elevated, but as the abscess becomes encapsulated, the ESR returns to normal. Inflammation of draining cavities such as the uterus and head sinuses may or may not be associated with an elevated ESR.

(d) Traumatic injury, including surgery involving much cutting of tissue, such as ear cropping and enucleation of the eyeball, extensive burns, and broken bones.

(e) Inflammation of the skin or alteration of skin structure as in hypothyroidism and Cushing's syndrome.

(f) Malignant neoplasia.

(g) Pregnancy.

(h) End stage kidney disease.

ESTIMATION OF TOTAL PLASMA PROTEIN BY REFRACTOMETER

The Goldberg refractometer or Total Solids (TS) meter (Fig. 2–22) was designed specifically for use in the medical and paramedical sciences to provide a simple, accurate measurement of total solids in urine, serum, and plasma. The instrument is also useful for estimating total proteins of transudates and exudates. The TS meter (number 10400 A, American Optical Co.) contains a direct reading scale for total protein in plasma or serum (range 2.5–15 g/dl, with an accuracy of 0.1 g/dl), for urine specific gravity, and for refractive index. The instrument is compensated for ambient temperature. For accurate readings, the refractometer should be calibrated periodically to zero reading with distilled water.

A single drop of plasma is placed on the platform of the refractometer and viewed through the eyepiece by natural or artificial illumination. The reading is made at the point where the dividing line between bright and dark fields crosses the scale. If the 75-mm capillary hematocrit tube is filled with blood to three-fourths its length, sufficient plasma is available after centrifugation to flood the platform of the refractometer. The capillary tube is broken immediately above the PCV column to transfer the plasma to refractometer. The refractometer platform and its covering plate should be thoroughly cleaned with distilled water after every use and wiped dry.

The protein scale has been compensated for certain common nonprotein constituents of plasma and serum. As long as the plasma or serum is clear, the prediction of total protein concentration is made with a high degree of accuracy. Cloudy or lipemic plasma and plasma containing free hemoglobin are not entirely suitable for total protein prediction (Wolf et al., 1962) because the instrument has not been compensated for these additional materials. The refractive index is increased markedly by lipids so that total protein values are erroneously high (Appendix Cases 1 and 7). It has been stated that an increase in bilirubin content does not affect refractive index significantly (Barry et al., 1960). Significantly elevated levels of glucose, cholesterol, and possibly other plasma constituents may lead to erroneously high protein readings. Protein concentrations obtained by the refractometer method and those by the biuret method are compared in Table 2–7. A close correlation was found between protein concentration by refractometry and the biuret method for equine serum and plasma samples (Carlson and Harrold, 1977). In our experience, plasma

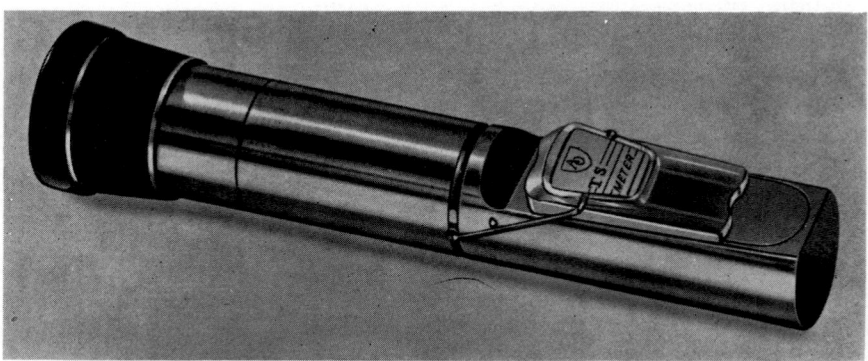

Fig. 2–22. The Goldberg refractometer, or TS meter.

Table 2–7. Comparison of Plasma Protein Concentrations as Predicted by Refractometer with the Biuret Method

Animal	Gross Appearance of the Plasma	Grams/dl Plasma Proteins		Grams/dl Difference of TS Meter over Biuret[a]
		TS Meter	Biuret Method	
Dog				
	Clear	3.1	3.0	0.10+
	Clear	5.7	5.8	0.10−
	Clear	8.0	7.95	0.05+
	Slightly pink (hemolysis)	6.0	5.95	0.05+
	Slightly pink (hemolysis)	6.4	5.95	0.45+
	Slightly pink (hemolysis)	6.7	7.1	0.40−
	Red (hemolysis)	6.9	6.1	0.80+
	Distinctly pink (hemolysis)	9.5	8.4	1.10+
	Slightly cloudy	8.6	8.3	0.30+
	Lactescent (lipemia)	7.7	6.6	1.10+
Horse				
	Clear	5.5	5.35	0.15+
	Clear	6.9	6.9	0.00
	Clear	7.2	6.9	0.30+
	Clear	7.2	7.0	0.20+
	Clear	7.4	7.4	0.00
	Clear	7.8	7.4	0.40+
	Clear	7.9	7.8	0.10+
	Clear	8.0	7.8	0.20+
	Clear	8.1	8.2	0.10−
	Clear	9.3	9.3	0.00
	Slightly pink (hemolysis)	5.9	5.9	0.00
	Distinctly pink (hemolysis)	7.8	7.35	0.45+
	Slightly cloudy	6.6	5.8	0.80+
	Lactescent (lipemia)	6.5	5.5	1.00+
	Strongly lactescent	8.3	6.0	2.30+
Cow				
	Clear	6.6	6.4	0.20+
	Clear	8.0	8.1	0.10−
	Clear	9.3	9.2	0.10+
	Slightly cloudy	6.9	6.7	0.20+
	Orange (icterus index over 100 units)	8.1	8.35	0.25−
	Brown (icterus index over 100 units)	7.7	8.0	0.30−

[a]0.2 gm% variation may be anticipated with the Biuret method.

protein concentrations obtained by the refractometer method are usually higher than total serum protein levels determined by an automated system, even after correcting for the amount of fibrinogen in the former samples.

Total plasma protein (TPP) concentration is lowest at birth (Table 34–5), being commonly less than 5.0 g/dl. Consumption of colostrum leads to an immediate small increase in TPP as the high globulin content is absorbed through the small intestine during the first few hours of life. Thereafter, TPP increases gradually with advancing age, ranging between 6.0 and 9.0 g/dl depending on the species involved. In old animals, the TPP often exceeds 7.5 g/dl as the globulin fraction increases throughout life in response to periodic exposure to antigens. Thus the low end of the normal range is characteristic of young growing animals, while the high end can be expected in mature animals. Age then becomes a factor in interpretation, especially in the dog (Schalm, 1970). For example, a dog 8 to 10 years of age with a TPP of 6.0 to 6.5 g/dl should be looked upon as being hypoproteinemic, whereas values of 7.5 to 8.0 g/dl in a dog less than 6 months of age would suggest hemoconcentration. The refractometer is useful for following progress of hydration as fluids are administered to combat water loss.

Plasma proteins are formed by lymphoid tissues and the liver. Major diseases involving these tissues may affect plasma protein production and result in either increases or decreases in TPP. The dog has presented the greatest variety of clinical conditions; Table 2–8 compares TPP with PCV in dogs with

Table 2–8. Plasma Protein Concentration Compared with PCV and the Nature of the Clinical Condition in the Dog

Age	Sex	Protein (g/dl)	PCV (%)	Nature of the Clinical Condition and Comments
6 yr	F	2.7	38	Chronic diarrhea and weight loss; sprue
1 yr	F	3.0	40	Chronic diarrhea and weight loss; sprue
9 mo	M	3.6	21	Suspected warfarin poisoning
14 mo	M	3.7	15	Liver cirrhosis, aplastic anemia, and ascites
1 yr	F	4.4	59	Passive congestion of the liver and ascites
4 yr	F	4.7	49	Hydrothorax following pneumonia
10 yr	F	4.8	38	Hepatic cell carcinoma and ascites
6 yr	M	4.8	46	Congestive heart failure
4½ yr	F	4.9	42	Cardiac problem and ascites
13 yr	F	5.0	27	Ruptured hemangioma of the spleen
1½ yr	M	5.0	17	Idiopathic thrombocytopenic purpura
3 mo	M	5.2	15	Suspected warfarin poisoning
10 mo	F	5.5	32	Ancylostomiasis
4 yr	M	5.6	18	Chronic blood loss from ulcerative colitis
3½ yr	M	5.8	34	Liver cirrhosis and ascites
1½ yr	F	6.5	58	Muscle pain; normal protein range, high PCV[a]
7 yr	M	6.7	56	History of convulsions; normal protein, high PCV[a]
7 yr	F	6.7	60	Bilateral alopecia; normal protein, high PCV[a]
2 yr	M	6.9	58	History of convulsions; normal protein, high PCV[a]
6 yr	F	7.1	60	Bleeding from the rectum; normal protein, high PCV[a]
2½ yr	M	7.7	19	Chronic interstitial nephritis, dehydration
3 yr	M	8.2	52	Leptospirosis, acute nephritis, and dehydration
2 yr	F	8.6	65	Paralysis (coonhound) and severe dehydration
2½ yr	M	8.9	53	Intussusception and dehydration
11 mo	M	9.4	58	Distemper and severe dehydration
4 yr	F	9.6	55	Cerebrocortical necrosis and dehydration
6 yr	M	9.9	43	Dermatitis and severe dehydration
9 mo	M	10.0	46	Leptospirosis and severe dehydration
11 yr	M	10.0	52	Chronic interstitial nephritis, extreme dehydration
9 mo	M	11.3	45	Acute nephritis and extreme dehydration

[a]Elevated PCV possibly due to excitement, with splenic contraction forcing a concentrated mass of erythrocytes into the circulation.

different diseases. Low plasma protein concentrations may be anticipated in *(a)* blood loss (Appendix Cases 20 and 33), *(b)* hepatopathy (Appendix Case 14), *(c)* malnutrition, *(d)* chronic glomerulonephritis (Appendix Case 4), and *(e)* generalized lymphosarcoma (Table 32–10). In dogs that are excitable, the PCV may be high because of contraction of the spleen. In such instances, the plasma protein concentration is unaffected. Hemoconcentration would increase both the PCV and TPP. Elevated plasma proteins occur in many chronic diseases. For example, hypergammaglobulinemia can be expected in infections as an expression of heightened immune response. Therefore an above-normal plasma protein concentration may be either relative (dehydration) or absolute (immune response) or a combination of both. Chapter 34 discusses the clinical application of TPP in detail.

ESTIMATION OF PLASMA FIBRINOGEN BY REFRACTOMETER

Fibrinogen is produced by the liver. It functions in the clotting of blood and plays a role in defense against injury to confine or localize an invasive disease process. An elevation of plasma fibrinogen may indicate the existence of disease in general.

Fibrinogen precipitates at 56–58°C, while the other plasma proteins remain in solution. This phenomenon can be used to measure fibrinogen concentration as the difference in plasma proteins before and after heating and centrifugation to remove the precipitated fibrinogen (Foster et al., 1959; Kaneko and Smith, 1967; Low et al., 1967). Heparinized blood is unsuitable for estimation of fibrinogen because it gives low values; therefore EDTA should be used as the anticoagulant when fibrinogen level is to be determined.

Method 1

Fill two 75-mm capillary tubes with blood to at least three-quarters capacity. Centrifuge both as in the microhematocrit test. Use one tube to determine total plasma proteins. Place the other capillary tube in a water bath at 56–58°C for 3 minutes and then recentrifuge

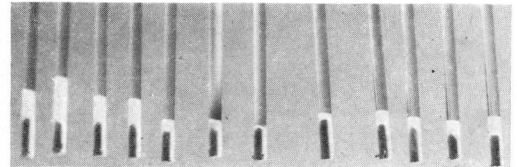

Fig. 2–23. Demonstration of removal of precipitated fibrinogen by centrifugation of 75-mm capillary tube containing plasma heated to 58°C. The fibrinogen is the white layer above the plug used to seal the tube.

to sediment the precipitated fibrinogen (Fig. 2–23). Break the capillary tube above the fibrinogen layer, transfer the fluid to the refractometer platform, and read the protein concentration. Fibrinogen concentration in g/dl is the difference between the protein content of the two tubes.

Method 2

Fill a Wintrobe hematocrit tube with blood, and centrifuge for 10 minutes to clear the plasma of cells. Estimate total plasma proteins, and then fill a 75-mm capillary tube with plasma from the Wintrobe tube to two-thirds capacity, seal the dry end, heat in a water bath, centrifuge, and test for protein, as in Method 1. Subtract plasma protein concentration in 75-mm tube from that in Wintrobe tube to obtain the fibrinogen concentration in g/dl.

Interpretation

Fibrinogen concentration in plasma, unlike total plasma proteins, is not affected by the age of the animal. The broad normal range of plasma fibrinogen in the dog, sheep, and pig is 0.1–0.5 g/dl. The cat appears to have a lower normal range of 0.05–0.3 g/dl, while the range for the cow is 0.3–0.7 g/dl and the horse and goat is 0.1–0.4 g/dl.

To compensate for dehydration, a plasma protein:fibrinogen ratio is developed by first subtracting the fibrinogen value from the TPP value and then dividing the fibrinogen value into the remainder. Ratios of 15:1 or greater are representative of normal and ratios of 10:1 or less reflect a true increase in plasma fibrinogen. (For further details, see Chapter 34; see also Tables 34–5 through 34–9.)

BLOOD EXAMINATION BY WET-FILM METHOD

Information not readily available from a stained blood film may be obtained by examination of a drop of blood under a coverslip, preferably between plastic surfaces (wet mount). This method permits the observation of erythrocyte morphology in three dimensions. It is the best method to see discoid biconcave shape of erythrocytes and any morphologic abnormality including crenation (Fig. 2–24:1). Rouleau formation is more obvious (Fig. 2–24:2). The presence of chylomicra is readily detected because of their brownian movement. The presence of platelets can also be detected. The neutrophil leukocyte can be observed to show ameboid movement, brownian movement of cytoplasmic granules, and cytolysis. When microfilariae are present in blood in sufficient number, they can be detected by this method.

STAINING BLOOD FILMS WITH NEW METHYLENE BLUE

This method is ideally suited to the needs of the busy practitioner for rapid examination of unfixed films of blood, bone marrow, body fluids, and other cytologic materials (Schalm, 1961, 1964). The staining solution consists of 0.5% new methylene blue (NMB) in 0.85% NaCl to which full-strength formalin is added as a preservative (1 ml/100 ml stain). Filtered stain can be kept at room temperature for several months.

The stain is applied to a dry unfixed blood film in the following manner: Use a round wood applicator stick or medicine dropper to transfer a large drop of stain to a clean glass slide, and then drop the coverslip film onto the stain, blood film facing the stain. If the film has been prepared on a slide, place the drop of stain on a clean coverslip and invert it on the slide or vice versa. Both the slide and the coverslip must be dust-free for the staining solution to spread evenly between the glass surfaces. The film is ready for microscopic examination as soon as the stain has been applied. Since the stain is contained in physiologic saline, the film is not permanent. Therefore the stain should not be applied

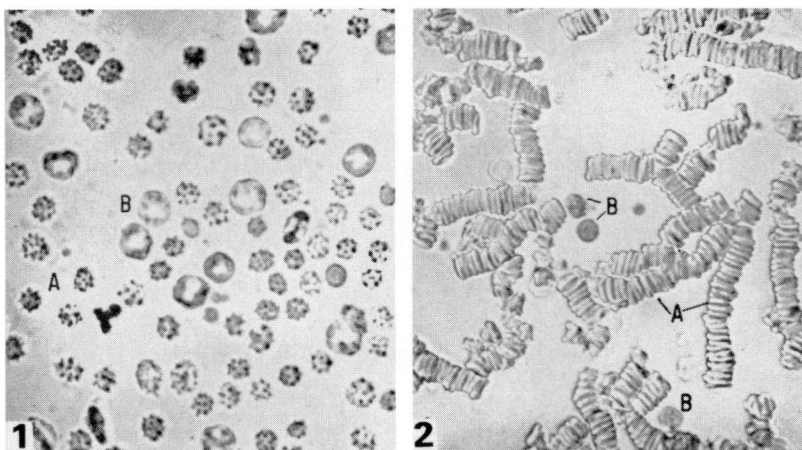

Fig. 2–24. Two examples of wet-film preparations observed under high dry magnification (×400). *1.* Canine blood in severe anemia with a marked reticulocyte response: *A,* crenated mature erythrocytes; *B,* all noncrenated, larger cells are reticulocytes. *2.* Feline blood with a low normal volume percent erythrocytes (PCV) exhibiting extensive rouleau formation (erythrocytes stacked like coins): *A,* rouleaux; *B,* leukocytes.

until time permits immediate examination. If the coverslip is ringed with immersion oil to prevent evaporation of the staining solution, the preparation can be retained for several days.

A variety of morphologic observations can be made from blood, bone marrow, and cytologic specimens stained with NMB. However, cellular identification and recognition of various abnormalities in NMB-stained films, compared to Wright-stained films, is difficult and requires experience.

Comments on Structures Discernible in Blood Films

1. Mature erythrocytes do not take the stain but appear as ghosts. The nuclei of immature erythrocytes, Howell-Jolly bodies, the infrequently encountered inclusion in immature erythrocytes in canine distemper (Fig. 36–1), and the reticulum of reticulocytes (Fig. 2–25:1) are readily demonstrated. This is the fastest method for the determination of a reticulocytosis.

2. Red blood cell parasites such as *Anaplasma* and *Piroplasma* (*Babesia,* Fig. 2–25:6) can be readily seen. Anaplasmosis on the Pacific coast is sometimes associated with parasites having loops and tail-like structures that are not visible in blood films stained by Roma-

nowsky methods; these are readily demonstrated with NMB (Fig. 2–25:6; Fig. 23–1). The method is generally not satisfactory for detection of *Haemobartonella felis* and other delicate parasites that can be confused with the reticulum in reticulocytes.

3. Heinz bodies are readily demonstrated (Fig. 2–25:3, 5; Plate XVIII–8). They appear as dense, unstained refractile structures within the red cells.

4. The chylomicra of lipemic blood appear as tiny refractile bodies on and surrounding many of the red blood cells (Fig. 2–25:2). There is some resemblance to reticulocytes, but the chylomicra are found along the cell periphery and are refractile, while the reticulum is not.

5. Some experience is needed to distinguish various leukocytes stained by NMB. The nuclei of leukocytes stain intensely, and the cytoplasm of each cell type has its own special characteristics. The eosinophil granules do not take the stain and appear refractile. Neutrophil cytoplasm does not reveal obvious granulation. Granules of basophils stain black in the horse and cow, while in the dog they tend to lose the stain quickly, perhaps because of their water-soluble nature. The cytoplasm of the lymphocyte and monocyte stains gray (Fig. 2–25:4). There may be a problem in dis-

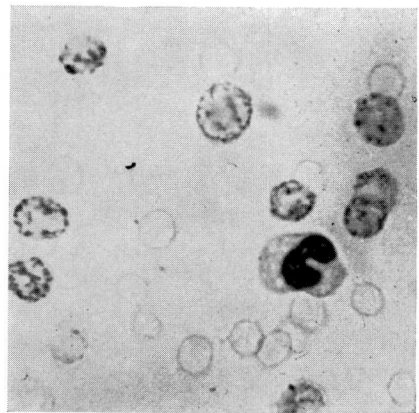

1. Dog. Reticulocytes in anemia in remission, also a band neutrophil.

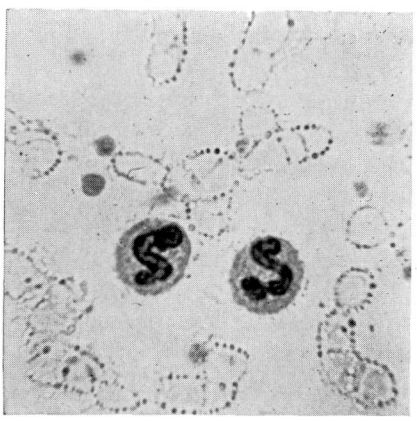

2. Dog. RBC are surrounded by chylomicra in lipemia. Two neutrophils and several thrombocytes are shown.

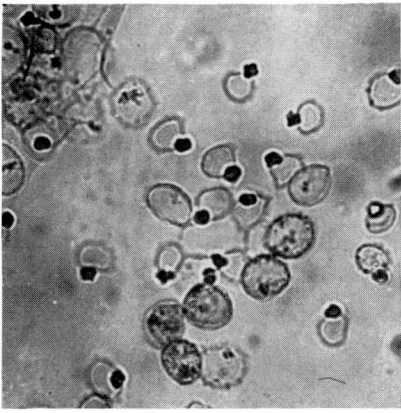

3. Cat. Heinz bodies in mature RBC. Reticulocytes are not involved in Heinz body formation.

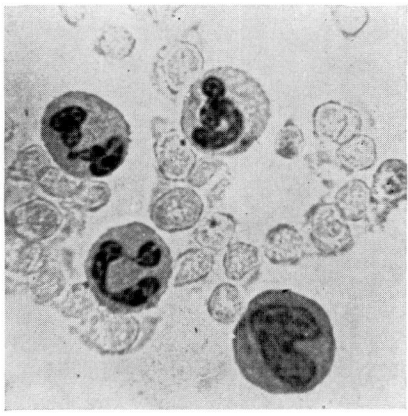

4. Cat. Three mature neutrophils and one monocyte at lower right.

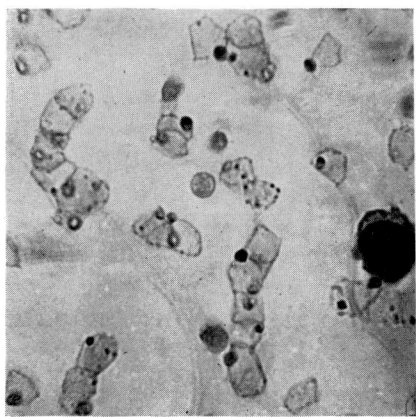

5. Horse. Heinz-body formation in the RBC in phenothiazine toxicosis.

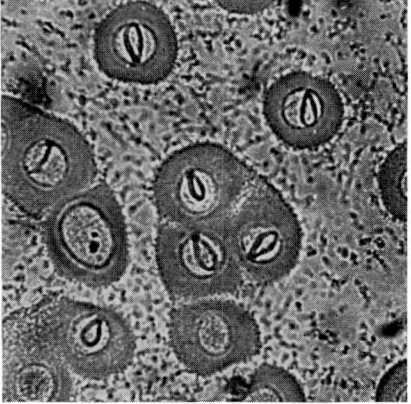

6. Cow. Tail-like loops in the RBC in a natural case of anaplasmosis. Precipitated protein surrounds the RBC.

Fig. 2–25. New methylene blue stain applied to dry unfixed blood films. (From Schalm, 1964; courtesy of the *Journal of the American Veterinary Medical Association.*)

tinguishing metamyelocytes from monocytes, especially when the cytoplasm of the former is basophilic as a result of the toxic effect of disease. However, monocytes can be distinguished by cytoplasmic vacuoles when present. Döhle bodies in neutrophils of the cat and horse can be demonstrated. NMB stain is helpful in distinguishing the heterophils from the eosinophils in the rabbit. Heterophil granules stain deep blue, while eosinophil granules are refractile as in the blood of other species.

6. Cytoplasmic inclusions in leukocytes— e.g., *Chlamydia*, *Ehrlichia* (Plate XIV–3), and bacteria—are demonstrable with NMB.

7. Thrombocytes appear as small, round, pale lavender structures of varying size (Fig. 2–25:2). Existence of thrombocytopenia is therefore detectable by this simple staining procedure.

Comments on Other Applications of New Methylene Blue Stain

1. NMB stain is useful for immediate examination of material aspirated from bone marrow to determine if it contains marrow cells. Detection of gross alterations in bone marrow cytology is possible with NMB.

2. Vaginal smears stained with NMB reveal good morphological features of epithelial cells. Neutrophils and bacteria stain well, while erythrocytes appear as ghosts.

3. Direct smears of cloudy body fluids or films prepared from sediments of clear fluids readily reveal the types of cells present. Inflammatory exudates can be distinguished from fluids of neoplastic origin. *Toxoplasma* and *Histoplasma* within cells can be detected, as well as intracellular and extracellular bacteria, yeasts, and fungi (Fig. 2–26). Rickettsial bodies in histiocytes of lymph nodes have been demonstrated in salmon poisoning of dogs.

4. Impression smears of tumors and lymph nodes or films from needle biopsy or aspirated fluid from lymph nodes stain well with NMB (Perman, 1966). Cells di-

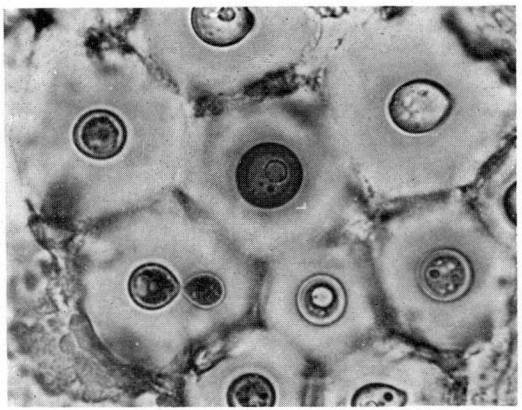

Fig. 2–26. *Cryptococcus neoformans* in an impression smear from the nasal chamber of a mouflon sheep. Note the wide, gelatinous refractive capsule and budding of one organism. (New methylene blue stain, ×2,200.)

agnostic of mastocytoma, lymphosarcoma, and other neoplasms can be identified.

5. Inclusion bodies of infectious canine hepatitis in liver smears have been demonstrated by NMB (Klopfer, 1969).

SPECIAL STAINING PROCEDURES

Staining and Counting Reticulocytes

Brilliant cresyl blue as 1.0% solution in 0.85% NaCl solution containing 0.4% sodium citrate has been used to stain reticulocytes. A commonly used reticulocyte stain consists of new methylene blue 0.5 g, potassium oxalate 1.6 g, and distilled water 100 ml (Brecher, 1949).

Two drops of blood and about an equal to double quantity of stain are mixed in a small test tube and allowed to interact for 5 to 20 minutes at room temperature. A film is prepared from the mixture in the usual manner. No counterstain is necessary. The mature erythrocytes appear yellowish or light green, while those containing dots, strings, or clumps of bluish material ("reticulum") are the reticulocytes. The reticulum develops from aggregation of ribosomes and may incorporate other cell organelles such as mitochondria (Fig. 18–9D). Cells containing strings and clumps of reticulum are referred to as "aggregate" or "reticulated" reticulocytes, while those with dots of bluish material are called "punctate" reticulocytes. The former type are characteristic in dogs, while the latter type with or without the former are often seen in cats during enhanced erythropoietic response to anemia. The reticulocyte count is made under oil-immersion lens by differentiation of at least 1,000 erythrocytes. Subjective criteria of reticulocyte identification is the major source of inaccuracy in reticulocyte counts (Peeble et al., 1981). The usual practice is to count aggregate reticulocytes, but a separate count of aggregate and punctate reticulocytes may be made on feline blood. For counting, it is helpful to employ an etched disc* in one ocular to divide the microscopic field into a number of small squares.

Results of the reticulocyte count are expressed as percentage of the erythrocytes. For interpretation, this value is converted to an "absolute count" or a "reticulocyte production index" (RPI). The absolute reticulocyte count is obtained by multiplying the red cell count by the percentile fraction of the reticulocyte count. For example, for an RBC count of $4.0 \times 10^6/\mu l$ and a reticulocyte count of 5%, the absolute reticulocyte count is $4.0 \times 10^6 \times 0.05 = 200,000/\mu l$ of blood. A reticulocyte count of greater than $60,000/\mu l$ of blood in the dog and cat is considered suggestive of reticulocytosis (Weiser, 1981). Calculation of the RPI as another approach to correction of the reticulocyte count is given in Chapter 18.

Blood films stained in the manner described above will also reveal Heinz bodies as blue spherical structures at one edge of erythrocytes containing them (Plate XVIII–8). Leukocytes and platelets are disrupted, and red cell parasites cannot be distinguished from the reticulum of reticulocytes.

Demonstration of Basophilic Stippling

Basophilic stippling in Wright-stained blood films is characteristically seen in chronic lead poisoning in the dog, during erythropoietic response to anemia and sometimes in chronic lead poisoning in the cow, and also occasionally during intense erythropoietic response to anemia in the dog and cat. The effect of sample preparation on the amount of basophilic stippling of erythrocytes was studied using blood from a calf with experimental lead poisoning (George and Duncan, 1981). The combination of EDTA anticoagulant and rapid drying of smears resulted in the most basophilic stippling. Alcohol prefixation reduced basophilic stippling, and better staining was achieved with Wright-Leishman stain than with Wright stain.

Permanent Stain for Heinz Bodies

This method was developed for staining Heinz bodies in cat blood (Jain, 1969), but it can be adapted for use on other species' blood.

1. Treat the dry unfixed blood smear with 0.5% copper sulfate solution for 15–20 seconds.
2. Briefly rinse and transfer to phosphate buffer solution (p. 32) for 1 minute.
3. Drain the excess buffer and place the film in Wright-Leishman stain for 2–3 minutes.
4. Transfer to buffer fortified with Wright-Leishman stain for 4–5 minutes (p. 34).
5. Rinse briefly in two changes of distilled water.
6. Drain, air-dry, and mount as usual.

Step 1 produces erythrocyte ghosts and makes the Heinz bodies apparent. Step 2 removes the copper sulfate solution and adjusts the pH of the blood cells for appropriate differential staining. Omission of exposure to buffer in step 2 results in inferior staining of leukocytes in the subsequent steps.

Staining for Sideroleukocytes

Rothenbacher et al. (1962) and Henson et al. (1967) have discussed use of the sideroleukocyte test as an aid to the diagnosis of equine infectious anemia (EIA). A sideroleukocyte is a white blood cell (neutrophil or monocyte) containing dark bluish-black particles within the cytoplasm (Plate XIV–2). The staining is done as follows:

1. Place 9 ml of fresh blood into a test tube

---

*A satisfactory disc is the American Optical eyepiece micrometer disc, 1421A. It is 20 mm in diameter and presents a 5-mm square subdivided into 25 smaller squares.

containing 1 ml of a 10% solution of sodium citrate.

2. Allow the tube to stand at room temperature for 1–2 hours for sedimentation of the erythrocytes.
3. Transfer the supernatant plasma to a conical centrifuge tube and centrifuge at 200 G for 3–4 minutes.
4. Discard the supernatant and mix the leukocyte plug with the remaining few drops of plasma using an applicator stick.
5. Prepare films of the leukocyte-plasma mixture in the same manner as for blood films.
6. Fix films for 5 minutes or more in absolute methyl alcohol and air-dry.
7. Freshly prepare acidified potassium ferrocyanide solution by dissolving 2 g in 10 ml of distilled water. Then slowly add concentrated HCl until a white precipitate forms. Filter the solution, and transfer to a Columbia jar.
8. Place the films in the above staining solution for 30 minutes, wash in running water for 2 minutes, counterstain with 0.2% aqueous safranin for 2 minutes, rinse in distilled water in two separate beakers, and then drain dry. Mount the film as usual for examination.

Iron Stain

Iron in mature red cells (siderocytes) and nucleated red cells (sideroblasts) in blood and bone marrow can be stained by following steps 6 through 8 of the method described above for staining sideroleukocytes.

Cytochemical Stains

Common cytochemical staining techniques for use on animal blood and bone marrow films are described in Chapter 33.

COUNTING EOSINOPHIL LEUKOCYTES

The direct counting of eosinophils is important in evaluating adrenocortical activity. In the presence of a normal adrenal gland, the eosinophil count in peripheral blood decreases upon administration of adrenocorticotropic hormone (ACTH) or cortisone. Counting of eosinophils following injection of ACTH is used as a screening test for adrenocortical insufficiency (Hopwood and Tibolla, 1958; Martin et al., 1954). This is referred to as the Thorn test (Thorn et al., 1948; Appendix Case 10). A direct eosinophil count may also be desired in cases of eosinophilias.

The diluting fluid contains propylene glycol to lyse erythrocytes and sodium carbonate to lyse all leukocytes except the eosinophils (Pilot, 1950). It is prepared as follows:

Propylene glycol	50 ml
Distilled water	40 ml
Aqueous phloxine (1%)	10 ml
Aqueous sodium carbonate (10%)	1 ml

The solution is stable at room temperature for at least 1 month. Mix and filter before use. Eosinophils stain red. An improved solution has been described for counting eosinophils in the dog blood (Farrington and Jetter, 1953). The staining solution is prepared as follows: Dissolve 0.25 g eosin Y and 0.25 g phloxine B in 50 ml of distilled water. Add 50 ml propylene glycol and mix. Add 0.5 ml each of concentrated formalin and 85% phenol as preservative. The stain can be used immediately without filtering.

The direct eosinophil count is made as follows: Draw blood to the 1.0 mark into the white-cell pipette, followed by the diluting fluid to the 11 mark. Shake the pipette for 2 minutes, discard the fluid in the capillary portion, and fill two hemocytometers for counting. Wait 15 minutes for complete lysing of cells before making the eosinophil count. To increase accuracy, it is recommended that two diluting pipettes be filled and a total of eight chambers on four hemocytometers be used; the eosinophils in all nine squares of each chamber should be counted. The average number of eosinophils per hemocytometer chamber multiplied by 11.1 gives the number of eosinophils per μl of blood.

Carper and Schalm (1962) compared the number of eosinophils per μl estimated from total leukocyte count and percentage of eosinophils in the differential count with the number obtained by the direct-counting method described above. This comparison was made on blood from 106 dogs, 133 horses, 128 cows, and 12 cats. The indirect method gave higher estimated numbers of eosinophils, but a statistically significant linear relationship was found between the two methods.

COUNTING PLATELETS

Direct and indirect methods for the estimation of platelet numbers have been devised.

Indirect Method

The indirect method is performed on the routinely stained blood smear. The simplest procedure is to note the number of platelets per oil-immersion field. The finding of three or fewer platelets indicates a count of less than 50,000/µl. The number of platelets encountered while scanning the film to count 100 leukocytes can be converted to an absolute platelet count as follows:

$$\frac{\text{Number of platelets}}{100} \times \text{WBC count}$$

$$= \text{number of platelets/µl}$$

This method has clinical application in thrombocytopenias when a direct counting method is not applicable. However, the error can be very high owing to uneven distribution or clumps of platelets in stained smears.

Direct Method

Enumeration of platelets can be done directly by using a hemocytometer and special diluent. The diluting fluid for platelet counting is prepared in advance and stored in a refrigerator; a small portion is filtered just before use. The formula given below is that proposed by Rees and Ecker (1923).

Sodium citrate	3.8 g
Formaldehyde (40%)	0.2 ml
Brilliant cresyl blue	0.1 g
Distilled water	100.0 ml

Blood in EDTA anticoagulant is preferred to avoid platelet aggregation. Thrombocytes tend to stick to glassware; to avoid as much error as possible from this source, the glassware must be clean and grease-free. The procedure is as follows:

1. Draw diluting fluid to the 1.0 mark of the red blood cell pipette and immediately expel. The purpose is to moisten the glass to reduce adherence of throm-

bocytes as blood is drawn into the stem of the pipette.
2. Draw well-mixed blood to the 0.5 mark and diluent to the 101 mark.
3. Hand mix the pipette as for the red or white cell count, or place it on a mechanical shaker for 5 minutes of mixing.
4. Expel about one-third of the fluid from the pipette, and immediately fill both sides of the hemocytometer chamber.
5. Allow 15 minutes for the platelets to settle before counting. To avoid evaporation during this period, place the hemocytometer in a Petri dish containing moistened filter paper. Rest the slide upon two wood applicator sticks to keep the underside from direct contact with the moistened paper.
6. Focus on the surface of the hemocytometer chamber with the high dry objective. Dim the light to make the thrombocytes visible, and while focusing up and down with the fine adjustment, count all the thrombocytes in the entire center 1.0-mm² area (erythrocyte-counting area) of both sides of the hemocytometer. This gives the number of thrombocytes in 0.2 µl of a 1:200 dilution of blood.
7. The number of thrombocytes counted × 1,000 = number of thrombocytes per µl of blood.

Platelet counts can also be determined by Unopette and electronic counting methods. Electronic counts on the basis of collection of platelet-rich plasma (PRP) after gravity sedimentation of red cells in whole blood, as done for human blood, are not possible on blood samples of cattle, sheep, goats, and other animals usually exhibiting little or no ESR. Dilution of the blood with isotonic cell counting medium (1:100 with 10 ml of Isoton) sufficiently accelerates ESR and collection of PRP and permits electronic counting of cattle and sheep platelets (Maxie, 1977; Steel, 1974). PRP obtained after gentle centrifugation of whole blood gives erroneous results. Electronic instruments utilizing whole blood for platelet counts circumvent this difficulty. As use of electronic instruments for platelet counts increases, new normal values have to be established; normal platelet counts given in this book and largely in the veterinary literature are based on the hemocytometer method.

COAGULATION TESTS

These tests are described in Chapter 14.

ASPIRATION OF BONE MARROW

The primary function of bone marrow is to produce erythrocytes, granulocytes, monocytes, and thrombocytes and to supply lymphoid precursor cells. Active bone marrow is red, while nonproductive resting marrow is yellow. In the adult, yellow marrow fills most of the shafts of the long bones. The flat bones, such as the ribs, pelvis, and bones of the head; the short bones, such as the vertebrae; and the ends of the long bones normally contain red marrow throughout life. To obtain bone marrow for study from living animals, it is necessary to select a readily accessible site for puncture of the marrow cavity. In humans, the sternum is frequently used, and it may also be used in animals such as the cow, horse, and dog (Melveger et al., 1969). The iliac crest is a convenient site (Fig. 2–27) for use in the dog (Meyer and Bloom, 1943), cat (Sawitsky and Meyer, 1947), horse (Archer, 1954), and cow. Techniques for aspiration of marrow from the rib have been described for the dog (West et al., 1971), cow (Lawrence et al., 1962), and horse (Calhoun, 1954). The dorsal femur is a readily accessible site for marrow aspiration in the cat (see below).

For best results, withdraw less than 0.5 ml of marrow fluid; otherwise dilution with blood will render the sample less satisfactory for study of marrow cytology. In the event blood dilution has occurred, centrifuge the sample and prepare films from the buffy coat, or place marrow spicules over a slide and tilt the latter to drain excessive fluid and then make smears. Marrow films are prepared and stained in the same manner as blood films. See Chapter 1 for evaluation of marrow films.

Marrow undiluted with blood does not clot readily; hence an anticoagulant is generally not required when marrow films can be prepared immediately after collection. When film

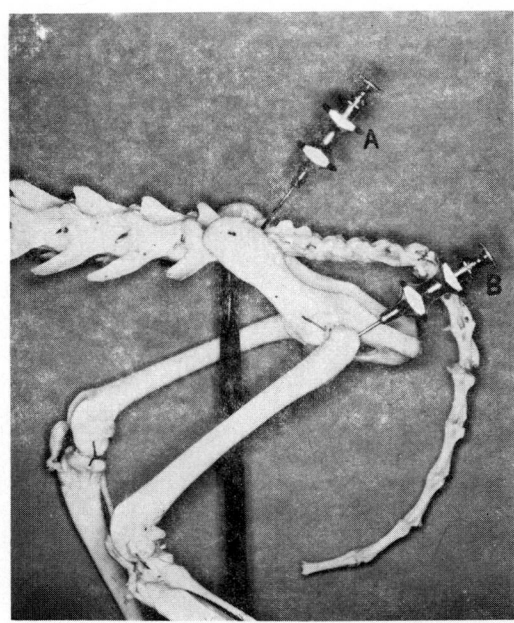

Fig. 2–27.   Bone marrow aspiration sites for use in the dog and cat. *A*, iliac crest; *B*, dorsal femur. (From Switzer and Schalm, 1968; courtesy of *The California Veterinarian*.)

preparation is to be delayed, the marrow should be transferred into a vial containing a minimum amount of anticoagulant (1.0-ml Vacutainer). If a problem arises because of difficulties in the procedure, coagulation can be prevented by first moistening the syringe with 0.25 ml of EDTA solution. The solution is prepared by adding 240 mg of dipotassium EDTA to 30 ml of sterile 0.85% NaCl solution. The solution keeps indefinitely at room temperature. Improved cell preservation and staining were achieved when bone marrow was aspirated directly into a syringe containing 0.5 ml of homologous serum fortified with disodium or dipotassium EDTA (2–4 mg/ml of serum) and smears were prepared after centrifugation and resuspension of the cells in a portion of the serum (Fluharty and Uhler, 1975).

Technique for the Dog

Outline the iliac crest with the finger, clip the hair at the immediate site of the puncture, usually the anterior-dorsal angle, and apply a suitable antiseptic. Infiltrate the area with 2% procaine or lidocaine. Make a short slit in the skin with a sharp scalpel to facilitate

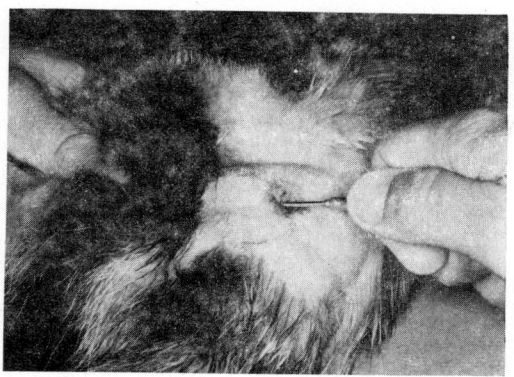

Fig. 2–28. Inserting bone marrow aspiration needle into the dorsal femur of a cat under light anesthesia. (From Switzer and Schalm, 1968. Courtesy of *The California Veterinarian.*)

needle penetration. A Jamshidi bone marrow biopsy needle is preferred.

Pass the sterile aspiration needle through the skin and muscle over the anterior-dorsal angle of the crest of the ilium (Fig. 2–28). When the needle reaches the periosteum, force it into the bone by steady pressure and back-and-forth rotation. When the needle is firmly embedded, it usually will have penetrated the medullary cavity. Use the stylet to free the needle of tissue or bone particles. Fit a dry 20-ml syringe to the needle, and pull the plunger to establish sufficient vacuum to withdraw marrow fluid. As soon as fluid appears, stop the suction process to avoid dilution of the marrow with blood.

Technique for the Cat

Aspiration of bone marrow from cats is more easily accomplished from the proximal femur (Fig. 2–27) via the trochanteric fossa than from the iliac crest (Conner et al., 1971; Schryver, 1963; Switzer and Schalm, 1968). A 16-gauge Rosenthal needle is used. Place the cat on its side, and clip a small area over the major trochanter. Anesthetize the area with 2% procaine or 2% lidocaine. If struggling is severe, administer a small sedative dose of thiamylal sodium (0.5–0.75 ml). Make a small stab incision over the trochanteric fossa. Grasp the hind leg in the mid-femur region, with the cat's knee resting firmly in the palm between the forefinger and the thumb. Insert the needle medial to the trochanter with firm pressure and an alternating rotating motion.

It is important at this step to keep the stylet in place to prevent bony material from plugging the needle. When the needle is well inserted into the femoral canal, about ½ inch, remove the stylet and aspirate the marrow with a 20-ml syringe. Withdraw only enough fluid to prepare the required number of films.

Technique for the Cow and the Horse

In adult cattle and horses, hematopoietically active marrow is accessible for aspiration from the sternum and the dorsal ends of the ribs. In cattle, the eighth through the eleventh ribs on each side of the body provide eight sites of sequential bone marrow aspirations, and when necessary, the twelfth rib may be used (Schalm and Lasmanis, 1976). In horses, the ninth through the fifteenth ribs can similarly be used.

Marrow aspiration is performed using the Westerman-Jensen biopsy needle (Becton Dickinson). Insert a sterile scalpel through the skin and underlying tissues until contact is made with the rib. Insert the trocar and cannula, using the scalpel as a guide to reach the rib. Penetrate the marrow cavity by placing pressure on the biopsy needle while producing a back-and-forth partial rotation of the needle. Attach a 10-ml syringe to the cannula, and withdraw approximately 0.5 ml of marrow fluid and immediately transfer it to a Vacutainer tube of 1.0-ml capacity containing dipotassium EDTA anticoagulant. The volume of fluid withdrawn should be limited to the smallest amount consistent with need in order to avoid excessive dilution of marrow with blood. The first 0.1 ml of marrow fluid from cattle was reported to be considerably more cellular than a 1.0-ml sample (Wilde, 1963). We have found a volume of 0.5 ml to be satisfactory, but less than that amount results in shrinkage of neutrophils by the anticoagulant contained in a 1.0-ml vial.

ESTIMATION OF TOTAL LEUKOCYTE COUNT BY DNA VISCOSITY TEST

Schalm and Noorlander (1957) described a test to be applied to milk for the detection of above-normal numbers of leukocytes and tissue cells. An anionic detergent was found to react with deoxyribonucleic acid of cell nuclei to produce a viscous mass or gel (Carroll and Schalm, 1962). The method was designated the California mastitis test, or CMT. The method was applied to blood by Schalm and Murray (1964) as a rapid screening procedure for estimating the level of leukocytes. Thirty ml of CMT concentrate reagent (Dairy Research Products) is diluted with tap water in quantity sufficient to make 1,000 ml. The dilute reagent solution should be light purple, indicating that it is slightly alkaline. Acid water is to be avoided. The bromcresol purple indicator in CMT reagent will cause the color to be other than purple when acid water is used.

The four steps in conducting the DNA viscosity test on blood are shown in Figure 2–29.

1. Measure diluted CMT reagent from a polyethylene wash bottle into a 15-ml graduated centrifuge tube to the 3.0-ml level. Other methods utilize a graduated pipette or burette to deliver 3.0 ml of

reagent into a test tube. It is important that the volume of reagent be exactly 3.0 ml and the total capacity of the tube 15 ml.

2. Add one full drop of well-mixed blood in EDTA or other anticoagulant by means of a straight-tip medicine dropper. It is best to allow two or three drops of blood to fall back into the blood vial before the one drop of blood is added to the 3.0 ml of reagent. This is to ensure a full drop of blood free of bubbles. Start a stopwatch immediately, and mix the blood and reagent by placing the thumb over the mouth of the tube and slowly inverting the tube exactly five times. This requires about 20 seconds.

3. Press the special glass funnel (Dairy Research Products) against a rubber stopper to close the stem. The same can be accomplished by holding the funnel between the thumb and index finger while

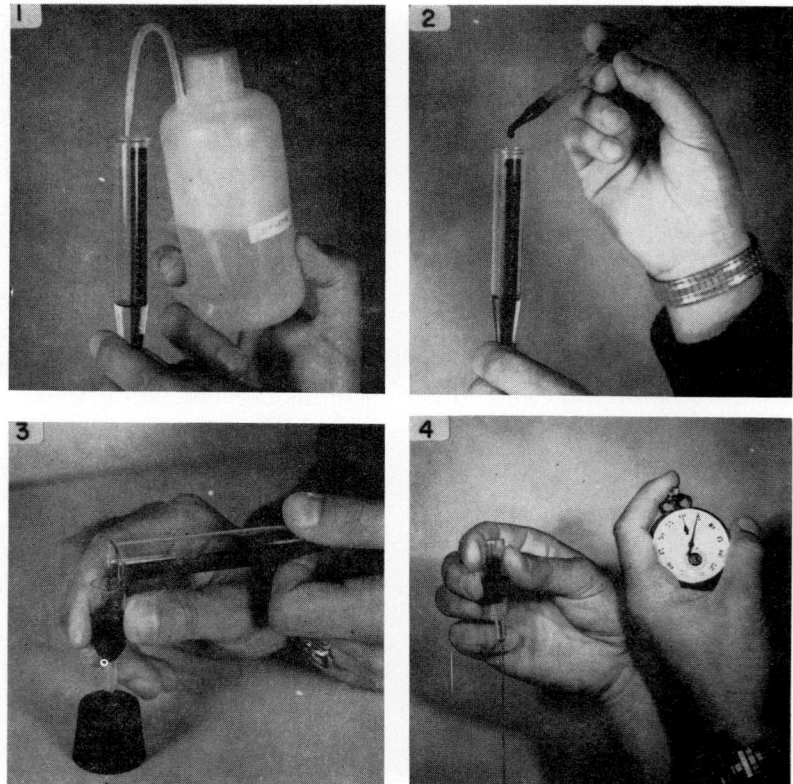

Fig. 2–29. Sequence of steps in estimation of leukocyte numbers in blood by DNA viscosity test as measured by flow time through a calibrated funnel stem. (From Schalm and Murray, 1964; courtesy of the *Journal of the American Veterinary Medical Association.*)

Table 2–9. Conversion of DNA Viscosity Test Flow Time to Estimated Mean Leukocyte Number per µl of Blood of Dog, Cat, Cow, and Horse

Flow Time (Seconds)	Estimated Mean Total Leukocyte Numbers/µl Blood			
	Dog	Cat	Cow	Horse
4.0	<5,000	<5,000	5,000	4,000
4.5	8,500	7,000	5,000	4,500
5.0	10,500	11,500	6,500	6,000
5.5	12,500	13,500	8,800	7,500
6.0	14,500	16,000	10,000	9,000
6.5	16,500	18,000	11,500	10,000
7.0	18,000	19,500	12,500	11,000
7.5	19,500	21,000	13,500	12,000
8.0	21,000	22,500	14,500	13,000
8.5	22,500	24,000	15,000	14,000
9.0	23,500	25,500	15,500	15,000
9.5	24,500	27,000	16,000	16,000
10.0	25,500	28,500	16,500	17,000
10.5	26,500	30,000	—	18,000
11.0	27,500	31,000	—	18,500
11.5	29,000	32,000	—	19,500
12.0	30,000	33,000	—	20,000
12.5	31,500	34,000		
13.0	32,750	35,000		
13.5	34,000	36,000		
14.0	35,000	37,000		
15.0	37,000	39,000		

pressing the tip of the stem against the side of the little finger of the same hand. Carefully pour the reagent blood mixture into the funnel.

4. Then at exactly 30 seconds from start of the watch, lift the funnel so that the fluid is permitted to flow. When the level of liquid falls to the bottom of the funnel (stem top), stop the watch, and record the flow time in seconds. Then convert the flow time to estimated leukocyte number from the reference Table 2–9. (Since the funnel and the CMT reagent used originally in developing the test have been replaced, the table developed to estimate the number of leukocytes by this method published in the third edition of this book no longer applies.) The content of DNA per somatic cell varies among animal species (Vendrely, 1955). For this reason, separate conversion tables for the cat, dog, horse, and cow are presented. Of these four species, the content of DNA per somatic cell is greatest for the cow and least for the cat.

When the fluid flows without interruption, the conversion of flow time to estimated leukocyte count is most accurate. With leukocyte counts in excess of 20,000, the mixture becomes increasingly more viscous. This results in discontinuous flow (by drops) of the latter half of the viscous mixture. To obtain a more accurate estimated count, repeat the test using 6, 9, 12, or 15 ml of reagent for one drop of blood, depending on degree of viscosity noted in the preliminary test. Divide the flow time by whatever multiple of 3 ml was used, estimate the leukocyte count employing the quotient, and multiply the result by the number of multiples of 3 ml employed. *Example:* 6 ml of reagent and one drop of dog blood gave a flow time of 14 seconds. Thus 14 ÷ 2 = 7 seconds = 18,000 leukocyte count (from Table 2–9) × 2 = 36,000 actual estimated count.

The DNA viscosity test is a rapid screening procedure for estimating the level of leukocytes in blood and is intended for use in veterinary practice where laboratory facilities are limited. Blood samples may be gathered and stored in the refrigerator until it is convenient to conduct the tests. A single medicine dropper may be used on a series of blood samples but must be rinsed with 0.85% saline solution between tests on different blood samples. The funnel and test tube are rinsed in running water and may be used immediately without drying for the next test. Speed and low cost are significant advantages of the method. Necessary materials are available from the manufacturer of CMT concentrate reagent (Dairy Research Products).

ERYTHROCYTE OSMOTIC FRAGILITY TEST

The erythrocyte cell membrane is flexible but essentially nonelastic. This means that the cell ruptures if water is taken into the cell beyond its critical volume. The resistance of the erythrocyte to hemolysis is measured by subjecting it to decreasing concentrations of NaCl solution. Minimum resistance is that concentration at which slight hemolysis is detectable, and maximum resistance is that concentration at which hemolysis of all cells has taken place.

Marked species variations exist in erythrocyte susceptibility to hemolysis in hypotonic saline (see p. 553). The susceptibility is related in part to red cell size, since increasing fragility correlates with decreasing red cell volume. Thus the canine erythrocyte in health, which measures about 70 fl, is the most resistant, and the goat erythrocyte, which measures only about 20 fl, is the most susceptible. Smaller size limits the capacity of the cell to expand without rupture.

Several extrinsic (pH, temperature, oxygenation) and intrinsic (age of animal, species, breed, lipemia, age of erythrocyte) factors influence the osmotic fragility (OF), and values obtained vary among laboratories. Each investigator should establish normal values in his own laboratory for comparative purposes. Resistance of the erythrocyte to hemolysis may be increased or decreased in disease. Reticulocytes and leptocytes have increased resistance, while spherocytes have decreased resistance. For further interpretation see Chapter 20.

Parpart et al. (1947) have shown that pH of the NaCl solution has a significant effect on the result of the OF test. They recommend preparation of a 10% buffered NaCl solution as follows: 180 g NaCl, 27.31 g Na_2HPO_4, and 3.74 g NaH_2PO_4 made up to 2 L with distilled water. This stock solution is stable for months. For each erythrocyte OF test, dilute 5 ml of the stock solution with distilled water to make 50 ml. This is a 1.0% salt solution. Place two series each of 16 test tubes of 7- to 10-ml capacity in a rack, and number each series sequentially from 1 to 16. In one series of tubes prepare the concentrations of NaCl solution shown in Table 2–10.

With the hemoglobin pipette, add 0.02 ml (20 μl) of blood to each tube. Mix by inversion and let stand at room temperature for 30 minutes. Centrifuge all tubes at 2,000 rpm for 10 minutes. Transfer 3.5 ml of supernatant to each of the empty tubes of the second series. Read the optical density of fluid from each tube of the second series using a spectrophotometer at 540 nm; use distilled water as a blank. The hemolysis in tube 16 is regarded as being 100%. Convert the optical density to percent hemolysis as follows:

$$\frac{\text{Optical density of unknown}}{\text{Optical density of tube 16}} \times 100 = 100\% \text{ hemolysis}$$

The results are graphed as shown in Figure 20–10. A *sigmoid curve* is obtained for normal blood when the percent hemolysis is plotted against the concentration of NaCl. It is a cumulative curve of percent hemolysis within a range of hypotonic saline. The mean corpuscular fragility (MCF) can be calculated by probit analysis to express the concentration of NaCl in which 50% hemolysis occurs (Parpart et al., 1947). A *derivative curve* (Fig. 8–14) can be plotted from percent hemolysis values obtained using the principle of "hemolytic increment" (Suess et al., 1948). In this case, the additional amount of hemolysis that occurs in each successive tube of solution of decreasing saline concentration is plotted against the NaCl concentration. These hemolytic increments yield a curve somewhat similar in configuration to the Price-Jones curve of red cell diameter. Such a curve makes apparent the different populations of red cells present in a

Table 2–10. Various Concentrations of NaCl Solution Utilized to Perform an Osmotic Fragility Test

Tube Number	ml of 1.0% NaCl	ml of Distilled Water	% NaCl Solution
1	4.25	0.75	0.85
2	4.00	1.00	0.80
3	3.75	1.25	0.75
4	3.50	1.50	0.70
5	3.25	1.75	0.65
6	3.00	2.00	0.60
7	2.75	2.25	0.55
8	2.50	2.50	0.50
9	2.25	2.75	0.45
10	2.00	3.00	0.40
11	1.75	3.25	0.35
12	1.50	3.50	0.30
13	1.25	3.75	0.25
14	1.00	4.00	0.20
15	0.50	4.50	0.10
16	0.00	5.00	0.00

particular sample. Thus an ordinary bimodal curve, due to two distinct populations of red cells, could be clearly resolved in two components (Figs. 20–10, 20–13; Jain, 1973). It was from these types of curves that two populations of red cells were distinctly demonstrated in the blood of young individuals of several animal species (Perk et al., 1964).

A special instrument—a fragiligraph—was invented to record the OF automatically (Danon et al., 1963).

Determination of the degree of hemolysis occurring after exposure of red cells to a standard degree of trauma in vitro is known as the *mechanical fragility test* (Shen et al., 1944). It is believed to be an index of the susceptibility of cells to destruction by wear and tear in the circulation.

CROSS-MATCHING BLOOD FOR TRANSFUSION

Experience in the practice of veterinary medicine has shown that, perhaps with exception of the horse (Gilman et al., 1960) and the cat (Auer et al., 1982), there is little danger from an initial transfusion of blood to domestic animals. However, severe and even fatal reactions may develop upon administration of a second transfusion at a later date or in cases of isosensitization resulting from transplacental immunization. For details concerning factors to be considered in giving blood transfusions to domestic animals, see Chapter 35.

Cross-Matching Donor and Recipient Bloods for Compatibility

Simple procedures involving a combination of tests for agglutination and hemolysis (lysis) are available and are within the scope of the veterinary practitioner. In cattle and sheep, the lytic test is required because erythrocytes of these species show little or no natural ability to agglutinate. In the dog and cat, the agglutination technique is applicable, but in the horse both lytic and agglutination testing methods are required, since most equine isoantibodies act as hemolysins.

The method for cross-matching to test for incompatibility by erythrocyte agglutination is outlined below:

1. Collect 2 ml of EDTA-anticoagulated blood from donor and recipient.
2. Centrifuge blood samples for 1 minute in Serofuge (Clay Adams; fixed speed of 1,000 G) or other appropriate centrifuge, and remove plasma to prelabeled 75 × 10 mm test tubes.
3. Make a 2% red cell suspension of each specimen in physiologic saline (0.85% NaCl) solution. This can be done by placing 0.02 ml of concentrated red cells in 0.98 ml of saline solution contained in a 75 × 10 mm test tube; mixing, centrifuging, and washing three times; and resuspending washed red cells in an equal volume of saline solution.
4. Place two drops of the recipient's plasma and two drops of the donor's cell suspension in a 10 × 75 mm test tube and mix (major system). In a second tube similarly place equal volumes of donor's plasma and recipient's cell suspension (minor system). To check for autoagglutination, set up controls in the same manner by mixing donor's red cells with its own plasma, and follow the same procedure with the recipient's red cells and plasma.
5. Shake rack of tubes and incubate for 30 minutes at room temperature; then centrifuge for 1 minute at 1,000 rpm.
6. Examine the supernatant for hemolysis. Shake the tubes gently by tapping with the finger to detect grossly visible agglutination of red cells.
7. If no agglutination is observed, transfer a small amount to a glass slide and examine under the low power of the microscope. A slight hemolysis in canine blood is nonspecific. Significant hemolysis and/or agglutination in one or both of the cross-matched tubes but not in the controls indicates an incompatibility and the need to choose a new donor.

Cross-Matching for Blood Transfusion in the Horse

Equine blood-typing reagents utilizing both isoimmune and rabbit antisera as sources of blood-typing antibodies have been developed (Stormont et al., 1964). A few of the blood-typing reagents act strictly as agglutinins. The majority, however, act primarily as hemolysins. Thus in cross-matching horse blood for the presence of isoantibodies, the lytic test is necessary. A similar procedure is used for cross-matching ruminant blood.

In the lytic test, fresh rabbit serum is used as complement. However, because all rabbits possess natural heterolysins and heteroagglutinins for horse red cells, it is necessary to remove those antibodies from the rabbit serum before using it as complement. To accomplish this, absorb the rabbit serum twice with horse red cells using a ratio of one part of washed, packed red cells to two parts of fresh rabbit serum per absorption. Wash the red cells three times in saline (0.90% NaCl) solution. Chill tubes of washed, packed red cells in an ice bath along with the rabbit serum. When the rabbit serum is thoroughly chilled, mix it with the red cells in one of the two tubes and allow to stand in the ice bath for 10 minutes; then centrifuge the tube (preferably in a refrigerated centrifuge). Transfer the supernatant serum to the second tube, mix with the red cells, and allow to stand for another 10 minutes. After centrifugation, dispense the supernatant serum, now called absorbed rabbit complement, in small volumes (e.g., 2 ml) into vials and keep frozen until needed.

For purposes of cross-matching, collect EDTA-anticoagulated blood from the recipient and several prospective donors. Centrifuge blood to remove plasma and transfer the plasma to properly labeled tubes. Then prepare 2% suspensions of washed red cells from each blood. This can be done by pouring some saline into each tube of blood, shaking the tubes, and then pouring some of the suspended red cells into freshly labeled tubes. Clotted blood can also be used as a source of serum and red cells for cross-matching. Wash the red cells twice, and adjust the button of red cells from the final washing to approximately 2% suspension.

The *agglutination* cross-matching tests are performed as follows: Add two drops of washed red cells to a series of 10 × 75 mm test tubes containing two drops of serum (or plasma) in such a manner that the red cells of each horse are tested against the serum of all other horses, including the homologous

serum, which serves as a negative control. Shake the tubes and allow them to stand at room temperature for 20 minutes, and then centrifuge them at about 1,000 rpm for 1 minute. Gently tap the tubes to resuspend the red cells and check for the presence or absence of agglutination. A donor's blood is declared incompatible when agglutinated by the serum of the recipient (the major cross-match). A recipient's blood is declared incompatible when agglutinated by the serum of a donor (the minor cross-match).

The *lytic* cross-matching tests are performed as follows: Prepare 1:4 and 1:16 dilutions in saline solution of each sample of serum. Heat the dilutions for about 15 minutes at 56°C to inactivate the complement. Add one drop of the washed 2% suspension of red cells to each of a series of tubes containing two drops of the appropriately diluted, heat-inactivated serum in such a manner that the red cells of each horse are tested with the 1:4 and 1:16 serum dilutions of all horses. Provide appropriate negative controls by adding one drop of the red cell suspension to two drops of saline solution. Shake the tubes. Then add one drop of the absorbed rabbit complement, thawed and properly mixed, to all tubes. Shake the tubes again and allow to stand for 30 minutes before recording hemolysis and/or agglutination. To facilitate reading these tests, it may be necessary to centrifuge the tubes to accommodate the less experienced eye. Hemolysis is evidenced by a red supernatant. Then flick each tube to resuspend any remaining red cells and record agglutination.

Incompatibility is indicated whenever the red cells of the recipient and those of a prospective donor are hemolysed and/or agglutinated in the presence of the other's serum.

It should be noted that the absorbed rabbit complement can be used to detect red cells sensitized with autoantibodies or with isoantibodies as in autoimmune hemolytic anemia or neonatal isoerythrolysis, respectively. To two drops of a 2% suspension of the washed red cells, add two drops of the absorbed rabbit complement. If the red cells are sensitized, they will lyse within 30 minutes (Stormont, 1975).

DETECTION OF ANTIBODIES TO ERYTHROCYTES

Coombs Tests

The detection of IgG antibodies active against erythrocytes, as in autoimmune hemolytic anemia (AIHA) and immune-mediated hemolytic anemia of the newborn, requires the use of a species-specific antiglobulin (Coombs et al., 1945). The test is designated the Coombs antiglobulin test or simply the Coombs test. The *direct Coombs test* is performed to demonstrate antierythrocyte antibodies directly on the surface of the patient's red cells, whereas the *indirect Coombs test* is performed to demonstrate the antibody in the patient's serum or in eluates prepared from the patient's red cells. Use of anticomplement in the direct Coombs test, to detect complement (particularly C3) on the surface of erythrocytes, significantly improves the diagnosis. These reagents can be obtained commercially. Animal Coombs reagents specifically for the dog, cat, and horse are available from Miles Laboratories.

The test is conducted as follows: A blood sample containing EDTA anticoagulant (or clotted blood) is used to prepare a 2% suspension of erythrocytes. Add about 0.5 ml of blood to 2 ml of 0.85% NaCl solution and centrifuge for 5 minutes. Discard the supernatant, resuspend the red cell button in 2 ml of saline, and recentrifuge for 1 minute. Repeat this washing process three times. When freshly clotted blood is used, hold two round applicator sticks close together and insert into the clot to break it up. Enough concentrated erythrocytes adhere to the sticks on withdrawal to serve in the test when transferred to 5 ml of saline solution.

For the *direct Coombs test,* add two drops of a 2% suspension of the patient's washed erythrocytes to a 75 × 10 mm test tube containing two drops of Coombs reagent. Mix the contents and incubate at 37°C. Use separate tubes for different Coombs reagents such as anti-IgG, anti-C, etc. Another tube containing an identical suspension of red cells in saline serves as the negative control. A duplicate set of tubes may be incubated at 10°C and another set at room temperature, if desired. After 30 minutes, centrifuge the suspension at 1,000 rpm for 1 minute. Then flick the tube with the finger to cause the erythrocytes to swirl upward, and at the same time observe the cells for agglutination. A magnifying glass may be used to observe fine red cell agglutination in the tube, or place a drop of the suspension on a slide and examine under the microscope at low power. The degree of agglutination is recorded from 1+ to 4+. Any agglutination is regarded as a positive test. Agglutination may sometimes be more prominent at 10°C, thereby indicating the presence of cold-reacting antibody. Red cells from a normal animal of the same species should be tested in parallel as a control.

For the *indirect Coombs test,* add two drops of a 2% suspension of normal washed erythrocytes to the patient's serum and incubate at 37°C for 30 minutes. Red cells for this purpose should be obtained from an animal that is potentially compatible with the patient, e.g., a dog that is blood group A negative. Heat patient's serum at 56°C for 30 minutes before use. Wash the red cells three times with physiologic saline, prepare a 2% cell suspension, and incubate two drops of red cells with four drops of patient's serum at 37°C for 30 minutes. This procedure sensitizes normal cells with antierythrocyte antibody in patient's serum. Rewash these red cells three times and use to perform the direct Coombs test as described above.

The Coombs test must be performed on blood anticoagulated with EDTA because EDTA is anticomplementary and prevents in vitro binding of C to erythrocytes. Clotted blood kept in the refrigerator will have red cells coated with C3, and such cells will give a false positive reaction with anti-C reagent. Enzyme-treated red cells are more susceptible to C-lysis and yield a higher degree of positivity in the indirect Coombs test (Jones and Darke, 1975). Titers or scores of a Coombs test may be helpful in following progress of an individual patient. In humans, remission is frequently associated with a decrease in antibody titer. With cold antibody, thermal reactivity of the antibody is more important than the titer (Petz, 1980). False positive or false negative reactions may sometimes be observed in the antiglobulin test (Chaplin, 1974). False positive reactions may be due to:

(a) The presence of cross-reactive antibodies in the Coombs reagent

(b) Nonimmune clumping of the patient's red cells secondary to particulate matter in the antiglobulin reagent

(c) Bacterial contamination of the patient's serum or the antiglobulin reagent

False negative reactions may be due to:

(a) A weak coating of erythrocytes by the antibody below the level of sensitivity of the method. Using a very sensitive technique, Gilliland et al. (1970) found that at least 500 or more molecules of IgG antibody per red cell are required to obtain a positive direct Coombs test in humans. Similarly, working with guinea pig erythrocytes, Schreiber and Frank (1972a, b) reported that 12,000 molecules of IgG and 50 molecules of IgM were necessary to obtain a positive direct Coombs test.

(b) Dissociation of antibody from the red cell surface under certain situations. The cold reacting IgM antibody elutes off the red cell surface at temperatures above 30°C, and the IgG antibody, but not the C components, can be eluted from the erythrocyte surface by heat, mild acid, or certain organic solvents (Leddy and Swisher, 1971).

(c) Failure to wash red cells properly.

(d) Unreliable reagents.

(e) A prozone phenomenon in a strong Coombs reagent. In such instances, the test is performed using serial twofold dilutions of the reagent and positive results are obtained at some higher dilution.

Interpretation

Three patterns of positive Coombs reactions are obtained when the test is performed with specific antiserums such as anti-IgG and anti-C. These patterns indicate that erythrocytes may be coated with either IgG alone, C alone, or both IgG and C. Most cases of AIHA in humans have both IgG and C, but as many as 25% of the cases may have either IgG or C alone. Hence, use of a polyspecific antiserum containing both anti-IgG and anti-C is recommended. Since IgM is capable of activating

Table 2–11. **Patterns of Results of Direct Coombs Tests for 32 Canine Patients with Autoimmune Hemolytic Anemia**

Anti-IgG and Anti-C3 Reagents*	Anti-IgG Reagent	Anti-C3 Reagent	Number of Cases	Percent of Total
+	+	+	16	50.0
+	+	−	10	31.2
+	−	+	6	18.8
100%	81.2%	68.8%		

From Switzer and Jain, 1981.
*All reagents from Miles Laboratories. Direct Coombs tests were performed at 37°C.

C, its role in AIHA can easily be assessed by using anti-C to detect C3 components on red cells. The identical situation prevails for animals, but it must be remembered that species-specific antiglobulin and anti-C3 reagents are needed. In a study involving 32 canine patients (Switzer and Jain, 1981), direct Coombs testing was done, simultaneously, using a polyspecific antiserum containing both anti-IgG and anti-C3 and monospecific anti-IgG and anti-C3 reagents (Table 2–11). It was interesting to note that (1) IgG was present on red cells of 81.2% of the dogs, (2) C was detected on red cells of 68.8%, (3) IgG alone was detected in 31.2%, and (4) C alone was detected in 18.8%.

Interpretation of the Coombs test results requires an understanding of the mechanisms of antibody and complement associations with the red cells, circumstances leading to and the types of immune responses, and therapeutic consequences (Jain, 1975; Petz, 1980). In cases of drug-induced AIHA, the offending drug must be incorporated in the test system, otherwise the test may yield negative results, whereas some normal individuals with no signs of anemia may give a weakly positive reaction. A positive direct Coombs test is also obtained in patients with hemolytic transfusion reaction and in neonatal isoerythrolysis. A patient's pattern of antiglobulin reaction may change during the course of disease and may become negative after prolonged therapy with corticosteroids or immunosuppressive drugs. In other cases, the direct Coombs test may remain positive even after complete remission from anemia. The direct Coombs test is sometimes positive during the clinical course, whereas the indirect Coombs test may or may not be positive. Both tests, however, are almost always positive at the onset of acute hemolysis. See Chapter 35 for additional information on the Coombs test and AIHA.

Agglutination of Papain-Treated Erythrocytes

Erythrocyte autoantibodies undetectable by the Coombs test can be demonstrated by more sensitive enzyme techniques (Lincoln and Dodd, 1978; Pirofsky, 1969) that modify the surface properties of erythrocytes so that the cells become highly reactive to anti–red cell antibodies and exhibit agglutination without the necessity of a Coombs reagent. It is presumed that the enzyme treatment alters the configuration of the red cell surface membrane by partially cleaving membrane proteins and glycoproteins, thereby reducing the surface charge and exposing cryptic antigens. Low ionic strength solution (LISS) may be used to wash and suspend red cells for use in enzyme techniques or the regular Coombs test. It reduces the electrostatic barrier (zeta potential) surrounding the red cells and enhances agglutination (Lincoln and Dodd, 1978; Moore and Mollison, 1976; Wicker and Wallas, 1976).

Papain-treated red cells have been used to detect canine erythrocyte autoantibodies (Feldman, 1982; Jones and Darke, 1975). The procedure has yielded evidence of the presence of autoantibodies in anemic dogs suspected of having immune-mediated hemolytic anemia on the basis of clinical and hematologic findings, but giving negative Coombs tests (Feldman, 1982). A procedure, as used in our laboratories, is given below.

Prepare 0.1 M phosphate buffers, pH 5.4 and 7.3. To prepare activated stock papain solution dissolve 1 g papain (Sigma P-3375) in 99.0 ml of a solution containing 10.0 ml phosphate buffer of pH 5.4 and 99.0 ml chilled 0.9% NaCl solution. Add 1.0 ml of 5.0% potassium EDTA, mix well, and store the solution overnight (12 hours) at 4°C. Then filter through Whatman No. 1 paper at 4°C and store in 1.0-ml aliquots at -40°C. A dilute working solution of papain is prepared by diluting 1.0 ml aliquot of the stock solution with 9.0 ml of the pH 7.3 phosphate buffer. Stock

solution is good for several months, but diluted solution should be used immediately.

Obtain patient's venous blood in anticoagulant (preferably using citrate, although EDTA or heparin may be used) and a small tube of serum. Wash red cells twice with 0.9% NaCl solution and discard the supernatant. Mix 2.0 ml of diluted, buffered papain solution with 0.5 ml of washed packed red cells. Incubate the mixture in a 37°C water bath for exactly 10 minutes. The timing is critical because longer incubation can induce nonspecific reaction and hemolysis. Wash the incubated red cells three times with 0.9% NaCl solution, and prepare a 5.0% suspension of red cells in the saline solution. Add 0.2 ml of red cell suspension to 0.2 ml of patient's serum in a small test tube, mix, and incubate in a 37°C water bath for exactly 1 hour. Immediately examine the tube for agglutination, macroscopically and, if necessary, microscopically at 37°C. Nonspecific agglutination can occur if the cells are allowed to remain at room temperature. Strengths of the agglutination reaction are recorded from trace to $4+$, with trace and $1+$ being negative and $2+$, $3+$ and $4+$ (complete) agglutination being positive.

The test should be performed in duplicate. A negative control (enzyme-treated A-negative red cells reacted with A-negative serum) should always be run simultaneously, and a positive control (enzyme-treated A-positive red cells reacted with A-positive serum) may be run if desired. LISS may be used for washing and resuspending red cells to enhance antigen-antibody interaction.

DETECTION OF ANTIPLATELET ANTIBODIES

Autoimmune thrombocytopenia (AITP) occurs in the dog and less frequently in the cat and the horse. Laboratory diagnosis is based on demonstration of antiplatelet antibody in serum, on platelets, or on megakaryocytes.

Platelet Factor 3 (PF-3) Test

The PF-3 test is used to detect antiplatelet antibody in serum (Jain and Kono, 1980; Joshi and Jain, 1976; Karpatkin et al., 1977). The test is based on the following principles: *(a)* the antiplatelet antibody causes immunologic injury to platelets and releases membrane-associated platelet phospholipid (PF-3) at an accelerated rate, and *(b)* the coagulation process is enhanced in the presence of PF-3. Thus an interaction of antiplatelet antibody with normal homologous platelets suspended in plasma promotes release of PF-3 which, in the presence of contact product (activated coagulation factors XII and XI) and calcium ions, causes accelerated coagulation of normal plasma as compared to a simultaneously run control test. When a particular drug is suspected as the cause of AITP, the PF-3 test must also be conducted in the presence of the drug; the test may otherwise be negative. See Chapter 35 for interpretation and clinical usefulness of the PF-3 test.

The PF-3 test, originally developed for use on human serums (Karpatkin and Siskind, 1969) was adapted for use on canine serums (Joshi and Jain, 1976; Wilkins et al., 1973). The procedure to detect canine antiplatelet antibody was further modified to read test results using a fibrometer rather than visually (Jain and Kono, 1980). The latter procedure is given below. A similar technique could be followed for use on other species serums.

Serum should be harvested within 2 hours of blood collection, heated at 56°C for 30 minutes, and tested immediately or stored frozen in aliquots of 2 ml at −30°C. Serums to be dispatched to a distant laboratory should be heated as above and sent frozen. Lipemic and hemolyzed serum samples give inconsistent test results. Plasma is unsuitable.

Platelet rich plasma (PRP), platelet poor plasma (PPP) and contact product (CP) are prepared from blood obtained from a clinically normal dog. Sodium citrate (3.8%, one part to nine parts blood) is used as the anticoagulant. The dog is fasted overnight to insure having a nonlipemic blood sample.

Fifty ml of anticoagulated blood is centrifuged immediately after collection at 650 G for 5 minutes at room temperature. The PRP is harvested carefully and either used immediately or stored in 2-ml aliquots in polypropylene or polystyrene tubes at −70°C after addition of dimethyl sulfoxide (DMSO) at a final concentration of 5%. Platelet counts are performed on each batch of PRP after addition

of DMSO and adjusted, if necessary, with PPP to 100,000 to 150,000 μl before storage.

PPP is obtained by centrifuging anticoagulated blood or PRP (prepared as above) at 1,000 G for 10 minutes and stored frozen in small aliquots at −30°C.

Contact product is prepared from PPP as described by Karpatkin and Siskind (1969) and stored in aliquots of 0.1 ml at −30°C. Briefly, 35 ml of anticoagulated blood is obtained to harvest PPP. The PPP is transferred into a 50-ml test tube and celite (20 mg/ml) is added and mixed. The suspension is kept at 37°C for 10 minutes while being mixed repeatedly. This is followed by centrifugation, harvesting the celite and washing it five times with distilled water, and then resuspending the celite in 10% NaCl solution equal to the original plasma volume. This suspension is then kept at 37°C for 10 minutes with repeated mixing to elute the CP off the celite. The preparation is then centrifuged and the supernatant fluid saved and dialyzed for 2–12 hours against physiologic saline at 4°C. Thereafter, 0.1-ml aliquots are stored at −30°C.

A fibrometer (BBL Fibrosystem, Becton Dickinson) equipped with an automatic syringe, heating block, and plastic cups with a cup holder, is used to perform the test. Both test section and heating block of the fibrometer are preheated (37°C) for 10 minutes before use. Remove one tube each of PRP, normal serum, and CP from storage and bring to room temperature by first placing them in the heating block for 5 minutes and then keeping at room temperature. Dilute the CP by adding 1.9 ml of physiologic saline. Place a tube of 0.025 M CaCl$_2$ in the heating block.

The PF-3 test is conducted as follows: To a test cup held at room temperature add 0.1 ml of PRP, 0.1 ml of test serum (normal or patient's serum), and 0.05 ml of CP. Place the cup in the test section of the fibrometer to warm up. After 5 minutes, add 0.1 ml of CaCl$_2$ with the automatic pipette to activate the fibrometer. Record the time taken for clot formation when the fibrometer count has stopped. Then reset the counter, clean probes, and remove the cup to place the next testing cup in position. Repeat this procedure on three aliquots of each test serum to obtain average coagulation time and to determine standared deviation (SD) of coagulation time for normal serum for interpretative purposes. When testing the patient's serum, always test a control normal serum simultaneously. The patient's serum is considered to be positive, i.e., to have antiplatelet antibody, if its coagulation time is shortened by more than double the SD of normal serum coagulation time. For example, in a test giving an average coagulation time of 50 seconds for patient's serum and average coagulation time of 70 seconds for normal serum with a 2 SD of 12 seconds, the patient serum would be considered positive since its coagulation time is shortened $(70 - 50 = 20$ seconds) by more than the 2 SD of normal serum coagulation time.

Direct Immunofluorescence of Megakaryocytes

The direct immunofluorescence technique can be used to demonstrate antiplatelet antibody associated with megakaryocytes (Joshi and Jain, 1976). The technique as applied to canine bone marrow smears is as follows:

Prepare bone marrow smears on coverslips and process immediately. Fix smears with 95% ethyl alcohol for 10 minutes, wash with distilled water for 5 minutes, and air-dry. Fixed smears can be stored at 4°C up to 1 month for processing later. Place rabbit anti-canine globulin conjugated with fluorescein isothiocyanate and diluted 1:20 with 0.01 M phosphate-buffered saline solution (PBSS; pH 7.2) on different smears, and place the smears in a moist Petri dish at room temperature. After 1 hour, wash the coverslips with PBSS for 20 minutes and with deionized water for a minimum of 45 minutes while stirring washing fluids constantly. Then rinse the smears with fresh deionized water, air-dry and mount on glass slides, using a drop of 10% buffered glycerin. Examine the preparations under a fluorescent microscope equipped with HBO 200 mercury vapor lamp, exciter filter BG-12, 340–480 nm, and barrier filter 50/44, 500–440 nm.

Apple green fluorescence of the megakaryocytes indicates a positive reaction. This technique is more sensitive than the PF-3 test for detection of antiplatelet antibody. However, its use in clinical practice is limited by the risk of performing marrow aspiration on a severely thrombocytopenic patient and because of the possibility that the marrow may be devoid of megakaryocytes.

An immunofluorescence microspectrophotometric method has been developed to detect antiplatelet antibody in serum and on the surfaces of platelets of humans with AITP (Van Boxtel et al., 1975). An enzyme-linked immunosorbent assay has been described for the detection of antiplatelet antibodies in dogs (Campbell et al., 1984).

DETECTION OF ANTINUCLEAR ANTIBODIES

Antinuclear antibodies (ANAs) are found in a variety of connective tissue disorders, particularly systemic lupus erythematosus (SLE). They may be seen as part of other immune-mediated disorders such as rheumatoid arthritis, AIHA, and drug-induced reactions, and in old age. ANAs are heterogenous with specificity for DNA, nucleoprotein, histones, and other nuclear components. Antibodies to double-stranded DNA are generally confined to SLE, while those to single-stranded DNA are found in many diseases (Talal, 1976). The most characteristic antinuclear antibody, antinucleoprotein, is responsible for the lupus erythematosus (LE) cell phenomenon (see below). ANAs are usually of IgG type, frequently of IgM type, and sometimes of IgA type. The presence of ANAs in a serum sample can be detected by various procedures, but the most sensitive and widely used is indirect immunofluorescence. LE cell test also is a measure of ANAs. These techniques are briefly outlined below along with some comments on their significance. The finding of ANAs and a positive LE cell test are not necessarily diagnostic of SLE. They form a component of an array of tests of major diagnostic significance for SLE and may be positive in some other diseases. In general, almost all human patients with a positive LE cell test give a positive ANA, but not the reverse. Such a relationship may or may not be seen in animals. See Chapter 35 for further discussion on interpretation of these tests.

Indirect Immunofluorescence Test

The test essentially consists of two steps. The first involves application of patient's serum to a substrate slide, which consists of either monolayers of certain tissue culture cell lines, e.g., HEp-2 (human epithelioid); frozen sections of mouse tissue, e.g., the liver and kidney; or blood leukocytes from buffy coat. During this step, ANAs in serum bind with the cell nuclei. Rinsing in buffered, physiologic saline removes the unbound serum globulins. The second step involves exposing the slides to a fluorescein-conjugated, species-specific anti-IgG. The latter binds to the substrate-antibody complexes formed in step one and makes them glow under the fluorescent microscope. Application of a nonspecific counterstain (Evans blue) enhances the contrast between nuclei (greenish yellow when positive) and cytoplasm (dark red). Patient's serum can be serially diluted (starting from 1:5 dilution) to determine the titer of ANAs therein, e.g., the highest dilution giving a positive fluorescence. A positive and a negative control serum of the species being tested should be run simultaneously. HEp-2 slides can be obtained commercially for use with species-specific, fluorescein-labeled antibody. ANAs are not species-specific, and so the species of origin of antigen (i.e., substrate slides) is not important. Instructions supplied by the manufacturer are followed, with some modifications if necessary, to perform the test.

Several patterns of immunofluorescence may be seen depending on the number or types of ANAs involved. These include: homogeneous—uniform staining of the entire nucleus; peripheral or shaggy—staining of the nuclear membrane; speckled—many distinct granules throughout the nucleus; and nucleolar. These different patterns have been related to various nuclear components (Friou, 1967). A homogenous pattern is indicative of the presence of antinucleoprotein, which is common in SLE. A peripheral or shaggy pattern is given by anti-DNA antibody, particularly reactive to double-stranded DNA, and is associated with active lupus nephritis. A speckled pattern is suggestive of antibody to phosphate-extractable antigen seen in SLE. A nucleolar pattern is given by nucleolar RNA.

Various patterns may change with the disease state. Higher titers are seen in patients with active lupus. Lower titers are associated with clinical improvement and remission, while rising titers may be a prodromal sign of developing crisis (Niejadlik, 1971). With canine serums, although a positive fluorescence may be detected in some cases at 1:5 dilution, a titer of 1:20 or above is of diagnostic significance. Highest titers obtained by us for canine samples were as follows: homogenous pattern, 1:1280; peripheral, 1:1280; speckled, 1:40; and nucleolar 1:40. See Chapter 35 for further discussion on ANA.

The Lupus Erythematosus (LE) Cell Test

The designation "LE cell" refers to a phenomenon first reported by Hargraves et al. (1948) as occurring in the bone marrow of persons suffering from lupus erythematosus.

Several laboratory techniques have been used to demonstrate LE cells in peripheral blood. A commonly used procedure is as follows: Ten ml of freshly drawn blood is permitted to clot and remain at room temperature for 2 hours. Press the serum and clot through a fine wire mesh screen into a Petri dish. With Pasteur pipette place 2–3 ml of strained mashed clot into a vial with glass beads. Continuously shake on a mechanical device for 15 minutes. Incubate at room temperature for 1 hour. Fill two Wintrobe hematocrit tubes with incubated mashed clot, and centrifuge at 2,000 G for 10 minutes. Discard the supernatant fluid, and prepare several films from the buffy coat and stain them by routine blood stains. Examine at least four films extensively for the typical LE cell.

The LE cell phenomenon results from the action of ANAs (Talal, 1976) upon nuclei of injured or nonviable leukocytes. Complement fixation is involved. The antibodies produce a depolymerization of the nuclear DNA of the cell nucleus (Klemperer et al., 1950). The nucleus swells, causing the cell to rupture and release an amorphous mass called an LE body. Viable neutrophils are attracted to the altered nuclear material to engulf it. Rarely, other leukocytes may also phagocytize such a material. The result is the appearance within the leukocyte cytoplasm of a round mass, about the size of a lymphocyte nucleus, that

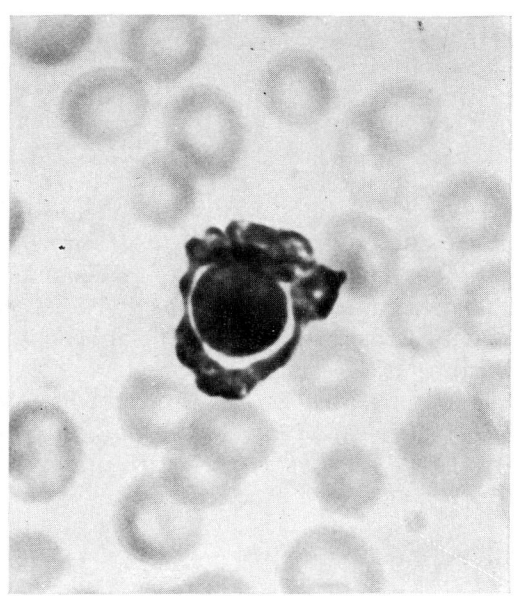

Fig. 2–30. LE cell in clotted blood preparation from a dog with myopathy. Wright-Leishman stain, ×4,000. (From Schalm and Ling, 1970; courtesy of *The California Veterinarian.*)

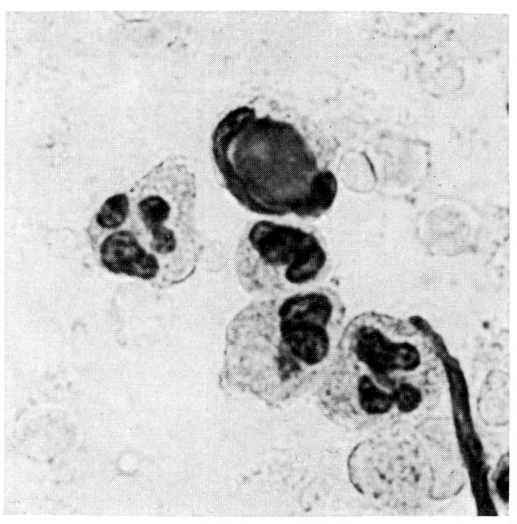

Fig. 2–32. A cluster of five neutrophils, one of which is an LE cell. New methylene blue stain, ×3,560. (From Schalm and Ling, 1970; courtesy of *The California Veterinarian.*)

takes the nuclear stain but lacks the normal chromatin pattern of a viable nucleus (Fig. 2–30). These cells are then recognized as LE cells. The engulfed mass is amorphous, which distinguishes it from simple nuclear phagocytosis (tart cell or pseudo-LE cell). Another feature that may occur is a rosette of neutro-

phils surrounding a mass of amorphous nuclear protein (Fig. 2–31 and Plate XIV–12). The rosette is not acceptable per se as evidence of a positive LE test. New methylene blue stain may be used to demonstrate LE cells (Fig. 2–32). A positive LE cell test is an abnormal finding. LE cells have been observed in specimens of blood from canine, feline, and equine patients and also in direct films of bone marrow of an occasional cat with myeloproliferative disorder (Schalm and Ling, 1970).

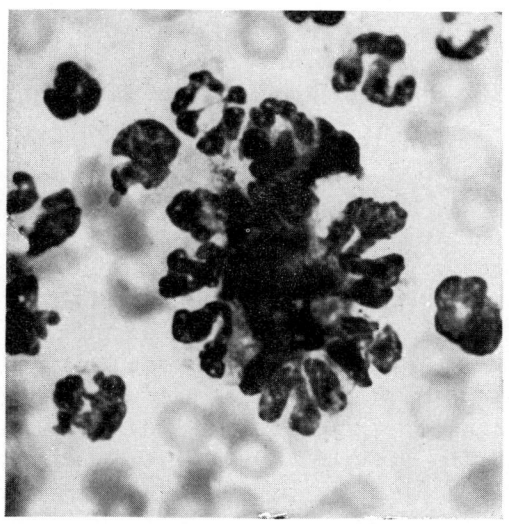

Fig. 2–31. Neutrophil leukocytes surrounding an amorphous nuclear mass to form the rarely encountered rosette. From a clotted-blood LE cell preparation. Wright-Leishman stain, ×2,350. (From Schalm and Ling, 1970; courtesy of *The California Veterinarian.*)

EXAMINATION OF CANINE BLOOD FOR MICROFILARIAE

Dirofilaria immitis, the heartworm of the dog, is an important cause of disease. The motile embryo, called microfilaria, circulates in the blood. *Dipetalonema reconditum* represents another form of filariasis in dogs in the United States. The microfilariae of *D. reconditum* and perhaps other *Dipetalonema* species also occur in the blood, but the adults are located in the subcutaneous tissues and fat. It is important to distinguish between *D. immitis* and species of *Dipetalonema* when microfilariae are detected on blood examination. Differentiation is based mainly on motility and morphologic characteristics (Jackson and Otto, 1974; Newton and Wright, 1957; Red-

Table 2–12. Characteristics of Microfilariae of *Dirofilaria immitis* and *Dipetalonema reconditum*

	D. immitis	D. reconditum
Number (per ml of blood)	Few to many (1–150,000)	Few (commonly <200)
Motility	Stationary	Progressive
Length (μm)	295–325 (mean, 308)	250–288 (mean, 263)
Width (μm)	5.0–7.5	4.5–5.5
Cephalic end	Tapered	Blunt
Caudal end	Mostly straight, rarely blunt, never button-hook	Usually curved or button-hook
Body	Usually straight	Usually curved
Annular striations	Present	Absent

Data from Jackson and Otto, 1974, and Redington et al., 1977.

ington et al., 1977). The characteristics of microfilariae of the two species are given in Table 2–12.

Several methods for detection of microfilariae in blood are available for routine use. Freshly drawn anticoagulated blood is used, particularly for observing motility. In fresh blood, the microfilariae of *D. immitis* undulate at one place in contrast to characteristic progressive movement of *D. reconditum*. Concentration techniques (see below) are used to obtain specimens for enumeration and morphologic studies; the modified Knott technique is commonly used (Jackson and Otto, 1974). The recommended method consists of adding 1.0 ml of fresh blood to 10.0 ml of 2% formalin solution, mixing a few minutes to lyse red cells, and centrifuging for 5 minutes at 1,000–1,500 rpm. The sediment is examined microscopically as a wet preparation after being mixed with an equal volume of 1:1,000 methylene blue. An alternative method for staining consists of adding a drop of new methylene blue (p. 59) to the sediment on a glass slide (Fig. 2–33). Vital (Rothstein and Brown, 1960) and cytochemical (Chalifoux and Hunt, 1971) staining for differentiation of microfilariae have been described. Permanent stained preparations of Knott sediment can be prepared using hematoxylin (Redington et al., 1977). More recently a very sensitive enzyme-linked immunosorbent assay (ELISA) and an indirect immunofluorescent antibody test have been developed for application to serum samples from dogs suspected of having heartworms (Wong, 1980). The former method has application particularly in detecting prepatent infection, the latter in patent and occult infections.

Direct Blood Film

Place a large drop of blood on a slide and cover with a coverslip. Scan the entire film under low magnification (100×). The larvae, when present, are viable and may be detected by their snake-like movement between the erythrocytes. *D. immitis* is characterized by a sluggish movement in a figure-eight pattern with little forward progress. *Dipetalonema* are considerably more active and commonly show a progressive movement.

Stained Blood Film

The routinely stained blood film may demonstrate the presence of microfilariae. Chances of finding a microfilaria in the film are nil when there are fewer than 1,000 microfilariae/ml of blood. Counts of 2,000 or more/ml commonly reveal one or more of the microfilariae when the entire coverslip blood film is scanned under low magnification (100×). The occurrence of microfilariae in the routinely stained blood film will generally be an indication that the parasite is *D. immitis*. *Dipetalonema* do not commonly occur in sufficient numbers in peripheral blood to make their presence known in the stained blood film.

Microcapillary Hematocrit Method

The Drummond microcapillary tube is ideal for this method (Schalm and Jain, 1966). The larger 75 × 1.0 mm tube may be used, but it is less satisfactory because its greater internal diameter gives greater depth to the plasma. After centrifugation as in the hematocrit procedure, affix the Drummond microcapillary tube to a microscope slide with cellophane tape or by other means. Lower the substage condenser of the microscope, and adjust the substage iris diaphragm so that the edges of the capillary tube appear dark while the center of the plasma column is light. By focusing up and down, examine the plasma while moving the mechanical stage to permit scanning of the entire length of the plasma column. The capillary hematocrit method for de-

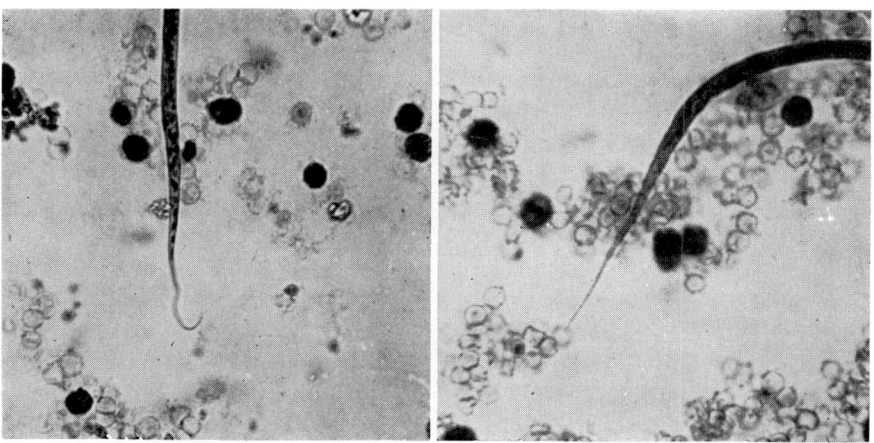

Fig. 2–33. Formalin-treated microfilariae stained with new methylene blue, showing buttonhook tail of *Dipetalonema* spp. *(left)* and straight tail of *Dirofilaria immitis (right)*. ×360.

tection of microfilariae is not satisfactory when there are fewer than 1,000 microfilariae/ml of blood. Immediately after centrifugation of the capillary hematocrit, the microfilariae are in or below the buffy coat, but with time, they emerge into the plasma (Fig. 2–34). It is best, therefore, to defer the examination until several hours after centrifugation has been completed. The larvae of *Dipetalonema* are actively mobile and tend to move throughout the plasma column. The microfilariae will remain viable in the plasma of the capillary hematocrit tube for several days.

Whole Blood Concentration Method

Because of the low frequency of microfilariae in blood, a concentration test is generally performed to detect microfilariae. Three commonly used methods are: the modified Knott test (described above), the polycarbonate or Nucleopore filter (Wallabs Inc.) method (Difil test), and the cellulose or Millipore filter (Millipore Corp.) method; the last two being available commercially (Jackson, 1977). Although the Millipore technique detected microfilariae in 112 out of 254 adult dogs compared to 109

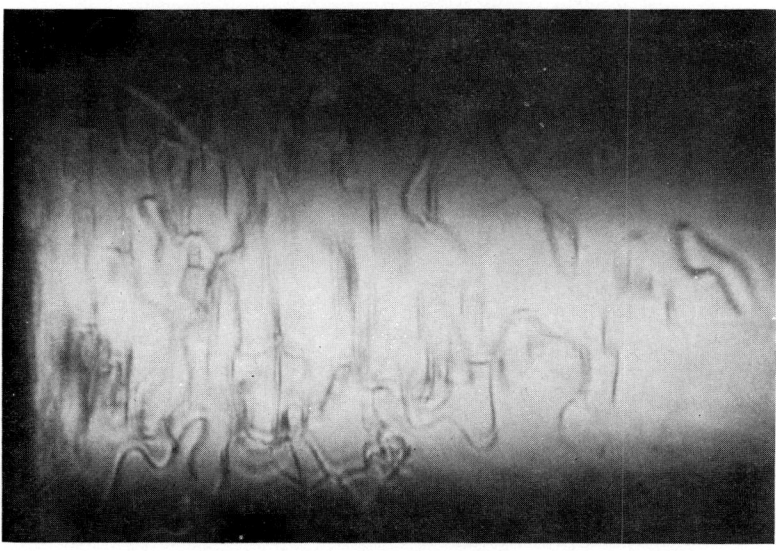

Fig. 2–34. Viable larvae of *Dirofilaria immitis* in the plasma immediately above the buffy coat in the capillary hematocrit tube. ×40.

positive samples each by the other two methods, the Knott test was considered the best because it yielded specimens suitable for morphologic differentiation of the microfilariae of *Dirofilaria immitis* and *Dipetalonema reconditum* (Jackson, 1977).

Serum Methods

Leave 3–5 ml of blood to clot at room temperature. After 3–4 hours, place a drop of serum under a coverslip and examine for viable larvae. Viable microfilariae have been observed for up to 15 days in serum of clotted blood held in the refrigerator (Stubbs and Live, 1935).

A serum-concentration method (Live and Stubbs, 1938), performed as follows, provides opportunity to detect many more microfilariae. Add serum from 3–5 ml of blood to 5 ml of 2–5% acetic acid and centrifuge at 1,500 rpm for 5 minutes. Carefully discard the supernatant, and resuspend the sediment in the few drops remaining in the test tube. Transfer the contents to a glass slide and examine under low power magnification.

Periodicity in Peripheral Blood

The number of circulating larvae of *Dirofilaria immitis* varies with time of day (Tongson and Romero, 1962). Peak counts occur generally between 11 P.M. and 1 A.M., while lowest counts are found between 6 A.M. and noon. The lowest counts are only 2–22% of the highest numbers of circulating larvae. A seasonal periodicity is also evident (Kume, 1974). It is directly related to the ambient temperature, maximum microfilariae being found in the summer and the lowest number during the winter.

Repeated blood examination for microfilariae may be negative in some dogs with adult worms in the heart as demonstrated at necropsy (occult dirofilariasis). Thus a negative finding does not necessarily mean that the patient is free of the parasite. Microfilariae are produced by gravid female adults, but are held back in the lungs from circulation by the presence of antibodies to microfilariae. Serologic tests must be performed to detect prepatent and occult infestations.

REFERENCES

Allen, B.V.: Method for the Automation of Equine Differential Leucocyte Counts. Equine Vet. J., *13*:115, 1981.

Anderson, A.C., and Gee, W.: Normal Values in the Beagle. Vet. Med., *53*:135, 1958.

Archer, R.K.: Bone Marrow Biopsy in the Horse: A Study of the Normal Marrow Cytology in Crossbred Ponies. Vet. Rec., *66*:261, 1954.

Auer, L., et al.: Blood Transfusion Reaction in the Cat. J. Amer. Vet. Med. Ass., *180*:729, 1982.

Baker, G.A., and Gorham, J.R.: A Technique for Bleeding Ferrets and Mink. Cornell Vet., *41*:235, 1951.

Barnett, C.W.: The Unavoidable Error in the Differential Count of the Leukocytes of the Blood. J. Clin. Invest., *12*:77, 1933.

Barry, K.G., et al.: A Practical Temperature-Compensated Hand Refractometer (the TS-meter): Its Clinical Use and Applications in Estimation of Total Serum Proteins. J. Lab. Clin. Med., *55*:803, 1960.

Benjaminsen, E., and Karlberg, K.: Blood Specimen Collection from Swine. Norsk Veterinaertidsskrift, *91*:15, 1979.

Berchelmann, M.L., et al.: Comparison of Hematologic Values from Peripheral Blood of the Ear and Venous Blood of Infant Baboons (Papio cynocephalus). Lab. Anim. Sci., *23*:48, 1973.

Berkson, J., et al.: The Error of Estimate of the Blood Cell Count as Made with the Hemocytometer. Amer. J. Physiol., *128*:309, 1940.

Brecher, G.: New Methylene Blue as a Reticulocyte Stain. Amer. J. Clin. Path., *19*:895, 1949.

Brecher, G., et al.: Evaluation of Electronic Red Blood Cell Counter. Amer. J. Clin. Path., *26*:1493, 1956.

Brown, C.M.: A Method for Taking Blood from the Internal Thoracic Vein in Swine. Point Vétérinaire, *9*:53, 1979.

Brown, J.R., et al.: Femoral Venipuncture for Repeated Blood Sampling in Miniature Swine. Lab. Anim. Sci., *28*:339, 1978.

Bunce, S.A.: Observations on the Blood Sedimentation Rate and the Packed Cell Volume of Some Domestic Farm Animals. Brit. Vet. J., *110*:322, 1954.

Calhoun, M.L.: Cytological Study of Costal Marrow. 1. The Adult Horse. Amer. J. Vet. Res., *15*:181, 1954.

Calvert, G.D., et al.: Percutaneous Cardiac Puncture in Domestic Pig. Aust. Vet. J., *53*:337, 1977.

Campbell, K.L., et al.: Application of the Immunosorbent Assay for the Detection of Platelet Antibodies in the Dog. Amer. J. Vet. Res., *45*:2561, 1984.

Carle, B.N., and Dewhirst, W.H., Jr.: A Method for Bleeding Swine. J. Amer. Vet. Med. Ass., *101*:495, 1942.

Carlson, G.P., and Harrold, D.R.: Relationship of Protein Concentration and Water Content of Equine Serum and Plasma Samples. Vet. Clin. Path., *6*:18, 1977.

Carper, H.A., and Schalm, O.W.: A Comparison of the Direct and Indirect Methods for Estimation of Eosinophil Numbers in Blood. Calif. Vet., *16*:16, Jan.–Feb., 1962.

Carroll, E.J., and Schalm, O.W.: Effect of Deoxyribonuclease on the California Test for Mastitis. J. Dairy Sci., *45*:1094, 1962.

Chalifoux, L., and Hunt, D.D.: Histochemical Differentiation of Dirofilaria immitis and Dipetalonema reconditum. J. Amer. Vet. Med. Ass., *158*:601, 1971.

Chaplin, H.: Clinical Usefulness of Specific Antiglobulin Reagents in Autoimmune Hemolytic Anemias. Prog. Hematol., *8*:25, 1974.

Conn, H.J.: Biological Stains. 8th ed. R.D. Lillie, ed. Williams & Wilkins, Baltimore, 1969.

Conner, G.H., et al.: A Technique for Bone Marrow Biopsy in the Cat. J. Amer. Vet. Med. Ass., *158*:1702, 1971.

Coombs, R.R.A., et al.: A New Test for the Detection of Weak and "Incomplete" Rh Agglutinins. Brit. J. Exp. Path. (London), *26*:255, 1945.

Cooper, R.W.: Personal communication, 1972.

Cornelius, C.E., et al.: Chromatographic Identification of Bile Pigments in Several Species. Cornell Vet., *50*:47, 1960.

Danon, D., et al.: An Instrument for Automatically Recording the Osmotic Fragility Curve of Red Cells and/or Its Derivative. Trans. Biomed. Electron., *10*:24, 1963.

Dole, V.P., and Cotzias, G.C.: A Nomogram for the Calculation of Relative Centrifugal Force. Science, *113*:553, 1951.

Doyle, C.T.: The Effect of Blood Volume and Choice of Anticoagulant on the PCV, MCHC and Total White Cell Count. Irish J. Med. Sci., *6*:429, 1967.

Drabkin, D.L., and Austin, J.H.: Spectrophotometric Studies. II. Preparation from Washed Blood Cells; Nitric Oxide Hemoglobin and Sulfhemoglobin. J. Biol. Chem., *112*:50, 1935.

Farrington, E.M., and Jetter, W.W.: An Improved Staining Solution for Counting Eosinophils in Dogs. Amer. J. Clin. Path., *23*:836, 1953.

Faulkner, M., et al.: Discrepancy between Haemocytometer and Electronic Leucocyte Counts in Neutrophilic Dogs. Vet. Rec., *110*:202, 1982.

Feldman, B.: Use of Low Ionic Strength Solution in Combination with Papain Treated Red Blood Cells for the Detection of Canine Erythrocyte Autoantibodies. J. Amer. Anim. Hosp. Ass., *18*:653, 1982.

Fluharty, D.M., and Uhler, S.P.: Aspiration of Bone Marrow Using EDTA Fortified Serum. Bull. Amer. Soc. Vet. Clin. Path., *4*:14, 1975.

Foster, J.B.T., et al.: Determination of Plasma Fibrinogen by Means of Centrifugation after Heating. Amer. J. Clin. Path., *31*:42, 1959.

Freeman, L.W., and Johnson, V.: The Hemolytic Action of Chyle. Amer. J. Physiol., *130*:723, 1940.

Friou, G.J.: Antinuclear Antibodies: Diagnostic Significance. Arthritis Rheumat., *10*:151, 1967.

George, J.W., and Duncan, J.R.: Effect of Sample Preparation on Basophilic Stippling in Bovine Blood Smears. Vet. Clin. Path., *10*:37, 1981.

Gilliland, B.C., et al.: The Detection of Cell-Bound Antibody on Complement-Coated Human Red Cells. Clin. Invest., *49*:898, 1970.

Gilman, M.A., et al.: Immunohematologic Studies of the Thoroughbred Horse. Amer. J. Vet. Res., *21*:393, 1960.

Gordon, C.M., and Wardley, J.R.: The Effect of the Plasma Proteins upon the Sedimentation Rate of Human Blood. Biochem. J., *37*:393, 1943.

Gray, S.J., and Mitchell, E.B.: The Effect of Purified Protein Fractions on Sedimentation Rate of Erythrocytes. Proc. Soc. Exp. Biol. Med., *51*:403, 1942.

Hargraves, M.M., et al.: Presentation of Two Bone Marrow Elements: "Tart" Cell and "L.E." Cell. Proc. Staff Meet. Mayo Clin., *23*:25, 1948.

Henson, J.B., et al.: The Diagnosis of Equine Infectious Anemia Using the Complement-Fixation Test, Siderocyte Counts, Hepatic Biopsies, and Serum Alterations. J. Amer. Vet. Med. Ass., *151*:1830, 1967.

Hoerlein, A.B., et al.: The Procurement and Handling of Swine Blood Samples of the Farm. J. Amer. Vet. Med. Ass., *119*:357, 1951.

Hopwood, R.T., and Tibolla, B.J.: The Effect of Adrenocorticotrophic Hormone on the Circulating Eosinophil Level: A Possible Screening Test for Adrenal Gland Function in the Cow. Amer. J. Vet. Res., *19*:833, 1958.

Hultsch, Von K.-H, and Ellendorff, F.: Ein neues Verfahren zur Blutentnahme beim Schwein (Kurzmitteilung). Dtsch. Tierärztl. Wschr., *86*:313, 1979.

Jackson, R.F.: Studies on the Filter Techniques for the Detection and Identification of Canine Microfilariae. Heartworm Symposium 1977, p. 38.

Jackson, R.F., and Otto, G.F.: Detection and Differentiation of Microfilariae. Heartworm Symposium 1974, p. 21.

Jain, N.C.: A Staining Technique to Demonstrate Erythrocyte Refractile Bodies in Cat Blood. Brit. Vet. J., *125*:437, 1969.

Jain, N.C.: Osmotic Fragility of Erythrocytes of Dogs and Cats in Health and in Certain Hematologic Disorders. Cornell Vet., *63*:411, 1973.

Jain, N.C.: Autoimmune Hemolytic Anemia. Canine Pract., *2*:30, 1975.

Jain, N.C., and Kono, C.S.: Erythrocyte Sedimentation Rate in the Dog and Cat: Comparison of Two Methods and Influence of Packed Cell Volume, Temperature and Storage of Blood. J. Small Anim. Pract., *16*:671, 1975.

Jain, N.C., and Kono, C.S.: The Platelet Factor-3 Test for Detection of Canine Antiplatelet Antibody. Vet. Clin Path., *9*:10, 1980.

Jasper, D.E., and Jain, N.C.: Effects of Lipemia upon Erythrocyte Fragility, Sedimentation Rate, and Plasma Refractometer Indexes in the Dog. Amer. J. Vet. Res., *26*:332, 1965.

Jones, D.R.E., and Drake, P.G.G.: Use of Papain for the Detection of Incomplete Erythrocyte Autoantibodies in Autoimmune Haemolytic Anemia of the Dog and Cat. J. Small Anim. Pract., *16*:273, 1975.

Joshi, B.C., and Jain, N.C.: Detection of Antiplatelet Antibody in Serum and on Megakaryocytes of Dogs with Autoimmune Thrombocytopenia. Amer. J. Vet. Res., *37*:681, 1976.

Kaneko, J.J., and Smith, R.: The Estimation of Plasma Fibrinogen and Its Clinical Significance in the Dog. Calif. Vet., *21*:21, Aug., 1967.

Karpatkin, M., et al.: The Platelet Factor 3 Immunoinjury Technique Re-evaluated. Development of a Rapid

Test for Antiplatelet Antibody: Detection in Various Clinical Disorders, Including Immunologic Drug-Induced and Neonatal Thrombocytopenias. J. Lab. Clin. Med., *89*:400, 1977.

Karpatkin, S., and Siskind, G.W.: In Vitro Detection of Platelet Antibody in Patients with Idiopathic Thrombocytopenic Purpura and Systemic Lupus Erythematosus. Blood, *33*:795, 1969.

Kassel, R., and Levitan, S.: A Jugular Technique for the Repeated Bleeding of Small Animals. Science, *118*:563, 1953.

Klemperer, P., et al.: Cytologic Changes of Acute Lupus Erythematosus. Arch. Path., *49*:503, 1950.

Klopfer, U.: A Quick Method for Demonstrating Inclusion Bodies of Infectious Canine Hepatitis in Liver Smears. Vet. Med. Small Anim. Clin., *64*:158, 1969.

Kume, S.: Experimental Observations on Seasonal Periodicity on Microfilariae. Heartworm Symposium 1974, p. 26.

Lawrence, W.C., et al.: A Simple Method for Bone Marrow Aspiration in the Cow. Cornell Vet., *52*:297, 1962.

Leddy, J.P., and Swisher, S.N.: Acquired Immune Hemolytic Disorders. *In* Immunological Diseases. Vol. 2, 2nd ed., Samter, M., ed. Little, Brown, Boston, 1971.

Lincoln, P.J., and Dodd, B.E.: The Use of Low-Ionic Strength Solution (LISS) in Elution Experiments and in Combination with Papain-Treated Cells for the Titration of Various Antibodies, Including Eluted Antibody. Vox Sang., *34*:221, 1978.

Live, I., and Stubbs, E.L.: The Diagnosis of Filariasis in the Dog. J. Amer. Vet. Med. Ass., *92*:686, 1938.

Lloyd, H.E.D.: Estimation of the Erythrocyte Sedimentation Rate of Capillary Blood: Description of a New Method. Ann. Rheum. Dis., *17*:234, 1958.

Loewy, A., et al.: Increased Erythrocyte Destruction on a High Fat Diet. Amer. J. Physiol., *138*:230, 1943.

Longworth, L.G., et al.: Electrophoretic Patterns of Normal and Pathological Human Blood Serum and Plasma. J. Exp. Med., *70*:399, 1939.

Low, E.M.Y., et al.: Simple Method for Detection of Abnormal Plasma Fibrinogen Levels. Amer. J. Clin. Path., *47*:538, 1967.

MacGregor, R.G.S., et al.: The Differential Leukocyte Count. J. Path. Bact., *51*:337, 1940.

Marshall, P.N.: Romanowsky Type Stains in Haematology. Histochem. J., *10*:1, 1978.

Marshall, P.N., et al.: Staining Properties and Stability of a Standardized Romanowsky Stain. J. Clin. Path., *31*:280, 1978.

Martin, J.E., et al.: The Action of Adrenocorticotrophic Hormone on Circulating Eosinophils in Dogs. A Proposed Screening Method for Evaluating Adrenal Cortical Function. Amer. J. Vet. Res., *15*:489, 1954.

Mattern, C.F.T., et al.: Determination of Number and Size of Particles by Electrical Grating: Blood Cells. J. Appl. Physiol., *10*:56, 1957.

Maxie, M.G.: Evaluation of Techniques for Counting Bovine Platelets. Can. J. Comp. Med., *41*:409, 1977.

Melveger, L.M., et al.: Sternal Bone Marrow Biopsy in the Dog. Lab. Anim. Care, *19*:866, 1969.

Meyer, L.M., and Bloom, F.: The Bone Marrow of Normal Dogs. Amer. J. Med. Sci., *206*:637, 1943.

Miale, J.B.: Laboratory Medicine: Hematology. 3rd ed. C.V. Mosby, St. Louis, 1967.

Moore, H.C., and Mollison, P.L.: Use of Low-Ionic Strength Medium in Manual Tests for Antibody Detection. Transfusion, *16*:291, 1976.

Moss, G., and Staunton, C.: Blood Flow, Needle Size and Hemolysis—Examining an Old Wives' Tale. New Eng. J. Med., *282*:967, 1970.

Newton, W.L., and Wright, W.H.: A Reevaluation of the Canine Filariasis Problem in the United States. Vet. Med., *52*:75, 1957.

Niejadlik, D.C.: Antinuclear Antibodies: Role in Diagnosing Systemic Lupus Erythematosus. Postgrad. Med., *50*:273, 1971.

Parpart, A.K., et al.: The Osmotic Resistance (Fragility) of Human Red Cells. J. Clin. Invest., *26*:636, 1947.

Peeble, D.A., et al.: Analysis of Manual Reticulocyte Counting. Amer. J. Clin. Path., *76*:713, 1981.

Pennock, C.A., and Jones, K.W.: Effect of Ethylene-Diamine-Tetra-Acetic Acid (Dipotassium Salt) and Heparin on the Estimation of Packed Cell Volume. J. Clin. Path., *19*:196, 1966.

Penny, R.H.C., et al.: Some Observations on the Effect of the Concentration of Ethylenediamine Tetraacetic Acid (EDTA) on the Packed Cell Volume of Domesticated Animals. Brit. Vet. J., *126*:383, 1970.

Perk, K., et al.: Osmotic Fragility of Red Blood Cells of Young and Mature Domestic and Laboratory Animals. Amer. J. Vet. Res., *25*:1241, 1964.

Perman, V.: Diagnostic Cytology in Canine Medicine. 16th Gaines Vet. Symp., Philadelphia, *16*:6, 1966. Gaines Dog Research Center, White Plains, N.Y.

Petz, L.D.: Acquired Immune Hemolytic Anemias. Churchill Livingstone, New York, 1980.

Pilot, M.L.: Use of Base in Fluids for Counting Eosinophils. Amer. J. Clin. Path., *20*:870, 1950.

Pirofsky, B.: Autoimmunization and the Autoimmune Haemolytic Anaemias. Williams & Wilkins, Baltimore, 1969.

Pruden, E.L., and Winstead, M.E.: Accuracy Control of Blood Cell Counts with the Coulter Counter. Amer. J. Med. Technol., *30*:1, 1964.

Ramsay, W.N.W.: Plasma Bilirubin in the Horse. Biochem. J., *39*:XXXII Proceedings Section, 1945.

Redington, B.C., et al.: The Various Microfilariae Found in Dogs in the United States. Heartworm Symposium 1977, p. 14.

Rees, H.M., and Ecker, E.E.: An Improved Method for Counting Blood Platelets. JAMA, *80*:621, 1923.

Reich, C.: Modified Wright Stain. Amer. J. Clin. Path., *24*:881, 1954.

Richar, W.J., and Breakell, E.S.: Evaluation of an Electronic Counter for the Counting of White Blood Cells. Amer. J. Clin. Path., *31*:384, 1959.

Riley, V.: Adaptation of Orbital Bleeding Technic to Rapid Serial Blood Studies. Proc. Soc. Exp. Biol. Med., *104*:751, 1960.

Rothenbacher, H.J., et al.: Equine Infectious Anemia. II. The Sideroleukocyte as an Aid in the Clinical Diagnosis. Vet. Med., *57*:886, 1962.

Rothstein, N., and Brown, M.L.: Vital Staining and Differentiation of Microfilariae. Amer. J. Vet. Res., 21:1090, 1960.

Sawitsky, A., and Meyer, L.M.: The Bone Marrow of Normal Cats. J. Lab. Clin. Med., 32:70, 1947.

Schalm, O.W.: Unpublished observations, 1961.

Schalm, O.W.: A Simple and Rapid Method for Staining Blood Films with New Methylene Blue. J. Amer. Vet. Med. Ass., 145:1184, 1964.

Schalm, O.W.: Clinical Significance of Plasma Protein Concentration. Amer. J. Vet. Med. Ass., 157:1672, 1970.

Schalm, O.W., and Jain, N.C.: Detection of Microfilariae Using the Capillary Hematocrit Tube. Calif. Vet., 20:14 (Sept.–Oct.), 1966.

Schalm, O.W., and Lasmanis, J.: Cytologic Features of Bone Marrow in Normal and Mastitic Cows. Amer. J. Vet. Res., 37:359, 1976.

Schalm, O.W., and Ling, G.V.: The L.E. Cell Phenomenon in the Dog. Calif. Vet., 24:20, (Dec.), 1970.

Schalm, O.W., and Murray, R.: Estimation of Blood Leukocyte Numbers by Means of a DNA Viscosity Test. J. Amer. Vet. Med. Ass., 145:1177, 1964.

Schalm, O.W., and Noorlander, D.O.: Experiments and Observations Leading to Development of the California Mastitis Test. J. Amer. Vet. Med. Ass., 130:199, 1957.

Schmidt, C.H., et al.: A New Anticoagulant for Routine Laboratory Procedures: A Comparative Study. U.S. Armed Forces Med. J., 4:1556, 1953.

Schreiber, A.D., and Frank, M.M.: Role of Antibody and Complement in the Immune Clearance and Destruction of Erythrocytes. I. In Vivo Effects of IgG and IgM Complement Fixing Sites. J. Clin. Invest., 51:575, 1972a.

Schreiber, A.D., and Frank, M.M.: Role of Antibody and Complement in the Immune Clearance and Destruction of Erythrocytes. II. Molecular Nature of IgG and IgM Complement Fixing Sites and Effects of Their Interaction with Serum. J. Clin. Invest., 51:583, 1972b.

Schryver, F.: The Bone Marrow of the Cat. Amer. J. Vet. Res., 24:1012, 1963.

Sears, P.M., et al.: Comparison between the Tail Vein and Jugular Vein Cannulation in Cattle. J. Dairy Sci., 61:947, 1978.

Shen, S.C., et al.: Experimental and Clinical Observations on Increased Mechanical Fragility of Erythrocytes. Science, 100:387, 1944.

Simms, B.T.: Erythrocyte Sedimentation Studies in Dogs. J. Amer. Vet. Med. Ass., 96:77, 1940.

Steel, E.G.: Evaluation of Electronic Blood Platelet Counting in Sheep and Cattle. Amer. J. Vet. Res., 35:1465, 1974.

Stier, H., and Leucht, W.: Blutentnahme aus dem Sinus venösus ophthalmicus beim Miniaturschwein. Zeit. Versuchstierkhunde, 22:161, 1980.

Stone, S.H.: Method for Obtaining Venous Blood from the Orbital Sinus of the Rat or Mouse. Science, 119:100, 1954.

Stormont, C.: Personal communication, 1975.

Stormont, C., et al.: Serology of Horse Blood Groups. Cornell Vet., 54:439, 1964.

Strumia, M.M., et al.: An Improved Microhematocrit Method. Amer. J. Clin. Path., 24:1016, 1954.

Stubbs, E.L., and Live, I.: The Diagnosis of Filariasis in the Dog. J. Amer. Vet. Med. Ass., 87:680, 1935.

Suess, J., et al.: A Quantitative Method for the Determination and Charting of the Erythrocyte Hypotonic Fragility. Blood, 3:1290, 1948.

Sunderman, F.W., et al.: Symposium on Clinical Hemoglobinometry. Amer. J. Clin.Path., 23:519, 1953.

Swank, R.L., and Roth, E.S.: Hemolysis and Alimentary Lipemia. Effects of Incubation, Heparin, and Protamine. Blood, 9:348, 1954.

Switzer, J.W., and Jain, N.C.: Autoimmune Hemolytic Anemia in Dogs and Cats. Vet. Clin. North Amer. (Small Anim. Pract.), 11:405, 1981.

Switzer, J.W., and Schalm, O.W.: Bone Marrow Disorders in Cats: Bone Marrow Sampling Techniques. Calif. Vet., 22:20, Aug., 1968.

Talal, N.: Antibodies to Nucleic Acids. Clin. Immunol., 3:375, 1976.

Theilen, G.H.: Personal communication. 1975.

Thorn, G.W., et al.: A Test for Adrenal Cortical Insufficiency: The Response to Pituitary Adrenocorticotrophic Hormone as a Test for Adrenal Cortical Insufficiency. JAMA, 137:1005, 1948.

Tongson, M.S., and Romero, F.R.: Observations on the Periodicity of Dirofilaria immitis in the Peripheral Circulation of the Dog. Brit. Vet. J., 118:299, 1962.

Vallejo-Freire, A.: A Simple Technique for Repeated Collection of Blood Samples from Guinea Pigs. Science, 114:524, 1951.

Valli, V.E., et al.: An Anticoagulant for Transport of Bovine Blood. Can. Vet. J., 21:252, 1980.

Van Boxtel, C.J., et al.: Immunofluorescence Microphotometry for the Detection of Platelet Antibodies. III. Demonstration of Autoantibodies against Platelets. Scand. J. Immunol., 4:657, 1975.

van Kampen, E.J., and Zijlstra, W.G.: Standardization of Hemoglobinometry. II. The Hemiglobincyanide Method. Clin. Chim. Acta, 6:538, 1961.

van Kampen, E.J., and Zijlstra, W.G.: Determination of Hemoglobin and Its Derivatives. Adv. Clin. Chem., 8:141, 1965.

Vendrely, R.: The Deoxyribonucleic Acid Content of the Nucleus. In Chargaff, E., and Davidson, J.M., eds.: The Nucleic Acids. Vol. 2, p. 155. Academic Press, New York, 1955.

Wallach, J.D.: A Simple Technique for the Collection of Blood for Small Zoo Animals. J. Amer. Vet. Med. Ass., 157:694, 1970.

Wartman, W.B.: Effect of Room Temperature on Sedimentation Rate of Blood Cells of Man. Amer. J. Med. Sci., 212:207, 1946.

Weide, K.D., et al.: Blood Cell Counting in Animals by Electronic Means. I. Erythrocyte Enumeration of Porcine, Ovine and Bovine Blood. Amer. J. Vet. Res., 23:632, 1962.

Weiser, M.G.: Hematologic Techniques. Vet. Clin. North Amer. (Small Anim. Pract.), 11:189, 1981.

Weiser, M.G.: Comparison of Two Automated Multi-

Channel Blood Cell Counting Systems for Analysis of Blood of Common Domestic Animals. Vet. Clin. Path., *12(2)*:25, 1983.

West, J.E., et al.: Serial Rib Marrow Aspiration Technique and Myelogram for Adult Beagles. AFRRI TN71–1. Armed Forces Radiobiology Research Institute, Bethesda, Maryland, January 1971.

Wicker, B., and Wallas, C.H.: A Comparison of a Low Ionic Strength Saline Medium with Routine Methods for Antibody Detection. Transfusion, *16*:469, 1976.

Wilde, J.K.H.: Bovine Bone Marrow. A Note on the Total Nucleated Cell Count. Res. Vet. Sci., *4*:160, 1963.

Wilkins, R.J., et al.: Immunologically Mediated Thrombocytopenia in the Dog. J. Amer. Vet. Med. Ass., *163*:277, 1973.

Wintrobe, M.M.: The Volume and Hemoglobin Content of the Red Blood Corpuscle. Amer. J. Med. Sci., *177*:513, 1929.

Wintrobe, M.M.: The Size and Hemoglobin Content of the Erythrocyte. Methods of Determination and Clinical Application. J. Lab. Clin. Med., *17*:899, 1932.

Wintrobe, M.M.: Macroscopic Examination of the Blood. Amer. J. Med. Sci., *185*:58, 1933.

Wintrobe, M.M.: Clinical Hematology. 6th ed., p. 414. Lea & Febiger, Philadelphia, 1967.

Wintrobe, M.M., et al.: Clinical Hematology. 8th ed. Lea & Febiger, Philadelphia, 1981.

Wisecup, W.G., and Crouch, B.G.: Evaluation and Calibration of an Electronic Particle Counter for Enumeration of Multi-Species Blood Cells. Amer. J. Clin. Path., *39*:349, 1963.

Wolf, A.V., et al.: New Refractometric Methods for Determination of Total Protein in Serum and in Urine. Clin. Chem., *8*:158, 1962.

Wong, M.M.: A Comparison of ELISA and IFA Titers in Dirofilariasis in Dogs. Heartworm Symposium 1980, p. 41.

Wong, S.Y.: Colorimetric Determination of Iron and Hemoglobin in Blood. J. Biol. Chem., *77*:409, 1928.

Wu, H.: Studies on Hemoglobin. I. The Advantage of Alkaline Solutions for Colorimetric Determination of Hemoglobin. J. Biochem., *2*:173, 1923.

COLOR PLATES

Blood and bone marrow cells from coverslip films stained with Wright-Leishman stain unless stated otherwise.

Plate I	Blood abnormalities in the Wintrobe hematocrit tube
Plate II	Blood abnormalities in the Wintrobe hematocrit tube
Plate III	Megakaryocytopoiesis in canine bone marrow
Plate IV	Erythropoiesis in canine and feline bone marrow and reticulocytes in feline blood
Plate V	Erythropoiesis and granulocytopoiesis in equine, canine, and feline bone marrow
Plate VI	Erythropoiesis and granulocytopoiesis in equine bone marrow
Plate VII	Leukocytes of various animal species
Plate VIII	Immature and mature monocytes, macrophages, and toxic neutrophils in canine blood
Plate IX	Feline leukocytes in health and in response to toxemic disease
Plate X	Cytochemical reactions of blood and bone marrow cells
Plate XI	Cells in blood and bone marrow, normal and abnormal
Plate XII	Blood and bone marrow cells of various animal species in health and disease
Plate XIII	Blood and bone marrow cells in diseases of the dog
Plate XIV	Parasites and abnormalities in leukocytes of various animal species
Plate XV	Abnormal blood and bone marrow cells of the cat
Plate XVI	Heinz bodies in feline blood
Plate XVII	Erythrocytes in various anemias
Plate XVIII	Hemoparasites and erythrocyte abnormalities
Plate XIX	Myeloproliferative disorders in the cat
Plate XX	Myeloproliferative disorders in the cat
Plate XXI	Lymphocytic leukemia in the dog and cat
Plate XXII	Granulocytic and mast cell leukemia in the cat
Plate XXIII	Granulocytic leukemia in the dog
Plate XXIV	Acute myelomonocytic leukemia in the dog
Plate XXV	Blood cells and parasites of birds

PLATE I. CANINE AND FELINE BLOOD ABNORMALITIES IN THE WINTROBE HEMATOCRIT TUBE

1. Comparison of the Wintrobe hematocrit with the small capillary microhematocrit. Blood from a case of lymphocytic leukemic leukemia with a total leukocyte count of 87,000/µl. A borderline anemia exists as shown by the PCV of 36%. The buffy coat of 5 mm reflects the high total leukocyte count. The reddish tinge to the buffy coat is imparted by admixture of some red cells, particularly reticulocytes and/or leptocytes.

2. A diphasic erythrocyte sedimentation (right) is indicated by the reddish plasma which clears upon centrifugation (center). The PCV of 29% reveals the existence of anemia, and the low icterus index as compared to the icterus index standard of 5 units (left) suggests an anemia of nonhemolytic origin.

3. Wintrobe hematocrit of a cat with polycythemia vera (center, PCV 67%) is compared with hematocrits of two normal cats (left, PCV 32% and right, PCV 36%). A small buffy coat is evident above the red cell column in the left and right tubes.

4. Buffy coat of an anemic cat (tube #2) is compared with that of an anemic dog (tube #3) to illustrate differences in blood elements that may comprise a rather grossly similar buffy coat. The cream-colored buffy coat of about 9 mm in tube #2 is made almost entirely of platelets (platelet count 1.2 million/µl, WBC count within normal range), whereas the reddish buffy coat of about 6 mm in tube #3 consists of primarily leukocytes (WBC count 100,000/µl, platelet count within normal range). Reddish tinge of the buffy coat in tube #3 is attributable to admixture of young erythrocytes produced in response to anemia.

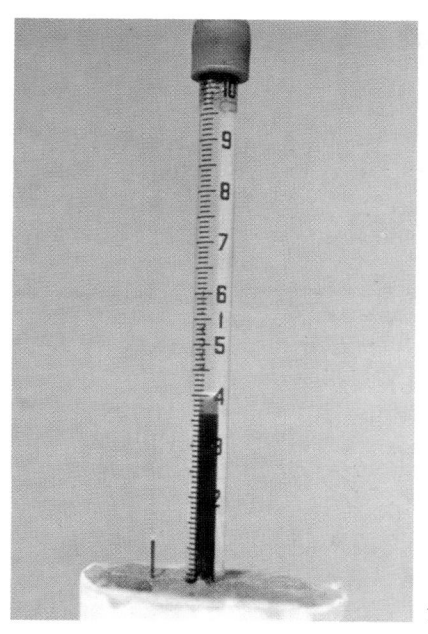

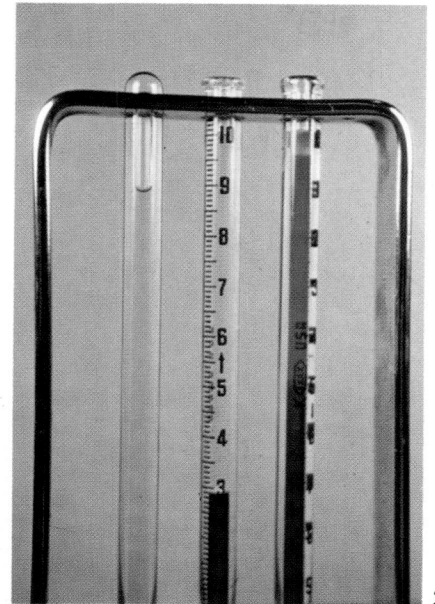

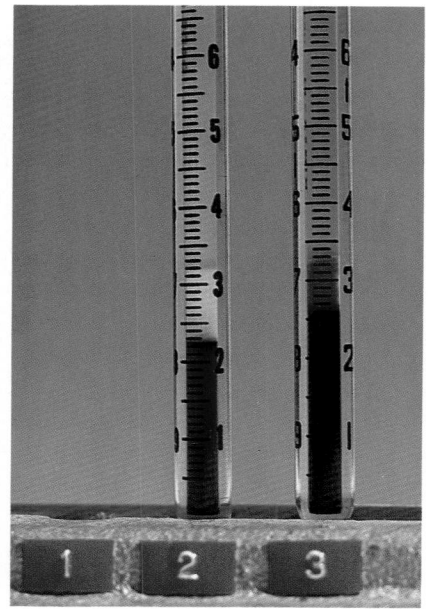

1

2

3

4

PLATE II. CANINE BLOOD ABNORMALITIES IN THE WINTROBE HEMATOCRIT TUBE

1. The left tube presents an icterus index value of 75 units due to retention of bilirubin from compression of the common bile duct in carcinoma of the pancreas. The blood in the center tube is typical of the anemia and low icterus index commonly observed in end stage kidney disease with uremia. The blood on the right also presents a colorless plasma. It is from a dog recently recovered from acute blood loss; the plasma is colorless because many of the erythrocytes are at the beginning of their life span. Daily destruction of overaged erythrocytes is too limited to contribute sufficient bilirubin to color the plasma.

2. Blood from two dogs with pyometra. The center tube is an icterus index standard of 5 units. The total leukocyte counts were 126,000/μl in the blood on the left and 82,500/μl in the blood on the right. These high leukocyte numbers are reflected in the buffy coats of 7 mm and 5 mm, respectively. The red tinge of these buffy coats is due to admixture of erythrocytes of low specific gravity (leptocytes) among the leukocytes. The PCV of each blood is 45%.

3. Lipemia is indicated in this hematocrit by the hazy plasma and the layer of neutral fat at the top of the plasma column. This hematocrit tube had been held overnight after centrifugation, which permitted a larger accumulation of fat at the top of the plasma column than had been present initially. Note that the plasma is clear immediately above the buffy coat and is increasingly opaque toward the top. The chylomicra are gradually rising to produce this effect.

4. A case of extreme lipemia. Hemolysis of erythrocytes, as shown by the red plasma that does not clear on centrifugation, often occurs with markedly lipemic blood. The hemolysis takes place after the blood is withdrawn and is enhanced by mechanical agitation of the sample or by forcing the blood from the syringe through the needle into the vial.

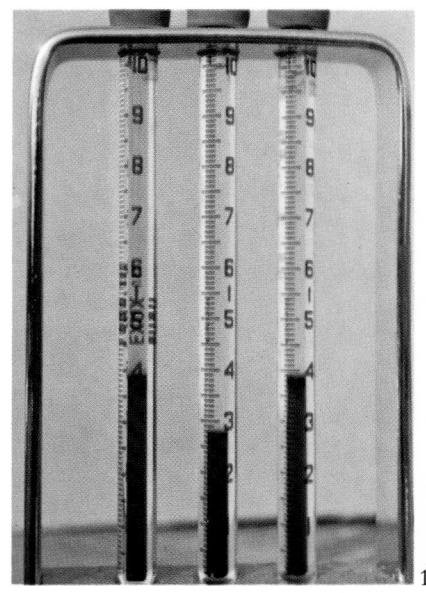

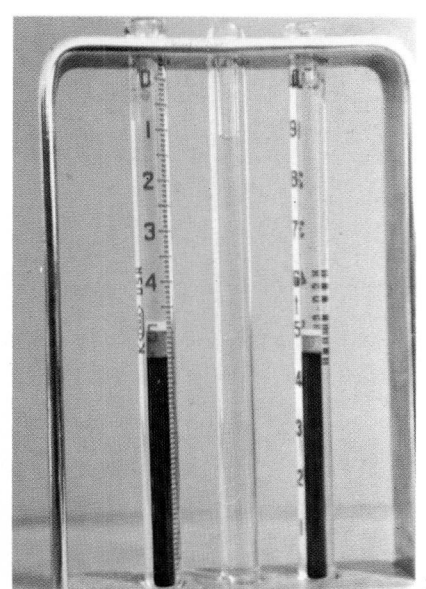

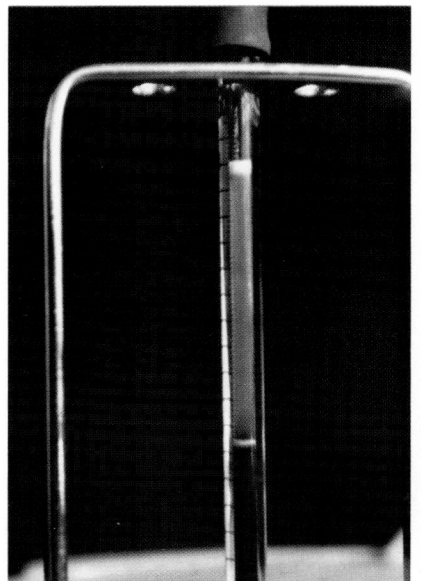

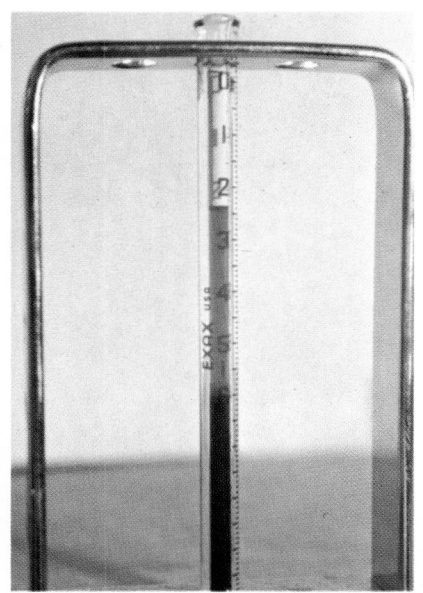

PLATE III. MEGAKARYOCYTOPOIESIS IN CANINE BONE MARROW

1. Megakaryoblast at the stage of first division of the nucleus. From a dog with autoimmune hemolytic anemia and thrombocytopenia. Cytoplasmic vacuolation is abnormal ($\times 1,800$).

2. Promegakaryocyte in mitotic division without cell division (endomitosis) ($\times 1,260$).

3. Megakaryoblast with four nuclei from the same marrow as Plate III–1. Cells with one to four nuclei are regarded by some hematologists as megakaryoblasts ($\times 1,800$).

4. Two promegakaryocytes (smaller cells) and two megakaryocytes (larger cells). The promegakaryocyte is distinguished from the megakaryoblast by the presence of a single mass of nuclear material with indistinct outline and larger cell size; it is distinguished from the megakaryocyte by its agranular blue cytoplasm ($\times 800$).

5. Megakaryocyte with a cytoplasmic process called a "proplatelet," which fragments into platelets ($\times 1,260$). See Fig. 15–6.

6. An osteoclast ($\times 800$).

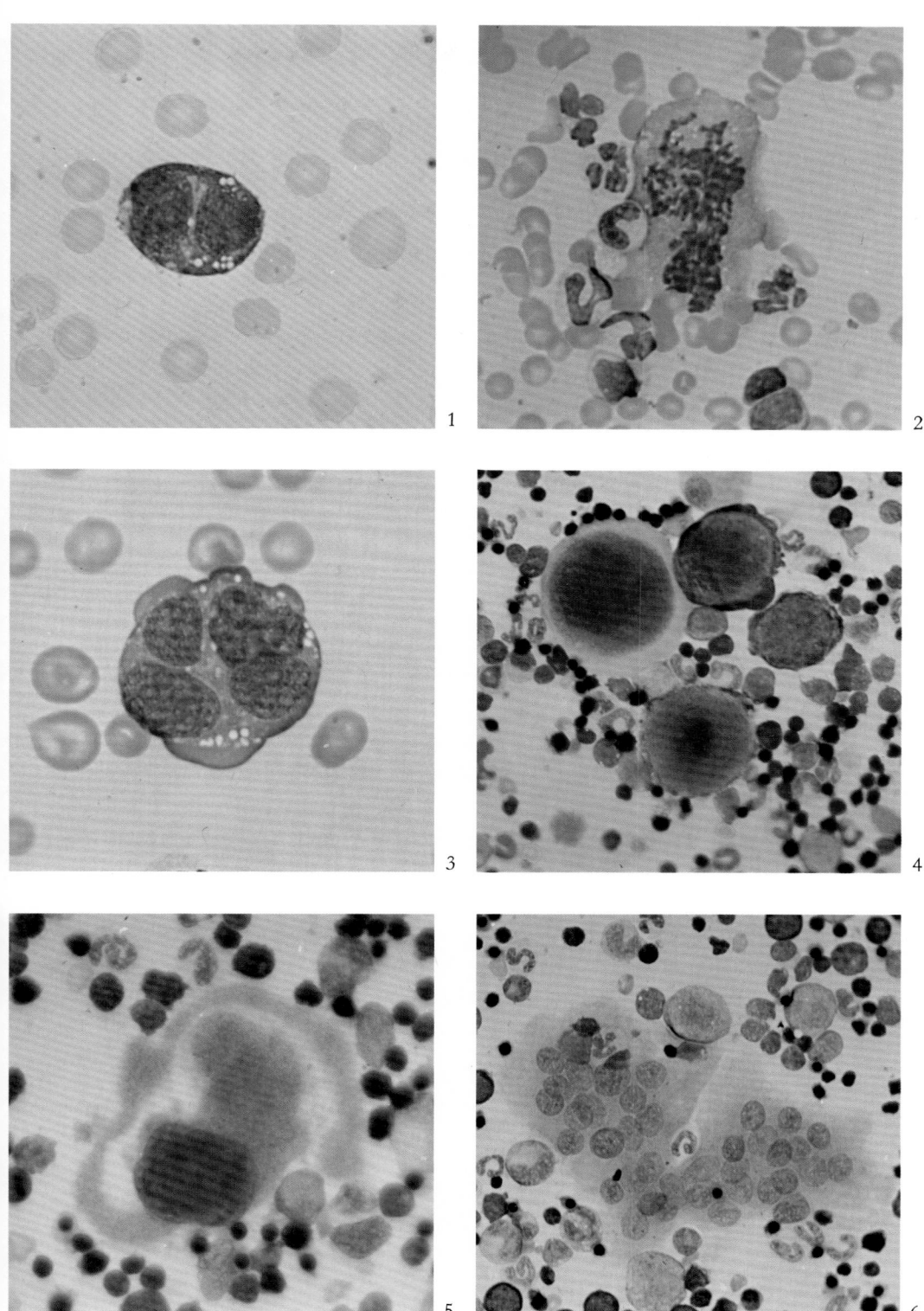

1

2

3

4

5

6

PLATE IV. ERYTHROPOIESIS IN CANINE AND FELINE BONE MARROW AND RETICULOCYTES IN FELINE BLOOD ($\times 1,800$)

1. The large cell in the center is a rubriblast with a prominent nucleolar ring, stippled chromatin, and deep blue cytoplasm. The ring of cells surrounding the rubriblast is comprised of polychromatic rubricytes in varying stages of hemoglobin synthesis and chromatin condensation. A portion of a naked nucleus of a reticuloendothelial cell is present in one corner. (Canine bone marrow in hemangiosarcoma.)

2. A metarubricyte and a hematogone (free nucleus of a metarubricyte) are present above the eosinophil. Below the eosinophil are one prorubricyte and four polychromatic rubricytes at various stages of hemoglobin synthesis and maturity. The prorubricyte has blue cytoplasm and stippled nuclear chromatin, but no nucleolus. Two large polychromatic red cells are present among mature discocytic red cells. (Canine bone marrow in responsive anemia.)

3. Canine bone marrow stained with new methylene blue. The large cell with two prominent nucleoli and deep blue cytoplasm is a rubriblast. The cell below the rubriblast and having a lightly stained coarse chromatin and grayish blue cytoplasm is a polychromatic rubricyte. The small cell to the right of the rubriblast and having a condensed nuclear chromatin and grayish cytoplasm is a late polychromatic rubricyte. Basophilic rubricytes (one above the rubriblast, one to the right of late polychromatic rubricyte and one at the lower margin) have a relatively coarser nuclear chromatin and darker cytoplasm than the polychromatic rubricyte. The anuclear cell with bluish granular cytoplasmic material situated near the mid-right margin is a reticulocyte, while red cell ghosts are present in the background. The cell to the left of the reticulocyte is a polychromatic rubricyte.

4. Bone marrow from a normal cat depicting two metarubricytes, two polychromatic rubricytes, a basophilic rubricyte, and a prorubricyte along cells of the neutrophilic series. A neutrophilic myelocyte is present at the upper margin and a band neutrophil is at the lower margin of the photomicrograph.

5. Bone marrow from a cat with regenerative hemolytic anemia. Intensified erythropoiesis was indicated by predominance of erythroid elements at various stages of maturation. Two rubriblasts, three polychromatic rubricytes, and three metarubricytes can be identified among the cells present.

6. Aggregate and punctate reticulocytes in the peripheral blood of a cat with regenerative hemolytic anemia. The large bluish objects near the margin of a few red cells are Heinz bodies. Reticulocyte stain.

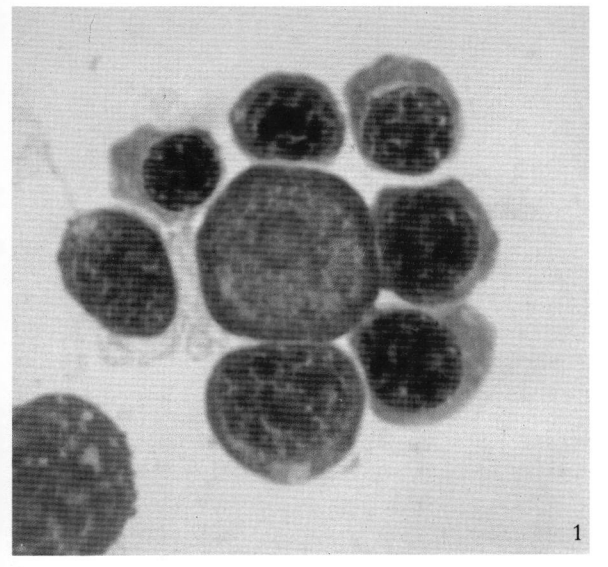

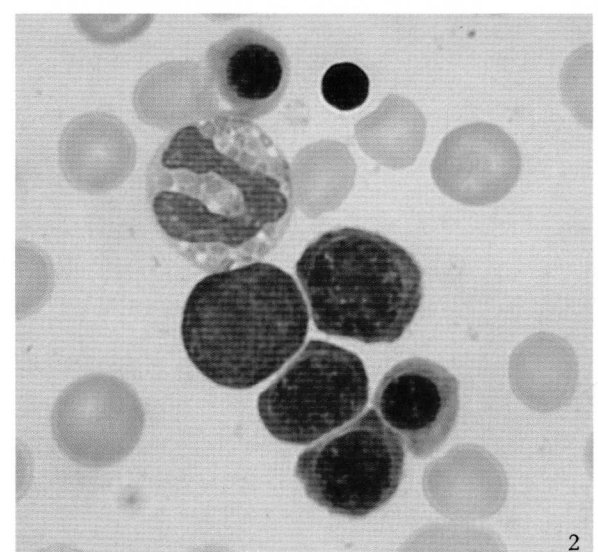

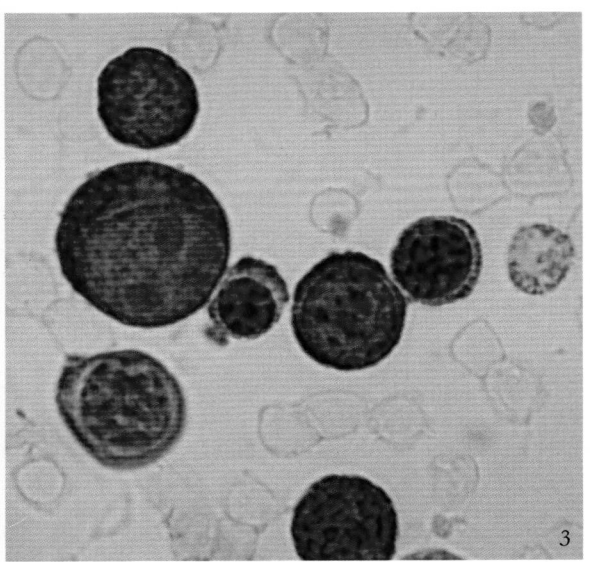

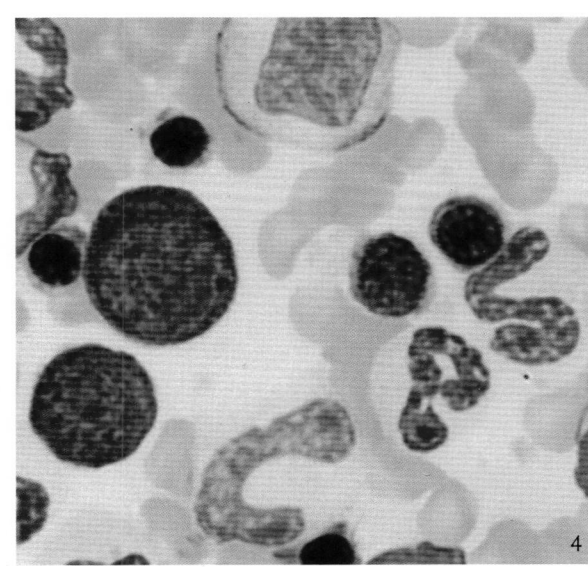

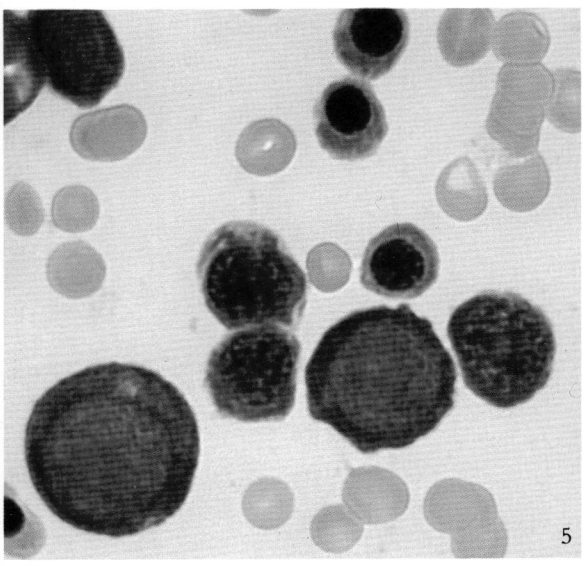

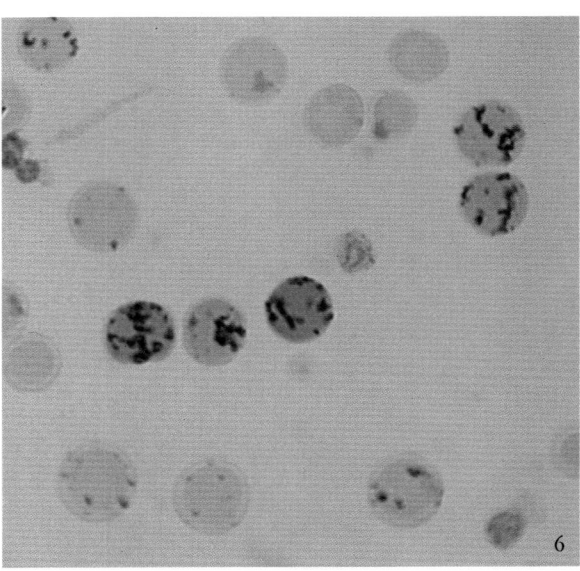

1.   Intensified erythropoiesis in a horse responding to an anemia. All nucleated cells are of the erythrocytic maturation seies. The cells, in descending order of size, are a rubriblast, four basophilic rubricytes, a polychromatophilic rubricyte, and several metarubricytes. Effective erythropoiesis is indicated particularly by the presence of large polychromatophilic erythrocytes.

2.   Cat bone marrow in feline infectious anemia. The largest cell is a basophilic myelocyte exhibiting many small, lightly stained cytoplasmic granules and fewer larger purple granules. The latter granules will disappear as the basophil matures, leaving the lightly stained granules in a grayish cytoplasm as characteristic of the mature feline basophil (see Plate VII–6). The remaining nucleated cells are, in decreasing order of size, a basophilic rubricyte, polychromatophilic rubricytes, and metarubricytes. The amorphous pinkish mass is a degenerating nucleus. A few polychromatophilic erythrocytes can be seen.

3.   Dog myeloblast with three nucleolar rings and a neutrophilic metamyelocyte. A free lymphocyte nucleus is next to the latter cell.

4.   A dog progranulocyte with azurophilic cytoplasmic granules. The nucleus presents a nucleolar ring, but the azurophilic granules take precedence in classifying the cell.

5.   Horse myeloblast (center) with several nucleolar rings, an eosinophilic myelocyte (largest cell), a basophilic metamyelocyte with purple granules, a degenerating neutrophilic metamyelocyte next to the basophil, and a small polychromatophilic rubricyte near the myeloblast.

6.   A cluster of horse neutrophilic granulocytes. A myelocyte (cell with round nucleus), several metamyelocytes, one of which is abnormally large, and a band neutrophil (lower cell with V-shaped nucleus) are seen. All cells with round, dark nuclei are either polychromatophilic rubricytes or metarubricytes.

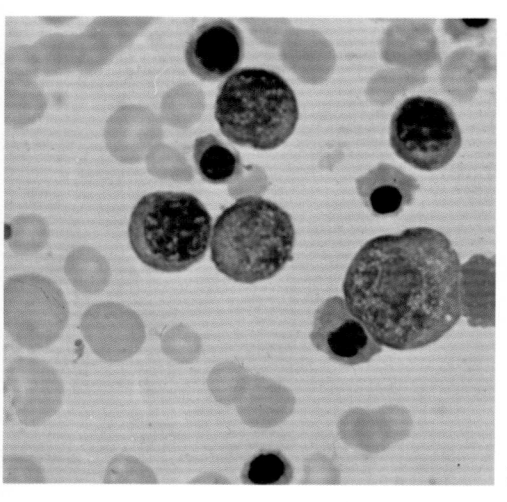

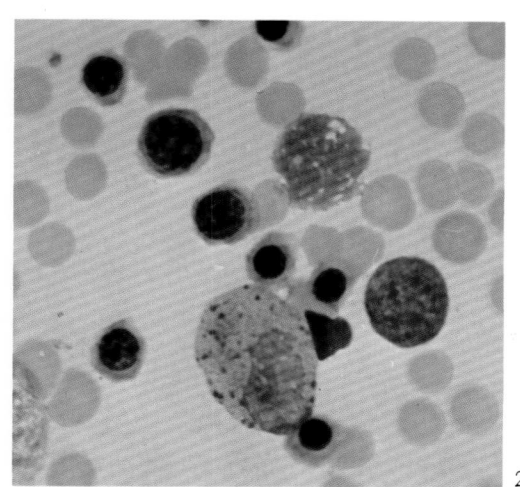

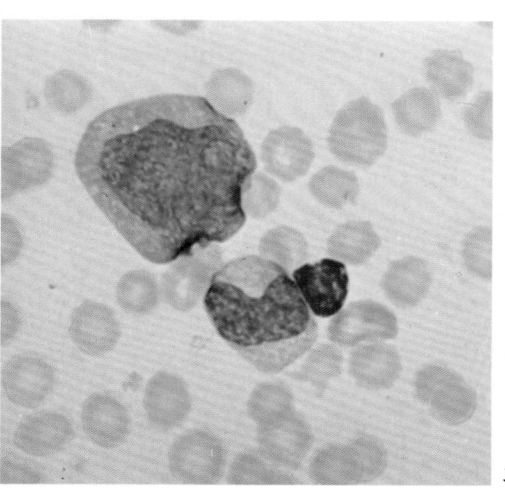

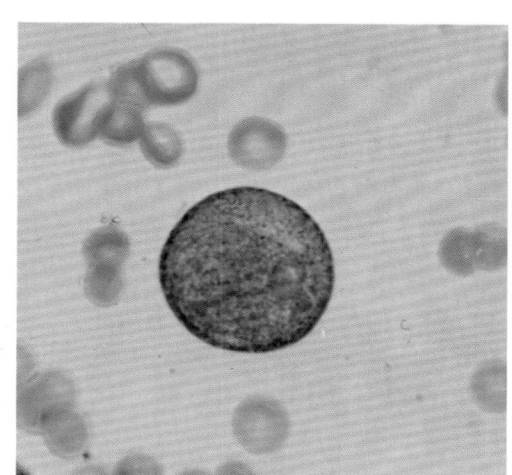

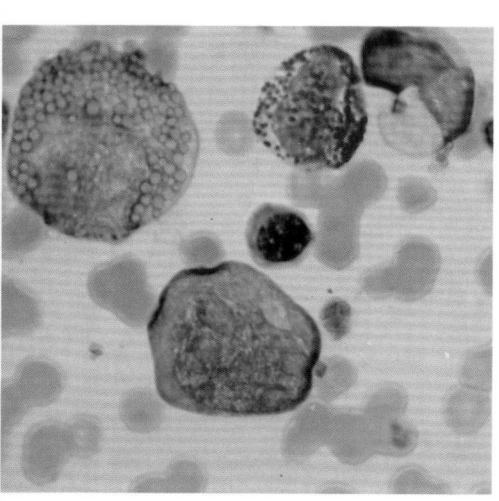

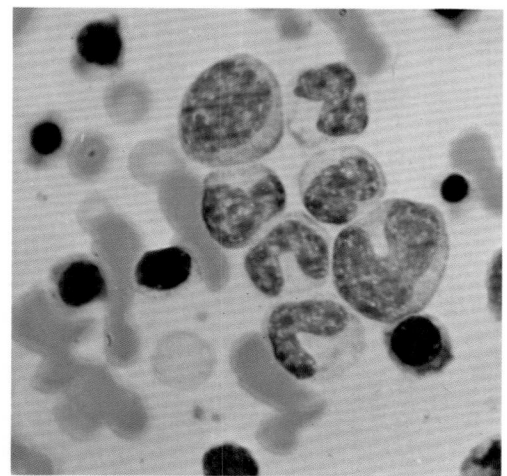

1. The lower large cell having a round nucleus with prominent nucleoli and finely stippled chromatin and a moderately blue cytoplasm is a myeloblast. The upper large cell having a round nucleus with somewhat coarse chromatin, a pale blue cytoplasm, and some indistinct reddish granules is a late promyelocyte. A metarubricyte is present to the left of the myeloblast, and two polychromatic rubricytes with nuclei at different stages of chromatin condensation are present to the right of the myeloblast.

2. The large cell with lightly stained, round nucleus and reddish purple granules in the light blue cytoplasm is a promyelocyte. A basophilic rubricyte, three polychromatic rubricytes, and two metarubricytes at various maturative stages are present. A free nucleus, probably from a degenerated leukocyte, is present to the left of the promyelocyte.

3. A basophil myelocyte with prominent, large, reddish purple granules somewhat masking the nucleus is present adjoining a neutrophilic metamyelocyte (upper right) and a mature monolobed neutrophil (lower right).

4. The large cell with distinct nucleoli, somewhat clumpy nuclear chromatin, and dark blue cytoplasm is a rubriblast. The nuclear chromatin in erythrocytic precursors, particularly rubriblasts and prorubricytes, is characteristically much coarser in the horse than in the dog and cat. An intermediate polychromatic rubricyte, two late polychromatic rubricytes, a neutrophilic metamyelocyte, and a neutrophilic band are present in the field.

5. Erythroid cells in various maturative stages in the bone marrow of a horse with lead poisoning. The largest cell is a prorubricyte and the two smaller cells with some clumpy chromatin and bluish cytoplasm are basophilic rubricytes. Among five cells with grayish cytoplasm, the smallest one with fully condensed nucleus is a metarubricyte, while the remaining cells are polychromatic rubricytes with varying degrees of nuclear chromatin condensation.

6. Erythroid cells in various maturative stages from rubriblast to metarubricytes and two neutrophilic granulocytes in bone marrow of a horse with responsive anemia.

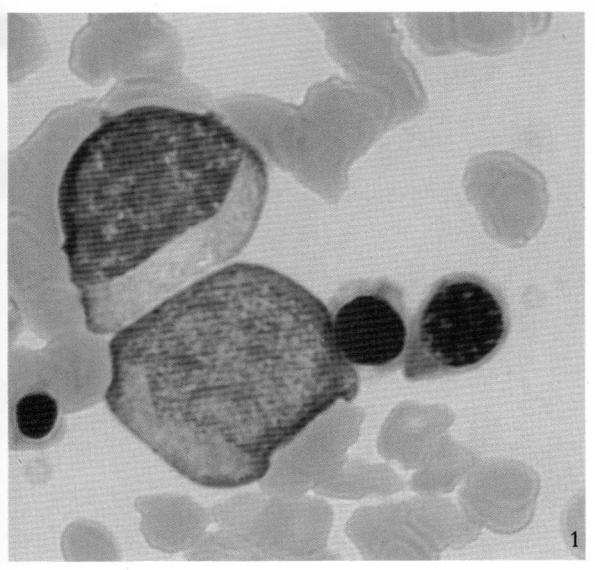

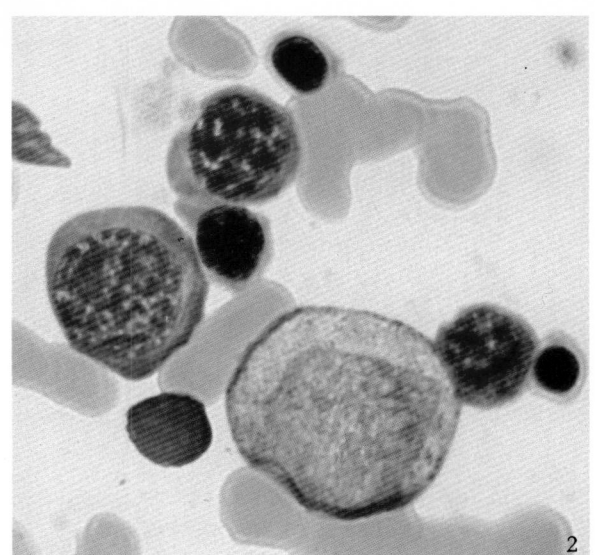

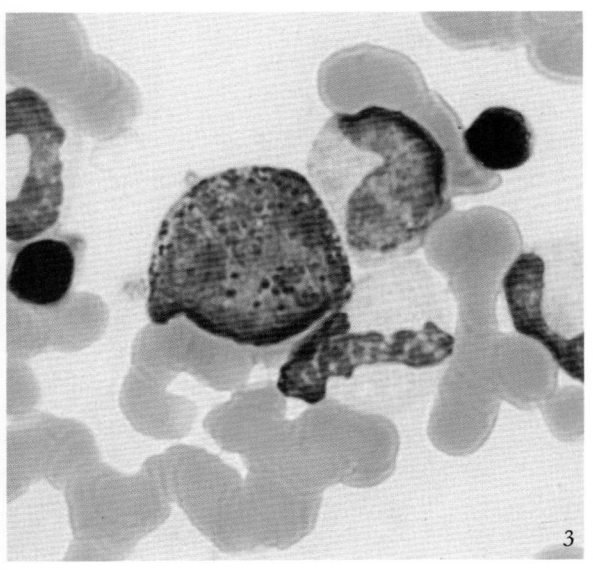

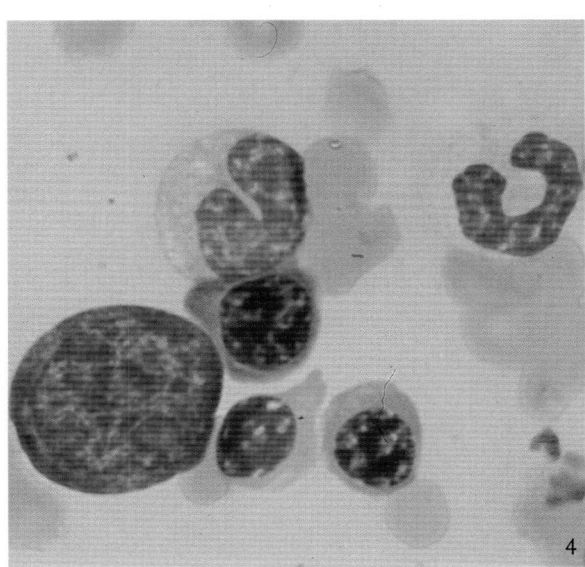

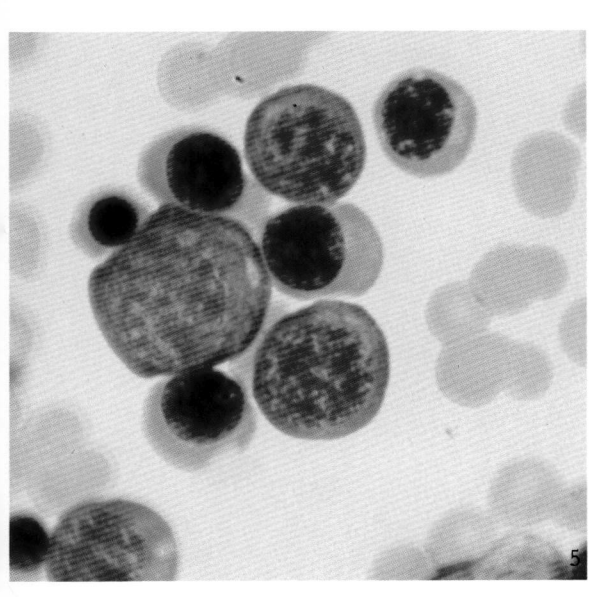

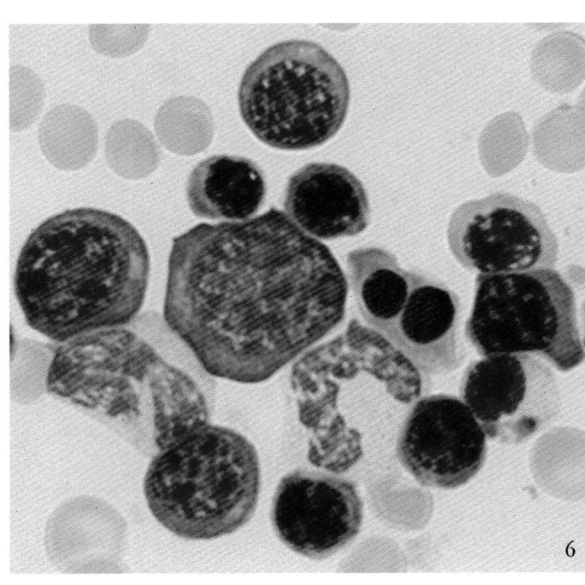

PLATE VII. LEUKOCYTES OF VARIOUS ANIMAL SPECIES ($\times 1{,}800$)

1. Mature bovine neutrophils. The rouleau formation of the erythrocytes is abnormal and is a response to an inflammatory disease.

2. A bovine lymphocyte (cell with round nucleus) and a monocyte.

3. A bovine monocyte and a lymphocyte with azurophilic cytoplasmic granules.

4. A bovine eosinophil containing distinct reddish granules and a monocyte. From the same blood as Plate VII–1.

5. A bovine basophil. Intensely stained metachromatic cytoplasmic granules usually mask the nucleus in basophils.

6. A feline eosinophil and two basophils. The eosinophil has reddish, rod-like granules, while the basophils have faintly stained, round granules. For morphology of immature basophil, see Plate XII–5.

7. An equine eosinophil and basophil.

8. Three mature equine neutrophils in a row and one band neutrophil on the left.

9. A mature neutrophil and an uncommon form of canine monocyte with a profuse number of reddish granules. For varied morphology of monocytes see Plate VIII.

10. Three typical canine monocytes. See also Plate VIII.

11. Two monocytes of the Indian elephant. Others have classified these cells as lymphocytes; however, they are peroxidase-positive (see next figure).

12. Peroxidase stain applied to leukocytes of the Indian elephant, a monocyte (left cell) and a neutrophil. Both are peroxidase-positive.

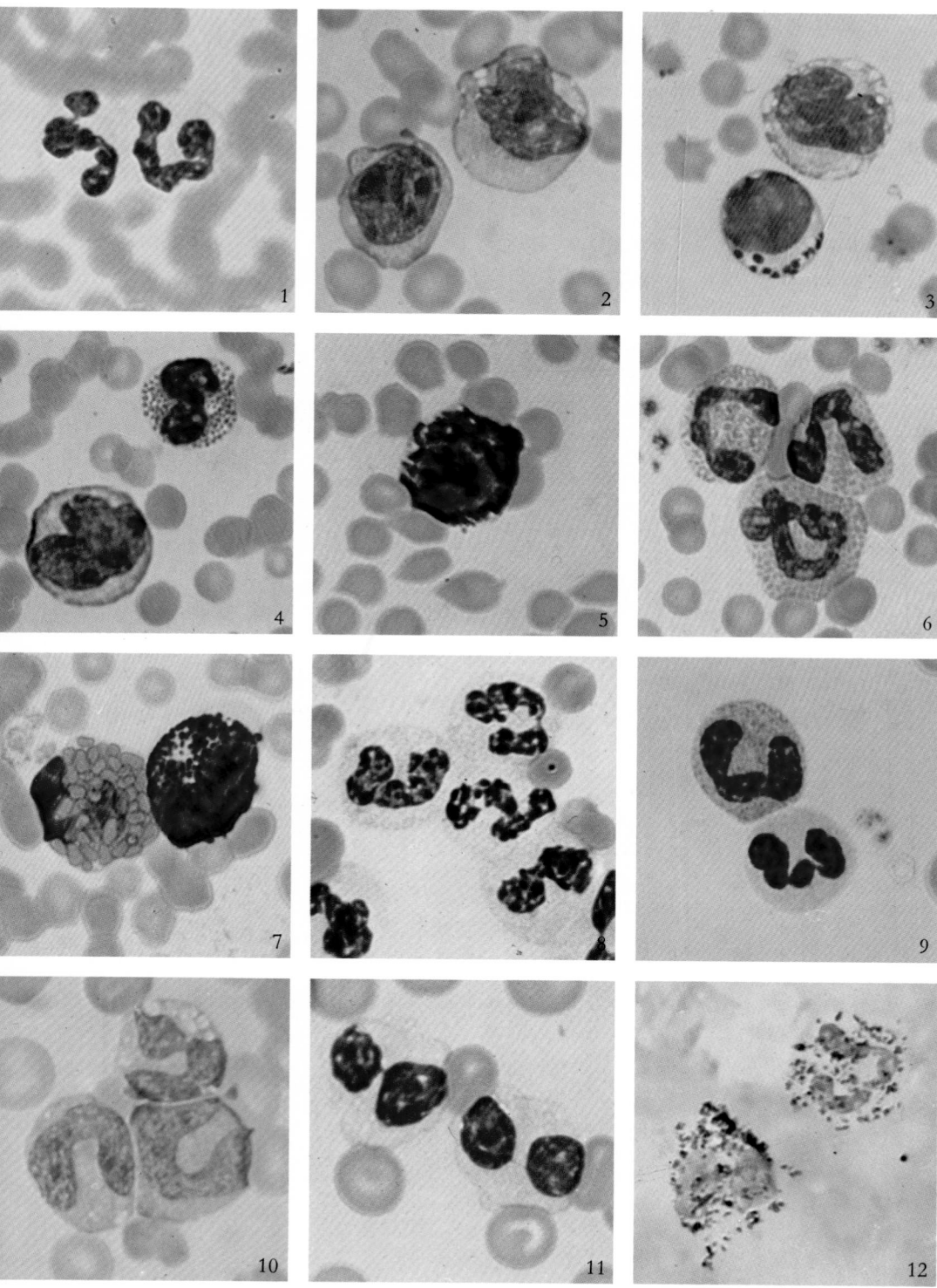

PLATE VIII.   IMMATURE AND MATURE MONOCYTES, MACROPHAGES, AND TOXIC NEUTROPHILS IN CANINE BLOOD ($\times 1,800$)

1. A monoblast with characteristic irregularly indented nucleus in blood of a dog with leukemoid reaction (WBC count 98,000/μl with left shift to myeloblast). The cell has finely stippled nuclear chromatin, inconspicuous nucleolus, moderately blue cytoplasm, and a high nucleus-to-cytoplasm ratio.

2. A monoblast and a polyploid monocytoid cell in blood of a dog with myelomonocytic leukemia. A platelet with distinct azurophilic granules is present above the two cells.

3. A promonocyte with undulated nuclear outline, incipient chromatin condensation, and vacuolated bluish cytoplasm.

4. An immature monocyte with round nucleus and bluish vacuolated cytoplasm. The nuclear shape may be suggestive of a neutrophilic myelocyte, but the coarse, lacy nuclear chromatin and cytoplasmic features distinguish this cell as monocytoid.

5. Two young monocytes with oblong or indented nuclei, reticular nuclear chromatin, and distinctive cytoplasmic features. Cytoplasmic vacuolation is evident in only one cell.

6. A monocyte with metamyelocyte-like nucleus, but unlike a neutrophilic metamyelocyte it has blue and vacuolated cytoplasm. A neutrophil with clear cytoplasm is also present.

7. A monocyte with a band-like nucleus and bluish cytoplasm tinged reddish with fine, indistinct azurophilic granules. The cytoplasmic features distinguish this cell from the nearby neutrophil.

8. A more mature monocyte with pale blue, ground-glass-like cytoplasm and band-like nucleus is compared with two mature neutrophils having clear cytoplasm.

9. A typical mature monocyte with ameboid nucleus and foamy blue, vacuolated cytoplasm and a mature neutrophil.

10. Two macrophages with highly vacuolated cytoplasm and ameboid nucleus in the peripheral blood of a dog with bacterial endocarditis. Monocyte to macrophage activation may sometimes occur in the circulation as in this patient. A medium-sized lymphocyte is present in the upper right area.

11. A neutrophilic metamyelocyte and two neutrophilic bands with toxic foamy blue cytoplasm. Pattern of nuclear chromatin (coarsely granular but not lacy or reticular) and cytoplasmic density and color (relatively clear and sky blue) distinguish these cells from monocytoid cells in Plates VIII–7 and VIII–8 above.

12. Highly vacuolated toxic bands cells with partially folded nuclei. Note the nuclear and cytoplasmic features of these cells and those in Plate VIII–11 for differentiation from macrophages in Plate VIII–10.

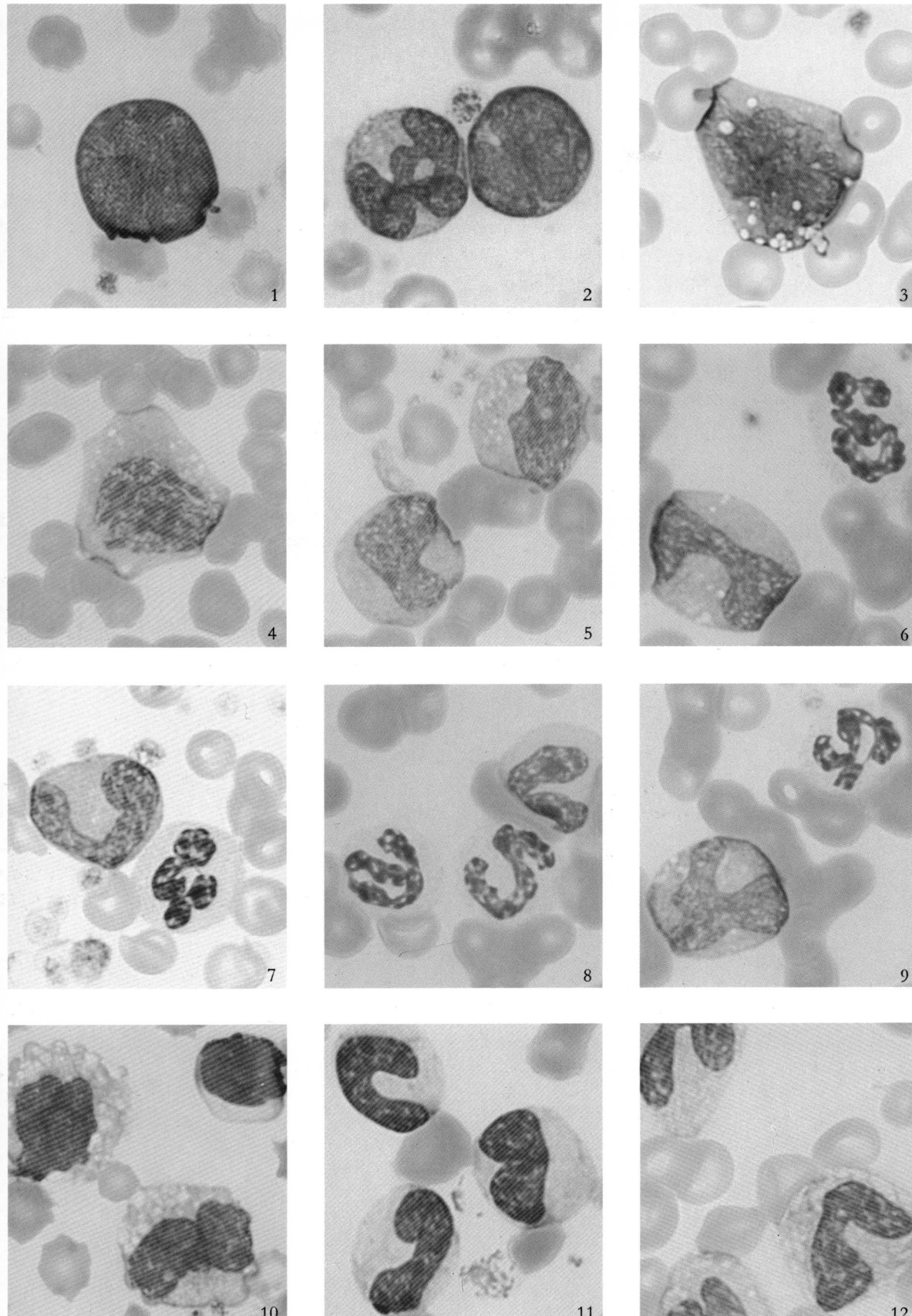

PLATE IX.   FELINE LEUKOCYTES IN HEALTH AND IN RESPONSE TO TOXEMIC DISEASE (×1,800)

1. An eosinophil, a lymphocyte, and three mature neutrophils are presented to show normal morphologic characteristics for comparison with Plate IX–2, 3, and 4; clusters of thrombocytes are also seen (Wright-Leishman stain).

2. Two mature neutrophils of greater than normal size are presented. A Döhle body (blue dot) appears in the cytoplasm at one edge of one of the cells. Döhle bodies appear to represent remnants of rough endoplasmic reticulum resulting from a minor interference in the maturation of the cytoplasm.

3. The four neutrophils arranged diagonally across the center of the figure are large and present a blue foamy cytoplasm. These cytologic features are signs of a defective maturation and characterize the cells as toxic neutrophils. A small lymphocyte of normal morphology is also present.

4. Giant neutrophils are seen in certain severe inflammatory diseases in the cat. One such giant neutrophil is presented here, together with four neutrophils of more normal morphology.

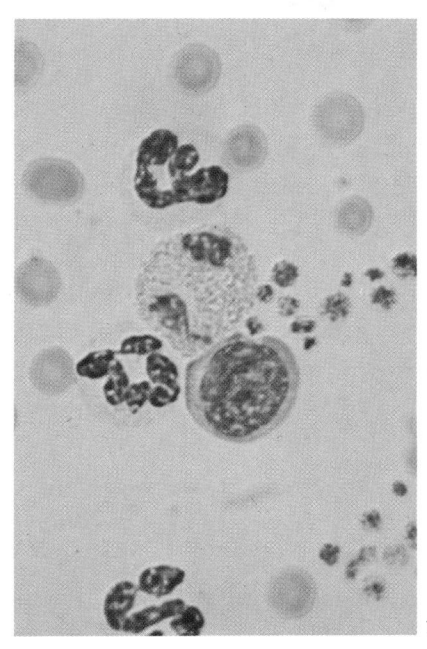

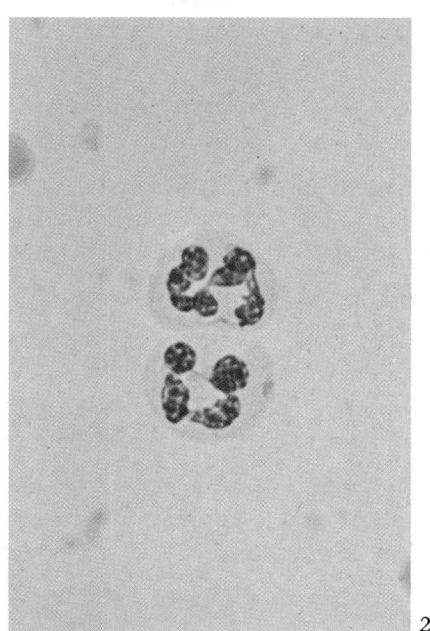

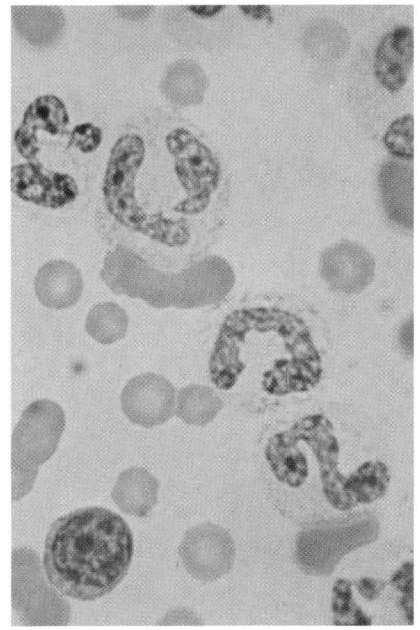

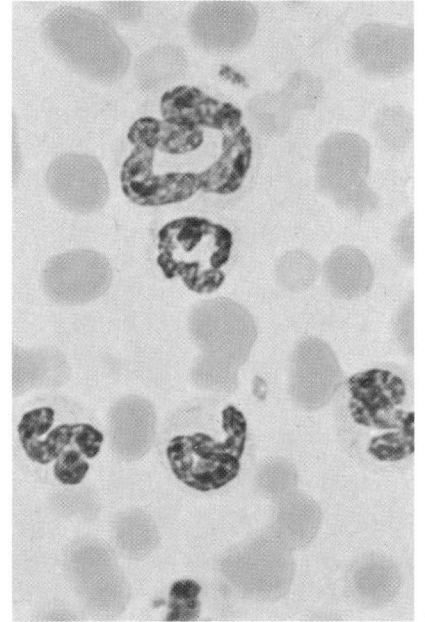

PLATE X.   CYTOCHEMICAL REACTIONS OF BLOOD AND BONE MARROW CELLS
($\times 1,800$)*

1. Two alkaline phosphatase-positive equine neutrophils. Stained by the method of Kaplow (1955).

2. Alkaline phosphatase activity in the intergranular cytoplasm of a canine eosinophil. Notice the absence of enzyme activity in specific granules of the eosinophil and in the adjacent neutrophil. Stained by the method of Kaplow (1955).

3. Alkaline phosphatase activity in the intergranular cytoplasm of a feline basophil. Notice the absence of enzyme activity in specific granules of the basophil and in the adjacent neutrophil. Stained by the method of Kaplow (1955).

4. Numerous peroxidase-positive orange granules in four canine neutrophils. 3-amino 9-ethylcarbazol method of Graham et al. (1965).

5. A peroxidase-positive canine neutrophil with abundant orange granules and folded nucleus (right) is compared with a canine monocyte with sparse, similarly-stained cytoplasmic granules (left). 3-amino 9-ethylcarbazol method of Graham et al. (1965).

6. A monocyte with few darkly stained, peroxidase-positive granules (left) is compared with a neutrophil containing numerous intensely stained, peroxidase-positive granules (right). Stained by the method of Kaplow (1965).

7. Sudan black B-positive granules in a bovine neutrophil. Sudanophilia in neutrophils generally parallels their peroxidase activity. Stained by the method of Sheehan and Storey (1947).

8. A lipase-positive monocyte with diffuse reddish cytoplasmic reaction and a chloroacetate esterase-positive band neutrophil with bluish cytoplasmic granules in feline bone marrow. Lipase staining by the method of Ansley and Ornstein (1970) and chloroacetate esterase staining by the method of Yam et al. (1971a).

9. A nonspecific esterase-positive monocyte with diffuse reddish cytoplasmic reaction (α-naphthyl acetate substrate) and a chloroacetate esterase-positive neutrophil with bluish cytoplasmic granules in human blood. Stained by the methods of Yam et al. (1971a).

10. A feline basophil exhibiting characteristic staining of its granules for naphthol AS-D chloroacetate esterase. Stained by the method of Bauer-Sic (1963).

11. Periodic acid Schiff (PAS) reactivity of canine neutrophils is indicated by diffuse magenta color in the cytoplasm. Methyl green was used as the nuclear stain. Stained by a modified method of Bauer-Sic (1963) and Hayhoe (1960).

12. Methyl green pyronin staining of canine bone marrow cells. Distinctive pyroninophilia is evident in a typical plasma cell. Stained by the method of Perry and Reynolds (1956).

*For complete listing of references, see Chapter 33.

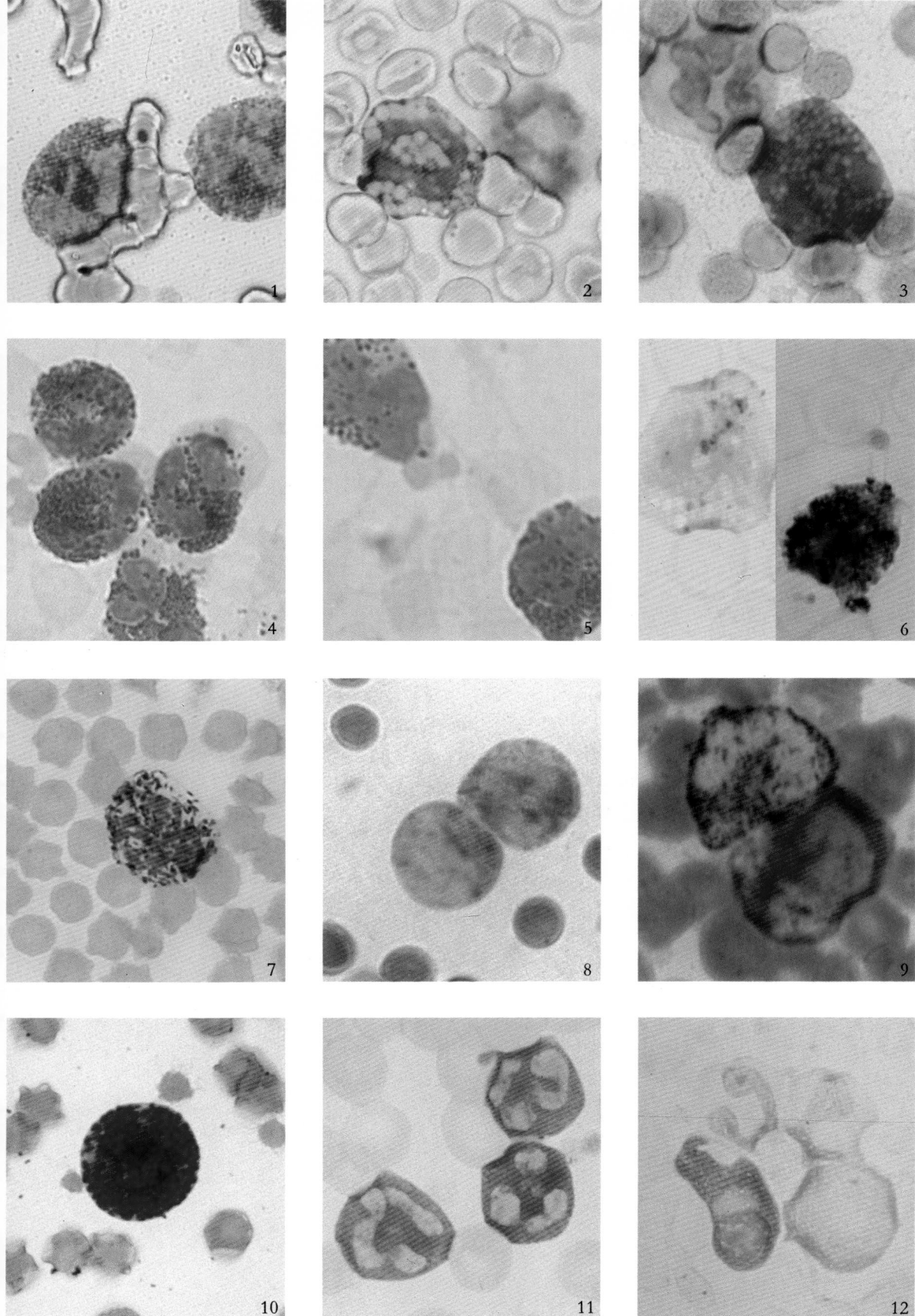

PLATE XI. CELLS IN BLOOD AND BONE MARROW, NORMAL AND ABNORMAL
(×1,800)

1. Macrophage with phagocytosed iron particles and erythrocyte debris from the bone marrow of a horse with anemia. Such a cell stains intensely for iron. See Plate XII-11.

2. Free nuclei of reticuloendothelial (RE) cells in aspirated bone marrow of a dog. The blue-staining nucleoli identify the structures as nuclei of RE cells. As the nucleus disintegrates, a net-like structure is formed, commonly referred to as a basket cell.

3. A neutrophil containing two circular masses of phagocytosed amorphous nuclear material typical of the lupus erythematosus (LE) cell. From the bone marrow of a cat with a myeloproliferative disease.

4. A cluster of four plasma cells, a neutrophilic myelocyte, and a polychromatophilic rubricyte from the bone marrow of a dog.

5. A plasma cell filled with vesicles called Russell bodies. A neutrophilic myelocyte is also present. From the bone marrow of a dog.

6. Monocytoid cells seen in peripheral blood of a dog with salmon poisoning (Appendix Case 36).

7. Neutrophil with a female sex chromatin lobe or drumstick (upper cell) from peripheral blood of a dog. Hypersegmented neutrophil of a cat (lower cell) in peripheral blood in suspected vitamin B_{12}-folate deficiency.

8. A monocyte of a dog with azurophilic cytoplasmic granules and a macrocytic erythrocyte in peripheral blood in suspected vitamin B_{12}-folate deficiency.

9. Two toxic metamyelocytes with foamy basophilic cytoplasm and a normal small lymphocyte in peripheral blood of a cow with acute coliform mastitis.

10. Toxic band neutrophils with foamy blue cytoplasm in peripheral blood of a cat with empyema of the thoracic cavity.

11. Toxic neutrophils (metamyelocyte and band) in blood of a foal with salmonellosis.

12. Neutrophils with toxic granulation in the blood of a horse with acute hepatitis.

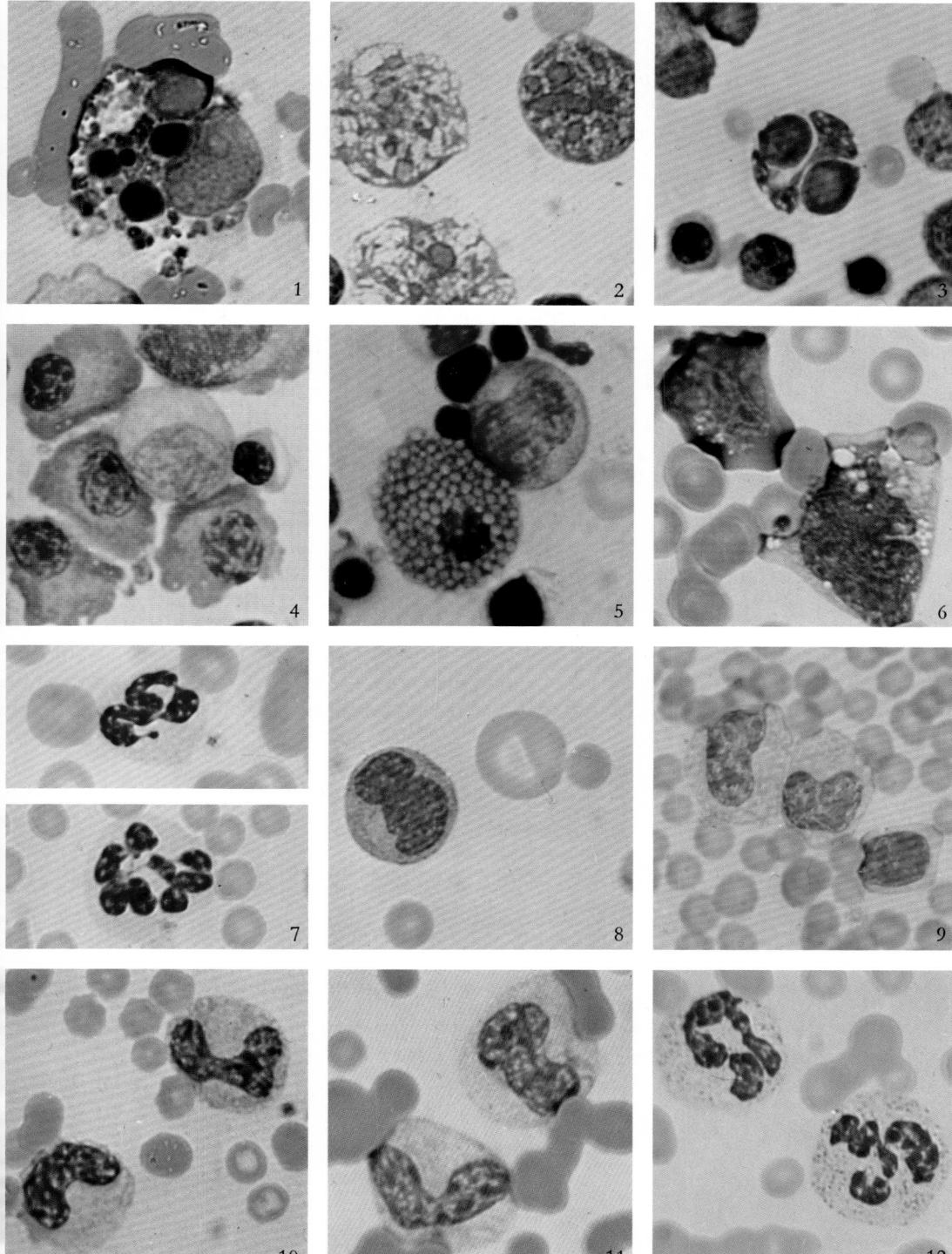

PLATE XII. BLOOD AND BONE MARROW CELLS OF VARIOUS ANIMAL SPECIES IN HEALTH AND DISEASE (×1,800)

1. An eosinophil and a basophil in the peripheral blood of a dog. The canine basophil characteristically contains sparse metachromatic granules in contrast to basophils in the horse and ruminants. Central pallor is evident in mature red cells.

2. The canine eosinophil differs from the eosinophils of other domestic animals in that the granules may vary considerably in number and size as depicted by the two eosinophils from blood of a dog with eosinophilia of undefined origin. A mature neutrophil is also present.

3. A canine eosinophilic promyelocyte with two types of cytoplasmic granules—some large azurophilic and many more light pink specific granules. Such a cell is extremely rare in normal bone marrow, but it is sometimes found in bone marrow with increased eosinophilopoiesis. A band neutrophil is also present.

4. A mast cell (upper right) studded with metachromatic granules is compared with a basophil myelocyte (lower right) having few metachromatic granules and many grayish specific granules. Bone marrow of a cat with mastocytoma.

5. An immature basophil in the peripheral blood of a cat. Notice the presence of both large, metachromatic granules and round, grayish granules as in the basophil myelocyte in the preceding photomicrograph. Compare this cell with the mature basophil in Plate VII–6.

6. Döhle bodies in somewhat foamy cytoplasm of toxic band neutrophils in the peripheral blood of a dog with chronic peritonitis.

7. Leukergy (clumping of neutrophils) in the peripheral blood of a horse; the cause of this rare phenomenon is obscure, but it is more frequent in horses with severe inflammatory conditions than in other conditions.

8. *Corynebacterium parvum* in a clump of platelets in blood of a dog given an intravenous injection of the bacteria in treatment of leukemia.

9. Three Howell-Jolly bodies (large, densely stained, marginal objects) and two Pappenheimer bodies (small, light blue, marginal structures) in the erythrocytes of a dog.

10. Siderocytes (red cells with dark blue specks) in the peripheral blood of a cat. Prussian blue stain for iron.

11. Macrophage 4+ iron in the bone marrow of a horse. Prussian blue stain for iron.

12. A brightly fluorescent (4+) megakaryocyte in the bone marrow of a dog with autoimmune thrombocytopenia. The bone marrow film was stained for direct immunofluorescence using anticanine IgG antibody.

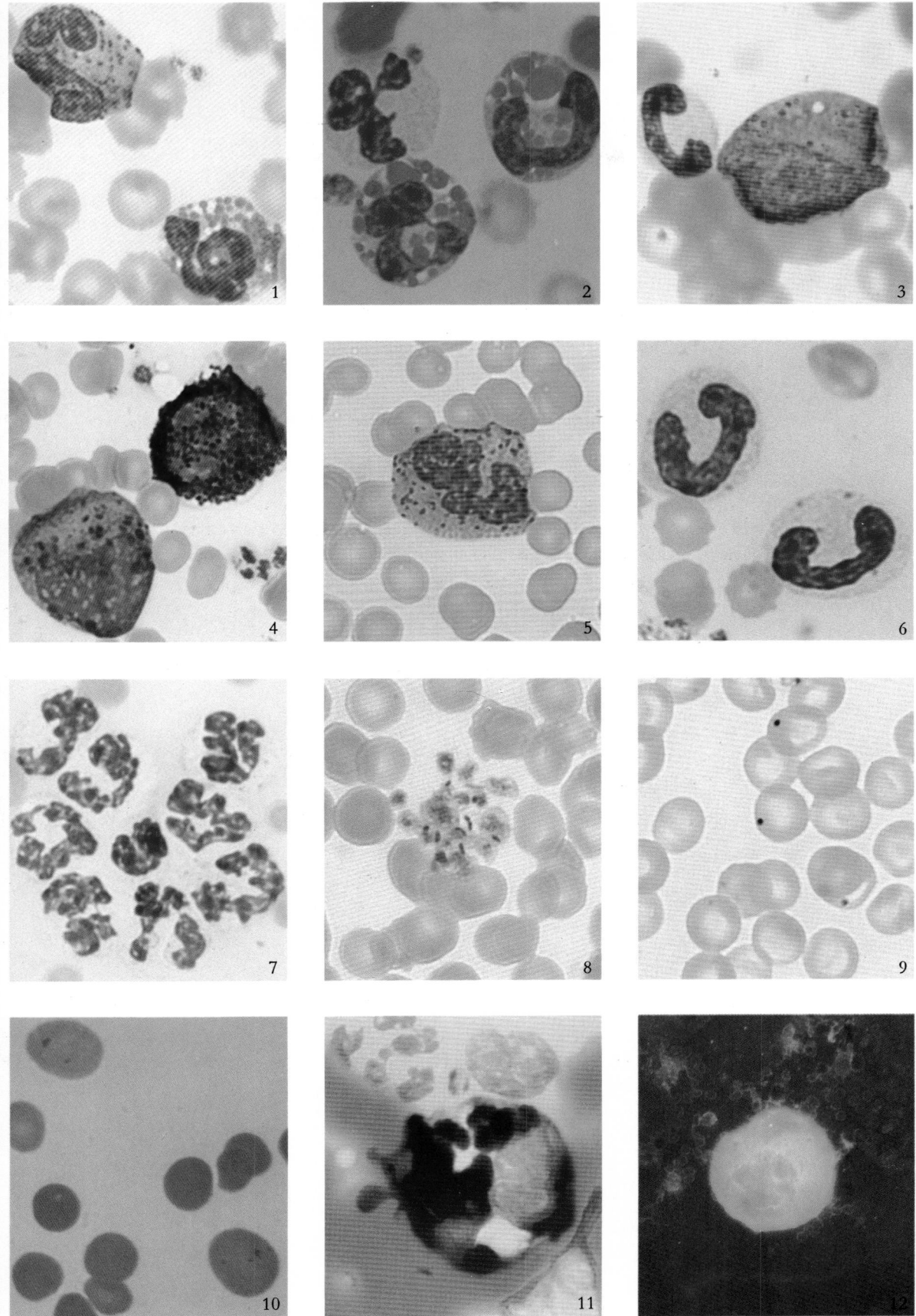

PLATE XIII. BLOOD AND BONE MARROW CELLS IN DISEASES OF THE DOG

1–4.   Prominent, coarse, azurophilic granules in two lymphocytes (1 and 2), a monocyte (3), and a neutrophil (4) in blood of a dog with mucopolysaccharidosis. Individual granules may appear to be within a clear vacuole or surrounded by a halo as seen in the lymphocytes ($\times$1,800). (From Schalm, O.W.: Canine Pract., pp. 28–32, Dec., 1977.)

5–6.   Morulae of *Ehrlichia canis* in a lymphocyte (5) and a neutrophil (6) in the peripheral blood of a dog ($\times$1,800). (From Schalm, O.W.: Canine Pract., pp. 13–17, Nov.–Dec., 1974.)

7–9.   Flame cells, i.e., plasma cells with abundant reddish cytoplasm, in the bone marrow of a dog with IgA myeloma (7, $\times$1,400; 8 and 9, $\times$800). (Courtesy of Dr. J.G. Zinkl. For details of this case see Zinkl et al.: Vet. Clin. Pathol., 12(3):15, 1983.)

10–12. A macrophage with phagocytosed polychromatic red cell and rubricytes (10) and a macrophage with phagocytosed red cells and band neutrophil (11) in bone marrow smears and erythrophagocytosis (12) in histologic section of the bone marrow from a dog with histiocytic medullary reticulosis or malignant histiocytosis (10 and 11, $\times$1,800; 12, $\times$1,260). (From Schalm, O.W.: Canine Pract., pp. 42–45, Aug. 1978.)

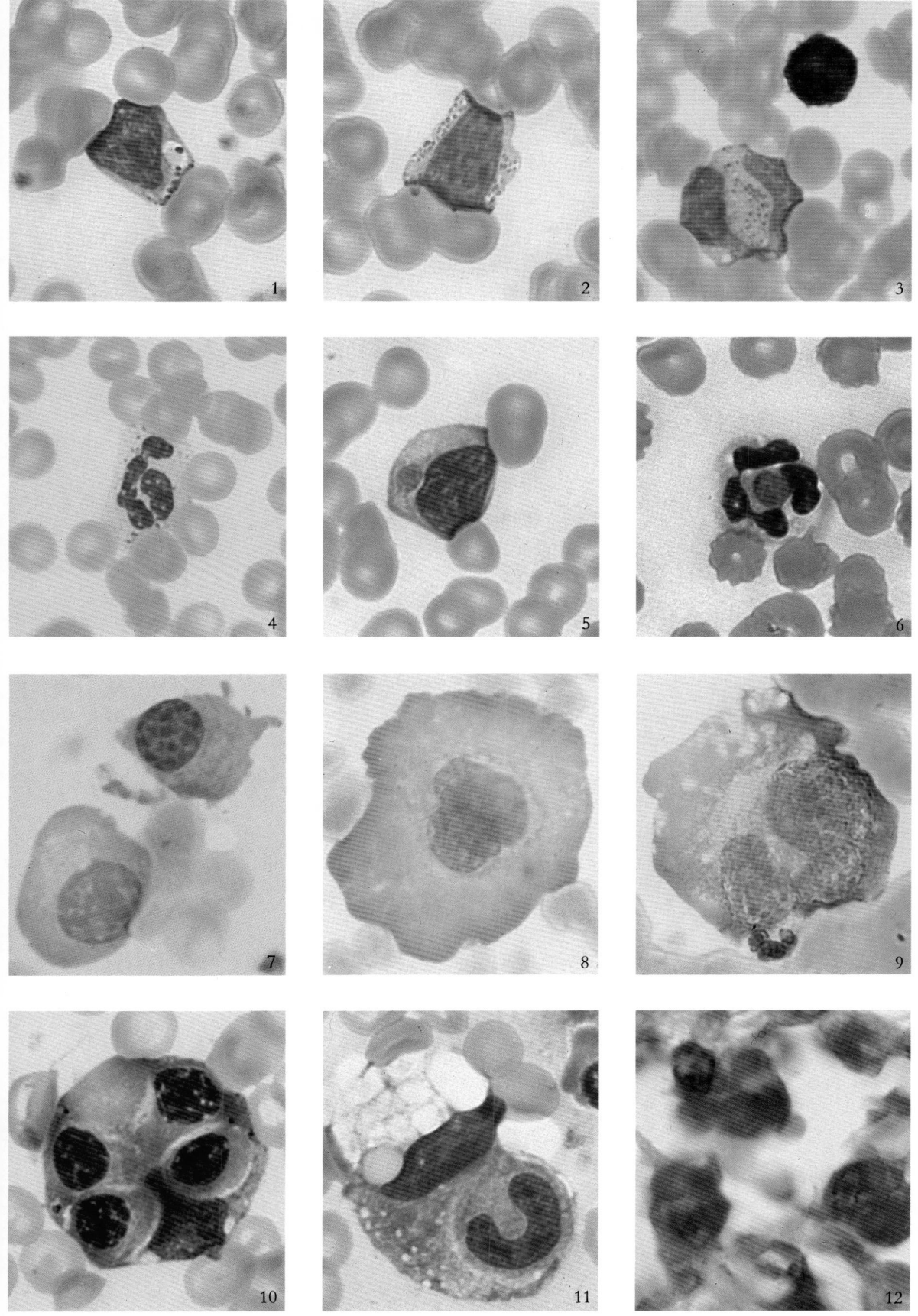

PLATE XIV. PARASITES AND ABNORMALITIES IN LEUKOCYTES OF VARIOUS ANIMAL SPECIES (×1,800)

1. Neutrophils in the blood of a horse. One neutrophil contains four morulae of *Ehrlichia equi*.

2. Band neutrophil in the blood of a horse containing two morulae of *Ehrlichia equi*.

3. A morula of *Ehrlichia equi* in a neutrophil of a horse stained with new methylene blue.

4. Morulae of *Ehrlichia* (arrow) in a monocytoid cell of the bone marrow of an experimentally infected dog.

5. A cytoplasmic inclusion with azurophilic granulation in the neutrophil of a cat with feline infectious peritonitis (Ward, J.M., Smith, R., and Schalm, O.W.: J. Amer. Vet. Med. Ass., *158*:348, 1970). The structure may possibly be a *Chlamydia* occurring coincidentally with infectious peritonitis.

6. Inclusion similar to that in Plate XIV-5 occurring in a mononuclear cell in peripheral blood of a cat presented with an idiopathic anemia. (Appendix Case 49.)

7. An inclusion in the cytoplasm of a lymphocyte in peripheral blood of a young dog with distemper (Appendix Case 37).

8. A blast cell, suggestive of a rubriblast, containing a cyst of *Toxoplasma gondii*. From the bone marrow of a cat in the terminal phase of erythroleukemia.

9. Trophozoites of *Toxoplasma gondii* in the same bone marrow as Plate XIV–8.

10. Neutrophil containing phagocytosed staphylococci from peripheral blood of a cat with staphylococcal septicemia.

11. A sideroleukocyte in the blood of a horse with an idiopathic anemia. The horse was negative to the immunodiffusion test for equine infectious anemia.

12. Lupus erythematosus cells in dog blood. A rosette of neutrophils surrounds amorphous nuclear material. Two of the neutrophils are typical LE cells, as shown by the filling of their cytoplasm with amorphous nuclear material (arrow).

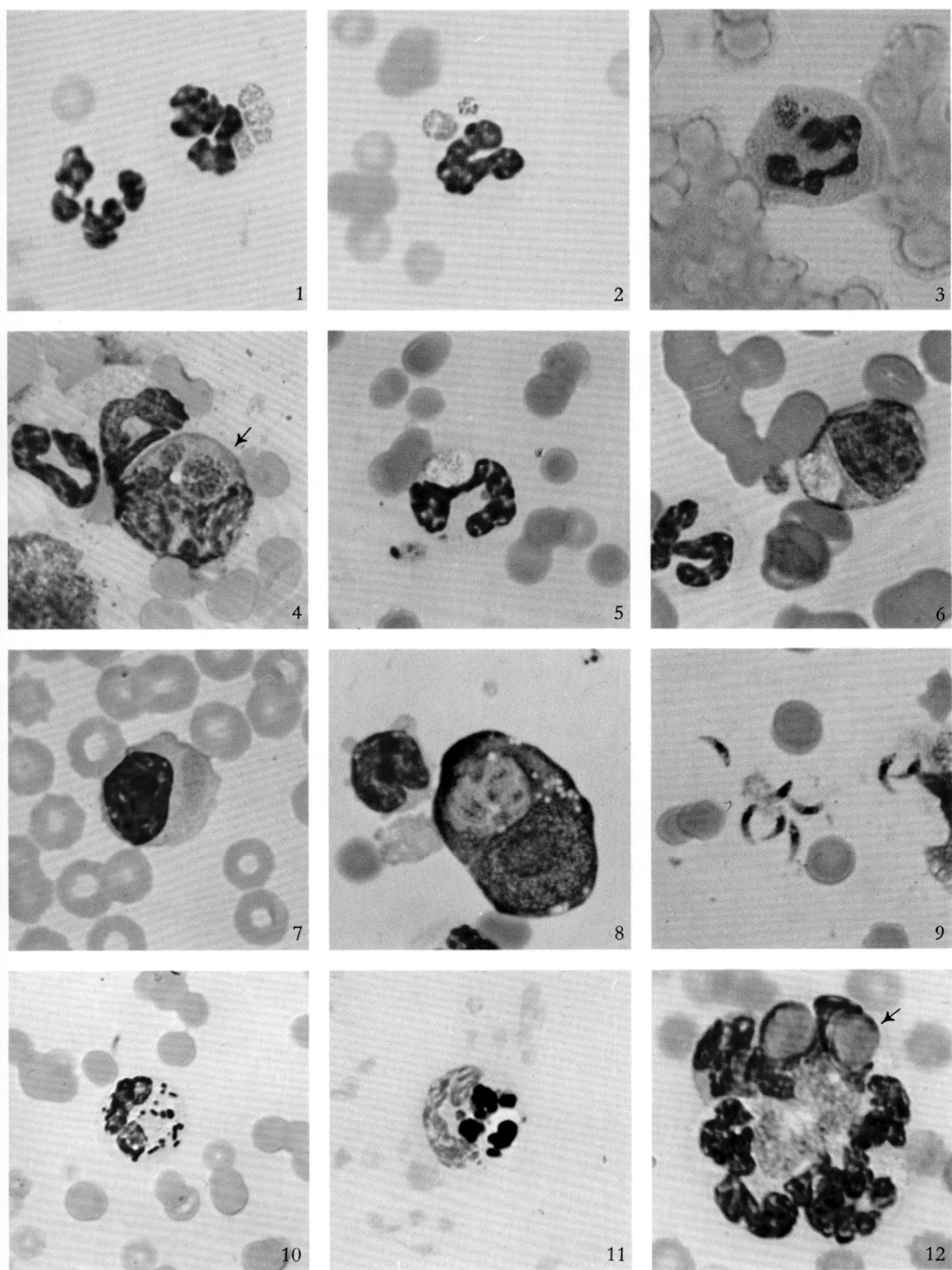

PLATE XV.   ABNORMAL BLOOD AND BONE MARROW CELLS OF THE CAT
(×1,800)

1. A blast cell in the blood in undifferentiated myeloproliferative disorder (reticuloendotheliosis).

2. Two unclassified cells in the blood in undifferentiated myeloproliferative disorder. One cell has reddish cytoplasmic granules.

3. An unclassified cell with a pseudopod and cytoplasmic granules in the bone marrow in undifferentiated myeloproliferative disorder.

4. Two megaloblastoid rubricytes in the bone marrow in erythremic myelosis. Notice the difference in cytoplasmic maturation.

5. A megaloblastoid rubricyte with iron granules (sideroblast) in the bone marrow in erythremic myelosis (iron stain).

6. A macrophage with two phagocytosed erythrocytes from the bone marrow of a cat with feline infectious anemia. Erythrophagocytosis is a common finding in anemias due to various causes in the cat. A lymphocyte and a metarubricyte are also seen.

7. A macrophage with a phagocytosed eosinophil from the bone marrow in a chronic disease associated with development of an aplastic marrow.

8. A giant metamyelocyte, a small lymphocyte, and a basophilic rubricyte in the bone marrow in panleukopenia. Maturation of the granulocyte has taken place directly from a primitive precursor cell without mitosis. Giant granulocytes with bizarre nuclear patterns are common in the bone marrow of the cat under conditions of depressed granulopoiesis.

9. A giant metamyelocyte in blood in depressed granulopoiesis.

10. Two giant, toxic band neutrophils in convalescent blood from panleukopenia.

11. An abnormal maturation form of a granulocytic precursor cell (myelocyte) in the blood in staphylococcal septicemia. (See also Plate XIV–10.)

12. Toxic granulation of neutrophils in blood of a 3-month-old kitten with pneumonitis. Toxic granulation is not a common finding in feline neutrophils. See Plate XI–10 for the more commonly encountered toxic signs in neutrophils of the cat.

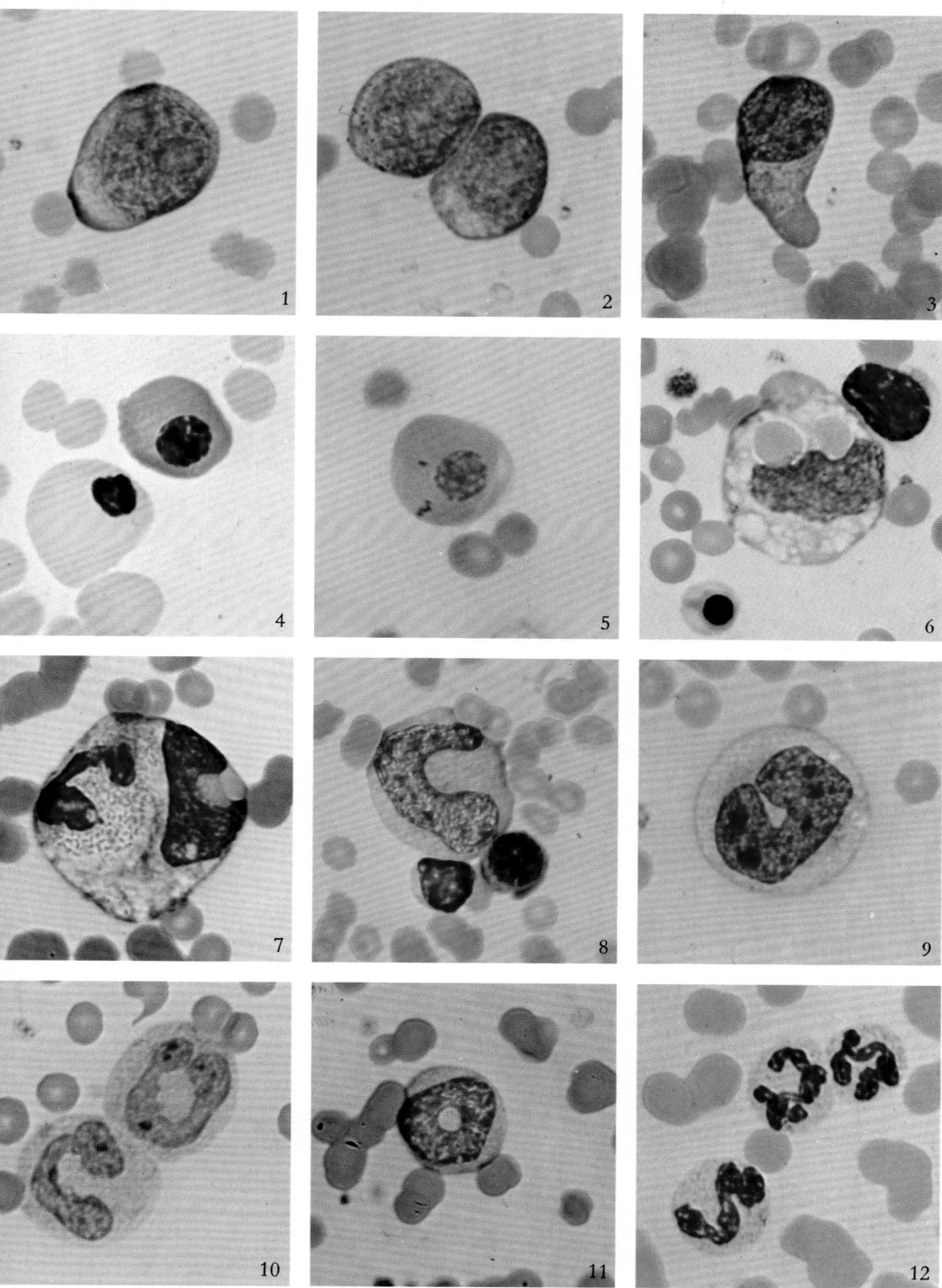

PLATE XVI.   HEINZ BODIES IN FELINE BLOOD ($\times 1,800$)

1. Anemia in remission. The large, grayish erythrocytes and the two nucleated cells are young red blood cells released to the circulation in response to anemia. Each small, mature red blood cell presents a pale structure near one edge that protrudes beyond the edge of some of the erythrocytes. These protruding structures are Heinz bodies. Destruction of Heinz body-laden erythrocytes, mainly by the spleen, leads to hemolytic anemia.

2. The appearance of Heinz bodies in a dry, unfixed blood film. Several of the white protrusions have broken away from the erythrocytes and are free between the cells.

3. Same blood as in Plate XVI-1 and 2 treated as a hanging drop stained with new methylene blue. The Heinz body in the red blood cell appears black (surface stain) when in focus, and it becomes refractile when the surface is out of focus. This characteristic suggested the name erythrocyte refractile body or ER body. (See Schalm, O.W., and Smith, R.: Small Anim. Clin., 3:311, 1963.)

4. Heinz bodies as they appear in a dry, unfixed blood film stained with new methylene blue. A metarubricyte and an unclassified cell are also present.

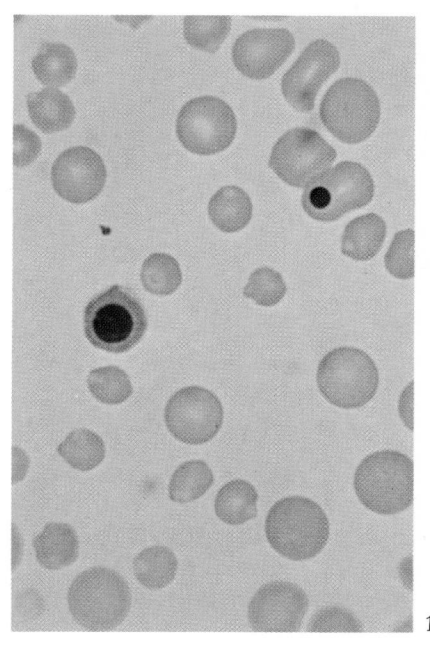

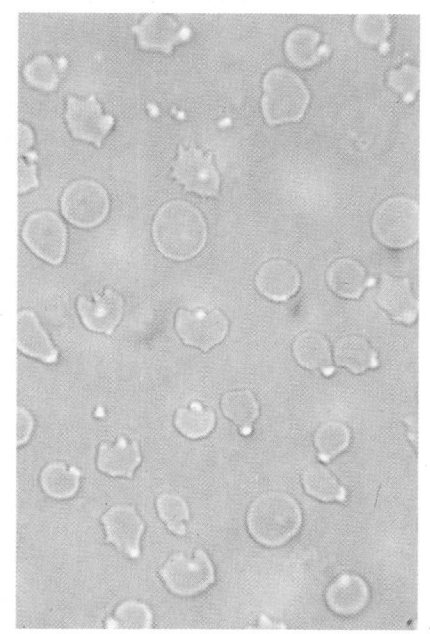

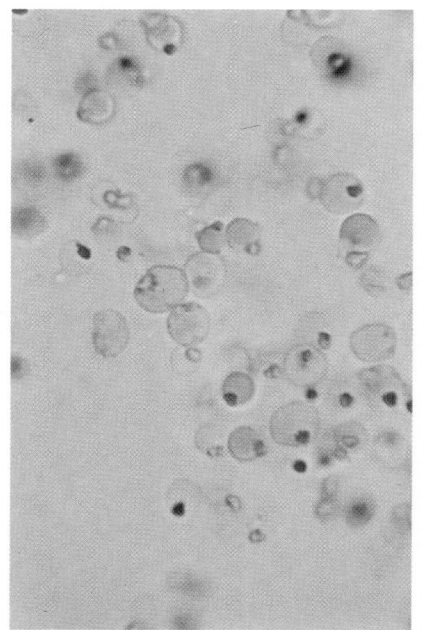

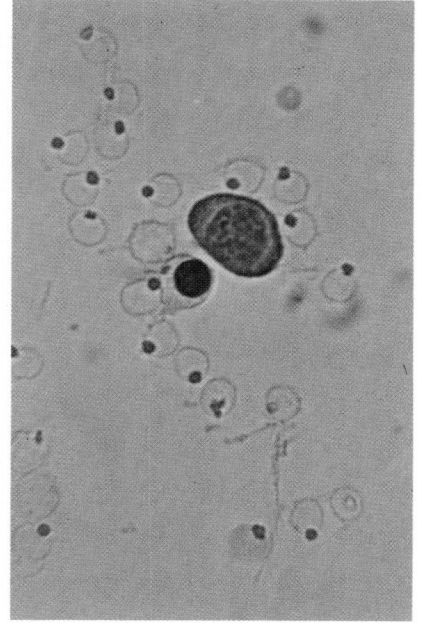

PLATE XVII. ERYTHROCYTES IN VARIOUS ANEMIAS ($\times 1,800$)

1. Microcytic hypochromic anemia from chronic blood loss in a dog. A blood transfus
    was given before the blood for this figure was taken. Normal transfused erythrocytes
    more deeply stained and are larger than some of the microcytic hypochromic cells.
    regularly shaped erythrocytes (poikilocytes) represent fragments of poorly formed ce

2. Bone marrow from the same dog represented in Plate XVII–1. A promyelocyte, two l
    rubricytes, and two metarubricytes are present. The metarubricytes increase in numb
    out of proportion to earlier maturative forms of rubricytes as they await hemoglo
    synthesis before extrusion of their nuclei.

3. Peripheral blood in anemia in remission in a dog. A metarubricyte, an erythrocyte w
    a Howell-Jolly body, and many polychromatophilic macrocytes are seen. Polychroma
    philic red cells will usually appear as reticulocytes when blood is stained with new me
    ylene blue or a reticulocyte stain. See Plate IV–6.

4. Peripheral blood of a dog with autoimmune hemolytic anemia in remission. The sm
    densely stained erythrocytes are spherocytes. A metarubricyte is seen. The majority
    cells are macrocytic erythrocytes, some of which present target-cell patterns and may
    polychromatophilic. Excessive surface membrane in relation to inner contents produ
    target-cell and bowl-shaped patterns in young red cells.

5. Blood in autoimmune hemolytic anemia in a cat. Note the cluster of agglutinated po
    chromatophilic erythrocytes. Polychromatophilic erythrocytes normally do not particip
    in the formation of clumps, and thus the phenomenon is indicative of action of an antibo
    A metarubricyte is seen. (Appendix case 51.)

6. Lymph node section of a cat with a myeloproliferative disease. Cells of the mononuc
    phagocyte system are engorged with erythrocytes (arrow) and hemosiderin. Extre
    erythrophagocytosis as seen in this figure may lead to a rapid fall of PCV. (Appen
    Case 50.)

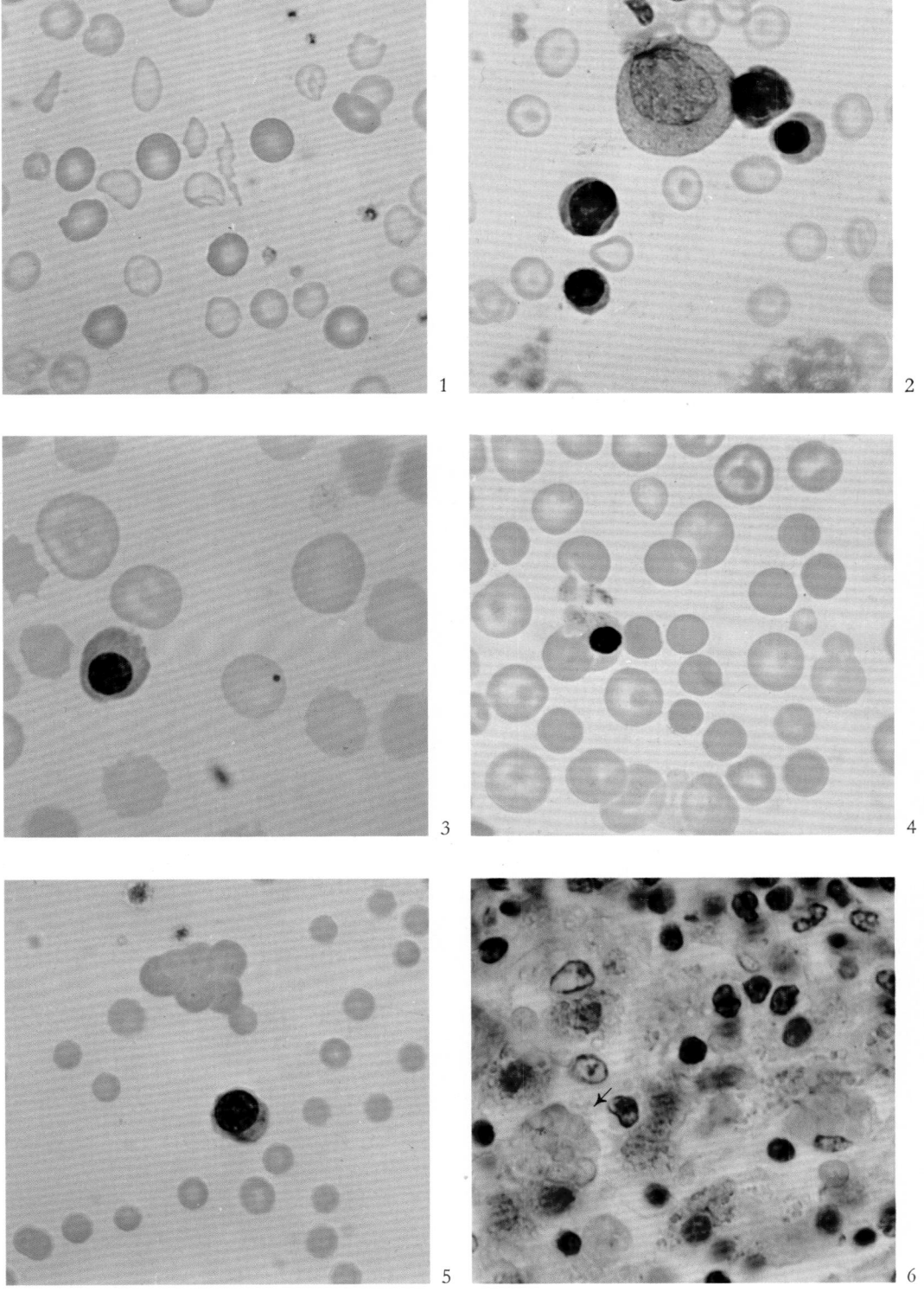

PLATE XVIII.   HEMOPARASITES AND ERYTHROCYTE ABNORMALITIES (× 1,800)

1. Blood in feline infectious anemia. One erythrocyte in the center area contains a round, deeply stained structure called a Howell-Jolly body. All other objects on the surface or at the margin of erythrocytes are *Haemobartonella felis*.

2. Blood in feline infectious anemia. *Haemobartonella felis* appears as faintly stained spheres on the surface of erythrocytes and as more deeply stained specks and short rods on the outside margin. (See also Fig. 23–4.)

3. Blood from a splenectomized dog showing isolated dots and chains of *Haemobartonella canis* on the surface of erythrocytes.

4. Bovine blood with both *Anaplasma marginale,* appearing as round, deeply stained structures in an eccentric position in two erythrocytes (arrows), and *Eperythrozoon wenyoni,* appearing as faintly stained objects on the surface or at the margin of several erythrocytes (see also Fig. 23–7).

5. Same blood as Plate XVIII–4, with a ring-like structure of *E. wenyoni* more clearly visible on the erythrocyte in the center (arrow). The same erythrocyte has another *E. wenyoni* on its margin. These structures are to be compared with the more deeply stained *A. marginale* located inside and at the margins of two erythrocytes.

6. Erythrocytes containing *Babesia canis.*

7. Bovine blood with many *Anaplasma marginale* in erythrocytes. A polychromatophilic rubricyte and a polychromatophilic erythrocyte are also present. The latter two cells indicate that the developing anemia is in a stage of beginning remission.

8. Heinz bodies in bovine erythrocytes in onion poisoning. Blood stained as for the routine reticulocyte count (see Chapter 2 for method).

9. Canine distemper inclusions in erythrocytes. These inclusions vary in size and staining characteristics and occur in young erythrocytes. They are seen only infrequently in canine distemper (see Fig. 36–1 and Appendix Case 37).

10. Basophilic stippling of a bovine erythrocyte. Stippled immature erythrocytes appear in peripheral blood in response to blood loss or hemolytic anemia in ruminants.

11. Two stippled polychromatophilic erythrocytes in the blood of a dog with lead poisoning.

12. A metarubricyte with a few punctate granules in peripheral blood of a horse with lead poisoning.

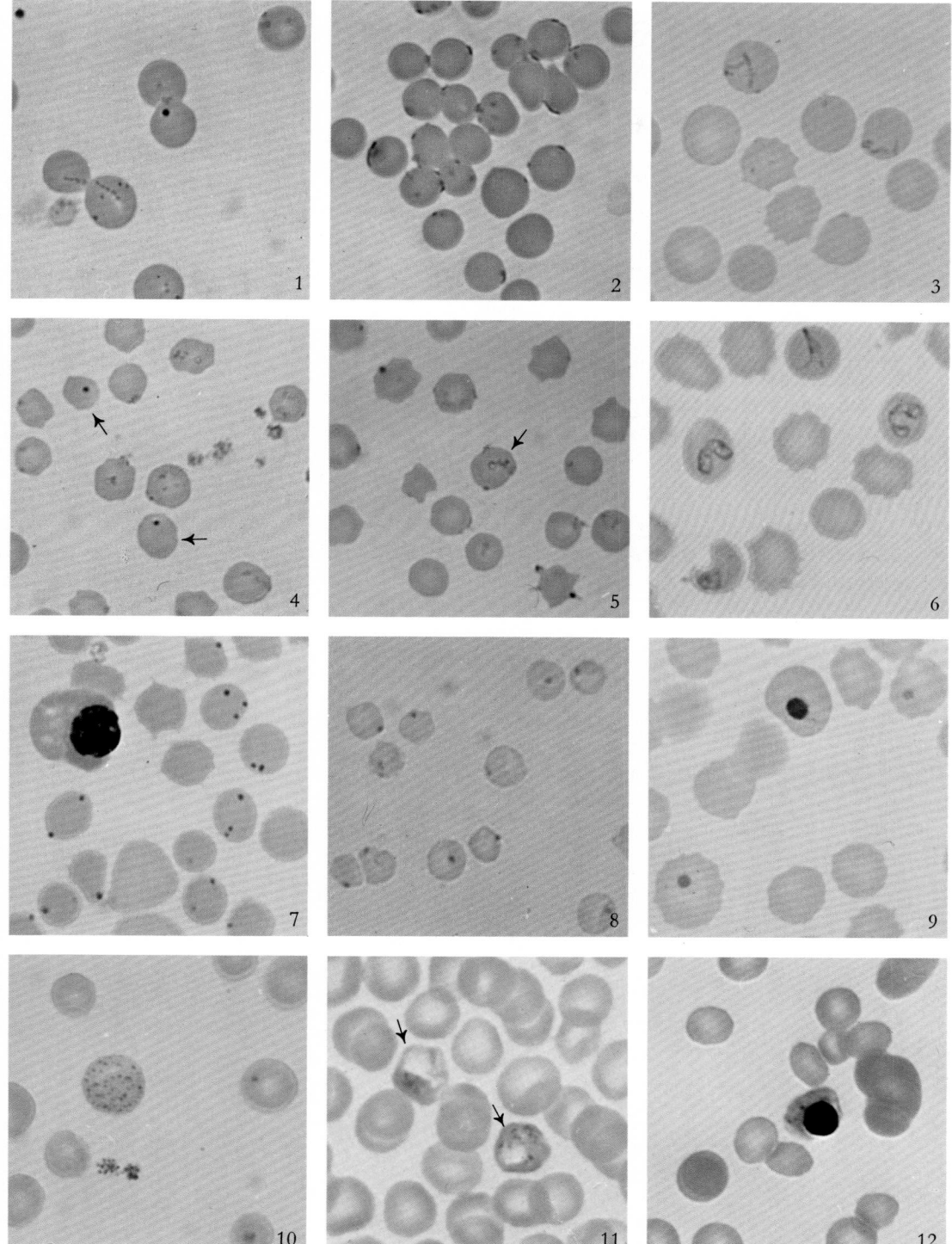

PLATE XIX.   MYELOPROLIFERATIVE DISORDERS IN THE CAT ($\times 1{,}800$)

1. Abnormal rubricytes in the bone marrow in suspected vitamin B_{12}-folate deficiency. Note the abnormal chromatin patterns of the two central cells.

2. Bone marrow cytology in a myeloproliferative disorder in which the primitive proliferating cells are of rubricytic origin. The nuclear chromatin patterns are similar to those of some cells seen in vitamin B_{12}-folate deficiency. Compare with Plate XIX–1.

3. Blood in erythremic myelosis exhibiting marked variation in size of fully hemoglobinized erythrocytes.

4. Blood in erythremic myelosis in which large numbers of nucleated erythrocytes are seen without accompanying anisocytosis or polychromasia. This pattern clearly indicates a myeloproliferative disorder involving the rubricytic series and leading to ineffective erythropoiesis.

5. Bone marrow of the same cat from which the blood was taken for Plate XIX–4. Primitive unclassified cells, possibly rubricytic in origin, two of which have cytoplasmic pseudopod-like projections. The more mature nucleated cells in the blood (Plate XIX–4) may have had their origin from extramedullary hematopoiesis in the greatly enlarged liver and spleen. See Plate XX–5 for liver histopathology.

6. Agglutinated polychromatophilic erythrocytes and metarubricytes in the bone marrow in a myeloproliferative disease. Also seen is a giant metarubricyte with two abnormal nuclei.

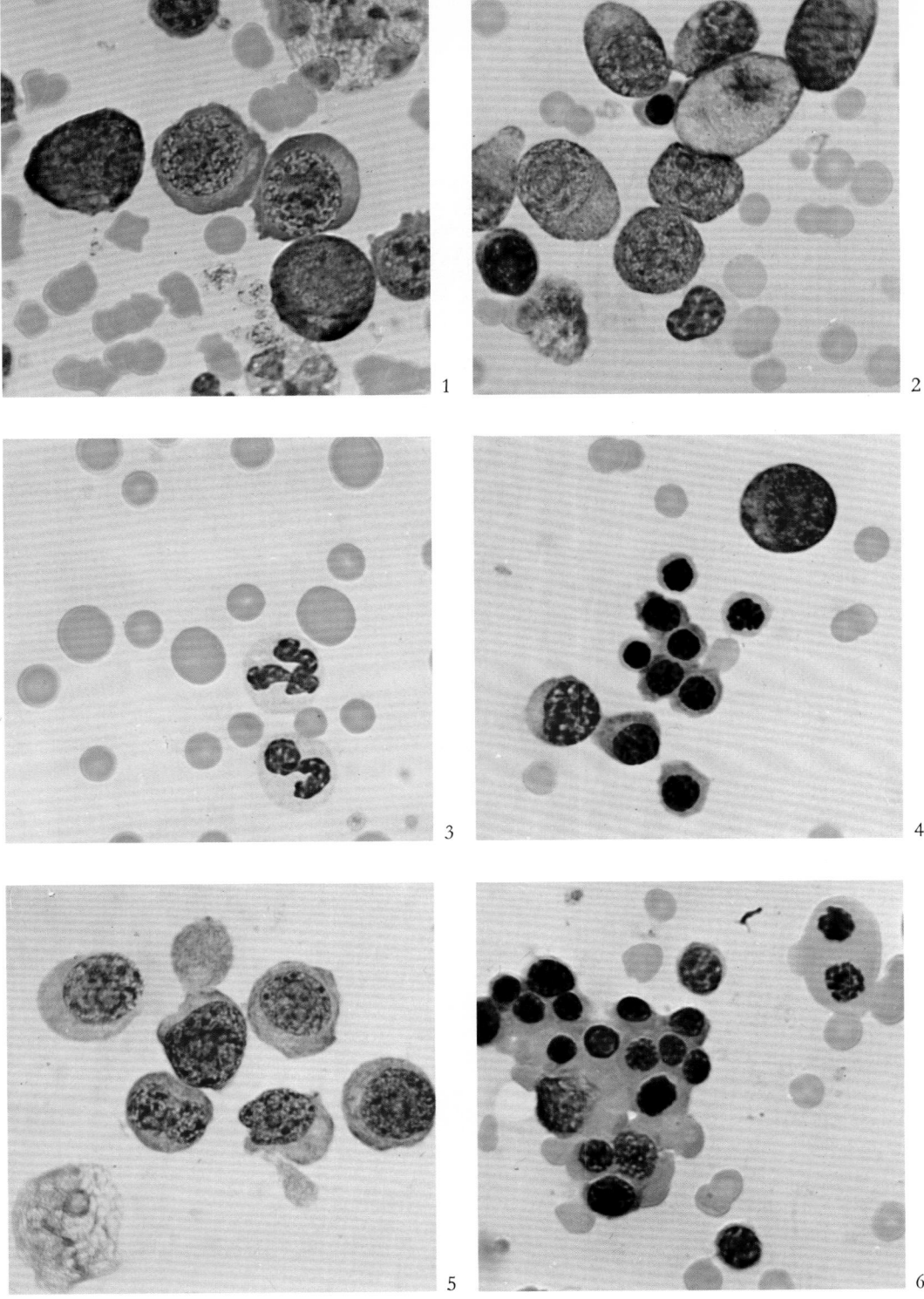

PLATE XX. MYELOPROLIFERATIVE DISORDERS IN THE CAT

1. Polyploidy involving polychromatophilic rubricytes in the bone marrow ($\times$1,800).

2. Erythrophagocytosis by a primitive cell of the bone marrow in erythremic myelos $(\times 1,800)$. See Cat 4, Table 32–4.

3. Bone marrow cytology in erythroleukemia at a time when megaloblastoid rubricytes we prominent. Marked asynchronism is seen between cytoplasm and nucleus of one rubricy $(\times 1,800)$. See Cat 6, Table 32–4.

4. Bone marrow of the same cat as in Plate XX–3 taken 10 days later. Granulocytic precurs cells are predominant, suggesting a change in the direction of granulocytic leukemia. O giant polychromatophilic rubricyte is at the right border ($\times$1,800).

5. A section of the liver in erythroleukemia demonstrating marked distention of sinusoi by proliferating hematopoietic cells. Two mitotic figures are seen in the central sinuso $(\times 1,260)$.

6. A section of bone marrow demonstrating myelofibrosis, which may be a terminal eve in myeloproliferative disease ($\times$900).

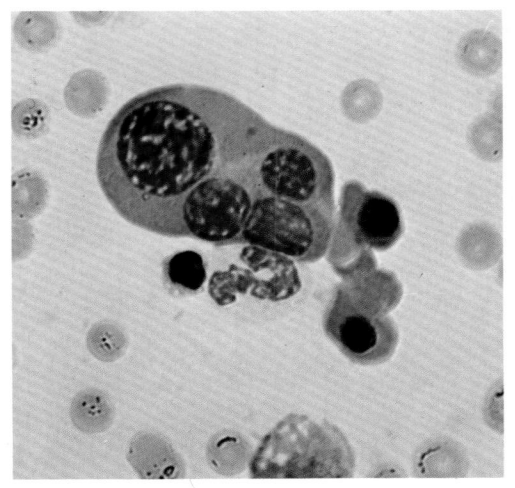

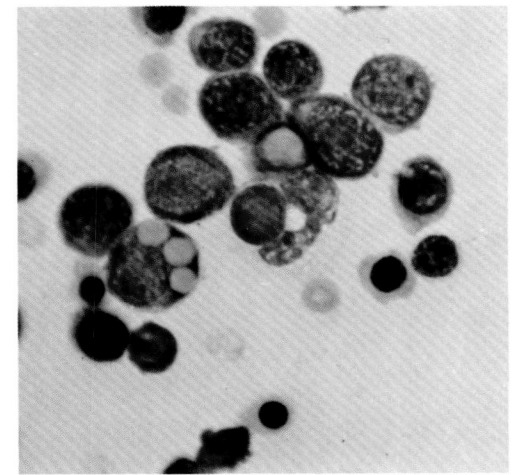

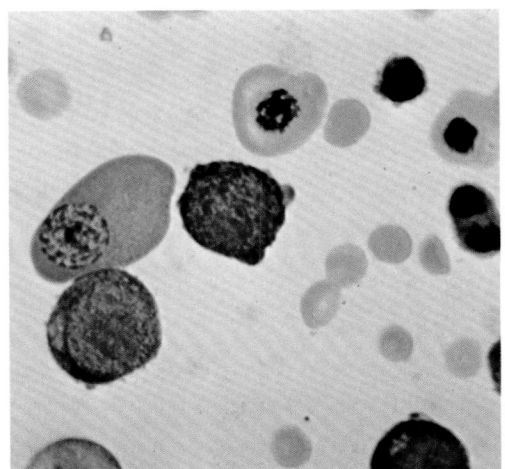

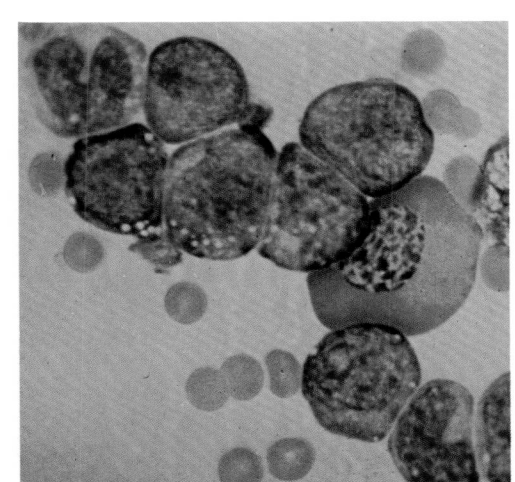

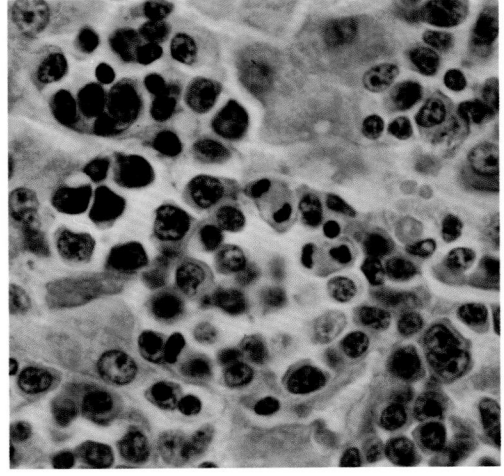

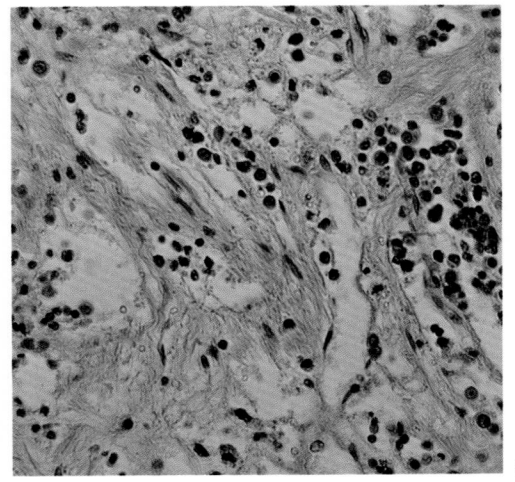

PLATE XXI.   LYMPHOCYTIC LEUKEMIA IN THE DOG AND CAT ($\times 1{,}800$)

1. Lymphoblasts and prolymphocytes in peripheral blood of a dog with lymphosarcoma. Note the single large nucleolus in the cell in center of field. Compare nuclear morphology with cells in Plate XXI–4.

2. Lymphoblasts in fluid aspirated from an enlarged lymph node of a dog with lymphosarcoma.

3. Prolymphocytes in peripheral blood of a cat with lymphosarcoma. Two neutrophils and a small mature lymphocyte are also present.

4. Bone marrow of a cat with lymphosarcoma. A basophil myelocyte is near the center, but most cells are prolymphocytes, some of which contain large vacuoles.

5. Bone marrow of a cat with large, vacuolated lymphoid cells. The diagnosis at necropsy was lymphosarcoma. Compare cell size and morphology with Plate XXI–4.

6. Bone marrow from the same cat as in Plate XXI–5 stained for peroxidase. A peroxidase-positive granulocyte is in center of field. The vacuolated lymphoid cells are peroxidase-negative.

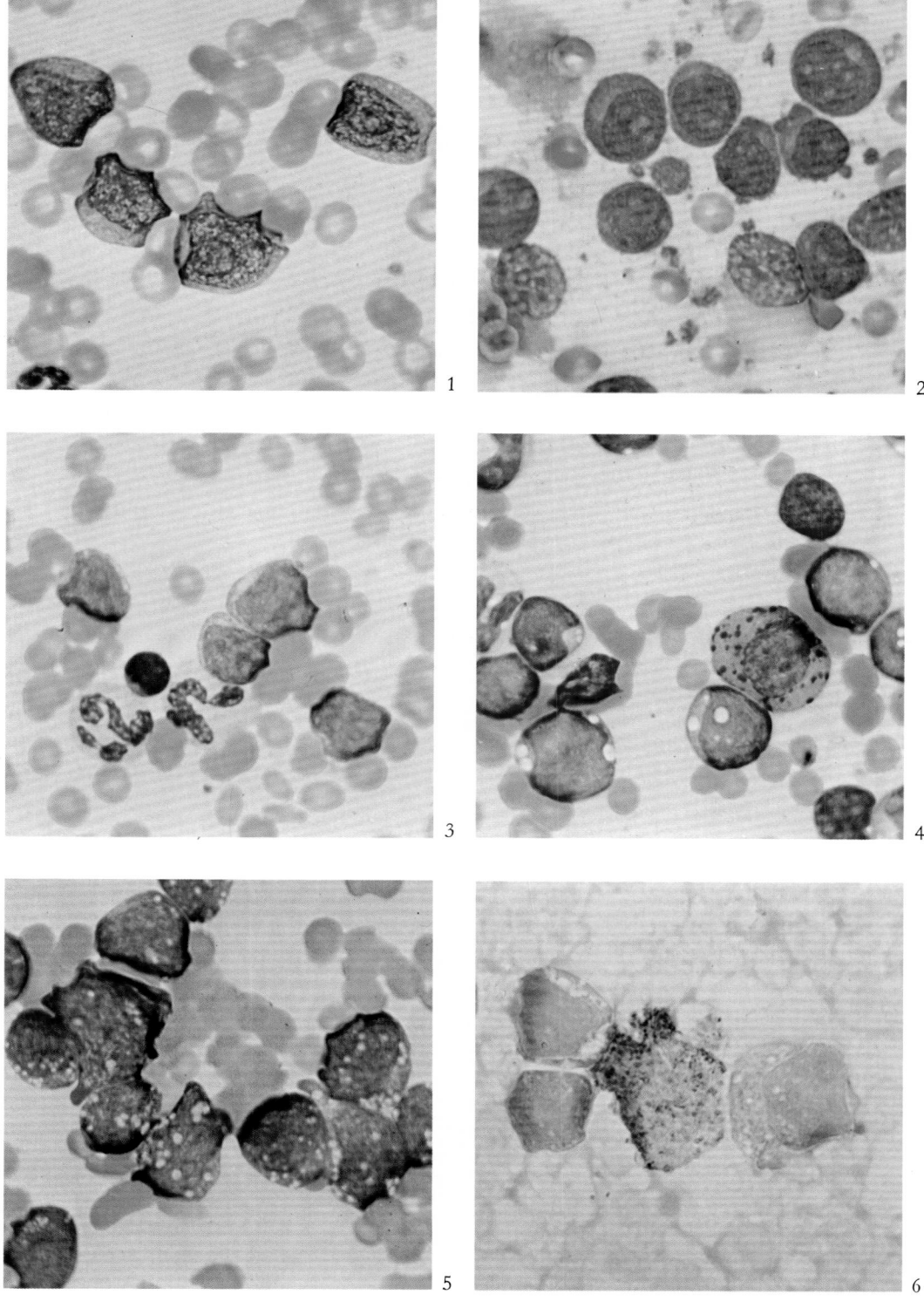

1   2

3   4

5   6

PLATE XXII.   GRANULOCYTIC AND MAST CELL LEUKEMIA IN THE CAT ($\times$ 1,800)

1. Blood in granulocytic leukemia in which the neoplastic cells are limited to myeloblasts, progranulocytes, and myelocytes. The total leukocyte count was 389,000/μl of blood.

2. Bone marrow from the same cat as in Plate XXII–1. The many cytoplasmic azurophilic granules permit identifying the cells as of granulocytic origin, namely, promyelocytes.

3. Bone marrow in subleukemic granulocytic leukemia. Progranulocytes are present, as are bizarre nuclear forms in the more mature granulocytes. See Table 32–6 for hemograms of this cat.

4. Bone marrow in subleukemic granulocytic leukemia. The granulocytes are neutrophilic myelocytes and metamyelocytes. One megaloblastoid normochromic rubricyte is present. See Cat 9, Table 32–4.

5. Bone marrow in eosinophilic leukemia. Two eosinophilic myelocytes and many band and segmented forms of eosinophils are present. See Table 32–7 for details on the blood and bone marrow cytology of this cat.

6. Bone marrow taken at necropsy from a cat with mast cell leukemia. The total leukocyte count in blood was 30,000/μl, of which 35% were mast cells (Fig. 32–23). The spleen was markedly enlarged.

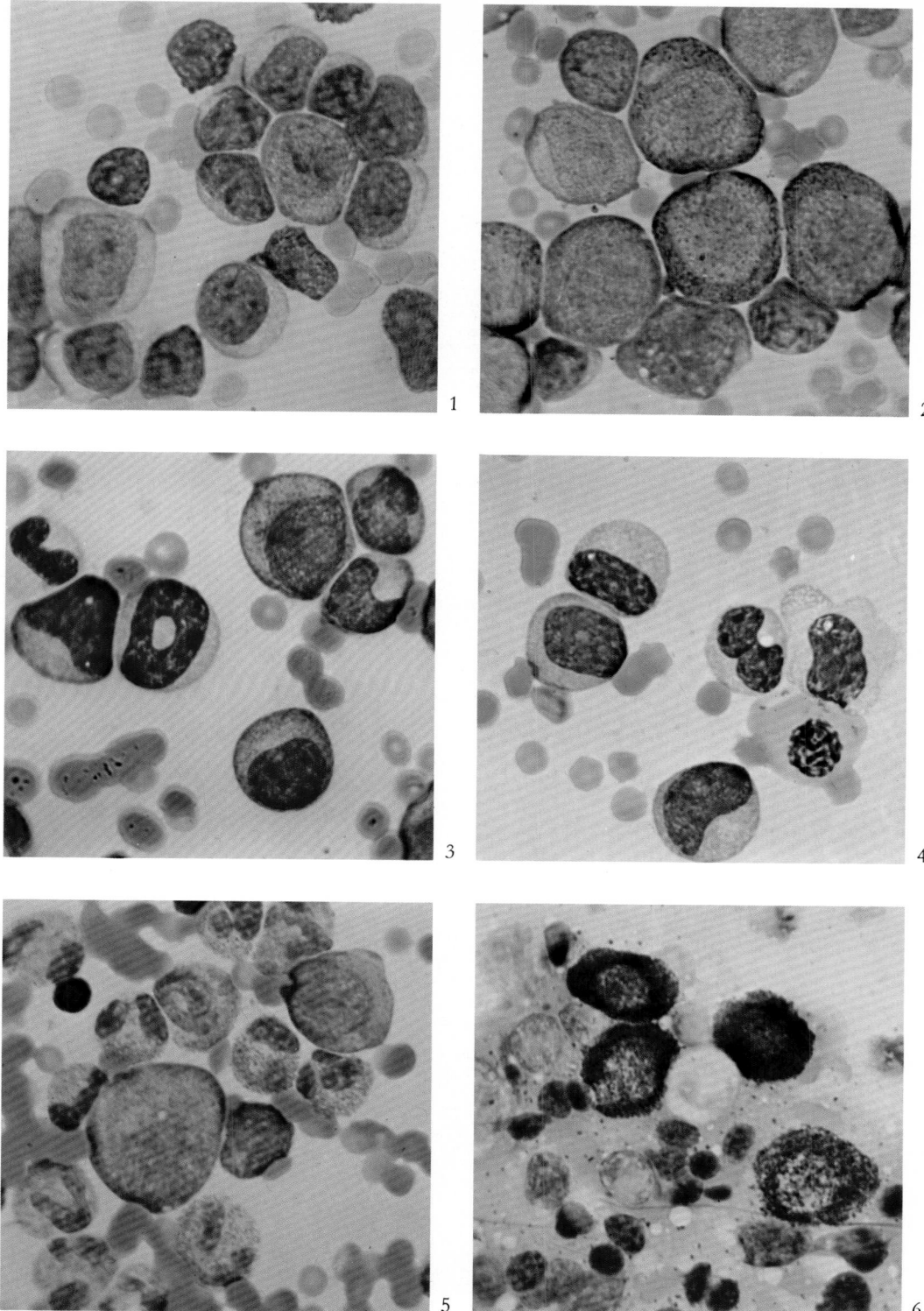

PLATE XXIII. GRANULOCYTIC LEUKEMIA IN THE DOG ($\times 1,800$)

1. Blood in granulocytic leukemia (305,000 leukocytes/μl) with many myeloblasts as well as more advanced maturation forms. The myeloblasts present multiple nucleoli.

2. Blood in granulocytic leukemia (29,900 leukocytes/μl) with myeloblasts and myelocytes. See Table 32–13, 7-year-old Irish Setter.

3. Bone marrow in granulocytic leukemia with giant, bizarre forms of neutrophilic granulocytes. See Table 32–13, 17-month-old German shepherd dog.

4. Bone marrow in granulocytic leukemia presenting myelocytes and metamyelocytes. See Appendix Case 16.

5. Blood with unclassified cells that were peroxidase-negative. The pathologist's study of gross and microscopic tissue changes led to a diagnosis of granulocytic leukemia. See comments for Plate XXIII–6.

6. Bone marrow from the dog from which the blood of Plate XXIII–5 was taken. One cell similar in morphology to the cells seen in the blood and another cell more typical of a bilobed granulocyte are shown to be positive for alkaline phosphatase. This reaction is interpreted as indicative of granulocytic leukemia in the dog. See Chapter 33 for a discussion of the alkaline phosphatase reaction in leukemic granulocytes.

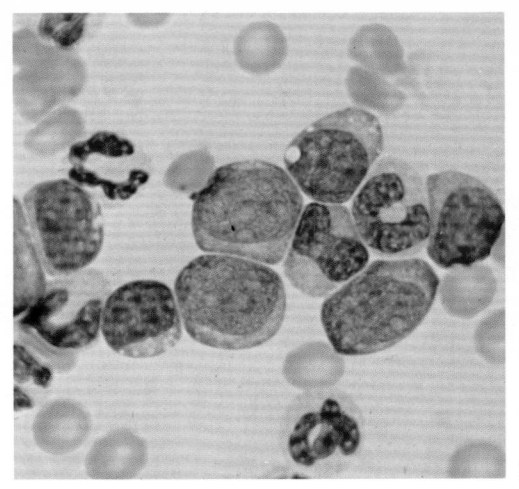

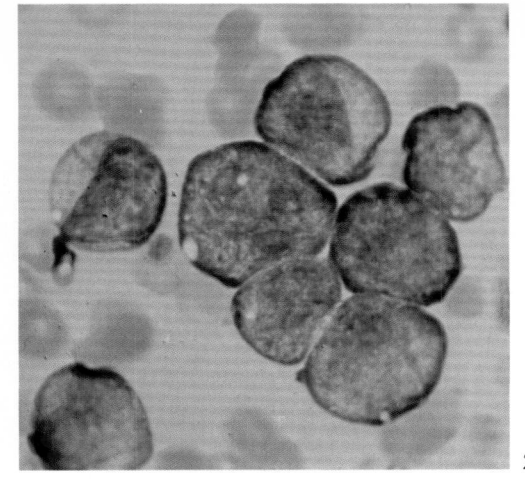

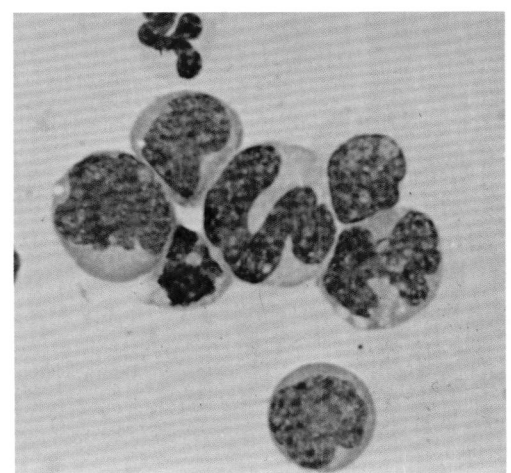

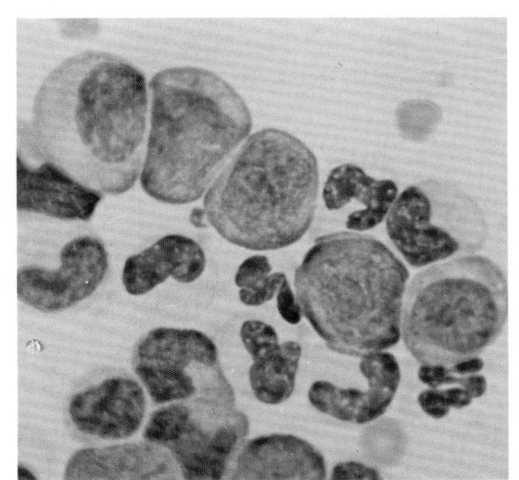

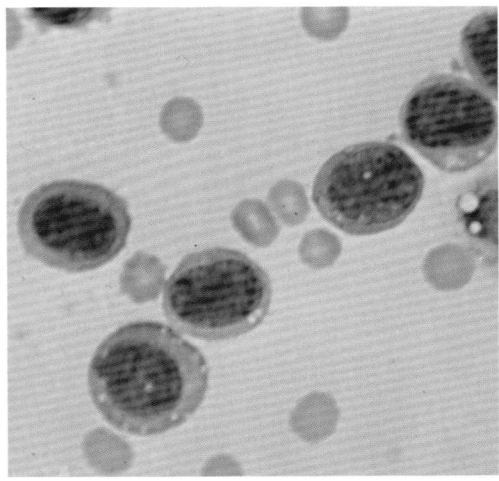

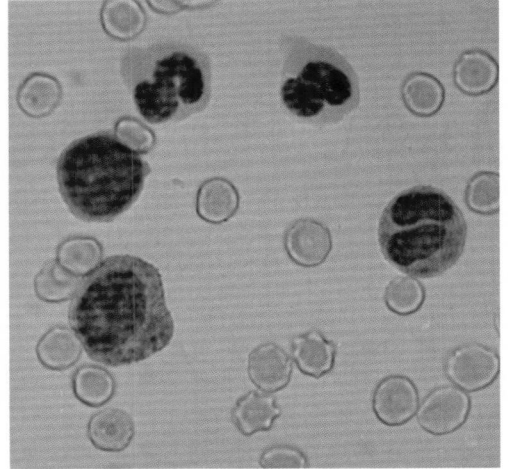

PLATE XXIV.   ACUTE MYELOMONOCYTIC LEUKEMIA IN THE DOG ($\times$1,800)

1. Myeloblasts are recognized by their round or almost round nucleus and other criteria
    cell immaturity such as stippled nuclear chromatin, indistinct nucleoli, and small amou
    of moderate blue cytoplasm giving a high nucleus-to-cytoplasm ratio. The promyeloc
    contains some small azurophilic granules. (Peripheral blood.)

2. A myeloblast in the middle of two monoblasts. With the exception of irregular or cleft
    nuclear outline, the monoblasts have morphologic features similar to those of myeloblas
    (Peripheral blood.)

3. A monoblast, three promonocytes, and a polyploid monocyte. Progressive cellular m
    turity is indicated by increasing nuclear indentation producing a pattern of radiating peta
    of a flower. (Peripheral blood.)

4. Bone marrow showing preponderance of immature monocytoid (cells with folded
    indented nuclei) and myeloid (round cells with regular nuclear outline) precursors.

5. Bone marrow cells stained for alkaline phosphatase (ALP), a cytochemical marker
    myeloid cells. Positive reaction is indicated by fine reddish orange granules in the cy
    plasm. Stained by the method of Kaplow (1955).

6. Bone marrow cells stained for nonspecific esterase (NSE, α-naphthyl acetate substrat
    a monocytic marker, and chloroacetate esterase (ChAcE), a myeloid marker. Positi
    reaction for NSE is indicated by localized reddish orange staining in the cytoplasm, wh
    bluish granular staining is indicative of ChAcE activity. Abnormally increased numbe
    of both ALP-positive (Plate XXIV–6) and NSE-positive immature cells confirmed the m
    phologic diagnosis of acute myelomonocytic leukemia. Stained by the methods of Ya
    et al. (1971a).

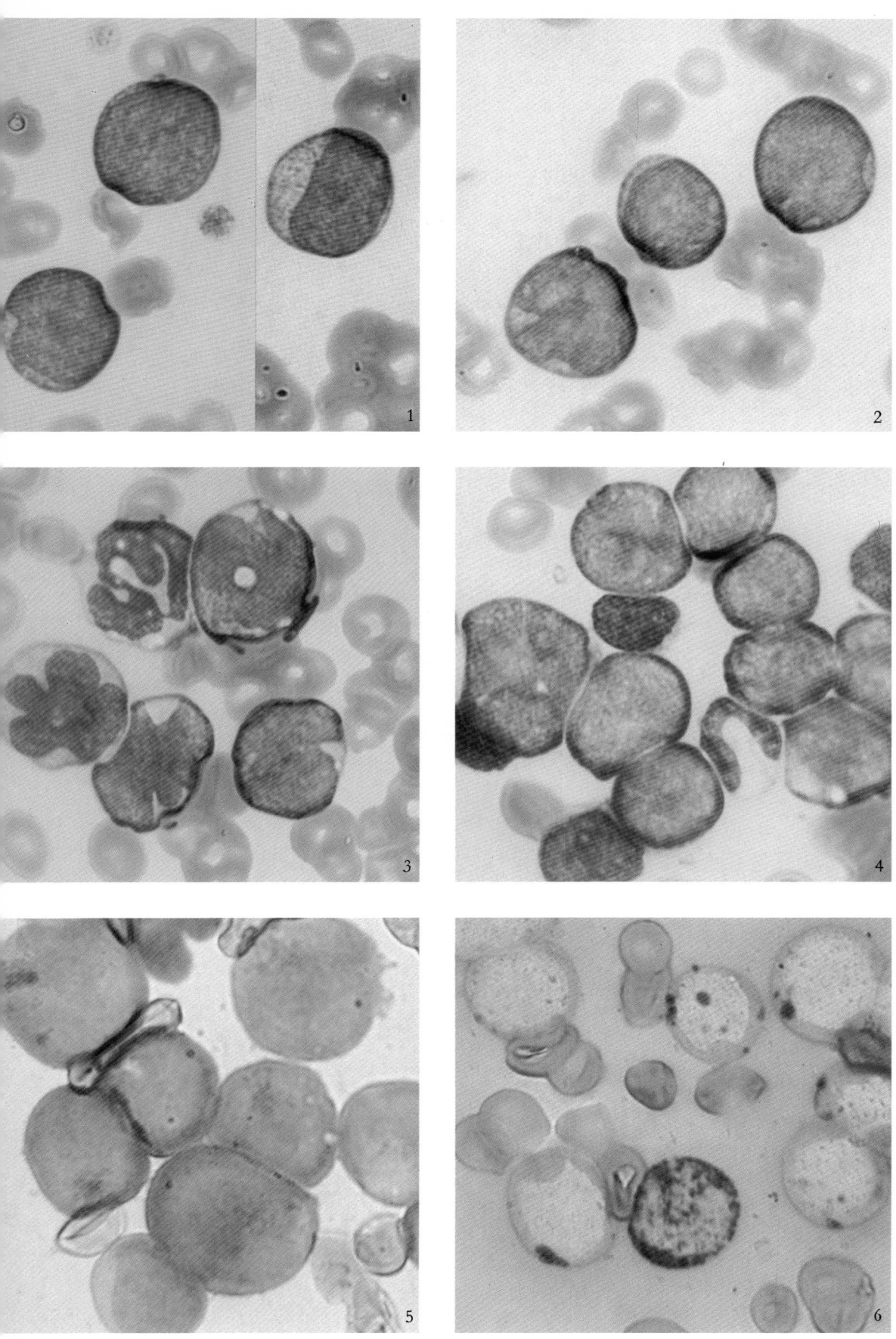

PLATE XXV. BLOOD CELLS AND PARASITES OF BIRDS
(×1,400 except XXV–8, which is ×560)

1. Heterophil, basophil, and two thrombocytes in the blood of a tawny eagle *(Aqu* *rapax).*

2. Eosinophil in the blood of a barn owl *(Tyro alba).*

3. Heterophil and monocyte in the blood of a tawny eagle.

4. Lymphocyte and thrombocyte in the blood of a barn owl.

5. Reticulocytes in the blood of a hyacinth macaw *(Anodorhynchus hyacinthus).* New me ylene blue stain.

6. Microfilaria of an unidentified species in the blood of an umbrella-crested cocka *(Kakatoe alba).*

7. *Borrelia anserina* in the blood of a domestic chicken *(Gallus gallus)* with spirochetos

8. Gametocyte of *Haemoproteus* sp. in an erythrocyte of a great horned owl *(Bubo virg anus).* Note pigment and the halter shape of the organism.

9. Immature gametocytes (trophozoites) of *Plasmodium* sp. in erythrocytes of a Swainso hawk *(Buteo swainsoni).* Note pigment and stained chromatin of the organisms.

10, 11. Gametocytes of *Leucocytozoon* sp. in leukocytes and immature gametocytes of *P modium* sp. in erythrocytes of a Swainson's hawk.

12. Gametocytes of *Leucocytozoon* sp. in a leukocyte of a great horned owl. Note the mark displacement of the host cell nucleus.

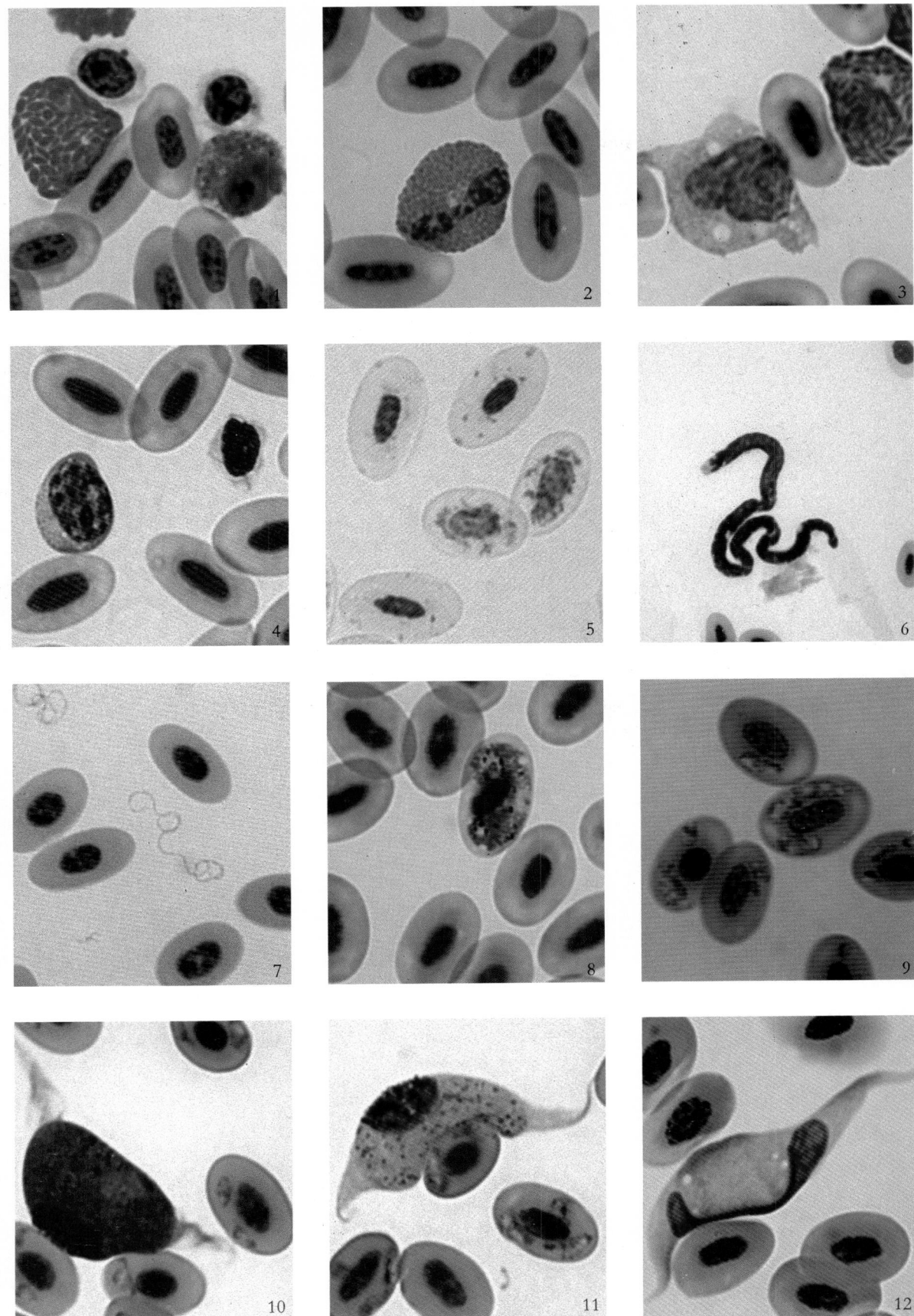

3

Blood Volume and Water Balance

BLOOD VOLUME DETERMINATIONS 87

THE RATIO OF BODY TO VENOUS
    HEMATOCRIT 93

BLOOD VOLUME IN ANIMALS 94

BLOOD VOLUME IN RELATION TO WATER
    BALANCE 96

HEMORRHAGE AND BLOOD
    RESTORATION 96

The total volume of circulating blood is a function of lean body weight. The volume of blood is so important to the dynamics of circulation that it is kept remarkably constant despite the periodic intake of water, the production of water of metabolism, and the continuous water loss via the skin, lungs, kidneys, mammary glands, and alimentary tract. Even in instances of sudden blood loss, the replacement of the lost volume by movement of interstitial fluid into the vascular system is initiated within minutes and continues until the original volume is restored and even exceeded within hours (Table 6–4). In comparison, the depleted erythrocyte volume requires a much longer period for restoration because the addition of a significant number of newly formed erythrocytes to the blood takes at least 72 hours and continues for days and even weeks, depending on the magnitude of the loss. The plasma volume serves as a buffer to maintain blood volume relatively constant, and as the circulating red cell volume is gradually restored, the plasma volume is correspondingly reduced. Even the addition of blood by transfusion does not alter the total volume of blood for long, for the plasma becomes reduced to accommodate the additional cell volume (Smith et al., 1965).

A reduction in blood volume below normal level is termed *hypovolemia* or *oligemia*, while a reduction in the red cell volume is termed *oligocythemia*. The converse are, respectively, *hypervolemia* and *polycythemia*.

BLOOD VOLUME DETERMINATIONS

An estimation of blood volume is desirable for appropriate therapeutic management of patients in circulatory shock resulting from a variety of causes precipitating severe acute blood loss, sequestration of blood in stagnant intravascular pools, and shift of fluids from the intravascular to the extravascular space. It is also valuable in evaluation of anemic and polycythemic patients. A variety of techniques have been used to determine plasma volume, erythrocyte volume, and total blood volume in humans and animals (Table 3–1). Granger (1977) summarized appropriate tracers and relevant principles involved in determination of blood volume in swine, cattle, dogs, rats, fowl, and humans. Based on reliability, reproducibility, and ease of operation in routine clinical use on human patients, the International Committee on Standardization in Haematology (1980) recommended measurement of red cell volume using sodium radiochromate (^{51}Cr) or sodium pertechnetate (^{99m}Tc) as a red cell label and measurement of plasma volume using human serum albumin labeled with radioiodine (^{131}I) as a plasma label. It was stated that the most common method of expressing blood volume is in terms of body weight (ml/kg), but this is theoretically unsatisfactory because the relationship between blood volume and body weight varies according to body composition; for example, in obese subjects blood volume tends to be low in relation to body weight. Blood volume is more closely correlated with lean body mass than with body weight, but the former determination is not practical. Predictions based on surface area are slightly more reliable than those based on body weight alone, especially in obese subjects.

Table 3–1. Selected Examples of Blood Volume Measurements in Animals from the Literature. (Some values were calculated from author's data or converted to ml/kg)

Species and References	Method Employed		Volume in ml/kg or % of Body Weight			Remarks
	Plasma	Erythrocytes	Plasma	Erythrocytes	Total Blood Volume	
Dog						
Reeve et al. (1953)	T-1824	32P	51.0	41.0	92.0	8 normal conscious dogs
	T-1824	32P	52.2	34.8	87.0	5 dogs under pentobarbital anesthesia
	T-1824	32P	46.9	30.9	77.8	16 splenectomized conscious dogs
Woodward et al. (1968)	—	59Fe	58.0± 7.0	44.6±7.7	102.6±12.0 SD	153 beagles, both sexes, 23 ± 11 months
	—	51Cr	56.7± 8.2	42.0±6.7	98.7±12.0 SD	30 beagles, both sexes, 29 ± 12 months
Dellenback et al. (1969)	131I	—	43.4± 4.4	41.3±4.5	84.9± 8.1 SD	10 beagles, 18 months and over
Lombardi (1972)	131I	51Cr	51.0± 5.0	24.0±5.0	75.0± 6.0	25 mongrel dogs, 9–28 kg, anesthetized
Sabourin et al. (1975)	131I	—	52.1± 6.6	39.4±5.8	98.1± 8.9 SD	39 dogs
Lee et al. (1976)	T-1824	59Fe	72.0±11.0	63.0±7.0	135.0±13.0 SD	1-day-old pups, 12 determinations
	T-1824	59Fe	66.0± 8.0	29.0±4.0	94.0±11.0 SD	dogs 1–5 weeks old, 35 determinations
	T-1824	59Fe	66.0± 8.0	27.0±3.0	93.0±10.0 SD	dogs 2–3 months old, 7 determinations
	T-1824	59Fe	49.0± 4.0	45.0± 2.0	94.0± 3.0 SD	dogs 8 months–2 years old, 6 determinations
Hood and Hightower (1976)	131I	—	55.1± 4.1	—	—	5 dogs; using labeled dog albumin
	131I	—	65.1± 4.8	—	—	Same 5 dogs; using labeled human albumin
Cat						
Da Silva et al. (1955)	T-1824	—	3.74%	—	6.71%	7 cats
Spink et al. (1966)	—	51Cr	46.8	19.9	66.7± 3.5 SE	10 cats
Reed et al. (1970)	—	51Cr	48.8	19.0	67.2	2 cats
Cow						
Reynolds (1953a)	T-1824	—	38.8± 1.4	18.6	57.4± 2.1 SD	10 nonlactating cows
Reynolds (1953b)	T-1824	—	38.5	20.7	59.2	20 nonlactating pregnant Guernseys
	T-1824	—	41.1	20.0	64.1	7 lactating nonpregnant Guernseys
Dale et al. (1956)	T-1824	—	39.0	22.2	61.2	3 nonlactating Jerseys, at 70–100°F ambient temperature
	T-1824	—	44.5	25.7	70.2	3 lactating Jerseys, at 70–100°F ambient temperature
	T-1824	—	55.5	29.7	85.2	3 lactating Holsteins, at 70–100°F ambient temperature
Dalton and Fisher (1961)	T-1824	—	—	—	110.0±20.0 SD	38 Ayrshire male calves, 1–3 weeks old
	T-1824	—	—	—	63.0± 8.3 SD	28 mainly nonlactating cows

Reference	Method					Description
Payne et al. (1967)	T-1824	—	54.3	27.9	82.2± 5.9 SD	6 grazing Herefords, 2 months old
	T-1824	—	47.7	26.5	74.2±13.7 SD	6 grazing Herefords, 6 months old
	T-1824	—	43.8	18.9	62.7± 3.8 SD	6 grazing Herefords, 14 months old
	T-1824	—	37.1	24.2	61.3± 6.4 SD	6 grazing Herefords, 38 months old
Mollerberg et al. (1975)	131I	—	54.0± 3.0	—	84.0± 5.0	9 Swedish red and white calves, at birth
	131I	—	63.0± 3.0	—	93.0± 4.0	above animals, at 1 day of age
	131I	—	58.0± 2.0	—	86.0± 4.0	above animals, at 8 days of age
	131I	—	57.0± 2.0	—	79.0± 2.0	above animals, at 30 days of age
	131I	—	50.0± 3.0	—	70.0± 3.0	above animals, at 60 days of age
Water Buffalo						
Pandey and Roy (1969)	T-1824	—	46.1	28.1	74.2± 1.2 SD	5 buffalo cows, nonlactating, nonpregnant
Sodhi and Singh (1975)	T-1824	—	51.8± 4.7	—	71.8± 5.8 SD	7 male buffalo calves, 1–1.5 years old, normal
	T-1824	—	48.4± 3.7	—	72.4± 4.3 SD	above animals, after exercise
	T-1824	—	43.5± 6.1	—	63.5± 6.8 SD	above animals, after 72-hour starvation and water deprivation
Sheep						
Hodgetts (1961)	T-1824	51Cr	46.7± 3.6	19.7±2.8	66.4± 5.4 SD	5 sheep, adrenalin IV to contract the spleen
Creasy et al. (1970)	131I	—	—	—	156.1± 2.9 SD	46 fetuses, 112–146 days in gestation
	—	—	—	—	110.0± 5.0 SD	17 neonatal lambs
	131I	51Cr	89.9± 2.0	44.8±1.8	134.7± 3.1 SD	46 fetuses as above
	131I	51Cr	72.4± 2.6	31.6±2.3	104.0± 4.2 SD	10 neonatal lambs
Wade and Sasser (1970)	59Fe	51Cr	53.2± 8.1	21.1±2.2	74.4± 8.7 SD	40 normal sheep, mean weight 32.6 kg
Sodhi and Sodhi (1976)	131I	—	59.1± 5.7	—	80.8± 5.4 SD*	7 rams, 7–8 years; *from whole blood
	—	—	—	—	86.0± 7.2 SD*	*after correction for trapped plasma (0.95)
	T-1824	—	60.3± 3.9	—	89.9± 6.3 SD*	*from whole blood
	T-1824	—	—	—	87.9± 6.1 SD*	*after correction for trapped plasma (0.95)
Goat						
Courtice (1943)	T-1824	—	53.0	17.0	70.0	30 normal goats
Klement et al. (1954)	131I	51Cr	5.96%	1.4%	7.37%	4 goats
Klement et al. (1955)	T-1824	51Cr	—	—	7.05%	20 goats, blood volume range 5.68–8.49%
Sodhi and Sodhi (1976)	131I		56.4± 0.4	—	70.9± 2.6 SD*	4 goats, 3 years old; *from whole blood
			—	—	76.2± 1.6 SD*	*after correction for trapped plasma (0.81)
	T-1824		60.2± 5.9	—	85.9± 5.9 SD*	*from whole blood
	T-1824		—	—	78.9± 6.0 SD*	*after correction for trapped plasma (0.81)

Table 3–1. *Continued*

Species and References	Method Employed Plasma	Method Employed Erythrocytes	Volume Plasma	Volume Erythrocytes	Total Blood Volume	Remarks
Horse						
Julian et al. (1956)	—	^{32}P	—	—	109.6	6 "hot-blooded" horses, blood volume range 84.5–136 ml/kg
Collery and Keating (1958)	—	^{32}P	—	—	71.7	4 Percherons, range 56.7–101.7 ml/kg
	—	^{32}P	43.0	25.8	68.8	5 ponies weighing 136–333 kg
Obara and Nakajima (1961)	T-1824	^{32}P	41.0	27.6	68.6	5 horses weighing 422–710 kg
	T-1824	—	42.5± 3.2	19.9±2.7	62.4± 4.2	9 horses, 1–2 years old
Dalton and Fisher (1963)	T-1824	—	49.0	24.0	73.0±10.5 SD	12 Clydesdales or Clydesdale crosses with lighter horses
Torten and Schalm (1964)	T-1824	—	42.2	23.9	66.1	2 quarter horse crossbred mares
	T-1824	—	34.7	19.3	54.0	Same 2 mares splenectomized
Marclese et al. (1964)	^{59}Fe	^{51}Cr	63.3± 8.8	39.8±6.5	103.1±13.5SD	31 English Thoroughbred racers
	^{59}Fe	—	52.5± 5.1	25.3±3.5	77.5± 3.8 SD	6 saddle horses
	—	^{51}Cr	43.5± 4.0	18.2±2.4	61.4± 5.9 SD	14 draft horses
Persson (1967)	T-1824	—	57.2	79.7	136.9	13 trotters, 4 years old, males
	T-1824	—	50.7	69.2	119.9	13 trotters, 4 years old, females
Deavers et al. (1973)	T-1824	^{51}Cr	50.8± 5.1	20.7±2.9	71.5± 6.2 SD	11 ponies, 68–147 kg
Burro						
Hansard et al. (1953)	^{131}I	^{32}P	—	—	190.0± 9.0 SE	2 burros, 1 day old
	^{131}I	—	—	—	95.0± 2.0 SE	4 burros, 1–3 months old
	—	^{32}P	—	—	66.0± 4.0 SE	9 burros, 4 years old
	—	—	—	—	62.0± 1.0 SE	13 burros, 4 years old
Pig						
Hansard et al. (1953)	—	^{32}P	—	—	74.0± 3.0 SE	3 piglets, 10 lbs, 2 weeks old
	—	^{32}P	—	—	67.0± 1.0 SE	4 piglets, 20 lbs, 4 weeks old
	—	^{32}P	—	—	63.0± 1.0 SE	8 pigs, 98 lbs, 3–4 months old
	—	^{32}P	—	—	46.0± 2.0 SE	4 pigs, 344 lbs, 2 years old
	—	^{32}P	—	—	35.0± 3.0 SE	3 pigs, 675 lbs, 3 years old
Bush et al. (1955)	^{59}Fe	^{32}P	62.5	32.5	95.0	At 10 kg body wt.
	^{59}Fe	^{32}P	52.3	31.3	83.5	At 20 kg body wt.
	^{59}Fe	^{32}P	48.3	30.0	78.3	At 30 kg body wt.
	^{59}Fe	^{32}P	44.3	28.8	73.0	At 40 kg body wt.
	^{59}Fe	^{32}P	41.9	27.5	69.4	At 50 kg body wt.
	^{59}Fe	^{32}P	40.3	25.8	66.2	At 60 kg body wt.
	^{59}Fe	^{32}P	38.9	24.6	63.6	At 70 kg body wt.
	^{59}Fe	^{32}P	37.8	23.7	61.5	At 80 kg body wt.
	^{59}Fe	^{32}P	37.2	22.5	59.7	At 90 kg body wt.
	^{59}Fe	^{32}P	36.0	22.0	58.0	At 100 kg body wt.
	^{59}Fe	^{32}P	35.4	21.1	56.5	At 110 kg body wt.

(Bush et al. rows:) 76 determinations on 31 swine under 5% pentobarbital anesthesia

Reference						Comments
Monkey						
Gregersen and Rawson (1959)	T-1824	^{32}P	36.4 ± 4.0	17.7 ± 1.7	54.0 ± 4.7 SD	18 *Macaca mulata*, 3.4–7.1 kg
Rabbit						
Armin et al. (1952)	—	^{32}P	—	17.2 ± 1.7	57.3 ± 4.8 SD	71 albino rabbits
	—	^{32}P	—	18.4 ± 2.4	64.7 ± 11.3 SD	9 brown rabbits
Guinea Pig						
Masouredis and Melcher (1951)	^{131}I	—	—	—	75.3 ± 7.1 SE	13 guinea pigs, weighing 414–543 g
Ancill (1956)	T-1824	—	—	—	72.0 ± 3.1 SD	18 normal males
Rat						
Belcher and Harriss (1957)	T-1824	^{59}Fe	53.8 ± 2.6	22.1 ± 1.4	75.9 ± 2.7 SE	Rats weighing 26–50 g
	T-1824	^{59}Fe	45.5 ± 2.5	24.7 ± 1.4	70.2 ± 2.5 SE	Rats weighing 101–125 g
	T-1824	^{59}Fe	30.3 ± 2.4	20.7 ± 2.2	51.0 ± 2.6 SE	Rats weighing 226–250 g
Wang (1959)	T-1824	^{32}P	40.4 ± 2.4	23.5 ± 2.2	63.9 ± 3.6 SD	11 normal Sherman rats, 254 g
	T-1824	^{32}P	38.2 ± 3.9	23.7 ± 1.9	61.9 ± 4.25 SD	10 splenectomized rats, 265 g
Yale and Torhorst (1972)	T-1824	—	36.1 ± 0.7	—	63.6 ± 1.1 SE	30 female germ-free Sprague-Dawley rats
	T-1824	—	32.6 ± 0.4	—	61.0 ± 1.5 SE	32 male germ-free Sprague-Dawley rats
Biewald and Billmeier (1978)	—	^{51}Cr	—	—	47.4 ± 8.0 SE	8 male Sprague-Dawley rats, 170–240 g
Mouse						
Wish et al. (1950)	T-1824	^{32}P	—	—	84.8	3 males, 2 females, anesthetized
	T-1824	^{32}P	—	—	72.0	6 males, anesthetized, dehydrated
Keighley et al. (1962)	T-1824	^{59}Fe	—	—	55.0	6 WB-B_6F_1 mice

Blood volume was found to vary with body surface area curvilinearly in men and linearly in women (Hurley, 1975).

Among the early methods for estimating blood volume by the injection of dyes or other substances into the blood stream, the blue azo dye, T-1824, commonly known as Evans blue, has remained the most popular (Dawson et al., 1920). It is an easy, rapid, and fairly accurate method. A known quantity of Evans blue (e.g., 5 ml of a 0.5% solution in sterile physiologic saline or autologous plasma) is injected intravenously after a preinjection anticoagulated blood sample has been collected, and then sequential blood samples are collected at short intervals over the next 15–30 minutes. Evans blue binds to the albumin fraction of blood plasma, and the quantity of dye per ml contained therein is measured spectrophotometrically at 620 nm; the preinjection plasma is used as the blank. Portions of blood samples are also processed by the hematocrit method to determine the packed cell volume (PCV). The plasma volume and total blood volume are calculated as follows:

$$\text{Plasma volume (ml)} = \frac{\text{mg dye injected}}{\text{mg/ml of dye in plasma}}$$

Blood volume (ml)

$$= \text{plasma volume} \times \frac{100}{100 - \text{PCV in percent}}$$

The Evans blue method overestimates the true total blood volume. The principal sources of error are the variations in the optical density of the plasma collected at different times from the same subject and the undefined in vitro alterations (Senn and Karlson, 1958, Nielson and Nielson, 1962). Extraction methods, in which the dye is extracted for quantitation, eliminate this error, but they are equally inaccurate. Measurement of the optical density of the plasma at both 620 and 740 nm apparently corrects for variations in the density of the plasma itself (Nielson and Nielson, 1962). Although results obtained in this way correlated well with those obtained by the radioiodinated (^{131}I) human serum albumin method, the Evans blue dye dilution method still overestimated the plasma volume of children in 19 out of 20 determinations by up to 10% (Linderkamp et al., 1977).

Another source of error resides in the trapping of plasma within the erythrocyte column in the hematocrit tube (Gregersen and Schiro, 1938). The completeness of packing of the erythrocytes is a function of the relative centrifugal force employed and the duration of centrifugation (Chapter 2). It is necessary, therefore, to employ approved methods of centrifugation to keep the trapping of plasma to a minimum. Factors affecting the amount and distribution of trapped plasma have been discussed (Hlad and Holmes, 1953). Owen and Powers (1953) have summarized trapped plasma values for humans and several animal species. A correction factor for trapped plasma may be introduced in the formula for blood volume determination; for the dog, a 4% (Reeve et al., 1953) or 5% (Billings and Brown, 1955) value has been used as a correction factor. Correction factors suggested for other species are 4–5% for pigs (Anderson, 1970), 6% for cows (Dalton and Fisher, 1961; Reynolds, 1953a), and 19% for goats (Klement et al., 1955). The following is an example of 4% correction factor introduced in the formula:

Blood volume (ml)

$$= \text{plasma volume} \times \frac{100}{100 - \text{PCV} \times 0.96}$$

The amount of trapped plasma in the erythrocyte column varies with the PCV, the size of the erythrocyte, and the degree of rouleau formation. The amount of trapped plasma in general decreases with reduction in PCV and increase in the MCV. Tighter packing of cells is enhanced by the presence of rouleaux and increasing erythrocyte size. Canine blood, characterized by large red cells and the tendency for rouleau formation, and equine blood, characterized by extreme rouleaux, will have less trapped plasma than bovine, ovine, or caprine blood, in which rouleau formation is essentially absent and erythrocyte size is small. A comparison of the Wintrobe and microhematocrit methods revealed 2–3% less trapped plasma by the microhematocrit method in human, canine, and elephant bloods, 5% less in ovine blood, and 9% less in caprine blood (Chien et al., 1965). Caprine blood centrifuged at 2,000 G for 30 minutes was found to have up to 20% trapped plasma;

the same blood centrifuged at 15,000 G for 7.5 minutes had only 2.0% trapped plasma (O'Brien et al., 1957). Hence a common practice to determine PCV for goat and sheep bloods is to perform centrifugation (in the microhematocrit method) for at least twice as long as for dog blood.

Other methods for measurement of blood volume involve the use of radioisotopes. ^{131}I-labeled human serum albumin is commonly used to determine plasma volume (Schultz et al., 1953; Sear et al., 1953) and is more accurate than the Evans blue method discussed above. The procedure is similar to that for the dye dilution technique. Indium (^{111}In) has also been used to determine plasma volume. It binds to transferrin and gives values about 5% higher than the above isotopic method (Campistron et al., 1979; Wintrobe et al., 1981).

[51]Cr-labeling of autologous red cells is the most reliable method for measuring red cell volume. The erythrocytes are labeled in vitro and injected into the subject, and the principle of isotope dilution is employed in determination of the erythrocyte volume. Since injected ^{51}Cr-labeled red cells can be trapped by the spleen, an exponential extrapolation of radioactivity to time zero is necessary to obtain correct values of circulating red cell volume in animals with intact spleen (Finsterer et al., 1973). After the erythrocyte volume is determined, the total blood volume is calculated from the following formula:

$$\text{Blood volume (ml)} = \text{erythrocyte volume} \times \frac{100}{\text{PCV}}$$

Because the concentration of red cells in capillary beds is lower than in the general circulation (see below), venous hematocrit slightly overestimates the total blood volume. A correction factor must be introduced to obtain a better estimate of total blood volume. Erythrocyte volume calculated from plasma volume and venous hematocrit, as by the dye dilution and labeled-albumin methods, is normally much lower than that calculated by radiochromate method (Persson et al., 1973). The best approach, though time-consuming, is to determine blood volume by double label method, i.e., ^{131}I-labeled albumin and [51]Cr-

labeled red cells, respectively, for plasma and red cell volumes.

The rate of elimination of Evans blue or ^{131}I-labeled albumin may affect blood volume determination. Both disappear more rapidly in the newborn than in the adult of several species (Deavers et al., 1971). This may exaggerate differences in blood volumes of the neonate and the adult. The rate of elimination of iodinated albumin in normal calves was similar in different age groups (birth to 90 days in age), but considerably more rapid in scouring calves (Mollerberg et al., 1975). An age-dependent faster rate of dye disappearance was seen in foals during the first month of postnatal life, but the effect on plasma volume (5% increase) was considered insignificant (Persson and Ullberg, 1979). The dye dilution method allows blood volume and red cell volume determinations in the horse with a precision of ±3%.

THE RATIO OF BODY TO VENOUS HEMATOCRIT

In early studies (Smith et al., 1921), significant differences were noted between total red cell volumes calculated from plasma volume and the hematocrit and that determined by a carbon monoxide tag. The explanation given was that the venous hematocrit is in error because the ratio of cells to plasma in peripheral venous blood does not reflect the ratio of cells to plasma throughout the vascular system. Blood in small vessels of the body has a significantly lower hematocrit value than blood in the heart or large vessels of the body. This difference is explained on the basis that red cells flow in an axial stream in small vessels and pass through the vessels more quickly than the plasma, which is partially stored in a marginal "still space."

The ratio of venous hematocrit to circulatory or body hematocrit, except that in the spleen, is generally slightly greater than 1 in most species. For example, a dog with a venous hematocrit of 43% was found to have PCV values of blood in different organs and tissues as follows (Gibson et al., 1946): spleen 80%, liver 40%, heart and skeletal muscles 20–25%, and kidney, gastrointestinal tract, and brain 15–20%. In another study on dogs,

31% and 49% fewer red cells were found in hepatic and renal blood, respectively, and 70% more red cells were found in splenic blood than in venous blood (Allen and Reeve, 1953). Observations on growing beagles, 4 hours to 7 months in age, showed that major internal organs, muscle, and skin contained a significantly larger volume of the total blood volume in the newborn than in the 3- to 7-month-old dogs (Smith et al., 1972). In a similar study on newborn piglets, most organs except the spleen were found to have hematocrit values lower than the venous hematocrit, the ratio being 0.84:1 (Linderkamp et al., 1980).

The ratio of total body hematocrit to venous hematocrit has been designated the F_{cells} by Reeve et al. (1953). The spleen plays a significant role in influencing the size of the circulating red cell mass and thus the ratio. When the spleen is engorged with erythrocytes, as may be the case with animals at rest or under the influence of tranquilizing drugs or sodium pentobarbital anesthesia, the venous hematocrit is less than the total body hematocrit (Baker and Remington, 1960; Hahn et al., 1943; Hausner et al., 1938). But in animals under severe stress, massive injection of erythrocytes into the circulation occurs as a result of splenic contraction, and the venous hematocrit tends to be greater than the total body hematocrit. Thus there is a pronounced overestimation of blood volume and erythroycte volume in an intact animal compared to a splenectomized animal, as was evident from observations on cats (Breznock and Strack, 1982). Splanchnic vasculature is also a potentially important reservoir of blood volume, contributing a 20–30% increase upon appropriate stimulation (Supple and Powell, 1981). Therefore, for greatest accuracy in deriving a value for total blood volume, the simultaneous direct measurement of both erythrocyte and plasma volumes is required. Total red cell volume and venous hematocrit followed a close linear relationship in normal and anemic persons (excluding those with splenomegaly) and a curvilinear relationship in polycythemic patients (Bentley and Lewis, 1976). Linear relationship was disturbed during dehydration and hemodilution.

BLOOD VOLUME IN ANIMALS

Selected examples of reports from the literature on blood volume in domestic and some laboratory animals are presented in Table 3–1. In order to make the data comparative in the table, values reported in the literature have been converted to ml/kg except in the few instances in which results were reported in percentage of body weight. For practical application to clinical veterinary medicine, the blood volumes of animals may be estimated on the basis of ml/kg or stated as percentage of body weight as follows: young dairy calves and "hot-blooded" horses, 88–110 ml/kg or 10–11%; dogs, 77–78 ml/kg or 8–9%; growing calves and lactating cows, 66–77 ml/kg or 7–8%; cats, yearling calves, nonlactating cows, "cold-blooded" horses, sheep, and goats, 62–66 ml/kg or 6–7%; and mature swine, 55 ml/kg or 5–6%. In general, the blood volumes of the common laboratory animals, from mice to monkeys, are approximately 6–7% of their body weights.

Blood volume in the neonate of various species is comparatively large in terms of body weight and decreases progressively with increasing body weight (Dalton and Fisher, 1961; Deavers et al., 1978; Turner and Herman, 1931). The time of cord severance immediately following birth can influence blood volume and erythrocyte mass in the neonate; blood volume of newborn piglets, lambs, and human babies may increase from placental blood transfusion (Linderkamp et al., 1981). During the first few days after birth, changes occur in both the red cell and plasma volumes, although the pattern and temporal sequence of changes vary among species. For example, the plasma volume increases in the dog within 12–24 hours of birth (Deavers et al., 1978), within 24 hours in the calf (Mollerberg et al., 1975), and within 24–48 hours in the pig (McCance and Widdowson, 1959) and the human neonate (Usher et al., 1963). This expansion of plasma volume is attributed to shift of fluid in body compartments (from intracellular location to the extracellular location) because of increases in total plasma protein concentration following ingestion of colostrum. Simultaneously, red cell volume decreases slightly by hemodilution. Subsequently, plasma volume diminishes and red cell volume continues to decline disproportionately because of rapid destruction of fetal erythrocytes (Lee et al., 1976). Thus reduction in blood volume continues over the next several weeks, during which it becomes exaggerated by rapid increase in body weight as shown by studies on pigs (Bush et al., 1955; Hansard et al., 1953; Setiabudi et al., 1976), rats (Belcher and Harriss, 1957), calves (Mollerberg et al., 1975), dogs (Lee et al., 1976), and horses (Persson and Ullberg, 1981). In pigs, this decrease in blood volume has been related to increase in body fat (Hansard et al., 1953). Thus the neonatal anemic state is a transient manifestation of physiologic adjustment of the newborn.

Blood volume is also influenced by factors such as body type, body size, climate, physical activity, pregnancy, lactation, and breed. In the cow, there is a difference in blood volume during dry and lactating states (Turner and Herman, 1931; Reynolds, 1953b; Dale et al., 1956). Breed differences in blood volumes of cattle may not be significant when the body weight is corrected for water content in the rumen (Brown et al., 1957). Blood volume determination on 18 normal male holstein-friesian calves showed a significant correlation to total body surface, but not to age and weight (Haxton, 1974). In fetal and newborn lambs, blood volume was found to be influenced by breed, gestation age, and body weight (Pipkin and Kirkpatrick, 1973). Blood volume was found to be greater in light versus draft horses (Julian et al., 1956; Marcilese et al., 1964). Increased metabolic activity leads to increase in size of the vascular bed, followed by an increase in blood volume (Gauer et al., 1970). A 10% increase in blood volume, from increase in plasma volume due to fluid shifts and in hematocrit due to splenic contraction, was seen in dogs during mild exercise (Sarelius and Sinclair, 1981; Sarelius, 1976). Such an increase constitutes part of the mechanism maintaining efficient oxygen supply to tissues during exercise. However, these changes in blood volume are usually transient, lasting for about 10 minutes. Insignificant changes occurred in plasma and blood volumes of exercised water buffalo calves, but starvation

and water deprivation of the calves for 72 hours caused significant reductions in both parameters (Sodhi and Singh, 1975). Stress in pigs induced hemoconcentration owing to a decrease in plasma volume (Steinhardt et al., 1972) and mobilization of red cell reserves from storage organs (Bergfeld et al., 1977).

Increases in blood volume and hematocrit of sheep after feeding for 20 minutes were associated with reduction in plasma volume and release of erythrocytes from the splenic reservoir; the latter manifested only partly in splenectomized sheep (Dooley and Williams, 1976). Total blood volume and plasma volume were studied in 14 nonpregnant sows and two sows during pregnancy (Jezkova et al., 1977). The plasma volume was found to decrease during the first 7–8 weeks of gestation, then increase over the next 4 weeks, and repeat a similar cycle during the last 10 days of parturition; opposite changes were noted in the PCV. Increase in plasma volume during the third trimester of pregnancy is a common cause of anemia in women (Wintrobe et al., 1981).

Changes in blood volume may also occur in pathologic conditions. Blood volume is increased significantly in polycythemia vera (Appendix Case 17) and tetralogy of Fallot (Appendix Case 18) because of a marked expansion of total erythrocyte mass. The plasma volume is lower than normal. Reduction in blood volume results from loss of water from the plasma as in severe dehydration and starvation (Chaiyabutr et al., 1980). Determination of red cell volume distinguishes hemoconcentration from polycythemia, but a distinction between primary and secondary polycythemia is not resolved. Total plasma protein concentration is usually increased in hemoconcentration, whereas it is normal in polycythemia.

Plasma volume was reduced in ponies developing severe metabolic acidosis from force-feeding of a high starch ration (Harkema et al., 1978), and in resting horses given intravenous injection of furosemide (Muir et al., 1978). A 31–35% decrease in plasma volume occurred in dogs during 5 days of intestinal obstruction, but RBC, Hb, or PCV, and total serum proteins were essentially unchanged (Herczeg et al., 1974). Plasma volume increased in dogs on high sodium intake (Gupta et al., 1981); in horses with equine infectious anemia (Maliska, 1973); in cattle, goats, and sheep infected with *Trypanosoma vivax* (Anosa and Isoun, 1976); and in sheep with schistosomiasis (Preston et al., 1973). Plasma volume is greater than normal in human patients with splenomegaly, multiple myeloma, macroglobulinemia or monoclonal gammopathy (Alexanian, 1977), and acute lymphocytic leukemia (Linderkamp et al., 1978). Total blood volume and plasma volume increased in persons living at high altitude (Kapoor and Chatterjee, 1978). Total blood volume and plasma volume were decreased in children with hypoproteinemia from nephrosis and malnutrition, while the reverse occurred in hypoproteinemia from cirrhosis (Lall et al., 1975). The cause of such diametrically opposite findings was unknown. These observations indicate that the anemia of cirrhosis has dual mechanisms—reduction in red cell mass (from decreased erythropoiesis) as well as hemodilution.

BLOOD VOLUME IN RELATION TO WATER BALANCE

Warm-blooded animals constantly eliminate water from the body via the respiratory tract and skin in the dissipation of body heat and via the urinary tract in the elimination of urea, salts, and other end products of metabolism. This water elimination takes place even when water intake has stopped and the animal is becoming progressively dehydrated. Thus a sick animal that refuses to eat and/or drink enters a state of anhydremia. Dehydration, which results in hemoconcentration and reduction in blood volume, is hastened when the illness is accompanied by an increase in body temperature, sweating, diuresis, vomiting and/or diarrhea. Therefore the data obtained from the analysis of a blood sample must be interpreted in light of the state of water balance of the animal. Dehydration is better judged clinically than from a hemogram. Although an increase in both PCV and total plasma protein concentration is highly suggestive of dehydration, these findings may be masked in an otherwise anemic and hypoproteinemic animal. For example, the se-

vere dehydration associated with adrenocortical insufficiency (Addison's disease) may mask anemia (Appendix Case 10) and hypoproteinemia (Keeton et al., 1972). Dehydration in this disease is primarily due to the failure to retain body water as a result of loss of NaCl via the urine (sodium diuresis) and partly due to intracellular movement of water (Reece, 1972). Experiments on acute and chronic dehydration in dogs revealed that dehydration resulted in gradual hemoconcentration, but toward the end of a 10-day period, when body water had been reduced by 25%, blood constituents decreased to slightly subnormal levels (DeBoer, 1945). Erythrocytes and plasma proteins may diminish through their actual destruction in severe dehydration (Marriott, 1923). In dogs experiencing dehydration, plasma volume was reduced by 17% on the fifth day and by 29% on the eleventh day of food and water deprivation (Painter et al., 1948). Dehydration of cats by water deprivation for 48 hours caused an 11.5% decrease in plasma volume and a 13.5% decrease in circulating proteins, while total plasma protein concentration and albumin:globulin ratio remained essentially unchanged (Schultze et al., 1972).

Skin and muscles are the principal depots of water. Under conditions of severe dehydration, the skin gives up a greater fraction of its water than other tissues. When puppies 27–55 days of age were deprived of water for periods of 2–7 days (Hamilton and Schwartz, 1935), the water loss per 100 g of fat-free dry substance compared with controls was as follows: skin, 43%; muscles, 35%; brain, 14%; liver, 13%; and kidneys, 9%. It has been stated that water loss resulting in a concentration of the blood exceeding 25% of normal is attended by grave signs and that a level maintained at 40% or more of normal is usually followed by death (Underhill and Kapsinow, 1922).

HEMORRHAGE AND BLOOD RESTORATION

Systemic, circulatory, and hematologic manifestations of blood loss vary with the degree and duration of hemorrhage. The rapid loss of blood may lead to death from hypovolemic shock. Shock is evidenced by fast, thready pulse, pale and dry mucous membranes, cold skin and extremities, depression or restlessness, hyperventilation, muscular weakness, and a subnormal body temperature. A healthy animal can tolerate as much as 20% reduction in blood volume, but signs of shock generally develop when blood volume is reduced to 60–70% of normal. In the dog, 60% of normal blood volume is the irreducible minimum compatible with survival (Walcott, 1945). In a study on 30 dogs with blood volume of 86–112 ml/kg, blood was removed at the rate of 32–46 ml/kg during a 15–20 minute period under ether anesthesia. At a blood volume of 59 ml/kg, 50% of these dogs survived, while at 69 ml/kg, 84% of the dogs survived (Wang et al., 1947). Similarly, among 24 splenectomized hemorrhaged dogs, 50% survival occurred at a residual blood volume of 61% (Rawson et al., 1959). Immediate restoration of blood volume is crucial to survival of patients with hypovolemic shock.

When blood loss occurs slowly, the animal's body may sustain a loss as great as 50% of the normal volume before grave signs appear. This is because the slow loss of blood provides time for movement of fluid from extravascular spaces into the circulation to maintain venous return at essentially normal levels. Clinical signs that begin to appear when 50% loss of the original blood volume has occurred are referable to the reduction of hemoglobin concentration leading to tissue hypoxia.

Compensatory mechanisms are triggered immediately after a significant hemorrhagic episode. Neurohormonal responses include increased secretion of catecholamines (vasoconstriction and increased cardiac output), cortisol (extracellular fluid maintenance), and antidiuretic hormone (water and sodium resorption). Major hematologic responses include replacement of blood volume—both red cell volume and plasma volume—and of other blood constituents such as plasma proteins. Other than release of stored red cells by the spleen as an emergency measure in hemorrhage, the body is incapable of replacing erythrocytes except through erythropoiesis in the bone marrow, which requires several days. Adjustments of plasma volume are made by withdrawal of fluid from the interstitial compartment and increased resorption of water through the kidneys. Absorption of fluid from the gastrointestinal tract also contributes significantly to restoration of plasma volume (Miller, 1976).

Splenic contraction leads to the injection of a concentrated mass of erythrocytes into the circulation in severe hemorrhage in most species, thereby masking the extent of the loss during the first few hours posthemorrhage (see Chapter 6, p. 142). The spleen may become reduced in size by about half following exercise and to an even smaller volume on death from severe hemorrhage (Barcroft et al., 1925; Barcroft and Stephens, 1927). The splanchnic region contains about 20–30% of the blood volume, which can be variedly mobilized depending on the extent of blood loss. Species variations are found in the amount of blood mobilized from different reservoirs. For example, in the dog the spleen exhibits the greatest ability to release blood in response to acute hemorrhage and the intestine the least (Carneiro and Donald, 1977). By contrast, in the cat the gastrointestinal tract makes the major contribution to the blood volume during hemorrhage, and the spleen plays a negligible role (Greenway and Lister, 1974). Observations on normal and splenectomized dogs indicated that anesthetized dogs of both groups can tolerate a greater degree of hemorrhagic hypotension than unanesthetized dogs and that dogs with spleens can sustain a larger loss of blood volume than splenectomized dogs (Chien et al., 1973). Studies on fetal and neonatal sheep indicated that the fetus can tolerate a greater degree of blood loss and that anesthesia and stress of surgery considerably modify circulatory response to blood loss (Nuwayhid et al., 1978).

Plasma volume is affected not only by intake and excretion of water and electrolytes, but also by movement of fluid among the vascular, interstitial, and intracellular compartments. Thus plasma volume can expand even in the absence of increased intake of water or electrolytes. The content of protein, particularly albumin, is of prime importance in regulating the distribution of fluid among various compartments. Recent studies on the restitution of blood volume and plasma proteins in dogs after 10% hemorrhage indicated a biphasic regulation (Gann, 1976). The first phase is initiated by the fall in capillary pressure as a result of arteriolar constriction and reduction in arterial pressure because of blood loss. The reduction in capillary pressure allows movement of protein-free fluid from the interstitium into the capillaries. This process may begin as early as 30 minutes and last as long as 6 hours after blood loss and may restore 20–50% of blood volume. The second phase is more complex and involves neuroendocrine mechanisms. Transmission of cardiovascular signals of blood loss to the central nervous system triggers release of multiple hormones (including cortisol) which, acting in concert, induce an increase in extracellular osmolarity (Gann and Pirkle, 1975). This leads to a shift of intracellular fluid to the interstitium and increases the interstitial volume and pressure. The latter events promote increased return of interstitial (preformed) albumin through lymphatics and of fluid through both lymphatics and capillaries. These events play an important role in restoration of both the plasma volume and protein concentrations (Gann, 1976).

Increasing plasma volume in acute hemorrhage as well as in chronically developing anemia serves to maintain the total blood volume within relatively constant limits. In hemorrhaged dogs, fluid moves in at the rate of 0.25 ml/kg/minute during the initial posthemorrhage state (Adolph et al., 1933). About 10–15% of the initial blood volume may be replaced within 5 minutes by fluid movement in splenectomized dogs (Allen et al., 1959). It has been observed that while the most pronounced hemodilution occurs in the first hour posthemorrhage, fluid movement into the vascular system continues at a decreasing rate for 72 hours (Elman et al., 1943). Replacement of plasma volume and plasma proteins was faster in dogs that were physically conditioned than in unconditioned dogs (Kirschner, 1971).

Replacement of fluid in excess of the amount of red cells and plasma proteins mobilized causes hemodilution as reflected in a falling PCV and decreasing plasma protein

concentration. No significant plasma protein replacement took place within the first 2 hours in splenectomized dogs when less than 35% of blood volume was removed, but when a greater volume was removed, replacement of plasma protein began within the first 2 hours (Chien, 1958). Studies on plasma albumin following hemorrhage in dogs revealed 50% replacement within 24 hours from albumin in the extravascular compartment (Wasserman et al., 1956). During the next 2–5 days, albumin replenishment resulted from synthesis as well as from reduced catabolism of the existing plasma albumin. Protein is also added to the circulation through the thoracic duct lymph (Cope and Litwin, 1962). The plasma globulin fraction was found to fall for the first 7 hours and then was rapidly restored over a period of 24–72 hours (Elman et al., 1943). Compensatory replacement may begin sooner, however, as shown by observations that at the end of 90 minutes in hemorrhaged dogs, 0.21 g of protein per kg of body weight had been added to the circulation and 76% of the added protein was globulin (Smith et al., 1965). A sevenfold increase in rate of lymph flow accompanied the reduction in blood volume and continued for 25 minutes after bleeding had stopped. Their data indicated that 0.6 g of protein per hour was returned to the circulation by the lymph during the control period, compared to 4.6 g/hour following massive hemorrhage.

Studies on massive blood withdrawal in a horse, first in the intact state and later in splenectomized state (Table 6–4), demonstrated that there was a masking of the extent of blood loss during the first few hours posthemorrhage as a result of massive injection of erythrocytes in the circulation by splenic contraction (Torten and Schalm, 1964). However, because movement of fluid into the vascular system begins immediately, as blood volume becomes reduced, plasma protein concentration decreases with hemodilution. The earliest decrease in PCV below the prebleeding value was seen at the fourth hour, and a marked reduction occurred by the twenty-fourth hour as a result of continuous hemodilution. Plasma proteins, however, increased by 24 hours. Therefore, an estimation of red cell values within 4 hours of blood loss is misleading with reference to the extent of blood loss; protein determinations hourly or at least 2 hours apart during the early period are most helpful. Others have also reported that as much as 2 L of the fluid loss in the horse may be made up before the end of the bleeding carried out over a 2-hour period (Dubois, 1973).

REFERENCES

(Titles in parentheses are English translations of foreign language titles.)

Adolph, E.F., et al.: The Rate of Entrance of Fluid into the Blood in Hemorrhage. Amer. J. Physiol., *104*:502, 1933.

Alexanian, R.: Blood Volume in Monoclonal Gammopathy. Blood, *49*:301, 1977.

Allen, T.H., et al.: Blood Volume, Bleeding Volume and Tolerance to Hemorrhage in the Splenectomized Dog. Amer. J. Physiol., *196*:176, 1959.

Allen, T.H., and Reeve, E.B.: Distribution of "Extra Plasma" in the Blood of Some Tissues in the Dog as Measured with P^{32} and T-1824. Amer. J. Physiol., *175*:218, 1953.

Ancill, R.J.: The Blood Volume of the Normal Guinea Pig. J. Physiol., *132*:469, 1956.

Anderson, D.M.: The Trapped Plasma Correction Factor in the Blood of Pigs. J. Comp. Path., *80*:163, 1970.

Anosa, V.O., and Isoun, T.T.: Serum Proteins, Blood and Plasma Volumes in Experimental Trypanosoma vivax Infections of Sheep and Goats. Trop. Anim. Health Prod., *8*:14, 1976.

Armin, J., et al.: The Plasma, Cell and Blood Volumes of Albino Rabbits as Estimated by the Dye (T-1824) and ^{32}P Marked Cell Methods. J. Physiol., *116*:59, 1952.

Baker, C.H., and Remington, J.W.: Role of the Spleen in Determining Total Body Hematocrit. Amer. J. Physiol., *198*:906, 1960.

Barcroft, J., et al.: A Contribution to the Physiology of the Spleen. J. Physiol., *60*:443, 1925.

Barcroft, J., and Stephens, J.G.: Observations upon the Size of the Spleen. J. Physiol., *64*:1, 1927.

Belcher, E.H., and Harriss, E.B.: Studies of Plasma Volume, Red Cell Volume and Total Blood Volume in Young Growing Rats. J. Physiol., *139*:64, 1957.

Bentley, S.A., and Lewis, S.M.: The Relationship between Total Red Cell Volume, Plasma Volume and Venous Haematocrit. Brit. J. Haematol., *33*:301, 1976.

Bergfeld, E., et al.: Changes in the Blood Volume of Pigs under Stress. Züchtungskunde, *49*:43, 1977.

Biewald, N., and Billmeier, J.: Blood Volume and Extracellular Space (ECS) of the Whole Body and Some Organs of the Rat. Experientia, *34*:412, 1978.

Billings, H.H., and Brown, E.B., Jr.: Effect of Splenectomy on Changes in Plasma and Blood Volume Produced by Inhalation of 30% and 40% CO_2 in Dogs. Amer. J. Physiol., *180*:363, 1955.

Breznock, E.M., and Strack, D.: Blood Volume of Nonsplenectomized and Splenectomized Cats before and after Acute Hemorrhage. Amer. J. Vet. Res., *43*:1811, 1982.

Brown, E., et al.: Blood Volume and Its Regulation. Ann. Rev. Physiol., *19*:231, 1957.

Bush, J.A., et al.: Blood Volume Studies in Normal and Anemic Swine. Amer. J. Physiol., *181*:9, 1955.

Campistron, G., et al.: The Measurement of Circulating Blood Volume and of the Blood Volume Impregnating Organs in Rats and Rabbits, Using ^{113}-In-Labelled Transferrin. Int. J. Nucl. Med. Biol., *6*:167, 1979.

Carneiro, J.J., and Donald, D.E.: Blood Reservoir Function of Dog Spleen, Liver, and Intestine. Amer. J. Physiol., *232*:H67, 1977.

Chaiyabutr, N., et al.: Effects of Starvation on the Cardiovascular System, Water Balance and Milk Secretion in Lactating Goats. Res. Vet. Sci., *28*:291, 1980.

Chien, S.: Quantitative Evaluation of the Circulatory Adjustment of Splenectomized Dogs to Hemorrhage. Amer. J. Physiol., *193*:605, 1958.

Chien, S., et al.: Plasma Trapping in Hematocrit Determinations: Differences among Animal Species. Proc. Soc. Exp. Biol. Med., *119*:1155, 1965.

Chien, S., et al.: Blood Volume, Hemodynamic, and Metabolic Changes in Hemorrhagic Shock in Normal and Splenectomized Dogs. Amer. J. Physiol., *225*:866, 1973.

Collery, L., and Keating, J.: Blood Volume Determination in Horses Using Radioactive Phosphorus. Vet. Rec., *70*:216, 1958.

Cope, O., and Litwin, S.B.: Contribution of the Lymphatic System to the Replenishment of the Plasma Volume following Hemorrhage. Ann. Surg., *156*:655, 1962.

Courtice, F.C.: The Blood Volume of the Normal Animals. J. Physiol., *102*:290, 1943.

Creasy, R.K., et al.: Determination of Fetal, Placental, and Neonatal Blood Volumes in Sheep. Circ. Res., *27*:487, 1970.

Dale, H.E., et al.: Environmental Physiology and Shelter Engineering. XXXIX. Environmental Temperature and Blood Volume (Cows). Mo. Exp. Sta. Res. Bull., 608, 1956.

Dalton, R.G., and Fisher, E.W.: Plasma and Blood Volumes in Ayrshire Cattle. Brit. Vet. J., *117*:115, 1961.

Dalton, R.G., and Fisher, E.W.: Plasma and Blood Volumes in Horses. Brit. Vet. J., *119*:384, 1963.

Da Silva, A.C., et al.: The Domestic Cat as a Laboratory Animal for Experimental Nutrition Studies. IV. Folic Acid Deficiency. J. Nutr., *56*:199, 1955.

Dawson, A.B., et al.: Blood Volume Studies. III. Behavior of a Large Series of Dyes Introduced into the Circulating Blood. Amer. J. Physiol., *51*:232, 1920.

Deavers, S., et al.: Extravascular-Vascular Distribution of ^{131}I-Tagged Albumin in the Growing Beagle. Amer. J. Vet. Res., *32*:1169, 1971.

Deavers, S., et al.: Blood Volumes and Total Body Water in the Domestic Pony. J. Appl. Physiol., *34*:341, 1973.

Deavers, S.I., et al.: Blood Volume Changes during the First Week after Birth in the Beagle and Pig. Proc. Soc. Exp. Biol. Med., *159*:152, 1978.

DeBoer, B.: Changes in the Blood during Chronic and Acute Dehydration. Amer. J. Physiol., *145*:154, 1945.

Dellenback, R.J., et al.: Effects of Splenectomy on Blood Picture, Blood Volume, and Plasma Proteins in Beagles. Amer. J. Physiol., *217*:891, 1969.

Dooley, P.C., and Williams, V.J.: Changes in Plasma Volume and Haematocrit in Intact and Splenectomized Sheep during Feeding. Aust. J. Biol. Sci., *29*:533, 1976.

DuBois, C.: (Haemodynamics of Bleeding in the Horse.) Thèse École Nationale Vétérinaire d'Alfort, 71 pp., 1973.

Elman, R., et al.: Plasma Proteins (Albumin and Globulin) and Red Cell Volume following a Single Severe

Non-Fatal Hemorrhage. Amer. J. Physiol., *138*:569, 1943.

Finsterer, U., et al.: The Role of the Spleen in Determination of Red Cell Volume with Cr_{51}-Labelled Erythrocytes in the Intact Dog. Pflügers Arch., *341*:73, 1973.

Gann, D.S.: Endocrine Control of Plasma Protein and Volume. Surg. Clin. North Amer., *56*:1135, 1976.

Gann, D.S., and Pirkle, J.C.: Role of Cortisol in the Restitution of Blood Volume after Hemorrhage. Am. J. Surg., *130*:565, 1975.

Gauer, O.H., et al.: The Regulation of Extracellular Fluid Volume. Ann. Rev. Physiol., *32*:547, 1970.

Gibson, J.G., 2nd, et al.: The Distribution of Red Cells and Plasma in Large and Minute Vessels of the Normal Dog, Determined by Radioactive Isotopes of Iron and Iodine. J. Clin. Invest., *25*:848, 1946.

Granger, W.: (Measurement of Blood Volume in Cattle.) Wiener Tierarztl. Monatssch., *64*:117, 1977.

Greenway, C.V., and Lister, G.E.: Capacitance Effects and Blood Reservoir Function in the Splanchnic Vascular Bed during Non-Hypotensive Haemorrhage and Blood Volume Expansion in Anaesthetized Cats. J. Physiol. (London), *237*:279, 1974.

Gregersen, M.I., and Rawson, R.A.: Blood Volume. Physiol. Rev., *39*:307, 1959.

Gregersen, M.I., and Schiro, H.: The Behavior of the Dye T-1824 with Respect to Its Absorption by Red Blood Cells and Its Fate in Blood Undergoing Coagulation. Amer. J. Physiol., *121*:284, 1938.

Gupta, B.N., et al.: The Influence of High and Low Sodium Intake on Blood Volume in the Dog. Q. J. Exp. Physiol., *66*:117, 1981.

Hahn, P.F., et al.: Removal of Red Cells from the Active Circulation by Sodium Pentobarbital. Amer. J. Physiol., *138*:415, 1943.

Hamilton, B., and Schwartz, R.: The Composition of Tissues in Dehydration. J. Biol. Chem., *109*:745, 1935.

Hansard, S.L., et al.: Blood Volume of Farm Animals. J. Anim. Sci., *12*:402, 1953.

Harkema, J.R., et al.: Cardiovascular, Acid-Base, Electrolyte and Plasma Volume Changes in Ponies Developing Alimentary Laminitis. Amer. J. Vet. Res., *39*:741, 1978.

Hausner, E., et al.: Roentgenologic Observations on the Spleen of the Dog under Ether, Sodium Amytal, Pentobarbital Sodium and Pentothal Sodium Anesthesia. Amer. J. Physiol., *121*:387, 1938.

Haxton, J.A., et al.: Blood Volume of the Male Holstein-Friesian Calf. Amer. J. Vet. Res., *35*:835, 1974.

Herczeg, B., et al.: Änderungen des Plasma volumes bei experimenteller Darmokklusion. Acta Chir. Acad. Sci. Hung., *15*:155, 1974.

Hlad, C.J., Jr., and Holmes, J.H.: Factors Affecting Hematocrit Determinations: Trapped Plasma, Its Amount and Distribution. J. Appl. Physiol., *5*:457, 1953.

Hodgetts, E.: The Dynamic Red Cell Storage Function of the Spleen in Sheep. III. Relationship to Determination of Blood Volume, Total Red Cell Volume, and Plasma Volume. Aust. J. Exp. Biol. Med. Sci., *39*:187, 1961.

Hood, D.M., and Hightower, D.: Evaluation of Radioiodinated Human Serum Albumin in the Dog for Assessment of Hemodynamic Function. Amer. J. Vet. Res., *37*:227, 1976.

Hurley, P.J.: Red Cell and Plasma Volumes in Normal Adults. J. Nucl. Med., *14*:46, 1975.

International Committee for Standardization in Haematology: Recommended Methods for Measurement of Red-Cell and Plasma Volume. J. Nucl. Med., *21*:793, 1980.

Jezkova, D., et al.: Changes in the Plasma Volume, Total Blood Volume and Haematocrit Values of Pregnant Sows. Acta Vet. Brno., *46*:203, 1977.

Julian, L.M., et al.: Blood Volume, Body Water and Body Fat of the Horse. J. Appl. Physiol., *8*:651, 1956.

Kapoor, S.C., and Chatterjee, A.K.: Haematological Response among New Arrival at High Altitude. Indian J. Med. Res., *67*:428, 1978.

Keeton, K.S., et al.: Adrenocortical Insufficiency in the Dog. Calif. Vet., *26*(6):12, 1972.

Keighley, G., et al.: Response of Normal and Genetically Anemic Mice to Erythropoietic Stimuli. Brit. J. Haematol., *8*:429, 1962.

Kirschner, H.: (Effect of Physical Training on Compensatory Increase of Plasma Volume after Blood Loss in Dogs.) Acta Physiol. Polonica, *22*:21, 1971.

Klement, A.W., Jr., et al.: Simultaneous Use of I^{131}-Albumin and Cr^{51}-Labelled Red Cells in Blood Volume Studies in the Goat. Proc. Soc. Exp. Biol. Med., *87*:81, 1954.

Klement, A.W., Jr., et al.: Simultaneous Use of Cr^{51} and T-1824 Dye in Blood Volume Studies in the Goat. Amer. J. Physiol., *181*:15, 1955.

Lall, A., et al.: Plasma and Blood Volume Changes during Hypoproteinemia. Indian Pediatr., *12*:165, 1975.

Lee, P., et al.: Blood Volume Changes and Production and Destruction of Erythrocytes in Newborn Dogs. Amer. J. Vet. Res., *37*:561, 1976.

Linderkamp, O., et al.: Plasma Volume Estimation in Severely Ill Infants and Children Using a Simplified Evans Blue Method. Europ. J. Pediatr., *125*:135, 1977.

Linderkamp, O., et al.: Blood Volume of Children with Leukemia. Acta Paediatr. Scand., *67*:281, 1978.

Linderkamp, O., et al.: Blood Volume and Hematocrit in Various Organs in Newborn Piglets. Pediatr. Res., *14*:1324, 1980.

Linderkamp, O., et al.: Blood Volume in Newborn Piglets: Effects of Time of Natural Cord Rupture, Intra-Uterine Growth Retardation, Asphyxia, and Prostaglandin-Induced Prematurity. Pediatr. Res. *15*:53, 1981.

Lombardi, M.H.: Radioisotopic Blood Volume and Cardiac Output in Dogs. Amer. J. Vet. Res., *33*:1825, 1972.

Maliska, C.: Studies of Equine Infectious Anaemia Using Radioisotopes. I. Half-Life of Labelled Erythrocytes in Thoroughbred Horses. II. Erythrocyte Mass and Blood Volume. Pesquisa Agropecuaria Brasileira, Serie Veterinaira, *8*:91, 1973.

Marcilese, N.A., et al.: Normal Blood Volumes in the Horse. Amer. J. Physiol., *207*:223, 1964.

Marriott, W.M.: Anhydremia. Physiol. Rev., *3*:275, 1923.

Masouredis, S.P., and Melcher, L.R.: Blood, Plasma and "Globulin" Space of Guinea Pigs Determined with I^{131} Rabbit Globulin. Proc. Soc. Exp. Biol. Med., *78*:264, 1951.

McCance, R.A., and Widdowson, E.M.: The Effect of Colostrum on the Composition and Volume of the Plasma of New-Born Piglets. J. Physiol., *145*:547, 1959.

Miller, W.L.: Plasma Volume Restoration by Intestinal Fluids following Acute Hemorrhage in the Dog. Diss. Abst., *36B*:4881, 1976.

Mollerberg, L., et al.: Plasma and Blood Volume in the Calf from Birth till 90 Days of Age. Acta Vet. Scand., *16*:178, 1975.

Muir, W.W., et al.: Effects of Furosemide on Plasma Volume and Extracellular Fluid Volume in Horses. Amer. J. Vet. Res., *39*:1688, 1978.

Nielsen, M.H., and Nielsen, N.C.: Spectrophotometric Determination of Evans Blue Dye in Plasma with Individual Correlation for Blank Density by a Modified Gaeblers Method. Scand. J. Clin. Lab. Invest., *14*:605, 1962.

Nuwayhid, B., et al.: Circulatory Shock in Pregnant Sheep. IV. Fetal and Neonatal Circulatory Responses to Hypovolemia—Influence of Anaesthesia. Amer. J. Obstet. Gynecol., *132*:658, 1978.

Obara, J., and Nakajima, H.: Iron Metabolism in Equine Infectious Anemia. III. Measurement of Blood Volume, Mean Corpuscular Volume, Mean Corpuscular Hemoglobin and Mean Corpuscular Hemoglobin Concentration and Estimation of Total Body Iron. Kachiku Eisei Shikenjo Bull., *42*:45, 1961.

O'Brien, W.A., et al.: Blood Volume Studies in Wounded Animals. J. Appl. Physiol., *11*:110, 1957.

Owen, C.A., Jr., and Powers, M.H.: Intercellular Plasma of Centrifuged Human Erythrocytes as Measured by Means of Iodo[131]-Albumin. J. Appl. Physiol., *5*:323, 1953.

Painter, E.E., et al.: Exchange and Distribution of Fluid in Dehydration in the Dog. Amer. J. Physiol., *152*:66, 1948.

Pandey, M.D., and Roy, A.: Variation in Volume and Composition of Body Fluids (Interstitial, Blood and Urine) as a Measure of Adaptability in Buffaloes to a Hot Environment. Brit. Vet. J., *125*:389, 1969.

Payne, E., et al.: Plasma, Blood and Extracellular Fluid Volumes in Grazing Hereford Cattle. Res. Vet. Sci., *8*:20, 1967.

Persson, S.: On Blood Volume and Working Capacity in Horses. Studies on Methodology and Physiological and Pathological Variations. Acta Vet. Scand. Suppl., *19*:1, 1967.

Persson, S.G.B., et al.: Circulatory Effects of Splenectomy in the Horse. I. Effect on Red-Cell Distribution and Variability of Haematocrit in the Peripheral Blood. II. Effect on Plasma Volume and Total and Circulating Red-Cell Volume. Zentralbl. Veterinaermed., *20A*:441, 456, 1973.

Persson, S.G.B., and Ullberg, L.E.: Blood Volume Determination with Evans Blue Dye in Foals. Acta Vet. Scand., *20*:10, 1979.

Persson, S.G.B., and Ullberg, L.E.: Blood Volume and Rate of Growth in Standardbred Foals. Equine Vet. J., *13*:254, 1981.

Pipkin, F.B., and Kirkpatrick, S.M.L.: The Blood Volume of Fetal and Newborn Sheep. Q. J. Exp. Physiol. Cog. Med. Sci., *58*:181, 1973.

Preston, J.M., et al.: Pathophysiology of Ovine Schistosomiasis. II. Some Observations on the Sequential Changes in Blood Volume and Water and Electrolyte Metabolism following a Single Experimental Infection of Schistosoma mattheei. J. Comp. Path., *83*:417, 1973.

Rawson, R.A., et al.: Determination of Residual Blood Volume Required for Survival in Rapidly Hemorrhaged Splenectomized Dogs. Amer. J. Physiol., *196*:179, 1959.

Reece, W.O.: Fluid Volume Changes Associated with Withdrawal and Restoration of Steroid Therapy in Adrenalectomized Dogs. Amer. J. Vet. Res., *33*:1493, 1972.

Reed, C., et al.: Polycythemia Vera in a Cat. J. Amer. Vet. Med. Ass., *157*:85, 1970.

Reeve, E.B., et al.: Distribution of Cells and Plasma in the Normal and Splenectomized Dog and Its Influence on Blood Volume Estimates with P[32] and T-1824. Amer. J. Physiol., *175*:195, 1953.

Reynolds, M.: Plasma and Blood Volume in the Cow Using the T-1824 Hematocrit Method. Amer. J. Physiol., *173*:421, 1953a.

Reynolds, M.: Measurement of Bovine Plasma and Blood Volume during Pregnancy and Lactation. Amer. J. Physiol., *175*:118, 1953b.

Sabourin, S., et al.: Normogramme hematologique et biochemique et variations quotidiennes des parametres de base chez le chien normal. Can. J. Comp. Med., *39*:397, 1975.

Sarelius, I.H.: Blood Volume and Exercise in Dogs. N.Z. Med. J., *84*:275, 1976.

Sarelius, I.H., and Sinclair, J.D.: Effect of Small Changes of Blood Volume on Oxygen Delivery and Tissue Oxygenation. Amer. J. Physiol., *240*:H177, 1981.

Schultz, A.L., et al.: A Critical Comparison of the T-1824 Dye and Iodinated Albumin Methods for Plasma Volume Measurement. J. Clin. Invest., *32*:107, 1953.

Schultze, G., et al.: Distribution and Circulation of Extracellular Fluid and Protein during Different States of Hydration in the Cat. Pflügers Arch., *337*:351, 1972.

Sear, H., et al.: Simultaneous Measurement in Dogs of Plasma Volume with I[131] Human Albumin and T-1824 with Comparisons of Their Long Term Disappearance from the Plasma. Amer. J. Physiol., *175*:240, 1953.

Senn, V.Y., and Karlson, K.E.: Methodologic and Actual Error of Plasma Volume Determination. Surgery, *44*:1095, 1958.

Setiabudi, M., et al.: Growth of the Pig: Changes in Red Cell and Plasma Volumes. Growth, *40*:127, 1976.

Smith, E.L., et al.: Effect of Blood Volume on Movement of Protein and Volume Distribution of Albumin in the Dog. Amer. J. Vet. Res., *26*:829, 1965.

Smith, E.L., et al.: Absolute and Relative Residual Organ Blood Volume and Organ Hematocrits in Growing Beagles. Proc. Soc. Exp. Biol. Med., *140*:285, 1972.

Smith, H.P., et al.: Blood Volume Studies. VII. Comparative Values of Welcher, Carbon Monoxide and Dye Methods for Blood Volume Determinations. Accurate Estimation of Absolute Blood Volume. Amer. J. Physiol., *56*:336, 1921.

Sodhi, S.P.S., and Singh, A.: Blood and Plasma Volumes and Changes in Electrolyte Content under Stress and Normal Conditions in Buffalo Calves. Indian J. Anim. Sci., *44*:305, 1975.

Sodhi, S.S., and Sodhi, J.S.: A Note on Simultaneous Use of RISA and T-1824 Dye in the Blood Volume Studies in Goats and Rams. Indian J. Anim. Sci., *46*:674, 1976.

Spink, R.R., et al.: Determination of Erythrocyte Half Life and Blood Volume in Cats. Amer. J. Vet. Res., *27*:1041, 1966.

Steinhardt, M., et al.: Studies on Plasma Volume, Blood Volume and Total Haemoglobin in Pigs. Arch. Exp. Veterinaermed., *26*:533, 1972.

Supple, E.W., and Powell, W.J., Jr.: Effect of Acetylcholine on Vascular Capacity in the Dog. J. Clin. Invest., *68*:64, 1981.

Torten, M., and Schalm, O.W.: Influence of the Equine Spleen on Rapid Changes in the Concentration of Erythrocytes in Peripheral Blood. Amer. J. Vet. Res., *25*:500, 1964.

Turner, C.W., and Herman, H.A.: A Determination of

the Blood and Plasma Volume of Dairy Cattle: A Study of the Blood and Plasma Volume during Growth, Pregnancy, and Lactation. Mo. Agr. Exp. Sta. Res. Bull., 159, 1931.

Underhill, F.P., and Kapsinow, R.: The Influence of Water Introduction upon Blood Concentration Induced by Water Deprivation. J. Biol. Chem., *54*:459, 1922.

Usher, R., et al.: The Blood Volume of the Newborn Infant and Placental Transfusion. Acta Paediatr., *52*:497, 1963.

Wade, L., Jr., and Sasser, L.B.: Body Water, Plasma Volume, and Erythrocyte Volume in Sheep. Amer. J. Vet. Res., *31*:1375, 1970.

Walcott, W.W.: Blood Volume in Experimental Hemorrhagic Shock. Amer. J. Physiol., *143*:247, 1945.

Wang, L.: Plasma Volume, Cell Volume, Total Blood Volume and F_{cells} Factor in the Normal and Splenectomized Sherman Rat. Amer. J. Physiol., *196*:188, 1959.

Wang, S.C., et al.: The Relation of Blood Volume Reduction to Mortality Rate in Hemorrhagic and Traumatic Shock in Dogs. Amer. J. Physiol., *148*:164, 1947.

Wasserman, K., et al.: Kinetics of Vascular and Extravascular Protein Exchange in Unbled and Bled Dogs. Amer. J. Physiol., *184*:175, 1956.

Wintrobe, M.M., et al.: Clinical Hematology. 8th ed. Lea & Febiger, Philadelphia, 1981.

Wish, L., et al.: Direct Determinations of Plasma, Cell, and Organ-Blood Volumes in Normal and Hypervolemic Mice. Proc. Soc. Exp. Biol. Med., *74*:644, 1950.

Woodward, K.T., et al.: Plasma, Erythrocyte, and Whole Blood Volume in the Normal Beagle. Amer. J. Vet. Res., *29*:1935, 1968.

Yale, C., and Torhorst, J.B.: Critical Bleeding and Plasma Volumes of the Adult Germfree Rat. Lab. Anim. Sci., *22*:497, 1972.

4

The Dog: Normal Hematology with Comments on Response to Disease

THE ERYTHROCYTES   103
   Erythrocyte Morphology   103
   Erythrocyte Parameters and Wintrobe
     Indexes in Relation to Age   104
   Breed Differences   107
   Sex Differences   107
   Interrelationship of PCV, Hb, and RBC   107
   Reticulocytes   108
   Erythrocyte Sedimentation Rate   108
   Erythrocyte Osmotic Fragility   108

THE LEUKOCYTES   109
   Influence of Age   109
   Effects of Corticosteroids   111
   Physiologic and "Emotional"
     Leukocytosis   111

   The Neutrophil   113
   The Eosinophil   118
   The Basophil   119
   The Lymphocyte   119
   The Monocyte   119

THE PLATELETS   119

THE PLASMA   122
   Icterus Index   122
   Total Plasma Proteins   122
   Plasma Fibrinogen   122

THE BONE MARROW   123
   The Myeloid:Erythroid Ratio   123

Normal blood values for the dog, as reported in the older literature, were commonly developed from small numbers of dogs used in the study of physiologic, pharmacologic, or medical problems. More recently, extensive use of the beagle dog in biomedical research and the use of the electronic cell counter and the microhematocrit have provided more reliable values (Andersen and Schalm, 1970). Mongrel dogs obtained from the pound are less reliable for normal data, unless carefully selected for freedom from occult disease and conditioned for several months before data collection (Porter and Canaday, 1971; Soave and Boyle, 1965). Similarly, red cell parameters may be lower in undernourished (but not anemic) dogs than in well-nourished dogs (Oduye, 1978). The veterinarian should be cognizant that normal values from a cross section of the population (see chart) may be too wide, while those from control animals or closed colonies used in experimental investigations may be too narrow for application to clinical situations (Tvedten, 1981).

Normal blood values for basenji (Table 4–1) and beagle (Table 4–2) dogs of various age groups are given. These values, although based on a limited number of observations, compare favorably with the more extensive reports on the beagle dogs. Blood values, particularly red cell parameters (RBC, Hb, and PCV), have been found to vary with age and nutritional status of the animal, and diurnal and seasonal variations may occur (Andersen and Gee, 1958; Andersen and Schalm, 1970; Tsessarskaya and Burkovskaya, 1976). Data on hematologic changes to 60 days of age in clinically normal beagles have been published (Earl et al., 1973; Shifrine et al., 1973). Selected recent references on normal hematologic values in the dog are given (Brunk and Becker-Berger, 1980; Konrad et al., 1980; Lumsden et al., 1979).

THE ERYTHROCYTES

Erythrocyte Morphology

Canine erythrocytes are typically biconcave discs about 7.0 μm in diameter and 1.7 μm

Normal Blood Values for the Dog

Erythrocytic Series	Range	Ave.	Leukocytic Series	Range	Ave.
Erythrocytes ($\times 10^6/\mu$l)	5.5– 8.5	6.8	Leukocytes/μl	6,000–17,000	11,500
Hemoglobin (g/dl)	12.0–18.0	15.0	Neutrophil (band)	0– 300	70
PCV (%)	37.0–55.0	45.0	Neutrophil (mature)	3,000–11,500	7,000
MCV (fl)	60.0–77.0	70.0	Lymphocyte	1,000– 4,800	2,800
MCH (pg)	19.5–24.5	22.8	Monocyte	150– 1,350	750
MCHC (%)			Eosinophil	100– 1,250	550
Wintrobe	31.0–34.0	33.0	Basophil	rare	0
Microhematocrit	32.0–36.0	34.0			
Reticulocytes (%)	0.0– 1.5	0.8	Percentage Distribution		
ESR (see Table 2–6) varies with PCV			Neutrophil (band)	0– 3	0.8
RBC diameter (μm)	6.7– 7.2	7.0	Neutrophil (mature)	60–77	70.0
RBC life span (days)	100–120		Lymphocyte	12–30	20.0
Resistance to			Monocyte	3–10	5.2
hypotonic saline (%)			Eosinophil	2–10	4.0
Min.	0.40–0.50	0.46	Basophil	rare	0.0
Max.	0.32–0.42	0.33			
Myeloid:erythroid ratio	0.75–2.5:1.0	1.2:1.0			

Other Data		
Thrombocytes ($\times 10^5/\mu$l)	2–5	
Icterus index (units)	2–5	
Total plasma proteins (g/dl)	6.0–8.0*	
Plasma fibrinogen (g/dl)		
Narrow range	0.2–0.4	
Broad range	0.1–0.5	

*Varies with age; see Table 4–1.

in thickness. They exhibit a distinct central pallor and slight anisocytosis (Plate XII–1). Minor artifactual crenation occurs frequently, but other shape transformations are abnormal. Slight rouleau formation is common. An occasional polychromic erythrocyte is a common finding that correlates well with the normal number (less than 2.0%) of reticulocytes in peripheral blood. An occasional nucleated erythrocyte and a rare red cell with a Howell-Jolly body may be encountered. Increased numbers of erythrocytes with Howell-Jolly bodies and, less commonly, nucleated erythrocytes appear in the blood of dogs on continuous corticosteroid therapy. These findings are a reflection of suppressed splenic function (Chapter 13; Fig. 13–21). Occasionally, hemoglobin crystals may be seen within and outside the red cells in the blood of young dogs (Lund, 1974; Spurling, 1977). This finding has been attributed to the immaturity of the mononuclear phagocyte system. Abnormalities of erythrocyte shape (Chapter 20) during disease are more often encountered in the dog and cat than in other animal species. Stomatocytic erythrocytes were found in Alaskan malamutes with hereditary hemo-lytic anemia (Pinkerton et al., 1974), and spheroechinocytes were observed in a basenji dog with anemia due to hereditary deficiency of pyruvate kinase (Chandler et al., 1975).

Erythrocyte Parameters and Wintrobe Indexes in Relation to Age

At birth, the erythrocytes of fetal origin are large; MCV is 95–100 fl (Andersen and Schalm, 1970; Ederstrom and DeBoer, 1946). As fetal erythrocytes are replaced by cells of smaller size, MCV becomes reduced, so that by 2–3 months of age, erythrocyte size is representative of the normal adult dog. Similarly, MCH is about 33 pg at birth and decreases to about 22 pg by 2 months of age (Shifrine et al., 1973). MCHC varies only slightly with age, being about 35% at birth and 33% at 2 months of age, and remaining constant at 32% irrespective of changes in PCV (Shifrine et al., 1973). MCHC may fluctuate within the normal range by 3–5% due to physiologic and technical variations.

Erythrocyte number, Hb, and PCV values are high at birth, but fall rapidly as the pup begins to nurse. Reduction of these values continues during the first month of life. These changes are related to increased destruction

Table 4–1. Influence of Age on the Canine Hemogram in Basenji Dogs[a] (means and 1 SD)

	Age				
	6–8 weeks	9–12 weeks	4–6 months	1–2 years	>2 years
Number of dogs	24	21	9	13	7
RBC ($\times 10^6/\mu l$)	4.73 ± 0.38	5.45 ± 0.54	6.56 ± 0.46	6.91 ± 0.60	7.19 ± 0.64
Hemoglobin (g/dl)	10.4 ± 0.58	11.8 ± 0.81	14.4 ± 0.82	15.9 ± 1.2	16.6 ± 1.1
PCV (%)	33.1 ± 2.2	37.2 ± 2.9	44.0 ± 2.4	49.3 ± 3.4	49.8 ± 3.4
MCV (fl)	70.1 ± 2.9	68.6 ± 2.9	67.2 ± 2.9	71.1 ± 4.0	69.6 ± 4.1
MCH (pg)	22.1 ± 1.4	21.8 ± 1.5	21.9 ± 0.9	23.0 ± 0.8	23.2 ± 1.8
MCHC (%)	31.5 ± 1.4	31.8 ± 1.3	32.7 ± 0.6	32.3 ± 1.2	33.3 ± 0.41
Icterus index units	1.3 ± 0.9	2.8 ± 1.9	0.66 ± 0.94	2.2 ± 2.3	2.0 ± 2.1
Plasma proteins (g/dl)	5.33 ± 0.29	5.87 ± 0.46	6.6 ± 0.25	7.03 ± 0.33	7.5 ± 0.24
Fibrinogen (g/dl)	0.18 ± 0.07	0.20 ± 0.08	0.22 ± 0.07	0.22 ± 0.08	0.20 ± 0.06
Reticulocytes (%)	3.4 ± 1.0	2.6 ± 1.8	0.24 ± 0.41	0.84 ± 0.9	0.84 ± 1.12
WBC/µl	13,433 ± 2,045	15,033 ± 2,077	13,589 ± 1,751	14,031 ± 2,270	12,157 ± 1,987
Percentage distribution of WBC					
Band neutrophils	0.65 ± 0.77	0.57 ± 1.1	0.61 ± 0.81	0.27 ± 0.42	0.07 ± 0.17
Segmenters	58.8 ± 10.9	56.4 ± 7.8	52.4 ± 5.5	58.1 ± 7.3	66.4 ± 6.7
Lymphocytes	30.1 ± 8.1	33.5 ± 8.1	36.9 ± 5.5	28.6 ± 7.7	23.1 ± 4.8
Monocytes	6.9 ± 2.6	6.7 ± 2.7	6.0 ± 1.8	5.2 ± 2.1	4.0 ± 1.4
Eosinophils	3.3 ± 1.9	2.3 ± 1.6	4.1 ± 1.9	7.3 ± 3.5	6.3 ± 2.3
Basophils	0.08 ± 0.24	0.07 ± 0.23	0.0 ± 0.0	0.12 ± 0.4	0.14 ± 0.22
Absolute numbers of WBC/µl					
Band neutrophils	85 ± 101	94 ± 186	88 ± 117	38 ± 62	8 ± 21
Segmenters	8,015 ± 2,387	8,463 ± 1,638	7,196 ± 1,509	8,169 ± 1,732	8,107 ± 1,864
Lymphocytes	3,965 ± 1,059	5,059 ± 1,555	4,948 ± 510	4,023 ± 1,207	2,805 ± 634
Monocytes	912 ± 325	986 ± 405	818 ± 311	715 ± 266	495 ± 191
Eosinophils	426 ± 239	341 ± 243	538 ± 225	990 ± 455	727 ± 229
Basophils	10 ± 29	10 ± 33	0 ± 0	17 ± 58	15 ± 23

[a]Normal basenji dogs reared by several commercial breeders. Data gathered in cooperation with Dr. G.O. Ewing, formerly at the Veterinary Medical Teaching Hospital, University of California, Davis. For additional data, see Ewing et al., 1972.

Table 4–2.   Blood Values in Normal Beagles to 2 Months of Age

	Age				
	0–3 days	14–17 days	28–31 days	40–45 days	56–59 days
Number of dogs	46	46	48	44	42
RBC ($\times 10^6$/μl)	4.8±0.8	3.5±0.3	3.9±0.4	4.1±0.4	4.7±0.4
Hemoglobin (g/dl)	15.8±2.9	9.9±1.1	9.6±0.9	9.2±0.7	10.3±0.9
PCV (%)	46.3±8.5	28.7±2.9	28.4±2.5	28.3±2.3	31.4±2.4
MCV (fl)	94.2±5.9	81.5±3.3	71.7±3.5	68.2±2.6	65.8±2.3
MCH (pg)	32.7±1.8	28.0±2.0	24.3±1.6	22.4±1.0	21.8±1.2
MCHC (%)	34.6±1.4	34.3±1.6	33.5±1.4	32.4±1.7	32.6±1.8
NucRBC/100 WBC	7.2±6.7	2.4±3.8	1.1±1.5	0.6±0.9	0.1±0.4
Reticulocytes (%)*	6.5	6.7	5.8	4.5	3.6
WBC/μl	16,800±5,700	13,600±4,400	13,900±3,300	15,300±3,700	15,700±4,400
Absolute number of WBC/μl					
Band neutrophils	600± 500	200± 200	100± 200	200± 200	300± 300
Segmenters	9,200±6,600	6,900±3,100	6,800±2,000	7,400±2,400	8,500±2,900
Lymphocytes	3,700±2,300	4,900±1,700	5,400±1,600	6,100±1,900	5,000±1,500
Monocytes	1,400±1,300	1,100± 600	1,100± 600	1,300± 600	1,400± 700
Eosinophils	400± 400	500± 500	400± 400	300± 300	400± 400
Platelets/μl*	302,000	290,000	287,000	321,000	411,000
M:E ratio*	1.6:1	1.7:1	1.7:1	1.8:1	1.4:1

Data from Shifrine et al., 1973, except as noted.
*Data from Earl et al. (1973); values were approximated for various age groups shown here; 5 males and 5 females were studied in each group.

of fetal erythrocytes as well as rapid growth of the pup whereby circulating red cell mass is significantly reduced (Lee et al., 1976). At about the beginning of the second month of life a gradual increase in RBC, Hb, and PCV takes place and continues until adult levels are attained at about 1 year of age (Andersen and Gee, 1958). In beagles, PCV was found to increase 43% from 2–8 months of age, after which it remained quite uniform, with RBC and Hb following the same pattern (Bulgin et al. 1970). In other studies, Hb and PCV increased at 42–52 days (Earl et al., 1973; Shifrine et al., 1973) and continued to increase until 18 months of age (Weiner and Bradley, 1972). Peak values were found between 13 months and 2 years of age (Abel and Schneider, 1973) with a steady decline thereafter (Dougherty and Rosenblatt, 1965). In a study of 73 German shepherd dogs between 6 months and 7 years of age, no age differences were found in RBC, WBC and differential leukocyte counts, Hb, MCV, MCH, and MCHC (Konrad et al., 1980).

Average life span of canine erythrocytes is about 115 days (range 110–120 days) and half-life of ^{51}Cr-labeled red cells is about 21–30 days (Spurling, 1977).

Breed Differences

Our experience with clinical specimens suggests that certain breeds of dogs tend to have high RBC, Hb, and PCV values, which may sometimes exceed the normal range for the species. Breeds most frequently involved have been poodles, German shepherds, boxers, beagles, dachshunds, and Chihuahuas and occasionally members of other common breeds. Greyhounds were found to have higher PCV and Hb values than other dogs of similar age (Doxey, 1966; Heneghan, 1977; Porter and Canaday, 1971). Hematologic and biochemical values in 36 purebred dalmatians were similar to values for beagles (Mazue et al., 1977). It is highly probable that the PCV of these breeds of dogs, which is normally between 50% and 55%, becomes elevated as a result of apprehension or fear. The dog that becomes apprehensive when being examined by a veterinarian may experience contraction of the spleen, forcing a concentrated mass of erythrocytes into the circulation. Such a

change is not seen in splenectomized dogs (Reece and Snodgrass, 1972). Hemoconcentration as a result of failure to drink water, in addition to excessive water loss when the dog is sick, will also result in increased red cell values.

The Japanese Akita generally exhibits MCV values of 55–65 fl, thereby indicating a tendency toward a smaller red cell than in other breeds. In contrast, certain poodles may normally have macrocytic (MCV over 80 fl) normochromic red cells and exhibit morphologic abnormalities such as nuclear fragmentation in nucleated erythrocytes and multiple Howell-Jolly bodies in mature red cells (Chapter 25).

Sex Differences

There is disagreement among investigators about sex differences in the circulating mass of erythrocytes. Slightly higher mean values for Hb in males (16.0 g/dl) than in females (15.6 g/dl) were found in a study of 46 male and 68 female beagle dogs (Michaelson et al., 1966). Similarly, higher levels of RBC, Hb, and PCV were found in male beagles under optimum conditions of nutrition and management (Andersen and Gee, 1958). It was also observed that during gestation PCV became gradually reduced from a mean of 53% to 32% at term, then increased to 42% during the next 6 weeks, and returned to normal level by the ninth week. In another study of 101 beagle dogs of each sex, the mean values of PCV were found to be 44.6% in females and 42.5% in males; RBC and Hb followed the same pattern (Robinson and Ziegler, 1968). The latter authors concluded that the differences between the sexes were of little practical value. In a more recent study involving 382 male and 382 female beagle dogs between 8 and 16 months of age, age-related changes in RBC, Hb, and PCV were seen, but no sex influence was noted (Brunk and Becker-Berger, 1980).

Interrelationship of PCV, Hb, and RBC

In a normal animal, the Hb occupies one-third of the volume of the red cell. Therefore it is possible to predict the Hb by dividing the PCV by 3 or to predict the PCV by multiplying the Hb by 3. A rough estimate of RBC number in millions can be obtained by dividing the PCV by 6 (Schalm and Wood, 1954; Uglialoro and Alder, 1957). This relationship does not hold during disease states and when laboratory errors occur in determination of various red cell parameters. In dwarfism in the Alaskan malamute, the PCV:Hb ratio is regularly 4:1 or 5:1 instead of 3:1 (Fletch et al., 1973). It also does not apply for certain animals (e.g., the family Camellidae).

Reticulocytes

Canine reticulocytes are mostly of the "aggregate" type, i.e., with strings and clumps of reticular material, and so they are easy to count. Their number correlates well with polychromatic red cells in Romanowsky-stained blood films (Laber et al., 1974). Circulating reticulocyte number is commonly less than 2% in the adult dog. In puppies, the reticulocyte count may be close to 7% (Table 4–2). Rapid replacement of fetal red cells and increased need to compensate for growth result in increased erythopoietic activity and release of more reticulocytes. In dogs younger than 16 months of age the reticulocyte count may be lower in females than in males (Brunk and Becker-Berger, 1980). In the adult dog, reticulocytes are released in blood with a periodicity of 14 days (Morley and Stohlman, 1969), and their average maturation time in circulation ranges from 19–43 hours with a mean of 31 hours (Nizet and Robscheit-Robbins, 1950). Increased erythropoietic response to anemia is associated with an elevation in reticulocyte numbers in the bone marrow, which precedes increase in the peripheral blood reticulocyte count by about 3 days (Sjöberg, 1978). The oscillatory nature of reticulocyte release, the release rate, and the intravascular maturation time may all change considerably during response to anemia. In such instances, a corrected reticulocyte count or reticulocyte production index (RPI) should be calculated before interpretations are made (Chapters 2 and 21). An absolute number of reticulocytes may be calculated by multiplying the percentile fraction by RBC count. A reticulocyte count of greater than 60,000/µl of blood is indicative of an erythropoietically more active marrow, and moderate to marked erythropoietic activity is indicated by counts

of 150,000–600,000 or more per µl (Weiser, 1981). Empirical observations suggest a normal RPI of 1.0 or less, and an RPI of 2.0 or more is indicative of responsive anemia.

Erythrocyte Sedimentation Rate

Erythrocyte sedimentation rate (ESR) may be performed on canine blood to gain some useful information for clinical evaluation of the patient. ESR is usually performed with the Wintrobe tube, although Westergreen (Spurling, 1977) and microhematocrit (Jain and Kono, 1975) tubes can also be used. The extent of ESR varies with the method used and is affected by a variety of factors. Most important, ESR varies inversely with the number of red cells or PCV. Hence, for proper evaluation of the influence of disease upon ESR, the observed ESR value must be corrected by subtracting from it the anticipated ESR due entirely to ratio of red cells to plasma. Table 2–6 provides anticipated ESR values obtained with the Wintrobe method for a wide range of PCV to correct observed ESR values, and a similar chart has been developed for correcting Westergreen ESR values (Spurling, 1977). No correction table or chart is available for microhematocrit ESR values. See Chapter 2 for factors affecting ESR and interpretation of ESR in various clinical situations in the dog.

Erythrocyte Osmotic Fragility

In a study of the pathogenesis of a hemolytic disease, determination of erythrocyte osmotic fragility may be helpful. Among common domestic animals, canine red cells are least susceptible to osmotic changes (Coldman et al., 1969), but they are more prone to lysis by change in pH than human or ovine red cells (Cruz and Baumgarten, 1957; Iampietro et al., 1967). Hence, osmotic fragility determinations should always be made with buffered NaCl solution (see Chapter 2 for technique). Maximum and minimum resistance to hypotonic NaCl solution has been measured, and although differences are apparent in published values, broad ranges are generally similar. In 34 determinations on 9 normal beagle dogs, initial hemolysis was seen at 0.450 ± 0.022% NaCl concentration, and complete hemolysis at 0.358 ± 0.025%. Observations on 26 male and 25 female dogs

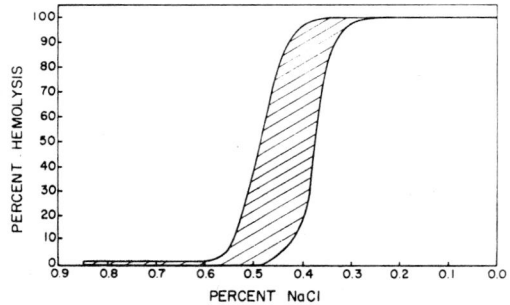

Fig. 4–1. Osmotic fragility curve for erythrocytes from 51 clinically normal dogs.

of various breeds and ages indicated beginning hemolysis (less than 5%) at a NaCl concentration of 0.45–0.55% and complete hemolysis at 0.4% or lower concentration (Fig. 4–1; Jain, 1973). The range and mean for the mean corpuscular fragility were, respectively, 0.36–0.48 and 0.43. Erythrocyte osmotic fragility essentially remains unchanged for canine blood kept for 3 days at 4°C. Mechanical fragility of canine erythrocytes is increased during lipemia (Jasper and Jain, 1964). The observation that newly formed red cells during response to anemia are osmotically more fragile than older red cells (Stewart et al., 1950) needs to be reconciled with common experience that reticulocytes are osmotically more resistant because of their greater surface area (Jain, 1973). See Chapter 20 for comments on changes in erythrocyte osmotic fragility of canine patients with hemolytic anemia.

THE LEUKOCYTES

The differential leukocyte count is expressed in both percentage and absolute number of each cell type per μl of blood. Responses to disease are more critically evaluated from absolute values (Schalm, 1963). Normal values of total leukocyte (WBC) and differential counts for the dog are summarized in Table 4–1 (basenji) and Tables 4–2 and 4–3 (beagles). Normal values are lower and the ranges are narrower for dogs maintained in colonies developed for research purposes than are similar values for small groups of dogs or the canine population at large.

There is little sex difference in WBC counts, but significant age differences are seen in both total and differential leukocyte counts. Some breed, diurnal, seasonal, and physiologic variations have been noted (Andersen and Gee, 1958; Andersen and Schalm, 1970). Beagles have somewhat higher lymphocyte numbers, and higher neutrophil numbers may be seen in older beagles than in other breeds (Spurling, 1977). Young beagles were found to have low WBC counts at 6 A.M. and gradually increasing counts during the day and night with highest level at 2 A.M. (Andersen and Schalm, 1970). These changes were related to physical activity of the animals. Adult dogs did not reveal such a pattern. A seasonal variation amounting to about 2,500 leukocytes/μl of blood was seen in beagles, with highest counts in early summer and lowest during fall and winter. Leukocyte counts increased, mainly due to changes in neutrophil numbers, during pregnancy to about 20,000/μl at term. Then a decline to normal level was seen after weaning.

Influence of Age

The normal range of 6,000–17,000 leukocytes/μl of blood for WBC count includes the effects of age and normal activity. WBC count is highest in young dogs and gradually decreases with age. This decrease is primarily due to changes in lymphocyte and neutrophil numbers. In a study of age-related hematologic changes in beagles up to 60 days in age, mean WBC, neutrophil, and lymphocyte numbers at birth were, respectively, 16,800, 9,200, and 3,700/μl of blood (Shifrine et al., 1973). The WBC count decreased during the first three weeks (12,300) and then gradually increased (15,700) until the eighth week. Neutrophil numbers followed a similar pattern. Lymphocyte numbers increased gradually to 6,100 by the sixth week and then declined to 4,000 by the sixtieth day. Observations on 193 beagles between 2 months and 4½ years in age, revealed a decrease in WBC count with age from a mean of 13,000/μl at 60 days to a mean of 10,000/μl at 4½ years, owing to decrease in both neutrophil and lymphocyte numbers (Bulgin et al., 1970). It was concluded that although a WBC count of 7,000 may be found in a clinically normal older dog, it would be representative of leukopenia in a dog less than 18 months of age. In other stud-

Table 4–3. Total and Differential Leukocyte Counts in Beagle Dogs (means ± 1 SD)

Reference	No of Dogs	Age	Sex	Total WBC (×10³/µl)	Neutrophils — Bands Absolute No./µl	Bands %	Neutrophils — Segmenters Absolute No./µl	Segmenters %	Lymphocytes Absolute No./µl	Lymphocytes %	Monocytes Absolute No./µl	Monocytes %	Eosinophils Absolute No./µl	Eosinophils %	Basophils Absolute No./µl	Basophils %
Michaelson (1966)	46	6 mo to 9 yr	Male	14.2± 3.3	—	2.0±1.7	—	57.5± 8.5	—	28.8± 7.0	—	4.5±1.7	—	7.1±5.2	—	—
	68		Female	14.8± 3.4	—	1.6±1.2	—	57.3± 7.3	—	31.9± 7.0	—	3.7±1.5	—	5.5±4.6	—	—
Robinson (1968)	101	6–12 mo	Male	13.8± 3.5	294±388	2.1±2.7	7,224± 2,652	52.5±12.1	5,007±1,969	37.3±13.2	563±449	4.1±3.0	590±658	4.2±4.2	20±73	0.1±0.5
	101	6–12 mo	Female	12.7± 3.5	247±600	1.7±2.5	6,623± 3,288	51.3±12.9	4,942±2,536	39.3±13.2	529±434	4.2±3.3	388±422	3.0±3.0	17±68	0.1±0.5
Andersen and Schalm (1970)	51	18 mo	Male	12.9	500	—	8,600	—	2,900	—	300	—	500	—	—	—
	47	18 mo	Female	12.1	400	—	7,900	—	2,900	—	300	—	600	—	—	—
Earl et al. (1973)	—	Adults	—	6.6±17.4 (12.0)	50	0.04%	1,700±12,000 (5,600)	26–69 (47)	1,700±12,000 (5,800)	25–71 (481)	0–1,000 (200)	0–6 (2.0)	0–1,700 (400)	0–10 (3.0)	0	0–0.02

ies conducted over a longer period (Andersen and Gee, 1958; Bulgin et al., 1970; Dougherty and Rosenblatt, 1965; Weisse et al., 1971), neutrophil and lymphocyte numbers were found to decrease from 6 months to 4 years of age and remain constant between 4 years and 7 years. Thereafter, an increase was seen in neutrophils. In a 10-year study that included 433 beagles (Dougherty and Rosenblatt, 1965), an age-dependent decrease in WBC, lymphocyte, and eosinophil counts and a slight increase in monocyte numbers were seen. The extent of decrease in lymphocytes is useful in the interpretation of the degree of stress imposed by the disease. It is our experience that lymphopenia may be said to exist when the absolute lymphocyte count is less than 2,000 in dogs 3–6 months of age, less than 1,500 in dogs 8–24 months of age, and less than 1,000 in dogs over 2 years of age.

Effects of Corticosteroids

The release of corticosteroids from the adrenal cortex in response to disease or stressful situations produces marked changes in the total number and differential distribution of circulating leukocytes. A hemogram developed from blood of an animal under treatment with corticosteroids may be misinterpreted when the effects due to the corticosteroids per se are not taken into consideration.

In the dog, in addition to the triad of neutrophilia, lymphopenia, and eosinopenia, a monocytosis results from exposure to synthetic corticosteroids or the injection of ACTH (Fig. 4–2; Jasper and Jain, 1965). Diurnal variations in WBC counts were determined 24 hours prior to exposure to 10 units of ACTH given intramuscularly and to 20 mg of prednisolone given orally (2.2 mg/kg body weight) 5 days later (Table 4–4). After ACTH administration, maximum changes in WBC counts occurred at the eighth hour. The WBC count increased threefold as a result of three- to fourfold increase in neutrophil and monocyte numbers. A marked decrease in lymphocyte and eosinophil numbers occurred by the fourth hour, with complete disappearance of eosinophils by the eighth hour. A normal pattern was reestablished by the twenty-fourth

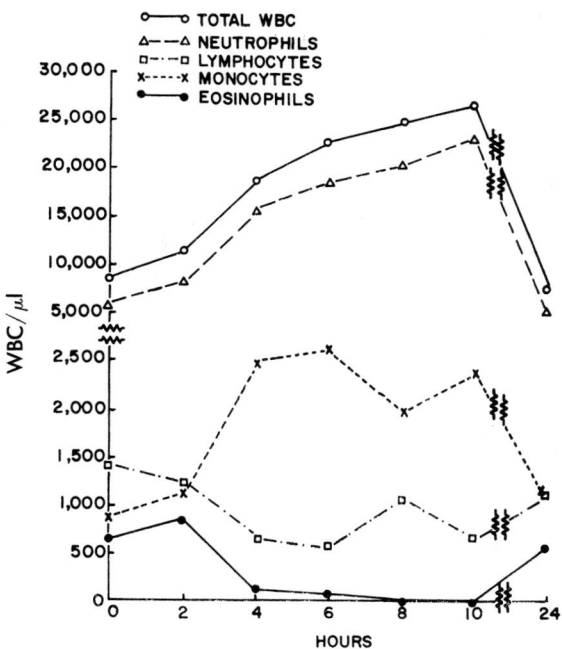

Fig. 4–2. Effect of 20 mg of oral prednisolone on leukocyte numbers in blood.

hour. Effects of prednisolone were similar to those of ACTH. In both instances, the neutrophil increase was accomplished essentially with mature cells. This increase is attributable to release of mature neutrophils from the marrow reserve and decrease in diapedesis of circulating neutrophils into the tissues (see Chapter 26 for details).

The occurrence of corticosteroid-induced monocytosis in the dog is significant in view of the opposite effect in the human, mouse, and rabbit (Fauci et al., 1976; Tompkins, 1952). Its cause is unknown. It probably involves: *(a)* a shift of marrow monocytes, although the existence of a marrow reserve of monocytes in the dog, unlike in the human and mouse, remains to be shown, or *(b)* a shift of monocytes from the marginal pool into the circulating pool, unlike the neutrophilic response. Some species differences can be anticipated in the effect of corticosteroids on circulating monocytes, as in the cat, horse, and cow.

Physiologic and "Emotional" Leukocytosis

Muscular activity, excitement, apprehension, and emotional stress may have a significant influence on total and differential leu-

Table 4–4.   Leukocyte Response in the Dog to ACTH[a] and Prednisolone

Clock Time	Elapsed Time (hr)	PCV (%)	Plasma Proteins (g/dl)	WBC /μl	Neutrophils Band	Neutrophils Mature	Absolute Leukocyte Number/μl Lymphocytes	Monocytes	Eosinophils	Other
				Control Hemograms						
8 a.m.	0	43	6.6	9,350	47	5,640	1,924	846	893	0
10 a.m.	2	40	6.3	9,800	0	6,125	1,568	1,078	931	98
Noon	4	39	6.5	9,750	0	6,338	1,268	1,414	730	0
2 p.m.	6	36	6.0	9,500	0	6,412	1,140	1,188	760	0
4 p.m.	8	42	6.9	13,400	0	9,380	1,608	1,340	1,072	0
6 p.m.	10	42	6.9	15,400	0	11,704	1,386	1,386	924	0
8 a.m.	24	40	6.9	11,400	0	7,980	1,482	798	798	342
				10 Units ACTH						
8 a.m.	0	40	6.9	11,400	0	7,980	1,482	798	798	342
10 a.m.	2	39	7.0	10,600	0	7,738	1,113	1,113	636	0
Noon	4	41	6.7	17,900	0	14,857	895	1,880	179	89
2 p.m.	6	37	7.2	16,900	0	14,312	835	1,670	83	0
4 p.m.	8	39	7.1	32,900	329	28,130	1,645	2,796	0	0
6 p.m.	10	39	6.6	20,400	102	17,748	1,020	1,530	0	0
8 a.m.	24	40	6.9	8,500	42	5,440	1,232	1,020	724	42
				20 mg of Prednisolone, Orally						
8 a.m.	0	42	6.9	8,500	42	5,440	1,488	935	595	0
10 a.m.	2	40	6.8	11,400	0	8,151	1,254	1,197	798	0
Noon	4	40	6.8	19,800	297	16,038	693	2,574	198	0
2 p.m.	6	41	7.1	22,700	227	19,068	567	2,724	114	0
4 p.m.	8	40	7.1	25,300	759	21,505	1,012	2,024	0	0
6 p.m.	10	45	7.4	27,000	405	23,490	675	2,430	0	0
8 a.m.	24	39	6.9	8,100	40	5,265	1,134	1,134	527	0

[a]Delta-Cortef, Upjohn.

Table 4–5. Physiologic Leukocytosis in a Clinically Normal 3-Month-Old Male Beagle; Comparison of the Hemogram at Rest (9 A.M.) and after Normal Activity in an Outside Run (4 P.M.)

	9 A.M.	4 P.M.
PCV%	36	46
Hemoglobin (g/dl)	11.9	15.4
ESR/1 hour (corrected)	14–	4–
Icterus index units	2	5
WBC/μl	13,100	18,900
Neutrophils	8,777	12,096
Lymphocytes	3,668	4,914
Monocytes	393	1,418
Eosinophils	262	472
Plasma proteins (g/dl)	5.6	5.9

kocyte numbers. In dogs at rest, the number of neutrophils sequestered in the capillary beds (marginal pool) on an average nearly equals the number circulating (see Chapter 26) and, similarly, lymphocytes are probably distributed in an extravascular pool of considerable magnitude (see Chapter 30). With increasing activity, circulation of blood and lymph increases leading to washing of sequestered leukocytes into large-vessel blood. An example of the effects of normal muscular activity on blood composition is presented in Table 4–5.

Another form of leukocytosis, which may have an emotional basis, is seen in young dogs under conditions of hospitalization or incarceration at a dog pound. There is an increase in number of several leukocyte types which may mask the leukocyte pattern commonly anticipated as a result of disease. Total and differential leukocyte counts of pound dogs are high, vary widely, and require several days or weeks for normalization (Soave and Boyle, 1965).

Table 4–6 presents data on several young dogs in which the normal pattern of lymphopenia and eosinopenia in response to stress of disease did not occur. Lymphocytosis or persistence of lymphocytes at the high normal range associated in some dogs with eosinophilia resulted in differential leukocyte patterns not common to disease. The dachshund developed a significant lymphocytosis during nine days of hospitalization, while the basset hound revealed a reduction in lymphocytes and monocytes during hospitalization. One might speculate that the dachshund failed to adjust to the hospital environment, while the basset hound became less "emotionally" disturbed under hospitalization. A lost dog (shepherd type) was found on necropsy to be positive for canine distemper, but the marked lymphopenia and eosinopenia common to distemper were masked by eosinophilia and persistence of lymphocytes in the high normal range. Thus significantly increased total leukocyte counts in young dogs, associated with persistence at high levels or increases above the maximum normal ranges of neutrophils, lymphocytes, monocytes, and eosinophils, is considered suggestive of an emotional crisis.

The Neutrophil

Canine neutrophils are produced in the bone marrow over a period of 3–5 days. Their release into the general circulation is regulated by neurohormonal mechanisms as well as need in body tissues. Once in blood, neutrophils distribute into the circulating and marginal pools almost equally or sometimes preferentially into the latter. They leave the circulation randomly, with a half-life of about 7 hours. Further information on granulokinetics is given in Chapter 26.

Mature Neutrophil

The nucleus of the mature neutrophil is irregularly lobed with rounded prominences. Filaments joining two lobes are occasionally seen, but simple narrowing between lobes without true filament formation is the rule. The chromatin is clumped or plaqued into large, deeply staining masses separated by lighter-staining ground substance (Plate VIII–8). The nuclear membrane is irregular or "moth-eaten." The cytoplasm is a faint pale gray with generally indistinct, diffuse, pinkish granulation.

Band Neutrophil

Band neutrophils are present in peripheral blood only in small numbers in health. The nucleus is a curved band having a smooth nuclear membrane and parallel sides for an appreciable length. The chromatin is somewhat less clumped than in the mature cell (Plate XII–3). The cytoplasm is characteristic of the mature neutrophil.

Table 4–6.   Examples of Leukocytosis in Young Dogs, Possibly Resulting from Emotional Stress

Breed	Age (mo)	Sex	Clinical Entity	PCV (%)	WBC/μl*	Neutrophils		Lymphocytes	Monocytes	Eosinophils	Basophils
						Band	Segmenter				
Dachshund	3	F	Sneezing and coughing (admission)	44	34,200	0	26,334	4,275	3,078	513	0
			9th day of hospitalization	42	42,900	214	24,338	13,514	4,719	214	0
Basset	2	F	Treated by owner for intestinal parasites	29	47,700	1,193	26,712	14,787	5,009	0	0
			After 4 days of hospitalization	32	24,300	1,337	19,926	2,430	486	121	0
Mongrel	2	F	Depression and anorexia. No distemper inclusions found	39	24,800	0	14,260	6,076	3,100	1,364	0
Mongrel	8	M	Fever of unknown origin	42	31,900	0	16,429	11,005	3,190	1,117	159
Shepherd type	8	F	Lost dog. Positive for distemper at necropsy	31	32,900	0	17,766	5,758	6,086	3,290	0

*All differential leukocyte values in absolute numbers per μl of blood.

Metamyelocyte Neutrophil

The metamyelocyte neutrophil is not found in the peripheral blood in health. Its nucleus varies in outline from round, with a slight indentation, to a kidney-bean shape. The chromatin is more diffuse and stains less intensely than that of the mature neutrophil. The cytoplasm tends to be bluer, but still essentially pale, and has indistinct granulation (Plate V–3). When metamyelocytes appear in peripheral blood, they are associated with a definite increase in the number of band neutrophils. The presence of more immature cells, myelocytes and promyelocytes, is an abnormal finding.

Shift to the Left and "Toxic" Neutrophils

The dog responds dramatically to the need for neutrophils to counteract bacterial infections and to participate in the inflammatory process. When need for neutrophils is greater than ability of the bone marrow pool to supply mature forms, bands, metamyelocytes, occasionally myelocytes, and, less frequently, promyelocytes appear together with mature neutrophils in peripheral blood. This is called "a shift to the left."

In severe toxemic states, granulopoiesis becomes suppressed and neutrophil morphology is altered by maturation defects. The most common alteration is inappropriate development of cytoplasmic granules, while the cytoplasm retains the bluish staining characteristic of the myelocyte. The primary granules retain their azurophilia through various maturative stages and become visible in mature neutrophils as reddish purple granules. This process is generally referred to as "toxic" granulation. In more severe toxemias, the cytoplasm stains a deeper blue and may be extensively vacuolated (Plate VIII–12). These characteristics permit the designation "toxic" neutrophils. Toxic granulation is not a common feature of canine neutrophils. Sometimes the nucleus of the neutrophil precursors may undergo beginning maturation without cell division (polyploidy). This results in the formation of occasional giant band forms and mature neutrophils presenting large, twisted, and bizarre nuclei. The nucleus undergoing maturation may divide, resulting in some instances in a cell with double nuclei. Infrequently, nuclear maturation begins with the formation of a central hole, leading to release of a giant cell with a doughnut-shaped nucleus (Plate XV–11).

In dogs, the nitroblue tetrazolium (NBT) reduction test is a useful indicator of the presence of bacterial infection or endotoxemia (Banas, 1974; Hallet and Wilson, 1973). NBT reduction is also increased after infection with *Dirofilaria immitis* (Farnes et al., 1972) and nonspecifically after blood transfusion (Hallet and Wilson, 1973).

Shift to the Right

Five or more lobes of the nucleus in the mature neutrophil commonly represent aging of the cell in the circulation. Corticosteroids have the effect of reducing neutrophil diapedesis into tissues. The circulating neutrophils may then become hypersegmented as a result of longer stay in the circulation. Hypersegmentation is also a feature of deficiency of vitamin B_{12} and folate. Reduced cell mitosis leads to larger definitive neutrophils with hypersegmentation (Plate XI–7). Hypersegmentation of leukocytes may occasionally be an artifact in stored blood (Figs. 4–3, 4–4).

Female Sex Chromatin

The nuclei of certain neutrophil leukocytes of the female characteristically reveal a chromatin appendage called the "drumstick" or "Barr body" (Fig. 4–5; Plate XI–7). Porter (1957) applied the criteria described for drumsticks in human neutrophils to the leukocytes of the dog. The typical drumstick was found in the female on an average of 1 in 22 cells (4.5%). Occasionally, the nucleus of the eosinophil will show a sex lobe. Most of the neutrophils in the blood films from male dogs showed nothing resembling a true drumstick. Occasionally, however, minor lobes and sessile nodules (Fig. 4–6) caused confusion on superficial examination. Small chromatin clumps, often multiple, were fairly frequent. Three hundred neutrophils were found to be a sufficient number to examine before concluding that the blood under study came from a male dog. In another study involving 77 female dogs (Irfan, 1961), the neutrophil with typical sex lobe occurred on an average only

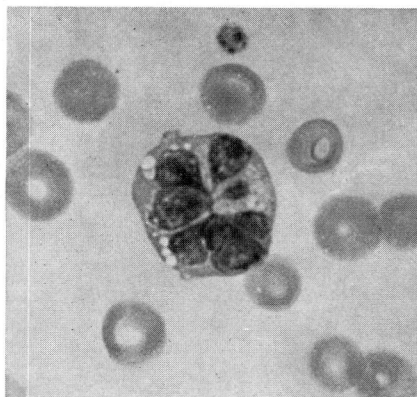

Fig. 4–3. Degenerating monocyte in old blood.

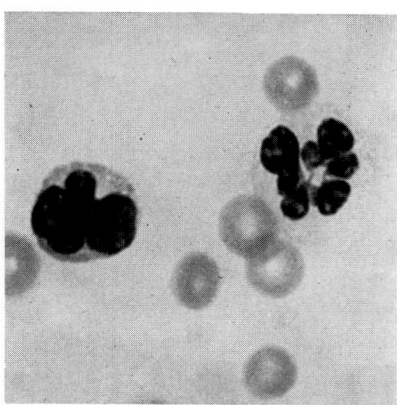

Fig. 4–4. Degenerating lymphocyte and neutrophil in old blood.

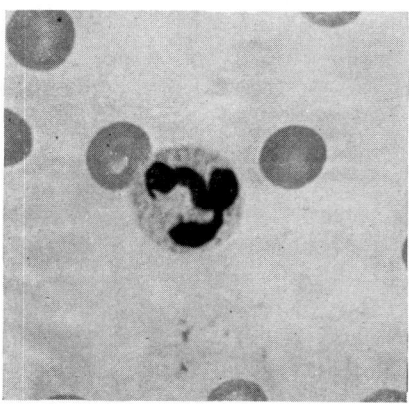

Fig. 4–5. Sex chromatin or "drumstick" lobe in a neutrophil of a female.

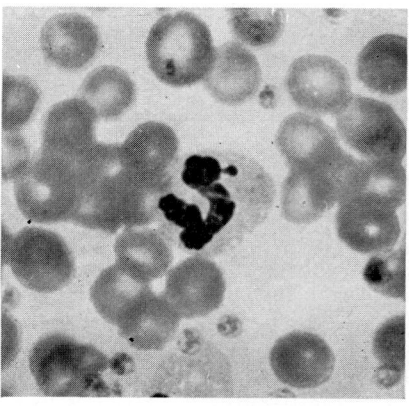

Fig. 4–6. Sessile nodules on the nucleus of a neutrophil of a male.

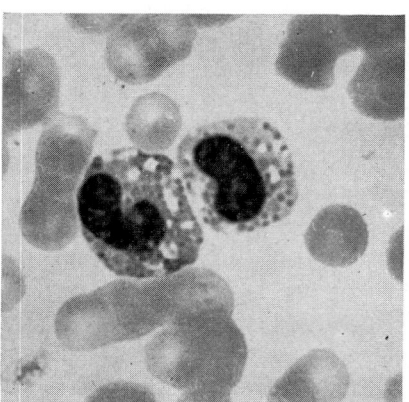

Fig. 4–7. Eosinophils in Pelger-Huët anomaly.

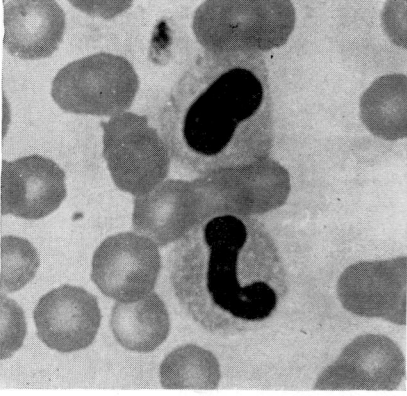

Fig. 4–8. Neutrophils in Pelger-Huët anomaly.

once in 51 cells, although in one female dog the sex lobe was present in 1 out of every 15 neutrophils and in another female in only 1 cell out of 95.

Pelger-Huët Anomaly

This is a hereditary trait in humans and is characterized by failure of the nucleus of granulocytes, especially the neutrophil leukocyte, to undergo normal maturation to the segmented form. This results in an apparent "pseudo" left shift in neutrophil leukocytes. Observations on the condition as it appears in humans have been briefly reviewed along with findings in a strain of rabbits discovered in Switzerland (Nachsheim, 1950; see also Chapter 12). In rabbits, the anomaly is lethal when a homozygous state is produced by selective breeding. The homozygous rabbit tends to die in fetal life, or if it survives to parturition, it usually dies within the first month of life. Surviving homozygous rabbits were stunted and presented a marked skeletal deformity. The Pelger-Huët anomaly in humans is benign when the condition is heterozygous. The total leukocyte count, phagocytic activity, and survival time are normal.

The first observation of the Pelger-Huët anomaly in the dog was as follows. A 6-year-old redbone hound was presented with a complaint of hind-leg stiffness. Radiographs revealed a chronic arthritis. Five hemograms developed between August 10 and December 13, 1961, revealed total leukocyte count to be in the normal range and the existence of a "permanent" shift to the left. This was not a true shift to the left, however, as the cytoplasm of the neutrophils and eosinophils appeared mature, while the nuclei were essentially nonsegmented and deeply stained as a result of the greater than normal condensation of chromatin (Figs. 4–7 and 4–8). A dif-

ferential leukocyte count from the December 13 hemogram is presented in Table 4–7 to show the unusual morphologic features of the neutrophils and eosinophils. The existence of the anomaly did not appear to have produced any effect on general health. An unsuccessful search was made for littermates for a study of their blood. Few other cases have been described in the literature (Bowles et al., 1979; Feldman and Ramans, 1976; Kiss and Kómár, 1957; Pace, 1977).

Blood from the redbone hound in question was transfused into a healthy female Walker hound of A-negative blood type to study in vivo survival time of neutrophils and eosinophils (Carper and Hoffman, 1966). Disappearance of the Pelger-Huët neutrophils from the blood of the recipient was exponential with a T½ value of 4.8 hours. Transfused Pelger-Huët eosinophils disappeared with a T½ value of 30 minutes, indicating that the circulating time is shorter for eosinophils than for neutrophils in the dog. Pelger-Huët canine neutrophils have chemotactic properties similar to normal neutrophils (Latimer and Prasse, 1982).

Acquired hyposegmentation of the granulocyte nucleus is referred to as pseudo-Pelger-Huët anomaly. It may occur during disturbed granulopoiesis from severe infection, leukemia, or idiopathic causes. Such cells were seen for 9 months in a dog with intermittent signs of prostatitis and were thought to have resulted from an idiosyncrasy to a chemotherapeutic agent (Shull and Powell, 1979).

Cyclic Hematopoiesis in Siver-Gray Collie Dogs

Canine cyclic hematopoiesis, previously known as canine cyclic neutropenia, is an autosomal recessive, semilethal condition of silver-gray collies (see reviews by Jones and

Table 4–7. Nuclear Abnormalities in Leukocytes of a Dog with Pelger-Huët Anomaly

| | | Number of Cells with Different Nuclear Shapes | | | | Differential Count (%) |
Cell	Round	Metamyelocyte type	Band type	2-lobed[a]	3-lobed[a]	
Neutrophils	5	15	40	5	4	69
Eosinophils	2	5	5	2	0	14
Lymphocytes						8
Monocytes						9

[a]No true filament formation, only slight indentation of the nuclear membrane.

Lang, 1983; and Lange and Jones, 1980). It was originally characterized by neutropenic cycles, occurring in both sexes and resulting in premature deaths most often from sudden overwhelming infection during a period of neutropenia (Ford, 1969; Lund et al., 1970). The affected pups are stunted or weak and less active at birth than their normal littermates. The first episode of neutropenia is observed within 12 days after birth. Observations on 92 affected pups showed that 62 pups died at birth or during the first week of life and only two pups lived to the age of one year (Ford, 1969). Survival of a female to 2½ years and a male to 3 years has been reported (Lund et al., 1970). The syndrome is remarkably similar to that of human cyclic neutropenia, which cycles at approximately 21 days.

Data on blood and bone marrow cytology in cyclic hematopoiesis have been reported (Cheville, 1968; Dale et al., 1972; Jones et al., 1974; Lange et al., 1976; Lund et al., 1967). A cyclic maturation arrest of granulocytes was demonstrated so that at times the bone marrow samples were nearly devoid of mature neutrophils. The conclusion was that the peripheral blood neutropenia resulted from a cyclic maturation arrest at the level of differentiation of the stem cell. The peripheral blood was characterized by: a marked cyclic neutropenia at 11- to 14-day intervals; a monocytosis peaking just as the neutropenia abates; a variable degree of thrombocytosis occurring 1–2 days before the neutropenia; and reticulocytosis (1.5–10%) occurring during the neutropenic phase. Neutrophil life span was normal, and so was the red cell survival. Erythrocyte parameters were often normal in mature dogs, although the affected pups may have had a mild anemia. Thrombocytopenia and anemia complicated the neutropenic episodes in terminal cases. Fever, septicemia, pneumonia, and enteritis may occur during neutropenic phases.

Recent studies have shown that the cytologic defect resides at the pluripotential stem cell level and is presumably due to an intrinsic marrow defect (Jones and Jolly, 1982). Because cyclic activity of other blood cells, including reticulocytes, platelets, monocytes, and lymphocytes, also appears to occur, the defect is termed canine cyclic hematopoiesis.

Levels of colony-stimulating factor (Yang et al., 1974), erythropoietin (Jones et al., 1975a), and thrombopoietin (McDonald et al., 1976) also show cyclic patterns in relation to changes in blood neutrophil, reticulocyte, and platelet numbers, respectively. Cyclic effect on erythrocyte parameters is not seen, probably because of the longer red cell life span (Lange et al., 1976). An abnormality of the lymphoid system has been demonstrated (Angus et al., 1978), and a periodic variation in lymphokine production has been observed (Lange and Jones, 1980). Functional abnormalities of platelets, e.g., defective adhesiveness and clot retractions, have also been detected (Reese et al., 1976).

Blood cell cycling can be induced in a normal gray collie dog by irradiation and infusion of marrow cells from an affected gray collie (Jones et al., 1975a; Weiden et al., 1974). Conversely, the disorder in an affected gray collie can be eliminated by total body irradiation followed by bone marrow transplantation from a normal gray collie (Dale and Graw, 1974; Jones et al., 1975b). Two of the bone marrow transplant chimeras were reported to be alive for 6 years without detectable signs of graft-versus-host reaction in the absence of any immunosuppressive therapy (Matsas and Yang, 1980). In this regard, it is noteworthy that bone marrow transplantation similarly corrected anemia in 3 basenji dogs with autosomal recessive deficiency of pyruvate kinase (Weiden et al., 1976). Cyclic changes in blood neutrophil, platelet, and reticulocyte numbers can be eliminated by daily administration of endotoxin over a period of several weeks (Hammond et al., 1979; Hammond et al., 1982). Also, treatment with lithium carbonate eliminated the recurrent neutropenia and normalized the other blood cell counts, probably by affecting the most primitive hematopoietic precursor cells (Hammond and Dale, 1980).

The Eosinophil

The granulation of the canine eosinophil is extremely variable. The granules may be numerous, small, and regular, or few and large, e.g., 3–4 μm in diameter (Plates XII–1, XII–2). Cells with extremely large granules are found infrequently. The granules have a weak affinity for the eosin stain. A better staining can be achieved with Wright-Leishman or May-Grünwald-Giemsa stain. Granule color is normally little more intense than that of the erythrocytes in the same blood film but is difficult to capture in color photographs. The nucleus may be partially obscured by granules, but commonly the granules are confined to the cytoplasm. The cytoplasm between the granules takes a light blue stain. Occasionally a few small vacuoles are seen in the cytoplasm, giving the impression of granule lysis; they correspond to electron-lucent, membrane-bound structures seen in electron microscopy (Fig. 27–2A). The eosinophil of the adult greyhound contains more vacuoles, which measure about 2 μm in diameter, than granules (Jones and Paris, 1963).

The Basophil

The granules in basophils vary in number and size. They are never enough to fill the cytoplasm, which stains a gray-blue (Plate XII–1). Basophil granules are water-soluble and tend to disappear in unfixed films stained with new methylene blue. In methanol-fixed films stained with Wright stain, basophil granules stain metachromatically (reddish purple), appear as partially vacuolated structures, and may become less numerous from dissolution. Basophils occur rarely in normal canine blood. They tend to appear in appreciable numbers in association with eosinophilia (Chapter 27). Sometimes they are seen in small numbers in the absence of eosinophils, as in Cushing's disease (Chapter 36).

The Lymphocyte

This leukocyte varies in size from small to large. The small lymphocyte is the most common. The nucleus of the small lymphocyte almost fills the cell, with only a narrow rim or crescent of cytoplasm being visible. The nuclear chromatin is clumped and stains deeply. The cytoplasm varies in color, but is usually pale blue. In the medium and large lymphocytes, the cytoplasm is more voluminous and encircles the nucleus. Occasionally a small lymphocyte with intensely blue-stained cytoplasm is found. An infrequent lymphocyte may present a cluster of a few small, reddish azurophilic granules in the cytoplasm.

Persistent lymphopenia in chronic disease is either a sign of direct action of the disease agent on lymphocytic tissue, as in canine distemper, or a sign of continuation of the depressing effect of corticosteroids. The return of lymphocytes in normal numbers to the circulation generally can be interpreted as a favorable sign.

The Monocyte

The monocyte is generally the largest of the mature leukocytes in the blood. Its most characteristic feature is a basophilic or blue-gray ground-glass cytoplasm. The cytoplasm commonly presents vacuoles that vary in size and frequently are clustered at one side of the cell (Plates VIII–5, VIII–9). An occasional vacuole may be within the nucleus. Another identifying feature, when present, is the occurrence of numerous dust-like, pinkish, azurophilic granules (Plates VII–9, XI–8). The nucleus is extremely variable and can assume any shape. It may at times resemble that of the early band neutrophil or late metamyelocyte (Plates VII–10, VIII–5 to VIII–8). However, the ends of the band-like nucleus of the monocyte are enlarged and knob-like. The nuclear chromatin pattern is characteristically diffuse or mesh-like; when clumping or condensation is present, it generally does not assume a uniform pattern seen in cells of the neutrophilic series. Because the nucleus tends to be ameboid in outline, slender processes suggesting pseudopodia represent another variation sometimes encountered in the monocyte nucleus.

This cell increases in number in peripheral blood in the dog in response to endogenous release of corticosteroids or exogenous administration of ACTH or synthetic corticosteroids (Fig. 4–2). Numbers are generally increased in all acute and chronic diseases of the dog, as shown in a majority of the appendix cases relating to this species.

THE PLATELETS

Platelets are cytoplasmic fragments of megakaryocytes (Plate III–5). They are pleomorphic, exhibiting noticeable variation in size and shape. Most commonly, they appear as roundish structures presenting a central cluster of fine, purplish azurophilic granules surrounded by a pale blue matrix enclosed in a delicate membrane (Plate VIII–2). Some platelets may appear agranular or have only a few granules. Occasionally, long, thread-like processes project outward in several directions. Round platelets measure about 2.5 μm in diameter, and oval forms are about 3.5 μm in length (Belleville et al., 1966). Clumping of platelets may occur in blood in which the clotting mechanism started to function before anticoagulation was complete. Giant forms, as large as the erythrocyte, may appear during remission from thrombocytopenia. Granular platelets are believed to be young platelets and often appear in increased numbers following blood loss (Ingram and Coopersmith, 1969).

Morphology of canine platelets has been studied with the transmission (Schultz, 1968) and scanning (Jain, 1975) electron microscopes. Their surface features are generally similar to those of other domestic animals, although there are species variations in shape and size and also variations within individuals of the same species. In critical point dried specimens prepared for scanning electron mi-

croscopy, canine platelets measure about 2.2–3.7 μm (mean 2.98) in diameter and about 0.5 μm in thickness. They present two morphological forms (Fig. 4–9). The majority are discoid, oval, or elongated, slightly biconvex or flat platelets with even contour. Their surface is less smooth or at times slightly rough when compared to that of mature erythrocytes, and sometimes exhibits few small shallow depressions or tiny protuberances. Few short pseudopods are seen on some platelets. The other variety is composed of irregular spheroidal platelets having many surface buds and few long pseudopods. Platelet morphology is markedly affected by temperature and time of storage of EDTA-anticoagulated blood; ideal storage time is less than 1 hour at 37°C.

The normal range of platelet count in the dog is 200,000–500,000/μl of blood. Venous blood has relatively less numerous platelets than the arterial blood, respective counts being 468,000 and 550,000/μl (Tocantins, 1938). In young beagle dogs, platelet counts are lower (280,000/μl at 6 months) than in adults (446,000/μl at 4 years) (Andersen and Gee, 1958). In another study on beagle dogs, the average platelet count was found to be 400,000/μl at 18 months of age and 300,000/

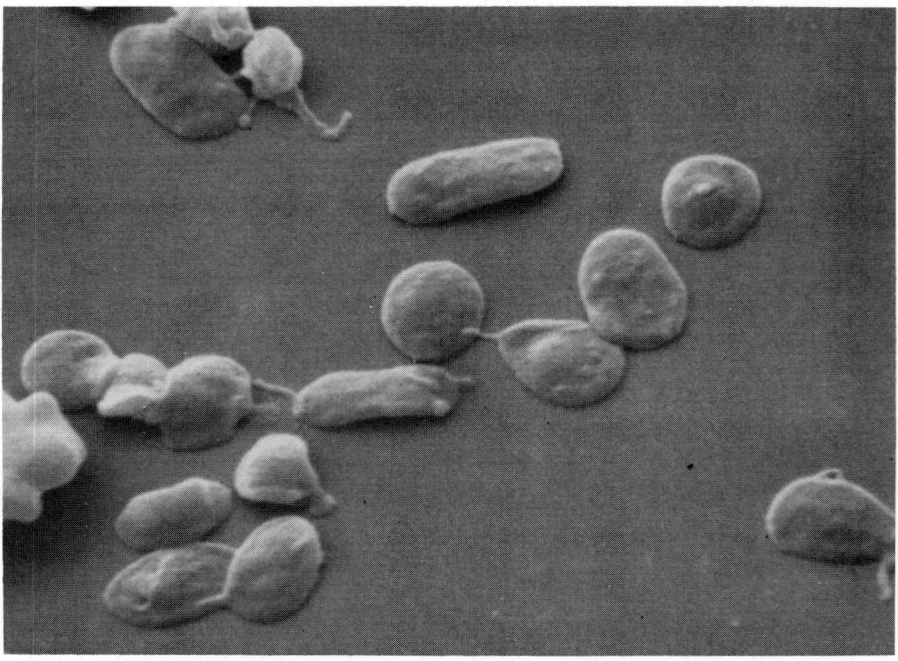

Fig. 4–9.   Scanning electron photomicrograph of canine platelets. × 5,600.

Table 4–8. Differential Cell Counts in Bone Marrow Aspirated from the Iliac Crest of the Same Normal Dog on Three Separate Days, Compared with Bone Marrow from a Dog with an Elevated Total Leukocyte Count in Blood

| | Percentage Distribution—500 Cells Differentiated | | | |
| | Normal Dog | | | Dog with |
	April 2	April 3	April 7	Otitis Externa
Erythrocytic Cells				
Rubriblasts	0.2	0.0	0.4	0.2
Prorubricytes	0.6	1.2	0.8	1.0
Basophilic rubricytes	11.6	9.6	8.2	5.2
Polychromatophilic rubricytes	17.0	19.0	13.6	11.6
Metarubricytes	9.6	9.8	8.2	1.8
Total erythrocytic cells	39.0	39.6	31.2	19.8
Granulocytic Cells				
Myeloblasts	0.8	1.2	1.2	1.0
Progranulocytes	0.6	2.0	1.6	2.6
Neutrophilic myelocytes	4.8	4.4	5.4	5.8
Eosinophilic myelocytes	2.0	0.8	1.0	1.0
Neutrophilic metamyelocytes	5.8	5.0	5.0	7.8
Eosinophilic metamyelocytes	1.6	1.4	1.2	0.6
Neutrophilic bands	17.0	10.4	10.6	14.2
Eosinophilic bands	1.4	1.2	2.4	1.4
Neutrophils	21.8	22.8	28.0	27.6
Eosinophils	1.6	1.4	0.8	0.4
Basophils	0.0	0.2	0.0	0.0
Total granulocytic cells	57.4	50.8	57.2	62.4
M:E ratio	1.5:1.0	1.3:1.0	1.8:1.0	3.27:1.0
Other Cells				
Hematogones	0.6	1.0	0.8	1.2
Lymphocytes	0.6	2.0	2.6	4.8
Monocytes	0.4	1.8	0.8	1.0
Mitotic cells	0.0	0.8	0.4	0.2
Plasma cells	0.2	0.4	2.2	5.0
Unclassified cells	0.2	0.0	0.0	0.2
Degenerated cells	1.8	1.8	2.8	2.4
Nuclei of RE cells	0.4	1.8	2.0	3.0
Peripheral Blood Values				
PCV	45.0	47.0	44.0	47.0
WBC (total leukocyte count/μl)	9,500	11,000	16,300	25,800

μl at 10 years of age (Dougherty and Rosenblatt, 1965). These findings may be a reflection of reduction in adrenocortical activity with advancing age since administration of corticosteroids generally stimulates thrombopoiesis.

Canine platelets are produced over a period of 3–4 days (Craddock et al., 1955). Their half-life in circulation was estimated at 2.2 days (Adelson et al., 1961) and exponential survival between 1.7 and 5.3 days (Rowsell et al., 1967). Platelet survival was prolonged by moderate doses of heparin, but with progressively increased doses it attained a maximum value and then declined. Recent studies suggest normal life span of canine platelets of about 5–6 days (see Chapter 15).

Functional studies of canine platelets have been performed, and some species differences have been found with regard to responses to aggregating agents. Canine platelets exhibit variable aggregation with adrenaline and marked and usually irreversible aggregation with thrombin (Calkins et al., 1974; Hall, 1972; MacMillan and Sim, 1970; Mason and Read, 1967), adenosine diphosphate (ADP), and collagen. Snake venom and ristocetin produce fine aggregation visible macroscopically. Dipyridamole inhibits ADP-induced aggregation of canine platelets as in humans (Calkins et al., 1974). Noradrenaline and serotonin do not induce platelet aggregation, but the latter potentiates the effect of ADP (Sinakos and Caen, 1967). Secondary response to adrenaline is also variable, and it is slower and follows disaggregation

Table 4–9.   Representative Differential Cell Counts in Marrow Aspirated from the Iliac Crest of the Dog in Normal and Disease States

		Percentage Distribution—500 Cells Differentiated			
	Normal	*Iron-Deficiency Anemia in Remission (Blood + Iron Therapy)*	*Chronic Ulcerative Colitis (Blood Loss)*	*End Stage Kidney Disease*	*Lymphocyte Leukemia*
Erythrocytic Cells					
Rubriblasts	0.2	1.3	0.0	0.2	0.0
Prorubricytes	3.9	2.7	2.3	5.2	1.1
Rubricytes	27.0	19.0	29.6	3.0	0.7
Metarubricytes	15.3	43.0	18.2	1.0	0.0
Total erythrocytic cells	46.4	66.0	50.1	9.4	1.8
Granulocytic Cells					
Myeloblasts	0.0	0.4	1.7	0.2	0.7
Progranulocytes	1.3	0.5	0.3	1.0	3.8
Neutrophilic myelocyte	9.0	1.1	3.3	0.2	9.8
Eosinophilic myelocyte	0.0	0.1	0.3	0.2	0.0
Neutrophilic metamyelocyte	7.5	2.4	6.0	7.0	25.5
Eosinophilic metamyelocyte	2.4	0.0	1.0	0.4	0.7
Neutrophilic bands	13.6	9.3	12.0	20.4	17.5
Eosinophilic bands	0.9	0.3	0.0	0.0	0.2
Neutrophils	18.4	8.8	23.0	34.4	11.8
Eosinophils	0.3	0.1	0.0	0.4	0.0
Basophils	0.0	0.0	0.0	0.2	0.0
Total granulocytic cells	53.4	23.0	47.6	64.4	70.0
M:E ratio	1.15:1.0	0.35:1.0	0.95:1.0	6.85:1.0	38.8:1.0
M:E, including degenerated cells	—	0.44	—	7.1	—
Other Cells					
Prolymphocytes	0.0	0.0	0.0	0.0	21.6
Lymphocytes	0.2	4.1	1.3	11.6	6.6
Monocytes	0.0	0.2	1.0	10.6	0.0
Unclassified cells	0.0	0.7	0.0	1.4	0.0
Degenerated cells	0.0	6.0	0.0	2.6	0.0
Peripheral Blood Values					
Total blood leukocytes/µl	12,000	9,100	19,850	13,500	58,000
Blood PCV (%)	45	29	15.5	22.5	21.3

(MacMillan and Sim, 1970). Adherence of canine platelets to glass bead column has been studied (Dodds, 1974); also see Chapter 16.

THE PLASMA

Icterus Index

The icterus index of the dog in health seldom exceeds 5 units. Plasma color equal to 7.5 units may occur in severe dehydration and always requires interpretation, while a reading of 10 units or greater is distinctly abnormal and clinically significant.

Total Plasma Proteins

Plasma protein concentration is lowest at birth, being commonly less than 5.0 g/dl, and is between 6.0 and 7.0 g/dl in dogs 4–6 months in age (Table 4–1). Dogs 1 year of age or older commonly have plasma proteins between 7.0 and 8.0 g/dl. The increase in plasma proteins with age is primarily due to the globulin fraction, which increases in response to foreign antigens. Influence of dehydration and disease on the plasma protein concentration is discussed in Chapter 34. Clinical significance of plasma protein concentration has been discussed (Schalm, 1970).

Plasma Fibrinogen

Plasma fibrinogen is not influenced by age. It normally ranges between 0.1 and 0.5 g/dl, but is most commonly between 0.2 and 0.4 g/dl (Table 4–1). Fibrinogen concentration increases in inflammatory and tissue-destroying diseases (see Chapter 34). An increase in plasma fibrinogen concentration, with total and differential leukocyte counts within the normal range, may be found in some diseased animals (Sutton and Johnstone, 1977). A two- to threefold increase in plasma fibrinogen may be seen in the pregnant bitch. This may be due partly to increases in plasma progesterone since its injection elevates plasma fibrinogen level (Gentry and Liptrap, 1981).

THE BONE MARROW

The Myeloid:Erythroid Ratio

The M:E ratio in clinically normal dogs is generally between 1.0 and 2.0:1. Published values have included a range of 0.75–2.53:1, with a mean of 1.25:1 (Bloom and Meyer, 1944) and a mean value of 1.20:1 from a study involving 187 dogs (Albritton, 1952). A comparison was made of marrow from the rib, femur, tibia, and humerus (Rekers and Coulter, 1948). Mean M:E ratio for the rib marrow from 36 mongrel dogs, 9–24 months of age and representing both sexes, was 1.89:1, while the M:E ratio for the long bones varied between 1.39 and 2.99:1. Similarly, a comparison of the cytology of aspirates from the sternum and ribs of 5 beagle dogs, 1–1½ years of age, revealed a mean M:E ratio of 1.66 ± 0.38 for sternal marrow and 1.53 ± 0.23 for rib marrow (Melveger, 1969).

Bone marrow was aspirated from the iliac crest of the same normal dog on three separate occasions (Table 4–8). The M:E ratios were 1.5, 1.3, and 1.8:1, demonstrating repeatability of results with aspirates made on different days from the same dog. Included in the study was a dog with a peripheral blood leukocytosis of 25,800/μl in response to otitis externa; the M:E ratio for that dog was 3.27:1 reflecting the intensification of granulopoiesis in response to infection.

Influence of a variety of disease entities on the M:E ratio is shown in Table 4–9. In iron deficiency in remission, the intensification of erythrogenesis is indicated by an M:E ratio considerably less than 1.0:1.0. In chronic ulcerative colitis with blood loss, an M:E ratio of 0.95:1.0 revealed a somewhat higher than normal erythrogenesis. In end stage kidney

disease, a depression of erythrogenesis was evident by a PCV of 22.5% and an M:E ratio of 6.85:1. The mean M:E ratio of 38.8:1 in lymphocytic leukemia indicates a depression of erythrogenesis, possibly as a result of massive infiltration of the bone marrow by neoplastic lymphocytes.

REFERENCES

Abel, H.H., and Schneider, B.: Einige "Normwerte" des Blutes für den Hundeauszechtstamm Brack: BEAGLE (Beagle/Brackwede). Zeit. Versuchstierkhunde, *15*:160, 1973.

Adelson, E., et al.: Platelet and Fibrinogen Survival in Normal and Abnormal States of Coagulation. Blood, *17*:267, 1961.

Albritton, E.C., ed.: Standard Values in Blood. W.B. Saunders, Philadelphia, 1952.

Andersen, A.C., and Gee, W.: Normal Blood Values in the Beagle. Vet. Med., *53*:135, 1958.

Andersen, A.C., and Schalm, O.W.: The Beagle as an Experimental Dog. pp. 261–281. *In* Hematology. Andersen, A.C., ed. Iowa State University Press, Ames, 1970.

Angus, K., et al.: Impaired Lymphocyte Response to Phytohemagglutinin in Dogs Affected with Cyclic Neutropenia. Clin. Immunol. Immunopathol., *11*:39, 1978.

Banas, D.A.: Experience with the Nitroblue Tetrazolium Test in Four Domestic Species. Bull. Amer. Soc. Vet. Clin. Path., *3*:17, 1974.

Belleville, J., et al.: Études des principaux tests de l'hémostase chez le chien normal. Path. Biol., *14*:41, 1966.

Bloom, F., and Meyer, L.M.: The Morphology of the Bone Marrow Cells in Normal Dogs. Cornell Vet., *34*:13, 1944.

Bowles, C.A., et al.: Studies of Pelger-Huët Anomaly in Foxhounds. Amer. J. Pathol., *96*:237, 1979.

Brunk, R., and Becker-Berger, S.: Statistiche Untersuchungen auf alters- und geschlechtsspezifische Unterschiede von Blutparametern an englishchen Beagle-Hunden. Berl. Münch. Tierärztl. Wochenschr., *93*:128, 1980.

Bulgin, M.S., et al.: Hematologic Changes to 4½ Years of Age in Clinically Normal Beagles. J. Amer. Vet. Med. Ass., *157*:1064, 1970.

Calkins, J., et al.: Comparative Study of Platelet Aggregation in Various Species. J. Med., *5*:292, 1974.

Carper, H.A., and Hoffman, P.L.: The Intravascular Survival of Transfused Pelger-Huët Neutrophils and Eosinophils. Blood, *27*:739, 1966.

Chandler, F.W., Jr., et al.: Surface Ultrastructure of Pyruvate Kinase–Deficient Erythrocytes in the Basenji Dog. Amer. J. Vet. Res., *36*:1477, 1975.

Cheville, N.F.: The Gray Collie Syndrome. J. Amer. Vet. Med. Ass., *152*:620, 1968.

Coldman, M.F., et al.: The Osmotic Fragility of Mammalian Erythrocytes in Hypotonic Solutions of Sodium Chloride. Comp. Biochem. Physiol., *31*:605, 1969.

Craddock, C.G., et al.: The Dynamics of Platelet Production as Carried Out by a Depletion Technic in Normal and Irradiated Dogs. J. Lab. Clin. Med., *45*:906, 1955.

Cruz, W.O., and Baumgarten, A.: Susceptibility of the Red Blood Cell of the Dog to Haemolysis in Alkaline Media. Brit. J. Haematol., *3*:359, 1957.

Dale, D., et al.: Studies of Neutrophil Production and Turnover in Grey Collie Dogs with Cyclic Neutropenia. J. Clin. Invest., *51*:2190, 1972.

Dale, D.C., and Graw, R.G., Jr.: Transplantation of Allogeneic Bone Marrow in Canine Cyclic Neutropenia. Science, *183*:83, 1974.

Dodds, W.J.: Blood Coagulation: Hemostasis and Thrombosis. *In* Handbook of Laboratory Animal Science. Vol. 2, p. 87. Melbey, E.C., Jr., and Altman, N.H., eds. C.R.C. Press, Cleveland, Ohio, 1974.

Dougherty, J.H., and Rosenblatt, L.S.: Changes in the Hemogram of the Beagle with Age. J. Gerontol., *20*:131, 1965.

Doxey, D.L.: Cellular Changes in the Blood as an Aid to Diagnosis. J. Small Anim. Pract., *7*:77, 1966.

Earl, F.L., et al.: The Hemogram and Bone Marrow Profile of Normal Neonatal, and Weanling Beagle Dogs. Lab. Anim. Sci., *23*:690, 1973.

Ederstrom, H.E., and DeBoer, B.: Changes in the Blood of the Dog with Age. Anat. Rec., *94*:663, 1946.

Ewing, G.O., et al.: Hematologic Values of Normal Basenji Dogs. J. Amer. Vet. Med. Ass., *161*:1661, 1972.

Farnes, P., et al.: N.B.T. Tests in Dog Neutrophils. Lancet, *1*(7740):47, 1972.

Fauci, A.S., et al.: Glucocorticosteroid Therapy: Mechanisms of Action and Clinical Considerations. Ann. Int. Med., *84*:304, 1976.

Feldman, B.F., and Ramans, A.U.: The Pelger-Huët Anomaly of Granulocytic Leukocytes in the Dog. Canine Pract., *3*:22, 1976.

Fletch, S.M., et al.: Clinical and Pathologic Features of Chondrodysplasia (Dwarfism) in the Alaskan Malamute. J. Amer. Vet. Med. Ass., *162*:357, 1973.

Ford, L.: Hereditary Aspects of Human and Canine Cyclic Neutropenia. J. Hered., *60*:293, 1969.

Gentry, P.A., and Liptrap, R.M.: Influence of Progesterone and Pregnancy on Canine Fibrinogen Values. J. Small Anim. Pract., *22*:185, 1981.

Hall, D.E.: Blood Coagulation and Its Disorders in the Dog. London, Baillière Tindall, 1972.

Hallett, J.W., Jr., and Wilson, J.W.: Nitroblue Tetrazolium Reduction by Neutrophils in Experimental Hemorrhagic Shock. Amer. J. Pathol., *73*:173, 1973.

Hammond, W.P., and Dale, D.C.: Lithium Therapy of Canine Cyclic Hematopoiesis. Blood, *55*:26, 1980.

Hammond, W.P., et al.: Cyclic Hematopoiesis: Effects of Endotoxin on Colony-Forming Cells and Colony-Stimulating Activity in Grey Collie Dogs. J. Clin. Invest., *63*:785, 1979.

Hammond, W.P., et al.: Canine Cyclic Haematopoiesis: The Effect of Endotoxin on Erythropoiesis. Brit.J. Haematol., *50*:283, 1982.

Heneghan, T.: Haematological and Biochemical Variables in the Greyhound. Vet. Sci. Commun., *1*:277, 1977.

Iampietro, P.F., et al.: pH-Dependent Lysis of Canine Erythrocytes. J. Appl. Physiol., *23*:505, 1967.

Ingram, M., and Coopersmith, A.: Reticulated Platelets following Acute Blood Loss. Brit. J. Haematol., *17*:225, 1969.

Irfan, M.: Studies on the Peripheral Blood Picture of the Dog and Cat in Health and Disease with Special Reference to Lymphatic Leukosis. Irish Vet. J., *15*:65, 1961.

Jain, N.C.: Osmotic Fragility of Erythrocytes of Dogs and Cats in Health and in Certain Hematologic Disorders. Cornell Vet., *63*:411, 1973.

Jain, N.C.: A Scanning Electron Microscopic Study of Platelets of Certain Animal Species. Thrombosis et Diathesis Haemaorrhogica, *33*:501, 1975.

Jain, N.C., and Kono, C.S.: Erythrocyte Sedimentation Rate in the Dog and Cat: Comparison of Two Methods and Influence of Packed Cell Volume, Temperature and Storage of Blood. J. Small Anim. Pract., *16*:671, 1975.

Jasper, D.E., and Jain, N.C.: Postprandial Lipemia in Dogs. Calif. Vet., *18*:27, May–June, 1964.

Jasper, D.E., and Jain, N.C.: The Influence of Adrenocorticotropic Hormone and Prednisolone upon Marrow and Circulating Leukocytes in the Dog. Amer. J. Vet. Res., *26*:844, 1965.

Jones, J.B., and Jolly, J.D.: Canine Cyclic Haematopoiesis: Bone Marrow Adherent Cell Influence of CFU-C Formation. Brit. J. Haematol., *50*:607, 1982.

Jones, J.B., and Lang, R.D.: Cyclic Hematopoiesis: Animal Models. Exp. Hematol., *11*:571, 1983.

Jones, J.B., et al.: Canine Cyclic Neutropenia: Erythropoietin and Platelet Cycles after Bone Marrow Transplantation. Blood, *45*:213, 1975a.

Jones, J.B., et al.: Canine Cyclic Haematopoiesis: Marrow Transplantation between Littermates. Brit. J. Haematol., *30*:215, 1975b.

Jones, J.B., et al.: Early-Life Hematologic Values of Dogs Affected with Cyclic Neutropenia. Amer. J. Vet. Res., *35*:849, 1974.

Jones, R.F., and Paris, R.: The Greyhound Eosinophil. J. Small Anim. Pract., *4*(suppl.):29, 1963.

Kiss, Von M., and Kómár, Gy., Jr.: Pelger-Huët'sche Kernanomalie der Leukozyten bei einem Hunde. Berl. Münch. Tierärztl. Wochenschr., *80*:474, 1967.

Konrad, J., et al.: Hematologie Klinicky Zdraveho Psa. Veterinarni Medicina, *25*:405, 1980.

Laber, J., et al.: Polychromasia of Reticulocytes: An Assessment of the Dog. J. Amer. Anim. Hosp. Ass., *10*:399, 1974.

Lange, R.D., et al.: Erythropoiesis and Erythrocytic Survival in Dogs with Cyclic Hematopoiesis. Amer. J. Vet. Res., *37*:331, 1976.

Lange, R.D., and Jones, J.B.: Canine Cyclic Hematopoiesis. *In* The Canine as a Biomedical Research Model: Immunological, Hematological, and Oncological Aspects. Shifrine, M., and Wilson, F.D., eds. pp. 278–295. Technical Information Center, U.S. Dept. of Energy, Springfield, Va., 1980.

Latimer, K.S., and Prasse, K.W.: Neutrophilic Movement of a Basenji with Pelger-Huët Anomaly. Amer. J. Vet. Res., *43*:525, 1982.

Lee, P., et al.: Blood Volume Changes and Production and Destruction of Erythrocytes in Newborn Dogs. Amer. J. Vet. Res., *37*:561, 1976.

Lumsden, J.H., et al.: Canine Hematology and Biochemistry Reference Values. Can. J. Comp. Med., *43*:125, 1979.

Lund, J.E.: Hemoglobin Crystals in Canine Blood. Amer. J. Vet. Res., *35*:575, 1974.

Lund, J.E., et al.: Cyclic Neutropenia in Grey Collie Dogs. Blood, *29*:452, 1967.

Lund, J.E., et al.: Additional Evidence on the Inheritance of Cyclic Neutropenia in the Dog. J. Hered., *61*:47, 1970.

MacMillan, D.C., and Sim, A.K.: A Comparative Study of Platelet Aggregation in Man and Laboratory Animals. Thrombosis et Diathesis Haemorrhagica, *24*:385, 1970.

Mason, R.G., and Read, M.S.: Platelet Response to Six

Agglutinating Agents: Species Similarities and Differences. Exp. Mol. Pathol., *6*:370, 1967.

Matsas, D.J., and Yang, T.J.: Karyotype Analysis of Leukocytes of Gray Collie (Cyclic Neutropenia): Normal Bone Marrow Transplant Chimeras Six Years after Transplantation. Amer. J. Vet. Res., *41*:1863, 1980.

Mazue, G., et al.: Étude des principales constantes sanguines du chien dalmate. Revue Med. Vet., *128*:639, 1977.

McDonald, T., et al.: Canine Cyclic Hematopoiesis: Platelet Size and Thrombopoietin Level in Relation to Platelet Count. Proc. Soc. Exp. Biol. Med., *153*:424, 1976.

Melveger, B.E., et al.: Sternal Bone Marrow Biopsy in the Dog. Lab. Anim. Care, *19*:866, 1969.

Michaelson, S.M., et al.: The Blood of the Normal Beagle. J. Amer. Vet. Med. Ass., *148*:532, 1966.

Morley, A., and Stohlman, F., Jr.: Erythropoiesis in the Dog: The Periodic Nature of the Steady State. Science, *165*:1025, 1969.

Nachsheim, H.: The Pelger Anomaly in Man and Rabbit, A Mendelian Character of the Nuclei of Leukocytes. J. Hered., *41*:131, 1950.

Nizet, A., amd Robscheit-Robbins, F.S.: Reticulocyte Ripening in Experimental Anemia and Hypoproteinemia. Blood, *5*:648, 1950.

Oduye, O.O.: Haematological Studies on Clinically Normal Dogs in Nigeria. Zentralbl. Veterinaermed., *25*:548, 1978.

Pace, E.M.: Pelger-Huët Anomaly Transmission. Canine Pract., *4*:33, 1977.

Pinkerton, P.H., et al.: Hereditary Stomatocytosis with Hemolytic Anemia in the Dog. Blood, *44*:557, 1974.

Porter, J.A., Jr., and Canaday, W.R., Jr.: Hematologic Values in Mongrel and Greyhound Dogs Being Screened for Research Use. J. Amer. Vet. Med. Ass., *159*:1603, 1971.

Porter, K.A.: A Sex Difference in Morphology of Neutrophils in the Dog. Nature, *170*:784, 1957.

Reece, W.O., and Snodgrass, R.R.: Effect of Splenectomy on Postfeeding Changes in Packed Cell Volume of Dogs. Amer. J. Vet. Res., *33*:635, 1972.

Reese, M.E., Jr., et al.: Platelet Function Studies in Dogs with Cyclic Hematopoiesis. Proc. Soc. Exp. Biol. Med., *153*:324, 1976.

Rekers, P.E., and Coulter, M.: A Hematological and Histological Study of the Bone Marrow and Peripheral Blood of the Adult Dog. Amer. J. Med. Sci., *216*:643, 1948.

Robinson, F.R., and Ziegler, R.F.: Clinical Laboratory Values of Beagle Dogs. Lab. Anim. Care, *18*:39, 1968.

Rowsell, H.C., et al.: Effect of Heparin on Platelet Economy in Dogs. Amer. J. Physiol., *213*:915, 1967.

Schalm, O.W.: Interpretation of Leukocyte Responses in the Dog. J. Amer. Vet. Med. Ass., *142*:147, 1963.

Schalm, O.W.: Clinical Significance of Plasma Protein Concentration. J. Amer. Vet. Med. Ass., *157*:1672, 1970.

Schalm, O.W., and Wood, M.: Observations on the Use of Certain Hematological Techniques in Canine Medicine. Proc. Book Amer. Vet. Med. Ass., 91st Ann. Meeting, p. 286, 1954.

Schultz, H.: Thrombocyten und Thrombose in elektronenmikroskopischen Bild. Springer Verlag, Berlin, p. 46, 1968.

Shifrine, M., et al.: Hematologic Changes to 60 Days of Age in Clinically Normal Beagles. Lab. Anim. Sci., *23*:894, 1973.

Shull, R.M., and Powell, D.: Acquired Hyposegmentation of Granulocytes (Pseudo-Pelger-Huët Anomaly) in a Dog. Cornell Vet., *69*:241, 1979.

Sinakos, Z., and Caen, J.P.: Platelet Aggregation in Mammalians (Human, Rat, Rabbit, Guinea-Pig, Horse, Dog): A Comparative Study. Thrombosis et Diathesis Haemorrhagica, *17*:99, 1967.

Sjöberg, A.E.: Vergleich de Erythrocytenstatus, insbesondere der Retikulocyten, in Venenblut und im Knochenmarksblut zweier Hunde nach Aderlass und bei physiologischer Blutmauserung. Inaug. diss. Freie Universität, Berlin. *In* Vet. Bull., *53*:73, 1978.

Soave, O.A., and Boyle, C.C.: A Comparison of the Hemograms of Conditioned and Non-Conditioned Laboratory Dogs. Lab. Anim. Care, *15*:359, 1965.

Spurling, N.: The Haematology of the Dog. *In* Comparative Clinical Haematology. Archer, R.K., and Jeffcott, L.B., eds. Blackwell Scientific Publications, Oxford, 1977.

Stewart, W.B., et al.: Age as Affecting the Osmotic and Mechanical Fragility of Dog Erythrocytes Tagged with Radioactive Iron. J. Exp. Med., *91*:147, 1950.

Sutton, R.H., and Johnstone, M.: The Value of Plasma Fibrinogen Estimations in Dogs: A Comparison with Total Leucocytes and Neutrophil Counts. J. Small Anim. Pract., *10*:277, 1969.

Tocantins, L.M.: The Mammalian Blood Platelet in Health and Disease. Medicine, *17*:155, 1938.

Tompkins, E.H.: The Response of Monocytes to Adrenal Cortical Extract. J. Lab. Clin. Med., *30*:365, 1952.

Tsessarskaya, T.P., and Burkovskaya, T.E.: Seasonal Variation in the Blood Leukocyte Count in Dogs. Bull. Exp. Biol. Med., *82*:1465, 1976.

Tvedten, H.W.: Hematology of the Normal Dog and Cat. Vet. Clin. North Amer. (Small Anim. Pract.), *11*:209, 1981.

Uglialoro, A., and Alder, H.L.: The Correlation between Packed Cell Volume and Erythrocyte Number in Canine Blood. Amer. J. Vet. Res., *18*:909, 1957.

Weiden, P.L., et al.: Canine Cyclic Neutropenia: A Stem Cell Defect. J. Clin. Invest., *53*:950, 1974.

Weiden, P.L., et al.: Severe Hereditary Haemolytic Anemia in Dogs Treated by Marrow Transplantation. Brit. J. Haematol., *33*:357, 1976.

Weiner, D.J., and Bradley, R.E.: The Hemogram and Certain Serum Protein Fractions in Normal Beagle Dogs. Vet. Med. Small Anim. Clin., *67*:393, 1972.

Weiser, M.G.: Hematologic Techniques. Vet. Clin. North Amer. (Small Anim. Pract.), *11*:189, 1981.

Weisse, I., et al.: Das Blutbild der englischen Beagle-Hunde in Abhängigkeit von Alter und Geschlecht. Arzneim. Forsch., *21*:1703, 1971.

Yang, T.J., et al.: Serum Colony-Stimulating Activity of Dogs with Cyclic Neutropenia. Blood, *44*:41, 1974.

5

The Cat: Normal Hematology with Comments on Response to Disease

THE ERYTHROCYTES 127
    Sex Differences 128
    Reticulocytes 128
    Howell-Jolly Bodies 130
    Nucleated Erythrocytes 130
    Heinz Bodies 130
    Basophilic Stippling 131
    Erythrocyte Sedimentation Rate 132
    Erythrocyte Osmotic Fragility 132

THE LEUKOCYTES 132
    The Neutrophil 133
    The Eosinophil 133
    The Basophil 133
    The Lymphocyte 134

    The Monocyte 134
    Influence of Corticosteroids on Total and
        Differential Leukocyte Counts 134
    Total Leukocyte Counts among Random
        Hospital Admissions 134
    Neutrophil Morphology in Toxemic
        Diseases 135

THE PLATELETS 136

THE PLASMA 136
    Icterus Index 136
    Total Plasma Proteins 136
    Plasma Fibrinogen 136

THE BONE MARROW 137
    The Myeloid:Erythroid Ratio 137

Several studies have been made on normal hematology of the cat (Anderson et al., 1971; Johnson and Perman, 1968; Lewis, 1941; Osbaldiston, 1978). The source of animals for our normal values (see chart) has been the occasional clinically normal cat rather than cats raised specifically for purposes of biomedical research. Part of the problem of establishing normal values for cats is that fright or "emotional" influences alter the total and differential leukocyte counts, causing neutrophil and lymphocyte numbers to be considerably elevated. This is particularly true for cats younger than 1 year of age and for cats introduced into a strange environment (Appendix Cases 53 and 54). This same effect may be encountered in young feline patients, thereby negating the value of the hemogram as an aid to understanding the disease process.

Another problem with cats is that large vessel blood is not as conveniently obtained as from other domestic animals, and for this reason routine blood studies are often limited to capillary blood obtained by puncturing a vessel of the ear. If the blood does not flow freely but is forced out by squeezing the tissues, the RBC and WBC counts will be erroneous. Large samples of blood can be obtained from the cephalic or jugular vein, but here also there may be some difficulty, leading to slow withdrawal of the sample. Platelets then begin to clump and present problems in the electronic counting of cells. In fact, we have been unsuccessful in obtaining good agreement between hemocytometer and Coulter electronic WBC counts in cat blood, and as a result WBC counts in our laboratory are made routinely by hemocytometer. Similarly, the Coulter electronic RBC counts in anemic blood are higher than the hemocytometer counts. It is conjectured that the source of disagreement lies in the counting of clumped platelets by the electronic counter. Collection of a smaller amount of blood than intended for the amount of EDTA present in a collection vial such as a Vacutainer tube results in shrinkage of red cells and erroneous PCV and MCV values. The size of feline erythrocytes may be considerably reduced when EDTA in excess of 4 mg/ml of blood is used (Penny et

Normal Blood Values for the Cat

Erythrocytic Series	Range	Ave.	Leukocytic Series	Range	Ave.
Erythrocytes ($\times 10^6/\mu l$)	5.0–10.0	7.5	Leukocytes/μl	5,500–19,500	12,500
Hemoglobin (g/dl)	8.0–15.0	12.0	Neutrophil (band)	0– 300	100
PCV (%)	24.0–45.0	37.0	Neutrophil (mature)	2,500–12,500	7,500
MCV (fl)	39.0–55.0	45.0	Lymphocyte	1,500– 7,000	4,000
MCH (pg)	12.5–17.5	15.5	Monocyte	0– 850	350
MCHC (%)			Eosinophil	0– 1,500	650
Wintrobe	31.0–35.0	33.0	Basophil	rare	0
Microhematocrit	30.0–36.0	33.2			
Reticulocytes (%)	0.2– 1.6	0.6	Percentage Distribution		
ESR (no data)	—	—	Neutrophil (band)	0– 3	0.5
RBC diameter (μm)	5.5– 6.3	5.8	Neutrophil (mature)	35–75	59.0
Resistance to			Lymphocyte	20–55	32.0
hypotonic saline (%)			Monocyte	1– 4	3.0
Min.	0.66–0.72	0.69	Eosinophil	2–12	5.5
Max.	0.46–0.54	0.50	Basophil	rare	0.0
Myeloid:erythroid ratio	0.6–3.9:1.0	1.6:1.0			

Other Data		
Thrombocytes ($\times 10^5/\mu l$)	3 – 8	4.5
Icterus index (units)	2 – 5	
Erythrocyte life span (days)	66 –78	
Plasma proteins (g/dl)	6.0 – 8.0	
Fibrinogen (g/dl)	0.05– 0.30	

al., 1970a). A false diagnosis of anemia, apparently from sequestration of erythrocytes in the spleen, may result when blood is collected from cats under anesthesia with ketamine hydrochloride and alphaxalone/alphadolone acetate (Frankel and Hawkey, 1980). Conversely, anemia may be masked by release of splenic mass of erythrocytes into the peripheral blood of cats experiencing emotional disturbance.

THE ERYTHROCYTES

An excellent study by Windle et al. (1940) clearly demonstrates changes in erythrocyte number, size, and hemoglobin concentration with advancing age (Table 5–1). The mean value for MCV at birth was 90.3 fl, in contrast to the erythrocyte of the adult cat, which had mean values of 45.0 for males and 49.2 for females. Replacement of large fetal red cells by smaller postnatal cells is brisk during the first few weeks after birth. This is reflected in marked reductions in PCV and Hb values with little changes in RBC counts and concomitant reductions in MCV and MCH. Hemoglobin and PCV values were lowest by the fourth week. As is common to other mammals, Hb concentration is reduced during the nursing period because of the low concentration of iron in milk; thus, although erythrocyte number gradually increases from the third week onward, Hb concentration may not keep pace. The adult level for erythrocyte number is attained by the third to fourth month of life, while the adult Hb level may not be attained until the fifth or sixth month, depending on availability of iron in the diet. Similar age-related changes in red cell parameters (RBC, Hb, and PCV) were reported in normal cats from 4 weeks to 1 year of age (Anderson et al., 1971), in 70 apparently normal kittens (38 females and 32 males) ranging from 8 to 30 weeks of age (Johnson and Perman, 1968), in kittens from birth to 17 weeks in age (Meyers-Wallen et al., 1984), and in kittens from birth to 60 days of age (Noguchi et al., 1981). The transient microcytosis and anemia observed in kittens during the first few weeks of life were attributed to iron deficiency based on findings of low serum iron in such kittens and significantly greater MCV and PCV and reduced microcytosis after injection of iron dextran at 2–3 weeks of age (Weiser and Kociba, 1983). It was also observed that erythrocyte volume distribution curves were more sensitive than the MCV in detecting microcytosis in kittens.

Table 5–1.   Some Aspects of Postnatal Changes in the Blood of the Cat[a]

Age	Number	RBC (×10⁶/μl)	Hb (g/dl)	PCV (%)	MCV[b] (fl)	MCH[b] (pg)	MCHC[b] (%)	MCD[c] (μm)	WBC (×10³/μl)
0– 6 hr	24; 24[d]	4.95	12.2	44.7	90.3	24.6	27.3	6.7	7.55
12–48 hr	23; 26	5.11	11.3	41.7	81.6	22.1	27.1	—	10.18
7 days	21; 21	5.19	10.9	35.7	68.8	21.0	30.5	6.7	7.83
14 days	18; 18	4.76	9.7	31.1	65.3	20.4	31.2	6.5	8.08
21 days	19; 19	4.99	9.3	31.3	62.7	18.6	29.7	6.1	8.82
28 days	20; 20	5.84	8.4	29.9	51.2	14.4	28.1	5.9	8.55
42 days	21; 20	6.75	9.0	35.4	52.4	13.3	25.4	5.9	8.42
56 days	19; 19	7.10	9.4	35.6	50.1	13.2	26.4	5.8	8.42
70 days	22; 22	7.33	9.9	—	—	13.5	—	—	9.18
80 days	21; 21	7.69	10.3	39.0	50.7	13.4	26.4	—	9.12
90 days	21; 21	8.26	10.4	43.1	52.2	12.6	24.1	—	9.01
120 days	21; 21	8.77	10.7	35.7	40.7	12.2	29.9	—	9.36
150 days	7; 7	9.27	11.4	41.5	44.7	12.3	27.7	—	11.66
Adult male	37; 35	9.02	12.2	40.6	45.0	13.5	30.0	5.7	12.4
Adult female	64; 64	8.39	12.0	41.3	49.2	14.3	29.1	5.8	10.5

[a]Modified from Windle et al., 1940.
[b]Estimated from the author's data.
[c]= Mean corpuscular diameter.
[d]= Number of cases averaged for RBC (first figure) and Hb (second figure).

Penny et al. (1970a) presented data on 128 blood samples from clinically normal cats of both sexes and over 6 months of age. Their data compare favorably with the values presented at the beginning of this chapter, the main differences being that the mean RBC count was somewhat lower (6.45 ± 0.87 × 10⁶/μl), the MCV somewhat higher (56.16 ± 6.22 fl), and the range for total WBC count considerably broader (3,500–24,000/μl). In comparison, data reported by Osbaldiston (1978) had higher upper limits for RBC, Hb, PCV, and WBC and lower limits for MCV than our values.

Red cell parameters of germfree cats were found to be similar to those of conventionally raised cats (Rohovsky and Griesemer, 1969). Cats maintained at an altitude of 7,200 feet (2,196 meters) had a mean Hb value of 14.2 ± 0.3 g/dl and a PCV of 46.5 ± 0.8% (Velasco et al., 1971). Means for Hb and PCV for the cat at near sea level are, respectively, 12.0 g/dl and 37.0%.

Pregnancy in the cat results in development of a normocytic normochromic anemia accompanied by an erythroid response by the bone marrow. In 6 queens, RBC, Hb, and PCV decreased during late pregnancy with marked reversal occurring during early postpartum period and return to early pregnancy values by the seventh day postpartum (Berman, 1974). The reticulocyte counts, comprised of both aggregate and punctate forms (discussed below), increased from 9.3 ± 4.9% to 26.5 ± 7.5% during late pregnancy, returned to early pregnancy values by 24 hours postpartum (15.5 ± 9.9%), and steadily decreased throughout lactation and thereafter (6.8 ± 4.3%). Plasma protein levels and WBC counts did not change remarkably during the entire period.

Sex Differences

Slightly higher values for RBC and WBC counts and Hb concentration for males were recorded in two studies on cats, although the differences were not great (Landsberg, 1940; Windle et al., 1940). A comparison of 23 males and 16 females in another study revealed slightly higher RBC counts and Hb concentration in males, but somewhat higher WBC counts in females (Lewis, 1941). In a study of 67 males and 82 females, respective mean values for RBC were 8.5 million and 8.1 million/μl of blood; for Hb, 13.9 and 12.5 g/dl; and for WBC, 10,400 and 11,000/μl (Hauser, 1963).

Reticulocytes

Reticulocyte counts are difficult to make in cat blood because some cells contain fine specks whose identification as true reticulocytes may be questionable. Such cells are particularly numerous in newborn kittens and probably comprise as many as 50% of the erythrocytes at 2–3 months of age. Using the standard new methylene blue stain formula for reticulocyte stain (Chapter 2), the erythrocytes with intracellular material taking the stain may be classified into three types: *type I*, cells containing faint blue stippling; *type II*, cells with distinct dark granules; and *type III*, cells with a heavy, dark granular network or reticulum. Among 37 cats having PCV values ranging from 24–44% (mean 35.5%), type I cells represented 0.4–4.2%, type II 0.2–2.2%, and type III 0.2–1.0%. The range for all three types was 0.4–6.4%, with a mean of 2.6%. Excluding type I, the range was 0.2–1.6% and the mean was 0.6%. Most published values on reticulocyte counts in cats appear to have included only the most obvious reticulated (type III) cells. For example, an average of 0.15% reticulocytes was found in 25 healthy kittens 1–6 months of age (Jennings, 1947); a range of 0.0–0.4% was found, with an average of 0.2% (Krumbhaar, 1922); and a mean of 0.05 ± 0.09% was found in 128 blood samples from cats of both sexes and over 6 months of age (Penny et al., 1970a). In view of the general principle that reticulocyte number in peripheral blood of animals correlates with life span of the erythrocyte, these literature values appear to be unreasonably low.

Recent studies on reticulocyte types and response in the cat have provided useful information concerning interpretation of a reticulocyte count in this species. In a study of 8 normal domestic cats (Cramer and Lewis, 1972), two morphologic forms of reticulocytes were identified—punctate (cells with variable amounts of reticulum in the form of punctate foci, i.e., both type I and type II cells) and aggregate (cells containing dense aggregates of reticulum, i.e., type III cells). In 28 blood samples from 4 normal cats, the reticulocyte count, comprised of both types of cells, ranged from 1.4–10.8%, with a mean of 4.6%. Most of the reticulocytes were of the punctate type, with only 0.0–0.4% being of the aggregate type. Studies on the erythropoietic response to blood withdrawal indicated that, in the cat, both types of reticulocytes form an integral part of the reticulocyte count and that a sustained reticulocytosis occurs during recovery from blood loss anemia. Removal of 30 ml of blood/kg body weight was associated with a consistent reticulocytosis in 5 of 6 cats. A rapid, sustained increase in the reticulocyte count to 50.0% occurred during the first 11 days, with a plateau for the next 9 days, and a gradual reduction to normal level in the next 5–9 days. It was concluded that both types of reticulocytes must be included in the reticulocyte count, but enumerated separately to determine accurately the past and present erythropoietic activities. Aggregate reticulocytes appear in large numbers in early response, while punctate reticulocytes are seen at a later stage and parallel the increase in PCV.

Similar observations were made in another study of reticulocyte response in cats in which types I, II, and III reticulocytes were counted following removal of 15%, 30%, and 45% blood volume (Fan et al., 1978). Response to removal of 15% blood volume was milder than when larger volumes were withdrawn, and more or less concomitant changes occurred in type II and type III reticulocytes. Regardless of the volume of blood withdrawn, increasing numbers of types II and III reticulocytes appeared in blood earlier (from the second day), peaked sooner (at 4–6 days), and decreased faster (by 12–14 days) than type I reticulocytes, which increased markedly after the fourth day, peaked by 10–12 days, and remained elevated even when PCV had returned to normal level. In addition, maturation time of types II and III cells was found to be about 12 hours and of type I cells about 3 days both in vivo and in vitro. It was concluded that lightly reticulated (type I) and heavily reticulated (types II and III) reticulocytes be counted separately to assess the response to anemia in the cat. Interestingly, all three types of reticulocyte numbers in nonsplenectomized anemic cats increased markedly after an injection of epinephrine. These findings indicate that excitement and struggling during blood sampling can markedly elevate the reticulocyte count in cats, particularly in those with responsive anemia.

The sustained reticulocytosis seen in anemic cats in the above studies was probably related to their increased circulating erythropoietin levels. In cats subjected to blood loss, erythropoietin levels were increased, proportional to the degree of blood loss, within 24 hours and remained higher than normal for 10 days (Dunn and Legendre, 1980).

Howell-Jolly Bodies

The occurrence of a small spherical body near the periphery of the feline erythrocyte was first described by Howell in 1890. He was making observations on a common phenomenon that occurs in some immature erythrocytes released to peripheral blood in response to anemia. The normal cat, however, presents a similar small structure in a few erythrocytes, unrelated to need for increased erythropoiesis. The inclusion, called the Howell-Jolly body, stains dark blue or black with Romanowsky stains and is present in 0.2–1.0% of feline erythrocytes (Hammon, 1940). Observations on 88 feline blood samples revealed mean occurrence of Howell-Jolly bodies to be 0.13 ± 0.28% (Penny et al., 1970a). The Howell-Jolly body is a nuclear remnant. It must not be mistaken for a red cell parasite such as *Haemobartonella felis*, which is relatively small and dense, presents varied morphology from coccoid to rod-shaped, and occurs singly or in small numbers often along the cell periphery.

Nucleated Erythrocytes

An occasional nucleated erythrocyte may be found in young cats up to 12 weeks of age (Anderson et al., 1971). Nucleated erythrocytes may appear in peripheral blood of adult cats without accompanying evidence of intensified erythrogenesis (Table 5–2, day 5).

Such occurrence appears to be a sign of systemic stress of disease and may be an expression of sluggish action of the spleen in removing these cells from the circulation. In some instances, many small metarubricytes appear in peripheral blood in acute disease without reference to need. Such a finding may indicate a derangement of bone marrow architecture. Thus the appearance of a few and sometimes numerous late forms of nucleated erythrocytes in peripheral blood of sick cats is a phenomenon unique to the cat. Nucleated red cells are frequently encountered in peripheral blood of cats with myeloproliferative disorders.

Heinz Bodies

A feature unique to the erythrocyte of the family Felidae is the occurrence in health of a small, eccentric refractile object called the Heinz body. This structure is usually not visible in blood films stained with routine Romanowsky stains. It is readily apparent in air-dried blood films treated with a vital stain such as 0.5% new methylene blue or 0.5% methyl violet in physiologic saline (Jain, 1973a). Heinz bodies are formed by aggregation of fine granules of precipitated denatured hemoglobin. The oxygen affinity of cat hemoglobin is much lower than that of other mammals, including humans (Taketa et al., 1967). Two hemoglobins exist in the cat, designated major and minor, and they differ from other mammalian hemoglobins in having the largest number (eight) of reactive

Table 5–2. An Example of Rapidly Changing Total and Differential Leukocyte Counts during Convalescence from Panleukopenia in the Cat

	Time since Admission to Clinic					
	Day 5		*Day 6*		*Day 8*	
	No.	*%*	*No.*	*%*	*No.*	*%*
PCV%		28		28		31
WBC/μl	1,100	(corrected)	6,900		36,100	
Blasts	44	4.0	0	0.0	0	0.0
Progranulocytes	11	1.0	69	1.0	0	0.0
Myelocytes	440	40.0	897	13.0	541	1.5
Metamyelocytes	55	5.0	1,518	22.0	2,166	6.0
Bands	22	2.0	2,001	29.0	9,205	25.5
Neutrophils	22	2.0	1,311	19.0	18,411	51.0
Lymphocytes	484	44.0	897	13.0	5,415	15.0
Monocytes	0	0.0	0	0.0	0	0.0
Eosinophils	22	2.0	69	1.0	361	1.0
Basophils	0	0.0	138	2.0	0	0.0
Nucleated RBC/100 WBC	8		0		0	

sulfhydryl groups. The physiologic occurrence of Heinz bodies in the erythrocytes of all members of the family Felidae indicates an unusual propensity for hemoglobin denaturation that may be related to the unique structure of feline hemoglobins.

Schmauch (1899) was the first to report the finding of these bodies in cat erythrocytes. Beritic (1965) reported observations on physiologic occurrence of "Schmauch" bodies in cats and considered that they were identical to Heinz bodies. The structures referred to as "erythroycte refractile bodies" in cat erythrocytes (Schalm and Smith, 1963) are now considered identical to Heinz bodies. The incidence of Heinz bodies, for some unknown reason, varies greatly among cat populations without evidence of hemolytic anemia. Values of <1.0% (Penny et al., 1970a) to more than 50.0% (Beritic, 1965; Jain, 1973b) have been reported.

The Heinz body in the blood of healthy cats is 0.5–1 μm in diameter, but on occasion, numerous erythrocytes, each with a single Heinz body up to 3.0 μm in diameter, have been found in so-called clinically normal cats. The larger structure may be detected in the routinely stained dry blood film as a round, pale area near the edge of the cell or protruding from its surface (Plate XVI–1). Permanent stained films of Heinz bodies can be prepared by the standard method for staining reticulocytes (Chapter 2). The Heinz body appears as a round blue object at the margin of the erythrocyte. Another method for permanent mounts is described on p. 63. Further details of morphology and method of study of Heinz body in cats can be found elsewhere (Jain, 1973a).

In some cats with large Heinz bodies, evidence of accelerated erythrocyte replacement may be found. Anisocytosis and polychromasia may be evident (Plate XVI–1), and some macrocytes may present a delicate basophilic stippling (Fig. 5–1). MCV does not always increase in proportion to the evidence of intensified erythrogenesis; this is because erythrocytes containing large Heinz bodies decrease in size as the Heinz body is extruded or removed by the mononuclear phagocyte system, while the erythrocyte may continue to circulate. Urinary antiseptics containing

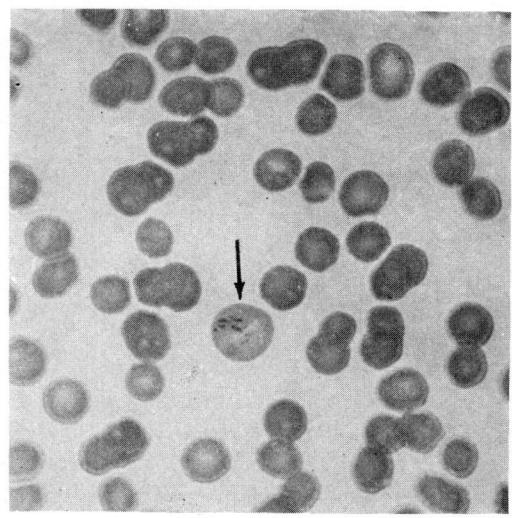

Fig. 5–1. Cat blood, with Heinz bodies appearing in some erythrocytes as a small unstained spot, and an immature erythrocyte with basophilic stippling (arrow). x2,700.

methylene blue have produced hemolytic anemia in some highly sensitive cats. The anemic process was related to a precipitous formation of Heinz bodies and rapid removal of affected cells by the mononuclear phagocyte system (Schechter et al., 1973). Methylene blue was found to produce Heinz bodies in early studies (Hänel, 1964; Spicer and Thompson, 1949).

When Heinz bodies are plentiful, Hb determination by the cyanmethemoglobin method becomes inaccurate unless the hemolysate is centrifuged to remove the suspended Heinz bodies before the reading is made in the spectrophotometer. Failure to remove the Heinz bodies leads to reduced transmission of light and a correspondingly increased value for Hb concentration. The inaccuracy in the Hb value results in erroneous elevation of MCH and MCHC values.

Basophilic Stippling

Delicate bluish stippling of some immature erythrocytes released to peripheral blood during response to anemia is a common finding. It is characteristic of the cat and is of no special significance insofar as etiology of the anemia is concerned (Fig. 5–1).

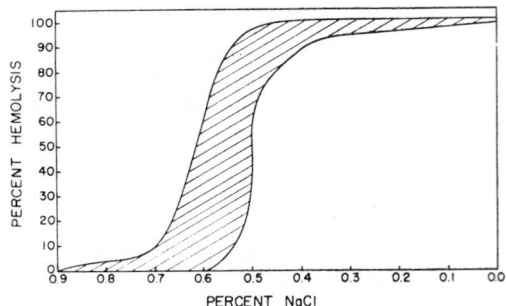

Fig. 5–2. Osmotic fragility curve for erythrocytes of the cat.

Erythrocyte Sedimentation Rate

Rouleau formation is a prominent feature of cat blood, and therefore erythrocyte sedimentation can be anticipated. The Wintrobe method is preferred, and the reading is taken at 1 hour. The observed ESR value, to be properly interpreted, requires correction for the number of red cells or PCV, as is done for ESR in the dog, but anticipated values of ESR in relation to PCV have not been developed for the cat. In our experience, the pattern of ESR in cats is generally similar to that in the dog, and so anticipated ESR values developed for the dog (Table 2–6) to calculate corrected ESR values, may be used to obtain a rough estimate of corrected ESR in cat blood when the need arises. However, a conservative approach should be taken in interpretation of such corrected ESR values.

Erythrocyte Osmotic Fragility

An erythrocyte osmotic fragility curve for 49 cats (35 males and 14 females) is shown in Figure 5–2. The cats had a PCV range of 27–45% and a reticulocyte count of 0.0–0.6%. The proportion of erythrocytes containing Heinz bodies varied from 1.0–56.0%; 10 cats had more than 20% Heinz body–laden cells, and 2 of these cats had more than 50% Heinz bodies. The occurrence of Heinz bodies is a normal finding in cats, as mentioned above. Osmotic fragility was related neither to PCV nor to the percentage of erythrocytes containing Heinz bodies. A small but insignificant sex difference was seen. "Beginning hemolysis" (less than 5%) was seen at 0.55–0.75% NaCl concentration, while "complete hemolysis" (over 95%) usually occurred at 0.5% or

lower concentration. Blood from a few cats did not seem to hemolyze completely even at 0.10% salt concentration. Thus there was a trailing of the osmotic fragility curve at the upper end. The range and mean for the mean osmotic fragility were, respectively, 0.46–0.64% and 0.54% saline concentration. Erythrocyte osmotic fragility is increased in cases of immune-mediated hemolytic anemia and anemia from haemobartonellosis.

THE LEUKOCYTES

Normal values for WBC counts and absolute numbers of neutrophils and lymphocytes in the cat have a broader range than in the dog. Physiologic factors such as fright and "emotional" disturbances have an immediate effect on leukocyte numbers and produce changes that often lack adequate interpretations (Table 5–3). The normal response to the stress of the disease is a decrease in lymphocyte and eosinophil numbers. In "emotional" leukocytosis, lymphocyte numbers are increased and equal or exceed elevations in neutrophil numbers, while eosinophils commonly are not decreased. The influence of physiologic leukocytosis is seen in the data of different authors in the broad ranges given as normal for the lymphocyte. This is especially true when cats less than a year of age have contributed significantly to the assembled data. Young cats normally have high lymphocyte counts and hence a greater tendency to develop lymphocytosis than the adult cats. Lymphocytes were found to increase in kittens from birth to 17 weeks of age (Meyers-Wallen et al., 1984).

Increases in neutrophil numbers due to physiologic influences are more pronounced in the cat than in the dog because of the differences in the intravascular distribution of neutrophils in this species. The mean marginal pool of neutrophils of clinically normal cats is about three times greater than the circulating pool (Prasse et al., 1973), whereas in the dog it is about equal or only slightly greater (Table 26–3). The existence of a large marginal pool of neutrophils contributes to the relative ease with which cats develop physiologic leukocytosis.

In a study of 28 juvenile germfree cats, lym-

Table 5–3. Examples of Leukocyte Counts in Young Cat Patients in Which "Emotional" Leukocytosis Was Suspected (in absolute numbers per μl)

Age (mo)	Sex	Clinical Entity	WBC/μl	Neutrophils		Lymphocytes	Monocytes	Eosinophils	Basophils
				Band	Segmenter				
4	M	Posterior ataxia	21,300	0	7,349	12,887	213	745	107
1½	F	Depression	36,800	368	10,856	24,104	920	552	0
6	F	Depression	35,600	0	22,962	11,214	1,424	0	0
6	M	Tongue erosion	24,300	729	10,449	10,813	1,458	729	121
12	XM	Anorexia, vomiting	22,000	330	9,020	11,990	0	660	0
14	XF	Dermatitis	27,400	274	13,974	10,686	1,918	274	274

phocytes ranged from 4,312–14,271, with a mean of 8,506 ± 2,162/μl and neutrophils from 1,584–5,921, with a mean of 3,163 ± 912/μl (Rohovsky and Griesemer, 1969). The data indicated that the absolute values of neutrophils and lymphocytes are reversed in the germfree cats compared to conventional laboratory cats. It was also found that following recovery from infections such as feline panleukopenia and feline rhinotracheitis, the neutrophil:lymphocyte ratio of germfree cats changed to that usually seen in conventional cats.

The Neutrophil

The nucleus of the neutrophil characteristically is a twisted coil with a pinching-in of the nuclear membrane to form lobes sometimes separated by true filaments (Plates IX–1, IX–2). Condensation of nuclear chromatin leads to formation of darker-staining plaques separated by delicate, light-staining areas. The cytoplasm is somewhat grayish with a delicate pink (but not prominent) granulation. A small nuclear sex bud or drumstick lobe is found in some neutrophils of the female. In a study of the occurrence of the sex chromatin lobe in cat leukocytes, the drumstick lobe was found in 4.2–11.4% neutrophils in blood of the female cats and in 0.0–1.9% neutrophils in both blood and bone marrow of the male cats (Loughman et al., 1970). In addition, mosaicism was found in three tricolor male cats; 1.9–4.0% of their neutrophils contained drumstick lobes. An occasional band neutrophil with drumstick may be found in the bone marrow (Penny et al., 1970a).

The *band neutrophil* is seen in blood in only small numbers in health. The cell is similar to the mature neutrophil, except that the nucleus is U-shaped or twisted, slender with smooth and almost parallel outline, and without distinct lobe formation. Less restrictive application of these criteria for identification could yield considerably greater numbers of band neutrophils in normal cats (Anderson et al., 1971; Osbaldiston, 1978).

The *metamyelocyte* is not seen in peripheral blood in health. Its nucleus is indented like a kidney bean, and the nuclear chromatin is lace-like, with early condensation to form plaques. The cytoplasm is somewhat basophilic with indistinct granulation.

The Pelger-Huët anomaly (see Chapter 4) involving neutrophils and eosinophils was found in two littermate cats (Weber et al., 1981). Chédiak-Higashi syndrome, in which morphologic as well as functional abnormalities occur in neutrophils of several species, was reported to occur also in cats (Chapter 26).

The Eosinophil

The reddish granules of eosinophils in Wright-stained blood films are typically rodlike and numerous (Plates VII–6, IX–1). The small amount of cytoplasm that may be seen between the granules may take a faint blue stain. The nucleus is similar to that of the mature neutrophil, with less tendency to lobulate. The nucleus may be partially covered by the granules. Figure 27–3 depicts the ultrastructure of a feline eosinophil.

The Basophil

The morphology of the cat basophil is unique compared to that of basophils of other domestic animals. Generally, the mature basophil contains numerous small, round, lightly stained (pinkish or orangish) granules in light gray cytoplasm (Plate VII–6). Some basophils may, in addition, contain few to many somewhat larger, darkly stained, purplish granules (Plate XII–5). It is believed that these cells represent less mature forms of basophils since in the bone marrow the basophil myelocyte of the cat distinctly contains the two types of granules (Plates V–2, XII–4). Infrequently such granules may also be seen in the basophil metamyelocyte and band cell. The nucleus of the mature basophil tends to coil with limited tendency toward lobe formation.

The Lymphocyte

The small lymphocyte is common in the cat. The nucleus is usually round, but occasionally it is indented like a kidney bean. The chromatin is condensed to a variable degree, and the nuclear outline is sharp. The cytoplasm is minimal, stains blue, and occasionally presents a perinuclear halo. Azurophilic granules are rarely seen. When observed, the granules are small, irregularly shaped, and scattered along the margin of the cytoplasm or clustered in the indentation of a kidney-bean nucleus (Plates IX–1, IX–3). Medium and large lymphocytes have a greater amount of light blue cytoplasm and nuclear chromatin as described for small lymphocytes. Large lymphocytes on average may form about 12–20% of the total circulating lymphocyte population in cats 4 weeks to 1 year of age (Anderson et al., 1971) and about 40% in adult cats (Penny et al., 1970a).

The Monocyte

The distinguishing feature of the monocyte is the gray-staining cytoplasm with rather frequent, well-defined vacuoles. A few reddish-purple, indistinct granules may sometimes be seen in some monocytes. The nuclear shape is irregular with no characteristic pattern. It may vary from rounded mass with some indentations to indented forms suggestive of a thick band or metamyelocyte nucleus. The nuclear chromatin is lacy with some condensation.

Influence of Corticosteroids on Total and Differential Leukocyte Counts

The effects on blood leukocytes of 5 mg of prednisolone given orally to a cat are shown in Figure 5–3. The response is similar to that described for the dog (Chapter 4); neutro-

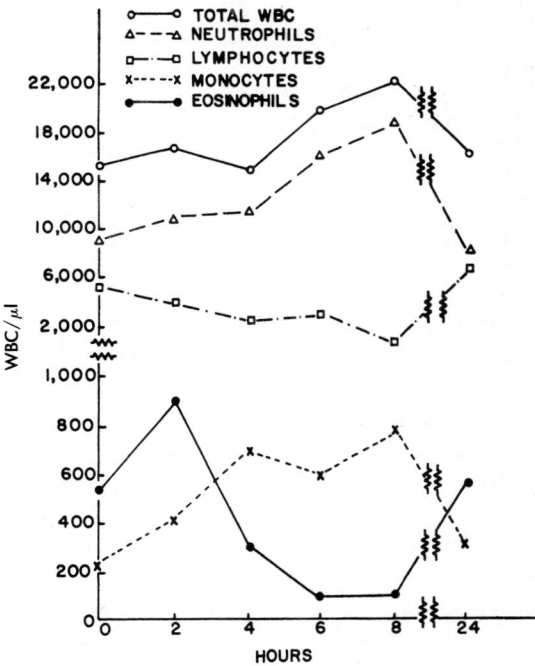

Fig. 5–3.   Blood leukocyte changes in a cat in response to oral administration of prednisolone (5 mg).

philia, monocytosis, lymphopenia, and eosinopenia develop within hours, with return to normal levels by the next day. Stress-induced monocyte response, however, may be variable among cats. Observations on cats responding to an acute disease have led to the conclusion that monocytosis is not a part of the initial response, as it is in the dog. The monocytes decrease in number in acute disease and return in numbers indicative of monocytosis somewhat later, when the disease becomes chronic.

Total Leukocyte Counts among Random Hospital Admissions

During a period of 12 months, 183 initial hemograms were conducted on feline patients. Leukocytosis was seen in 58 cats (31.7%), with 64% of the elevated counts between 21,000 and 30,000, 22% between 31,000 and 40,000, and 13.3% above 40,000/μl of blood. WBC counts in excess of 75,000/μl are uncommon in the cat, except in some forms of leukemia. Only an occasional cat has presented a WBC count in excess of 100,000/μl in nonleukemic disease.

WBC counts of less than 5,500/μl or neutrophil numbers less than 3,500/μl were observed in 43 cats (23.5%). Less than half of these were regarded as due to panleukopenia. Panleukopenia is the most frequent cause of low WBC counts in young cats (Appendix Case 54; Table 5–2). This results from destruction of mitotically active precursors of blood cells by the panleukopenia virus (Rohovsky and Fowler, 1971). Systemic diseases associated with high fever, but not otherwise characteristic of panleukopenia may depress granulopoiesis and lead to a significant leukopenia in cats of all ages. Other reports on hematologic observations in feline patients may be consulted for additional information (Osbaldiston, 1978; Sutton, 1980). It has been suggested that a ratio of segmented to band neutrophils may have a useful application in feline medicine as an index of neutrophil response to injury (Osbaldiston, 1978). This suggestion is worth exploring further.

Neutrophil Morphology in Toxemic Diseases

The most common abnormality of neutrophils encountered in the cat is the occurrence of one or more round or angular, bluish, granular objects in the cytoplasm (Plate IX–2). Similar structures were described by Döhle (1911) as occurring in neutrophils of humans in scarlet fever. Later, Döhle bodies were found in neutrophils of persons suffering from severe burns (Weiner and Topley, 1955). Döhle bodies are now known to be remnants of rough endoplasmic reticulum resulting from defective maturation of the cytoplasm (Fig. 26–11).

Another sign of defective maturation of neutrophils is failure of nuclear division at the proper time. The cell remains large while the nucleus undergoes maturation (Plate XV–9), leading to bizarre patterns and giant forms (Schalm and Smith, 1963).

Cellular patterns in blood and bone marrow in convalescence from panleukopenia (Table 5–2) are typical of changes that may occur in a variety of diseases in which leukopenia is produced. An occasional myeloblast or promyelocyte (Fig. 5–4) makes its appearance in peripheral blood accompanied by a few myelocytes, metamyelocytes, and band forms of large size with basophilic cytoplasm and bi-

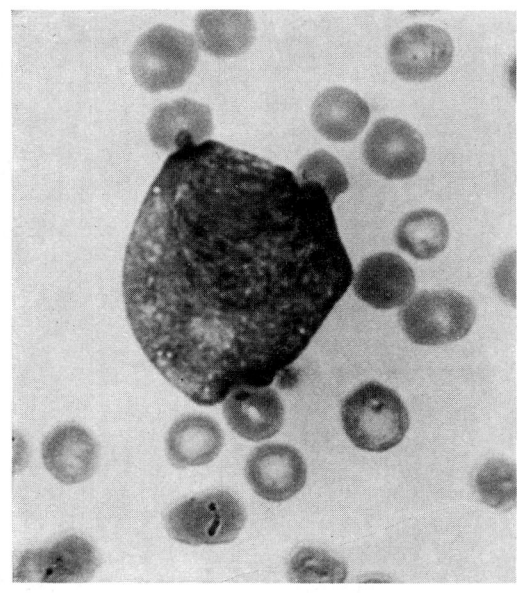

Fig. 5–4. Promyelocyte in cat blood with leukopenia and left shift. ×3,200.

zarre nuclear patterns (Fig. 5–5; Plates IX–3, XV–11). Examination of bone marrow at this stage reveals that the bizarre giant forms originated as precursor cells undergoing nuclear maturation without cell division (Plate XV–8). With each passing day, the WBC count increases in blood, and, although at first the neutrophils remain large and have basophilic cytoplasm (Plates XI–10, XV–10), within 4 or

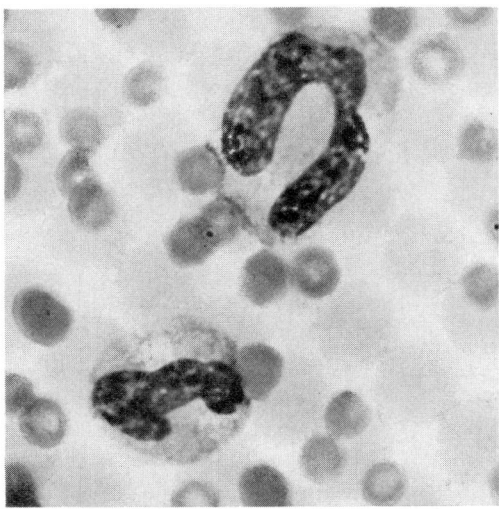

Fig. 5–5. Same blood as in Fig. 5–4, showing a giant band neutrophil with bizarre nucleus and a somewhat smaller band neutrophil. Both leukocytes have retained a bluish staining of the cytoplasm (toxic forms). ×3,200.

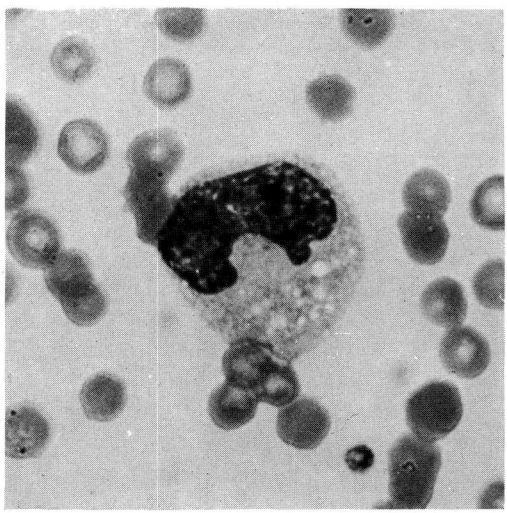

Fig. 5–6. Same blood as in Fig. 5–4, showing a giant metamyelocyte with vacuolation of the cytoplasm (toxic form). ×3,200.

5 days most neutrophils in blood are mature and of normal morphology. Giant neutrophils with bizarre nuclear patterns as well as large neutrophils with basophilic cytoplasm are referred to as "toxic" cells (Fig. 5–5). "Toxic" (reddish purple) granulation of neutrophils (Plate XV–12) is not a common finding in the cat, but cytoplasmic vacuolation is seen with some frequency (Fig. 5–6). An occasional giant neutrophil may be encountered in association with leukocytosis due to neutrophilia (Plate IX–4).

THE PLATELETS

Platelets in the cat commonly are small, spherical bodies with a central cluster of purple azurophilic granules surrounded by a pale blue background enclosed in a delicate membrane (Plate IX–1). The size is variable, and giant forms equal in size to the erythrocyte may occur. Sometimes the platelets appear as elongated structures, and the tendency to clump results in formation of amorphous masses.

The ratio of erythrocyte number to platelets in the cat is about 20:1 (Tocantins, 1938). Platelet counts ranged from 200,000 to more than 600,000, with an average of 422,000/µl of blood in 121 counts made on 55 normal cats (Lawrence and Valentine, 1947). Mean counts

of 232,000 ± 10,600/µl (Landsberg, 1940) and 245,000 ± 60,000 (Osbaldiston et al., 1970) have been reported in other studies. Electronic platelet counts correlated well with manual counts done by phase microscopy over a wide range. Observations on 25 healthy adult cats yielded platelet counts of 296,000 to 850,000/µl and mean platelet volume of 11.0–18.0 fl (Weiser and Kociba, 1984). Platelets of the cat clump readily, and this clumping may account for the lower mean values of some authors. Platelet counts on blood of 7 cats in which clumping did not occur have ranged from 355,000 to 828,000/µl. As mentioned previously, clumping of platelets in cat blood interferes with accuracy of WBC counts with the electronic particle counter. Excitement of normal cats for as short a time as 3 minutes caused a sudden increase in platelet counts, while a slight decrease occurred in sympathectomized cats, and a somewhat greater decrease occurred in splenectomized cats (Field, 1930).

THE PLASMA

Icterus Index

The yellow color of the plasma of cats in health gives an icterus index of 2–5 units. In severe dehydration, plasma color may increase to 7.5 units. In the absence of hemoconcentration, 7.5 units of color is indicative of an absolute increase in bilirubin concentration, and 10 units is clinically significant regardless of the state of water balance.

Total Plasma Proteins

The normal range for total plasma proteins in cats, as determined by means of the refractometer, is 6.0–7.5 g/dl of plasma. As with other animals, the lower value is characteristic of young cats. Some apparently normal cats, particularly aged cats, may have a total plasma protein concentration of 8.0–8.5 g/dl as a result of an increase in the gamma globulin fraction.

Plasma Fibrinogen

The normal level of plasma fibrinogen in the cat ranges from 0.05–0.30 g/dl of plasma. Elevation of fibrinogen in response to traumatic or inflammatory injury is not as great in cats as in other domestic animals, although levels as high as 1.0 g/dl have been recorded.

THE BONE MARROW

The Myeloid:Erythroid Ratio

Cellular composition of normal bone marrow of the cat has been described (Gilmore et al., 1964; Lawrence et al., 1940; Penny et al., 1970a; Sawitsky and Meyer, 1947; Schryver, 1963). Mean values for each cell type, as reported in these studies, are presented in Table 5–4. The data were based on histologic sections taken from the rib, vertebra, femur, or humerus as biopsy or necropsy material (Lawrence et al., 1940) or on aspirated marrow from the iliac crest (Gilmore et al., 1964; Penny et al., 1970a; Sawitsky and Meyer, 1947) or the dorsal femur (Schryver, 1963). The M:E ratio in these studies ranged between 1.45 and 3.5:1. A lower M:E ratio (1.16–1.23:1, mean 1.20 ± 0.02:1) was found in germfree cats (Rohovsky and Griesemer, 1969). Bone marrow cytology of aspirates taken by us from iliac crest of 7 normal adult cats is presented in Table 5–5. The average M:E ratio in these samples was 1.63 ± 0.35:1.

The effect of drug administration on bone marrow cytology of the cat has been determined in some studies. Five adult cats given aspirin were found to have M:E ratios of 2.1–12.2:1 compared to 4 normal cats with ratios of 1.75–2.72:1 (Penny et al., 1967a). Marrow hypoplasia developed in 3 of the 5 cats. Four cats died and one was destroyed *in extremis* after an average of 7 doses were given daily at the rate of 0.11 g/kg of body weight. Observations were also made on changes in blood and bone marrow of 4 cats given chloramphenicol intramuscularly for 21 days at a daily dose of 50 mg/kg body weight (Penny et al., 1967b, 1970b). Marrow examination revealed vacuolation of precursor cells of both the erythrocytic and granulocytic series by the fourteenth day. Such changes were not seen in 2 normal cats. The M:E ratios of the 4 cats receiving chloramphenicol ranged between 7.66 and 19.71:1, compared to ratios of 2.42 and 2.65:1 for 2 control cats. In another study on chloramphenicol toxicosis (Watson and Middleton, 1978), 6 cats were given 120 mg of the drug per kg per day orally in 3 divided doses for 14 days, and 5 cats were given half that dose for 21 days. A dose-dependent, reversible marrow suppression was

Table 5–4.   Cellular Composition (percent) of the Bone Marrow of Normal Cats as Reported in the Literature

	Lawrence et al. (1940)	Sawitsky and Meyer (1947)	Schryver (1963)	Gilmore et al. (1964)	Penny et al. (1970a)
Number of samples	13	15	10	15	60
Myeloblasts	1.3	0.82	0.34	1.1	1.74
Progranulocytes	7.6	—	1.11	2.8	0.88
Neutrophilic myelocytes	4.6	5.22	6.13	5.9	9.76
Eosinophilic myelocytes	—	1.10	—	0.3	1.47
Neutrophilic metamyelocytes	9.8	7.96	16.01	15.0	7.32
Eosinophilic metamyelocytes	—	—	—	0.2	1.52
Band neutrophils	13.4	30.59	—	14.7	25.80
Band eosinophils	—	—	—	0.3	—
Neutrophils, mature	5.3	22.52	32.51	14.0	9.24
Eosinophils	1.5	1.71	2.90	1.3	0.81
Basophils	—	—	0.26	—	0.002
Total granulocytic cells	43.5	69.9	59.32	55.6	58.53
Rubriblasts	0.7	0.35	0.62	1.2	1.71
Prorubricytes and rubricytes	6.3	1.24	6.74	18.9	12.50
Metarubricytes	8.3	18.52	33.34	18.2	11.68
Total erythrocytic cells	15.3	20.1	40.70	38.4	25.88
Lymphocytes	7.8	9.05	3.51	5.1	7.63
Plasma cells	0.3	0.75	0.62	0.5	1.61
Reticulum cells or RE nuclei	—	0.02	—	0.3	0.13
Monocytes	—	—	0.56	—	—
Mitotic cells	—	—	0.48	—	0.61
Unclassified cells	6.2	—	—	—	1.62
Disintegrated cells	26.3	—	—	—	4.60
Vacuolated myeloid cells	—	—	—	—	0.21
Myeloid:erythroid ratio	2.8:1.0	3.5:1.0	1.5:1.0	1.4:1.0	2.3:1.0

Table 5–5. Cellular Composition (percent distribution based on 500 cells) of the Bone Marrow of Normal Adult Cats

Cat Number	1	2	3	4	5	6	7	Mean ± SD
WBC/μl of blood	13,400	12,100	7,500	9,700	6,400	5,700	16,800	10,200 ± 4,000
PCV (%)	32	34	36	42	35	32	41	36 ± 4
Rubriblast	0.2	0.0	0.2	0.0	0.8	0.0	0.0	0.17±0.29
Prorubricyte	0.6	1.2	1.0	0.0	1.2	1.6	1.4	1.00±0.54
Basophilic rubricyte	6.2	4.0	5.4	1.6	4.0	2.6	4.4	4.02±1.56
Polychromic rubricyte	17.6	17.0	23.2	8.6	17.8	20.2	18.6	17.57±4.48
Metarubricyte	1.0	7.4	5.2	10.4	7.4	2.8	4.6	5.54±3.15
Mitotic rubricyte	0.8	0.4	0.4	0.0	0.4	0.4	0.6	0.43±0.24
Total erythrocytic cells	26.4	30.0	35.4	20.6	31.6	27.6	29.6	28.74±4.64
Myeloblast	0.4	0.0	0.2	0.0	0.0	0.0	0.0	0.08±0.16
Promyelocyte	3.0	3.0	1.6	0.0	1.2	1.8	1.6	1.74±1.04
Myelocyte, neutrophilic	8.0	3.2	5.2	0.6	2.8	3.8	6.6	4.31±2.49
Myelocyte, eosinophilic	1.4	0.6	0.6	0.0	0.6	0.6	0.4	0.60±0.42
Myelocyte, basophilic	0.2	0.2	0.2	0.0	0.2	0.0	0.0	0.11±0.11
Metamyelocyte, neutrophilic	13.2	10.4	11.0	4.4	7.0	12.4	12.0	10.06±3.20
Metamyelocyte, eosinophilic	1.0	0.8	0.8	0.0	0.2	0.8	0.2	0.54±0.39
Metamyelocyte, basophilic	0.0	0.2	0.0	0.0	0.0	0.0	0.0	0.03±0.07
Band, neutrophilic	13.4	15.0	15.0	16.6	12.8	13.4	14.6	14.4 ±1.30
Band, eosinophilic	0.2	0.2	1.0	0.4	1.0	0.6	0.0	0.49±0.40
Band, basophilic	0.0	0.0	0.0	0.0	0.0	0.0	0.0	0.0
Neutrophil	9.4	11.0	6.8	22.0	13.6	15.0	12.2	12.86±4.85
Eosinophil	0.6	0.8	0.4	0.4	0.8	0.8	0.4	0.60±0.20
Basophil	0.0	0.0	0.0	0.0	0.0	0.0	0.0	0.0
Total granulocytic cells	50.8	45.4	42.8	44.4	40.2	49.2	48.0	45.86±3.78
Myeloid:erythroid ratio	1.92:1	1.51:1	1.21:1	2.16:1	1.27:1	1.78:1	1.62:1	1.63±0.35:1
Hematogones	0.0	0.8	0.8	0.8	0.6	2.4	0.4	0.83±0.75
Lymphocytes	17.2	14.0	11.6	21.6	17.4	10.6	18.8	16.13±2.92
Plasma cells	1.8	1.4	0.6	0.2	0.2	0.8	0.6	0.80±0.60
Monocytes	0.6	1.2	1.6	0.2	0.4	1.0	0.4	0.77±0.51
Mitotic cells	0.4	0.0	0.6	0.0	0.0	0.4	0.0	0.20±0.26
Macrophage	0.0	0.0	0.0	0.2	0.2	0.0	0.0	0.06±0.10
Unclassified cells	0.4	0.8	0.4	0.6	0.8	0.4	0.0	0.49±0.28
Degenerated cells	2.0	6.4	6.2	11.2	8.6	7.6	2.2	6.31±3.32
Total other cells	22.4	24.6	21.8	34.8	28.2	23.2	22.4	25.40±4.75

seen along with marrow hypoplasia, maturation arrest of erythroid cells, inhibition of mitosis, and vacuolation of early erythroid and myeloid cells and lymphocytes. Hematologic changes included decreases in neutrophil, lymphocyte, reticulocyte, and platelet numbers. Abnormalities in the bone marrow were evident after 1 week and in the peripheral blood by the second week. The M:E ratios in cats given the higher dose were as follows: 0 day, 1.39 ± 0.69; day 7, 29.01 ± 18.56; day 14, >100; day 21, 2.75 ± 1.36; and day 35, 1.31 ± 0.61:1.0. Additional observations on chloramphenicol toxicosis in cats have been reported (Watson, 1980).

REFERENCES

Anderson, L., et al.: Haematological Values in Normal Cats from Four Weeks to One Year of Age. Res. Vet. Sci., 12:579, 1971.

Beritic, T.: Studies on Schmauch Bodies. I. The Incidence in Normal Cats (Felis domestica) and the Morphologic Relationship to Heinz Bodies. Blood, 25:999, 1965.

Berman, E.: Hemogram of the Cat during Pregnancy and Lactation and after Lactation. Amer. J. Vet. Res., 35:457, 1974.

Cramer, D.V., and Lewis, R.M.: Reticulocyte Response in the Cat. J. Amer. Vet. Med. Ass., 160:61, 1972.

Döhle, B.: Leukocyteneinschlusse bei Scharlach. Zentralbl. Bakteriol., 61:63, 1911.

Dunn, C.D.R., and Legendre, A.: Humoral Regulation of Erythropoiesis in Cats: Preliminary Report. Amer. J. Vet. Res., 41:779, 1980.

Fan, L.C., et al.: Reticulocyte Response and Maturation in Experimental Acute Blood Loss Anemia in the Cat. J. Amer. Anim. Hosp. Ass., 14:219, 1978.

Field, M.E.: The Effect of Emotion on the Blood Platelet Count. Amer. J. Physiol., 93:245, 1930.

Frankel, T., and Hawkey, C.M.: Haematological Changes during Sedation in Cats. Vet. Rec., 107:512, 1980.

Gilmore, C.E., et al.: Bone Marrow and Peripheral Blood of Cats: Technique and Normal Values. Path. Vet., 1:18, 1964.

Hammon, W.D.: Cellular Blood Elements of Normal Kittens. Anat. Rec., *76*:259, 1940.

Hänel, A.: Über die toxischen Wirkungen von Methylenblau auf Erythrozyten in vivo. Acta Biol. Med. German., *12*:644, 1964.

Hauser, P.: Quantitatives und Qualitatives Blutbild der Gesunden Katze. Schweiz. Arch. Tierheilkd., *105*:438, 1963.

Howell, W.H.: The Life-History of the Formed Elements of the Blood, Especially the Red Blood Corpuscles. J. Morphol., *4*:57, 1890.

Jain, N.C.: Demonstration of Heinz Bodies in Erythrocytes of the Cat. Bull. Amer. Soc. Vet. Clin. Path., *2*:13, 1973a.

Jain, N.C.: Studies on the Occurrence and Persistence of Heinz Bodies in Erythrocytes of the Cats. Folia Haematol., *99*:28, 1973b.

Jennings, A.R.: Haematology of Healthy Kittens. Brit. Vet. J., *103*:234, 1947.

Johnson, K.H., and Perman, V.: Normal Values for Jugular Blood in the Cat. Vet. Med. Small Anim. Clin., *63*:851, 1968.

Krumbhaar, E.B.: Reticulosis-Increased Percentage of Reticulated Erythrocytes in the Peripheral Blood. J. Lab. Clin. Med., *8*:11, 1922.

Landsberg, J.W.: The Blood Picture of Normal Cats. Folia Haematol., *64*:169, 1940.

Lawrence, J.S., et al.: Infectious Feline Agranulocytosis. Amer. J. Pathol., *16*:333, 1940.

Lawrence, J.S., and Valentine, W.N.: The Blood Platelets: The Rate of Their Utilization in the Cat. Blood, *2*:40, 1947.

Lewis, L.A.: The Blood Picture of Adrenalectomized Animals Treated iwth Different Adrenal Fractions. Endocrinology, *28*:821, 1941.

Loughman, W.D., et al.: Bone Marrow Mosaicism in Three Male Tricolor Cats. Amer. J. Vet. Res., *31*:307, 1970.

Meyers-Wallen, V.N., et al.: Hematologic Values in Healthy Neonatal, Weanling, and Juvenile Kittens. Amer. J. Vet. Res., *45*:1322, 1984.

Noguchi, J., et al.: Fluctuations in Some Blood Constituents of Kittens from Birth to Sixty Days of Age. B. Azabu Univ. Vet. Med., *2*:91, 1981.

Osbaldiston, G.W.: Haematological Values in Healthy Cats. Brit. Vet. J., *134*:524, 1978.

Osbaldiston, G.W., et al.: Blood Coagulation: Comparative Studies in Dogs, Cats, Horses, and Cattle. Brit. Vet. J., *126*:512, 1970.

Penny, R.H.C., et al.: Effects of Aspirin (Acetylsalicylic Acid) on the Haemopoietic System of the Cat. Brit. Vet. J., *123*:154, 1967a.

Penny, R.H.C., et al.: Effects of Chloramphenicol on the Haemopoietic System of the Cat. Brit. Vet. J., *123*:145, 1967b.

Penny, R.H.C., et al.: The Blood and Marrow Picture of the Cat. Brit. Vet. J., *126*:459, 1970a.

Penny, R.H.C., et al.: Further Observations on the Effect of Chloramphenicol on the Haemopoietic System of the Cat. Brit. Vet. J., *126*:453, 1970b.

Prasse, K.W., et al.: Blood Neutrophilic Granulocyte Kinetics in Cats. Amer. J. Vet. Res., *34*:1021, 1973.

Rohovsky, M.W., and Fowler, E.H.: Lesions of Experimental Feline Panleukopenia. Jour. Amer. Vet. Med. Ass., *158*:872, 1971.

Rohovsky, M.W., and Griesemer, R.A.: Hematology of the Germ Free Cat. Lab. Anim. Care, *19*:60, 1969.

Sawitsky, A., and Meyer, L.M.: The Bone Marrow of Normal Cats. J. Lab. Clin. Med., *32*:70, 1947.

Schalm, O.W., and Smith, R.: Some Unique Aspects of Feline Hematology in Disease. Small Anim. Clin., *3*:311, 1963.

Schechter, R.D., et al.: Heinz Body Hemolytic Anemia Associated with the Use of Urinary Antiseptics Containing Methylene Blue in the Cat. J. Amer. Vet. Med. Ass., *162*:37, 1973.

Schmauch, G.: Ueber endoglobulare Körperchen in den Erythrozyten der Katze. Virchow Arch. (Path. Anat.), *156*:201, 1899.

Schryver, H.F.: The Bone Marrow of the Cat. Amer. J. Vet. Res., *24*:1012, 1963.

Spicer, S.S., and Thompson, E.C.: Heinz Body Formation in Vivo: A Property of Methylene Blue. J. Indus. Hyg. Toxicol., *31*:206, 1949.

Sutton, R.H.: The Value of a Single Haematological Examination in the Diagnosis of Disease in the Cat. J. Small Anim. Pract., *21*:339, 1980.

Taketa, F., et al.: Studies on Cat Hemoglobin and Hybrids with Human Hemoglobin A. Biochemistry, *6*:3809, 1967.

Tocantins, L.M.: The Mammalian Blood Platelet in Health and Disease. Medicine, *17*:155, 1938.

Velasco, M., et al.: Some Constituents in Normal Cats. J. Amer. Vet. Med. Ass., *158*:763, 1971.

Watson, A.D.J.: Further Observations on Chloramphenicol Toxicosis in Cats. Amer. J. Vet. Res., *41*:293, 1980.

Watson, A.D.J., and Middleton, D.J.: Chloramphenicol Toxicosis in Cats. Amer. J. Vet . Res., *39*:1199, 1978.

Weber, S.E., et al.: Pelger-Huët Anomaly of Granulocytic Leukocytes in Two Feline Littermates. Feline Pract., *11*:44, 1981.

Weiner, W., and Topley, E.: Döhle Bodies in the Leucocytes of Patients with Burns. J. Clin. Pathol., *8*:324, 1955.

Weiser, M.G., and Kociba, G.J.: Sequential Changes in Erythrocyte Volume Distribution and Microcytosis Associated with Iron Deficiency in Kittens. Vet. Path., *20*:1, 1983.

Weiser, M.G., and Kociba, G.J.: Platelet Concentration and Platelet Volume Distribution in Healthy Cats. Amer. J. Vet. Res., *45*:518, 1984.

Windle, W.F., et al.: Some Aspects of Prenatal and Postnatal Development of the Blood of the Cat. Anat. Rec., *78*:321, 1940.

6

The Horse: Normal Hematology with Comments on Response to Disease

DYNAMICS OF CIRCULATING
        ERYTHROCYTE VOLUME   140
    Role of the Spleen   140
    Influence of Splenectomy and Acute Blood
        Loss   142

THOROUGHBRED AND QUARTER HORSE
        FOALS   144
    Erythrocyte Number and Size   146
    Blood Volume   146
    Total and Differential Leukocyte
        Counts   147
    Icterus Index   147
    Plasma and Serum Proteins   149
    Plasma Fibrinogen   149

MATURE HOT-BLOODED HORSES   149
    Influence of Age   151
    Sex Differences   151
    Influence of Pregnancy and Lactation   151
    Seasonal Differences   151

Influence of Training   154
Breed Differences   154
Cold-Blooded versus Hot-Blooded
    Horses   155
The Erythrocytes   155
The Leukocytes   158
The Platelets   159
The Plasma   159
The Bone Marrow   161

EFFECTS OF EXOGENOUS
        CORTICOSTEROIDS AND NATURAL
        STRESS   163
    Effect of Corticosteroid Administration   163
    Effect of Sustained Muscular Activity   166
    Physiologic Leukocytosis in Young
        Horses   166

COMMENTS ON RESPONSE TO
        DISEASE   169

For interpretation of equine hematology, it is necessary to know whether the animal is classed as "hot-blooded" or "cold-blooded." Horses with considerable Arabian ancestry are commonly referred to as hot-blooded, and these are essentially the Arabians per se and the Thoroughbreds. American horses of Arabian ancestry are the American saddle horse, the Morgan horse, and the Standardbred trotter. The cow ponies and wild mustangs of the western United States, from which the quarter horse developed, are also of Arabian ancestry. Normal blood values in the horse are presented in the chart.

DYNAMICS OF CIRCULATING ERYTHROCYTE VOLUME

Role of the Spleen

The spleen serves as a large reservoir of erythrocytes that can be released to the cir-

culation within minutes during excitement or strenuous exercise. The red cell parameters (RBC, Hb, and PCV) of the horse increase promptly upon excitement, twitching, handling, exertion, and racing (Archer and Clabby, 1965; Cardinet et al., 1964; Keenan, 1980; Meagher and Tasker, 1972; Persson et al., 1973; Stewart et al., 1977; Torten and Schalm, 1964). Slight increase in WBC count may also occur upon exertion (Archer, 1974). The slight excitement caused by venipuncture by a stranger may result in an increase in RBC counts of 10–15% (Irvine, 1958). Greater elevations are found with increase in the degree and duration of physical stress, although individual variations may be found. Larger differences may be seen with increase in age of the horse (Persson and Ullberg, 1979). Horses in training exhibit a more pronounced change than those not in training (Catling, 1975).

Normal Blood Values for the Horse

	Hot-Blooded Breeds (based on 147 clinically normal horses)		Cold-Blooded Breeds (from the literature)	
	Range	Mean ± SD	Range	Ave.
Erythrocytic Series				
Erythrocytes ($\times 10^6/\mu l$)	6.8 –12.9	9.0 ±1.2	5.5– 9.5	7.5
Hemoglobin (g/dl)	11.0 –19.0	14.4 ±1.7	8.0–14.0	11.5
PCV (%)	32.0 –53.0	41.0 ±4.5	24.0–44.0	35.0
MCV (fl)	37.0 –58.5	45.5 ±4.3	—	—
MCH (pg)	12.3 –19.7	15.9 ±1.5	—	—
MCHC (%)	31.0 –38.6	35.2 ±1.4	—	—
RBC diameter (μm)	5.0 – 6.0	5.5 —	—	—
Resistance to hypotonic saline (%)	0.34– 0.56	0.45 —	—	—
Leukocytic Series				
Total Leukocytes/μl	5,400–14,300	9,050±1,800	6,000–12,000	8,500
Neutrophil (band)	0– 1,000	36± 104	—	—
Neutrophil (segmenter)	2,260– 8,580	4,745±1,235	—	—
Lymphocyte	1,500– 7,700	3,500±1,120	—	—
Monocyte	0– 1,000	388± 288	—	—
Eosinophil	0– 1,000	305± 244	—	—
Basophil	0– 290	45± 62	—	—
(See Table 6–6 for influence of age on total and differential leukocyte counts.)				
Percentage Distribution				
Neutrophil (band)	0– 8.0	0.35±0.97	0– 2.0	0.5
Neutrophil (segmenter)	22.0–72.0	52.62±8.73	35–75.0	54.0
Lymphocyte	17.0–68.0	38.73±8.66	15–50.0	35.0
Monocyte	0–14.0	4.32±2.42	2–10.0	5.0
Eosinophil	0–10.0	3.35±2.55	2–12.0	5.0
Basophil	0– 4.0	0.49±0.65	0– 3.0	0.5
Other Data				
Plasma proteins (g/dl)	5.8– 8.7	6.9 ±0.6	—	—
Fibrinogen (g/dl)	0.1– 0.4	0.26±0.08	—	—
Icterus index (units)	7.5–20	(influenced by plant pigments and PCV)		
Thrombocytes ($\times 10^5$)	1.0– 3.5	2.25	—	—
Erythrocyte life span (days)	140–150			
Myeloid:erythroid ratio	0.5–1.5:1.0	—	—	—

Normalization of red cell parameters may take about 40–60 minutes or several hours depending on the extent of excitement.

Examples of the effect of strenuous exercise on circulating erythrocyte parameters are presented in Table 6–1. Blood samples were taken on 5 occasions by the student owner of a Thoroughbred horse in the early morning, both before and immediately after running the horse about 1 mile. On 4 occasions, the PCV values at rest ranged from 36.5% to 47%, and after exercise they were between 50% and 56%. On these 4 occasions, the increase in PCV during exercise varied between 15% and 37% (ave. 28%). A slight elevation in WBC counts was also evident at these times. On

Table 6–1.   Effect of Strenuous Exercise in the Horse on Red Cell Mass and Total Leukocyte Count

Date	Condition	RBC ($\times 10^6/\mu l$)	PCV (%)	Hb (g/dl)	WBC (/μl)
Jan. 13	Rest	7.97	40	13.3	8,050
	Exercise	11.28	52	17.5	10,700
Jan. 26	Rest	7.90	36.5	13.5	8,500
	Exercise	10.80	50	17.0	10,200
Feb. 10[a]	Rest	10.60	53	17.0	9,250
	Exercise	9.43	51.5	16.9	8.650
Feb. 25	Rest	9.42	47	15.8	8,800
	Exercise	11.02	54	17.5	9,550
Mar. 10	Rest	8.32	43	14.5	9,000
	Exercise	11.40	56	18.6	11,450

[a]Stranger present.

one occasion (Feb. 10), the PCV was 53% before and 51.5% after exercise. On that occasion another student, strange to the horse, was present when the resting blood sample was drawn. It was conjectured that the horse developed an apprehensive attitude, with consequent splenic contraction, as a result of the presence of a stranger. This event served as a demonstration of the rapidity of elevation of the circulating erythrocyte mass merely as a result of a psychologic influence.

The increase in red cell parameters seen after exertion is attributable largely to splenic contraction and partly to reduction in plasma volume. The splenic release of red cells is considered an epinephrine effect. For example, within 3 minutes of epinephrine injection into the horse, RBC count increased by 38%, Hb by 37%, and PCV by 40%, all values gradually returning to preinjection level by 1 hour (Lumsden et al., 1976). No effect was seen on total and differential leukocyte counts, red cell indexes, and total plasma proteins. Physical stress or epinephrine injection does not cause an increase in PCV in a splenectomized horse (Persson et al., 1973; also see next section).

Additional evidence for the effect of excitement and of anesthesia upon PCV was obtained on horses before and after being placed on the operating table for experimental surgery (Table 6–2). The average increase in PCV resulting from restraining was 18.3%, although the increase in individual horses ranged from 14% to 64%. The PCV decreased to slightly less than the resting value after anesthetization. This decrease suggested that the relaxing effect of anesthesia caused erythrocytes to become sequestered in the spleen. In two other horses, tranquilization with promazine hydrochloride (350 mg) caused the PCV to decrease from 51% to 35% and from 46% to 35%, respectively, within 30 minutes. Others have also reported a substantial decrease in PCV and slight reduction in total plasma protein levels in horses injected with promazine hydrochloride (Moor et al., 1978). A similar decline in PCV was observed after administration of acetylpromazine maleate (Dalton, 1972; Jeffcott, 1974; Lumsden et al., 1976; Meagher and Tasker, 1972). Ether and nitrous oxide anesthesia caused an increase

in PCV, whereas barbiturates followed by halothane or halothane alone caused a decrease in PCV, the opposing effects presumably arising from a reduction or increase in size of the splenic reservoir, respectively (Gillespie et al., 1976). These responses in the horse are similar to those observed in the dog.

A slight increase in plasma protein concentration was observed with the increase in PCV in horses restrained for surgery (Table 6–2). This increase indicated that water left the vascular system in partial compensation for the sudden increase in circulating red cell mass. A sharp decrease in plasma volume, accompanied by a modest increase in plasma protein concentration, was observed in horses undergoing exertion-induced increase in red cell parameters (Catling, 1975). Similar observations have been reported by others (Littlejohn, 1969; Persson, 1967). Increases in red cell mass and plasma proteins are associated with a concomitant increase in plasma viscosity (Jeffcott, 1974).

These observations have practical implications. It is not possible for a stranger to obtain a resting blood sample from an excitable horse. In fact, it has been stated that the normal values for PCV, RBC, and Hb reported in the literature for hot-blooded horses are in some instances not representative of true resting values (Irvine, 1958). Even when conditions are carefully standardized to ensure that the horse has been at rest and to prevent apprehension, considerable variations can be expected in RBC parameters in blood collected on different days (Persson, 1969).

Influence of Splenectomy and Acute Blood Loss

Two crossbred quarter horse mares in excellent physical condition, estimated to be 15 and 8 years of age, and identified as horses 1 and 2, respectively, were splenectomized (Torten and Schalm, 1964). Comparisons of their PCV values before and after excitation revealed no significant change (Table 6–3).

The two horses were also subjected to massive phlebotomies, both before and after recovering from the splenectomy. The purpose was to compare PCV values during the first few hours of massive blood loss in intact and splenectomized states. Approximately one-

Table 6–2.   Blood Values of Mixed-Breed Horses, Both Sexes, Aged 2 Years and Over, at Rest in the Stall, on Operating Table before Administration of Anesthesia, and 11–12 Days after Thoracotomy (means and 1 SD)

| Condition | Number of Horses | PCV (%) | Plasma Protein (g/dl) | WBC (μl) | Differential Leukocyte Count in Absolute Numbers/μl | | | N:L ratio |
| | | | | | Neutrophils | | Lymphocytes | |
					Band	Mature		
At rest in stall	65	38.2 ± 4.4	7.28 ± 0.41	9,775 ± 1,980	20 ± 48	5,842 ± 1,530	2,810 ± 941	2.28 ± 0.88:1.0
Preanesthetic on surgery table	24	45.2 ± 5.7[a]	7.54 ± 0.45	10,426 ± 2,423	64 ± 116	6,451 ± 2,135	3,080 ± 1,100	2.35 ± 0.59:1.0
Anesthetized presurgery	32	37.0 ± 4.7	7.04 ± 0.38	8,239 ± 1,965	56 ± 30	5,546 ± 1,825	2,646 ± 1,025	2.42 ± 1.23:1.0
11–12 days after surgery	24	30.2 ± 5.3	7.64 ± 1.0	16,875 ± 6,782	298 ± 480	12,711 ± 6,180	2,547 ± 1,200	5.76 ± 4.34:1.0

[a]Average increase over resting value, 18.3%

Table 6–3. A Demonstration of the Stability of the Circulating Erythrocyte Volume (PCV) under Excitation in the Splenectomized Horse

Trial No.[a]	PCV (%) Before Excitation	PCV (%) 15 minutes after Excitation
Horse No. 1		
1	37	37
2	36.5	37
3	36.5	37
4	33	33
5	33.5	34
6	34	33.5
Horse No. 2		
1	48	48
2	47	47
3	31	32
4	29	30
5	30	30.5
6	31	31

[a]1, 2, 3: Excitation accomplished by placing the horse on the operating table. 4, 5, 6: Excitation accomplished by frightening the horse in the corral.

third of the blood volume was removed rapidly from the jugular vein. The initial plasma volume and subsequent dilution by movement of extravascular fluid into the blood were measured with Evans blue (T-1824) before bleeding, at the end of blood withdrawal (called the 0-hour), and at 1, 4, and 24 hours post bleeding.

The RBC, PCV, and Hb values were greater in the intact horse at the 0-hour than at the prebleeding period (Table 6–4; Figs. 6–1, 6–2). In contrast, all erythrocyte parameters were reduced at the 0-hour in the splenectomized state. Thus the increase in PCV immediately after removal of a large volume of blood in the intact horse was due to erythrocytes entering the circulation by forceful contraction of the spleen. The two horses withstood the acute blood loss when normal and when splenectomized, although in the latter state a brief temporary weakness was apparent at the 0-hour.

The dilution of the plasma with tissue fluid began almost immediately. In the splenectomized condition, the PCV decreased by 2–3% between the prebleeding period and the end of blood withdrawal (0-hour). This clearly demonstrates the rapidity with which fluid is mobilized into the vascular system following massive hemorrhage. In the intact horse, the movement of fluid into the bloodstream to compensate for the blood loss was masked during the first 4 hours by the massive injection of erythrocytes by splenic contraction (Figs. 6–1 and 6–2). Thus response of the spleen of the horse to massive hemorrhage precludes an estimation of the magnitude of blood loss at least during the first 4–5 hours post hemorrhage.

Measurement of plasma protein concentration would reflect the influx of fluids into the plasma compartment. Two analyses 1 or 2 hours apart should provide information on the movement of fluid into the circulation during the early period following hemorrhage when PCV is elevated rather than decreased. For example, a male horse, 6 years old, had its carotid artery exteriorized in preparation for an experiment. Before surgery, the PCV was 32% and plasma proteins 7.0 g/dl. The exteriorized vessel was injured sometime during the following night, perhaps in the early morning hours, with considerable loss of blood. At the time of discovery of the injury, PCV and plasma proteins were, respectively, 35% and 5.5 g/dl. The low value for plasma proteins indicated that extensive movement of fluid into the circulation had taken place. Twenty-four hours later, the PCV was 19% and the plasma proteins 5.3 g/dl.

In summary, splenic contraction, whether from physiologic or pathologic causes, forces its reservoir of red cells into the circulation and quickly raises the RBC, Hb, and PCV values. However, under physiologic conditions, simultaneously with the increase in red cell parameters, a slight increase in total plasma protein concentration occurs from a compensatory movement of fluid out of the vessels into the tissues. In contrast, following acute blood loss, intravascular movement of fluid from extravascular locations begins within minutes and results in lowering of total plasma protein concentration within hours. In an intact animal, a reduction in red cell parameters or anemia is appreciated by 12–24 hours when plasma volume has expanded beyond the initial compensatory effort of the spleen to raise the circulating red cell mass.

THOROUGHBRED AND QUARTER HORSE FOALS

Normal hematology of foals from birth to 1 year of age has been described (Aldous,

Table 6–4. Effect of Massive Hemorrhage in the Normal and Splenectomized Horse on Circulating Red Blood Cell Mass and on Plasma Volume as Measured by the T-1824 Dye Dilution Method

Horse Number	Status and Weight[a]	Amount of Blood[b] Withdrawn and Time	Sampling Time in Hours[c]	PCV (%)	RBC (×10^6/μl)	Hb (g/dl)	Plasma Proteins[d] (g/dl)	Plasma Volume (ml)	Plasma Volume (%)
1	Normal; 364 kg	9.05 liters withdrawn in 40 min	Prebleeding	35	6.8	12.8	—	15,788	100
			0	37	7.3	13.6	—	10,722	68
			1	37.5	—	—	—	13,424	85
			4	34	6.7	12.4	—	14,974	95
			24	27	5.16	9.8	—	18,202	115
1	Splenectomized; 334 kg	7.3 liters withdrawn in 28 min	Prebleeding	35	7.05	12.1	6.95	12,230	100
			0	32	6.25	11.5	6.35	8,459	69
			1	30	—	—	5.9	9,275	76
			4	28	5.35	9.8	5.8	10,610	87
			24	25	4.47	9.1	6.35	15,541	127
2	Normal; 452 kg	11.2 liters withdrawn in 53 min	Prebleeding	43	8.05	15.8	—	18,669	100
			0	47	8.1	16.8	—	14,954	80
			1	43	—	—	—	15,765	84
			4	41	7.5	14.7	—	20,410	109
			24	34	6.45	12.2	—	21,577	116
2	Splenectomized; 419 kg	9.3 liters withdrawn in 28 min	Prebleeding	40	7.7	13.9	7.3	13,950	100
			0	38	7.2	12.3	6.85	10,752	77
			1	36	—	—	6.8	11,743	84
			4	33	6.65	11.5	6.7	13,018	93
			24	28	5.20	9.8	6.65	16,483	118

[a]Hemorrhage was produced in normal state in summer. Horses were splenectomized in the fall, and the second blood loss trials were conducted in the following spring when the horses were completely recovered.

[b]Volume of blood withdrawn was estimated to be approximately 30% of total blood volume.

[c]0-hour represents the time at the end of blood withdrawal.

[d]Predicted from Goldberg refractometer.

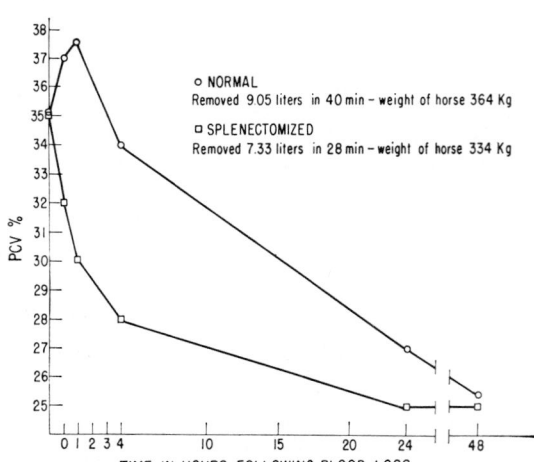

Fig. 6–1. Packed cell volume changes from induced blood loss in horse 1 both before and after splenectomy. (From Torten and Schalm, 1964; courtesy of the *American Journal of Veterinary Research.*)

1970; Allen and Archer, 1973; Ferraro et al., 1979; Hansen et al., 1950b; Harvey et al., 1984a; Jeffcott, 1971; Sato et al., 1979; Todd et al., 1951). Hematologic observations have also been made on premature foals (Jeffcott et al., 1982).

Erythrocyte Number and Size

In general, red cell parameters are high at birth and decrease sharply within 12–24 hours as a result of colostrum consumption. They continue to decline for 2 weeks (Table 6–5) to 1 month (Aldous, 1970) or longer (Jeffcott, 1971) and then increase to attain highest values from 1–2 years of age. Fetal erythro-

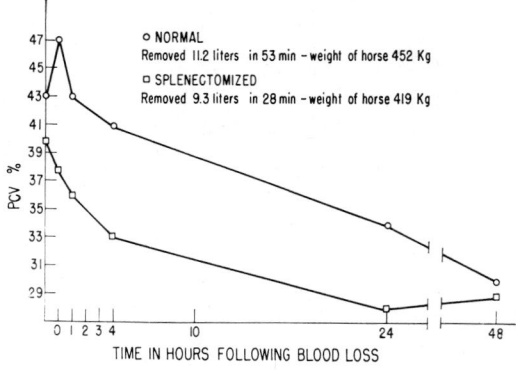

Fig. 6–2. Packed cell volume changes from induced blood loss in horse 2 before and after splenectomy. (From Torten and Schalm, 1964; courtesy of the *American Journal of Veterinary Research.*)

cytes are larger, and so MCV is high at birth (Table 13–5). It decreases during the first 9–12 weeks of life as fetal erythrocytes are replaced and then increases with age.

Jeffcott (1971) made a detailed study of age-related changes in red cell parameters of 8 pony foals from birth to 1 year of age. After an initial decline by 12 hours of life followed by a gradual decrease for 10 days, varied responses occurred in different red cell parameters. RBC counts increased after 10 days of age to peak at 2 months and then gradually decreased to a mean of 8.63 million/μl of blood at 1 year. Hb levels decreased to 11.29 g/dl by 3 months of age and then stabilized at 12 g/dl. PCV values continued to decline for 9 months, followed by a slight increase to near 33% at 1 year of age. A marked decrease was observed in MCV from a value of 37.8 fl at 2 weeks to 31.9 fl at 9 weeks of age. The MCV remained low for 4 months and then increased gradually to 38.0 fl at 1 year of age. The MCH decreased in a similar manner but less dramatically, while MCHC fluctuated unremarkably for 2 months and then increased to a peak of 37.9% at 10 months of age.

Our observations on foals from birth to 3 months of age are presented in Table 6–5. The mean RBC count of 10.5 million/μl, observed on the day of birth, diminished to 9.0 million between the eighth and fourteenth day and then increased to 11.9 million at the average age of 51 days. PCV and Hb followed this fall and rise pattern, but did not exceed the mean birth values as was the case with the RBC counts. This was due to a marked reduction in erythrocyte size from a mean MCV of 39–40 fl up to 2 weeks of age to 32.4 fl at the average age of 51 days. With the reduction in RBC size, MCH fell from a mean of 13.6 pg to 11.2 pg over the same period, while MCHC increased slightly. Studies on 34 foals, from birth to one year of life, at Sao Paulo, Brazil, revealed mean MCV values of 40.95 fl at birth, 34.97 fl at 5 months of age, and 42.58 fl at 12 months of age (Medeiros, 1970). Others have observed a similar trend for red cell indexes (Todd et al., 1951; Ferraro et al., 1979).

Blood Volume

Blood volume in 45 Standardbred foals during the first 400 days of life decreased pro-

Table 6–5. Normal Blood Values of Thoroughbred and Quarter Horse Foals of Both Sexes (means and 1 SD)[a]

Age	1st Day	2–7 Days (ave. 5)	8–14 Days (ave. 9)	21–30 Days (ave. 28)	1–3 Months (ave. 51 days)
Number of foals	34	16	15	8	14
RBC ($\times 10^6/\mu$l)	10.5 ± 1.4	9.5 ± 0.8	9.0 ± 0.8	11.2 ± 1.3	11.9 ± 1.3
Hb (g/dl)	14.2 ± 1.3	12.7 ± 0.9	11.8 ± 1.2	13.1 ± 1.1	13.4 ± 1.6
PCV (%)	41.7 ± 3.6	37.1 ± 2.8	34.9 ± 3.7	37.8 ± 3.3	38.3 ± 4.1
MCV (fl)	40.1 ± 3.8	39.2 ± 2.8	39.1 ± 2.2	34.0 ± 2.4	32.4 ± 1.9
MCH (pg)	13.6 ± 1.2	13.4 ± 1.0	13.1 ± 0.8	11.8 ± 0.8	11.2 ± 0.6
MCHC (%)	33.9 ± 1.6	34.2 ± 1.2	33.6 ± 0.9	34.5 ± 1.0	34.9 ± 1.2
Icterus index units	40 ± 30 (30)	29 ± 21	19 ± 6	12.5 ± 5.6	15 ± 5
Plasma protein (g/dl)	6.2 ± 0.9 (32)	6.4 ± 0.5	6.1 ± 0.6	6.2 ± 0.4	6.4 ± 0.4
Fibrinogen (g/dl)	0.27 ± 0.06 (15)	0.33 ± 0.13 (6)	0.30 ± 0.05 (9)	0.40 ± 0.05 (5)	0.46 ± 0.07 (10)
Total leukocytes/μl	9,602 ± 3,372	9,300 ± 2,346	9,483 ± 2,196	9,688 ± 1,940	10,893 ± 2,977
Band neutrophils	138 ± 198	29 ± 37	48 ± 125	19 ± 33	10 ± 28
Mature neutrophils	6,824 ± 2,757	6,448 ± 2,128	6,338 ± 1,849	5,501 ± 1,346	5,315 ± 2,437
Lymphocytes	2,192 ± 891	2,420 ± 739	2,633 ± 933	3,823 ± 863	5,086 ± 1,419
Monocytes	414 ± 373	308 ± 172	302 ± 124	266 ± 192	348 ± 175
Eosinophils	0	30 ± 34	21 ± 38	48 ± 53	115 ± 88
Basophils	14 ± 78	41 ± 44	29 ± 50	11 ± 29	12 ± 26
Leukocytes (%)					
Band neutrophils	1.5 ± 1.8	0.3 ± 0.4	0.5 ± 1.1	0.2 ± 0.3	0.1 ± 0.3
Mature neutrophils	68.9 ± 10.7	68.2 ± 9.4	66.2 ± 9.0	56.8 ± 7.4	46.9 ± 12.1
Lymphocytes	25.1 ± 10.3	27.0 ± 9.8	28.5 ± 9.4	39.6 ± 6.5	48.5 ± 11.5
Monocytes	3.9 ± 2.9	3.4 ± 1.9	3.3 ± 1.5	2.6 ± 2.0	3.3 ± 1.8
Eosinophils	0	0.3 ± 0.4	0.2 ± 0.4	0.4 ± 0.5	1.0 ± 0.8
Basophils	0.02 ± 0.08	0.4 ± 0.4	0.3 ± 0.5	0.1 ± 0.3	0.1 ± 0.3
N:L ratio (mean)	2.8:1.0	2.5:1.0	2.3:1.0	1.4:1.0	1.1:1.0

[a]Numbers in parentheses indicate number of foals when less than total for series.

portionately with age, and, consequently, the plasma and red cell volumes as functions of the body weight were high at birth (mean 93 ml/kg and 59 ml/kg, respectively), decreased during the first few months, and became relatively stable at 57 mg/kg and 44 ml/kg from the age of 100 days (Persson and Ullberg, 1981). (See also Table 3–1.)

Total and Differential Leukocyte Counts

The total leukocyte count was found to remain at about 9,600/μl for the first month of life and then to increase to 10,900/μl between 1 and 3 months of age (Table 6–5). The neutrophil:lymphocyte (N:L) ratio changed over the first 3 months from 2.8:1.0 at birth to 1.1:1.0 at an average age of 51 days, because of a substantial increase in lymphocyte numbers and some decrease in neutrophil numbers. A similar ratio was attained at 9–12 weeks of age in 14 Thoroughbred foals (Todd et al., 1951), at 3 months of age in 8 pony foals (Jeffcott, 1971), and at 5 months of age in 34 Thoroughbred foals (Medeiros et al., 1973). Lymphocyte numbers continue to increase resulting in N:L ratios below unity between 6 and 8 months and a peak lymphocyte count at 7 months (Jeffcott, 1971). The lymphocyte

numbers then decline to reverse the trend (Allen et al., 1984). Thus, the approximate 1.0:1.0 ratio attained during early life of the foal persists through the first 1–2 years of life, and then, the ratio increases as lymphocyte numbers are reduced, while neutrophil numbers remain stable (Table 6–6).

Some band neutrophils may be seen at all ages. Basophils were not found through the first year of life, while eosinophils were absent or rare during the first week, very low for 1 month, and <400/μl up to 1 year of age (Medeiros et al., 1973). Some have reported eosinophils to reach a peak level at 3–5 months (Aldous, 1970) or 5–6 months of age (Jeffcott, 1971).

Foals respond to infection and stress in a manner similar to adult horses. Leukopenia with degenerative left shift is seen in septicemia; neutrophilia and lymphopenia are a common response to a variety of disorders, with WBC counts of 15,000–20,000; less frequently, in chronic suppurative diseases, the total count may exceed 25,000, characterized by a regenerative left shift and monocytosis.

Icterus Index

Icterus index is generally elevated at birth (25–100 units) and gradually declines over a

Table 6–6.   Influence of Age on Normal Blood Values of Hot-Blooded Horses (means and 1 SD)

No. of Horses	Age	RBC (×10⁶/μl)	Hb (g/dl)	PCV (%)	MCV (fl)	MCH (pg)	MCHC (%)	Protein (g/dl)	Fibrinogen (g/dl)[a]	WBC/μl	Band No.	Band %	Segmenter No.	Segmenter %	Lymphocytes No.	Lymphocytes %	Monocytes No.	Monocytes %	Eosinophils No.	Eosinophils %	Basophils No.	Basophils %	N:L Ratio
8	8–18 mo	8.60 ±0.58	11.8 ±1.6	34.5 ±3.8	40.1 ±2.9	13.7 ±1.3	34.1 ±1.4	7.3 ±0.9	0.29 ±0.04 (7)	10,812 ±1,874	16 ±28	0.1 ±0.2	4,658 ± 745	43.8 ± 7.0	5,210 ±1,250	47.9 ± 6.0	398 ±278	3.6 ±2.0	478 ±403	4.1 ±2.9	43 ±47	0.4 ±0.5	0.9:1.0
27	2 yr	9.88 ±1.34	14.7 ±1.6	41.4 ±4.2	42.7 ±2.8	14.9 ±1.1	34.9 ±1.3	6.8 ±0.5	0.29 ±0.07 (14)	9,678 ±1,883	39 ±81	0.4 ±1.1	4,805 ±1,196	50.1 ±10.1	4,059 ±1,456	41.4 ±10.5	445 ±255	4.7 ±2.8	278 ±232	2.8 ±2.1	33 ±58	0.3 ±0.5	1.2:1.0
50	3–4 yr	9.10 ±1.16	14.3 ±1.4	40.8 ±4.3	44.8 ±3.4	15.7 ±1.2	35.2 ±1.5	6.8 ±0.5	0.24 ±0.08 (30)	8,666 ±1,560	48 ±153	0.4 ±1.2	4,568 ±1,189	52.5 ± 8.0	3,376 ± 787	39.3 ± 7.7	360 ±176	4.2 ±2.0	278 ±218	3.2 ±2.6	34 ±46	0.4 ±0.5	1.3:1.0
62	5+ yr	8.57 ±0.98	14.4 ±1.6	40.8 ±4.1	47.8 ±4.0	16.8 ±1.3	35.4 ±1.4	7.0 ±0.5	0.26 ±0.07 (36)	8,822 ±1,760	22 ±57	0.3 ±0.7	4,877 ±1,316	55.0 ± 7.7	3,146 ± 826	36.0 ± 7.4	385 ±240	4.4 ±2.6	316 ±231	3.6 ±2.6	60 ±72	0.7 ±0.8	1.5:1.0

[a]Number in parentheses indicates number of samples, when less than total for all other values.

period of 2 weeks, at which time it is generally 25 units or less. Mean values of icterus index of foals from birth to the first 3 months of life are presented in Table 6–5.

Plasma and Serum Proteins

Blood taken from 4 foals within 1 hour of birth had 5.2 ± 0.5 g/dl total plasma proteins. In 7 foals bled 4–9 hours after birth, protein concentration was 6.4 ± 1.2 g/dl, and in 16 foals bled 10–16 hours after birth the total proteins were 6.2 ± 0.7 g/dl. The rapid increase in plasma proteins during the day of the birth appears to reflect consumption of colostrum rich in γ-globulins. The mean total plasma proteins remained between 6.1 and 6.4 g/dl during the first 3 months of life.

Serum protein concentration was very low (3.6–5.2 g/dl) in 33 foals at birth and increased precipitously, within 3–10 hours of colostrum consumption, because of increases in β- and γ-globulins. A slight decrease in serum proteins occurred from 3 days to 28 days of age, and then a gradual increase to more than 6.0 g/dl by 140 days of age was seen (Morgan and Mock, 1976). Similar trends in total serum protein levels were observed in normal Thoroughbreds from birth to 4–6 years of age (Jeffcott, 1974). Postcolostral decline in serum proteins occurred for 14 days, and then levels increased to 5.9 g/dl by 6–9 months and again to 6.4 g/dl by 4–6 years of age. Albumin decreased during the first week and then increased after the second month; α- and β-globulins in general increased for 6 months to 1 year and then decreased, while γ-globulins continued to increase.

The serum of the newborn foal, with rare exception, is devoid of IgG, but contains IgM, which is detectable in fetal serum at least during the latter part of gestation (Morgan and Mock, 1976). In Arabian foals with combined immune deficiency, both IgG and IgM are absent in prenursing serum (McGuire et al., 1974). After ingestion of colostrum, serum immunoglobulin levels approach those of the mare owing to absorption of immunoglobulins as in normal foals. The absorption is usually complete within 24 hours. Subsequently, serum immunoglobulin levels decline from catabolism of maternal immunoglobulins, while the foal begins to synthesize its own immunoglobulins. See Chapter 34 for details of immunodeficiency disorders of the horse.

Plasma Fibrinogen

Plasma fibrinogen levels of foals from birth to 3 months of age are given in Table 6–5. At birth, mean plasma fibrinogen value was 0.27 ± 0.06 g/dl. There was a gradual increase over the first 3 months of life to 0.46 ± 0.07 g/dl. This increase may have been in response to subclinical respiratory infections. A total of 8 foals were excluded from the data in Table 6–5 because of the presence of a mild respiratory disorder in which fibrinogen became elevated to 0.6–0.8 g/dl. Fibrinogen levels of 0.8–1.1 g/dl were recorded in pneumonia, 0.8–1.2 g/dl in response to fractures, and 1.5–1.6 g/dl in foals with acute disease from which *Salmonella typhimurium* was obtained on culturing of fecal material.

MATURE HOT-BLOODED HORSES

Normal values for hot-blooded breeds of horses—the Thoroughbred, the quarter horse, the Appaloosa, the Standardbred, and the Arabian—have been developed from data gathered from horses presented for routine physical examination (Tables 6–6, 6–7, and chart at beginning of chapter). A number of clinicians collected the blood samples from horses brought to the School of Veterinary Medicine, University of California, Davis, or from horses on farms or at a racetrack. In each instance, sampling was conducted in a manner least likely to excite the animal. The conditions under which our normal values were acquired were similar to those facing the veterinary practitioner who is called to make a physical examination of a hot-blooded horse.

Normal values of mature horses of various breeds have been reported by numerous investigators (Allen and Archer, 1973; Alonso, 1981; Archer, 1959; Gill and Kownacka, 1979; Hansen et al., 1950a, c, d, 1951; Hansen and Todd, 1951; Jeffcott, 1977; Jones, 1976; Knill et al., 1969; Littlejohn, 1968; Lumsden et al., 1980; Marbach, 1978; Miller and Campbell, 1983; Stewart et al., 1970, 1977; Stewart and Holman, 1940; Trum, 1952). Selected data are presented in Table 6–8. Similar data for some

Table 6-7. Blood Composition of Clinically Normal Horses of the Thoroughbred, Quarter Horse, Standardbred, Arabian, and Appaloosa Breeds (means and 1 SD)

Breed and Number	Sex	RBC (×10⁶/μl)	Hb (g/dl)	PCV (%)	MCV (fl)	MCH (pg)	MCHC (%)	Protein (g/dl)	Fibrinogen (g/dl)[a]	WBC/μl	Band No.	Band %	Segmenters No.	Segmenters %	Lymphocytes No.	Lymphocytes %	Monocytes No.	Monocytes %	Eosinophils No.	Eosinophils %	Basophils No.	Basophils %
Thoroughbred 26	F	9.64 ±1.06	15.2 ±1.4	43.6 ±3.9	45.6 ±5.2	15.8 ±1.7	35.1 ±1.2	7.0 ±0.7	0.29 ±0.08 (13)	9,815 ±1,449	39 ±67	0.4 ±0.7	5,326 ±989	54.2 ±7.1	3,684 ±975	37.6 ±8.0	371 ±215	3.8 ±2.2	310 ±208	3.1 ±2.0	31 ±56	0.3 ±0.3
34	Mᵇ	9.35 ±1.05	14.8 ±1.3	41.6 ±3.8	44.7 ±3.8	15.9 ±1.4	35.8 ±1.4	6.7 ±0.4	0.26 ±0.06 (16)	8,782 ±2,022	56 ±184	0.5 ±1.5	4,788 ±1,430	54.5 ±9.4	3,193 ±1,155	36.5 ±9.4	297 ±219	4.6 ±2.4	293 ±258	3.2 ±2.6	43 ±54	0.5 ±0.6
Quarter Horse 15	F	9.10 ±1.35	13.8 ±1.7	40.0 ±5.0	44.3 ±4.6	15.3 ±1.6	34.6 ±1.4	6.9 ±0.5	0.26 ±0.07 (7)	9,673 ±1,302	30 ±65	0.3 ±0.5	5,121 ±1,053	52.8 ±7.6	3,855 ±972	39.9 ±8.6	320 ±162	3.4 ±1.6	287 ±197	3.0 ±2.0	57 ±89	0.6 ±1.0
17	Mᵇ	8.26 ±1.02	13.3 ±1.6	38.0 ±4.0	46.2 ±3.9	16.1 ±1.7	34.9 ±1.6	7.2 ±0.6	0.29 ±0.08 (14)	8,894 ±1,927	44 ±97	0.6 ±1.3	4,573 ±1,101	51.7 ±8.1	3,429 ±1,152	38.2 ±7.5	386 ±242	4.3 ±2.4	408 ±281	4.6 ±2.9	44 ±55	0.5 ±0.7
Standardbred 8	F	8.32 ±0.72	13.7 ±0.9	39.3 ±2.5	47.3 ±3.4	16.5 ±1.3	34.8 ±1.6	6.8 ±0.2	0.27 ±0.08	7,913 ±988	27 ±49	0.3 ±0.6	4,429 ±740	56.4 ±9.0	2,933 ±818	36.7 ±7.7	397 ±240	4.9 ±2.8	84 ±63	1.1 ±1.0	42 ±46	0.5 ±0.6
18	Mᵇ	8.37 ±1.00	13.6 ±1.6	38.3 ±3.5	46.1 ±4.0	16.3 ±1.4	35.5 ±1.6	6.8 ±0.5	0.23 ±0.06	7,828 ±1,592	8 ±19	0.1 ±0.2	4,158 ±1,052	52.9 ±6.8	2,957 ±591	38.2 ±5.6	452 ±327	5.4 ±3.1	223 ±220	2.9 ±2.7	42 ±48	0.5 ±0.5
Appaloosa 12	Both	8.60 ±1.11	13.3 ±1.6	38.4 ±4.7	44.8 ±4.4	15.5 ±1.3	34.5 ±0.8	7.1 ±0.7	0.23 ±0.05 (12)	8,817 ±1,450	8 ±17	0.1 ±0.2	4,226 ±1,111	47.5 ±6.9	3,776 ±833	43.1 ±7.5	337 ±187	3.7 ±1.9	415 ±200	4.9 ±2.7	58 ±78	0.6 ±0.8
Arabian 6	Both	8.41 ±1.21	13.8 ±2.1	39.3 ±5.0	46.9 ±1.9	16.4 ±0.9	34.9 ±1.0	7.0 ±0.4	0.20 ±0.10 (2)	9,533 ±2,349	18 ±26	0.2 ±0.2	4,751 ±1,528	49.3 ±7.2	4,011 ±1,346	41.9 ±7.2	421 ±151	4.7 ±1.8	266 ±113	3.2 ±1.6	67 ±63	0.7 ±0.7

aNumbers in parentheses indicate number of horses when less than total for series.
bMainly geldings.

cold-blooded horses are given in Table 6–9 and the chart at the beginning of the chapter.

Influence of Age

Age-related changes in red cell values continue to occur after 1 year of life. In general, red cell parameters decrease and MCV and MCH increase with age. Allen and Archer (1973) determined normal values for 1,000 Thoroughbreds, aged younger than 1 month to older than 4 years. RBC counts were higher at 1–9 months of age than at less than 1 month of age and then decreased gradually. Hb and PCV values were lowest at 1–9 months and then increased to 4 years of age; MCH and MCV followed a similar trend. MCHC and plasma viscosity generally remained consistent. The decrease in the RBC count with age, accompanied by an increase in PCV and Hb values, may reflect compensatory increases in the red cell size and the amount of hemoglobin within the red cell. Such an age-related decline in red cell numbers was not seen in older horses (9 years or older) in training (Allen and Archer, 1976).

Our data on 147 horses of several age groups revealed peak RBC, Hb, and PCV values in the 2-year-olds and then declining values with advancing age (Table 6–6). MCV, MCH, and MCHC consistently increased from youngest through oldest group of horses. WBC counts were highest in the youngest group, $10,812 \pm 1,874/\mu l$, compared with a progressive decline with age to $8,822 \pm 1,760/\mu l$ among horses 5–17 years of age. The N:L ratio was 0.9:1.0 in the youngest group and increased gradually to 1.5:1.0 in the oldest group. Among 16 horses 10–17 years of age the N:L ratio was 1.9:1.0, representing a mean of 59.2% neutrophils and 31.3% lymphocytes. It is obvious that age of the horse must be taken into consideration in interpretation of its hemogram.

Sex Differences

Our observations indicated that females of both Thoroughbreds and quarter horses had somewhat greater mean values for RBC counts, Hb concentration, and PCV values than males (Table 6–7). For example, the mean RBC counts for females and males were, respectively, 9.64 and 9.35 million/μl

for Thoroughbreds and 9.10 and 8.26 million/μl for quarter horses. On the other hand, males of both breeds had a greater Hb concentration in erythrocytes than females, as evident by MCH and MCHC.

Literature reports on sex differences in red cell parameters in the horse indicate higher values for the male. Hansen et al. (1950c, d, 1951) found Thoroughbred stallions to have slightly higher RBC, Hb, and PCV levels than mares, regardless of whether the mares were pregnant, lactating, or barren (Table 6–8). Archer (1959), reporting on the English Thoroughbred, found geldings to have higher values for RBC, Hb, and PCV than mares, but mares had larger erythrocytes with more hemoglobin per cell by weight (MCH) and volume (MCHC). Stewart et al. (1970) found higher values in stallions than in geldings and mares. Miller and Campbell (1983) reported higher RBC counts and lower MCV in stallions than in gelding or mares.

In our study females had higher mean WBC counts than males because they had slightly more neutrophils and lymphocytes. The mean values for WBC count for females versus males were, respectively, 9,815 and 8,782/μl for Thoroughbreds and 9,673 and 8,894/μl for quarter horses. Differences between females and males for both erythrocyte and leukocyte parameters were not as great for Standardbred horses.

Influence of Pregnancy and Lactation

Mares in foal and barren mares exhibited slight differences in their erythrocyte parameters, while lactating mares tended to have lower mean values for erythrocyte parameters than nonlactating mares (Table 6–8; Trum, 1952). Thoroughbred mares in foal were reported to have a mean RBC count of 10.75 million/μl, while barren mares had counts of 8.8 million/μl (MacLeod et al., 1947).

Seasonal Differences

In a study of hematological values in 10 pregnant Thoroughbred mares over a period of 1 year in Poland, RBC counts and PCV were found to be highest in autumn and winter and lowest in late spring and summer, while Hb levels were high in winter and early spring (Gill and Kownacka, 1979). WBC counts were

Table 6–8. Hematology of the Thoroughbred and Arabian Horse[a] as Reported in the Literature

Reference	Class	Number	RBC (×10⁶/μl)	Hb (g/dl)	PCV (%)	MCV (fl)	MCHC (%)	MCH[c] (pg)	WBC (×10³/μl)	Differential Leukocyte Count (%)				
										Neutrophils	Lymphocytes	Monocytes	Eosinophils	Basophils
Thoroughbred														
Todd et al. (1951)	Foals 1–4 wk	10; 10[b]	9–14 (11)	11–14 (12)	33–44 (36)	27–38 (33)	32–35 (33)	10.9	4.8–11.3 (8.36)	38–81 (59)	19–62 (39)	0–3.5 (1.5)	0–1.0 (0.29)	0 (0)
	Foals 5–8 wk	14; 9	9–15 (12)	11–14 (12.6)	33–44 (38)	27–36 (31.5)	31–36 (33)	10.5	6.3–15.7 (10.61)	42–74 (59)	24–55 (39)	0–4 (1.9)	0–1.5 (0.4)	0–0.5 (0.04)
	Foals 9–12 wk	19; 14	10–1.5 (12.8)	11–16 (12.9)	32–49 (39)	26–34 (30.4)	30–36 (33)	10.1	9.4–21.6 (13.64)	33–63 (49)	35–64 (48)	0–4 (1.9)	0–9.5 (1.12)	0–0.5 (0.1)
	Foals 13–19 wk	18; 17	9–15 (11.8)	10–16 (12.2)	31–47 (36)	28–35 (30.8)	29–43 (34)	10.3	9.3–19.2 (13.67)	26–71 (53)	27–74 (42)	0–7.5 (2.4)	0–7.0 (2.4)	0–0.5 (0.05)
	Foals 20–26 wk	11; 9	9–14 (11)	10–14 (11.7)	29–42 (35)	25–37 (31.7)	30–37 (33)	10.6	9.9–20.5 (14.53)	30–82 (53)	15–67 (41)	0–14 (2.9)	0–10 (3.0)	0–1.0 (0.12)
Hansen et al. (1950b)	Weanlings	70	9–13 (11)	10–14 (12)	30–42 (37)	30–36 (33.7)	30–35 (33)	10.9	7.6–18.6 (13.64)	21–74 (45)	23–79 (50)	0.5–7.6 (2.7)	0.5–7.0 (2.3)	0–1.0 (0.1)
Hansen et al. (1950a)	Mares in foal	65	9–13 (10.5)	13–17 (14.9)	38–51 (45)	38–48 (42.9)	31–36 (33)	14.2	6.8–13.5 (9.97)	30–66 (49)	24–65 (44)	0.5–6.5 (2.7)	0.5–9.5 (3.7)	0–3.5 (0.7)
	Nonlactating mares	17	7–11 (9.7)	11–16 (13.5)	37–49 (42)	37–55 (43.7)	29–35 (32)	13.9	7.3–14.0 (10.8)	25–61 (44)	35–72 (50)	0–4.5 (1.3)	0.5–8.0 (3.9)	0–2 (0.5)
Hansen et al. (1950d)	Lactating mares	17	7–10 (8.3)	10–14 (11.9)	32–45 (37)	42–48 (43.8)	31–34 (33)	14.3	7.4–11.7 (9.58)	23–54 (42)	36–72 (51)	0–4.0 (1.5)	2.5–11 (5.0)	0–0.5 (0.5)
Hansen et al. (1951)	Barren mares	70	8–11 (9.9)	12–16 (13.8)	35–49 (43)	37–49 (43)	29–35 (32)	13.9	7.1–14.1 (10.37)	25–63 (48)	30–72 (46)	0.5–6.0 (1.7)	0.5–11.5 (4.6)	0.5–2.5 (0.5)
Hansen et al. (1950c)	Stallions	36	8–13 (10.8)	12–18 (14.7)	38–59 (47)	39–46 (43)	30–34 (31)	13.6	5.1–11.9 (8.27)	35–65 (51)	30–58 (44)	0.5–7.0 (2.0)	0.5–7.0 (4.0)	0–2.0 (0.5)
Arabian														
Hansen and Todd (1951)	Barren mares	5	7–11 (9.6)	10–15 (13)	30–45 (40)	40–43 (41)	32–34 (33)	13.5	6.1–11.8 (9.42)	52–58 (56)	36–40 (39)	0–3.5 (2.2)	2.5–4.5 (3.5)	— (0.5)
	Mares in foal	4	8–10 (9.2)	12–13 (12.4)	33–43 (37)	40–42 (41)	31–35 (34)	13.5	6.5–9.6 (8.11)	37–52 (46)	41–57 (48)	1–1.5 (1.2)	2.5–8.0 (4.9)	—
	Stallions	7	9–11 (10)	12–15 (13)	35–46 (39)	38–42 (39)	33–34 (33.5)	13.0	6.4–10.9 (8.65)	43–71 (58)	28–51 (38)	0–3.5 (2.1)	1–3 (2.3)	0

[a]For data on English Thoroughbred horse, see the report by Archer, 1954.
[b]Number of foals for erythrocytic series; number of foals for leukocytic series.
[c]From author's mean RBC and Hb values.

Table 6-9. Hematology of the Cold-Blooded Horse from Some Literature Reports

| Reference | Type | No. of Horses | RBC ($\times 10^6/\mu l$) | Hb (g/dl) | PCV (%) | MCV (fl) | MCHC (%) | WBC ($\times 10^3/\mu l$) | Differential Leukocyte Count (%) | | | | | |
									Band Neutrophils	Mature Neutrophils	Lymphocytes	Monocytes	Eosinophils	Basophils
Neser (1923)	Mixed	26	5.2–11.45 (7.76)	—	23–48.5 (32.9)	— (42.3)	—	b	—	52.0	39.0	4.0	4.0	1.0
Stewart and Holman (1940)	Clydesdale	36	5.7–8.8 (6.96)	8.1–11.0 (9.55)	24–34 (27)	— (38.8[a])	35.3[a]	6.6–12.4 (8.8)	0.5–8 (3)	34–78 (52)	13–56 (31.5)	1–8 (5)	1–28 (8)	0.3 (0.5)
Morris (1942)	Army (?)	10	7–9.49 (7.3)	—	—	—	—	5.7–10.3 (8.9)	0.5	55.9	35.0	3.4	4.3	0.8
Trum (1952)	Percherons	11	5.7–9.55 (7.39)	10.1–14.5 (11.67)	—	—	—	6–10.5 (8.01)	—	36–74 (52.2)	20–59 (41.1)	0–5 (1.5)	2–13 (4.7)	—
Geiser et al. (1984)	Clydesdale	70	6.23–9.03 (7.3)	10.7–14.6 (12.4)	28–39 (32.6)	— (44.6)	— (38.1)	3.9–12.4 (7.9)	— (0.3)	— (63.5)	(30.8)	(3.3)	(1.4)	(0.2)

[a]Calculated from the author's data.
[b]Neser presented considerable data on total leukocyte counts, but it is difficult to obtain ranges and means.

highest in February and August/September and lowest in October and May. Eosinophil numbers were very low in January and February, the periods of stress such as those associated with birth and lactation. Neutrophil numbers increased to 70% at the time of parturition.

Blood samples taken from horses on coastal farms of Australia before and after the wet season in two consecutive years were analyzed (Miller and Campbell, 1983). Seasonal changes were detected in all parameters except PCV and lymphocyte and eosinophil numbers. Neutrophil and monocyte numbers were greater in summer than in autumn or winter. Serum protein levels were higher in autumn than in winter.

Influence of Training

Thoroughbreds in training were reported to have no detectable differences in their blood values (Archer, 1959), or to have somewhat lower RBC counts (Brenon, 1958; MacLeod et al., 1947) than those not in training. Irvine (1958) found a slight drop in erythrocyte parameters with increasing fitness of horses in training. From his observations on 184 racehorses, he came to the conclusion that horses with a low basal RBC count that could be increased by 60% under stress performed best. The best performing horses in his study had the following mean resting blood values: PCV 35%, Hb 12.0 g/dl, and MCHC 34%. Another study on 185 racehorses in training concluded that the hematologic parameters of top performing horses have a narrow range (Marbach, 1978): RBC, 9.0–11.5 million/μl; Hb, 14.8–15.8 g/dl; PCV, 40–49%; MCV, 39–47 fl; total plasma proteins, 6.0–8.0 g/dl; and ESR between 3 and 51 mm/hour. The MCV was a valuable indicator of racing potentialities; values greater than 47 fl indicated insufficient training experience, while values less than 39 fl indicated fatigue.

Other reports indicate a positive influence of training on red cell values. Training of racehorses was found to increase total blood volume and elevate total hemoglobin concentration by 30% within 2 years (Persson, 1976). RBC counts in 8 Thoroughbreds in training increased an average 4% per month over a period of 6 months (Archer, 1974). Intensive exercise over a 6-month period significantly increased PCV values in 30 English Thoroughbred racehorses (Allen, 1978). In addition, serum folate levels decreased and serum bilirubin increased significantly in these horses. A decrease in red cell 2,3-diphosphoglycerate (2,3-DPG) levels was observed during training, and this may have had significant influence on hemoglobin oxygen transport (Lewis and McLean, 1975). Red cell 2,3-DPG levels correlated negatively with Hb concentrations in the Thoroughbreds; the levels were higher in mares than stallions and geldings and were not affected by age. A significant decrease in ESR was observed during the first 3 months of training of Thoroughbred racehorses (Szarska, 1981).

Stewart et al. (1970) made interesting observations on 15 Thoroughbreds in training for about 2 months and not receiving hematinics. Horses with resting PCV of less than 40% exhibited an increase in red cell parameters after 10–12 weeks of training, whereas horses with PCV of greater than 40% developed no such change.

Breed Differences

RBC counts of horses of both sexes were 9.41 ± 1.03 million/μl of blood for 60 Thoroughbreds, 8.65 ± 1.26 for 32 quarter horses, 8.60 ± 1.11 for 12 Appaloosas, 8.41 ± 1.21 for 6 Arabians, and 8.35 ± 0.93 for 26 Standardbreds. Thus the Thoroughbreds had greater RBC counts than the four other breeds and also more Hb (15.0 g/dl versus 13.3–13.8 g/dl for the others) and a higher PCV (42.5% versus 38.4–39.3% for the others). Similar observations regarding higher red cell parameters in Thoroughbreds have been reported by others (Alonso, 1981; Neser, 1923; Stewart et al., 1970).

It has been stated that the better bred the horse, the smaller the MCV; e.g., Thoroughbreds have lower MCV than draught horses (Gerber et al., 1976b). In Thoroughbreds and quarter horses, the MCV was similar—45.4 fl versus 45.3 fl, respectively—but Hb concentration was greater for Thoroughbreds— MCH, 16.1 pg versus 15.7 pg; MCHC 35.5% versus 34.7%, respectively.

The Thoroughbreds have significantly more and the saddle horses significantly less total blood volume in relation to body weight than trotters (Persson, 1976).

Some differences were apparent in WBC counts of various breeds. The Standardbred horses had the lowest mean WBC count (7,850/μl) and the other breeds in order of increasing mean WBC count were Appaloosas (8,800), Thoroughbred (9,200), quarter horse (9,250), and Arabian (9,530).

Hematologic values have been determined on American Miniature horses of mixed ages and both sexes (Harvey et al., 1984b).

Cold-Blooded versus Hot-Blooded Horses

The literature reports on hematology of cold-blooded horses indicate that RBC counts range from 5 million to 10 million, with a mean of 7.5 million/μl (Table 6–9; MacLeod and Ponder, 1946; MacLeod et al., 1947; Marcilese et al., 1965; Jones, 1976). In comparison with hot-blooded horses, therefore, the cold-blooded horses have lower RBC counts. Similarly, lower Hb and PCV values are found in the cold-blooded horses. Cold-blooded draught horses have much less blood volume relative to their body dimensions in comparison with the hot-blooded horses (Persson, 1976). The mean N:L ratio was 1.7:1.0 compared to 1.0:1.0 in Thoroughbreds and Arabians (MacLeod et al., 1947).

The Erythrocytes

Morphology

Rouleau formation is the most prominent feature of the erythrocytes in drawn blood of the horse. This marked natural aggregation of erythrocytes leads to separation of cells and plasma within minutes; this characteristic necessitates repeated mixing of horse blood whenever a portion is removed from a sample vial for examination. Individual erythrocytes of the horse are discocytic, biconcave cells, about 5–6 μm (ave. 5.5 μm) in diameter.

Howell-Jolly bodies occur in health in a small number of erythrocytes. They vary somewhat in size and staining, but generally appear dark purple and in an eccentric position. It has been stated that the erythrocyte with the Howell-Jolly body is not a young cell (Sonoda, 1960); on average 10 such cells were found per 10,000 erythrocytes.

Erythrocyte Life Span

The life span of the red cells of the horse is similar to that of the adult cow. Labeling with glycine-2-^{14}C revealed erythrocyte survival in 2 Thoroughbred stallions, 7 and 2 years of age, to be 140 and 150 days, respectively (Cornelius et al., 1960). A mean red cell life span of 136 ± 17 days was found using DF^{32}P in 5 Shetland ponies (McGuire et al., 1960). DF^{32}P was used as a label to determine the erythrocyte life span in 10 adult crossbred Percheron draft horses (Marcilese et al., 1966). Results varied from 137 to 162 days, with a mean of 147.2 ± 8.2 days. Half-time of survival of ^{51}Cr-labeled erythrocytes in 4 normal horses of undefined breed was 14.96 ± 1.98, and it was significantly reduced in 2 horses with equine infectious anemia (Obara and Nakajima, 1961).

A mean red cell life span of 155 ± 10 days was found using ^{75}Selenomethionine as a protein marker for developing marrow cells in 3 normal Shetland ponies, and a mean of 148 ± 7.8 days was obtained using ^{3}H-DFP as a marker in 3 other ponies (Valli et al., 1976). In this study, overall platelet production time was estimated at 4 days, platelet life span at 7 days, granulocyte production time at 5.54 days, and fibrinogen clearance half-time of about 6 days.

Erythrocyte Sedimentation Rate

Sedimentation of equine erythrocytes has been determined using the Cutler method (Hammersland et al., 1938), the Westergreen method (Van Zijl, 1948; Gilman, 1952), and the Wintrobe method (Torten and Schalm, 1962). Because of the natural rapid settling of erythrocytes in drawn anticoagulated blood, the erythrocyte sedimentation rate (ESR) has not been found useful in clinical medicine. This rapid settling of the horse red cells is also evident when they are suspended in sheep or dog plasma (Osbaldiston, 1971). Some breed differences in ESR have been reported (Hammerl and Kraft, 1983).

The rate of settling is dependent on the ratio of erythrocytes to plasma. Experimental observations (Torten and Schalm, 1962) on reconstituted normal blood of different PCV values were made to obtain ESR values at 10-

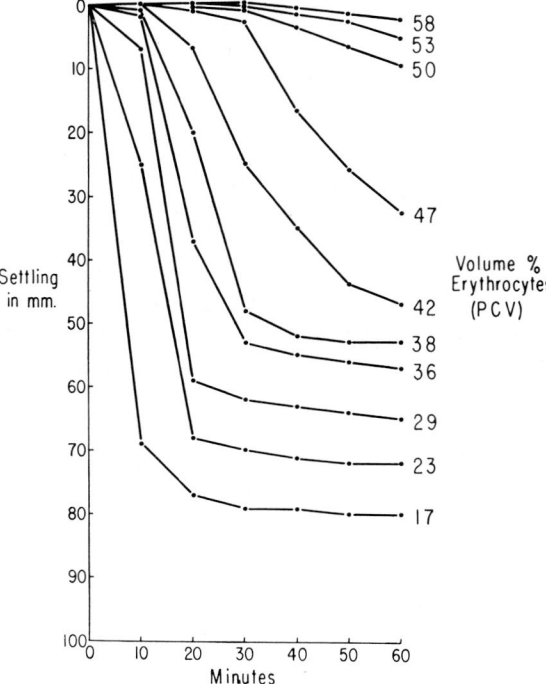

Fig. 6–3. An example of erythrocyte sedimentation rates in Wintrobe tubes in relation to PCV in horse blood. Volume of erythrocytes (PCV) in horse plasma was established artificially. Different PCV values were obtained by recombining erythrocytes and plasma from a single centrifuged blood sample. (From Torten and Schalm, 1962; courtesy of *The California Veterinarian.*)

minute intervals over a period of 60 minutes (Fig. 6–3). With PCV values of 30% or below (anemic level), rapid sedimentation occurred within the first 10–20 minutes. In contrast, with PCV values of 50% or greater, no settling of erythrocytes occurred during the first 30 minutes, and it was limited to less than 10 mm during the next 30 minutes. The results of separate trials to establish anticipated ESR for different PCV values led to the conclusion that the 20-minute reading would be the most useful. ESRs to be anticipated at 20 minutes (ESR-20) for PCV increments from 10–50% are given in Table 6–10. In application of these data to blood taken from equine patients, it appeared that in disease ESR-20 was more often less than anticipated rather than greater, even during inflammatory disease, in which a marked increase above anticipated rate would normally occur in the blood of the dog, cat, and human. It appeared, therefore, that *erythrocyte sedimentation is slowed, rather*

than increased, in inflammatory diseases of the horse.

In comparison to ESR, plasma viscosity was considered a simpler and more reproducible nonspecific test yielding abnormal values in horses with organic diseases (Archer and Allen, 1970; Jeffcott, 1977). Normal plasma viscosity for 80 Thoroughbreds had a range of 1.43–1.74, with a mean of 1.58 ± 0.076 centipoises. Values above 1.8 centipoises were considered clinically significant and were seen after surgery and in cases of chronic inflammation, parasitic infections, neoplasia, and paraproteinemia. Plasma and serum viscosity has been correlated with plasma protein concentrations (Allen and Blackmore, 1984).

Erythrocyte Osmotic Fragility

Initial hemolysis for cold-blooded Clydesdale horses was found to occur on an average at 0.55% saline concentration and complete hemolysis at 0.40% (Stewart and Holman, 1940). Others have reported beginning hemolysis and complete hemolysis, respectively, at average saline concentrations of 0.54% and 0.34% (Perk et al., 1964) and 0.56% and 0.30% (Scarborough, 1930–1931).

Reticulocytes

The erythrocytes are released to peripheral blood in a mature state, so reticulocytes are not present in health. The horse is unique among domestic animals in the response of the erythropoietic tissue to acute blood loss or hemolytic anemia. Reticulocytes or polychromatic erythrocytes are absent or extremely rare in the circulation during anemia in remission. Hence reticulocyte count on peripheral blood of an anemic horse is of little help in assessing erythropoietic response. However, reticulocyte counts in marrow aspirates may be performed to evaluate erythropoietic response of an anemic patient. An increase in reticulocyte numbers of more than 5% indicates increased erythropoietic activity (Schalm, 1975). Erythrocyte production time in the horse is estimated at 4 days (Valli et al., 1976), and more time is needed for optimal generation. At the peak of intensified erythropoiesis, younger erythrocytes may be released in circulation and occasional macro-

Table 6–10.   Anticipated 20-Minute Erythrocyte Sedimentation Rates in Horse Blood (ESR-20) for PCV Increments from 10 to 50%

PCV (%)	Anticipated ESR-20 (mm)	PCV (%)	Anticipated ESR-20 (mm)	PCV (%)	Anticipated ESR-20 (mm)
10	86 ± 1	26	58 ± 4	41	8 ± 4
11	85 ± 1	27	55 ± 4	42	5 ± 4
12	84 ± 1	28	53 ± 4	43	4 ± 4
13	83 ± 1	29	50 ± 4		
14	82 ± 1				
15	80 ± 1	30	47 ± 5	44	3.0 ± 1
16	78 ± 1	31	44 ± 5	45	2.5 ± 1
17	76 ± 1	32	40 ± 5	46	2.0 ± 1
		33	36 ± 5	47	1.5 ± 1
18	74 ± 2			48	1.0 ± 1
19	72 ± 2	34	32 ± 15	49	0.5 ± 1
20	70 ± 2	35	28 ± 15	50	0.0 ± 1
21	68 ± 2	36	24 ± 15		
		37	20 ± 15		
22	66 ± 3				
23	64 ± 3	38	17 ± 8		
24	62 ± 3	39	14 ± 8		
25	60 ± 3	40	11 ± 8		

cytes may be seen in blood films, but increase in MCV rarely exceeds 10–15 fl (Appendix Case 55).

Measurement of certain red cell enzymes or substances, e.g., adenosine-5-triphosphatase (Smith and Agar, 1976) and creatine levels (Wu et al., 1983), may be helpful to assess the erythropoietic response.

Recovery from hemolytic anemia is faster than from hemorrhagic anemia, although in the horse both may take several weeks. For example, RBC counts reached initial levels 37–54 days after induction of a severe hemolytic anemia by intravenous injection of 4 mg/kg of acetyl phenylhydrazine, while prebleeding levels were attained after 63–98 days of 63% removal of blood volume during a 3-day period (Lumsden et al., 1975). This faster recovery was related to the higher rate of erythropoiesis in hemolytic than in hemorrhagic anemia. Recovery from a less severe degree of blood loss anemia or a responsive anemia of unknown cause may occur within 2–4 weeks (Carlson, 1976a).

The Leukocytes

As discussed earlier, total and differential leukocyte counts are influenced by age (Jeffcott, 1971; Kielstein, 1960; Medeiros et al., 1973; Miller and Campbell, 1983; Todd et al., 1951). With advancing age, the absolute neutrophil count remains essentially unchanged, but lymphocyte numbers decline progressively (Table 6–6). Thus, on the percentage basis, the neutrophils exhibit a relative increase with age. Numbers of monocytes, eosinophils, and basophils do not seem to be greatly influenced by age. The mean WBC count declines with advancing age in proportion to the decline in numbers of lymphocytes.

The Neutrophil

The nuclear chromatin is heavily plaqued, causing the nuclear membrane to be jagged (Plate VII–8). Lobulation is common, but true filaments are rare. The female sex chromatin or drumstick lobe occurs in some neutrophils. Because of the heavy chromatin plaques at the nuclear margin, the nuclear outline of the band neutrophil is more irregular than in other domestic animals. In comparison with the mature neutrophil, the nucleus of the band form is thicker, less jagged, and usually not coiled (Plate VII–8). The cytoplasm of the mature and band neutrophils presents dustlike, pink granules. Under conditions of toxemia, the cytoplasm fails to complete its maturation and appears light blue and often foamy. Less frequently, the toxemic state is expressed in the neutrophil by so-called toxic granulation (Plate XI–12). Signs of toxemia are seen in neutrophils in diseases accompanied by depression of granulopoiesis, e.g., severe gastrointestinal disorders. Metamyelocytes and band neutrophils may appear in peripheral blood in numbers greater than mature neutrophils, producing what is generally referred to as a "degenerative left shift." Occasionally, the left shift may include a few myelocytes; this is seen at times in acute salmonellosis. Under these circumstances, there is commonly a marked leukopenia, and the immature neutrophils are larger than normal. The nucleus appears swollen, and the lighter parachromatin seems to be more abundant, giving the nucleus a more reddish coloration while the cytoplasm remains diffusely basophilic (Plate XI–11). In some instances, the nucleus assumes bizarre shapes. An incidental but persistent finding in a horse was that of hypersegmented neutrophils (Prasse et al., 1981). We have observed occasional hypersegmented neutrophils in horses with neutrophilia accompanying diseases presumably associated with increased levels of corticosteroids in circulation.

The Eosinophil

This leukocyte characterizes the horse blood. Eosinophil granules are very large and tightly packed, and they almost completely fill the cytoplasm. Because of the larger size of the granules, the cell outline conforms to the granule contour, giving the cell a raspberry-like appearance (Plate VII–7). The granules stain a bright reddish orange and frequently are so numerous that they partially obscure the nucleus. A pale blue cytoplasm may show between the granules and along the edge of the cell. Archer and Hirsch (1963) have made motion picture studies of degranulation of horse eosinophils during phagocytosis.

The Basophil

The granules of the basophil are purple and irregular in size and shape and may be tightly packed or scattered irregularly in the cytoplasm. Some granules may be over the nucleus, and others may cause the cell wall to bulge (Plate VII–7). The basophil nucleus is less segmented than that of mature neutrophils.

The Lymphocyte

The majority of lymphocytes are small with darkly stained nucleus and limited amount of cytoplasm. Lymphocytes as large as the monocyte may be encountered, and these have a smooth nuclear chromatin and a considerable quantity of pale blue, smooth cytoplasm. Azurophilic granules, when present, are sparse, small, irregularly shaped, and not necessarily evenly dispersed.

The Monocyte

The nucleus of the monocyte is characteristically in the form of a broad kidney bean, and some folding and partial formation of lobes may be seen. The chromatin is lacy or stringy and at times may appear clumped. The cytoplasm is blue-gray and granular; pinpoint, pinkish azurophilic granules may be scattered throughout the cytoplasm, and an occasional small vacuole may be seen.

The Platelets

Of the common domestic animals, the horse has the lowest normal number of platelets. Reported ranges and mean values (when given) of platelet counts include: 90,000–410,000/μl, with a mean of 210,000/μl, in 36 Clydesdale horses (Stewart and Holman, 1940); 98,000–199,000/μl, with a mean of 138,000, in 46 German trotters (Stolpe, 1970); 92,500–377,500/μl in 93 horses of mixed ages and breeds (Finocchio et al., 1970); 132,000–226,000/μl in 7 Thoroughbreds and 223,000–276,000/μl in 3 Shetland ponies (Bell and Tomlin, 1955); and 114,000–160,000/μl for 8 Thoroughbreds and 184,000–312,000 for 4 Shetland ponies (Barkhan et al., 1957). Data of the last two reports indicate higher platelet numbers in Shetland ponies than in Thoroughbreds. Splenectomy results in a substan-

tial and persistent increase in the platelet count (Catling and Jeffcott, 1975).

Equine platelets typically stain lightly; the cytoplasm is light blue and contains fine azurophilic granules (Plate VII–7). Their shape varies from the more common oval form to elongated structures (Fig. 16–2A), and giant forms as large as the erythrocyte may be observed. Their surface is generally smooth, although some surface invaginations may be present (Fig. 16–3B). Their ultrastructure is similar to that of human platelets, except with regard to storage organelles (White et al., 1976). There are fewer and smaller dense bodies than in human platelets, and the granules present a striped appearance. Horse platelets differ from human platelets in their response to certain aggregating agents, e.g., epinephrine and serotonin.

The Plasma

Icterus Index

The plasma of the horse normally contains a greater quantity of bilirubin than that of other domesitc animals. A mean bilirubin concentration of 1.57 ± 0.86 mg/dl was found in 77 plasma samples from 51 horses, with lowest concentration of 0.48 mg/dl and 5 samples containing more than 3 mg/dl (Ramsay, 1946). A range of 0.6–1.7 mg/dl, mean 0.98 mg/dl, was found in 30 horses (Jennings and Mulligan, 1953). Breed differences have been found in serum bilirubin values, with Thoroughbreds having higher values than draught horses (Gerber et al., 1976a). Certain horses, perhaps as many as 15% of the population, have plasma bilirubin levels of 2.0 mg/dl or more (Tennant et al., 1976). In addition to the natural yellow color due to bilirubin, the plasma of a horse on green feed may have yellow pigment contributed by carotenoids from the feed (Palmer, 1916).

Fasting a horse for 48 hours caused marked increase in plasma bilirubin (Ramsay, 1946). In fasted horses and ponies, bilirubin concentration begins to increase rapidly, exceeding baseline values by 15 hours and leveling off by 2–3 days (Grownwall and Mia, 1975; Naylor et al., 1980). Fasting may result in frank clinical icterus in horses with normally higher levels of plasma bilirubin. An extreme example was seen in a horse with an initial level of 1.96 mg/dl; the level rose to 5.12 mg/dl during fasting and then returned to 1.86 mg/dl in 4 days after the fast was broken. The fasting hyperbilirubinemia in the horse was shown to be essentially of hepatic origin because bilirubin synthesis or redistribution did not change, but bilirubin excretion decreased by 50–80% during fasting and increased markedly following refeeding (Grownwall, 1976; Grownwall and Mia, 1975; Grownwall et al., 1980). The efficiency of the liver in removing plasma bilirubin in certain other species is also decreased during fasting, resulting in increased plasma bilirubin levels. Factors involved in decreased hepatic transport of bilirubin remain unknown.

Observations on plasma color in horses on low plant pigment intake have revealed that the icterus index score varied in direct proportion to circulating erythrocyte volume as measured by PCV:

PCV %	Icterus Index (Units)
25	2 – 5
25–30	5 – 7.5
30–35	7.5–15
35–40	10 –15
40–55	15 –25

Similar observations have been made by others (Gerber et al., 1976a).

A PCV of 25% or less and an icterus index of 20 units or more should excite suspicion of the existence of a hemolytic process to explain the anemic state (Appendix Case 56). On the other hand, icterus index scores of 50, 75, and 100 units or more are not per se indicative of hemolytic disease (Tables 6–16 and 6–17). Diseases associated with anorexia, and especially acute and peracute diseases involving the gastrointestinal tract, characteristically lead to the retention of bilirubin and generally an elevated PCV as a result of hemoconcentration.

A comparison in equine patients of icterus index units in plasma with direct-acting (bilirubin glucuronide), indirect-acting (prehepatic or free bilirubin), and total bilirubin in serum, determined by the van den Bergh test, is shown in Table 6–11. Icterus index scores increased proportionately with increasing amounts of total bilirubin primarily because of indirect-acting bilirubin. It has been stated

that the interpretation of van den Bergh test results is somewhat different in the horse than in other animal species (Tennant et al., 1976). Even in complete extrahepatic bile duct obstruction, less than half of the plasma bilirubin is direct-acting. However, when the direct-reacting bilirubin represents 25–35% of the plasma bilirubin, regardless of the total concentration, there is good reason to suspect either intrahepatic or extrahepatic cholestasis.

Plasma and Serum Proteins

Total plasma proteins were found to range from 6.0–8.5 g/dl in 147 clinically normal horses. Racehorses 2–3 years of age were found to have commonly less than 7.0 g/dl total plasma proteins; the range for 14 such horses in training or racing was 6.1–7.1 g/dl, with a mean of 6.5 ± 0.4 g/dl. Although an increase in total plasma proteins with age ordinarily would be anticipated as in other animals, it did not appear to be the case for horses grouped by increasing age (Tables 6–5, 6–6). For example, a gelding Standardbred horse at 21 years of age had 7.2 g/dl total plasma proteins. In a study of 475 trotting horses of both sexes 1–27 years of age (Salutini and Biagi, 1977) albumin tended to increase in male and decrease in female horses, while α_1- and α_2-globulins decreased and γ-globulins increased sharply between 2 and 6 years of age and then slowly in both sexes.

Literature values on serum proteins include a mean of 6.47 ± 0.28 g/dl for 11 healthy mature horses (Mattheeuws et al., 1966); a mean of 7.3 g/dl in 70 normal horses (Irfan, 1967); a range of 5.4–7.2 g/dl, with a mean of 6.6, for 7 Thoroughbreds at an altitude of 8,600 feet (Mussman and Rubiano, 1970); a range of 4.0–10.8 g/dl, with a mean of 6.4 ± 0.7, for 540 clinically normal horses of all ages, the lower values being characteristic of horses younger than 1 year of age (Pierce, 1976); a range of 5.84–7.96 g/dl, with a mean of 7.14 ± 0.21, for 94 racehorses at the Madras Racecourse (Viswanathan and Gopalakrishnan, 1979); and a mean of 6.39 ± 0.41 g/dl, as determined by a modified biuret method, for 60 normal racehorses in training (Rudolph and Venegas, 1979).

Table 6–11. Comparison of Plasma Icterus Index Units with Serum Bilirubin Levels in the Horse

Number of Samples	Plasma Icterus Index Units	Bilirubin in Serum (mg/dl) (mean and 1 SD)		
		Direct-Acting Bilirubin	Indirect-Acting Bilirubin	Total Bilirubin
5	5	0.10 ± 0.0	0.56 ± 0.24	0.71 ± 0.26
10	7.5–10	0.17 ± 0.08	0.80 ± 0.30	0.96 ± 0.27
2	15	0.17 ± 0.10	1.97 ± 0.10	2.15 ± 0.20
3	20–25	0.30 ± 0.26	3.20 ± 0.26	3.50 ± 0.40
5	50	0.74 ± 0.88	4.74 ± 0.88	5.48 ± 1.11
6	75	0.45 ± 0.33	5.36 ± 0.79	5.80 ± 0.93
11	100 +	2.80 ± 2.20	10.90 ± 3.6	13.70 ± 3.90

Fibrinogen

The normal range of fibrinogen is 0.1–0.4 g/dl of blood. Plasma fibrinogen concentration is not influenced by age except slightly during the first 3 months of life (Table 6–6). It increases in inflammatory, neoplastic, and traumatic disorders. Low fibrinogen levels were observed in galloping and trotting horses subject to epistaxis (Stolpe and Wiesner, 1970).

A heat-precipitation method, in which length of the precipitated fibrinogen column was measured and converted into plasma fibrinogen concentration, correlated well with a chemical method of fibrinogen estimation and gave slightly higher results than the method described in Chapter 2 (Campbell et al., 1981). With this method, 100 healthy horses of different breeds were found to have fibrinogen levels of 0.297–0.631 g/dl, with a mean of 0.387 ± 0.074. No breed differences were observed. Horses with bacterial pneumonia and abscesses had greater fibrinogen values than those with colic, fractures, and nonsuppurative wounds.

Lipemia

Occurrence of lipemia in Equidae is clinically significant. We have encountered it in cases of severe hepatitis, in a case of carcinoma of the stomach, and in diabetes mellitus. Lipemia and hypercholesterolemia in a horse with diabetes mellitus have been reported (Tasker et al., 1966).

Lipemia is prominent in the blood of fasted ponies (Baetz and Pearson, 1972). Ponies appear to be particularly susceptible to lipemia in association with certain disease states. Observations have been made of hyperlipemia in Danish ponies, all mares in the last trimester of pregnancy or mares that had just foaled and had recently been transfused (Eriksen and Simesen, 1970). The initial sign of the disorder was anorexia, and 8 of the ponies had diarrhea. Coagulation time was increased, and sulfobromophthalein (Bromsulphalein; BSP) clearance was decreased. Blood samples left standing for a few minutes developed a milky white top layer of lipids. There was a marked increase in total lipids, especially serum triglycerides, cholesterol, and, to a lesser degree, phospholipids. At necropsy, there was fatty infiltration of the liver and most other ogans. A report on lipemia in ponies of the Netherlands revealed association of hyperlipemia with anorexia and its frequent occurrence in periparturient mares (Schotman and Kroneman, 1969). Prognosis was usually poor. Appendix Case 64 presents a case of icterus and lipemia associated with hepatic lipidosis in a horse.

The Bone Marrow

The iliac crest, sternum, or ribs are sites for aspiration of bone marrow in the horse. A detailed description of erythropoiesis, granulopoiesis, monocyte production, and thrombopoiesis in bone marrow from the iliac crest and of lymphocyte production in the bone marrow and lymph node preparations has been published along with 32 excellent color photomicrographs (Tschudi et al., 1975).

Calhoun (1946, 1954, 1955) and Archer (1954) reviewed the literature on bone marrow cytology of the horse and presented observations on marrow differential cell counts (Table 6–12). The former investigator employed 7 old, cold-blooded horses and aspirated marrow from the rib under local anesthesia. The latter investigator used 12 "mongrel" ponies representing crosses be-

Table 6–12. Cellular Composition of the Bone Marrow of the Horse

Cell Type	Archer (1954) (12 ponies)		Calhoun (1954) (7 horses)		Tschudi et al. (1976) (15 horses)		Franken et al. (1982a) (24 horses)	
	Range (%)	Mean (%)	Range (%)	Mean (%)	Range (%)	Mean (%)	Range (%)	Mean (%)
Myeloblast	0.0 – 0.66	0.237	—	—	0.3– 2.0	1.19	0.0– 5.0	1.0
Promyelocyte	0.14– 0.99	0.502	0.0– 5.0	1.83	0.0– 3.0	1.27	0.5– 3.5	1.7
Neutrophilic myelocyte	11.14–28.60	17.94	26.2–56.0	38.06	1.0– 5.0	3.28	1.0– 7.5	3.2
Eosinophilic myelocyte	0.69– 2.35	1.43	0.4– 3.6	2.34	0.0– 0.3	0.05		
Neutrophilic metamyelocyte	17.90–29.40	21.80	—	—	5.0–11.0	7.91	1.5–15.0	5.6
Eosinophilic metamyelocyte	1.05– 6.95	3.46	—	—	0.0– 0.3	0.1		
Basophilic metamyelocyte	0.14– 5.39	0.99	—	—	0.0– 0.3	0.08		
Band neutrophils			—	—	—		6.0–26.5	15.7
Neutrophil	7.83–25.30	14.70	1.8–20.2	13.31	11.0–30.0	20.40	3.0–16.5	8.4
Eosinophil	0.52– 5.95	2.63	0.2– 1.2	0.60	0.0– 0.6	0.20	0.0– 5.0	1.8
Basophil	0.0 – 0.33	0.05	0.0– 1.0	0.60	0.0– 0.5	0.14	0.0– 1.0	0.3
Total myeloid		63.73		56.74		34.53		37.9
Rubriblast	0.0 – 0.87	0.34	0.4– 3.4	1.6[a]	0.6– 4.0	2.18	0.0– 2.0	0.7
Prorubricyte	0.16– 4.35	1.88	—	—	2.0– 9.0	5.78	1.0– 9.5	3.6
Rubricyte	2.21–13.00	6.34	8.0–32.0	20.94	10.0–23.0	16.20	14.5–44.0	28.2
Metarubricyte	4.20–39.20	17.60	5.0–24.2	13.71	25.0–45.0	34.90	14.0–36.0	23.2
Total erythroid		26.16		34.66		60.48		55.9
Monocyte		—	1.2– 4.8	2.46	0.0– 2.0	0.82	0.0– 1.0	0.2
Lymphocyte	2.46–20.90	9.71	2.0– 5.6	3.91	1.0– 6.0	3.76	1.5– 8.5	3.8
Plasma cell	0.0 – 1.66	0.50	0.0– 0.8	0.63	0.0– 2.0	0.72	0.0– 2.0	0.6
Megakaryocyte			—	—	—		0.0– 1.0	0.3
Mitotic figure			—	—	0.4– 2.0	1.2	0.0– 3.5	0.8
Myeloid:erythroid ratio	1.1–10.20:1	2.43:1	0.9–3.76:1	1.64:1	0.34–0.85:1	0.60:1	0.48–0.91:1	0.71:1

[a]Calhoun called this group "stem cell" and did not include it in the total erythroid count.

tween two or more breeds. Marrow aspiration was made from the tuber coxae under local anesthesia. In foals, only ⅛-inch penetration of the needle was required, but in ponies 10 years of age or older, the needle had to be inserted 2 inches or more to obtain marrow. The M:E ratios reported by these two investigators, respectively, ranged from 0.9–3.76:1.0, with a mean of 1.64:1.0, and from 1.1–10.2:1.0 with a mean of 2.43:1.0. The higher range of M:E ratio in these reports may reflect at least partly the influence of significant hemodilution since a narrower range and mean values below unity were obtained by us and in subsequent reports (Franken et al., 1982a; Tschudi et al., 1976).

The M:E ratio on sternal marrow of 15 horses, 4–27 years of age, ranged from 0.34–0.85:1.0, with a mean of 0.60 ± 0.13:1.0 (Tschudi et al., 1976). The M:E ratio increased in 4 cases of anemias associated with chronic purulent infection and/or heavy intestinal parasites and decreased in 3 cases of anemias of unknown etiology and with a high rate of mitosis, presumably involving the erythroid series. Recent observations on sternal bone marrow of 24 clinically normal, warm-blooded horses yielded a range of 0.48–0.91:1.0 and a mean of 0.71 ± 0.11:1.0 for the M:E ratio (Franken et al., 1982a). A considerable amount of stainable iron (2 + to 3 +) was found in the bone marrow of 17 of 24 horses. Marrow examination of 66 anemic horses indicated that increased erythroid activity was not always present in anemia (M:E <0.49:1.0 in 8 horses, within the normal range in 38 horses, and greater than normal in 20 horses) (Franken et al., 1982b). The iron concentration in the bone marrow of anemic horses was usually normal.

Our own differential cell counts, representing normal bone marrow cytology, have been limited to 4 clinically normal, mixed-breed horses. Their PCV ranged from 29–36% and WBC counts from 8,250–12,500/μl of blood. The M:E ratios were 0.52, 0.62, 1.13, and 1.45:1.0. The range of 0.52–1.45:1.0, along with the differential marrow cell counts, has served well for evaluating the status of hematopoiesis in equine patients. A comparison of the bone marrow cytology in several clinical states associated with anemia

is shown in Table 6–13. These observations on anemic horses indicate that *a low M:E ratio by itself does not necessarily reflect effective erythrogenesis.* The finding of polychromatic erythrocytes or reticulocytes in ample numbers in bone marrow films (Plate V–6) is a more certain sign of effective erythropoiesis than an M:E ratio of less than unity. Staining horse bone marrow films for reticulocytes by new methylene blue stain as well as by routine staining methods can be helpful in evaluating the effectiveness of erythropoiesis in this species (see p. 156).

EFFECTS OF EXOGENOUS CORTICOSTEROIDS AND NATURAL STRESS

Effect of Corticosteroid Administration

A mature male quarter horse and a mature Thoroughbred gelding were used to observe the effect on PCV and leukocyte numbers of the intravenous injection of dexamethasone. The quarter horse was given a single injection of 10 mg, and the Thoroughbred received 3 injections of 5 mg each at 24-hour intervals (Table 6–14). No significant changes in PCV were seen, other than the anticipated variations related to differing degrees of splenic contraction. Changes in both total and differential leukocyte numbers were evident within 2 hours, with maximum effects appearing as early as the fourth hour. The response to 10 mg of the steroid was no greater than that produced by a single 5-mg dose. WBC counts increased by twofold, while neutrophils increased two- to threefold. Band neutrophils appeared briefly and in small numbers after each injection of the steroid, indicating their release along with mature neutrophils from the bone marrow pool into peripheral blood. The major effect, however, was the increase in mature neutrophils. Lymphocytes decreased by 30% by the tenth hour following the single injection of the steroid, while about 50–60% reduction was evident at 5–7 hours following the second and third injection of the 5-mg dose. Eosinopenia developed after each injection, while monocytes revealed no clear response.

Injection of ACTH and dexamethasone

Table 6–13. Differential Cell Counts (in Percent) and Myeloid:Erythroid Ratios in Normal and Patient Horses

Cell Type	(1) Range in 4 Normal Horses	(2) Lead Poisoning Horse A	(2) Lead Poisoning Horse B	(3) Pheno-thiazine Toxicosis	(4) Chronic Bleeding	(5) Hemolytic Anemia and Purpura	(6) Progressive Anemia Pyrexia	(7) Emaciated	(8) Stomach Carcinoma
PCV (%) in blood	29–36	24	21	28	16	23	20	27	24
WBC/μl in blood	8,250–12,500	9,900	13,300	14,100	8,800	10,000	7,300	11,000	9,300
No. cells differentiated	1,000	500	500	500	500	500	500	500	500
Myeloblast	0.3– 1.5	1.2	0.6	0.8	1.8	1.2	1.2	2.4	1.8
Progranulocyte	1.0– 1.9	0.0	1.2	2.0	1.0	1.2	1.0	1.6	4.8
Neutrophilic myelocyte	1.9– 3.2	1.4	2.0	0.8	3.0	1.6	3.4	2.6	3.0
Eosinophilic myelocyte	0.2– 0.8	0.6	0.6	0.2	0.8	0.2	0.0	0.0	1.0
Basophilic myelocyte	0.0– 0.1	0.0	0.0	0.0	0.0	0.0	0.0	0.0	0.2
Neutrophilic metamyelocyte	2.1– 7.3	1.2	3.2	3.2	5.0	2.6	7.8	3.2	12.4
Eosinophilic metamyelocyte	0.2– 1.8	0.4	0.4	0.4	0.0	0.0	0.6	0.0	0.0
Band neutrophil	6.8–14.7	6.8	6.6	4.0	12.8	8.8	8.0	11.2	19.4
Band eosinophil	0.6– 1.2	0.2	0.0	0.0	0.2	0.4	0.0	0.0	0.2
Neutrophil	9.6–21.0	4.4	5.2	7.8	6.6	3.8	10.6	19.2	20.0
Eosinophil	1.8– 3.0	0.2	0.0	0.6	0.4	0.2	0.0	2.0	0.4
Basophil	0.0– 1.4	0.6	0.2	0.2	0.2	0.6	0.4	2.8	0.2
Total myeloid	28.1–48.4	17.0	20.0	20.0	31.8	20.6	33.0	45.2	63.0
Rubriblast	0.6– 1.1	0.8	0.0	0.4	2.2	0.4	0.6	0.4	0.4
Prorubricyte	1.0– 2.0	1.8	1.0	1.6	2.2	1.2	1.4	1.2	0.6
Rubricyte, basophilic	4.5–11.1	3.4	7.2	17.0	9.4	12.4	5.6	3.6	3.2
Rubricyte, polychromatic	14.7–26.0	36.0	33.8	33.4	28.8	34.0	25.4	14.6	10.4
Rubricyte, normochromic	0.7– 4.3	0.0	0.0	0.4	1.0	0.0	0.0	0.0	0.0
Metarubricyte	10.7–15.4	30.8	29.0	13.4	11.4	25.0	15.8	8.2	6.4
Mitotic rubricyte	0.0– 1.9	2.0	2.8	1.4	1.2	0.0	0.6	1.0	0.0
Total erythroid	33.2–56.2	74.8	73.8	67.6	56.2	73.0	49.4	29.0	21.0
Lymphocyte	1.8– 6.7	2.6	2.2	6.8	2.6	1.4	8.8	19.8	6.2
Plasma cell	0.2– 1.8	0.0	0.2	0.2	1.8	0.2	0.8	0.8	1.0
Monocyte	0.0– 1.0	0.2	0.2	0.2	0.4	0.0	3.2	2.4	1.0
Mitotic cell	0.0– 0.2	0.4	0.0	0.2	0.8	0.8	0.0	0.0	0.2
RE nucleus	0.2– 1.6	0.0	0.0	0.0	0.6	0.6	1.4	0.2	2.4
Hematogone	0.2– 1.4	1.4	0.2	2.2	2.6	0.0	0.8	0.2	0.6
Unclassified cell	0.2– 1.7	0.0	0.0	0.2	0.0	0.4	0.0	0.4	0.0
Degenerated cell	2.3– 9.0	3.4	3.4	2.6	3.0	2.0	1.8	2.0	4.2
Macrophage	0.0– 0.0	0.2	0.0	0.0	0.0	0.0	0.8	0.0	0.0
Myeloid:erythroid ratio	0.52–1.45:1.0	0.23:1.0	0.27:1.0	0.30:1.0	0.57:1.0	0.28:1.0	0.67:1.0	1.56:1.0	3.00:1.0

Table 6–14. Leukocyte Responses in the Horse to Intravenous Administration of 9α-fluoro-16α-methylprednisoline (Dexamethasone-Schering)[a]

Horse	Date	Dose	Clock Time	Elapsed Time (hr)	PCV (%)	WBC/μl	Neutrophils Band	Neutrophils Mature	Lymphocytes	Monocytes	Eosinophils	Disintegrated Cells
									Absolute Leukocyte Numbers/μl			
I	June 10		9 am	(control)	44	8,700	44	4,959	2,349	392	870	87
Mature male	June 11	10 mg	9 am	(control)	42	9,000	0	4,995	2,835	225	900	45
Quarter horse	June 11		11 am	2	41	15,200	152	10,488	3,876	304	304	76
	June 11		1 pm	4	42	16,700	584	13,193	2,422	418	84	0
	June 11		4:30 pm	7½	46	16,400	82	13,612	2,132	574	0	0
	June 11		7:30 pm	10½	43	16,500	330	13,695	1,980	412	82	0
	June 12		9 am	24	40	11,600	0	8,236	2,900	464	0	0
	June 12		3 pm	30	43	10,200	0	7,140	2,601	357	102	0
	Sept. 14		9 am	(control)	44	8,800	0	5,324	2,860	308	264	44
	Sept. 14		3:30 pm	(control)	41	10,800	0	6,048	3,456	756	486	54
	Sept. 15	5 mg	7 am	0	—	—	—	—	—	—	—	—
	Sept. 15		8 am	1	35	6,600	0	4,191	1,881	198	165	165
	Sept. 15		9 am	2	41	17,800	267	13,261	3,115	979	178	0
	Sept. 15		10 am	3	42	17,000	170	12,920	2,890	510	170	340
	Sept. 15		1 pm	6	41	15,900	398	12,482	2,544	477	0	0
II	Sept. 15		4 pm	9	44	19,300	96	15,440	3,184	579	0	0
Mature	Sept. 16	5 mg	8 am	25	37	12,000	0	7,560	3,180	1,200	60	0
Thoroughbred	Sept. 16		1 pm	5	41	15,800	237	12,719	1,738	1,106	0	0
Gelding	Sept. 16		4 pm	8	40	18,700	94	14,960	3,179	468	0	0
	Sept. 17	5 mg	9 am	25	41	10,700	0	6,046	3,852	749	54	122
	Sept. 17		10:30 am	1½	—	12,200	122	7,442	3,782	732	0	0
	Sept. 17		2:30 pm	5½	40	18,800	376	16,168	1,598	658	0	0
	Sept. 17			7	38	12,500	62	10,875	1,250	312	0	0
	Sept. 18		9 am	24	38	11,000	0	6,875	3,685	275	110	55
	Sept. 18		4 pm	31	32	11,900	0	6,069	4,998	536	238	60

[a]These data obtained in cooperation with Dr. John D. Wheat.

caused leukocytosis, neutrophilia, eosinopenia, and lymphopenia of variable degree and duration (Osbaldiston and Johnson, 1972). A dose-dependent response was evident, with dexamethasone producing more pronounced effects. No significant changes were observed in RBC counts, platelet counts, and monocyte numbers. Prolonged corticosteroid therapy in horses was associated with persistent but fluctuating leukocytosis, neutrophilia, lymphopenia, and eosinopenia (Straub and Gerber, 1976).

That the leukocytic response to corticosteroids may be somewhat age-related was shown in a recent study (Burguez et al., 1983). Plasma cortisol and total and differential leukocyte counts were measured in 6 horses (2–19 years old) and 6 foals (about 2–4 days old) given cortisol (0.75 mg/kg) intramuscularly. Plasma cortisol levels increased more in horses and persisted for 8 hours in horses as compared to 4 hours in foals. The N:L ratio almost doubled in foals at 2 hours, while it tripled in horses by 4 hours and remained over twice normal for 8 hours. These changes were associated with an increase in neutrophil numbers and a simultaneous decrease in lymphocyte numbers. All values returned to normal by 24 hours post injection.

Effect of Sustained Muscular Activity

A 12-year-old mare of mixed breeding that had not been subjected to exercise for the preceding 2 years was employed in this demonstration. Her general condition was what could be expected in a horse that had been maintained on good pasture without supplemental concentrate feeding. Though somewhat overweight, she was not obese.

The exercise consisted of a 32-mile course traversed in 8 hours from 8 A.M. to 4 P.M., with 15-minute rest periods given at 10 A.M. and 2 P.M. and 1 hour of rest between noon and 1 P.M. The total actual time at work was 6½ hours, and the overall average working speed was 4.9 miles per hour, ranging from 6.0 miles per hour initially to 2.5 miles per hour at the end of the period. Approximately one-third (12 miles) of the total distance was covered during the first 2 hours, between 8 A.M. and 10 A.M. General signs of fatigue were quite evident at 2 P.M. Blood samples were collected at 2-hour intervals during exercise and compared with control hemograms developed the day before when the horse was at rest. The 24-hour water consumption was 15 gallons on the control day and 18 gallons on the day of exercise. The ambient temperature was high on both days, rising from 77°F at 8 A.M. to 96°F at 2 P.M. on the control day, compared to 79°F and 99°F, respectively, on the day of the exercise. The comparative hemograms are depicted in Figure 6–4.

Variations in PCV (A) and plasma proteins (B) on the control day were probably a reflection of dilution by water intake. On the day of the exercise, the marked increases in both PCV and plasma proteins were attributable primarily to dehydration from shifting of intravascualr fluid to extravascular fluid compartments and from loss of water through profuse sweating. A portion of the rise in PCV was attributable to splenic contraction. The WBC count (C) and changes in absolute numbers of various leukocyte types (D–H) were similar to those of the horses given dexamethasone (Table 6–14). This response of the leukocytes to sustained muscular exercise in the horse was interpreted, therefore, as a response to the physiologic release of adrenocorticoid hormones. Plasma levels of corticosteroids were found to increase after exercise (James et al., 1970) and endurance rides (Dybdal et al., 1980). Horses in endurance races exhibit clinical dehydration and metabolic alkalosis (Carlson, 1976b; Rose et al., 1979). Acidosis develops in most speedy horses (Rose et al., 1979), and most severely exhausted horses may exhibit partially compensated acidosis and slight left shift (Carlson, 1976b).

Physiologic Leukocytosis in Young Horses

Hemograms of young, vigorous horses are likely to be affected by physiologic leukocytosis under conditions requiring restraint, such as the collection of blood. This can be seen from data collected on 16 quarter horse yearlings to be wormed and vaccinated (Table 6–15). The horses were unbroken and ordinarily stayed out on pasture. They were brought into a corral, where they remained for an hour before the veterinarian and students arrived for the vaccination and worm-

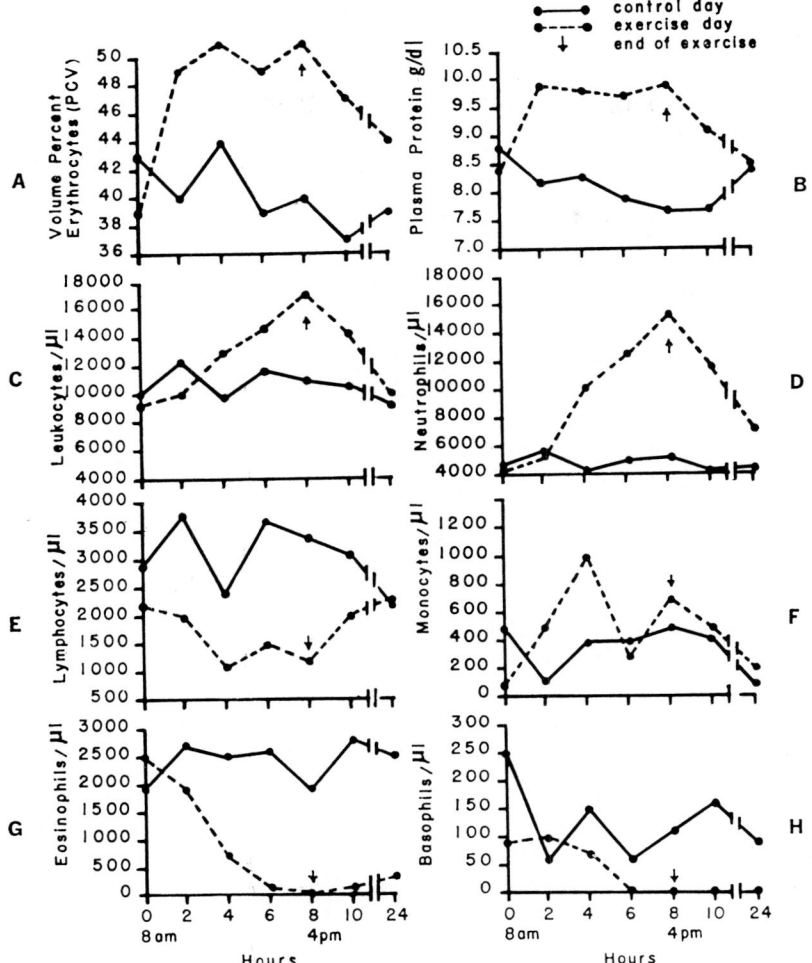

Fig. 6–4. Sequential hemograms of a 12-year-old mare during no exercise (control day) and during exercise in covering a 32-mile distance. (From Cardinet, et al., 1964; courtesy of *The California Veterinarian.*)

ing procedure. The horses were approached quietly and haltered. A blood sample was taken from the jugular vein before the vaccination and worming. The entire procedure required about 1½ hours, and during this time the more excitable and aggressive horses were able to avoid being caught until the very last. The least excitable horses, which were mostly females, were caught first, and there was little opportunity for muscular activity or fear to influence the hemogram, while the last horses to be caught had been milling about for an hour or more. The effect of excitement and muscular activity can be seen to be greatest among these.

Female yearling horses 1, 4, 6, and 9 (Table 6–15) revealed the least excitement, and their

blood values may be used as within group controls for purposes of comparison with the more apprehensive horses. A PCV of 40% or greater possibly reflects splenic contraction. A WBC count of 18,000 is significantly in excess of normal resting values, and an N:L ratio of less than 0.9:1.0 or greater than 1.0:1.0 would reflect a significant disturbance in the normal balance between the circulating numbers of these two leukocyte types (see Table 6–6). A most interesting observation was the marked increase in lymphocyte numbers in 6 of the 16 horses.

Garrey and Butler (1929), reporting on physiologic lymphocytosis in humans, stated that the increase in count is proportional to the severity of the muscular exercise. A mod-

Table 6–15. Effect of Strenuous Muscular Activity and Excitement on the Circulating Erythrocyte Volume (PCV), the Total Leukocyte Count, and the Differential Leukocyte Count in Yearling Horses[a]

Sequence of Being Caught	Sex[a]	Signs of Excitement	PCV (%)	WBC/μl	Differential Leukocyte Count in Absolute Numbers/μl					N:L Ratio
					Neutrophils	Lymphocytes	Monocytes	Eosinophils	Basophils	
1[c]	F	No comment	37	13,900	6,046	7,158	418	278	0	0.84:1.0
2	F	No comment	42	17,700	6,372	9,205	1,150	796	177	0.69:1.0
3	F	Slight excitement	41	16,100	6,279	8,694	483	644	0	0.72:1.0
4[c]	F	No comment	37	13,630	5,822	6,918	274	616	0	0.84:1.0
5	F	Slight excitement	43	18,000	7,110	9,720	540	630	0	0.73:1.0
6[c]	F	No comment	38	11,700	5,148	5,616	468	468	0	0.92:1.0
7	F	No comment	45	19,200	4,920	11,870	770	1,544	96	0.41:1.0
8	XM[b]	Excited	42	19,100	12,572	5,568	96	864	0	2.26:1.0
9[c]	F	No comment	39	16,700	6,596	8,100	584	1,420	0	0.81:1.0
10	XM	No comment	40	14,400	4,896	8,712	288	504	0	0.56:1.0
11	XM	Excited	44	22,800	7,296	14,022	570	798	114	0.52:1.0
12	XM	Excited	42	23,200	14,384	7,076	1,160	580	0	2.03:1.0
13	XM	Excited	43	26,300	11,572	13,544	790	394	0	0.85:1.0
14	F	No comment	44	20,300	7,410	11,164	914	812	0	0.66:1.0
15	XM	No comment	44	16,600	3,735	10,956	1,079	830	0	0.34:1.0
16	XM	Excited	40	20,200	6,666	12,625	606	303	0	0.53:1.0

[a]From Schalm and Hughes, 1964; courtesy of *The California Veterinarian*.
[b]XM = gelding
[c]Hemograms approximating normal control values.

est leukocytosis is chiefly due to a rise in neutrophils, whereas a marked leukocytosis may show preponderance of lymphocytes. Similar exercise-related changes in lymphocyte and neutrophil numbers have been described in horses (Snow et al., 1983).

As the blood circulates through the capillaries at rest, the erythrocytes flow in the central stream, while the leukocytes roll along the walls and readily become sequestered in the capillary beds. Flushing of the leukocytes into the major blood vessels takes place with strenuous exercise or increased heart action resulting from fright or apprehension. Furthermore, lymph flow may increase, leading to dumping of increased numbers of lymphocytes into the circulation from vast reserves in peripheral lymphoid organs (see Chapter 30 for details). This redistribution of leukocytes leads to increased numbers in large-vessel blood. The leukocytosis produced by fear and muscular activity is called "physiologic leukocytosis" as opposed to "reactive leukocytosis" in response to disease (see Chapter 26).

COMMENTS ON RESPONSE TO DISEASE

Hematologic changes in diseases of the horse are summarized in Tables 6–16, 6–17, and 6–18.

The N:L ratio in blood varies from 0.9:1.0 in yearlings to 2.0:1.0 in aged horses. The ability of the horse to increase circulating neutrophils in response to disease is limited by its characteristic N:L ratio. Among 870 horse patients, 71.9% of WBC counts fell within the range of 7,000–14,000/μl, and only 1.6% had WBC counts in excess of 30,000. The highest WBC count recorded by us in the horse was 65,000 in a patient with a pleural effusion associated with infarcts in the heart and kidneys. Moderate leukocytosis is 14,000–20,000, marked leukocytosis is 21,000–30,000, and extreme leukocytosis exists when counts are greater than 30,000.

In peracute and acute diseases of the gastrointestinal tract (impaction, torsions, intussusceptions, perforations, and salmonellosis), the extremely serious nature of the disease may be reflected in a leukogram characterized by a degenerative left shift. WBC count is generally decreased. In the more severe cases, a left shift to include myelocytes may be seen, with immature granulocytes exceeding mature forms. The cytoplasm of all neutrophil types is basophilic (Plate XI–11) and foamy, indicating the toxemic nature of the disease. Leukograms characterized by leukopenia and degenerative left shift call for an unfavorable or guarded prognosis. In some instances, marked and even extreme WBC counts are associated with "toxic" neutrophils. In rare instances the neutrophils exhibit a "toxic" granulation characterized by irregularly shaped, reddish cytoplasmic granules (Plate XI–12).

The extent of leukocytic changes in salmonellosis depends on severity of the disease process and clinical manifestations of the disease as shown in natural (Dorn et al., 1975) and experimental (Smith et al., 1979) salmonellosis. Leukopenia due mainly to neutropenia and slight to marked degenerative left shift are characteristic findings. Administration of endotoxin intravenously into ponies was found to produce an immediate neutropenia with a marked degenerative left shift and toxic changes, lymphopenia, monocytopenia, eosinopenia, and thrombocytopenia (Burrows, 1976). Rebound neutrophilia and monocytosis were seen during the recovery phase, 24–48 hours post injection.

Lymphocyte numbers are readily depressed to low levels by corticosteroids of stress. This is especially true in young horses in which lymphocytes comprise 45–50% of the normal differential leukocyte count. Perhaps lymphopenia should be regarded as present in yearlings and 2-year-olds when absolute lymphocyte numbers fall below 2,000/μl and in older horses when the count is less than 1,500/μl. As systemic stress becomes more and more severe, the absolute lymphocyte count of horses of any age will be reduced to less than 1,000/μl. Arabian foals with combined immune deficiency generally have an absolute lymphocyte count of less than 1,000/μl (McGuire et al., 1974).

The monocyte is not especially responsive to disease in the horse. It is commonly reduced in numbers in the circulation during the early acute stage of disease. In diseases

Table 6–16.   Hemograms of the Horse in a Variety of Diseases

Breed	Sex	Age (yr)	PCV (%)	Plasma Proteins (g/dl)	Icterus Index (units)	WBC/μl	Neutrophils			Lympho-cytes	Mono-cytes	Eosino-phils	Baso-phils	Other	Clinical Entity
							Metamyelo-cytes	Band	Mature						
QH	M	4	34	7.0	10	16,500	0	82 (0.5%)	7,507 (45.5%)	7,507 (45.5%)	1,155 (7%)	82 (0.5%)	165 (1%)	0	Parasitism: 2,450 ova per gram of feces
QH	F	13	35	6.8	7.5	13,000	—	65 (0.5%)	6,435 (49.5%)	3,120 (24%)	325 (2.5%)	2,990 (23%)	0	0	Chronic dermatitis
QH	F	17	29	11.9	10	20,900	0	314 (1.5%)	18,496 (88.5%)	1,568 (7.5%)	522 (2.5%)	0	—	—	Chronic nephritis, BUN = 100+
QH	XM	2	29	6.4	7.5	62,500	0	312 (0.5%)	51,563 (82.5%)	6,875 (11%)	3,750 (6%)	0	—	—	Abscesses
QH	XM	6	29	Lipemic plasma		9,900	0	297 (3%)	6,683 (67.5%)	2,029 (20.5%)	792 (8%)	99 (1%)	—	—	Carcinoma of stomach
Pony	F	10	40	Lipemic plasma		10,650	0	1,278 (12%)	6,869 (64.5%)	2,236 (21%)	266 (2.5%)	0	—	—	Necrotic hepatitis
Grade	F	25	40	8.8	60	19,800	0	297 (1.5%)	17,325 (87.5%)	1,287 (6.5%)	891 (4.5%)	0	—	—	Tetanus
Grade	XM	4	61	9.6	75	7,800	0	1,326 (17%)	4,368 (56%)	546 (7%)	1,560 (20%)	0	—	—	Aspiration pneumonia
Grade	F	?	38	7.6	20	7,400	0	37 (0.5%)	3,626 (49%)	2,960 (40%)	370 (5%)	370 (5%)	37 (0.5%)	0	Nigropallidal encephalomalacia (star thistle poisoning)
Same horse 2 days later			43	8.3	100	5,700	28 (0.5)	1,425 (25%)	1,368 (24%)	2,508 (44%)	314 (5.5%)	28 (0.5%)	0	28 (0.5%)	
QH	M	2	35	7.1	100	17,100	4,617 (27)	4,617 (27%)	3,933 (23%)	2,907 (17%)	1,026 (6%)	0	—	0 (0.5%)	Third-degree burns covering body
Thor.	F	8	60	—	100	33,330	333 (1)	765 (2.3%)	28,538 (85.7%)	3,230 (9.7%)	432 (1.3%)	0	—	—	Ovarian tumor (post-surgery-moribund)
QH	F	2	57	9.3	100	31,550	473 (1.5%)	473 (1.5%)	28,237 (89.5%)	1,577 (5.0%)	789 (2.5%)	0	—	0	Rabies
Pony	M	14	47	—	100	13,400	0	67 (0.5%)	11,792 (88%)	1,005 (7.5%)	536 (4%)	0	—	—	Rabies

Differential Leukocytes in Absolute Values/μl and in Percent

Table 6–17. Hemograms in Acute Diseases of the Gastrointestinal Tract of the Horse

						Neutrophils								
				Icterus		*Differential Leukocytes in Absolute Values/μl and in Percent*								
Breed	Sex	Age	PCV (%)	Index Units	WBC/μl	Metamyelo-cytes	Band	Mature	Lympho-cytes	Mono-cytes	Eosino-phils	Baso-phils	Other	Clinical Entity
Thor.	F	2 yr	69	50	26,850	0	537 (2%)	23,091 (86%)	2,953 (11%)	268 (1%)	0	0	0	Intussusception (died)
Thor.	F	?	56	50	10,200	–	1,428 (14%)	6,681 (65.5%)	1,173 (11.5%)	867 (8.5%)	0	0	51 (0.5%)	Intussusception (died)
Pony	M	2 yr	39	10	10,700	–	1,017 (9.5%)	6,527 (61%)	2,675 (25%)	428 (4%)	0	53 (0.5%)	0	Torsion of the colon (died)
Grade	M	?	63	100	5,800	348 (6%)	1,044 (18%)	3,828 (66%)	580 (10%)	0	0	0	0	Volvulus (died)
QH	XM	3 yr	64	25	13,100	0	1,834 (14%)	8,712 (66.5%)	2,227 (17%)	328 (2.5%)	0	0	0	Strangulated inguinal hernia (died)
QH	F	13 yr	51	15	1,100	–	55 (5%)	297 (27%)	737 (67%)	0	0	11 (1%)	–	Ruptured stomach (died)
Grade	F	20 yr	75	–	2,000	0	0	360 (18%)	980 (49%)	540 (27%)	20 (1%)	0	100 (5%)	Impaction and rupture of the colon (died)
Grade	F	10 mo	45	75	5,700	57 (1%)	1,340 (23.5%)	1,454 (25.5%)	2,308 (40.5%)	484 (8.5%)	0	0	57 (1%)	Ruptured intestine (died)
Pony	F	20 mo	49	20	5,600	336 (6%)	2,464 (44%)	1,288 (23%)	1,176 (21%)	336 (6%)	0	0	0	Perforated rectum (died)
QH	F	14 yr	57	50	3,400	170 (5%)	714 (21%)	1,938 (57%)	408 (12%)	136 (4%)	34 (1%)	0	0	Perforated rectum (died)
QH	F	8 yr	57	100	7,600	0	456 (6%)	5,852 (77%)	760 (10%)	532 (7%)	0	0	0	Prolapsed rectum (died)
QH	F	5 yr	46	100	33,250	–	1,330 (4%)	30,590 (92%)	665 (2%)	665 (2%)	0	0	0	Colic and impaction (died)

Table 6–18. Examples of the Effects of Various Diseases in the Horse on Plasma and Serum Protein Concentration and the Albumin:Globulin Ratio[a]

Accession	Age (yr)	Sex	Clinical Condition	PCV (%)	Plasma Proteins (g/dl)[b]	Serum Proteins (g/dl)[c]	Albumin (g/dl)	Globulin (g/dl)	A:G Ratio[d]	Comments
62L2669	2	F	Acute colic	65	—	8.0	3.9	4.1	0.95	Dehydration, normal A:G
62L2603	19	XM	Carpal fracture	49	8.1	6.9	3.6	3.3	1.09	Normal A:G
63L475	5	M	Leg lameness	—	—	6.0	3.3	2.7	1.22	Normal A:G
63L589	8	M	Abscess (spleen)	33	8.9	7.6	1.07	6.53	0.16	Hyperglobulinemia
62L2418	6	F	Hepatic abscesses	34	10.3	9.0	1.2	7.8	0.15	Hyperglobulinemia
63L317	9	M	Pneumonia (chronic)	30	11.5	10.5	1.0	9.5	0.10	Hyperglobulinemia
63L262	—	F	Dermatitis	33	11.6	10.0	1.2	8.8	0.14	Hyperglobulinemia
64L735	14	F	Fistula (chronic infection)	—	—	9.1	2.2	6.9	0.32	Hyperglobulinemia
62L2690	17	F	Nephritis	29	11.9	11.0	2.0	9.0	0.22	Hyperglobulinemia

[a] Extreme normal range for A:G ratio established at 0.75–1.50.
[b] From refractive index.
[c] From biuret method of chemical analysis.
[d] From paper electrophoresis.

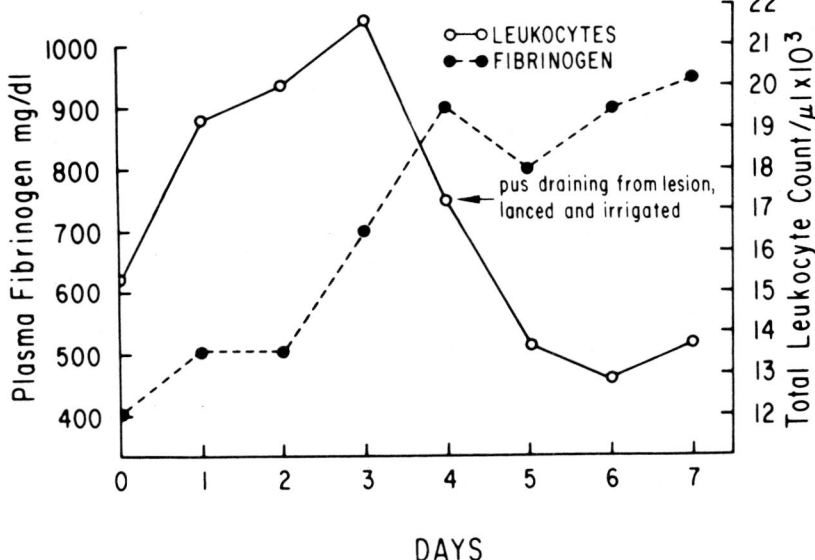

Fig. 6–5. Total leukocyte counts and plasma fibrinogen levels in a 2-year-old pony during development of an acute localized inflammation following inoculation of live *Corynebacterium pseudotuberculosis* into the pectoral muscles. The developing abscess was drained and irrigated daily from day 4 on. (From Schalm, 1979; courtesy of *Equine Practice*.)

leading to necrosis and in chronic inflammatory diseases, the number of monocytes increases. A monocytosis is reflected by absolute monocyte counts of greater than 1,000/µl.

Eosinophils are commonly depressed in all acute diseases by the activity of the adrenal cortex. Reaction to foreign protein in the hypersensitive state will lead to eosinophilia, as in other domestic animals. Eosinophilia exists when the absolute number is greater than 1,000/µl. The majority of horses with strongyloidiasis, with egg counts of 1,000–5,000/g of feces, have not exhibited eosinophilia. For example, 24 horses having 1,340 ± 326 *Strongylus* eggs/g of feces had absolute eosinophil counts of 469 ± 316, and 8 horses with 5,150 ± 800 eggs/g had eosinophil counts of 120 ± 103/µl. The low eosinophil numbers among the latter 8 horses may have been a reflection of the stress of the heavy worm burden.

The influence of worm burden on erythrocyte parameters was studied in weanlings from two Kentucky farms (Hansen et al., 1950b). The infestations were considered light to moderate and representative of all weanlings in the study. RBC counts of 11.5 million and Hb levels of 12 g/dl were found; thus the observed level of parasitism did not appear to have a significant effect. Heavy parasitic burden may be associated with anemia as shown in a study of the blood picture of two groups of crossbred ponies (Archer and Poynter, 1957); one group was regularly treated with anthelmintics and the other was left to acquire a considerable parasite burden naturally. In the latter group of ponies, anemia, with Hb levels dropping to as low a 5–6 g/dl of blood, developed in association with erythrocytic hypoplasia of the bone marrow. In another study, it was commented that anemia in the Thoroughbred is frequently associated with parasitic infestation, particularly with the larger *Strongylus* species (Archer and Miller, 1959).

Additional features of the hemogram of the horse in acute diseases associated with anorexia include the retention of bilirubin leading to plasma icterus index scores of 50–100 units (Tables 6–16 and 6–17). Acute pain results in splenic contraction and, when compounded by dehydration, a relative polycythemia develops, with PCV values in excess of 50%. PCV values of 60–75% are to be anticipated in severe gastrointestinal disorders. Plasma or serum proteins increase in disorders leading to dehydration or in infections resulting in antibody production (Table 6–18).

Estimation of plasma fibrinogen as part of the hemogram provides information relative to the probable nature of a disease (inflammatory) and its severity. Fibrinogen levels may increase within 1 or 2 days of infection, but peak levels are not attained until 3 or 4 days later (Fig. 6–5). Thus fibrinogen levels of 0.5–0.6 g/dl may represent an early or peracute stage of the disease, while levels of 1.0 g/dl or more reflect a more advanced stage as well as serious nature of the disease. Values as high as 1.7 g/dl hve been observed by us in a case of suppurative pleuritis (Schalm, 1979). Hyperfibrinogenemia was found to be more indicative of the severity of a disease process than WBC count in one-third to one-half of equine patients (Schalm, 1975). However, many horses with hyperfibrinogenemia and normal WBC counts had significant left shift. The frequency of death or need to destroy the horse was found to increase in parallel with increasing plasma fibrinogen (greater than 1.0 g/dl) levels (Schalm, 1979). Gradual reductions in the WBC counts and fibrinogen levels signify recovery from the disease process.

A recent publication summarizes abnormalities in blood and bone marrow cytology of the horse (Schalm, 1984).

Significantly elevated levels of serum prealbumin were found in horses with acute infections, acute laminitis, and malignant tumors, and such values showed a positive correlation with leukocyte counts and a negative correlation with serum albumin content (Ek, 1980).

REFERENCES

Aldous, H.M.J.: Hematology of Foals. 16th Annu. Conv. Amer. Ass. Equine Pract., p. 37, 1970.

Allen, B.V.: Serum Folate Levels in Horses, with Particular Reference to the English Thoroughbred. Vet. Rec., *103*:257, 1978.

Allen, B.V., and Archer, R.K.: Studies with Normal Erythrocytes of the English Thoroughbred Horse. Equine Vet. J., *5*:135, 1973.

Allen, B.V., and Archer, R.K.: Some Hematological Values in English Thoroughbred Horses. Vet. Rec., *98*:195, 1976.

Allen, B.V., and Blackmore, D.L.: Relationship Between Paired Plasma and Serum Viscosity and Plasma Proteins in the Horse. Res. Vet. Sci., *36*:360, 1984.

Allen, B.V., et al.: Leucocyte Counts in the Healthy English Thoroughbred in Training. Equine Vet. J., *16*:207, 1984.

Alonso, F.P.-I.: El analisis de sangre en clinica equina. Hygia Pecoris, *3*:37, 1981.

Archer, G.T., and Hirsch, J.G.: Motion Picture Studies on the Degranulation of Horse Eosinophils during Phagocytosis. J. Exp. Med., *118*:2287, 1963.

Archer, R.K.: Bone Marrow Biopsy in the Horse: A Study of the Normal Marrow Cytology in Cross-Bred Ponies. Vet. Rec., *66*:261, 1954.

Archer, R.K.: The Normal Haemograms and Coagulograms of the English Thoroughbred Horse. J. Comp. Path., *69*:390, 1959.

Archer, R.K.: Haematology in Relation to Performance and Potential: A General Review. J. S. Afr. Vet. Assoc., *45*:273, 1974.

Archer, R.K., and Allen, B.V.: The Viscosity of Equine Blood Plasma: A New Nonspecific Test. Vet. Rec., *86*:360, 1970.

Archer, R.K., and Clabby, J.: The Effect of Excitation and Exertion on the Circulating Blood of Horses. Vet. Rec., *77*:689, 1965.

Archer, R.K., and Miller, W.C.: The Interpretation of Haematological Examinations in Thoroughbred Horses. Vet. Rec., *71*:273, 1959.

Archer, R.K., and Poynter, D.: Anaemia and Eosinophilia Associated with Helminthiasis in Young Horses. J. Comp. Path., *67*:196, 1957.

Baetz, A.L., and Pearson, J.E.: Blood Constituent Changes in Fasted Ponies. Amer. J. Vet. Res., *33*:1941, 1972.

Barkhan, P., et al.: Comparative Coagulation Studies on Horse and Human Blood. J. Comp. Path., *67*:358, 1957.

Bell, W.N., and Tomlin, S.C.: The Coagulation Mechanism of the Blood of the Horse with Particular Reference to Its "Haemaphilioid" Status. J. Comp. Path., *65*:255, 1955.

Brenon, H.C.: Further Erythrocyte and Hemoglobin Studies in Thoroughbred Racing Horses. J. Amer. Vet. Med. Ass., *133*:102, 1958.

Burguez, P.N., et al.: Changes in Blood Neutrophil and Lymphocyte Counts following Administration of Cortisol to Horses and Foals. Equine Vet. J., *15*:58, 1983.

Burrows, G.E.: Hematologic Alterations Associated with Acute E. coli Endotoxemia. *In* Proceedings of the First International Symposium of Equine Hematology. Kitchen, H., and Krebhiel, J.D., eds. Amer. Ass. Equine Pract., Golden, Colorado, p. 505, 1976.

Calhoun, M.L.: Bone Marrow of Horses and Cattle. Science, *104*:423, 1946.

Calhoun, M.L.: A Cytological Study of Costal Marrow. I. The Adult Horse. Amer. J. Vet. Res., *15*:181, 1954.

Calhoun, M.L.: A Cytological Study of Costal Marrow. III. Hemograms of the Horse and Cow. Amer. J. Vet. Res., *16*:297, 1955.

Campbell, M.D., et al.: Determination of Plasma Fibrinogen Concentration in the Horse. Amer. J. Vet. Res., *42*:100, 1981.

Cardinet, G.H., III., et al.: Effects of Sustained Muscular Activity upon Blood Morphology in the Horse. Calif. Vet., *18*:31, Nov.–Dec., 1964.

Carlson, G.P.: Evaluation of Responsive Anemia in Horses. *In* Proceedings of the First International Symposium of Equine Hematology. Kitchen, H., and Krebhiel, J.D., eds. Amer. Ass. Equine Pract., Golden, Colorado, p. 327, 1976a.

Carlson, G.P.: Hematologic Alterations in Endurance-Trained Horses. *In* Proceedings of the First International Symposium of Equine Hematology. Kitchen, H., and Krebhiel, J.D., eds. Amer. Ass. Equine Pract., Golden, Colorado, p. 444, 1976b.

Catling, S.J.: Studies on Hematology of Exertion in Horses. Brit. J. Haematol., *30*:123, 1975.

Catling, S.J., and Jeffcott, L.B.: Personal communication, 1975. (Cited in Jeffcott, 1977.)

Cornelius, C.E., et al.: Erythrocyte Survival Studies in the Horse, Using Glycine-2-C¹⁴. Amer. J. Vet. Res., *21*:1123, 1960.

Dalton, R.G.: The Significance of Variations with Activity and Sedation in the Hematocrit, Plasma Protein Concentration, and Erythrocyte Sedimentation Rate of Horses. Brit. Vet. J., *128*:439, 1972.

Dorn, C.R., et al.: Neutropenia and Salmonellosis in Hospitalized Horses. J. Amer. Vet. Med. Ass., *166*:65, 1975.

Dybdal, N.O., et al.: Alterations in Plasma Corticosteroids, Insulin and Selected Metabolites in Horses Used in Endurance Rides. Equine Vet. J., *12*:137, 1980.

Ek, N.: Concentration of Serum Prealbumin (Pr) Protein in Sick Horses and Its Correlation to Blood Leucocyte Count and Albumin Content in Serum. Acta Vet. Scand., *21*:482, 1980.

Eriksen, L., and Simesen, M.G.: Hyperlipaemia hos ponier. Nord. Vet. Med., *22*:273, 1970.

Ferraro, L., et al.: Hematology and Serum Protein Values in Arabian and Non-Arabian Foals. J. Equine Med. Sur., *3*:411, 1979.

Finocchio, E.J., et al.: Platelet Counts in Horses. Cornell Vet., *60*:518, 1970.

Franken, P., et al.: The Bone Marrow of the Horse. I. The Technique of Sampling and Examination and Values of Normal Warm-Blooded Horses. Zentralbl. Veterinaermed., *29A*:16, 1982a.

Franken, P., et al.: The Bone Marrow of the Horse. II. Warm-Blooded Horses with Anaemia. Zentralbl. Veterinaermed., *29A*:23, 1982b.

Garry, W.E. and Butler, V.: Physiological Leukocytosis. Amer. J. Physiol., *90*:355, 1929.

Geiser, D.R., et al.: Normal Hematology and Serology of the Clydesdale Draft Horse. Equine Pract., *6*(10):7, 1984.

Gerber, H., et al.: Total Bilirubin in Different Breeds of Horses. *In* Proceedings of the First International Symposium of Equine Hematology. Kitchen, H., and Krebhiel, J.D., eds. Amer. Ass. Equine Pract., Golden, Colorado, p. 241, 1976a.

Gerber, H., et al.: "Normal" Values for Different Breeds of Horses. *In* Proceedings of the First International Symposium of Equine Hematology. Kitchen, H., and Krebhiel, J.D., eds. Amer. Ass. Equine Pract., Golden, Colorado, p. 266, 1976b.

Gill, J., and Kownacka, M.: Seasonal Changes in Erythrocyte, Hemoglobin and Leukocyte Indexes in Pregnant Mares of Thoroughbred Horses. Bull. Acad. Pol. Sci. (Biol.), *27*:143, 1979.

Gillespie, J.R., et al.: Hematologic Response of the Horse to General Anesthesia: A Review and New Data. *In* Proceedings of the First International Symposium of Equine Hematology. Kitchen, H., and Krebhiel, J.D., eds. Amer. Ass. Equine Pract., Golden, Colorado, p. 490, 1976.

Gilman, A.R.: The Blood Sedimentation Rate in the Horse. Amer. J. Vet. Res., *13*:77, 1952.

Grownwall, R.: Bilirubin Metabolism. *In* Proceedings of the First International Symposium of Equine Hematology. Kitchen, H., and Krebhiel, J.D., eds. Amer. Ass. Equine Pract., Golden, Colorado, p. 237, 1976.

Grownwall, R., and Mia, A.S.: Fasting Hyperbilirubinemia in Horses. Amer. J. Dig. Dis., *17*:473, 1975.

Grownwall, R., et al.: Direct Measurement of Biliary Bilirubin Excretion in Ponies during Fasting. Amer. J. Vet. Res., *41*:125, 1980.

Hammerl, J., and Kraft, W.: Blut Körperchen sen Kungs Reaktion Beim Pferd. Berl. Münch. Tierarztl. Wochenschr., *96*:145, 1983.

Hammersland, H.L., Herrin, H.S., and Haynes, C.F.: A Study of the Blood of Horses Infected with Infectious Anemia. J. Amer. Vet. Med. Ass., *93*:320, 1938.

Hansen, M.F., and Todd, A.C.: Preliminary Report on the Blood Picture of the Arabian Horse. J. Amer. Vet. Med. Ass., *118*:26, 1951.

Hansen, M.F., et al.: Studies on the Hematology of the Thoroughbred Horse. I. Mares in Foal. Amer. J. Vet. Res., *11*:296, 1950a.

Hansen, M.F., et al.: Studies on the Hematology of the Thoroughbred Horse. II. Weanlings. Amer. J. Vet. Res., *11*:393, 1950b.

Hansen, M.F., et al.: Studies on the Hematology of the Thoroughbred Horse. III. Stallions. Amer. J. Vet. Res., *11*:397, 1950c.

Hansen, M.F., et al.: Blood Pictures of Lactating and Non-lactating Thoroughbred Mares. Vet. Med., *45*:228, 1950d.

Hansen, M.F., et al.: Studies on the Hematology of the Thoroughbred Horse. IV. Barren Mares. Amer. J. Vet. Res., *12*:31, 1951.

Harvey, J.W., et al.: Haematology of Foals up to One Year Old. Equine Vet. J., *16*:347, 1984a.

Harvey, J.W., et al.: Clinical Biochemical and Hematologic Values of the American Miniature Horse: Reference Values. Amer. J. Vet. Res., *45*:987, 1984b.

Irfan, M.: The Electrophoretic Pattern of Serum Proteins in Normal Animals. Res. Vet. Sci., *8*:137, 1967.

Irvine, C.H.G.: The Blood Picture in the Race Horse. I. The Normal Erythrocyte and Hemoglobin Status. A Dynamic Concept. J. Amer. Vet. Med. Ass., *133*:97, 1958.

James, V.H.T., et al.: Adrenocortical Function in the Horse. J. Endocrinol., *48*:319, 1970.

Jeffcott, L.B.: Perinatal Studies in Equidae with Special Reference to Passive Transfer of Immunity. Ph.D. thesis, Univ. of London, 1971.

Jeffcott, L.B.: Haematology in Relation to Performance and Potential. 2. Some Species Aspect. J. S. Afr. Vet. Assoc., *45*:278, 1974.

Jeffcott, L.B.: Clinical Haematology of the Horse. *In* Comparative Clinical Haematology. Archer, R.K., and Jeffcott, L.B., eds. Blackwell Scientific Publications, Oxford, 1977.

Jeffcott, L.B., et al.: Haematological Changes in the Neonatal Period of Normal and Induced Premature Foals. J. Reprod. Fertil. [Suppl.], *32*:537, 1982.

Jennings, F.W., and Mulligan, W.: Levels of Some Chemical Constituents in Normal Horse Sera. J. Comp. Path., *63*:286, 1953.

Jones, D.M.: The Husbandry and Veterinary Care of Wild Horses in Captivity. Equine Vet. J., *8*:140, 1976.

Keenan, D.M.: Changes in Packed Cell Volume of Horses during Races. Aust. Vet. Pract., *10*:125, 1980.

Kielstein, P.: Der Einfluss des Alters auf das Differentialblutbild des Pferdes. Vet. diss., Univ. of Leipzig, 1959. (Abstr. in J. Amer. Vet. Med. Ass., *137*:59, 1960; abstr. in Die Vetmed. (in German), *12*:567, 1959.

Knill, L.M., et al.: Hemogram of the Arabian Horse. Amer. J. Vet. Res., *30*:295, 1969.

Lewis, I.N., and McLean, J.G.: Physiological Variations in Levels of 2,3-Diphosphoglycerate in Horse Erythrocytes. Res. Vet. Sci., *18*:186, 1975.

Littlejohn, A.: PCV, Hb and Plasma Electrolyte Studies in Horses. I. Mean Values in Clinically Normal Horses. Brit. Vet. J., *124*:529, 1968.

Littlejohn, A.: PCV, Hb and Plasma Electrolyte Studies in Horses. II. The Effect of Surgical Operations under Chloroform Anesthesia on PCV, Hb and Plasma Electrolyte Concentrations in Horses. Brit. Vet. J., *125*:1, 1969.

Lumsden, J.H., et al.: The Kinetics of Hematopoiesis in the Light Horse. II. The Haematological Response to Hemorrhagic Anemia. III. The Hematological Response to Hemolytic Anemia. Can. J. Comp. Med., *39*:324, 332, 1975.

Lumsden, J.H., et al.: The Comparison of Erythrocyte and Leukocyte Response to Epinephrine and Acepromazine Maleate in Standardbred Horses. *In* Proceedings of the First International Symposium of Equine Hematology. Kitchen, H., and Krebhiel, J.D., eds. Amer. Ass. Equine Pract., Golden, Colorado, p. 516, 1976.

Lumsden, J.H., et al.: Hematology and Biochemistry Reference Values in the Light Horse. Can. J. Comp. Med., *44*:32, 1980.

MacLeod, J., et al.: The Blood Picture of the Thoroughbred Horse. Cornell Vet., *37*:305, 1947.

MacLeod, J., and Ponder, E.: An Observation on the Red Cell Content of the Blood of the Thoroughbred Horse. Science, *103*:73, 1946.

Marbach, W.: Haematological Parameters of the Fitness of Racehorses and the Effect of Coforta/Catosal on the Fatigued Horse. Vet. Med. Rev., no. *1*:82, 1978.

Marcilese, N.A., et al.: Erythrokinetics in the Horse. Amer. J. Physiol., *209*:727, 1965.

Marcilese, N.A., et al.: Red Cell Survival Time in the Horse, Determined with Di-isopropyl-phosphorofluoridate-P^{32}. Amer. J. Physiol., *211*:281, 1966.

Mattheeuws, D.R.G., et al.: Compartmentalization and Turnover of ^{131}I-labeled Albumin and Gamma Globulin in Horses. Amer. J. Vet. Res., *27*:699, 1966.

McGuire, T.C., et al.: Virus-Induced Hemolysis in Equine Infectious Anemia. Amer. J. Vet. Res., *30*:2091, 1960.

McGuire, T.C., et al.: Combined (B- and T-lymphocyte) Immunodeficiency: A Fatal Genetic Disease in Arabian Foals. J. Amer. Vet. Med. Ass., *164*:70, 1974.

Meagher, D.M., and Tasker, J.B.: Effects of Excitement and Tranquilization on the Equine Hemogram. Mod. Vet. Pract., *53*:41, 1972.

Medeiros, L.O.: Contribuicao ao Estudo do Quadro Hematico de Equinos Puro Sangue Ingles Durante o Desenvolvimento Etario. Doctoral Diss., Universidade de Sao Paulo, Faculdade de Medicina-Veterinaria, Sao Paulo, Brasil, 1970.

Medeiros, L.O., et al.: Changes in Leucocyte Distribution Associated with Age in Thoroughbred Horses, Zentralbl. Veterinaermed., *20A*:166, 1973.

Miller, R.I., and Campbell, R.S.F.: Haematology of Pastured Horses in Tropical Queensland. Aust. Vet. J., *60*:31, 1983.

Moor, A. De, et al.: Influence of Promazine on the Venous Haematocrit and Plasma Protein Concentration in the Horse. Zentralbl. Veterinaermed., *25*:189, 1978.

Morgan, D.O., and Mock, R.E.: Serum Proteins of the Neonatal Foal. *In* Proceedings of the First International Symposium of Equine Hematology. Kitchen, H., and Krebhiel, J.D., eds. Amer. Ass. Equine Pract., Golden, Colorado, p. 183, 1976.

Morris, P.G.D.: Comparative Blood Picture of Army Mules and Horses. Vet. J., *98*:224, 1942.

Mussman, H.C., and Rubiano, A.: Serum Protein Electrophoregram in the Thoroughbred in Bogota, Colombia. Brit. Vet. J., *126*:574, 1970.

Naylor, J., et al.: Fasting Hyperbilirubinemia and Its Relationship to Free Fatty Acids and Triglycerides in the Horse. Proc. Soc. Exp. Biol. Med., *165*:86, 1980.

Neser, C.P.: The Blood of Equines. 9th and 10th Rep., Dir. Vet. Educ. Res., p. 479. Pretoria, Union of South Africa, 1923.

Obara, J., and Nakajima, H.: Life Span of ^{51}C-Labeled Erythrocytes in Equine Infectious Anemia. Jap. J. Vet. Sci., *23*:207, 1961.

Osbaldiston, G.W.: Erythrocyte Sedimentation Rate: Studies in Sheep, Dog, and Horse. Cornell Vet., *61*:386, 1971.

Osbaldiston, G.W., and Johnson, J.H.: Effect of ACTH and Selected Glucocorticoids on Circulating Blood Cells in Horses. J. Amer. Vet. Med. Ass., *161*:53, 1972.

Palmer, L.S.: The Physiological Relation of Plant Carotenoids to the Carotenoids of the Cow, Horse, Sheep, Goat, Pig, and Hen. J. Biol. Chem., *27*:27, 1916.

Perk, K., et al.: Osmotic Fragility of Red Blood Cells of Young and Mature Domestic and Laboratory Animals. Amer. J. Vet. Res., *25*:1241, 1964.

Persson, S.G.B.: On Blood Volume and Working Capacity in Horses. Acta Vet. Scand. Suppl., *19*:42, 1967.

Persson, S.G.B.: Value of Haemoglobin Determination in the Horse. Nord. Vet. Med., *21*:513, 1969.

Persson, S.G.B.: Blood Volume and Work Performance. *In* Proceedings of the First International Symposium of Equine Hematology. Kitchen, H., and Krebhiel, J.D., eds. Amer. Ass. Equine Pract., Golden, Colorado, p. 321, 1976.

Persson, S.G.B., and Ullberg, L.E.: Blood Volume Distribution with Evans Blue Dye in Foals. Acta Vet. Scand., *20*:10, 1979.

Persson, S.G.B., and Ullberg, L.E.: Blood Volume and Rate of Growth in Standardbred Foals. Equine Vet. J., *13*:254, 1981.

Persson, S.G.B., et al.: Circulatory Effects of Splenectomy in the Horse. 1. Effect on Red-Cell Distribution and Variability in the Horse. Zentralbl. Veterinaermed., *20A*:441, 1973.

Pierce, K.R.: Assay of Equine Serum Proteins by Chemical and Electrophoretic Methods. *In* Proceedings of the First International Symposium of Equine Hematology. Kitchen, H., and Krebhiel, J.D., eds. Amer. Ass. Equine Pract., Golden, Colorado, p. 144, 1976.

Prasse, K.W., et al.: Idiopathic Hypersegmentation of Neutrophils in a Horse. J. Amer. Vet. Med. Ass., *178*:303, 1981.

Ramsay, W.N.M.: Plasma Bilirubin in the Horse. Brit. Vet. J., *102*:206, 1946.

Rose, R.J., et al.: Blood-Gas, Acid-Base and Haematological Values in Horses during an Endurance Ride. Equine Vet. J., *11*:56, 1979.

Rudolph, W., and Venegas, R.: Proteinas sericas del equino finasangre de carrera determinadas por biuret, electroforesis y bromo-cresolsulfon-ftaleina. Arch. Med. Vet. (Chile), *11*:9, 1979.

Salutini, E., and Biagi, G.: Il quadro sieroprotidemico del

cavallo sportiva clinicamente sano, in rapporto all'eta' ed al sesso. Ann. Fac. Med. Vet., *30*:307, 1977.

Sato, T., et al.: Haematological and Biochemical Values of Thoroughbred Foals in the First Six Months of Life. Cornell Vet., *69*:3, 1979.

Scarborough, R.A.: The Blood Picture of Normal Laboratory Animals: Horse. Yale J. Biol. Med., *3*:431, 1930–1931.

Schalm, O.W.: Equine Haematology. IV. Erythroid Marrow Cytology in Response to Anemia. Calif. Vet., *29*:8, Oct., 1975.

Schalm, O.W.: Equine Hematology. III. Significance of Plasma Fibrinogen Concentration in Clinical Disorders in Horses. Equine Pract., *1*:24, 1979.

Schalm, O.W.: Manual of Equine Hematology. Veterinary Practice Publishing Co., Santa Barbara, 1984.

Schalm, O.W., and Hughes, J.P.: Some Observations on Physiologic Leukocytosis in the Cat and Horse. Calif. Vet., *18*:23, Sept.–Oct., 1964.

Schotman, A.J.H., and Kroneman, J.: Hyperlipemia in Ponies. Neth. J. Vet. Sci., *2*:60, 1969.

Smith, B.P., et al.: Equine Salmonellosis: Experimental Production of Four Syndromes. Amer. J. Vet. Res., *40*:1072, 1979.

Smith, J.E., and Agar, N.S.: Studies on Erythrocyte Metabolism following Acute Blood Loss in the Horse. Equine, Vet. J., *8*:34, 1976.

Snow, D.H., et al.: Haematological Response to Racing and Training Exercise in Thoroughbred Horses with Particular Reference to the Leucocyte Response. Equine Vet. J., *15*:149, 1983.

Sonoda, M.: Clinical and Experimental Studies on the Erythrocytes Which Include Jolly's Bodies in Horses. Jap. J. Vet. Res., *8*:1, 1960.

Stewart, G.A., et al.: Hematology of the Racehorse and Factors Affecting Interpretation of the Blood Count. Proc. 16th Ann. Conv. Amer. Ass. Equine Pract., p. 17, 1970.

Stewart, G.A., et al.: Haematology of the Racehorse: A Recent Study of Thoroughbreds in Victoria. Aust. Vet. J., *53*:353, 1977.

Stewart, J., and Holman, H.H.: The "Blood Picture" of the Horse. Vet. Rec., *52*:157, 1940.

Stolpe, J.: Untersuchungen zur Thrombozytenzahl der Trabrennpferde. Mh. Veterinaermed., *25*:510, 1970.

Stolpe, J., and Wiesner, E.: Das Fibrinogen bei nasenblutenden Galopbrennpferden und Trabern. Arch. Exp. Veterinaermed., *24*:903, 1970.

Straub, R., and Gerber, H.: Effects of Prolonged Use of Corticoids. *In* Proceedings of the First International Symposium of Equine Hematology. Kitchen, H., and Krebhiel, J.D., eds. Amer. Ass. Equine Pract., Golden, Colorado, p. 536, 1976.

Szarska, E.: An Attempt to Establish Metabolic Indices Useful in Evaluating the Training of Thoroughbred Racehorse. Zentralbl. Veterinaermed., *28*:750, 1981.

Tasker, J.B., et al.: Diabetes Mellitus in the Horse. J. Amer. Vet. Med. Ass., *149*:393, 1966.

Tennant, B., et al.: Clinical Significance of Hyper Bilirubinemia in the Racehorse. *In* Proceedings of the First International Symposium of Equine Hematology. Kitchen, H., and Krebhiel, J.D., eds. Amer. Ass. Equine Pract., Golden, Colorado, p. 246, 1976.

Todd, A.C., et al.: Studies on the Hematology of the Thoroughbred Horse. V. Sucklings. Amer. J. Vet. Res., *12*:364, 1951.

Torten, M., and Schalm, O.W.: The Relation of Sedimentation Rate of Erythrocytes to Packed Cell Volume (PCV) in the Horse. Calif. Vet., *16*:34, Sept.–Oct., 1962.

Torten, M., and Schalm, O.W.: Influence of the Equine Spleen on Rapid Changes in the Concentration of Erythrocytes in Peripheral Blood. Amer. J. Vet. Res., *25*:500, 1964.

Trum, B.F.: Normal Variances in Horse Blood Due to Breed, Age, Lactation, Pregnancy and Altitude. Amer. J. Vet. Res., *13*:514, 1952.

Tschudi, P., et al.: The Cells of Equine Blood and Their Development. Equine Vet. J., *7*:141, 1975.

Tschudi, P., et al.: Secondary Anemia in the Horse. *In* Proceedings of the First International Symposium of Equine Hematology. Kitchen, H., and Krebhiel, J.D., eds. Amer. Ass. Equine Pract., Golden, Colorado, p. 362, 1976.

Valli, V.E., et al.: The Kinetics of Haematopoiesis in the Normal Light Horse: The Life Span of Peripheral Blood Cells and Plasma Proteins. *In* Proceedings of the First International Symposium of Equine Hematology. Kitchen, H., and Krebhiel, J.D., eds. Amer. Ass. Equine Pract., Golden, Colorado, p. 91, 1976.

Van Zijl, W.J.: Blood Sedimentation Rate in the Horse and the Cow. Tijdschr. Diergeneeskd., *73*:485, 1948.

Viswanathan, S., and Gopalakrishnan, L.V.: Total Protein and Pherogram Pattern of Sera of Indian Horse. Cherion, Tamil Nadu J. Vet. Sci. Anim. Husb., *8*:210, 1979.

White, J.G., et al.: Platelet Studies in Normal and a Bleeder Horse. *In* Proceedings of the First International Symposium of Equine Hematology. Kitchen, H., and Krebhiel, J.D., eds. Amer. Ass. Equine Pract., Golden, Colorado, p. 209, 1976.

Wu, Ming-Jeong, et al.: Using Red Cell Creatine Concentration to Evaluate the Equine Erythropoietic Response. Amer. J. Vet. Res., *44*:1427, 1983.

7

Cattle: Normal Hematology with Comments on Response to Disease

THE INFLUENCE OF AGE ON BLOOD
   COMPOSITION   178
   Erythrocyte Parameters   179
   Erythrocyte Osmotic Fragility   181
   Total and Differential Leukocyte
      Numbers   185
   Plasma Proteins   187
   Plasma Fibrinogen   188

INFLUENCE OF METHODS AND
   ENVIRONMENTAL AND
   PHYSIOLOGICAL FACTORS ON THE
   HEMOGRAM   188
   The Hematocrit   188
   Icterus Index   188
   Muscular Activity and Psychologic
      Factors   189
   Water Balance   189
   Environmental Temperature and Seasonal
      Variation   189

Pregnancy   191
Parturition   191
Influence of Lactation   191
Influence of Sex and Breed   191
Influence of Altitude   193

MORPHOLOGY OF BOVINE BLOOD
   CELLS   194
   The Erythrocytes   194
   The Neutrophil   195
   The Eosinophil   195
   The Basophil   195
   The Lymphocyte   196
   The Monocyte   196
   The Platelets   197

THE BONE MARROW   197

CLINICAL INTERPRETATIONS   198
   Response to Corticosteroids   198
   Leukocyte Response to Disease   201

Normal values for cattle have been reported by many investigators. Disagreements in these values obtained by various workers relate mainly to physiologic differences such as animal excitement, muscular activity, time of day of sampling, ambient temperature and water balance, altitude, quality of nutrition, average age of the groups sampled, and possibly breed and sex. Differences referable to technique result from type and concentration of anticoagulant and methods employed for estimation of hemoglobin concentration and PCV. Improper packing of erythrocytes renders the mean corpuscular volume (MCV) and mean corpuscular hemoglobin concentration (MCHC) invalid. However, despite the variety of physiologic and technical influences affecting the data of different investigators, there remains an amazing uniformity in the mean values for the various blood components of adult cattle (Table 7–1). Modest

diurnal changes and circadian rhythms in blood values have been reported (Abt et al., 1966; Stampfli et al., 1980a; Zielinski and Machoy, 1981). Additional information on bovine hematology can be found elsewhere (Doxey, 1977; Schalm, 1977, 1980–1981, 1984; Straub et al., 1981).

THE INFLUENCE OF AGE ON BLOOD COMPOSITION

The influence of age has been stressed in several studies (Canham, 1930; Fraser, 1929–1930; Greatorex, 1954, 1957; Holman, 1956; Lumsden et al., 1980; Meneses et al., 1980; Reece, 1984; Stampfli et al., 1980b; Wingfield and Tumbleson, 1973; Wittwer and Bohmwald, 1974). Data gathered at Davis, California, on calves, growing cattle, and mature dairy cows of the Jersey and Holstein breeds are summarized in Tables 7–2 to 7–5.

Normal Blood Values for Cattle

Erythrocytic Series	Range	Ave.	Leukocytic Series	Range	Ave.
Erythrocytes ($\times 10^6/\mu l$)	5.0–10.0	7.0	Leukocytes/μl	4.000–12,000	8,000
Hemoglobin (g/dl)	8.0–15.0	11.0	Neutrophil (band)	0– 120	20
PCV (%)	24.0–46.0	35.0	Neutrophil (mature)	600– 4,000	2,000
MCV (fl)	40.0–60.0	52.0	Lymphocyte	2,500– 7,500	4,500
MCH (pg)	11.0–17.0	14.0	Monocyte	25– 840	400
MCH (%)			Eosinophil	0– 2,400	700
Wintrobe	26.0–34.0	31.0	Basophil	0– 200	50
Microhematocrit	30.0–36.0	32.7			
Reticulocytes (%)	0	0	Percentage Distribution	0– 2	0.5
ESR (mm)			Neutrophil (band)	15–45	28.0
1 hour	0	0	Neutrophil (mature)	45–75	58.0
8 hours	0–3		Lymphocyte	2– 7	4.0
RBC diameter (μm)	4.0–8.0	5.8	Monocyte	0–20	9.0
Resistance to saline (%)			Eosinophil	0– 2	0.5
Min			Basophil		
Max	0.52–0.66				
Myeloid:erythroid ratio	0.44–0.52				
	0.31–1.85:1.0	0.71:1.0			

Other Data		
Thrombocytes ($\times 10^5$)	1.0–8.0	5.0
Icterus index (units)	2–15	5–10
Erythrocyte life span (days)	160	
Plasma proteins (g/dl)	7.0–8.5	
Fibrinogen (g/dl)	0.3–0.7	

Erythrocyte Parameters

An investigation (Hubbert and Hollen, 1971) on 79 fetuses of several breeds of cattle from 100 days of gestation to term revealed that RBC and WBC counts, Hb concentration, PCV value, and neutrophil and lymphocyte numbers increased throughout gestation, while reticulocytes and nucleated erythrocytes declined to almost zero near term. Erythrocyte osmotic fragility decreased slightly so that fetal erythrocytes seemed to be more resistant than those in adult cattle. The number of eosinophils and neutrophils increased markedly between day 180 and day 210 of gestation. No significant age-related changes were detected in platelet numbers estimated from distribution on blood films. Similar observations with regard to red cell parameters were made earlier by Winqvist (1954), who also found an average platelet count of 500,000/μl in 14 fetuses. Total and differential leukocyte counts differed in the 2 studies, although similar trends were noticed.

Data presented in Figures 13–8 to 13–14 and Tables 13–2 and 13–3 demonstrate changes in blood values of developing bovine fetuses. The mean size of the fetal erythrocyte (MCV) decreases throughout gestation from a high of 90–100 fl to half that size (46.2 ± 4.8 fl) at birth. During this period, RBC counts decrease twofold, while inconsistent fluctuations occur in Hb and PCV values. Erythrocyte size continues to decrease for the first 3–4 months in the neonatal calf, reaching a value of 37.8 ± 3.2 fl. This gradual reduction in MCV coincides with the disappearance of fetal hemoglobin and its replacement by hemoglobin A (Grimes et al., 1958; Lee et al., 1971). Erythrocyte size gradually increases again after the fourth month in parallel with a gradual decrease in erythrocyte number (Table 7–3). In the negative correlation between size and number of erythrocytes, a compensatory mechanism exists whereby PCV and MCHC remain essentially stabilized (Holman, 1952). PCV commonly falls to between 34% and 38%, and the mean value for MCHC remains at approximately 32%, but MCH increases and decreases in unison with the changes in erythrocyte size. The common range for MCH is 11.0–17.0 pg, but in young cattle with exceptionally high erythrocyte numbers, MCH may be as low as 8.5 pg (Table 7–3). Macrocytosis associated with a reduction in RBC count was found to be present in 25–30% of Danish cattle (Veirup, 1977).

Table 7-1. Blood Values of Cattle as Reported in the Literature

Reference	No. of Cattle	RBC ($\times 10^6/\mu l$)	PCV (%)	Hb (g/dl)	WBC ($\times 10^3/\mu l$)	Differential Leukocyte Count (%)				
						Neutrophils	Lymphocytes	Monocytes	Eosinophils	Basophils
Greatorex (1957)	49	5.7±1.3	37.4±4.0	12.0±1.5	9.1±1.4	12–54 (30)	36–72 (57)	0–8 (2)	2–30 (11)	0
Norris and Chamberlin (1929)	27 (ave. age 7 yr)	7.8	—	—	4.9	27.0	54.0	9.0	8.0	0–1.0
Canham (1930)	35	5.4–8.0	—	—	9.7	33.0	53.0	4.0	9.0	1.0
Fraser (1929–1930)	—	6.5±0.74	—	—	7.8±1.2	30.7±7.4	50.7±7.4	7.2±2.7	11.2±4	0.24±0.18
Scarborough (1931–1932)	—	5.0–8.0 (6.62)	—	8.9–11.0	6.0–12.0 (9.25)	20–40 (31.9)	45–65 (55.4)	3–15 (5.2)	3–15 (7.7)	0–1 (0.62)
Holman (1955)	81 (Ayrshire)	5.95±0.765	33.7±4.14	11.3±1.49	7.03±1.96	29.1±9.15	51.4±11.8	8.32±2.7	9.87±11.9	0
Braun (1946)	25	6.66	34.4	11.8	9.263	28.6	52.4	8.9	9.3	0.8
Dimock and Thompson (1906)	21	4.8–7.9 (6.15)	—	—	2.3–10.6 (5.48)	13.2–45.8 (30.5)	31–76 (54.2)	0.2–3.3 (1.47)	3.9–26.5	0.1–1.2 (0.6)
Moore (1946)	15	5.433	—	8.73	6.38	33.2	58.3	2.9	4.33	0.6
Benjamin (1953)	100 (beef)	8.26	—	—	9.094	27.17	61.79	7.11	3.90	—
Ferguson et al. (1945)	25	4.1–10.0 (6.32)	—	—	3.3–18.7 (8.9)	34.7	41.2	7.9	14.9	0.6
Bell and Irwin (1938)	35	6.12	—	—	9.57	34.8	42.3	9.5	12.4	1.0
Brody et al. (1949)	7	6.95	36.6	12.7	8.57	32.2	59.2	0.7	6.4	0.5
Calhoun (1955)	14	4.53–7.94 (6.28)	—	8.7–16.5 (11.87)	4.26–14.14 (7.75)	17.3–51.0 (31.0)	35–67.3 (58.2)	0.7–13.3 (6.6)	3.7–14.3 (9.3)	0.1–1.3 (0.68)

Table 7-2. Influence of Age on the Hemogram of Cattle (means and 1 SD)

	Fetuses 7–8½ Mo	Calves Day of Birth	Calves 3–16 Weeks	Yearlings[a]	Adult Cows[a]
Number of animals	7	37	15	35	42
Erythrocytes ($\times 10^6/\mu l$)	5.86 ± 0.63	7.72 ± 1.73	9.5 ± 1.0	8.36 ± 1.05	6.36 ± 0.8
Hemoglobin (g/dl)	8.5 ± 0.05	10.2 ± 1.8	11.2 ± 1.5	11.4 ± 1.7	10.9 ± 1.7
PCV (%)	31.4 ± 1.4	34.5 ± 7.7	35.9 ± 3.8	35.9 ± 4.3	33.6 ± 5.2
MCV (fl)	53.9 ± 5.1	46.2 ± 4.8	37.8 ± 3.2	43.2 ± 7.1	52.8 ± 4.4
MCH (pg)	14.7 ± 1.5	13.3 ± 1.3	11.8 ± 1.6	13.6 ± 1.7	17.0 ± 1.6
MCHC (g/dl)	27.3 ± 0.8	28.7 ± 1.5	31.2 ± 2.8	32.3 ± 1.7	32.5 ± 1.2
Icterus index units	4.8 ± 2.1	7.7 ± 11.7	4.4 ± 2.3	—	—
Plasma proteins (%)	4.4 ± 0.3	5.0 ± 0.8	6.2 ± 0.6	—	—
Fibrinogen (g/dl)	0.10 ± 0.08	0.16 ± 0.13	0.08 ± 0.20	—	—
Total leukocytes/μl	6,743 ± 2,114	9,623 ± 3,453	10,713 ± 3,047	—	—
Band neutrophils	10 ± 25	123 ± 184	24 ± 56	—	—
Mature neutrophils	1,389 ± 646	4,869 ± 3,439	2,872 ± 1,331	—	—
Lymphocytes	4,762 ± 1,364	3,931 ± 1,744	6,861 ± 2,179	—	—
Monocytes	323 ± 209	497 ± 374	794 ± 270	—	—
Eosinophils	227 ± 150	124 ± 167	106 ± 342	—	—
Basophils	31 ± 38	33 ± 53	54 ± 76	—	—
Leukocytes (%)					
Band neutrophils	0.29 ± 0.7	1.2 ± 1.5	0.23 ± 0.5	—	—
Mature neutrophils	19.3 ± 6.9	47.2 ± 18.8	26.2 ± 8.8	—	—
Lymphocytes	72.1 ± 7.9	44.5 ± 19.2	64.1 ± 8.6	—	—
Monocytes	4.7 ± 2.9	4.8 ± 2.8	8.2 ± 4.2	—	—
Eosinophils	3.1 ± 1.9	1.4 ± 1.9	0.7 ± 2.0	—	—
Basophils	0.5 ± 0.6	0.4 ± 0.6	0.5 ± 0.6	—	—
Neutrophil:lymphocyte ratio	0.27:1.0	1.1:1.0	0.41:1.0	—	—

[a]Blood samples from clinical patients whose erythrocyte parameters were within normal ranges.

The general trend is that RBC, Hb, and PCV values are high at birth and decline with age over the first 6 months to 1 or 2 years of life (Greatorex, 1957; Holman, 1956; Wingfield and Tumbleson, 1973), although considerable differences are found in values reported by various investigators, and inconsistent or no significant changes have been observed in these parameters, particularly RBC and Hb values, in a certain group of animals (Greatorex, 1954; Tennant et al., 1975a; Tables 7–2 and 7–3). By 2–4 years of age, various red cell parameters tend to increase slightly and then stabilize. However, RBC counts may continue to decline for 5–6 years of age before becoming stabilized, while Hb and PCV may remain constant irrespective of age (Straub et al., 1981). An age-related slight decline in RBC, Hb, and PCV values was seen in Holstein dairy cattle between 1 and 10 years of age (Wingfield and Tumbleson, 1973) and in female Hereford cattle between 1.5 and 11 or 12 years of age (Noonan et al., 1978), whereas these parameters were found to increase slightly in Friesian bulls between 2 and 8 years of age (Penny et al., 1966). MCH and MCHC increased, while MCV changed inconsistently

with age in the Hereford cattle. Red cell counts have been found to decline with age to anemic levels in a few animals, particularly in high-producing dairy cows (Whitlock et al., 1974).

Veal calves raised solely on milk or a milk replacer diet show a rapid and considerably greater reduction in RBC, Hb, and PCV values than conventionally raised calves and may be considered anemic rather than "normal" (Breukink et al., 1974; Doxey, 1977). Similarly, calves and cattle raised on a low protein diet have lower RBC and PCV values as well as low serum albumin levels (Manston et al., 1975). Some newborn calves may be anemic (PCV <25%) and have low levels of serum iron suggestive of a congenital iron deficiency anemia (Tennant et al, 1975b). It has been observed that anemia in growing calves in the first few weeks of life is due mainly to iron deficiency responsive to iron supplementation (Bunger et al., 1982).

Erythrocyte Osmotic Fragility

Osmotic resistance of erythrocytes to hypotonic saline is greatest at birth, decreases with growth over the next 3–5 months, and

Table 7-3.　Mean Blood Values in Purebred Jersey Female Cattle as Influenced by Age

No. of Animals	Age	RBC ($\times 10^6/\mu l$)	Hb (g/dl)	PCV (%)	MCV (fl)	MCH (pg)	MCHC[a] (%)	WBC/μl	Differential Leukocyte Count (%)				
									Neutrophils	Lymphocytes	Monocytes	Eosinophils	Basophils
6	3½–4½ mo	13.10	11.07	36.16	27.6	8.45	30.6	7,567	28.2	62.9	8.0	0.8	0.1
5	7½–9 mo	10.65	10.10	30.40	28.5	9.48	33.2	8,000	8.8	82.2	8.0	1.0	0.0
8	11–12 mo	8.62	9.60	28.10	32.6	11.13	34.0	8,281	12.9	78.4	6.9	1.5	0.3
5	15–19 mo	9.15	10.97	34.80	38.0	11.99	31.5	8,840	26.2	63.0	3.4	6.6	0.8
11	20–36 mo	7.50	10.70	34.80	46.4	14.30	30.7	8,050	24.0	64.5	5.0	6.0	0.5
7	3–4 yr	8.70	11.30	40.00	46.0	13.00	28.2	7,063	25.0	60.5	3.8	9.7	1.0
6	4–6 yr	7.89	11.20	38.70	49.2	14.20	28.8	6,950	21.0	64.2	5.0	8.8	1.0
7	6–14 yr	7.47	11.10	37.40	50.0	14.86	29.7	6,630	18.5	65.8	3.2	12.0	0.5

[a]Determined from the PCV of the Wintrobe hematocrit. The microhematocrit PCV gives higher values because of more complete packing of the erythrocytes.

Table 7-4. Normal Absolute Values for Leukocytes/μl in Female Jersey Cattle (means and 1 SD)

Age	No. of Cattle	Total Leuko-cyte Count	Band Neutrophils	Mature Neutrophils	Lymphocytes	Monocytes	Eosinophils	Basophils
1–6 mo	16	8,750 ± 2,500	50 ± 75	3,000 ± 1,750	4,650 ± 1,300	680 ± 370	170 ± 520	50 ± 60
6–12 mo	10	7,750 ± 1,800	0	800 ± 450	6,300 ± 1,500	600 ± 170	80 ± 50	0
1–2 yr	14	9,000 ± 2,500	0	2,350 ± 1,400	5,900 ± 1,600	420 ± 170	500 ± 380	60 ± 60
2–3 yr	31	9,400 ± 1,750	25 ± 125	2,150 ± 930	5,300 ± 1,200	475 ± 220	1,300 ± 1,000	70 ± 100
3–4 yr	28	7,700 ± 1,900	0	1,900 ± 950	4,600 ± 1,050	325 ± 150	900 ± 650	50 ± 50
4–6 yr	29	7,500 ± 1,100	15 ± 45	1,800 ± 650	4,000 ± 850	450 ± 200	1,200 ± 700	60 ± 50
>6 yr	21	7,700 ± 2,500	5 ± 30	1,800 ± 900	4,250 ± 2,050	350 ± 200	1,300 ± 700	20 ± 30

Table 7–5. Normal Absolute Values for Leukocytes/µl in Female Holstein Cattle (means and 1 SD)

Age (yr)	No. of Cattle	Total Leuko- cyte Count	Band Neutrophils	Mature Neutrophils	Lymphocytes	Monocytes	Eosinophils	Basophils
1–2	9	11,000 ± 3,200	0	2,260 ± 630	6,880 ± 1,250	350 ± 100	620 ± 400	30 ± 50
2–3	16	11,400 ± 2,100	10 ± 40	3,900 ± 1,350	5,800 ± 2,100	860 ± 300	750 ± 550	60 ± 70
3–4	34	9,350 ± 2,000	25 ± 20	3,450 ± 1,350	4,900 ± 1,250	300 ± 350	630 ± 525	25 ± 40
4–6	44	8,150 ± 2,000	30 ± 100	2,800 ± 1,100	4,200 ± 1,500	550 ± 300	550 ± 350	35 ± 25
>6	17	7,900 ± 1,700	15 ± 25	3,000 ± 1,250	3,750 ± 950	450 ± 200	650 ± 500	40 ± 30

then increases to reach adult level by 2 years of age. This is illustrated by observations made in two studies. In one, resistance to hypotonic saline was greatest at birth, beginning hemolysis occurring in 0.346% NaCl solution (Holman, 1956). Resistance then decreased, reaching a point of greatest fragility in calves 5 months of age (0.532% NaCl); from this point resistance increased up to 2 years of age (0.483% NaCl). For mature cows, the mean value for complete hemolysis was 0.474% NaCl. In the other study (Greatorex, 1954, 1957), osmotic resistance of erythrocytes decreased with age, as follows: beginning hemolysis occurred at a saline concentration of 0.30–0.35% during the first 4 weeks of life, decreasing to 0.40–0.45% during the next 4 months; beginning hemolysis occurred at 0.5% saline concentration from the twentieth week onward during the first year of life, and complete hemolysis of red cells of adult cattle occurred at a mean saline concentration of 0.45%. In other studies on adult cattle, initial hemolysis and complete hemolysis were seen, respectively, at 0.5% and 0.38% saline concentrations (Perk et al., 1964).

A correlation is found between the type of hemoglobin and fragility of the total erythrocyte population (Frei et al., 1963). At birth, HbF constitutes about 60–90% of total hemoglobin. With advance in age, HbF diminishes at a fairly steady rate, until it disappears completely after 8–12 weeks. Erythrocytes containing HbF are osmotically more resistant than erythrocytes containing HbA. Thus osmotic fragility of bovine erythrocytes increases as the larger fetal erythrocytes are replaced by smaller, postnatal erythrocytes.

The natural occurrence of water intoxication associated in some instances with hemoglobinuria is a unique phenomenon occurring in young calves (see Hannan, 1965 for review). When the only liquid intake has been milk or when calves are deprived of water, they may drink excessive amounts of water when suddenly given free access to it. Hemoglobinuria has been reported to occur among calves 2–10 months of age, but is found most frequently in calves 3–5 months of age. It is during this period that the mean red cell size is at its lowest. Lysis of the more susceptible small erythrocytes apparently re-

sults as the plasma becomes hypotonic coincident with water overloading and failure of rapid development of diuresis (Kirbride and Frey, 1967).

Erythrocytes of cattle with double-muscling trait, in which body muscle mass is highly developed, were found to have a greater osmotic fragility than those of normal cattle, and the fragility was related to the degree of phenotypic expression of the trait (Basarab et al., 1980). Similarly, increased erythrocyte osmotic fragility was seen in calves with white muscle disease (Kursa and Kroupova, 1976).

Total and Differential Leukocyte Numbers

Circulating leukocyte numbers vary considerably among calves and cows. This variation may be ascribed to several factors in addition to age (Tables 7–4 and 7–5)—in particular, to muscular activity and the emotional state of the animal (stress) at the time of blood sampling. For this reason, blood samples should be drawn with as little disturbance of the animal as possible.

The general trend is for WBC counts to be high at birth and in calves and growing animals (1–2 years of age), followed by a gradual reduction with advancing age (Moberg, 1955; Wittwer and Bohmwald, 1974; Penny et al., 1966). Neutrophils exceed lymphocytes at birth, but their ratio is reversed within the first week to persist for life as a species-specific characteristic. Lower WBC values were found in veal calves than in conventionally raised calves, although a similar pattern of changes in neutrophils and lymphocytes was noted (Scheidegger et al., 1974). Higher and irregular leukocyte values observed in adult dairy cattle, with peaks at 5–7 years of age (Wingfield and Tumbleson, 1973), do not seem to be entirely age-dependent; environmental and physiologic factors as well as udder health may also have been involved.

Among 37 calves on the day of birth, the mean WBC count was one-third greater than the mean recorded in 7 fetuses in late gestation (Table 7–2). The increase was due to a threefold increase in neutrophils accompanied by a slight reduction in lymphocyte numbers. Marked differences between individual calves were apparent in WBC counts (5,000–18,600/μl) and in neutrophil: lymphocyte (N:L) ratios (6:1 to 1:4). The N:L ratio changes in response to stress of birth; blood levels of corticosteroids increase at birth, and calves delivered after cesarean have an N:L ratio similar to that in the adult cattle (Tennant et al., 1974). The cortisol level of the fetus increases during the last days of pregnancy (Comline et al., 1974; Hunter et al., 1977), is high at birth (94–121 ng/dl), and decreases progressively after birth for 11–20 days to reach adult level (about 3 ng/dl) (Cabello, 1979; Eberhart and Patt, 1971; Hudson et al., 1976; Massip, 1980). The neonatal hypercortisolimeia results from secretion by the fetal adrenals (Comline et al., 1974), although a minor portion may be that from increased cortisol secretion in the dam at parturition. Cortisol level is higher in calves delivered after dystocia than in those after normal delivery or cesarean (Massip, 1980) and also in calves experiencing further stress after birth such as from diarrhea or exposure to cold (Hudson et al., 1976). These changes may be reflected in circulating leukocyte counts. For example, a calf taken forcefully from a cow with dystocia had a WBC count of 43,000/μl with a modest left shift. By the next day, the WBC count had diminished to 15,600. That the stress factor is involved to a varying degree in newborn calves is indicated by the common finding that neutrophils exceed lymphocytes on the day of the birth and that within 24 hours the number of neutrophils falls and the number of lymphocytes increases. The neutrophils then continue to decrease and lymphocytes continue to increase throughout the first year of life (Fig. 7–1). The crossover takes place during the first week, usually about the fourth day of life (Holman, 1956; Tennant et al., 1974), so that the N:L ratio falls below unity and at times is as low as 0.3:1.0. See Chapter 26 for mechanisms of corticosteroid-induced changes in blood leukocyte numbers.

Circulating eosinophil numbers also change with age. A mean count of 1.5% during the first 6 months, with a steady increase thereafter to 10.0% at the age of 22 months was reported in one study (Holman, 1956). In another study, a marked increase in circulating eosinophils was observed between 4 and 8 months of age in parasite-free calves, and in adults the eosinophils made 2–30% of the differential leukocyte count (Greatorex, 1957). A fairly steep increase in eosinophil numbers during the first 2–6 years of life, starting at very low numbers (70–400/μl) and leveling off at a plateau of about 680 (range 450–1,000/μl) was seen in a recent study (Straub et al., 1981). High eosinophil counts in lactating dairy cows might be in response to a phenomenon in which some cows become allergic to their own milk (Brewer, 1957; Campbell, 1970).

The basophil leukocyte occurs in numbers too low to allow detection of any influence of age.

Monocytes increase during the first weeks of life to about double their value at birth, but thereafter a slight decline (Straub et al., 1981) or no influence of advancing age has been noted.

A persistent lymphocytosis in cattle is considered to be a possible prodromal sign of impending lymphocytic leukemia. To establish upper limits of the normal absolute lymphocyte number in relation to age, studies have been conducted on comparatively large numbers of mature cattle in leukemia-free herds. An age-related decrease was observed for total leukocytes, neutrophils, and lymphocytes in 849 Holstein-Friesian cows, 2–13 years of age, in 36 Minnesota herds (Perman et al., 1970). A hematologic survey was conducted on 434 Jersey cattle from 71 herds on the island of Jersey, where lymphocytic leukemia is a rarity (Theilen et al., 1967). Age-related decreases were found for WBC counts and absolute lymphocyte numbers, but not for other leukocyte types, after the first year of life (Table 7–6). In a report on 706 cattle, below and above 3 years of age and of several breeds in two herds in Australia (Granzien, 1968), values for WBC counts and lymphocytes, neutrophils, and monocytes decreased with age, while values for eosinophils increased. The decrease in lymphocytes contributed the most to the total decrease noted. In a recent study of total and differential leukocyte counts on several European cattle breeds, changes in absolute numbers of neutrophils were found to be age-independent, whereas an age-dependent decrease was noted in lymphocyte numbers, particularly during the first 6 years of life (Straub et al.,

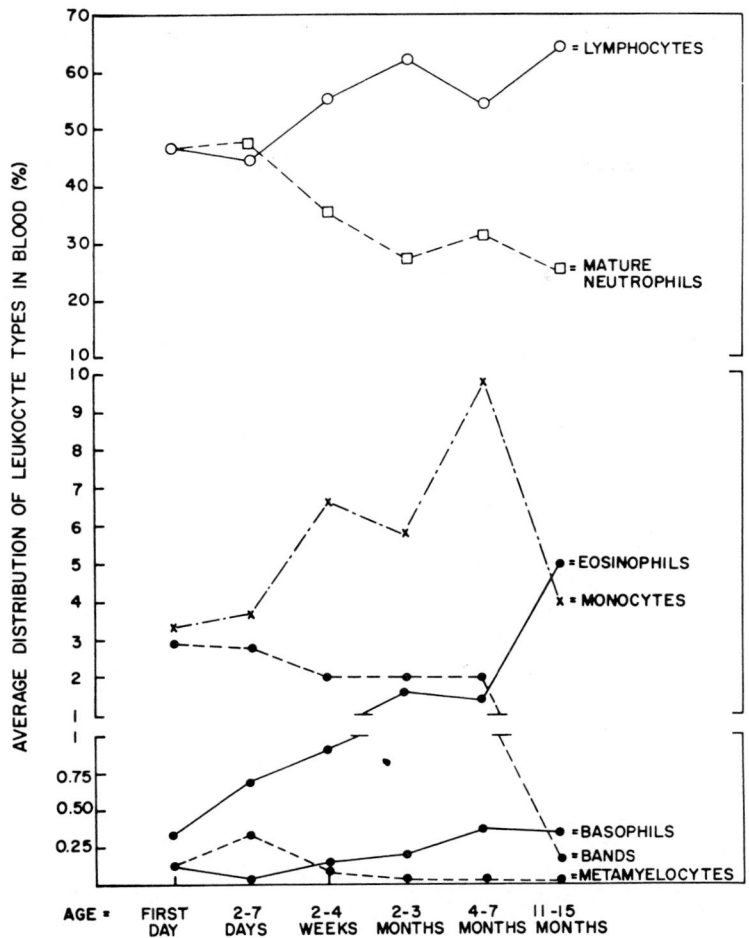

Fig. 7–1. A demonstration of the changes occurring in the differential distribution of leukocytes in blood during the first year of life of cattle. (From Straub, 1956; courtesy of Dr. O.C. Straub.)

Table 7–6. Age-Related Changes in Total and Absolute Differential Leukocyte Counts/μl of Blood in Cattle

Cell Type	Cows 1–2 Years of Age	Cows over 5 Years of Age
Total leukocytes	8,840 ± 2,110	6,180 ± 1,890
Lymphocytes	6,340 ± 1,610	3,260 ± 1,100
Neutrophils	1,420 ± 670	1,660 ± 990
Monocytes	580 ± 280	560 ± 370
Eosinophils	440 ± 440	640 ± 440
Basophils	80 ± 10	50 ± 60

Data from Theilen et al. (1967).

1981). The latter change was used as a basis to develop a new "leukosis" key for detection of hematologically leukosis-positive cattle.

Plasma Proteins

Plasma protein concentration is low during the fetal life and at birth. An immediate increase is seen after colostrum consumption followed by a gradual increase during the first year of life. The total plasma proteins of 7 fetuses, at the late trimester of gestation, was 4.4 g/dl. In 16 colostrum-deprived calves, mostly taken by cesarean section, the range of plasma proteins was 4.0–5.3 g/dl, with an average value of 4.7 g/dl (Schalm et al., 1970). Among 37 calves during the first day of postnatal life, the total plasma protein concentration was 5.0 ± 0.8 g/dl (Table 7–2). Serum protein concentration was found to increase from 4.4 g/dl to 7.0 g/dl among 5 colostrum-fed calves (McEwan et al., 1968). Colostrum, with its high concentration of gamma globulin, is quickly absorbed, thereby elevating the plasma protein levels (Tumbleson et al., 1973). Serum globulins in 6 colostrum-fed calves increased from 1.95 g/dl at birth to 7.62 g/dl within 24 hours despite hemodilution taking place during this period as indicated by a 20–25% decline in serum albumin and PCV values (McMurray et al., 1978). Plasma protein concentration was found to be lower in septicemic calves (5.8 ± 0.69 g/dl) because of hypogammaglobulinemia than in calves with primary enteric infection and clinical evidence of dehydration (8.6 ± 1.5 g/dl), but PCV was similar in both groups of animals (Tennant et al., 1975a).

Plasma proteins increase early in the neonatal life from the low level at birth. Among 15 calves, 3–16 weeks of age, the mean value was 6.2 ± 0.6 g/dl (Table 7–2). By 1 year of age, a common range is 6.8–7.5 g/dl and for mature cattle, it is 7.0–8.5 g/dl. Plasma protein concentration may exceed 8.5 g/dl in normal cows during periods of high environmental temperature. In sick cows, refusal of food and water leads to rapid hemoconcentration with elevation of plasma proteins to between 10 and 12 g/dl. High total plasma proteins in sick cows may also be due in part to increase in fibrinogen.

Plasma Fibrinogen

Fetuses in late gestation and newborn calves may lack or have very low levels of circulating fibrinogen. The mean value at birth of 37 calves was 0.16 ± 0.13 g/dl, and there was little change during the first 3–16 weeks of life (Table 7–2). Calves developing gastrointestinal disease or pneumonia, however, commonly have plasma fibrinogen levels in excess of 1.0 g/dl. The normal range for plasma fibrinogen in growing and adult cattle is 0.3–0.7 g/dl. There is no age-related increase in plasma fibrinogen once the neonatal period is over. Physiologic factors such as changes in water balance and parturition, as well as disease prevention procedures such as injection of strain 19 *Brucella abortus* vaccine, may temporarily elevate plasma fibrinogen. Disease has a marked influence on circulating fibrinogen level (McSherry et al., 1970; Schalm, 1970), values of 1.0–1.5 g/dl being common. In fact, high plasma fibrinogen values are more indicative of the severity of a disease process in the cow than the WBC count during the early stages of disease and

in many chronic inflammatory diseases (see Table 34–9). A plasma protein:fibrinogen ratio is calculated to differentiate an absolute increase in fibrinogen due to disease from that due to hemoconcentration, which is associated with an increase in both plasma protein and fibrinogen levels without affecting their ratio (Schalm, 1970). A plasma protein:fibrinogen ratio of less than 10:1 (Chapter 34) and more precisely 8:1 (Sutton and Hobman, 1975) is considered indicative of an increase in fibrinogen due to disease.

INFLUENCE OF METHODS AND ENVIRONMENTAL AND PHYSIOLOGICAL FACTORS ON THE HEMOGRAM

Variations in reported normal values for the blood of cattle may result in part from methods employed in sampling and processing blood and in part from environmental and physiological factors.

The Hematocrit

The small size of the bovine erythrocyte and absence of rouleau formation result in considerable trapping of plasma unless the relative centrifugal force and time of centrifugation are adequate. MCV and MCHC are significantly influenced by variations in PCV due to inadequate centrifugation. Bovine blood requires centrifugation for 1 hour at 3,000 rpm for complete packing of erythrocytes in the Wintrobe tube (Bunce, 1954). With the microhematocrit method, 12,000 G for 10 minutes is required to pack bovine erythrocytes with a minimum of trapped plasma (Fisher, 1962). In the latter study, PCV of the jugular blood was found to be higher than that of the mammary vein blood by 2% in dry cows and by 4.2% in lactating cows.

Icterus Index

The bovine liver possesses a very large fundamental reserve for excretion of bilirubin. Even in generalized liver disease, the maximum serum bilirubin concentration was found not to exceed 3.5 mg/dl (Garner, 1953). Cattle on dry feed have an almost colorless plasma as a result of the efficient excretion of bilirubin diglucuronide by the liver. Cattle on green feed develop a yellow plasma because of plant pigments, carotenoids (Palmer, 1916). The plasma color of plant origin may measure as much as 25 units on the icterus index scale. Normal icterus index in cattle ranges from 5 to 15 units.

Muscular Activity and Psychologic Factors

The influence of such factors as rest, exercise, and apprehension on the hemogram of 16 cattle, mostly Hereford steers, was investigated (Gartner et al., 1965). Comparisons were made between nontranquilized and tranquilized (chlorpromazine hydrochloride) intact and splenectomized animals. Red cell values were found to be considerably higher in nontranquilized intact animals than in tranquilized intact animals at rest, after exercise, or after audiovisual stimulation. The difference was much less in the splenectomized animals. In tranquilized, splenectomized animals, there were no significant changes following exercise or rest.

Fear or excitement at the time blood samples are collected may cause splenic contraction resulting in elevation of PCV, Hb, and RBC values. Increased rate and force of the heart tends to elevate WBC count by flushing sequestered cells into large-vessel blood. Familiarizing cattle for 1 week with the environment in which they were subsequently bled resulted in relatively stable values by the second week (Gartner et al., 1969). An example of the influence of conditioning was observed in a 1-year-old female Holstein cow. During the first week, it was necessary to chase the cow in order to restrain her for sampling. By the second week, the cow was considerably less fractious. Differences were noted in the hemograms between the first and second weeks (Table 7–7).

Water Balance

Effects of water restriction on blood composition of steers was investigated (Bianca et al., 1965). In one trial, dehydration took place over 4 days at 15°C, and in another trial, during 2 days at 40°C. The erythrocyte parameters increased linearly with time. PCV, for example, at 15°C increased from a mean of 30.5% to 36.1%, and at 40°C, from 27.6% to 30.8%. Following ingestion of water, the PCV

exhibited a transient rise, with peak values up to 44.4%. This transient rise was considered a result of splenic contraction in response to excitement of having access to water under conditions of extreme thirst. These studies were followed by more extensive observations in which 4 oxen, kept at 20°C, were subjected to (a) deprivation of water for 3 days, (b) rehydration by drinking, (c) rehydration by infusion of water through a rumen canula, and (d) overhydration by infusion of water into the rumen of normally hydrated cattle (Bianca, 1970). Deprivation of water for 3 days caused a 34% increase in blood viscosity. PCV increased by 3.93%, MCHC by 2.26%, and plasma total solids from 7.81 g/dl to 8.84 g/dl. These findings indicated that water is lost from both the plasma and erythrocytes (minimal increase in PCV) during dehydration. Upon rehydration by drinking, the marked transient elevation of PCV mentioned above occurred again, and heart rate increased from 60 beats per minute to 100 beats per minute. There was an increase in erythrocyte osmotic fragility during rehydration of dehydrated animals by drinking. In two instances of rehydration by drinking, intravascular hemolysis led to hemoglobinuria. When rehydration was accomplished by infusion of water into the rumen, the sharp transient rise in PCV did not occur and cardiac rate did not increase. Overhydration of normally hydrated cattle imposed a mild stress indicated by slight elevation of PCV and heart rate. Despite pronounced diuresis in overhydrated animals, two instances of hemoglobinuria were noted.

Acutely ill cattle lose weight rapidly as a result of water loss. It is not unusual to encounter severe dehydration under such illness. Simultaneous elevation of both PCV and total plasma proteins, which occurs in hemoconcentration, may indicate the degree of dehydration in sick cattle (Appendix Case 68).

Environmental Temperature and Seasonal Variation

Moisture loss by sweating in cattle is relatively low (Brody et al., 1949). When drinking water is cooler than the air temperature, animals increase their water consumption. Con-

Table 7–7.   Changes in Blood Composition of a 1-Year-Old Female Holstein Cow as a Result of Conditioning to Blood Sampling (means and 1 SD of four blood samples taken each week)

	First Week	Second Week	Change
PCV (%)	44.5 ± 2.3	37.0 ± 1.8	7.5 −
Hemoglobin (g/dl)	14.7 ± 0.8	11.5 ± 0.1	3.2 −
Plasma proteins (g/dl)	7.5 ± 0.4	7.2 ± 0.2	0.3 −
Total leukocytes/μl	13,275 ± 838	9,175 ± 1,621	4,100 −
Band neutrophils	0	56 ± 46	56 +
Mature neutrophils	1,392 ± 875	938 ± 160	454 −
Lymphocytes	10,555 ± 1,286	7,450 ± 1,288	3,105 −
Monocytes	657 ± 307	566 ± 234	91 −
Eosinophils	636 ± 547	56 ± 21	580 −
Basophils	17 ± 35	81 ± 84	64 +

sequently, with rising ambient temperatures, the concentration of blood constituents tends to decrease, provided cool water is available. In this study, hemoglobin level was not influenced significantly by an ambient temperature range of 10.0–37.8°C. However, a significant influence of environmental temperature was observed on the hemoglobin level of native and imported cattle in the Philippines (Manresa et al., 1934, 1939). A close reciprocal but negative relationship was found between hemoglobin indexes and atmospheric temperature. The hemoglobin was highest during the coolest months and lowest during warmest months of the year. Observations made every 3–4 hours throughout the day revealed hemoglobin levels to follow a regular pattern of being highest in the mornings and evenings and lowest in the late morning or early afternoon when atmospheric temperatures were highest. A sample of their data on Indian Nellore oxen is given in Table 7–8. The daily fluctuations in the hemoglobin of native cattle probably can be attributed to changes in water balance, more water being consumed as the temperature rises.

An increase in PCV, hemoglobin, and WBC count was seen in studies on mature breeding bulls of the Jersey, Guernsey, and Holstein breeds during summer months when environmental temperatures rose to more than 27°C (Rusoff et al., 1954). In general, Hb, PCV, and total protein concentration are somewhat lower during the winter than in the spring and summer (Doxey 1977; Hewett, 1974; Rowlands et al., 1974). In Hereford cattle, autumn values for RBC, PCV, Hb, and MCV were higher than spring values, whereas platelet counts were often higher in the spring than in the autumn (Noonan et al., 1978). Environmental and genetic effects on hematologic characteristics of beef cows were studied in the northeastern United States (Fisher et al., 1980); lowest PCV, RBC, and Hb values were found during April through June and highest values during the winter and fall months. No changes were seen in RBC and WBC counts of cows kept at a constant temperature of 32°C, but a significant decrease occurred in cows kept at fluctuating day and night temperatures (Paape et al., 1973). The decrease in RBC was ascribed to hemodilution from increased water intake during periods of high temperature. A slight decrease in total serum protein with an increase in environmental temperature ranging from 17–37°C has been reported (Saksena et al., 1980).

Table 7–8.   Hemoglobin Levels in Cattle in Relation to Time of Sampling Reflecting Changes Due to Ambient Temperature

10 animals 1–3 years of age					
Time of day	6:30 A.M.	9:00 A.M.	11:30 A.M.	2:00 P.M.	4:30 P.M.
Mean Hb (g/dl)	9.41	8.70	8.53	8.70	8.72

7 animals 6–10 years of age					
Time of day	2:00 A.M.	6:00 A.M.	10:00 A.M.	2:00 P.M.	6:00 P.M.	10:00 P.M.
Mean Hb (g/dl)	11.12	10.17	10.2	9.69	10.4	10.45

Pregnancy

The stage of gestation did not have a noticeable effect on WBC count, eosinophil number, or PCV (Conner et al., 1967). Erythrocyte numbers increased slightly as pregnancy advanced. Some age-related differences were noted in blood values of pregnant cows. Lymphocytes were significantly higher and neutrophils lower for cows 2–4 years of age, with no significant fluctuation due to month of pregnancy. A decrease in WBC count, due primarily to a reduction in number of lymphocytes, was noted in advanced gestation in an earlier study (Moberg, 1955).

Parturition

Changes typical of stress response are seen in total and differential leukocyte counts of cows at parturition (Holman, 1956; Straub et al., 1959). WBC counts are significantly elevated, mainly through a marked increase in neutrophils, with or without left shift. Changes in lymphocyte numbers may depend on the degree of stress involved, and changes in other leukocyte types are variable depending also on the degree of stress and status of fetal membranes. These changes are evident within 12–24 hours post partum and subside over the next few days. RBC, Hb, and PCV values may also change similarly.

The WBC count in 11 cows at the moment of delivery of the calf was 11,800–24,700/μl, with a mean of 17,700/μl of blood (Table 7–9, group B). In 24 hours, the WBC count had fallen to 5,700–18,000/μl, with a mean of 10,000 (Table 7–9, group C). The stress pattern was evident in the differential count; there was a marked increase in neutrophils and a decrease in lymphocytes (Fig. 7–2, group C). The mean lymphocyte value was above normal for cows not under stress, but since observations were not made on the differential leukocyte count on the day prior to parturition, it could not be determined from the data whether the lymphocyte count was dropping or increasing. A decrease in the lymphocyte count is to be anticipated in response to stress.

Blood studied on the second day post partum of cows with fetal membranes dropped or retained (Table 7–9 and Fig. 7–2, groups D and E) show a depression of WBC count as well as depression of all leukocyte types, the greatest effect being on the neutrophils. In addition, a shift to the left appeared, with band and metamyelocyte neutrophils entering peripheral blood from the second to the fifth days (Table 7–9, groups F, G, and H). The absolute monocyte count was elevated at all times, and this elevation may be related to the need for removal of tissue debris associated with retained placenta. Monocytosis in the condition of retained fetal membranes has been reported (Moore, 1946). Bone marrow of cows with retained placenta contains a very low percentage of mature neutrophils (Winqvist, 1959). This could be due to depletion of the neutrophil pool as these cells are drained from blood and bone marrow into the uterus.

Influence of Lactation

Lactation-related changes may be irregular and vary from herd to herd. In general, nonlactating cows have higher RBC, Hb, and PCV values than lactating cows (Noonan et al., 1978). Hb and PCV values decline during lactation, while globulins may increase or change variably (Hewett, 1974; Rowlands et al., 1977). This decline in red cell values may be related to milk yield (Hewett, 1974); high producers tend to develop anemia more frequently than low producers, particularly during the winter (Whitlock et al., 1974). WBC counts may also decrease, primarily due to decline in neutrophil numbers (Paape et al., 1974a).

PCV, RBC, Hb, serum iron, total iron binding capacity, and serum albumin levels decreased during early lactation and rose to prelactation levels by mid-lactation; PCV and Hb remained low for 4 months and RBC for 1 month (Esievo et al., 1979). The reduction in Hb and PCV values was greater in cows on a low protein diet than in those on a medium to high protein diet for a long period of time (Manston et al., 1975).

Influence of Sex and Breed

It has been reported that bulls have erythrocyte counts 1 million to 1.5 million/μl greater than females (Scarborough, 1931–1932). A greater difference has also been

Table 7–9.   Effect of Parturition and Retention of the Fetal Membranes on the Hemogram in Cattle

Group Identification	No. of Cows	History of the Blood Samples	RBC ($\times 10^6/\mu l$)	Hb (g/dl)	PCV (%)	WBC ($\times 10^3/\mu l$)	Meta-myelo-cytes	Band Neutro-phils	Mature Neutro-phils	Lympho-cytes	Mono-cytes	Eosino-phils	Baso-phils
A	—	Normal range and mean	5.0–10.0 (7.0)	8.0–14.0 (11.0)	24–48 (35)	4.0–12.0 (8.0)	0	0.0–2.0 (0.5)	15–45 (28.0)	45–75 (58.0)	2.0–7.0 (4.0)	2.0–20.0 (9.0)	0.2 (0.5)
B	11	Blood drawn at parturition	5.5–9.3 (7.4)	8.7–15.3 (13.2)	24–44 (40)	11.8–24.7 (17.7)	0	0.0–2.0 (0.8)	13–68 (55.4)	25–67 (34.6)	2.0–12.0 (7.4)	0.0–9.0 (1.8)	0
C	12	One day postpartum, membranes dropped	6.0–8.9 (7.1)	11.8–15.4 (13.4)	35–45 (40)	5.7–18.0 (10.0)	0	0.0–3.5 (0.9)	29–61 (47.3)	28–59 (39.8)	2.5–11.5 (7.7)	1.0–12.0 (3.9)	0–1
D	8	2 days postpartum, membranes dropped	5.6–6.8 (6.2)	10.5–14.3 (12.6)	32–43 (37)	4.9–14.7 (10.0)	0	0.0–3.0 (0.9)	15–55 (38.6)	26–61 (41.8)	6.0–16.0 (10.9)	0.5–17.0 (7.2)	0–2 (0.5)
E	21	2 days postpartum, membranes retained	4.9–12.0 (6.9)	9.5–21.0 (12.1)	30–68 (38)	3.3–9.2 (5.7)	0–5 (0.6)	0.0–24.0 (6.0)	3–35 (14.5)	30–87 (61.3)	1.0–32.0 (11.7)	0.0–21.0 (5.3)	0–2 (0.3)
F	32	3 days postpartum membranes retained	4.9–7.9 (6.4)	9.6–14.9 (11.7)	28–46 (34)	3.4–14.6 (6.6)	0–4[a] (1.0)	0.0–22.0 (7.5)	2–46 (17.5)	24–90 (55.9)	2.0–29.0 (13.9)	0.0–10.0 (3.7)	0–2 (0.3)
G	7	4 days postpartum, membranes retained	4.9–7.1 (6.1)	8.8–11.9 (10.6)	28–36 (33)	3.4–9.4 (6.7)	0–3 (0.7)	1.0–10.0 (4.3)	5–47 (17.6)	28–60 (55.7)	2.0–38.0 (15.0)	0.0–32.0 (6.7)	0
H	7	5 days postpartum, membranes retained	5.8–10.0 (7.1)	10.6–11.9 (11.3)	32–37 (35)	3.6–8.0 (6.1)	0	0.0–13.0 (2.7)	4–25 (20.3)	41–89 (62.2)	2.0–26.0 (10.0)	1.0–8.0 (4.8)	0
J	10	About 2 months postpartum following retained membranes	5.8–8.2 (6.5)	10.9–13.3 (11.6)	31–42 (36)	6.0–11.1 (8.5)	0	0.0–4.0 (0.5)	17–46 (34.7)	30–66 (47.7)	2.0–10.0 (7.2)	0.0–26.0 (9.9)	0–1 (0.2)

[a]Myelocytes were also present in four cows in 0.5–2.0% of the differential count.

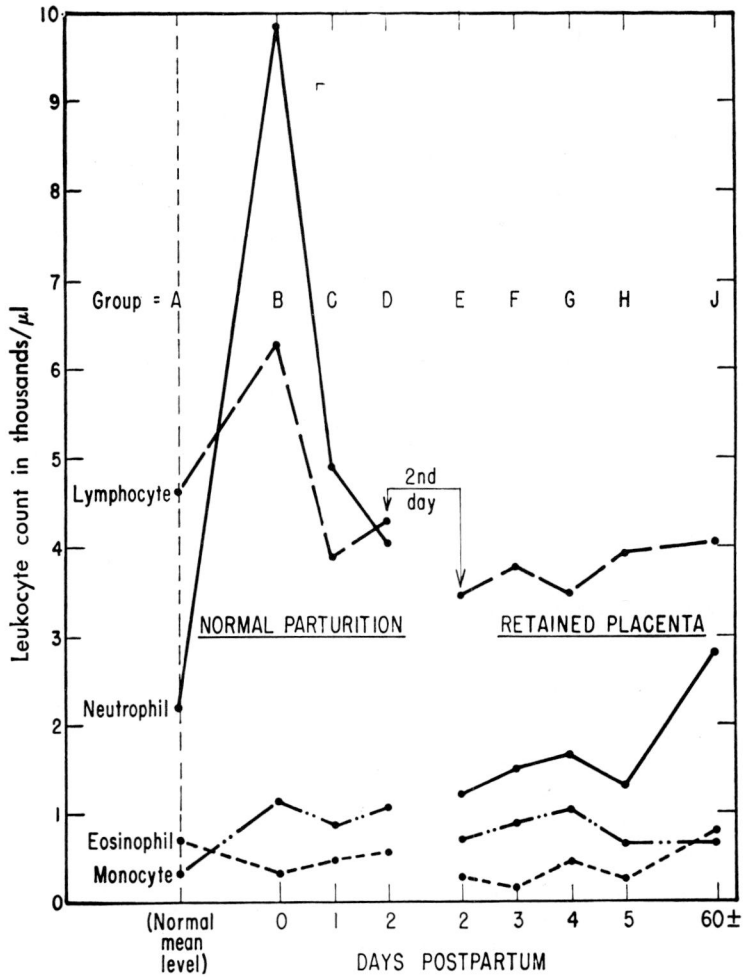

Fig. 7–2.   Absolute leukocyte numbers as influenced by normal parturition or parturition with retained placenta. See Table 7–9 for the description of groups A through J.

found, e.g., a mean count of 8.4 million/μl for bulls and 5.69 million/μl for dairy cows (Fraser, 1929–1930).

Statistically significant breed differences have been claimed by several authors. The differences are not large enough to cause concern in clinical interpretation of hemograms in cattle. In general, the Jersey (Ryan, 1971a, b; Straub et al., 1981) and Guernsey (Penny et al., 1966; Wingfield and Tumbleson, 1973) cattle have lower RBC and WBC counts; the "Braunvieh" (Brown Swiss) have a lower RBC count (Straub et al., 1981), while Charlais (Ryan, 1971a; Straub et al., 1981) have higher RBC, Hb, and PCV values than most other breeds. Higher WBC, neutrophils, and lymphocytes were found in Hereford and Char-

lais cattle, while lower values were observed in the Jersey (Ryan, 1971b). Higher WBC and lymphocytes were seen in the Jersey than in the Holstein (Meneses et al., 1980).

Influence of Altitude

It is well known that reduced oxygen tension leads to increased production and release of erythropoietin, thereby stimulating erythropoiesis. Cattle grazing high in mountain ranges would naturally experience an increase in circulating erythrocyte number, hemoglobin, and PCV. A report on cattle in Colorado gave mean RBC counts of 9.3 million/μl in early summer and 8.6 million/μl in late summer (Clawson, 1914). When 11 cattle were studied at an elevation of 5,000 feet

(1,524 m) in early summer, their mean count was 8.7 million/μl. These cattle were transferred to an elevation of 9,000 feet (2,743 m) in late summer; at that altitude their mean RBC count was 9.2 million/μl. It was stated that the effect of altitude was much greater than the data indicated at first glance, since the latter counts were made in late summer, when previous experience had shown that RBC count normally declined. Increases in RBC, Hb, and PCV values, along with alterations in some other blood values and physiological and behavioral changes, were observed in cattle kept at simulated altitude of 4,000 m (Bianca and Näf, 1978) and in calves kept at simulated altitude of 5,000 m (Bianca and Espinosa, 1975).

MORPHOLOGY OF BOVINE BLOOD CELLS

The Erythrocytes

Anisocytosis of slight to moderate degree is normal; an occasional cell may appear twice the size of the smallest erythrocyte. Erythrocyte diameter ranges from 4.0–8.0 μm, with an average of 5.8 μm (Blount, 1939). In health, bovine erythrocytes are generally biconcave with an occasional cell appearing uniconcave (Fig. 20–16). They are found singly dispersed without rouleau formation. Small size and absence of rouleaux confer suspension stability. Gross sedimentation of erythrocytes does not take place even after a sample has been stood for many hours. In the Wintrobe hematocrit tube, a range of 2.2–4.0 mm of sedimentation in 24 hours has been observed in blood of normal cattle (Bunce, 1954). In tubes held at a 45° angle, ESR of 2–7 (mean 3.78 ± 1.63) mm at 1 hour was observed for blood from 36 cattle with PCV of 28–42% (Olsen, 1966). A curvilinear relationship was seen between PCV and ESR, and a chart was developed to correct ESR to a standard PCV of 36%. Rouleau formation occurs and suspension stability of erythrocytes is reduced in bovine blood as fibrinogen levels become significantly increased in disease (Plates VII–1, VII–4).

Central pallor of the bovine erythrocyte in health tends to be minimal. In acute disease, however, the erythrocyte may increasingly assume a bowl shape and the resulting deep central concavity causes the cell's center to have a sharply "punched-out" appearance (Appendix Case 68). This phenomenon is best seen in the thicker areas of the blood film where depth is sufficient for the red cell to retain its assumed shape. We have observed acanthocytes (Fig. 20–2D) in some clinically normal cows. Poikilocytosis of unknown origin was observed in 7 newborn calves (Sato and Mizuno, 1982).

Reticulocytes and nucleated red cells are not seen in bovine blood during health except during fetal life and probably the first few days of postnatal life. The absence of immature erythrocytes (polychromatic cells) in the circulation of normal cattle parallels the long life span of the bovine red cell. Erythrocyte life span has been reported to be 70–126 days in calves 3–4 months of age (Johnson and Schwartz, 1970) and 160 days in the adult cow (Kaneko, 1963).

In anemia in remission, immature erythrocytes are released to the circulation in proportion to the severity of blood loss or erythrocyte destruction. Macrocytosis, polychromasia, nucleated erythrocytes, and Howell-Jolly bodies are common. A significant additional feature is the appearance of a variable number of erythrocytes with basophilic stippling (Plate XIII–10). This is a normal feature of anemia in remission in cattle and should not be confused with the basophilic stippling that may occur in chronic lead poisoning (Christian and Tryphonas, 1971). Basphilic stippling is most prominent in EDTA-anticoagulated blood and rapidly dried blood films stained with Wright-Leishman stain without prior fixation with alcohol (George and Duncan, 1981; also see Chapter 2). Hematologic changes in 4 clinically normal splenectomized calves included increased RBC counts, PCV, platelet numbers, and morphological changes in various formed elements of blood (Rodriguez et al., 1973). Red cell size increased and basophilic stippling, Howell-Jolly bodies, and nucleated erythrocytes appeared in variable numbers. Pleokaryocytes (giant or hypersegmented neutrophils) and both small and large platelets were found.

The Neutrophil

The *mature neutrophil* ranges in size from 10–15 μm, averaging about 11.5 μm. Its nucleus usually presents a relatively smooth but highly irregular membrane with one or more points of partial pinching-in without true filament formation (Plate VII–1). True lobe formation is mostly limited to a single lobe separated from the main portion of the nucleus by a filament. The cytoplasm contains numerous dust-like, pinkish granules, and under some conditions of staining, the granules may appear reddish.

The *band neutrophil* is an immature cell of rare occurrence in normal bovine blood. In a study of 152 bulls of several breeds, the band neutrophil occurred in 46.7% of samples, but only 5 samples had more than 5% band forms (Penny et al., 1966). We regard 1–2% bands to be the upper limit in normal adult bovine blood. The band cell has a nucleus that is considerably thicker than that of the mature neutrophil. Its nuclear membrane is smooth throughout its length, with no constriction in any part. The cytoplasm is similar in appearance to the mature neutrophil.

The *metamyelocyte neutrophil* is not seen in health in peripheral blood of the adult cattle. Its nucleus is short and thick with variable indentation, but rarely has a true kidney-bean shape. The nuclear membrane is smooth. Cytoplasm tends to be bluish and less granular than the more mature cells of the neutrophil series.

Left Shift and "Toxic" Neutrophils

Ability to identify immature neutrophils and to recognize "toxic" signs is a prerequisite to use of the leukogram as an aid to diagnosis and prognosis in the cow. In the initial stages of acute inflammatory diseases such as peritonitis, mastitis, and metritis, the mature neutrophils readily leave the blood to enter the lesion. The bone marrow of the cow does not have a large reserve of neutrophils, and therefore immature neutrophils quickly make their appearance in peripheral blood and often exceed in number the mature forms. A marked fall in WBC count is a common finding during the developmental stage of an acute localizing inflammatory process (Fig. 7–3).

The degree of generalized toxemia is reflected in the morphology and staining characteristics of neutrophils, both mature and immature. In severe toxemia, basophilia of the cytoplasm is retained by metamyelocyte (Plate XI–9) and band neutrophils; the cytoplasm may be vacuolated and appear devoid of specific granules. Sometimes a few large, reddish granules may be present, and then the condition is referred to as "toxic" granulation. Such granules may also be found interspersed among the pinkish specific granules of mature neutrophils. A finding of this nature limited to mature neutrophils may be an expression of minimal effect of toxemia.

In rare instances of acute suppurative disease, toxemia is so severe that granulopoiesis is depressed, and precursor cells in the bone marrow may become severely vacuolated and fail to divide, thereby contributing additionally to the existing neutropenia. In other instances, the precursor cell nucleus undergoes an attempt at maturation although the cell fails to divide. This leads to appearance in peripheral blood of an occasional giant form with bizarre nuclear pattern and a basophilic cytoplasm that may contain toxic granules.

The Eosinophil

The average size of the bovine eosinophil is 12–13 μm, and some cells attain a diameter of 15 μm. The eosinophil leukocyte is readily identifiable by its numerous small, round, jewel-like, intensely red, refractile granules of uniform size. The granules nearly fill the cytoplasm (Plate VII–4) and may partially cover the nucleus. Light blue cytoplasm is barely visible. The nucleus may be bilobate, but more commonly it retains a band form.

The Basophil

The basophil varies in size from 11–14 μm. The cell commonly appears as a dense and dark-staining granular object because the nucleus is mostly masked by granules (Plate VII–5). The true shape of the nucleus is not readily apparent. Basophils are rare in the peripheral blood of the cow; they were seen in 19.7% of 152 healthy bulls of several breeds (Penny et al., 1966).

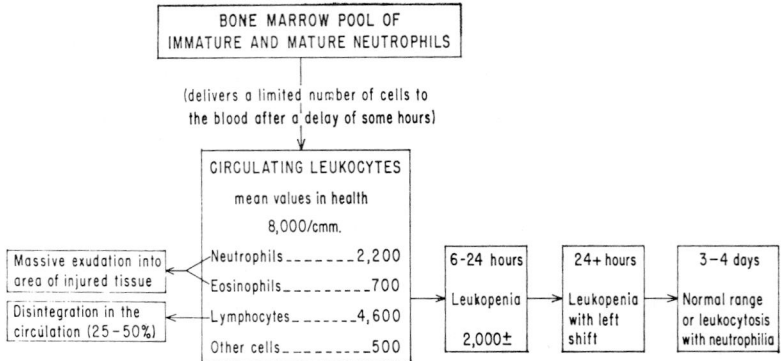

Fig. 7–3. Dynamics of leukocyte responses in localized acute bacterial infection in the bovine.

The Lymphocyte

The lymphocyte is the major leukocyte of bovine blood. It may constitute 70–80% of the differential count of yearling cattle. The lymphocyte count decreases significantly with advancing age and takes on clinical significance in the diagnosis of the preleukemic and leukemic states. The lymphocyte of the cow varies from 8–15 μm in diameter. The largest forms have been called transitional cells because they may be confused with monocytes.

The *small lymphocyte* has a round, densely stained nucleus that fills the cell so that little or no cytoplasm is apparent. The *medium lymphocyte* has a nucleus that stains somewhat lighter and presents a chromatin pattern characterized by darker-staining blobs separated by lighter-staining parachromatin. The nucleus is round but may have a slight indentation. The cytoplasm is represented by a narrow rim, but it may be more to one side of the cell due to eccentric location of the nucleus. The cytoplasm generally stains pale blue and tends to be somewhat dark at the very edge. The *large lymphocyte* has a much lighter-staining nucleus and cytoplasm; the nucleus has a smooth chromatin pattern, although darker blobs may occur. The nucleus is commonly round and is placed eccentrically in the cell. Some large lymphocytes may present a kidney-bean nucleus, or a deep cleft may tend to divide the nucleus into two lobes. A cell with the latter form of nucleus is called a Rieder cell; it is seen more commonly in lymphocytic leukemia (Fig. 32–37). The cytoplasm is pale blue, usually surrounds the nucleus completely, and occasionally pre-

sents a few small, round vacuoles. The finding of an occasional lymphocyte with a nucleolus or faint nucleolar rings in bovine blood should be viewed with extreme caution as a sign of lymphocytic leukemia since such cells may be found in health. Ultrastructure studies of peripheral blood lymphocytes of normal and leukemic cows have been made (Hammer and Weber, 1974; Wever et al., 1967).

Azurophilic granules are seen relatively frequently in the cytoplasm, but such lymphocytes may not be encountered in every film of bovine blood (Plate VII–3). These granules vary considerably in size, shape, and number. Their size ranges from small to large. Some are rod-like, others are round; and they stain reddish or dark purple. When present, they occur in clusters rather than being evenly distributed throughout the cytoplasm. Occurrence of azurophilic granules in large lymphocytes will definitely identify the lymphocytic origin of the cell.

The Monocyte

The monocyte varies considerably in size from 13–19 μm, with an average diameter of about 16 μm. The nucleus is variable in shape from round to convoluted, the latter shape being more common. The chromatin is usually diffuse and appears stringy (Plate VII–2), but darker blobs (Plate VII–4) may be present. The cytoplasm tends to stain somewhat darker than that of lymphocytes and appears more granular. True azurophilic granules are not commonly seen; when present, they appear indistinct, giving the cytoplasm a patchy, slightly pinkish color. Vacuoles occur in the cytoplasm with considerable frequency and tend to be more numerous and less regular in size (Plate VII–3) than those that may occur in some lymphocytes. The agranulocytes that appear to be large lymphocytes by light microscopy are classified as monocytes by ultrastructural criteria (Hammer and Weber, 1974). Monocytes tend to disappear from blood during the acute phase of disease, returning in increasing numbers as the disease becomes chronic.

The Platelets

The individual platelet is usually small, but giant forms equal in size to the erythrocyte may be present. Pseudopodia-like projections may extend from larger forms. Commonly, the platelets occur in small or large clusters, and individual platelets may appear superimposed upon erythrocytes. The latter must be distinguished from blood parasites. The usual appearance of platelets is that of a rosette of reddish-purple granules within a light blue cytoplasm enclosed by a delicate membrane. Normal platelet survival time in the circulation was found to be about 10 days (Mizuno et al., 1959).

Platelet counts on 32 male Holstein-Friesian calves, 9–15 weeks of age, were 192,000–892,000/µl of blood with a mean of 542,000 ± 175,000 (Nelson et al., 1974). Platelet number in adult cattle has been variously reported to be between 100,000 and 800,000/µl of blood. Changes in platelet numbers with age were minimal, and no consistent seasonal influence was noticed, although higher counts were found in the spring than in the autumn in 8 of 12 years (Noonan et al., 1978). Platelet counts may vary considerably during the estrus cycle (Rota and Cristofori, 1975); minimum values were seen on the day of the estrus (274,000 ± 41,462/µl) and on the eighth day (319,500 ± 43,681/µl) and the fifteenth day (294,000 ± 37,435/µl) postestrus.

Reports of platelet abnormalities in cattle are few. A transient occurrence of megathrombocytes (80–90% platelets with a mean diameter of 12.5 µm) with a below normal platelet count was seen in a 3-year-old Ayrshire cow with traumatic reticulitis (Dixon et al., 1980). Platelet count and size became normal after clinical recovery. Platelets from cattle with the Chédiak-Higashi syndrome were found to have a dense granule storage pool deficiency (Meyers et al., 1979).

THE BONE MARROW

Methods of obtaining fresh bone marrow from cattle have been described (Lawrence et al., 1962; Lewis, 1967; Schalm and Lasmanis, 1976; Wilde, 1961). The differential distribution of bone marrow cells reported in these studies is given in Table 7–10. Winqvist (1954) conducted an extensive study of bone marrow in bovine embryos, calves, and adult cattle. He found cellular composition of marrow of various bones to be similar. The M:E ratio was found to be 0.47 ± 0.06:1.0 in calves 3–36 days old and 0.64 ± 0.13:1.0 in cattle between 2 months and 10 years of age. In 5 adult cows, the mean M:E ratio was 0.79 ± 0.18:1.0. A similar mean M:E ratio of 0.68:1.0 was found for rib marrow of 12 cows (Calhoun, 1946). Myelograms of 50 normal young adult cattle developed from sternal marrow aspirates had a similar mean M:E ratio of 0.71 ± 0.29:1.0 (Wilde, 1964). The mean M:E ratio of less than 1.0 in normal cattle points to the fact that bovine bone marrow is more productive of erythrocytes than of granulocytes. This correlates with the low neutrophil numbers in peripheral blood in healthy cattle and the rapidity with which bone marrow reserve of neutrophils is drained and immature neutrophils appear in the circulation in response to acute inflammatory disease such as mastitis (Schalm and Lasmanis, 1976; Table 7–11).

The need for a particular cell type may modify the cellular composition of the bone marrow. This was shown in studies on bone marrow cultures of endotoxin-treated and anemic calves (Kaaya and Maxie, 1980). Marrow aspirates of calves given *Pseudomonas aeruginosa* endotoxin developed an increased number of granulocyte/macrophage progenitors and a reduced number of erythroid progenitor cells. In contrast, the reverse was seen in marrow aspirates of calves made anemic by repeated bleeding.

Table 7–10. The Cellular Composition of the Bone Marrow of Adult Cattle as Reported by Different Investigators

	Calhoun (1946) (12 cows)		Winqvist (1954) (5 cows)		Wilde (1964) (50 cows)	
	%	Range	%	Range	% ± S.D.	Range
Myeloblasts	—	—	—	—	2.3±1.39	0.6– 7.4
Progranulocytes	1.51	0.0– 6.8	0.79	0.2– 1.4	1.5±0.81	0.2– 4.0
Neutrophilic myelocytes and metamyelocytes	19.39	10.4–32.0	7.04	2.3–12.4	6.5±2.42	2.8–12.4
Eosinophilic myelocytes and metamyelocytes	6.69	1.8–10.4	2.82	0.8– 4.8	4.9±1.89	0.6–12.2
Band neutrophils	—	—	8.2	5.0–12.8	9.7±3.70	4.4–21.6
Band eosinophils	—	—	—	—	3.0±1.40	0.6– 7.4
Neutrophils	5.73	1.2–12.2	11.46	4.9–19.0	6.2±2.62	1.2–14.0
Eosinophils	1.92	0.0– 7.6	5.67	2.4–10.8	0.4±0.46	0.0– 1.0
Basophils	0.34	0.0– 1.0	0.19	0.0– 0.8	0.3±0.27	0.0– 1.0
Prorubricytes and blasts	—	—	1.23	0.6– 1.7	2.3±1.25	0.8– 7.2
Rubricytes	30.26	11.8–42.8	25.73	16.3–30.8	9.0±3.29	3.4–12.0
Metarubricytes	21.69	7.2–39.2	23.28	10.4–35.3	40.3±8.07	24.6–55.2
M:E ratio	0.68:1	0.27–2.5:1	0.79:1	0.4–1.84:1	0.71±0.29:1	0.31–1.85:1
Lymphocytes	6.68	1.4–16.8	10.69	5.6–16.3	7.2±2.88	2.4–17.4
Plasma cells	0.79	0.2– 2.0	0.99	0.4– 2.3	0.2±0.27	0.0– 1.0
Monocytes	2.64	0.0– 7.6	0.16	0.0– 0.4	0.4±0.39	0.0– 2.0
Reticulum cells	—	—	1.27	0.2– 2.9	0.9±0.63	0.0– 2.4
Megakaryocytes	—	—	0.05	0.0– 0.2	0.1±0.16	0.0– 0.8
Stem cells	2.14	0.0– 5.0	0.43	0.2– 0.8	—	—
Mitotic cells	—	—	—	—	0.2±0.26	0.0– 0.8
Unclassified and damaged cells	—	—	—	—	4.6±2.67	1.0–14.4

CLINICAL INTERPRETATIONS

Response to Corticosteroids

Principal corticosteroids in cattle are cortisol and corticosterone, occurring in the ratio of 7:1 (Paape et al., 1974a). Corticosteroid levels are lower in nonlactating cows than in lactating cows (Wagner and Oxenreider, 1972), while similar levels are found in lactating cows free of intramammary mastitis pathogens and cows infected with mastitis pathogens (Paape et al., 1974a). The average corticosteroid level in the last two groups of cattle was 4.7 ng/ml of plasma. Secretion of corticosteroids is increased two- to threefold after neurohormonal stimulation, e.g., preparation for milking or vasopressin injection (Wagner and Oxenreider, 1972) and after injection of ACTH (Paape et al., 1974a). A diurnal variation with lowest values between 6 P.M. and 2 A.M. was seen in one study (Wagner and Oxenreider, 1972), but not in another (Paape et al., 1974a).

Corticosteroid-induced changes have been studied in cattle after injection of ACTH (Paape et al., 1974a; Pehrson and Wallin, 1966) and various corticoid preparations (Schalm et al., 1965; Schillinger and Bucher,

1980). In our studies on corticosteroid-induced hematologic changes, mature lactating cows were administered 9-α-fluoroprednisolone acetate intramuscularly in single doses of 50, 100, and 500 mg (Table 7–12). The 50-mg dose produced a twofold increase in WBC count and a threefold increase in mature neutrophils. These changes were demonstrated between 12 and 18 hours after administration. Lymphocytes were at their lowest levels (30% below the preinjection level) between 36 and 60 hours after injection. A monocytosis was observed within 12 hours, and both eosinopenia and basopenia appeared at the same time. Larger doses appeared to extend the effects over a longer period of time. Cow 1249 was not normal; her circulating lymphocyte count was elevated to the point that she was a lymphosarcoma suspect. Although her lymphocytes remained comparatively high, there was a 50% decrease at the thirty-sixth hour. Her monocytes revealed a fivefold increase by the twelfth hour and remained elevated through the ninetieth hour, when the last blood sample was taken.

Five cows in advanced pregnancy were given an intramuscular injection of 20 mg of

Table 7–11. Bone Marrow Differential Cell Counts in Normal and Mastitic Cows (percentage of 500 Cells) (Schalm and Lasmanis, 1976)

	Normal Cows			Mastitic Cows*			
Cell Classification	No. 1	No. 2	No. 3	No. 4	No. 5	No. 6	No. 7
Erythroid series							
Rubriblast	0.2	0	0	0.2	0.2	0	0
Prorubricyte	1.2	0.4	0.8	0.6	0.4	0	1.0
Basophil rubricyte	4.8	5.2	8.4	3.2	3.6	1.4	6.0
Polychromic rubricyte	29.6	36.4	23.0	20.4	16.2	26.4	29.0
Metarubricyte	16.8	9.2	12.6	11.8	14.6	11.0	4.6
Mitotic rubricyte	1.0	0	0.4	1.0	0	0.4	1.0
Total	53.6	51.2	45.2	37.2	35.0	39.2	41.6
Myeloid series							
Myeloblast	0.2	0	0	0.8	0.2	0	0
Promyelocyte	1.4	1.4	0	5.6	1.8	2.2	1.6
Myelocyte, neutrophilic	3.2	3.4	2.8	5.2	2.4	5.2	3.6
Metamyelocyte, neutrophilic	2.8	6.2	3.2	12.2	4.2	5.8	2.0
Band, neutrophilic	6.6	4.6	8.4	10.4	10.0	9.2	7.8
Neutrophil	12.6	11.2	22.6	3.0	14.2	18.0	18.4
Metamyelocyte, eosinophilic	0.4	0.6	0.4	0.6	0.8	1.4	0.6
Band, eosinophilic	1.8	2.6	1.0	1.8	3.2	2.2	2.2
Eosinophil	0.6	0.6	1.6	0.8	0.6	1.2	0.2
Basophil (all)	0.4	1.0	0	0.6	0.6	0.4	0.6
Total	32.6	34.8	44.0	41.8	40.0	50.4	39.2
Other cells							
Hematogone	2.6	2.0	0.2	3.4	1.8	0.8	3.0
Lymphocyte	3.6	4.2	6.0	7.0	13.2	3.0	8.6
Plasma cell	1.2	1.0	0.2	1.2	0.8	1.0	0.6
Monocyte	2.2	1.2	0.4	2.4	3.2	1.6	3.8
Macrophage	0.8	0	0.2	0	0.8	0.2	0
Mitotic cell	0.2	0	0	0	0	0	0
Unclassified cell	0.8	0.2	0	1.6	0.2	0.4	0
Degenerated cell	2.4	5.4	3.8	5.4	5.0	3.4	3.2
Total	13.8	14.0	10.8	21.0	25.0	10.4	19.2
Myeloid:erythroid ratio	0.61:1.0	0.68:1.0	0.97:1.0	1.12:1.0	1.14:1.0	1.28:1.0	0.94:1.0

*Cow 4 had naturally acquired *Streptococcus agalactiae* infection of unknown duration in right front (RF), right rear (RR), and left front (LF) quarters, with acute flare-up in RR. Cow 5 had experimentally induced *Staphylococcus aureus* infection of 40 days' duration in RF and LF and naturally acquired *Pseudomonas aeruginosa* infection of 5 months' duration in RR. Cow 6 had naturally acquired *S. aureus* infection of unknown duration (chronic mastitis) in RR, LF, and left rear (LR) quarters. Cow 7 had experimentally induced *S. aureus* infection of 186 and 300 days' duration (mild chronic mastitis), respectively, in LF and RR.

dexamethasone to induce labor. Mean values and standard deviations of WBC and differential leukocyte counts, before and 24 hours after injection, are shown in Table 7–13.

Normal adrenocortical function is indicated in cattle when an intravenous injection of 200 IU of ACTH produces a more than 50% decrease in eosinophil numbers, more than 100% increase in neutrophil numbers, and more than 10% increase in WBC counts within 6–10 hours (Pehrson and Wallin, 1966). Paape et al. (1974a) made a detailed study relating endogenous corticosteroid levels in blood and associated hematologic changes following an intravenous injection of 250 IU of ACTH in cows. About a sevenfold

increase in corticosteroid level occurred after 1 hour, with high levels persisting for 8 hours and returning to normal by 10 hours. The WBC count increased after 2 hours, peaked at 10 hours, and remained increased for the next 24 hours. The increase in WBC was due primarily to increase in neutrophil numbers. Lymphocyte and monocyte numbers did not change significantly. Eosinophil numbers decreased after 4 hours, remained depressed for 10 hours, and returned to normal level after 24 hours. Corticosteroid and WBC responses were significantly influenced by the stage of lactation and milk yield in that cows in late lactation and those producing more than 18 kg/day exhibited a lower response.

Table 7–12. Leukocyte Responses in the Lactating Cow to Intramuscular Administration of 9-α-Fluoroprednisolone Acetate (Upjohn)[a]

Cow	Dose	Elapsed Time (hr)	WBC /μl		Differential Leukocyte Counts in Absolute Numbers/μl					
					Neutro-phils	Lympho-cytes	Mono-cytes	Eosino-phils	Baso-phils	Other
44	50 mg	0	6,200		3,069	2,418	372	310	31	0
		12	11,800		8,850	2,065	885	0	0	0
		18	13,350		9,745	2,737	868	0	0	0
		36	9,000		6,750	1,890	270	45	45	0
		60	7,500		4,950	1,800	488	225	37	0
		66	7,200		3,924	2,700	396	114	36	0
		72	7,900		4,187	2,805	710	118	0	80
		78	6,000		2,520	2,520	510	60	90	0
1249	100 mg	0	14,200		4,118	8,662	355	923	142	0
		12	22,800		12,198	8,664	1,710	228	0	0
		18	19,900		12,239	5,671	1,692	298	0	0
		36	15,100		9,211	4,530	1,208	151	0	0
		42	18,500	(Band) 68	10,175	6,382	1,758	185	0	0
		60	13,600		6,392	6,052	952	68	68	0
		66	11,800		6,077	5,074	590	59	0	0
		84	14,400		7,488	5,328	1,440	144	0	0
		90	14,500		6,380	6,815	1,015	290	0	0
2208	500 mg	0	8,400		2,688	4,284	504	840	84	0
		5	11,550		7,392	2,945	578	578	57	0
		9	13,900		9,730	3,267	486	278	0	139
		24	13,600		10,132	2,448	952	68	0	0
		30	13,200	(Band) 113	9,768	2,112	1,254	66	0	0
		35	11,300		7,910	2,260	904	0	0	113
		48	14,600		10,366	2,336	1,898	0	0	0
		54	14,180		9,784	2,411	1,914	71	0	0
		72	11,100		7,381	2,553	1,166	0	0	0
		78	8,000		5,320	1,680	1,000	0	0	0

[a]Italics = Major change in cell numbers.

Hematologic changes in normal cattle and cattle affected with lymphocytic leukemia were compared after intramuscular injection of 0.25 IU of ACTH/kg body weight (Jovanovic, 1972). Eosinopenia was evident at 8 hours postinoculation in all animals of both groups, but responses differed with regard to other leukocytes and WBC counts; neutrophilia was seen in 97% and 77%, leukocytosis in 100% and 57%, and lymphopenia in 63–80% and 50–63% of the normal and leukemic cattle, respectively. An interesting observation was that the absolute number of lymphocytes *increased* in 20–37% of normal and 37–50% of leukemic cattle. A similar lymphocytosis was observed by us in two water buffalo calves given prednisolone or dexamethasone (Chapter 12). The cause of such a variable response of lymphocytes to corticosteroids remains unknown and may involve differences in cell surface binding and clearance half-time of circulating corticosteroids (Bloom et al., 1980). Lymphocyte surface marker studies in lymphosarcomatous cattle revealed that there was an increase in B-lymphocytes (antibody-complement rosette-forming cells) and a decrease in T-lymphocytes (erythrocyte rosette-forming cells) and nonrosette-forming cells, and that corticosteroids caused an overall reduction of all lymphocyte types (Wilkie et al., 1979).

Responses to exogenous corticosteroids

Table 7–13. Effect of Intramuscular Injection of Dexamethasone (20 mg) on Peripheral Blood Leukocytes of a Cow

	Preinjection	24 Hours Postinjection	Difference
Total leukocytes	6,960 ± 1,432	13,000 ± 344	87% increase
Band neutrophils	9 ± 21	65 ± 77	—
Neutrophils	2,578 ± 882	9,575 ± 1,438	240% increase
Lymphocytes	3,370 ± 837	2,418 ± 663	22% decrease
Monocytes	336 ± 216	903 ± 529	170% increase
Eosinophils	666 ± 620	38 ± 58	Marked decrease

and ACTH were studied in dry, nonpregnant German Simmental cows injecte intramuscularly with 15 mg dexamethasone-21-isonicotinate, 200 mg prednisolone actetate, or 300 IU ACTH (Schillinger and Bucher, 1980). All cows developed leukocytosis, the greatest increase occurring with dexamethasone. The mean increase was 122% above initial values. WBC counts returned to normal by 70–96 hours after dexamethasone, 66 hours after prednisolone, and 54 hours after ACTH injections. The proportion of neutrophils increased by 94–117%, the greatest increase being caused by prednisolone. Lymphocytes decreased by 39–67%, the greatest decrease being caused by dexamethasone. In all experiments, the proportion of eosinophils fell to zero at the time of maximum hormonal effect.

Thus corticosteroid-induced leukocytosis, neutrophilia, eosinopenia, and lymphopenia may develop in cattle, as in other species. The extent and duration of changes observed vary with the health of the animal and with the dose and type of drug administered. Although cattle develop monocytosis in response to exogenous corticosteroids, this leukocyte is commonly observed to disappear initially from the circulation in peracute and acute inflammatory diseases in the cow. In fact, from a clinical point of view, return of monocytes to the blood is conjectured to be a sign that the disease has entered the chronic phase.

Leukocyte Response to Disease

Inflammatory Response

Recent studies on responses of the cow to intramammary inoculation of a variety of inflammatory agents have provided some insight into hematologic changes during inflammatory response in this species (Griel et al., 1975; Jain et al., 1978; Paape et al., 1974a, b; Schalm, 1981; Schalm and Lasmanis, 1976). The general trend observed is briefly conceptualized here; the interested reader should look into cited publications and pertinent references therein.

The WBC count in the early stage of inflammatory diseases in the cow generally does not reflect the seriousness of the disease. This is because lymphocytes exceed the neutrophils in health, and are decreased in response to corticosteroids of stress. Eosinophil numbers also become reduced. Simultaneously, neutrophils and monocytes leave the blood to participate in the developing inflammatory lesion. Although mature neutrophils from the bone marrow pool now enter the circulation, they are also attracted to the site of injury. Thus neutrophilic response to corticosteroids is masked by the rapidity of emigration of neutrophils into the inflammatory lesion, the net effect being a precipitous fall in the WBC count to leukopenic levels. As the bone marrow reserve of mature neutrophils becomes depleted, immature neutrophils enter the circulation in increasing numbers during the first 24–48 hours (Fig. 7–3). Subsequently, stimulation of bone marrow stem cells leads to intensification of neutrophil production so that as the disease passes into a more chronic phase, the left shift disappears and is replaced by neutrophilia consisting of mostly mature forms. Monocytes also increase and may exceed their maximum normal range. The WBC count now increases above normal, with counts of 20,000–30,000/μl being representative of an extreme leukocytosis. Thus transitory leukopenia with marked left shift is the common initial response to severe inflammatory disease in the cow. The persistence of leukopenia beyond the third or fourth day is a sign of inadequacy of granulopoiesis to meet the demands for neutrophils. The incidence of leukopenia was 6.9% in 4,287 hemograms on 3,639 cows, and the average duration of leukopenia was 3.8 days (Andresen, 1970). Myeloid hypoplasia may develop in certain chronic infections and thereby contribute to a persistent neutropenia or leukopenia (Valli et al., 1979).

Response to Endotoxemia and Septicemia

Leukocytic changes are generally similar in septicemia and endotoxemia except for differences in magnitude depending on extensiveness of the lesion and the amount of toxin in circulation. Experimental studies in humans and animals including cows (Griel et al., 1975; Jain and Lasmanis, 1978; Lumsden et al., 1974) and calves (Tennant et al., 1975a) have shown that endotoxin given in minute amounts systemically produces a transient neutropenia (hence leukopenia) followed by a "rebound" neutrophilia. The former is attributed to shift of circulating neutrophils into the marginal pool and the latter to accelerated release of cells from the marrow reserve (Chapter 26). However, neutrophil response as well as changes in other leukocytes in blood depend on the amount and route of endotoxin administration (Jain and Lasmanis, 1978; Lumsden et al., 1974). For example, neutropenia may not develop at low doses, while lymphopenia and slight to marked left shift may manifest at relatively higher doses (Table 7–14). Nucleated erythrocytes may also appear in blood, and death may follow within a few hours of injection of a large dose (Tennant et al., 1975a).

Endotoxin induces an acute inflammatory reaction in the mammary gland causing massive mobilization of neutrophils into the mammary parenchyma and milk. This and systemic absorption of endotoxin leads to quantitative changes in blood and bone marrow myeloid cells (Jain et al., 1978). Similar responses may be anticipated from endotoxin absorption from other lesions such as coliform mastitis and enteritis. For example, leukopenia was evident in terminal cases of septicemia, while a variable degree of leukocytosis was seen in calves with primary coliform enteritis (Tennant et al., 1975a). Leukocytic changes may be evident within hours of infection as shown by experimental studies of acute salmonellosis in calves (Hoerstke et al., 1982). Lymphopenia and neutrophilia were evident with the onset of fever within a few hours of infection before diarrhea was appar-

Table 7–14. **Changes in Peripheral Blood Leukocyte Numbers of Cows Given an Intravenous Injection of** *Escherichia coli* **Endotoxin**

Endotoxin (μg)	Time (h)	Cells/μl of blood			
		Leukocyte count	Immature neutrophils*	Mature neutrophils	Lymphocytes
5	0	7,200	0	2,376	3,924
	1	6,300	0	1,922	3,348
	2	5,500	0	2,117	3,080
	4	10,500	0	6,247	3,150
	6	10,500	0	5,652	3,780
	8	10,500	0	5,774	3,622
	10	8,100	0	3,888	3,280
	24	7,600	0	2,584	3,914
20	0	7,100	71 B	2,023	4,012
	1	6,000	0	1,920	3,600
	2	5,600	0	2,352	2,968
	4	7,600	0	3,876	2,850
	6	8,500	0	3,995	3,570
	8	8,600	0	3,569	4,042
	10	8,000	40 B	2,920	4,120
	24	6,800	0	1,530	4,352
50	0	8,100	0	3,078	4,212
	1	4,000	0	1,480	2,420
	2	2,300	58 B	402	1,610
	4	2,400	24 B	588	1,584
	6	3,500	70 B	1,015	2,152
	8	4,700	47 B	1,692	2,585
	10	5,300	26 B	1,404	3,418
	24	5,800	29 B	1,218	3,973
100	0	8,900	0	1,691	5,295
	1	1,700	0	68	1,496
	2	2,300	80 Mt	69	1,898
	4	1,600	16 B	80	1,336
	6	1,700	17 B	153	1,317
	8	3,900	468 Mt	643	2,281
	10	6,800	1632 Mt	1,088	3,366
	24	11,600	2088 Mt	3,422	5,104

From Jain and Lasmanis, 1978; courtesy of *Research in Veterinary Science.*
*Left shift involving: B, band cells; Mt, metamyelocytes

Table 7-15. Blood Values in Cattle in Acute Indigestion with Toxemia

Breed	Age (mo)	PCV (%)	WBC/μl	Differential Leukocyte Counts in Absolute Numbers/μl			Lymphocytes	Monocytes	Eosinophil	Basophil
				Neutrophil						
				Metamyelocytes	Band	Segmenter				
Hereford	Mature	35	9,400	94	1,504	3,901	3,055	188	517	141
Hereford	Mature	39	19,500	878	3,705	8,580	6,645	195	98	0
Hereford	18	31	18,250	0	182	12,684	5,110	182	91	0
Hereford	24	44	14,300	2,646	2,288	3,504	5,362	500	0	0
Angus	6	43	23,400	0	936	16,965	5,031	351	117	0
Angus	6	39	10,900	0	3,379	2,180	4,796	545	0	0
Angus	6	39	25,700	514	7,839	8,995	6,168	1,670	385	129
Angus	6	38	17,100	0	1,026	10,602	5,045	427	0	0

ent, while plasma proteins decreased with the onset of watery-fibrinous diarrhea (13 hours postinfection).

Effect of Acute Indigestion

The stress induced by acute indigestion in cattle was found to result in a left shift without accompanying leukopenia. A herd of 15 Hereford crossbred cattle on poor pasture and poor-quality oat and alfalfa hay was abruptly switched to about 114 kg of bread daily. Several cattle developed acute indigestion characterized by recumbency, weakness, cessation of rumination, pulse rates of 110–130, and normal body temperature. A second herd of 50 Angus crossbred cattle was assembled for a feeding trial. The cattle were placed on a ration of 57% concentrates on July 20. On August 7, at 4 P.M., feed and water were withheld as part of a 12-hour shrinking process prior to weighing the animals and placing them on an experimental ration. The next day, the cattle were given a ration consisting of 90% concentrates. Approximately 20 hours later, some cattle were ataxic and weak and exhibited a stiff gait and diarrhea. Physical examination of several cattle revealed respiratory distress, hyperpnea, increased heart rate, body temperatures of 39.4–40.0°C, and tympanic rumen sounds on percussion. Hemograms were developed for 4 cows in each of the 2 herds (Table 7–15). Leukocytosis occurred in 6 of the 8 cows, primarily due to neutrophilia and persistence of lymphocytes near high normal levels. The significant neutrophilia can perhaps be explained on the basis of increased heart rate (physiologic leukocytosis) and the effect of corticosteroids of stress. The variable degree of left shift, including metamyelocytes in half of the cattle, was a unique finding. Numbers of monocytes, eosinophils, and basophils were variable. The left shift indicated the acute nature of the disease, while the neutrophilia and absence of lymphopenia indicated that the stress was distinctly different from that commonly associated with inflammatory disease. Fibrinogen level ranged from 0.7–1.0 g/dl of plasma, which was lower than commonly encountered in inflammatory diseases of cattle (see Table 36–15).

REFERENCES

Abt, D.A., et al.: Circadian and Seasonal Variations in the Hemogram of Mature Dairy Cattle. Cornell Vet., 56:479, 1966.

Andresen, H.A.: Evaluation of Leukopenia in Cattle. J. Amer. Vet. Med. Ass., 156:858, 1970.

Basarab, J.A., et al.: Erythrocyte Fragility in "Doubled-Muscled" Cattle. Can. J. Anim. Sci., 60:869, 1980.

Bell, F.N., and Irwin, M.R.: Studies of the Variation of the Blood Cells of Cattle in Health and during Brucella Infections. J. Infect. Dis., 63:251, 1938.

Benjamin, M.M.: Blood Cytology of Shipping Fever in Beef Cattle. J. Amer. Vet. Med. Ass., 123:209, 1953.

Bianca, W.: Effects of Dehydration, Rehydration and Overhydration on the Blood and Urine of Oxen. Brit. Vet. J., 126:121, 1970.

Bianca, W., and Espinosa, J.P.: Untersuchungen Uber dio hohan toleranz von kalboun. Zeitschrift für Tierzuentung und Züchtungs biologic, 92:282, 1975.

Bianca, W., and Näf, F.: Reaktionen von rindern owl 4000m simulierte Hobe in Abhan gig keil rom after Schweiza. Arch. Tierheilkunde, 120:615, 1978.

Bianca, W., et al.: Responses of Steers to Water Restriction. Res. Vet. Sci., 6:38, 1965.

Bloom, J.C., et al.: Glucocorticoid Receptors in Peripheral Blood Lymphocytes from Bovine Leukemia Virus-Infected Cows with Persistent Lymphocytosis. Cancer Res., 40:2240, 1980.

Blount, W.P.: Normal Blood Cells in the Bovine. Vet. J., 95:222, 1939.

Braun, W.: Average Levels of Various Constituents, Physical Properties and Formed Elements of the Blood of Cows on Pasture. Amer. J. Vet. Res., 7:450, 1946.

Breukink, H.J., et al.: Variations in the Composition of the Blood in Veal Calves Solely Fed on a Milk Replacer during a Fattening Period of Eighteen Weeks. Tijdschr. Diergeneeskd., 99:1219, 1974.

Brewer, R.L.: An Allergic Condition in Jersey Cows. J. Amer. Vet. Med. Ass., 130:181, 1957.

Brody, S., et al.: Environmental Physiology. III. Influence of Ambient Temperature, 50–100°F, on the Blood Composition of Jersey and Holstein Cows. Mo. Agr. Exp. Sta. Bull., 433, 1949.

Bunce, S.: Observations on the Blood Sedimentation Rate and the Packed Cell Volume of Some Domestic Farm Animals. Brit. Vet. J., 110:322, 1954.

Bunger, U., et al.: Referenzwerte des Hämoglobingehalts, des Hämatokrits und der mittleren korpuskularen Hämoglobinkonzentration bei Aufzuchtkalbern ohne Eisensubstitution. 3. Vergleich der beobachteten Altersabhangigkeiten mit Literaturangaben. Arch. Tierernaehr., 32:137, 1982.

Cabello, G.: Neonatal Changes in the Plasma Levels of Cortisol, Cortisone and Aldosterone in the Calf. Biol. Neonate, 36:35, 1979.

Calhoun, M.L.: Bone Marrow of Horses and Cattle. Science, 104:423, 1946.

Calhoun, M.L.: A Cytological Study of Costal Marrow. III. Hemograms of the Horse and Cow. Amer. J. Vet. Res., 16:297, 1955.

Campbell, S.G.: Milk Allergy and Autoallergic Disease of Cattle. Cornell Vet., 60:684, 1970.

Canham, A.S.: Blood of Cattle. 16th Rep. Div. Vet. Serv. Anim. Ind., p. 531. Pretoria, Union of South Africa, 1930.

Christian, R.G., and Tryphonas, L.: Lead Poisoning in Cattle: Brain Lesions and Hematologic Changes. Amer. J. Vet. Res., 32:203, 1971.

Clawson, A.B.: Some Results of Blood Counting on Cattle. Amer. Vet. Rev., 45:527, 1914.

Comline, R.S., et al.: Parturition in the Cow: Endocrine Changes in Animals with Chronically Implanted Catheters in the Foetal and Maternal Circulation. J. Endocrinol., 63:451, 1974.

Conner, G.H., et al.: Effect of Pregnancy and Age on Hemograms of Holstein-Friesian Cattle in a Herd with No Evidence of Leukemia. Amer. J. Vet. Res., 28:1303, 1967.

Dimock, W.W., and Thompson, M.C.: Clinical Examination of the Blood of Normal Cattle. Amer. Vet. Rev., 30:553, 1906.

Dixon, P.M., et al.: Bovine Megathrombocytosis. Vet. Rec., 106:311, 1980.

Doxey, D.L.: Haematology of the Ox. In Comparative Clinical Haematology. Archer, R.K., and Jeffcott, L.B., eds. Blackwell Scientific Publications, Oxford, p. 215, 1977.

Eberhart, R.J., and Patt, J.A.: Plasma Cortisol Concentrations in Newborn Calves. Am. J. Vet. Res., 32:1921, 1971.

Esievo, K.A.N., and Moore, W.E.: Effect of the Dietary Protein and Stage of Lactation on the Haematocytology and Erythrocytes Enzyme Activity of High Producing Dairy Cattle. Res. Vet. Sci., 26:53, 1979.

Ferguson, L.C., et al.: On Variation in the Blood Cells of Healthy Cattle. J. Infect. Dis., 76:24, 1945.

Fisher, D.D., et al.: Environmental and Genetic Effects on Hematologic Characteristics of Beef Cows. Amer. J. Vet. Res., 41:1533, 1980.

Fisher, E.W.: Observations on the Bovine Hematocrit. Brit. Vet. J., 118:513, 1962.

Fraser, A.C.: A Study of the Blood of Cattle and Sheep in Health and Disease. Rep. Dir. Inst. Anim. Path., Cambridge, 1:114, 1929–1930.

Frei, Y.F., et al.: Correlation between Osmotic Resistance and Fetal Hemoglobin in Bovine Erythrocytes. Exp. Cell Res., 30:561, 1963.

Garner, R.J.: Bile Pigment Metabolism in Cattle: Disturbances in Bile Pigment Metabolism in Disease. J. Comp. Path., 63:247, 1953.

Gartner, R.J.W., et al.: Variations in the Concentration of Blood Constituents in Relation to the Handling of Cattle. Res. Vet. Sci., 10:7, 1969.

Gartner, R.J.W., et al.: The Influence of Degree of Excitation on Certain Blood Constituents in Beef Cattle. Aust. J. Exp. Biol. Med. Sci., 43:713, 1965.

George, J.W., and Duncan, J.R.: Effect of Sample Preparation on Basophilic Stippling in Bovine Blood Smears. Vet. Clin. Path., 10:37, 1981.

Granzien, C.K.: Leucocyte Values in Queensland Cattle. Res. Vet. Sci., 9:544, 1968.

Greatorex, J.C.: Studies on the Haematology of Calves from Birth to One Year of Age. Brit. Vet. J., 110:120, 1954.

Greatorex, J.C.: Observation on the Haematology of Calves and Various Breeds of Adult Dairy Cattle. Brit. Vet. J., 113:29, 65, 469, 1957.

Griel, L.C., Jr., et al.: Clinical and Clinico-Pathological Effects of Escherichia coli Endotoxin in Mature Cattle. Can. J. Comp. Med., 39:1, 1975.

Grimes, R.M., et al.: Bovine Fetal Hemoglobin. I. Postnatal Persistence and Relation to Adult Hemoglobin. J. Dairy Sci., 41:1527, 1958.

Hammer, R.F., and Weber, A.F.: Ultrastructure of Agranular Leukocytes in Peripheral Blood of Normal Cows. Amer. J. Vet. Res., 35:527, 1974.

Hannan, J.: Water Intoxication of Calves. Irish Vet. J., 19:211, 1965.

Hewett, C.: On the Causes and Effects of Variations in the Blood Profile of Swedish Dairy Cattle. Acta Vet. Scand. Suppl., 50:1, 1974.

Hoerstke, M., et al.: Verlaufskontrolle von verschiedenen Blutparametern bei der akuten Salmonellose des Kalbes. Tierarz. Umschau, 37:500, 1982.

Holman, H.H.: A Negative Correlation between Size and Number of the Erythrocytes of Cows, Sheep, Goats and Horses. J. Path. Bact., 64:379, 1952.

Holman, H.H.: The Blood Picture of the Cow. Brit. Vet. J., 111:440, 1955.

Holman, H.H.: Changes Associated with Age in the Blood Picture of Calves and Heifers. Brit. Vet. J., 112:91, 1956.

Hubbert, W.T., and Hollen, E.J.: Cellular Blood Elements in the Developing Bovine Fetus. Amer. J. Vet. Res., 32:1213, 1971.

Hudson, S., et al.: Plasma Corticoid Levels in Healthy and Diarrheic Calves from Birth to 20 Days of Age. Brit. Vet. J., 132:551, 1976.

Hunter, J.T., et al.: Foetal and Maternal Hormonal Changes preceding Normal Bovine Parturition. Acta Endocrinol., 84:653, 1977.

Jain, N.C., and Lasmanis, J.: Leucocytic Changes in Cows Given Intravenous Injections of Escherichia coli Endotoxin. Res. Vet. Sci., 24:386, 1978.

Jain, N.C., et al.: Neutrophil Kinetics in Endotoxin-Induced Mastitis. Amer. J. Vet. Res., 39:1662, 1978.

Johnson, L.W., and Schwartz, S.: Isotopic Studies of Erythrocyte Survival in Normal and Porphyric Cattle: Influence of Light Exposure, Blood Withdrawal, and Splenectomy. Amer. J. Vet. Res., 31:2170, 1970.

Jovanovic, M.J.: Investigation by the Thorn Test of Adrenocortical Function in Cattle Affected with Lymphatic Leukemia. Acta Vet., Beograd, 22:309, 1972.

Kaaya, G.P., and Maxie, M.G.: The Kinetics of Haemopoietic Differentiation Assessed by in Vitro Bone Marrow Culture in Endotoxin-Treated and in Anaemic Calves. Res. Vet. Sci., 29:63, 1980.

Kaneko, J.J.: Erythrokinetics and Iron Metabolism in Bovine Porphyria Erythropoietica, Ann. N.Y. Acad. Sci., 104:689, 1963.

Kirbride, C.A., and Frey, R.A.: Experimental Water Intoxication in Calves. J. Amer. Vet. Med. Ass., 151:742, 1967.

Kursa, J., and Kroupova, V.: Osmotic and Oxidative Haemolysis of Erythrocytes in Calves with White Muscle Disease. Res. Vet. Sci., 20:97, 1976.

Lawrence, W.C., et al.: A Simple Method for Bone Marrow Aspiration in the Cow. Cornell Vet., 52:297, 1962.

Lee, C.K., et al.: Postnatal Loss of Bovine Fetal Hemoglobin. Amer. J. Vet. Res., 32:1039, 1971.

Lewis, H.B.: Bone Marrow Biopsy in Cattle. Vet. Rec., 80:452, 1967.

Lumsden, J.H., et al.: The Piromen Test as an Assay of Bone Marrow Granulocyte Reserve in the Calf. I. Studies on Bone Marrow and Peripheral Blood. Can. J. Comp. Med., 38:56, 1974.

Lumsden, J.H., et al.: Hematology and Biochemistry Reference Values for Female Holstein Cattle. Can. J. Comp. Med., 44:24, 1980.

Manresa, M., et al.: Hematological Studies on Cattle in the Philippines. Philipp. Agri., 23:588, 1934; 28:79, 1939; 28:187, 1939.

Manston, R., et al.: The Influence of Dietary Protein upon Blood Composition in Dairy Cows. Vet. Rec., 96:497, 1975.

Massip, A.: Relation between the Type of Delivery and the Acid-Base and Plasma Cortisol Levels of the Newborn Calf. Brit. Vet. J., *136*:488, 1980.

McEwan, A.D., et al.: The Effect of Colostrum on the Volume and Composition of the Plasma of Calves. Res. Vet. Sci., *9*:284, 1968.

McMurray, C.H., et al.: Sequential Changes in Some Blood Components in the Normal Neonatal Calf. Brit. Vet. J., *134*:590, 1978.

McSherry, B.J., et al.: Plasma Fibrinogen Levels in Normal and Sick Cows. Can. J. Comp. Med., *34*:191, 1970.

Meneses, G.A., et al.: Comportamiento de las Constantes Sanguineas en Costa Rica: Efecto de la Raza y Edad en Vacas Holstein y Jersey. Ciencias Veterinarias, Costa Rica, *2*:29, 1980.

Meyers, K.M., et al.: Storage Pool Deficiency in Platelets from Chédiak-Higashi Cattle. Am. J. Physiol., *237*:R239, 1979.

Mizuno, N.S., et al.: Life Span of Thrombocytes and Erythrocytes in Normal and Thrombocytopenic Calves. Blood, *14*:708, 1959.

Moberg, R.: The White Blood Picture in Sexually Mature Female Cattle with Special Reference to Sexual Conditions: A Clinical Experimental Study. Thesis, Kungliga Veterinarhogskolan, Stockholm, Sweden, 1955.

Moore, G.R.: The Blood Picture in Cases of Retained Fetal Membranes in Cattle. J. Amer. Vet. Med. Ass., *109*:39, 1946.

Nelson, J.H., et al.: Blood Characteristics of the Holstein Calf Relevant in Cardiopulmonary Studies. J. Appl. Physiol., *37*:145, 1974.

Noonan, T.R., et al.: Effects of Age, Season and Reproductive Activity of Hemograms of Female Hereford Cattle. Am. J. Vet. Res., *39*:433, 1978.

Norris, J.H., and Chamberlin, W.E.: A Chemical and Histological Investigation in Victoria (Australia) of the Blood of Cattle and Sheep. Aust. J. Exp. Biol. Med. Sci., *6*:285, 1929.

Olsen, R.E.: Determination of Erythrocyte Sedimentation Rate of Cattle. J. Amer. Vet. Med. Ass., *148*:801, 1966.

Paape, M.J., et al.: Thermal Stress and Circulating Erythrocytes, Leucocytes and Milk Somatic Cells. J. Dairy Sci., *56*:84, 1973.

Paape, M.J., et al.: Corticosteroid, Circulating Leukocytes and Erythrocytes in Cattle. Diurnal Changes and Effects of Bacteriologic Status, Stage of Lactation and Milk Yield on Response to Adrenocorticotropin. Am. J. Vet. Res., *35*:355, 1974a.

Paape, M.J., et al.: Plasma Corticosteroid, Circulating Leukocyte and Milk Somatic Cell Responses to Escherichia coli Endotoxin-Induced Mastitis. Proc. Soc. Exp. Biol. Med., *145*:553, 1974b.

Palmer, L.S.: The Physiological Relations of Plant Carotenoids to the Carotenoids of the Cow, Horse, Sheep, Goat, Pig, and Hen. J. Biol. Chem., *27*:27, 1916.

Pehrson, B., and Wallin, O.: A Test of Adrenal Cortical Function in Dairy Cows by ACTH Administration. Acta Vet. Scand., *7*:35, 1966.

Penny, R.H.C., et al.: Hematological Values for the Clinically Normal Bull. Brit. Vet. J., *122*:239, 1966.

Perk, K., et al.: Osmotic Fragility of Red Cells of Young and Mature Domestic and Laboratory Animals. Amer. J. Vet. Res., *25*:1241, 1964.

Perman, V., et al.: Statistical Evaluation of Lymphocyte Values on Minnesota Dairy Cattle. Amer. J. Vet. Res., *31*:1217, 1970.

Reece, W.O.: Acid-Base Balance and Selected Hemato-

logic, Electrolytic, and Blood Chemical Variables in Cows Nursing Calves: One Week Through Fifteen Weeks. Amer. J. Vet. Res., *45*:666, 1984.

Rodriguez, O.N., et al.: Cuadro Hematologico en Bovinos Posteplenctomizodos. Revista Cubana de Ciencias Veterinarias, *4*:159, 1973.

Rota, E., and Cristofori, F.: Numerical Variations in the Platelets in Blood Taken from the Jugular Vein of Cattle in Relation to the Stage of the Oestrous Cycle. Folia Vet. Latina, *5*:191, 1975.

Rowlands, G.J., et al.: The Effect of Season on the Composition of the Blood of Lactating and Non-Lactating Cows as Revealed from Repeated Metabolic Profile Tests on 24 Dairy Herds. J. Agric. Sci. (Camb.), *83*:27, 1974.

Rowlands, G.J., et al.: Relationship between Blood Composition and Sterility in Dairy Cows: A Field Study. J. Dairy Res., *44*:1, 1977.

Rusoff, L.L., et al.: Blood Studies of Breeding Bulls. J. Dairy Sci., *37*:30, 1954.

Ryan, G.M.: Blood Values in Cows: Erythrocytes. Res. Vet. Sci., *12*:572, 1971a.

Ryan, G.M.: Blood Values in Cows: Leukocytes. Res. Vet. Sci., *12*:576, 1971b.

Saksena, S.K., et al.: Effect of Environmental Temperature on Certain Characteristics of Blood Serum in Zebu and Its Cross-Bred Male Cattle. Indian J. Anim. Sci., *50*:947, 1980.

Sato, T., and Mizuno, M.: Poikilocytosis of Newborn Calves. Jap. J. Vet. Sci., *44*:801, 1982.

Scarborough, R.A.: The Blood Picture of Normal Laboratory Animals. Yale J. Biol. Med., *4*:69, 1931–1932.

Schalm, O.W.: Plasma Protein: Fibrinogen Ratios in Routine Clinical Material from Cats, Dogs, Horses, and Cattle. Part III. Calif. Vet., *24*:6, June, 1970.

Schalm, O.W.: Bovine Hematology. Mod. Vet. Pract., *58*:923, 1977.

Schalm, O.W.: The Bovine Leukocytes. Bovine Pract., *1(6)*:8, 1980; *2(1)*:28, 1981; *2(2)*:32, 1981; *2(4)*:14, 1981.

Schalm, O.W.: Manual of Bovine Hematology. Veterinary Practice Publishing Co., Santa Barbara, 1984.

Schalm, O.W., and Lasmanis, J.: Cytologic Features of Bone Marrow in Normal and Mastitic Cows. Am. J. Vet. Res., *37*:359, 1976.

Schalm, O.W., et al.: The Use of a Synthetic Corticoid on Experimental Coliform (Aerobacter aerogenes) Mastitis in Cattle. The Response of Leukocytes and the Effect of Hormone-Induced Neutrophilia. Am. J. Vet. Res., *26*:851, 1965.

Schalm, O.W., et al.: Plasma Protein: Fibrinogen Rations in Dogs, Cattle and Horses. I. Influence of Age on Normal Values and Explanation of Use in Disease. Calif. Vet., *24*:9, Feb., 1970.

Scheidegger, H.H., et al.: Das Weiss Blutbild von Aufzucht und Milchmastkalbern. Schweiz. Arch. Tierheilkd., *116*:87, 1974.

Schillinger, D., and Bucher, W.: Untersuchungen uber den Einfluss von Glukokortikoiden und von ACTH auf das Blutbild des Rindes. Tierarz. Umschau, *35*:651, 1980.

Stampfli, G., et al.: Hämatologische und klinisch-chemische Blutwerte bei Aufzuchtrindern. Schweiz. Arch. Tierheilkd., *122*:363, 1980a.

Stampfli, G., et al.: Der Eifluss der Tageszeit auf hämatologische und klinisch-chemische Parameter bei der Milchkuh. Schweiz. Arch. Tierheilkd., *122*:327, 1980b.

Straub, O.C.: Uber das Blutbild von gesunden kalbern leukosefrier Herkunst in den ersten 3 Lebensmonaten und vergleichende Untersuchungen an gleichaltrigen klinisch gesunden Kalbern aus Leukosebestanden. Inaug. diss., Tierärztl. Hochsch., Hannover, Germany, 1956.

Straub, O.C., et al.: Bovine Hematology. II. Effect of Parturition and Retention of Fetal Membranes on Blood Morphology. J. Amer. Vet. Med. Ass., *135*:618, 1959.

Straub, O.C., et al.: Bovine Hematology. Verlag Paul Parey, Berlin, 1981.

Sutton, R.H., and Hobman, B.: The Value of Plasma Fibrinogen Estimations in Cattle: A Comparison with Total Leucocytes and Neutrophil Counts. N.Z. Vet. J., *23*:21, 1975.

Tennant, B.C., et al.: Hematology of the Neonatal Calf: Erythrocyte and Leukocyte Values of Normal Calves. Cornell Vet., *64*:516, 1974.

Tennant, B., et al.: Hematology of the Neonatal Calf. II. Response Associated with Acute Enteric Infections, Gram-Negative Septicemia, and Experimental Endotoxemia. Cornell Vet., *65*:457, 1975a.

Tennant, B., et al.: Hematology of the Neonatal Calf. III. Frequency of Congenital Iron Deficiency Anemia. Cornell Vet., *65*:543, 1975b.

Theilen, G.H., et al.: Hematologic Survey of Cattle on the Island of Jersey, with Reference to the Reported Incidence of Lymphosarcoma (Leukemia). Amer. J. Vet. Res., *28*:1313, 1967.

Tumbleson, M.E., et al.: Serum Protein Concentrations as a Function of Age, in Female Dairy Cattle. Cornell Vet., *63*:65, 1973.

Valli, V.E.O., et al.: The Pathogenesis of Trypanosoma congolense Infection in Calves. III. Neutropenia and Myeloid Response. Vet. Path., *16*:96, 1979.

Veirup, N.H.: Makrocytose hos kvaeg. Fortsatte undersogelser. Dansk Veterinaertidsskrift, *60*:833, 1977.

Wagner, W.C., and Oxenreider, S.L.: Adrenal Function in the Cow. Diurnal Changes and the Effects of Lactation and Neurohypophyseal Hormones. J. Anim. Sci., *34*:630, 1972.

Wever, A.F., et al.: Electron Microscopic Studies of Agranulocytes of Peripheral Blood from Clinically Normal and Preleukemic Cows. Anat. Rec., *157*:340, 1967.

Whitlock, R.H., et al.: The Incidence of Anemia in Dairy Cows in Relation to Season, Milk Yield and Age. Res. Vet. Sci., *16*:122, 1974.

Wilde, J.K.: A Technique of Bone Marrow Biopsy in Cattle. Res. Vet. Sci., *2*:315, 1961.

Wilde, J.K.H.: The Cellular Elements of the Bovine Bone Marrow. Res. Vet. Sci., *5*:213, 1964.

Wilkie, B.N., et al.: Bovine Lymphocytes: Erythrocyte Rosettes in Normal Lymphomatous and Corticosteroid-Treated Cattle. Can. J. Comp. Med., *43*:22, 1979.

Wingfield, W.E., and Tumbleson, M.E.: Hematologic Parameters, as a Function of Age, in Female Dairy Cattle. Cornell Vet., *63*:72, 1973.

Winqvist, G.: Morphology of the Blood and the Hemopoietic Organs in Cattle under Normal and Some Experimental Conditions. Acta. Anat. Suppl., *21*:1, 1954.

Winqvist, G.: Bone Marrow Changes in Cows in Connection with Normal Parturient, Paresis, and Retained Foetal Membranes. Acta Vet. Scand., *1*:27, 1959.

Wittwer, F., and Bohmwald, H.: Leucocyte Count in Normal Female Friesian Cattle of Various Ages in the Valdivia Area, Chile. Arch. Med. Vet., *6*:32, 1974.

Zielinski, J., and Machoy, H.: Proba okreslenia dobowych zmian ilosci krwinek bialych oraz hematokrytu we krwi zylnej doroslego bydla. Medycyna Weterynaryjna, *37*:568, 1981.

8

The Sheep: Normal Hematology with Comments on Response to Disease

FETAL BLOOD VALUES   208

EFFECT OF AGE ON BLOOD VALUES   208

BLOOD VALUES IN ADULT SHEEP   209
The Erythrocytes   209
The Leukocytes   215
The Platelets   216
The Plasma   216

MORPHOLOGY OF BLOOD CELLS   218
The Erythrocytes   218

The Neutrophil   218
The Eosinophil   218
The Basophil   218
The Lymphocyte   220
The Monocyte   222
The Platelets   222

THE BONE MARROW   222
The Myeloid:Erythroid Ratio   222

The hematology of the sheep is in general similar to that of the cow, with the exception of size and number of erythrocytes. Because of the type of husbandry, sheep harbor gastrointestinal parasites much more commonly than cattle. Literature references on normal blood values, summarized in Tables 8–1 and 8–2, no doubt reflect to some extent the influence of parasitism. Several authors state that the sheep were in good physical condition but not necessarily free from internal parasites. Modest variations due to season and nutritional state have also been observed, particularly in parasitized sheep.

FETAL BLOOD VALUES

Data relative to various erythrocyte parameters in sheep, from 62 days of gestation to birth, are summarized in Table 13–4. In general, RBC, Hb, and PCV values increase progressively during gestation and are highest at birth. MCV and MCH decrease gradually to 122–128 days of gestation and then stabilize, while MCHC fluctuates inconsistently within a narrow range. Nucleated erythrocytes are prominent during early gestation, but then decrease and are absent by 136 days. Plasma protein concentration is low throughout gestation except the week before parturition,

when a marked increase is observed. Additional data, derived from 23 normal fetuses, at 122–145 days of gestation, are presented in Table 8–3. Mean values for 10 females indicated a somewhat greater RBC count, PCV value, Hb concentration, and WBC count than in 13 male fetuses of similar ages. Average reticulocyte counts ranged from 0.9–2.4%. Neutrophil:lymphocyte ratios ranged from 0.24–0.43:1.0. Mean plasma fibrinogen levels were below 0.2 g/dl in normal fetal lambs at 114–140 days of gestation and slightly increased in growth-retarded fetuses of similar age (Pickart et al., 1976).

EFFECT OF AGE ON BLOOD VALUES

Changes occurring with age follow the same general trends as for cattle. Ullrey et al. (1965) made more than 9,000 determinations relative to erythrocyte parameters on the blood of 316 Hampshire, Shropshire, and Suffolk sheep from birth to maturity. RBC, Hb, and PCV values were found to decline from birth to a low level at approximately 14 days of age and then increase to be highest at 3 months of age (Table 8–4). MCV and MCH were greatest at birth and declined subsequently, reaching low points at 5 and 3 months, respectively. MCHC increased from

Normal Blood Values for the Sheep

Erythrocytic Series	Range	Ave.	Leukocytic Series	Range	Ave.
Erythrocytes ($\times 10^6/\mu l$)	9–15	12.0	Leukocytes/μl	4,000–12,000	8,000
Hemoglobin (g/dl)	9–15	11.5	Neutrophil (band)	Rare	—
PCV (%)	27.0–45.0	35.0	Neutrophil (mature)	700– 6,000	2,400
MCV (fl)	28–40	34.0	Lymphocyte	2,000– 9,000	5,000
MCH (pg)	8–12	10.0	Monocyte	0– 750	200
MCHC (%)	31–34	32.5	Eosinophil	0– 1,000	400
Reticulocytes (%)	0	0	Basophil	0– 300	50
ESR (mm)	0	0			
RBC diameter (μm)	3.2–6.0	4.5	Percentage Distribution		
Resistance to hypotonic saline (%)			Neutrophil (band)	Rare	—
Min.	0.58–0.76		Neutrophil (mature)	10–50	30.0
Max.	0.40–0.55		Lymphocyte	40–75	62.0
Myeloid:erythroid ratio	0.77–1.68:1.0	1.1:1.0	Monocyte	0– 6	2.5
	(Grunsell, 1951)		Eosinophil	0–10	5.0
			Basophil	0– 3	0.5

Other Data		
Thrombocytes ($\times 10^5/\mu l$)	2.5–7.5	4.0
Icterus index (units)	Normally <5	
Plasma proteins (g/dl)	6.0–7.5	
Fibrinogen (g/dl)	0.1–0.5	
Erythrocyte life span (days)	140–150	

birth to 12 months of age. Reticulocyte number was generally low at birth, but an increase was seen during the first two weeks coincident with the decrease in RBC count. Similar age-related observations on various erythrocyte parameters were made in other studies on growing lambs (Littleton et al., 1968; Upcott et al., 1971). Mean RBC counts in lambs up to 1 year of age are generally between 11 million and 13 million/μl of blood; values for adult sheep are about 1 million to 2 million less.

The decline in erythrocyte parameters during the first two weeks appeared to be, at least in part, a consequence of an inadequate supply of iron for hemoglobin synthesis. Anemic lambs and lambs with low PCV responded quickly to parenteral administration of 300–375 mg iron dextran (Ullrey et al., 1965; Bostedt, 1979). For example, mean Hb value in 4 lambs given 375 mg iron dextran intramuscularly rose from 7.8 g/dl at 14 days of age to 10.8 g/dl at 21 days, and during the same period PCV increased from 23.8% to 33.6%. Untreated lambs would take about 7 weeks to attain similar values (Holz et al., 1961).

Ullrey et al. (1965) also made more than 10,000 observations relative to total and differential leukocyte counts on the same 316 sheep from birth to maturity (Table 8–4). The WBC count was found to double by 12 hours after birth, declined at 24 hours, and then increased to a peak at 3 months of age. Segmented neutrophils comprised 34% of the leukocytes at birth, but increased to 52% at 12 hours after birth and then declined to 16% at 12 months of age. Increases in WBC count and neutrophil numbers shortly after birth appear to be stress-related, as in newborn calves. Another study also reported a significant increase in WBC count between 20 and 40 days after birth and to a lesser extent between 60 and 90 days of age (More and Sahni, 1979). In some earlier studies, a downward trend in mean WBC count with advancing age was observed due to a reduction in lymphocytes (Grunsell, 1955b; Hackett et al., 1957). Variations in monocyte numbers were unrelated to age. Eosinophils show a modest increase with advancing age, from a mean value of about 1.0% in lambs to 4.0% in adults.

BLOOD VALUES IN ADULT SHEEP

The Erythrocytes

The mean RBC count in adult sheep is about 12.0 million/μl of blood, with a range of 9.0 million to 15.0 million. Mean PCV values as reported for sheep in Great Britain fall

Table 8–1. RBC and WBC Counts in Lambs and Adult Sheep from the Literature

Reference	No. of Animals	Breed	Age	RBC (×10⁶/μl)	WBC (×10³/μl)	Neutrophils (%)	Lymphocytes (%)	Monocytes (%)	Eosinophils (%)	Basophils (%)
Reda et al. (1957)	60	Egyptian	1–60 days	9.08–12.78 (10.92)	10.0	64.5	44.0	1.2	0.2	0.1
		Egyptian	2–12 mo	9.24–11.92 (10.59)	8.5	39.0	55.0	3.0	2.5	0.5
		Egyptian	1–2 yr	9.02–10.45 (9.73)	9.2	43.0	48.5	4.3	4.0	0.2
		Egyptian	2–5 yr	7.6–9.21 (8.58)	8.0	41.0	50.0	3.0	5.7	0.3
Hackett et al. (1957)	200+	Suffolk	Lambs and ewes	10.89	9.95	29.9	64.6	2.5	2.4	0.5
Holman (1944a)	100–116	Scottish Hill	Mostly adult	6.2–15.5 (11.5)	1.1–17.5 (9.2)	11–47 (24)	41–83 (67.3)	0–13 (2.3)	0–15 (4.2)	0–3 (0.5)
Todd et al. (1952)	55	Southdown	Pregnant ewes	8.27–15.5 (12.65)	3.15–11.88 (7.26)	10–53.9 (27.6)	34.8–77.0 (62.4)	0.5–7.5 (2.4)	1.8–25.0 (6.2)	0–4.0 (1.4)
	35	Hampshire	Pregnant ewes	9.52–17.8 (12.47)	4–13.62 (7.74)	15–49.3 (28.5)	45.8–77.5 (62)	0.3–6.5 (2.2)	1.0–18.5 (5.5)	0.5–4.5 (1.9)
Hudson and Osborn (1954)	20	Hampshire	11–36 mo	4.8–12.2 (8.9)	3.2–10.2 (5.1)	37.0 (1.0% band)	52.0	2.5	7.2	0.5

Table 8-2. Erythrocyte Parameters in Sheep from the Literature

Reference	No. of Animals	Breed	Age	RBC ($\times 10^6/\mu l$)	PCV (%)	Hb (g/dl)	MCV (fl)	MCH (pg)	MCHC (%)
Becker and Smith (1950)	6 each	Corriedale, Hampshire, Dorset	1–14 wk	10.9–13.7 (12.23)	37.9	12.09	27–36 (31)	8.6–11.0 (9.8)	29.2–34.1 (31.5)
			Yearlings	9.6–13.3 (11.88)	37.0	12.23	27–36 (31)	9–11.3 (10.1)	30.6–34.2 (32.2)
			Mature	10.1–13.2 (11.63)	38.8	12.91	28–37 (33.8)	8.8–11.9 (10.8)	30.8–33.3 (32.1)
Hackett et al. (1957)	200+	Suffolk	Lambs and ewes	10.89	35.0	10.78	32.1[a]	9.9[a]	30.8[a]
Holman (1944a)	100–114	—	Mostly adults	6.2–15.5 (11.5)	22–39 (30.5)	8.6–15.8 (12.4)	19–35 (27.4)	10.8[a]	41.2
Todd et al. (1952)	55	Southdown	Pregnant ewes	8.27–15.51 (12.65)	32.3–47.2 (40.38)	10.3–16.0 (13.4)	23.6–48.6 (32.23)	10.6[a]	33.2[a]
	35	Hampshire	Pregnant ewes	9.52–17.8 (12.47)	31.3–45.2 (38.35)	10.4–14.7 (12.34)	26.7–41.9 (39.07)	9.9[a]	32.2[a]
Overas (1969)	29	Norwegian breeds	3–3½ mo	11.7±1.0	34.5±2.6	11.4±1.0	29.7±2.2	9.8±0.8	32.9±1.2
	18		5 mo	13.5±0.9	39.4±2.3	12.4±1.1	29.4±2.3	—	—
	11		6–10 mo	11.0±0.9	34.5±2.1	10.8±0.6	31.7±2.0	9.9±0.6	31.1±0.7
	10		2 yr[b]	9.9±0.9	35.1±3.1	10.6±0.8	35.5±2.1	—	—
			2 yr[c]	12.9±1.2	38.5±2.9	11.7±0.7	30.1±3.2	—	—
Mackenzie et al. (1970)	99	Rhodesian fat-tail	Lambs and adults	8.72–15.6 (12.0)	25–44.5 (35.6)	9–15.7 (12.4)	25–41.8 (30.1)	8–12.5 (10.5)	29.8–39.5 (34.6)

[a]Estimated from author's data.
[b]On farm leys.
[c]On return from mountain pasture.

Table 8–3. Hemograms of Ovine Fetuses in Advanced Gestation (means and 1 SD)

Age (days)	122–129	122–129	131–145	131–145
Sex	Male	Female	Male	Female
Number	6	5	7	5
RBC ($\times 10^6/\mu$l)	6.5 ± 0.9	7.9 ± 0.6	7.4 ± 1.2	8.4 ± 0.4
Hb (g/dl)	8.8 ± 1.5	10.4 ± 0.4	9.9 ± 2.1	10.5 ± 0.8
PCV (%)	30.2 ± 5.4	37.4 ± 1.2	34.0 ± 6.7	37.4 ± 3.1
MCV (fl)	46.3 ± 2.8	47.3 ± 2.2	44.7 ± 4.2	44.4 ± 2.4
MCH (pg)	13.5 ± 0.8	13.2 ± 1.0	13.2 ± 1.0	12.4 ± 0.7
MCHC (%)	29.3 ± 0.6	27.8 ± 1.1	29.2 ± 1.4	28.0 ± 1.2
Plasma proteins (g/dl)	3.5 ± 0.4	3.9 ± 0.3	3.7 ± 0.2	4.1 ± 0.3
Fibrinogen (g/dl)	0.25 ± 0.24	0.16 ± 0.08	0.17 ± 0.07	0.20 ± 0.16
Reticulocytes (%)	1.6 ± 1.7	2.4 ± 3.0	1.0 ± 1.4	0.9 ± 1.1
WBC/μl	2,217 ± 467	2,870 ± 635	2,485 ± 925	3,040 ± 706
Band neutrophils	76 ± 129	0	17 ± 42	0
Mature neutrophils	467 ± 299	890 ± 498	654 ± 456	627 ± 445
Lymphocytes	1,542 ± 461	1,893 ± 288	1,664 ± 599	2,306 ± 409
Monocytes	102 ± 44	29 ± 6	106 ± 194	42 ± 46
Eosinophils	12 ± 12	34 ± 12	31 ± 30	46 ± 26
Basophils	17 ± 20	24 ± 13	14 ± 16	19 ± 27
Leukocytes (%)				
Band neutrophils	4.0 ± 6.0	0	1.6 ± 3.8	0
Mature neutrophils	20.5 ± 13.6	29.4 ± 11.2	25.1 ± 12.0	19.0 ± 10.9
Lymphocytes	69.3 ± 10.7	67.6 ± 11.5	67.6 ± 12.8	77.8 ± 12.2
Monocytes	5.0 ± 2.9	1.0 ± 0	3.9 ± 5.5	1.2 ± 1.2
Eosinophils	0.5 ± 0.5	1.2 ± 0.4	1.1 ± 1.0	1.4 ± 0.5
Basophils	0.7 ± 0.7	0.8 ± 0.4	0.7 ± 0.7	0.6 ± 0.8
Thrombocytes ($\times 10^5/\mu$l)	534 ± 126	414 ± 69	719 ± 140	—

between 30 and 35%, while in the United States, values are between 35 and 40%. The small size of the sheep erythrocyte places special demands on centrifugation in order to ensure complete packing of RBC to obtain a valid PCV (see Chapter 2). The mean Hb value is 11.5 g/dl, but in individual sheep levels may reach 16.0 g/dl (Holman, 1944a; Todd et al., 1952). The effect of high altitude in raising the Hb concentration has been reported (Watson, 1953). Sheep at sea level in Peru were observed to have Hb concentrations of 8.0–10.0 g/dl; after 3–4 months at altitudes of 3,353–4,572 m (11,000–15,000 ft), the Hb ranged from 12–16 g/dl. Hb concentration of sheep on mountain pasture in Norway was found to be 3.0 g/dl greater than that when the same sheep were maintained at a lower altitude (Overas, 1969).

Hemoglobin has been observed to decrease appreciably during and after lambing (Hackett et al., 1957). A slight decrease in RBC, Hb, and PCV values was observed during gestation and 14 days after parturition in another study (Ullrey et al., 1965). Total plasma protein concentration declines during pregnancy, and plasma volume is increased by 23% during the last third of gestation (Mackie, 1977).

No evidence has been found in the literature to the effect that significant sex or breed differences exist in various erythrocyte parameters. Significant seasonal variations have been reported (Holman, 1944a; Singh and Rattan, 1981), and parasitic infection and nutritional state also contribute to such variations. Hemoglobin values in adult sheep may vary as follows: spring, 9.6 g/dl of blood; summer, 11.7 g/dl; autumn, 10.6 g/dl; and winter, 11.7 g/dl (Holman, 1944a). The low levels of Hb in fall and spring were attributed to inanition. A decided decrease in nematode egg counts in fecal samples from sheep was observed over a period of 5 years, during which time an increase in the Hb concentration occurred during the winter months in ewes and yearling lambs (Hawkins and De Freitas, 1947). A diet providing half maintenance had no effect on hematopoiesis in worm-free sheep; when parasites were present, however, Hb and PCV values fell (Grunsell, 1955b). A significant association between lower RBC counts and a rise in worm burden was found in late winter and early spring. However, in the summer months, the period of nutritional abundance, the RBC counts increased, suggesting that a high level of nutrition partly offsets the effect of the worm

Table 8–4. Hemograms of Growing Lambs (Means ± SE)[a]

Age	RBC (10⁶/µl)	Hb (g/dl)	PCV (%)	MCV (fl)	MCH (pg)	MCHC (%)	Reticulocytes (%)	WBC (10⁶/µl)	Neutrophils (%)	Lymphocytes (%)	Monocytes (%)	Eosinophils (%)	Basophils (%)
Birth	11.08 ± 0.20	12.9 ± 0.02	41.9 ± 0.06	36.5 ± 0.7	12.1 ± 0.2	30.9 ± 0.4	0.08 ± 0.1	3,032 ± 207	34.0 ± 3.0	64.0 ± 3.0	0.40 ± 0.13	0.20 ± 0.07	0.05 ± 0.03
12 hr	9.55 ± 0.25	11.4 ± 0.2	35.80 ± 0.08	36.8 ± 0.8	12.2 ± 0.3	32.0 ± 0.5	0.11 ± 0.02	6,129 ± 378	52.0 ± 3.0	46.0 ± 3.0	0.30 ± 0.30	0.40 ± 0.10	0.02 ± 0.02
24 hr	9.93 ± 0.25	11.6 ± 0.2	36.2 ± 0.8	35.9 ± 0.6	11.9 ± 0.2	32.0 ± 0.4	0.08 ± 0.02	3,349 ± 273	48.0 ± 3.0	50.0 ± 3.0	0.40 ± 0.13	0.60 ± 0.13	0.09 ± 0.04
48 hr	9.74 ± 0.25	11.1 ± 0.2	33.4 ± 0.8	33.5 ± 0.6	11.5 ± 0.2	33.6 ± 0.4	0.16 ± 0.03	4,262 ± 219	37.0 ± 2.0	62.0 ± 2.0	0.90 ± 0.16	0.20 ± 0.07	0.16 ± 0.06
5 days	10.04 ± 0.29	10.4 ± 0.3	30.9 ± 0.9	32.0 ± 0.5	11.0 ± 0.2	33.8 ± 0.4	0.33 ± 0.08	6,342 ± 247	36.0 ± 2.0	62.0 ± 2.0	1.30 ± 0.21	0.20 ± 0.07	0.08 ± 0.04
8 days	8.79 ± 0.16	9.6 ± 0.2	29.2 ± 0.3	31.6 ± 0.1	11.1 ± 0.1	33.9 ± 0.3	0.31 ± 0.05	7,809 ± 145	38.0 ± 2.0	60.0 ± 2.0	1.30 ± 0.21	0.20 ± 0.10	0.08 ± 0.04
14 days	8.91 ± 0.03	8.9 ± 0.2	27.2 ± 0.5	30.8 ± 0.4	9.9 ± 0.2	32.2 ± 0.4	0.72 ± 0.10	7,404 ± 366	36.0 ± 2.0	60.0 ± 2.0	1.30 ± 0.17	1.20 ± 0.18	0.09 ± 0.03
1 mo	11.39 ± 0.14	10.4 ± 0.1	31.5 ± 0.3	28.0 ± 0.5	9.1 ± 0.2	33.0 ± 0.4	0.31 ± 0.07	7,892 ± 224	29.0 ± 1.0	68.0 ± 1.0	0.80 ± 0.50	2.00 ± 0.22	0.25 ± 0.05
2 mo	12.43 ± 0.14	11.6 ± 0.1	34.0 ± 0.2	27.6 ± 0.3	9.3 ± 0.1	33.9 ± 0.7	0.02 ± 0.01	9,014 ± 221	22.0 ± 1.0	76.0 ± 1.0	0.50 ± 0.06	1.10 ± 0.11	0.19 ± 0.04
3 mo	12.95 ± 0.17	11.8 ± 0.1	34.2 ± 0.4	26.2 ± 0.3	9.0 ± 0.1	34.6 ± 0.2	0.03 ± 0.02	9,525 ± 186	23.0 ± 1.0	76.0 ± 1.0	0.60 ± 0.07	0.70 ± 0.12	0.30 ± 0.05
5 mo	12.35 ± 0.13	11.3 ± 0.3	31.4 ± 0.7	26.1 ± 0.3	9.0 ± 0.1	34.6 ± 0.2	0.02 ± 0.01	9,097 ± 219	20.0 ± 1.0	78.0 ± 1.0	0.60 ± 0.11	1.40 ± 0.17	0.33 ± 0.07
8 mo	10.96 ± 0.27	10.9 ± 0.2	31.8 ± 0.5	29.2 ± 0.5	10.3 ± 0.2	34.5 ± 0.4	0.03 ± 0.01	6,637 ± 291	25.0 ± 1.0	71.0 ± 1.0	0.80 ± 0.14	2.50 ± 0.33	0.45 ± 0.10
12 mo	11.85 ± 0.23	11.8 ± 0.2	33.8 ± 0.5	26.5 ± 0.5	9.3 ± 0.2	35.0 ± 0.3	0.02 ± 0.01	7,341 ± 552	16.0 ± 1.0	78.0 ± 3.0	1.80 ± 0.53	2.60 ± 0.51	0.16 ± 0.05

[a]Compiled from Ullrey et al., 1965.

burden. Statistically analyzed hematologic data on more than 700 sheep have been presented (Jones and Krebs, 1972).

The potential life span of erythrocytes of adult sheep was found to be about 150 days irrespective of the type of hemoglobin within the erythrocytes and high-K+ (HK) or low-K+ (LK) type of red cells (Tucker, 1963, 1966). In comparison, the potential life span of erythrocytes of newborn lambs was estimated at 75 days. Some seasonal influence on red cell life span was observed; mean life span in autumn was 155.5 ± 10.6 days and in spring 135 ± 5.6 days. Red cells deficient in glutathione exhibited a shortened life span (Tucker, 1974).

Influence of the Spleen

The circulating red cell mass in the sheep is significantly influenced by the spleen, which contains as much as one-fourth of the total red cell mass (Turner and Hodgetts, 1959). The jugular PCV was found to vary over a wide range, depending on whether the sheep were excited or tranquil. Removing a sheep from the companionship of the flock may increase the PCV, RBC, and Hb values significantly until it has adjusted to the new environment. PCV of blood collected 1 hour after isolation of a sheep from its penmates was often considerably less than that in samples collected immediately after isolation. The PCV was observed to vary as much as 25% under conditions of excitement or emotional stress. Removal of the spleen resulted in stabilization of the PCV. It was suggested that to avoid excessively high PCV values when collecting blood from sheep, the sheep should be made accustomed to the personnel, environment, and manipulation routine and should be handled with gentleness. After being caught, the sheep should be held for 15 minutes by a sympathetic attendant to produce a psychological tranquilization before the blood is drawn. The normal values for RBC, PCV, and Hb as reported in the literature are probably higher than the true resting levels for sheep since it is not conceivable that any great care was taken to reduce excitement or emotional stress before collecting the blood for establishment of normal values by the various investigators.

Stress of handling and restraining and of blood collection by venipuncture, particularly by a stranger, was found to cause marked elevations in RBC, Hb, and PCV values (Gohary, 1978; Gohary and Bickhardt, 1979). Significant increases were also seen in eosinophil numbers and many blood chemistry values. Exercise and adrenalin administration caused considerable increase in the PCV in intact sheep and goats, but not in splenectomized sheep (Anosa and Isoun, 1978). A long-term effect of splenectomy was decrease in RBC, Hb, and PCV values (Bolbol et al., 1982).

Reticulocytes

A few reticulocytes (<1.0%) may be found at birth (Table 8–4), as indicated by their presence in small numbers in late-gestation blood (Table 8–3), but they generally disappear within 2 weeks (Ullrey et al., 1965; Upcott et al., 1971). However, a higher percentage (up to 9.0%) has been reported in lambs 2–7 days of age when erythrocytes containing a few scattered granules with little or no reticulum were included in the reticulocyte count (Overas, 1969). Counting such punctate reticulocytes, the count was generally less than 0.5% in adult sheep. Reticulocytes appear in greater numbers in peripheral blood after hemorrhage or hemolytic destruction of erythrocytes.

Erythrocyte Sedimentation Rate

Erythrocyte rouleaux may be found to a limited extent, and therefore some sedimentation may be anticipated in sheep blood. When the erythrocyte sedimentation level is observed at the end of 1 hour, less than 1.0 to 2.5 mm of fall may be noted (Reda and Hathout, 1957; Osbaldiston, 1971), and when observed after a period of 24 hours, 3.0–10.0 mm of settling may have taken place (Bunce, 1954). Increased sedimentation was observed in an apparently healthy ewe as a result of undefined red cell factor (Osbaldiston, 1971).

Erythrocyte Osmotic Fragility

It is generally stated that hemolysis begins at 0.65% saline, but beginning hemolysis at higher saline concentrations has been observed, e.g., at 0.76% (Rossouw, 1930) and at 0.80% level (Wirth, 1950). Fifty percent hemolysis occurs at 0.65–0.70% saline (Overas, 1969). Complete hemolysis occurs at 0.55% saline or lower. Two populations of red cells, one osmotically more fragile and the other more resistant, were demonstrated in blood of newborn lambs on the basis of erythrocyte osmotic fragility peaks (Perk et al., 1964). Young ovine erythrocytes, although more resistant to hypotonic lysis, were more susceptible to virus-induced lysis (by Newcastle disease virus) than were older erythrocytes (Sziegoleit et al., 1980).

Hemoglobin Types

Common hemoglobin types in sheep are A, B, and AB. The existence of two genetic variants of hemoglobin in sheep of different breeds was demonstrated on the basis of electrophoretic mobility. The hemoglobin moving more rapidly toward the anode at pH 8.6 was called HbA or HbII, and the slow-moving hemoglobin was called HbB or HbI (Evans et al., 1956; van der Helm et al., 1957). The inheritance of hemoglobins A and B is not related to that of HK and LK type (Evans et al., 1956). The mean maximum hemoglobin values for sheep of each hemoglobin type form a series in which A is greater than AB and AB is greater than B (Evans and Whitlock, 1964).

A new hemoglobin was found to appear in sheep of type A after severe blood loss due to parasitism (Blunt and Evans, 1963), in anemic lambs (Braend et al., 1964), and after experimental bleeding of sheep of type A and AB but not of type B (van Vliet and Huisman, 1964; Moore et al., 1966). The new hemoglobin was named HbN for Norway in one report (Braend et al., 1964) and HbC in another report (van Vliet and Huisman, 1964); the latter designation is currently in vogue. HbC occurs in lambs in relatively higher amounts than in adult sheep (Efremov and Braend, 1966); in 1-month-old lambs, it constitutes about 10–30% of the hemoglobin. It is observed most often in sheep of type A, less often in type AB, and not at all in type B. In extreme blood loss, HbA is replaced entirely by HbC, while production of HbB is not affected. A direct relationship was found between the severity of anemia and the amount of HbC produced, and HbC was found to per-

sist in peripheral blood for 120–150 days (Tucker, 1966; Kitchen et al., 1968). HbC was found to be produced under natural conditions of development of anemia in sheep fed on kale, but only in sheep of genotypes AA and AB. Although sheep of type BB also developed Heinz bodies and anemia of kale feeding, no HbC was produced (Tucker, 1969).

Hemoglobin A has a higher affinity for molecular oxygen than does HbB because of differences in the dissociation rates (Kernohan, 1961). This factor may be partly responsible for higher Hb and PCV values reported in sheep with HbA (Evans and Whitlock, 1964). The affinity for molecular oxygen was found to be identical for HbA and HbC (van Vliet and Huisman, 1964), but a higher oxygen affinity for HbC than for HbA and HbB was reported recently (Vaccaro-Torracca et al., 1980). It appears, however, that HbC releases oxygen more readily than HbA and therefore may be advantageous under conditions of tissue hypoxia (Huisman and Kitchen, 1968). This finding is corroborated by a finding of increased synthesis of HbC in sheep at high altitude (Boyer et al., 1968) and in sheep subjected to simulated altitude of 7,010 m (23,000 ft) for 3 weeks in a decompression chamber (Blunt et al., 1970). The observation of increased synthesis of HbC in sheep exposed to the hypoxia of high altitude supported a concept of biologic similarity between erythropoietin and the factor(s) responsible for hemoglobin A-to-C switching (Boyer et al., 1968). Later, a correlation was found between the degree of A-to-C switching and the concentration of erythropoietin administered to sheep of HbA type (Thurmon et al., 1970). See Chapter 19 for additional observations.

The Leukocytes

The normal range for total leukocyte count, 4,000–12,000/µl of blood, is similar to that of the cow. Considerable disagreement exists regarding the mean count, but most investigators have reported it to be 7,000–8,000/µl. The WBC count increases with age during the first few weeks after birth. In the adult sheep, a count of 13,000/µl is regarded as indicative of slight leukocytosis and 20,000/µl as indicative of marked leukocytosis (Holman, 1944b).

The differential count reflects a high lymphocyte:neutrophil ratio as in cattle. Table 8–5 presents patterns of differential counts associated with increasing levels of WBC counts in blood from lambs and sheep presented with a variety of clinical problems. Significant left shift occurred when WBC counts were less than 5,000/μl (leukopenia). This reflected depression of granulopoiesis in association with systemic toxemia. A modest left shift accompanied some instances of marked leukocytosis (>20,000/μl). Neutrophil percentage increased in parallel with WBC counts, and this increase was associated with a corresponding percentage decrease in lymphocytes. Changes in percentage distribution of monocytes, eosinophils, and basophils did not appear to be influenced by the WBC count. Eosinophil counts rarely increase in response to parasitic infection in sheep, although eosinophil number is lower in lambs than in adult sheep (Greenwood, 1977). Parturition in sheep resulted in an increase in red cell parameters and typical corticoid-induced leukocytic changes, e.g., neutrophilia, lymphopenia, and eosinopenia (Anosa and Ogbogu, 1979). Red cell parameters attained prepartum levels by the seventh day and leukocytes by the fourteenth day post partum. Exposure of 2- to 3-year-old Merino sheep to intermittent artificial rainfall for 7 days was associated with an increase in WBC count and percentage of neutrophils and a decrease in lymphocyte percentage (Hay et al., 1982).

The Platelets

Platelet counts reported in the literature include ranges and means (in parentheses) of: 540,000–700,000/μl of blood (620,000) in lambs and 250,000–750,000/μl (490,000) in adults (Fraser, 1929–1930); 284,000–659,000/μl (441,000) (Tocantins, 1938); 130,000–690,000/μl (340,000 ± 123,000) (Overas, 1969); and 260,000–740,000/μl (457,000 ± 121,000) (Gajewski and Povar, 1971). Our range and mean are, respectively, 250,000–750,000/μl and 400,000/μl of blood.

The Plasma

Icterus Index

The plasma color is not affected by the yellow pigments of the ration, as is the case with cattle. Thus the icterus index normally does not exceed 5 units in health; in dehydration it may reach 7.5 units.

Total Plasma Proteins

The total plasma protein value of male fetuses in late gestation was 3.7 ± 0.2 g/dl, and in female fetuses it was 4.1 ± 0.3 g/dl (Table 8–3). A marked increase in plasma proteins was observed during the last week of gestation. At birth, total plasma proteins may be anticipated to range between 4.0 and 5.0 g/dl with a slight increase following ingestion of colostrum. Total plasma proteins continue to increase gradually, attaining a level of 6.0 g/dl at approximately 3 months of age. The normal level for mature sheep commonly falls within the range of 6.5–7.5 g/dl.

In a recent study, plasma protein concentration of 2.47–7.70 g/dl was reported in fetuses between 124 and 146 days of gestation, and it was found to decrease during the first 10 days after birth (Nathanielsz et al., 1980). The higher level in fetuses may reflect a greater antigenic stimulation during the intrauterine life.

The mean serum protein concentration, using the Kjeldahl method, was found to be 6.69 ± 0.23 g/dl (Mehrotra and Mullick, 1959). Serum proteins were found to increase with age from 5.78 g/dl in female lambs 3 months old to 7.36 g/dl in lactating ewes 3 years old (Perk and Lobl, 1960). The mean serum protein level of 100 ewes, 3–7 years of age, was reported to be 6.78 ± 0.79 g/dl (Egan and Cuill, 1971). Serum protein concentration is slightly lower than total plasma protein value because the fibrinogen is removed during clotting of the blood. Agarose gel electrophoresis of serum proteins has been performed (Keay and Doxey, 1984).

In diseases affecting general health, food and water intake is reduced and hemoconcentration develops. The plasma proteins become elevated, attaining levels of 8.0–10.0 g/dl. Infrequently, in generalized disease, plasma proteins may exceed 10.0 g/dl, thereby

Table 8-5. Percentage Differential Leukocyte Distribution at Various Levels of Total Leukocytes in Blood from Sheep of All Ages Exhibiting a Variety of Clinical Problems

Number of Samples	Total WBC/μl	Percentage Distribution								
		Neutrophils				Lymphocytes	Monocytes	Eosinophils	Basophils	
		Myelocytes	Metamyelo- cytes	Band	Mature					
11	<5,000 3,850±450	0.4±1.5	2.4±5.1	16.9 ±14.4	17.3±13.3	57.1±19.0	2.8±2.3	0.7 ±1.5	0.3 ±0.6	
23	5,000–12,000 7,250±1,800	0	0	0.34± 0.95	45.5±18.0	47.6±17.0	4.3±3.0	1.8 ±3.7	0.23±0.42	
20	12,100–15,000 13,100±1,000	0	0	0.5 ± 1.0	60.6±12.5	33.9±12.9	3.4±2.7	1.3 ±2.5	0.1 ±0.3	
12	15,100–20,000 17,700±1,400	0	0	1.0 ± 0.9	72.9±13.7	20.7±10.9	4.2±4.8	1.0 ±2.3	0.1 ±0.3	
15	>20,000 25,800±5,500	0	0.2±0.5	4.0 ± 6.3	75.0±13.0	16.2±10.7	3.9±2.0	0.23±0.41	0.1 ±0.3	

reflecting extreme dehydration. Elevation of plasma proteins should also be anticipated in response to chronic infections as a result of an increase in γ-globulins. For example, plasma protein levels of 10–11 g/dl were observed in sheep with actinobacillosis. Hypoproteinemia is a common finding in parasitism leading to blood loss as in haemonchosis and fascioliasis. In chronic blood loss, it is not uncommon for total plasma protein concentration to fall below 5.0 g/dl. Plasma protein levels decrease during pregnancy (Mackie, 1977) and after splenectomy (Bolbol et al., 1982).

Fibrinogen

The broad normal range for fibrinogen is 0.1–0.5 g/dl. Plasma fibrinogen levels of 1.0–1.5 g/dl have been recorded in some instances of pneumonia, encephalitis, intestinal obstruction, and polyarthritis. In one instance, a fibrinogen concentration of 1.6 g/dl was recorded in a 6-month-old lamb with signs of central nervous system disease. More commonly, increases of plasma fibrinogen in disease have been in the range of 0.6–0.9 g/dl, both in lambs and adult sheep.

MORPHOLOGY OF BLOOD CELLS

The Erythrocytes

Sheep erythrocytes are uniformly biconcave with a small central concavity (Fig. 8–3D; also see Fig. 20–1E), which imparts a faint suggestion of central pallor to erythrocytes seen in stained blood films (Fig. 8–1). In disease, when the erythrocytes assume a uniconcave shape with a deep central concavity, the central area may frequently appear "punched out." A slight anisocytosis may be seen, with an occasional giant cell measuring twice the normal diameter. Short chains of rouleaux are to be anticipated in health, with more marked rouleau formation in severe disease. Polychromasia and basophilic stippling of immature erythrocytes represent the normal response to blood loss or hemolytic disease. Nucleated erythrocytes and Howell-Jolly bodies are also commonly found in peripheral blood during anemia in remission.

Individual erythrocytes may be as small as 3.2–3.8 μm in diameter or as large as 6.5 μm or greater. Price-Jones curves on 3 sheep revealed erythrocyte diameter to vary from 3.5–6.0 μm, the mean sizes being 4.5, 4.7, and 4.9 μm (Holman, 1944a). Erythrocyte diameters of 500 cells were measured in blood films of 33 fetuses, 2 lambs, and 6 ewes (Karvonen, 1954). In fetuses at 60 and 125 days of gestation, the mean diameter was 6.51 μm and 5.3 μm, respectively; in lambs 3–6 weeks of age, 4.5 μm; and in ewes, 4.31–4.65 μm.

The Neutrophil

The *mature neutrophil* has a nucleus that is frequently multilobed, has short filaments, and exhibits plaqued chromatin. In the female, a small nuclear sex chromatin lobe may be observed in some cells. The cytoplasm stains faintly, usually slightly pinkish. A few larger and more deeply stained granules superimposed on the diffusely stained pinkish background are a common feature of the ovine neutrophil. Both primary and secondary granules are visible with the transmission electron microscope (Fig. 8–2A).

The *band neutrophil* has a nucleus that may be fat and U-shaped with occasional elongation to the S form. Chromatin plaques are not as condensed as in the mature cell. The cytoplasm is slightly bluer and less granular. Band neutrophils are rarely present in peripheral blood in health.

The Eosinophil

The eosinophil granules are uniform in size, ovoid, and refractile and stain orange-red. The cytoplasm is densely packed with granules, some of which may be scattered over the nucleus (Fig. 8–1). A small amount of pale blue cytoplasm is sometimes apparent, especially near the margin of the cell. The ultrastructure of sheep eosinophil (Fig. 8–2B) is similar to that of the cat eosinophil (Fig. 27–3) in that the eosinophil granules appear crystalloid.

The Basophil

This cell presents a variable number of dark granules that contrast well with the lighter blue–staining lobulated nucleus (Fig. 8–1). Mature granules are generally electron dense (Fig. 8–2C).

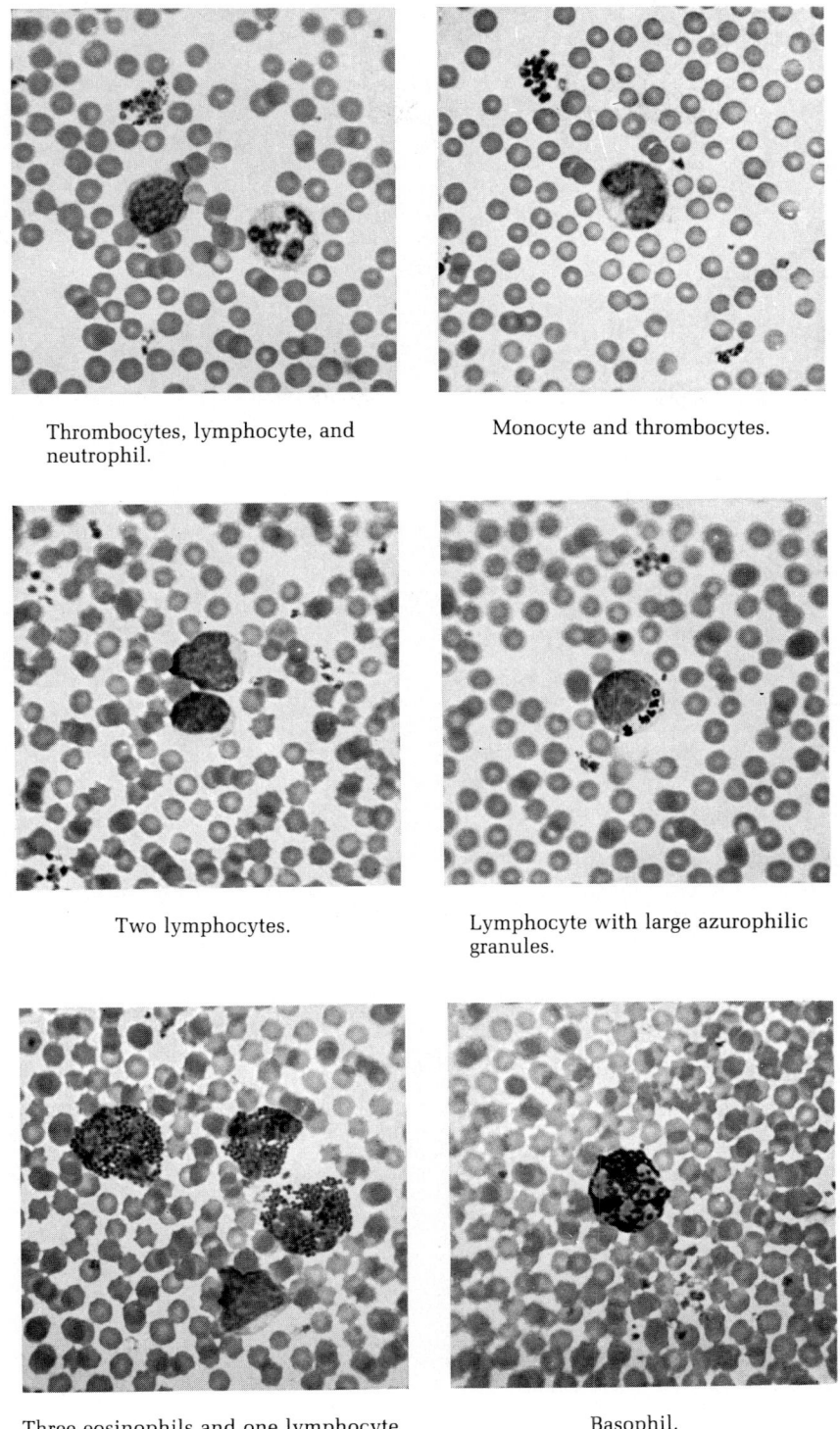

Thrombocytes, lymphocyte, and neutrophil.

Monocyte and thrombocytes.

Two lymphocytes.

Lymphocyte with large azurophilic granules.

Three eosinophils and one lymphocyte.

Basophil.

Fig. 8–1. Ovine blood cells (×600, original magnification).

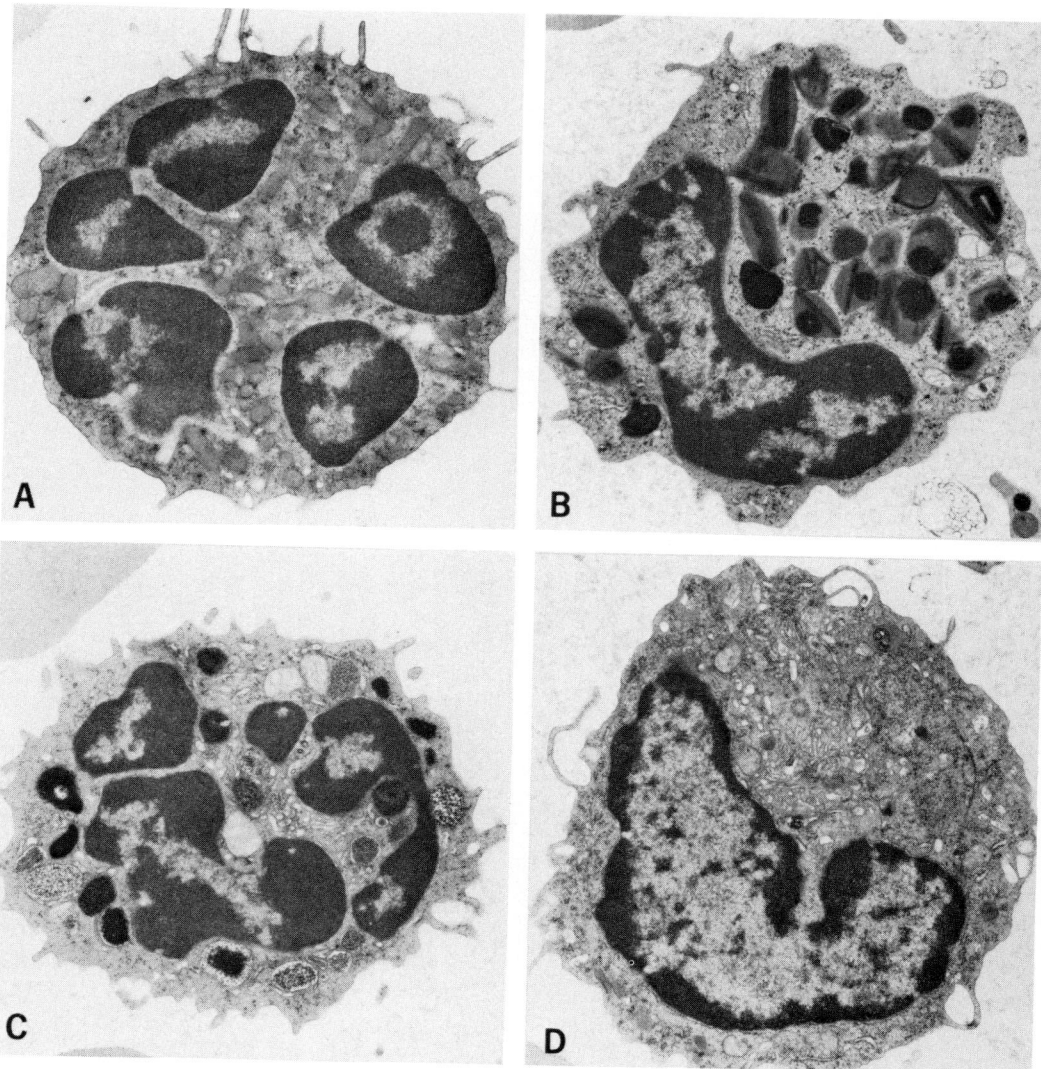

Fig. 8–2.   An ovine neutrophil *(A)*, eosinophil *(B)*, basophil *(C)*, and monocyte *(D)* prepared from the buffy coat of peripheral blood. The neutrophil *(A)* has a multilobed nucleus, and its cytoplasm is filled with larger, electron-dense primary granules and smaller, less dense specific granules. Few other cellular organelles are seen. ×14,000. The eosinophil *(B)* of the sheep is characterized by pleomorphic granules that contain crystalloid rods and membranous whorls. Cellular organelles are sparse. ×12,000. The basophil *(C)* also contains a diverse population of cytoplasmic granules. Maturation of granules proceeds from lightly to densely stippled structures. ×13,000. The cytoplasm of the monocyte *(D)* has granules, vesicles, and abundant ribosomes. Rough endoplasmic reticulum, mitochondria, and Golgi bodies are prominent. ×13,000. (Photographs courtesy of Drs. Kurt H. Albertine and Norman C. Staub.)

The Lymphocyte

Cell size is variable, but the cells are not easily divided into small and large types as in the cow (Fig. 8–1). The larger lymphocytes are few and do not have characteristics that would cause them to be confused with monocytes. The nucleus of all forms is round or oval, has smooth margin and chromatin, and occasionally stains slightly reddish. Infrequently, large, bizarre, binucleated forms may be seen. The cytoplasm stains distinctly blue and often extends completely around the nucleus. A perinuclear halo is commonly observed. The cytoplasm of large lymphocytes is lighter in color and more homogeneous. Azurophilic granules that vary in number, size, and shape may be observed occasionally (Fig. 8–1). In some instances, the azurophilic granules may overlie the nucleus, but more commonly they are in the cytoplasm near one edge of the cell. The ultrastructure of small

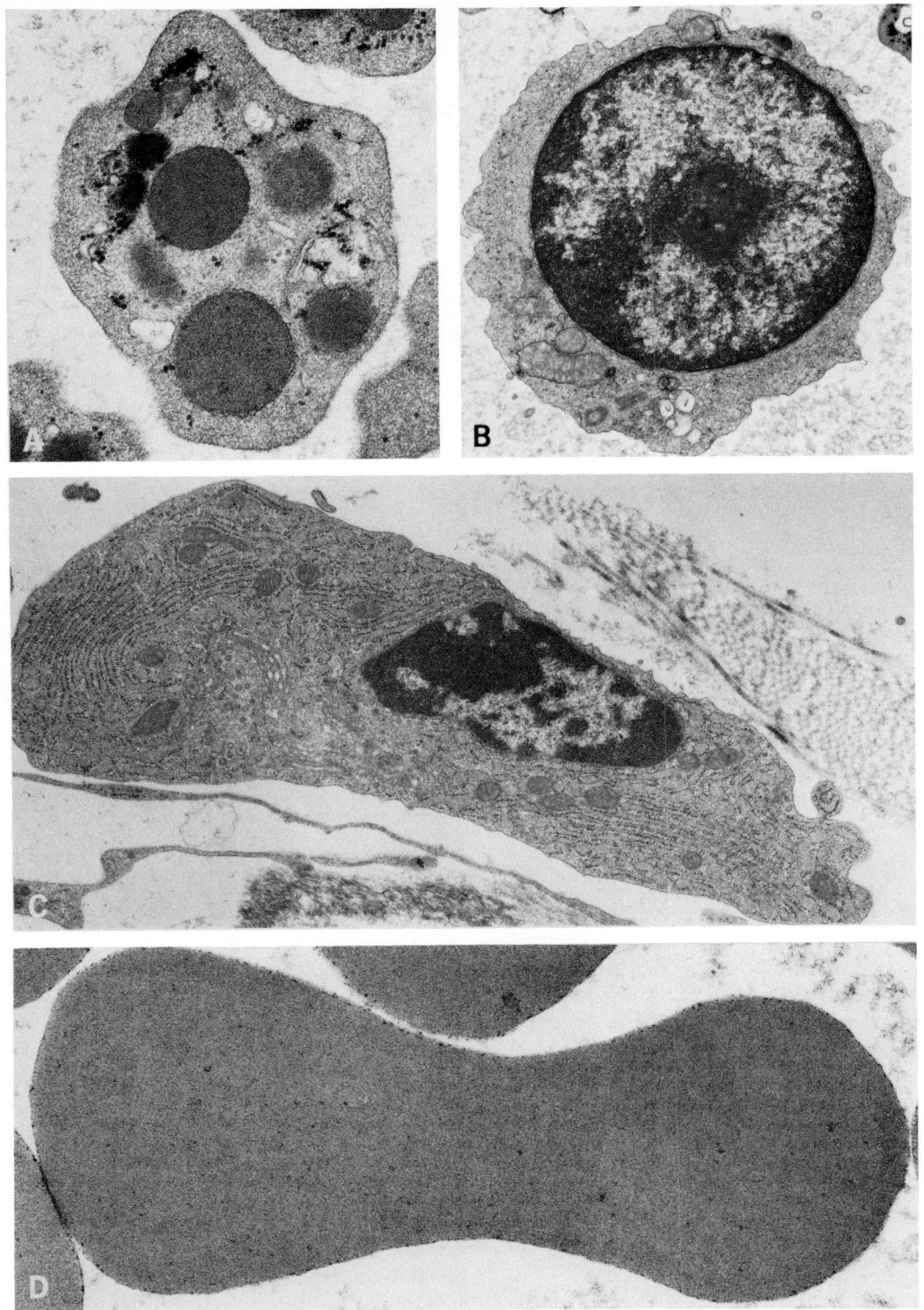

Fig. 8–3. A platelet *(A)*, lymphocyte *(B)*, plasma cell *(C)*, and erythrocyte *(D)* from the sheep. The platelet *(A)* is from a peripheral blood sample prepared for electron microscopy, and so its shape is irregular. Circulating platelets in fixed blood vessels are disc-shaped. The cytoplasm contains large, round alpha granules, smaller granules, and occasional organelles. ×36,800. The peripheral blood small lymphocyte *(B)* has an open-faced vesicular nucleus that occupies most of the cell's volume. Contained within the cytoplasmic rim are occasional mitochondria, a poorly developed Golgi complex, free ribosomes, and, in the fortuitous section, a pair of perpendicularly oriented centrioles. ×15,000. The nucleus of the plasma cell *(C)* is usually eccentric, and the chromatin is clumped peripherally. The hallmark of the plasma cell is an abundant array of densely packed rough endoplasmic reticulum. Numerous Golgi bodies and mitochondria are present. ×15,120. The mature erythrocyte *(D)* has the familiar biconcave disc shape and electron-dense hemoglobin. ×41,600. (Photographs courtesy of Drs. Kurt H. Albertine and Norman C. Staub.)

Table 8–6. Nucleated Cells in Aspirated Marrow of the Sheep

Cell Type	Range (%)	Mean (%)	Mean Cell Size (μm)
Hemocytoblasts	0.0– 0.2	0.005	33.00
Myeloblast	0.1– 1.4	0.47	19.18
Progranulocyte	0.0– 0.6	0.24	19.60
Neutrophilic myelocyte	1.5– 8.1	4.60	20.30
Neutrophilic metamyelocyte	2.1– 6.0	4.33	14.63
Band	10.6–22.8	16.38	—
Neutrophil	1.4– 6.9	4.58	—
Eosinophilic myelocyte	3.3– 6.2	4.85	20.57
Eosinophilic metamyelocyte	7.8–15.0	10.84	15.87
Eosinophil	0.8– 5.1	2.80	—
Basophil	0.3– 2.3	1.04	15.73
Total myeloid		50.13	
Rubriblast	0.5– 1.4	0.96	15.60
Prorubricyte	1.5– 4.9	3.30	13.40
Rubricyte	27.2–37.3	31.86	9.19
Metarubricyte	4.9–15.1	9.91	5.37
Total erythroid		46.03	
Plasma cell	0.0– 1.0	0.35	
Lymphocyte	0.6– 3.1	1.73	
Monocyte	0.0– 0.7	0.26	
Mitotic forms	0.2– 1.6	0.84	

M:E ratio = mean   1.103:1.0
              range   0.77–1.68:1.0

Modified from Grunsell (1951). The author has included the plasma cells, etc. in the myeloid series to obtain the M:E ratios. Actual mean M:E ratio would be 1.09:1.

lymphocytes and plasma cells (Fig. 8–3B, C) is similar to that in other species.

The Monocyte

The nucleus of the monocyte shows a chromatin pattern of lacy strands that stain relatively intense. Nuclear shape is usually ameboid, often with two or three lobes that are always of wide dimension (Fig. 8–1). The cytoplasm is rather coarse, blue-gray, and of ground-glass texture. The staining of the cytoplasm is more intense than that of the large lymphocyte. The ultrastructure of the ovine monocyte (Fig. 8–2D) is similar to that in other species.

The Platelets

Platelets are represented by small clusters of deep purple granules surrounded by a delicate membrane that is not always visible (Fig. 8–1). Several granule types are seen with the electron microscope (Fig. 8–3A). There is a marked tendency for platelets to form compact masses that vary considerably in size. Giant platelets larger than an erythrocyte may be encountered occasionally.

THE BONE MARROW

The Myeloid:Erythroid Ratio

Bone marrow is usually obtained from the sternum or iliac crest. A detailed description of marrow cells of sheep has been given along with the response of the marrow to anemia (Grunsell, 1951: 1955a, b). The M:E ratio of sternal marrow from 10 Cheviot ewes, 3–6 years of age, was 0.77–1.68:1, with a mean of 1.09:1 (Table 8–6). The M:E ratio of 8 normal lambs was $0.61 \pm 0.28:1$ (Overas, 1969). Blood values and myelograms of 18 clinically healthy, essentially parasite-free mature Merino wethers and ewes based on 112 separate samplings have been published (Winter, 1964, 1967). A higher proportion of eosinophils was found in marrow of sheep than in other species; this was thought to be a result of parasitic infection (Grunsell, 1951) or a species characteristic (Winter, 1964).

REFERENCES

Anosa, V.O., and Isoun, T.T.: Haematological Studies on Domestic Animals in Nigeria. I. Factors Influencing the Haematocrit of Sheep and Goats. Zentralbl. Veterinaermed., 25:640, 1978.
Anosa, V.O., and Ogbogu, D.A.: The Effect of Parturition

on the Blood Picture of Sheep. Res. Vet. Sci., *26*:380, 1979.

Becker, D.E., and Smith, S.E.: A Chemical and Morphological Study of Normal Sheep Blood. Cornell Vet., *40*:350, 1950.

Blunt, M.H., and Evans, J.V.: Changes in the Concentration of Potassium in Erythrocytes and in Haemoglobin Type in Merino Sheep under Severe Anaemic Stress. Nature, *200*:1215, 1963.

Blunt, M.H., et al.: The Production of Haemoglobin C by Sheep at Simulated High Altitude. Res. Vet. Sci., *11*:191, 1970.

Bolbol, A.E., et al.: Long Term Haematological and Serum Protein Changes following Splenectomy in Sheep. Vet. Res. Comm., *5*:383, 1982.

Bostedt, H.: Effect of Parenteral Administration of Iron Dextran on the Development of the Haemogram in Artificially Reared Lambs. Berl. Müench. Tierärztl. Wochenschr., *92*:236, 1979.

Boyer, S.H., et al.: Hemoglobin Switching in Non-Anemic Sheep. II. Response to High Altitude. Johns Hopkins Med. J., *123*:92, 1968.

Braend, M., et al.: Abnormal Haemoglobin in Sheep. Nature, *204*:700, 1964.

Bunce, S.: Observation on the Blood Sedimentation Rate and the Packed Cell Volume of Some Domestic Farm Animals. Brit. Vet. J., *110*:322, 1954.

Efremov, G., and Braend, M.: Haemoglobin N of Sheep: Age, Breed and Seasonal Distribution. Anim. Prod., *8*:161, 1966.

Egan, D.A., and Cuill, T.O.: Some Biochemical and Haematological Parameters of Inwintered Sheep. Brit. Vet. J., *127*(6):XV, 1971.

Evans, J.V., et al.: Genetics of Haemoglobin and Blood Potassium Differences in Sheep. Nature, *178*:849, 1956.

Evans, J.V., and Whitlock, J.H.: Genetic Relationship between Maximum Hematocrit Values and Hemoglobin Type in Sheep. Science, *145*:1318, 1964.

Fraser, A.C.: A Study of the Blood of Cattle and Sheep in Health and Disease. Rep. Dir. Inst. Anim. Path., Cambridge, *1*:114, 1929–1930.

Gajewski, J., and Povar, M.L.: Blood Coagulation Values of Sheep. Amer. J. Vet. Res., *32*:405, 1971.

Gohary, G.S.: Influence of Blood Sampling Stress on Some Blood Values of Sheep. Inaug. diss., Tierärztl. Hochsch., Hannover, Germany, 53 pp., 1978.

Gohary, G.S., and Bickhardt, K.: Influence of Blood Sampling Stress on Blood Values of Sheep. Dtsch. Tierärztl. Wochenschr., *86*:225, 1979.

Greenwood, B.: Haematology of the Sheep and Goat. *In* Comparative Clinical Haematology. Archer, R.K., Jeffcott, L.B., eds. Blackwell Scientific Publications, Oxford, p. 305, 1977.

Grunsell, C.S.: Marrow Biopsy in Sheep. I. Normal. Brit. Vet. J., *107*:16, 1951.

Grunsell, C.S.: The Marrow Cells of Normal Sheep. J. Comp. Path., *65*:8, 1955a.

Grunsell, C.S.: Seasonal Variation in the Blood and Bone Marrow of Scottish Hill Sheep. J. Comp. Path., *65*:93, 1955b.

Hackett, P.L., et al.: Blood Constituents in Suffolk Ewes and Lambs. Amer. J. Vet. Res., *18*:338, 1957.

Hawkins, P.A., and De Freitas, M.C.: Studies of Sheep Parasites. VIII. Overwintering of Nematode Larvae. J. Parasitol., *33*:Section 2, Abstr. 55, 1947.

Hay, J.B., et al.: The Effect of Exposure to Rainfall on White Blood Cell Counts in Sheep. Aust. Vet. J., *59*:60, 1982.

Holman, H.H.: Studies on the Haematology of Sheep. I. The Blood-Picture of Healthy Sheep. J. Comp. Path., *54*:26, 1944a.

Holman, H.H.: Studies on the Haematology of Sheep. III. Leucocytic Reactions. J. Comp. Path., *54*:207, 1944b.

Holz, R.C., et al.: Hemoglobin Levels of Lambs from Birth to Eight Weeks of Age and the Effects of Iron-Dextran on Suckling Lambs. J. Anim. Sci., *20*:415, 1961.

Hudson, A.E.A., and Osborn, J.C.: A Note on Certain Blood Values of Adult Sheep. Vet. Med., *49*:423, 1954.

Huisman, T.H.J., and Kitchen, J.: Oxygen Equilibria Studies of the Hemoglobins from Normal and Anemic Sheep and Goats. Amer. J. Physiol., *215*:140, 1968.

Jones, D.C.L., and Krebs, J.S.: Hematologic Characteristics of Sheep. Amer. J. Vet. Res., *33*:1537, 1972.

Karvonen, M.J.: The Diameter of Foetal Sheep Erythrocytes. Acta Anat., *20*:53, 1954.

Keay, G., and Doxey, D.L.: Serum Protein Values from Healthy Ewes and Lambs of Various Ages Determined by Agarose Gel Electrophoresis. Brit. Vet. J., *140*:85, 1984.

Kernohan, J.C.: Kinetics of the Reaction of Two Sheep Haemoglobins with Oxygen and Carbon Monoxide. J. Physiol., *155*:580, 1961.

Kitchen, H., et al.: Rapid Production of a Hemoglobin by Induced Hemolysis in Sheep: Hemoglobin C. Amer. J. Vet. Res., *29*:281, 1968.

Littleton, C.A., et al.: Organ Weight and Hematologic Studies during Neonatal Development of Lambs. Amer. J. Vet. Clin. Path., *2*:145, 1968.

Mackenzie, P.I.I., et al.: Some Blood Values for Indigenous Sheep under Natural Conditions in Rhodesia. Rhod. Vet. J., *1*:31, 1970.

Mackie, W.S.: Changes in the Concentration of Plasma Protein in Intensively Bred Ewes. J. Agric. Sci., *88*:283, 1977.

Mehrotra, P.M., and Mullick, D.N.: Studies on Physiological Reactions of Sheep. II. Seasonal Variation in the Blood Composition. Indian J. Vet. Sci., *29*:62, 1959.

Moore, S.L., et al.: The Production of Hemoglobin C in Sheep Carrying the Gene for Hemoglobin A.: Hematologic Aspects. Blood, *28*:314, 1966.

More, T., and Sahni, K.L.: Some Haematological Changes during Three Months after Birth of Chokla Lambs under Semi-Arid Conditions. Indian Vet. J., *56*:646, 1979.

Nathanielsz, P.W., et al.: Circulating Plasma Protein Concentrations in the Fetal and Neonatal Sheep. Biol. Neonate, *38*:126, 1980.

Osbaldiston, G.W.: Erythrocyte Sedimentation Rate Studies in Sheep, Dog, and Horse. Cornell Vet., *61*:386, 1971.

Overas, J.: Studies on *Eperythrozoon ovis*-Infection in Sheep. Acta Vet. Scand. Suppl., *28*:7, 1969.

Perk, K., et al.: Osmotic Fragility of Red Blood Cells of Young and Mature Domestic and Laboratory Animals. Amer. J. Vet. Res., *25*:1241, 1964.

Perk, K., and Lobl, K.: Chemical and Paper Electrophoretic Analysis of Normal Sheep Serum Proteins and Lipoproteins. Brit. Vet. J., *116*:167, 1960.

Pickart, L.R., et al.: Hyperfibrinogenemia and Polycythemia with Intrauterine Growth Retardation in Fetal Lambs. Amer. J. Obstet. Gynecol., *124*:168, 1976.

Reda, H., and Hathout, A.F.: The Haematological Examination of the Blood of Normal Sheep. Brit. Vet. J., *113*:251, 1957.

Rossouw, S.D.: A Short Study of the Isotonicity of Sheep Blood. 16th Rep. Dir. Vet. Serv. Anim. Ind. p. 525, 1930.

Singh Chakal, A., and Rattan, P.J.S.: Seasonal Variations in the Contents of Haemoglobin and the Packed-Cell Volume in the Blood of Corriedale Rams. J. Res. Punjab Agric. Univ., *18*:344, 1981.

Sziegoleit, A., et al.: Influence of the Age of Sheep Red Blood Cells on Virus-Induced Hypotonic Hemolysis. Med. Microbiol. Immunol., *168*:211, 1980.

Thurmon, R.F., et al.: Hemoglobin Switching in Nonanemic Sheep. III. Evidence for Presumptive Identity between the A-C Factor and Erythropoietin. Blood, *36*:598, 1970.

Tocantins, L.M.: The Mammalian Blood Platelet in Health and Disease. Medicine, *17*:155, 1938.

Todd, A.C., et al.: On the Blood Picture of Healthy Southdown and Hampshire Ewes. Amer. J. Vet. Res., *13*:74, 1952.

Tucker, E.M.: Red Cell Life Span in Young and Adult Sheep. Res. Vet. Sci., *4*:11, 1963.

Tucker, E.M.: The Life Span and Other Physiological Properties of Sheep Red Cells Containing Type A, B, or C (N) Haemoglobin. Res. Vet. Sci., *7*:368, 1966.

Tucker, E.M.: The Onset of Anaemia and the Production of Haemoglobin C in Sheep Fed on Kale. Brit. Vet. J., *125*:472, 1969.

Tucker, E.M.: A Shortened Life Span of Sheep Red Cells with a Glutathione Deficiency. Res. Vet. Sci., *16*:19, 1974.

Turner, A.W., and Hodgetts, V.E.: The Dynamic Red Cell Storage Function of the Spleen in Sheep. I. Relationship to Fluctuations of Jugular Haematocrit. Aust. J. Exp. Biol. Med. Sci., *37*:399, 1959.

Ullrey, D.E., et al.: Sheep Hematology from Birth to Maturity. J. Anim. Sci., *24*:141, 1965.

Upcott, D.H., et al.: Erythrocyte and Leukocyte Parameters in Newborn Lambs. Res. Vet. Sci., *12*:474, 1971.

Vaccaro-Torracca, A.M., et al.: Higher Oxygen Affinity of Sheep Hb C Compared to Hb A and Hb B. Experientia, *36*:559, 1980.

van der Helm, H.J., et al.: Investigations on Two Different Hemoglobins of the Sheep. Arch Biochem. Biophys., *72*:331, 1957.

van Vliet, G., and Huisman, T.H.J.: Changes in the Haemoglobin Types of Sheep as a Response to Anaemia. Biochem. J., *93*:401, 1964.

Watson, D.F.: Studies on the Hemoglobin Content of Sheep Blood in the Sierra of Peru. Amer. J. Vet. Res., *14*:405, 1953.

Winter, H.: The Myelogram of Normal Sheep. J. Comp. Path., *74*:457, 1964.

Winter, H.: Myelogram of Sheep in Posthemorrhagic Anemia. Amer. J. Vet. Res., *28*:1389, 1967.

Wirth, D.: Grundlagen einer Klinischen Hämatologie der Haustiere. Urban und Schwarzenberg, Vienna, 1950.

9

The Goat: Normal Hematology with Comments on Response to Disease

THE ERYTHROCYTES 225
    Age-Related Changes 225
    Packed Cell Volume and Hemoglobin 225
    Influence of Season, Sex, Pregnancy, and
        Lactation 229
    Reticulocytes 229
    Erythrocyte Sedimentation Rate 229
    Erythrocyte Osmotic Fragility 229
    Hemoglobin Types 230

THE LEUKOCYTES 231

THE PLATELETS 231

THE PLASMA 232
    Icterus Index 232
    Total Plasma Proteins and Fibrinogen 232

MORPHOLOGY OF BLOOD CELLS 232
    The Erythrocytes 232
    The Neutrophil 236
    The Eosinophil 236
    The Basophil 238
    The Lymphocyte 238
    The Monocyte 238
    The Platelets 238

THE BONE MARROW 238

Data from the literature on hematology of the goat are presented in Tables 9–1 and 9–2. Holman and Dew (1963, 1964, 1965a, b, 1966a, b) have performed extensive studies on the blood of the normal goat from birth to maturity. Greenwood (1977) has provided a comprehensive description of goat hematology, and observations on pigmy goats have been described by Castero et al. (1977).

THE ERYTHROCYTES

Age-Related Changes

The data of Holman and Dew (1964, 1965a) indicate that erythrocyte numbers from birth (8.14 million/μl of blood) fall during the first week of life (7.3 million), then rapidly increase to peak levels at 3 months (20.05 million), and thereafter decline gradually to reach adult levels (11–12 million) at 3 years of age (Table 9–1). Similar trends were reported by other workers (DeShaw et al., 1969; Edjtechade, 1978; Wilkins and Hodges, 1962).

Age-related changes have been observed in MCV. At birth, mean MCV was 45.1 fl, followed by a decline to 16.9 fl at 3 months of age. Between 3 and 30 months, erythrocyte

size increased, attaining adult values of 23–24 fl. Our own data, for 18 nonanemic goats presenting various clinical problems, gave a mean MCV of 19.6 ± 2.5 fl and MCHC of 32.6 ± 2.2 g/dl. MCH is influenced by erythrocyte size and hemoglobin concentration. It varies little with age within the narrow range of 5.0–8.0 pg.

Packed Cell Volume and Hemoglobin

The small size of the goat erythrocyte places special requirements on centrifugation for a valid PCV. The Wintrobe method, which employs 2,250 G for 30 minutes, leaves an average of 20% plasma trapped within the column of packed red cells (see Chapter 3). When the PCV is significantly influenced by trapped plasma, MCV and MCHC are also spurious, i.e., the MCV is larger and the MCHC is smaller than the true value. PCV, MCV, and MCHC of goat erythrocytes as influenced by degree of relative centrifugal force and time are shown in Table 9–3. It is conjectured that proper centrifugation of normal blood of the goat should provide an MCHC value not less than 30% or more than 36%. MCHC values in excess of 36% may re-

Normal Blood Values for the Goat

Erythrocytic Series	Range	Ave.	Leukocytic Series	Range	Ave.
Erythrocytes ($\times 10^6/\mu$l)	8.0–18.0	13.0	Leukocytes/μl	4,000–13,000	9,000
Hemoglobin (g/dl)	8.0–12.0	10.0	Neutrophil (band)	Rare	—
PCV (%)			Neutrophil (mature)	1,200–7,200	3,250
Wintrobe			Lymphocyte	2,000–9,000	5,000
(2,250 G $\times$ 30 min)	24.0–48.0	35.0	Monocyte	0–550	250
Microhematocrit			Eosinophil	50–650	450
(14,000 G $\times$ 10 min)	22–38	28.0	Basophil	0–120	50
MCV (fl)					
(Wintrobe)	19.5–37	27	Percentage Distribution		
(Microhematocrit)	16–25	19.5	Neutrophil	30–48	36.0
MCHC (%)			Lymphocyte	50–70	56.0
(Wintrobe)	28–34	31.5	Monocyte	0–4	2.5
(Microhematocrit)	30–36	33	Eosinophil	1–8	5.0
MCH (pg) (Microhematocrit)	5.2–8.0	6.5	Basophil	0–1	0.5
Reticulocytes (%)	none	—			
ESR (mm)	none	—			
RBC diameter (μm)	2.5–3.9	3.2			
Resistance to hypotonic saline (%)					
Min.	0.74	—			
Max.	0.44	—			
Myeloid:erythroid ratio	0.69:1.0				

Other Data		
Thrombocytes ($\times 10^5/\mu$l)	3.0–6.0	4.5
Icterus index (units)	2–5	
Plasma proteins (g/dl)	6.0–7.5	
Fibrinogen (g/dl)	0.1–0.4	
Erythrocyte life span (days)	125	

sult from (a) use of excessive centrifugal force, (b) shrinkage of erythrocytes due to excessive EDTA anticoagulant, or (c) hemolysis (see Chapter 2).

It has been reported that PCV is high at birth (36.6%), initially declines by 1 month (23.7%), then rises by 3 months (33.9%), and attains adult levels (28.7%) by 2 years of age (Holman and Dew, 1964). Age-related changes also occurred in Hb concentration. It was found to be 11.6 ± 1.32 g/dl at birth and decreased to 10.1 g/dl by the second day, possibly owing mainly to hemodilution through nursing. However, a gradual reduction in Hb concentration took place in the growing kid, reaching a low level of 8.27 ± 1.59 g/dl at 1 month of age. Thereafter, Hb concentration increased again to 12.1 ± 1.1 g/dl at 3 months of age. At 2 years of age, hemoglobin of 50 females was 11.09 ± 1.78 g/dl and for goats 3 years and over, a reduction to 9.85 ± 1.31 g/dl was observed. Hb values for goats in the Philippines were found to range from 7.31–11.03 g/dl, with a mean of 9.69 ± 0.13 (Gonzaga and DeGuman, 1964). Only minor differences were found in PCV and Hb values

of venous and arterial blood (Houchin et al., 1939).

The rapid fall of Hb concentration in neonatal goats was found to be due to iron deficiency. Due to the low iron content of milk, the growing nursing kid becomes deficient in iron as its blood volume expands to accommodate the increasing body size. Injection of 150 mg of iron dextran into newborn kids prevented the decrease in Hb and PCV values observed in the untreated kids (Holman and Dew, 1966b). The difference between treated and untreated kids was greatest at 1 month of age and disappeared by 3 months of age. In addition, the erythrocytes were smaller in the untreated kids than in those receiving iron dextran. On the basis of normal values proposed in this book, values reported for normal goats by some investigators (Table 9–1; Murty and Kehar, 1951; Mukherjee and Bhattacharya, 1952; Vaidya et al., 1970) would be considered suggestive of anemia. Recent observations (Bhargava, 1980) on 50 healthy Marwari goats, 1.75–2 years of age, from India, were found to have higher mean Hb (10.09 g/dl) than reported earlier.

Table 9-1. Red Blood Cell Parameters of Apparently Normal Goats as Reported in the Literature (means and 1 SD or range)

Reference	No. of Goats	Sex and Age	RBC ($\times10^6/\mu l$)	PCV (%)	Hb (g/dl)	MCV (fl)	MCH (pg)	MCHC (%)
Murty and Kehar (1951)	30	Males, 9–30 mo	12.70±0.35	29.8±0.8	6.7±0.2	23.5±0.5	5.3±0.1	22.7±0.4
Mukherjee and Bhattacharya (1952)[a]	8	Males (August)	—	27.7±0.7	5.9±0.1	—	—	—
		Males (February)	—	31.7±1.3	6.6±0.7	—	—	—
Millson et al. (1960)	10	8 castrated males, 2 females, 20 mo	12–18	26–39	9.5–13.6	—	—	—
Wilkins and Hodges (1962)	48	Female adults	13.94±2.80	28.9±5.1	11.4±1.6	21.1±3.1	8.4±1.6	39.6±4.4
	6	Male adults	14.95±2.40	27.2±5.2	10.6±1.6	18.1±1.7	7.2±0.8	39.5±3.6
	6	Castrated male adults	16.34±2.10	34.8±3.8	13.1±1.2	21.4±0.8	8.1±0.5	37.7±2.1
	6	Male kids	19.15±1.17	31.9±1.9	11.7±0.7	16.7±1.7	6.1±0.7	36.7±2.8
Holman and Dew (1963)	50	Females, 2–3 yr	12.73±2.63	28.7±4.5	11.1±1.8	22.7±3.8	—	40.2±4.6
Holman and Dew (1964, 1965a)	40	1st day of life	8.14±1.32	36.6±5.1	11.6±1.3	45.1±4.3	—	31.3±2.3
	33	1 week	7.30±0.73	27.7±3.7	9.6±1.1	38.1±5.0	—	33.9±3.2
	33	1 mo	11.33±1.19	23.7±4.5	8.3±1.6	20.4±3.3	—	34.5±3.0
	34	3 mo	20.05±2.69	33.9±3.6	12.1±1.1	16.9±1.6	—	35.1±3.0
	60	2 yr	12.73±2.63	28.7±3.6	11.1±1.8	22.7±3.7	—	40.2±4.6
	35	3 yr and over	11.20±1.33	27.7±4.1	9.9±1.3	24.3±2.1	—	34.4±2.8
DeShaw et al. (1969)	5	1–2 mo	11.86±0.52	22.2±0.6	8.8±0.3	18.8±0.7	7.7±0.2	—
		3–12 mo	17.77±0.15	27.2±0.3	10.5±0.1	15.3±0.1	5.9±0.1	—
Vaidya et al. (1970)	—	Male kids	11.10±0.65	—	7.8±0.2	—	—	—
		Female kids	12.60±0.44	—	8.0±0.4	—	—	—
		Male adult	12.40±0.78	—	8.5±0.2	—	—	—
		Female adult	8.80±0.49	—	6.7±0.1	—	—	—
Schalm (1975)	18	Mature, nonanemic; variety of clinical problems	15.56±2.28	30.3±4.5[b]	10.0±1.1[c]	19.6±2.5	6.5±0.8	32.9±1.8
Bhargava (1980)	10	Mature, anemic	9.74±1.69	19.8±2.4[b]	6.4±0.7[c]	20.3±3.2	6.6±0.9	32.6±2.2
	50	Marwari, 1.75–2 yr	8.5–12.6 (10.1)	27–35 (32)	7.1–11.2 (10.1)	27.4–35.4 (31.1)	8.3–11.5 (8.4)	21.1–35.7 (26.7)
Pyne et al. (1982)	42	Black Bengal, 11–14 mo	12.35±0.35	—	10.0±0.6	—	—	—

[a] Monthly PCV and Hb values were reported; data shown represent lowest and highest PCV values only.
[b] 14,000 G for 10 min.
[c] Cyanmethemoglobin method.

Table 9–2. Leukocyte Values of Apparently Normal Goats as Reported in the Literature (means and 1 SD or range)

Reference	No. of Goats	Sex and Age	WBC (/μl)	Differential Leukocyte Count									
				Neutrophils		Lymphocytes		Monocytes		Eosinophils		Basophils	
				No./μl	%	No./μl	%	No./μl	%	No./μl	%	No./μl	%
Millson et al. (1960)	10	8 castrated males, 2 females, 20 mo	9,000–15,000	—	21–44	—	53–79	—	0–2	—	0–4	—	0–1
Wilkins and Hodges (1962)	48	Female adults	8,200±2,400	—	42.4±13.9	—	54.1±15.1	—	1.7±1.4	—	2.3±1.9	—	—
	6	Male adults	9,200±3,500	—	51.9±11.7	—	40.3±9.1	—	2.7±1.1	—	3.3±3.9	—	—
	6	Castrated male adults	7,700±1,200	—	30.5±8.3	—	65.9±9.4	—	2.6±0.9	—	0.9±0.4	—	—
	6	Male kids	11,700±3,100	—	29.8±5.4	—	68.1±6.7	—	1.3±0.8	—	0.7±0.5	—	—
Holman and Dew (1963)	50	Females 2–3 yr	8,083±2,511	3,980±1,550	49.0±10.7	3,713±1,601	42.3±10.4	229±164	3.1±2.5	148±141	1.9±1.6	7±24	0.09±0.29
Holman and Dew (1965b)	40	1st day of life	7,523±2,947	4,481±2,813	55.2±17.9	2,780±1,008	41.3±14.9	—	2.0±1.3	—	1.6±0.7	—	0.2
	33	1 week old	8,904±4,140	3,491±1,117	42.9±11.8	4,575±950	52.4±11.9	—	2.6±1.2	—	0.2	—	0.5
	33	1 mo	9,239±2,416	3,357±1,809	32.7±10.8	5,786±1,880	62.5±9.4	—	2.1±1.7	—	1.0	—	0.1
	34	3 mo	18,180±3,835	4,053±2,830	22.5±5.8	13,236±1,203	72.6±11.5	—	2.0±3.7	—	1.1	—	0.4
	60	2 yr	8,083±2,511	3,980±1,550	49.0±10.7	3,713±1,601	42.3±10.4	—	3.1±2.5	—	1.9	—	0.9
	35	3 yr and over	9,731±2,507	4,614±1,973	47.7±12.2	4,642±1,313	48.2±12.0	—	2.2±1.0	—	1.5	—	0.2
DeShaw et al. (1969)	5	1–2 mo	12,240±840	1,400±200	10.2±0.8	10,840±690	89.8±0.8	—		—		—	—
		3–12 mo	13,530±240	4,440±160	32.5±1.0	9,130±210	67.5±1.0	—		—		—	—
Vaidya et al. (1970)	—	Male kids	15,900±800	—	37.9±1.6	—	56.5±1.6	—	3.1±0.3	—	2.5±0.8	—	—
	—	Female kids	15,700±710	—	37.7±2.1	—	54.7±2.4	—	3.3±0.3	—	4.3±0.9	—	—
		Male adult	13,800±910	—	47.8±2.1	—	45.9±2.7	—	2.0±0.3	—	4.3±0.6	—	—
		Female adult	13,900±810	—	48.0±2.5	—	45.0±2.5	—	2.2±0.2	—	4.8±0.6	—	—
Bhargava (1980)	50	Marwari, 1.75–2 yr	6,900–14,000 (10,090)	—	28–66 (39)	—	29–69 (57.7)	—	1–4 (2.1)	—	1–4 (1.1)	—	0–0.5 (0.04)
Pyne et al. (1982)	42	Black Bengal, 11–14 mo	10,180±240	—	34.6±0.7	—	60.3±0.1	—	3.1±0.2	—	2.0±0.1	—	0.04±0.02

Table 9–3. Several Examples of the Effect of Centrifugation of Goat Blood at Different Combinations of Centrifugal Force and Time

| Specimen | Erythrocyte Values | | | Wintrobe Method 2,250 G for 30 min | Microhematocrit Method, 14,000 G | |
	RBC (×10⁶/μl)	Hb (g/dl)	Other		2 min	10 min
Mature	13.6	8.5	PCV (%)	27	25	23
female			MCV (fl)	19.3	17.8	16.4
(normal)			MCHC (%)	30.0	32.4	35.2
Mature	13.6	10.8	PCV (%)	—	34.0	30.0
female			MCV (fl)	—	25.0	22.0
(infection)			MCHC (%)	—	30.7	36.0
Female	15.15	9.6	PCV (%)	32	30	27
2 yr old			MCV (fl)	21.1	19.8	17.8
(mastitis)			MCHC (%)	30	32.0	35.5
Kid	11.3	10.8	PCV (%)	38	33	33
12 days old			MCV (fl)	33.6	29.2	29.2
(infection)			MCHC (%)	28.4	32.7	32.7
Kid	12.6	9.5	PCV (%)	35	31	30
6 weeks old			MCV (fl)	27.8	24.6	23.8
(infection)			MCHC (%)	27.1	30.6	31.6

Influence of Season, Sex, Pregnancy, and Lactation

Higher RBC, Hb, and PCV values were found in the late summer and autumn than in the winter and spring (Holman and Dew, 1966a). A similar pattern was detected for blood viscosity. With the increase in ambient temperature, humidity, and rainfall, a concomitant decrease in the Hb and PCV values was noted (Mukherjee and Bhattacharya, 1952).

Sex differences in erythrocyte parameters have been observed in some studies. After 3 months of age, male goats were found to have a higher RBC count than females, although PCV and Hb concentration remained the same because of the smaller size of male erythrocytes (Holman and Dew, 1966a). Significantly greater values for both RBC count and Hb concentration were found for adult male goats than for adult female goats in India (Table 9–1; Vaidya et al., 1980). In an earlier study (Wilkins and Hodges, 1962), slightly greater Hb and PCV values were found in adult females than in adult males, and all three red cell parameters were significantly higher in 6 male castrated goats than in either of the intact sexes.

Pregnancy was not found to influence red cell parameters significantly, but PCV values decreased over the first 5 months of lactation mainly because of a decrease in cell size.

Reticulocytes

No reticulocytes are found in peripheral blood of goats in health. Small numbers appear in the circulation during anemia in remission, but reticulocytosis in response to anemia is not as prominent as in cattle. A 40% and 36% reduction in Hb concentration of 2 goats by periodic bleeding over a 3-week period was associated with a maximal reticulocytosis of 5.2% and 5.7%, respectively (Tables 9–4, 9–5).

Erythrocyte Sedimentation Rate

Rouleau formation is absent in health or present only to a minor degree in thicker areas of the film. This absence of significant rouleaux correlates with lack of sedimentation during the usual observation period of 1 hour. However, 2–3 mm of settling may take place over a period of 24 hours (Bunce, 1954; Holman and Dew, 1963).

Erythrocyte Osmotic Fragility

When animals are listed in the order of their red cell volumes, they are also arranged in order of the degree of hypotonicity that produces beginning hemolysis (Ponder, 1935). On this basis, among red cells of common domestic and laboratory animals the small red cells of the goat appear to be the most sensitive to hypotonic saline (see Table 20–2). Minimum resistance is reported at 0.66%

Table 9–4. Hematological Changes in Goat 6773 as a Result of Blood Loss Anemia

Week after Start of Bleeding[a]	RBC (10⁶/μl)	Hb (g/dl)	PCV (%)	Plasma Proteins (g/dl)	MCV (fl)	MCHC (%)	MCH (pg)	Reticulocytes (%)[b]	Erythrocyte Types (%)		
									Fusiform	Other Forms	Discoid
0	17.88	11.75	29.0	7.5	16.2	40.5	6.6	0	50	10	40
3	10.29	7.00	20.0	6.0	19.4	35.0	6.8	1.8	26	13	61
5	8.24	7.25	19.5	6.0	23.7	37.2	8.8	2.5	13	40	47
8	8.10	6.00	16.0	6.1	19.7	37.5	7.4	1.3	4	82	14
13	17.31	11.00	29.0	7.1	16.7	37.9	6.3	3	3	69	28
17	17.43	10.50	28.0	7.1	16.1	37.5	6.0	0	17	24	59
21	17.82	10.50	29.0	7.5	16.3	39.5	6.5	0	27	12	61
25	17.64	10.50	26.0	7.5	14.7	40.4	6.0	0	32	16	52
28	15.45	10.25	26.0	7.7	16.8	39.4	6.6	0	49	14	37

From Jain et al., 1980.
[a]Bleeding to induce anemia discontinued after the eighth week.
[b]Highest count of 5.7% recorded at the fourth week.

saline solution and maximum resistance at 0.44% (Perk et al., 1964). Erythrocytes of 50 female goats, 2 years of age, exhibited complete hemolysis at a mean saline concentration of $0.634 \pm 0.065\%$, with a range between 0.500 and 0.725% saline (Holman and Dew, 1963). Osmotic fragility was found to increase from birth to 2 years of age and then decline slightly; complete hemolysis was observed at a mean saline concentration of $0.382 \pm 0.051\%$ at birth; at $0.414 \pm 0.055\%$ at 4 weeks of age; at $0.500 \pm 0.035\%$ at 12 weeks of age; at $0.634 \pm 0.065\%$ at 2 years of age; and at $0.540 \pm 0.043\%$ at the age of 3 years or older (Holman and Dew, 1965b).

Osmotic and mechanical fragilities of erythrocytes were determined for 7 goats having 3.4–71.0% fusiform erythrocytes (Jain et al., 1980). The osmotic fragility, but not mechanical fragility, was related to the red cell shape in that the osmotic resistance was consider-

ably higher for bloods containing more than 26% fusiform erythrocytes than for bloods with less than 10% such cells. The former exhibited 50% hemolysis at 0.56–0.58% saline concentration, while the latter exhibited 50% hemolysis at 0.69–0.77%.

Hemoglobin Types

Hemoglobin types in normal adult goats are A, B, and AB (Holman and Dew, 1965a). In addition, fetal hemoglobin is present in the neonate but disappears by the second month of life. HbA was found to be replaced by HbC in goats made anemic by weekly bleeding for 5–7 weeks (Blunt et al., 1969). In the more severely anemic goat, reticulocytes increased to 5% concurrently with the increase in HbC. Although the number of reticulocytes bore no relationship to the amount of HbC, in general reticulocytosis seemed to occur before HbC could be measured accurately. It was con-

Table 9–5. Hematological Changes in Goat 6828 as a Result of Blood Loss Anemia

Week after Start of Bleeding[a]	RBC (10⁶/μl)	Hb (g/dl)	PCV (%)	Plasma Proteins (g/dl)	MCV (fl)[b]	MCHC (%)	MCH (pg)	Reticulocytes (%)[c]	Erythrocyte Types (%)		
									Fusiform	Other Forms	Discoid
0	17.91	11.0	29.0	7.2	16.2	37.9	6.1	0	1	1	98
3	10.14	7.0	21.0	6.2	20.7	33.3	6.9	3.6	1	11	88
5	8.24	7.0	20.5	6.0	24.9	34.1	8.5	4.2	1	36	63
8	8.76	7.0	19.5	5.6	21.7	36.8	8.0	2.5	1	37	62
13	15.30	11.5	30.0	7.0	19.6	38.3	7.5	0	0	21	79
17	16.44	11.5	29.0	6.9	17.3	39.6	7.0	0	1	6	93
21	16.74	10.5	28.0	6.6	16.7	37.5	6.3	0	1	5	94
25	17.13	11.0	28.0	7.2	16.3	39.3	6.4	0	2	7	91
28	17.55	10.5	27.5	7.2	15.7	38.2	6.0	0	1	3	96

From Jain et al., 1980.
[a]Bleeding to induce anemia discontinued after the eighth week.
[b]Highest value of 27.4 fl recorded at the sixth week.
[c]Highest count of 5.2% recorded at the sixth week.

cluded that the switch from HbA to HbC was easier to induce through bleeding of goats than through bleeding of sheep. Furthermore, for comparable degrees of anemia, goats apparently produced more HbC than did sheep, and the rate of elimination of HbC from peripheral blood was slower in goats than in sheep. In a study of 208 Iranian nomadic goats, 3 hemoglobin types giving 4 phenotypes (B, AB, BC, and ABC) were found (Mostaghni, 1979). The distribution of various phenotypes was as follows: HbB predominated (61.5%) and had the highest gene frequency; HbBC comprised 23.0%, HbAB 9.6%, and HbABC 5.7%.

THE LEUKOCYTES

Literature values are given in Table 9–2. WBC counts were found to be 8,083 ± 2,511/µl of blood for 50 adult female goats (Holman and Dew, 1963), and 8,200 ± 2,400/µl for 48 adult female and 9,200 ± 3,500/µl for 6 adult male goats (Wilkins and Hodges, 1962). An age influence was found in total and differential leukocyte counts, primarily because of lymphocyte numbers. The WBC count increased from birth to peak about the third or fourth month, then decreased to levels seen at birth. The WBC count averaged 7,523 ± 2,947/µl over the first 24 hours, was below 10,000/µl for the first 4 weeks of life, increased to 18,180 ± 3,835/µl at 3 months of age, and subsequently fell to 8,083 ± 2,511/µl at 2 years of age (Table 9–2; Holman and Dew, 1965b). Average neutrophil number was 4,481 ± 2,813/µl during the first 24 hours, decreased to 2,240 ± 1,022/µl by the second week, and then increased to 4,053 ± 2,830/µl at 3 months of age, after which it fluctuated between 3,500 and 5,000/µl of blood. In comparison, lymphocytes gradually increased from 2,780 ± 1,008/µl at birth to 13,236 ± 1,203/µl at 3 months of age, then declined to 3,713 ± 1,601/µl at 24 months of age and almost equaled neutrophils at 3 years of age.

On a percentage basis, neutrophils exceeded (55.2 ± 17.9%) lymphocytes (41.3 ± 14.9%) at birth, with reversal of the ratio occurring at 1 week and attaining respective values of 22.5 ± 5.8% and 72.6 ± 11.5% at 3 months of age. Subsequent reduction in lym-

phocyte numbers without similar changes in neutrophils brought the ratio near unity in goats aged 3 years and over. Immature neutrophils (band forms) in peripheral blood rose from an average of 0.42% to 2.5% on the fourth day of life, then fell to 1.0% in the second week, and were absent thereafter. Significant changes were not seen in monocytes, eosinophils, and basophils. The differential leukocyte count in most reports on the normal mature goat places neutrophils at 47–48% and lymphocytes at 42–45%. Others have given a slight edge to the lymphocytes (Millson et al., 1960; Wilkins and Hodges, 1962). Higher eosinophil and basophil numbers were found in adult goats than in juvenile Mexican goats, probably as a result of changes in immunologic experience (Earl and Carranza, 1980). In this study, small lymphocytes were found to be about twice as frequent in kids as in adult goats. In one study, lymphocytes were about 92% at 1 month of age, 76% at 3 months, and 58% at 11 months (DeShaw et al., 1969).

Band neutrophils are fairly common in peripheral blood in association with neutrophilia in response to disease. A left shift to metamyelocytes is infrequent, and myelocytes have rarely been encountered. WBC counts in disease have been observed to attain levels of 22,000–27,000/µl, mainly as a result of neutrophilia. The highest WBC count so far recorded by us was 36,300/µl of blood in a 7-year-old female goat with a kidney abscess. Leukopenia was not observed in 32 goats presented with a variety of clinical problems, some of which were inflammatory in nature.

THE PLATELETS

Platelet counts reported in the literature include an average value of 500,000/µl for the goat (Wirth, 1950), a representative value of 421,000 ± 134,000/µl for 60 adult goats and of 517,000 ± 88,000/µl for 6 male kid goats (Wilkins and Hodges, 1962). Holman and Dew (1963, 1965b) reported platelet numbers in kids and mature goats considerably lower than counts reported above and considered normal.

THE PLASMA

Icterus Index

Color of the plasma is not influenced by plant pigments, as in the cow. The color in health is comparable to 2–5 units of icterus index.

Total Plasma Proteins and Fibrinogen

Total plasma proteins of 6.7–7.85 g/dl in 8 castrated males and 2 intact female goats have been reported (Millson et al., 1960). The total plasma protein of 10 mature goats considered to be clinically normal ranged from 6.6–7.5 g/dl (mean, 7.1 ± 0.5). Among 23 mature goats, presented with various clinical problems, total plasma proteins ranged from 4.8 (Johne's disease) to 8.3 g/dl (mean 6.8 ± 0.8). Total plasma proteins decreased from 7.0 ± 0.15 g/dl to 5.7 ± 0.12 g/dl within 8 days of normal parturition or cesarian section (Verma and Tyagi, 1974). A decrease in total plasma protein concentration was observed between 10 and 50 days after experimental infection with cysticerci of *Taenia hydatigena* (Pathak and Gaur, 1981). Hyperproteinemia, princi-

pally due to increase in γ-globulins, occurred in goats chronically infected with *Corynebacterium pseudotuberculosis* (Desiderio et al., 1979).

Plasma fibrinogen appears from our limited data to have a normal range of 0.1–0.4 g/dl. Two goats with Johne's disease had fibrinogen values of 0.2–0.4 g/dl. A goat presenting abnormal central nervous system signs and another goat with enteritis each had 0.7 g/dl of fibrinogen. Another goat with abnormal central nervous system signs had 1.1 g/dl, and a goat with kidney abscess had plasma fibrinogen of 1.0 g/dl. These limited findings may indicate that the goat is not as responsive as the cow in elevating plasma fibrinogen in response to disease.

MORPHOLOGY OF BLOOD CELLS

The Erythrocytes

The red blood cells of the goat are the smallest among the domestic animals. Erythrocytes of the adult goat may be fairly discocytic and slightly biconcave or bluntly triangular (Fig.

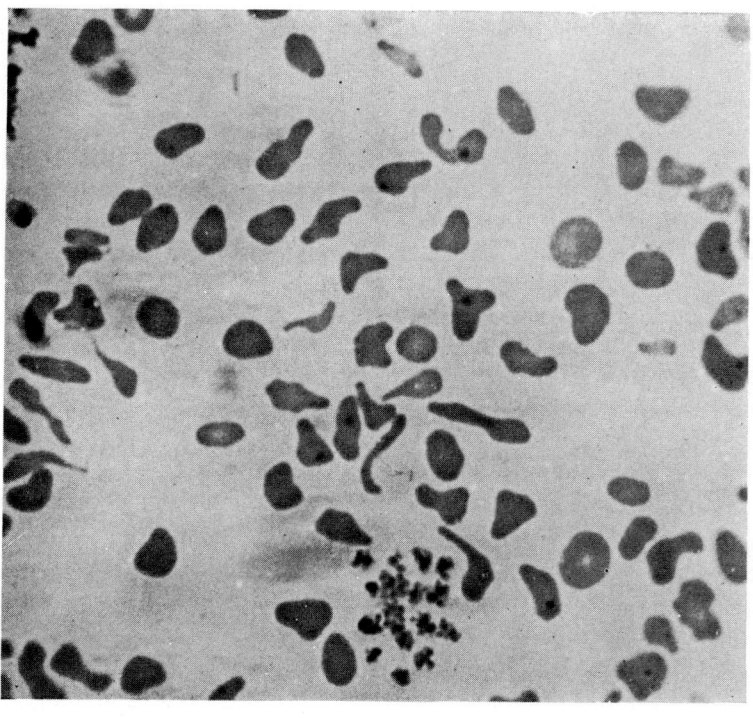

Fig. 9–1.   Poikilocytes (irregularly shaped erythrocytes) in the blood of a goat kid 2 months of age. The dark spherical body in each of several poikilocytes may be a Howell-Jolly body. A cluster of thrombocytes is seen at bottom center.

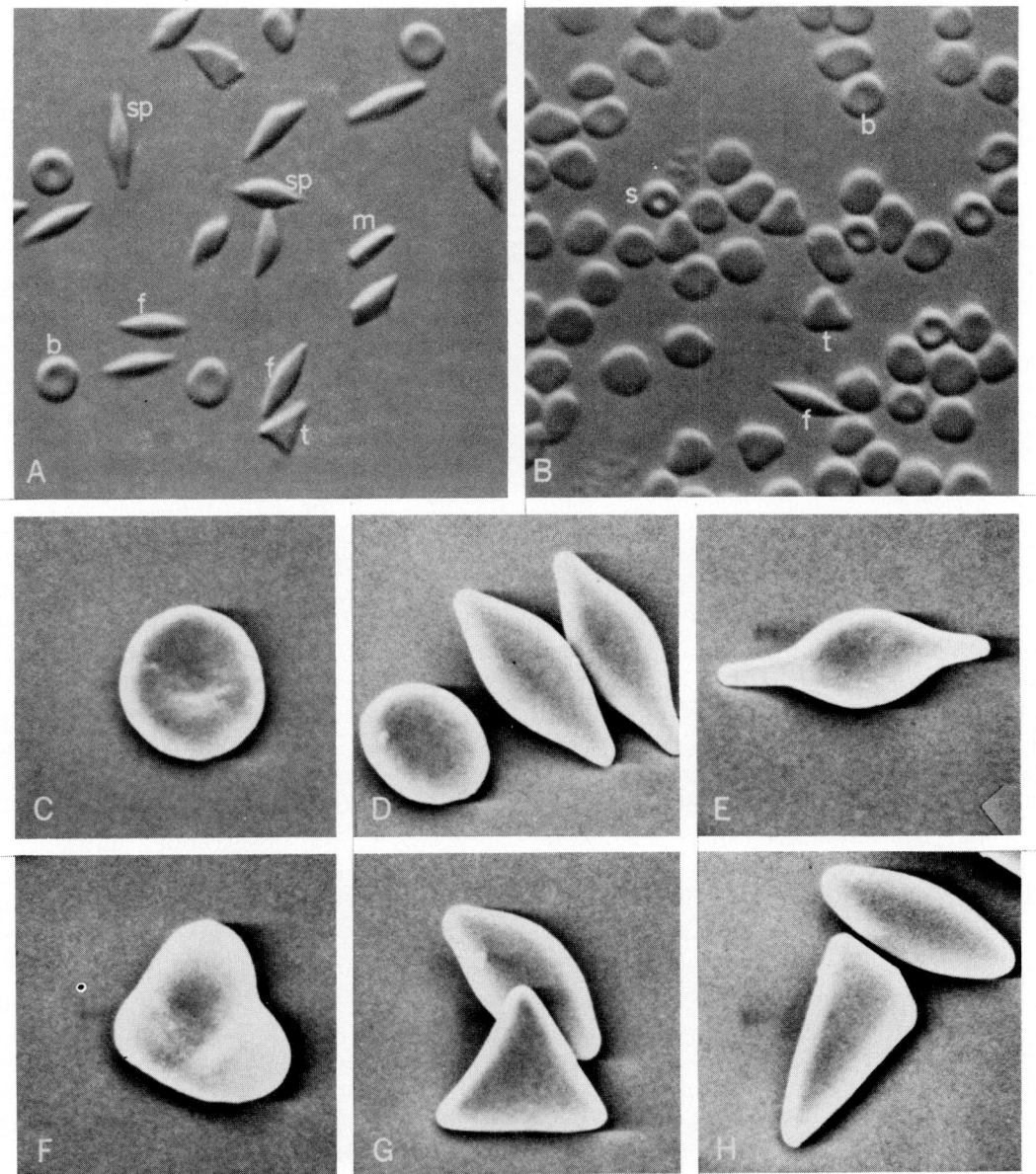

Fig. 9–2. Morphology of erythrocytes from two Angora goats, one with nearly 60% fusiform cells *(A, C–H)* and another with only 2% such cells *(B)*. *A* and *B* are from wet preparations of fresh blood examined with Nomarski interference-contrast optics; various forms of fusiform (f), spindle-shaped (sp), matchstick (m), and triangular (t) cells are compared with stomatocytes (s) and normal discoid cells (b). Scanning electron photomicrographs (C–H) of glutaraldehyde-fixed cells show their distinctive morphology. *A* and *B,* ×1,450; C–H, ×4,500. (From Jain and Kono, 1977a.)

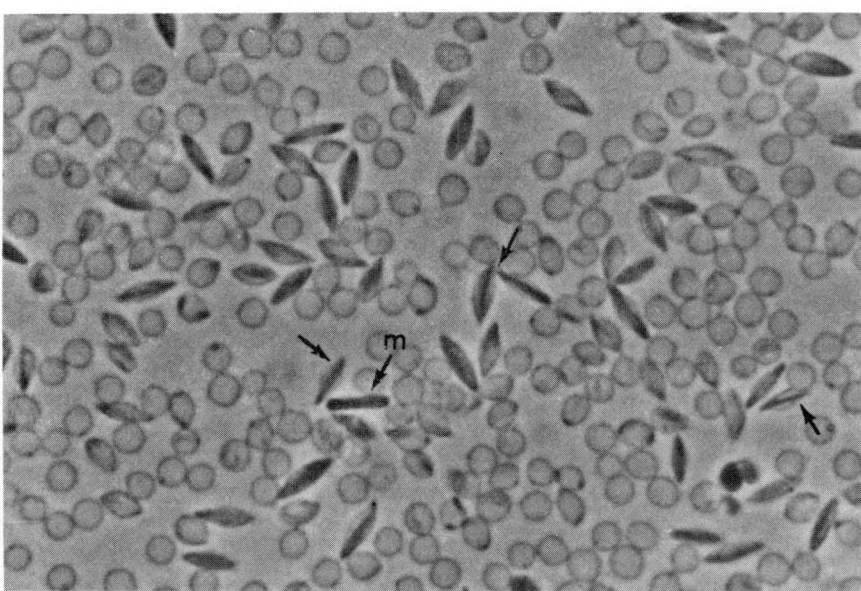

Fig. 9–3. Blood film stained with new methylene blue. Partially lysed fusiform erythrocytes containing a dense bar of polymerized hemoglobin *(arrows)* can be seen among spheroidal erythrocytic ghosts. A matchstick form (m) with a dense hemoglobin rod is also present. Many spheroidal ghost cells contain one or two granules representing precipitated hemoglobin. ×425. (From Jain and Kono, 1977a.)

9–2*B*). They lack a central pale area and do not normally exhibit rouleau formation. Prominent anisocytosis is seen during the first month of life of the goat kid (Holman and Dew, 1964) and infrequently in a mature goat. Poikilocytosis is striking in goat kids under 3 months of age and may be prominent in some mature goats of certain breeds. Elliptical cells, which somewhat resembled sickle cells, were found to be characteristic of the goat kid between 1 and 3 months of age (Holman and Dew, 1964). The phenomenon was said to be similar to sickling of deer erythrocytes in that it was pH-dependent and could be eliminated by lowering the pH to 6.0. We have observed in blood samples of sick goat kids, 1–3 months of age, extremes of poikilocytosis (Fig. 9–1). In view of the observations on erythrocyte morphology of kid goats, such a finding was considered to be an influence of age rather than of disease.

Varying numbers of aberrant red cells were encountered in peripheral blood of 12 clinically normal, mature Angora goats (Jain and Kono, 1977a, b). Spindled, fusiform, matchstick form, oblong, triangular, and pear-shaped erythrocytes were observed along with some discocytic red cells and bizarre

forms (Fig. 9–2). The number of spindle-shaped and fusiform erythrocytes varied from 2–69% with 2 goats having such cells in excess of 50%. Such morphology was evident in Wright-stained blood films, but it was better appreciated in wet mounts of fresh blood or cells fixed in 1% buffered glutaraldehyde. Light (Fig. 9–3) and electron microscopic (Figs. 9–4, 9–5) observations indicated that polymerization of hemoglobin in the form of longitudinal tubular filaments was responsible for conferring the fusiform and spindle shapes to the red cells, a phenomenon akin to that seen in sickle-shaped human and deer erythrocytes. However, hemoglobin and globin electrophoresis on starch gel failed to reveal any gross abnormality of hemoglobin in goats with many fusiform and spindle-shaped erythrocytes. Variations in the morphology of fusiform and spindle-shaped cells with pH and oxygen tension indicated partial reversibility of the cell shape in vitro and a similarity to sickling phenomenon of deer erythrocytes. The cell shape was also influenced by temperature of blood storage; it was better preserved at 40°C (normal body temperature of the goat) and room temperature than at 4°C.

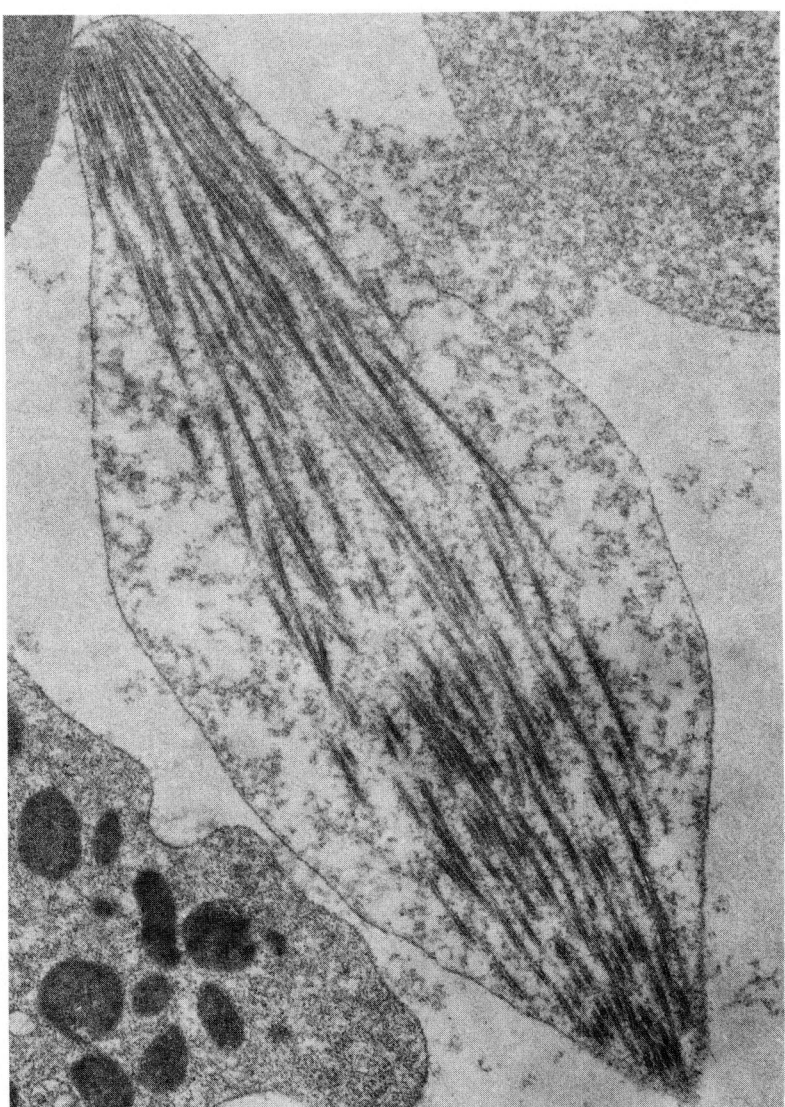

Fig. 9–4. Transmission electron photomicrograph of a partially lysed fusiform erythrocyte having many long tubular filaments of polymerized hemoglobin. Notice that the filaments seem to extend through the entire cell length even though there is a filament discontinuity at many places. ×42,000. (From Jain and Kono, 1977a.)

Erythrocyte morphology may be significantly altered by anemia because of formation of HbC as was shown in experiments with Angora goats (Jain et al., 1980). The development of anemia was associated with a gradual reduction in the proportion of fusiform erythrocytes and a simultaneous increase in the production of erythrocytes exhibiting distinct poikilocytosis not evident before (Tables 9–4, 9–5; Fig. 9–6). Severe blood loss anemia in goats is known to induce synthesis of HbC (see Hemoglobin Types, above), and formation of such a hemoglobin in these Angora

goats was demonstrated by electrophoresis and column chromatographic analyses. Peak changes in red cell morphology were apparent by 5–8 weeks after bleeding, when a very high to maximal level of HbC would be expected to have been synthesized. The reversal of these changes occurred gradually with the decrease in synthesis of HbC during the post-bleeding recovery phase.

Erythrocyte size varies inversely with number. Price-Jones curves developed for goat erythrocytes revealed mean cell diameters as follows: 5.1 μm at birth, 4.2 μm at 1 week,

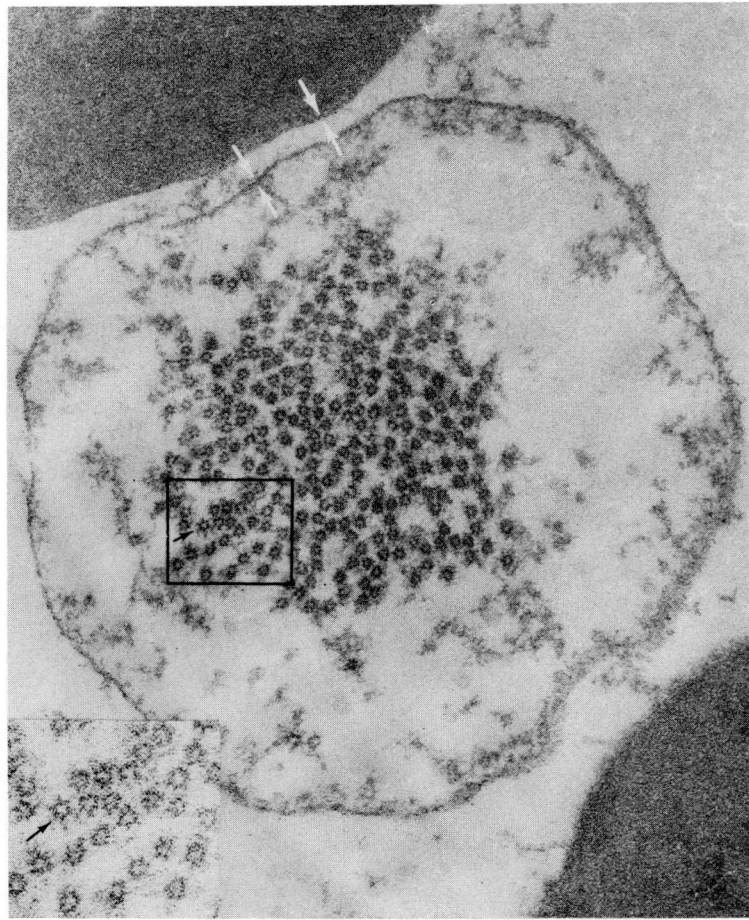

Fig. 9–5. Transmission electron photomicrograph of a transverse section of a partially lysed fusiform erythrocyte. The tubular nature of polymerized hemoglobin filaments is apparent, particularly in the inset, which also shows their hexagonal form at some places *(arrow)*. Notice the bilamellar erythrocyte membrane between white arrows. × 84,000; inset, × 163,000. (From Jain and Kono, 1977a.)

3.3 μm at 1 month, 2.7 μm at 2–3 months, and 2.2–3.9 μm in mature goats (Holman and Dew, 1964). Others have reported means of 3.1–4.1 μm for mature goats. An occasional erythrocyte may be as small as 1.5 μm or as large as 5 μm in diameter.

Examination of blood films from 39 kids each day for 8 days and then once weekly for 8 weeks revealed the presence of a few nucleated erythrocytes in 15 kids on the day of birth and during the first week and only an occasional nucleated erythrocyte in 1 or 2 samples through the seventh week (Holman and Dew, 1964). Polychromasia was not a common feature, but punctate basophilia was seen in about half of the kids up to the sixth week of age.

The Neutrophil

The nucleus of the mature neutrophil in the goat tends to have fewer lobes than in the sheep. The nuclear chromatin is irregular because of knob-like projections of condensed chromatin. A blunt sex chromatin or "drumstick" lobe can be found in some females. The cytoplasm is similar to the sheep neutrophil in that it stains pink without clearly demonstrating granules. However, some mature neutrophils may present a few distinct and deeply stained granules. Band neutrophils are rare in the peripheral blood in health.

The Eosinophil

The nucleus of the mature eosinophil may be of band form or may present 2 or 3 lobes.

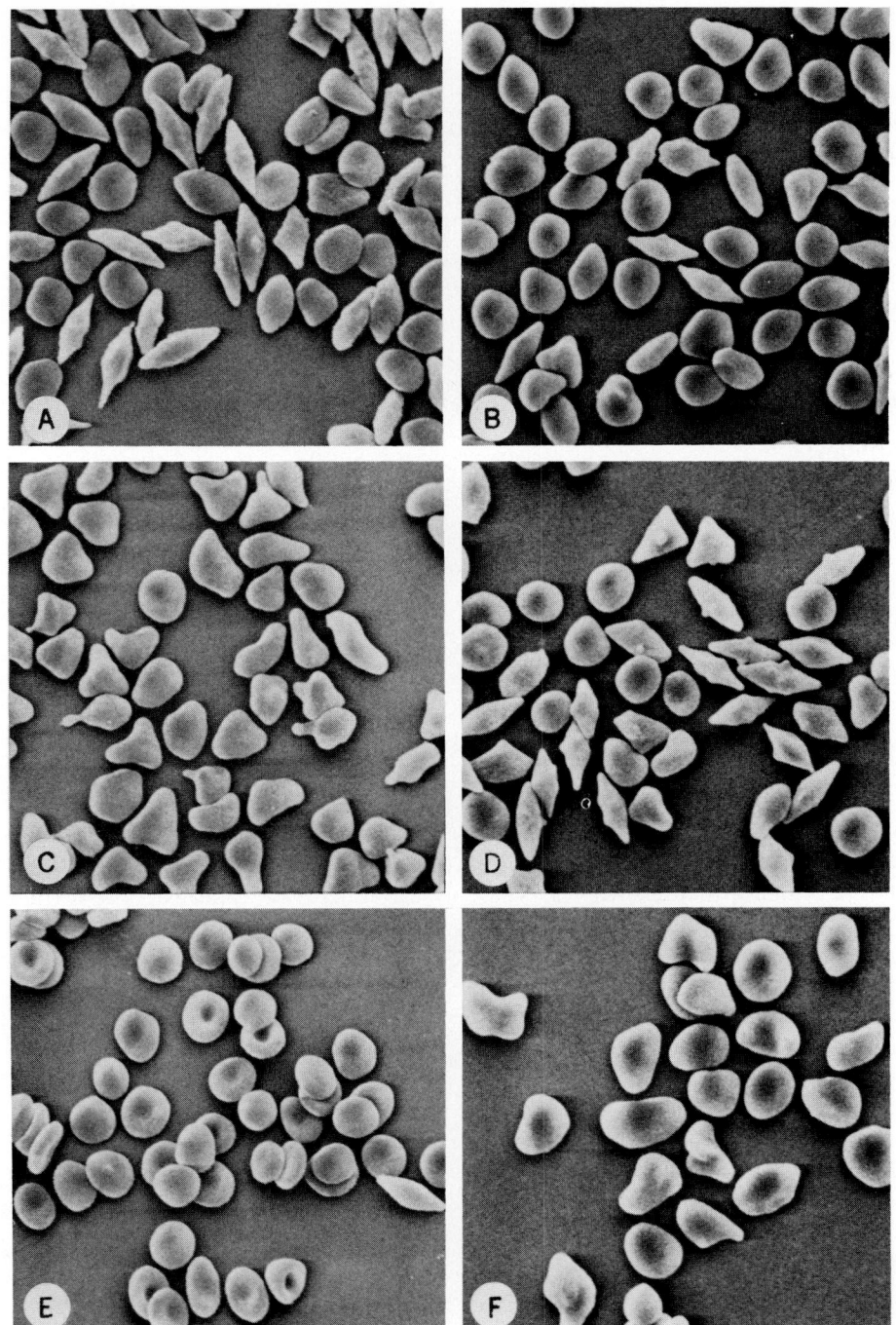

Fig. 9-6. Scanning electron photomicrographs of goat 6773 *(A–D)* and goat 6828 *(E, F)* before, during, and after recovery from experimentally induced blood loss anemia. The former goat had more than 50% fusiform erythrocytes, while the latter had nearly 98% discoid cells. (So that the reader can follow the effect of anemia on the erythrocyte morphology, hemoglobin value for each sampling time is given in parentheses; see Tables 9–4 and 9–5 and text for details). *A*, prebleeding sample (Hb 11.75 g/dl) containing many fusiform and discoid erythrocytes and a few odd-shaped cells; *B*, three weeks postbleeding sample (Hb 7.0 g/dl) showing a decrease in the proportion of fusiform erythrocytes and an increase in the discoid cells; *C*, eight weeks postbleeding sample (Hb 6.0 g/dl) depicting a marked poikilocytosis, but the absence of typical fusiform cells; *D*, 28 weeks postbleeding sample (Hb 10.5 g/dl) showing the return of fusiform erythrocytes and many discoid cells essentially identical to those in *A*; *E*, prebleeding sample (Hb 11.0 g/dl) containing predominantly discoid, slightly concave erythrocytes, a few stomatocytic forms, and a fusiform cell; *F*, five weeks postbleeding sample (Hb 7.0 g/dl) depicting a marked poikilocytosis and a few macrocytes; this erythrocyte morphology reverted to prebleeding type by 28 weeks as in the other goat. ×2000. (From Jain et al., 1980.)

237

The granules are small, round, numerous, and strongly acidophilic. They nearly fill the cytoplasm, which stains pale blue.

The Basophil

Basophils contain numerous densely packed, round granules. The granules stain purple with a reddish halo that gives the cytoplasm an overall reddish tinge. The nucleus is often in eccentric position and stains diffusely purple.

The Lymphocyte

The lymphocytes can be classified as small, medium, and large. The nucleus is surrounded by a variable amount of pale blue cytoplasm. Some cells stain a darker blue at the periphery and lighter blue near the nucleus. A few small to large, reddish purple azurophilic granules appear in the cytoplasm of some lymphocytes. An occasional lymphocyte may have some small cytoplasmic vacuoles. The nucleus is round to oval with an occasional cell exhibiting a kidney-bean indentation, and infrequently a binucleated cell may be encountered. The chromatin pattern is important in distinguishing the very large lymphocyte from the monocyte. The chromatin is condensed in comparatively large, irregularly shaped masses separated by narrow bands of lighter parachromatin. A few of the medium to large lymphocytes may contain 1 or 2 ring-like patterns within the nucleus that are somewhat suggestive of nucleolar remnants. The chromatin pattern of easily classified lymphocytes should be kept in mind and applied to the occasional large cell with ovoid nucleus that might be confused with a monocyte. When in doubt, classify the cell as a lymphocyte.

The Monocyte

The monocyte is a large cell with distinctly blue cytoplasm having a ground-glass appearance. Several vacuoles, usually clustered to one side of the cell, are commonly present. Another distinctive feature, although not present in every monocyte, is the occurrence of dust-like, reddish azurophilic granules in the cytoplasm. These are smaller, more numerous, and more evenly distributed than the azurophilic granules seen occasionally in lymphocytes. The nucleus of the monocyte may be almost any shape, e.g., ovoid, band form, or three-pronged. The chromatin is commonly stringy and diffuse with only limited condensation. When condensation does occur, however, it tends to be in smaller masses than described for the lymphocyte, and the condensed material is separated by a greater quantity of lighter-staining parachromatin.

The Platelets

The platelets in peripheral blood films are usually distributed in small to large aggregates. They vary in size and shape, but most are small, round structures with uniformly distributed, prominent azurophilic granules within lightly stained, pale blue cytoplasm. An occasional platelet exhibits somewhat peripheral distribution of granules. Cytoplasmic projections are very rare.

THE BONE MARROW

A mean M:E ratio of 0.69:1.0 was found in sternal bone marrow of 10 goats (Winqvist, 1954). This ratio indicates that the bone marrow of the goat is more active in the production of erythrocytes than of granulocytes. In this respect, the M:E ratio of the goat is similar to that of the cow.

REFERENCES

Bhargava, S.C.: Haematological Studies in Goats. Indian Vet. J., *57*:485, 1980.

Blunt, M.H., et al.: The Production of Haemoglobin C in Adult Sheep and Goats. Aust. J. Exp. Biol. Med. Sci., *47*:601, 1969.

Bunce, S.: Observations on the Blood Sedimentation Rate and the Packed Cell Volume of Some Domestic Farm Animals. Brit. Vet. J., *110*:322, 1954.

Castero, A., et al.: Hematologic Values in Normal Pigmy Goats. Amer. J. Vet. Res., *38*:2089, 1977.

DeShaw, J.R., et al.: Hematology of the Developing Juvenile Spanish Goat. Southwestern Vet., *22*(4):287, 1969.

Desiderio, J.V., et al.: Serum Proteins of Normal Goats and Goats with Caseous Lymphadenitis. Amer. J. Vet. Res., *40*:400, 1979.

Earl, P.R., and Carranza, B.A.: Leukocyte Differential Counts of the Mexican Goat. International Goat and Sheep Research, *1*(1):6, 1980.

Edjtechade, M.: Age-Associated Changes in the Blood Picture of the Goat. Zentralbl. Veterinaermed., *25A*:198, 1978.

Gonzaga, A.C., and De Guman, V.A., Jr.: Observation on the Blood Sugar, Iron and Hemoglobin of Philippine Native Goats. Nutr. Abstr. Rev., *34*:103(554), 1964.

Greenwood, B.: Haematology of the Sheep and Goat. *In* Comparative Clinical Haematology. Archer, L.K., and Jeffcott, L.B., eds. Blackwell Scientific Publications, Oxford, p. 305, 1977.

Holman, H.H., and Dew, S.M.: The Blood Picture of the Goat. I. The Two-Year-Old Female Goat. Res. Vet. Sci., *4*:121, 1963.

Holman, H.H., and Dew, S.M.: The Blood Picture of the Goat. II. Changes in Erythrocytic Shape, Size and Number Associated with Age. Res. Vet. Sci., *5*:274, 1964.

Holman, H.H., and Dew, S.M.: The Blood Picture of the Goat. III. Changes in Haemoglobin Concentration and Physical Measurements Occurring with Age. Res. Vet. Sci., *6*:245, 1965a.

Holman, H.H., and Dew, S.M.: The Blood Picture of the Goat. IV. Changes in Coagulation Times, Platelet Counts, and Leucocyte Numbers Associated with Age. Res. Vet. Sci., *6*:510, 1965b.

Holman, H.H., and Dew, S.M.: The Blood Picture of the Goat. V. Variations Due to Season, Sex, and Reproduction. Res. Vet. Sci., *7*:276, 1966a.

Holman, H.H., and Dew, S.M.: Effect of an Injection of Iron-Dextran Complex on Blood Constituents and Body Weight of Young Kids. Vet. Rec., *78*:772, 1966b.

Houchin, O.B., et al.: The Chemical Composition of the Blood of the Dairy Goat. J. Dairy Sci., *22*:241, 1939.

Jain, N.C., et al.: Fusiform Erythrocytes Resembling Sickle Cells in Angora Goats: Observations on Osmotic and Mechanical Fragilities and Reversal of Cell Shape during Anaemia. Res. Vet. Sci., *28*:25, 1980.

Jain, N.C., and Kono, C.S.: Fusiform Erythrocytes Resembling Sickle Cells in Angora Goats: Light and Electron Microscopic Observations. Res. Vet. Sci., *22*:169, 1977a.

Jain, N.C., and Kono, C.S.: Fusiform Erythrocytes in Angora Goats Resembling Sickle Cells: Influence of Temperature, pH, and Oxygenation on Cell Shape. Amer. J. Vet. Res., *38*:983, 1977b.

Millson, G.C., et al.: Biochemical and Hematological Observations on the Blood and Cerebralspinal Fluid of Clinically Healthy and Scrapie-Affected Goats. J. Comp. Path., *70*:194, 1960.

Mostaghni, K.: A Note on Haemoglobin Types and Some Blood Minerals of Goats (Capra hircus) in Iran. Indian J. Anim. Sci., *49*:857, 1979.

Mukherjee, D.P., and Bhattacharya, P.: Seasonal Variation in Haemoglobin and Cell-Volume Contents in Rams and Goats. Indian J. Vet. Sci., 23, Part 3:191, 1952.

Murty, V.N., and Kehar, N.D.: Physiological Studies on the Blood of Domestic Animals. Part II. Goats. Indian J. Physiol. Allied Sci., *5*:71, 1951.

Pathak, K.M.L., and Gaur, S.N.S.: Serum Proteins in Goats Experimentally Infected with Cysticercus tenuicollis of Taenia hydatigena. Haryana Vet., *20*:109, 1981.

Perk, K., et al.: Osmotic Fragility of Red Blood Cells of Young and Mature Domestic and Laboratory Animals. Amer. J. Vet. Res., *25*:1241, 1964.

Ponder, E.: The Measurement of Red Cell Volume. VI. The Different "Fragility" of the Red Cells of Various Mammals. J. Physiol., *83*:352, 1935.

Pyne, A.K., et al.: Physiological Studies on Blood of Goats. Indian Vet. J., *59*:597, 1982.

Schalm, O.W.: Unpublished data, 1975.

Vaidya, M.B., et al.: Hematological Constituents of Blood of Goats. Indian Vet. J., *47*:642, 1970.

Verma, S.K., and Tyagi, R.P.S.: The Effect of Caesarian Section and Normal Parturition upon the Concentration of Blood Electrolytes, Glucose and Total Proteins in Goats. Res. Vet. Sci., *16*:162, 1974.

Wilkins, J.H., and Hodges, R.E.D.H.: Observations on Normal Goat Blood. Royal Army Vet. Corps. J., *3*:37, 1962.

Winqvist, G.: Morphology of the Blood and the Hemopoietic Organs in Cattle under Normal and Some Experimental Conditions. Acta Anat. Suppl., *21*:1, 1954.

Wirth, D.: Grundlagen einer Klinischen Hämatologie der Haustiere. 2nd ed. Urban and Schwarzenberg, Vienna, 1950.

10

The Pig: Normal Hematology with Comments on Response to Disease

THE FETUS 240

NEONATAL PIGS 241
   Iron Requirement of Suckling Pigs 243
   Vitamin E and Selenium Deficiency 244

GENERAL PORCINE HEMATOLOGY 244
   Influence of Age 244
   Observations on Miniature Swine 245
   Influence of Pregnancy, Parturition, and
      Lactation 245
   Sex and Breed Differences 247
   The Erythrocytes 247
   The Leukocytes 248

The Platelets 249
The Plasma 250
The Bone Marrow 250

MORPHOLOGY OF BLOOD CELLS 250
   The Erythrocytes 250
   The Neutrophil 252
   The Eosinophil 252
   The Basophil 252
   The Lymphocyte 252
   The Monocyte 252
   The Platelets 252

A comprehensive description of swine hematology and hematopoietic organs is given by Calhoun and Brown (1975), and hematology of the pig is described by Imlah and McTaggart (1977). These publications will give the reader additional information on swine hematology.

THE FETUS

Cell population and serum proteins of 124 fetuses taken by cesarian section at 30, 51, 72, and 93 days of gestation were studied (Waddill et al., 1962). Umbilical cord blood was sampled at 30 days, cardiac blood at 51 days, and anterior vena cava blood was withdrawn from older fetuses and pigs at birth. In an-

Normal Blood Values for the Pig

Erythrocytic Series			Leukocytic Series		
	Range	Ave.		Range	Ave.
Erythrocytes ($\times 10^6/\mu l$)	5.0–8.0	6.5	Leukocytes/μl	11,000–22,000	16,000
Hemoglobin (g/dl)	10.0–16.0	13.0	Percentage Distribution		
PCV (%)	32–50	42.0	Neutrophil (band)	0–4	1.0
MCV (fl)	50–68	60	Neutrophil (mature)	28–47	37.0
MCH (pg)	17.0–21	19.0	Lymphocyte	39–62	53.0
MCHC (%)	30.0–34.0	32.0	Monocyte	2–10	5.0
Reticulocytes (%)	0.0–1.0	0.4	Eosinophil	0.5–11	3.5
ESR (mm in 1 hr.)	variable		Basophil	0–2	0.5
RBC diameter (μm)	4.0–8.0	6.0			
RBC life span (days)	86 ± 11.5		*Other Data*		
Resistance to hypotonic			Thrombocytes ($\times 10^5/\mu l$)	5.2 ± 1.95	
saline (%)			Icterus index (units)	<5	
Min		0.70	Plasma proteins (g/dl)	6.0–8.0	
Max.		0.45	Fibrinogen (g/dl)	0.1–0.5	
Myeloid:erythroid ratio	1.77 ± 0.52:1				
	(Lahey et al., 1952)				

other study, fetal blood was examined at 98, 102, and 110 days of gestation (Brooks and Davis, 1969). Erythrocyte and leukocyte values were obtained for 240 fetuses and piglets aged 30–144 days after conception (Upcott et al., 1973). The average gestation period in pigs is 114 days.

Erythrocyte number increased from approximately 0.5 million/μl at 30 days of gestation to between 5.6 million and 6.4 million at birth. Corresponding similar increases were seen in PCV and Hb values. The increase in red cell parameters was greater during the first half of gestation. The majority (more than 90%) of erythrocytes were nucleated at 30 days of gestation, but were rapidly replaced by nonnucleated cells as gestation progressed, and nucleated erythrocytes were less than 200/μl of blood at birth. MCV was 148 ± 16.4 fl at 35–45 days, 117 fl at 51 days of gestation, and decreased to 66 fl at birth. Reticulocytes were 3.85 ± 0.37% at 70–109 days (maximum 6.5% on day 70) and decreased to 1.49 ± 0.36% or less at birth. Serum proteins remained within the narrow range of 2.25–2.83 g/dl throughout gestation.

Leukocytes were usually absent or very low in number at 35–40 days of gestation. Leukocyte numbers fluctuated between 500 and 2,500/μl of blood from 40–109 days of gestation and increased at birth to 4,200–6,200/μl (Waddill et al., 1962) or to 9,000/μl (Brooks and Davis, 1969). Most of the cells were mature lymphocytes with some immature forms evident after 85 days. During this period, neutrophils comprised about 10% of the cells and increased to outnumber lymphocytes at birth. Differential distribution of leukocytes at birth was: 60% neutrophils, 38% lymphocytes, 1.0% monocytes, 0.2% eosinophils, and 0.1% basophils. Similar patterns of changes with somewhat higher cell counts were described in a later study (Gabris, 1974).

NEONATAL PIGS

Blood values for newborn piglets and changes occurring within the first few weeks of life have been described (Olowookorun and Makinde, 1980; Upcott et al., 1973). A sharp transient decrease in red cell parameters occurs within a few days after birth, MCV continues to decrease to near 50 fl by 3–4 weeks of life, and an increase in reticulocytes and nucleated erythrocytes (about 5%) may be seen by 25–29 days.

Blood values on a single litter of five males and four females, bled 6 times during the first 36 days of life, are given in Table 10–1. The litter was farrowed and kept inside on concrete for the first 10 days and then transferred outside to soil. Mean weights revealed a near doubling in 1 week and a fourfold increase by the third week. The means for the erythrocyte parameters (RBC, Hb, and PCV) diminished by 30–33% during the first 10 days.

Colostrum consumption during the first 24 hours of life is associated with a decrease in erythrocyte parameters and an increase in total plasma protein and globulin levels. The former is a result of hemodilution by expanded blood volume and the latter a result of absorption of globulins through the gut. A comparison of blood values of fasting pigs and nursing pigs was made during the first 24 hours after birth (McCance and Widdowson, 1959). The fasted pigs revealed almost no change in blood composition, while pigs receiving colostrum experienced a reduction in PCV from 38% to 28% and an increase in plasma volume of 30%. Serum globulins in nursing pigs increased from 0.93 g/dl to 3.58 g/dl during the same period. Similar results were reported for 20 nursing pigs in a subsequent study (Ramirez, et al., 1963); PCV dropped from 36% to 27% during the first 24 hours of life, while total plasma proteins increased from 2.4 g/dl to 5.3 g/dl. An increase in γ-globulins from 6.5% of total serum proteins to 44.7% by the end of the first 24 hours of life of suckling pigs has been reported (Miller et al., 1961b). Albumin diminished during the same period from 16.7% to 8.9% of the total serum proteins, probably as a result of dilution in expanding plasma volume. Immunoelectrophoresis of serum proteins of newborn piglets revealed that the adult pattern was evident within 2 hours of colostrum ingestion, whereas the fetal pattern was retained in piglets raised without colostrum and under germ-free conditions; in these latter animals the adult pattern was reached progressively within 3 weeks (Metzger et al., 1978). In piglets deprived of colostrum and reared

Table 10-1. Influence of Age and Husbandry on the Hematology of Young Duroc-Jersey Pigs. Ranges and Means for a Single Litter of 5 Males and 4 Females. Pigs Kept on Concrete Until 10 Days of Age and Then Placed on Soil[a]

Age (days)	Value	Wt. (lb)	RBC ($\times 10^6/\mu l$)	Hb (g/dl)	PCV (%)	MCV (fl)	MCHC (%)	MCH (pg)	Retic. (%)	Nuc. RBC/100 WBC	Sed. Rate (1 hr)	WBC ($\times 10^3/\mu l$)[b]	Differential Leukocyte Count (%)					
													Band	Neutrophil	Lymphocyte	Monocyte	Eosinophil	Basophil
1	Min.	1.7	4.3	8.4	27.0	57	28.9	18.0	4.5	0.5	0	7.6	1.0	64.5	16.0	0.5	0	0
	Max.	3.3	6.4	12.3	42.5	71	31.3	21.0	10.0	4.0	4	15.3	7.0	75.5	31.0	7.5	2.0	1.0
	Ave.	2.4	5.3	10.5	35	67	30.5	20	6.7	2	2	11.5	3.6	71	20	4.7	0.9	0.2
3	Min.	2.4	3.3	7.8	26.5	70	29.1	21.0	6.9	7	2	6.3	1.0	38.0	23.5	6.0	0	0
	Max.	4.0	5.2	11.0	36.5	81	30.3	24.0	16.6	57	12	13.4	5.5	61.5	54.0	9.5	1.5	0
	Ave.	3.2	4.5	9.8	33	73	29.5	22	12.0	17	5	9.4	3.3	51	37.6	6.8	0.8	0
6	Min.	3.5	3.4	6.4	22.0	60	26.4	17.0	4.5	5	12	7.4	1.0	33.0	32.5	2.0	0	0
	Max.	5.0	4.7	9.4	31.0	74	30.9	23.0	13.0	54	33	10.5	3.3	60.5	55	10.5	1.0	0
	Ave.	4.5	4.0	8.0	26.7	67	29.1	20	7.7	14	22.6	8.2	2	45.4	45.3	4.9	0.3	0
10	Min.	5.2	2.1	4.2	15.0	62	29.0	19.0	6.0	3	1	5.6	0	8.0	36.5	1.0	0	0
	Max.	7.1	4.3	8.7	20.0	78	31.0	24.0	12.0	30	35	19.1	2.0	51.0	82.0	10.0	0.5	0.5
	Ave.	6.4	3.5	7.0	24	68	29.6	20	10	11	12	10.9	1	27	64	7	0.1	0.05
20	Min.	8.5	4.4	9.0	35.5	70	26.0	19.0	9.0	1	0	6.2	0	13.5	55.0	2.0	0	0
	Max.	11.5	5.3	11.2	40.5	82	29.0	23.0	13.0	25	1	10.5	3.5	39.5	82.0	7.0	2.0	0.5
	Ave.	10.5	4.9	10.2	37	76	27.6	21	10.6	11.5	0	7.7	1.4	25.7	66.8	4.3	0.8	0.05
36	Min.	—	5.9	11.3	37.0	62	28.0	18.8	1.6	0	0	12.7	0	28.0	40.0	3.0	3.5	0
	Max.	—	6.8	13.3	44.0	68	32.0	20.0	6.8	1	2	20.9	5.0	43.0	68.0	10.5	14.0	1.5
	Ave.	—	6.2	12.1	39.7	64	30.5	19.4	3.0	0.5	0.5	16.3	1.8	33	52	6	7	0.5

[a]These data were developed in cooperation with Dr. Otto Straub.
[b]Corrected for nucleated red cells.

away from sows, increases in total plasma protein concentration and RBC and WBC counts were delayed, and the neutrophil:lymphocyte ratio did not reverse (Marx, et al., 1974a, b).

A significant increase in the erythrocyte parameters occurred between 10 and 20 days, when the litter was removed from concrete to contact with soil (Table 10–1). Intense erythrogenesis during the first 3 weeks of life was reflected in high levels of reticulocytes, nucleated erythrocytes, Howell-Jolly bodies, and polychromasia in peripheral blood. The number of nucleated erythrocytes in some piglets may exceed 50/100 WBC. Crenation of erythrocytes was a constant feature, erythrocyte rouleau formation was variable, and slight poikilocytosis was noted after the sixth day. RBC count and Hb concentration were low at weaning and increased to adult levels by 5 months of age (Miller et al., 1961b). Adult levels of red cell parameters were reached at 45 days of age for 5 litters of piglets raised under improved husbandry practices (Saror and Santiago, 1981). Hemoconcentration from diarrhea can raise red cell parameters in piglets (Kofer et al., 1981).

Erythrocyte sedimentation was nil or slight at birth, but it increased and reached a peak at the end of the first week of life and then tapered off to zero by the end of the third week (Table 10–1). Diphasic sedimentation rates were consistently observed and were a reflection of the high level of reticulocytes in peripheral blood.

The icterus index was uniformly 5 units or less, and the plasma often appeared opalescent or cloudy.

The WBC count must be corrected for nucleated erythrocytes (see Chapter 2). At 1 day of age, the WBC count was slightly higher than during the next 3 weeks. The most significant change with growth was in the differential count. At birth, the neutrophils were 71% and the lymphocytes 20%. The neutrophils decreased quickly, while the lymphocytes increased, so that by the tenth day, the proportion of the two cell types was reversed. Similar observations were reported by others (Gardiner et al., 1953). WBC counts as high as $26,000 \pm 1,710/\mu l$ have been recorded within a few days of birth (Upcott et al., 1973).

These changes in total and differential leukocyte counts seem to be a reflection of high circulating corticosteroid levels in piglets at birth, as in other species, and markedly diminished levels during the next few days of life (Brenner and Gurtler, 1977).

Iron Requirement of Suckling Pigs

Newborn piglets have mean hemoglobin levels of 10–12 g/dl of blood, and their mean total iron content of the body is about 50 mg (Venn et al., 1947). Less than one-tenth of this iron is in reserve and available for new blood formation. Milk is notoriously low in iron, and the iron content of sow's milk has been reported to be only 0.009% (McGowan and Crichton, 1923).

Suckling pigs grow rapidly. Their weight is doubled by the end of the first week of life, and a gain of four times the birth weight can be expected by the end of the third or fourth week. It has been estimated that a baby pig will obtain 6 mg of iron from milk during the first week and a total of about 23 mg in the first 3 weeks of life. However, the need for iron to supply hemoglobin for the expanding blood volume approaches 7 mg/day. A physiologic drop in the Hb concentration occurs during the first week of life as the body doubles in size and plasma volume increases by 30%. A 25–30% reduction in the Hb level is to be anticipated (Table 10–1). Unless a source of iron is available, the pigs become severely anemic during the next 2–3 weeks, leading to stunting, lowered resistance to disease, and some deaths. Spontaneous recovery begins about the fifth or sixth week of life, when the pigs begin to take nourishment in addition to milk.

Contact with soil early in the life of the pig is important in the prevention of anemia. Soil may contain as much as 1.5% iron, and pigs begin to root and eat dirt about the third or fourth day (Kernkamp, 1932, 1935). Washings of the gut were shown to contain as much as 500 mg of iron. If inclement weather necessitates raising the pigs indoors on concrete floors, it is important to bring soil into the farrowing house. Pigs raised outdoors on concrete are less anemic than pigs raised indoors (Doyle et al., 1928).

Supplementing the ration of the sow with

iron during pregnancy and lactation may lead to a slight increase in the iron content of the milk, but is not sufficient to prevent the development of anemia in the baby pigs (Hart et al., 1929). Pigs receiving no added iron developed microcytic hypochromic anemia within 6 weeks; 125 parts per million of oral iron appeared adequate to maintain RBC count and Hb concentration at normal levels in growing pigs (Ullrey et al., 1960). Iron may be supplied to suckling pigs by the daily application of a saturated solution of iron sulfate to the teats of the sow or by daily dosing pigs during the second week of life with 30 mg of iron pyrophosphate (Foot and Thompson, 1947). A less tedious procedure was a single intramuscular injection of 100 mg of iron in the form of an iron-dextran complex, administered on the fourth day of life (Barber et al., 1955; Kernkamp, 1957; Swenson et al., 1957).

Early literature on anemia of young pigs has been reviewed (Seamer, 1956). Studies on iron metabolism and anemia in piglets have been reported (Furugouri and Tohara, 1970, 1971; Larkin and Hannan, 1983). Both iron- and copper-deficient pigs develop microcytic anemia, the former as a result of decreased hemoglobin synthesis and the latter from shortened red cell survival; the red cell life span of iron-deficient pigs is said to be normal (Calhoun and Brown, 1975). In newborn piglets developing microcytic hypochromic anemia during the first 25 days, copper levels peaked by 9 days of age, and a marked increase occurred in ceruloplasmin activity (Mader et al., 1980). Piglets raised without iron supplementation were found to develop anemia and metabolic acidosis between 4 and 32 days of age, while those given iron showed no anemia and complete compensation of metabolic acidosis by 13 days of age (Schlerka, 1981).

Vitamin E and Selenium Deficiency

Swine with vitamin E deficiency have been reported to develop anemia, leukocytosis, and bone marrow abnormalities such as multinucleation of erythroid cells and increase in megakaryocytes (Bustad and Nafstad, 1972; Nafstad, 1965). Blood and bone marrow examinations were performed up to 56 days of age on pigs deficient in selenium and vitamin E that were born of sow fed Se–vitamin E depletion ration during gestation and lactation (Niyo et al., 1980). Anemia was not detected, although defective erythroid maturation was evident at 21 and 56 days of age. Binucleated erythroid precursor cells were found in newborn and control pigs, whereas erythroid cells with three or more nuclei were seen mainly in bone marrow from pigs deficient in selenium and vitamin E and less frequently in pigs with vitamin E deficiency. Experimental vitamin E deficiency in nonhuman primates and swine causes a normocytic normochromic anemia, but it takes months to more than 2 years for the anemia to develop (Drake and Fitch, 1980). The anemia is thought to be due to defective erythropoiesis, reduced red cell life span, or both.

GENERAL PORCINE HEMATOLOGY

Muscular activity and physical stress during blood collection can affect red and white cell parameters. For example, PCV increased by 9.7% and Hb by 2.3 g/dl within 5 minutes of the beginning of stress in pigs (Brenner and Gurtler, 1981). "Stress-susceptible" pigs have higher total leukocyte and lymphocyte numbers and exhibit greater stress-induced changes in total and differential leukocyte counts than "stress-resistant" pigs (Ellersieck et al., 1979).

Influence of Age

RBC, Hb, and PCV values vary with age and husbandry (see Neonatal Pigs, above). Newborn pigs experience 30% reduction in RBC count and about 38% decrease in red cell mass during the first week of life that is attributed to expansion of plasma volume from absorbed colostrum (McCance and Widdowson, 1959; Setiabudi et al., 1976). This state of anemia stimulates erythropoiesis leading to appearance of polychromasia and nucleated erythrocytes in blood during the first few weeks of life (Miller et al., 1961b). The larger size of the immature erythrocytes is reflected in a modest increase in MCV (Table 10–1). Age-related changes also occur in leukocytes (see The Leukocytes, below).

Blood volume is greatest in young pigs and decreases with growth (Table 3–1); blood volume decreased from 74 ml/kg in Hampshire pigs weighing 4.5 kg (2 weeks of age) to 35 ml/kg in pigs weighing more than 307 kg (3 years of age) (Hansard et al., 1951, 1953) and from 95 ml/kg in young pigs to 56 ml/kg in pigs of the Chester White breed weighing about 91 kg (Bush et al., 1955b). Higher plasma volume was estimated with ^{59}Fe than with ^{32}P method, particularly in anemic swine with a faster rate of iron utilization (Bush et al., 1955b). With growth, plasma volume was found to decrease more rapidly than the erythrocyte volume; hence the large pigs have a greater volume percent of erythrocytes. In anemic swine, the reduction of red cell volume was not compensated by a comparable increase in plasma volume. Thus a slightly lower total blood volume was observed in anemic swine, compared to normal swine of the same weight.

Observations on Miniature Swine

Normal hematologic and biochemical parameters for miniature swine of various age groups have been described (Burks et al., 1977; Gregor, 1979; Kircher, 1976; Mandel and Travnicek, 1982; McClellan et al., 1966; Tegeris et al., 1966; Travnicek and Mandel, 1982). From weaning to 9 months of age, PCV and Hb values increased slightly and then stabilized at about 42% and 14–15 g/dl of blood, respectively. RBC counts increased slightly during this period and stabilized at about 7 million/μl. The MCV, MCH, and MCHC increased slightly from weaning to 42 months of age, stabilizing at 64 fl, 22 pg, and 34–35%, respectively. Reticulocyte numbers declined progressively from weaning to 3 years of age, stabilizing at 30,000/μl of blood. WBC counts, reflecting changes in neutrophil and lymphocyte numbers, increased from weaning to 3 months of age, then progressively declined and finally stabilized at 3 years of age at about 12,000, with about 50% lymphocytes and 40% neutrophils. Eosinophil numbers increased slowly from weaning to a plateau of about 700/μl at 2 years of age. Monocyte and basophil numbers were variable, generally 300–600/μl and about 100/μl, respectively. Platelet counts decreased progressively from weaning to 9 months of age and stabilized at 200,000–250,000/μl.

Influence of Pregnancy, Parturition, and Lactation

Pregnancy-associated changes in erythrocyte parameters are presented in Table 10–2. A comparison of RBC, Hb, and PCV values in nine nonpregnant 1-year-old females with those of sows at various stages of pregnancy revealed a slight increase in these parameters between the third and eighth week of pregnancy. A slight decline in the erythrocyte parameters occurred during late gestation, about 2 weeks or less before parturition, and continued thereafter so that slight anemia was evident by 15–49 days postpartum. The Hb values continue to decrease and reach lowest levels at the end of the lactation, and Hb levels decrease in sows with age, from the first to the fifth litter (Petersen et al., 1979). Increase in reticulocyte counts (6.3–7.4%) has been reported in sows at mid-to-late lactation and near farrowing, as compared to values of less than 1% in nonpregnant older animals (Miller et al., 1961b).

The changes in red cell parameters during pregnancy and lactation are largely attributed to changes in blood volume (Jezkova et al., 1977; Steinhardt et al., 1981). Both plasma volume and total blood volume decreased by the eighth week of gestation. Hence, the increase in erythrocyte parameters between the third and eighth weeks of gestation is probably related to a comparatively larger reduction in plasma volume than in red cell mass during early stages and to an increase in erythrocyte mass from enhanced production in later stages. The decline in erythrocyte parameters during the last part of gestation is a hemodilution effect from increased plasma volume. The increase in reticulocyte count probably reflects response to tissue hypoxia as body weight and need for oxygen increase with advancing gestation. A negative linear relationship between Hb level and plasma volume was found in 113 multiparous sows in the 14th week of pregnancy and in 88 sows at 28–35 days in lactation (Steinhardt et al., 1981). A thorough study of pregnancy-related changes in red cell parameters, reticulocytes, and blood volume is, however, needed to arrive at a unifying concept.

Changes in total and differential leukocyte

Table 10–2. The Hematology of Duroc-Jersey Swine as Influenced by Age, Sex, Castration, Pregnancy, and Parturition[a]

Classification	No.	Value	RBC (×10⁶/µl)	Hb (g/dl)	PCV (%)	MCV (fl)	MCHC (%)	Sed. Rate (1 hr.)	WBC (×10³/µl)	Myelocyte	Metamyelocyte	Band	Neutrophil	Lymphocyte	Monocyte	Eosinophil	Basophil
																	Differential Leukocyte Count (%)
Both sexes 3½ to 4 months	10	Min.	6.4	11.5	38	53	28	0	18.9	—	—	1.0	17	46	1.0	0.5	0.0
		Max.	8.0	13.3	44	61	31	6	33.8	—	—	3.0	42	77	8.0	8.5	1.5
		Ave.	7.1	12.0	40	57	30	2.6	26.9	0.0	0.0	2.0	27	63	5.0	2.5	0.5
Castrated males 3 to 6 months	16	Min.	6.0	9.8	31	54	28	0	11.1	—	—	0.5	17	44	2.0	0.0	0.0
		Max.	8.0	13.0	44	68	32	25	28.3	—	—	4.5	45	73	10.0	10.0	1.0
		Ave.	7.0	11.7	39	59	30	5	19.5	0.0	0.0	2.0	29	60	6.0	2.5	0.5
Males 6 to 12 months	9	Min.	6.3	11.5	37	55	29.5	1	13.4	—	—	0.0	30	51	4.0	0.5	0.0
		Max.	8.6	13.5	44	68	33	14	25.3	—	—	2.5	41	61	9.0	4.5	1.0
		Ave.	7.0	12.4	41	59	31	5	18.9	0.0	0.0	1.5	33	57	6.0	2.2	0.3
Males 1 year and older	8	Min.	5.8	12.8	41	62	30	0.5	10.0	—	—	0.0	11	36	5.0	2.0	0.0
		Max.	7.5	15.3	50	72	33	31	17.4	—	—	2.0	49	76	12.0	5.5	3.0
		Ave.	6.7	14.1	45	66	31	13	13.3	0.0	0.0	0.6	32	55	8.0	3.5	0.9
Females 6 to 12 months; not pregnant	10	Min.	5.4	10.4	36	53	30	5	14.5	—	—	0.5	19	53	3.5	0.0	0.0
		Max.	7.9	13.8	46	67	34	27	21.6	—	—	3.5	37	67	10.5	5.5	2.0
		Ave.	7.0	12.9	41	59	32	15	15.3	0.0	0.0	1.2	33	57	5.5	2.7	0.6
Females 1 year and over; not pregnant	9	Min.	4.7	9.6	31	56	30	24	11.6	—	—	0.0	28	38	0.0	0.5	0.0
		Max.	7.7	14.3	48	69	33	55	21.0	—	—	2.0	42	61	9.0	10.0	1.5
		Ave.	6.0	12.1	38	64	31	26	16.4	0.0	0.0	0.7	36	54	5.0	4.0	0.3
Females 1 year and over; pregnant 3 to 8 weeks	20	Min.	5.6	11.5	37	58	30	1	11.3	—	—	0.0	31	39	2.5	1.0	0.0
		Max.	8.0	14.7	48	68	32	30	22.3	—	—	2.5	48	61	11.0	12.0	2.0
		Ave.	6.4	13.3	43	63	31	7	16.3	0.0	0.0	1.0	37	51	6.0	4.0	1.0
Females 1 year and over; pregnant 2½ to 3½ months	38	Min.	5.1	11.2	35	59	29	3	9.8	—	0.0	0.0	23	30	0.5	0.0	0.0
		Max.	8.0	15.3	50	69	33	53	20.9	—	0.5	4.5	58	68	12.0	9.0	2.0
		Ave.	6.4	12.8	42	65	31	20	14.4	0.0	0.1	1.1	35	55	5.0	3.0	0.8
Females 2 weeks or less before parturition	14	Min.	4.9	11.0	34	63	30	0	11.5	—	—	0.0	25	34	1.5	0.0	0.0
		Max.	6.3	14.5	46	75	33	47	21.9	—	—	3.5	55	57	9.0	2.5	1.5
		Ave.	5.7	12.6	40	70	31.6	21	15.6	0.0	0.0	1.7	39	52	6.0	0.7	0.6
Females 1 to 6 hours postpartum	5	Min.	4.9	11.2	35	57	31	21	15.1	—	0.0	0.0	43	17	0.5	0.5	0.0
		Max.	6.5	12.8	42	73	32	45	19.2	—	1.0	5.5	67	48	9.0	11.5	0.0
		Ave.	5.7	12.1	38	66	31.8	33	17.3	0.0	0.2	2.8	52	33	5.0	7.0	0.0
Females 10 to 24 hours postpartum	8	Min.	4.5	10.0	30	57	31	10	7.0	—	0.0	0.0	8	34	2.5	1.0	0.0
		Max.	7.3	14.5	46	70	33	54	17.2	4.0	6.0	42.0	45	72	11.0	6.0	1.5
		Ave.	5.8	12.0	37	63	32	47	10.3	0.5	1.8	10.0	30	46	7.0	4.0	0.7
Females 2 to 10 days postpartum	13	Min.	4.5	9.8	30	59	31	0	7.8	—	—	0.0	4	29	2.5	0.5	0.0
		Max.	6.9	15.1	47	71	34	28	21.0	—	—	7.5	58	57	30.0	9.5	3.0
		Ave.	5.5	12.7	39	66	32	12	15.0	0.0	—	3.0	43	40	9.0	4.0	1.0
Females 15 to 49 days postpartum	10	Min.	2.4	5.1	15	61	29	3	8.8	—	0.0	0.5	36	31	2.0	2.0	0.0
		Max.	6.0	12.3	42	79	35	55	24.4	—	3.0	14.0	59	52	11.5	10.0	3.5
		Ave.	4.9	10.4	32	66	32	35	18.7	0.0	0.6	4.0	46	37	6.0	5.0	1.4

[a]These data were developed in cooperation with Dr. Otto Straub.

counts have been reported for sows during gestation (Tewes et al., 1979) and periparturient periods (Fraser, 1938; Gabris, 1975; Luke, 1953a, b). WBC counts and lymphocyte numbers were greater at 30 and 60 days of gestation than on day 90, but the reverse was found with regard to nonsegmented neutrophils, while segmented neutrophils did not change significantly (Nachreiner and Ginther, 1972a). Eosinophil number was greater on day 30. Marked neutrophilia and lymphopenia were evident at 1–6 hours postpartum (Table 10–2). Similar changes were reported by others (Fraser, 1938; Gabris, 1975; Luke, 1953a, b). Plasma corticosteroid levels increased 1–24 hours postpartum and were associated with increases in WBC count and numbers of segmented and nonsegmented neutrophils and decreases in lymphocyte and eosinophil numbers (Nachreiner and Ginther, 1972b). Neutrophilia and lymphopenia may be apparent 6–10 hours prior to parturition and exceptionally as early as 9 days before farrowing (Luke, 1953a). A left shift that included myelocytes, metamyelocytes, and band neutrophils was observed 10–24 hours postpartum. An example of the leukocyte picture observed in one sow at parturition is given in Table 10–3.

Sex and Breed Differences

No consistent influence of sex on erythrocytes was observed, although RBC count was slightly less and cell size slightly greater in females than in castrated males (Miller et al., 1961b). A study on 1559 piglets, 1–48 days old, revealed no significant sex differences in blood values (Gabris, 1973). In a 1-year study of 11 male and 14 female pigs 4–67 months of age, significantly higher RBC count, percentage of segmented neutrophils, and prothrombin time were found in males, whereas

females had significantly higher MCV, MCH, and percentage of lymphocytes (Crookshank et al., 1975). No significant breed differences are described.

The Erythrocytes

For normal values of erythrocyte parameters see chart at the beginning of this chapter and Tables 10–1 and 10–2. The erythrocytes of the pig at birth are about 10 fl larger than those of the mature pig except when the latter is responding to physiologic anemia of pregnancy (McDonald et al., 1955; Miller et al., 1961b; also compare data in Tables 10–1 and 10–2). MCV of the newborn pig is 65–67 fl. After a brief increase to 70 fl during physiologic adjustment of erythrocyte mass and plasma volume, erythrocyte size decreases to 50–55 fl between 2 and 6 months of age and then increases to the mean adult size of 60 fl. Diameter of the erythrocytes of the mature pig ranges from 4–8 μm, with a mean of about 6 μm.

Changes in red cell size (microcytosis) and shape (poikilocytosis) were observed in piglets with gastrointestinal disorders (Stamatovic and Varga, 1979).

The life span of red cells of 5 normal growing pigs was studied using glycine-2-^{14}C as the red cell label (Bush et al., 1955a). The mean survival time was estimated to be 62 days, while the corrected average potential life span was 86 ± 11.5 days. Half-survival time of autologous ^{51}Cr-labeled erythrocytes was 28 ± 4 days and that of homologous red cells 13.8 ± 5.7 days (Talbot and Swenson, 1963).

Reticulocytes and Nucleated Erythrocytes

Reticulocytes, nucleated erythrocytes, and polychromasia are prominent features of blood of suckling pigs. Reticulocytes varied

Table 10–3.   Total and Differential Leukocyte Counts in a Sow at Parturition

Stage	WBC (× 10³)	Differential Leukocyte Count (%)						
		Meta-myelocyte	Band Neutro-phil	Neutro-phil	Lympho-cyte	Mono-cyte	Eosino-phil	Baso-phil
Just before parturition	11.8	0	2.5	55.0	34.0	5.0	2.0	0
2 hr postpartum	15.1	0	0	45.5	39.5	4.5	11.5	0
12 hr postpartum	8.9	1.0	25.0	27.5	39.0	6.5	1.0	0
24 hr postpartum	8.55	4.0	6.0	41.5	33.5	6.0	1.0	0

from 5.6 ± 2.3% at 6–18 hours of age to 5.1 ± 2.3% at 8 weeks of age, with a high of 11.4 ± 5.7% at 3 weeks of age (Swenson and Talbot, 1963). A range of 0.6–7.9% was found in 1270 pigs from 3 months to 2 years of age (Miller et al., 1961b). Absolute reticulocyte counts of 471,000 ± 22,000/µl were reported for 65 Pitman-Moore pigs 1.5 to 24 months of age (Hackett et al., 1961) and of 30,000/µl for miniature swine 3 years or more in age (McClellan et al., 1966). When the RBC count approaches the normal adult level of 6.5 million to 7.0 million/µl, the reticulocytes are commonly less than 1.0%. They appear again only during response to anemia. A few nucleated erythrocytes may be found in normal swine blood (Calhoun and Brown, 1975).

Erythrocyte Sedimentation Rate

The pig erythrocytes exhibit a tendency to rouleau formation and sedimentation. A diphasic sedimentation is observed in suckling pigs during the period of most intense erythrogenesis. It appears from the limited data reported in Table 10–2 that rather high ESR can be anticipated in normal swine blood. Observed values of ESR vary widely and fluctuate from day to day (Imlah and McTaggart, 1977). Observations on mature swine blood need to be extended before conclusions can be drawn regarding the anticipated ESR for normal swine blood compared to that of the dog and horse.

Erythrocyte Osmotic Fragility

The pig erythrocyte is highly susceptible to hemolysis by hypotonic saline. Osmotic fragility of erythrocytes is greater for pigs less than 3 days old than for pigs 7 months old (Hudson, 1955). Of 20 samples from suckling pigs, 65% showed initial hemolysis in 0.80% saline, whereas only 15% of bloods of 7-month-old pigs revealed initial hemolysis in that concentration of saline. Erythrocytes of newborn pigs, in which 85% of the cells appeared to be fetal-type, exhibited complete hemolysis at 0.18% saline, whereas normal adult erythrocytes revealed minimum resistance at 0.52% saline and maximum resistance at 0.29% saline concentration (Perk et al., 1964). These data indicate much greater resistance of pig erythrocytes to hypotonic saline than was previously found by others.

The Leukocytes

The WBC counts, as determined in one litter of 9 pigs, ranged beween 5,600 and 19,100/µl during the first 3 weeks of life. Nine other pigs, 2 months of age, selected at random from a larger group, revealed WBC counts of 16,000–25,000/µl, with one pig having a count of 44,800. Excluding the latter count, the mean was 21,500/µl. WBC counts on the blood of 32 sows revealed a range of 11,300–22,250/µl, with a mean of 15,900. WBC counts on 1,671 normal pigs, 6–12 weeks of age, revealed a range of 10,000–40,000/µl, with a mean of 21,000 (Dunne, 1963). In this study, 3.5% of counts were over 40,000 and considered to be abnormal, while 0.6% counts were below 10,000 and were considered not representative of the normal. It was concluded that in pigs 6 weeks of age or older, any count lower than 10,000 would indicate a definite leukopenia. The WBC count in general is high at birth, decreases by the second day to remain stabilized for 3–4 weeks, and then increases slightly by 6–7 weeks. During this period eosinophil numbers increase from 15/µl to 105 ± 72/µl (Dvorak, 1969).

Differential leukocyte counts are characterized by a high percentage of neutrophils at birth. By the end of the first week of life, the neutrophils and lymphocytes are present in about equal numbers (45%), but the former continue to drop and the latter continue to rise until 3 weeks of age and then stabilize by 6 months to a neutrophil:lymphocyte ratio of about 1:2 (Tables 10–1 and 10–2). A transient lymphocytosis was observed at 3 months of age in a closed herd of normal miniature pigs (McClellan et al., 1966). One or occasionally two distinct peaks of lymphocytes, with mean counts of 16,034 ± 3,837/µl and occasional counts as high as 30,000/µl, were observed in a "minimal disease" (MD) herd of pigs between 9 and 15 weeks of age (McTaggart, 1975). At such times, lymphocytes constituted about 80% of the differential count, and most of them were small lymphocytes. It was concluded that a high WBC count and a high lymphocyte percentage are not in themselves diagnostic of hereditary lymphosarcoma seen in pigs between 4 and 18 weeks of age. An abnormally high proportion of lymphoblasts and poorly differentiated cells must be present to make the diagnosis.

ACTH (25 mg) and adrenal cortical extract (200–300 mg), when injected into young pigs (40–50 lb), produced a leukocytosis associated with marked neutrophilia and lymphopenia within 2 hours with a return of cell counts to normal levels by 24 hours (Luke, 1953b). Injection of ACTH or stress-induced release of ACTH produced, within a few hours, eosinopenia and neutrophilia but not lymphopenia (Dvorak et al., 1967, 1969; Mutsumi, 1974). On the other hand, adrenalectomy was associated with marked eosinophilia and lymphocytosis within 2–6 days (Dvorak et al., 1967; Dvorak, 1969). Stress of feeding may also increase leukocyte counts (Bickhardt and Wirtz, 1978; Slesinger, 1967). Corticosteroid levels in peripheral blood of swine were 3.4 ± 0.3 μg/dl by competitive protein binding, and 2.4 ± 0.2 μg corticosterone/dl was measured by a fluorimetric method (Favre and Moatti, 1977). These levels underwent diurnal variations, increased after ACTH administration, and decreased after dexamethasone treatment.

The influence of exposure of pigs to the challenge of environmental bacteria has been studied by comparison of blood values of MD and "conventionally reared" (CR) bacon pigs (McTaggart and Rowntree, 1969). The CR pigs exhibited reduced growth rate and diminished erythrocyte parameters. Most remarkable changes were in leukocyte numbers. The WBC count was higher in the CR pigs ($19,627 \pm 844$) than in the MD pigs ($15,948 \pm 430$). The difference was principally due to the presence of twice as many neutrophils in the CR pigs ($6,310 \pm 555$) as in the MD pigs ($3,080 \pm 178$). Lymphocyte numbers were similar in both groups of pigs, while monocytes, eosinophils, and basophils were more numerous in the CR pigs. From these and subsequent observations, it was concluded that an increase in neutrophil numbers is a sensitive indicator of infection in pigs and that such an increase often precedes clinical appearance of the disease (Imlah and McTaggart, 1977).

Experimental hog cholera was character-ized by leukopenia (developing within 24–48 hours but most marked after 5–6 days), neutropenia with left shift, and thrombocytopenia (Sorensen et al., 1961a, b). The latter was associated with gross hemorrhages seen in various organs, and both leukopenia and thrombocytopenia were attributed to bone marrow hypoplasia. Lymphocyte and eosinophil numbers also diminished. Concomitant infection with *Salmonella choleraesuis* altered the leukocytic response in that a leukocytosis was seen instead of typical leukopenia (Sorensen, 1961b).

Pig husbandry is not common in our area of veterinary medicine. As a result, our experience with hematology of sick pigs has been limited. Of 77 hemograms on sick pigs, mostly less than 6 months of age, WBC counts have varied from a low of 1,700 to a high of 82,000/μl. In 17% of the pigs, the WBC count was less than 10,000 and in 24% it was greater than 30,000. A degenerative left shift was common in counts of less than 10,000. Several pigs with septicemia due to *Erysipelothrix rhusiopathiae* had absolute eosinophil numbers above 2,000/μl. Otherwise eosinophil numbers were generally depressed by the corticoids of stress, as were lymphocytes. Basophils were not commonly observed in sick pigs. Monocytes tended to be depressed in the leukopenic state and to increase, together with neutrophils, in leukocytosis.

The Platelets

Platelet counts in the pig seem to be age-dependent. A mean platelet count of $337,000 \pm 79,000$/μl of blood at birth was found to decrease during the first 2 days, then increase to a peak level of $578,000 \pm 128,000$ on the 10th day, and decrease slightly to $492,000 \pm 115,000$ on the 15th day (Lie, 1968). A similar pattern was observed in other studies carried out to 3–5 weeks of life (Linklater, 1971; Linklater and McTaggart, 1972), but not in some other reports. For examples, platelet counts at 1 day and 1, 2, and 3 weeks of age were, respectively, $524,000 \pm 94,000$, $630,000 \pm 114,000$, $717,000 \pm 132,000$, and $710,000 \pm 135,000$/μl of blood (Olowookorun and Makinde, 1980). A range of 220,000–665,000, with a mean of 407,000/μl, was found in pigs 2–3 months in age (Blecher and Gunstone, 1969).

A normal range of 250,000–850,000 was found in normal pigs, with young animals sometimes exceeding the higher limits and most pigs 3 months or older having counts between 400,000 and 500,000/μl (Sorensen et al., 1961a). Platelet counts in 10 normal swine, 84 ± 19.6 days in age, were found to be 520,000 ± 195,000/μl (Lahey et al., 1952). In contrast to above observations, an age-dependent decrease in platelet counts was observed in miniature swine with values of just over 600,000 at weaning, 330,000 at 6 months, and a stable value of 200,000–250,000/μl at 9 months of age and older (McClellan et al., 1966).

A hematologic feature of hog cholera is thrombocytopenia, developing from the second day of infection, with platelet counts decreasing usually to below 50,000 by 6–7 days and essentially to zero thereafter (Sorensen et al., 1961a). A marked thrombocytosis (1.311 million ± 0.509 million) was seen in iron-deficient pigs, but not in copper-deficient animals, although both groups developed microcytic hypochromic anemia (Lahey et al., 1952). A less prominent increase occurred in pigs deficient in both elements.

The Plasma

Total Plasma and Serum Proteins

Pigs under 1 month of age normally have total plasma proteins less than 5.5 g/dl, while pigs 2–6 months of age have 5.5–7.0 g/dl, and pigs over 1 year of age have 7.0–8.0 g/dl of blood. Mean plasma protein concentration was found to increase from 4.7 g/dl at 30 days of age to 7.29 g/dl at 240 days of age (Stekel and Smith, 1969). Plasma protein levels may be affected by weaning, growth rate, food intake, and hormone action (Dvorak, 1979; Marx et al., 1974b). Colostrum-deprived pigs failed to develop early increase in γ-globulins and had lower total plasma protein levels than suckled pigs until about 40 days of life (Marx et al., 1974b). Faster growing pigs show a greater reduction in total protein concentration after weaning than those growing slowly. The plasma protein values may vary during pregnancy; plasma proteins of eight sows were 7.3 ± 0.18 g/dl before breeding, 6.9 ± 0.06 at 21 days of pregnancy and

7.9 ± 0.08 at 112 days of pregnancy (Jezkova and Padalikova, 1977).

Observations on serum protein levels from birth through 2 years of age revealed the following mean values: at birth, 2.22 g/dl; at 1–5 weeks of age, 4.75; at 2–3 months, 5.5; at 4–6 months, 6.8; at one year, 7.51; and at 2 years 7.97 (Miller et al., 1961a).

Among pigs of various ages, but mostly under 6 months of age, presented for various clinical problems, total plasma proteins have varied from a low of 3.9 to a high of 10.7 g/dl. Values in excess of 8.0 g/dl in young pigs should be considered abnormal.

Fibrinogen

A gravimetric analysis of fibrinogen concentration in pigs 2–3 months of age revealed the normal range to be 0.2–0.4 g/dl (Blecher and Gunstone, 1969). Normal values by the refractometer method (Chapter 2) is 0.1–0.5 g/dl. In sick pigs, we have observed plasma fibrinogen levels of 0.6–1.2 g/dl.

Icterus Index

Icterus index is 2–5 units in health and may attain 7.5–10 units in some pigs. Plant pigments in the diet do not add color to the plasma of pigs (Palmer, 1916).

The Bone Marrow

The myeloid:erythroid ratio in 10 normal swine was found to be 1.77 ± 0.52:1 (Lahey et al., 1952).

A report in German provides details of bone marrow puncture, histologic examination, and cellular composition (Kohler, 1956). An electron microscopic study of bone marrow cells is available (Nafstad and Nafstad, 1968).

MORPHOLOGY OF BLOOD CELLS

The Erythrocytes

Rouleau formation is characteristic, and sharp-pointed crenation is a commonly seen artifact in pig blood films (Fig. 10–1). Central pallor may be absent or variable. In disease, the red cells may become bowl-shaped and reveal a deep concavity that appears in stained films as a sharply "punched out" cen-

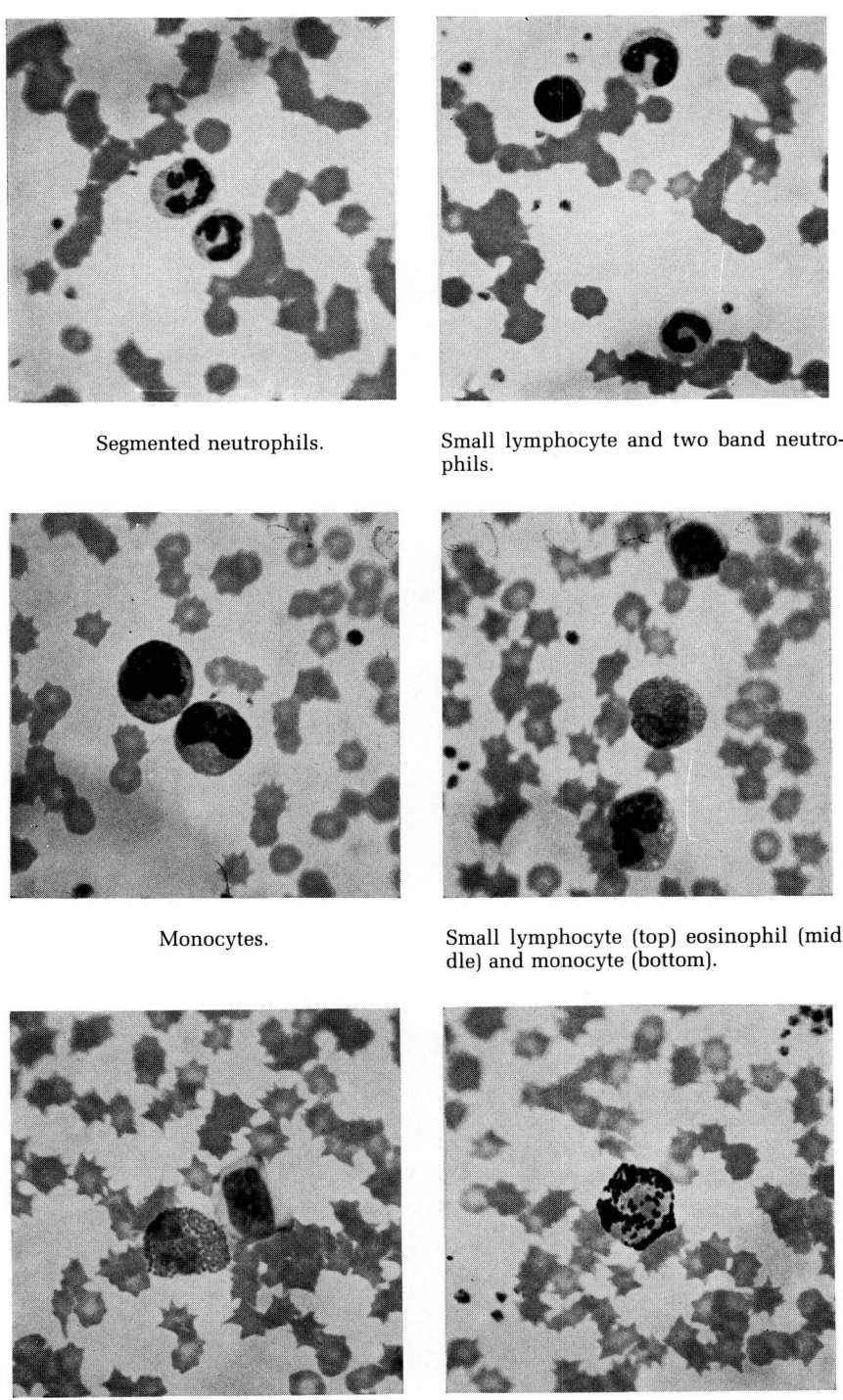

Segmented neutrophils.

Small lymphocyte and two band neutrophils.

Monocytes.

Small lymphocyte (top) eosinophil (middle) and monocyte (bottom).

Eosinophil and large lymphocyte.

Basophil and thrombocytes.

Fig. 10–1.   Porcine blood cells (×600, original magnification).

tral portion. Polychromasia, nucleated erythrocytes, and erythrocytes with Howell-Jolly bodies are to be anticipated in the blood of piglets and growing swine up to 3 months of age and during anemia in remission at any age.

The Neutrophil

Mature Neutrophil. The nuclear chromatin is well plaqued and stains intensely (Fig. 10–1). The nucleus is often coiled, and the nuclear outline is very irregular, but filaments are commonly absent. The cytoplasm is diffusely filled with dust-like pink granules. The overall color of the cytoplasm varies somewhat from pale blue to pink, depending on the intensity of staining of the granules.

Band Neutrophil. The nucleus is U- or S-shaped, with a smooth nuclear membrane (Fig. 10–1). Otherwise the cell is similar to the mature neutrophil. Band neutrophils may make up 1–2% of the differential leukocyte count in health. A higher percentage, particularly in young pigs, has been reported by some workers. This may be due partly to subjective criteria used in classification of this cell.

Metamyelocyte Neutrophil. It may appear in peripheral blood in health during stress as in a sow on the first day postpartum. The nuclear shape is a fat band. The metamyelocyte also occasionally appears as a doughnut form and not uncommonly as a band with enlarged or clubbed ends. The chromatin is neatly plaqued, and the nuclear membrane is smooth. The cytoplasm tends to be pale blue or basophilic because the specific granules do not stain prominently.

The Eosinophil

The eosinophil granules are round to ovoid, stain a dull orange, and completely fill the cytoplasm, with a few granules also over the nucleus (Fig. 10–1). The cell margin may present a cobblestone appearance because of the marked concentration of specific granules. The nucleus tends toward immaturity in that oval, kidney-bean, and band forms are commonly present.

The Basophil

The nucleus takes a lavender stain, and the chromatin is smooth. The granules may stain like the nucleus, or they may take a much darker stain (Fig. 10–1). They are generally limited to the cytoplasm, with a few scattered over the nucleus. The shape of the granules is coccoid to dumbbell.

The Lymphocyte

The small lymphocyte presents an oval nucleus that nearly fills the cell so that there is minimum evidence of cytoplasm (Fig. 10–1). The nuclear chromatin is smooth, but shows some condensation. The large lymphocyte has a nucleus that stains somewhat lighter and shows some plaquing of the chromatin. The cytoplasm is generally pale blue. Occasionally, ring-like structures appear in the nucleus representing nucleolar remnants, but the cell is not immature in other respects. Azurophilic granules are occasionally observed in the cytoplasm. The granules are small, tend to be elongated, and lie near the margin of the cell.

The Monocyte

The nucleus is irregular in outline, and its surface is folded and convoluted (Fig. 10–1). The chromatin is lacy or stringy, with uniformly distributed condensations. The cytoplasm is fairly voluminous and has a blue-gray, ground-glass, somewhat mottled appearance due to variation in intensity of staining. Azurophilic granulation is generally inconspicuous, and cytoplasmic vacuoles may be observed occasionally. It has been stated that some monocytes may be difficult to differentiate from large lymphocytes or early neutrophils (Imlah and McTaggart, 1977).

The Platelets

Platelets predominantly appear as small oval structures consisting of a cluster of deeply stained purplish granules surrounded by a pale blue cytoplasm (Fig. 10–1). They are frequently gathered into irregular masses of varying size. Giant forms with finger-like extensions are occasionally seen. Platelet morphology of pigs with von Willebrand's disease is similar to that of normal pigs (Lewis and Bowie, 1978).

REFERENCES*

Barber, R.S., et al.: Studies on Anaemia in Pigs. I. The Provision of Iron by Intramuscular Injection. Vet. Rec., 67:348, 1955.

Bickhardt, K., and Wirtz, A.: (Influence of Restraint Stress and of Feeding on Blood Values of Pigs.) Dtsch. Tierarztl. Wochenschr., 85:457, 1978.

Blecher, T.E., and Gunstone, M.J.: Fibrinolysis, Coagulation and Haematological Findings in Normal Large White/Wessex Cross Pigs. Brit. Vet. J., 125:74, 1969.

Brenner, K.V., and Gurtler, H.: (Concentrations of Cortisol, Glucose and Free Fatty Acids in Blood Plasma of Swine, Depending on Age, and in Sows Close to Farrowing.) Arch. Exp. Veterinaermed., 31:741, 1977.

Brenner, K.V., and Gurtler, H.: Further Investigations on Metabolic and Haematological Reactions of Pigs to Restraint by Means of a Rope Round the Upper Jaw. Arch. Exp. Veterinaermed., 35:401, 1981.

Brooks, C.C., and Davis, J.W.: Changes in Hematology of the Perinatal Pig. J. Anim. Sci., 28:517, 1969.

Burks, M.F., et al.: Age and Sex Related Changes of Hematologic Parameters in Sinclair (S–1) Miniature Swine. Growth, 41:51, 1977.

Bush, J.A., et al.: Erythrocyte Life Span in Growing Swine as Determined by Glycine-2-C14. J. Exp. Med., 101:451, 1955a.

Bush, J.A., et al.: Blood Volume Studies in Normal and Anemic Swine. Amer. J. Physiol., 181:9, 1955b.

Bustad, B., and Nafstad, I.: Hematologic Response to Vitamin E in Piglets. Brit. J. Nutr., 28:183, 1972.

Calhoun, M.L., and Brown, E.M.: Hematology and Hematopoietic Organs. In Diseases of Swine. Dunne, H.W., and Lemane, A.D., eds. Iowa University Press, 4th ed., Ames, Iowa, p.. 38, 1975.

Crookshank, H.R., et al.: Hematological Parameters of American-Essex Swine. J. Anim. Sci., 40:190, 1975.

Doyle, L.P., et al.: Anemia in Young Pigs. J. Amer. Vet. Med. Ass., 72:491, 1928.

Drake, J.R., and Fitch, C.D.: Status of Vitamin E as an Erythropoietic Factor. Amer. J. Clin. Nutr., 33:2386, 1980.

Dunne, H.W.: Field and Laboratory Diagnosis of Hog Cholera. Vet. Med., 58:222, 1963.

Dvorak, M.: Eosinophil Levels in the Blood of Piglets with Normal and Retarded Development. Doc. Vet. Brno., 7:199, 1969.

Dvorak, M.: (Effects of Different Growth Rates, Starvation and Hormone Actions on Some Metabolic Measures in the Blood Plasma of Weaned Piglets.) Vet. Med., 24:301, 1979.

Dvorak, M., et al.: Adrenalectomy in Piglets. I. Clinical, Hematological and Pathophysiological Studies. Doc. Vet. Brno., 6:229, 1967.

Ellersieck, M.R., et al.: Response of Stress-Susceptible and Stress-Resistant Hampshire Pigs to Electrical Stress. II. Effects on Blood Cells and Blood Minerals. J. Anim. Sci., 48:453, 1979.

Favre, B., and Moatti, J.P.: (Determination of Plasma Corticosteroids in the Piglet.) Ann. Rech. Vet., 8:111, 1977.

Foot, A.S., and Thompson, S.Y.: Preventing Anemia in Young Pigs. G.B.J. Min. Agr., 54:308, 1947.

Fraser, A.C.: A Study of the Blood of Pigs. Vet. J., 94:3, 1938.

Furugouri, K., and Tohara, S.: Studies on Iron Metabolism and Anemia in the Piglets. I. Relationship between Growth and Anemia. Bull. Natl. Inst. Anim. Ind., no. 21 (March), 1970.

Furugouri, K., and Tohara, S.: Studies on Iron Metabolism and Anemia in the Piglets. II. Blood Volume and Mean Corpuscular Constants. Bull. Natl. Inst. Anim. Ind., no. 24 (July), 1971.

Gabris, J.: (Differences between the Sexes and during Summer and Winter in the Blood Picture of Unweaned Piglets.) Folia Vet., 17:303, 1973.

Gabris, J.: (Changes in the Relationship between Leucocytes, Neutrophil and Lymphocyte Counts in the Blood of Pig Fetuses and Unweaned Piglets.) Vet. Med., 19:591, 1974.

Gabris, J.: (Relationship between the Numbers of Leucocytes, Neutrophil, Granulocytes, and Lymphocytes in Sows before and during Parturition and during Lactation.) Folia Vet., 19:151, 1975.

Gardiner, M.R., et al.: The Blood Picture in Newborn Pigs. Amer. J. Vet. Res., 14:68, 1953.

Gregor, G.: (Haematological and Biochemical Studies on MINI-MINI-LEWE Miniature Swine. I. Blood Picture and Serum Proteins.) Zeit. Versuchstierkd., 21:92, 1979.

Hackett, P.L., et al.: Blood Constituents in Pittman-Moore, Palouse and Hormel Swine. Biol. Res. Ann. Rept., p. 146, 1961.

Hansard, S.L., et al.: Blood Volume of Farm Animals. J. Anim. Sci., 12:402, 1953.

Hansard, S.L., et al.: Blood Volume of Swine. Proc. Soc. Exp. Biol. Med., 78:544, 1951.

Hart, E.B., et al.: Anemia in Suckling Pigs. Wis. Agr. Exp. Sta. Bull., 409, 1929.

Hudson, A.E.A.: Fragility of Erythrocytes in Blood from Swine of Two Age Groups. Amer. J. Vet. Res., 16:120, 1955.

Imlah, P., and McTaggart, H.S.: Haematology of the Pig. In Clinical Haematology. Archer, R.K., and Jeffcott, L.B., eds. Blackwell Scientific Publications, Oxford, p. 271, 1977.

Jezkova, D., and Padalikova, D.: Proteins and Free Amino Acids in the Blood Plasma of Sows before Breeding, during Gestation and after Farrowing. Acta Vet. Brno, 46:217, 1977.

Jezkova, D., et al.: Changes in the Plasma Volume, Total Blood Volume and Haematocrit Values of Pregnant Sows. Acta Vet. Brno, 46:203, 1977.

Kernkamp, H.C.H.: The Blood Picture of Pigs Kept under Conditions Favorable to the Production and to the Prevention of So-Called "Anemia of Suckling Pigs." Minn. Agr. Exp. Sta. Tech. Bull., 86, 1932.

Kernkamp, H.C.H.: Soil, Iron, Copper and Iron in the Prevention and Treatment of Anemia in Suckling Pigs. J. Amer. Vet. Med. Ass., 87:37, 1935.

Kernkamp, H.C.H.: A Parenteral Hematinic for the Control of Iron-Deficiency Anemia in Baby Pigs. North Amer. Vet., 38:6, 1957.

Kircher, G.H.: (Determination of Haematological and Biochemical Normal Profiles for the Hanford Miniature Swine and German Landrace in Relation to Age.) Inaug. diss., Fachbereich Tiermedizin, Munich, 248 pp., 1976. (Abst. in Vet. Bull., 48(2):1281, 1978.)

Kofer, J., et al.: (Changes in Blood Gases and the Acid-Base Equilibrium and Measurement of Haemoglobin and Haematocrit in Piglets. III. During the First Three Weeks after Weaning.) Dtsch. Tierärztl. Wochenschr., 88:89, 1981.

---

*Titles in parentheses are English translations of foreign language titles.

Kohler, H.: The Bone Marrow and Blood Picture of the Piglet I. The Healthy Piglet. Vet. Med., 3:359, 1956.

Lahey, M.E., et al.: Studies on Copper Metabolism. II. Hematologic Manifestation of Copper Deficiency in Swine. Blood, 7:1053, 1952.

Larkin, H.A., and Hannan, J.: Gastric Structure and Function in Iron-deficient Piglets. Res. Vet. Sci., 34:11, 1983.

Lewis, J.C., and Bowie, F.J.W.: Ultrastructural Studies of Platelets of von Willebrand and Normal Swine. Mayo Clinic Proc., 53:179, 1978.

Lie, H.: Thrombocytes, Leucocytes and Packed Red Cell Volume in Piglets during the First Two Weeks of Life. Acta Vet. Scand., 9:105, 1968.

Linklater, K.A.: A Study of Some Blood Cellular Antigenic Factors and Isoimmunization in the Pig. Thesis, Univ. of Edinburgh, 1971, p. 153. Cited by Imlah and McTaggart, 1977.

Linklater, K.A., and McTaggart, H.S.: Unpublished observations, 1972. Cited by Imlah and McTaggart, 1977.

Luke, D.: The Reaction of the White Blood Cells at Parturition in the Sow. Brit. Vet. J., 109:241, 1953a.

Luke, D.: The Effect of Adrenocorticotrophic Hormone and Adrenal Cortical Extract on the Differential White Cell Count in the Pig. Brit. Vet. J., 109:434, 1953b.

Mader, H., et al.: (Behaviour of Blood Parameters of Iron and Copper Metabolism in Piglets before Weaning.) Vet. Med., 27A:70, 1980.

Mandel, L., and Travnicek, J.: Haematology of Conventional and Germfree Miniature Minnesota Piglets. I. Blood Picture. Zeit. Versuchstierkd., 24:299, 1982.

Marx, D., et al.: (Blood Examination on Piglets up to 6 Weeks after Separation from the Sow at Birth (Kept in Cages till 30 Days Old). I. GOT, Glucose, Blood Status.) Berl. Müench. Tierärztl. Wochenschr., 87:290, 1974a.

Marx, D., et al.: (Blood Examination on Piglets up to 6 Weeks after Separation from the Sow at BIrth (Kept in Cages till 30 Days Old). II. Plasma Protein Fraction and Total Protein Content.) Berl. Müench. Tierärztl. Wochenschr., 87:317, 1974b.

McCance, R.A., and Widdowson, E.M.: The Effect of Colostrum on the Composition and Volume of the Plasma of Newborn Piglets. J. Physiol., 145:547, 1959.

McClellan, R.O., et al.: Age-related Changes in Hematological and Serum Biochemical Parameters in Miniature Swine. In Swine in Biomedical Research. Bustad, L.K., et al., eds. Battell-Northwest, Richland, Wash., p. 597, 1966.

McDonald, F.F., et al.: An Effective Treatment for Anaemia of Piglets. Brit. Vet. J., 111:403, 1955.

McGowan, J.P., and Crichton, A.: On the Effect of Deficiency of Iron in the Diet of Pigs. Biochem. J., 17:204, 1923.

McTaggart, H.S.: Lymphocytosis in Normal and Young Pigs. Brit. Vet. J., 131:574, 1975.

McTaggart, H.S., and Rowntree, P.G.M.: The Haematology of "Minimal Disease" Bacon Pigs: A Comparison with Genetically-Related Conventionally-Reared Pigs. Brit. Vet. J., 125:240, 1969.

Metzger, J.J., et al.: Serum Protein Profiles in the Suckling and Nonsuckling Piglet: The Importance of Colostrum. Ann. Rech. Vet., 9:301, 1978.

Miller, E.R., et al.: Swine Hematology from Birth to Maturity. I. Serum Proteins. J. Anim. Sci., 20:31, 1961a.

Miller, E.R., et al.: Swine Hematology from Birth to Maturity. II. Erythrocyte Population, Size and Hemoglobin Concentration. J. Anim. Sci., 20:890, 1961b.

Mutsumi, M.: Influence of Adrenocorticotropic Hormone upon the Circulating Leukocyte Count of Peripheral Blood in Pigs. Natl. Inst. Anim. Health Q. (Tokyo), 14:104, 1974.

Nachreiner, R.F., and Ginther, O.J.: Gestational and Periparturient Periods of Sows: Serum Chemical and Hematologic Changes during Gestation. Amer. J. Vet. Res., 33:2215, 1972a.

Nachreiner, R.F., and Ginther, O.J.: Gestational and Periparturient Periods of Sows: Serum Chemical, Hematologic and Clinical Changes during the Periparturient Period. Amer. J. Vet. Res., 33:2233, 1972b.

Nafstad, I.: Studies of Hematology and Bone Marrow Morphology in Vitamin E Deficient Pigs. Path. Vet., 2:277, 1965.

Nafstad, H.J., and Nafstad, I.: An Electron Microscopic Study of Normal Blood and Bone Marrow in Pigs. Path. Vet., 5:451, 1968.

Niyo, Y., et al.: Effects of Intramuscular Injection of Selenium and Vitamin E on Peripheral Blood and Bone Marrow of Selenium-Vitamin E Deficient Pigs. Amer. J. Vet. Res., 41:474, 1980.

Olowookorun, M.O., and Makinde, M.O.: Thrombocytes, Clotting Time, Haemoglobin Value and Packed Cell Volume in Nigerian Piglets during the First Four Weeks of Life. Vet. Med., 27A:508, 1980.

Palmer, L.S.: The Physiological Relation of Plant Carotenoids to the Carotenoids of the Cow, Horse, Sheep, Goat, Pig, and Hen. J. Biol. Chem., 27:27, 1916.

Perk, K., et al.: Osmotic Fragility of Red Blood Cells of Young and Mature Domestic and Laboratory Animals. Amer. J. Vet. Res., 25:1241, 1964.

Petersen, E.S., et al.: Sow Haemoglobin Values: Influence of Sow Age and Reproductive Performance Effect. Acta Agri. Scand., 29:45, 1979.

Ramirez, C.G., et al.: Swine Hematology from Birth to Maturity. III. Blood Volume of the Nursing Pig. J. Anim. Sci., 22:1068, 1963.

Saror, D.I., and Santiago, F.: Haematological Parameters of Large White Pigs in Nigeria. Bull. Anim. Health Prod. Africa, 29:129, 1981.

Schlerka, G., et al.: (Changes in Blood Gases and Acid-Base Equilibrium and Measurement of Haemoglobin and Haematocrit in Piglets.) Dtsch. Tierarztl. Wochenschr., 88:50, 1981.

Seamer, J.: Piglet Anemia. Vet. Rev. Annotations, 2:79, 1956.

Setiabudi, M., et al.: Growth of the Pigs: Changes in Red Cell and Plasma Volumes. Growth, 40:127, 1976.

Slesinger, L.: (Hematological Results in Healthy Pigs Kept in Balance Pens.) Berl. Müench. Tierärztl. Wochenschr., 80:291, 1967.

Sorensen, D.K., et al.: Clinical and Hematological Manifestations of Hog Cholera. In Symposium on Hog Cholera. Manwaring, G.T., and Sorensen, D.K., eds. Univ. Minnesota, St. Paul, Minn., p. 29, 1961a.

Sorensen, D.K., et al.: Clinical and Hematological Manifestations of Hog Cholera. In Symposium on Hog Cholera. Manwaring, G.T., and Sorensen, D.K., eds. Univ. Minnesota, St. Paul, Minn., p. 109, 1961b.

Stamatovic, S., and Varga, F.: (Erythrocyte Values of Piglets up to Ten Days of Age as an Indicator of Dehydration.) Vet. Glasnik, 33:359, 1979.

Steinhardt, M., et al.: Relationships between Certain Values for Blood Concentration and Blood Volume in Sows. Arch. Exp. Veterinaermed., 35:707, 1981.

Stekel, A., and Smith, N.J.: Hematologic Studies of Severe Undernutrition of Infancy. I. The Anemia of Prolonged Caloric Deprivation in the Pig. Pediatr. Res., *3*:320, 1969.

Swenson, M.J., et al.: A Preliminary Report on the Effects of Iron-Dextran, Injected Intramuscularly on the Growth of Newborn Pigs. J. Amer. Vet. Med. Ass., *131*:146, 1957.

Swenson, M.J., and Talbot, R.B.: Unpublished observations, 1963. Cited by Calhoun and Brown, 1975.

Talbot, R.B., and Swenson, M.J.: Survival of Cr⁵¹ Labelled Erythrocytes in Swine. Proc. Soc. Exp. Biol. Med., *112*:573, 1963.

Tegeris, A.S., et al.: Normal Hematological and Biochemical Parameters of Young Miniature Swine. *In* Swine in Biomedical Research. Bustad, L.K., et al., eds. Battell-Northwest, Richland, Wash., p. 575, 1966.

Tewes, H., et al.: Investigations on the Blood Composition of Sows during the Reproductive Cycle. II. Blood Changes during Pregnancy. Zuchthygiene, *14*:111, 1979.

Travnicek, J., and Mandel, L.: Haematology of Conventional and Germfree Miniature Minnesota Piglets. II. Serum Proteins and Immunoglobulins. Zeit. Versuchstierkd., *24*:308, 1982.

Ullrey, D.E., et al.: The Requirement of the Baby Pig for Orally Administered Iron. J. Nutr., *70*:187, 1960.

Upcott, O.M., et al.: Erythrocyte and Leukocyte Parameters in Fetal and Neonatal Piglets. Res. Vet. Sci., *15*:8, 1973.

Venn, J.A.J., et al.: Iron Metabolism in Piglet Anaemia. J. Comp. Path., *57*:314, 1947.

Waddill, D.G., et al.: Blood Cell Populations and Serum Protein Concentrations in the Fetal Pig. J. Anim. Sci., *21*:583, 1962.

11

Avian Hematology

Joseph G. Zinkl

AVIAN BLOOD   256
  Normal Blood Values in Chickens   256

FUNCTIONS OF BLOOD ELEMENTS   258

HEMATOLOGIC TECHNIQUES   259
  Blood Sampling   259
  Anticoagulants   260
  Laboratory Techniques   260

HEMATOPOIESIS IN AVIAN MARROW   263

AVIAN HEMATOPOIETIC NEOPLASIAS   264
  Marek's Disease   264
  Leukosis/Sarcoma Complex   266
  Reticuloendotheliosis and Other
    Lymphoproliferative Diseases   267

Leukosis-like Disease in Birds Other Than
  Chickens and Turkeys   267

BLOOD PARASITES   268
  Plasmodium species   268
  Haemoproteus and *Parahaemoproteus*
    species   269
  Leukocytozoon species   269
  Microfilariae   270

SPIROCHETOSIS   270

HEINZ BODY ANEMIA DUE TO INGESTION
  OF CRUDE OIL   270

LEAD POISONING   271

The use of hematology to aid in the diagnosis of diseases of birds is increasing rapidly. This can be attributed to several factors including the increase in the number of pet birds being kept and their monetary and sentimental values. Naturally the traditional necropsy examination for diagnosing poultry diseases cannot be used when an individual bird's health rather than that of the flock is concerned. The interest of many environmentally minded people, including veterinarians, also has increased the use of laboratory investigations for studying blood samples taken from ill and wounded wild birds designated for rehabilitation. Additionally, the pivotal role that chickens have had in defining the immunologic system and in the research and understanding of viral etiology of hematologic neoplasia emphasizes the importance of avian hematology. Furthermore, the importance of avian malaria in causing catastrophic losses in some bird populations of remote islands indicates the severe consequences that can occur due to hematologic diseases.

A general description of blood elements and some common hematologic diseases of avian species follows. Selected hematologic techniques applicable to avian blood are discussed. Other publications may be consulted for more details on various aspects of avian hematology (Archer, 1971; Gee et al., 1981; Hodges, 1977; Leonard, 1982; Lucas and Jamoroz, 1961; Olson, 1965; Rosskopf et al., 1982).

AVIAN BLOOD

The major differences in the blood of birds and mammals are that birds have nucleated erythrocytes and nucleated thrombocytes (Plate XXV–1). The erythrocytes are generally elliptical and quite large. The nucleus is condensed and in the center of the cell. Hemoglobin concentration (MCHC) is lower in avian cells than in mammalian erythrocytes, probably because of the space occupied by the nucleus.

Thrombocytes appear to function in hemostasis in birds analogously to the platelets of mammals. Although the terms thrombocyte and platelet are synonymous in mammalian hematology, only the term thrombocyte should be used in descriptions pertaining to avian species. Birds and mammals also differ in coagulation, particularly in the intrinsic system where birds appear to lack coagulation factors XI and XII (Doerr and Hamilton, 1981a).

Normal Blood Values In Chickens

Although many species of birds exist, we used the domestic chicken, *Gallus gallus domesticus*, for the basic discussion of blood parameters and in the presentation of normal values (Table 11–1). Although many generalities concerning avian blood can be obtained from such a discussion, moderate-to-marked species differences should be expected. In Wright-stained blood films, mature avian erythrocytes in the chicken are elliptical and measure about 12 μm in length. The nucleus is also elliptical and has condensed chromatin that stains moderately basophilic. The cytoplasm appears orange-pink. A few large erythrocytes that have a slight-to-moderate polychromatic cytoplasm, are nearly round, and have fewer condensed nuclei, are found in low numbers in most blood films. These cells are immature erythrocytes and would appear as reticulocytes when stained with new methylene blue (Plate XXV–5). Occasionally, immature erythrocytic precursor cells can be seen in blood films of anemic birds. These cells are larger, have a more basophilic cytoplasm, and show little nuclear

condensation compared to mature erythrocytes (Lucas and Jamoroz, 1961).

Leukocytes of various types are found in avian blood. Differentiating heterophils from eosinophils can be difficult, and differentiating lymphocytes, monocytes, and thrombocytes can cause confusion. Both heterophils and eosinophils are segmented cells having similarly stained reddish-orange granules. In both cells, the segmented nucleus may be obscured by overlying intensely stained granules. In chickens, heterophils often have rod-shaped granules, and eosinophils have round granules (Plates XXV–1, XXV–2, XXV–3). As stated by Dein (1982), however, this distinction is not always clear with light microscopy. In Wright-stained blood films, heterophil granules stain lighter than eosinophil granules, giving the cell a slightly faded appearance. This difference is quite subtle, however, and may vary among laboratories. When two distinctly eosinophilic-staining granulocytes are found in a blood smear, the most numerous type is usually the heterophil. This criterion for differentiating heterophils and eosinophils should be used as a last resort and with caution when performing differential leukocyte counts.

Two types of lymphocytes exist in avian blood: small lymphocytes and large or medium lymphocytes (Dein, 1982; Hodges, 1977). Small lymphocytes have a thin rim of basophilic cytoplasm around an oval nucleus

Table 11–1. Normal Blood Values for the Chicken (*Gallus gallus domesticus*)

Erythrocytic Series			Leukocytic Series		
	Range	*Ave.*		*Range*	*Ave.*
Erythrocytes ($\times 10^6/\mu l$)	2.5– 3.5	3.0			
Hemoglobin (g/dl)	7.0– 13.0	9.0	Leukocytes/μl	12,000–30,000	12,000
PCV (%)	22.0– 35.0	30.0	Heterophil (band)	Rare	—
MCV (fl)	90.0–140.0	115.0	Heterophil (mature)	3,000– 6,000	4,500
MCH (pg)	33.0– 47.0	41.0	Lymphocyte	7,000–17,500	14,000
MCHC (%)	26.0– 35.0	29.0	Monocyte	150– 2,000	1,500
Reticulocytes (%)	0– 0.6	0.0	Eosinophil	0– 1,000	400
ESR* (mm)	3.0– 12.0	7.0	Basophil	Rare	—
RBC size (μm)	7.0 × 12.0				
Other Data					
Thrombocytes ($\times 10^3/\mu l$)	20.0–40.0	30.0	Percentage Distribution		
Icterus index (units)	2 – 5	2	Heterophil (band)	Rare	—
Plasma proteins (g/dl)	4.0– 5.5	4.5	Heterophil (mature)	15.0–40.0	28.0
Fibrinogen (g/dl)	0.1– 0.4	0.2	Lymphocyte	45.0–70.0	60.0
Erythrocyte life span (days)	20–35 days		Monocyte	5.0–10.0	8.0
			Eosinophil	1.5– 6.0	4.0
			Basophil	Rare	—

*ESR determined after 1 hour at 45° angle.

(Plate XXV–4). The deeper staining of the cytoplasm and its sparse amount are usually sufficient to distinguish lymphocytes from thrombocytes. Sometimes, however, thrombocytes do not appear to have abundant cytoplasm, especially in thick smears or when thrombocyte aggregation has occurred. Because it is difficult to differentiate between monocytes and large lymphocytes, they are frequently misclassified. Monocytes are usually the largest of the leukocytes seen in blood smears of birds. Their nuclei are usually round or oval, but may be elongated with an indentation on one side. Their cytoplasm usually is abundant and frequently vacuolated or foamy (Plate XXV–3). Since some monocytes may be small and may not be vacuolated, they can appear similar to large lymphocytes. Because some monocytes may not be easily distinguishable from large lymphocytes by light microscopy, the microscopist must be consistent when classifying these cells. Some large lymphocytes may have a few large, azurophilic granules within their homogeneous cytoplasm. These granules are larger and less numerous than granules with similar staining qualities seen in some thrombocytes. Such granules are not seen in monocytes.

As previously stated, thrombocytes can be misclassified as lymphocytes. Typical thrombocytes are oval. They usually have oval nuclei and a moderate amount of lightly stained cytoplasm. (Plates XXV–1, XXV–4). Occasionally, small-to-large groups of oval nuclei with a homogeneous cytoplasmic background can be found in blood smears. These groups are aggregates of thrombocytes and are found more frequently in blood samples that were difficult to obtain allowing time for thrombocyte aggregation to begin before anticoagulation.

FUNCTIONS OF BLOOD ELEMENTS

The blood cells of birds have the same general functions as their mammalian counterparts. Erythrocytes transport oxygen from the lungs; heterophils and monocytes have phagocytic functions; lymphocytes act in the immune mechanisms; thrombocytes act in hemostasis; and the plasma proteins are important in osmotic regulation, coagulation,

immunity, and transport of many substances. Nevertheless, some of these elements differ in some respects from those of mammals because of the anatomic and physiologic differences between birds and mammals.

In birds, the transport of oxygen to the developing embryo must contend with the eggshell, which acts as a barrier. Oxygen transport is accomplished by diffusion through micropores of the eggshell and the underlying shell membranes (Paganelli et al., 1978). Oxygen affinity of embryonic chicken blood increases between 8 and 16 days of development (Po_250 drops from 75 mmHg at day 8 to 35 mmHg at day 16). During this time there is an almost complete replacement of embryonic hemoglobins by adult hemoglobins (Baumann and Baumann, 1978). Oxygen consumption also increases during incubation, although there is a variability in the patterns of oxygen consumption between birds (Hoyt et al., 1978). The oxygen-hemoglobin dissociation curve of adult birds is similar to that of mammals and is influenced by phosphorylated compounds. In the chicken, myo-inositol pentaphosphate appears to be the major phosphorylated compound causing increased Po_250 and right shifting of the hemoglobin-O_2 dissociation curve (Bauer et al., 1978).

Respiration in birds is markedly different from that of mammals. The major differences are that birds have numerous large air sacs and their lungs have a "flow-through" system rather than the "blind-sac" construction of mammalian lungs. The air sacs act as air reservoirs in the respiratory circuit rather than as air terminals. Bird lungs are provided with a system of interconnecting tubes and sacs that allows a continuous flow of air across respiratory surfaces. Thus air is not drawn into the lungs during inhalation, but through these tubes and sacs. Because of their large air sacs and because air passes through the lungs during both inhalation and exhalation, birds have a larger capacity of air per breath, and do not need to breathe as rapidly as mammals of comparable size to obtain the same supply of oxygen (Welty, 1982). Perhaps mammals have adapted to the increased oxygen demands necessitated by homeothermic metabolism by increasing their blood-oxygen carrying capacity through evolutionary development of anucleated erythrocytes, and birds have acquired a more effective respiratory system although maintaining the nucleated erythrocyte.

Although the experimental and clinical evidence in birds is sparse compared to mammals, it is likely that the white blood cells of birds function similarly to their counterparts in mammals. Note that in birds, the heterophil is the counterpart of the mammalian neutrophil. This designation refers to the staining quality of the cell and does not imply different functional activities.

Investigations of the lymphatic system of birds set the foundation for the modern concept of the T- and B-lymphocytes. It was in bursectomized chickens that the first indication of a separate population of lymphocytes involved in humoral immunity was discovered (Glick et al. 1956). Eventually the acceptance of the concepts that cellular and humoral immunities coexist and interact developed from this model.

Perhaps the major difference between mammals and birds in the functions of blood elements is in the hemostatic mechanism. Differences exist in both protein and cellular elements. It is apparent that the major coagulation mechanism in birds is the extrinsic system combined with the common pathway. Apparently birds lack the mammalian contact initiator factors XII and XI. This does not imply, however, that contact initiation of coagulation does not occur in birds, rather, it is probable that an undiscovered mechanism for contact initiation of coagulation is present in birds since avian blood and decalcified plasma coagulate more rapidly when contacted by surface activators such as kaolin or glass. Furthermore, partial thromboplastin time and activated partial thromboplastin time tests demonstrated clotting, and intrinsic thromboplastin could be generated from dilute whole chicken blood (Doerr and Hamilton, 1981a). In addition, factor IX deficiency could be demonstrated in chickens fed aflatoxin. Addition of factor IX reagent partially restored whole blood coagulation time, but addition of both factors XI and XII had no effect (Doerr and Hamilton, 1981b). The experimental evidence suggests that birds have strong extrinsic and common pathways, but that their intrinsic pathway is weak and does not involve the usual contact factors of mammals.

Birds also differ from mammals in that their cellular element of coagulation is the thrombocyte, a nucleated cell, rather than the anucleated platelet. The differences in size and the presence or absence of a nucleus are not the only differences. Bird thrombocytes and mammalian platelets also differ in origin, subcellular morphology and, at least in part, in function. The mammalian platelet arises from cytoplasmic fragmentation of megakaryocytes, but the origin of the avian thrombocyte remains elusive.

Recent observations indicate that the avian thrombocyte should be regarded as a cell with multiple capabilities, one of which is hemostatic activity. Such a cell may be in transition from the first primitive cell in the hemolymph of invertebrates which, in addition to other functions, has a platelet-like capacity for spreading. This function is one of the most ancient, life-saving functions of blood cells (Janzarik, 1981). Thrombocytes have also been reported to have remarkably good phagocytic abilities (Chang and Hamilton, 1979; Hamilton and Weeks, 1978). A close relationship between thrombocytes and lymphocytes has been suggested in some recent studies (Janzarik, 1981; Janzarik and Morgenstein, 1979). Such similarities, however, do not necessarily suggest that thrombocytes and lymphocytes are derived from the same precursor cell.

HEMATOLOGIC TECHNIQUES

Blood Sampling

Many methods have been used to obtain blood from birds. Before taking a blood sample the clinician should know the minimal volume necessary to perform the procedures being done. For routine hematologic techniques, only a few drops are needed. The consequences of blood loss or injury at the site of sampling should be considered before drawing blood. Occasionally peculiarities of the species may preclude obtaining blood from some sites, and it is often difficult to run every test desired in many smaller species.

For pet birds, one of the most commonly used methods for obtaining blood for hematologic examination is to clip the toenail until a small amount of blood flows from the wound (Leonard, 1982; Rosskopf and Woerpel, 1982). This technique, however, is not recommended by all clinicians (Dein, 1982). Although this method is generally useful for collecting the few drops of blood needed for routine hematologic studies, the samples must be processed rapidly by smearing and dilution to prevent coagulation and aggregation of thrombocytes. The clipped-nail method cannot be used when collecting blood for testing hemostatic mechanisms because tissue thromboplastin is released from trauma to the nail. Another disadvantage is that permanent damage to the nail bed can occur (Dein, 1982). Thus this method is not recommended for birds in which nail damage could decrease their functional capabilities; for example, for raptors that are being rehabilitated.

Small blood samples (<0.5 ml) can be collected after lancet wounding of vascular structures, e.g., the wing veins and the comb of chickens (Archer et al., 1977). Such samples can be collected in microhematocrit tubes. Recently a new capillary collecting apparatus (Microvette Capillary Vessels, Sarstedt, W. Germany), which can be used to collect about 30 μl of blood, has been introduced. These devices can be purchased precoated with EDTA or heparin or without an anticoagulant. They can be centrifuged without transferring blood to another container.

Larger blood samples can be obtained from a variety of veins. A commonly used vein is the wing vein or cutaneous ulnar or brachial vein (Archer et al., 1977; Dein, 1982; Fredrickson et al., 1957). Bleeding from these veins often occurs after sampling, with formation of a subcutaneous hematoma. Application of pressure to the venipuncture site can reduce the size of the hematoma but usually will not completely eliminate it. Using the smallest needle available and applying restraint adequate to prevent wing movement, will often reduce the size or prevent formation of hematoma. Serial samples can be obtained from these veins if performed carefully. A major advantage of this method is that the sampling site is relatively featherless and only a few feathers need to be plucked.

Birds usually have only the right jugular vein which, in many larger birds, can be used to obtain blood. This vein can be used in mallards to obtain blood daily without serious complications (Zinkl, unpublished observations).

The medial metatarsal vein, which runs along the inside of the lower leg, is a good site for obtaining moderate amounts of blood. This site is usually surrounded by supporting muscle that assists in hemostasis (Dein, 1982; Murdock and Lewis, 1964).

Cardiac puncture can be used to obtain large volumes of blood, but is a dangerous procedure and should not be used unless the bird is to be sacrificed after bleeding.

Anticoagulants

Small, nonanticoagulated blood samples must be processed soon after they are obtained; they should be diluted immediately for cell counts or smeared for differential cell counts.

Heparin, EDTA, and sodium citrate can be used to prevent coagulation of avian blood. Blood can be drawn into heparinized capillary tubes from open wounds such as clipped toenails. Such samples can be stored for 2–3 hours. Excessive powdered EDTA can cause sufficient red cell shrinkage to alter the hematocrit value. Liquid anticoagulants decrease the hematocrit and total cell counts by diluting the blood samples. Samples taken for coagulation studies should be collected in 3.8% sodium citrate in a ratio of 1 part citrate solution to 9 parts blood (Doerr and Hamilton, 1981a, 1981b). For increased precision, the needles, syringes, and tubes should be siliconized, particularly when the samples are to be used for studies of the intrinsic coagulation system.

Laboratory Techniques

Several characteristics of avian blood present difficulties when performing hematologic examination by techniques routinely used to study mammalian blood. These characteristics include the presence of nucleated erythrocytes, nucleated thrombocytes, and intensely red heterophil granules similar in color to those in eosinophils. When proper procedures are used to minimize the effects of these properties of avian blood, however, reliable hematologic data can be obtained. See Chapter 2 for routine hematologic techniques most of which can be applied to study avian blood. The following sections provide brief comments on techniques specifically applicable to hematologic examination of birds.

Hemoglobin Concentration

Hemoglobin concentration determined by the cyanmethemoglobin method will be erroneously elevated because the nuclei of the erythrocytes scatter light and increase optical density readings. This problem can be corrected by simply centrifuging the cyanmethemoglobin reagent-blood mixture before determining the optical density as is recommended for blood containing Heinz bodies (see Chapter 2). Failure to make this correction causes the hemoglobin concentration to be overestimated, and consequently the MCHC and MCH values to be erroneously high.

Total Leukocyte Counts

The presence of nucleated erythrocytes in avian blood precludes the application of leukocyte counting methods used in mammals. Routine leukocyte counting techniques, as applied to mammalian blood, depend on lysing the erythrocytes and leaving the leukocytes or their nuclei intact. These structures are then counted in a hemocytometer or by automated counting machines. With avian blood, two different approaches to counting leukocytes have been used. The first is to determine the ratio of leukocytes to erythrocytes on blood smears and calculate the WBC count from a previously determined RBC count. The second approach is to differentially stain the leukocytes in suspension and count them in a hemocytometer. Counting by automated machines is not recommended because these methods depend on size to differentiate cells and in most birds there is relatively little difference in the size of erythrocytes and most leukocytes.

Indirect determination of WBC counts based on the ratio of leukocytes to erythrocytes in stained blood smears is subject to inaccuracies. Variations in distribution of the leukocytes, variations in the number of erythrocytes in the smear, and lysis of cells during preparation of blood films are some factors that can cause inaccuracy. Several indirect methods have been used to obtain WBC counts (Lucas and Jamoroz, 1961), some of which are briefly described in the following paragraphs.

The most rapid but inaccurate method is to count leukocytes in 8 oil immersion fields and multiply the count by 1000 to obtain the total WBC count. This method is without merit and should not be used.

Another method is to perform the RBC count first and then estimate the average number of erythrocytes per microscopic field of a stained blood film. Then the number of leukocytes per field is determined similarly. From these data, the WBC count is determined as follows:

$$\text{WBC count}/\mu l = \frac{\text{RBC count}/\mu l \times \text{Leukocytes/field}}{\text{Erythrocytes/field}}$$

A variation of this method is to determine the actual number (rather than an estimate) of erythrocytes and leukocytes per microscopic field for calculation of the WBC count by the given formula.

Many semidirect and direct methods have been described to obtain WBC counts. These methods depend on the vital staining of all or certain populations of leukocytes, which are then counted in a hemocytometer chamber (Lucas and Jamoroz, 1961). A semidirect method depends on counting eosin-stained cells in a hemocytometer chamber and using this count in conjunction with the percentage of eosin-colored cells on a stained smear to calculate the total WBC count. The original method, using phloxine as a leukocyte stain, was described by Wiseman (1931) and modified by Lucas and Jamoroz (1961). A simplified method (Costello, 1970; Dein, 1982) consists of using the Eosinophil Unopette (Becton-Dickinson) to obtain hemocytometer cell counts. Our experience has been that both heterophils and eosinophils stain by the

Unopette method. The WBC count is obtained using the following formula:

WBC count/μl

$$= \frac{\text{Eosin-colored cells/μl} \times 100}{\text{Percentage of eosin-colored cells}}$$

Direct methods depend on staining leukocytes and counting stained cells in the hemocytometer chamber. Many methods have been described including those using solutions developed by Natt and Herrick (1952) and Stroud (1964) and a modification of the Rees and Ecker (1923) method (De Eds, 1927). Ferris and Bacha (1984) recently described a direct method of counting chicken heterophils and eosinophils using a solution of 0.1% phloxine B in 50% propylene glycol. Leonard (1982) suggests diluting 5 parts Natt-Herricks's solution with 4 parts distilled water for staining budgerigar heterophils in a counting chamber. This method is a semidirect method and requires a differential count before the total WBC count can be determined using the above formula by substituting data for eosin-colored cells with data for heterophils.

We have found that 0.01% toluidine blue in saline stains leukocytes in a manner that allows easy visualization in the counting chamber to obtain a direct WBC count. A 1:100 dilution using a red cell pipette is used. All leukocytes in the large central primary square of a hemocytometer are counted. In addition, the erythrocytes in 5 secondary squares of the central primary square are counted. Multiplication of the leukocytes counted by 100 and of the erythrocytes by 400 gives the WBC and RBC counts per μl of blood, respectively.

Differential Leukocyte Counts

Accurate leukocyte differential counts require that the cell distribution be uniform on the slide to be examined. The method of making a smear probably has the greatest influence on the distribution of the cells. Leonard (1982) suggests that the push-slide method does not adversely affect the distribution of avian leukocytes but may increase the disruption of some cells, especially lymphocytes. Dein (1982) suggests that the slide and coverslip method, i.e., when a coverslip is pulled across a drop of blood on a slide, results in even distribution of leukocytes.

Romanowsky stains are commonly used for staining blood smears. Wright and Wright-Leishman stains have been successfully used for staining avian blood films in our laboratories. Dein (1982) criticized rapid stains in that they result in significant cell rupture. Leonard (1982) found that a pH of 5.0 in the third (buffer) phase of Wright's staining is necessary to properly stain avian blood cells, and reported that a pH of 7.0, used for staining mammalian cells, does not properly stain avian cells. Our experience, however, has been that staining techniques used for mammalian cells stain avian cells satisfactorily. Limited experience with Harleco Diff-Quik stain (Curtis Matheson Scientifc, Inc.) also suggests that it works well.

Cell distinction is more difficult in avian blood than in mammalian blood. Immature erythrocytes can occasionally be difficult to distinguish from thrombocytes and lymphocytes because immature erythrocytes have a bluish tinge to their cytoplasm. However, experienced persons generally can make this distinction easily. Similarly, differentiating thrombocytes from lymphocytes may be confusing to people beginning to study avian leukocytes, but with experience the distinction can easily be made because thrombocytes have clear cytoplasm whereas lymphocytes have basophilic cytoplasm. In addition, thrombocytes frequently contain a few small reddish-purple granules that do not appear in lymphocytes. A clear line of demarcation between lymphocytes and monocytes does not exist. Both are mononuclear cells with basophilic cytoplasm. Perhaps size is the best characteristic for distinguishing lymphocytes from monocytes. Monocytes may have an irregular nucleus, but this feature is variable.

Differentiating heterophils from eosinophils can be difficult, even for the experienced observer. The ease of distinction probably also varies with the species being examined. Both heterophils and eosinophils have lobed nuclei, although lobulation is more prominent in heterophils. Granules in both cells stain red with Romanowsky stains, and the intensity of staining is variable and cannot be used as a differential feature. Granule shape is usually round in eosinophils and elongated in heterophils, although round granules can be found in heterophils of some species. Thus there are no exclusive distinguishing characteristics of either types of cells. Familiarity and experience with the leukocyte characteristics of normal birds of each species of interest is the best way to establish confidence in distinguishing heterophils and eosinophils. With normal birds the most numerous segmented leukocytes with red granules are likely to be heterophils and provide a basis for recognizing heterophils in diseased birds. Criteria for recognizing eosinophils can be established by being familiar with the features of the less numerous segmented cells having reddish granules in normal birds.

Generally basophils are not a problem in the differential count. Their basophilic granules easily distinguish them from other mature leukocytes (Plate XXV–1). Most basophils of birds do not have segmented nuclei.

HEMATOPOIESIS IN AVIAN MARROW

A unique feature of avian species is that erythropoiesis and possibly thrombopoiesis occur within the vascular sinuses (see Fig. 13–18), and granulopoiesis takes place outside the vascular sinuses. This distribution of hematopoietic cells can be recognized easily in histologic sections of bone marrow. The marrow of the radius and ulna of young pigeons can be simplified or rendered hypoplastic by subjecting the birds to starvation (Doan et al., 1925). After 10 days to 2 weeks, during which only water is allowed, the marrow becomes essentially devoid of hematopoietic activity. Food is then permitted, and the birds are sacrificed at 24-hour intervals to remove marrow for fixation and sectioning. Within 24 hours, considerable cellular activity is apparent, and separate foci of erythropoiesis and granulopoiesis can be distinguished (see Fig. 13–18). In histologic sections, the developing granulocytes are easily distinguished by the eosin-colored granules common to heterophils and eosinophils of avian species. Electron microscopy (Campbell, 1967) reveals that the wall of the vascular sinus is formed by elongated lining cells, lacking basement membrane, and is continuous

except where granulocytes appear to be passing through. The immature erythroid cells appear to adhere to the sinus wall, while the more mature cells containing hemoglobin are found in the central area of the lumen. Thrombopoiesis is difficult to recognize. The marrow of avian species does not have megakaryocytes.

Cellular events of erythropoiesis in birds are similar to those of mammals (Lucas and Jamoroz, 1961). Rubriblasts, prorubricytes, basophilic rubricytes, and polychromatophilic rubricytes can be found in avian marrow. Nuclear condensation also occurs during the maturation of erythroid precursors, but it is not as marked as in mammals. Reticulum can be found with vital stains such as new methylene blue in polychromic erythrocytes and some normochromic erythrocytes. In addition to the location of erythropoiesis, the second difference between avian and mammalian erythropoiesis is that the nucleus remains in avian erythrocytes and is extruded in mammalian erythrocytes.

The granulocytic series in birds is similar to that of mammals. Lucas and Jamoroz (1961) reported that a stage between the myeloblast and promyelocyte, which they called metagranuloblast, can be recognized in avian marrow. This cell is similar to the myeloblast (granuloblast) but the cytoplasm contains small vacuolated spaces of approximately equal size. As a result, the cytoplasm stains lightly basophilic. The vacuoles may be early stages of primary (azurophilic) granule formation that characterizes the promyelocyte. Monoblasts have not been recognized in avian marrow. It is likely that precursors of monocytes and heterophils are similar at early stages, as in mammals, and cannot be distinguished by light microscopy. The suggestion that monocytes in birds develop in lymphoid organs (Lucas and Jamoroz, 1961) seem incongruous with recent observations in mammals indicating that monocytes and neutrophils are closely related in origin (see Chapter 13).

In adult birds, blood lymphocytes probably arise mostly from "peripheral" lymphoid tissues including the spleen, caecal tonsils, and other gut-associated lymphoid tissue. It is well known that experiments in birds provided the functional basis for separation of morphologically similar populations of lymphocytes. The bursa of Fabricius was established as the site for processing B-lymphocytes responsible for humoral immunity, and the thymus for processing T-lymphocytes. The origin of the lymphocytic progenitor cells in birds, as in mammals, however, is probably the bone marrow. Also, it is likely that in some mammalian species the marrow acts as a peripheral lymphoid organ in the adult, helping to supply lymphocytes to the circulation. For additional information on lymphocytes see Chapter 30.

The origin of the thrombocyte is unclear. Thrombocytes may develop in the marrow sinuses along with the erythrocytes from cells that closely resemble erythrocytic precursors (Lucas and Jamoroz, 1961).

Routine bone marrow examination in avian clinical medicine is not feasible at present. On necropsy examination of freshly killed birds marrow should be obtained and smears made rapidly to prevent disintegration of marrow elements. This approach to marrow examination can be used only when the bird has little monetary or sentimental value.

AVIAN HEMATOPOIETIC NEOPLASIAS

A complex group of neoplastic conditions of the hematopoietic system occurs in poultry. Viral etiology has been established for most of these neoplasias. These hematopoietic neoplasias have been characterized best in chickens, but natural and experimental neoplasias have been found in other gallinaceous birds. Morphologically similar tumors have been found in nongallinaceous birds; however, the etiology of these tumors is unknown. Classification of the leukemogenic viruses and the diseases they produce in chickens and turkeys is given in Table 11-2. Herpes virus of Group B, a DNA virus, causes Marek's disease in chickens; the other leukemia viruses are RNA retroviruses that produce a variety of tumors and other abnormalities in chickens and turkeys.

Hematopoietic neoplasias, particularly Marek's disease, have posed serious economic threats to the poultry industry for years. Beyond their economic importance, these neoplasias have provided us with the earliest and most comprehensive understanding of the viral etiology of cancer. The best studied of these conditions are Marek's disease and the leukosis/sarcoma complex. In 1907 Marek described a polyneuritis in chickens. Over the years the syndrome of lymphoid tumors of nerves and other tissues caused by a Herpes virus has become known as Marek's disease. Nearly simultaneously with Marek's description, Ellerman and Bang (1908) described a lymphoid leukosis which after years of confusion with Marek's disease was found to have a different etiologic basis. Lymphoid leukosis was found to be a part of a complex of diseases with an RNA retrovirus etiology. These diseases ar now called leukosis/sarcoma complex.

The establishment of the etiologic bases of avian hematopoietic neoplasias has led to a classification scheme based on etiology rather than on pathologic findings. Etiologic classification provides a basis for clarifying many confusing aspects of Marek's disease and the leukosis/sarcoma complex (Table 11–2). Hematologic manifestations may occur in both groups, but are not usually the basis for diagnosis. Diagnosis is usually established by the age of the birds, the tissues and organs involved, and epidemiologic factors.

Marek's Disease

Marek's disease usually occurs in young chickens and it may be epinoric. The most common signs are neurological (Allan et al., 1982; Biggs, 1968; Calnek and Witter, 1977). Affected birds are often between 12 and 24 weeks old but older and younger birds can be affected. Mortality in acute Marek's disease may be up to 80% of the flock, but it is usually about 10–15%. The signs of Marek's disease are dependent on the nerves involved. Paresis progressing to paralysis is the most common course of the disease. Birds are often unable to stand; one leg may extend forward while the other lags behind, with a disorder involving the sciatic nerve. Brachial nerve lesions may cause the wings to droop. Torticollis, crop impaction, head tilt, and respiratory dysfunction may also occur. When the iris is involved, blindness may occur. In acute Marek's disease some birds may die suddenly

Table 11–2. Classification of Avian Leukemia Viruses

Virus Group	Virus	Disease	Lesions/Conditions
Herpes virus	Herpesviridae	Marek's disease	Lymphoid proliferation in peripheral nerves and other tissues and organs. Inflammation in CNS and peripheral nerves.
Leukosis/Sarcoma complex	Retroviridae	Leukosis of the fowl	Lymphoid leukosis Erythroblastosis Myeloblastosis Myelocytomatosis Osteopetrosis Other tumors Decreased production
Reticuloendotheliosis	Retroviridae	Sporadic miscellaneous disease in fowl	Wasting, anemia, neuropathy, and feather defects in young birds. Lymphoid tumors in peripheral nerves in older birds.
Reticuloendotheliosis	Retroviridae	Leukosis of the turkey	Lymphoid tumors
Lymphoproliferative	Retroviridae	Lymphoproliferative lesions in the turkey	Lymphoproliferative lesions

Modified from Allan et al., 1982; courtesy of Baillière Tindall Ltd.

before exhibiting any clinical signs. Comparative features that differentiate Marek's disease from lymphoid leukosis are presented in Table 11–3.

The lesions of Marek's disease can be found in a variety of organs. In *classic Marek's disease,* enlargement of the peripheral nerves usually occurs. The nerves are grayish, edematous, and thickened. The normal striations and the white glistening appearance become inapparent. Lymphomatous tumors may be found in the ovary, lungs, heart, liver, and kidneys. In

Table 11–3. Features Useful in Differentiating Marek's Disease from Lymphoid Leukosis

Feature	Marek's Disease	Lymphoid Leukosis
Age of birds	6 weeks or older	Not less than 16 weeks
Signs	Frequent paralysis	Nonspecific
Incidence	Frequently more than 5%	Rarely more than 5%
Macroscopic lesions		
Neural enlargement	Frequent	Absent
Bursa of Fabricius	Diffuse enlargement or atrophy	Nodular tumors
Tumors in skin, muscle, and proventriculus	May be present	Usually absent
Microscopic lesions		
Neural involvement	Yes	No
Liver tumors	Often perivascular	Focal or diffuse
Bursa of Fabricius	Interfollicular tumor and/or atrophy of follicles	Intrafollicular tumor
Central nervous system involvement	Yes	No
Lymphoid proliferation in skin and feather follicles	Yes	No
Cytology of tumors	Pleomorphic lymphoid cells including lymphoblasts; small, medium, and large lymphocytes; and reticulum cells	Lymphoblasts, extensively pyroninophilic
Origin of tumor cells	Primarily T-cells	Almost exclusively B-cells

From Allan et al., 1982; courtesy of Baillière Tindall Ltd.

acute Marek's disease lymphomatous involvement of these and other tissues including the skin may occur. Visceral lesions may be indistinguishable from the lesions of lymphoid leukosis (see Leukosis/Sarcoma Complex).

Hematologic changes that are specific for Marek's disease have not been recognized. The leukocyte count may be increased, largely due to the presence of many large lymphocytes and lymphoblasts (Evans and Patterson, 1971). Some birds may become anemic. Cytologic examination of lesions can be helpful in diagnosis (see differential diagnosis of Marek's disease and lymphoid leukosis; and Table 11–3).

Marek's disease virus spreads rapidly throughout a flock, and infection is ubiquitous among chickens. Feather follicle epithelium is the most important source of infection. The virus proliferates in epithelial cells of feather follicles which, when exfoliated and sloughed, contaminate the litter, dander, and dust of poultry houses. Airborne transmission through the respiratory tract is the most important route of infection (Beasley et al., 1970). The incidence of disease depends on a variety of factors including genetic resistance to development of the disease, the sex of the birds (females are more susceptible), and the virus strain including the presence or absence of nonpathogenic or mild strains that can induce immunity to more virulent strains (Allan et al., 1982).

Leukosis/Sarcoma Complex

The leukosis/sarcoma complex is a group of neoplastic diseases that are caused by related RNA viruses (Allan et al., 1982; Purchase and Burmester, 1977). These diseases generally have a sporadic occurrence and are usually found in adult birds. The most common of the leukosis/sarcoma diseases is lymphoid leukosis.

Clinical signs of the leukosis/sarcoma complex are nonspecific and usually only a small percentage of adult birds develop the disease. The liver, spleen, bursa, kidneys, lungs, gonads, heart, bone marrow, and mesentery may be involved in lymphoid leukosis. The liver may be enlarged and extend throughout the abdominal cavity. Tumors are white and may be nodular, miliary, or diffuse. Leukemia

is rare. Diagnosis is based on finding appropriate lesions (see below).

Viruses of the leukosis/sarcoma group can be transmitted vertically or horizontally. Congenital transmission in eggs and subsequent horizontal spread usually result in a high percentage of infections. Most birds will not develop the disease, however, but subclinical effects such as reduced production and decreased weight gains can occur (Garwood et al., 1981; Govora et al., 1982). The economic loss caused by lymphoid leukosis virus infection is probably much greater than just the economic loss from death or condemnation due to the viral induced tumors.

Lymphoid leukosis and Marek's disease are often difficult to distinguish, although they are etiologically distinct. Both produce tumors of lymphoid cells and similar tissues may be involved. Necropsy examination of a sufficient number of birds and a study of flock records often provide enough evidence to determine which condition is present. The most important differentiating factors are the age of the affected birds, the epidemiology, the presence or absence of paralysis, and the distribution of lesions. Detailed histologic and cytologic examinations, however, may be necessary to differentiate the disease (Table 11–3). Cytologic examination of impression smears of tumors stained with methyl green-pyronine technique reveals extensive pyroninophilia in lymphoid leukosis and little pyroninophilia in Marek's disease (Cooper et al., 1968; Siccardi and Burmester, 1970). Wright-Giemsa stained smears reveal lymphoblasts primarily in lymphoid leukosis, whereas a variety of lymphoid cells are found in Marek's disease, including lymphocytes, lymphoblasts, and plasma cells (Allan et al., 1982).

The leukosis/sarcoma viruses cause various other diseases and conditions besides lymphoid leukosis (Table 11–2). Osteopetrosis, which most commonly involves long bones, frequently accompanies lymphoid leukosis. Anemia is also often present. Sometimes an increased lymphocyte count is found. Primary tumors of other hematopoietic cells are caused by some strains of leukosis/sarcoma viruses. Erythroblastosis, myeloblastosis, and myelocytomatosis are found sporadically. Chickens with erythroblastosis may be anemic and often have circulating erythroid precursor cells. The birds are usually weak. The liver and sometimes the spleen, kidneys, and bone marrow are bright red owing to sinusoidal congestion caused by the leukemic cells. In anemic birds the bone marrow may be thin and watery. In addition to marked erythropoietic immaturity and abnormality, myelocyte and thrombocyte immaturity may be found (Allan et al, 1982; Purchase and Burmester, 1977).

Myeloblastosis and myelocytomatosis are most likely variations of myeloid neoplasia affecting different tissues. In myeloblastosis, signs of weakness, emaciation, and diarrhea are found. Myeloid proliferation in the liver and spleen causes these organs to be greatly enlarged. Frequently, marked leukemia is found with the cells being mostly myeloblasts although promyelocytes and myelocytes may also be present. Myelocytomatosis is also caused by the proliferation of myeloid cells, but in this condition cellular proliferation occurs most often on the visceral surface of the flat bones. The tumorous growths are nodular, yellowish-white, and friable with a cheesy or chalky consistency. These growths occur most often on the sternum; the ribs, especially at the costochondral junction; the pelvis; and the bones of the skull and mandible. The tumors are comprised primarily of cells with characteristics of myelocytes containing eosinophilic or heterophilic granules (Allan et al., 1982; Darcel, 1979; Purchase and Burmester, 1977).

Many strains of the leukosis/sarcoma viruses are multipotential and can cause a variety of other tumors including hemangiomas, renal tumors, hepatocarcinomas, and a variety of connective tissue tumors (Purchase and Burmester, 1977). Virus strains that produce a consistent tumor type in chickens may cause a different tumor in another species. For example, a virus causing erythroblastosis in chickens induced myeloid leukemia in Japanese quail (Moscovici et al., 1981).

Reticuloendotheliosis and Other Lymphoproliferative Diseases

Reticuloendotheliosis viruses, a distinct group of retroviruses, cause sporadic diseases in chickens and turkeys. Chickens infected early in life show poor growth, emaciation, and anemia. Nerve swelling owing to edema and infiltration by lymphocytes and plasma cells may occur and can be confused with Marek's disease (Sharma, 1976). This confusion is of particular concern because some vaccines for Marek's disease are of turkey origin and inadvertent transmission of the reticuloendotheliosis virus could occur during vaccination. Disease resulting in such cases might be interpreted as a "vaccine break." The major problem with reticuloendotheliosis is in turkeys in which a leukosis-like disease occurs (Paul et al., 1976). A variety of tissues including the liver and spleen may have lymphoid tumors (Allan et al., 1982). Intestinal ulceration owing to reticuloendotheliosis virus has been reported in ducks (Purchase et al., 1973).

Another lymphoproliferative disease caused by a retrovirus distinct from those implicated in leukosis/sarcoma complex and reticuloendotheliosis occurs in turkeys. This disease is found most commonly in young turkeys. Splenomegaly and tumors of the peripheral nerves and other tissues are found. The lesions contain pleomorphic lymphoid cells including lymphocytes, lymphoblasts, plasma cells, and macrophage-like cells.

Leukosis-like Disease in Birds Other Than Chickens and Turkeys

Leukosis-like disease has been found in birds other than chickens and turkeys. Experimentally, tumors of hematopoietic cells and other body cells have been produced by several of the leukosis viruses in other gallinaceous birds and in a few birds of other families. Naturally occurring leukosis-like diseases have also been found in wild birds. In these cases, however, a viral etiology has not been established. The disease is sporadic and has been found in several orders including Galliformes, Columbiformes (doves and pigeons), Psittaciformes (parrots and parakeets), Passeriformes (perching birds) and Stigiformes (owls) (Fowler, 1978a; Halliwell, 1971; Palmer and Stauber, 1981; Wadsworth et al., 1981). Lesions comprised of immature lymphoid cells were found in the liver, spleen, and other tissues. Although classification of poultry leukosis complexes is based on etiology, labelling morphologically similar diseases in other birds with terms used in chickens and turkeys cannot be justified until specific etiology is determined even though pathologic descriptions may suggest similarity to a specific poultry leukosis disease.

BLOOD PARASITES

Several protozoan parasites occur in the blood of birds. The most important are *Plasmodium*, *Haemoproteus* and *Leukocytozoon* species, but *Trypanosoma*, *Lankesterella* (syn. *Atoxoplasma)* species and *Piroplasma* organisms *(Nuttallia* and *Aegyptianella* species) may also be found. The hematozoan parasites require two hosts, with schizogony (asexual replication) occurring in the bird and sporogony (sexual replication) occurring in an invertebrate host. Often the organisms can be present without evidence of disease, perhaps having a commensal rather than a parasitic relationship with the host. These organisms can cause disease, however, particularly when the host becomes debilitated or stressed. Furthermore, naive and aberrant hosts may be seriously affected by such organisms.

Plasmodium Species

Plasmodium species cause avian malaria. Numerous species are described. Their differentiation is not as important as recognizing the genus *Plasmodium*. Furthermore, classification of the organisms by species is difficult and often authorities are not in agreement. It should be recognized, however, that these organisms can cause serious effects in some bird species.

Avian malaria parasites are transmitted by mosquitos, particularly of the *Culex* and *Aedes* genera. The mosquito ingests gametocytes contained in erythrocytes. In the mosquito gamete formation, oocyte development, sporogony and sporozoite formation occur. Sporozoites injected into a bird by a mosquito, during a subsequent blood meal, invade cells of the mononuclear phagocyte system. After two generations of development, merozoites invade erythrocytes. Merozoites develop in erythrocytes to form trophozoites. During intraerythrocytic development, hemoglobin is used and iron pigment is deposited in the cell. The erythrocytic forms may develop into gametocytes or they may be released from ruptured erythrocytes to undergo further exoerythrocytic development in macrophages and infect other erythrocytes. Iron pigment and developing schizonts in erythrocytes are important criteria for differentiating *Plasmodium*, *Haemoproteus*, and *Leukocytozoon* species.

Plasmodium species are found in many species of birds. Disease due to these parasites is unusual except in certain species of birds or in unusual circumstances. *P. gallinaceum* produces anemia in chickens, and its exoerythrocytic stages may cause capillary blockage in the brain and produce neurologic signs leading to death (Kemp, 1977). Ducks and geese of Eastern Canada have also been found to be infected with *Plasmodium* species (Bennett et al., 1975). The significance of the parasite is unknown, however, penguins in zoos are highly susceptible to parasitism with plasmodia. *Plasmodium* species which are relatively nonpathogenic to North American birds may cause severe disease in penguins (Herman et al., 1968). Canaries are highly susceptible to infection by *Plasmodium* species and are often used for experimental infection. Psittacines seem to be rarely infected and relatively resistant to avian malaria (Keymer, 1982).

Apparently, malaria due to *Plasmodium relictum* has caused the extinction of several native passerine birds in Hawaii. It has been suggested that extinctions that have occurred in the twentieth century have been due to malaria, while those occurring in the nineteenth century were due to causes other than malaria (van Riper et al., 1982). Although the mosquito vector *Culex quinquefasciatus* has been present in Hawaii since 1826, it seems likely that malaria parasites did not become established until the early twentieth century when they were introduced with exotic birds such as painted quail, Japanese white-eye, American cardinals, and others. Apparently many of the remaining native Hawaiian birds are susceptible to malaria and severe disease and devastating effects could still occur. This has not yet occurred, however, because the remaining native bird populations have adapted behaviorally to the mosquito. The birds appear to migrate altitudinally each day feeding at lower elevations in the day and roosting at high elevations during the night, thus avoiding the mosquitos that live primarily at lower altitudes and feed at night. The native birds also appear to inhabit drier areas, which are less suitable habitats for mosquitos (van Riper et al., 1982). If the range of the mosquitos expands, further severe effects on the native avifauna of Hawaii could occur.

Clinical signs of malaria are nonspecific, and the presence of malarial organisms does not mean a bird has the disease. The birds may be anorexic, depressed and weak, and may die suddenly. Intense and severe anemia may occur. Splenomegaly and hepatomegaly are found (Fowler, 1978b; Kemp, 1977; Keymer, 1982). Reticuloendothelial hyperplasia with mature schizonts in the cells is found on histopathology (Fowler, 1978b; Keymer, 1982). Erythrocytes containing schizonts are found in blood smears. If schizonts are not found, infection with *Plasmodium* species cannot be easily separated from infection with with *Haemoproteus* infections. Organisms of both of these parasites have iron pigment in the erythrocytes, while organisms of *Leukocytozoon* species do not (Keymer, 1982).

Antimalarial drugs have been used to treat malaria with some success. It is possible to prevent the disease in domestic and pet birds through isolation from mosquito vectors by housing, screening, and nets. For susceptible wild populations, vector control should be considered including the elimination of breeding sites by removing standing waters in gutters and around construction sites. Insecticides may be necessary where standing water cannot be eliminated.

Haemoproteus and *Parahaemoproteus* Species

Haemoproteus and *Parahaemoproteus* species are common blood parasites of birds (Keymer, 1982; Wobeser, 1981). Numerous species of the parasite exist. They appear to be nonpathogenic or have low pathogenicity to birds. It is possible however that infection in an aberrant, naive host could cause severe disease. The life cycle of the parasite is similar to other hematozoan parasites requiring an avian host and an intermediate insect host-vector. The insect vectors are midges (*Culicoides* sp.) and louse flies (*Hippoboscidae*) (Cook, 1971a). The intermediate host ingests infected blood and a series of developmental stages occur in the insect. The sporozoites reach the lumen of the salivary gland where they are discharged when the insect feeds on another host. The sporozoites are carried in the blood to the vascular endothelial cells where they undergo multiplication. Schizogony occurs in endothelial cells only, unlike *Plasmodium* species in which schizogony occurs in endothelial cells as well as erythrocytes. Gametocytes are found in erythrocytes. They are usually halter shaped and contain pigment (Plate XXV–9). Disease due to *Haemoproteus* infection is unusual suggesting that the parasites and host are well adapted to each other. Differentiation of *Haemoproteus* and *Parahaemoproteus* species from *Plasmodium* and *Leukocytozoon* species is necessary (Plates XXV–8 to XXV–12).

Leukocytozoon Species

Leukocytozoon species infect many species of birds and can cause severe disease in some birds. *Leukocytozoon* species are transmitted by black flies (*Simulium* spp.) and perhaps by midges (*Culicoides* spp.). Sporozoites injected into the bloodstream of a bird invade cells of the liver, heart, spleen, and other tissues, and develop into schizonts. The schizonts rupture upon maturation and release merozoites and multinucleated fragments. The merozoites may reinfect tissue cells or develop into round gametocytes in leukocytes and erythrocytes. Multinucleated fragments enter macrophages and develop into megaloschizonts which release merozoites; the latter develop into elongated gametocytes in the leukocytes (Keymer, 1982; Wobeser, 1981).

Leukocytozoon simondi can cause severe losses in wild ducklings and goslings. The birds become weak, listless, and dyspneic. They may die suddenly. Anemia and leukocytosis are present and splenomegaly and hepatomegaly may be evident. Liver necrosis with diffuse lymphocytic infiltration can be found. Megaloschizonts in various tissues may cause severe enough damage to organs to cause death (Cook, 1971b; Keymer, 1982; Springer, 1977; Wobeser, 1981).

Leukocytozoon species have been found in weaver bird nestlings, parakeets, various grouse, turkeys (wild and domestic), chickens, pigeons, and doves, and a variety of passerine birds (Bennett et al., 1978; Cook, 1971b; Keymer, 1982; Kucera, 1981; Springer, 1977).

Leukocytozoon infection is diagnosed by finding gametocytes in stained blood films or schizonts in tissue sections. The gametocytes may be round or elongated. The elongated forms may be dark-staining macrogametocytes or light-staining microgametocytes (Plates XXV–10, XXV–11). Pigment granules are not found. This is an important characteristic for distinguishing leukocytozoonosis from *Plasmodium* or *Haemoproteus* infection (Plates XXV–8 to XXV–12). Schizogony does not occur in the blood, but megaloschizonts are found in tissues such as the liver and heart.

Microfilariae

Microfilariae, larval forms of filarial roundworms, are frequently found in the blood of birds but for the most part are an incidental finding. These long, thin worms can be found in blood smears or wet mount preparations (Plate XXV–6). The microfilariae are over 200 μm in length and can be easily seen at lower magnification. In wet mounts, they can be seen wiggling about the smear.

The life cycles of most of the species of avian filarial worms is unknown, and many unnamed species likely exist. If they are similar to other filarial worms, it is likely that blood-feeding insects play an important role in development and transmission.

The effects of most filarial worms in birds are unknown but it is likely they are minimal. Huizinga et al. (1971) have suggested that *Splendidofilaria passerina* may be pathogenic to house sparrows (*Passer domesticus*). The adult worms cause enlargement and thickening of the arterial wall, producing fibrosis, necrosis, and stenosis.

SPIROCHETOSIS

Spirochetosis, due to *Borrelia anserina*, may occur in many species of birds. In fowl, it is

an acute disease characterized by fever, depression, weakness, cyanosis, and diarrhea. Anemia may develop. The disease is transmitted by the tick *Argas persicus* (Gross, 1977). The organism can be transmitted directly from bird to bird, suggesting that mechanical transmission can also occur. At necropsy the spleen and liver are enlarged, although shrunken spleens have been reported in ring-necked pheasants with spirochetosis (Mathey and Siddle, 1955). In birds that survive several days, response to anemia with reticulocytosis, macrocytosis, and polychromasia becomes evident. Diagnosis is based on finding organisms in fresh blood by dark field microscopy or in Giemsa-stained blood films on light microscopy (Plate XXV–7). Inoculation of young chicks with suspected blood and finding spirochetes three to four days later in blood of such chicks may be necessary when demonstration of organisms in blood has not been possible.

Spirochetosis may affect passerine species (Fowler, 1978a; Yakunin, 1962). The birds may be anemic (Fowler, 1978a). It is possible that infected wild birds could be carriers of the organisms, but it is unknown if they have a role in disease of domestic fowl.

HEINZ BODY ANEMIA DUE TO INGESTION OF CRUDE OIL

A primary toxic manifestation of ingestion of crude oil is hemolytic anemia associated with the production of Heinz bodies. Young herring gulls (*Larus argentatus*) and Atlantic puffins (*Fratercula arctica*) developed severe hemolytic anemia after several days of oral dosing with a Prudhoe Bay crude oil. The herring gulls had markedly reduced hematocrit values after 5 days of dosing with 10 or 20 ml oil/kg body weight. In addition, their reticulocyte percentages were 3 to 4 times those of undosed control birds. Atlantic puffins showed a similar response 4 days after receiving 10 ml oil/kg body weight. In erythrocytes of both groups of birds many Heinz bodies were found. Doses of 1 and 4 ml oil/kg body weight in herring gulls and 5 ml oil/kg body weight in Atlantic puffins produced neither anemia nor Heinz bodies (Leighton et al., 1983). The amount of oil ingested by oil-covered wild birds when preening is unknown, making it difficult to evaluate the implications of the preceding study. The observations indicate, however, that it is important to perform hematologic evaluation of birds contaminated with oil. Furthermore, it is possible that lesions seen in birds dying after ingestion of oil may be secondary to the effects on the erythron.

LEAD POISONING

Many wild waterfowl die of lead poisoning each year (Wobeser, 1981). These birds obtain lead by ingesting spent lead shot. Other birds may also die of lead poisoning by ingesting other sources of lead. Raptors may be poisoned secondarily by eating tissues of lead-poisoned birds or by ingesting lead shot embedded in tissues. (Usually, the lead shot obtained in the latter manner will be eliminated when the raptor casts indigestible substances.) Captured pet or wild birds may be poisoned by ingesting lead-based paints on cages or other objects (Zook et al., 1972) or by eating lead or lead-containing objects (Feldman and Kruckenberg, 1975). Lead-poisoned birds show gastrointestinal and nervous system signs. Waterfowl are anorexic, weak, and have greenish diarrhea (Wobeser, 1981). The birds may have drooping wings, ataxia, trembling, paralysis or paresis of exterior muscles, and convulsions (Hartung, 1971). Impaction of the crop, gizzard, and esophagus may occur, and the lining of the gizzard may slough.

Hematologically, mild hypochromic anemia with reticulocytosis may occur (Roscoe et al., 1979). Lead causes aberrant erythrocyte metabolism, and detection of such abnormalities may be helpful in diagnosing lead poisoning and determining the extent of lead exposure in birds. Erythrocyte delta-aminolevulinic acid dehydratase (ALAD) was inhibited in mallard ducks (*Anas platyrhynchos*) given lead shot (Finley et al., 1976). ALAD activity was inversely correlated to blood lead levels in the mallards (Burch and Siegel, 1971). Wild canvasback ducks (*Aythya valisineria*) sampled at two locations (Chesapeake Bay and upper Mississippi River) in 1974 and 1975 showed a similar inverse relationship of ALAD activity and blood lead concentrations (Dieter, 1979). Increased protoporphyrin production occurs in lead-poisoned mallards (Roscoe et al., 1979). The concentrations of erythrocytic protoporphyrin in lead-poisoned ducks may be low in fresh blood because under *in vivo* situations red cell protoporphyrin diffuses into plasma and is excreted by the liver. Refrigeration of blood for 2 days after sampling allows sufficient free protoporphyrin to be produced so that it may be detected using a specially modified hematofluorometer (AVIA Associates).* Experimentally, elevated protoporphyrin concentrations (greater than 40 μg/dl) are detectable 2 days after dosing birds with lead shots and high levels persist for 22 to 36 days after dosing (Roscoe and Nielsen, 1979; Roscoe et al., 1979).

REFERENCES

Allan, W.H., et al.: Viral Diseases. *In* Poultry Diseases, 2nd ed. Gordon, R.F., and Jordon, F.T.W., eds. Baillière Tindall, London, pp. 76–159, 1982.

Archer, R.K.: Blood Coagulation. *In* Physiology and Biochemistry of the Domestic Fowl. Bell, D.T., and Freeman, B.M., eds. Academic Press, London, pp. 897–911, 1971.

Archer, R.K., et al.: Technical Methods. *In* Comparative Clinical Haematology. Archer, R.K., and Jeffcott, L.B., eds. Blackwell Scientific Publications, Oxford, pp. 557–610, 1977.

Bauer, C., et al.: Mechanisms Controlling the Oxygen Affinity of Bird and Reptile Blood: A Comparison Between the Functional Properties of Chicken and Crocodile Hemoglobin. *In* Respiratory Functions in Birds, Adult and Embryonic. Piiper, J., ed. Springer-Verlag, New York, pp. 61–66, 1978.

Baumann, R., and Baumann, F.H.: Respiratory Function of Embryonic Chicken Hemoglobin. *In* Respiratory Functions in Birds, Adult and Embryonic. Piiper, J., ed. Springer-Verlag, New York, pp. 292–297, 1978.

Beasley, J.N., et al.: Transmission of Marek's Disease by Poultry House Dust and Chicken Dander. Am. J. Vet. Res., *31*:339, 1970.

Bennett, G.F., et al.: Hematozoa of the Anatidae of the Atlantic Flyway. II. The Marotime Provenceo of Canada. J. Wildl. Dis., *11*:280, 1975.

Bennett, G.F., et al.: Blood Parasites of Some Birds from Senegal. J. Wildl. Dis., *14*:67, 1978.

Biggs, P.M.: Marek's Disease—Current Status of Knowledge. Curr. Top. Microbiol. Immunol., *143*:92, 1968.

Burch, H.B., and Siegel, A.L.: Improved Methods for Measurement of delta-Aminolevulinic Acid Dehydratase Activity in Human Erythrocytes. Clin. Chem., *17*:1038, 1971.

---

*The hematofluorometer is modified by substituting an emission filter with a band pass of 620 nm for the factory installed filter with a band pass of 594 nm.

Calnek, B.W., and Witter, R.L.: Marek's Disease. *In* Diseases of Poultry, 7th ed. Hofstad, M. S., ed. Iowa State University Press, Ames, pp. 385–418, 1977.

Campbell, F.: Fine Structure of the Bone Marrow of the Chicken and Pigeon. J. Morphol., 123:405, 1967.

Chang, C.F., and Hamilton, P.B.: The Thrombocyte as a Primary Phagocyte in Chickens. J. Reticuloendothel. Soc., 25:585, 1979.

Cook, R.S.: Haemoproteus Kruse, 1890. *In* Infectious and Parasitic Diseases of Wild Birds. Davis, J.W., et al., eds. Iowa State University Press, Ames, pp. 300–308, 1971a.

Cook, R.S.: Leukocytozoon Danelewsky, 1890. *In* Infectious and Parasitic Diseases of Wild Birds. Davis, J.W., et al., eds. Iowa State University Press, Ames, pp. 291–299, 1971b.

Cooper, M.D., et al.: Pathogenesis of Avian Lymphoid Leukosis. I. Histogenesis. J. Natl. Cancer Inst., 41:373, 1968.

Costello, R.T.: A Unopette for Eosinophil Counts. Amer. J. Clin. Path., 54:249, 1970.

Darcel, C. Le Q.: Pathology and Pathogenesis of the Avian Leucosis Complex and its Diagnosis. *In* Comparative Clinical Haematology. Archer, R.K., and Jeffcott, L.B., eds. Blackwell Scientific Publications, Oxford, pp. 519–536, 1979.

De Eds, F.: Normal Blood Counts in Pigeons. J. Lab. Clin. Med., 12:437, 1927.

Dein, F.J.: Avian Clinical Hematology. Proc. Ass. Avian Vet., pp. 5–29, 1982.

Dieter, M.D.: Blood delta-Aminolevulinic Acid Dehydratase (ALAD) to Monitor Lead Contamination in Canvasback Ducks (Aythya valisineria). *In* Animals as Monitors of Environmental Pollutants. National Academy of Sciences, Washington, D.C., 1979, pp. 177–191.

Doan, C.A., et al.: Experimental Studies on the Origin and Maturation of Avian and Mammalian Red Blood Cells. Contrib. Embryol., 16:163, 1925.

Doerr, J.A., and Hamilton, P.B.: New Evidence for Intrinsic Blood Coagulation in Chickens. Poult. Sci., 60:237, 1981a.

Doerr, J.A., and Hamilton, P.B.: Aflatoxin and Intrinsic Coagulation Function in Broiler Chickens. Poult. Sci., 60:1406, 1981b.

Ellerman, V., and Bang, O.: Experimentelle Leukemie bei Hühnern. Zbl. Bakt., Abt. I (Orig.), 46:595, 1908.

Evans, D.L., and Patterson, L.T.: Serum Lysozyme Determinations in Marek's Disease-Infected Chickens. Poult. Sci., 50:1575, 1971.

Feldman, B.F., and Kruckenberg, S.M.: Clinical Toxicities of Domestic and Wild Caged Birds. Vet. Clin. North Amer., 5:653, 1975.

Ferris, M., and Bacha, W.J., Jr.: A New Method for the Identification and Enumeration of Chicken Heterophils and Eosinophils. Avian Dis., 28:179, 1984.

Finley, M.T., et al.: delta-Aminolevulinic Acid Dehydratase: Inhibition in Ducks Dosed with Lead Shot. Environ. Res., 12:243, 1976.

Fowler, M.E. (ed.): Infectious and Zoonotic Diseases. *In* Zoo and Wild Animal Medicine. W.B. Saunders, Philadelphia, pp. 367–374, 1978a.

Fowler, M.E. (ed.) Penguins, Cranes. Storks and Flamingos. *In* Zoo and Wildlife Animal Medicine. W.B. Saunders, Philadelphia, pp. 157–158, 1978b.

Fredrickson, T.N., et al.: Preliminary Investigations on the Hematology of Broiler Flocks. Avian Dis., 1:67, 1957.

Garwood, V.A., et al.: Association of Lymphoid Leukosis Virus and Performance in a Randombred Layer Population. Poult. Sci., 60:2619, 1981.

Gee, G.F., et al.: Species Differences in Hematological Values of Captive Cranes, Geese, Raptors, and Quail. J. Wildl. Management, 45:463, 1981.

Glick, B., et al.: The Bursa of Fabricius and Antibody Production in the Domestic Fowl. Poult. Sci., 35:224, 1956.

Govora, J.S., et al.: Performance of Meat-Type Chicken Test-Positive and -Negative for Lymphoid Leukosis Virus Infection. Avian Pathol., 11:29, 1982.

Gross, W.B.: Spirochetosis. *In* Diseases of Poultry. Holstad, M.S., ed. Iowa State University Press, Ames, pp. 330–334, 1977.

Halliwell, W.H.: Lesions of Marek's Disease in a Great Horned Owl. Avian Dis., 15:49, 1971.

Hamilton, P.B., and Weeks, B.A.: Phagocytosis and Intracellular Killing of Candida albicans by Avian Leukocytes and Thrombocytes. Annu. Meet. Amer. Soc. Microbiol., 78:323, 1978.

Hartung, R.: Effects of Toxic Substances. *In* Infectious and Parasitic Diseases of Wild Birds. Davis, J.W., et al. eds. Iowa State University Press, Ames, pp. 325–335, 1971.

Herman, C.M., et al.: Plasmodium elongatum from a Penguin. Bull. Wildl. Dis. Ass., 4:132, 1968.

Hodges, R.D.: Normal Avian (Poultry) Haematology. *In* Comparative Clinical Haematology. Archer, R.K., and Jeffcott, L.B., eds. Blackwell Scientific Publications, Oxford, pp. 483–517, 1977.

Hoyt, D.V., et al.: Metabolism of Avian Embryos; Comparative Ontogeny. *In* Respiratory Functions in Birds, Adult and Embryonic. Piiper, J., ed. Springer-Verlag, New York, pp. 237–238, 1978.

Huizinga, H.W., et al.: Pulmonary Arterial Filariasis in the House Sparrow. J. Wildl. Dis., 7:205, 1971.

Janzarik, H.: Nucleated Thrombocytoid Cells. II. Phase- and Interference-Contrast Microscopic Studies on Blood Cells of the Domestic Fowl. Cell Tissue Res., 219:497, 1981.

Janzarik, H., and Morgenstein, E.: The Nucleated Thrombocytoid Cells. I. Electron Microscopic Studies on Chicken Blood Cells. Thromb. Haemost., 41:608, 1979.

Kemp, R.L.: Avian Malaria. *In* Diseases of Poultry, 7th ed. Holstad, M.S., ed. Iowa University Press, Ames, pp. 830–832, 1977.

Keymer, I.F.: Parasitic Diseases. *In* Diseases of Cage and Aviary Birds, 2nd ed. Petrak, M.L., ed. Lea & Febiger, Philadelphia, pp. 535–598, 1982.

Kucera, J.: Blood Parasites of Birds in Central Europe. 2. Leucocytozoon. Folia Parasitol. (Praha), 28:193, 1981.

Leighton, F.A., et al.: Heinz-body Hemolytic Anemia from the Ingestion of Crude Oil: A Primary Toxic Effect in Marine Birds. Science, 220:871, 1983.

Leonard, J.L.: Clinical Laboratory Examinations. *In* Diseases of Cage and Aviary Birds, 2nd ed. Petrak, M.L., ed. Lea & Febiger, Philadelphia, pp. 269–303, 1982.

Lucas, A.M., and Jamoroz, C.: Atlas of Avian Hematology. Agriculture Monograph 25. U.S. Department of Agriculture, Washington, D.C., 1961, 271 pp.

Marek, J.: Multiple Neroenentzundung bei Hühnern. Dt. Tierärztl. Wochenschr., 15417, 1907.

Mathey, W.J., and Siddle, P.J.: Spirochetosis in Pheasants. J. Amer. Vet. Med. Ass., 126:123, 1955.

Moscovici, C., et al.: Myeloid and Erythroid Neoplastic Responses to Avian Defective Leukemia Viruses in Chickens and Quail. Virology, 113:765, 1981.

Murdock, H.R., and Lewis, J.O.D.: A Simple Method for

Obtaining Blood From Ducks. Proc. Soc. Exp. Biol. Med., *116*:51, 1964.

Natt, M.P., and Herrick, C.A., A New Blood Diluent for Counting Erythrocytes and Leukocytes in Chickens. Poult. Sci., *31*:735 1952.

Olson, C.: Avian Hematology. *In* Diseases of Poultry, 5th ed. Biester, H.E., and Schwarte, L.H., eds. Iowa State University Press, Ames, pp. 100–119, 1965.

Paganelli, C.V., et al.: The Avian Egg: In Vitro Conductance to Oxygen, Carbon Dioxide, and Water Vapor in Late Development. *In* Respiratory Functions In Birds, Adult and Embryonic. Piiper, J., ed. Springer-Verlag, New York, pp. 212–218, 1978.

Palmer, G.H., and Stauber, E.: Visceral Lymphoblastic Leukosis in an African Grey Parrot. Vet. Med. Small Anim. Clin., *76*:1355, 1981.

Paul, P.S., et al.: Naturally Occurring Reticuloendotheliosis in Turkey: Transmission. J. Natl. Cancer Inst., *56*:419, 1976.

Purchase, H.G., and Burmester, B.R.: Leukosis/Sarcoma Group. *In* Diseases of Poultry. 7th ed. Holstad, M.S., ed. Iowa University Press, Ames, pp. 418–468, 1977.

Purchase, H.G., et al.: A New Group of Oncogenic Viruses: Reticuloendotheliosis, Chick Syncytial, Duck Infectious Anemia, and Spleen Necrosis Viruses. J. Natl. Cancer Inst., *51*:489, 1973.

Rees, M., and Ecker, E.E.: An Improved Method for Counting Blood Platelets. JAMA, *80*:621, 1923.

Roscoe, D.E., and Nielsen, S.W.: Lead Poisoning in Mallard Ducks (Anas platyrhynchos). *In* Animals as Monitors of Environmental Pollutants, National Academy of Sciences, Washington, D.C., 1979, pp. 165–176.

Roscoe, D.E., et al.: A Simple Quantitative Test for Erythrocytic Protoporphyrin in Lead-Poisoned Ducks. J. Wildl. Dis., *15*:127, 1979.

Rosskopf, W.J., and Woerpel, R.W., Jr.: The Use of Hematologic Testing Procedures in Caged Bird Medicine: An Introduction. Calif. Vet., *36(3)*:19, 1982.

Rosskopf, W.J., et al.: Hematologic and Blood Chemistry Values for Common Pet Avian Species. Vet. Med., Small Anim. Clin., *77*:1233, 1982.

Sharma, J.M.: Reticuloendotheliosis in Chickens (Abstract).*In* Differential Diagnosis of Avian Lymphoid Leukosis and Marek's Disease. Payne, L.N., ed. Directorate-General, Scientific and Technical Information and Information Management, Luxenburg, p. 94, 1976.

Siccardi, F.J., and Burmester, B.R.: The Differential Diagnosis of Lymphoid Leukosis and Marek's Disease. USDA Tech. Bull. No. 1412, 1970, 25 pp.

Springer, W.T.: Leucocytozoonosis. *In* Diseases of Poultry, 7th ed. Hafstad, M.S., ed. Iowa State University Press, Ames, pp. 825–830, 1977.

Stroud, R.: Stroud's Digest on the Diseases of Birds. T.F.H. Publications, Inc. Jersey City, N.J., 1964, 476 pp.

Van Riper, C., III, et al.: The Impact of Malaria on Birds in Hawaii Volcanoes National Park. Technical Report 47, Cooperative National Park Resources Studies Unit, University of Hawaii at Manoa, 73 pp., 1982.

Wadsworth, P.F., et al.: Some Cases of Lymphoid Leukosis in Captive Wild Birds. Avian Pathol., *10*:499, 1981.

Welty, J.C.: Blood, Air and Heat. *In* The Life of Birds, 3rd ed. Saunders College Publishing, San Francisco, pp. 130–155, 1982.

Wiseman, B.K.: An Improved Method for Obtaining White Cell Counts in Avian Blood. Proc. Soc. Exp. Biol. Med., *28*:1030, 1931.

Wobeser, G.A.: Diseases of Wild Waterfowl. Plenum Press, New York, 1981, 300 pp.

Yakunin, M.P.L.: Spirochetes in Wild Birds. Trudy. Insti. Akad. Nauk. Koz. kl. SSR., *16*:15, 1962. Cited by T-W-Fiennes, R.N.: Infectious Diseases. *In* Diseases of Cage and Aviary Birds. 2nd ed. Petrak, M.L., ed. Lea & Febiger, Philadelphia, pp. 497–515, 1982.

Zook, B.C., et al.: Lead Poisoning in Captive Wild Animals. J. Wildl. Dis., *8*:264, 1972.

12

Normal Values in Blood of Laboratory, Fur-Bearing, and Miscellaneous Zoo, Domestic, and Wild Animals

THE RABBIT 276
    The Erythrocytes 276
    The Leukocytes 280
    The Platelets 282
    The Plasma or Serum 282
    The Myeloid:Erythroid Ratio 282

THE GUINEA PIG 282
    The Erythrocytes 282
    The Leukocytes 283
    The Platelets 288
    The Plasma or Serum 288
    The Myeloid:Erythroid Ratio 288

THE RAT 288
    The Erythrocytes 289
    The Leukocytes 296
    The Platelets 297
    The Plasma or Serum 297
    The Myeloid:Erythroid Ratio 298

THE MOUSE 298
    The Erythrocytes 299
    The Leukocytes 306
    The Platelets 307
    The Plasma 307
    The Myeloid:Erythroid Ratio 307
    Splenic Hematopoiesis 307

THE GERBIL 308

THE GOLDEN HAMSTER 308
    The Erythrocytes 308
    The Leukocytes 310
    The Platelets 310
    The Plasma 310
    The Myeloid:Erythroid Ratio 310

WILD RODENT SPECIES 310

THE MONKEY 311
    The Erythrocytes 311
    The Leukocytes 313
    The Platelets 314
    The Plasma or Serum 314
    The Myeloid:Erythroid Ratio 314
    Age-Related Hematologic Values 315

FUR-BEARING ANIMALS 315
    Mink 315
    Raccoon 318
    Muskrat 318
    Chinchilla 319
    Fox 320

THE DEER 322

THE WATER BUFFALO 322

**OTHER WILD AND DOMESTICATED
    ANIMALS 329**
    Bovidae 329
    Camellidae 336
    Canidae 337
    Cervidae 337
    Elephantidae 338
    Equidae 339
    Felidae 340
    Giraffidae 341
    Hyaenidae 341
    Tayassuidae 341
    Ursidae 341

Veterinarians are involved in the control of diseases of a great variety of animals other than the common domestic types, namely, laboratory animals used in research, animals in zoos and certain wild animals. A knowledge of normal hematology of these animals is essential for evaluation of their health status.

Normal values gathered by investigators in different laboratories may vary significantly. Many factors influence the composition of drawn blood—capillary versus large-vessel or heart blood, time of day, genetic factors (breed, strain), age, sex, anesthesia and type of anesthetic, nutrition, environmental conditions, and physiologic status including state of excitation of the animal. All such factors that may influence blood composition should be stated when normal values are being reported.

Early literature on normal blood values of common laboratory animals was reviewed by Scarborough (1930–1931, 1931–1932) and Gardner (1947). Details of blood morphology of laboratory animals are provided in texts by Schermer (1954, 1967) and Sanderson and Phillips (1981). Hematologic and biochemical reference values of various experimental animals are given by Mitruka and Rawnsley (1977). Cellular composition and blood coagulation of captive wild animals are described by Hawkey (1975). Normal hematologic values of certain arctic mammals are summarized by Dieterich (1970). Blood collection techniques and normal blood values for several species of laboratory animals are described by Wechsler (1983).

Many species characteristics have been observed in erythrocyte, leukocyte, and platelet morphology among wild and laboratory animals. A brief description of major differences follows; the interested reader is referred to Hawkey (1975, 1977) for details of normal and abnormal hematology of wild animals. Mammalian erythrocytes are nonnucleated and, with rare exception, discocytic cells with varying degrees of biconcavity. Erythrocytes of the camel are typically elliptical, and so are the red blood cells of other members of the family Camellidae. Deer blood often reveals erythrocyte sickling, usually as an in vitro phenomenon. The erythrocyte of the Malay chev-

rotain is the smallest erythrocyte (about 1.5 μm in diameter), while that of the elephant is the largest (about 9.0–10.0 μm) among mammals. Nucleated, elliptical erythrocytes characterize the blood of reptiles, amphibians, fish, and birds. Nucleated red blood cells are usually absent or very rare in the adult mammal. However, 4–40% nucleated erythrocytes are normal in koala blood. Red blood cell life span of some reptiles may be as long as 3 years and appears to be temperature-dependent (Frye, 1978). Heinz bodies are common in the Felidae and white rhino. Cabot's rings are occasionally found in the normal Bactrian camel (Hawkey, 1975). Basophilic stippling is common in gerbils. Reticulocyte percentage is higher in rodents, reflecting a rapid erythrocyte turnover due to a shorter life span than that of common domestic animals (see Table 20–1).

In general, RBC count varies inversely with erythrocyte size, but Hb, PCV, and MCHC are remarkably constant. MCHC is more than 40% in the camel, while in other mammals it fluctuates around the mean value of 33%.

Thrombocytes are nucleated structures in species exhibiting nucleated erythrocytes, whereas they are nonnucleated in mammals. In reference to mammalian blood, the term *platelet* has become synonymous with the thrombocyte. Platelet number is very high in laboratory animals, often exceeding 1 million/ μl of blood. Platelet shape may vary from round, oval, oblong, or cigar-shape to elongated. Spiny anteaters present elongated platelets in addition to regular forms. Species variations have been demonstrated in platelet aggregation and blood-clotting factors (Hawkey, 1975). For example, birds lack coagulation factors V, VII, X, XI, and XII.

Leukocyte count and morphology vary among species. Neutrophils vary with regard to granule color, shape, size, and nuclear morphology. The neutrophil leukocyte in peripheral blood of common laboratory animals, e.g., the rabbit, guinea pig, rat, and mouse, is often referred to as a *heterophil* because its granules do not display neutral staining reaction in blood films stained with Romanowsky stain. The granules often stain a strong pink similar in color to eosinophil granules; hence the cell is sometimes also called a pseudo-eosinophil. For all practical purposes, the heterophil of laboratory animals is equivalent to the neutrophil leukocyte seen in common domestic animals and humans. Heterophils are also observed in other animal species, e.g., birds and elephants. Heterophil granules appear elongated in some species (birds). Heterophils of the ring-tailed lemur are unique in that their granules stain dark purple to almost black. Nuclear segmentation also varies among species. Most nonhuman primates have hypersegmented neutrophils, whereas rodents often display U-shaped, doughnut, and distorted nuclei. Eosinophilic granules are generally round, but may sometimes be rod-shaped (guinea pig) as in the cat. Eosinophil number is high in normal owl monkeys, and the granules are cigar-shaped. Basophil number in blood is generally inversely proportional to the number of tissue mast cells. Lymphocytes and monocytes do not present any unusual features. The neutrophil:lymphocyte ratio varies widely in health and disease.

We have investigated the influence of age and sex on blood composition of New Zealand White rabbits, guinea pigs of mixed strain, 2 strains of mice, and 2 strains of rats. Heart blood was collected in EDTA anticoagulant, between 8 and 9 A.M. from animals fasted overnight. Each animal was bled only once during its lifetime. Ether anesthesia was used on the mice, rats, and guinea pigs but not on the rabbits. These animals were bred and maintained by the Department of Animal Science, University of California, Davis. They were kept under ideal conditions, and epizootic disease was not present during the 3-year period required for the study. It was rare that a blood sample had to be rejected because of disease.

RBC and WBC counts were obtained with the Coulter counter. Hb concentration was determined as cyanmethemoglobin. The Drummond microhematocrit method provided PCV values. Total plasma proteins and plasma fibrinogen were estimated using a refractometer. Blood platelets were counted in the hemocytometer, and 200 leukocytes were differentiated for differential leukocyte counts. Reticulocyte percentage was determined on 500 erythrocytes. Icterus index of

the plasma was obtained by comparison with potassium dichromate standards. The data were subjected to computer analysis. The results of our studies are presented in the sections that follow.

THE RABBIT

Blood specimens may be collected from the marginal ear vein, jugular vein, or heart. Large volumes of blood to harvest serum (40–190 ml) may be collected from the auricular artery or cardiac puncture (Stickrod et al., 1981).

New Zealand White (NZW) rabbits, 138 females and 107 males, ranging in age from 35 days to 26 months, were bled by cardiac puncture without use of anesthesia. The data are presented in Tables 12–1, 12–2, and 12–3. Sex was not found to influence the composition of blood significantly. Wild jackrabbits, 12 younger than 1 year old and 17 adults, were bled from an ear vein (Fetters, 1972). The data are summarized in Table 12–4. Major differences observed in blood composition between jackrabbits and laboratory raised NZW rabbits were, perhaps, influenced only to a minor degree by the different sites for blood collection, that is, ear vein as opposed to cardiac blood.

Literature references may be consulted for published hematologic values of the rabbit (Burns and de Lannoy, 1966; Bushnell and Bangs, 1926; Dougherty and White, 1944; Gardner, 1947; Hinton et al, 1982; Jones, 1975, MacNamee and Sheehy, 1952; Mitruka and Rawnsley, 1977; Pearce and Casey, 1930; Pintor and Grassini, 1957; Sabin et al., 1936; Scarborough, 1930–1931; Schermer, 1967; Scott and Simon, 1924; Srinivasan et al., 1979). Reports on blood volume in rabbits are presented in Table 3–1.

The Erythrocytes

The red blood cell of the rabbit is similar in size and shape to the erythrocyte of the dog. It is a biconcave disc having an average diameter of 6.7–6.9 μm. MCV was 68.3 ± 3.6 fl in adults (Table 12–1). Age had a minor influence on erythrocyte parameters in NZW rabbits. Erythrocyte counts at all ages (both sexes) were 5.55 million to 6.33 million/μl,

Table 12–1. Erythrocyte Parameters and Plasma Composition in New Zealand White Rabbits—Sex and Age Influence (means and 1 SD)[a]

Number of Rabbits	Sex	Age	PCV (%)	RBC (×10^6/μl)	Hb (g/dl)	MCV (fl)	MCHC (%)	MCH (pg)	Reticulocytes (%)	Icterus Index (units)	Plasma Proteins (g/dl)	Fibrinogen (g/dl)
31	male	35–60 days	40.5±2.4	5.64±0.49	11.8±0.8	72.2±5.1	28.4±4.2	21.0±1.3	6.3±3.6	2.2±1.2	5.5±0.6	0.16±0.05
23	male	65–85 days	40.6±3.2	5.92±0.54	12.1±0.9	68.9±5.4	30.0±1.3	20.6±1.5	4.2±2.0	3.7±2.1	5.5±0.5	0.26±0.09
8	male	3 mo	42.5±1.6	6.24±0.24	13.4±0.5	68.1±1.9	31.4±0.9	21.5±0.6	3.7±1.6	3.6±1.9	6.4±0.2	0.25±0.05
23	male	4–6 mo	43.3±2.6	6.34±0.39	13.9±1.1	68.2±4.1	32.0±1.2	21.9±1.5	3.3±1.1	3.3±3.0	6.3±0.3	0.21±0.07
16	male	7–12 mo	42.4±1.6	6.03±0.30	13.7±0.6	70.9±2.3	32.0±0.8	22.7±0.8	3.8±1.5	2.2±1.5	6.2±0.4	0.23±0.08
6	male	13–23 mo	42.7±1.8	6.34±0.70	13.2±1.0	67.9±5.6	31.0±1.8	21.0±1.1	3.2±1.1	3.9±2.1	6.9±0.5	0.33±0.13
29	female	35–60 days	40.3±2.2	5.50±0.62	11.5±0.8	73.9±6.4	28.5±0.9	21.1±1.6	8.0±5.1	2.5±1.3	5.4±0.5	0.19±0.07
12	female	65–85 days	41.9±1.6	5.87±0.20	12.7±0.5	71.5±2.4	30.3±1.3	21.6±0.5	3.0±1.0	3.7±2.1	5.8±0.2	0.22±0.07
12	female	3 mo	41.4±2.5	6.02±0.23	12.6±0.7	68.7±2.5	30.4±1.0	20.9±0.8	3.7±1.9	3.7±2.1	6.0±0.2	0.30±0.09
40	female	4–6 mo	43.0±2.3	6.32±0.43	13.5±0.9	68.2±3.0	31.4±1.1	21.4±1.2	3.8±2.1	3.3±2.7	6.4±0.5	0.22±0.08
27	female	7–12 mo	41.7±3.2	5.95±0.43	13.1±1.0	70.2±3.1	31.4±1.2	22.1±1.1	3.7±1.2	2.7±3.1	6.2±0.6	0.21±0.10
18	female	13–26 mo	40.8±3.5	5.96±0.54	12.7±1.3	68.5±2.7	31.3±1.4	21.4±1.0	2.9±1.4	3.4±1.9	6.6±0.6	0.24±0.12
60	both	35–60 days	40.3±2.4	5.55±0.56	11.6±0.8	73.0±5.8	28.4±3.0	21.0±1.4	7.4±4.7	2.4±1.3	5.4±0.6	0.19±0.07
35	both	65–85 days	41.1±2.9	5.90±0.46	12.3±0.8	69.8±4.8	30.1±1.3	20.9±1.4	3.8±1.8	3.7±2.1	5.6±0.5	0.24±0.09
20	both	3 mo	41.9±2.2	6.11±0.26	12.9±0.7	68.5±2.3	30.8±1.1	21.1±0.8	3.9±1.8	3.7±2.0	6.1±0.3	0.26±0.05
63	both	4–6 mo	43.1±2.4	6.33±0.41	13.6±1.0	68.2±3.4	31.6±1.2	21.6±1.3	3.6±1.8	3.3±2.9	6.4±0.4	0.21±0.08
43	both	7–12 mo	42.0±2.7	5.98±0.39	13.3±0.9	70.4±2.9	31.7±1.1	22.3±1.1	3.7±1.3	2.4±2.6	6.2±0.5	0.21±1.00
24	both	13–26 mo	41.2±3.2	6.05±0.61	12.9±1.3	68.3±3.6	31.2±1.5	21.3±1.1	3.0±1.3	3.5±2.0	6.7±0.6	0.26±0.13

[a]Heart blood collected without anesthesia.

Table 12-2. Total and Differential Leukocyte Numbers in New Zealand White Rabbits—Sex and Age Influence (means and 1 SD)[a]

Number of Rabbits	Sex	Age	WBC/μl	Neutrophils Band	Neutrophils Mature	Lymphocytes	Monocytes	Eosinophils	Basophils
				Differential Leukocyte Count in Absolute Numbers/μl					
31	male	35–60 days	5,997 ± 1,977	19 ± 59	2,250 ± 1,538	3,281 ± 676	332 ± 425	50 ± 36	120 ± 100
23	male	65–85 days	7,821 ± 2,402	0	2,396 ± 1,377	5,081 ± 2,051	200 ± 274	69 ± 66	71 ± 61
8	male	3 mo	8,450 ± 1,341	7 ± 17	2,370 ± 800	5,449 ± 1,369	421 ± 536	128 ± 58	77 ± 47
23	male	4–6 mo	7,713 ± 1,083	0	2,165 ± 945	5,243 ± 975	140 ± 122	55 ± 55	107 ± 99
16	male	7–12 mo	8,994 ± 1,753	0	2,593 ± 1,040	5,620 ± 1,897	210 ± 169	66 ± 50	254 ± 179
6	male	13–23 mo	10,000 ± 2,849	0	4,669 ± 1,394	4,343 ± 1,107	605 ± 661	168 ± 128	205 ± 164
29	female	35–60 days	5,379 ± 1,851	1 ± 5	1,917 ± 1,265	3,095 ± 736	192 ± 144	47 ± 38	128 ± 120
12	female	65–85 days	8,060 ± 3,723	0	1,893 ± 760	5,145 ± 3,476	121 ± 183	134 ± 97	96 ± 86
12	female	3 mo	9,108 ± 3,539	0	2,521 ± 1,020	6,252 ± 3,219	112 ± 72	99 ± 126	125 ± 87
40	female	4– 6 mo	7,687 ± 1,601	2 ± 14	2,236 ± 1,169	4,740 ± 1,386	200 ± 173	110 ± 72	183 ± 131
27	female	7–12 mo	7,696 ± 1,787	0	2,238 ± 706	4,913 ± 1,721	264 ± 206	94 ± 82	185 ± 131
18	female	13–26 mo	9,722 ± 3,314	4 ± 16	4,683 ± 3,084	4,128 ± 1,122	433 ± 297	178 ± 124	296 ± 192
60	both	35–60 days	5,647 ± 1,936	10 ± 63	2,068 ± 1,405	3,170 ± 713	258 ± 326	47 ± 37	121 ± 111
35	both	65–85 days	7,899 ± 2,898	0	2,224 ± 1,225	5,103 ± 2,628	173 ± 250	92 ± 84	80 ± 71
20	both	3 mo	8,765 ± 2,900	3 ± 11	2,460 ± 941	5,931 ± 2,668	235 ± 376	111 ± 105	106 ± 77
63	both	4– 6 mo	7,697 ± 1,431	1 ± 11	2,210 ± 1,093	4,924 ± 1,275	178 ± 159	90 ± 71	156 ± 126
43	both	7–12 mo	8,179 ± 1,882	0	2,350 ± 858	5,176 ± 1,821	245 ± 195	83 ± 73	211 ± 154
24	both	12–26 mo	9,792 ± 3,207	3 ± 15	4,680 ± 2,769	4,182 ± 1,122	476 ± 425	176 ± 125	273 ± 189

[a]Heart blood collected without anesthesia.

Table 12–3. Leukocyte and Platelet Counts in New Zealand White Rabbits—Sex and Age Influence (means and 1 SD)[a]

Number of Rabbits	Sex	Age	WBC/μl	Differential Leukocyte Count (%)						Platelets (×10³/μl)
				Neutrophils		Lympho-cytes	Mono-cytes	Eosino-phils	Basophils	
				Band	Mature					
31	male	35–60 days	5,997 ± 1,977	0.2 ± 0.7	34.7 ± 11.7	57.7 ± 13.1	5.5 ± 7.0	0.8 ± 0.6	2.0 ± 1.7	428 ± 178
23	male	65–85 days	7,821 ± 2,402	0	30.3 ± 12.5	65.4 ± 13.5	2.4 ± 2.9	0.9 ± 0.8	1.0 ± 0.7	418 ± 146
8	male	3 mo	8,450 ± 1,341	0.06 ± 0.2	28.9 ± 8.4	65.7 ± 9.2	5.6 ± 7.5	1.6 ± 0.8	0.8 ± 0.6	360 ± 117
23	male	4– 6 mo	7,713 ± 1,083	0	27.6 ± 10.4	68.5 ± 11.1	1.7 ± 1.4	0.8 ± 0.8	1.4 ± 1.3	291 ± 91
16	male	7–12 mo	8,994 ± 1,753	0	27.9 ± 8.0	62.0 ± 16.9	2.5 ± 2.4	0.8 ± 0.7	3.0 ± 2.6	290 ± 98
6	male	13–23 mo	10,000 ± 2,849	0	47.0 ± 5.9	44.5 ± 7.0	4.9 ± 4.5	1.5 ± 1.0	2.3 ± 2.3	303 ± 168
29	female	35–60 days	5,379 ± 1,851	0.02 ± 0.1	31.9 ± 12.2	61.1 ± 12.5	3.7 ± 2.6	0.9 ± 0.9	2.3 ± 2.2	474 ± 195
12	female	65–85 days	8,060 ± 3,723	0	27.8 ± 5.8	67.0 ± 5.7	1.8 ± 3.1	1.9 ± 0.9	1.4 ± 0.9	395 ± 202
12	female	3 mo	9,108 ± 3,539	0	28.8 ± 10.0	67.5 ± 10.3	1.4 ± 0.9	0.9 ± 0.8	1.5 ± 0.8	385 ± 145
40	female	4– 6 mo	7,687 ± 1,601	0.03 ± 0.2	28.9 ± 10.4	63.9 ± 10.4	2.7 ± 2.3	1.5 ± 0.9	2.5 ± 1.8	347 ± 93
27	female	7–12 mo	7,696 ± 1,787	0	30.0 ± 9.7	62.8 ± 11.8	3.5 ± 2.6	1.2 ± 1.1	2.4 ± 2.0	351 ± 110
18	female	13–26 mo	9,722 ± 3,314	0.03 ± 0.1	44.7 ± 14.6	45.6 ± 14.4	4.8 ± 2.5	2.0 ± 1.6	3.3 ± 2.2	354 ± 101
60	both	35–60 days	5,647 ± 1,936	0.09 ± 0.5	33.4 ± 11.9	59.5 ± 12.8	4.5 ± 5.4	0.9 ± 0.8	2.1 ± .19	460 ± 196
35	both	65–85 days	7,899 ± 2,898	0	29.5 ± 10.8	66.0 ± 11.4	2.2 ± 3.0	1.2 ± 0.9	1.1 ± 0.8	409 ± 169
20	both	3 mo	8,765 ± 2,900	0.03 ± 0.1	28.8 ± 9.4	66.8 ± 9.9	3.1 ± 5.2	1.2 ± 0.9	1.3 ± 0.8	372 ± 131
63	both	4– 6 mo	7,697 ± 1,431	0.02 ± 0.1	28.4 ± 10.4	65.6 ± 10.9	2.4 ± 2.1	1.2 ± 0.9	2.1 ± 1.7	326 ± 96
43	both	7–12 mo	8,179 ± 1,882	0	29.2 ± 9.1	62.5 ± 13.9	3.2 ± 2.6	1.1 ± 1.0	2.7 ± 2.2	331 ± 110
24	both	13–26 mo	9,792 ± 3,207	0.02 ± 0.1	45.2 ± 13.1	45.3 ± 13.0	4.6 ± 3.1	1.9 ± 1.5	3.0 ± 2.3	343 ± 120

[a]Heart blood collected without anesthesia.

Table 12–4. The Hemogram of the Wild Jackrabbit (Lepus californicus) (means and 1 SD)[a]

Item	12 Rabbits <1 Year of Age			17 Adults Rabbit		
	No.		%	No.		%
Erythrocytes ($\times 10^6/\mu l$)	7.73 ± 0.78		—	7.79 ± 0.51		—
Hemoglobin (g/dl)	15.97 ± 1.30		—	15.98 ± 1.18		—
PCV (%)	49.08 ± 3.98		—	47.58 ± 2.89		—
MCV (fl)	63.62 ± 2.47		—	61.08 ± 2.45		—
MCH (pg)	20.70 ± 1.07		—	20.48 ± 1.10		—
MCHC (%)	32.52 ± 1.04		—	33.54 ± 1.20		—
Icterus index (units)	2.5 ± 1.1		—	4.1 ± 1.4		—
Reticulocytes (%)	0.3 ± 0.74		—	1.3 ± 2.1		—
Plasma proteins (g/dl)	5.9 ± 0.68		—	5.5 ± 0.56		—
Fibrinogen (g/dl)	0.28 ± 0.10		—	0.27 ± 0.10		—
WBC/μl	4,908 ± 2,193		—	7,459 ± 3,146		—
Band neutrophils	4 ±	14	0.08 ± 0.28	2 ±	7	0.03 ± 0.12
Mature neutrophils	1,721 ±	874	34.6 ± 11.4	3,638 ± 2,580		50.4 ± 21.4
Lymphocytes	2,598 ± 1,202		54.2 ± 11.6	3,300 ± 2,401		42.7 ± 19.8
Monocytes	334 ±	294	6.3 ± 3.5	294 ±	223	4.3 ± 3.0
Eosinophils	229 ±	237	4.5 ± 3.6	190 ±	219	2.2 ± 2.0
Basophils	23 ±	35	0.4 ± 0.6	36 ±	51	0.4 ± 0.5
Blood platelets ($\times 10^3/\mu l$)	447 ±	215	—	449 ±	179	—

[a]Blood taken from an ear vein.

agreeing with literature reports. Hemoglobin concentration was lowest in NZW rabbits at 35–60 days of age (11.6 ± 0.8 g/dl), increased to a peak of 13.6 ± 1.0 g/dl at 4–7 months of age, and declined to 12.9 ± 1.3 g/dl in adults. The PCV exhibited a similar pattern, with the highest value of 43.1 ± 2.4% at 4–6 months of age. MCHC was 28.4 ± 3.0% at 35–60 days of age and did not exceed 32.0 ± 1.2% in older rabbits. Wild jackrabbits presented considerably higher values for RBC, Hb, and PCV and had somewhat smaller erythrocytes (Table 12–4). NZW rabbits had reticulocyte counts of 7.4 ± 4.7% at 35–60 days of age, followed by a 50% reduction during the third month of life and a further smaller decrease to 3.0 ± 1.3% in adult rabbits. Both young and adult jackrabbits had considerably fewer reticulocytes than NZW rabbits. A mean reticulocyte count of 2.64 ± 1.22% was reported for 111 male rabbits (Pintor and Grassini, 1957). Short chains of rouleaux occur in stained blood films, and some polychromasia is commonly present. Anisocytosis, polychromasia, nucleated erythrocytes, and Howell-Jolly bodies characterize the peripheral blood in anemia in remission. Osmotic fragility begins at 0.50% NaCl and is complete at 0.30% (Perk et al., 1964). Life span of the normal rabbit erythrocyte has been variously reported to be 45–70 days (Table 20–1).

The Leukocytes

Leukocyte counts (Table 12–2) were lowest in the youngest rabbits and increased with advancing age, with 2 distinct peaks. The first peak (8,765 ± 2,900/μL) at 3 months of age was followed by a modest decline between 4 and 6 months of age and then an increase to a second and higher peak (9,792 ± 3,207) in rabbits over 1 year of age. Differential leukocyte counts revealed neutrophil leukocytes to remain between 1,800 and 2,500/μl through the first year of life, followed by a 100% increase (4,680 ± 2,769) in rabbits over 1 year of age. Lymphocyte numbers were lowest (3,170 ± 713/μl) in the youngest rabbits, increased to highest levels (5,931 ± 2,668) in rabbits at 3 months of age, and then gradually declined to 4,182 ± 1,122 in rabbits over 1 year of age. Thus an increase in lymphocytes was mainly responsible for the first peak in WBC count at 3 months of age, while a marked increase in neutrophils produced the second and highest counts in rabbits over 1 year of age.

Differential leukocyte counts in percentage are presented in Table 12–3. Neutrophil:lymphocyte ratios, expressed as percentages, changed from 33:60 in the second month of life to 45:45 in rabbits over 1 year of age. Monocytes, eosinophils, and basophils contributed less than 500 cells each to the WBC count during the first year of life and exhibited a slight to modest increase in older rabbits. Although WBC counts were lower in wild jackrabbits than in NZW rabbits, a shift in N:L ratio with age was noted in both species. Leukocyte counts varied be-

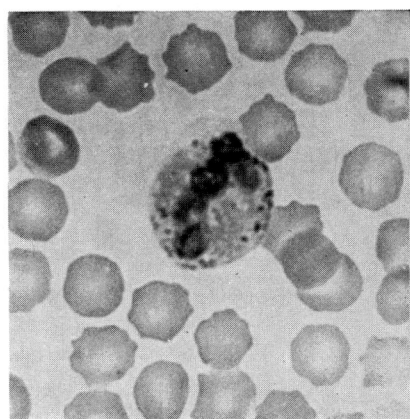

Fig. 12–1.   Rabbit pseudo-eosinophil (heterophil).

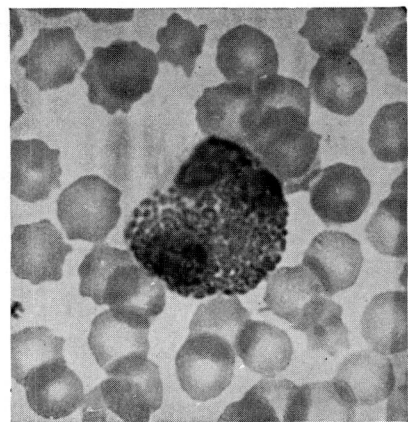

Fig. 12–2.   Rabbit eosinophil.

tween 3,200 and 23,500/μl in normal rabbits (Pearce and Casey, 1930), and most investigators have reported mean values of 7,000–9,000. Average WBC counts in relation to age were found to be 2,000/μl in the first week of life; 3,500 at 30 days; 4,500 at 60 days; 4,500–6,000 between 100 and 200 days; and 2,000–12,000 with a mean of 7,000 for adult rabbits (Cheng, 1930). A diurnal variation of circulating leukocyte numbers was reported, with peak counts in the early afternoon followed by a rapid decline (Jackson and Stovall, 1930). Variations due to sex and breed may also occur. Trapped cottontail rabbits were found to have high corticosteroid levels, PCV, and neutrophil numbers and low lymphocyte numbers (Jacobson et al., 1978). Pelger-Huët anomaly may be encountered in leukocytes of certain rabbits (see Chapter 4).

The Neutrophil (Heterophil)

The unique feature of rabbit blood is the leukocyte comparable to the neutrophil of large domestic animals. Pseudo-eosinophil and amphophil are other terms applied to this cell. The nucleus is polymorphous and stains with a combination of light purple and light blue, the latter color following the outline of the nuclear membrane. The cytoplasm is diffusely pink, apparently because of fusion of many small acidophilic specific granules, with a variable number of large, reddish granules superimposed upon the diffusely pink background (Fig. 12–1). These larger granules stain darkly with new methylene blue applied to an unfixed, dry blood film. Two types of

granules are also defined by the electron microscope; the larger granules correspond to primary or azurophilic granules and the smaller to secondary or specific granules (Bainton and Farquhar, 1966).

The Lymphocyte

This cell has the typical morphology described for other species of animals. Both small and large forms are found, and an occasional large lymphocyte presents a few azurophilic granules in the cytoplasm.

The Monocyte

Under conditions of health, the monocyte is a large cell that is identified by its ameboid nuclear patterns, diffuse and lightly staining nuclear chromatin, and blue cytoplasm, which commonly presents a few distinct vacuoles. Witts and Webb (1927) described the occurrence of large, dark red to purple granules, about the size of the eosinophil granule, in the cytoplasm of the monocyte in rabbits infected wih *Bacterium monocytogenes (Listeria monocytogenes)*.

The Eosinophil

This cell is readily distinguishable from the heterophil by its larger size and characteristic granules (Fig. 12–2). The granules are three to four times the size of those of the heterophil, fill the cytoplasm, and are intensely acidophilic.

The Basophil

The rabbit is unique among the common laboratory animals in that the basophil leukocyte is regularly present in the circulation in small to modest numbers. The nucleus takes a light purple stain, and the cytoplasm is packed with purple to black metachromatic granules. It is not infrequent to find rabbits with 8–10% basophils, (Gardner, 1947; Pearse and Casey, 1930; Sabin et al., 1936; Scarborough, 1930–1931), and rarely counts up to 30% have been found (Schermer, 1967).

The Platelets

The individual platelet presents a small cluster of azurophilic granules surrounded by a pale blue cytoplasm. Platelets appear both singly and in groups throughout the blood film. Platelet counts reported in the literature include a range of 200,000 to 1 million/μl, with an average of 540,000 (Sarborough, 1930–1931); a range of 126,000 to 1 million (Schermer, 1967); and a mean of 251,000 (Sutherland et al., 1958). In NZW rabbits, the platelets were more numerous (460,000 ± 196,000) at 35 to 60 days of age than in older rabbits. In rabbits over 1 year of age, platelet counts were 343,000 ± 120,000.

The Plasma or Serum

Icterus index varied between 2 and 7.5 units. Total plasma protein concentration increased with age in NZW rabbits from 5.4 ± 0.6 g/dl at 35–60 days of age to 6.7 ± 0.6 g/dl in adults. Plasma fibrinogen was generally less than 0.2 g/dl in the youngest rabbits and ranged between 0.2 and 0.4 g/dl in older rabbits (Table 12–1). Total plasma protein was somewhat lower in wild jackrabbits (Table 12–4) than in the laboratory-raised NZW rabbits, but fibrinogen levels were similar in both strains of rabbits.

A mean plasma protein value of 5.8 g/dl was reported for rabbits (Sutherland et al., 1958). Serum proteins in NZW rabbits were found to range from 2.87 to 10.13 g/dl, with a mean of 4.96 ± 1.39 (Burns and de Lannoy, 1966) and from 4.4 to 6.3 g/dl in males and 4.3 to 7.3 in females, with respective means of 5.2 and 5.7 g/dl (Kozma et al., 1967).

The Myeloid:Erythroid Ratio

Sabin et al., (1936) investigated the M:E ratio in rabbits from birth to 5 months of age with the following results: at birth, 0.72; 1 week, 0.19; 4 weeks, 1.09; 2 months, 0.61; 3 months, 0.81; 4 months, 1.42: and 5 months, 0.89:1.0. Dikovinova (1957) investigated the myelograms of 26 normal rabbits (Table 12–5) and reported a mean M:E ratio of 1.01:1.0.

Bone marrow biopsy may be obtained from an anesthetized rabbit from the shaft of the ilium (Wilson, 1971) or from the humerus or femur using an 18-gauge Rosenthal pediatric needle (Horan et al., 1980).

THE GUINEA PIG

Blood may be obtained from the ear by puncturing a capillary vessel and filling pipettes directly from free-flowing blood. Blood may also be collected from the thigh vein, jugular vein, or orbital sinus. Methods for obtaining repeated blood samples have been described (Vallejo-Freire, 1951; Lopez and Navia, 1977). When a larger quantity of blood is needed, heart puncture is employed. We employed heart puncture under ether anesthesia to collect blood from 144 male and 189 female mixed strain guinea pigs, 2 days to 28 months of age. The data on blood composition by age and sex are summarized in Tables 12–6, 12–7, and 12–8.

Selected references on hematology of the guinea pig are Bilbey and Nicol, 1955; Burnett, 1917; Burns and de Lannoy, 1966; Quillec et al., 1977; King and Lucas, 1941; MacNamee and Sheehy, 1952; Mahadevan et al., 1981; Mitruka and Rawnsley, 1977; Pattison and McDiarmid, 1943; Sawitsky and Meyer, 1948; Scarborough, 1930–1931; Schermer, 1967.

The Erythrocytes

During the first 3 months of life there was no evidence of sex differences (Table 12–6). Erythrocyte numbers increased by 1 million/μl from the first month (4.62 ± 0.57 million/μl) through the third month (5.58 ± 0.37 million/μl) of life. Hemoglobin concentration and PCV increased along with the RBC count. A slight decline in values of the erythrocyte parameters occurred in males beginning with the fourth month of life, compared to a somewhat greater decline of the same values in females. Mean values for RBC, Hb, and PCV for male guinea pigs 13–28 months of age

Table 12–5.   Differential Cell Distribution (%) in the Marrow of Normal Rabbits[a]

Cell Type	Min.	Max.	Ave.
Erythroid Series			
Rubriblasts	0.2	0.8	0.2
Prorubricytes	0.2	2.0	0.6
Basophilic rubricytes	0.4	10.8	5.5
Polychromatophilic rubricytes	10.9	26.6	18.9
Metarubricytes	6.6	24.3	16.7
Total erythrocytic cells	—	—	41.9
Granulocytic Series			M:E = 1.01:1.0
Myeloblasts	0.2	1.6	0.7
Progranulocytes	0.1	1.6	0.6
Myelocytes	1.1	6.1	3.1
Metamyelocytes	2.8	10.0	7.4
Band pseudo-eosinophils	10.8	33.6	23.2
Segmenter pseudo-eosinophils	2.0	9.0	5.3
Basophils	0.1	2.4	0.7
Eosinophils	0.2	2.4	1.4
Total granulocytic cells			42.4
Other Cells in the Marrow			
Megakaryocytes	0.1	0.3	0.1
Lymphocytes	4.1	21.3	12.6
Monocytes	0.4	3.6	1.6
Plasma cells	0.1	1.2	0.2
RE nuclei	0.2	1.7	1.0
Hemocytoblasts	0.1	0.8	0.2

[a]Data from Dikovinova, 1957.

were, respectively, 5.37 million/μl, 13.6 g/dl, and 43.9%. For female guinea pigs, they were 4.67 million/μl, 11.8 g/dl, and 39.8%. The greater reduction of erythrocyte numbers in females beginning with the fourth month of life was compensated in part by a larger MCV. The MCV of adult males was 81.8 ± 3.5 fl and for adult females, 85.4 ± 4.5 fl. The MCHC of both sexes varied between 29.5% and 31.6%. The diameter of the guinea pig erythrocyte has a range of 7.2–7.8 μm, and mean of 7.5 μm (Burnett, 1917; Scarborough, 1930–1931). The guinea pig erythrocyte is the largest RBC among the more common laboratory animals.

Short chains of rouleaux occur in the thicker areas of blood films and polychromasia is slight to moderate, depending on the age of the guinea pig. Neonates may have as many as 25% polychromatic red cells (Schermer, 1967). During the first month of life, reticulocytes were most numerous, with counts averaging 6.1 ± 3.8%. Reticulocyte numbers fell during the second month of life to 2.6 ± 1.5%, while the count in adult guinea pigs was 1.8 ± 2.2%. Reticulocyte numbers increase in peripheral blood in anemia in remission, as reflected by anisocytosis and polychromasia ac-

companied by nucleated erythrocytes and Howell-Jolly bodies.

Hemolysis in buffered hypotonic saline begins at 0.52% NaCl solution and is complete at 0.30% (Perk et al., 1964). Respective values reported earlier were 0.42% and 0.32% (Scarborough, 1930–1931).

The Leukocytes

There is considerable variation among reports concerning the normal range and mean for WBC counts in the guinea pig. A comparison of RBC and WBC counts in peripheral blood and heart blood was made (Roofe et al., 1950). The heart blood was taken under sodium pentobarbital anesthesia, while the peripheral blood was drawn before administration of the anesthetic. The mean values for peripheral blood were 7,558/μl for leukocytes and 6.26 million/μl for erythrocytes, compared with 5,763/μl and 5.49 million/μl, respectively, for heart blood. These data cannot be considered as representing a valid comparison between peripheral and heart blood because of the possible effect of anesthesia on the cellular composition of heart blood. Sodium pentobarbital anesthesia causes a reduction of circulating erythrocytes through

Table 12–6. Erythrocyte Parameters and Plasma Protein Concentration in Guinea Pigs—Sex and Age Influence (means and 1 SD)[a]

Number of Guinea Pigs	Sex	Age	PCV (%)	RBC (×10⁶/μl)	Hb (g/dl)	MCV (fl)	MCHC (%)	Reticulocytes (%)	Plasma Proteins (g/dl)
54	male	2–30 days	38.3 ± 4.5	4.67 ± 0.65	11.36 ± 1.5	82.4 ± 4.0	29.7 ± 1.4	6.3 ± 3.7	4.7 ± 0.5
46	male	31–60 days	42.9 ± 2.9	5.18 ± 0.47	13.06 ± 1.0	82.9 ± 3.9	30.3 ± 0.9	2.6 ± 1.3	5.1 ± 0.4
16	male	63–90 days	46.3 ± 2.3	5.64 ± 0.38	14.04 ± 0.9	82.2 ± 2.7	30.3 ± 1.2	2.7 ± 1.6	5.7 ± 0.4
8	male	4– 6 mo	45.1 ± 4.5	5.81 ± 0.62	14.07 ± 1.0	77.7 ± 3.8	31.2 ± 1.2	1.9 ± 0.9	6.0 ± 0.5
9	male	7–12 mo	44.0 ± 3.7	5.55 ± 0.51	13.90 ± 1.4	79.4 ± 3.7	31.6 ± 1.1	1.3 ± 0.4	5.8 ± 0.3
11	male	13–28 mo	43.9 ± 3.7	5.37 ± 0.46	13.56 ± 1.1	81.8 ± 3.5	30.9 ± 1.4	1.5 ± 0.6	6.2 ± 0.3
75	female	2–30 days	37.5 ± 3.5	4.58 ± 0.52	11.07 ± 1.2	82.1 ± 4.6	29.5 ± 1.1	5.8 ± 3.9	4.6 ± 0.4
42	female	31–60 days	43.5 ± 3.1	5.19 ± 0.40	13.30 ± 0.8	84.0 ± 4.7	30.7 ± 1.0	2.5 ± 1.7	5.4 ± 0.4
15	female	63–90 days	46.2 ± 2.8	5.52 ± 0.35	14.20 ± 0.9	83.7 ± 1.9	30.8 ± 1.6	1.9 ± 1.4	5.9 ± 0.3
18	female	4– 6 mo	44.1 ± 3.8	5.27 ± 0.49	13.55 ± 1.4	83.7 ± 3.1	30.7 ± 1.0	2.4 ± 2.2	6.1 ± 0.8
19	female	7–12 mo	41.2 ± 2.4	4.87 ± 0.24	12.40 ± 0.7	84.6 ± 3.0	30.1 ± 0.9	2.7 ± 2.2	5.7 ± 0.4
20	female	13–28 mo	39.8 ± 2.6	4.67 ± 0.39	11.76 ± 0.8	85.4 ± 4.5	29.6 ± 0.8	1.9 ± 2.7	5.4 ± 0.5
129	both	2–30 days	37.9 ± 4.0	4.62 ± 0.57	11.20 ± 1.3	82.2 ± 4.3	29.6 ± 1.2	6.1 ± 3.8	4.6 ± 0.4
88	both	31–60 days	43.2 ± 3.1	5.19 ± 0.44	13.20 ± 0.9	83.5 ± 4.3	30.5 ± 1.0	2.6 ± 1.5	5.2 ± 0.4
31	both	63–90 days	46.2 ± 2.6	5.58 ± 0.37	14.10 ± 0.9	83.0 ± 2.5	30.5 ± 1.4	2.3 ± 1.6	5.8 ± 0.4
26	both	4– 6 mo	44.4 ± 4.1	5.44 ± 0.59	13.70 ± 1.3	81.8 ± 4.3	30.9 ± 1.1	2.3 ± 1.9	6.1 ± 0.7
28	both	7–12 mo	42.1 ± 3.1	5.09 ± 0.47	12.90 ± 1.2	83.0 ± 4.0	30.6 ± 1.2	2.3 ± 1.9	5.7 ± 0.4
31	both	13–28 mo	41.2 ± 3.6	4.92 ± 0.54	12.40 ± 1.3	84.1 ± 4.5	30.1 ± 1.2	1.8 ± 2.2	5.7 ± 0.6

[a]Heart blood collected under ether anesthesia.

Table 12-7. Total and Differential Leukocyte Numbers in Guinea Pigs—Sex and Age Influence (means and 1 SD)[a]

Differential Leukocyte Count in Absolute Numbers/μl

Number Guinea Pigs	Sex	Age	Total WBC/μl	Neutrophils Band	Neutrophils Mature	Lymphocytes	Monocytes	Eosinophils	Basophils	Lymphocytes with Kurloff Bodies
54	male	2–30 days	3,735 ± 938	11 ± 2	947 ± 548	2,618 ± 688	79 ± 86	83 ± 102	9 ± 19	14 ± 27
46	male	31–60 days	5,520 ± 1,832	0	1,677 ± 1,196	3,595 ± 1,125	113 ± 84	53 ± 45	8 ± 18	30 ± 45
16	male	63–90 days	5,938 ± 1,225	4 ± 10	1,910 ± 845	3,902 ± 912	74 ± 58	36 ± 32	10 ± 21	90 ± 106
8	male	4– 6 mo	9,575 ± 3,172	0	1,952 ± 723	7,201 ± 2,373	210 ± 186	94 ± 64	15 ± 20	348 ± 203
9	male	7–12 mo	11,500 ± 2,020	0	2,625 ± 531	8,248 ± 1,669	300 ± 128	328 ± 625	0	526 ± 112
11	male	13–28 mo	13,527 ± 2,465	0	4,153 ± 2,577	8,654 ± 2,423	385 ± 318	310 ± 459	26 ± 36	418 ± 239
75	female	2–30 days	4,087 ± 1,004	2 ± 10	865 ± 315	3,062 ± 860	58 ± 62	76 ± 71	5 ± 16	148 ± 188
42	female	31–60 days	7,043 ± 2,099	2 ± 11	1,934 ± 1,475	4,912 ± 1,294	117 ± 123	71 ± 61	5 ± 14	594 ± 435
15	female	63–90 days	7,973 ± 2,270	2 ± 8	2,163 ± 989	5,559 ± 1,480	123 ± 135	110 ± 99	9 ± 18	373 ± 220
18	female	4– 6 mo	10,239 ± 1,869	0	2,576 ± 1,613	7,198 ± 1,385	217 ± 154	217 ± 215	31 ± 51	400 ± 249
19	female	7–12 mo	10,926 ± 3,206	3 ± 15	2,443 ± 1,344	7,904 ± 2,857	319 ± 292	249 ± 261	9 ± 21	460 ± 225
20	female	13–28 mo	9,879 ± 2,101	5 ± 14	2,315 ± 1,361	6,496 ± 2,446	341 ± 436	206 ± 193	23 ± 29	342 ± 201
129	both	2–30 days	3,940 ± 992	2 ± 11	899 ± 430	2,876 ± 822	67 ± 74	79 ± 86	7 ± 18	92 ± 159
88	both	31–60 days	6,247 ± 2,106	1 ± 7	1,800 ± 1,343	4,224 ± 1,376	115 ± 105	62 ± 54	7 ± 16	299 ± 413
31	both	63–90 days	6,923 ± 2,074	3 ± 10	2,032 ± 926	4,703 ± 1,475	98 ± 106	72 ± 81	9 ± 19	227 ± 222
26	both	4– 6 mo	10,035 ± 2,368	0	2,384 ± 1,430	7,199 ± 1,749	215 ± 164	179 ± 190	26 ± 45	384 ± 237
28	both	7–12 mo	11,111 ± 2,891	2 ± 12	2,501 ± 1,150	8,014 ± 2,541	312 ± 251	274 ± 416	6 ± 18	481 ± 199
31	both	13–38 mo	11,217 ± 2,848	3 ± 11	2,967 ± 2,080	7,261 ± 2,648	357 ± 399	243 ± 319	24 ± 32	369 ± 218

[a]Heart blood collected under ether anesthesia.

Table 12–8. Leukocyte and Platelet Counts in Guinea Pigs—Sex and Age Influence (means and 1 SD)[a]

Number Guinea Pigs	Sex	Age	WBC/μl	Neutrophils		Lymphocytes	Monocytes	Eosinophils	Basophils	Platelets (×10³/μl)	Lymphocytes with Kurloff Bodies (%)
				Band	Mature						*Differential Leukocyte Count (%)*
54	male	2–30 days	3,737 ± 938	0.06 ± 0.30	27.9 ± 10.8	70.7 ± 11.7	2.1 ± 1.9	2.2 ± 2.1	0.22 ± 0.48	537 ± 127	0.4 ± 0.7
46	male	31–60 days	5,520 ± 1,832	0	29.0 ± 10.7	66.2 ± 13.6	2.1 ± 1.5	1.0 ± 0.8	0.13 ± 0.28	504 ± 149	0.5 ± 0.8
16	male	63–90 days	5,938 ± 1,225	0.06 ± 0.16	31.9 ± 10.7	65.9 ± 10.6	1.3 ± 1.1	0.6 ± 0.6	0.19 ± 0.39	489 ± 109	1.5 ± 1.7
8	male	4–6 mo	9,575 ± 3,172	0	20.8 ± 6.1	75.3 ± 6.7	1.9 ± 1.4	1.2 ± 1.0	0.19 ± 0.24	563 ± 131	4.1 ± 2.9
9	male	7–12 mo	11,500 ± 2,020	0	23.2 ± 5.1	71.4 ± 4.0	2.8 ± 1.4	2.6 ± 4.5	0	506 ± 112	4.7 ± 1.4
11	male	13–28 mo	13,527 ± 2,465	0	30.3 ± 15.7	64.8 ± 16.1	2.7 ± 1.6	2.1 ± 2.4	0.18 ± 0.24	443 ± 155	3.1 ± 1.7
75	female	2–30 days	4,087 ± 1,004	0.05 ± 0.28	21.2 ± 6.4	74.9 ± 7.7	1.4 ± 1.4	1.9 ± 1.7	0.13 ± 0.40	570 ± 152	3.4 ± 4.2
42	female	31–60 days	7,043 ± 2,099	0.02 ± 0.10	25.8 ± 11.7	71.5 ± 12.5	1.6 ± 1.5	1.0 ± 0.8	0.08 ± 0.21	499 ± 173	8.2 ± 4.2
15	female	63–90 days	7,973 ± 2,270	0.03 ± 0.12	26.3 ± 7.1	70.5 ± 7.1	1.7 ± 2.0	1.4 ± 1.2	0.10 ± 0.20	549 ± 113	5.0 ± 3.1
18	female	4–6 mo	10,239 ± 1,869	0	24.3 ± 11.3	71.3 ± 11.9	2.2 ± 1.6	2.0 ± 1.8	0.31 ± 0.47	628 ± 152	4.1 ± 2.8
19	female	7–12 mo	10,926 ± 3,206	0.03 ± 0.11	23.5 ± 11.0	71.4 ± 11.3	2.7 ± 2.2	2.3 ± 2.5	0.08 ± 0.18	559 ± 175	4.2 ± 1.8
20	female	13–28 mo	9,879 ± 2,101	0.05 ± 0.15	24.7 ± 10.6	69.4 ± 13.2	3.4 ± 3.6	2.3 ± 2.1	0.22 ± 0.29	573 ± 124	3.8 ± 1.9
129	both	2–30 days	3,940 ± 992	0.05 ± 0.28	22.8 ± 8.7	73.1 ± 9.8	1.7 ± 1.6	2.0 ± 1.9	0.17 ± 0.44	556 ± 143	2.2 ± 3.6
88	both	31–60 days	6,247 ± 2,106	0.01 ± 0.07	27.5 ± 11.3	68.7 ± 13.4	1.8 ± 1.5	1.0 ± 0.8	0.11 ± 0.25	502 ± 160	4.2 ± 4.9
31	both	63–90 days	6,923 ± 2,074	0.05 ± 0.15	29.2 ± 9.6	68.1 ± 9.3	1.5 ± 1.6	1.0 ± 1.0	0.14 ± 0.32	518 ± 115	3.2 ± 3.1
26	both	4–6 mo	10,035 ± 2,368	0	23.2 ± 10.2	72.5 ± 10.7	2.1 ± 1.5	1.8 ± 1.6	0.27 ± 0.42	608 ± 149	4.1 ± 2.9
28	both	7–12 mo	11,111 ± 2,891	0.02 ± 0.09	23.4 ± 9.5	71.4 ± 9.6	2.7 ± 1.9	2.4 ± 3.3	0.05 ± 0.15	545 ± 162	4.4 ± 1.7
31	both	13–28 mo	11,217 ± 2,848	0.03 ± 0.12	26.7 ± 12.9	67.8 ± 14.4	3.1 ± 3.1	2.2 ± 2.2	0.21 ± 0.28	530 ± 149	3.5 ± 1.9

[a]Heart blood collected under ether anesthesia.

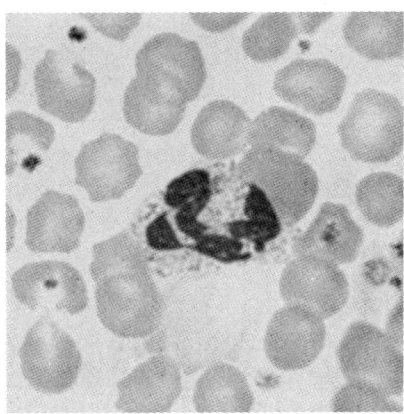

Fig. 12–3.   Guinea pig pseudo-eosinophil.

sequestration in the spleen, while ether has the opposite effect (Hausner et al., 1938).

No significant sex differences were noted in either the total or differential distribution of leukocyte types (Tables 12–7 and 12–8). WBC counts increased with age from 3,940 ± 992/µl during the first month of life to 11,217 ± 2,848 in guinea pigs over 1 year of age. All leukocyte types, with the possible exception of the basophil leukocyte, increased gradually with age. In the different age groups, mean values for neutrophils ranged from 22.8 ± 8.7% to 29.2 ± 9.6%, and the values for lymphocytes ranged from 67.8 ± 14.4% to 73.1 ± 9.8%, but there was no consistent pattern reflecting an influence of age.

Young germfree guinea pigs were found to have lower WBC counts and fewer neutrophils than conventional guinea pigs of the same age (Gordon, 1959).

Leukemia has been reported to occur in guinea pigs (Congdon and Lorenz, 1954; Ediger and Rabstein, 1968).

The Neutrophil (Heterophil)

The guinea pig neutrophil differs from the rabbit neutrophil in that the granules are more distinct and generally round, and they stain more intensely red. The granules are separated one from another so that a considerable amount of nonstaining cytoplasm is visible (Fig. 12–3). The nucleus tends to be multilobed and more polymorphous than the comparable cell of the rabbit. A "drumstick" sex chromatin lobe may occur in this cell in the female.

The Lymphocyte

The small lymphocyte is about the size of the red blood cell or smaller and presents a deeply stained nucleus and a narrow crescent of cytoplasm. The larger lymphocyte presents a pale blue cytoplasm that may extend completely around the nucleus and sometimes contains a cluster of azurophilic granules.

The Monocyte

The morphologic characteristics of this cell are similar to those of the monocyte in the rabbit. Cells classified as monocytes by us do not contain Kurloff bodies (see The Kurloff Body).

The Eosinophil

The nucleus of this cell is frequently monolobed and may be partially covered by granules. The cytoplasm is packed with comparatively large, round, and strongly acidophilic granules. The cell is readily distinguishable from the heterophil.

The Basophil

The nucleus of the basophil leukocyte takes a light purple stain, while the granules are reddish-purple to black. The granules are oval and larger than the granules of the eosinophil. This cell is not as prevalent in guinea pig blood as in rabbit blood. An increase in the basophil leukocyte in guinea pigs experimentally infected with swine lungworms has been reported (Porter, 1937).

The Kurloff Body

A unique feature of guinea pig blood is the occurrence of a variable number of cells in the lymphocyte series that contain a single large cytoplasmic inclusion or, more rarely, several masses. The material is diffusely red or vacuole-like, with reddish granulation. These unique cytoplasmic inclusions are called Kurloff bodies (Fig. 12–4). Ledingham (1940) called the inclusions Foa-Kurloff bodies because they were described independently by Foa in Italy and Kurloff in Germany. The cell is also referred to as the Kurloff cell. Joyner (1938), employing a supravital stain, identified the cell containing the Kurloff body as a lymphocyte. Ledingham (1940) proposed a

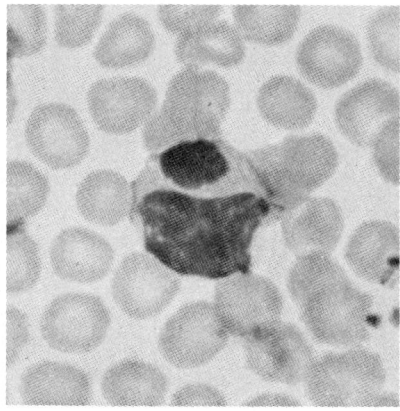

Fig. 12–4. Guinea pig lymphocyte with Kurloff body.

relationship between the number of lymphocytic cells containing Kurloff bodies and the sex hormones. That such may be the case was apparent in our data only during the first 3 months of life (Table 12–7). Kurloff bodies were lowest in number during the first month of life in both sexes, although females had 10 times as many Kurloff cells. From the second month of life onward, the number of cells containing Kurloff bodies in females attained their maximum number, while only a modest increase occurred in males at 2 and 3 months of age. Thereafter, no significant differences were apparent between the sexes.

Schermer (1967) concluded that the Kurloff body represents a manifestation of a phagocytic activity of the monocyte leukocyte. Similarly, Izard et al. (1976) concluded that the Kurloff cell belongs to the macrophage system as far as ultrastructure, adhesiveness, and relationship to Kupffer cells are concerned. Large numbers of Kurloff cells are found in the spleen, liver, and lung blood, but not in lymph nodes and diffuse lymphoid tissues, although they are found in the thymus. Recently the Kurloff cell was identified as a T-lymphocyte because it formed rosettes with rabbit red cells (Revell, 1974). Kurloff bodies were not found in blood of the cuis (*Galea musteloides*), a relative of the domestic guinea pig (Watson and Hawkey, 1976).

The above indicates that further studies are needed to define the cellular origin of the Kurloff cell. The significance of the inclusion itself also remains to be determined. It consists of glycoprotein complexes rich in neutral muco-

polysaccharides and stains metachromatically with toluidine blue (Izard et al., 1976).

The Platelets

These are small, are usually round but sometimes spindle-shaped, and consist of a cluster of azurophilic granules within a pale blue cytoplasm. Sex and age had no influence on numbers, which varied between 489,000 ± 109,000 and 628,000 ± 152,000/μl (Table 12–8). Considerably lower platelet numbers, with a range of 120,000–182,000 were reported earlier (Schermer, 1967).

The Plasma or Serum

Plasma volume expressed as a percentage of body weight decreases from birth to maturity. This decrease is reflected in blood volume changes from 11.5% of the body weight at birth to 5.9% at maturity (Constable, 1963). Plasma proteins were found to average 4.6 ± 0.4 g/dl during the first month of life and to increase to 6.1 ± 0.7 g/dl at 4–6 months of age (Table 12–6). Thereafter, there was a slight decrease to 5.7 ± 0.6 g/dl at maturity. Serum proteins were reported to range from 4.2–5.3 g/dl in males and from 4.7 to 5.1 g/dl in females, with means of 4.8 and 5.1 g/dl, respectively (Kozma et al., 1967).

The Myeloid:Erythroid Ratio

The mean M:E ratio in 17 guinea pigs was found to be 1.53:1.0 in the right humerus and 1.45:1.0 in the left humerus (Harris et al., 1954). Supravital staining revealed the M:E ratio to be 1.2:1.0 in films of bone marrow and 1.6:1.0 in tissue sections of marrow from the same guinea pig (Epstein and Tompkins, 1943). Total nucleated cell counts of 48,100–377,000/μl were found in marrow samples from 17 guinea pigs (Sawitsky and Meyer, 1948). Lymphocytes ranged from 10.8–48.0%, with a mean of 25.42% of total nucleated cells.

THE RAT

Blood is commonly obtained from rats by clipping the tip of the tail, puncturing a tail vessel, or puncturing the heart. Orbital sinus (Chapter 2) may be used to obtain repeated blood samples. Cardiac puncture may be per-

Table 12-10. Total and Differential Leukocyte Numbers in Long-Evans Rats—Sex and Age Influence (means and 1 SD)[a]

Number of Rats	Sex	Age	WBC/μl	Neutrophils		Differential Leukocyte Count in Absolute Numbers/μl			
				Bands	Mature	Lymphocytes	Monocytes	Eosinophils	Basophils
10	male	26–30 days	4,000 ± 944	0	646 ± 368	3,159 ± 883	151 ± 80	38 ± 32	5 ± 11
23	male	37–75 days	8,543 ± 2,231	2 ± 8	1,435 ± 649	6,681 ± 1,772	284 ± 205	127 ± 155	84 ± 365
11	male	3 mo	8,809 ± 2,342	9 ± 20	1,776 ± 336	6,661 ± 2,124	200 ± 118	159 ± 161	5 ± 16
41	male	4– 6 mo	10,249 ± 2,794	5 ± 25	2,027 ± 680	7,807 ± 2,355	181 ± 150	222 ± 192	8 ± 27
70	male	7–12 mo	9,591 ± 1,961	7 ± 25	2,585 ± 1,054	6,366 ± 1,401	295 ± 222	333 ± 275	9 ± 25
21	male	13–15 mo	9,595 ± 3,433	6 ± 19	3,379 ± 1,540	5,330 ± 1,732	534 ± 368	319 ± 262	23 ± 63
10	female	26–30 days	3,800 ± 865	6 ± 17	527 ± 264	3,120 ± 689	135 ± 71	11 ± 18	2 ± 5
25	female	37–82 days	7,100 ± 2,423	2 ± 8	1,136 ± 689	5,709 ± 1,891	118 ± 74	133 ± 137	3 ± 10
13	female	3 mo	8,315 ± 1,868	2 ± 8	1,469 ± 520	6,464 ± 1,596	201 ± 129	176 ± 106	3 ± 11
36	female	4– 6 mo	8,478 ± 3,126	11 ± 25	1,512 ± 677	6,525 ± 2,691	93 ± 110	332 ± 390	6 ± 17
75	female	7–12 mo	7,079 ± 2,045	4 ± 19	1,593 ± 761	4,773 ± 1,708	197 ± 204	270 ± 269	5 ± 15
6	female	13–15 mo	6,983 ± 1,293	10 ± 22	1,495 ± 426	4,881 ± 1,228	207 ± 124	391 ± 513	0
20	both	26–30 days	3,900 ± 911	3 ± 12	586 ± 326	3,139 ± 792	143 ± 76	25 ± 29	3 ± 9
48	both	37–82 days	7,792 ± 2,442	2 ± 8	1,279 ± 687	6,175 ± 1,898	197 ± 193	130 ± 146	42 ± 256
24	both	3 mo	8,542 ± 2,113	5 ± 15	1,610 ± 470	6,554 ± 1,859	200 ± 124	168 ± 134	4 ± 14
77	both	4– 6 mo	9,421 ± 3,084	8 ± 25	1,786 ± 725	7,207 ± 2,597	139 ± 140	273 ± 306	7 ± 23
145	both	7–12 mo	8,309 ± 2,365	6 ± 22	2,075 ± 1,041	5,548 ± 1,757	244 ± 219	301 ± 274	6 ± 20
27	both	13–15 mo	9,015 ± 3,274	7 ± 19	2,960 ± 1,581	5,230 ± 1,644	461 ± 357	335 ± 336	20 ± 56

[a]Heart blood collected under ether anesthesia.

Table 12-11. Leukocyte and Platelet Counts in Long-Evans Rats—Sex and Age Influence (means and 1 SD)[a]

Number of Rats	Sex	Age	WBC/µl	Differential Leukocyte Count (%)						Platelets (×10³/µl)
				Neutrophils		Lymphocytes	Monocytes	Eosinophils	Basophils	
				Band	Mature					
10	male	26–30 days	4,000± 944	0	16.1±8.2	78.8±7.7	4.2±2.9	0.9±0.7	0.1 ±0.20	1,099±145
23	male	37–75 days	8,543±2,231	0.02±0.10	16.6±5.7	78.3±7.1	3.4±2.5	1.5±1.9	0.6 ±2.70	923±294
11	male	3 mo	8,809±2,342	0.09±0.19	21.3±5.6	74.6±5.7	2.2±1.2	1.7±1.5	0.1 ±0.30	840±155
41	male	4– 6 mo	10,249±2,794	0.05±0.24	20.1±5.4	75.9±5.9	1.8±1.5	2.1±1.5	0.06 ±0.20	882±173
70	male	7–12 mo	9,591±1,961	0.07±0.30	26.6±7.8	66.8±9.1	3.1±2.2	3.4±2.4	0.1 ±0.24	953±194
21	male	13–15 mo	9,595±3,433	0.07±0.20	35.3±7.8	56.0±7.6	5.2±3.3	3.1±2.1	0.2 ±0.60	980±193
10	female	26–30 days	3,800± 865	0.20±0.60	13.4±4.3	82.5±5.5	3.7±2.0	0.3±0.4	0.05±0.15	1,089±123
25	female	37–82 days	7,100±2,423	0.04±0.20	15.3±5.7	80.9±5.7	1.6±1.0	2.1±2.4	0.04±0.14	949±149
13	female	3 mo	8,315±1,868	0.04±0.13	17.9±6.1	77.5±5.9	2.5±1.6	2.0±1.2	0.04±0.13	969±156
36	female	4– 6 mo	8,478±3,126	0.10±0.23	18.5±6.8	76.3±8.9	1.3±1.5	3.7±3.4	0.08±0.25	1,016±196
75	female	7–12 mo	7,079±2,045	0.09±0.40	23.2±7.4	69.8±8.9	2.9±2.4	3.9±3.6	0.07±0.20	984±175
6	female	13–15 mo	6,983±1,293	0.17±0.40	22.7±9.4	69.2±9.6	2.8±1.4	5.3±6.0	0	1,038±136
20	both	26–30 days	3,900± 911	0.10±0.40	14.8±6.7	80.6±7.0	3.9±2.5	0.6±0.7	0.08±0.20	1,093±133
48	both	37–82 days	7,792±2,442	0.03±0.20	15.9±5.7	79.7±6.5	2.5±2.1	1.8±2.2	0.3 ±1.90	936±234
24	both	3 mo	8,542±2,113	0.06±0.20	19.4±6.1	76.2±6.0	2.3±1.5	1.9±1.4	0.06±0.20	907±169
77	both	4– 6 mo	9,421±3,084	0.07±0.20	19.4±6.1	76.1±7.4	1.6±1.5	2.8±2.7	0.07±0.20	946±196
145	both	7–12 mo	8,309±2,365	0.08±0.30	24.9±7.6	68.3±9.1	3.0±2.3	3.6±3.1	0.08±0.20	969±185
27	both	13–15 mo	9,015±3,274	0.09±0.30	32.5±9.7	58.9±9.8	4.7±3.2	3.6±3.5	0.17±0.50	993±183

[a]Heart blood collected under ether anesthesia.

Table 12–12. Erythrocyte Parameters and Plasma Composition in Sprague-Dawley Rats—Sex and Age Influence (means and 1 SD)[a]

Number of Rats	Sex	Age	PCV (%)	RBC (×10⁶/μl)	Hb (g/dl)	MCV (fl)	MCHC (%)	MCH (pg)	Reticulocytes (%)	Icterus Index Units	Plasma Proteins (g/dl)	Fibrinogen (g/dl)
22	male	25–35 days	36.6±2.4	5.15±0.57	10.8±0.8	71.2±3.8	29.4±0.9	20.9±1.1	16.2±7.5	2.0±2.0	5.7±0.4	0.27±0.05
28	male	50–77 days	46.6±1.8	7.04±0.50	14.6±0.6	66.6±5.0	31.3±0.9	20.9±1.6	4.6±3.1	5.0±2.0	7.0±0.4	0.21±0.08
29	male	3 mo	48.7±2.2	7.95±0.49	15.4±1.1	61.3±2.3	31.6±1.5	19.4±1.2	2.8±1.8	4.6±1.9	7.1±0.4	—
29	male	4– 6 mo	48.1±1.9	8.53±0.47	15.3±0.6	56.4±2.4	31.8±0.9	17.9±1.0	2.3±1.6	4.4±2.2	7.3±0.4	—
67	male	7–12 mo	47.1±2.6	8.20±0.56	15.0±0.9	57.6±3.4	31.9±1.2	18.3±1.1	2.1±1.3	4.0±2.2	7.3±0.5	0.28±0.08
26	male	13–15 mo	46.5±1.6	8.28±0.59	15.1±1.0	56.3±3.3	32.4±1.6	18.3±1.6	2.1±0.7	3.3±1.8	7.9±0.5	0.37±0.06
20	female	25–35 days	37.4±2.0	5.19±0.61	11.0±0.8	72.5±5.3	29.5±1.3	21.4±1.7	16.2±8.1	3.0±2.0	5.7±0.3	0.20±0.06
24	female	50–77 days	45.6±1.6	7.05±0.38	14.8±0.6	64.9±3.5	32.3±0.9	21.0±1.4	2.5±1.5	4.0±1.5	7.2±0.3	0.25±0.05
12	female	3 mo	45.3±2.0	7.14±0.63	14.7±0.7	63.8±4.8	32.4±1.0	20.7±1.7	3.4±1.5	4.0±2.0	7.3±0.5	0.17±0.06
30	female	4– 6 mo	46.0±1.5	7.60±0.34	15.2±0.7	60.4±2.3	33.0±1.1	19.9±0.9	2.8±1.2	3.0±1.7	7.7±0.5	—
67	female	7–12 mo	45.1±1.8	7.46±0.43	14.5±0.7	60.4±2.4	32.1±0.9	19.5±0.9	2.4±1.0	2.6±2.0	8.1±0.5	0.17±0.06
29	female	13–15 mo	44.7±2.2	7.27±0.40	14.5±0.8	61.5±2.4	32.5±0.8	20.0±0.9	2.6±1.1	3.7±2.4	8.6±0.5	0.20±0.09
42	both	25–35 days	37.0±2.2	5.18±0.59	10.9±0.8	71.8±4.6	29.4±1.1	21.2±1.5	16.2±7.8	2.7±1.9	5.7±0.4	0.24±0.06
52	both	50–77 days	46.2±1.8	7.04±0.45	14.7±0.6	65.7±4.5	32.0±1.0	20.9±1.5	3.6±2.7	4.5±2.1	7.1±0.4	0.23±0.07
41	both	3 mo	47.7±2.6	7.71±0.65	15.2±1.0	62.0±3.4	31.8±1.4	19.8±1.5	3.0±1.7	4.3±2.0	7.1±0.4	0.17±0.06
59	both	4– 6 mo	47.0±2.0	8.06±0.62	15.2±0.7	58.4±3.1	32.4±1.2	19.0±1.4	2.6±1.5	3.7±2.1	7.5±0.5	—
134	both	7–12 mo	46.1±2.5	7.83±0.62	14.8±0.8	59.0±3.2	32.5±1.1	18.9±1.2	2.2±1.2	3.4±2.2	7.7±0.7	0.23±0.09
55	both	13–15 mo	45.5±2.1	7.75±0.70	14.8±1.0	59.0±3.9	32.5±1.3	19.2±1.5	2.3±1.0	3.5±2.2	8.3±0.6	0.26±0.12

[a]Heart blood collected under ether anesthesia.

Table 12–13. Total and Differential Leukocyte Numbers in Sprague-Dawley Rats—Sex and Age Influence (means and 1 SD)[a]

Number of Rats	Sex	Age	WBC/μl	Differential Leukocyte Count in Absolute Numbers/μl					
				Neutrophils		Lymphocytes	Mono-cytes	Eosino-phils	Baso-phils
				Bands	Mature				
22	male	25–35 days	8,377 ± 2,896	9 ± 24	1,212 ± 570	6,859 ± 2,402	251 ± 174	36 ± 56	3 ± 13
28	male	50–77 days	12,457 ± 3,506	3 ± 13	1,715 ± 659	10,407 ± 2,988	247 ± 185	82 ± 79	4 ± 15
29	male	3 mo	15,255 ± 3,536	17 ± 39	2,471 ± 1,142	12,425 ± 2,892	219 ± 179	117 ± 110	7 ± 22
29	male	4– 6 mo	11,983 ± 3,111	9 ± 28	2,436 ± 982	9,231 ± 2,484	181 ± 135	109 ± 102	18 ± 33
67	male	7–12 mo	11,585 ± 2,269	8 ± 27	2,975 ± 1,207	8,146 ± 1,697	262 ± 211	182 ± 135	12 ± 41
26	male	13–15 mo	15,076 ± 13,280	15 ± 32	4,524 ± 3,912	9,069 ± 9,225	678 ± 522	172 ± 133	5 ± 17
20	female	25–35 days	7,430 ± 2,963	0	1,048 ± 470	6,117 ± 2,557	243 ± 193	22 ± 33	0
24	female	50–77 days	12,479 ± 2,689	12 ± 27	1,898 ± 760	10,274 ± 2,468	173 ± 154	114 ± 69	9 ± 24
12	female	3 mo	11,458 ± 2,567	7 ± 24	1,501 ± 1,217	9,568 ± 1,489	253 ± 347	129 ± 113	0
30	female	4– 6 mo	9,810 ± 1,789	2 ± 10	1,529 ± 613	7,697 ± 1,493	230 ± 189	106 ± 94	9 ± 20
67	female	7–12 mo	8,366 ± 2,011	3 ± 13	1,976 ± 1,026	5,994 ± 1,677	232 ± 172	152 ± 118	5 ± 21
29	female	13–15 mo	7,417 ± 1,624	3 ± 18	2,137 ± 813	4,910 ± 1,135	222 ± 123	131 ± 96	13 ± 28
42	both	25–35 days	7,926 ± 2,966	5 ± 18	1,134 ± 531	6,506 ± 2,505	247 ± 183	29 ± 47	2 ± 10
52	both	50–77 days	12,467 ± 3,156	7 ± 21	1,799 ± 713	10,346 ± 2,761	213 ± 175	97 ± 77	6 ± 20
41	both	3 mo	14,143 ± 3,709	14 ± 35	2,187 ± 1,245	11,589 ± 2,873	229 ± 241	120 ± 111	5 ± 19
59	both	4– 6 mo	10,878 ± 2,750	5 ± 21	1,975 ± 933	8,589 ± 2,137	206 ± 167	108 ± 98	13 ± 27
134	both	7–12 mo	9,975 ± 2,680	5 ± 21	2,475 ± 1,226	7,070 ± 2,001	247 ± 193	167 ± 128	8 ± 33
55	both	13–15 mo	10,963 ± 9,882	9 ± 26	3,265 ± 3,000	6,876 ± 6,724	438 ± 434	150 ± 117	9 ± 23

[a]Heart blood collected under ether anesthesia.

Table 12–14. Leukocyte and Platelet Counts in Sprague-Dawley Rats—Sex and Age Influence (means and 1 SD)[a]

| Number of Rats | Sex | Age | WBC/µl | Differential Leukocyte Count (%) | | | | | | Platelets ($\times 10^3/\mu l$) |
| | | | | Neutrophils | | Lympho-cytes | Mono-cytes | Eosino-phils | Basophils | |
				Band	Mature					
22	male	25–35 days	8,377 ± 2,896	0.14±0.43	14.4±4.5	81.9±5.5	2.9±1.7	0.4±0.7	0.02±0.10	1,173±261
28	male	50–77 days	12,457 ± 3,506	0.02±0.09	13.7±3.9	83.6±4.1	2.0±1.3	0.7±0.7	0.04±0.13	1,051±178
29	male	3 mo	15,255 ± 3,536	0.12±0.28	16.0±5.6	81.5±5.7	1.5±1.4	0.8±0.7	0.05±0.15	998±183
29	male	4– 6 mo	11,983 ± 3,111	0.07±0.21	20.1±5.6	77.3±6.0	1.4±1.0	1.0±0.9	0.13±0.24	1,031±201
67	male	7–12 mo	11,585 ± 2,269	0.06±0.20	25.3±7.3	70.6±8.0	2.3±1.8	1.6±1.2	0.10±0.31	1,108±193
26	male	13–15 mo	15,076 ± 13,280	0.10±0.30	31.3±6.4	61.9±6.9	5.0±2.7	1.3±0.9	0.04±0.13	1,179±257
20	female	25–35 days	7,430 ± 2,963	0	14.2±4.9	82.3±5.4	3.2±2.2	0.3±0.5	0	1,038±254
24	female	50–77 days	12,479 ± 2,689	0.08±0.19	15.4±6.0	82.0±6.6	1.5±1.4	0.9±0.5	0.06±0.17	1,135±202
12	female	3 mo	11,458 ± 2,567	0.04±0.14	12.1±6.8	84.8±8.3	2.0±2.5	1.1±0.9	0	1,112±135
30	female	4– 6 mo	9,810 ± 1,789	0.02±0.09	15.4±4.5	81.3±5.1	2.3±1.6	1.2±1.1	0.08±0.19	1,139±258
67	female	7–12 mo	8,366 ± 2,011	0.04±0.16	23.6±8.6	71.6±9.3	2.8±2.1	1.8±1.4	0.05±0.23	980±187
29	female	13–15 mo	7,417 ± 1,624	0.05±0.27	28.4±7.2	66.4±7.5	3.0±1.5	1.9±1.5	0.17±0.35	1,120±220
42	both	25–35 days	7,926 ± 2,966	0.07±0.32	14.3±4.6	82.1±5.6	3.1±1.8	0.4±0.6	0.01±0.07	1,111±266
52	both	50–77 days	12,467 ± 3,156	0.05±0.15	14.5±5.1	82.9±5.4	1.8±1.4	0.8±0.6	0.05±0.15	1,089±194
41	both	3 mo	14,143 ± 3,709	0.10±0.25	14.9±6.2	82.5±6.7	1.7±1.8	0.9±0.8	0.04±0.13	1,026±179
59	both	4– 6 mo	10,878 ± 2,750	0.04±0.16	17.7±5.6	79.3±5.9	1.9±1.5	1.1±1.0	0.11±0.21	1,085±237
134	both	7–12 mo	9,975 ± 2,680	0.05±0.18	24.5±8.0	71.1±8.7	2.5±2.0	1.7±1.3	0.08±0.28	1,043±200
55	both	13–15 mo	10,963 ± 9,882	0.09±0.29	29.8±7.0	64.3±7.6	4.0±2.2	1.6±1.3	0.11±0.28	1,148±239

[a] Heart blood collected under ether anesthesia.

(Tables 12–9 and 12–12). The somewhat larger erythrocyte in the female partially compensates for the somewhat smaller number in that sex compared to males. In both Long-Evans and Sprague-Dawley rats, the PCV and Hb values were slightly lower in females than in males. The values were lowest during the first month of life, attained peak levels at approximately 4–6 months of age, and then decreased slightly. MCH and MCHC were slightly greater in females than in males, correlating with the slightly larger MCV of the erythrocyte in females. PCV decreases during pregnancy, but recovers 20 days after parturition (Remesar et al., 1981).

Numbers of reticulocytes in peripheral blood are high in the very young and decrease rapidly with age. It has been reported that rats have an average of 98.7% reticulocytes at birth, 25% at weaning at 21 days of age, 3.0% at 70 days of age and 1.7% to 2.8% in older rats (Orten and Smith, 1934). These observations were confirmed, and strain differences were noted in rats 100 days of age or older (Drabkin and Fitz-Hugh, 1934). Reticulocyte numbers in relation to age were similar in Long-Evans and Sprague-Dawley rats, and no sex difference was noted (Tables 12–9 and 12–12). In the youngest rats, reticulocytes ranged from 6–40% with averages of 16.2% ± 7.5% to 21.1 ± 9.8%, while in rats 3 months of age or older, reticulocytes averaged approximately 2.5 ± 0.1%. Wistar albino rats, aged 4 months or older, had 4.0% reticulocytes as an average in females and 4.5% in males. Polychromasia is a constant feature of normal rat blood that reflects the presence of reticulocytes. Life span of the rat erythrocyte ranges from 45 of 68 days (Table 20–1) compared with 100 to 120 days in the dog. The shorter life span of the rat erythrocyte correlates well with the larger number of reticulocytes in peripheral blood.

Hemolysis in hypotonic saline is reported to begin at 0.47% to 0.42% NaCl solution and to be complete at 0.30% (Perk et al., 1964).

The Leukocytes

The considerable variation in WBC counts as reported by different investigators (about 5,000–26,000/µl) may be due in part to strain differences (Reich and Dunning, 1943), but more likely is due to the conditions of sampling and the excitable nature of the animals. For example, Hulse (1964) anesthetized adult rats with sodium pentobarbital, opened the chest, and withdrew blood from the heart. He reported mean WBC counts of 6,040/µl in one series of rats and 7,130/µl in another. Kozma et al. (1969) anesthetized rats with ether and withdrew blood by heart puncture; he reported WBC counts of 13,479 ± 3,291/ µl in rats 8 months of age and 9,425 ± 3,187/ µl in rats 2 years of age. Free-flowing tail blood had mean WBC counts of 20,400 in females and 21,400 in males (Cameron and Watson, 1949). Age differences have been noted in diurnal variations with regard to total and differential leukocyte counts (Bubna-Littitz et al., 1981).

Our data on Long-Evans and Sprague-Dawley rats are representative of heart blood collected under ether anesthesia. WBC counts were greater at all ages in Sprague-Dawley rats than in Long-Evans rats (Tables 12–10, 12–13). In both strains, WBC counts increased with age, with highest counts between 3 and 6 months of age, followed generally by a slight decline in older rats. Both strains of rats had higher WBC counts in males than in females, especially in rats 3 months of age and older. The higher counts in males were due to greater numbers of both neutrophils and lymphocytes. The neutrophil number increased gradually with age and generally attained highest values in rats over 1 year of age. Numbers of lymphocytes increased with age, attaining a peak between 3 and 6 months, and then declined somewhat with advancing age. Monocytes and eosinophils were lowest in the first month of life and generally attained highest levels in rats over 1 year of age. Eosinophil numbers, however, decreased by 50% in rats of advanced age (762 days average) over the values recorded at an average age of 326 days (Everitt and Webb, 1958). The basophil leukocyte was present in small numbers and did not appear to vary under the influence of sex or age.

Neutrophil:lymphocyte ratios were widest in young rats and gradually narrowed with advancing age. The change with age was greater in male than in female rats, the result of a greater increase in neutrophil numbers

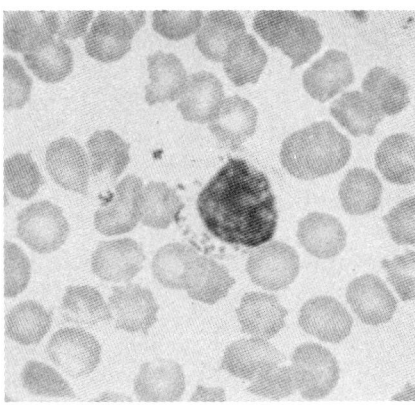

Fig. 12–5. Rat lymphocyte with azurophilic granules.

and smaller decrease in lymphocyte numbers with advancing age in male rats. The average N:L ratios (stated in percentages; Table 12–11) for Long-Evans rats at 26–30 days of age and at 13–15 months of age were 16.1:78.8 and 35.3:56.0, respectively, for males and 13.4:82.5 and 22.7:69.2 for females. Similar ratios existed in the Sprague-Dawley rats between the youngest and oldest groups (Table 12–14).

The Neutrophil (Heterophil)

The nucleus of the neutrophil is polymorphous, but younger cells have a nucleus in the form of a ring or a twisted coil. The cytoplasm is essentially colorless and presents tiny, dust-like, reddish granules that do not seem to be abundant.

The Lymphocyte

Both small and large lymphocytes are seen, the former about the size of the erythrocyte and the latter attaining a size comparable to the neutrophil. The cytoplasm is light blue, and the larger cells often present clusters of large, dark-staining azurophilic granules (Fig. 12–5).

The Monocyte

The nucleus of the monocyte is of variable shape, although a kidney-bean form is not uncommon. The cytoplasm is basophilic and often vacuolated and may contain a few azurophilic granules.

The Eosinophil

This leukocyte is generally larger than the neutrophil, and its nucleus is commonly U-shaped. The nucleus stains a combination of light purple and pale blue. The granules are small, round, and strongly acidophilic, and they fill the cytoplasm. A trace of blue-staining background outlines the cell.

The Basophil

This cell is present only in small numbers and may be absent from many individual blood films. It is readily identified by its many basophilic, metachromatic granules of uniform size. It should be distinguished from the much larger mast cell that may be present on rare occasions in blood taken by heart puncture.

The Platelets

Platelet numbers do not appear to be influenced by age or sex. In Long-Evans rats (Table 12–11) their average numbers varied from 840,000 ± 155,000 to 1,099,000 ± 145,000/μl, and in Sprague-Dawley rats (Table 12–14) their numbers varied from 980,000 ± 187,000 to 1,179,000 ± 257,000/μl. Platelet counts by the indirect method of comparing numbers on blood films with erythrocytes gave a ratio of platelets to erythrocytes of 1.0:7.5 and yielded an average platelet count of 1,275,000 for an RBC count of 9.6 million (Gunn and Vaughan, 1930). A mean platelet count of 838,000/μl was found in Albino rats (Hulse, 1964; Roofe et al., 1955) and of 502,100 ± 30,000/μl in Wistar rats (Kiczak et al., 1976). Platelets are considerably more numerous in rats than in rabbits and guinea pigs.

The Plasma or Serum

Icterus index varied from colorless plasma to 7.5 units, with an average value approaching 5 units. Plasma proteins increased with advancing age from 5.7 ± 0.4 g/dl at 25–35 days of age in Sprague-Dawley rats to 8.3 ± 0.6 g/dl in rats 13–15 months of age (Table 12–12). In Long-Evans rats (Table 12–9), the plasma proteins increased from 5.6 ± 0.4 g/dl at 26–30 days of age to 7.7 ± 0.6 g/dl in rats 13–15 months of age. Plasma fibrinogen ranged between 0.1 and 0.4 g/dl and did not exhibit an influence of advancing age.

An age-related increase in total plasma protein concentration, associated with an increase in γ-globulins and a decrease in albumin, was found in Albino rats 4–34 weeks in age (Frolke et al., 1974). Serum proteins in 4 strains of rats ranged from 4.6–6.5 g/dl for males and from 4.8–7.2 g/dl for females. In 1 strain, serum proteins ranged from 3.9–5.0 g/dl in the males and from 4.7–8.6 g/dl in the females (Kozma et al., 1967).

The Myeloid:Erythroid Ratio

Hematopoiesis in the adult rat occurs in the bone marrow and the spleen. Bone marrow studies appear to have been conducted more frequently in the rat than in other laboratory animals. The granulocytic series is of particular interest from the point of view of maturation of the nucleus. Some cells in this series develop a hole in the nucleus that gradually enlarges, giving the nucleus a "ring" or "donut" appearance, The hole may be found in an intermediate position between the myelocyte and metamyelocyte (Vogel, 1947) and may appear as early as in the progranulocyte (Hulse, 1964). Ring forms occurred in neutrophils and eosinophils but were not found in the few basophil leukocytes encountered.

Ramsell and Yoffey (1961) reviewed the reports of 17 investigations on the M:E ratio in the rat and found the mean values to vary from 0.62–2.7:1.0. Age of the rats at the time of bone marrow sampling may influence the M:E. ratio. A ratio of 1.62:1.0 was found in rats at 1 month of age and 1.93:1.9 at 2 months of age (Endicott and Ott, 1945). A comparison of the M:E ratios in marrow of the femur and rib yielded a mean of 1.75:1.0 and 1.40:1.0, respectively (Stasney and Higgins, 1936). An M:E ratio of 1.66 ± 0.22 was found in adult Wistar rats (Kiczak et al., 1976). Table 12–15 presents the differential distribution of bone marrow cells on 12 albino rats, 6–8 months in age (Vogel, 1947) and 130 adult Wistar rats (Kiczak et al., 1976).

Lymphocytes are present in considerable numbers in normal rat bone marrow. Lymphocyte counts of 13.4–20.0% were found in 10 rats having a mean M:E ratio of 1.9 ± 0.46 (Ramsell and Yoffey, 1961). Mean lymphocyte counts of 18.0% and 24.2% were found in two series of rat bone marrows (Hulse, 1964).

Lymphocyte numbers as high as 45% were obtained in rats at 3 weeks of age, with a rapid decline thereafter to attain a mean of 4.9 ± 2.6% of marrow cells at 50 weeks of age (Harris and Burke, 1957). Lymphocyte counts of about 5% were reported in bone marrow of adult Wistar rats (Kiczak et al., 1976).

Rats deficient in folate develop granulocytopenia from decreased granulopoiesis as indicated by a mean M:E ratio of 0.45 ± 0.48 in 13 folate-deficient rats, compared with 1.93 ± 0.93 in 22 normal rats (Endicott et al., 1945).

THE MOUSE

Blood is commonly obtained from the mouse by cutting the tip of the tail, incising a tail vein, or puncturing the heart. Various techniques have been developed to collect blood from the tail (Lewis et al., 1976; Fields and Cunningham, 1976). A simple technique for repeated collection of blood samples from the tail was described (Stoltz and Bendall, 1975). Blood may also be collected from the jugular vein (Kassel and Levitan, 1953). Collecting blood from the orbital sinus is described in Chapter 2. We obtained heart blood under ether anesthesia from 132 males and 126 females of Parkes strain mice and 125 males and 130 females of Regular yellow A^y strain mice, 1–12 months of age. The data from these two strains of mice are presented in Tables 12–16 through 12–21. Selected references on hematology of the mouse may be consulted for additional data (Berger, 1979; DeKock, 1931; Dougherty and White, 1944; Feher and Moza, 1974; Finch and Foster, 1973; Frith et al., 1980; Gardner, 1947; Greenman et al., 1982; Harrison et al., 1978; Heinecke, 1961, 1962, 1963; MacNamee and Sheehy, 1952; Mitruka and Rawnsley, 1977; Russell et al., 1951; Scarborough, 1930–1931; Schermer, 1967).

The composition of mouse blood is significantly influenced by genetic strain, in some aspects by sex, and by the site and time of blood withdrawal (Heinecke, 1963). Age exerts an important influence; both red cell parameters and leukocyte numbers increase with age in young mice (Rugh and Somogyi, 1968).

Table 12–15. Differential Cell Distribution in the Bone Marrow of Rats

Cell Type	Vogel (1947) Range (%)	Kiczak et al. (1976) Range (%)	Mean (%)
Blast cells	2.3– 6.1	2.2– 8.0	3.3±0.3
Progranulocytes	0.3– 1.8	4.0–10.0	5.8±0.2
Myelocytes, neutrophilic	1.6– 4.0	3.2– 7.8	5.5±0.2
Myelocytes, eosinophilic	0.1– 0.5	—	—
Ring cells	4.2– 9.0	—	—
Metamyelocytes, neutrophilic	2.4– 4.8	5.3–10.0	6.2±0.3
Metamyelocytes, eosinophilic	0.6– 1.9	—	—
Bands, neutrophilic	7.6–22.0	5.8–15.0	11.0–0.4
Band, eosinophilic	1.2– 6.0	—	—
Neutrophils	16.2–28.1	10.1–20.2	12.4±1.1
Eosinophils	2.5– 7.0	0.5– 8.0	4.0±1.3
Basophils	0.0– 0.2	0.0– 2.2	0.2±0.04
Erythroblasts[a]	8.0–16.0	5.8–14.0	8.8±0.8
Normoblasts[b]	18.9–30.0	13.5–30.7	21.4±0.2
Lymphocytes	1.8– 5.3	0.5– 2.0	0.5±0.03
Monocytes	0.0– 0.6	—	—
Plasma cells	0.4– 1.0	2.5– 6.0	3.5±0.3
Megakaryocytes	0.0– 1.6	0.4– 1.6	1.0±0.05
Macrophages	0.0– 0.4	—	—
Unclassified cells	0.0– 0.2	5.0–15.0	8.0±0.5
Mast cells	—	0.4– 1.6	1.0±0.05
Reticulum cells	—	1.4– 7.0	3.4±0.4

[a]Possibly includes rubriblasts, prorubricytes, and basophilic rubricytes.
[b]Possibly includes polychromatic rubricytes and metarubricytes.

The Erythrocytes

Cellular composition of mouse fetal blood at 17 days gestation and of postnatal blood from birth to 24 months of age has been investigated (Rugh and Somogyi, 1968). In fetal blood, RBC counts were about 3.3 million/µl, of which half contained nuclei, and Hb concentration was 8.3 g/dl in the female and 8.9 g/dl in the male. Erythrocyte numbers increased rapidly after birth to attain levels of 9 million to 10 million by the ninth week of life, with a reduction to 8 million to 9 million at 12 months of age and 7 million to 8 million at 24 months of age. Hb concentration followed a similar pattern, with the exception of an initial reduction at 2 weeks of age from the birth value and then a rapid rise to a peak of 14.5–15.5 g/dl at 9 weeks of age, followed by a gradual reduction to 12.0–13.5 g/dl at 24 months of age. From the fourth week onward, female mice had slightly higher RBC and Hb values than male mice. Erythrocyte parameters of C57BL/6Jax male mice at intervals between 4 and 24 months of life were studied, and a significant negative linear regression of Hb, RBC, MCV, and MCH with age was found (Ewing and Tauber, 1964). In a comparison of 18 inbred strains of virgin mice, 2–3 months of age, significant genetic differences were found among strains with respect to erythrocyte parameters (Russell et al., 1951).

Our studies on Regular Yellow A[y] (Table 12–16) and Parkes (Table 12–19) strains of mice did not reveal any large strain differences in erythrocyte parameters. Sex differences were minimal, but an influence of age on erythrocyte number and size was evident. RBC, PCV, and Hb values increased to peak at 2–3 months of life, followed by gradual reductions during the remainder of the first year of life. Erythrocytes were large (MCV 53.6 to 56.0 fl) at 1 month of age and gradually decreased in size by 7–12 months of age (MCV 48.1–50.0 fl). MCHC varied between 29.4% and 31.9% at 1 month and between 30.7% and 33.2% for the remainder of the first year of life.

Both strains of mice had reticulocyte counts of 11.1 ± 3.7% to 16.9 ± 4.0% at 1 month of age, with rapid reduction by the second month to levels characteristic of the strain as follows: In the Regular Yellow A[y] strain (Table 12–16), reticulocyte counts varied between 3.3 ± 0.9% and 5.2 ± 2.0%, while in the Parkes strain (Table 12–19) counts varied between 2.2 ± 1.3% and 7.3 ± 3.4%. Mean reticulocyte counts of 1.5% to 3.5% were found among 18

Table 12–16. **Erythrocyte Parameters and Plasma Composition in Mice, Regular Yellow A^y Strain—Sex and Age Influence (means and 1 SD)**[a]

Number of Mice	Sex	Age (mo)	PCV (%)	RBC (×10⁶/μl)	Hb (g/dl)	MCV (fl)	MCHC (%)	MCH (pg)	Reticulocytes (%)	Icterus Index Units	Plasma Proteins (g/dl)	Fibrinogen (g/dl)
12	male	1	38.7±1.2	6.94±0.58	12.3±0.8	56.0±4.3	31.7±1.5	17.8±1.5	12.7±4.8	2.9±1.9	6.0±0.4	0.16±0.05
12	male	2	42.0±1.6	8.62±0.49	13.9±0.8	49.1±1.9	32.7±0.8	16.1±0.8	4.3±1.7	—	6.6±0.3	0.20±0.00
10	male	3	42.6±1.1	8.90±0.44	13.6±0.9	47.9±2.5	31.9±1.6	15.3±1.2	3.3±0.9	2.3±2.0	6.7±0.5	—
39	male	4–6	42.1±2.0	8.69±0.61	13.6±0.8	48.6±2.9	32.2±1.1	15.6±1.0	4.0±1.4	2.3±2.7	6.9±0.6	0.20±0.08
52	male	7–12	38.6±3.5	8.04±0.79	12.3±1.3	48.1±2.8	31.9±1.2	15.4±1.0	4.8±3.5	2.2±2.3	7.1±0.6	0.26±0.12
11	female	1	37.7±1.6	7.01±0.49	12.1±0.6	53.9±2.1	31.9±1.2	17.2±0.8	13.3±2.8	2.1±2.2	5.9±0.4	0.18±0.08
12	female	2	42.7±2.0	8.76±0.47	14.2±0.7	48.7±1.6	33.2±0.9	16.2±0.5	4.1±2.4	—	6.9±0.3	0.18±0.06
10	female	3	43.7±1.6	9.00±0.42	14.5±0.6	48.0±1.8	33.2±0.8	16.1±0.6	5.2±2.0	—	7.2±0.3	—
38	female	4–6	42.6±2.4	8.61±0.76	14.0±0.9	49.7±4.0	32.8±1.0	16.3±1.4	3.4±1.7	1.9±2.2	7.0±0.5	0.26±0.13
59	female	7–12	42.0±3.4	8.44±0.95	13.8±1.4	50.0±3.6	32.7±1.5	16.4±0.9	4.7±3.2	1.6±2.2	7.0±0.5	0.20±0.10
23	both	1	38.2±1.5	6.97±0.54	12.2±0.7	55.0±3.6	31.8±1.4	17.5±1.2	13.0±4.0	2.6±2.1	5.9±0.4	0.17±0.06
24	both	2	42.3±1.8	8.69±0.49	14.0±0.7	48.9±1.8	33.0±0.9	16.2±0.6	4.2±2.1	—	6.8±0.3	0.18±0.06
20	both	3	43.2±1.5	8.95±0.43	14.1±0.9	48.0±2.1	32.5±1.4	15.7±1.1	4.3±1.8	1.2±1.8	6.9±0.5	—
77	both	4–6	42.4±2.2	8.65±0.69	13.8±0.9	49.2±3.5	32.5±1.1	16.0±1.3	3.7±1.6	2.1±2.5	6.9±0.5	0.22±0.10
111	both	7–12	40.4±3.8	8.25±0.90	13.1±1.5	49.1±3.4	32.3±1.4	15.9±1.1	4.7±3.3	1.9±2.3	7.1±0.5	0.22±0.11

[a]Heart blood collected under ether anesthesia.

Table 12-17. Total and Differential Leukocyte Numbers in Mice, Regular Yellow A^y Strain—Sex and Age Influence (means and 1 SD)[a]

Number of Mice	Sex	Age (mo)	WBC/μl	Neutrophils		Lymphocytes	Monocytes	Eosinophils	Basophils
				Band	Mature	Differential Leukocyte Count in Absolute Numbers/μl			
12	male	1	3,658 ± 843	4 ± 13	475 ± 187	3,062 ± 749	114 ± 92	3 ± 9	2 ± 6
12	male	2	4,717 ± 1,907	0	588 ± 292	4,030 ± 1,621	30 ± 35	61 ± 83	0
10	male	3	4,730 ± 2,192	0	690 ± 420	3,867 ± 1,788	115 ± 119	51 ± 60	6 ± 15
39	male	4–6	4,972 ± 1,710	8 ± 20	777 ± 322	4,037 ± 1,524	82 ± 75	62 ± 59	3 ± 11
52	male	7–12	6,408 ± 2,706	4 ± 15	1,484 ± 919	4,608 ± 2,649	144 ± 125	107 ± 114	1 ± 2
11	female	1	4,027 ± 826	0	442 ± 170	3,401 ± 611	152 ± 242	32 ± 29	0
12	female	2	4,917 ± 1,233	0	778 ± 377	4,026 ± 1,171	80 ± 62	28 ± 31	0
10	female	3	5,410 ± 902	6 ± 18	562 ± 186	4,688 ± 925	103 ± 86	46 ± 56	0
38	female	4–6	5,338 ± 1,743	13 ± 27	774 ± 648	4,213 ± 1,362	136 ± 165	54 ± 57	7 ± 23
59	female	7–12	6,268 ± 4,426	5 ± 19	945 ± 510	5,077 ± 4,229	142 ± 166	60 ± 56	6 ± 25
23	both	1	3,835 ± 855	2 ± 9	459 ± 180	3,224 ± 707	132 ± 181	17 ± 25	1 ± 4
24	both	2	4,817 ± 1,609	0	683 ± 350	4,028 ± 1,414	55 ± 56	45 ± 65	0
20	both	3	5,070 ± 1,710	3 ± 13	626 ± 331	4,277 ± 1,481	109 ± 104	49 ± 58	3 ± 11
77	both	4–6	5,150 ± 1,736	10 ± 24	776 ± 510	4,124 ± 1,449	108 ± 130	58 ± 58	5 ± 18
111	both	7–12	6,333 ± 3,721	5 ± 17	1,197 ± 779	4,858 ± 3,584	143 ± 148	82 ± 91	3 ± 18

[a]Heart blood collected under ether anesthesia.

Table 12–18. Leukocyte and Platelet Counts in Mice, Regular Yellow Av Strain—Sex and Age Influence (means and 1 SD)[a]

Number of Mice	Sex	Age (mo)	WBC/μl	Neutrophils		Lymphocytes	Monocytes	Eosinophils	Basophils	Platelets ($\times 10^3$/μl)
				Band	Mature					
12	male	1	3,658 ± 843	0.08 ± 0.30	13.3 ± 4.4	83.5 ± 4.5	3.0 ± 2.0	0.08 ± 0.30	0.08 ± 0.30	1,286 ± 429
12	male	2	4,717 ± 1,907	0	12.8 ± 3.7	85.3 ± 3.5	0.7 ± 0.8	1.0 ± 1.1	0	1,372 ± 295
10	male	3	4,730 ± 2,192	0	14.0 ± 4.9	82.5 ± 6.0	2.5 ± 2.5	1.0 ± 1.9	0.15 ± 0.30	1,162 ± 171
39	male	4– 6	4,972 ± 1,710	0.20 ± 0.60	16.2 ± 5.9	80.4 ± 6.7	1.8 ± 1.6	1.3 ± 1.3	0.05 ± 0.20	1,135 ± 239
52	male	7–12	6,408 ± 2,706	0.06 ± 0.20	24.9 ± 13.7	69.5 ± 13.7	2.5 ± 2.3	1.9 ± 2.0	0.01 ± 0.07	1,224 ± 395
11	female	1	4,027 ± 826	0	11.1 ± 4.0	84.9 ± 4.4	3.3 ± 4.2	0.7 ± 0.6	0	1,257 ± 148
12	female	2	4,917 ± 1,233	0	16.2 ± 7.0	81.5 ± 7.3	1.6 ± 1.2	0.6 ± 0.6	0	932 ± 340
10	female	3	5,410 ± 902	0.10 ± 0.30	10.7 ± 4.1	86.3 ± 5.3	2.0 ± 1.9	0.8 ± 1.0	0	1,236 ± 204
38	female	4– 6	5,338 ± 1,743	0.30 ± 0.60	14.0 ± 5.6	81.9 ± 7.2	2.7 ± 3.5	1.0 ± 0.9	0.10 ± 0.30	1,035 ± 271
59	female	7–12	6,268 ± 4,426	0.10 ± 0.40	17.5 ± 7.7	78.5 ± 8.1	2.4 ± 1.8	1.1 ± 1.0	0.10 ± 0.60	1,090 ± 352
23	both	1	3,835 ± 855	0.04 ± 0.20	12.2 ± 4.3	84.2 ± 4.5	3.1 ± 3.3	0.4 ± 0.6	0.04 ± 0.20	1,275 ± 349
24	both	2	4,817 ± 1,609	0	14.5 ± 5.8	83.4 ± 6.0	1.2 ± 1.1	0.8 ± 0.9	0	1,183 ± 383
20	both	3	5,070 ± 1,710	0.05 ± 0.20	12.3 ± 4.8	84.4 ± 6.0	2.2 ± 2.3	0.9 ± 0.9	0.08 ± 0.20	1,197 ± 191
77	both	4– 6	5,150 ± 1,736	0.30 ± 0.60	15.1 ± 5.8	81.2 ± 7.0	2.2 ± 2.8	1.1 ± 1.1	0.08 ± 0.30	1,084 ± 261
111	both	7–12	6,333 ± 3,721	0.09 ± 0.30	21.0 ± 11.5	74.3 ± 13.1	2.4 ± 2.0	1.5 ± 1.6	0.08 ± 0.40	1,163 ± 382

Differential Leukocyte Count (%)

[a] Heart blood collected under ether anesthesia.

Table 12–19. Erythrocyte Parameters and Plasma Composition in Mice, Parkes Strain—Sex and Age Influence (means and 1 SD)[a]

Number of Mice	Sex	Age (mo)	PCV (%)	RBC (×10⁶/μl)	Hb (g/dl)	MCV (fl)	MCHC (%)	MCH (pg)	Reticulo-cytes (%)	Icterus Index (units)	Plasma Proteins (g/dl)	Fibrinogen (g/dl)
12	male	1	41.4±1.4	7.73±0.49	12.6±0.5	53.6±2.4	29.4±4.0	16.4±0.8	16.9±4.0	0.2±0.6	5.6±0.3	0.18±0.04
10	male	2	44.7±1.8	9.03±0.53	13.8±0.7	49.5±1.7	30.7±0.9	15.2±0.8	4.5±2.1	0.5±1.5	6.1±0.2	0.18±0.08
12	male	3	44.4±1.6	8.84±0.39	14.0±0.6	50.3±1.5	31.6±0.8	15.9±0.2	6.5±2.3	0.4±1.4	5.6±0.4	0.20±0.06
31	male	4–6	43.9±3.3	8.69±0.59	13.7±1.2	50.5±2.2	31.2±0.8	15.8±0.9	4.7±2.0	3.0±2.0	5.8±0.4	0.15±0.05
67	male	7–12	41.2±2.9	8.44±0.57	13.1±1.0	48.9±2.4	31.7±1.1	15.5±0.8	7.3±3.4	1.3±1.8	5.9±0.6	0.17±0.07
12	female	1	41.2±0.9	7.87±0.28	12.9±0.5	53.7±0.4	30.2±0.6	16.3±0.3	11.1±3.7	2.0±0.0	5.7±0.3	0.23±0.08
12	female	2	45.4±1.4	8.99±0.45	14.7±0.5	50.5±2.2	32.3±0.7	16.3±0.7	5.1±3.6	0.4±1.4	6.0±0.3	0.15±0.05
4	female	3	46.0±3.5	9.06±0.52	14.9±1.2	49.0±0.7	32.4±0.6	15.8±0.1	2.2±1.3	1.0±1.0	6.2±0.4	0.20±0.00
35	female	4–6	42.7±2.6	8.47±0.50	13.6±0.8	50.3±1.9	31.8±1.2	16.0±0.8	6.0±3.2	1.7±1.9	5.8±1.0	0.14±0.06
63	female	7–12	42.4±2.9	8.47±0.67	13.8±1.1	49.2±5.3	31.2±4.0	16.3±0.9	6.1±4.3	1.6±3.6	6.0±0.5	0.17±0.09
24	both	1	41.3±1.2	7.80±0.40	12.7±0.5	53.6±1.9	29.7±3.2	16.4±0.6	14.0±4.8	1.1±1.0	5.7±0.3	0.21±0.07
22	both	2	45.1±1.6	9.01±0.49	14.3±0.8	50.1±2.1	31.5±1.1	15.8±0.2	4.8±3.0	0.5±1.4	6.1±0.3	0.16±0.07
16	both	3	44.8±2.4	8.88±0.43	14.3±0.9	49.9±1.4	31.7±0.9	15.9±0.2	5.5±2.9	0.7±1.3	5.8±0.4	0.20±0.06
66	both	4–6	43.2±3.0	8.57±0.55	13.6±1.0	50.4±2.1	31.5±1.1	15.9±0.9	5.4±2.8	2.3±2.1	5.8±0.8	0.15±0.06
130	both	7–12	41.8±3.0	8.45±0.62	13.4±1.1	49.0±4.0	31.5±2.9	15.9±1.0	6.7±4.0	1.4±2.8	6.0±0.6	0.17±0.08

[a]Heart blood collected under ether anesthesia.

Table 12–20.   Total and Differential Leukocyte Numbers in Mice, Parkes Strain—Sex and Age Influence (means and 1 SD)[a]

Number of Mice	Sex	Age (mo)	WBC/µl	Neutrophils		Lymphocytes	Monocytes	Eosinophils	Basophils
				Band	Mature				
12	male	1	5,061±1,825	7±16	832± 395	4,045±1,505	145±135	27± 28	5±16
10	male	2	7,440±2,131	0	1,187± 462	5,827±2,120	39± 53	107±114	0
12	male	3	7,933±1,627	0	1,477± 586	6,244±1,264	127±141	85± 48	0
31	male	4– 6	7,110±2,739	4±17	1,548± 826	5,347±2,382	126±124	97±153	10±37
67	male	7–12	7,555±2,632	5±26	1,804±1,102	5,524±2,007	148±143	75± 83	1± 5
12	female	1	6,908±1,867	0	791± 314	5,957±1,798	120±106	41± 57	0
12	female	2	7,808±2,479	8±25	1,047± 401	6,542±2,234	98± 63	114± 94	0
4	female	3	6,900±2,331	0	1,026± 351	5,631±2,075	108± 68	135±102	0
35	female	4– 6	10,031±4,453	0	1,097± 465	8,588±4,439	101±106	83± 99	0
63	female	7–12	7,476±3,364	3±20	1,250± 866	6,099±2,768	85± 93	86± 87	0± 2
24	both	1	5,983±2,064	4±12	811± 358	5,000±1,914	132±122	34± 46	2±11
22	both	2	7,641±2,334	4±19	1,111± 436	6,217±2,212	72± 66	111±103	0
16	both	3	7,675±1,883	0	1,364± 572	6,091±1,532	122±127	98± 70	0
66	both	4– 6	8,659±4,021	2±12	1,309± 697	7,066±3,966	113±116	90±127	5±26
130	both	7–12	7,517±3,009	4±23	1,538±1,033	5,800±2,420	118±126	80± 85	0± 4

Differential Leukocyte Count in Absolute Numbers/µl

[a]Heart blood collected under ether anesthesia.

Table 12-21. Leukocyte and Platelet Counts in Mice, Parkes Strain—Sex and Age Influence (means and 1 SD)[a]

Number of Mice	Sex	Age (mo)	WBC/μl	Neutrophils		Lymphocytes	Monocytes	Eosinophils	Basophils	Platelets (×10³/μl)
				Band	Mature					
12	male	1	5,061±1,825	0.13± 5.3	16.6± 5.3	79.9± 6.4	2.8±2.2	0.6±0.7	0.08±0.28	1,194± 169
10	male	2	7,440±2,131	0	15.8± 5.2	77.4±13.3	0.5±0.6	1.4±1.4	0	1,513± 402
12	male	3	7,933±1,627	0	18.4± 6.0	79.0± 7.0	1.5±1.5	1.1±0.7	0	1,571± 73
31	male	4– 6	7,110±2,739	0.08±0.36	22.6±10.0	74.4±10.6	1.7±1.3	1.4±1.9	0.13±0.47	1,125± 193
67	male	7–12	7,555±2,632	0.05±0.25	23.6±10.4	73.4±10.8	2.0±1.6	1.0±1.0	0.01±0.06	2,152± 745
12	female	1	6,908±1,867	0	12.0± 6.2	85.7± 6.5	1.8±1.7	0.6±0.8	0	1,473± 197
12	female	2	7,808±2,479	0.08±0.28	13.9± 4.8	83.4± 4.7	1.3±0.9	1.4±0.9	0	1,125± 123
4	female	3	6,900±2,331	0	15.4± 4.8	80.9± 5.3	2.0±1.4	1.8±0.8	0	1,249± 205
35	female	4– 6	10,031±4,453	0	11.6± 4.3	84.2±14.0	1.2±1.3	0.9±1.1	0	1,339± 279
63	female	7–12	7,476±3,364	0.03±0.18	16.9± 7.4	80.6± 7.9	1.2±1.1	1.3±1.6	0.01±0.06	1,684±1,250
24	both	1	5,984±2,064	0.06±0.22	14.3± 6.2	82.8± 7.1	2.3±2.0	0.6±0.8	0.04±0.20	1,276± 218
22	both	2	7,641±2,334	0.05±0.21	14.8± 5.1	80.6±10.1	0.9±0.9	1.2±1.1	0	1,300± 344
16	both	3	7,675±1,883	0	17.7± 5.9	79.5± 6.4	1.6±1.5	1.3±0.8	0	1,442± 212
66	both	4– 6	8,659±4,021	0.04±0.25	16.7± 9.3	79.6±13.4	1.4±1.3	1.1±1.5	0.06±0.33	1,234± 264
130	both	7–12	7,517±3,009	0.04±0.21	20.4± 9.7	76.9±10.1	1.6±1.5	1.1±1.3	0.01±0.06	1,950±1,022

Differential Leukocyte Count (%)

[a]Heart blood collected under ether anesthesia.

inbred strains of virgin mice at 2–3 months of age (Russell et al., 1951). Polychromasia is a constant feature of mouse blood correlating with the short life span (20–45 days) of the mouse erythrocyte (Table 20–1).

The red cell life span in several strains of mice was found to be 38.6–42.3 days with ^{14}C-labeled glycine and 47.4 ± 1.0 days in one strain when DF^{32}P was used as a label (Horky et al., 1978). Erythrocyte osmotic fragility begins at 0.50% and is complete at 0.30% buffered NaCl solution (Perk et al., 1964).

The Leukocytes

Total WBC count is significantly influenced by the site of blood withdrawal and the time of day. Leukocyte numbers in tail blood may be 1.5–5 times greater than in large-vessel blood (DeKock, 1931). A marked diurnal variation was found in tail blood of mice (Brown and Dougherty, 1956). Total counts increased during the day from a mean of 14,000/μl at 6 A.M. to 21,150/μl at 3 P.M., followed by a fall to lowest levels of 7,000/μl at 9 P.M. These changes could be correlated with activity of the mice in that highest counts occurred during periods of relative inactivity. When blood flows more slowly through capillaries, the leukocytes become sequestered, and capillary blood under such circumstances contains more leukocytes than large-vessel or heart blood. Similar diurnal variations were found in eosinophil numbers in tail blood (Halberg et al., 1957). Furthermore, it was observed that females had lower eosinophil counts than males without any overlap of mean counts through a 24-hour period. Significant differences were found in WBC counts among mice representing 18 inbred lines (Russell et al., 1951). Furthermore, the percentage of granulocytes tended to be greater in males than females; also, the mean WBC counts within each strain were said to be negatively correlated wtih the percentage of granulocytes (Russell et al., 1951). Significant influence of age on WBC counts was not found in mice at 6, 12, and 18 months of age (Talbot et al., 1965), but counts were found to increase with age in young mice (Rugh and Somogyi, 1968). WBC counts of 1,500 and 1,700/μl were found in female and male fetal mice, respectively, at 17 days gestation. At birth, the counts av-

eraged 3,000–3,500/μl and then dropped to less than 1,500/μl at 2 weeks of age, followed by a rapid rise to 9,000–10,000 by the ninth week of life. Males tended to have higher WBC counts than females after the fourth week of life.

We have recorded total and differential leukocyte counts in heart blood at 1, 2, 3, 4–6, and 7–12 months of life for mice of the Regular Yellow A^y strain (Tables 12–17 and 12–18) and the Parkes strain (Tables 12–20 and 12–21). WBC counts for Parkes strain mice were approximately 2,000 cells greater for males and 2,500 cells greater for females than for the Regular Yellow A^y strain of mice. Females tended to have slightly higher WBC counts than males within each strain. WBC counts appeared to increase with age when the data for both sexes within a strain were combined. For the Regular Yellow A^y strain, the WBC count at 1 month of age was 3,835 ± 855/μl, and at 7–12 months, it was 6,333 ± 3,721/μl. In comparison. Parkes strain mice at 1 month of age had an average WBC count of 5,984 ± 2,064/μl with an increase to 8,659 ± 4,021/μl at 4–6 months of age and slight reduction thereafter. In both strains of mice, neutrophils increased and lymphocytes decreased with advancing age during the first year of life. Very little influence of age was apparent with respect to numbers of monocytes and eosinophils. Basophils were not commonly present.

The Neutrophil (Heterophil)

The cytoplasm of the neutrophil stains diffusely pink and at first sight appears to be nongranular. Close inspection reveals delicate pink, dust-like granules. The nucleus is commonly polymorphous but may be elongated and coiled to form a ring or other configuration (Simonds, 1925). A "drumstick" chromatin lobe, indicating the sex to be female, may be seen in some neutrophils.

The Lymphocyte

This leukocyte comprises more than 80% of the differential leukocyte count in young mice and between 70% and 80% in older mice. Both small and large varieties are seen. The cytoplasm of the small lymphocyte may stain a dark blue, while the larger lymphocytes have

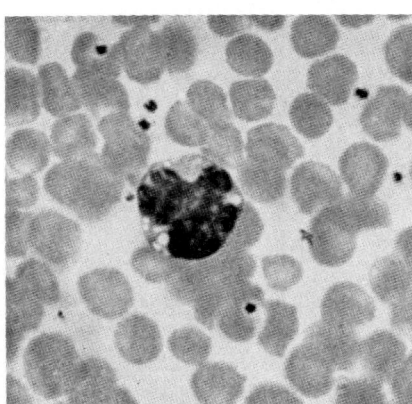

Fig. 12–6. Mouse monocyte with ameboid nuclear outline and typical cytoplasmic vacuoles.

a paler blue cytoplasm, and some cells may present scattered azurophilic cytoplasmic granules. The nucleus is commonly round and assumes a somewhat eccentric position. The chromatin pattern consists of clumps of darker-staining basichromatin separated by streaks of lighter-staining perichromatin.

The Monocyte

The cytoplasm of the monocyte takes a grayish-blue stain and commonly contains a few small vacuoles and reddish-purple azurophilic granules. The nucleus is ameboid with pale chromatin strands (Fig. 12–6).

The Eosinophil

The nucleus of this leukocyte is commonly elongated and coiled to form U-shaped and ring-like patterns. The cytoplasm is basophilic with small, scanty acidophilic granules arranged in clumps or patches.

The Basophil

The granules of the basophil are large, stain a deep purple, and often obscure the nucleus. A tissue mast cell may be encountered occasionally in blood drawn by cardiac puncture. The mast cell is larger than the basophil and presents numerous dark-staining cytoplasmic granules.

The Platelets

Literature values on platelets range from 157,000–1,536,000/μl, with most counts falling between 260,000 and 500,000 (Heinecke,

1963), and from 100,000–400,000/μl, with a mean of 200,000 (Schermer, 1967). Our counts (Tables 12–18 and 12–21) were considerably in excess of the previously mentioned reports and were similar to the high platelet numbers we found in 2 strains of rats. Platelet numbers were not influenced by age or sex and ranged from 932,000 ± 340,000 to 2,152,000 ± 745,000/μl. It is noteworthy that the maximum platelet counts were obtained in males 7–12 months of age in the Parkes strain. Platelet counts of 450,000/μl in fetal mice at 17 days of gestation, 600,000 at birth, and 1.2 million to 1.5 million from the second week of life onward were reported (Rugh and Somogyi, 1968).

The Plasma

Icterus index varied between colorless plasma and 5 units of color. The influence of age on plasma proteins was more apparent among Regular Yellow A^y strain mice than among Parkes strain mice. In the former, the plasma proteins at 1 month of age averaged 5.9 ± 0.4 g/dl, and at 7–12 months of age the average was 7.1 ± 0.5 g/dl. In the Parkes strain, values of 5.6 ± 0.3 to 6.2 ± 0.4 g/dl were found. Plasma fibrinogen varied between 0.1 and 0.4 g/dl (Tables 12–16 and 12–19).

The Myeloid:Erythroid Ratio

Differential counts were performed on femoral marrow of 15 mature mice taken after killing by decapitation (Quittner et al., 1951). The M:E ratios ranged from 0.8–2.4:1.0, with a mean of 1.49 ± 0.47:1.0. Maturation of the nucleus of the neutrophil and eosinophil is similar to that described for the rat. Ring forms occur as an intermediate stage between the myelocyte and metamyelocyte. The ring may break with separation of the ends, or, instead of breaking in one place, the ring may begin to form constrictions at several points, leading to segmentation (Simonds, 1925). Ring forms in the neutrophil series ranged from 7.6–14.4%, and in the eosinophil series from 0–4.8% in bone marrow differential cell counts (Quittner et al., 1951).

Splenic Hematopoiesis

The spleen of the adult mouse is actively engaged in hematopoiesis. Schermer (1967)

described the occurrence of erythrocytes in all stages of maturation in the spleen. He also noted that the granulocytic maturation series was less numerous in the spleen than in bone marrow and that, in particular, there were fewer granulocytes with ring-shaped nuclei in the spleen. Numerous megakaryocytes were also found in the spleen, which further emphasized the hematopoietic function of this organ in the mouse. Early erythrocyte production after irradiation and injection of bone marrow may occur preferentially in the spleen (Gurney and Rosett, 1968).

THE GERBIL

Up to 40% of the red cells of fetal and newborn gerbils were found to exhibit basophilic stippling, which decreased with age. In the adult, basophilic stippling was seen in 5.4 ± 2.4% red cells in blood compared to 26.1 ± 7.6% red cells in bone marrow (Smith et al., 1976). Blood values have been reported for the Mongolian gerbil (Dillon and Glomski, 1975; Gattermann, 1979). Sex differences were found in PCV and Hb values and WBC and lymphocyte numbers (Dillon and Glomski, 1975). Bone marrow cytology was studied, and an M:E ratio of 1.6 ± 0.75:1.0 (range 0.6–3.6:1) was found (Weeks and Glomski, 1978). Cell morphology was similar to that of other rodents, and ring heterophils, characteristically found in the rat and mouse, were also seen in gerbil marrow. Lymphocytes in marrow ranged from 1.4–20.1%, with a mean of 8.4 ± 4.2%.

THE GOLDEN HAMSTER

Blood is commonly taken under light anesthesia by cardiac puncture. Up to 2 ml can be withdrawn safely from a 100-g hamster. A ⅜-inch, 25-gauge needle is adequate (Desai, 1968). The tail or paw may be used for taking a smaller amount of blood (Stein and Carrier, 1945). The jugular or femoral vein may also be used. The orbital sinus has been employed successfully using a tuberculin syringe and a 23-gauge needle (Pansky et al., 1961). The orbital sinus offers several advantages as a source of blood. A method is described for obtaining a volume of blood up to 4.5% of the

body weight in terminal experiments (Manning and Giannina, 1966). Blood volume has been determined (Silverman and Chavannes, 1977). Selected reports from the literature are listed in Table 12–22.

The Erythrocytes

In the newborn, 10–30% of circulating erythrocytes were found to be nucleated, while in the adult hamster, nucleated red cells either were absent or comprised less than 2.0% (Desai, 1968). The erythrocytes are biconcave and commonly measure 6.2–7.0 μm (Stewart et al., 1944; Gardner, 1947) or 5.0–7.0 μm, with a mean of 6.0 μm (Schermer, 1967). MCV was found to be 72.4 ± 3.0 fl (Sherman and Patt, 1956) and 71.2 ± 3.2 fl (Desai, 1968). RBC count increased from 5 million/μl at 20 days of age to 9 million/μl at 100 days (Stein and Carrier, 1945). At the same time, the MCV decreased from approximately 70 fl at 33 days of age to 57 fl at 100 days. A 25–30% decrease in RBC counts and size occurred in castrated male hamsters (Stewart et al., 1944). Splenectomy was also followed by a decrease in erythrocyte numbers. Testosterone restored the RBC number in castrates but not in splenectomized hamsters.

Blood values of hamsters kept at 23°C (active) were compared with those kept at 5°C (hibernating) (Lyman et al., 1957). Blood volume, as well as RBC, Hb, and PCV, increased during hibernation. Hematopoiesis was suppressed as indicated by a reduction in circulating reticulocytes and failure of a reticulocyte response to massive blood withdrawal. When hibernation was terminated, the long-delayed reticulocyte response took place. In hibernating hamsters, RBC senescence was retarded and random erythrocyte destruction was virtually absent; the former was associated with an increased potential erythrocyte life span to 160 days (Brock, 1960) compared to normal erythrocyte life span of 60–70 days (Rigby et al., 1961). During hibernation WBC counts were found to be low, averaging about 2,500/μl with a neutrophil:lymphocyte ratio of 1.0:1.0 (Schermer, 1967). Platelet counts were also reduced (Reznik et al., 1975).

Reticulocyte numbers were found to vary from 2.0–12.5%, with a mean of 4.9% (Trincao et al., 1949). A mean of 2.5 ± 1.2% reticulo-

Table 12–22. Compilation from the Literature of Hemograms for the Golden Hamster

Source	RBC (×10⁶/μl)	Hb (g/dl)	PCV (%)	MCD (μm)	MCV (fl)	WBC (×10³/μl)	Differential Leukocyte Count (%)				
							Neutrophils	Lymphocytes	Monocytes	Eosinophils	Basophils
Stewart et al. (1944)	7.5±0.5	17.6±1.0	47.4±2.4	6.2–7.0 (6.6)	—	8.56±1.54	29±11.0	67.9±11.9	2.43	0.68	0.0
Stein and Carrier (1945)	5.0–9.0	15.6–18.9	41–53	—	57–70	—	—	—	—	—	—
Gardner (1947)	5.0–9.2	15.0–20.0	47.4	6.2–7.0	—	8.5–10.0	16–29	68–81	0.0–2.5	0.7–2.8	0.0
Trincao et al. (1949)	5.55–7.90 (6.67)	14.6–18.0 (16.5)	—	—	—	2.5–12.5 (7.40)	15–51 (33.2)	44–79 (60.4)	3.2–9.5 (5.63)	0.0–2.5 (0.72)	0.0
MacNamee and Sheehy (1952)	7.2	17.4	46.2	—	—	7.6–8.4	28.0	68.2	2.2	0.8	0.8
Fulton et al. (1954)	6.96±1.5	16.0±7.0	49±5	—	—	4.64±1.9	26.0±8.0	70.0±13.0	2.5±0.7	1.3±1.4	0.0
Sherman and Patt (1956)	6.96±0.70	16.2±1.3	50.7±1.3	—	72.4±3.0	5.78±1.29	29.9±5.5	66.4±5.9	2.6±0.8	1.1±0.02	0.0
Desai and Fulton (1960)	7.1±1.7	15.5±4.1	—	—	—	5.24±1.20	20±6.0	61±7.5	3.0±0.5	1.8±0.2	0.0
Desai (1968)	7.5±2.4	16.8±1.2	52.5±2.3	—	71.2±3.2	7.62±1.3	29.9±8.0	73.5±9.4	2.5±0.8	1.1±0.02	0.0
Schermer (1967)	6.0–9.0 (7.0)	—	—	5.0–7.0 (6.0)	—	3.4–7.6 (6.2)	3–43	50–96	0.0–1.0	0.0–2.0	0.0

cytes was given for adult hamsters (Desai, 1968). Polychromatophilic erythrocytes are present in small to moderate numbers in normal hamster blood, and a marked reticulocytosis occurs following massive blood loss.

Erythrocyte fragility begins at 0.51% and is complete at 0.30% of buffered saline solution (Perk et al., 1964).

The Leukocytes

Ranges for WBC counts, as reported by different authors (Table 12–22), have varied considerably. House et al. (1961) observed no significant variation with age and reported mean counts at various ages; at 4 to 5 weeks, 7.78 ± 2.27 × $10^3/\mu$l; at 8 to 9 weeks, 7.62 ± 2.39; at 6 months, 8.10 ± 2.5; and at 1 year, 7.31 ± 2.2. WBC counts as well as RBC counts were found to be lowest in laboratory-bred European hamsters (Emminger et al., 1975). A marked leukopenia (1,160 ± 360/μl) was observed in hibernating hamsters (Lyman et al., 1957). Neutrophils of hamsters exhibit extremely high alkaline phosphatase activity (Desai, 1968).

Hu and Pai (1938) differentiated 50 neutrophils in each of 10 hamsters and found the frequency of different nuclear forms to be as follows: ring-shape, 8%; figure-eight, 53%; U-shape, 20%; and two to four distinct lobes, 19%. The most frequent leukocyte in peripheral and heart blood is the lymphocyte, with mean values as reported by various authors (Table 12–22) ranging from 60–73.5%. House et al. (1961) reported the mean neutrophil:lymphocyte ratios, stated in percentages, to be 30.9:66.1 at 4–5 weeks of age; 21.9:75.5 at 8–9 weeks; 21.3:76.3 at 6 months; and 28.6:68.0 at 1 year. The lymphocyte appears in both small and large forms, and the latter may present a few azurophilic cytoplasmic granules. The monocyte exhibits the stringy chromatin pattern characteristic of this leukocyte in all species and a clear blue cytoplasm with fine reddish granules clumped in the indentation of the nucleus. The granules of the eosinophil are large and strongly acidophilic. Basophils were not found in peripheral or cardiac blood by any investigators except MacNamee and Sheehy (1952). They reported 0.8% basophil leukocytes, but these may have been tissue mast cells that have been reported occasionally in hamster blood (Fulton et al., 1954; Desai, 1968). Basophil leukocytes (0.1%) were found in the bone marrow (Trincao et al., 1949).

The Platelets

Platelet counts ranging from 250,000–1 million/μl have been reported. A mean of 296,000 ± 73,000 was found in 40 hamsters 8–10 weeks of age (Sherman and Patt, 1956) and of 338,000 ± 89,000 in 80 hamsters 5–8 weeks of age (Fulton et al., 1954). A range of 504,000–880,000 was found in 12 females (Ottis and Tauber, 1952). Platelet counts of 902,000 ± 50,000 were found in 11 normal hamsters (Desai and Fulton, 1960), but a mean of 310,000 ± 62,800 was given as characteristic of hamster blood (Desai, 1968). Schermer (1967) gave the range as 336,000–587,000/μl. Platelet counts were lower in older than in younger European hamsters (Emminger et al., 1975).

The Plasma

Plasma protein concentration is lower than in the mouse and rat. A mean of 4.5 ± 0.73 g/dl was reported for 14 normal hamsters (House et al., 1962). A range of 2.4 to 5.7 g/dl, with a mean of 4.5 ± 0.73 g/dl, was given for hamster blood (Desai, 1968).

The Myeloid:Erythroid Ratio

Desai (1968) reported the M:E ratio to be 8–10:1.0 and stated that neutrophils with ring-shaped nuclei were commonly seen in bone marrow films. Trincao et al. (1949), however, reported, the mean M:E ratio of 20 hamsters to be 1.7:1.0 and the mean differential cell counts in normal hamster marrow as presented in Table 12–23.

WILD RODENT SPECIES

Dieterich (1973) presented the erythrocyte parameters and total and differential leukocyte counts for six standardized wild rodent species maintained at the Institute of Arctic Biology, University of Alaska. The species were *Acomys cahirinus* (spiny mouse), *Calomys ducilla* (vesper mouse), *C. callosus* (Bolivian field mouse), *Peromyscus maniculatus borealis* and *P. maniculatus bairdii* (deer mouse), and

Table 12–23. Mean Differential Cell Distribution in the Marrow of Normal Hamsters

Erythrocytic Series		Granulocytic Series	
Rubriblast	0.41%	Myeloblast	1.22%
Prorubricyte	1.94	Promyelocyte	3.03
Basophilic rubricyte	9.34	Myelocyte (neut)	13.72
Polychrom rubricyte	22.10	Myelocyte (eos)	0.29
Metarubricyte	2.39	Metamyelocyte (neut)	29.56
Total erythroid cells	36.18%	Metamyelocyte (eos)	0.55
		Metamyelocyte (bas)	0.05
Other Cells		Neutrophil	12.69
Lymphocyte	0.04%	Eosinophil	0.20
Monocyte	0.07	Basophil	0.10
Plasma cell	0.47	Total granulocytic cells	61.41%
RE cell	1.91		
Other	0.03		
	M:E = 1.696:1.0		

From Trincao et al., 1949.

Lemmus trimucronatus alascensis (brown lemming). PCV values varied from 44 ± 3% to 50 ± 3%. Erythrocyte number varied from 7.58 ± 1.35 × 10⁶/μl for *Acomys cahirinus* to 13.62 ± 2.10 × 10⁶/μl for *Peromyscus maniculatus bairdii*. Mean values for the remaining four species fell between these extremes. Total leukocyte counts also varied greatly among the six species, e.g., 16.79 ± 4.39 × 10³/μl for *Acomys cahirinus* and 2.50 ± 0.97 × 10³/μl for *Lemmus trimucronatus alascensis*. Lymphocytes were considerably in excess of neutrophils in five of the species, while the neutrophil:lymphocyte ratio was 1.09:1 in *L. trimucronatus alascensis*.

THE MONKEY

Hematology of the macaque has received the most attention, although the decade of the sixties saw an expansion of investigations to include New World monkeys and higher primates. Reviews of older literature, including tables of data, have been presented (Gardner, 1947; Hall, 1929; Krise, 1960; Scarborough, 1931–1932; Schermer, 1967; Shuckers et al., 1938; Williams, 1962). This section briefly summarizes information on the hematology of the genus *Macaca*, particularly the rhesus monkey, *Macaca mulatta*. Readers interested in information on a greater variety of nonhuman primates are referred to the *Atlas of Comparative Primate Hematology* by Huser (1970) and *Comparative Mammalian Haematology* by Hawkey (1975).

In the older literature, hematologic data were based on capillary blood obtained from a marginal ear vein. The more recent data are based on large-vessel blood (femoral vein) and the use of sophisticated methods of cell counting, hemoglobin determination, and the capillary hematocrit procedure. These methods permit a more reliable calculation of the erythrocytic indices MCV, MCH, and MCHC (Table 12–24).

Monkeys have often been caught in the wild, imported, and made available to laboratories by handlers. Allen and Carstens (1965) found that a period of 90 days was required to establish normal blood values despite extensive therapy and efficient nursing care. Stabilization of hematologic values depends upon freeing monkeys of parasites, providing a diet adequate in protein, minerals, and vitamins, and training the monkey to be handled and bled without fear.

The Erythrocytes

The diameter of the erythrocyte was reported to range from 6.4–7.1 μm (Scarborough, 1931–1932) and from 6.6–7.5 μm (Gardner, 1947). The mean diameter was found to be 8.0 μm in wet films and 7.3 μm in dry films for *M. mulatta* (Ponder et al., 1929). A mean MCV of 78.6 ± 4.8 fl was found for 200 young *M. mulatta* monkeys (Melville et al., 1967), and it averaged 72–74 fl for males and 73–74 fl for females of the species (Stanley and Cramer, 1968). Thus, the erythrocyte was found by most investigators to be somewhat smaller than the red cell of humans. The finding of high values for MCV (89.57–93.52 fl) of *M. mulatta* (Robinson and Zeigler, 1968) may have involved some technical error.

Table 12–24. Selected Hemograms from the Literature for Monkeys of the Genus Macaca (means and 1 SD)

Source	Species	Number, Sex, Age	RBC ($\times 10^6/\mu l$)	Hb (g/dl)	PCV (%)	MCV (fl)	MCHC (%)	MCH (pg)	WBC ($\times 10^3/\mu l$)	Differential Leukocyte Count (%)				
										Neutrophils	Lymphocytes	Monocytes	Eosinophils	Basophils
Krise and Wald (1958)	M. mulatta	538	5.37 ±0.73	11.72 ±3.02	37.0 ±6.7	—	—	—	15.15 ±5.98	35.8 ±16.7	60.5 ±17.3	0.7 ±0.4	2.63 ±2.37	0.21 ±0.18
Usacheva and Raeva (1963–1964)	M. rhesus	45	4.6–7.3 (5.5)	10.7–14.4 (12.9)	—	—	—	—	5.5–19.5 (10.95)	52.3	38.5	4.0	2.0	0.15
King and Gargus (1967)	M. mulatta	15 females	5.19 ±0.57	13.4 ±1.4	41.1 ±3.2	—	—	—	12.8 ±4.8	43.0 ±17.0	52.0 ±17.0	1.0 ±1.0	4.0 ±4.0	0
Melville et al. (1967)	M. mulatta	200	5.38 ±0.41	12.2 ±0.6	42.1 ±2.2	78.6 ±4.8	28.9 ±1.3	22.8 ±1.7	10.95 ±2.87	41.1 ±11.4	55.7 ±11.5	0	2.7 ±1.8	0
Switzer (1967a)	M. mulatta	20 female 6 males	5.78 ±0.39	14.1 ±1.1	44.4 ±2.9	77.0 ±4.0	32.0 ±1.0	25.0 ±2.0	10.8 ±3.6	29.0 ±15.0	63.0 ±14.0	3.0 ±2.0	5.0 ±3.0	0.4 ±0.6
Stanley and Cramer (1968)	M. mulatta	22 females <3 yr	5.57 ±0.55	13.4 ±1.1	40.9 ±3.0	73.0	32.9	24.0	8.50 ±3.18	37.0 ±15.3	57.8 ±14.3	—	—	—
		36 males <3 yr	5.70 ±0.59	14.1 ±0.9	41.9 ±2.6	74.0	33.6	25.0	7.88 ±2.35	32.5 ±13.5	63.8 ±13.3	—	—	—
		34 females >3 yr	5.60 ±0.57	13.5 ±1.0	41.1 ±2.8	74.0	33.0	24.0	7.57 ±2.37	38.7 ±13.0	56.7 ±12.3	—	—	—
		38 male >3 yr	5.85 ±0.62	13.8 ±1.0	42.1 ±2.8	72.0	32.8	24.0	8.20 ±3.21	34.5 ±14.3	61.3 ±14.3	—	—	—
Huser (1970)	M. mulatta	?	5.60 ±0.6	12.3 ±1.1	42.1 ±3.2	76.0 ±6.5	29.1 ±2.0	22.0 ±2.4	10.1 ±3.6	40.0 ±17.0	55.0 ±16.5	1.1 ±1.6	3.5 ±3.0	0.3 ±0.5
Oser et al. (1970)	M. arctoides	79 females	—	12.0 ±1.4	40.0 ±5.2	—	—	—	14.13 ±5.05	31.4 ±15.2	61.9 ±16.9	0.52 ±1.56	5.2 ±5.2	0.22 ±0.57
		76 males	—	12.2 ±1.2	39.3 ±5.8	—	—	—	14.69 ±5.46	28.3 ±15.2	67.3 ±15.2	0.54 ±1.39	3.6 ±3.5	0.20 ±0.60

Mean values for PCV have been reported to vary from $37.0 \pm 6.7\%$ to $44.4 \pm 2.9\%$, RBC from $5.19 \pm 0.57 \times 10^6$ to $5.85 \pm 0.62 \times 10^6/\mu l$, and Hb from 11.7 ± 3.0 g/dl to 14.1 ± 1.1 g/dl (Table 12–24). The erythrocytes have been hypochromic, with MCHC falling below 30% in some colonies (Melville et al., 1967; Huser, 1970), while others have found MCHC to be 32.0–33.6%. When the mean MCHC falls below 30%, methods for Hb and PCV determination should be checked for errors; if none are found, the diet should be improved to preclude iron deficiency.

Nucleated erythrocytes are rarely found in peripheral blood of the normal monkey, but after blood loss, immature erythrocytes appear in the circulation in large numbers. A normal monkey can withstand an abrupt loss of a third of the average blood volume without irreversible ill effects and with apparent return to normal within 28 days (Krise and Wald, 1959). A prompt increase in circulating reticulocytes was noted, with peak numbers being attained at 4 days after blood loss. In the normal state, circulating reticulocytes ranged between 0.1% and 3.4%, with a mean of 0.35% (Krise and Wald, 1958). A mean value of $1.15 \pm 0.57\%$ reticulocytes was found in 200 normal young *M. mulatta* monkeys (Melville et al., 1967). On this basis, polychromasia would not be a prominent feature of normal monkey blood.

Hemolysis of *M. mulatta* erythrocytes was found to begin at 0.46% and to be complete at 0.33% NaCl solution (Krumbhaar and Musser, 1920). Ponder et al. (1929) found erythrocyte resistance to hypotonic saline to be greater than that of the red blood cell of humans in 8 of 12 species of primates investigated. Complete hemolysis for *M. mulatta* was found to occur at 0.27% saline.

Erythrocyte sedimentation rate (ESR) at 1 hour was found to be minimal (0–2 mm; Switzer, 1967a) and 0–13 mm with a mean of 1.3 mm (King and Gargus, 1967). The ESR in the female was reported to accelerate at about day 120 of gestation and to continue to increase until delivery, with a rapid decline thereafter (Allen and Siegfried, 1966). ESR continued to increase after parturition to a maximum at 72 hours with a return to normal

by the fourteenth day postpartum (Switzer et al., 1970).

The life span of the erythrocyte, as determined with ^{59}Cr, ranged from 52–128 days, with a mean of 85 days (Huser, 1970). Using ^{52}Cr and DF^{32}P, a range of 86–105 days, with a mean potential life span of 99.9 ± 1.0 days, was found for erythrocytes of *M. mulatta* (Kreier et al., 1970). Half-life of ^{51}Cr-tagged autologous erythrocytes of *M. mulatta* was found to be 17.0 days (Glomski et al., 1971).

The Leukocytes

All investigators have found wide differences in WBC counts among individual monkeys. Mean values as low as $7,570 \pm 2,370$ and as high as $15,150 \pm 5,980$ have been reported (Table 12–24). Ives and Dack (1956) stressed the importance of training monkeys to be handled and bled to avoid the "alarm reaction" that elevates WBC count and alters the differential distribution of leukocyte types. They found the total WBC count in capillary blood from an ear vein of 36 normal untrained rhesus monkeys to be $15,822 \pm 846$; after 3 months of conditioning to the procedure of restraint and bleeding, the mean count was $8,061 \pm 216$ leukocytes/μl. The ratio of neutrophils to lymphocytes, stated in percent, was 28:64 in untrained and 54:42 in trained monkeys and subsequently became 42:56. Fox (1927) stressed the importance of diurnal variations in WBC counts and stated that the neutrophil was mainly responsible for extreme counts. The majority of investigators have found the lymphocyte to be present in peripheral blood in greater numbers than the neutrophil, with the former between 50% and 60% and the latter between 35% and 45% of the differential leukocyte count.

The Neutrophil

Krumbhaar and Musser (1920) were the first to call attention to the increased number of lobes of the neutrophil of the rhesus monkey. Although subsequent investigators have reported as many as 10–15 lobes, the nucleus commonly presents 5–6 lobes, with extremes of 2–8 lobes (Hall, 1929). However, 2.5–4.0 lobes, with a mean of 3.21, which fell within the range of lobes of the normal human neutrophil, have been reported (Huser, 1970).

The "drumstick" chromatin lobe, indicative of the female sex, was found in 1.6% of 500 neutrophils of *M. mulatta* (Chiarelli and Barberis, 1964). The cytoplasmic granules are a delicate pink and vary from dust-like to being considerably more prominent between individual leukocytes as well as between neutrophils of individual monkeys.

The Lymphocyte

Lymphocytes were classified as small (5–6%), medium (80–85%), and large (10–12%) (Hall, 1929). The small and medium-sized cells have the typical features of lymphocytes, namely, eccentric nucleus with dense chromatin clumping and a narrow rim or crescent of pale blue cytoplasm. The large lymphocytes, some of which have been referred to as "atypical" lymphocytes by some authors, present nuclei of varying shape, such as round, oval, or bean-form, and not infrequently a nucleus may be bizarre and polymorphous in shape. A mitosis resulting in cells with double nuclei may be encountered. Some lymphocytes may have the characteristics ascribed to the plasma cell. The nucleus is small, round, or oval, with deeply staining chromatin masses, and the cytoplasm is basophilic at the cell periphery with a lighter-stained area near the center and next to the margin of the nucleus. Azurophilic granules occur in the cytoplasm of some lymphocytes and more particularly in the larger cells.

The Monocyte

The shape of the nucleus in the typical monocyte is subject to considerable variation. Bean-shaped forms are common, but deep indentations also occur frequently. The chromatin takes a lighter stain than that of the large lymphocyte, and it is characteristically arranged in fine, thin strands, giving a reticulated appearance. The cytoplasm is grayish-blue and may contain fine azurophilic granules.

The Eosinophil

The nucleus of the eosinophil is much less segmented than that of the neutrophil; the mean lobe count was found to be 1.96 compared to 3.21 for the neutrophil of the rhesus monkey (Huser, 1970). The granules are large and round and stain a bright red. The granules are distributed unevenly, and a pale sky-blue cytoplasm appears in areas of the cell devoid of granules. In the majority of cells, however, the granules fill the cytoplasm completely and may be superimposed upon the nucleus.

The Basophil

The nucleus of the basophil may be U-shaped, bilobed, or polymorphous. The nuclear outline is sharply defined and rarely obscured by the granules. Most granules are the same size as or slightly larger than the granules of the eosinophil, but some basophils have both large and small granules. The smaller granules are round, while the larger ones are oval or spindle-shaped. Staining varies from pale violet to dark purple. The cytoplasm is seen as a contrasting bluish-gray color between the violet to dark purple granules.

The Platelets

Mean platelet counts for *M. mulatta* have been 454,000 ± 104,000 (Melville et al., 1967), 560,000 ± 174,000 (Stanley and Cramer, 1968), and 417,000 ± 114,700/μl (Huser, 1970). Platelet counts for *M. arctoides* were reported to be 353,000 ± 93,900/μl (Vondruska, 1970).

The Plasma or Serum

The plasma protein concentration ranged from 6.4–9.6 g/dl in males and from 6.9–9.1 g/dl in females of *M. mulatta*, with a mean of 8.0 g/dl in both sexes (Rollins et al., 1970). Serum protein concentration was 8.3 ± 0.7 g/dl in males less than 3 years of age and 8.2 ± 0.8 g/dl in females over 3 years of age (Stanley and Cramer, 1968).

The Myeloid:Erythroid Ratio

Switzer (1967a,b) conducted bone marrow studies on 20 adult female and 5 adult male *M. mulatta* monkeys with material aspirated from the ischial tuberosity. Mean values were, for the nucleated erythrocytic cell, 39.12 ± 4.67%; for the granulocytic series, 53.04 ± 4.13%; and for M:E ratio, 1.36 ± 0.26:1.0. No correlation of M:E ratios with age, sex, or hematocrit values was noted. Considerable numbers of large, irregular, band-like neutrophils that were difficult to classify were seen. Since these cells were more immature than typical band neutrophils, they were classified as metamyelocytes; others (Huser and Beard, 1969) have also noted the presence of giant metamyelocytes in the bone marrow of several species of nonhuman primates. It was concluded that the presence of these macrometamyelocytes was a natural characteristic and not secondary to acquired deficiencies of vitamin B_{12} or folate.

Stasney and Higgins (1936) studied histologic sections and imprints of bone marrow taken from different bones of 6 adult *M. rhesus* monkeys immediately after death. They reported the M:E ratios for the sternum to be 1.37; vertebra, 1.36; rib, 1.28; femur, 1.11; and tibia, 0.92:1.0. Usacheva and Raeva (1963–1964) studied the bone marrow cells in 14 *M. mulatta* monkeys and reported for the erythroid series a range of 10.6–38.2%, with a mean of 30.87%, and for the myeloid series, a range of 43.5–71.6%, with a mean of 68.9%. Using these means, the average M:E was 1.91:1.0. Lymphocytes in the marrow ranged from 0.8% to 23.0% with a mean of 8.6%.

Age-Related Hematologic Values

Martin et al. (1973) have reported on changes occurring in 170 hand-reared *M. mulatta* from birth through 2 years of age. The PCV at birth was 49.1 ± 7.21% and rapidly declined by 2 weeks to 37.2 ± 3.59%. Thereafter, there was a gradual rise in PCV to 39.7 ± 2.34% at 24 weeks, 41.1 ± 2.40% at 36 weeks, and 42.7 ± 2.1% at 2 years of age. The WBC count was more variable in the infant than in the adult, but by 12 weeks of age, the mean values had attained adult levels of 8,000–9,000/μl. The neutrophil:lymphocyte ratio, expressed as percentages, was 72.4:22.7 at birth and changed gradually over the first 8 weeks of life, attaining a ratio of 22.6:70.4, which is comparable to the adult ratio.

FUR-BEARING ANIMALS (Table 12–25)

Certain fur-bearing animals are bred and raised in large numbers as a commercial endeavor; prevention of disease becomes a major effort. Although raised under domestication, the fur-bearing animals are resentful of handling and will bite if given the opportunity. Considerable thought must be given to the method of extracting blood in sufficient quantity for complete examination.

Mink

A technique has been described for bleeding ferrets and minks by cardiac puncture under ether anesthesia (Baker and Gorham, 1951). Ether-soaked cotton was held in a heavy leather glove and forced over the muzzle. As soon as the animal was completely relaxed, which was usually within 1 minute, it was placed flat on its back with the cotton laid over its muzzle to maintain anesthesia. A 10- or 20-ml syringe and a 1-inch, 20-gauge needle were used. The point of the needle was inserted on the midline immediately posterior to the xiphoid cartilage, and while the rib cage was squeezed to center the heart and prevent it from rolling, the needle was pushed forward at an angle of about 35° for a distance of approximately 1 inch, or until blood appeared. Ten to 15 ml of blood could be taken with no apparent ill effect. Death attributed to mechanical injury with the needle was reported to have occurred in 3 out of 150 bleedings.

Cardiac puncture, using a 2-inch, 18-gauge needle, was performed to obtain blood, but after 5 minks died after bleeding, blood was taken by cutting off a half inch of the tail (Kubin and Mason, 1948). Differences between the means for hemograms of mink in the two reports cited in Table 12–25 may be referable to the use of pentobarbital sodium by Kubin and Mason. Excitement can alter chemical and cellular composition of blood, and so anesthesia or sedation is recommended to collect a large volume of blood (Jepsen et al., 1981).

Descriptive morphology of the individual blood cells is taken from the work of Kennedy (1935a). Blood was taken from conscious mink. A small net and thick leather gloves were used in catching and handling the mink. A mink was held in restraint by having an assistant grip it firmly around the neck with one hand while holding the foot from which the blood was to be extracted with the other.

Table 12-25. Compilation from the Literature of Hemograms for Some Fur-Bearing Animals

Source	Species	Number, Sex, Age	Erythrocytic Series RBC ($\times 10^6/\mu l$)	Hb (g/dl)	PCV (%)	MCD (μm)	MCV (fl)	WBC ($\times 10^3/\mu l$)	Leukocytic Series—Total and Differential Counts Neutrophils No.	Neutrophils %	Lymphocytes No.	Lymphocytes %	Monocytes No.	Monocytes %	Eosinophils No.	Eosinophils %	Basophils No.	Basophils %
Lord et al. (1954)	Muskrat	71	4.3–8.0 (6.4±0.8)	6.6–19.8 (13.6±2.8)	34–68[a] (50±6)	—	65–119[a] (80±11.6)	3.3–25.0 (7.5±3)	—	33–93 (70.1)	—	5–46 (24.9)	—	0.0–10.0 (2.84)	—	0.0–2.5 (0.61)	—	0.0–15.0 (1.66)
Kennedy (1935a)	Raccoon	6 adult males	9.6–13.3 (11.2)	11–12 (11.5)	—	5.0–9.0 (6.5)	—	12.2–16.2 (14.3)	—	19.5–37.5 (27.8)	—	59.0–78.5 (66.8)	—	0.0–2.0 (1.25)	—	1.5–7.0 (4.1)	—	0.0
		10 adult females	9.5–13.6 (11.1)	8.2–11.5 (10.4)	—	—	—	10.6–26.8 (16.1)	—	30.5–60.5 (45.7)	—	35.0–65.5 (49.3)	—	0.0–3.5 (0.8)	—	1.5–8.0 (4.3)	—	0.0
Kennedy (1935a)	Mink	10 adult males	8.9–10.4 (9.68)	9.5–15.6 (11.9)	—	6.0–9.5 (7.8)	—	3.8–10.2 (6.38)	—	18.5–69.0 (47.1)	—	22.5–57.5 (43.5)	—	0.0–5.5 (1.1)	—	2.5–16.0 (7.2)	—	0.0–2.5 (0.8)
		9 adult females	7.5–11.3 (9.72)	11.4–17.3 (15.0)	—	—	—	5.2–12.2 (7.80)	—	26.5–65.5 (46.3)	—	30.0–68.5 (47.5)	—	0.0–5.0 (1.5)	—	0.0–13.0 (4.0)	—	0.0–1.5 (0.8)
Kubin and Mason (1948)	Mink	15	5.7–9.3 (7.50)	13.5–17.5 (14.7)	41–57 (48)	—	62–82 (68)	3.2–11.2 (6.0)	—	45–88 (66.0)	—	14–50 (32.0)	—	0.0–3.0 (1.0)	—	0.0–3.0 (1.0)	—	0.0–1.0 (0.0)
Kennedy (1935b)	Silver black fox	6–48 mo	6.0–12.0 (8.80)	8.3–14.2 (11.0)	—	—	—	4.2–15.8 (9.26)	2.0–12.5 (4.5)	—	2.2–8.5 (3.8)	—	0.0–0.4 (0.2)	—	0.0	—	0.0–2.0 (0.9)	—
Spitzer et al. (1941)	Silver fox	12 (mature)	7.4–8.5 (8.0)	13.9–16.1 (15.0)	53–64[a] (59)	—	61–84[a] (74.8)	—	—	—	—	—	—	—	—	—	—	—
Strike (1970)	Chinchilla lanigera	41 males, 1–8 yr	5.8–10.3 (7.3)	8.0–15.1 (11.7)	27–54 (38.7)	—	(53)[b]	1.6–39.9 (7.6)	—	9.0–75 (42.4)	—	19–86 (54.7)	—	0.0–5.0 (1.3)	—	0.0–7.0 (0.4)	—	0.0–10.0 (0.4)
		52 females, 1–8 yr	5.2–9.9 (6.6)	8.8–15.4 (11.7)	25–52 (38.3)	—	(58)[b]	2.2–45.1 (8.0)	—	1.0–78 (44.6)	—	19–98 (53.6)	—	0.0–5.0 (1.2)	—	0.0–9.0 (0.5)	—	0.0–11.0 (0.4)

[a] Probably invalid owing to inadequate centrifugation.
[b] Estimated from the mean values for RBC and PCV.

The blood vessel found in the integument between the toes was the most suitable place for extracting blood from mink.

The Erythrocyte

Mink erythrocytes are biconcave cells having a distinct central pallor; poikilocytosis is observed in mink of all ages. Nucleated erythrocytes were present in peripheral blood of mink at all ages, but most frequently at 3–4 months of age. Reticulocytes are common in mink blood and were reported to range from 0–10% (Kubin and Mason, 1948).

The Lymphocyte

Lymphocytes and neutrophils may be present in equal percentage (Kennedy, 1935a) or found in a ratio of 2:1 (Kubin and Mason, 1948). Both small and large forms are present. In the larger forms, the nuclei are round, oval, bean-shaped, or slightly lobed, situated in the center or to one side of the cell, and usually surrounded by a comparatively wide band of cytoplasm.

The Neutrophil

The cytoplasm has a faint blue color and contains a large number of very small, reddish-brown granules that in many instances are difficult to observe. Band forms comprise 2–8% and are more common in younger mink; metamyelocytes may contribute 0.5–2.0% to the count. The mature neutrophil presents 2–7 lobes, which may be separated quite widely although connected by filaments. Portions of the nuclear chromatin stain a dark blue and are separated by bands staining the same color as the cytoplasm.

The Monocyte

Nuclear shape is variable in the monocyte. The chromatin stains dark blue with bands of lighter parachromatin. The cytoplasm has a slightly granular appearance, is gray-blue, and apparently is devoid of azurophilic granules.

The Eosinophil

The nucleus takes a lighter blue stain than the neutrophil nucleus; it also has fewer segments or lobes than the neutrophil, and filaments are distinct. Numerous dark red granules, about 0.5 μm in diameter, loosely fill the cytoplasm and may partially obscure the nucleus. The cytoplasm stains so lightly as to be almost colorless.

The Basophil

The cytoplasm is pale blue with large (1.0 μm), dark blue to purple granules that appear to project above the surface of the cell membrane.

The Platelet

A range of 194,000–380,000/μl was reported in 15 mink (Kubin and Mason, 1948). The cytoplasm is light blue and contains fine, deep blue granules that are irregular in outline and are usually situated in the center of the cytoplasm in the form of a crescent or circle. When massed together in stained films, the platelets lose their individual identity.

The Serum

Total serum proteins of 29 normal mink were found to be 7.53 ± 0.69 g/dl. Other data were albumin, 4.17 ± 0.61 g/dl; α-globulin, 0.7 ± 0.28 g/dl; β-globulin, 1.25 ± 0.27 g/dl; γ-globulin, 1.37 ± 0.32 g/dl; and an albumin:globulin ratio of 1.2:1.0 (Henson et al., 1963). Serum proteins are important in the study of Aleutian disease of mink because hypergammaglobulinemia is a constant feature.

Aleutian Disease of Mink

Aleutian disease of mink is a spontaneously transmissible viral disease having a genetic disposition as well as a familial occurrence. The importance of this disease to medical sciences is that it may serve as a model for studying the pathogenetic mechanisms of certain similar connective-tissue diseases of humans, e.g., Chédiak-Higashi syndrome.

Mink with Chédiak-Higashi syndrome were found to have prolonged bleeding times with normal platelet counts. Functional and biochemical abnormalities of platelets included impaired aggregation in response to collagen, markedly reduced ATP and ADP levels, and lower content of calcium, magnesium, and serotonin (Meyers et al., 1979).

Some information about bone marrow cells for 29 mink was obtained by Avram et al. (1982a). Unusual cytoplasmic granules were found in peripheral-blood leukocytes of mink homozygous recessive for the Aleutian gene *aa* (Leader et al., 1963). The granules in question were much larger than normal neutrophilic granules, although their staining pattern was similar. The greatest frequency was 4 abnormal cells to 51 normal cells in the neutrophilic series. The eosinophils in these cases revealed small numbers of large granules; normally, smaller granules are numerous. A few lymphocytes and monocytes revealed a single granule. These morphologic abnormalities in mink leukocytes were compared with leukocyte abnormalities seen in Chédiak-Higashi syndrome of children (see also Chapter 26).

Raccoon

The data reported here are based on the observations of Kennedy (1935a). Raccoons were caught in a net, and a large funnel about 2 feet long, 12 inches across at one end, and tapering to about 3 inches at the other was placed over the head. The raccoon was forced into the funnel, from which a hind foot could readily be drawn out and held in position for bleeding. A metacarpal blood vessel was the most suitable for this purpose. Although the vessel is not visible, plenty of blood was readily obtained by puncturing the skin between the metacarpal bones with a No. 11 Bard Parker blade.

The Erythrocyte

Staining characteristics give the appearance of a biconcave shape. Nucleated cells are rare, and anisocytosis is not generally observed. The average diameter is 6.5 μm with a range of 5.0–9.0 μm.

The Neutrophil

The cytoplasm stains a very light blue, and small, faintly stained, reddish-blue granules may be discerned, especially in the blood of the young. The nuclei stain deep blue to purple; they are segmented and sharply divided into bands by the oxyphil portion of the nuclear material. The nuclear segments vary in number from 2 to 7. Occasionally a myelocyte and more frequently metamyelocytes may appear in peripheral blood.

The Lymphocyte

Variation in size from small to large cells is common; the smaller form is the most numerous. In the larger cells, the nucleus may be rounded, bean-shaped, or irregular in outline. The cytoplasm is pale blue, and azurophilic granules may be present.

The Monocyte

The cytoplasm takes a light blue stain, and azurophilic granules are not seen. The nucleus is ameboid in outline, so shapes described as kidney, band, horseshoe, L, and three-lobed may be observed.

The Eosinphil

This is a large cell with bold outline and a tendency to have slightly frayed or roughened borders. The granules are numerous, large, and bright red to pink; they fill the cell almost obscuring the cytoplasm and portions of the nucleus. The nucleus is frequently oval, S-shaped, or in the form of a curved bar or divided into two or three lobes.

The Basophil

This cell is seldom in peripheral blood. Two types of granules are seen, and these occur in different individual cells. Most common is a basophil with numerous granules staining a very faint light blue which are about the size of the granules of the eosinophil. The other type of basophil contains much larger and fewer granules that stain a bright purple, while the cytoplasm stains lilac or light mauve.

The Platelets

Platelets often appear in large masses, but single ones are round, oblong, or irregular in outline. A pale blue cytoplasm surrounds a cluster of dark blue azurophilic granules.

Muskrat

Lord et al. (1954) reported on hemograms from cardiac blood taken from 71 muskrats under sodium pentobarbital anesthesia. There appears to be some disparity between their reported data on Hb concentration and PCV, with the latter being greater than anticipated for the Hb levels. If the PCV is invalid owing to inadequate centrifugation, then the reported MCV would be greater than the true values. That this is probably the case is indicated by their statement that centrifugation was at 2,500 rpm for 1 hour at 15-cm radius (1,000 G). The Wintrobe method requires 2,260 G to approach complete packing.

The Erythrocyte

These are biconcave discs averaging 6.79 μm in diameter and staining pale orange. Polychromasia, Howell-Jolly bodies, and nucleated red cells were common. Target cells were frequently encountered.

The Neutrophil

The nucleus has poorly defined lobulations, with as many as 8 lobes in a single cell. Frequently the nucleus was folded on itself to form a figure-8, and sometimes it appeared in cloverleaf pattern. There were numerous pink cytoplasmic granules.

The Lymphocyte

The cytoplasm was strongly basophilic and the nuclear chromatin coarse and dense. Immature lymphocytes were numerous, and some contained nucleoli. Azurophilic granules, 4 to 12 in number, were sometimes observed in mature lymphocytes.

The Monocyte

The nucleus was irregular and frequently folded on itself, creating a lobular appearance. Nucleoli were rarely observed. The cytoplasm was homogeneous, pale blue, and stuffed with fine, bluish-purple granules. These granules were much smaller than the azurophilic granules of the lymphocyte.

The Eosinophil

The nucleus was rarely segmented, but a doughnut-shaped structure was common. The granules were large and filled the central and peripheral cytoplasmic spaces.

The Basophil

This leukocyte type was not observed in any of the 71 muskrat bloods examined.

Chinchilla

Blood can be obtained from the orbital sinus (Brookhyser et al., 1977). Strike (1970) obtained cardiac blood, after the chest was opened surgically under ether anesthesia, from 41 males and 52 females, 1–8 years old (Table 12–25). The data of five other workers were tabulated for comparative purposes. The only significant difference between hemograms of the sexes was a lower RBC count in females. The means for RBC counts were $7.3 \times 10^6/\mu l$ for males and $6.6 \times 10^6/\mu l$ for females; for PCV, the values were 38.7% for males and 38.3% for females. On the basis of these data, the erythrocytes of females would be somewhat larger than those of males. Reticulocytes varied from 0–2.8% with an average of 0.3% in males and 0.2% in females. It would appear from these data that polychromasia would not be a prominent feature of chinchilla blood. The chinchilla erythrocyte is typically round and has a diameter of 6.7–7.3 μm (Kraft, 1959).

Mean WBC counts as reported by several authors (Strike, 1970) varied from 7,600–13,900/μl, with no differences between the sexes. Lymphocytes were more numerous than neutrophils (heterophils). The neutrophil is described as having a "Pelger-like" nucleus (meaning that lobe formation was not a common feature) and eosinophilic cytoplasmic granules (pseudo-eosinophil) (Kraft, 1959). Typical "drumstick" nuclear appendages, indicative of the female sex, were not found, although structures suggesting sessile nodules or appendages were described. Granules of the eosinophil were described as round to elongated oval. Basophils may be absent (Kraft, 1959) or range from 0–11.0% (Strike, 1970).

Platelet counts were found to be 254,000 ± 21,000/μl in males and 298,000 ± 20,600/μl in females (Strike, 1970). Mean platelet counts from 90 males and 38 females, all 1 year old, were reported to be 490,000 ± 55,700/μl and 498,000 ± 58,600/μl, respectively (Casella, 1963).

The myeloid:erythroid ratios of bone marrow differential counts were 1.1 ± 0.2:1.0 for 20 males and 0.9 ± 0.2:1.0 for 20 females (Strike, 1970).

Fox

Kennedy (1935b) reported on the blood of the silver black fox, 6–48 months of age, and Spitzer et al. (1941) presented data on the erythrocyte parameters of 12 mature silver foxes (Table 12–25). The data of the latter investigators relative to PCV and MCV appear to be in error, probably as a result of inadequate centrifugation in the hematocrit test, leading to an excessive amount of trapped plasma (see Chapter 3).

We had the opportunity to develop hemograms on two 5-month-old, clinically normal, female gray foxes and on a 4-year-old male gray fox presented with an abscess due to a penetrating plant awn (foxtail). These hemograms are presented in Table 12–26.

We observed erythrocyte morphology similar to that of the dog. There was slight anisocytosis, a small number of polychromatic cells, and an occasional nucleated erythrocyte. A reticulocyte count of 2.2% was recorded for the mature fox with an abscess. Erythrocyte sedimentation at 1 hour for foxes 1 and 2 was 7 mm and 4 mm, respectively, which was less than anticipated for the PCV value (dog data, Table 2–6) but correlated with the low normal plasma protein concentration. The ESR was significantly increased in the mature fox in response to the abscess, and the total and differential leukocyte counts were typical of a response to a chronic suppurative process. Plasma fibrinogen concentration, however, was not elevated, as would be anticipated in an active inflammatory process.

McCue (1984) developed hematologic values from the jugular blood of 92 San Joaquin kit foxes (*Vulpes macrotis mutica*), 65 adults and 27 puppies (3–6 months of age). Mean values (± one standard deviation) for the adults were: RBC, 8.4 ± 0.8 million/μl; Hb, 14.9 ± 1.5 g/dl; PCV, 46.9 ± 3.9%; MCV, 56.4 ± 3.6 fl; MCH, 18.2 ± 0.9 pg; MCHC, 32.0 ± 2.1%; reticulocytes, 0%; WBC, 6,900 ± 2,100/μl; neutrophils, 80.3 ± 8.1% or 5,771 ± 1,652/μl; lymphocytes, 15.6 ± 7.8% or 1,095 ± 546/μl; monocytes, 2.8 ± 1.9% or 203 ± 154/μl; eosinophils, 0.4 ± 0.7% or 27 ± 51/μl; and basophils, 0%. No significant sex differences were found, but RBC, Hb, and PCV of the puppies were lower than those of the adults. Plasma protein values of 5 red foxes (*Vulpes fulva*) and 2 gray foxes *Urocyon cinereoargenteus*) were between 5.3 and 6.8 g/dl (Brooks and Morris, 1979). Bone marrow cytology for 20 adult silver foxes has been described (Avram et al., 1982b).

Table 12–26. Hemograms of Two Clinically Normal Gray Fox Pups and One Mature Gray Fox with an Abscess

	Normal Fox Pup No. 1	Normal Fox Pup No. 2	Mature Fox with Abscess
RBC ($\times 10^6$/μl)	6.91	7.05	4.76
Hb (g/dl)	12.7	12.7	10.8
PCV (%)	41.0	41.0	34.0
MCV (fl)	59.3	58.1	71.4
MCH (pg)	18.3	18.0	22.6
MCHC (%)	30.9	30.9	31.7
Nucleated RBC/100 WBC	0	1	2
RBC sedimentation rate at 1 hour (observed less anticipated = corrected rate)[a]	7/9 = 2−	4/9 = 5−	51/18 = 33+
Icterus index (units)	2	2	2
Plasma proteins (g/dl)	5.8	6.3	7.6
Plasma fibrinogen (g/dl)	0.10	0.10	0.30
WBC ($\times 10^3$/μl)	8.1	6.6	20.1
Band neutrophils	0 (0.0%)	0.066 (1.0%)	1.005 (5.0%)
Neutrophils	4.293 (53.0%)	3.432 (52.0%)	12.361 (61.5%)
Lymphocytes	2.794 (34.5%)	2.046 (31.0%)	2.010 (10.0%)
Monocytes	0.567 (7.0%)	0.396 (6.0%)	2.713 (13.5%)
Eosinophils	0.445 (5.5%)	0.660 (10.0%)	2.010 (10.0%)
Anisocytosis	slight	slight	slight
Polychromasia	slight	slight	slight

[a]See correction for canine ESR, Table 2–6.

THE DEER

Deer are of interest to veterinarians because they may serve as a natural reservoir for the hemoparasite *Anaplasma marginale,* transmissible between deer and cattle occupying the same range (see Chap. 23). The erythrocytes of deer belonging to the family Cervidae are of special interest because of a sickling phenomenon (Figs. 12–7 and 12–8) that was first described by Gulliver in 1840. The erythrocytes circulate as round cells and are similar in size to the erythrocytes of cattle.

O'Roke (1936) associated sickled erythrocytes with the possibility of disease leading to winter losses of deer in Michigan. Shortly thereafter, however, Whitlock (1939) concluded that the sickling phenomenon was a physiologic characteristic of the blood of certain deer. The normal deer erythrocyte is not sickled when first removed from the body, but sickling takes place as the sample stands at either room or refrigerator temperature. Undritz et al. (1960) observed that sickling could be prevented by acidifying the blood, whereas there was a relatively sharp transition from normal to sickle shape between pH 7.0 and 7.5, with nearly all cells sickling at pH 7.4. Sickling was enhanced when oxygen gas was passed through the blood. Transient alkalosis and oxygenation of blood in vivo enhanced sickling (Parasall et al., 1975). Pritchard et al. (1963) reported the presence of several hemoglobins with different electrophoretic properties in the blood of the white-

tailed deer *(Odocoileus virginianus).* Kitchen et al. (1964) identified four hemoglobins designated I, II, III, and V, and later added types IVa, IVb, and VII (Kitchen et al., 1966). The number of hemoglobins in an individual deer was found to vary from 1 to 3. Sickling was prevented when hemoglobin V or VII was present (Kitchen et al., 1967). Hemoglobins I and III were present in 53.4% of 47 deer. Hemoglobin II, either alone or in combination with hemoglobins I, III, or IVb, was associated with the final development of a matchstick appearance (Fig. 12–9) after passing through the sickled stage. In a small percentage of deer, the erythrocytes assumed a burr shape associated with hemoglobin type IVa. Blood from a sick barking deer *(Muntiacus muntjak)* was submitted to us for study, and we observed marked sickling of the erythrocytes.

Data from various herds of white-tailed deer (Table 12–27) indicate that this species presents values for RBC, Hb, and PCV that are considerably greater than those found in normal domestic cattle, while WBC counts are lower than those of cattle (see Chapter 7). White-tailed deer weakened by malnutrition also had RBC counts on the order of $20 \times 10^6/\mu l$, with WBC counts falling in the range of 5.2–$6.2 \times 10^3/\mu l$ (Teeri et al., 1958). Mule deer as well as black-tailed deer including those from California (Table 12–27) have lower values for RBC, Hb, and PCV than white-tailed deer from Florida, but somewhat higher values than domestic cattle.

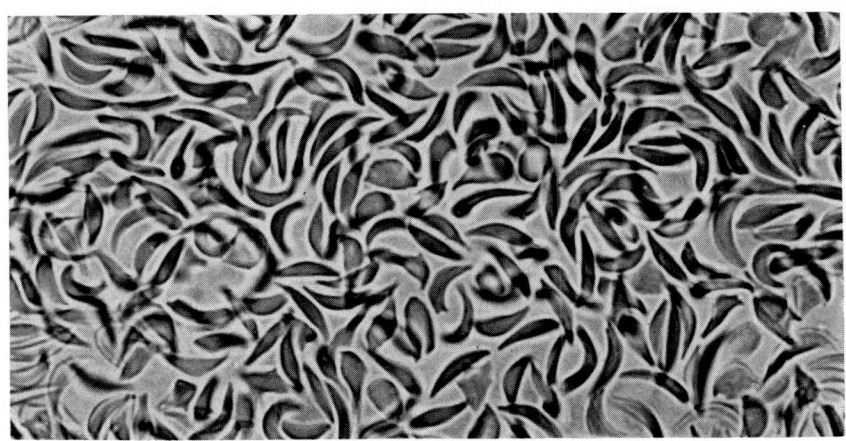

Fig. 12–7.   Classic sickle-shaped deer erythrocytes. (From Kitchen et al., 1964; courtesy of AAAS.)

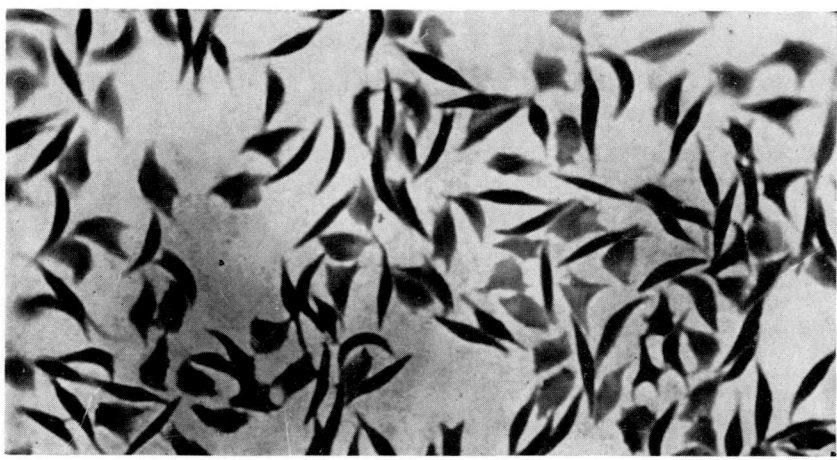

Fig. 12–8. Crescent and holly-leaf forms of sickled deer erythrocytes. (From Kitchen et al., 1964; courtesy of AAAS.)

Age- and sex-related changes in hematologic parameters were studied in suckling black-tailed deer, 80 males and 105 females (Table 12–28). A distinct pattern of increase in RBC, Hb, and PCV with age was evident regardless of sex. Males had higher values than females only after 140 days of age. Total plasma protein concentration was also greater in older deer, while fibrinogen concentration was essentially similar. An age-related increase in RBC, Hb, and to a lesser extent in PCV, is also apparent from data presented in Table 12–27.

THE WATER BUFFALO (BUBALIS BUBALIS)

Selected data on hematology of water buffaloes are presented in Table 12–29, and the following references may be consulted for additional details: Hafez and Anwar, 1954; Hafez et al., 1983; Hamza and El-Abdin, 1976; Hassan et al., 1981; Kehar and Murty, 1951; Kohli and Singh, 1975; Malik et al., 1974; Moustafa et al., 1964; Murthy, 1980; Oshiro et al., 1978; Purushotham and Mahendar, 1963; Sharma et al., 1973; Singh et al, 1981; Timmaiah et al., 1976; Vogel and Vogel, 1967. Various blood values obtained for 50 clinically normal, lactating Murrah water buffaloes are presented in Table 12–30 (Jain et al., 1981). Prominent features in the normal hemogram included average size (MCV) of the erythrocytes similar to that in cattle, low icterus index, conspicuous ESR, absence of reticulocytes, and predominance of lymphocytes over neutrophils.

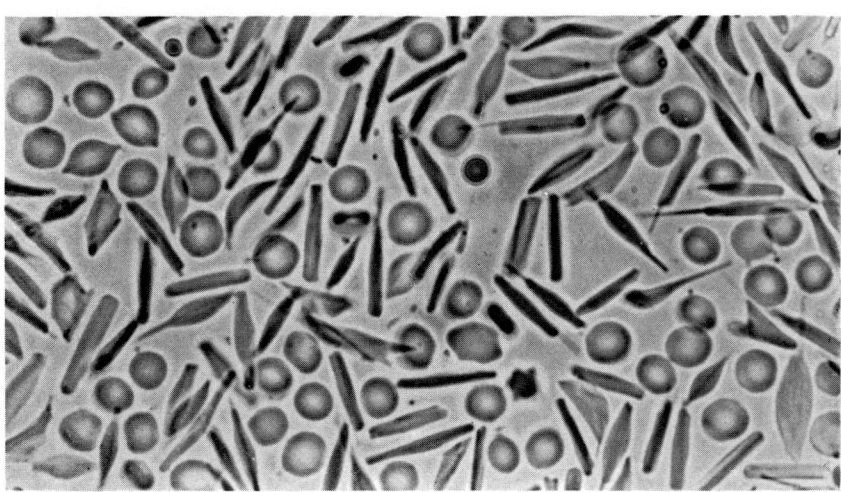

Fig. 12–9. Sickled erythrocytes of the deer, matchstick form, associated with hemoglobin II, either alone or in combination with hemoglobins I, III, or IVb. (From Kitchen et al, 1964; courtesy of AAAS.)

Table 12–27.   Hematologic Values in Members of the Cervidae Family

| Source | Animal | Number, Age, Sex | RBC ($\times10^6/\mu l$) | Hb (g/dl) | PCV (%) | MCV (fl) | MCH (pg) | MCHC (%) | WBC ($\times10^3/\mu l$) | Differential Leukocyte Count (%) | | | | |
										Neutrophils	Lymphocytes	Monocytes	Eosinophils	Basophils
Cowan and Bandy (1969)	Blacktail* (Vancouver)	26 females, 2–21 days	5.5±0.3	10.3±0.3	33.8±1.4	—	—	—	5.04±0.43	41±1.8	39±2.0	15.8±1.1	2.1	0.8
	Blacktail* (Vancouver)	23 males, 2–21 days	5.5±0.3	9.8±0.4	35.1±1.7	—	—	—	5.52±0.45	—	—	—	—	—
	Blacktail† (Vancouver)	11 males and females, 24–57 days	11.6±0.7	14.2±0.2	36.8±3.5	—	—	—	5.52±0.40	37±3.5	57±2.6	5.9±1.7	0	0.2
	Blacktail† (Alaska)	9 males and females, 40–45 days	10.4±0.6	14.0±0.2	36.2±1.2	—	—	—	5.45±0.44	34±1.9	60±1.9	4.0±0.5	0	0.7
	Blacktail† (California)	16 males and females, 65–117 days	14.2±0.6	15.7±0.2	43.0±1.2	—	—	—	4.42±0.29	41±1.7	52±1.8	4.0±4.0	0.1	0.4
	Mule deer	8 males and females, 23–68 days	8.8±0.7	13.5±0.3	34.1±1.4	—	—	—	5.83±0.70	49±3.2	45±2.7	4.0±0.3	0.1	0.4
Rosen and Bischoff (1952)	Mule deer	368 males and females, mature	10.1	17.0	44.8	—	—	—	—	—	—	—	—	—
Bowman and Sears (1955)	Mule deer	8 males and females, 1–6.5 yr	5.2–12.7 (9.19)	10.2–16.5 (12.8)	32.1–45.7 (39.6)	—	—	—	1.8–5.0 (3.3)	—	—	—	—	—
Anderson et al. (1970)	Mule deer	170–175 males and females, 1–162 mo	8.8±0.2	16.4±0.3	46.7±0.6	—	—	—	3.0±0.1	40.6±1.2	43.4±1.1	6.2±0.5	8.3±0.6	0.4±0.1
Kitchen and Pritchard (1962)	Whitetail (Florida)	>500 males and females, >1 yr	17.0–20.0	17–21	55–61	—	—	—	1.5–3.0	30–35	55–70	2	2–15	0–2
Johnson et al. (1968)	Whitetail (Michigan)	126 males and females, birth to 6 mo	16.9±0.4	17.5±0.4	46.3±0.8	30.2±0.5	11.1±0.1	35.8±0.3	3.7±0.1	—	—	—	—	—
	Whitetail (Michigan)	258 males and females, 7 mo–5 yr	17.0±0.2	20.8±0.1	56.3±0.4	33.0±0.4	12.2±0.1	37.2±0.2	3.2±0.1	—	—	—	—	—
Seal and Erickson (1969)	Whitetail (Minnesota)	18 males, >1 yr	10.8±1.9	13.5±1.9	40.0±5.7	—	—	—	—	—	—	—	—	—
	Whitetail (Minnesota)	33 females, >1 yr	11.2±1.6	14.7±2.6	44.0±7.4	—	—	—	—	—	—	—	—	—

*Wild animals.

†Captive animals revealed higher RBC parameter than wild animals.

Table 12-28. **Changes in Blood Components with Growth of Suckling Black-Tailed Deer (*Odocoileus hemionus columbianus*) (mean ± standard error and range)[a]**

Parameter	Sex	1–9 days	10–29 days	30–89 days	90–139 days	>140 days	Probability Value[b]
RBC (×10^6/µl)	M	7.51±1.22 (15)[c] (5.52–10.02)	7.79±1.00 (18) (6.36–9.66)	9.67±1.54 (23) (8.00–12.96)	10.60±1.39 (9) (6.01–12.35)	10.46±1.80 (15) (6.52–13.28)	***
	F	7.32±0.85 (20) (5.85–9.03) NS[d]	7.10±0.52 (16) (6.30–8.30) *	9.65±1.26 (24) (7.47–12.16) NS	10.03±1.62 (13) (8.12–13.82) **	8.96±1.25 (32) (7.20–11.56)	***
Hb (g/dl)	M	9.33±0.93 (15) (8.10–11.00)	11.32±1.45 (18) (8.20–14.40)	13.45±2.17 (23) (8.80–18.10)	14.04±1.08 (9) (12.70–15.80)	15.43±2.63 (15) (10.80–22.00)	***
	F	9.38±1.08 (20) (9.30–12.70) NS	10.93±1.13 (16) (9.30–12.70) NS	13.73±1.42 (24) (10.10–16.20) NS	13.44±1.06 (13) (12.30–16.40) NS	12.90±1.29 (32) (9.90–15.20) **	***
PCV (%)	M	29.7±3.5 (15) (24.0–37.0)	32.2±3.7 (18) (26.0–40.0)	37.4±5.9 (23) (25.0–50.0)	38.7±2.9 (9) (34.0–42.0)	42.1±7.4 (15) (31.0–61.0)	**
	F	29.1±3.7 (20) (21.0–35.0) NS	32.3±2.9 (16) (28.0–37.0) NS	37.9±3.6 (24) (30.0–44.0) NS	37.6±2.8 (13) (35.0–45.0) NS	35.4±3.4 (32) (29.0–44.0) **	***
MCV (fl)	M	39.9±4.0 (15) (32.7–47.1)	41.6±4.7 (18) (35.8–49.0)	38.9±6.0 (23) (31.0–59.9)	36.8±3.6 (9) (32.4–43.8)	40.8±5.9 (15) (32.5–49.2)	NS
	F	40.1±3.4 (20) (33.9–46.5) NS	45.6±3.0 (16) (40.6–49.7) **	39.6±2.7 (24) (34.6–44.6) NS	38.0±3.7 (13) (30.3–43.1) NS	39.8±3.6 (32) (32.0–45.8) NS	*

							p[b]
MCHC (%)	M	31.7±1.7 (15) (27.4–34.3)	35.2±1.45 (18) (31.5–37.6)	36.1±1.5 (23) (34.1–39.7)	36.3±0.8 (9) (35.3–37.6)	36.1±2.5 (15) (28.1–39.0)	**
	F	32.4±1.5 (20) (30.9–36.2)	33.8±1.0 (16) (32.2–35.2)	36.3±1.2 (24) (33.7–38.8)	35.7±0.6 (13) (34.9–36.4)	36.5±1.1 (32) (34.2–38.3)	***
	p[d]	NS	**	NS	NS	NS	***
MCH (pg)	M	12.6±1.4 (15) (10.8–14.7)	14.6±1.6 (18) (12.3–17.6)	14.1±2.5 (23) (10.9–23.5)	13.4±1.3 (9) (11.7–15.9)	15.0±2.1 (15) (11.6–17.8)	*
	F	13.0±1.3 (20) (10.8–16.1)	15.4±1.1 (16) (13.6–17.3)	14.3±1.1 (24) (12.8–16.7)	13.6±1.3 (13) (10.9–15.3)	14.5±1.3 (32) (12.0–16.9)	**
	p[d]	NS	NS	NS	NS	NS	
Protein (g/dl)	M	6.1±0.6 (15) (5.4–7.5)	5.8±0.6 (18) (5.0–7.0)	5.8±0.5 (23) (4.9–6.4)	6.1±0.3 (9) (5.7–6.5)	6.6±0.5 (15) (5.4–7.5)	*
	F	6.0±0.3 (20) (5.6–6.6)	6.0±0.4 (16) (5.2–6.5)	6.0±0.4 (24) (5.5–6.8)	6.0±0.3 (13) (5.6–6.5)	6.7±0.5 (32) (5.7–8.0)	*
	p[d]	NS	NS	NS	NS	NS	
Fibrinogen (g/dl)	M	0.3±0.15 (15) (0.1–0.6)	0.29±0.12 (18) (0.1–0.5)	0.28±0.14 (23) (0.1–0.6)	0.27±0.11 (9) (0.1–0.4)	0.27±0.12 (15) (0.1–0.5)	NS
	F	0.25±0.14 (20) (0.1–0.6)	0.37±0.20 (16) (0.1–0.7)	0.32±0.17 (24) (0.1–0.9)	0.25±0.10 (13) (0.1–0.4)	0.23±0.11 (32) (0.1–0.6)	NS
	p[d]	NS	NS	NS	NS	NS	
WBC ($\times 10^3$/µl)	M	5.3±1.8 (15) (3.2–9.3)	5.0±2.5 (18) (2.7–10.5)	4.5±2.4 (23) (1.3–11.1)	2.8±1.1 (9) (1.2–4.5)	3.6±8.6 (15) (1.9–5.3)	**
	F	5.1±2.2 (20) (2.4–12.5)	4.4±1.1 (16) (2.7–5.9)	4.1±9.7 (24) (2.3–6.1)	3.7±1.0 (13) (2.6–5.7)	5.0±1.7 (32) (2.7–9.3)	**
	p[d]	NS	NS	NS	NS	***	

[a] From Dr. Nadine K. Jacobsen, unpublished observations.
[b] Probability value of unbalanced, one-way ANOVA by sex class. NS = nonsignificant difference, * = <0.05, ** = <0.01, *** = <0.001.
[c] Number in parentheses = number of deer.
[d] Probability value of unpaired t-test of differences between sexes within an age class.

Table 12–29.   Selected Published Hematologic Values of Water Buffaloes (Bubalis bubalis)

Source	Species	Number, Age, Sex	RBC (×10⁶/μl)	Hb (g/dl)	PCV (%)	WBC (×10³/μl)	Differential Leukocyte Count (%)				
							Neutrophils	Lymphocytes	Monocytes	Eosinophils	Basophils
Hafez and Anwar (1954)	Egyptian water buffaloes	20 females	6.8	11.0–15.2 (13.0)	38–52 (44.3)	6.7	36.0	51.0	8.0	5.0	1.0
Karram et al. (1981)	Egyptian water buffaloes	5 (1 day)	9.34±0.46	—	—	11.12±2.75	51.4±8.6	39.2±0.8	4.6±0.6	0.8±1.9	—
		11 (2–7 days)	8.18±1.28	—	—	11.09±0.42	43.1±2.3	49.2±2.2	7.1±0.3	0.6±0.8	—
		6 (2 wks)	10.07±1.75	—	—	9.87±4.33	39.7±1.2	55.7±0.8	4.0±1.3	0.5±0.6	0.3±0.8
		6 (3 wks)	9.24±1.50	—	—	4.72±0.77	39.5±1.1	54.0±1.9	4.5±1.2	0.8±1.0	0.2±0.4
		6 (4 wks)	9.44±1.77	—	—	4.34±1.28	31.0±2.1	62.2±5.0	5.8±1.4	0.4±0.7	—
		56 (1.5–2 mo)	10.07±1.22	—	—	8.85±1.43	27.0±3.4	67.3±6.0	5.3±0.9	0.3±0.4	—
		18 (2.5–3 mo)	9.45±0.98	—	—	9.01±1.55	22.4±4.6	72.5±6.2	5.4±1.2	0.1±0.3	—
		14 (3.5–4 mo)	9.28±1.14	—	—	11.95±0.84	18.9±1.4	73.4±1.7	7.8±0.8	—	—
		14 (4.5–5 mo)	9.26±0.78	—	—	10.76±0.78	19.7±2.3	71.1±2.9	8.6±0.6	—	—
		14 (5.5–6 mo)	8.57±2.26	—	—	11.16±0.63	20.6±1.1	70.4±1.5	5.7±0.8	—	—
Thangaraj et al. (1979)	Indian water buffaloes	Birth	8.07±1.22	20.66±2.18	50.9±6.88	9.09±2.56	60.0	39.7	0.08	0	—
		1 day	6.50±2.0	—	—	7.30±2.24	—	—	—	—	—
		28 days	—	17.31±1.3	43.46±4.43	8.39±1.65	32.15	66.4	0.77	0.62	—
Murthy (1980)	Indian water buffaloes	192 (4–8 yr)	5.7±0.1	10.3±0.2	37.9±0.5	9.1±0.1	24.1±1.0	67.9±1.2	—	4.4±0.1	—
Sulong et al. (1980)	Malaysian swamp buffaloes	50 (2–4 yr)	8.8	13.4	39.2	10.7	35.2	54.2	3.7	6.6	0.3

Table 12–30. Hematologic Values in 50 Clinically Normal, Lactating Murrah Buffaloes[a]

Parameter	Range	Mean	Standard Deviation
RBC ($\times 10^6/\mu$l)	5.07–8.27	6.54	0.77
Hb (g/dl)	9–13.5	11.1	0.96
PCV (%)	26–34	31.0	2.0
MCV (fl)	40.6–55.2	48.2	4.60
MCHC (%)	30.5–38.5	35.2	2.34
MCH (pg)	13.5–20.5	17.10	1.85
Icterus index (units)	2–5	2	1.25
ESR (mm at 1 hr)	17–69	53	12.30
Plasma protein (g/dl)	6–9	7.8	0.70
Fibrinogen (g/dl)	0.2–0.8	0.37	0.20
Reticulocytes (%)	0	0	0
WBC (number/μl)	6,250–13,050	9,676	1,789
Bands	0–106	18	40
Neutrophils	1,285–6,893	3,257	1,262
Lymphocytes	2,554–9,637	5,065	1,595
Monocytes	63–1,349	584	301
Eosinophils	170–1,471	592	452
Basophils	0–326	131	98
WBC, percentages			
Bands	0–1	0.2	0.34
Neutrophils	13–54	32.9	8.74
Lymphocytes	26–75	52.7	12.0
Monocytes	1–11.5	5.9	2.63
Eosinophils	2–14.0	6.9	4.64
Basophils	0–3.5	1.4	1.02

[a]Modified from Jain et al., 1981.

Morphologic features of red cells and leukocytes are similar to those of cattle cells. A brief description of blood cells as seen in 50 Murrah water buffaloes follows.

Erythrocytes generally exhibit slight to marked rouleau formation, slight anisocytosis, and uniform staining. Individual erythrocytes, however, appear as slightly biconcave discs with distinct or indistinct central pallor. Biconcave discocytic morphology of the erythrocytes is distinctly visible in blood samples processed for scanning electron microscopy (Fig. 12–10). Polychromasia is absent, as are reticulocytes in the new methylene blue–stained films. Howell-Jolly bodies are rare.

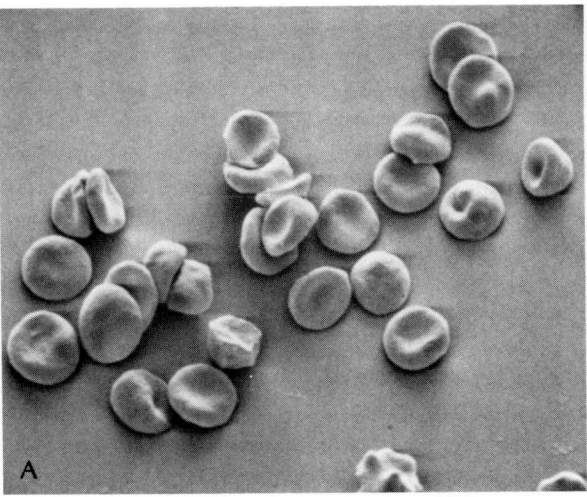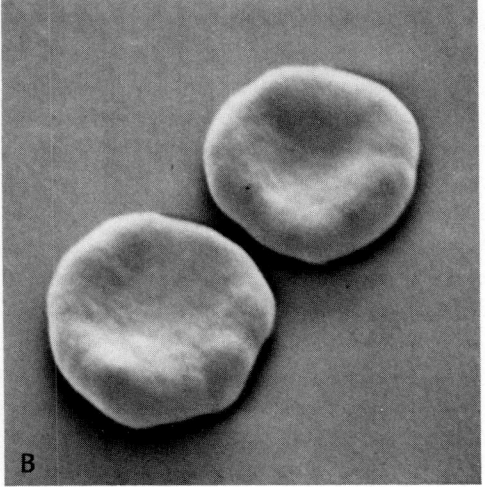

Fig. 12–10. Scanning electron photomicrographs of buffalo blood depicting discocytic erythrocytes with typical concave surface and two erythrocytes with narrow concavity (arrows in *A*). *A*, ×1,800; *B*, ×4,000. (From Jain et al., 1981; courtesy of *Research in Veterinary Science*.)

Platelets are abundant and usually distribute in small to large clumps. Individual platelets are pleomorphic with rounded to elongated shapes, measure about a quarter to half the size of an erythrocyte, and contain small but distinct azurophilic granules.

Small, medium, and large lymphocytes are present in varying numbers, with only one type predominating in an individual animal. Their nuclei are typically round or oval with an occasional slight indentation and contain coarsely granular and/or plaqued chromatin. The cytoplasm stains pale to dark blue. Some lymphocytes contain a few azurophilic granules (0.5–2 μm) in loose clusters. Rarely, binucleated lymphocytes, lymphocytes with nucleolar rings, and lymphocytes with a few cytoplasmic vacuoles are observed. An occasional large lymphocyte may appear monocytoid, but it can be distinguished by the absence of ameboid nucleus and lack of foamy or distinctly vacuolated cytoplasm characteristic of monocytes.

Monocytes are usually larger than lymphocytes. Their nuclei are ameboid in shape and contain finely granular, "lacy" or "stringy" and sometimes plaqued chromatin. The cytoplasm stains moderately blue and appears grainy or foamy and vacuolated. Rarely, a few fine azurophilic granules may be observed in the cytoplasm.

Neutrophils generally have coiled, multilobed and sometimes monolobed nuclei and pale to slightly pink, fine, indistinct cytoplasmic granules. The multilobed nuclei have two to four lobes with plaqued chromatin, a few clear areas of euchromatin, and irregular outline. The monolobed nuclei exhibit one or two shallow constrictions, slight membrane roughness, and relatively less chromatin condensation than multilobed neutrophils. In comparison, band cells are infrequent and have an obviously smooth nuclear outline without definite constrictions.

Eosinophils contain small, uniformly round, bright pink granules almost filling the clear or pale cytoplasm. Their nuclei are generally smoother and less lobulated than those of neutrophils.

Basophils contain numerous large, dark purple granules almost masking the nuclear lobes. The water-soluble nature of the granules may be apparent in some smears that show basophils with lightly stained, inconspicuous granules, smeared nuclear staining, and "leached out" granular contents in the vicinity.

Hematologic examination was carried out on buffalo fetuses, 3–10 months of gestation age (El-Naggar et al., 1982). RBC, Hb, PCV, and WBC increased with age; reticulocytes were present in significant numbers at 3–4 months of age, after which their number decreased to be nil by the ninth month. Lymphocytes increased gradually until 6 months, when a sharp increase occurred. Neutrophils decreased between 3 and 10 months, and eosinophils, basophils, and monocytes were not seen before 5 months.

Hematologic changes with age have been studied in water buffaloes at birth to 28 days of life (Thangaraj, 1979; Table 12–29). The RBC count at birth was 8.07 ± 1.22 million/μl, decreased to 6.50 ± 2.0 million on day 1, and fluctuated between 6.79 ± 1.44 million and 7.42 ± 1.48 million up to 28 days. Hemoglobin and PCV values were higher at birth than in adults, being 20.1 ± 2.2 g/dl and 50.9 ± 6.9%, respectively, and decreased to 17.3 ± 1.3 g/dl and 43.5 ± 4.4% on day 28. The WBC count was 9,090 ± 2,561/μl at birth, fell to 7,300 ± 2,247 on day 1, increased to 8,812 ± 1,850 on day 14, and was 8,392 ± 1,650 on day 28. The differential leukocyte count consisted of 60% neutrophils and 39.7% lymphocytes at birth and changed to 32.2% and 66.4%, respectively, by day 28. Monocytes and eosinophils increased during the 28-day period but were still below 1%. Similar studies were performed on buffalo calves from birth to 6 months of age (Karram et al., 1981; Table 12–29). Lymphocytes increased from birth to a peak at 4 months, while eosinophils were generally below 1% until 4 months, when they were nearly absent. In 6 buffalo calves, plasma fibrinogen concentration was lower (0.53 g/dl) at 2 weeks of age than at 6 months of age (0.82 g/dl) and it was positively correlated with ESR and negatively correlated with PCV (Nangia and Garg, 1982).

Experimental withdrawal of about one-third blood volume from two water buffalo calves resulted in typical blood loss anemia and hypoproteinemia, but reticulocytes were not seen at any stage during recovery from anemia (Jain et al., 1979b). These preliminary observations need to be extended because of their importance in interpretation of erythropoietic response of anemic buffaloes. Injection of *Escherichia coli* endotoxin (intravenously) induced leukopenia, whereas administration of prednisolone and dexamethasone (intramuscularly) induced leukocytosis in two water buffalo calves (Jain et al., 1979a). Changes in total and differential leukocyte numbers were generally similar to those reported in cattle given endotoxin (Jain and Lasmanis, 1978) and corticosteroids (see Chapters 7, 26, and 36). However, a slight lymphocytosis preceded reduction in lymphocyte numbers following corticosteroid administration.

Malaysian swamp buffaloes were found to have higher RBC, Hb, PCV, and WBC values than river buffaloes and cattle (Sulong et al., 1980). Similar hematologic values were reported for mature Australian swamp buffaloes (Canfield et al., 1984). RBC, Hb, and PCV values were lower in spray-cooled or wallowing water buffaloes than in those at normal environmental temperature (Bahga et al., 1980). Exercise, load carrying, and starvation were associated with increases in blood volume and PCV (Sodhi and Singh, 1975). Fasting of seven buffalo calves for 6 days (on water only) resulted in increased RBC, Hb, and PCV for 3 days and then decreased values for the rest of the period (Singh and Malik, 1979). Seasonal changes in blood values and serum proteins have been reported (Anwar and Chaudhri, 1984; Moustafa et al., 1978; Salem, 1980). Serum electrophoresis (Nahani et al., 1976; Vihan et al., 1973) and immunoelectrophoresis have been performed (Satija et al., 1979). A significant correlation was found between red cell glutathione peroxidase activity and plasma selenium in 89 Egyptian water buffaloes (Gazia and Wegger, 1980).

OTHER WILD AND DOMESTICATED ANIMALS

Values of blood taken from animals captured or killed in the wild or taken from animals in zoos may be expected to vary in composition characteristic of the resting state due to the effects of fright resulting from capture and methods of restraint. The resulting stress may elevate RBC counts through splenic contraction, and WBC count in large-vessel blood may be increased by flushing of cells from capillary beds as heart rate and force of blood flow increase. The differential leukocyte count may also be altered from the normal resting pattern by the effect of stress.

Difficulties arising in collecting the blood may result in significant hemolysis of erythrocytes, leading to a reduction of PCV and an increase of MCH and MCHC values. Too little blood in EDTA anticoagulant results in shrinkage of erythrocytes with reduction of the PCV and MCV and an increase in MCHC.

Hemograms of certain wild and domesticated large animals, as reported in literature, are recorded in Tables 12–31 through 12–33. Hemograms of individual animals in California zoos are presented in Table 12–34.

Bovidae

We found blood composition of the zebu (*Bos indicus*) (Table 12–34) to be similar to that of domestic cattle. Greater RBC, PCV, and Hb values were found for bison (*Bison bison*) than for cattle of similar age (Hawley and Peden, 1982).

Data on springbok, oryx, and yaks are presented in Table 12–31. Hemograms of a yak, an impala, 2 Barbary sheep (aoudads), and 3 blackbucks are included in Table 12–34. Erythrocyte number of the yak was similar to that of domestic cattle, while numbers of RBC of the other Bovidae were more characteristic of the domestic goat (12–20 × 10^6/μl). Similar high RBC counts (15.7 ± 3.46 × 10^6/μl) were reported for the adult aoudad by Tumbleson et al. (1970). Hematologic values were measured for 10 healthy yaks, aged 3–6 years, kept at an altitude of 11,000 feet (Sahu et al., 1981); average RBC count was 6.13 million/μl; Hb, 13.2 g/dl; and WBC, 8,100/μl. The WBC count and the percentage of lymphocytes were much greater than values reported for yaks from the California zoo (Table 12–34). Yaks sedated with xylazine had significantly lower RBC, PCV, and Hb values, fewer lymphocytes, and higher monocyte counts than those bled while restrained manually (Hawkey et

Table 12-31.   Selected Published Hematologic Values of Certain Wild and Domesticated Large Animals

Source	Species	Number	RBC (×10⁶/μl)	Hb (g/dl)	PCV (%)	WBC (×10³/μl)	Differential Leukocyte Count (% or no./μl)				
							Neutrophils	Lymphocytes	Monocytes	Eosinophils	Basophils
Gibbs (1960)	Barren Ground caribou	7	9.5–11.8 (10.8)	11.5–16.5 (14.5)	—	2.25–5.40 (4.20)	38–70 (57.3)	26–57 (38.3)	1.0–4.0 (3.0)	1.0–3.0 (2.1)	0–1.0 (0.8)
Simon (1961)	Indian elephant	15	1.98–4.0 (2.81)	12.0–15.5 (13.4)	30–43.3 (38.2)	6.4–14.0 (10.2)	22–50 (36.5)	40–60 (51.7)	0.0–5.0 (2.2)	6.0–15.0 (9.4)	0–2.0 (0.5)
Jainudeen and Jayasinghe (1971)	Asian elephant	42	3.18±1.01	12.1±2.2	33.3±1.99	14.7±6.15	40.3±8.7	52.7±10.9	5.3±3.4	2.4±1.9	0.2
Debbie and Clausen (1975)	African elephant	8–23	3.77±0.25	7.08±0.44	—	11.4±0.98	20.2±0.6	69.1±1.9	8.2±0.03	1.3±0.03	0.1±0.08
Bush et al. (1980)	Giraffes	37–38	12.4±3.4	13.5±2.4	38.8±5.8	13.5±4.2	9,400±3,700	3,000±1,500	200±300	300±300	400±600
Raphael et al. (1982)	Springbok	34	6.1–9.9 (8.0)	—	36–54 (43.4)	3.6–20.1 (10.2)	42–76 (55.3)	11–46 (26.4)	1.0–11 (4.9)	3–30 (11.6)	0–5 (0.7)
Bush et al. (1983)	Oryx	27–31	10.0±2.4	13.9±2.0	39.8±6.0	7.24±2.89	4,700±2,150	2,420±1,260	180±220	220±420	220±420
Hawkey et al. (1983)	Yak	6–7[a]	6.4±0.9	13.7±1.7	38.0±4.0	6.6±1.2	42.0±12.0	46.0±10.0	0.4	10.7	0.5
		7–18[b]	5.4±0.66	10.9± 0.9	31.0±4.0	5.8±1.6	45.0±9.6	41.0±8.4	1.7	13.0	0.9±0.2

[a]Manually restrained adult females.
[b]Sedated with xylazine.

Table 12-32. Selected Published Hematologic Values of Members of the Family Camellidae

Source	Species	Number, Age, Sex	RBC (×10⁶/μl)	Hb (g/dl)	PCV (%)	WBC (×10³/μl)	Differential Leukocyte Count (%)				
							Neutrophils	Lymphocytes	Monocytes	Eosinophils	Basophils
Soni and Agarwala (1958)	Camelus dromedarius	95	3.8–12.6 (8.2)	10.6–20.3 (15.5)	—	12.9–27.2 (20.1)	21.1–56.3 (38.7)	26.5–65.4 (46.0)	0.0–12.3 (5.7)	0.0–18.9 (9.5)	0.0–1.0
Banerjee et al. (1962)	Camelus dromedarius	20	6.1–9.3 (7.24)	10.6–15.1 (13.1)	20–33 (27)	10.5–28.3 (18.1)	30–60 (50.6)	33–58 (40)	1.5–6.0 (3.0)	2.0–17.5 (6.5)	0.0–0.5 (0.05)
Nassar et al. (1977)	Camelus dromedarius (Egypt)	46 adult males	9.1	14.0	32.0	22.0	43.0	49.3	4.5	3.3	0.2
		42 adult females	3.0	12.0	29.6	17.5	50.0	43.8	2.8	1.2	0.3
Khan and Kohli (1978)	Camelus dromedarius (India)	15 males before rut	7.0–11.5 (8.8)	11.0–14.0 (12.6)	—	6.5–13.6 (10.5)	23–34 (27)	43.0–59.0 (51.0)	7–18 (13)	5–11 (9)	1–3 (1.9)
		During rut	6.6–6.9 (8.4)	9.6–11.8 (10.8)	—	10.5–19.2 (14.2)	24–34 (29)	47.0–59.0 (53.0)	5–11 (7)	4–15 (9)	1–3 (1.8)
Majeed et al. (1980)	Camelus dromedarius (Pakistan)	10 males 10 females	6.7±0.2	11.1±0.3	—	10.6± 0.4	44.7±1.4	47.5±1.4	1.2±0.1	7.2±0.4	<0.1
Kraft (1957)	Young mature Llamas										
	Lama glama	7	8.3–12.5 (9.91)	11.6–14.5 (12.8)	—	8.9–22.0 (16.2)	6–37[a] 22–48	15–59	0.5–2.0	3.5–6.0	0.5–3.0
	Lama guanicoe	8	8.9–11.7 (10.4)	14.6–19.2 (16.4)	—	6.4–17.0 (8.82)	27–58[a] 14–35	15–27	0.5–2.5	4.0–16.5	1.0–2.0
	Lama pacos	8	7.8–10.8 (9.52)	7.5–16.7 (12.2)	—	6.9–15.5 (11.8)	27–47[a] 16–32	14–27	0.0–0.5	9.0–33.5	0.0–1.5
	Lama vicugna	6	9.4–11.5 (10.3)	9.8–14.8 (12.2)	—	6.4–19.2 (11.7)	16–38[a] 25–55	11–40	0.0–0.5	5.5–18.0	0.5–3.0
Schalm (unpublished, 1975)	Lama guanicoe	3	12.1–17.8 (15.5)	13.2–20.5 (17.3)	31–45	8.6–19.0 (12.6)	0.5–2.0[a] 57–76 (64)	16–30 (24)	2–3.5 (3)	3–8 (5)	0–0.5

[a]Immature neutrophils.

Table 12–33. Hematologic Values of Donkeys and Mules

Source	Class	Number, Sex	RBC (×10⁶/μl)	Hb (g/dl)	PCV (%)	MCV[a] (fl)	MCH (pg)	MCHC (%)	WBC (×10³/μl)	Neutrophils	Lymphocytes	Monocytes	Eosinophils	Basophils
										Differential Leukocyte Count (%)				
Neser (1923)	So. African donkeys	14 (RBC), 32 (WBC)	4.6–8.5 (6.4)	—	30–40 (37)	— (57.8)	—	—	11.5–21.9 (14.4)	15–57 (34)	33–71 (53)	2–15 (4)	1–14 (8)	0–1 (1)
Wilding et al. (1952)	S.W. U.S. burros	16 males	5.65–8.58 (6.91)	9.3–15.5 (11.61)	31–45 (36)	— (52.1)	— (16.8)	— (32.2)	7.0–17.7 (12.6)	26–65 (43)	18–64 (42)	1–13.5 (6)	0–18 (7.5)	—
	S.W. U.S. burros	12 females	4.9–10.27 (7.1)	8.0–16.7 (12.11)	26–51 (37)	— (52.1)	— (17.0)	— (32.7)	9.3–28.5 (14.4)	28–64 (43)	24–59 (24)	0–11.5 (5.5)	0.5–26 (8)	—
Neser (1923)	So. African mules	15 (RBC), 28 (WBC)	4.86–10.60 (8.04)	—	30–42 (35)	— (43.5)	—	—	9.0–18.3 (12.9)	32–70 (49)	22–60 (41)	1–5 (3)	2–13 (6)	0–2 (1)
Morris (1942)	English army mules	20	6.17–9.93 (7.37)	—	—	—	—	—	6.0–10.75 (8.94)	33–60 (43)	36–60 (47)	2–7 (4)	2–11 (5)	0–1 (0.6)
Sharma et al. (1981)	Indian mules	8 males	6.46	13.76	38.87	62.1	22.4	35.5	10.25	47.75	45.38	1.63	4.13	—
		15 females	6.75	13.62	37.46	66.1	20.4	38.9	10.55	53.87	39.87	1.40	4.00	—

[a]Estimated from the author's means.

Table 12-34. Hematologic Values from Individual Clinically Normal Herbivores, Omnivores, and Carnivores in California Zoos[a]

Animal	Age	Sex	RBC (×10⁶/μl)	Hb (g/dl)	PCV (%)	MCV (fl)	MCH (pg)	MCHC (%)	Icterus Index Units[b]	Plasma Protein (g/dl)	Fibrinogen (g/dl)	WBC/μl	Neutrophils	Lymphocytes	Monocytes	Eosinophils	Basophils
Elephas maximus (elephant)	6 yr	F	3.08	12.3	34.0	110	39.9	36.1	2	7.1	0.5	12,700	18.0	29.5	51.5	1.0	0.0
Elephas maximus (elephant)	8 yr	M	4.08	15.2	48.0	118	37.2	31.6	2	8.9	0.6	20,800	34.5	18.5	47.0	0.0	0.0
Hippotigris sp. (zebra)	—	—	12.0	14.8	43.0	35.8	12.3	34.4	5	6.7	0.2	12,200	66.5	25.5	5.5	2.5	—
Giraffa camelopardalis (giraffe)	neonate	M	12.52	14.1	44.0	35.1	11.2	32.0	5	6.0	0.3	8,700	55.0	38.0	7.0	—	—
Giraffa camelopardalis (giraffe)	5 mo	M	18.24	18.1	51.0	27.9	9.9	35.5	5	6.7	0.3	10,300	37.5	56.5	2.5	3.0	0.5
Giraffa camelopardalis (giraffe)	4 yr	F	12.82	15.1	43.0	33.5	12.3	35.1	7.5	9.1	0.1	14,400	65.0	30.5	1.5	2.5	0.5
Okapia johnstoni (okapi)	2 yr	M	12.36	11.9	36.0	29.1	9.6	33.0	2	7.8	0.5	5,500	36.0	60.0	2.0	1.0	1.0
Camelus dromedarius (camel)	1 day	—	8.36	12.5	28.0	33.4	14.9	44.6	7.5	4.8	0.3	6,000	61.0	35.0	3.5	0.0	0.5
Lama peruana (llama)	—	F	17.92	19.4	44.0	24.6	11.5	44.1	hemo	7.1	0.3	10,600	53.0	32.0	3.5	11.5	0.0
Lama glama (llama)	1 yr	M	9.55	10.4	23.0	24.1	10.9	45.2	2	5.0	0.4	17,000	76.5	13.5	3.0	7.0	—
Bos grunniens (yak)	35 yr	M	6.21	12.8	36.0	58.0	20.6	35.6	7.5	7.8	0.7	4,500	67.0	23.0	3.0	7.0	0.0
Bos grunniens (yak)	40 yr	M	5.81	12.7	36.0	61.9	21.8	35.2	5	7.0	0.5	4,000	59.0	30.0	2.0	9.0	—
Bos indicus (zebu)	3 yr	M	9.04	12.5	40.0	44.2	13.8	31.2	5	6.9	0.3	6,600	25.0	62.0	5.0	8.0	0.0
Bos indicus (zebu)	8 yr	F	5.83	11.6	36.0	61.7	19.8	32.2	5	7.8	0.4	3,500	25.0	68.0	0.0	7.0	0.0
Aepyceros melampus (impala)	5 yr	F	20.25	13.5	40.0	19.7	6.6	33.7	2	5.9	0.6	10,100	75.5	23.5	1.0	0.0	0.0
Ammotragus lervia (barbary sheep)	2½ yr	M	20.86	16.1	46.0	22.1	7.7	35.0	5	7.8	0.3	10,700	65.0	30.0	3.0	2.0	0.0
Ammotragus lervia (barbary sheep)	9 yr	M	17.56	17.0	44.0	25.0	9.6	38.6	hemo	7.8	0.4	9,000	80.0	10.0	9.0	1.0	0.0
Antilope cervicapra (blackbuck)	1 yr	F	12.92	17.1	48.0	37.1	13.2	35.6	hemo	7.1	0.3	3,500	34.0	64.0	2.0	0.0	0.0
Antilope cervicapra (blackbuck)	1 yr	M	14.38	18.0	49.0	34.0	13.0	38.3	hemo	7.6	0.2	3,900	14.0	82.0	2.0	1.0	1.0
Antilope cervicapra (blackbuck)	5 yr	M	13.28	17.4	49.0	36.8	13.1	35.5	hemo	7.8	0.3	5,900	77.0	20.0	3.0	0.0	0.0
Gazella subgutturosa (gazelle)	—	M	9.27	16.0	44.0	47.5	17.3	36.4	5	6.3	0.3	4,000	53.0	38.0	8.0	—	1.0
Tayassu sp (peccary)	2 yr	F	8.27	14.1	47.0	56.8	17.0	30.0	hemo	8.9	0.3	7,100	20.0	77.0	2.0	1.0	0.0
Tayassu sp (peccary)	3½ yr	F	8.17	13.5	43.0	52.6	16.5	31.3	5	8.9	0.3	7,400	43.0	53.5	1.5	1.5	0.5
Papio sp (baboon)	—	M	6.3	15.4	52.0	82.5	24.4	29.6	5	9.2	—	15,700	88.0	8.0	3.5	0.5	—
Papio sp (baboon)	—	F	5.65	14.6	48.0	84.9	25.8	30.4	2	8.3	0.2	8,900	45.0	48.0	5.5	1.5	—

Table 12-34. *Continued*

Animal	Age	Sex	RBC (×10⁶/µl)	Hb (g/dl)	PCV (%)	MCV (fl)	MCH (pg)	MCHC (%)	Icterus Index Units[b]	Plasma Protein (g/dl)	Fibrinogen (g/dl)	WBC/µl	Differential Leukocyte Count (%)				
													Neutrophils	Lymphocytes	Monocytes	Eosinophils	Basophils
Pan sp (chimpanzee)	—	F	5.08	13.8	44.0	86.6	27.1	31.3	2	7.5	0.3	7,000	44.5	51.0	2.5	1.5	0.5
Pan sp (chimpanzee)	—	M	5.46	15.0	45.0	82.4	27.4	33.3	2	7.2	0.4	9,700	49.0	26.0	4.0	1.0	—
Gorilla gorilla (gorilla)	—	M	5.34	13.1	43.0	80.5	24.5	30.5	10	8.1	0.3	5,600	84.0	24.0	10.0	2.0	—
Pongo pygmaeus (orangutan)	Newborn	M	5.95	16.3	46.0	77.3	27.3	35.4	—	—	—	8,700	50.0	45.0	5.0	—	—
(orangutan)	Adult	M	5.70	14.3	44.0	76.4	24.8	32.5	10	8.2	0.4	9,300	67.5	26.5	4.5	1.0	0.5
Cercocebus sp (mangabey)	—	F	6.15	14.0	46.0	74.8	22.8	30.4	5	8.1	0.2	8,900	25.0	67.0	6.0	1.0	1.0
(mangabey)	—	M	4.72	11.7	38.0	80.5	24.8	30.8	5	7.0	0.3	5,300	32.0	62.0	4.0	2.0	—
Cebus capucinus (capuchin)	7 mo	M	4.96	12.6	37.0	74.5	25.4	34.0	2	7.0	0.1	9,500	32.5	61.5	4.0	2.0	—
Ateles sp (spider monkey)	15 yr	M	5.29	11.4	38.0	73.7	21.6	29.2	mod hemo	7.5	0.4	13,000	89.0	11.0	—	—	—
Lemur catta (ring-tailed lemur)	—	M	8.30	15.0	52.0	62.6	18.0	28.8	hemo	8.8	0.2	9,200	44.5	48.0	5.0	1.5	1.0
Panthera leo (African lion)	8 mo	—	7.85	11.5	36.0	46.0	14.6	31.9	—	—	—	4,500	59.5	31.0	9.0	0.0	0.5
Panthera leo (African lion)	20 yr	F	8.12	13.9	41.0	50.5	17.1	33.9	2	8.0	0.1	20,500	73.0	9.0	17.0	6.0	—
Panthera leo (African lion)	20 yr	M	7.19	13.1	36.0	50.1	18.2	36.4	2	8.3	0.2	13,400	90.0	7.0	2.0	1.0	—
Panthera tigris (Bengal tiger)	6 mo	M	6.18	9.8	31.0	50.1	15.8	31.6	2	6.7	0.2	20,900	69.0	18.5	8.0	4.5	0.0
Panthera tigris (Bengal tiger)	3 yr	M	6.59	12.1	37.0	56.1	18.3	32.7	—	8.0	0.3	16,600	78.0	17.5	2.5	1.0	1.0
Panthera tigris (Bengal tiger)	—	F	7.43	14.9	45.0	60.6	20.0	33.1	5	7.7	0.2	12,600	73.5	15.0	8.0	3.5	—
Panthera pardus (leopard)	7 yr	F	—	—	46.0	—	—	—	—	8.8	—	15,000	84.0	9.0	3.0	4.0	0.0
Panthera pardus (leopard)	—	M	7.93	13.1	39.0	49.2	16.5	33.6	5	8.1	0.1	10,300	79.0	17.0	3.0	1.0	—
Panthera onca (jaguar)	5 yr	M	—	—	44.0	—	—	—	—	8.3	—	12,300	74.0	15.0	1.0	3.0	0.0
Felis concolor (mountain lion)	2 yr	M	10.52	15.4	47.0	44.7	14.6	32.8	2	8.8	0.4	22,000	86.0	10.0	4.0	0.0	0.0
Felis pardalis (ocelot)	10 yr	M	9.36	13.8	45.0	48.0	14.7	30.6	hemo	9.8	0.2	13,650	60.0	35.0	2.5	2.0	0.5

Species	Age	Sex															
Felis serval (serval cat)	6 mo	M	5.29	10.3	34.0	64.2	19.4	30.2	2	6.4	0.5	13,600	81.5	12.0	4.5	2.0	0.0
Felis serval (serval cat)	6 yr	F	6.73	13.3	36.0	53.4	19.7	36.9	hemo, lipemic	7.9	0.4	22,500	44.0	49.0	5.5	1.5	0.0
Felis (Lynx) caracal (caracal)	—	F	9.89	13.4	40.0	40.4	13.5	33.5	2	8.1	0.1	7,900	63.0	16.0	3.0	18.0	—
Felis (Lynx) rufus (bobcat)	3 yr	F	9.26	14.4	45.0	48.5	15.5	32	2	8.1	0.1	8,300	40.5	54.5	2.5	2.5	—
Acinonyx jubatus (cheetah)	1½ yr	F	—	—	46.0	—	—	—	—	6.9	—	11,600	52.0	33.0	2.5	12.5	0.0
Acinonyx jubatus (cheetah)	10 yr	M	—	—	35.0	—	—	—	—	7.1	—	13,300	74.5	16.0	3.0	6.5	0.0
Felis uncia (snow leopard)	4 mo	M	9.06	11.1	34.0	37.5	12.2	32.6	2	6.7	0.2	12,500	73.0	21.5	4.5	1.5	0.0
Euarctos americanus (American black bear)	15 yr	M	7.32	18.2	55.0	75.1	24.8	33.0	2	7.3	0.2	8,900	73.0	13.5	12.0	1.5	0.0
Thalarctos maritimus (polar bear)	8½ yr	M	8.67	21.3	57.0	65.7	24.5	37.3	hemo	9.2	0.3	11,200	82.5	6.0	6.5	5.0	0.0
Thalarctos maritimus (polar bear)	8½ yr	F	8.00	18.1	52.0	65.0	22.6	34.8	5	9.3	0.2	11,800	71.5	12.5	5.5	10.5	0.0
Melursus ursinus (sloth bear)	8 yr	F	6.31	17.5	49.0	72.9	27.7	35.7	2	8.0	0.3	9,500	81.0	17.0	1.0	1.0	0.0
Hyaena hyaena (striped hyena)	6 yr	M	—	—	43.0	—	—	—	—	7.1	—	19,300	72.0	15.0	4.0	4.0	—
Crocuta crocuta (spotted hyena)	3 mo	M?[c]	5.65	9.0	28.0	49.5	15.9	32.1	—	6.5	—	17,100	—	—	—	—	—
Potos flavus (kinkajou)	—		—	—	—	—	—	—	—	—	—	—	—	—	—	—	—
Canis lupus (wolf)		F	8.88	16.8	49.0	55.2	18.9	34.3	—	8.9	0.1	7,100	31.0	66.0	2.0	1.0	—
Canis lupus (wolf)		M	8.42	14.8	45.0	53.4	17.6	32.9	—	8.4	0.1	19,200	15.0	76.0	1.0	7.5	0.5
Vulpes fulva (fox)	5 mo		5.48	11.8	35.0	63.9	21.5	33.7	2	6.0	0.3	7,900	85.0	11.0	1.0	3.0	—
Vulpes fulva (fox)			5.21	9.2	34.0	65.2	17.6	27.0	—	6.8	0.2	11,400	44.0	34.0	9.0	10.5	1.0
Grison vittata (grison)	2 yr	M	6.25	14.4	44.0	70.4	23.0	32.7	—	8.5	0.3	5,400	41.0	36.0	13.0	10.0	—

[a] These data collected in cooperation with Drs. Murray Fowler and C.J. Sedwick.
[b] hemo = hemolyzed.
[c] See Figure 12-18.

al., 1983). Eosinophilia may be seen in yaks with asymptomatic intestinal nematode infection (Hawkey et al., 1983).

Camellidae

This family of ruminants includes camels, guanacos, llamas, alpacas, and vicunas (Table 12–32). The erythrocytes are elliptical and thin (Fig. 12–11; see also Fig. 20–2*E* and *F*). Reticulocytes and nucleated red cells are said to be round (Hawkey, 1975). The MCHC of *Camelus dromedarius* and *Lama peruana* (Table 12–34) of 44% is considerably in excess of the range of 30–36% common to animals with disc-shaped erythrocytes. A similar high value for MCHC is obtained when calculated for *Lama guanicoe* (Schalm, 1975) and the Indian camel (Banerjee et al., 1962) from Table 12–32. A higher MCHC and a significantly lower electrolyte concentration were found in erythrocytes of 40 camels than in those of other mammals (Little et al., 1970). It appears from the latter study that the high MCHC of camel erythrocytes is a species characteristic and not a technical artifact.

The size of 1,250 erythrocytes from 50 Indian camels *(Camelus dromedarius)* was measured, and ranges and means for length and width were reported to be 7.2–8.4 µm (7.7) by 3.7–4.7 µm (4.2) (Kohli, 1963). Literature values indicate greater numbers (10–19 × 10⁶/µl) of slightly smaller (7.2 × 3.5 µm) erythrocytes in the two-humped Asian camel (*Camelus bactrianus*) than in the Indian camel (Banerjee et al., 1962). Erythrocyte sedimentation is approximately 1.0 mm in 1 hour (Banerjee et al., 1962), with an increase to several millimeters of fall over a period of 7 hours (Bhatt and Kohli, 1959). Fetal hematopoiesis was studied in 120 dromedary fetuses; it was found to occur in the spleen, liver, thymus, and bone marrow and to vary with fetal growth (Farahat et al., 1980).

Perk (1963) commented on the camel's ability to regain body water losses (about 30 gallons) within 10 minutes without producing intravascular hemolysis of its erythrocytes. In a comparative study of osmotic fragility of mammalian erythrocytes, the camel erythrocytes were found to be most resistant to hemolysis in hypotonic saline solution (Perk et al., 1964). Initial hemolysis was observed at 0.30% NaCl solution and complete hemolysis at 0.21% saline solution. In another

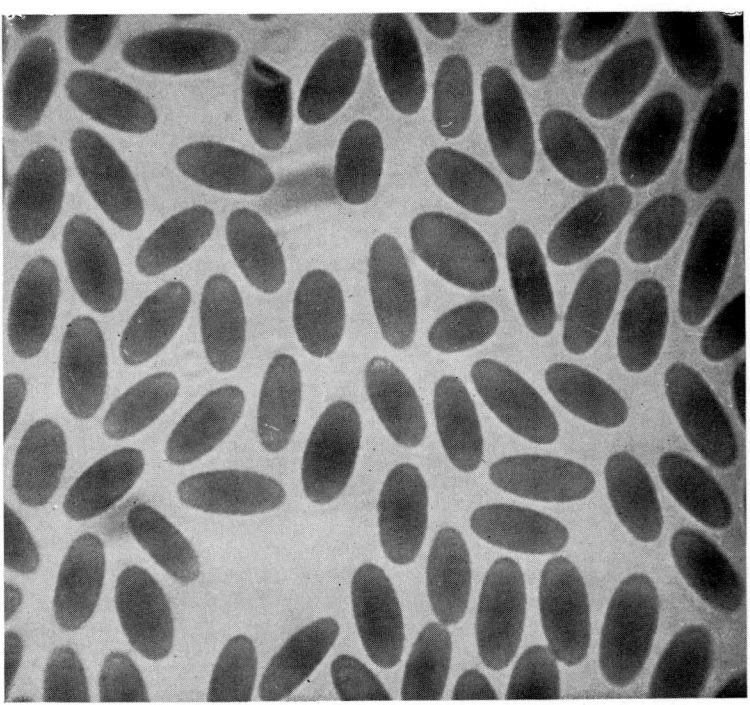

Fig. 12–11.   Elliptical erythrocytes (from *Lama guanicoe*) typical of the family Camellidae.

study (Soliman and El Amrousi, 1966), beginning hemolysis occurred at 0.37 ± 0.04% and complete hemolysis at 0.25% ± 0.03% saline for 40 female camels 4–6 years of age. This unique property of the camel erythrocyte may be related to its membrane structure (Eitan et al., 1976).

Cornelius and Kaneko (1962), using the isotope ^{14}C, estimated the median erythrocyte life span in 2 mature guanacos to be 225 days, with maximal destruction at 235 days.

Seasonal (Ghosal et al., 1974; Majeed et al., 1980) and sex (Majeed et al., 1980; Nassar et al., 1977) variations in blood values of camel have been reported. Influence of the rutting season in the male has been noted in increased WBC counts (Khan and Kohli, 1978). Blood examination of 99 apparently normal dromedaries under 1 year, 1–5 years, and over 5 years in age revealed highest leukocyte counts in older animals (Ghodsian et al., 1978).

The female sex chromatin or "drumstick" lobe was found in the neutrophil of *Lama guanicoe* (Kraft, 1957). Hematologic observations of 30 alpacas *(Lama pacos)* between 6 months and 10 years of age revealed significantly higher Hb and PCV values in adult males than in females and animals younger than 2 years of age, higher total plasma protein concentration in animals older than 2 years of age, and no age-related changes in WBC counts and fibrinogen concentrations (Montes et al., 1983).

Canidae

Hematologic and serum chemistry analyses have been reported for conditioned, captive wild coyotes *(Canis latrans)* (Gates and Goering, 1976), 18-month-old pen-raised coyotes (Rich and Gates, 1979), and wild, free-ranging coyotes (Smith and Rongstad, 1980). No significant sex-related differences were found in blood values of conditioned wild coyotes or pen-raised coyotes. WBC counts and neutrophil numbers were higher in coyotes soon after capture than in conditioned coyotes. Higher eosinophil numbers than those in normal dogs were found in wild coyotes and attributed to light to moderate parasitic burden. Significantly higher lymphocyte and monocyte numbers and lower neutrophil numbers

were found in pen-raised coyotes than in captive wild coyotes, while no significant differences were found between mean PCV values. Stress of capture and restraint may cause increases in WBC counts and PCV values in coyotes as in other animal species, and nutritional differences may be reflected in higher PCV and hemoglobin values of adults compared to those of juveniles (Smith and Rongstad, 1980). Nutritional and dietary differences were similarly associated with lower red cell parameters of wolf *(Canis lupus)* pups compared to dogs in the same age group (Seal et al., 1975).

Cervidae

Blood values of 42 fallow deer *(Dama dama)* were analyzed with respect to age, season, and sex (Chapman et al., 1982). Hematologic parameters were measured of 100 male and female red deer *(Cervus elaphus)* aged 3 months and over (Wilson and Pauli, 1982). Normal blood values for elk belonging to the family Cervidae have been reported (Pedersen and Pedersen, 1975; Vaughn et al., 1973; Wolfe et al., 1982).

Gibbs (1960) collected blood from the Barren Ground caribou (reindeer) immediately after killing by shooting (Table 12–31). Significant alterations in cellular composition of the blood from resting normal values should be anticipated as a result of the method for obtaining the blood samples. Handling stress in reindeer caused significant changes in blood picture and cortisol and urea values, with marked increases in neutrophils and immature cells and moderate increases in PVC and RBC (Rehbinder and Edqvist, 1981). Hematologic studies on reindeer from 1 day to 5 years of age have been reported (Timisjärvi et al., 1981). Erythrocyte parameters were lowest at birth and increased by 5–6 months to near adult level. For example, Hb concentration was 10.8 g/dl in newborns and increased to a maximum of 18.06 g/dl by 5 months. WBC count ranged from 6,100–7,800/μl and increased during the first week. Hb concentration decreased slightly during pregnancy, and a further decrease occurred after parturition.

Elephantidae

Blood is obtained from a vessel on the underside of the ear.

The Indian elephant, *Elephas maximus*, is of interest to the hematologist because of its large red blood cell and unusual differential leukocyte pattern. The erythrocyte is a biconcave disc that measures about 8.8–10.6 μm in diameter and forms rouleaux in drawn blood. Simon (1961) reported the RBC count to range from 1.98 million to 4.0 million/μl, with a mean of 2.81 million (Table 12–31). Nirmalan et al. (1967) reported means of 2.42 ± 0.44 million/μl for baby elephants; 2.47 ± 0.42 for tuskers; 2.40 ± 0.51 for nonpregnant females; and 1.84 ± 0.43 for pregnant females. The low number of erythrocytes compared with other large animals is compensated for by the large cell size (MCV) and hemoglobin concentration (MCH). Others (Dhindsa et al., 1972; Jainudeen and Jayasinghe, 1971; Lewis, 1974) have reported similar mean RBC counts, but MCV of 117–127 fl and MCH of 42–47 pg. No sex or age difference was found (Jainudeen and Jayasinghe, 1971). Anemia is suspected when the RBC count is less than 2 million/μl, and xylazine injection tends to reduce the count (Kuntze and Hunsdorff, 1981).

Our data (Table 12–34) on two Indian elephants revealed RBC counts of 3.08×10^6/μl for the female and 4.08×10^6/μl for the male. The MCV and MCH values for the female and the male were, respectively, 110 fl and 39.9 pg and 118 fl and 37.2 pg. An anteater, *Myrmecophaga tridactyla*, was observed by us to have a similarly low RBC count (3.27×10^6/μl) and large red cell size (MCV, 148 fl).

Mean WBC counts have been reported to be 6,400–18,956/μl, and our values on the two elephants were 12,700 and 20,800. The differential leukocyte count of the Indian elephant presents a problem in classification of a cell having a bilobed or, less commonly, a trilobed nucleus with clumped chromatin (Fig. 12–12, Plate VII–11). Bilobed cells are also seen in African elephants (Hawkey et al., 1983). The nuclear lobes are connected by a thin filament. This cell is present in prominent numbers and was classified as a variation of the lymphocyte by Simon (1961) (Table 12–31). Nirmalan et al. (1967) also reported

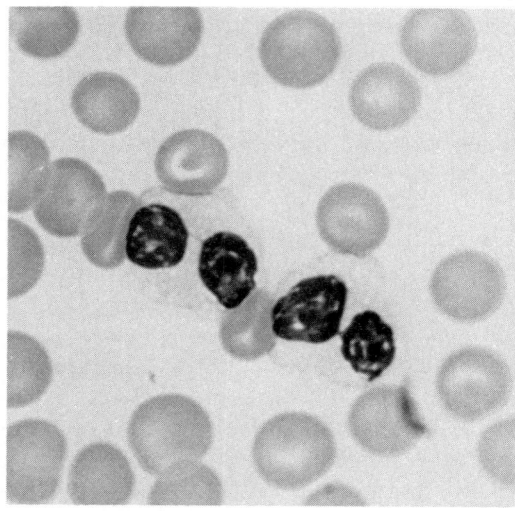

Fig. 12–12. Bilobed monocytes of *Elephas maximus*. ×2,700.

the cell as a lymphocyte, as indicated by their differential leukocyte counts, which assigned 50.6–59.0% of the count to lymphocytes. The cytoplasm of the cell in question is similar in staining quality to the typical monocyte, and both cell types may have small cytoplasmic vacuoles (compare Figs. 12–13 and 12–14). Furthermore, both the typical monocyte and the cell in question are peroxidase-positive. The bilobed cell is distinctly different from the peroxidase-positive neutrophil (heterophil or pseudoeosinophil) (Plate VII–12). On the basis of these morphologic and staining char-

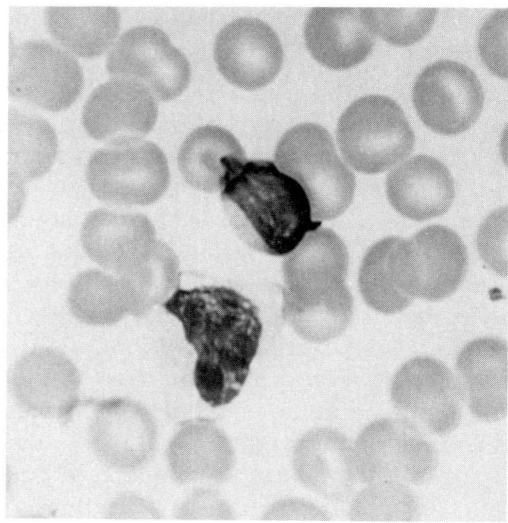

Fig. 12–13. Typical lymphocyte (small cell) and typical monocyte of *Elephas maximus*. ×2,700.

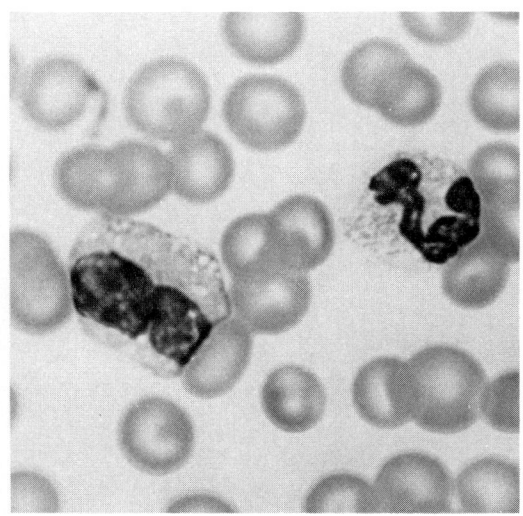

Fig. 12–14. A bilobed monocyte (large cell) and a heterophil leukocyte in the blood of *Elephas maximus.* ×2,700.

acteristics, we have classified the bilobed leukocyte as a monocyte (Table 12–34), making the monocyte the most numerous leukocyte in normal elephant blood. The eosinophil is characterized by numerous round granules that fill the cytoplasm. Leukopenia may develop during viral infecton (Kuntze and Hunsdorff, 1981).

Lewis (1974) reported platelet counts of 491,000–975,000/µl, with a mean of 637,000, and made observations on blood coagulation and ultrastructure of leukocytes and platelets of 4 Indian elephants.

Some data on blood composition of the African elephant *(Loxodonta africana)* have been presented (Debbie and Clausen, 1975; Dhindsa et al., 1972; Riegel et al., 1967; Woodford, 1979). WBC counts are lower in blood collected from domesticated African elephants (Woodford, 1979) than in samples from shot (Debbie and Clausen, 1975) or immobilized (Young and Lombard, 1967) African elephants. RBC counts and MCV are similar to those of Indian elephants (Table 12–31).

Fetal red cells were studied by Riegel et al. (1967). Gestation period in elephants is about 21 months. A 5-month-old fetus characteristically had numerous nucleated red cells (160/100 WBC), 15% fetal hemoglobin, MCV of 142.3 fl, and red cell diameter of 9.96 µm. Nucleated red cells and fetal hemoglobin

were absent in blood of a 12-month-old fetus, and its red cell size was smaller than that in the adult elephant. MCV and red cell diameter for the 12-month-old fetus and adult elephants were, respectively, 107.2 fl and 8.63 µm and 131.4 fl and 9.34 µm. A lactating female had lower red cell parameters than 2 pregnant females.

Equidae

A limited number of observations have been made on the hematology of the donkey and mule (Table 12–33).

The diameter of erythrocytes of the donkey was found to range from 4.8–7.2 µm, with a mean of 6.2 µm; in the mule the range was 4.8–8.8 µm, with a mean of 6.23 µm (Neser, 1923). The data in Table 12–33 indicate that RBC counts of mules and donkeys are similar to those of the cold-blooded horses (Table 6–9), but the MCV is somewhat larger. The larger erythrocytes lead to a generally higher mean PCV than is observed in cold-blooded horses, but is considerably lower than is commonly found in hot-blooded horses. Mean values for MCHC are higher in the burro foal than in the adult (Davis et al., 1978).

In a comparison of the blood values of 50 female and 50 male donkeys, 2–5 years of age, females were found to have higher mean values for RBC and ESR and lower values for Hb, WBC, absolute lymphocyte and monocyte numbers, platelet counts, and red cell diameter (Nayeri, 1978). Platelet counts were reported at 135,400 ± 27,200/µl in females and 136,400 ± 29,300/µl in males. No significant sex differences were found in blood values of 8 male and 15 female mules (Sharma et al., 1981).

Erythrocyte sedimentation rate was conducted on the blood of the burro by the Wintrobe method and read at 1 hour (Wilding et al., 1952). For males, the range was 21.0–63.0 mm, with a mean of 54.3 mm; for females, the range was 4.0–67.0 mm, with a mean of 47.5 mm.

Serum bilirubin content is much lower (0.4 mg/dl) in the donkey as well as in Przewalski and zebra than in the horse (Jeffcott, 1977). Total serum lipid level is higher in the donkey than in various breeds of horses (Straub et al., 1975).

A comparison was made of several hematological and biochemical values of 10 normal mules and 10 horses, all kept at an elevation of 7,500 feet (Sastry and Dhanda, 1953). The blood of mules was characterized by slightly larger erythrocytes; higher PCV, MCV, and MCH; longer prothrombin time; lower icterus index and bilirubin; lower serum calcium and phosphorus; and higher γ-globulin. The absence of reticulocytes in the blood of the horse was confirmed. The range for total serum proteins in the mule was 6.3–7.7 g/dl, with a mean of 7.12 g/dl. The albumin:globulin ratio ranged from 0.81–1.26:1.0, with a mean of 0.96:1.0. Similarly, higher RBC counts than normal for horses were found in 44 mules, 10–25 years old, and were attributed to their being at higher altitudes (Lemmer et al., 1980); no sex difference was noted.

The donkey has one hemoglobin type and the mule has three, compared to one or two in the horse (Jeffcott, 1977). Studies on equine serum immunoglobulins revealed homologues of horse IgGa, IgGb, IgGc, and IgA in normal donkey, mule, hinny, and zebra serums (Allen and Dalton, 1975).

The mean WBC count for donkeys was 12,600–14,400/μl. This is considerably higher than the means for mature hot- or cold-blooded horses. In the case of mules, means of 12,900 (Neser, 1923) and 8,940/μl (Morris, 1942) have been reported. The relative differential leukocyte count of both donkeys and mules is similar to that of hot-blooded horses in that the N:L ratio approximates 1:1. In one report on the donkey (Neser, 1923), however, lymphocytes were found to outnumber neutrophils, giving an N:L ratio of 3:5.

Felidae

Hemograms of several individuals representing the genera *Panthera, Felis, Uncia,* and *Acinonyx* are presented in Table 12–34. In general, blood composition was similar to that of the domestic cat, with the exception of a greater plasma protein concentration and somewhat higher PCV values for several of the large cats. All of the cats presented a few erythrocytes containing a single refractile structure (Heinz body) when stained with new methylene blue (see Chapter 2). In this respect, the erythrocytes of all the large cats

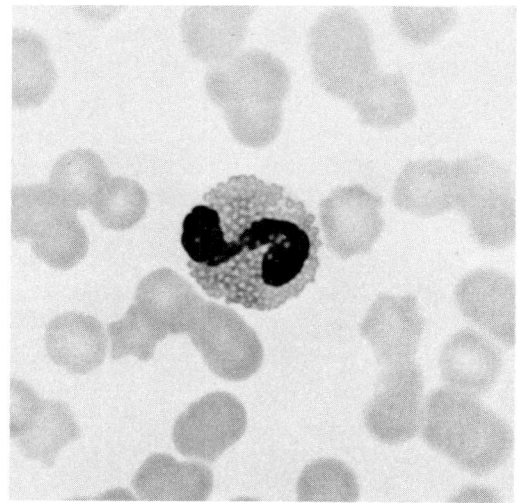

Fig. 12–15. Eosinophil of *Panthera leo.* ×3,600.

were similar to those of the domestic cat. A male mountain lion had many Heinz bodies associated with chronic nephritis from which the animal died 2 days after the blood sample was taken. An occasional erythrocyte containing a Howell-Jolly body was seen in two cheetahs and one leopard, indicating an additional similarity to the normal domestic cat. The granules of the eosinophil are rod-like in the domestic cat. Similar rod-like eosinophilic granules were seen in the cheetah, while round granules were characteristic of eosinophils of the lion (Fig. 12–15), mountain lion (Fig. 12–16), and leopard. The eosinophil leu-

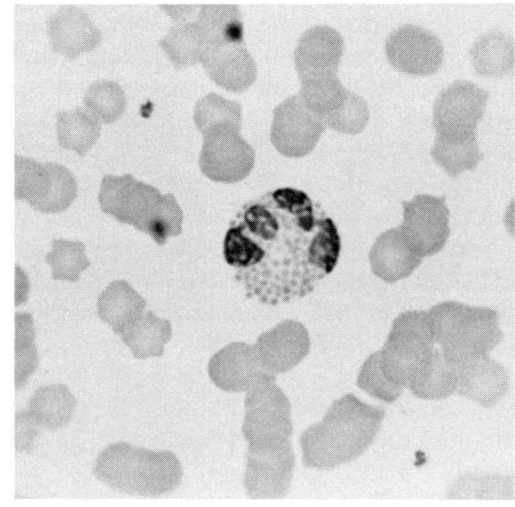

Fig. 12–16. Eosinophil of *Felis concolor.* ×2,700.

kocyte of the mountain lion was further characterized by a reduced number of granules, with blue cytoplasm visible between the granules.

In a hematologic study of wild and captive mountain lions *(Felis concolor)* higher PCV was found in the former (46.9%) than in the latter (41.8%) (Currier and Russell, 1982).

Giraffidae

This family consists of the two genera, *Giraffa* and *Okapia*. Hemograms of *Giraffa camelopardalis*, a male 5 months old and its mother 4 years old, are presented in Table 12–34. The small, round erythrocytes (MCV 27.9 fl in male and 33.5 fl in female) readily formed prominent rouleaux in drawn blood; they numbered 18.24 million and 12.82 million/μl, respectively. The cytoplasm of the neutrophil contained dust-like, faintly pinkish granules. A "drumstick" nuclear appendage, characteristic of the female sex, was present in an occasional neutrophil of the 4-year-old giraffe. Granules of the eosinophil were lens-shaped, stained intensely red, and nearly filled the cytoplasm. Additional data are given in Table 12–31.

One hemogram of a 2-year-old male *Okapia johnstoni* is presented in Table 12–34. Small, round erythrocytes forming prominent rouleaux characterized the blood film. Neutrophils were prominently lobed, with distinct filaments between lobes, and the cytoplasm was diffusely pink because of the presence of numerous small granules. Granules of the eosinophil were small, round, and intensely acidophilic, and they filled the cytoplasm. Lymphocytes outnumbered neutrophils.

Hyaenidae

Examples of blood composition of a mature male striped hyena *(Hyaena hyaena)* and a young spotted hyena *(Crocuta crocuta)* of debatable sex are presented in Table 12–34. The eosinophil of both the spotted hyena and striped hyena presented distinct round vacuoles in the place of granules in a gray cytoplasm (Fig. 12–17). In that respect, the eosinophil of the spotted hyena was somewhat similar to the vacuolated eosinophil of the greyhound (see Chapter 4). The neutrophil leukocyte may be of some value in dis-

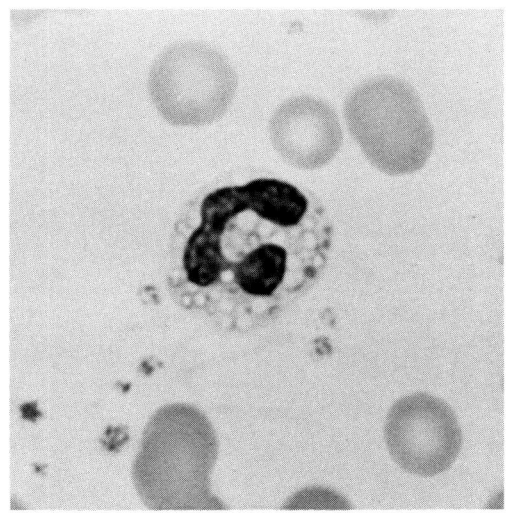

Fig. 12–17. Eosinophil of *Hyaena hyaena.* ×4,500 as shown.

tinguishing between the sexes of the spotted hyena, especially at a young age. The external genitalia of *Crocuta crocuta* are so similar in appearance in young animals that it is difficult to distinguish a male from a female. The similarity decreases with further sexual development (Davis and Story, 1949). It is possible that the presence of the "drumstick" nuclear appendage on a sufficient number of neutrophils would aid in indicating the sex to be female. Fig. 12–18 is that of a neutrophil with a typical female sex chromatin lobe found in the 3-month-old spotted hyena (Table 12–34) that was considered to be a male. Information as to the true sex of the individual did not become available later.

Tayassuidae

The peccary is a pig-like animal that is classifed separately from swine. Hemograms of two mature females are presented in Table 12–34. Cellular composition, including erythrocytes and leukocytes, was similar to that of the domestic pig. The erythrocytes were not crenated, as is common with pig blood. Rouleau formation was a prominent feature, and an occasional polychromatophilic erythrocyte and nucleated erythrocyte were seen. More lymphocytes were present than neutrophils, and they appeared as small, medium, and large cells. The small lymphocytes were densely stained and only slightly larger than

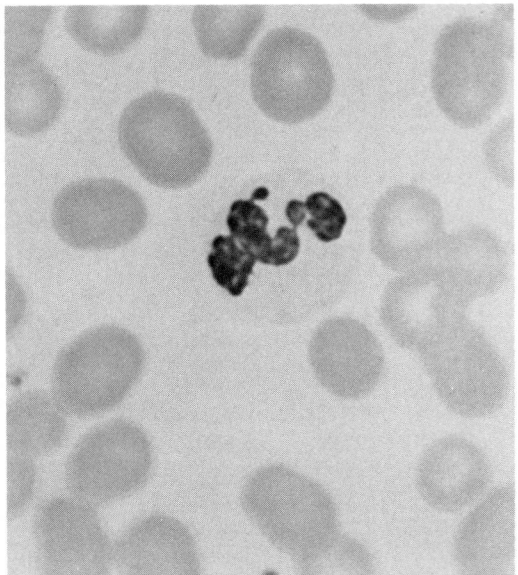

Fig. 12–18. Neutrophil with typical female sex chromatin lobe in the blood of a 3-month old spotted hyena that was considered to be a male from the appearance of the external genitalia. ×3,600 as shown.

the erythrocytes. Black azurophilic granules were present in the cytoplasm of some medium and large lymphocytes. A "drumstick" nuclear appendage, characteristic of the female sex, was present in some neutrophils. The eosinophil leukocyte presented many small, round, intensely stained cytoplasmic granules, and the nucleus was round or kidney-bean shape in some cells. The basophil leukocyte presented a moderate number of round, black granules in the cytoplasm and partly over the nucleus. The monocyte was similar to that of other mammals.

Ursidae

Hemograms of the American black bear and polar bear were characterized by high values for RBC, Hb, and PCV; high plasma protein concentration was seen in two polar bears (Table 12–34). In other respects, blood composition was similar to that of the domestic dog. The bears were under anesthesia when the blood was drawn. A comparison was made of some hematologic values of wild and captive polar bears (Lee et al., 1977). Blood values of 6 captive polar bears, 4 to over 14 years old, were similar to those in free living polar bears (Seidel, 1980). The MCV is largest in the Alaskan brown bear (80–98 fl) and sloth

bear (82–88 fl), while it is smallest in spectacled bear (less than 60 fl) and some black bears (as low as 52 fl) (Fowler, 1978).

REFERENCES

General References

Burnett, S.H.: The Clinical Pathology of the Blood of Domesticated Animals. 2nd ed. Macmillan, New York, 1917.

Burns, K.F., and de Lannoy, C.W., Jr.: Compendium of Normal Blood Values of Laboratory Animals, with Indication of Variations. Toxicol. Appl. Pharmacol., *8*:429, 1966.

Dieterich, R.A.: Hematologic Values of Some Arctic Mammals. J. Amer. Vet. Med. Ass., *157*:604, 1970.

Dougherty, T.F., and White, A.: Influence of Hormones on Lymphoid Tissue Structure and Function. Endocrinology, *35*:1, 1944.

Fowler, M.W.: Zoo and Wild Animal Medicine. W.B. Saunders Co. Philadelphia, 1978.

Frye, R.: Hematology of Captive Reptiles. *In* Zoo and Wild Animal Medicine. Fowler, M.E., ed. W.B. Saunders, Philadelphia, p. 146, 1978.

Gardner, M.V.: The Blood Picture of Normal Laboratory Animals; A Review of the Literature 1936–1946. J. Franklin Inst., *243*:77 (rat), 172 (mouse), 251 (rabbit), 434 (hamster), 498 (guinea pig), and *244*:155 (monkey), 1947.

Hausner, E., et al.: Roentgenologic Observations on the Spleen of the Dog under Ether, Sodium Amytal, Pentobarbital Sodium and Pentothal Sodium Anesthesia. Amer. J. Physiol., *121*:387, 1938.

Hawkey, C.M.: Comparative Mammalian Haematology. William Heinemann Medical Books, London, 1975.

Hawkey, C.M.: The Haematology of Exotic Mammals. *In* Comparative Clinical Haematology. Archer, R.K., and Jeffcott, L.B., eds. Blackwell Scientific Publications, Oxford, Chap. 4, p. 103, 1977.

Kozma, C.K., et al.: Electrophoretic Determination of Serum Proteins of Laboratory Animals. J. Amer. Vet. Med. Ass., *151*:865, 1967.

MacNamee, J.K., and Sheehy, R.W.: The Use of the Small Laboratory Animal for Repeated Clinical Pathological Studies. Proc. Book Amer. Vet. Med. Ass., 89th Ann. Session, 138, 1952.

Mitruka, B.M., and Rawnsley, H.M.: Clinical Biomedical and Haematological Reference Values in Normal Experimental Animals. Masson, New York, 1977.

Perk, K. et al.: Osmotic Fragility of Red Blood Cells of Young and Mature Domestic and Laboratory Animals. Amer. J. Vet. Res., *25*:1241, 1964.

Sanderson, J.H., and Phillips, C.E.: An Atlas of Laboratory Animal Haematology. Clarendon Press, Oxford, 1981.

Scarborough, R.A.: The Blood Picture of Normal Laboratory Animals; A Compilation of Published Data. Yale J. Biol. Med., *3*:64 (rabbit), 169 (guinea pig), 267 (rat), 272 (mouse), 1930–1931, and *4*:199 (monkey), 1931–1932.

Schermer, S.: Die Blutmorphologie der Laboratoriumstiere. Barth, Leipzig, 1954.

Schermer, S.: The Blood Morphology of Laboratory Animals. 3rd ed. F.A. Davis, Philadelphia, 1967.

Wechsler, S.J.: Blood Collection Techniques and Normal

Values for Ferrets, Rabbits, and Rodents. A Review. Vet. Med. Small Anim. Clin., 78:713, 1983.

Wintrobe, M.M., and Schumacer, H.B., Jr.: Erythrocyte Studies in the Mammalian Fetus and Newborn. Amer. J. Anat., 58:313, 1936.

The Rabbit

Bainton, D.F., and Farquhar, M.G.: Origin of Granules in Polymorphonuclear Leukocytes. J. Cell. Biol., 28:277, 1966.

Bushnell, L.D., and Bangs, E.F.: A Study of the Variation in Number of Blood Cells of Normal Rabbits. J. Infect. Dis., 39:291, 1926.

Cheng, S.C.: Leucocytic Counts in Rabbits; Observations on the Influence of Various Physiologic Factors and Pathological Conditions. Amer. J. Hyg., 11:449, 1930.

Dikovinova, N.V.: The Absolute Number of Cells in the Bone Marrow and Myelograms of Normal Rabbits. Bull. Exp. Biol. Med., 44:1129, 1957.

Fetters, M.D.: Hematology of the Black-Tailed Jack Rabbit (Lepus californicus californicus). Lab. Anim. Sci., 22:546, 1972.

Hinton, M., et al.: Haematological Findings in Healthy and Diseased Rabbits: A Multivariate Analysis. Lab. Anim., 16:123, 1982.

Horan, P.K., et al.: Aseptic Aspiration of Rabbit Bone Marrow and Enrichment for Cycling Cells. Lab. Anim. Sci., 30:77, 1980.

Jackson, J.W., and Stovall, W.D.: Normal Blood Count of the Rabbit. J. Lab. Clin. Med., 16:82, 1930.

Jacobson, H.A., et al.: Hematologic Comparisons of Shot and Live Trapped Cottontail Rabbits. J. Wildl. Dis., 14:82, 1978.

Jones, R.T.: Normal Values of Some Biochemical Constituents in Rabbits. Lab. Anim., 9:143, 1975.

Pearce, L., and Casey, A.E.: Studies in the Blood Cytology of the Rabbit J. Exp. Med., 51:83, 1930; 52:23, 39, 145, 167, 1930.

Pintor, P.P., and Grassini, V.: Individual and Seasonal Spontaneous Variations of Haematological Values in Normal Male Rabbits: Statistical Survey. Acta Haematol., 17:122, 1957.

Sabin, F.R., et al.: Changes in the Bone Marrow and Blood Cells of Developing Rabbits. J. Exp. Med., 64:97, 1936.

Scott, J.M., and Simon, C.E.: Experimental Measles. I. The Thermic and Leucocytic Response of the Rabbit to Inoculation with the Virus of Measles, and Their Value as a Criteria of Infection. Amer. J. Hyg., 4:559, 1924.

Srinivasan, R., et al., A Study of the Normal Hematology of Rabbits. Indian Vet. J., 56:550, 1979.

Stickrod, G., et al.: Use of Mini-Peristaltic Pump for Collection of Blood from Rabbits. Lab. Anim. Sci., 31:87, 1981.

Sutherland, G.B., et al.: Cold Adapted Animals. II. Changes in the Circulating Plasma Proteins and Formed Elements of Rabbit Blood under Various Degrees of Cold Stress. J. Appl. Physiol., 12:362, 1958.

Wilson, P.: Bone Marrow Biopsy in the Rabbit. Lab. Anim., 5:203, 1971.

Witts, L.J., and Webb, R.A.: The Monocytes of the Rabbit in B. monocytogenes Infection: A Study of Their Staining Reactions and Histogenesis. J. Path. Bact., 30:687, 1927.

The Guinea Pig

Bilbey, D.L.J., and Nicol, T.: Normal Blood Picture of the Guinea Pig. Nature. 176:1218, 1955.

Congdon, C.C., and Lorenz, E.: Leukemia in Guinea Pigs. Amer. J. Pathol., 30:337, 1954.

Constable, B.J.: Changes in Blood Volume and Blood Picture during the Life of the Rat and Guinea-Pig from Birth to Maturity. J. Physiol., 167:229, 1963.

Ediger, R.D., and Rabstein, M.M.: Spontaneous Leukemia in a Hartley Strain Guinea Pig. J. Amer. Vet. Med. Ass., 153:954, 1968.

Epstein, R.D., and Tompkins, E.H.: A Comparison of Techniques for the Differential Counting of Bone Marrow Cells (Guinea Pig). Amer. J. Med. Sci., 206:249, 1943.

Gordon, H.A.: Morphological and Physiological Characterization of Germfree Life. Ann. N.Y. Acad. Sci., 78:208, 1959.

Harris, R.S., et al.: A Quantitative Comparison of the Nucleated Cells in the Right and Left Humeral Bone Marrow of the Guinea Pig. Blood, 9:374, 1954.

Izard, J., et al.: The Kurloff Cell: Its Differentiation in the Blood and Lymphatic Tissue. Cell Tissue Res., 173:237, 1976.

Joyner, A.L.: A Study of the White Blood Cells of the Normal Guinea Pig. Amer. J. Anat., 62:497, 1938.

King, E.S., and Lucas, M.: A Study of the Blood Cells of Normal Guinea Pigs. J. Lab. Clin. Med., 26:1364, 1941.

Ledingham, J.C.G.: Sex Hormones and the Foa-Kurloff Cell. J. Path. Bact., 50:201, 1940.

Lopez, H., and Navia, J.M.: A Technique for Repeated Collection of Blood from the Guinea Pig. Lab. Anim. Sci., 27:522, 1977.

Mahadevan, S., et al.: Normal Haematological and Serum Biochemical Parameters of Guinea Pigs (Cavia porcellus). Indian Vet. J., 58:359, 1981.

Pattison, I.H., and McDiarmid, A.: Differences in the Cellular Elements of Blood Obtained from the Right and Left Ventricles of Healthy Guinea Pigs. J. Path. Bact., 55:217, 1943.

Porter, D.A.: An Increase in the Proportion of Basophilic Leucocytes in Guinea Pigs Experimentally Infected with Swine Lungworms. J. Parasitol., 23:73, 1937.

Quillec, M., et al.: Red Cell and White Cell Counts in Adult Guinea-Pigs. Pathol. Biol., 25:443, 1977.

Revell, P.A.: Kurloff Cell Levels in the Peripheral Blood of Normal and Oestrogen Treated Guinea-Pigs. Brit. J. Exp. Path., 55:525, 1974.

Roofe, P.G., et al.: Comparison of Peripheral Blood with Heart Blood in Guinea Pigs. Science, 111:337, 1950.

Sawitsky, A., and Meyer, L.M.: Bone Marrow of Normal Guinea Pigs. Blood, 3:1050, 1948.

Vallejo-Freire, A.: A Simple Technique for Repeated Collection of Blood Samples from Guinea Pigs. Science, 114:524, 1951.

Watson, P.F., and Hawkey, C.M.: The Effects of Age and Anaesthetic on the Blood Picture of the Cuis, Galea musteloides. Lab. Anim., 10:279, 1976.

The Rat

Archer, R.K., et al.: Haematology of Conventionally-Maintained Lac:P Outbred Wistar Rats during the 1st Year of Life. Lab. Anim., 16:198, 1982.

Bickhardt, K., et al.: Influence of Bleeding Procedure and Some Environmental Conditions on Stress-dependent Blood Constituents of Laboratory Rats. Lab. Anim., 17:161, 1983.

Bruckner-Kardoss, E., and Wostmann, B.S.: Blood Volume of Adult Germfree and Conventional Rats. Lab. Anim. Sci., 24:633, 1974.

Bubna-Littitz, H., et al.: Untersuchungen zu den Tageschwankungen der Konzentration von Blutzellen bei jungen und alten Ratten. Wiener Tierärztl. Monatsschr., *68*:383, 1981.

Burns, K.F., et al., Serum Chemistry and Hematological Values for Axenic (Germfree) and Environmentally Associated Inbred Rats. Lab. Anim. Sci., *21*:415, 1971.

Cameron, D.G., and Watson, G.M.: The Blood Counts of the Adult Albino Rat. Blood, 4:816, 1949.

Choubey, B.J., et al.: Some Aspects of Haematology of a Common Indian Field Rat, Rattus rattus arborius (Linn.) in Relation to Sex and Size. Folia Haematol., *105*:779, 1978.

Crafts, R.C.: Effects of Ether Anesthesia upon Total Erythrocytes and White Cell Counts of Adult Female Rats. J. Lab. Clin. Med., 29:1070, 1944.

Drabkin, D.L., and Fitz-Hugh, T., Jr.: A Comparison of the Normal Blood Picture of Rats of Two Different Colonies Reared upon Different Stock Rations. Amer. J. Physiol., *108*:61, 1934.

Endicott, K.M., and Ott, M.: The Normal Myelogram in Albino Rats. Anat. Rec., *92*:61, 1945.

Endicott, K.M., et al.: The Bone Marrow in Folic Acid Deficiency and Its Response to Crystalline Lactobacillus Casei Factor (Folic Acid). Arch. Path., *40*:364, 1945.

Everitt, A.V., and Webb, C.: The Blood Picture of the Aging Male Rat. J. Gerontol., *13*:255, 1958.

Frolke, Von. W., et al.: Blutwerte der Ratte in Abhängigkeit von Alter und Greschlecht. Arzneim. Forsch., *24*:1262, 1974.

Guenard, E., et al.: Blutwerte der Ratte in Abhängigkeit von Alter und Geschlecht. Arzneim. Forsch., *24*:1542, 1974.

Gunn, F.E., and Vaughan, S.L.: Bone Marrow Reactions. II. The Blood Count in the Albino Rat: Blood Platelets. Anat. Rec., *45*:59, 1930.

Harris, C., and Burke, W.T.: The Changing Cellular Distribution in Bone Marrow of the Normal Albino Rat between One and Fifty Weeks of Age. Amer. J. Pathol., *33*:931, 1957.

Hulse, E.V.: Quantitative Cell Counts of the Bone Marrow and Blood and Their Secular Variations in the Normal Adult Rat. Acta Haematol., *37*:50, 1964.

Jin Ja Kim, et al.: Masseentwicklung und hämatologische Werte waschsender Ratten bei unterschiedicher Fe- und Cu-Versorgung. Zentralbl. Veterinärmed., *28A*:516, 1981.

Kast, A., and Nishikawa, J.: The Effect of Fasting on Oral Acute Toxicity of Drugs on Rats and Mice. Lab. Anim., *15*:359, 1981.

Kiczak, J., et al.: Normal Values of Blood Morphotic Elements, Haematocrit and Bone Marrow Cell Pattern in Adult Wistar Rats. Acta Physiol. Pol., *27*:183, 1976.

Kozma, C.K., et al.: Normal Biological Values for Long-Evans Rats. Lab. Anim. Care, *19*:(Part II):746, 1969.

McCord, C.P., and Bradley, W.R.: Basophilic Aggregations in the Blood of the Newly Born. Amer. J. Clin. Path., *9*:329, 1939.

Nichols, J., and Miller, A.T., Jr.: A Comparison of the Total Leukocyte Count in Heart Blood and Peripheral Blood of the Rat. Science, *108*:378, 1948.

Orten, J.M., and Smith, A.H.: The Proportion of Reticulocytes in the Blood of Albino Rats. Amer. J. Physiol., *108*:66, 1934.

Quimby, F.H., et al.: Total White Cell Counts of Peripheral and Heart Blood of the Rat. Science. *107*:447, 1948.

Ramsell, T.B., and Yoffey, J.M.: The Bone Marrow of the Adult Rat. Acta Anat., *47*:55, 1961.

Reich, C., and Dunning, W.F.: Studies on the Morphology of the Peripheral Blood of Rats. Cancer Res., *3*:248, 1943.

Remesar, X., et al.: Body and Organ Size and Composition during the Breeding Cycles of Rats (Rattus norvegicus). Lab. Anim. Sci., *31*:67, 1981.

Roofe, P.G., et al.: A Quantitative Study of Normal Hemopoiesis in the Albino Rat. Anat. Rec., *121*:495, 1955.

Smith, C.J., and McMahon, J.B.: Method for Collecting Blood from Fetal and Newborn Rats. Lab. Anim. Sci., *27*:112, 1977.

Stasney, J., and Higgins, G.M.: A Quantitative Cytologic Study of the Bone Marrow of the Adult Albino Rat. Anat. Rec., *63*:77, 1935.

Thewlis, E.W., and Meyer, O.O.: The Blood Count of Normal White Rats. Anat. Rec., *82*:115, 1942.

Upton, P.K., and Morgan, D.J.: The Effect of Sampling Technique on Some Blood Parameters of the Rat. Lab. Anim., *9*:85, 1975.

Vogel, M.: The Femoral Bone Marrow Cells of the Albino Rat. Amer. J. Med. Sci., *213*:456, 1947.

Wrieg, H.-H.: Hämatologische Parameter von Sprague-Dawley Ratten in Abhängigkeit von Alter und mikrobieller Definition. 96 pp. Inaug. diss., Freie Univ., Berlin, 1978. (Vet. Bull. 49, Abstract no. 4237, 1979.)

Yamauchi, C., et al.: Effects of Room Temperature on Reproduction, Body and Organ Weights, Food and Water Intake, and Hematology in Rats. Lab. Anim. Sci., *31*:251, 1981.

The Mouse

Berger, J.: Seasonal Variations in Blood Pictures of Mice of H Strain. Zeit. Versuchstierkd., *21*:33, 1979.

Brown, H.E., and Dougherty, T.F.: The Diurnal Variations of Blood Leukocytes in Normal and Adrenalectomized Mice. Endocrinology, *58*:365, 1956.

DeKock, G.W.: Studies on the Blood of Mice. 17th Rep. Dir. Vet. Sci. Anim. Ind., Union of South Africa, August 1931, p. 573.

Dougherty, T.F., and White, A.: Influence of Hormones on Lymphoid Tissue Structure and Function. Endocrinology, *35*:1, 1944.

Ewing, K.L., and Tauber, O.E.: Hematologic Changes in Aging Male C57BL/6Jax Mice. J. Gerontol., *19*:165, 1964.

Feher, L., and Moza, S.: Correlations between Haematological Parameters and Age in Inbred Strain C57BL/10ScSn Mice. Acta Biol. Acad. Sci. Hung., *25*:173, 1974.

Fields, B.T., Jr., and Cunningham, D.R.: A Tail Artery Technic for Collecting One-half Milliliter of Blood from a Mouse. Lab. Anim. Sci., *26*:505, 1976.

Finch, C.E., and Foster, J.R.: Hematologic and Serum Electrolyte Values of the C57BL/6J Male Mouse in Maturity and Senescence. Lab. Anim. Sci., *23*:339, 1973.

Frith, C.H., et al.: Hematologic and Clinical Chemistry Findings in Control BALB/C and C57Bl/C Mice. Lab. Anim. Sci., *30*:835, 1980.

Greenman, D.L., et al.: Clinical Chemistry and Hematology of Mice: A Comparison of Cereal-Based and Semipurified Diets. Lab. Anim. Sci., *32*:414, 1982.

Gurney, C.W., and Rosett, W.: Splenic Erythropoiesis in the Mouse. Exp. Hematol., *15*:94, 1968.

Halberg, F., et al.: Sex Difference in Eosinophil Counts in Tail Blood of Mature B₁ Mice. Science, *125*:73, 1957.

Harrison, S.D., Jr., et al.: Hematology and Clinical Chemistry Reference Values for C57BL/6XDBA 12F1 Mice. Cancer Res., *38*:2636, 1978.

Heinecke, von, H.: Das Blutbild der Maus. I. Das Normale Quantitative und Qualitative Weisse Blutbild. Zeit. Versuchstierkd., *1*:16, 1961.

Heinecke, von, H.: Das Blutbild der Maus: II. Das Normale Rote Blutbild. Zeit. Versuchstierkd., *1*:141, 1962.

Heinecke, von, H.: Das Blutbild der Maus. III. Thrombozyten Normalwerte. Zeit. Versuchstierk., *3*:77, 1963.

Horky, J., et al.: Comparison of Lifespan of Erythrocytes In Some Inbred Strains of Mouse Using ^{14}C-Labelled Glycine. Physiol. Bohemoslov., *27*:209, 1978.

Kassel, R., and Levitan, S.: A Jugular Technique for the Repeated Bleeding of Small Animals. Science, *118*:563, 1953.

Lewis, V.J., et al.: A New Technic for Obtaining Blood from Mice. Lab. Anim. Sci., *26*:211, 1976.

Quittner, H., et al.: The Effect of Massive Doses of Cortisone on the Peripheral Blood and Bone Marrow of the Mouse. Blood, *6*:513, 1951.

Rugh, R., and Somogyi, C.: Pre- and Postnatal Normal Mouse Blood Cell Counts. Proc. Soc. Exp. Biol. Med., *127*:1267, 1968.

Russell, E.A., et al.: Comparison of Normal Blood Picture of Young Adults from 18 Inbred Strains of Mice. Proc. Soc. Exp. Biol. Med., *78*:761, 1951.

Simonds, J.P.: The Blood of Normal Mice. Anat. Rec., *30*:99, 1925.

Stoltz, D.R., and Bendall, R.D.: A Simple Technic for Repeated Collection of Blood Samples from Mice. Lab. Anim. Sci., *25*:354, 1975.

Talbot, R.B., et al.: Age Changes in Blood Parameters of C57BL Mice. Lab Anim. Care, *15*:392, 1965.

The Gerbil

Dillon, W.G., and Glomski, C.A.: The Mongolian Gerbil: Qualitative and Quantitative Aspects of the Cellular Blood Picture. Lab. Anim., *9*:283, 1975.

Gattermann, R.: Hematological and Clinical Chemical Normal Ranges in the Mongolian Gerbil (Meriones unguiculatus). Zeit. Versuchstierkd., *21*:273, 1979.

Smith, R.A., et al.: Erythrocyte Basophilic Stippling in the Mongolian Gerbil. Lab. Anim., *10*:379, 1976.

Weeks, A.M., and Glomski, C.A.: Cytology of the Bone Marrow in the Mongolian Gerbil. Lab. Anim., *12*:195, 1978.

The Golden Hamster

Brock, M.A.: Production and Life Span of Erythrocytes during Hibernation in the Golden Hamster. Amer. J. Physiol., *198*:1181, 1960.

Desai, R.G.: Hematology and Microcirculation. *In* The Golden Hamster: Its Biology and Use in Medical Research. Hoffman, R.A., Robinson, P.F., and Magalhaes, H., eds. Iowa State Univer. Press, Ames, p. 185, 1968.

Desai, R.G., and Fulton, G.P.: Evidence for a Vessel Wall Defect in Immuno-Thrombocytopenic Hamsters. Blood, *15*:675, 1960.

Emminger, A., et al.: Differences in Blood Values Depending on Age in Laboratory-Bred European Hamsters (Cricetus cricetus L.). Lab. Anim., *9*:33, 1975.

Fulton, G.P., et al.: Hematologic Findings in the Total Body X-Irradiated Hamster. Blood, *9*:622, 1954.

House, E.L., et al.: Age Changes in Blood of the Golden Hamster. Amer. J. Physiol., *200*:1018, 1961.

House, E.L., et al.: Blood Volume, Total Protein and Total Cholesterol in Normal and Diabetic Hamsters. Anat. Rec., *144*:25, 1962.

Hu, C.H., and Pai, H.C.: Further Study on the White Blood Cells of Hamsters Experimentally Infected with Kala-Azar. Chin. Med. J., Suppl. 2, 131, 1938.

Lyman, C.P., et al.: The Effect of Hibernation on the Replacement of Blood in the Golden Hamster. J. Exp. Zool., *136*:471, 1957.

Manning, J.P., and Giannina, T.: A Simple Method for Obtaining Blood from Hamsters in Terminal Experiments. Lab. Anim. Care, *16*:523, 1966.

Ottis, K.A., and Tauber, O.E.: Blood Platelet Counts of the Golden Hamster, Cricetus auratus. Blood, *7*:948, 1952.

Pansky, B., et al.: The Orbital Region as Source of Blood in the Golden Hamster. Anat. Rec., *139*:409, 1961.

Reznik, G., et al.: Comparative Studies of Blood from Hibernating and Nonhibernating European Hamsters (Cricetus cricetus L.). Lab. Anim. Sci., *25*:210, 1975.

Rigby, P.G., et al.: Erythrocyte Survival in Hamsters Using Intraperitoneal Na$_2$Cr^{51}O$_4$. Proc. Soc. Exp. Biol. Med., *106*:313, 1961.

Sherman, J.C., and Patt, D.I.: Blood Cell Factors and Tumor Growth in the Cheek Pouch of the Golden Hamster. Cancer Res., *16*:394, 1956.

Silverman, J., and Chavannes, J.-M.: Biological Values of the European Hamster (Cricetus cricetus). Lab. Anim. Sci., *27*:641, 1977.

Stein, K.F., and Carrier, E.: Changes in Erythrocytes of Hamsters following Castration, Splenectomy, and Subsequent Liver, Iron, and Testosterone Injections. Proc. Soc. Exp. Biol. Med., *60*:313, 1945.

Stewart, O.M. et al.: Hematological Findings in the Golden Hamster. J. Exp. Med., *80*:189, 1944.

Trincao, C., et al.: Blood and Bone Marrow of the Golden Hamster (title trans. from Portuguese). Anais Inst. Med. Trop., *6*:41, 1949.

Wild Rodent Species

Dieterich, R.A.: Hematologic Values for Six Standardized Wild Rodent Species. Amer. J. Vet. Res., *34*:431, 1973.

The Monkey

Allen, J.R., and Carstens, L.A.: Hematologic Alterations Observed in Newly Acquired Monkeys during a Period of Their Isolation. Lab. Anim. Care, *15*:103, 1965.

Allen, J.R., and Siegfried, L.M.: Hematologic Alterations in Pregnant Rhesus Monkeys. Lab. Anim. Care, *16*:465, 1966.

Chiarelli, B., and Barberis, L.: Drumsticks in the Leucocytes of Primates. Experientia, *20*:679, 1964.

Fox, H.: The Blood Count of Macacus rhesus. Folia Haematol., *35*:416, 1927.

Glomski, C.A., et al.: Survival of Chromium-51-Labeled Erythrocytes in the Rhesus Monkey. Amer. J. Vet. Res., *32*:149, 1971.

Hall, B.E.: The Morphology of the Cellular Elements of the Blood of the Rhesus Monkey, Macacus rhesus. Folia Haematol., *38*:30, 1929.

Huser, H.J.: Atlas of Comparative Primate Hematology. Academic Press, New York, 1970.

Huser, H.J., and Beard, M.E.J.: Studies on Folate and Vitamin B Metabolism in Primates. I. Blood and Bone

Marrow Morphology, Folate and Vitamin B Levels. Folia. Primatol., *10*:172, 1969.

Ives, M., and Dack, G.M.: "Alarm Reaction" and Normal Blood Picture in Macaca mulatta. J. Lab. Clin. Med., *47*:723, 1956.

King, T.O., and Gargus, J.L.: Normal Blood Values of the Adult Female Monkey (Macaca mulatta). Lab. Anim. Care, *17*:391, 1967.

Kreier, J.P., et al.: Erythrocyte Life Span and Label Elution in Monkeys (Macaca mulatta) and Cats (Felis catus) Determined with Chromium-51 and Diisopropyl Fluorophosphate-32. Amer. J. Vet. Res., *31*:1429, 1970.

Krise, G.M., Jr.: Hematology of the Normal Monkey. Ann. N.Y. Acad. Sci., *85*:803, 1960.

Krise, G.M., Jr., and Wald, N.: Normal Blood Picture of the Macaca mulatta Monkey. J. Appl. Physiol., *12*:482, 1958.

Krise, G.M., Jr., and Wald, N.: Hematological Effects of Acute and Chronic Experimental Blood Loss in the Macaca mulatta Monkey. Amer. J. Vet. Res., *20*:1081, 1959.

Krumbhaar, E.B., and Musser, J.H., Jr.: Studies on the Blood of Normal Monkeys. J. Med. Res., *42*:105, 1920.

Martin, D.P., et al.: Age Related Changes of Hematologic Values in Infant Macaca mulatta. Lab. Anim. Sci., *23*:194, 1973.

Melville, G.S., Jr., et al.: Hematology of the Macaca mulatta Monkey. Lab. Anim. Care, *17*:189, 1967.

Oser, F. et al.: Blood Values in Stumptailed Macaques (Macaca arctoides) under Laboratory Conditions. Lab. Anim. Care, *20*:462, 1970.

Ponder, E., et al.: Studies in Comparative Haematology. II. Primates. Q. J. Exp. Physiol., *19*:181, 1929.

Robinson, F.R., and Ziegler, R.F.: Clinical Laboratory Data Derived from 102 Macaca mulatta. Lab. Anim. Care, *18*:50, 1968.

Rollins, J.B., et al.: Hematologic Studies of the Rhesus Monkey (Macaca mulatta). Lab. Anim. Care, *20*(Part I):681, 1979.

Shuckers, C.F., et al.: The Normal Blood Picture of the Young Rhesus Monkey. Folia Haematol., *60*:416, 1938.

Stanley, R.E., and Cramer, M.B.: Hematologic Values of the Monkey (Macaca mulatta). Amer. J. Vet. Res., *29*:1041, 1968.

Stasney, J., and Higgins, G.M.: The Bone Marrow of the Monkey (Macacus rhesus). Anat. Rec., *67*:219, 1936.

Switzer, J.W.: Bone Marrow Composition in the Adult Rhesus Monkey (Macaca mulatta). J. Amer. Vet. Med. Ass., *151*:823, 1967a.

Switzer, J.W.: A New Technique for Sampling Bone Marrow in Monkey. Lab. Anim. Care, *17*:255, 1967b.

Switzer, J.W., et al.: Hematologic Changes Associated with Pregnancy and Parturition in Macaca mulatta. Lab. Anim. Care, *20*:930, 1970.

Usacheva, N., and Raeva, N.V.: Normal Indices of the Peripheral Blood and Bone Marrow of the Monkey Macacus rhesus. Bull. Exp. Biol. Med. (English edition), *54*:1285, 1963–1964.

Vondruska, J.F.: Certain Hematologic and Blood Chemical Values in Adult Stumptailed Macaques (Macaca arctoides). Lab. Anim. Care, *20*:97, 1970.

Williams, R.A.: The Blood Pictures of Monkeys (New and Old World). Southeastern Vet., *13*:88, 1962.

Fur-Bearing Animals

(Titles in parentheses are translations of foreign language titles.)

Avram, N., et al.: (Normal Haematological Values in Mink and Coypu). Lucrările Institutului de Cercetări Veterinare si Biopreparate "Pasture," *16*:271, 1982a.

Avram, N., et al.: (Normal Haematological Values of the Silver Fox [*Vulpes fulvus*]. Lucrările Institutului de Cercetări Veterinare si Biopreparate "Pasture," *16*:279, 1982b.

Baker, G.A., and Gorham, J.R.: A Technique for Bleeding Ferrets and Mink. Cornell Vet., *41*:235, 1951.

Brookhyser, K.M., et al.: Adaptation of the Orbital Sinus Bleeding Technique to the Chinchilla (Chinchilla laniger). Lab Anim. Sci., *27*:251, 1977.

Brooks, C., and Morris, K.D.: Blood Values and the Use of Ketamine HCl in the Fox. Vet. Med. Small Anim. Clin., *74*:1179, 1979.

Casella, R.L.: Blood Platelets of the Chinchilla. Mod. Vet. Pract., *44*(10):51, 1963.

Henson, J.B, et al.: Hypergammaglobulinaemia in Mink Initiated by a Cell-Free Filtrate. Nature, *197*:206, 1963.

Jepsen, O.R., et al.: Collection of Blood and Anesthesia in Mink. Nord. Vet. Med., *33 (Suppl. 1)*:99 pp. 1981.

Kennedy, A.H.: Cytology of the Blood of Normal Mink and Raccoon. Can. J. Res., *12*:479, 1935a. I. Morphology of Mink's Blood, 479. II. The Numbers of the Blood Elements in Normal Mink, 484. III. Morphology and Numbers of the Blood Elements in Racoon, 495.

Kennedy, A.H.: A Graphical Study of the Blood of Normal Foxes. Can. J. Res., *12*:796, 1935b.

Kraft, V.H.: Das Morhphologische Blutbild von Chinchilla velligera (Prell 1934). Blut, *5*:386, 1959.

Kubin, R., and Mason, M.M.: Normal Blood and Urine Values for Mink. Cornell Vet., *38*:79, 1948.

Leader, R.W., et al.: Studies of Abnormal Leukocyte Bodies In Mink. Blood, *22*:477, 1963.

Lord, G.H., et al.: The Blood Picture of Muskrats under Pentobarbital Sodium. Amer. J. Vet. Res., *15*:79, 1954.

McCue, P.M.: Hematologic Values of San Joaquin Kit Fox *(Vulpes macrotis mutica)*. Unpublished Observations, 1984.

Meyers, K.M., et al.: Characteristics of Platelets from Normal Mink and Mink with the Chédiak-Higashi Syndrome. Amer. J. Hematol., *7*:137, 1979.

Spitzer, E.H., et al.: Preliminary Studies on the Blood Chemistry of the Fox. Amer. J. Vet. Res., *2*:193, 1941.

Strike, T.A.: Hemogram and Bone Marrow Differential of the Chinchilla. Lab. Anim. Care, *20*:33, 1970.

The Deer

Anderson, A.E., et al.: Erythrocytes and Leukocytes in a Colorado Mule Deer Population. J. Wildl. Management, *34*:2, 1970.

Bowman, L.G., and Sears, H.S.: Erythrocyte Values and Alimentary Canal pH Values in Mule Deer. J. Mammal., *36*:474, 1955.

Cowan, I.M., and Bandy, P.J.: Observations on the Haematology of Several Races of Black-Tailed Deer (Odocoileus hemionus). Can. J. Zool., *47*:1021, 1969.

Johnson, H.E., et al.: Hematological Values of Michigan White-Tailed Deer. J. Mammal., *49*:749, 1968.

Kitchen, H., and Pritchard, W.R.: Physiology of Blood. *In* Proceedings of the First National White-Tailed Deer Disease Symposium. University of Georgia,

Center for Continuing Education, Athens, Georgia, p. 109, 1962.

Kitchen, H., et al.: Hemoglobin Polymorphism: Its Relation to Sickling of Erythrocytes in White-Tailed Deer. Science, *144*:1237, 1964.

Kitchen, H., et al.: The Structural Basis for the Polymorphic Hemoglobins of White-Tailed Deer (Odocoileus virginianus): A Comparison of the Hemoglobins Associated with Sickled and Nonsickled Erythrocytes, p. 73. *In* International Symposium on Comparative Hemoglobin Structure. Thessaloniki, 1966.

Kitchen, H., et al.: Hemoglobin Polymorphism in White-Tailed Deer: Subunit Basis. Blood, *29*:867, 1967.

O'Roke, E.C.: Sickle Cell Anemia in Deer. Proc. Soc. Exp. Biol. Med., *34*:738, 1936.

Parasall, C.J., et al.: Erythrocyte Sickling in the Japanese Sika Deer (Cervus nippon). Amer. J. Vet. Res., *36*:749, 1975.

Pritchard, W.R., et al.: Studies on the Mechanism of Sickling of Deer Erythrocytes. Exp. Mol. Pathol., *2*:173, 1963.

Rosen, M.N., and Bischoff, A.I.: The Relation of Hematology to Condition in California Deer, p. 482, Transaction, 17th North American Wildl. Conf., 1952.

Seal, U.S., and Erickson, A.W.: Hematology, Blood Chemistry and Protein Polymorphisms in the White-Tailed Deer (Odocoileus virginianus). Comp. Biochem. Physiol., *30*:695, 1969.

Teeri, A.E., et al.: Blood Composition of the White-Tailed Deer. J. Mammal., *39*:269, 1958.

Undritz, E., et al.: Sickling Phenomenon in Deer. Nature, *187*:333, 1960.

Whitlock, S.C.: Studies on the Blood of White-Tailed Deer. J. Wildl. Management, *3*:14, 1939.

The Water Buffalo

Anwar, M., and Chaudhri, A.Q.: Haematology of Buffalo During Summer and Winter. Pakistan Vet. J., *4*:5, 1984.

Bahga, G.S., et al.: Effect of Spray Cooling and Wallowing on Blood Composition in Buffaloes during Summer. Indian J. Dairy Sci., *33*:294, 1980.

Canfield, P.J., et al.: Normal Haematological and Biochemical Values for the Swamp Buffalo *Bubalus bubalis*) in Australia. Aust. Vet. J., *61*:89, 1984.

El-Naggar, M.A., et al.: Haematological parameters of Buffalo Foetus. Assiut Vet. Med. J., *9*:167, 1982.

Gazia, N., and Wegger, I.; Glutathione Peroxidase and Selenium in Blood from Egyptian Water Buffaloes. Acta Vet. Scand., *21*:137, 1980.

Hafez, E.S.E., and Anwar, A.: Normal Haematological Values in the Buffalo. Nature, *174*:611, 1954.

Hafez, A.M., et al.: Enzymatic and Haematological Studies on Buffaloes at Periparturient Periods. Assiut Vet. Med. J., *11*:173, 1983.

Hamza, S.M., and El-Abdin, Y.Z.: Studies on Some Biochemical Constituents and Enzymes in the Serum of Normal Non-Pregnant Dairy Egyptian Buffaloes. J. Egypt. Vet. Med. Ass., *36*:169, 1976.

Hassan, A., et al.: Seasonal Variations in Lactational Performance and Blood Haematological Characteristics of Cross-Bred (Egyptian X Holstein) and Buffalo (Bubalus bubalis) Cows under Subtropical Conditions. World Rev. Anim. Prod., *17*:65, 1981.

Jain, N.C., and Lasmanis, J.: Leucocytic Changes in Cows Given Intravenous Injections of Escherichia coli Endotoxin. Res. Vet. Sci., *24*:386, 1978.

Jain, N.C., et al.: Hematologic Changes in Buffalo Calves Inoculated with Escherichia coli Endotoxin and Corticosteroids. Unpublished observations, 1979a.

Jain, N.C., et al.: Absence of Reticulocytosis during Acute Blood Loss Anemia in Buffalo Calves. Unpublished observations, 1979b.

Jain, N.C., et al.: Haematological Studies on Normal Lactating Indian Water Buffaloes. Res. Vet. Sci., *32*:52, 1981.

Karram, M.H., et al.: Studies on the Red and White Blood Cells of Buffalo Calves from Birth up to 6 Months Age. J. Egypt. Vet. Med. Ass., *39*:133, 1981.

Kehar, N.D., and Murty, V.N.: Physiological Studies on the Blood of Domestic Animals. II. Male Buffaloes. Indian J. Vet. Sci. Anim. Hus., *21*:13, 1951.

Kohli, R.N., and Singh, S.M.: Studies on Erythrocyte Sedimentation Rate in Buffaloes. I. Evaluation of Various Techniques. Indian Vet. J., *52(12)*:915, 1975.

Malik, J.K., et al.: Hematology of Male Buffalo Calves. Indian Vet. J., *51*:95, 1974.

Moustafa, I.H., et al.: Some Peculiarities of Buffaloes Blood. Vet. Med. J., *10*:263, 1963.

Moustafa, T.H., et al.: The Effect of Climatic Changes on Haemoglobin Content and Corpuscular Constituents of Blood in Cattle and Buffaloes. Assiut Vet. Med. J., *4(7)*:229, 1977.

Murthy, T.S.: A Note On Certain Cellular Constituents of Blood in Buffaloes. Livestock Adviser, Bangoler, India, *5*:44, 1980. (Vet. Bull., *51*:368, 1980.)

Nahani, D., Comparison Electrophoretique des Fractions Proteiniques de Serum des Bovins Laitiers et des Buffles à l'état Normal, par Acétate et Nitrate de Cellulose. Revue de Médecine Vétérinaire, *127(5)*:807, 1976.

Nangia, O.P., and Garg, S.L.: Age-Related Changes in Plasma Fibrinogen and Related Parameters in Buffalo-Calves. Indian J. Anim. Sci., *52*:1024, 1982.

Oshiro, S., et al.: Comparative Studies on the Blood Composition of Water Buffaloes, Cattle and Goats. Sci. Bull. College Agri., Univ. Ryukyus, Okinawa, No. 25:383, 1978. (Abstract Vet. Bull., *49*:985, 1979.)

Purushotham, N.P., and Mahendar, M.: A Note on the Comparative Study of the Blood Picture in Domestic Animals. Indian Vet. J., *40*:553,. 1963.

Salem, I.A.: Seasonal Variations in Some Body Reactions and Blood Constituents in Lactating Buffaloes and Friesian Cows with Reference to Acclimatization. J. Egypt. Vet. Med. Ass., *40*:63, 1980.

Satija, K.C., et al.: Electrophoresis of Buffalo (Bos bubalis) Serum Proteins Including Immunoglobulins. Infect. Immun., *24*:567, 1979.

Sharma, D.P., et al.: Age-Wise and Species-Wise Haematological Studies in Farm Animals. Indian J. Anim. Sci., *43*:289, 1973.

Singh, S.P., and Malik, J.K.: A Note on Haematological Changes in Buffalo Calves during Fasting. Indian J. Anim. Sci., *49*:63, 1979.

Singh, S.P., et al.: Note on the Effect of Anticoagulants and Storing Time on Erythrocyte Sedimentation Rate of Buffalo Blood. Indian J. Anim. Sci., *51*:363, 1981.

Sodhi, S.P.S., and Singh, A.: Blood and Plasma Volumes and Changes in the Electrolyte Content under Stress and Normal Conditions in Buffalo Calves. Indian J. Vet., *44(5)*:305, 1975.

Sulong, A., et al.: Haematology of the Malaysian Swamp Buffalo (Bubalus bubalis). Pertanika, *3*:66, 1980. (Vet. Bull., *51*:688 1981.)

Thangaraj, T.M., et al.: Haematological Changes in Neonate of Bubalus bubalis. Indian J. Dairy Sci., 32:240, 1979.

Thimmaiah, K., et al.: Iron Content of the Buffalo Blood and Its Effect on Erythrocyte Sedimentation Rate, Packed Cell Volume and Hb Content at Different Ages. Meysore J. Agric. Sci., 10(2):290, 1976.

Vihan, V.S., et al.: A Note on Electrophoretic Pattern of Serum Protein in Some Disease Conditions among Buffaloes. Indian J. Anim. Sci., 43:546, 1973.

Vogel, J., and Vogel, L.: Some Haematological Indices of the Buffalo (Bubalus bubalis). Veterinaria (Rio de Janeiro), 20:166, 1967.

Other Wild and Domesticated Animals

(Titles in parentheses are translations of foreign language titles.)

Allen, P.Z., and Dalton, E.J.: Studies on Equine Immunoglobins. IV. Immunoglobins of the Donkey. Immunology, 28:187, 1975.

Banerjee, S., et al.: Hematological Studies in the Normal Adult Indian Camel (Camelus dromedarius). Amer. J. Physiol., 203:1185, 1962.

Bhatt, P.L., and Kohli, R.N.: A Preliminary Study on Camel's Blood Sedimentation Rate. Indian Vet. J., 36:376, 1959.

Bush, M., et al.: Hematology and Serum Chemistry Profiles for Giraffes (Giraffa camelopardalis): Variations with Sex, Age, and Restraint. J. Zoo Anim. Med., 11:122, 1980.

Bush, M., et al.: Hematologic and Serum Chemistry Values of Captive Scimitar-Horned Oryx (Oryx tao): Variations with Age and Sex. J. Zoo Anim. Med., 14:51, 1983.

Chapman, D.I., et al.: Some Haematological Data for Fallow Deer (Dama dama) in England. Res. Vet. Sci., 33:205, 1982.

Cornelius, C.E., and Kaneko, J.J.: Erythrocyte Life Span in the Guanaco. Science, 137:673, 1962.

Currier, M.J.P., and Russell, K.R.: Hematology and Blood Chemistry of the Mountain Lion (Felis concolor). J. Wildl. Dis., 18:99, 1982.

Davis, D.D., and Story, H.E.: The Female External Genitalia of the Spotted Hyena. Fieldiana Zool., 31:277, 1949.

Davis, T.P., et al.: Hormonal, Hematologic, and Other Biochemical Constituents in the Burro, Equinus asinus. J. Equine Med. Surg., 2:389, 1978.

Debbie, J.G., and Clausen, B.: Some Hematological Values of Free-Ranging African Elephants. J. Wildl. Dis., 11:79, 1975.

Dhindsa, D.S., et al.: Comparative Studies of the Respiratory Functions of Mammalian Blood. VIII. Asian Elephant (Elephas maximus) and African Elephant (Loxodonta africana africana). Respir. Physiol., 14:332, 1972.

Eitan, A., Aloni, B., and Livne, A.: Unique Properties of the Camel Erythrocyte Membrane. II. Organization of Membrane Proteins. Biochim. Biophys. Acta, 426(4):647, 1976.

Farahat, A.A., et al.: Studies on Foetal Haemopoiesis of Camel (Camelus dromedarius). J. Egypt. Vet. Med. Ass., 38:45, 1980.

Gates, N.L., and Goering, E.K.: Hematologic Values of Conditioned Captive Wild Coyotes. J. Wildl. Dis., 12:402, 1976.

Ghodsiam, I., et al.: A Study of Some Haematological Parameters in the Iranian Camel. Trop. Anim. Health Prod., 10(2):109, 1978.

Ghosal, A.K., et al.: Studies on the Seasonal Variation in the Blood Contituents of Indian Camels (Camelus dromedarius). Indian J. Anim. Sci., 43(7):642, 1974.

Gibbs, H.C.: Some Haematological Values for the Barren-Ground Caribou. Can. J. Comp. Med. Vet. Sci., 24:150, 1960.

Hawkey, C.M., et al.: Normal and Clinical Haematology in the Yak (Bos grunniens). Res. Vet. Sci., 34:31, 1983.

Hawley, A.W.L., and Peden, D.G.: Effects of Ration, Season and Animal Handling on Composition of Bison and Cattle Blood. J. Wildl. Dis., 18:321, 1982.

Jainudeen, M.R., and Jayasinghe, J.B.: Hemogram of the Domesticated Asiatic Elephant (Elephas maximus). J. Zoo Anim. Med., 2(3):5, 1971.

Jeffcott, L.B.: Clinical Haematology of the Horse. In Comparative Clinical Haematology. Archer, R.K., and Jeffcott, L.B., eds. Blackwell Scientific Publications, Oxford, p. 161, 1977.

Kehar, N.D., and Murty, V.N.: Physiological Studies on the Blood of Domestic Animals. II. Male Buffaloes, Indian J. Vet. Sci. Anim. Husb., 21:13, 1951.

Khan, A.A., and Kohli, I.S.: A Note on Some Haematological Studies on Male Camel (Camelus dromedarius) before and during Rut. Indian. J. Anim. Sci., 48:325, 1978.

Kohli, R.N.: Cellular Micrometry of Camel's Blood. Indian Vet. J., 40:134, 1963.

Kraft, H.: Untersuchungen über das Blutbild der Cameliden. Münch. Tierärztl. Wschr., 70:371, 1957.

Kuntze, A., and Hunsdorff, P.: Evaluation of Haematological and Biochemical Findings Obtained from Healthy and Diseased Female Elephants (Elephas maximus). Internationalen Symposiums über die Erkrankungen Zootiere, Berlin, p. 337, 1981.

Lee, J., et al.: Some Blood Values of Wild Polar Bears. j. Wildl. Management, 41:520, 1977.

Lemmer, B. et al.: Laboratory Diagnostic Examinations of Haflinger Horses and Mules (Pack-Animals of the German Federal Armed Forces). I. Haematology. Tierärztl. Prax., 8:245, 1980.

Lewis, J.H.: Comparative Hematology: Studies on Elephants, Elephas maximus. Comp. Biochem. Physiol., 49A:175, 1974.

Little, A., et al.: Blood Electrolytes in the Australian Camel. Aust. J. Exp. Biol. Med. Sci., 48:17, 1970.

Majeed, M.A., et al.: Effects of Sex and Season on 10 Haematological Values of Normal Adult One-humped Camel. Rev. Elev. Med. Vet. Pays Trop., 33:135, 1980. (Vet Bull., 51:592(4262).

Montes, G., et al.: (Haematological Values, Total Blood Protein and Fibrinogen in Alpacas (Lama pacos) in Parinacota Province, Chile). Arch. Med. Vet. Chile, 15:37:1983.

Morris, P.G.D.: Comparative Blood Picture of Army Mules and Horses. Vet. J., 98:224, 1942.

Nassar, S.M., et al.: Influence of Sex on the Normal Blood Picture of Adult Egyptian Camel (Camelus dromedarius). Assiut Vet. Med. J., 4:43, 1977.

Nayeri, G.D.: Blood Characteristics of the Adult Donkey. Zentralbl. Veterinärmed., 25A:541, 1978.

Neser, C.P.: The Blood of Equines. 9th and 10th Rep., Dir. Vet. Educ. Res., p. 479. Pretoria, Union of South Africa, 1923.

Nirmalan, G., et al.: Hematology of the Indian Elephant (Elephas maximus). Canad. J. Physiol. Pharmacol., 45:985, 1967.

Pedersen, R.J., and Pedersen, A.A.: Blood Chemistry and Hematology of Elk. J. Wildl. Management, 39:617, 1975.

Perk, K.: The Camel's Erythrocyte. Nature, *200*:272, 1963.

Raphael, B.L., et al.: Hematologic and Serum Chemistry Values for Captive Springbok (Antidorcas marsupialis). J. Zoo Anim. Med., *13(2)*:65, 1982.

Rehbinder, C., and Edqvist, L.-E.: Influence of Stress on Some Blood Constituents in Reindeer (Ragiferi tarandus). Acta Vet. Scand., *22*:480, 1981.

Rich, J.E., and Gates, N.L.: Hematologic and Serum Chemistry Values of Pen-Raised Coyotes. J. Wildl. Dis., *15*:115, 1979.

Riegel, K., et al.: Comparative Studies on the Respiratory Functions of Mammalian Blood. IV. Fetal and Adult African Elephant Blood. Respir. Physiol., *2*:182, 1967.

Sahu, R.N., et al.: Blood Studies in Yaks of Sikkim. Indian Vet. J., *58*:614, 1981.

Sastry, G.A., and Dhanda, M.R.: Studies on the Blood of Mules. Indian Vet. J., *29*:395, 478, 1953.

Seal, U.S., et al.: Blood Analyses of Wolf Pups and Their Ecological and Metabolic Interpretation. J. Mammal., *56*:64, 1975.

Seidel, B.: Klinischer Beitrag zur Hämatologie bei Eisbären, Thalarctos maritimus. Milu, Berlin, 5:298, 1980. (Vet. Bull., *51*:127, 1981.)

Sharma, M.C., et al.: Normal Blood Values of Indian Mules. Indian Vet. J., *58(11)*:874, 1981.

Simon, K.J.: Haematological Studies on Elephants. Indian Vet. J., *38*:241, 1961.

Smith, G.J., and Rongstad, O.J.: Serological and Haematological Values of Wild Coyotes in Wisconsin. J. Wildl. Dis., *16*:491, 1980.

Soliman, M.K., and El Amrousi, S.: Erythrocyte Fragility of Healthy Fowl, Dog, Sheep, Cattle, Buffalo, Horse and Camel Blood. Vet., Rec., *78*:429, 1966.

Soni, B.K., and Aggarwala, A.C.: Studies in the Physiology of the Camel (Camelus dromedarius). Indian Vet. J., *35*:209, 1958.

Straub, R., et al.: Serum-Lipids in Horses, Ponies, Donkeys and Mules. Proc. First Int. Symposium on Equine Hematology, Amer. Ass. Equine Pract., p. 232, 1975.

Timisjärvi, J., et al.: Haematological Values for Reindeer. J. Wildl. Management, *45*:976, 1981.

Tumbleson, M.E., et al.: Serum Biochemic and Hematologic Parameters of Adult Aoudads (Ammotragus lervia) in Captivity. Lab. Anim. Care, *20 (Part 1)*:242, 1970.

Vaughn, H.W. et al.: A Study of Reproduction, Disease and Physiological Blood and Serum Values in Idaho Elk. J. Wildl. Dis., *9*:296, 1973.

Wilding, J.L., et al.: Some Blood Values of the Southwestern Burro (Equus asinus asinus). Amer. J. Vet. Res., *13*:509, 1952.

Wilson, P.R., and Pauli, J.V.: blood Constituents of Farmed Red Deer (Cervus elaphus). I. Haematological Values. N.Z. Vet. J., *30*:174, 1982.

Wolfe, G., et al.: Hematologic and Serum Chemical Values of Adult Female Rocky Mountain Elk from New Mexico and Oklahoma. J. Wildl. Dis., *18*:223, 1982.

Woodford, M.H.: Blood Characteristics of the African Elephant (Loxodonta africana cyclotis). J. Wildl. Dis., *15*:111, 1979.

Young, E., and Lombard, C.J.: Physiological Values of the African Elephant (Loxodanta africana). The Veterinarian, *4*:169, 1967.

13

The Hematopoietic System

HEMATOPOIESIS IN PRENATAL AND
EARLY POSTNATAL LIFE   350
Dog   350
Cat   351
Cow   352
Fetal and Early Postnatal Erythrocyte
Morphology   355

HEMATOPOIESIS IN GROWING AND
ADULT ANIMALS   359
The Bone Marrow   359
Transit of Cells from Marrow to Blood   362
Hematopoiesis in Avian Marrow   364

The Hematopoieic Stem Cells   365
Factors Regulating Hematopoiesis   368

LYMPHOID (LYMPHATIC) TISSUES   372
The Thymus   373
The Spleen   375
The Lymph Nodes and Follicles   379

OTHER TISSUES AND ORGANS   380
The Mononuclear Phagocyte System   380
The Liver   380
The Stomach   381
The Intestinal Mucosa and Iron Stores   382
The Kidney   383

Hematopoiesis, or hemopoiesis, means making blood, particularly blood cells. The hematopoietic system is widely distributed and includes organs having functions other than contributing to blood formation (Table 13–1).

HEMATOPOIESIS IN PRENATAL AND EARLY POSTNATAL LIFE

During intrauterine life, hematopoietic cells are first recognized in the yolk sac both in mammalian and avian embryos. Liver and spleen successively become hematopoietically active in the mammalian fetus, the liver usually being more active than the spleen. Finally, in both birds and mammals, the bone marrow becomes the major site of hematopoiesis. This progression in sites of hematopoiesis is believed to result from in situ differentiation of circulating stem cells (Douaren et al., 1975). Stem cells to the bursa of Fabricius in birds and the thymus in mammals and birds are also supplied through the circulation. During postnatal life, hematopoiesis is restricted almost exclusively to the bone marrow, while the spleen and liver are usually inactive but retain hematopoietic potential to be expressed at times of need generally as-

sociated with bone marrow hypoplasia or aplasia.

Dog

Prenatal and postnatal hematopoiesis in the beagle dog has been described (Andersen and Goldman, 1970; Andersen and Schalm, 1970). The gestation period in the beagle ranged from 60–65 days. Extraembryonic erythropoiesis was observed in the allantois of a 5-mm embryo at 23 days postcoitum (Fig. 13–1). Intraembryonic erythropoiesis was seen in a 10.5-mm embryo at 24 days postcoitum (Fig. 13–2). Erythropoiesis was a prominent feature of the liver by the fortieth day. In the spleen, slight evidence of early red and white pulp differentiation was present in a 45-day-old fetus. Bone marrow from the mid-diaphysis of a humerus at 48 days was characterized by poorly defined sinusoids and beginning myelopoiesis. By the fifty-eighth day, bone marrow presented well-defined sinusoids and organized hematopoietic tissue.

During the first week of postnatal life, scattered hematopoietic foci remained in the liver, but disappeared by the forty-fifth day. Splenic hematopoiesis was active at birth and continued at gradually reduced levels up to 175 days. Developing lymphocytic nodules were present in the spleen at birth and were dis-

Table 13-1. Hematopoietic Organs and Tissues and Their Related Functions

Organ or Tissue		Functions
Bone marrow	1.	Hematopoiesis—production of erythrocytes, granulocytes, monocytes, platelets, and B-lymphocytes; supplies stem cells for lymphocyte production elsewhere.
	2.	Stores iron.
Thymus	1.	A central lymphoid organ concerned with differentiation of bone marrow-derived precursor cells into immunologically competent T-lymphocytes involved in cellular immunity, and production of lymphokines.
Lymph nodes and follicles	1.	Produce lymphocytes and plasma cells.
	2.	Actively engage in antibody synthesis.
Spleen	1.	Produces lymphocytes and plasma cells.
	2.	Antibody synthesis.
	3.	Reservoir of erythrocytes and platelets.
	4.	Destroys senescent and abnormal erythrocytes and degrades hemoglobin.
	5.	Stores iron.
	6.	Pitting function—removes Howell-Jolly bodies, Heinz bodies, nuclei, and parasites from erythrocytes and possibly returns the purged cells to the circulation.
	7.	Retains its embryonic potential for hematopoiesis.
Mononuclear phagocyte system (reticuloendothelial system)	1.	A major phagocytic system of the body concerned with cellular defense in microbial infection.
	2.	Destroys various blood cells.
	3.	Degrades hemoglobin into iron, globin, and free bilirubin.
	4.	Stores iron.
	5.	Secretes macromolecules of biologic importance, e.g., colony-stimulating factor, complement, etc.
Liver	1.	Stores vitamin B_{12}, folate, and iron.
	2.	Produces most of the coagulation factors, albumin, and some globulins.
	3.	Converts free bilirubin to bilirubin glucuronide for excretion into bile and participates in enterohepatic circulation of urobilinogen.
	4.	Produces a precursor (an α-globulin) of erythropoietin or some actual erythropoietin.
	5.	Retains its embryonic potential for hematopoiesis.
Stomach and intestine	1.	Stomach produces (*a*) HCl for release of iron from complex organic molecules and (*b*) intrinsic factor to facilitate absorption of vitamin B_{12}.
	2.	Intestinal mucosa is involved in absorption of vitamin B_{12} and folates and controls the rate of iron absorption in relation to body needs.
Kidney	1.	Produces erythropoietin and also thrombopoietin.
	2.	Degrades excessively filtered hemoglobin to iron and bilirubin for excretion into urine.

tinct by the forty-fifth day. The bone marrow was hypercellular in the young pup as a result of active erythropoiesis, granulopoiesis, and megakaryocytopoiesis (Fig. 13–3).

Prenatal development of the canine thymus and secondary lymphoid tissue has been investigated (Kelly, 1963). Beginning formation of the thymus was observed in an embryo at 25 days, with rapid development to nearly adult structure by the fortieth day. Lymph node formation had begun by the forty-eighth day, and lymphocytes were appearing in the spleen by the fifty-fourth day. At birth, Peyer's patches were present in the gut, and the structure of lymphoid organs was well advanced toward adult form.

Cat

The liver is the major center for hematopoiesis during the greater portion of fetal life. A liver-impression film from a 35-day-old feline fetus (average gestation, 61 days) contained large clusters of erythropoietic cells. Some fully hemoglobinized metarubricytes were megaloblastoid (Fig. 13–4). Granulopoiesis was less prominent but was in evi-

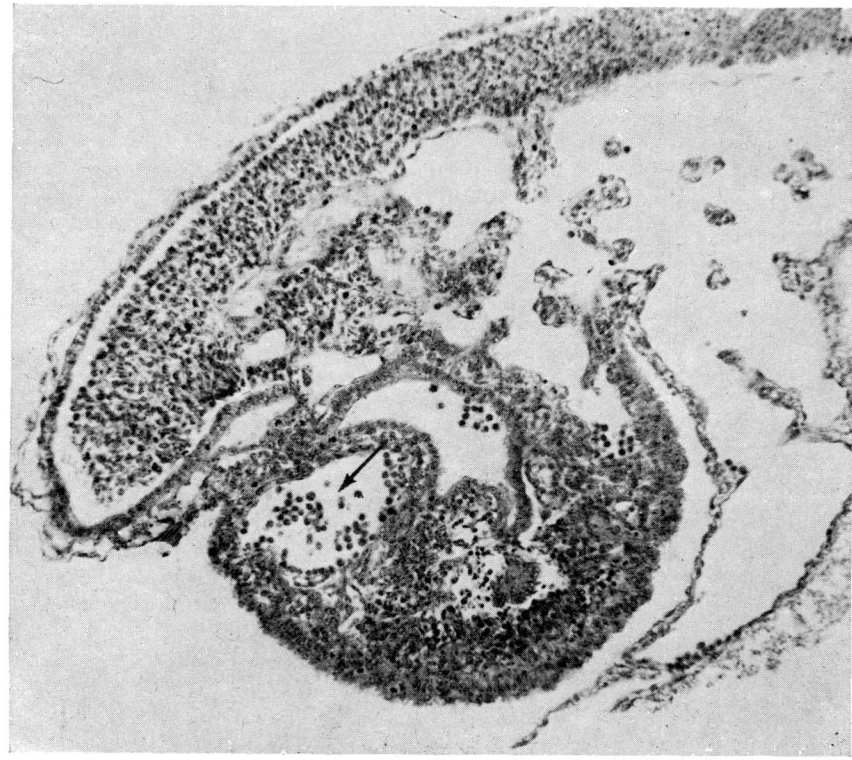

Fig. 13–1.   Allantois from a 5-mm canine embryo, 23 days postcoitum, demonstrating extraembryonic erythropoiesis. Blood-forming tissue consists of tubules or cords of endothelial cells with primitive nucleated erythrocytes in the lumen *(arrow)*. H and E stain, ×80. (From Andersen and Schalm, 1970, p. 262; courtesy of Iowa State University Press.)

dence. A band neutrophil with female sex chromatin lobe (drumstick or Barr body) was seen (Fig. 13–5A), as was a megakaryocyte (Fig. 13–5B).

Hematopoiesis in 65 embryos of 22 cats was investigated by Tiedemann and Ooyen (1978). Relative hematopoietic contributions of the yolk sac, liver, spleen, and bone marrow during intrauterine life are depicted in Figure 13–6. Erythropoiesis in the yolk sac was evident up to a period of 30 days, with peak erythropoietic activity on the nineteenth day. Neutrophils and platelets were seen on the seventeenth day and eosinophils and lymphocytes on the twenty-fifth day. Hepatic hematopoiesis began with erythropoiesis on the twentieth day and granulopoiesis on the twenty-fifth day. Splenic hematopoiesis began about the thirty-sixth day, but contributed little to the blood. Bone marrow activity commenced at mid-term and supplied about 50% of the blood cells by the forty-fifth day. PCV increased from 22% on the thirty-sixth

day to 47% at birth, exceeding normal adult values. RBC count increased from 0.8 million/µl on the twenty-fifth day to 3.8 million on the forty-fifth day and 6.3 million at birth. WBC count was 880/µl of blood on the forty-fifth day and 6,400 at birth. Nucleated erythrocytes were 98% on the nineteenth day and predominated from the thirty-sixth through forty-fifth days, but were exceeded by leukocytes at birth. It was shown that the yolk sac of the cat produces definitive red cells and megakaryocytes, in comparison to the production almost exclusively of primitive erythroid cells in the mouse, rat, and human.

Cow

Hematopoiesis in the bovine embryo and fetus has been described (Winqvist, 1954). The smallest embryo examined (4 mm) presented primitive nucleated erythrocytes that developed extravascularly. Circulating nucleated erythrocytes of various sizes are shown in Figure 13–7. The first evidence of

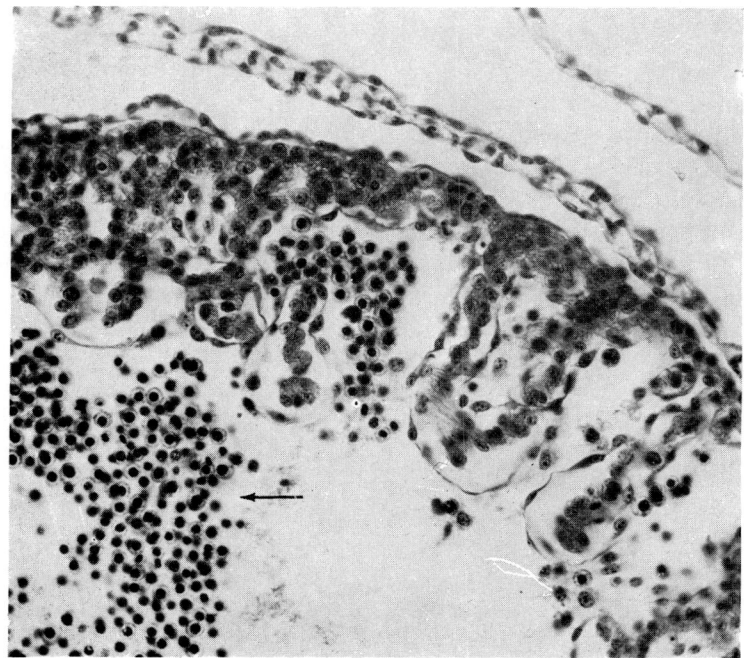

Fig. 13–2. Intraembryonic erythropoiesis in the primitive liver of a 10.5-mm Beagle embryo, 24 days postcoitum. The liver at this state is a hollow organ with its boundary consisting of hepatic cells and forming laminae; and it contains nucleated erythroblastic cells suspended in plasma *(arrow)*. H and E stain, × 600. (Courtesy of A.C. Andersen.)

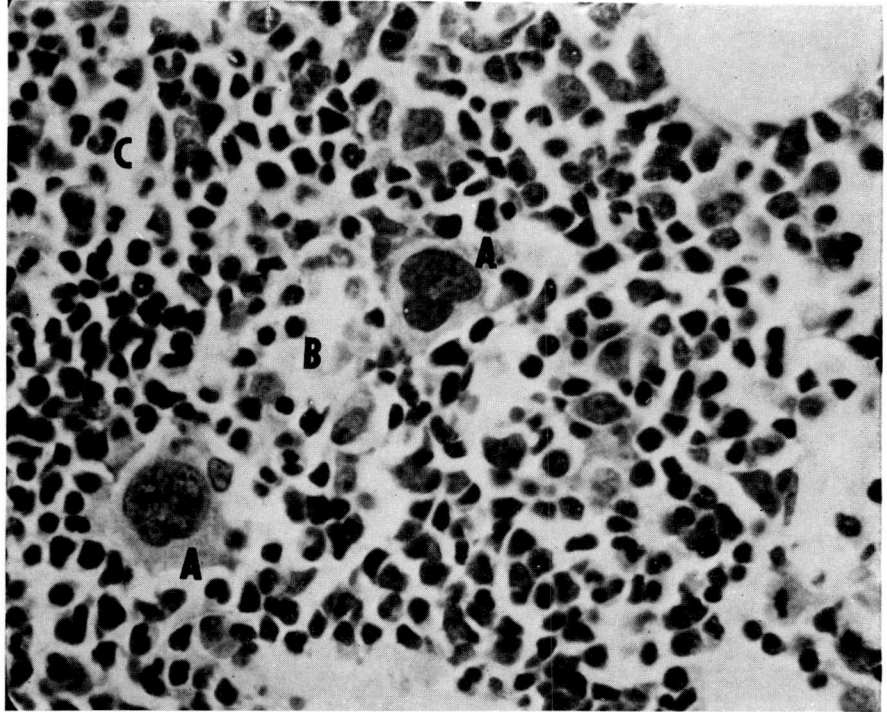

Fig. 13–3. Histologic section of bone marrow from the mid-diaphysis of the femur of a 14-day-old beagle pup. *A,* megakaryocyte; *B,* nucleated erythrocytes; and *C,* band neutrophils. H and E stain, × 650. (Courtesy of A.C. Andersen.)

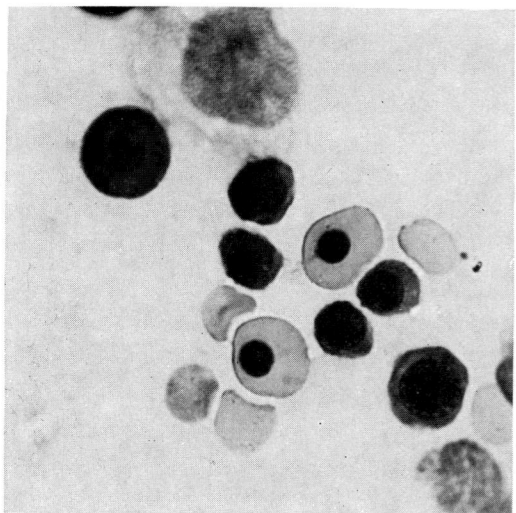

Fig. 13–4. Liver-impression film of a 35-day feline fetus showing erythropoiesis. Dark-staining cells are rubricytes in various stages of maturation. Two megaloblastoid normochromic metarubricytes are present. ×3,200.

extravascular erythrocyte formation was observed in the liver of embryos 4–8 mm in length (about 28 days of gestation). Megakaryocytes at various stages of development were also observed. A few neutrophilic myelocytes were detected in both the circulating blood and the hematopoietic foci of the liver in 1.2- to 1.3-cm embryos (about 33 days). Hepatic hematopoiesis remained a prominent feature in fetuses up to 35 cm in length (about 140 days), followed by a gradual decrease with complete disappearance by birth. Gestation period in the cow varies from 273–290 days.

Splenic hematopoiesis began at about the 7.0-cm stage (about 60 days) and was prominent in fetuses up to 60 cm in length (about 200 days), after which it gradually subsided until birth. Erythrocytes, granulocytes, lymphocytes, and megakaryocytes were formed in the spleen as well as in other lymphocytic foci. Even in newborn calves, the prefemoral lymph nodes were observed to be a site of lively formation of neutrophils. Phagocytosis of erythrocytes by fixed reticulum cells of hemolymph nodes occurred in calves and became a characteristic feature of adult cattle.

The newly formed marrow cavity of an 18-cm (about 100 days) bovine embryo contained erythropoietic foci, megakaryocytes of varying maturity, and a small number of immature eosinophils and neutrophils. All hematopoietic cells were situated extravascularly. Erythropoiesis predominated, as shown by a myeloid:erythroid ratio of less than 0.1:1.0. Extrusion of nuclei from metarubricytes was common at this as well as later stages. At the 30-cm stage (about 120 days), considerable numbers of neutrophilic myelocytes and metamyelocytes were present, and in the 50-

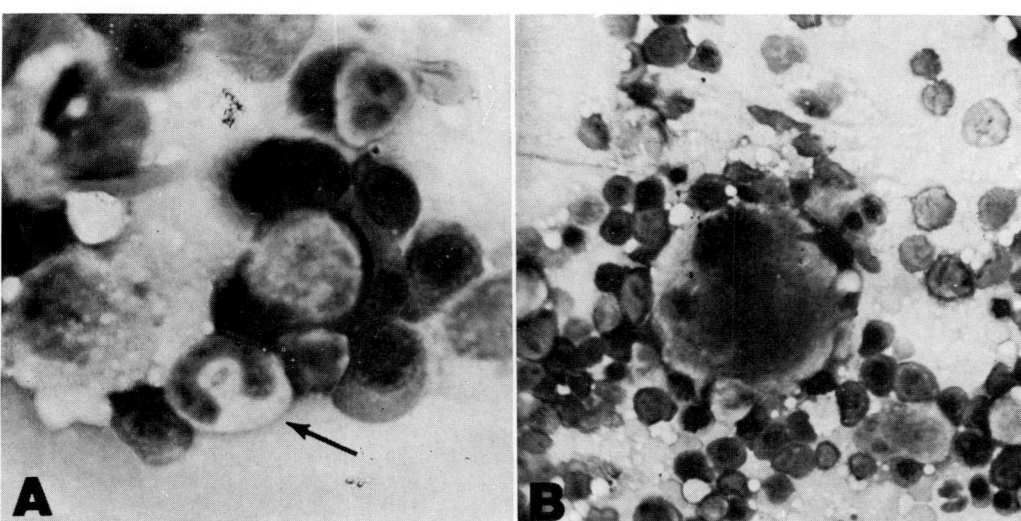

Fig. 13–5. *A,* Liver-impression film of a 35-day feline fetus. *Arrow* points to a neutrophilic band cell with a female sex chromatin lobe showing faintly between the arms of the U-shaped nucleus. ×3,200. *B,* Liver-impression film of a 35-day feline fetus presenting a megakaryocyte (giant cell in picture center). ×1.070.

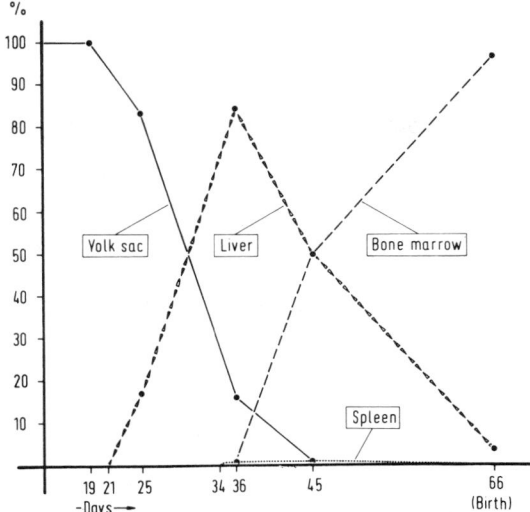

Fig. 13–6. Contribution of hematopoietic organs to prenatal blood formation in the cat. (From Tiedemann and Ooyen, 1978; courtesy of *Anatomy and Embryology.)*

cm fetus (about 6 months), the marrow contained an appreciable number of fat cells. Lymphocytic foci were not found in the bovine bone marrow, although nodule-like aggregations of lymphocytes have been described in human bone marrow.

Fetal and Early Postnatal Erythrocyte Morphology

Bovine, ovine, and equine fetal blood samples, provided from several research projects

were analyzed. Included were blood samples from calves on the day of birth through the first 16 weeks of life. The majority of the *bovine* fetal blood samples originated from a study in which either the cow or the fetus had been inoculated with the virus of bovine viral diarrhea (BVD). The changes in MCV with advancing gestation and during postnatal life are shown in Figure 13–8. Details relative to erythrocyte number and morphology and certain plasma characteristics for 6 normal fetuses and 8 others that had mild histologic lesions of BVD are presented in Table 13–2. Total and differential leukocyte counts for the same 14 fetuses, ranging from 90–280 days of development, are summarized in Table 13–3. The opinion of the pathologist was that lesions of BVD were so mild that blood morphology may not have been adversely affected.

Erythrocyte morphology in the youngest fetuses parallels that seen in acute blood loss in the calf or cow. Macrocytosis, marked anisocytosis, polychromasia, and a large number of nucleated erythrocytes characterized early fetal blood (Fig. 13–9). Erythrocyte size gradually decreased as gestation advanced (Figs. 13–9 to 13–14) so that at birth the mean erythrocyte volume was half that of fetal blood at 90–110 days of development. In fetuses over 200 days of age, polychromasia and

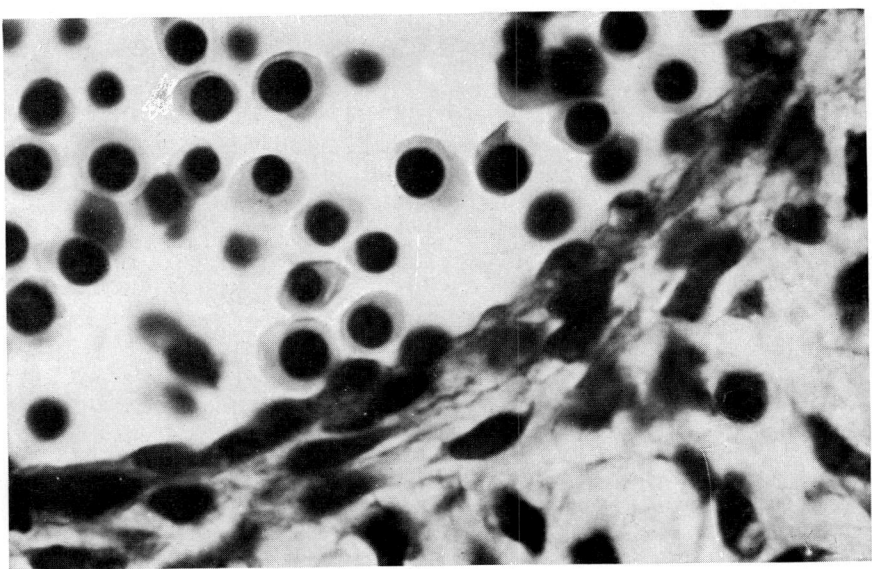

Fig. 13–7. Histologic section of the heart of a 1.0-cm bovine embryo. All erythrocytes are nucleated. ×3,600.

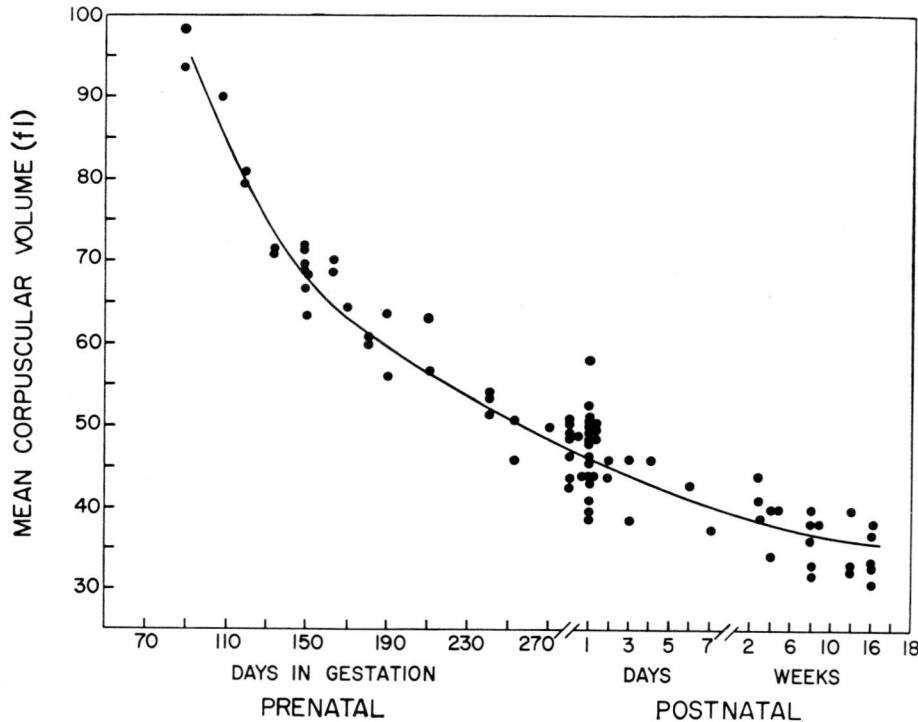

Fig. 13–8. Influence of advancing gestation and early postnatal life on the mean corpuscular volume of bovine erythrocytes.

nucleated erythrocytes were rare or absent. After birth, erythrocyte size continued to decrease to a mean MCV of 35.5 fl for calves 6–16 weeks of age (Fig. 13–8). The MCHC of fetal erythrocytes varied between 23.0 and 28.5%, and MCH decreased from 22.7 to 12.1 pg in parallel with the decreasing size of the erythrocytes. Plasma proteins increased from 3.0 g/dl in the youngest fetuses to 4.7–5.0 g/dl at birth. Fibrinogen was 0–0.1 g/dl during most of fetal life, but increased to 0.3–0.4 g/dl just before birth.

Total leukocyte counts varied from 1,600–4,600/μl between 90 and 180 days of fetal development (Table 13–3). The lymphocyte was the major leukocyte type, although

Table 13–2. Erythrocyte and Plasma Values in Bovine Fetal Blood of Normal Controls (N) and Fetuses Showing Mild Lesions of Bovine Viral Diarrhea (V)

Age (days)	RBC (×10⁶/μl)	Hb (g/dl)	PCV (%)	MCV (fl)	MCH (pg)	MCHC (%)	Icterus Index (units)	Plasma Proteins (g/dl)	Fibrin-ogen (g/dl)	Nucleated RBC No./ 100 WBC	Nucleated RBC Absolute No./μl
90 (N)	3.61	8.2	35	97.0	22.7	23.4	hemo[a]	3.2	0.10	376	6,016
110 (N)	3.00	7.5	27	90.0	25.0	27.8	hemo	3.0	0	59	2,537
135 (V)	4.21	8.2	30	71.3	19.4	27.3	5	3.0	0.10	49	980
150 (N)	5.97	10.9	40	67.0	18.2	27.3	7.5	3.7	0.10	85	2,805
150 (N)	6.09	10.7	42	69.0	17.5	25.5	5	3.5	0.10	58	1,450
150 (V)	5.99	10.0	40	66.8	16.7	25.0	7.5	3.6	0	205	5,330
165 (N)	4.70	7.6	33	70.2	16.2	23.0	5	3.6	0	90	1,620
165 (V)	4.84	9.4	33	68.2	19.4	28.5	7.5	3.8	0	51	1,122
180 (V)	5.82	9.1	35	60.1	15.6	26.0	10	3.8	0.30	68	3,128
210 (V)	5.27	7.8	30	56.9	14.8	26.2	2	4.0	0	3	219
225 (V)	5.65	8.1	31	54.4	14.3	26.1	7.5	4.0	0	0	0
255 (V)	6.99	8.6	32	45.8	12.3	26.9	2	4.9	0.10	0	0
280 (N)	8.20	11.2	41	50.0	13.6	27.3	2	4.7	0.40	0	0
280 (V)	7.55	9.1	32	42.4	12.1	28.4	15	5.0	0.30	0	0

[a]Hemo = hemolyzed

Table 13–3. Total and Differential Leukocyte Counts in Bovine Fetal Blood of Normal Controls (N) and Fetuses Showing Mild Lesions of Bovine Viral Diarrhea (V)

Age (days)	Total Leukocytes/μl	Neutrophils								Lymphocytes		Monocytes		Eosinophils		Basophils		Unclassified Cells	
		Myelocytes		Metamyelocytes		Bands		Segmenters											
		No.	%	No.	%	No.	%	No.	%	No.	%	No.	%	No.	%	No.	%	No.	%
90 (N)	1,600	0	—	0	—	0	—	0	—	512	32.0	704	44.0	0	—	0	—	384[a]	24.0
110 (N)	4,300	0	—	0	—	0	—	43	1.0	1,161	27.0	0	—	0	—	0	—	3,053[a]	71.0
135 (V)	2,000	0	—	0	—	40	2.0	260	13.0	1,640	82.0	0	—	40	2.0	0	—	20[a]	1.0
150 (N)	3,300	198	6.0	0	—	99	3.0	330	10.0	2,508	76.0	66	2.0	66	2.0	33	1.0	0	—
150 (N)	2,500	0	—	0	—	50	2.0	25	1.0	2,550	94.0	0	—	0	—	0	—	75[a]	3.0
150 (V)	2,600	0	—	0	—	52	2.0	78	3.0	2,392	92.0	78	3.0	0	—	0	—	0	—
165 (N)	1,800	252	14.0	0	—	0	—	90	5.0	1,314	73.0	0	—	18	1.0	18	1.0	108[b]	6.0
165 (V)	2,200	220	10.0	0	—	0	—	154	7.0	1,826	83.0	0	—	0	—	0	—	0	—
180 (V)	4,600	0	—	0	—	0	—	506	11.0	3,588	78.0	138	3.0	368	8.0	0	—	0	—
210 (V)	7,300	0	—	0	—	0	—	1,898	26.0	4,818	66.0	73	1.0	511	7.0	0	—	0	—
225 (V)	9,500	0	—	0	—	0	—	1,995	21.0	6,650	70.0	475	5.0	285	3.0	95	1.0	0	—
255 (V)	7,300	0	—	0	—	0	—	1,533	21.0	5,183	71.0	438	6.0	146	2.0	0	—	0	—
280 (N)	9,900	0	—	0	—	49	0.5	5,197	52.5	3,564	36.0	693	7.0	297	3.0	99	1.0	0	—
280 (V)	5,800	0	—	0	—	174	3.0	3,364	58.0	1,682	29.0	493	8.5	0	—	87	1.5	0	—

[a] Possibly myeloid cell precursors.
[b] Degenerated cells.

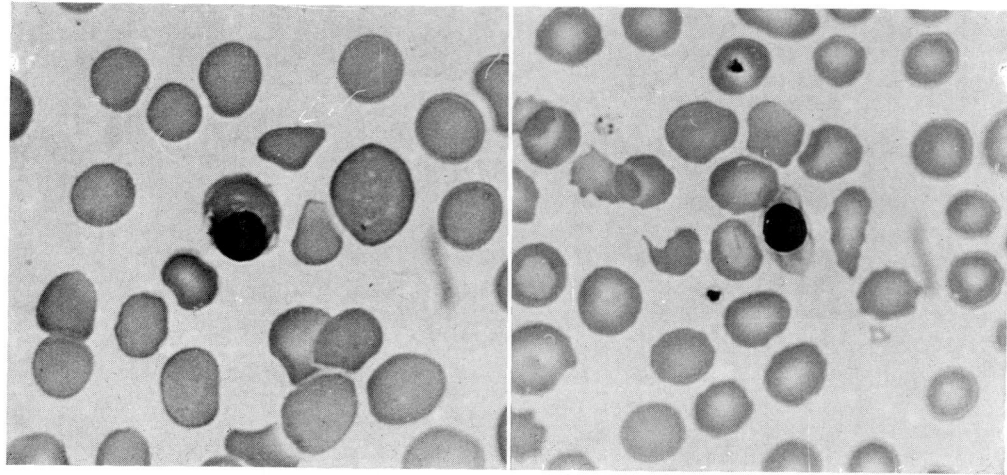

Fig. 13–9. Erythrocytes of a 90-day-old bovine fetus. MCV, 97 fl. ×3,060.

Fig. 13–10. Erythrocytes of a 5-month-old bovine fetus. MCV, 68.5 fl. ×3,060.

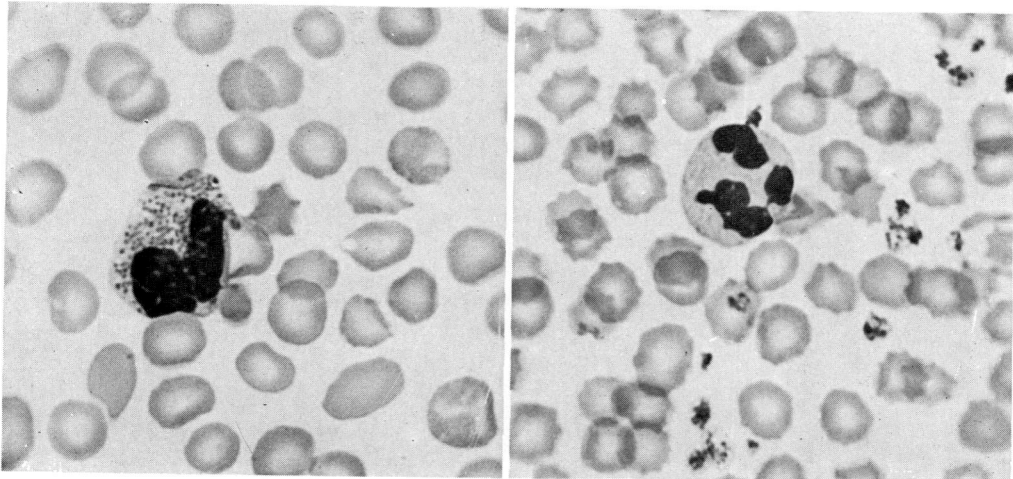

Fig. 13–11. Erythrocytes (MCV, 68.5 fl) and eosinophil of a 5-month-old bovine fetus. ×3,060.

Fig. 13–12. Erythrocytes (MCV, 56.9 fl), a neutrophil leukocyte, and platelets of a 7-month-old bovine fetus. ×3,060.

in the 2 youngest fetuses, unclassified cells were a prominent feature. A few eosinophils were first seen in a 135-day-old fetus, and a few basophils were seen at 150 days. Neutrophils, both mature and immature forms, were present in small numbers from day 110 onward. A change came at about 200 days of fetal life, when numbers of mature neutrophils and lymphocytes increased significantly, although neutrophils remained limited to between 21% and 26%. At birth, neutrophils exceeded lymphocytes. See Chapter 7 for additional data on neonatal

changes in differential leukocyte counts in calves; see also Hubbert and Hollen (1971).

Blood from *ovine* embryos and fetuses was obtained during several experiments. The youngest fetuses had been inoculated with bluetongue virus, while the fetuses in the final trimester of gestation (122–143 days) had catheters placed into the ascending vena cava and into the bladder via the urethra for renal clearance studies. Blood samples from the latter fetuses were taken at the time of initial surgery. Erythrocyte morphology and plasma characteristics are summarized in Table 13–4.

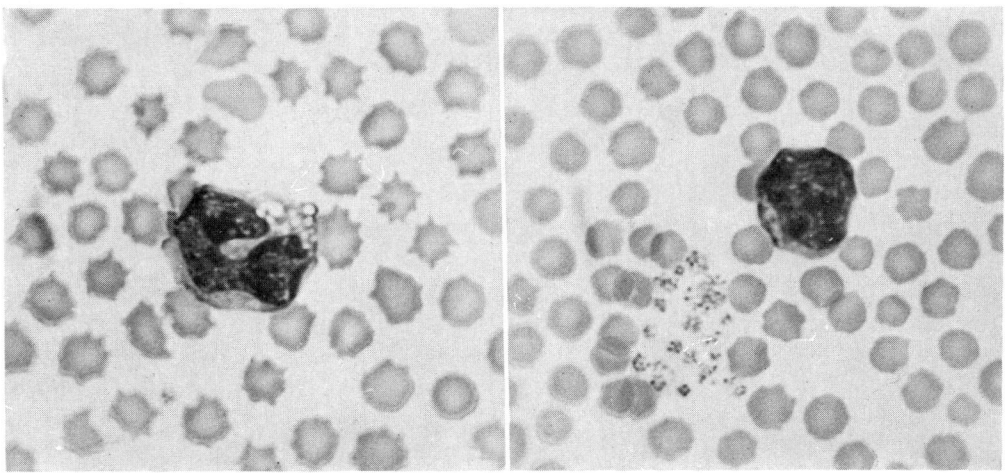

Fig. 13–13. Erythrocytes (MCV, 50 fl) and a monocyte of a newborn calf. ×3,060.

Fig. 13–14. Calf blood at 16 weeks of age. MCV, 32.7 fl. Lymphocyte and platelets. ×3,060.

The data were similar to those for bovine embryos and fetuses (Table 13–2), except that MCV was not as great in the youngest ovine embryos, while at birth the MCV was similar in lambs and calves.

The hemograms from 5 normal *equine* fetuses between 242 and 303 days of age (gestation, average 335 days) are summarized in Table 13–5. Nucleated erythrocytes were present in the blood of only 1 fetus. Icterus index tended to be somewhat higher in these late equine fetuses than those recorded for late bovine and ovine fetuses. Lymphocytes characteristically exceeded neutrophils, monocytes were rare, and eosinophils were observed in only 1 of the fetuses.

HEMATOPOIESIS IN GROWING AND ADULT ANIMALS

The Bone Marrow

Hematopoiesis during postnatal life occurs principally in the bone marrow. At first, the marrow of all bones is hematopoietically active. This activity involves a vigorous production of erythrocytes, granulocytes, monocytes, and megakaryocytes and a variable production of progenitors of T- and B-lymphocytes and plasma cells. During the phase of rapid growth of the young, blood volume is expanding and placing heavy demand for erythrocytes on the marrow. In addition, the fetal erythrocytes must be replaced by red

cells most suited to serve the air-breathing mammal. This strain on erythropoiesis is dramatically illustrated in the piglet during the first weeks of life (Table 10–1). As demand for erythrocytes decreases with approaching maturity, hematopoiesis recedes from the shafts of the long bones. Red, hematopoietically active marrow is replaced by resting yellow marrow. Active hematopoiesis continues throughout life in all flat bones, such as the sternum, ribs, pelvis, vertebrae, and skull, as well as in the epiphyses of the long bones.

Bone marrow consists of various blood cells and their precursors, reticular cells and reticular fibers, endothelial-lined sinusoids, and fat cells or adipocytes. The yellow marrow is limited to three types of cells: reticular cells, which are connected with the endosteum and blood capillaries; the endothelial cells forming the walls of capillaries and sinusoids; and the fat cells. The fat cells occupy space as hematopoiesis recedes and give up space as demand for expansion of red marrow occurs in response to continuous blood loss or hemolytic anemia. Transition from yellow to red marrow takes place in response to the hormone erythropoietin.

Blood supply to the marrow consists of a nutrient artery system that extends through the longitudinal axis of the bone and gives off radial branches that terminate at the periphery of the marrow to form vascular sinuses

Table 13–4.   Erythrocyte Morphology and Blood Plasma Characteristics of Ovine Embryos and Fetuses[a]

Age (days)	RBC (×10⁶/μl)	PCV (%)	Hb (g/dl)	MCV (fl)	MCH (pg)	MCHC (%)	Nucleated RBC/μl	Anisocytosis	Polychromasia	Poikilocytosis	Basophilic Stippling	Icterus Index (units)	Plasma Protein (g/dl)	Fibrinogen (g/dl)
62[b]	3.35	25	6.2	74.6	18.5	24.8	4,400	++	+++	++	—	hemo[c]	2.2	—
62[a]	4.10	32	8.8	78.0	21.4	27.5	9,240	++	+++	+	—	hemo	2.3	—
82[b]	5.05	31	7.6	61.4	15.1	24.5	2,925	+	++	+	—	hemo	3.0	—
100	5.20	34	9.3	65.4	17.9	27.3	620	++	++	++	++	—	—	—
100[b]	6.30	34	9.3	54.0	14.7	27.4	1,990	++	++	+	—	5	3.4	—
122	7.23	36	10.7	49.8	14.8	29.7	51	+	+	+	—	5	3.5	0.10
128	8.30	38	10.7	45.8	12.9	28.2	252	++	+	+	—	15	3.8	0.10
136	8.92	42	11.2	47.0	12.5	26.7	0	++	+	+	—	15	3.7	0.10
143	7.42	36	10.0	48.5	13.4	27.8	0	+	—	+	—	2	3.4	0.10
Birth	8.65	39	13.1	45.1	15.1	33.6	0	+	—	++	—	10	5.6	—

[a]—, not seen; +, slight or few; ++, moderate amount; +++, prominent or marked.
[b]Inoculated with bluetongue virus.
[c]hemo = hemolyzed.

Table 13–5. Hemograms of Five Normal Equine Fetuses in the Final Trimester of Gestation

Age (days)	242	244	244	291	303
RBC ($\times 10^6/\mu l$)	6.94	6.48	6.18	6.20	9.07
Hemoglobin (g/dl)	12.3	12.5	11.5	10.4	13.2
PCV (%)	40	37	36	33	39
MCV (fl)	57.6	57.1	58.3	53.2	43.0
MCH (pg)	17.8	19.2	18.6	16.7	14.5
MCHC (%)	30.8	33.8	31.9	31.5	33.8
Icterus index (units)	20	15	15	25	100
Plasma proteins (g/dl)	4.0	3.7	3.5	3.4	4.6
Fibrinogen (g/dl)	0.10	0.20	0.20	0.20	0.20
Nucleated RBC/100 WBC	0	64	0	0	0
Leukocytes/μl	4,000	1,890	1,700	1,600	3,700
Neutrophils	560	529	612	256	1,258
	(14.0%)	(28.0%)	(36.0%)	(16.0%)	(34.0%)
Lymphocytes	3,240	1,323	1,054	1,296	2,294
	(81.0%)	(70.0%)	(62.0%)	(81.0%)	(62.0%)
Monocytes	200	37	34	48	74
	(5.0%)	(2.0%)	(2.0%)	(3.0%)	(2.0%)
Eosinophils	0	0	0	0	74
					(2.0%)

that carry the blood back to a central vein (Fig. 13–15). The hematopoietic marrow of mammals lies between these broad radial sinuses (Fig. 13–16). The sinusoidal microcirculation is designed specifically to serve hematopoiesis, and when it is irreversibly injured, as demonstrated in locally irradiated bone marrow of the rat (Knospe et al., 1966), hematopoietic regeneration initially takes place, but 2–6 months later, aplasia develops as the

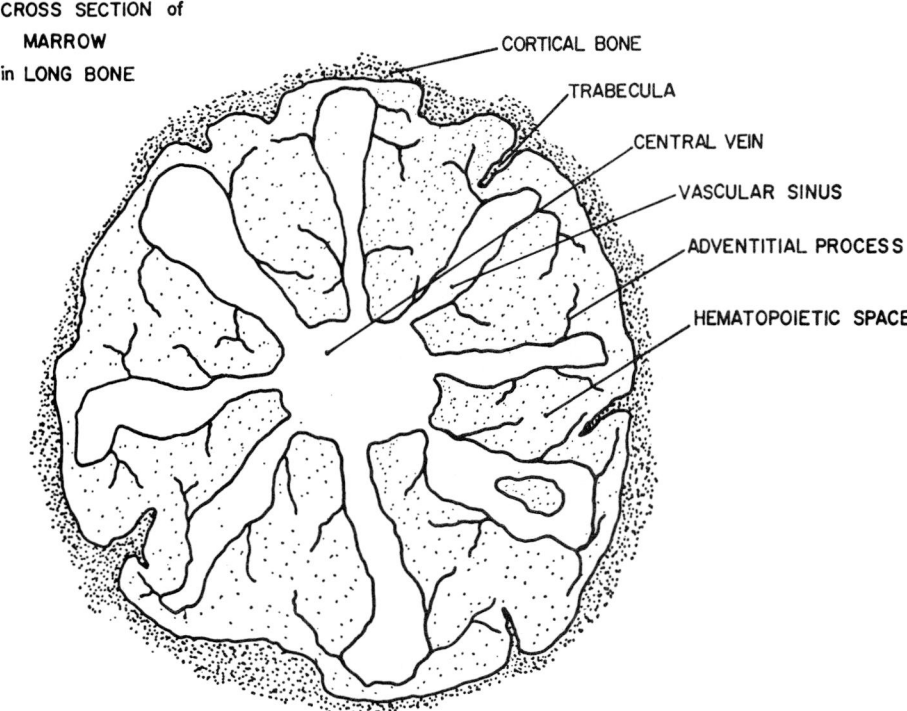

CROSS SECTION of
MARROW
in LONG BONE

CORTICAL BONE
TRABECULA
CENTRAL VEIN
VASCULAR SINUS
ADVENTITIAL PROCESS
HEMATOPOIETIC SPACE

Fig. 13–15. Organization of the venous vasculature of the marrow of a long bone. Thin-walled vascular sinuses originate at the periphery from termination of transverse branches of the nutrient artery (not shown). The vascular sinuses run transversely toward the center to join the central vein. Hematopoiesis takes place in the space between the vascular sinuses. Adventitial processes project into the hematopoietic space, producing partial compartmentalization. (From Weiss, 1967: courtesy of the author and J.B. Lippincott Co.)

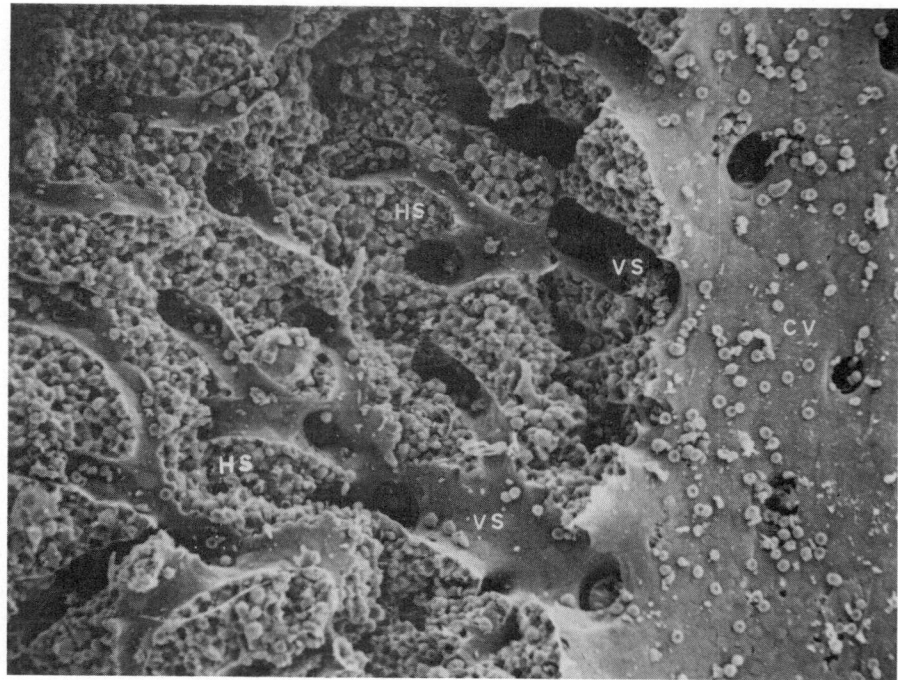

Fig. 13–16. A scanning electron micrograph of a rat bone marrow showing developing cells in hematopoietic spaces (HS), anastomosing venous sinusoids (VS), and central vein (CV). ×290. (Prepared with assistance of Dr. Prem Handagama.)

sinusoidal microcirculation becomes disrupted by chronic changes in bone marrow structure.

The bone marrow, while widely distributed, constitutes an organ about two-thirds the size of the liver. In 2 adult canine female littermates, the marrow volumes were found to be 289 ml and 319 ml, or 2.4% and 1.9% of body weight, respectively (Fairman and Whipple, 1933). In these dogs, the marrow weights were 61% and 67%, respectively, of the liver weights. Marrow volume in 2 rabbits was estimated at 2.0% and 2.5% of body weights (Nye, 1931), and functional bone marrow constituted 2% of body weight in guinea pigs (Yoffey, 1954).

Transit of Cells from Marrow to Blood

The process by which the extravascularly produced mammalian hematopoietic cells enter the blood has been investigated with the electron microscope (Aoki and Tavassoli, 1981; De Bruyn, 1981; Pease, 1956; Tavassoli, 1978, 1981; Weiss, 1965, 1967, 1970, 1981; Zamboni and Pease, 1961). The walls of the venous sinuses are remarkably thin (1–2 μm),

consisting of an inner endothelial lining, a basement membrane, and an outer adventitial cell layer in areas of maximum development (Fig. 13–17). In some areas the adventitial layer seems to be incomplete, with only the endothelial cells forming the wall structure. The endothelial lining may present varied anatomic features. It may appear discontinuous so that the hematopoietic cells appear to be exposed to an open sinus; it may appear continuous with or without preexisting pores; or the cytoplasmic extensions of the endothelial cells at places appear attenuated and show fenestrations spanned by thin diaphragms (De Bruyn, 1981). At places ends of the endothelial cells may overlap or interdigitate without forming tight junctions so that the cells can slide over each other in response to various stimuli and thereby change the luminal size and allow or disallow transmural passage of cells (Tavassoli, 1981). The endothelial cells are highly equipped with organelles essential for synthetic activity and exhibit endocytotic activity; both kinds of activities may be functionally important.

Recent studies on dynamics of red cell de-

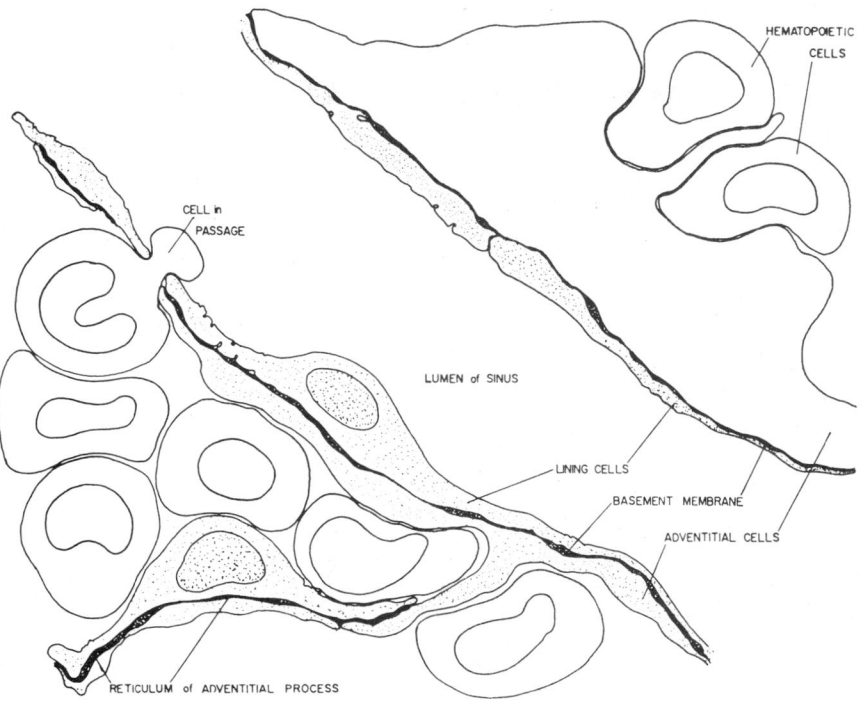

Fig. 13–17. Segment of the wall of a vascular sinus, including an adventitial process. The sinus wall is trilaminar in most places, consisting of a lining (or endothelial) cell, a basement membrane, and an adventitial cell. In places apertures may occur in the wall, and free cells may pass through such apertures. Elsewhere, the basement membrane and/or adventitial layer may be absent, resulting in a wall of one or two layers. The adventitial cells are commonly very voluminous and rarefied, extending deeply into the contiguous hematopoietic space and displacing hematopoietic cells. (The upper labeled adventitial cell exemplifies this.) An adventitial process is of the same structure as the sinus wall. (From Weiss, 1967; courtesy of the author and J.B. Lippincott Co.)

livery from the bone marrow into the blood indicate that the cell egress across the sinus wall is transcellular, not intercellular, and depends on the interaction between the migratory cell and the endothelium (Aoki and Tavassoli, 1981: De Bruyn, 1981; Tavassoli, 1981). This migration necessitates constant formation and repair of small apertures in the sinus wall. Cell migration is selective and depends on a variety of factors including deformability and surface characteristics of the migratory cells, surface characteristics of the endothelial cells, and the permissiveness of the endothelial wall. The adventitial layer modulates the rate of cell egress into circulation by its coverage of the sinus endothelium and by its dynamic contractile nature. For example, an increase in the rate of cell delivery is associated with a decrease in the coverage of endothelium by the adventitial layer or a reduction in the luminal size by contraction of adventitial cells. The adventitial cells may also project

cytoplasmic processes into the mass of maturing blood cells to partially encircle them at the same time that a portion of the venous sinus wall drops out, placing the encircled maturing hematopoietic cells within the circulation. The venous sinus and adventitial processes appear to form a reciprocating system whereby sinusoidal walls are "constantly in a state of dynamic flux and readjustment" (Zamboni and Pease, 1961). Branemark (1959) conducted in situ studies of living bone marrow in the rabbit and observed that the marrow sinuses exhibited rhythmic dilatations, with an increase in width of about 2–3 times normal occurring within a few minutes, and poured their contents into the circulation. Dilated sinuses dominated in highly hematopoietic marrow, and sinus dilatation occurred in response to reduced oxygen-carrying capacity of blood, as from severe blood loss.

The terminal stage of erythrocyte maturation occurs next to the venous sinus wall, and metarubricytes and reticulocytes can be seen pressing against the sinus wall. The nucleus is at the opposite end of the cell and can be seen to be extruded and then phagocytosed (Fig. 18–8). The reticulocytes, by pressing on the sinus wall, may create an opening in the endothelial cell through which they pass, or they may enter the sinus through an existing aperture; the diameter of these openings does not exceed 2 μm (Tavassoli, 1981). Reticulocytes may be held in the marrow by a stickiness of their surface membrane resulting from a coating of transferrin or a transferrin-like component (Jandl, 1960) or sialic acid residues, or both. This sticky surface coating diminishes as the reticulocytes mature, and then they are released through gaps in the sinus wall. In response to the need for increased erythropoiesis and release of erythrocytes to the blood, large clusters of early reticulocytes and rubricytes may press upon the sinus wall and may be incorporated into the circulation by disappearance of that portion of the wall structure. Erythropoietin not only enhances erythropoiesis, but also accelerates delivery of reticulocytes into the circulation. A disruption of marrow architecture such as by granulomatous inflammation, tumor metastasis, or leukemia is usually associated with inappropriate release of nucleated erythrocytes and/or appearance of deformed erythrocytes in the circulation.

Leukocytes are endowed with the ability of ameboid movement. Leukocytes are produced in the interior of the bone marrow parenchyma. These cells move into the sinus lumen by their own locomotion, passing through newly created apertures into the sinus wall. Leukocyte movement is influenced by cellular deformability, which increases with cell maturation. Leukocyte release into the circulation is influenced by surface charge, which decreases with cell maturation, and by hormonal factors such as neutrophil releasing factor (see Chapter 26). Under conditions of excessive need for granulocytes, immature as well as mature neutrophils enter the circulation in large numbers (left shift). A massive delivery of mature and immature granulocytes may occur as a result of breakage in the sinus wall followed by displacement of cells into vascular spaces.

Megakaryocytes are found adjacent to the sinus wall or may be seen where the wall structure is lacking. In the latter situation, the large size of the cell serves to complete the continuity of the sinus wall. The megakaryocyte is in a position to readily shed its platelets directly into the sinus lumen, or it extends long cytoplasmic extensions (proplatelets) through the sinus wall that subsequently break into platelets. Occasionally a megakaryocyte may enter the circulation as an intact cell and shed its platelets there or in the lungs (see Chapter 15).

Hematopoiesis in Avian Marrow

In birds, erythropoiesis and thrombopoiesis occur intravascularly while granulopoiesis takes place extravascularly. These processes can be readily demonstrated experimentally. The marrow of the radius and ulna of young pigeons can be simplified or rendered hypoplastic by subjecting the birds to starvation (Doan et al., 1925). After 10 days to 2 weeks, during which only water is allowed, the marrow becomes essentially devoid of hematopoietic activity. Food is then permitted and the birds are sacrificed at 24-hour intervals to remove marrow for fixation and sectioning. Within 24 hours considerable cellular activity is apparent, and separate foci of erythropoiesis and granulopoiesis can be distinguished. Erythropoiesis occurs within the vascular sinuses, while granulopoiesis takes place outside the vascular sinuses (Fig. 13–18). In histologic sections, the developing granulocytes are easily distinguished by the eosin-colored granules common to the heterophils of avian species. Electron microscopy (Campbell, 1967) reveals the wall of the vascular sinus to be formed by elongated lining cells, lacking basement membrane, which are continuous except where granulocytes are seen to be passing through. The immature erythroid cells appear to adhere to the sinus wall, while the more mature cells containing hemoglobin occur in the central area of the lumen. The marrow of avian species does not have megakaryocytes, but instead a nucleated cell line produces a definitive nucleated thrombocyte that serves the same function in hemostasis and blood clotting as the anuclear platelets of mammals.

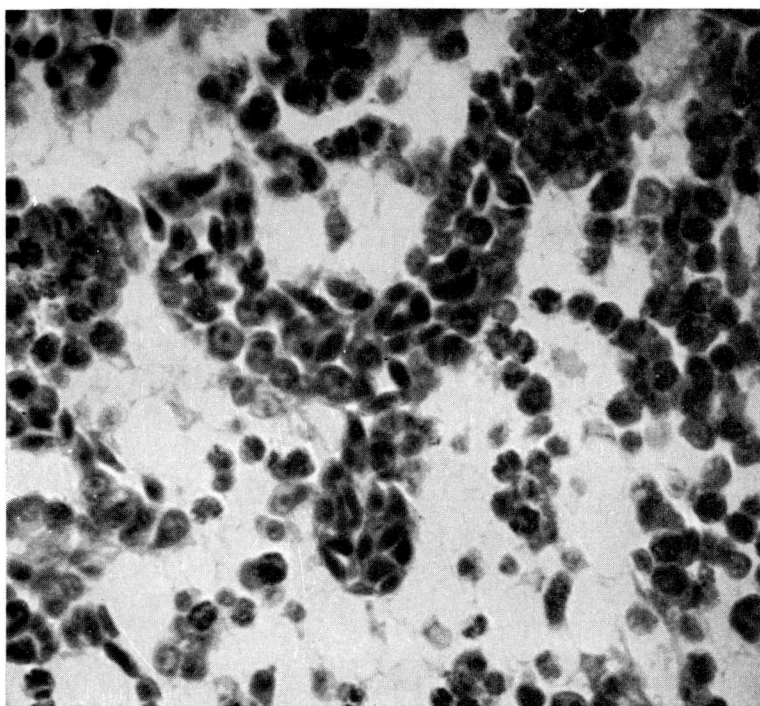

Fig. 13–18. Bone marrow section from the ulna of a young pigeon in which the marrow was first simplified by starvation. The Y-shaped cellular mass in the center is a site of active intravascular erythropoiesis.

Studies of hematopoiesis in the Japanese quail and chick indicated that the whole hematopoietic population of the bursa of Fabricius, bone marrow, and thymus is derived from blood-borne extrinsic stem cells originating in the yolk sac (Douaren et al., 1975).

The Hematopoietic Stem Cells

In the normal animal, numbers of erythrocytes and of each of the various leukocyte types remain relatively constant. Production and utilization of various cells remain in delicate balance. When this steady state is disturbed by reduced erythrocyte numbers, as in hemorrhage or hemolytic anemia, or by increased utilization or destruction of neutrophil leukocytes, as in inflammatory diseases, or by increased destruction of platelets, as in immune-mediated thrombocytopenia, the hematopoietic centers are stimulated to increase production of the needed cells. This means that for each cell type a stimulatory feedback mechanism exists that responds to the decreased cell population. It is believed that a compartment of primitive stem cells exists in the bone marrow that responds to

these demands and initiates production of additional precursor cells for the specific cell line that requires expansion.

In vitro and in vivo studies have revealed a structured hierarchy of multipotential, oligopotential, and unipotential stem cells of the formed elements of blood (see reviews by Ogawa et al., 1983; Lichtman, 1983). The most primitive pluripotential hematopoietic stem cells are capable of differentiating into oligopotential progenitor cells (cells capable of producing progenitors of two or more cell lines) which in turn differentiate into unipotential cells committed to produce a single lineage under appropriate environmental and humoral stimuli. The morphologic identity of these three types of stem cells is uncertain, but they appear to be lymphocyte-like (Fliedner et al., 1968, 1970; Richman et al., 1978; Thomas et al., 1965; Yoffey, 1964). The unipotential progenitor cells than develop into morphologically recognizable precursor cells, e.g., rubriblast, myeloblast, and megakaryoblast, which ultimately give rise to mature cells of the series under specific stimuli. Recent observations indicate existence of subsets of the pluripotential stem cells and committed progenitor cells of various cell lineages.

The Pluripotential Stem Cell

From the various theories proposed by early histologists regarding the origin of various blood cells, the one that has found support in the past and in recent years is that of Maximow (1924), who proposed that the myeloid and lymphoid cells originate separately but from a common progenitor cell. The current concept of hematopoiesis (Fig. 13–19) has evolved from a varied set of experimental observations such as in vivo studies on normal, irradiated, and mutant mice, in vitro culture studies of murine and human blood and bone marrow cells, in vivo cultures of bone marrow cells in diffusion chambers, chromosomal and enzymatic abnormalities in leukemic human patients, and chromosomal chimeric studies in mice. With the exception of basophils and mast cells, whose ancestry remains rather speculative, pathways for the development of recognizable lymphoid and myeloid elements have been fairly well delineated, although some modifications of the schema may be anticipated as active research in this field continues.

It is envisioned that erythrocytes, all leukocyte types, macrophages, mast cells, and megakaryocytes originate from a pluripotential stem cell (Cline and Golde, 1979; Metcalf, 1981; Miura, 1980; Quessenbery and Levitt,

1979). This progenitor cell is termed *the hematopoietic stem cell.* Its existence was demonstrated by Till and McCulloch (1961) in experiments in which normal mouse bone marrow cells were transplanted into heavily irradiated syngeneic mice. Macroscopic colonies, comprised of either pure or mixed populations of erythroid, neutrophilic, megakaryocytic, and undifferentiated cells were found to develop after 8–10 days on the surface of the spleen. Reinjection of cell suspensions from individual splenic colonies into irradiated mice again produced similar colonies. By clonal and chromosomal analysis (Becker et al., 1963), these colonies were found to originate from a single progenitor cell designated the colony forming unit in the spleen (CFU-S). The CFU-S is capable of self-renewal and differentiation into various types of progenitor cells; thus it has attributes of a pluripotential stem cell. Dedifferentiation of a progenitor cell into the pluripotential stem cell has not been found to occur (Metcalf, 1981). The presence of a small number of cells more primitive than CFU-S has been demonstrated in normal marrow (Abramson et al., 1977; Quessenberry and Levitt, 1979); these cells are capable of differentiating into myeloid and lymphoid progenitor cells. These observations are supported by the finding, although rare, of transformation of a myeloproliferative disorder into a lymphocytic leukemia (Barton et al., 1980).

Studies on human leukemias provide ad-

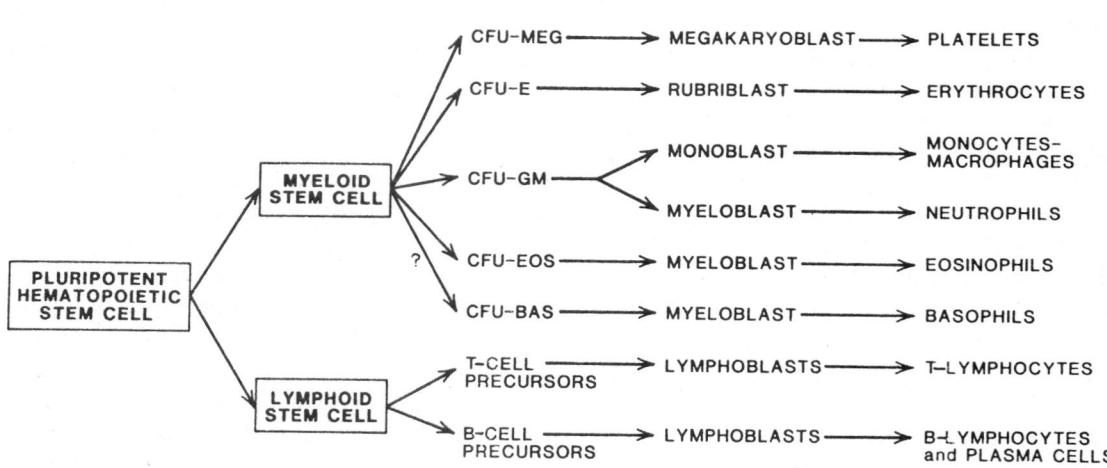

Fig. 13–19. Schematic diagram of hematopoietic differentiation of myeloid and lymphoid cells. CFU = colony forming unit.

ditional evidence for the existence of the various stem cells. A chromosomal abnormality is found in chronic granulocytic leukemia in humans (Nowell and Hungerford, 1961). The abnormal chromosome was designated Ph[1] for Philadelphia chromosome because of the location of the laboratory where the chromosome was first observed (Tough et al., 1961). The Ph[1] chromosome was demonstrated in erythroid, granulocytic, and possibly megakaryocytic cells of patients with chronic granulocytic leukemia (Whang et al., 1963). This finding implicated a common progenitor cell (clonal origin) for each of the three cell lines. Ph[1] was not found in lymphoid cells. Glucose-6-phosphate dehydrogenase (G-6-PD) has also been a useful marker. G-6-PD occurs in two isoenzyme forms, A and B. Females heterozygous for G-6-PD contain both isoenzymes in their somatic cells, including fibroblasts and bone marrow cells, although only one isoenzyme is found in an individual cell line because of random inactivation of the other isoenzyme during embryonic life. In such females, clonal proliferation of marrow cells, such as during chronic granulocytic leukemia, could be detected by the presence of one or the other isoenzyme in various myeloid cells. In chronic granulocytic leukemia patients with G-6-PD heterogeneity, the same isoenzyme is found in erythrocytes, neutrophils, monocytes, eosinophils, and platelets (Beutler et al., 1967; Douver et al., 1981).

The hematopoietic stem cell is considered to be a primitive cell of mesenchymal origin. During intrauterine life, such stem cells are first supplied by the embryonic yolk sac and then by the fetal liver, spleen, and bone marrow. In the adult life, bone marrow is the principal source in most species, although a small number of such stem cells can be found in the circulating blood (see literature review by Zwaan, 1982). Loutit (1967) postulated a stem cell concentration of 1:1,000 cells in bone marrow and 1:100,000 leukocytes in blood. Normal beagles were found to have 40–400 committed stem cells per milliliter of peripheral blood, and a 10 times greater number was found after repeated injection of dextran sulfate, a stem cell mobilizing agent (Fliedner, 1978). Migration of granulocytic progenitor

cells into blood can be induced by a variety of stimuli or agents, e.g., exercise, ACTH, dexamethasone, epinephrine, endotoxin, antigenic exposure, hypoxia, and localized irradiation (Barrett et al., 1978; Barton, 1981; Morra et al., 1981; Raghavachar et al., 1982). A high number of committed erythroid and granulocyte-macrophage stem cells is found in fetal blood (Barker, 1980; Linch et al., 1982; Roodman and Zanjani, 1979). Experimental evidence suggests that myeloid metaplasia involves colonization of migrating bone marrow stem cells at suitable extramedullary sites (Wang and Tobin, 1982).

Neoplastic and nonneoplastic disorders of stem cells have been uncovered in recent years. Neoplastic disorders include acute and chronic myelogenous leukemia (Douver et al., 1981; Lichtman, 1983), erythroleukemia (Roggli and Saleem, 1982), essential thrombocythemia (Fialkow et al., 1981), and polycythemia vera (Lichtman, 1983). Nonneoplastic disorders include cyclic hematopoiesis in gray collie dogs (Chapter 4) and pure red cell aplasia and aplastic anemia in humans. Some success has been achieved in correcting nonneoplastic disorders by proper marrow transplantation (Quessenberry and Levitt, 1979).

The Committed Hematopoietic Progenitor Cells

Provision for a committed unipotential progenitor cell between the primitive multipotential stem cell and the differentiated blast cell of a specific series serves to explain the selective depression of a specific cell series under experimental as well as certain natural conditions of disease. As an example, vinblastine administered to dogs was found to produce marked suppression of erythropoiesis and granulopoiesis, but megakaryocytopoiesis was little affected (Boggs et al., 1964). Both the multipotential and unipotential stem cell compartments must be self-perpetuating to be able to supply large numbers of cells on demand without exhaustion of the compartment (Lajtha et al., 1964; Morse and Stohlman, 1966). Under physiologic conditions, the replacement of mature blood cells as they become effete occurs possibly within the compartment of differentiated progenitor cells, with limited supplementation of each cell line from the undifferentiated stem cell compartment (Loutit, 1967). The stem cells are generally resting and require a serious insult to the hematopoietic tissue to increase their mitotic activity and furnish more progenitor cells. The latter, under appropriate growth conditions, could be diverted to differentiate into progenies of a particular cell line. For example, bone marrow cultures of endotoxin-treated and anemic calves exhibited a preferential increase of granulocyte-macrophage and erythroid progenitors, respectively, thereby indicating a directional proliferation of stem cells in response to the need for a particular cell type (Kaaya and Maxie, 1980).

Information on the committed stem cells and their regulators has come primarily from in vitro studies of bone marrow cultures in a variety of semisolid media including soft agar, plasma clot, and methyl cellulose. Bradley and Metcalf (1966) and Pluznik and Sachs (1966) were independently able to culture neutrophil-macrophage colonies in agar, and the progenitor cell was named the colony forming unit in culture (CFU-C); it is also referred to as colony forming unit granulocyte-macrophage (CFU-GM). These observations suggested that neutrophils and monocyte-macrophages have a common progenitor.

Subsequently, erythroid colony formation was reported to occur in vitro (Stephenson et al., 1971). It involved development from two progenitor cells termed the burst forming unit erythroid (BFU-E) and the colony forming unit erythroid (CFU-E) (Iscove and Sieber, 1975). The BFU-E is the progenitor of the CFU-E, probably with some intermediate progenies. The BFU-E produces large erythroid colonies over several days (8 days in mice and 14 days in humans) in the presence of a large amount of erythropoietin or a humoral factor termed the burst promoting activity (BPA) (Gregory, 1976). The CFU-E forms small erythroid colonies within a few days (2 days in mice and 7 days in humans) in the presence of a small amount of erythropoietin.

The progenitor for megakaryocytes is designated the colony forming unit megakaryocyte (CFU-M or CFU-Meg) (Metcalf et al., 1975; Nakeff et al., 1975).

Some cultural studies have been conducted on hematopoietic, lymphopoietic, and stromal stem or progenitor cells of the dog (reviewed by Wilson and Shifrine, 1980); myeloid and erythroid stem cells of the cow (Kaaya et al., 1979, 1982); myeloid and erythroid elements of the cat (Boyce et al., 1981); and granulocyte-macrophage precursors of the sheep (Chandra et al., 1983).

Variations of the aforementioned concept of the origin of hematopoietic cells have been put forward, although basically all carry the same theme. Some other theories state that there is a common progenitor of erythroid and megakaryocytic (CFU-E-Meg) lines originating from the CFU-S; that a common progenitor cell for B-lymphocytes and myeloid stem cells (CFU-GM) and a separate progenitor cell for T-lymphocytes originate from the pluripotential stem cell; and that T- and B-lymphocytes have a common origin independent of myeloid stem cells. Ontogenic relationships between T-lymphocytes and basophils, between basophils and mast cells, and between mast cells and macrophages have been proposed (see Chapter 28).

Factors Regulating Hematopoiesis

A variety of endogenous and exogenous factors influence hematopoiesis in vitro and in vivo (Table 13–6). These factors include the microenvironment and many humoral substances capable of stimulating or suppressing proliferation of single or multiple cell lineages. In general, multispecific growth factors such as interleukin-3 stimulate early progenitor cells, whereas monospecific factors such as erythropoietin act on differentiated specific cell lineages. These two types of growth factors may sometimes act in concert with an additive effect. Specific poietins have been described for certain cell lines; these include erythropoietin, thrombopoietin, eosinophil-opoietin, granulocytopoietin, and monocytopoietin. Certain lymphokines such as lymphocyte mitogenic factor (Geha and Merler, 1974) and T-cell growth factor (interleukin-1) (Smith, 1980) have a similar function in modulating lymphopoiesis. Often a humoral regulator is required to be present continuously for colony growth in vitro. Abnormal hematopoiesis may involve pathologic disturbances of one or more humoral regulators, and immune suppression may occur in certain

Table 13–6. Factors Influencing Hematopoiesis

Hematopoietic Process	Stimulators	Inhibitors
Stem cell differentiation	HIM; "short-range" hormonal factors	
Erythropoiesis	Burst promoting activity (Il-3) Erythropoietin Certain lymphokines Macrophages PGE_1 and PGE_2 PGI_2 Erythroblast enhancing factor Erythropoietic stimulating cofactor Androgens Corticosteroids Growth hormone Thyroxine Cobalt GM-Colony-stimulating factor	Estrogen A factor in urine A factor in plasma Lithium Feline leukemia virus Suppressor T-lymphocytes
Granulopoiesis	GM-Colony-stimulating factor G-Colony-stimulating factor (Syn. granulocytopoietin ?) Antichalone Certain lymphokines Eosinophilopoietin Basophilopoietin Lithium PGI_2 Corticosteroids	Colony-inhibiting factor Chalone Lactoferrin; transferrin Acidic isoferritins Certain lymphokines PGE_1 and PGE_2 Macrophage products Unidentified plasma factors
Monocytopoiesis	M-Colony-stimulating factor Monocytopoietin	A serum inhibitor PGE_1 and PGE_2 Corticosteroids
Megakaryocytopoiesis and thrombopoiesis	Meg-Colony-stimulating factor Thrombopoietin Iron Lithium A factor in bovine bile	A splenic factor Iron in different amounts
Lymphopoiesis	Specific microenvironment Thymic hormones Antigens Il-1 and Il-3 Lymphokines such as Il-2, B-cell growth factor, and B-cell differentiation factors	Corticosteroids

GM, granulocyte-macrophage; HIM, hematopoietic inductive microenvironment; Il, interleukin; M, macrophage; Meg, megakaryocyte; PG, prostaglandin.

cases (Cline and Golde, 1978). Inhibition of both granulopoiesis and erythropoiesis by cytotoxic/suppressor T-lymphocytes has been demonstrated in vitro and in clinical situations (Bagby, 1981; Burakoff et al., 1983).

Regulation of the Pluripotential Stem Cell

The differentiation of the pluripotential hematopoietic stem cells into committed hematopoietic progenitor cells and that of the latter into recognizable precursor cells and their progenies is influenced by a variety of stimulatory and inhibitory factors acting at different levels of cellular development (Metcalf, 1981; Riches et al., 1981; Wright and Lord,

1978). Proliferation of the hematopoietic stem cell compartment is regulated by the microenvironment and the elaboration of locally produced humoral factors.

The concept that the hematopoietic inductive microenvironment (HIM) influences the differentiation of the hematopoietic stem cell was borne of experimental studies of Wolf and Trentin (1968). In normal mice, bone marrow is engaged primarily in granulopoiesis, while the spleen is concerned with lymphopoiesis and erythropoiesis. Splenic colony assays in mice implanted with irradiated bone marrow stroma into the spleen showed that granulocytic colonies still develop in marrow stroma localized within the spleen, while erythroid colonies develop in the adjacent splenic tissue. This concept is supported by other observations. Human marrow fibroblasts have been found to produce a stimulator of CFU-S and an inhibitor of CFU-GM (Blackburn and Goldman, 1982). A genetically transmitted (recessive) macrocytic anemia is found in certain mutant (Sl/Sl^d) mice as a result of defective HIM (Bernstein, 1970). Cells from these mice grow well in unaffected but not in mutant littermates (Lai et al., 1979). Also, splenic transplantation corrects anemia in the mutant mice, while reconstitution with the hematopoietic stem cells has no effect. Hypoplastic anemia in a human patient was attributed to an unfavorable microenvironment in the bone marrow (Ershler et al., 1980). Chloramphenicol was found to have a suppressive effect on HIM in mice. thereby providing an explanation for aplastic anemia seen in certain patients receiving this drug (Nara et al., 1982).

The influence of microenvironment on lymphopoiesis is well known; the thymus influences commitment of marrow-derived lymphoid progenitor cells to differentiate into subsets of T-lymphocytes, whereas the bursa of Fabricius in birds and probably bone marrow in mammals similarly direct development into B-lymphocytes.

Regulation of Committed Progenitor Cells

The committed progenitor cells of the erythrocyte, granulocyte-macrophage, eosinophil, and megakaryocyte are regulated by specific stimulators all of which in the mouse are neuraminic acid–containing glycoproteins (Metcalf, 1981). The erythroid progenitor cells are stimulated by erythropoietin (Graber and Krantz, 1978), BPA (Iscove, 1978), and other recently characterized specific factors (Table 13–6). Differentiation of the pluripotential stem cell into the BFU-E is enhanced by BPA and certain diffusible growth factors produced by T-lymphocytes as well as other cells. Macrophages stimulate erythrocyte production by promoting growth of both early (BFU-E) and late (CFU-E) committed erythroid progenitors, and this stimulation is mediated by soluble substances and through cell-to-cell interaction (Gordon et al., 1980).

Differentiation of the pluripotential stem cell into the BFU-E is enhanced by certain diffusible growth factors produced by T-lymphocytes. Proliferation of late erythroid precursor cells in vitro and in vivo was stimulated by factors distinct from erythropoietin; these factors were called erythroblast enhancing factor (Krystal, 1983) and erythropoietic stimulating cofactor (Blanchet et al., 1984).

Corticosteroids and prostaglandins have stimulatory effects, whereas estrogen and lithium have an inhibitory influence on erythropoiesis (Table 13–6). Prostaglandins of the E series and PGI$_2$ are believed to be involved in the production of erythropoietin by the kidney as well as in the activation of erythropoietin-responsive cells (Fisher et al., 1980). Thyroid hormones have a definite effect on proliferation of erythroid precursors (Golde et al., 1977a). Androgens stimulate erythropoiesis in animals and humans in various ways: by direct stimulation of the pluripotential stem cell and of early and late erythroid progenitor cells and indirectly by stimulation of erythropoietin production (Besa and Bullock, 1981). Small doses are said to be more "erythropoietic" (Molinar, 1982). Growth hormone causes species-specific stimulation of erythropoiesis in vitro and possibly in vivo (Golde et al., 1977b). An inhibitor of erythropoiesis is found in the urine of humans and sheep (Kotwica et al., 1978) and in the plasma of sheep, goats, and rabbits (Neal et al., 1979). Feline leukemia virus-induced erythroid aplasia is associated with a rapid and selective suppression of erythroid progenitor cells (Boyce et al., 1981). For further discussion of factors controlling erythropoiesis, see Chapter 18.

The committed myeloid cells are stimulated by colony-forming activity (CFA) or colony-stimulating factor (CSF) and antichalones, whereas they are reciprocally inhibited by colony-inhibiting factor (CIF) and chalones (see Chapter 26). Considerable experimental and clinical evidence indicates that CSF regulates in vivo granulopoiesis. For example, an inverse relationship exists between blood levels of CSF and neutrophil numbers in cyclic neutropenia (hematopoiesis) in dogs and humans (Dale et al., 1971; Guerry et al., 1974). Nude mice injected subcutaneously with CSF-producing human pancreatic carcinoma cells developed tumors accompanied by a rise in serum CSF activity, granulocytosis, and expanded marrow granulocyte pools, the extent of all of which correlated with tumor size. Resection of the tumor resulted in restoration of normal granulocyte levels (Yunis et al., 1984).

Three major forms of CSF are produced by mouse and human cells (Burakoff et al., 1983; Dexter, 1983; Stanley and Jubinsky, 1984). CSF-1 or M-CSF (macrophage-CSF) is a lineage-specific glycoprotein with a MW of 40,000 to 60,000; CSF-2 or GM-CSF (granulocyte-macrophage-CSF) is a multispecific glycoprotein with a MW of about 23,000 that stimulates macrophage production in low concentration and granulocyte production in high concentration; and G-CSF (granulocyte-CSF) is a glycoprotein with a MW of about 24,000 that stimulates production of granulocytes as well as other myeloid cells, namely megakaryocytic and erythrocytic lineages. A CSF may stimulate various progenitor cells directly or indirectly via its action on cells of the mononuclear phagocyte system. The type and amount of CSF is believed to govern the lineage of cell differentiation, and under certain circumstances a CSF may act synergistically with other stimuli of hematopoiesis. For example, GM-CSF may act synergistically with erythropoietin in stimulating proliferation of erythroid colonies (Metcalf, 1981).

Lithium enhances granulopoiesis and megakaryocytopoiesis, while it inhibits erythropoiesis (Barr and Galbraith, 1983; Gallicchio and Chen, 1982; Gamba-Vitalo et al., 1983). The granulopoietic effect was reported to be mediated through stimulation of CFU-S and CFU-C and increased production of CSF or only by the latter process. Lactoferrin, a glycoprotein of 80,000–100,000 MW, from neutrophils inhibits granulopoiesis by suppressing elaboration of CSF by mnonuclear phagocytes (Broxmeyer et al., 1978) or by inhibiting the production of monokines which stimulate T-lymphocytes to elaborate CSF (Bagby, 1981). A CIF from phagocytosing neutrophils suppresses granulopoiesis in vitro (Philip et al., 1982). Acidic isoferritins of varied cellular origin have been shown to directly inhibit differentiation of CFU-GM

(Broxmeyer, 1982). T-lymphocytes promote growth of pluripotent stem cells and interact with marcophages to regulate granulopoiesis in vitro (Bagby, 1981).

Although PGE_1 and PGE_2 have been implicated in inhibition of both granulopoiesis and monocytopoiesis (Kurland et al., 1978), observations on marrow cultures from gray collie dogs and humans have shown that PGEs produced from monocytes and macrophages preferentially regulate progenitor cells destined to become monocytes, but not those leading to production of neutrophils or eosinophils (Hammond et al., 1983; Pelus et al., 1981). CFU-GM from human patients with chronic myelogenous leukemia was found to be insensitive (Aglietta et al., 1981) or stimulated (Taelte and Mendelsohn, 1981) by PGE_1. A monocytopoiesis inhibitor, affecting the number of bone marrow colonies and macrophage proliferation in vitro, was found in the serum of mice during the terminal stage of an inflammatory reaction. Corticosteroids stimulate early differentiation of CFU-GM inducing granulocytopoiesis and inhibiting production of monocyte/macrophage populations (Suda et al., 1983). See Chapter 26 for further discussion of factors governing granulopoiesis and Chapter 29 for factors influencing monocyte production.

Eosinophil production is regulated by eosinophilopoietin (identical to eosinophil colony-stimulating factor, or Eo-CSF) and products from T-lymphocytes (Mahmoud et al., 1975; see Chapter 27). In short-term cultures, basophil production was found to be antigen-specific and required soluble factors termed "basophilopoietins" derived from splenic T-lymphocytes (Denburg et al., 1980).

Studies of megakaryocytopoiesis in mice made thrombocytopenic or thrombocytotic indicated that CFU-Meg is not immediately responsive to acute changes in platelet demand, although megakaryocyte ploidy and size are affected, and that megakaryocytopoiesis is structured on at least two levels that are independently regulated, the early stage being rather insensitive to changes in platelet numbers or thrombopoietin levels (Burstein et al., 1981). These observations may be considered suggestive of an early CFU-Meg analogous to BFU-E and a late CFU-Meg analogous to CFU-E. It is postulated that a megakaryocyte colony-stimulating factor (Meg-CSF) affects the early progenitor cells, while thrombopoietin influences the megakaryocyte development (Williams and Levine, 1982).

Production of B- and T-lymphocytes is influenced by specific microenvironment as mentioned in the preceding section. In addition, lymphopoiesis is regulated by several humoral factors such as thymic hormones, interleukin-1, and lymphokines specific for T- and B-lymphocytes (see Table 13–6). In vitro studies have shown that interleukin-1 (MW 12,000–16,000) increases proliferation of both T- and B-lymphocytes; interleukin-2 (MW 15,000-26,000) is essential for proliferation of activated T-lymphocytes; interleukin-3 (MW 28,000) induces maturation of T-cells and also differentiation of various myeloid cells; B-cell growth factor is required for proliferation of activated B-lymphocytes; and B-cell differentiation factors act at the terminal stage of B-cell differentiation leading to increased synthesis and release of immunoglobulins (reviewed by Izaguirre, 1984). Antigenic stimulation of lymphopoiesis and lympholytic effects of corticosteroids are well-known.

Sources of Various Hematopoietic Humoral Factors

Erythropoietin is produced primarily by the kidney and to a small extent by the liver (see Chapter 18). Burst promoting activity (BPA) can be obtained from T-lymphocytes (Nathan et al., 1978) and macrophages (Zuckerman, 1981). Colony stimulating factor (CSF) is found in serum and urine, and is produced by a variety of cells and tissues including monocytes, macrophages, lymphocytes, fibroblasts, endothelial cells, and placenta (Burakoff et al., 1983; Moore, 1979). Injection of endotoxin induces increased production of CSF in laboratory animals and dogs, and bacteria and bacterial products including endotoxin appear to be major stimuli and regulators of CSF production in vivo. Dogs given endotoxin (0.01–0.02 mg/kg body weight) have increased serum levels of CSF within 1 hour, with a peak activity at 2–3 hours post-injection (Hinterberger et al., 1979). Serum CSF levels and marrow CFU-C were signifi-

cantly reduced in the dog by a reduction in intestinal gram-negative flora (MacVittie and Walker, 1978). Also, clearance of bacteria by mature neutrophils infiltrating at the site of infection exerts a negative feedback influence (Hartmann et al., 1981). Eosinophilopoietin is produced by lymphoid cells and also by the placenta, marrow cells, and monocytes. The kidneys are at least one source of thrombopoietin (McDonald, 1981; Williams and Levine, 1982). Meg-CSF is produced by lymphoid cells and can be obtained from other sources including culture filtrate of mouse splenic cells, serums and urines from patients with aplastic anemia and idiopathic thrombocytopenia, and serums of patients receiving intensive antileukemic cytotoxic therapy (Kawakita et al., 1983; Mazur et al., 1981, 1984). The production of Meg-CSF is regulated by the number of megakaryocytes or their progenitor cells in bone marrow. Interleukin-1 is derived from mononuclear phagocytes, while stimulated T-lymphocytes are the source of interleukin-2, interleukin-3, B-cell growth factor, and B-cell differentiation factors (Izaguirre, 1984). Interleukin-3 is produced also by myeloid cells. Recent studies have shown BPA and interleukin-3 activity may reside in a single macromolecule (Stanley and Jubinsky, 1984).

LYMPHOID (LYMPHATIC) TISSUES

Lymphoid organs and accumulations of lymphoid cells in loose connective tissue throughout the body constitute the lymphoid or lymphatic tissues. The thymus and the bursa of Fabricius are the primary lymphoid organs. Their parenchyma is composed of diffuse lymphoid tissue essentially containing T- and B-lymphocytes, respectively. In comparison, the secondary lymphoid organs such as the spleen and lymph nodes contain both diffuse and nodular lymphoid tissue. The diffuse lymphoid tissue is composed primarily of T-lymphocytes and the nodular tissue of B-lymphocytes. The stroma of secondary but not primary lymphoid organs is rich in reticular fibers and phagocytic reticular cells (macrophages). The primary lymphoid organs are well developed at birth, while secondary lymphoid organs develop fully after birth in parallel with immunocompetence. Significant antigenic exposure is required to stimulate lymphopoiesis in the secondary lymphoid organs. A brief description of the structure and immunologic functions of the thymus, spleen, and lymph nodes is given below; see a standard histology or immunology text for further details of the appropriate subject matter.

The Thymus

Structure

The thymus develops from an epithelial analogue of the third pharyngeal pouch and is seeded by lymphoid progenitor cells from the bone marrow during fetal life. It is fully developed at birth and involutes with age, probably under the influence of sex and adrenocortical hormones. The thymic lobes have a thin connective tissue capsule from which trabeculae extend inward dividing the parenchyma into partially separated lobules. Each lobule appears to have a peripheral cortex and a central medulla which is confluent with adjacent, incompletely separated lobes. The cortex is rich in large to small T-lymphocytes and stains densely, whereas the medulla is lightly stained and contains many more epithelial reticular cells, a significant number of macrophages, and relatively few lymphocytes. Thymic or Hassall's corpuscles, whose function remains unknown, are scattered throughout the medulla. Lymphoid cells enter and leave the thymus via postcapillary venules and veins in the medulla or at the corticomedullary junction, while the capillaries in the cortex are impervious to cells and macromolecules (this constitutes the so-called blood-thymus barrier). The thymic parenchyma is devoid of lymph vessels. It is the first organ in which lymphocytes develop during fetal life.

In the chicken, the thymus consists of a series of lobes, and the spleen is similar to that of mammals; there are no lymph nodes, but foci of lymphocytes are located in the gut wall, and there is a lymphoid organ, called the bursa of Fabricius, associated with the cloaca. The bursa is a primary lymphoid organ and histologically resembles the thymus, but is more completely lobulated and has a clear separation into cortex and medulla.

Function

The mammalian thymus is the central lymphoid organ in control of initiating the immunologic potentialities of the body. In addition, nonlymphoid hematopoiesis has been demonstrated in the developing human thymus, from 14 weeks of gestation to 15 months after birth (Bourgeois et al., 1981). Granulopoietic foci observed in the thymus of young rats have served as a model for studying granulopoiesis at extravascular locations (see Chapter 26). Thymic enlargement in birds during the breeding season has been related to increase in thymic erythropoietic activity (Kendall, 1981).

The thymus receives committed lymphoid progenitor cells from bone marrow and acts upon them to initiate differentiation into precursor cells whose descendants are commonly known as T-lymphocytes. Most of the precursor cells die in situ, but a minority enter the circulation and preferentially localize in the spleen, lymph nodes, and other foci of lymphocytic tissues. At these locations, T-lymphocytes are produced in response to appropriate antigenic stimulation. Lymphoid differentiation toward T-cell lineage in the thymus is influenced by the thymic microenvironment, stromal contact, thymic hormones, particularly thymosins, lymphokines, and macrophages (see Chapter 30). A humoral component from the calf thymus has been reported to confer immunologic competence to neonatally thymectomized mice (Trainin and Small, 1970). This finding would suggest that the thymus hormone is not species-specific. Further support for the hypothesis of a thymus hormone is found in results with thymus implants in cell-tight diffusion chambers (Miller, 1967).

Thymectomy in neonatal mice results in marked reduction in lymphocytes in the blood, lymphoid hypoplasia of the bone marrow, and minimal development of lymphocytic cells in the spleen, lymph nodes, and Peyer's patches. Mild anemia in athymic (nude) and thymectomized mice may be related to erythroid hypoplasia of the bone marrow, as a result of lymphoid hypoplasia, a reflection of the absence of thymocyte-derived factors promoting increase in erythrocyte production (Bamberger et al., 1977).

Thymectomized mice will accept allogeneic skin grafts, thereby indicating failure of development of the immunologic graft rejection reaction. Such mice live for about 3 months and then exhibit weight loss and diarrhea that lead to death. The syndrome has been referred to as runt disease. Thymectomized neonatal germ free mice do not exhibit the runt disease, indicating the possibility that the wasting, diarrhea, and death of neonatally thymectomized conventional mice is the result of failure to develop protective immune response to bacteria and viruses of the environment. Thymectomy of mice after 3 weeks of age does not lead to immediate failure of immunogenesis; this failure becomes evident only after a number of months (Miller, 1962, 1966). Disappearance of the ability to elicit an immune response after a lapse of 6–9 months in thymectomized older mice is an indication that within the first few days and weeks after birth the thymus gland releases immunologically competent cells to the secondary lymphoid tissues, which then can function independently of the thymus. The observation also indicates a life span of months for these lymphocytes, since the delay or failure of immunogenesis must be related to eventual depletion of the immunocytes. Furthermore, it indicates that the function of the thymus is not limited to the neonatal period, but is required throughout life to maintain an adequate pool of immunologically competent cells. It is apparent that the thymus is required for development of antigen-sensitive cells from precursor cells; after release from the thymus, however, these cells no longer depend directly on the thymus but rather are stimulated to proliferate by contact with antigen (Miller et al., 1967). Involution of the thymus is followed by a loss in the functional integrity of the immune system.

For an immune response to take place, an antigen must be recognized as foreign. The immunologically competent small lymphocytes in the spleen and lymph nodes have been observed to enlarge under the stimulus of antigen and to become cells exhibiting pyroninophilia. It is conjectured that these pyroninophilic cells proliferate to produce progenies committed to interact with the specific antigen.

It is apparent that immunogenesis is the result of the functional activity of at least two different populations of lymphocytes, the T-cells and the B-cells. The circulating pool of T-lymphocytes has an important function in cellular immunity leading to tissue graft rejection and delayed hypersensitivity reactions. B-lymphocytes are responsible for the immunoglobulin production associated with most humoral antibody responses. Neonatally thymectomized rats were given a series of injections of horse serum at 2 months of age and were sacrificed 3 weeks later. A rise in serum globulin was demonstrated, but the rats failed to form a precipitating antibody against horse serum. Numerous plasma cells were present in the spleen and other lymphoid tissues (Azar et al., 1963). Plasma cells (Plate XI–4) function in the production of immunoglobulins. They originate from B-lymphocytes derived from precursor cells in the bursa of Fabricius in birds and its mammalian equivalent, bone marrow and probably the Peyer's patches. See Chapter 30 for further comments on immunologic functions of T- and B-lymphocytes.

Surgical removal of the bursa or thymus in day-old chicks, followed by sublethal x-irradiation, has demonstrated the separate functions of different populations of lymphocytes (Cooper et al., 1966); humoral antibody production is curtailed, while cellular immunity remains unaltered in bursectomized chicks. As in mammals, the T-lymphocytes of the chicken are the small lymphocytes of the circulation and white pulp of the spleen. These morphologically distinct lymphocytes are responsible for cellular immunity in the chicken as in mammals. They play a less clearly defined role in antibody response to at least some antigens. The large lymphocytes of germinal centers were shown to be B-cells, and after transformation to plasma cells, they were responsible for immunoglobulin production.

Immunologic tolerance is the natural state in which the antigens of the animal's own tissues do not stimulate antibody production that would lead to destruction of the normal animal. Production of "mutant," immunologically competent cells could lead to proliferation of such cells en masse and the production of a lymphoma or lymphocytic leukemia, or other aberrations leading to automimmune disease, such as autoimmune hemolytic anemia and systemic lupus erythematosus. In the normal state, it is assumed that mutant antibody-forming cells are destroyed. Under abnormal conditions leading to dysfunction of the thymus, it is possible that aberrant, immunologically competent cells are tolerated (Burnet, 1962; Fudenberg, 1966). Thymic tumors in humans have been reported to result in pure erythrocyte agenesis, with a marked predominance of occurrence in the female (Schmid et al., 1965).

The thymus is sensitive to natural stress-inducing situations and to administered corticosteroids. Complete depletion of lymphocytes from the thymic cortex may occur in one or two days (Burnet, 1962). A severe reaction of the thymus to stress may provide in part a basis for understanding the marked and persistent lymphopenia commonly associated with chronic diseases of the dog and cat.

The Spleen

Throughout postnatal life, the spleen constitutes the largest single mass of lymphocytic cells in the body. Its unique structure and location in the systemic blood circulation bestow upon it the important function of filtering the blood. It is an important immunocompetent organ reacting to blood-borne infections. Its nonimmunologic functions include storage of erythrocytes and platelets; removal of senescent, defective, and damaged erythrocytes; removal of foreign substances from blood and of inclusions from within the red cells; processing hemoglobin to bilirubin and salvaging iron; and lymphocyte production and recirculation.

Structure

The splenic capsule is made of a thick layer of dense connective tissue from which numerous trabeculae branch into the splenic tissue (Fig. 13–20). The capsule and trabeculae contain an appreciable number of elastic fibers and smooth muscles which significantly modulate splenic size under neurohormonal influences. The thickness of the capsule and its composition vary among species; e.g., spleens of the dog, cat, and horse have a significant number of smooth muscles. The splenic pulp or parenchyma is composed of white pulp, red pulp, and the intervening marginal zone. The white pulp is composed of diffuse and nodular lymphoid tissue, while the red pulp is composed primarily of splenic or venous sinuses filled with erythrocytes and splenic cords located between the sinuses. The splenic cords are highly cellular, being composed of a variety of cells including macrophages, lymphocytes, other leukocytes, plasma cells, and erythrocytes enmeshed in a network of reticular fibers. The marginal zone is composed of a dense reticular network and constitutes an efficient filter for blood flowing through the spleen. Species differences are found in histologic composition of the spleen (Dellmann and Brown, 1981).

Blood circulation through the spleen contributes a great deal to various functions of this organ. Blood vessels enter and leave the spleen following the path within trabeculae. The splenic artery enters at the hilus and travels through the organ, branching off into trabecular arteries, which in turn give rise to nodular or central arteries. The latter are surrounded by diffuse lymphoid tissue termed the "periarterial lymphoid sheath" (PALS) and by adjacent lymphoid nodules at scattered locations. The diffuse lymphoid tissue is composed predominantly of T-lymphocytes and the nodular areas are rich in B-lymphocytes. In the red pulp, the central arteries branch into several penicilliary arteries whose segments later become sheathed capillaries (ellipsoids) and end as terminal capillaries opening into the meshwork of reticular fibers and macrophages in the marginal zone ("open circulation") or directly into venous sinuses ("closed circulation"). Blood from the marginal zone enters the venous sinuses through openings in their walls. The red pulp contains cords of diffuse lymphoid tissue surrounded by anastomosing venous sinuses which are drained by red pulp veins and trabecular veins. The venous sinuses are discontinuously lined by endothelial cells running parallel to their long axis and having slits or gaps between adjacent endothelial cells.

SPLEEN

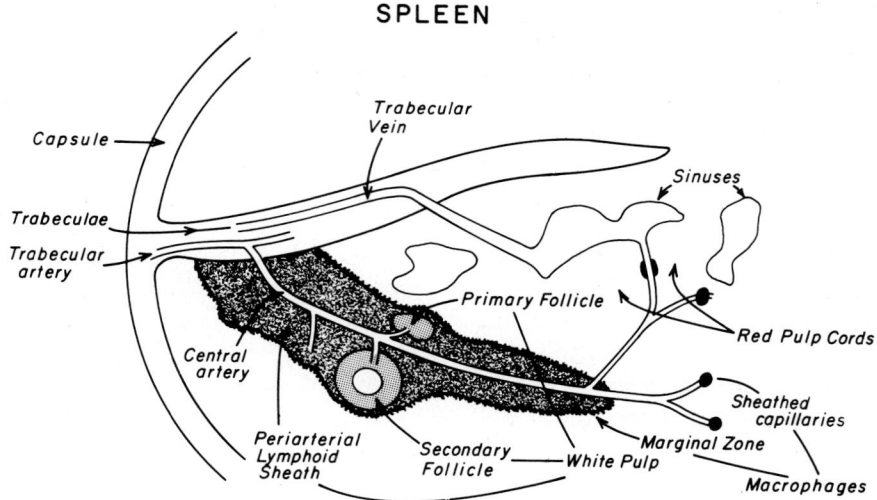

Fig. 13–20.   Diagrammatic cross section of the spleen. (Courtesy of Dr. J.G. Zinkl.)

These slits open and close with relaxation and contraction of the sinus wall. This unique arrangement allows for migration of pliant erythrocytes from the splenic cords into the sinus lumen and also provides a means by which perisinusoidal macrophages can have access to blood flowing through the sinuses.

Function

The spleen functions briefly in hematopoiesis during fetal life and in some instances (e.g., the dog) for a short period neonatally (Table 13–1). The spleen is most active in lymphopoiesis, although it retains potential for nonlymphoid hematopoiesis into adult life. When need arises, the spleen becomes active again in the production of erythrocytes, granulocytes, and megakaryocytes (myeloid metaplasia). In the mouse, the spleen is normally active in adult life in the production of erythrocytes (Hummel et al., 1966). In a study on the response to hemorrhage, it was calculated that 50% of the increase in erythropoiesis in bled mice took place in the spleen (Boggs et al., 1969). The normal mouse spleen contains stem cells capable of proliferation and differentiation into erythroid, myeloid, and megakaryocytic cells in the bone marrow and spleen of irradiated mice.

The *immunologic function* of the spleen relates to antigenic exposure through a hematogenous route. It functions in both humoral and cellular immune responses. Antigens

trapped and processed by macrophages in the marginal zone and elsewhere within the spleen provide stimulus to lymphoid cells in the white pulp, in both the PALS and lymphoid nodules, to undergo mitosis and respond immunologically. During an immune response, increased numbers of plasma cells are found in the marginal zone and the red pulp and are associated with an increase in immunologlobulin production.

The spleen in most species functions as a *reservoir of erythrocytes*. In certain animals, e.g., the dog, cat, horse, and sheep, the reservoir capacity is significant, and upon excitement or muscular activity, the spleen contracts, forcing a concentrated mass of erythrocytes into the circulation; this is apparently not the case in humans (Wintrobe et al., 1981). This splenic function is related to the relative amount of smooth muscle in the splenic capsule and trabeculae. Ascertaining the actual normal resting volume of circulating erythrocytes as expressed by erythrocyte count, hemoglobin level, or PCV is not possible in animal species with contractile spleen, particularly when the animals are apprehensive or emotionally disturbed. In response to hemorrhage in the cat, about 8% of the blood volume was contributed by the spleen (Barcroft et al., 1925). It was estimated in both the dog and cat that in exercise, shrinkage of the spleen corresponded with a 6–15% increase in circulating blood volume. Anesthetics that produce an initial period of excitement, e.g., ether, cause splenic contraction and a marked increase in the circulating red cell mass. An opposite effect, splenic engorgement by erythrocytes, is produced by tranquilizing drugs and anesthetics such as sodium amytal and pentobarbital sodium (Hauser et al., 1938). One-third of the red cell mass was found to be sequestered in the spleen of anesthetized dogs (Motulsky, 1958). For additional discussion of the influence of splenic contraction on the circulating erythrocyte mass, see Chapter 4 for the dog, Chapter 6 for the horse, and Chapter 8 for the sheep.

The spleen also serves as a *reservoir of platelets, but not of leukocytes,* with the possible exception of lymphocytes. The spleen concentrates blood platelets to the extent that one-third of the total available platelets are retained by the spleen for dynamic exchange with circulating platelets (Aster, 1966). The platelets are found adherent to the reticular cells of the red pulp and sinus endothelial cells (Weiss, 1974). Splenectomy leads to a reactive thrombocytosis (see Chapter 17), while hypersplenism may result in thrombocytopenia as the enlarged organ places greater demands for its share of available platelets (Appendix Case 26). That there is no reserve of neutrophils in the spleen became evident from studies in which in vivo distribution of DF^{32}P-labeled neutrophils was found to be similar before and after splenec-f71tomy in dogs (Raab et al., 1964) and from studies in which WBC counts were similar after epinephrine injection in normal and splenectomized persons (Storti et al., 1967). That the spleen may serve as a reservoir of mononuclear cells is apparent from observations made on splenectomized persons, namely, the occurrence of lymphocytosis and monocytosis, a decrease in the recirculating pool of lymphocytes, and an increase in recovery of labeled lymphocytes (Scott and Davidson, 1970: Wintrobe et al., 1981).

The spleen functions in *destruction of aging, damaged, and defective erythrocytes.* Erythrocytes that have lost their ability to change shape (deformability), which facilitates rapid passage through the tortuous microcirculation of the spleen, are retained in the spleen and rapidly destroyed by macrophages that protrude through the sinus walls (Weiss and Tavassoli, 1970). The erythrocyte membrane can distort with little resistance but cannot stretch much without rupture. Thus deformability is very important for erythrocyte survival in the spleen. Erythrocytes that become spherical (spherocytes) have a rigid membrane that resists deformation (Burton, 1966). It is believed that most spherocytes of autoimmune hemolytic anemia are produced by partial erythrophagocytosis by the mononuclear phagocyte system (MPS) and are destroyed in the spleen. Experimental observations indicate that slightly damaged erythrocytes are removed by the spleen, while severely damaged erythrocytes are destroyed by the mononuclear phagocytes of the liver and the body as a whole (Weiss, 1962; see Chapter 20). Damaged leukocytes and platelets are also removed by the spleen.

The slowing of passage of erythrocytes through the spleen subjects them to a specialized action called the *"pitting function"* by Crosby (1959). This concept visualizes removal of particles from erythrocytes, such as siderotic (iron) granules, Howell-Jolly bodies, nuclei, and Heinz bodies, possibly followed by release of the "cleansed" cell to the circulation. In addition, red cell parasites are also removed by this mechanism (see below). Some examples indicating the absence of the "pitting function" or its partial suppression have been encountered in animals. Following removal of the spleen in 2 horses, Heinz bodies appeared spontaneously and were present constantly in 10–20% of erythrocytes over a period of 5 years (Torten and Schalm, 1964). Perhaps in the normal aging process of red cells, a natural Heinz body-like structure is formed that is removed by the spleen. One might speculate that the pitting function of the spleen of cats is less aggressive than in other animals. Splenectomy in the cat was not associated with an increase in Heinz body formation. By the use of new methylene blue stain on blood films of cats, a single Heinz body can be demonstrated in a small number of erythrocytes as a refractile object (Plates XVI–3, XVI–4). Hence these red cell inclusions have also been called erythrocyte refractile (ER) bodies. They are found under normal conditions in all members of the fam-

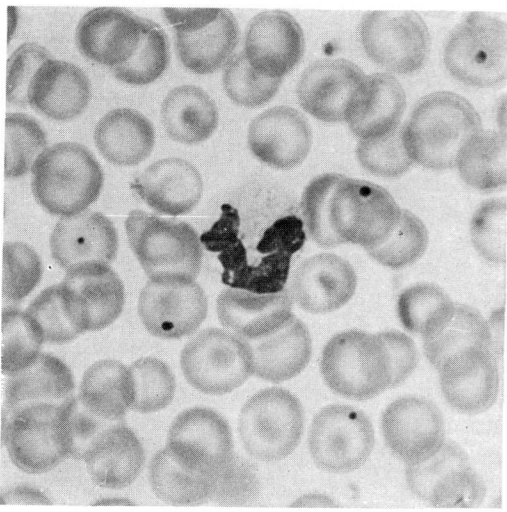

Fig. 13–21. Blood film from a dog receiving corticosteroids and cytotoxic drugs for the treatment of lymphosarcoma. Depression of splenic activity is indicated by the occurrence of numerous Howell-Jolly bodies and also possibly by the presence of target cells. ×3,150.

ily Felidae (Chapter 5). Heinz bodies in cats often increase in size and number in response to still-undetermined causes. Small Heinz bodies have been found to appear in erythrocytes of some canine patients given continuous corticosteroid therapy, and some such dogs have also exhibited increased numbers of erythrocytes containing Howell-Jolly bodies (Fig. 13–21); sometimes nucleated erythrocytes appeared in blood in numbers out of proportion to any evidence of need for intensified erythrogenesis. These findings are interpreted as an expression of hyposplenism brought about by the action of corticosteroids upon normal splenic function.

The spleen exerts some *influence on erythrocyte morphology*. Remodeling of reticulocytes into mature erythrocytes is believed to occur in the spleen since reticulocytes labeled with glycine-^{14}C and ^{32}P have been found to selectively lose labeled lipid and some membrane protein and then circulate as mature erythrocytes (see Wintrobe et al., 1981, for references). In the absence of the spleen in the dog, erythrocyte morphology changes within a few days to target cell types, and reticulocyte number increases in the circulation (Lorber, 1958). Crosby (1963) conjectured that the spleen normally sequesters reticulocytes until they mature, and during sequestration the

surface area may decrease. Reticulocytes are slightly larger than mature erythrocytes. Without sequestration, there may be insufficient reduction that results in the appearance of postsplenectomy target cells and other leptocytic forms with increased osmotic resistance (see Fig. 20–7L).

The spleen functions in the *control of bacteria and certain blood parasites* gaining access to the circulation. It is the first line of defense in cleansing the body of microorganisms gaining access to the circulation. Calves are resistant to *Anaplasma marginale* but become susceptible after splenectomy. Splenectomy may be followed by an acute flare-up of haemobartonellosis in several species of animals, the parasite having been present in such animals as a latent infection. Occurrence of haemobartonellosis in a dog following splenectomy and blood transfusion has been reported (Brodey and Schalm, 1963). Splenectomy of prospective blood-donor cats is advised in order to bring forth evidence of a carrier state of *Haemobartonella felis*, since this parasite renders the cat unsuitable for use as a donor. *Eperythrozoon wenyonii* is a blood parasite producing a silent infection in calves and growing cattle. Occasionally it is observed in considerable numbers in the plasma and on the surface of erythrocytes of animals severely sick from other causes. Following splenectomy, and in one instance following injection of blood from a carrier into a splenectomized calf, *E. wenyonii* produced a mild anemia and fever within 7 days.

The spleen exercises some *control over hematopoiesis*—erythropoiesis, thrombopoiesis, and granulopoiesis. As mentioned earlier, the spleen has been shown to contain stem cells capable of repopulating depleted bone marrow in the mouse. A 30% decrease in nucleated erythrocytes and 50% decrease in reticulocytes in the bone marrow of dogs was observed following splenectomy (Alexanian et al., 1965; Waldmann et al., 1960). It has been reported that splenectomy in the dog resulted in a significant reduction in circulating erythrocytes due to reduced erythrocyte production; life span of erythrocytes was not significantly altered. Erythrocyte life span before and after splenectomy of dogs was found to be 113 and 105 days, respectively (Singer and Weisz, 1945). Partial and total splenectomy in mice is associated with an increase in platelet numbers, respectively, of 60% and 87% and an increased incorporation of ^{75}Se-methionine, thereby indicating increased platelet production (Bessler et al., 1981). These observations were consistent with the view that splenic lymphocytes exert an inhibitory influence on thrombopoiesis. Splenic control of leukocyte production is suggested from several observations (Wintrobe et al., 1981); the degree of leukocytosis seen after splenectomy is greater than that observed after other surgeries; partial splenectomy and splenic transplants (as little as 10% spleen) prevent leukocytosis; leukocytosis does not develop in a splenectomized rat after parabiosis with an intact rat; and a humoral factor from splenic transplants is found to affect leukocyte number in splenectomized individuals.

The Lymph Nodes, and Follicles

Structure

Lymph nodes (Fig. 13–22) are scattered throughout the body along lymph channels and are the main source of lymphocytes. A lymph node is enclosed in a dense connective tissue capsule from which trabeculae extend into the organ. The trabeculae are surrounded by cortical and marginal sinuses lined by endothelial cells. The parenchyma is divided into an outer cortex and inner medulla. The cortex is composed of lymphoid nodules with indistinct (primary lymphoid follicles) or distinct (secondary lymphoid follicles) germinal centers surrounded by diffuse lymphoid tissue (the paracortical region). The medulla is made of anastomosing cord-like structures of diffuse lymphoid tissue separated by medullary sinuses and some connective tissue trabeculae. The stroma and sinuses of the lymph node are supported by a network of reticular fibers in which both fixed and free macrophages can be found. Blood enters the lymph node through arteries in the hilus. Postcapillary venules, through which lymphocytes enter the lymph node, are located in the diffuse cortex (thymus-dependent area) and are lined with a cuboidal type of endothelium; hence they are often called "high endothelial venules" (HEVs). Lymph drains from afferent lymphatics entering the lymph node at the outer aspect of the cortex into the subcapsular sinus, trickles down the cortex through lymphoid tissue or through the cortical or trabecular and marginal sinuses, and enters the medulla, from which it leaves the node via the efferent lymphatics located at the hilus. Immune response in the lymph nodes is directed uniquely against antigens presented through the lymphatic circulation.

The histologic structure of the lymph node is distinctive in the pig; the cortex and medulla have reverse locations.

Function

The diffuse lymphoid tissue is composed primarily of T-lymphocytes, while the nod-

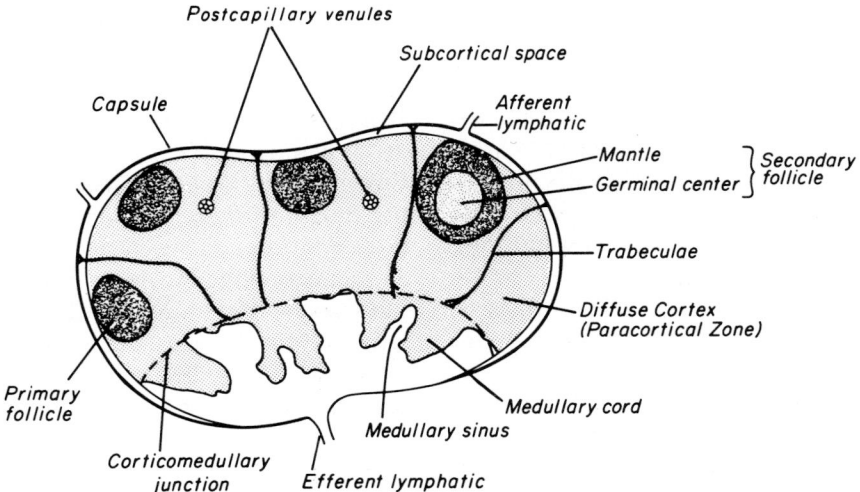

Fig. 13–22. Diagrammatic cross section of a lymph node. (Courtesy of Dr. J.G. Zinkl.)

ules contain primarily B-lymphocytes. Neonatal thymectomy or bursectomy (in birds) is associated with impaired growth of lymphoid areas, whereas antigens stimulating cellular or humoral immunity cause proliferation of appropriate cell types. Antigens drained via the lymph induce appropriate immune responses. Macrophages and dendritic cells trap antigen and present it to lymphocytes to induce an immune response. Germinal centers become prominent after immune stimulation, and increased numbers of plasma cells are found in the lymph node, primarily in medullary cords and sinuses.

The lymphocytes migrate into sinuses of the nodes and are carried via the lymphatics to the thoracic duct, from which they are dumped into the bloodstream. Lymphopoiesis and immunologic response are the major functions of the lymph nodes. This aspect is discussed in detail in Chapter 30. The lymph nodes may serve as extramedullary sites of granulopoiesis. Lymphocytic tissue is depressed by adrenocortical activity; on the other hand, hypertrophy of lymphocytic tissue results when there is hypofunctioning of the adrenal glands. Atrophy of lymphocytic tissue resulting in lymphopenia is seen in chronic interstitial nephritis (end stage kidney disease) and distemper in the dog.

OTHER TISSUES AND ORGANS

The Mononuclear Phagocyte System

The mononuclear phagocyte system (MPS), previously known as the reticuloendothelial system (RES), is widely scattered and is composed of macrophages of the loose connective tissue, the spleen, the lymph nodes, and the bone marrow and the Kupffer cells of the liver and similar cells in the adrenal glands, lungs, brain, and other locations. Monocytes in the bone marrow and blood form an important component of the MPS.

The MPS cells engulf and destroy cellular debris and particulate foreign material entering the body. They play a significant role in the catabolism of hemoglobin, especially in the spleen. The macrophages are capable of engulfing whole erythrocytes (Plate XVII–6), but usually the overaged erythrocytes go through a process of fragmentation to hemoglobin dust that is engulfed by the macrophages. They are the major site of iron storage in the body. Macrophages play an important role in the body's defense against microbial infection and in immune response. They secrete a variety of molecules of diverse biologic significance and are implicated in regulation of hematopoietic activity (see Chapter 29 for details).

The Liver

The liver functions in a number of ways in support of hematopoiesis. It is the main depot for vitamin B_{12} and folic acid and serves in the storage of excess iron. It produces all coagulation factors with the exception of Factor VIII. Albumin is synthesized by the liver, and in chronic hepatopathy, the synthesis of albumin is curtailed, resulting in a reduction of total plasma proteins. Liver also produces α- and some β-globulins. The liver produces an $α_2$-globulin that is the precursor of erythropoietin (Fig. 18–12).

The liver functions in removing from the body the useless pigment bilirubin, which is an end product of hemoglobin catabolism. The free bilirubin is derived from the degradation of hemoglobin within the MPS, especially in the spleen. The free bilirubin is brought by the blood plasma to the liver, where it is conjugated with glucuronic acid and excreted in the bile. Free bilirubin does not pass through the kidney to appear in the urine, but the conjugated form is capable of passing through the kidney. The presence of bile pigment in the urine reflects either occlusion of biliary canaliculi, as often occurs in hepatitis, or extrahepatic bile duct closure. Bilirubinuria may also be seen in dogs with an acute hemolytic episode. The kidney threshold for conjugated bilirubin is low in the dog, and therefore bile (1+) in the urine is a common finding in normal dogs as well as in dogs with a variety of diseases. Bilirubinuria of a higher degree (2+ to 3+) is considered significant, particularly in dilute urine, and may be unaccompanied by bilirubinemia. Bile is normally absent in the urine of the cat, horse, sheep, and pig, and bilirubinuria is not a consistent finding in cattle with hepatic disease (Cornelius, 1980).

"Cloudy swelling" of liver cells may lead to a partial occlusion of biliary canaliculi and interference with excretion of the conjugated bilirubin via the normal route through the common bile duct into the lumen of the intestine. Inability of the liver to conjugate free bilirubin or to excrete bilirubin glucuronide leads to retention of bilirubin in the blood plasma, resulting in elevation of the icterus index. See Chapter 19 for further comments on bilirubin metabolism.

The Stomach

In humans, the stomach plays an important role in preparing Vitamin B_{12} for absorption by the intestinal mucosa. Vitamin B_{12} is a water-soluble vitamin and is commonly referred to as cobalamin because it contains cobalt. It is present in foods of animal origin (e.g., meat, fish, eggs, and milk) and is synthesized by bacteria in the gastrointestinal tract of animals. Cooking and acid-peptic hydrolysis in gastric juice frees vitamin B_{12} bound to proteins in food, and then the vitamin binds with "intrinsic factor," or "R-proteins" (proteins with rapid electrophoretic mobility; also called cobalophilins) (Stenman, 1975), or both, in the gastrointestinal tract. Both intrinsic factor and R-proteins are glycoproteins, but the former has a MW of 50,000–60,000 and the latter, about 60,000–120,000. The intrinsic factor, but not R-proteins, facilitates absorption of vitamin B_{12}. The latter bind about 20% of the vitamin B_{12} in gastric fluid and then probably transfer it to the intrinsic factor for absorption. The intrinsic factor–vitamin B_{12} complex binds to specific receptors located on the brush border of the mucosal cells of the ileum and is absorbed. The complex is broken down within the ileal cells, and free vitamin B_{12} is released into blood where it binds to transcobalamin II for delivery to body tissues. Transcobalamins I (origin unknown) and III (from granulocytes) do not actually function as transport proteins for vitamin B_{12}. Malabsorption in the small intestine is a common cause of cobalamin and folate deficiency.

Castle and Townsend (1929) discovered the intrinsic factor that is produced by the parietal cells of the gastric mucosa in humans and by the pyloric region and the Brunner glands of the duodenum in the pig. When this factor is absent in humans, the condition called pernicious anemia develops. Partial or complete gastrectomy and, more commonly, diseases of the stomach are associated with reduced production of intrinsic factor. Intrinsic factor is readily obtainable for therapeutic purposes from the gastric mucosa of the pig (Robbins and Shields, 1957). Pernicious anemia has not been found in animals, and removal of the stomach, duodenum, and first 30 cm of the jejunum of dogs did not lead to development of pernicious anemia (Bachrach and Fogelson, 1938). The dog and other carnivores neither produce nor need the intrinsic factor for absorption of vitamin B_{12} (Okuda, 1969). An occasional dog of the poodle breed has been encountered in which maturation defects are seen in the erythrocytic series and less frequently in the granulocytic series (see Chapter 25). These changes may be considered suggestive of a possible deficiency of vitamin B_{12} or folate or a defect in utilization of these substances by the involved hematopoietic cells. Such a relationship remains to be proved, however.

Folates in food are absorbed primarily in the upper third of the small intestine (the duodenum and jejunum). Dietary folates occur primarily as polyglutamates; in the intestine, they are enzymatically broken down to the monoglutamate form for transportation in the blood (Butterworth and Krumdieck, 1975). In humans, dietary deficiency of folate is more common than that of vitamin B_{12} because body stores of folate become depleted within a few weeks because of its high excretory rate and the body's daily requirements for it. Hematologic changes appear after several weeks of continued folate deficiency, and anemia develops after $4\frac{1}{2}$ months (Wintrobe et al., 1981). Humans on a strict vegetarian diet take 2–12 years to develop dietary deficiency of vitamin B_{12} because the body stores are large, particularly in the liver, and daily need is low. Deficiency of vitamin B_{12} in humans results primarily in defective synthesis of DNA and myelin, which are, respectively, associated with hematologic and neurologic disorders. The latter manifestation does not occur with folate deficiency.

Another function of the stomach in hematopoiesis is the production of HCl. Food iron is ionized by HCl to ferric iron, which passes into the duodenum and there it is reduced to ferrous iron, in which form it can be taken up by the intestinal mucosa. Iron absorption is influenced by the availability of reducing agents in the gut, such as ascorbic acid. Iron becomes unavailable for absorption if a high level of phosphates is present in the gut. Iron bound to phytates or phosphoproteins (egg yolk) or oxalates is not absorbed. Lack of HCl is called achlorhydria, and the abnormality leads to development of iron deficiency in humans. Achlorhydria is not common in animals.

The Intestinal Mucosa and Iron Stores

The amount of iron absorbed by mucosal cells of the intestine is regulated by need. Studies have been conducted with radioiron in normal and anemic dogs (Hahn et al., 1943). Normal dogs were found to absorb little iron, but the rate of iron absorption was increased 6-fold to 15-fold in dogs with chronic blood loss anemia. The term "physiologic saturation" with iron was applied to explain the acceptance or refusal of ingested iron by the intestinal mucosal epithelium. It was observed that the unlabeled iron given 1–6 hours before the radioactive iron produced a "mucosal block." It was postulated that a protein, such as ferritin or apoferritin, functions to take up iron from the intestinal lumen and pass it on to the blood plasma when the iron level of the plasma is lowered. The "mucosal block" hypothesis was challenged (Brown et al., 1958; Chodos et al., 1957), but more recent studies lend strong support. Studies were conducted regarding the absorption of ^{59}Fe from intestinal loops produced surgically in rats (Wheby et al., 1964). The data supported the concept of intestinal mucosal regulation of iron absorption. In the normal rat, iron absorption was most active in the proximal duodenum, but the area was increased to include the proximal jejunum in iron-deficient rats. It was concluded that the intestinal mucosal cells possess an absorptive mechanism responsive to body iron requirements that, within limits, is capable of regulating iron absorption. Increased need for iron, as during increased erythropoiesis, enhances iron absorption. In humans, 5–10% of dietary iron is absorbed normally, and this absorption increases about threefold to fivefold in iron deficiency and decreases during iron overload.

Using radioautographic methods and ^{59}Fe in rats, Conrad and Crosby (1963) found that the columnar epithelial cells of the duodenal villi incorporated iron from the body's iron stores, the amount depending on the body's requirement for the new iron. This incorporation of the intrinsic iron into villus cells occurred as the cells formed in the crypts of Lieberkühn. In the iron-replete rat, the iron remained in the epithelial cells as they were pushed upward along the villus by newly forming cells, and the iron-containing epithelial cells were finally pushed off the tip of the villus into the lumen of the gut. The duodenal mucosa of iron-loaded rats was found to block the absorption of dietary iron almost completely, while in iron-deficient rats, there was less radioactivity in mucosal epithelial cells, indicating acceptance of dietary iron and passage into the body.

Iron in the body is essentially in a closed cycle; there is only a small amount of daily loss into the gut. Excess iron is stored as ferritin and hemosiderin in the liver, spleen, and bone marrow. Iron markedly in excess of normal needs is irritating and leads to hemochromatosis and development of cirrhosis. Repeated blood transfusions may overburden the body with iron when anemia is not the result of blood loss. The mechanism of the mucosal block is the natural means whereby the body protects itself against an overload of dietary iron.

Ferritin is visible only on electron microscopy, whereas hemosiderin is visible on light microscopy as golden brown granules in cells of the MPS (Plate XVII–6). When hemorrhage occurs into the tissues or hemoglobin is released in massive amounts, the iron appears in the macrophages of the immediate area as hemosiderin. Both ferritin and hemosiderin are available for use in the production of hemoglobin. When hemoglobin is degraded in the destruction of erythrocytes, heme iron is released and becomes immediately available for conversion into hemoglobin again, but iron in excess of immediate need is stored.

Heme iron in foods of animal origin is absorbed as hemin (ferric form) by mucosal cells.

See Chapter 25 for comments on iron levels in plasma, erythrocytes, and bone marrow and iron metabolism in various types of anemias.

The Kidney

Erythropoietin (Ep) is well established as a plasma factor elaborated in increasing amounts in response to hypoxia and capable of stimulating erythropoiesis. A search for the organ or tissue of origin focused attention on the kidney (Erslev, 1971; Jacobson et al., 1957). Rats subjected to removal of the pituitary, thyroid, spleen, adrenals, or gonads retained the capacity to produce Ep, as did rats from which seven-eighths of the liver had been removed. After bilateral nephrectomy, neither rats nor rabbits had the capacity to produce Ep. Ureter-ligated rats, whose blood urea nitrogen concentration equaled that of nephrectomized animals, responded nearly as normal controls did to bleeding or phenylhydrazine anemia, and Ep activity was demonstrated in their plasma.

Before attention was focused on the kidney as the source of Ep, polycythemia in humans had in some instances been associated with hypernephroma, hydronephrosis, and benign adenoma of the kidney; the polycythemia disappeared upon surgical removal of the involved kidney (Cooper and Tuttle, 1957). The kidney appears to be the sole source of Ep in the dog (Naets, 1960; Murphy et al., 1970), but Ep in blood plasma had been demonstrated after removal of both kidneys in humans (Naets and Wittek, 1968), baboons (Murphy et al., 1970), rats (Fried et al., 1969), and rabbits. In humans and some animals, however, other tissue sites or organs such as the liver may take over the function of producing Ep in the absence of the kidneys. Evidence has been presented from experiments conducted with cats that the carotid body secretes one or more erythropoiesis-controlling hormones (Tramezzani et al., 1971). Erythropoietin production is increased in cats responding to blood loss anemia (Dunn and Legendre, 1980). Prevalent views regarding the mode of elaboration of Ep and its action on erythropoiesis are discussed in Chapter 18 and summarized in Figure 18–12.

Recently, the kidney has been designated as a source of thrombopoietin (McDonald, 1981; Williams and Levine, 1982).

REFERENCES

Abramson, S., et al.: The Identification in Adult Bone Marrow of Pluripotent and Restricted Stem Cells of the Myeloid and Lymphoid Systems. J. Exp. Med., *145*:1567, 1977.

Aglietta, M., et al.: Prostaglandins and Myelopoiesis: Effects of Prostaglandin E_1 on Normal and Chronic Myeloid Leukemia Colony Forming Cells (CFU-GM) Subpopulations. Cell Biol. Int. Rep., *5*:836, 1981.

Alexanian, R., et al.: Effect of Splenectomy upon Bone Marrow Cellularity in the Dog. Clin. Res., *13*:38, 1965.

Andersen, A.C., and Goldman, M.: Growth and Development. *In* The Beagle as an Experimental Dog. Andersen, A.C., ed. Iowa State University Press, Ames, p. 43, 1970.

Andersen, A.C., and Schalm, O.W.: Hematology. *In* The Beagle as an Experimental Dog. Andersen, A.C., ed. Iowa State University Press, Ames, p. 261, 1970.

Aoki, M., and Tavassoli, M.: Dynamics of Red Cell Egress from Bone Marrow after Blood Letting. Brit. J. Haematol., *49*:337, 1981.

Aster, R.H.: Pooling of Platelets in the Spleen: Role in the Pathogenesis of "Hypersplenic" Thrombocytopenia. J. Clin. Invest., *45*:645, 1966.

Azar, H.A., et al.: Dissociation between Serum Gamma Globulin and Precipitin Antibody in Rats Thymectomized at Birth. Fed. Proc., *22*:600, 1963.

Bachrach, W.H., and Fogelson, S.J.: The Role of the Upper Gastrointestinal Tract in the Etiology of Pernicious Anemia: An Experimental Study in Dogs. J. Lab. Clin. Med., *24*:249, 1938.

Bagby, G.G., Jr.: T Lymphocytes Involved in Inhibition of Granulopoiesis in Two Neutropenic Patients Are of the Cytoxic/Suppression (T3+ T8+) Subset. J. Clin. Invest., *68*:1597, 1981.

Bamberger, E.G., et al.: Haematopoiesis in Hereditary Athymic Mice. Lab. Anim. Sci., *27*:43, 1977.

Barcroft, J., et al.: A Contribution to the Physiology of the Spleen. J. Physiol., *60*:443, 1925.

Barker, J.E.: Haemoglobin Switching in Sheep: Characteristics of BFU-E-Derived Colonies from Fetal Liver. Blood, *56(3)*:495, 1980.

Barr, R.D., and Galbraith, P.R.: Lithium and Hematopoiesis. Can. Med. Ass. J., *128*:123, 1983.

Barrett, A.J., et al.: Mobilization of CFU-C by Exercise and ACTH Induced Stress in Man. Exp. Hematol., *6*:590, 1978.

Barton, J.C.: Comments on Hematopoietic Stem Cells. Alabama J. Med. Sci., *18*:233, 1981.

Barton, J.C., et al.: Acute Lymphblastic Leukemia in Idiopathic Refractory Sideroblastic Anemia; Evidence for a Common Lymphoid and Myeloid Progenitor Cell. Amer. J. Hematol., *9*:109, 1980.

Becker, A.J., et al.: Cytological Demonstration of the Clonal Nature of Spleen Colonies Derived from Transplanted Mouse Marrow Cells. Nature, *197*:452, 1963.

Bernstein, S.E.: Tissue Transplantation as an Analytic

and Therapeutic Tool in Hereditary Anemias. Amer. J. Surg., 119:448, 1970.

Besa, E., and Bullock, L.P.: The Role of the Androgen Receptor in Erythropoiesis. Endocrinology, 109:1983, 1981.

Bessler, H., et al.: The Effect of Partial Splenectomy on Platelet Production in Mice. Thromb. Haemost., 46:602, 1981.

Beutler, E., et al.: Value of Genetic Variants of Glucose-6-Phosphate Dehydrogenase in Tracing the Origin of Malignant Tumors. New Engl. J. Med., 276:389, 1967.

Blackburn, M.J., and Goldman, J.M.: Inhibitor of CFU-GM Produced by Human Marrow Fibroblasts. Brit. J. Haematol., 52:144, 1982.

Blanchet, J.P., et al.: A Factor in Normal Mouse Serum Stimulates Late Erythroid Precursor Proliferation. Exp. Hematol., 12:595, 1984.

Boggs, D.R., et al.: Leukokinetic Studies. VII. Morphology of the Bone Marrow and Blood of Dogs Given Vinblastine Sulfate. Blood, 23:53, 1964.

Boggs, D.R., et al.: Contribution of the Mouse Spleen to Post-Hemorrhagic Erythropoiesis. Life Sci., 8:587, 1969.

Bourgeois, N., et al.: The Thymus as Haematopoietic Tissue on Non-Lymphoid Cells. Virchows Arch. (Pathol. Anat.), 391:81, 1981.

Boyce, J.T., et al.: Feline Leukemia Virus-Induced Erythroid Aplasia: In Vitro Hemopoietic Culture Studies. Exp. Hematol., 9:990, 1981.

Bradley, T.R., and Metcalf, D.: The Growth of Mouse Bone Marrow Cells in Vitro. Aust. J. Exp. Biol. Med. Sci., 44:287, 1966.

Branemark, P.I.: Vital Microscopy of Bone Marrow in Rabbit. Scand. J. Clin. Lab. Invest., Suppl., 38:1, 1959.

Brodey, R.S., and Schalm. O.W.: Hemobartonellosis and Thrombocytopenic Purpura in a Dog. J. Amer. Vet. Med. Ass., 143:1231, 1963.

Brown, E.B., Jr., et al.: Studies on Iron Transportation and Metabolism. XI. Critical Analysis of Mucosal Block by Large Doses of Inorganic Iron in Human Subjects. J. Lab. Clin. Med., 52:335, 1958.

Broxmeyer, H.E.: Acidic Isoferritins and E-type Prostaglandins in Sources of Colony-Stimulating Factors Mask Detection of Cycling Granulocyte-Macrophage Progenitor. Cells, 60:1042, 1982.

Broxmeyer, H.E., et al.: Identification of Lactoferrin as the Granulocyte-Derived Inhibitor of Colony-Stimulating Activity. J. Exp. Med., 148:1052, 1978.

Burakoff, S.J., et al.: Recapitulation of the Immune Response and Haematopoietic System in Bone Marrow Transplantation. Clin. Haematol., 12:695, 1983.

Burnet, M.: Role of the Thymus and Related Organs in Immunity. Brit. Med. J., 2:807, 1962.

Burstein, S.A., et al.: Megakaryocytopoiesis in the Mouse: Response to Varying Platelet Demand. J. Cell. Physiol., 109:333, 1981.

Burton, A.C.: Role of Geometry of Size and Shape of the Microcirculation. Fed. Proc., 25:1753, 1966.

Butterworth, C.E., and Krumdieck, C.L.: Intestinal Absorption of Folic Acid Monoglutamates and Polyglutamates; A Brief Review of Some Recent Developments. Brit. J. Haematol., 31(Suppl.):111, 1975.

Campbell, F.: Fine Structure of the Bone Marrow of the Chicken and Pigeon. J. Morphol., 123:405, 1967.

Castle, W.B., and Townsend, W.C.: Observations on the Etiologic Relationship of Achylia Gastrica to Pernicious Anemia. II. The Effect of the Administration to Patients with Pernicious Anemia of Beef Muscle after Incubation with Normal Human Gastric Juice. Amer. J. Med. Sci., 178:764, 1929.

Chandra, P., et al.: Growth of Ovine Granulocyte-Macrophage Precursors In Vitro Without Exogenous Colony-Stimulating Activity. Amer. J. Vet. Res., 44:2070, 1983.

Chodos, R.B., et al.: The Absorption of Radioiron Labelled Foods and Iron Salts in Normal and Iron-Deficient Subjects and an Idiopathic Hemochromatosis. J. Clin. Invest., 36:314, 1957.

Cline, M.J., and Golde, D.W.: Immune Suppression of Hematopoiesis. Amer. J. Clin. Path., 64:301, 1978.

Cline, M.J., and Golde, D.W.: Cellular Interactions in Haematopoiesis. Nature, 277:177, 1979.

Conrad, M.E., Jr., and Crosby, W.H.: Intestinal Mucosal Mechanisms Controlling Iron Absorption. Blood, 22:406, 1963.

Cooper, M.D., et al.: The Functions of the Thymus System and the Bursa System in the Chicken. J. Exp. Med., 123:75, 1966.

Cooper, W.M., and Tuttle, W.B.: Polycythemia Associated with a Benign Kidney Lesion: Report of a Case of Erythrocytosis with Hydronephrosis with Remission of Polycythemia following Nephrectomy. Ann. Intern. Med., 47:1008, 1957.

Cornelius, C.E.: Liver Function. In Clinical Biochemistry of Domestic Animals. Kaneko, J.J., ed. 3rd Ed. Academic Press, New York, p. 201, 1980.

Crosby, W.H.: Normal Function of the Spleen Relative to Red Blood Cells: A Review. Blood, 14:399, 1959.

Crosby, W.H.: Hyposplenism: An Inquiry into Normal Functions of the Spleen. Ann. Rev. Med., 14:349, 1963.

Dale, D.C., et al.: Cyclic Urinary Leukopoietic Activity in Gray Collie Dogs. Science, 173:152, 1971.

De Bruyn, P.H.: Structural Substrates of Bone Marrow Function. Semin. Hematol., 18:179, 1981.

Dellmann, H.-D., and Brown, E.M.: Textbook of Veterinary Histology. Lea & Febiger, Philadelphia, 1981.

Denburg, J.A., et al.: Basophil Production. J. Clin. Invest., 65:390, 1980.

Dexter, T.M.: The Regulation of Haemopoietic Stem Cells, Progenitor Cells and Macrophage Development. Trans. R. Soc. Trop. Med. Hyg., 77:597, 1983.

Doan, C.A., et al.: Experimental Studies on the Origin and Maturation of Avian and Mammalian Red Blood Cells. Contrib. Embryol., 16:163, 1925.

Douaren, N.M. Le, et al.: Origin of Hematopoietic Stem Cells in Embryonic Bursa of Fabricius and Bone Marrow Studied through Interspecies Chimeras. Proc. Natl. Acad. Sci., 72:2701, 1975.

Douver, D., et al.: Chronic Myelocytic Leukaemia: A Pleuripotent Haemopoietic Cell Is Involved in the Malignant Clone. Brit. J. Haematol., 49:615, 1981.

Dunn, C.D., and Legendre, A.: Humoral Regulation of Erythropoiesis in Cats: Preliminary Report. Amer. J. Vet. Res., 41:779, 1980.

Ershler, W.B., et al.: Bone Marrow Microenvironment Defect in Congenital Hypoplastic Anemia. New Eng. J. Med., 302:1321, 1980.

Erslev, A.J.: The Search for Erythropoietin. New Engl. J. Med., 284:849, 1971.

Fairman, E., and Whipple, G.H.: Bone Marrow Volume in Adult Dogs. Amer. J. Physiol., 101:352, 1933.

Fudenberg, H.: Immunologic Deficiency, Autoimmune Disease and Lymphoma: Observations, Implications and Speculations. Arthritis Rheum., 9:464, 1966.

Fialkow, P.J., et al.: Evidence That Essential Thrombocythemia is a Clonal Disorder with Origin in a Multipotent Stem Cell. Blood, *58*:916, 1981.

Fisher, J.W., et al.: Prostaglandin Activation of Erythropoietin Production and Erythroid Progenitor Cells. Exp. Hematol., Suppl., *8*:65, 1980.

Fliedner, T.M.: Hematopoietic Stem Cells in Blood: Characteristic and Potentials. *In* Hematopoietic Cell Differentiation. D.W. Golde, et al., eds. Academic Press, New York, p. 193, 1978.

Fliedner, T.M., et al.: Complete Labelling of All Cell Nuclei in Newborn Rats with H³-Thymidine: A Tool for the Evaluation of Rapidly and Slowly Proliferating Cell Systems. Lab. Invest., *18*:249, 1968.

Fliedner, T.M., et al.: Morphologic and Cytokinetic Aspects of Bone Marrow Stroma. *In* Hemopoietic Cellular Proliferations. F. Stohlman, Jr., ed. Grune & Stratton, New York, p. 67, 1970.

Fried, W., et al.: Studies on Extrarenal Erythropoietin. J. Lab. Clin. Med., *73*:244, 1969.

Gallicchio, V.S., and Chen, M.G.: Cell Kinetics of Lithium-Induced Granulopoiesis. Cell Tissue Kinet., *15*:179, 1982.

Gamba-Vitalo, C., et al.: Lithium Stimulated In Vitro Megakaryocytopoiesis. Exp. Hematol., *11*:382, 1983.

Geha, R.S., and Merler, E.: Human Lymphocyte Mitogenic Factor: Synthesis by Sensitized Thymus-Derived Lymphocytes; Dependence of Expression on the Presence of Antigen. Cell Immunol., *10*:86, 1974.

Golde, D.W., et al.: Thyroid Hormones Stimulate Erythropoiesis in Vitro. Brit. J. Haematol., *37*:173, 1977a.

Golde, D.W., et al.: Growth Hormone: Species-Specific Stimulation of Erythropoiesis in Vitro. Science, *196*:1112, 1977b.

Gordon, L.I., et al.: Regulation of Erythroid Colony Formation by Bone Marrow Macrophages. Blood, *55(6)*:1046, 1980.

Graber, S., and Krantz, S.: Erythropoietin and the Control of Red Cell Production. Ann. Rev. Med., *29*:51, 1978.

Gregory, C.J.: Erythropoietin Sensitivity as a Differentiation Marker in the Hemopoietic System: Studies of the Erythropoietic Colony Responses in Culture. J. Cell. Physiol., *89*:289, 1976.

Guerry, D., et al.: Human Cyclic Neutropenia: Urinary Colony-Stimulating Factor and Erythropoietin Levels. Blood, *44*:257, 1974.

Hahn, P.F., et al.: Radioactive Iron Absorption by Gastro-Intestinal Tract. J. Exp. Med., *78*:169, 1943.

Hammond, W.P., et al.: Mechanism of Canine Cyclic Hematopoiesis: The Role of Prostaglandin E in Feedback Regulation. Amer. J. Hematol., *14*:27, 1983.

Hartmann, D.W., et al.: Regulation of Granulopoiesis and Distribution of Granulocytes in Early Phase of Bacterial Infection. J. Cell. Physiol., *109*:17, 1981.

Hauser, E., et al.: Roentgenologic Observations on the Spleen of the Dog under Ether, Sodium Amytal, Pentobarbital Sodium and Pentothal Sodium Anesthesia. Amer. J. Physiol., *121*:387, 1938.

Hinterberger, W., et al.: Endotoxin-Induced Myeloid Reactions in Dogs. Exp. Pathol., *17*:113, 1979.

Hubbert, W.T., and Hollen, E.J.: Cellular Blood Elements in the Developing Bovine Fetus. Amer. J. Vet. Res., *32*:1213, 1971.

Hummel, K.P., et al.: Anatomy. *In* Biology of the Laboratory Mouse. Green, E.L., ed. McGraw-Hill, New York, Chap. 13, p. 247, 1966.

Iscove, N.N.: Erythropoietin-Independent Stimulation of Early Erythropoiesis in Adult Marrow Cultures by Conditioned Media from Lectin Stimulated Mouse Spleen Cells. *In* ICN-UCLA Symposia on Molecular and Cellular Biology. Golde, D.W., et al., eds. Vol. 10. Academic Press, New York, p. 37, 1978.

Iscove, N.N., and Sieber, F.: Erythroid Progenitors in Mouse Bone Marrow Detected by Macroscopic Colony Formation in Culture. Exp. Haematol., *3*:22, 1975.

Izaguirre, C.A.: Colony Formation by Lymphoid Cells. Clin. Haematol., *13*:405, 1984.

Jacobson, I.O., et al,: Role of the Kidney in Erythropoiesis. Nature, *179*:633, 1957.

Jandl, J.H.: The Agglutination and Sequestration of Immature Red Cells. J. Lab. Clin. Med., *55*:663, 1960.

Kaaya, G.P., and Maxie, M.G.: The Kinetics of Haemopoietic Differentiation Assessed by in Vitro Bone Marrow Culture in Endotoxin-Treated and in Anaemic Calves. Res. Vet. Sci., *29*:63, 1980.

Kaaya, G.P., et al.: Bovine Granulocyte/Macrophage and Erythroid Colony Cultures Characteristics of the Colonies and the Assay Systems. Can. J. Comp. Med., *43*:448, 1979.

Kaaya, G.P., et al.: Characteristics of Erythroid Colonies Formed by Bovine Marrow Progenitor Cells in Methyl Cellulose Cultures. Res. Vet. Sci., *32*:213, 1982.

Kawakita, M., et al.: Characterization of Human Megakaryocyte Colony-Stimulating Factor in the Urinary Extracts from Patients with Aplastic Anemia and Idiopathic Thrombocytopenic Purpura. Blood, *61*:556, 1983.

Kelly, W.D.: The Thymus and Lymphoid Morphogenesis in the Dog. Fed. Proc., *22*:600, 1963.

Kendall, M.D.: The Thymus and Haemopoiesis. Prog. Clin. Biol. Res., *59B*:221, 1981.

Kessel, R.G., and Kardon, R.H.: Tissues and Organs: A Text-Atlas of Scanning Electron Microscopy. W.H. Freeman, San Francisco, 1979.

Knospe, W.H., et al.: Regeneration of Locally Irradiated Bone Marrow. I. Dose Dependent, Long-Term Changes in the Rat, with Particular Emphasis upon Vascular and Stromal Reaction. Blood, *28*:398, 1966.

Kotwica, G., et al.: Presence of Erythropoiesis Inhibitor in the Urine of Normal Sheep and Those with Transfused Polycythemia. Acta Physiol. Pol., *29*:37, 1978.

Krystal, G.: Physical and Biological Characterization of Erythroblast Enhancing Factor (EEF), a Late Acting Erythropoietic Stimulator in Serum Distinct from Erythropoietin. Exp. Hematol., *11*:18, 1983.

Kurland, J.I., et al.: Role for Monocyte-Macrophage-Derived Colony Stimulating Factor and Prostaglandin E in the Positive and Negative Feedback Control of Myeloid Stem Cell Proliferation. Blood, *52*:388, 1978.

Lai, K., et al.: The Hematopoietic Microenvironment as Studied on Intraperitoneal Cell Coated Cellulose Acetate Membranes. Conference on Aplastic Anemia, San Francisco, National Institute of Health Publications, p. 17, June 1979.

Lajtha, L.G., et al.: Kinetics of a Bone-Marrow Stem-Cell Population. Ann. N.Y. Acad. Sci., *113(Art. 2)*:742, 1964.

Lichtman, M.A.: Hemopoietic Stem Cell Disorders. Amer. J. Med. Technol., *49*:97, 1983.

Linch, D.C., et al.: Studies of Circulating Hemopoietic Progenitor Cells in Human Fetal Blood. Blood, *59*:976, 1982.

Lorber, M.: The Effects of Splenectomy on the Red Blood Cells of the Dog with Particular Emphasis on the Reticulocyte Response. Blood, *13*:972, 1958.

Loutit, J.P.: Grafts of Haemopoietic Tissue: The Nature

of the Haemopoietic Stem Cells. J. Clin. Path., *20(Suppl.)*:535, 1967.

MacVittie, T.J., and Walker, R.I.: Canine Granulopoiesis: Alterations Induced by Suppression of Gram-Negative Flora. Exp. Hematol., *6*:639, 1978.

Mahmoud, A.A.F., et al.: Eosinophilopoietic Activity in Mouse Serum. Clin. Res., *23*:524, 1975.

Maximow, A.A.: Relation of Blood Cells to Connective Tissues and Endothelium. Physiol. Rev., *4*:533, 1924.

Mazur, E.M., et al.: Regulation of Human Megakaryocytopoiesis: An in Vitro Analysis. J. Clin. Invest., *68*:733, 1981.

Mazur, E.M., et al.: Human Serum Megakaryocyte Colony-Stimulating Activity Increases in Response to Intensive Cytotoxic Chemotherapy. Exp. Hematol., *12*:624, 1984.

McDonald, T.P.: Assay and Site of Production of Thrombopoietin. Brit. J. Haematol., *49*:493, 1981.

Metcalf, D.: Control of Hemopoietic Cell Proliferation and Differentiation. Prog. Clin. Biol. Res., *66A*:473, 1981.

Metcalf, D., et al.: Growth of Mouse Megakaryocyte Colonies in Vitro. Proc. Natl. Acad. Sci. U.S.A., *72*:1744, 1975.

Miller, J.F.A.P.: Part I. The Role of the Lymphoid System in Hemotransplantation Reactions. Role of the Thymus in Transplantation Immunity. Ann. N.Y. Acad. Sci., *99(Art. 3)*:340, 1962.

Miller, J.F.A.P.: The Thymus in Relation to the Development of Immunological Capacity. *In* Ciba Symposium on the Thymus: Experimental and Clinical Studies. Little, Brown, Boston, p. 153, 1966.

Miller, J.F.A.P.: The Thymus, Yesterday, Today, and Tomorrow. Lancet, *2*:1299, 1967.

Miller, J.F.A.P., et al.: Cellular Basis of the Immunological Defects in Thymectomized Mice. Nature, *214*:992, 1967.

Miura, Y.: Regulatory Mechanisms of Erythrocyte Differentiation in the Early Embryonic Yolk Sac: Cell Structure and Function, *5*:285, 1980.

Molinar, P.F.: Erythropoietic Mechanism of Androgens: A Critical Review and Clinical Implications. Haematologica, *67*:442, 1982.

Moore, M.A.S.: Humoral Regulation of Granulopoiesis. Clin. Haematol., *8*:287, 1979.

Morra, L., et al.: Influence of the Spleen on the Blood Distribution of the Colony-Forming Cells (CFU-C) in Man. Acta Haematol., *66*:81, 1981.

Morse, B.S., and Stohlman, F., Jr.: Regulation of Erythropoiesis. XVIII. The Effect of Vincristine and Erythropoietin on Bone Marrow. J. Clin. Invest., *45*:1241, 1966.

Motulsky, A.G.: Anemia and the Spleen. New Engl. J. Med., *259*:1164, 1958.

Murphy, G.P., et al.: Extrarenal and Renal Erythropoietin Levels in Human Beings and Experimental Animals in Intact, Anephric, or Renal Allotransplanted State. J. Urol., *103*:686, 1970.

Naets, J.P.: The Role of the Kidney in Erythropoiesis. J. Clin. Invest., *39*:102, 1960.

Naets, J.P., and Wittek, M.: Erythropoiesis in Anephric Man. Lancet, *1*:941, 1968.

Nakeff, A., et al.: Megakaryocytes in Agar Cultures of Mouse Bone Marrow. Ser. Haematol., *8*:4, 1975.

Nara, N., et al.: Effects of Chloramphenicol on Hematopoietic Inductive Microenvironment. Exp. Hematol., *10*:20, 1982.

Nathan, D.G., et al.: Human Erythroid Burst Forming

Unit: T Cell Requirement for Proliferation in Vitro. J. Exp. Med., *147*:324, 1978.

Neal, W.A., et al.: Inhibition of Erythropoiesis by Plasma Component(s) from Sheep, Goat, and Rabbits. Amer. J. Vet. Res., *40*:493, 1979.

Nowell, P.C., and Hungerford, D.A.: Chromosome Studies in Human Leukemia. II. Chronic Granulocytic Leukemia. J. U.S. Natl. Cancer Inst., *27*:1013, 1961.

Nye, R.N.: Bone Marrow Volume in Rabbits. Proc. Soc. Exp. Biol. Med., *29*:34, 1931.

Ogawa, M., et al.: Renewal and Committment to Differentiation of Hemopoietic Stem Cells (An Interpretive Review). Blood, *61*:823, 1983.

Okuda, K.: On Intrinsic Factor and the Dog. Gastroenterology, *52*:614, 1969.

Pease, D.C.: An Electron Microscopic Study of Red Bone Marrow. Blood, *11*:501, 1956.

Pelus, L.M., et al.: Regulation of Human Myelopoiesis by Prostaglandin E and Lactoferrin. Cell Tissue Kinet., *14*:515, 1981.

Philip, M.A., et al.: Phagocytosing Neutrophils Rapidly Release a Factor Which Inhibits Granulopoiesis in Vitro. Acta Haematol., *67*:20, 1982.

Pluznik, D.H., and Sachs, L.: The Cloning of Normal "Mast" Cells in Tissue Culture. J. Cell. Comp. Physiol., *66*:319, 1966.

Quessenberry, P., and Levitt, L.: Hematopoietic Stem Cells. New Eng. J. Med., *301*:755, 819, 868, 1979.

Raab, S.O., et al.: Granulokinetics in Normal Dogs. Amer. J. Physiol., *206*:83, 1964.

Raghavachar, A., et al.: Granulocytic Progenitor Cells (CFU-C) in Canine blood: Mobilization by Dexamethasone. Blut, *441*:107, 1982.

Riches, A.C., et al.: The Control of Haematopoietic Stem Cell Proliferation by Humoral Factors. Prog. Clin. Biol. Res., *59B*:269, 1981.

Richman, C.M., et al.: Purificatl and Characterization of Granulocytic Progenitor Cells (CFU-C) from Human Peripheral Blood Using Immunologic Surface Markers. Blood, *51*:1, 1978.

Robbins, K.R., and Shields, J.: Preparation of Partially Purified Porcine Intrinsic Factor. Proc. Soc. Exp. Biol. Med., *95*:781, 1957.

Roggli, V.L., and Saleem, A.: Erythroleukemia: A Study of 15 Cases and Literature Review. Cancer, *49*:101, 1982.

Roodman, G.D., and Zanjani, E.D.: Endogenous Erythroid Colony Forming Cells in Fetal and Newborn Sheep. J. Lab. Clin. Med., *94*:699, 1979.

Schmid, J.R., et al.: Thymoma Associated with Pure Red Cell Agencies: Review of Literature and Report of 4 Cases. Cancer, *18*:216, 1965.

Scott, J.L., and Davidson, J.G.: Normal Lymphocyte Kinetics: Influence of Splenectomy and Epinephrine. Proc. XIII Annu. Meeting, Amer. Soc. Hematol., Puerto Rico, Dec. 6–8, p. 42, 1970.

Singer, K., and Weisz, L.: The Life Cycle of the Erythrocyte after Splenectomy and Problems of Splenic Hemolysis and Target Cell Formation. Amer. J. Med. Sci., *210*:301, 1945.

Smith, K.A.: T-Cell Growth Factor. Immunol. Rev., *51*:337, 1980.

Stanley, E.R., and Jubinsky, P.T.: Factors Affecting the Growth and Differentiation of Haematopoietic Cells in Culture. Clin. Haematol., *13*:329, 1984.

Stenman, U.H.: Characterization of the R-Type Vitamin B_{12} Binding Proteins by Isoelectric Focusing. Scand. J. Haematol., *13*:129, 1974; *14*:19, 1975.

Stephenson, J.R., et al.: Induction of Colonies of Hemo-globin-Synthesizing Cells by Erythropoietin in Vitro. Proc. Natl. Acad. Sci. U.S.A., *68*:1542, 1971.

Storti, E., et al.: Biological and Clinical Significance of the Adrenalin Test in Haematology. Haematologia, *1*:27, 1967.

Suda, T., et al.: The Effect of Hydrocortisone on Human Granulocytes In Vitro with Cytochemical Analysis of Colonies. Exp. Hematol., *11*:114, 1983.

Taelte, R., and Mendelsohn, J.: An Emerging Role for Prostaglandin E_1 in Regulation of Granulopoiesis. Leuk. Res., *5*:511, 1981.

Tavassoli, M.: Red Cell Delivery and the Function of the Marrow-Blood Barrier: A Review. Exp. Hematol., *6*:257, 1978.

Tavassoli, M.: Structure and Function of Sinusoidal Endothelium of Bone Marrow. Prog. Clin. Biol. Res., *59B*:249, 1981.

Thomas, E.D., et al.: The Problem of the Stem Cell: Observation in Dogs following Nitrogen Mustard. J. Lab. Clin. Med., *65*:794, 1965.

Tiedemann, K., and Ooyen, B. Van: Prenatal Hemato-poiesis and Blood Characteristics of the Cat. Anat. Embryol., *153*:243, 1978.

Till, J.E., and McCulloch, E.A.: A Direct Measurement of the Radiation Sensitivity of Normal Mouse Bone Marrow Cells. Radiat. Res., *14*:213, 1961.

Torten, M., and Schalm, O.W.: Influence of the Equine Spleen on Rapid Changes in the Concentration of Erythrocytes in Peripheral Blood. Amer. J. Vet. Res., *25*:500, 1964.

Tough, I.M., et al.: Cytogenetic Studies in Chronic My-eloid Leukaemia and Acute Leukaemia Associated with Mongolism. Lancet, *1*:411, 1961.

Trainin, N., and Small, M.: Studies on Some Physico-chemical Properties of a Thymus Humoral Factor Conferring Immunocompetence on Lymphoid Cells. J. Exp. Med., *132*:885, 1970.

Tramezzani, J.H., et al.: The Carotid Body as a Neu-roendocrine Organ Involved in Control of Erythro-poiesis. Proc. Natl. Acad. Sci. U.S.A., *68*:52, 1971.

Waldmann, T.A., et al.: The Effect of Splenectomy on Erythropoiesis in the Dog. Blood, *15*:873, 1960.

Wang, J.C., and Tobin, M.S.: Mechanism of Extra-medullary Haematopoiesis in Rabbits with Sapon-Induced Myelofibrosis and Myeloid Metaplasia. Brit. J. Haematol., *51*:277, 1982.

Weiss, L.: The Role of the Spleen in the Removal of Nor-mally Aged Red Cells. Amer. J. Anat., *111*:175, 1962.

Weiss, L.: The Structure of Bone Marrow. Functional Interrelationships of Vascular and Hematopoietic Com-partments in Experimental Hemolytic Anemia: An Electron Microscopic Study. J. Morphol., *117*:467, 1965.

Weiss, L.: The Histophysiology of Bone Marrow. Clin. Orthop., *52*:13, 1967.

Weiss, L.: Transmural Cellular Passage in Vascular Si-nuses of Rat Bone Marrow. Blood, *36*:189, 1970.

Weiss, L.: A Scanning Electron Microscopic Study of the Spleen. Blood, *43*:665, 1974.

Weiss, L.: Haemopoiesis in Mammalian Bone Marrow. Ciba Found. Symp., *84*:5, 1981.

Weiss, L., and Tavassoli, M.: Anatomical Hazards to the Passage of Erythrocytes through the Spleen. Semin. Hematol., *7*:372, 1970.

Whang, J., et al.: The Distribution of the Philadelphia Chromosome in Patients with Chronic Myelogenous Leukemia. Blood, *22*:664, 1963.

Wheby, M.S., et al.: Studies on Iron Absorption. Intes-tinal Regulatory Mechanisms. J. Clin. Invest., *43*:1433, 1964.

Williams, N., and Levine, R.F.: The Origin, Development and Regulation of Megakaryocytes. Brit. J. Haema-tol., *52*:173, 1982.

Wilson, F.D., and Shifrine, M.: The Canine as a Model for Studies on Stem and Progenitor Cells of Lym-phodermatopoiesis. *In* The Canine as a Biomedical Research Model: Immunological, Hematological and Oncological Aspects. Shifrine, M., and Wilson, F.D., eds. Tech. Inf. Center/U.S. Dept. of Energy, Spring-field, Va., p. 3, 1980.

Winqvist, G.: Morphology of the Blood and the Hemo-poietic Organs in Cattle under Normal and some Experimental Conditions. Acta Anat., *22*(Suppl. 21):1, 1954.

Wintrobe, et al.: Clinical Hematology. 8th ed. Lea & Febiger, Philadelphia, 1981.

Wolf, N.S., and Trentin, J.J.: Hemopoietic Colony Stud-ies. V. Effect of Hemopoietic Organ Stroma on Dif-ferentiation of Pluripotent Stem Cells. J. Exp. Med., *127*:205, 1968.

Wright, E.G., and Lord, B.I.: Production of Stem Cell Proliferation Stimulators and Inhibitors by Haema-topoietic Cell Suspensions. Biomedicine. *28*:156, 1978.

Yoffey, J.M.: Bone Marrow. Brit. Med. J., *2*:193, 1954.

Yoffey, J.M.: The Lymphocyte. Ann. Rev. Med., *12*:125, 1964.

Yunis, A.A., et al.: Further Evidence Supporting an In Vivo Role for Colony-Stimulating Factor. Exp. Hem-atol., *12*:838, 1984.

Zamboni, L., and Pease, D.C.: The Vascular Bed of Red Bone Marrow. J. Ultrastruct. Res., *5*:65, 1961.

Zuckerman, K.S.: Human Erythroid Burst Forming Units. Growth in Vitro Is Dependent on Monocytes, but Not T Lymphocytes. J. Clin. Invest., *67*:702, 1981.

Zwaan, F.E.: Haematopoietic Progenitor Cells in Periph-eral Blood. Blut, *45*:87, 1982.

14

Coagulation and Its Disorders

B.F. Feldman, E.J. Carroll, and N.C. Jain

PRIMARY HEMOSTASIS 389

ROLE OF THE PLATELETS 391

COAGULATION 392
Coagulation Factors and Their
Interactions 393
Summary of Coagulation and Platelet
Interactions During Hemostasis 396

**BIOSYNTHESIS OF CLOTTING FACTORS
AND THE ROLE OF VITAMIN K 397**

**REGULATION OF THE CLOTTING
PROCESS 398**

FIBRINOLYSIS 399
Mechanisms 399
Measurements 401
Clinical Observations 402

DISORDERS OF COAGULATION 402
Hereditary Coagulopathies 402
Acquired Coagulopathies 402

**DISSEMINATED INTRAVASCULAR
COAGULATION (DIC) 410**
Conditions Associated with DIC 411
Pathophysiology 411
Diagnosis 412
Therapy 413

THROMBOSIS 415
Pathogenesis 415
Diagnosis 416
Therapy 417

DIAGNOSTIC METHODS 419
Screening Tests of Hemostasis 420
Routine Tests of Hemostasis 420
Hemostatic Tests for DIC and
Fibrinolysis 423
Protamine Sulfate Test 425
Hemostatic Tests of Fibrin Stabilization 425
Platelet Tests 425

As more complex species evolved in nature, more complex mechanisms of blood coagulation arose. These mechanisms were necessitated in part by increasing blood pressures in thicker-walled vessels. At the same time, increasing complexities required the evolution of several safety devices by which blood is prevented from clotting within the vessels. Naturally occurring anticoagulants exist as well as a complex system for dissolving clotted blood.

Blood, when removed from normal endothelium-lined blood vessels, clots. Clotting is more rapid in glass vessels than in vessels coated with silicone or similar materials, which indicates that when blood comes in contact with glass, the clotting mechanism is activated. This phenomenon is called *contact activation* and indicates that all components

necessary for clotting are present in normal blood. This type of clotting is brought about by the so-called *intrinsic* or endogenous system. On the other hand, clotting is accelerated greatly if thromboplastins, which arise from damaged tissues, are added to the plasma. The clotting system involving tissue factors is called the *extrinsic* or exogenous system. Both systems are necessary to maintain normal hemostasis, i.e., prevention of blood loss from damaged vessels.

This chapter discusses the process of hemostasis, as well as aberrations of the hemostatic mechanisms leading to disease. Additional information is available in several excellent publications on these topics (Colman et al., 1982; Dodds, 1980; Fishbach and Fogdall, 1981; Hall, 1972; Hirsh and Brain, 1983; Jones, 1979; Moake and Funicella, 1983; Thompson and Harker, 1983).

Table 14–1.   Pathogenesis of Defective Hemostasis

Vascular Defects
   Structural
   Immune-mediated
   Inflammation

Quantitative Platelet Abnormalities
   Failure of production
   Reduced survival
   Increased sequestration

Qualitative Platelet Abnormalities
   Failure to adhere or release adenosine diphos-
      phate (ADP)
   Failure to aggregate
   Failure to make phospholipid available

Coagulation Factor Defects
   Absolute failure of synthesis
   Production of abnormal molecule
   Excessive destruction of coagulation factors
   Circulatory inhibitors

PRIMARY HEMOSTASIS

Hemostasis involves a complex series of physiologic and biochemical events involving both promotors and inhibitors of blood coagulation. The hemostatic process is designed to maintain blood within the confines of blood vessels. Primary hemostasis is initiated when vascular injury disrupts endothelium, exposing subendothelial connective tissue to flowing blood. Essentially three functional components of hemostasis act in concert to arrest bleeding, namely, blood vessels, platelets, and coagulation proteins or factors. Acquired or hereditary disorders of any of these three components can lead to defective hemostasis (Tables 14–1 and 14–2).

The mechanism of arrest of bleeding differs somewhat, depending on the size of the vessels involved. During the first minutes after a small cut is made in the skin, the axon reflex leads to transient vasoconstriction. The interaction of platelets and vascular endothelium may be sufficient to arrest bleeding. Severing of a larger vessel involves a more complex mechanism of platelet plug formation and activation of the blood coagulation system. The basic hemostatic mechanism is rapid and localized but the system is not without risk—

too much hemostasis at the site of injury leads to thrombosis with resultant vascular obstruction and ischemia, whereas too little hemostasis leads to persistent bleeding (Thompson and Harker, 1983).

Platelets do not adhere to normal intact endothelium. Intact endothelium does not activate hemostasis. This property of endothelium is attributed to both active and passive processes. Active mechanisms are associated with direct or indirect participation of intact endothelial cells and include synthesis of prostacyclin (PGI_2) (see Chapter 16), plasminogen activators, and thrombomodulin; uptake and degradation of adenosine diphosphate (ADP) and proaggregating vasoactive amines; and inactivation of thrombin. Passive mechanisms involve endothelial proteoglycans, primarily heparin sulfate with anticoagulant properties, and net negative surface charge repelling similarly charged blood cells. PGI_2 stimulates membrane adenylcyclase and increases platelet cyclic adenosine monophosphate (cAMP) concentrations. Increased cAMP concentration impairs platelet-to-platelet cohesion (aggregation) and inhibits release of ADP and other platelet contents. A cAMP stimulated, protein kinase mediated phosphorylation of platelet membrane or cytoplasmic protein can cause these inhibitory effects (Moake and Funicella, 1983). Injury to endothelial cells results in loss of resistance to platelet adherence as well as exposure of collagen promoting coagulation. As blood escapes from the larger vessels and passes the damaged vessel walls, platelets adhere to the subendothelial collagen through interaction of their surface receptors with endothelial or subendothelial factor VIII-related von Willebrand's factor (factor VIII:vWF). This process is referred to as *platelet adhesion* (Fig. 14–1). Collagen must be present in appropriate fibrillar configuration to promote binding of platelets (Ruggeri et al, 1982) and to activate coagulation (Gentry et al., 1975). Fibronectin

Table 14–2.   Clinical Signs in Vascular, Platelet, or Coagulation Defects

Vascular or Platelet Defect	Coagulation Defect
Petechiae, superficial bruising	Deep-spreading hematoma
Bleeding in skin and mucous membranes	Hemarthroses or retroperitoneal bleeding
Immediate bleeding	Recurrent and late bleeding

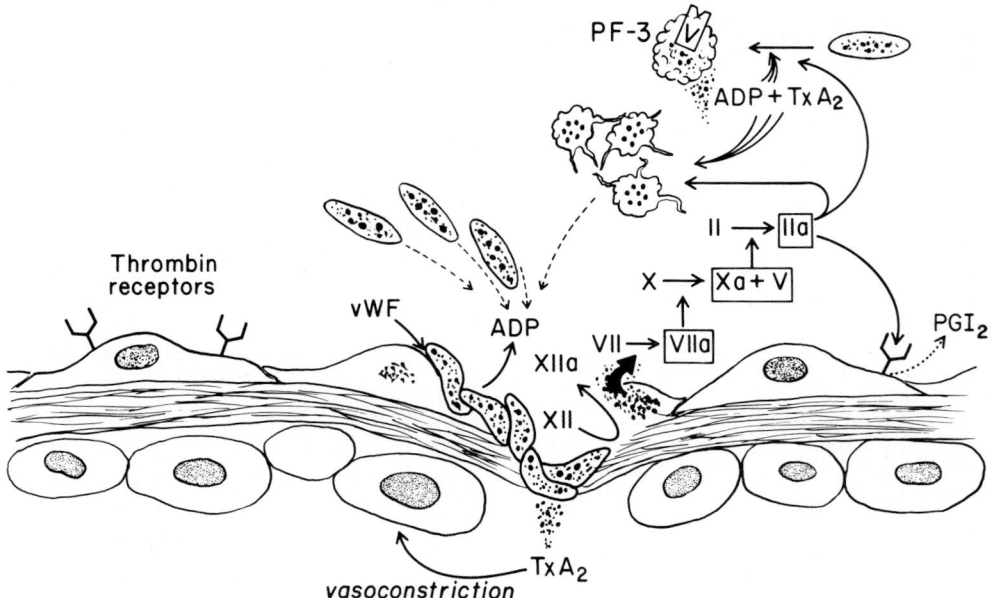

Fig. 14–1. Hemostatic events associated with vessel wall injury. Collagen-induced activation of platelets by adenosine diphosphate (ADP) and thromboxane (Tx)A$_2$ and initiation of clotting through activation of intrinsic system (beginning at factor XII) and extrinsic system (begininng at factor VII). See text for details. (Prepared with the assistance of Dr. R. Slappendel.)

and thrombospondin, released from platelet alpha-granules, may also be involved in the process of platelet adhesion. The adhered platelets undergo shape change from discs to irregular spheres and begin to release their internal contents. This release reaction attracts other platelets from the passing stream and induces *platelet aggregation*, which eventually forms a large mass over the injured area; within a short time, the opening in the vessel is filled, and blood ceases to escape. Platelet aggregation up to a certain point may be reversible (White and Gerrard, 1982). These reversible platelet aggregates often become detached and are carried away; new aggregates then form. The irreversible phase of platelet aggregation is called *viscous metamorphosis* (Zucker, 1980).

The interaction of platelets with collagen fibers concomitantly initiates a contractile process aided by centripetal movement of a circumferential band of microtubules herding platelet storage granules toward the center of the platelet, and finally extruding the granular contents through the open canalicular system. During this process of platelet activation and release reaction, many factors are released into the microenvironment. These factors are either stored preformed in various

platelet organelles or newly synthesized as a result of metabolic stimulation (see Table 16–1) and include ADP, adenosine triphosphate (ATP), serotonin, platelet factors 3 and 4, platelet fibrinogen, thromboxane (Tx) A$_2$, platelet-derived growth factor, β-thromboglobulin, and acid hydrolases. The release of ADP and the generation of TxA$_2$ attract more platelets to the area to enlarge the hemostatic plug. ADP interacts with platelet membranes to expose a specific fibrinogen binding receptor site associated with the glycoprotein IIb–IIIa complex on the platelet membrane. Bound fibrinogen serves as a primary recognition site for platelet-to-platelet interaction during aggregation (White and Gerrard, 1982; Zucker, 1980).

The next step, which is the most important factor in the induction of viscous metamorphosis, occurs when prothrombin in the plasma is converted to thrombin. Platelet adherence and aggregation create favorable conditions for localized activation of the clotting system. Platelets can activate the intrinsic clotting system through interactions with a factor XII receptor and high-molecular-weight (HMW) kininogen, through release of platelet factor 3 (PF-3) and through trapping of coagulation factors on their surfaces. The release of tissue thromboplastin from injured endothelium and subendothelial connective tissue presumably activates the extrinsic clotting system on the platelet surface (Fig. 14–2; Deykin and Moake, 1983). Thrombin generated by activation of coagulation pathways amplifies platelet aggregation and release responses.

The next stage involves fibrin formation, enmeshing platelets, and the production of a compact mass (Fig. 14–2). Evidence suggests that an actomysin-like contractile protein, thrombosthenin, present within platelet microfilaments, produces contraction of platelets that tends to tense the fibrin strands, thereby reinforcing and sealing the hemostatic plug.

Thrombin activity is limited to the area of hemostasis by the action of plasma protease inhibitors, thrombin-antithrombin III complex formation, and endothelial activation of protein "C," which destroys coagulation factors V and VIII (Thompson and Harker, 1983). Dissolution of the hemostatic plug, after it has served its purpose, occurs after activation of the fibrinolytic system (see Fibrinolysis). Fibrinolysis remains localized as does thrombin activation.

For additional information on platelets in hemostasis see Chapter 16 and Figure 16–7.

ROLE OF THE PLATELETS

Platelets have been described as being "spongy" in that they "soak up" plasma constituents. At least 15 plasma proteins are known to have been adsorbed to platelet surfaces including coagulation factors II, V, VIII, IX, X, XI, XII, and XIII (White and Gerrard, 1982). In addition, the following three platelet coagulation factors (distinguished by Arabic numerals) are considered unique to the platelets, although 10 such factors have been described (Wintrobe et al., 1981). Platelet factor 1 (PF-1) is probably plasma coagulation factor V; PF-5 is fibrinogen adsorbed from the plasma; and PF-6 is a plasmin inhibitor associated with platelet membrane. Other platelet factors are poorly defined.

PF-2: A heat-stable protein that accelerates the conversion of fibrinogen to fibrin by thrombin. It also inhibits antithrombin III and induces platelet aggregation.

PF-3: A thermostable lipoprotein closely associated with the platelet membrane. It becomes "available" or is "activated" following platelet activation and release re-

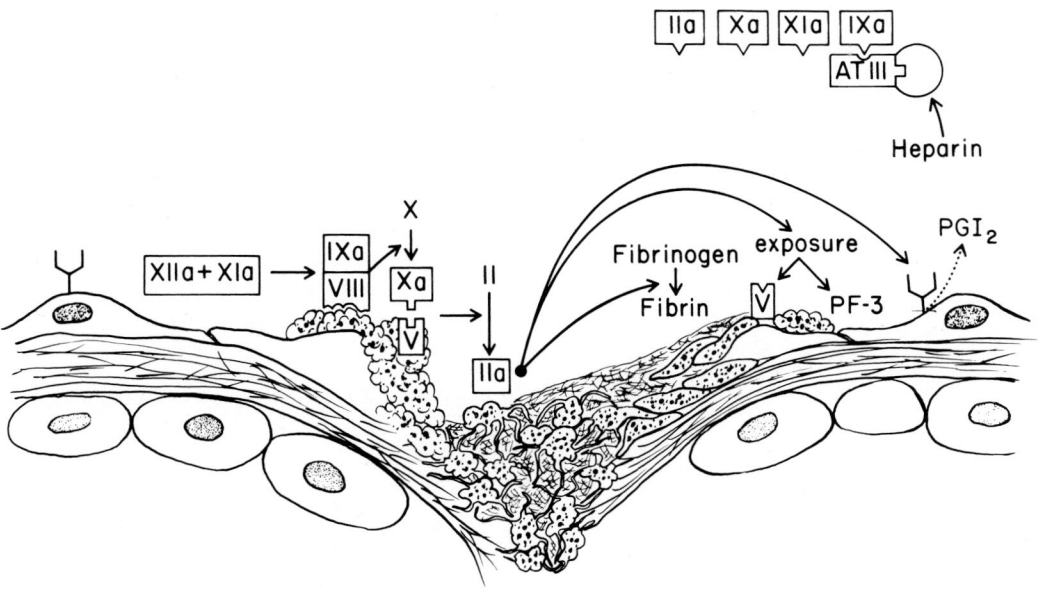

Fig. 14–2. Hemostatic events associated with vessel wall injury. Organization of platelet plug, fibrin deposition, and regulatory actions of prostacyclin (PGI₂) and heparin-antithrombin III (ATIII) complex. See text for details. (Prepared with the assistance of Dr. R. Slappendel.)

action. It is required for the activation of factor X by factors IXa and VIIIa and for the conversion of prothrombin to thrombin by factors Xa and Va (Fig. 14–3).

PF-4: A thermostable glycoprotein (MW 9,600–21,000) present in alpha-granules and on the membrane. It neutralizes heparin, inhibits collagenase from skin and neutrophils, and facilitates ADP-induced platelet aggregation.

The primary role of platelets in hemostasis is adhesion, aggregation, and viscous metamorphosis as discussed and depicted in Figures 14–1 and 14–2. Defective hemostasis results when thrombocytopathies and thrombocytopenias occur. See Chapter 16 for details on platelet structure and function, and Chapter 17 for details on thrombocytopenias and thrombocytopathies.

COAGULATION

Blood coagulation can be described as a series of reactions in which the product of reaction A is an enzyme that catalyzes reaction B, and the product of reaction B is the enzyme that catalyzes reaction C and so on, where A, B, and C are present initially as inactive or precursor proenzymes and at most steps, activation occurs by limited proteolytic cleavage and protein-to-protein complexing reactions. This type of activity is common to several biologic systems such as the complement cascade and kinin formation. The series of step-like

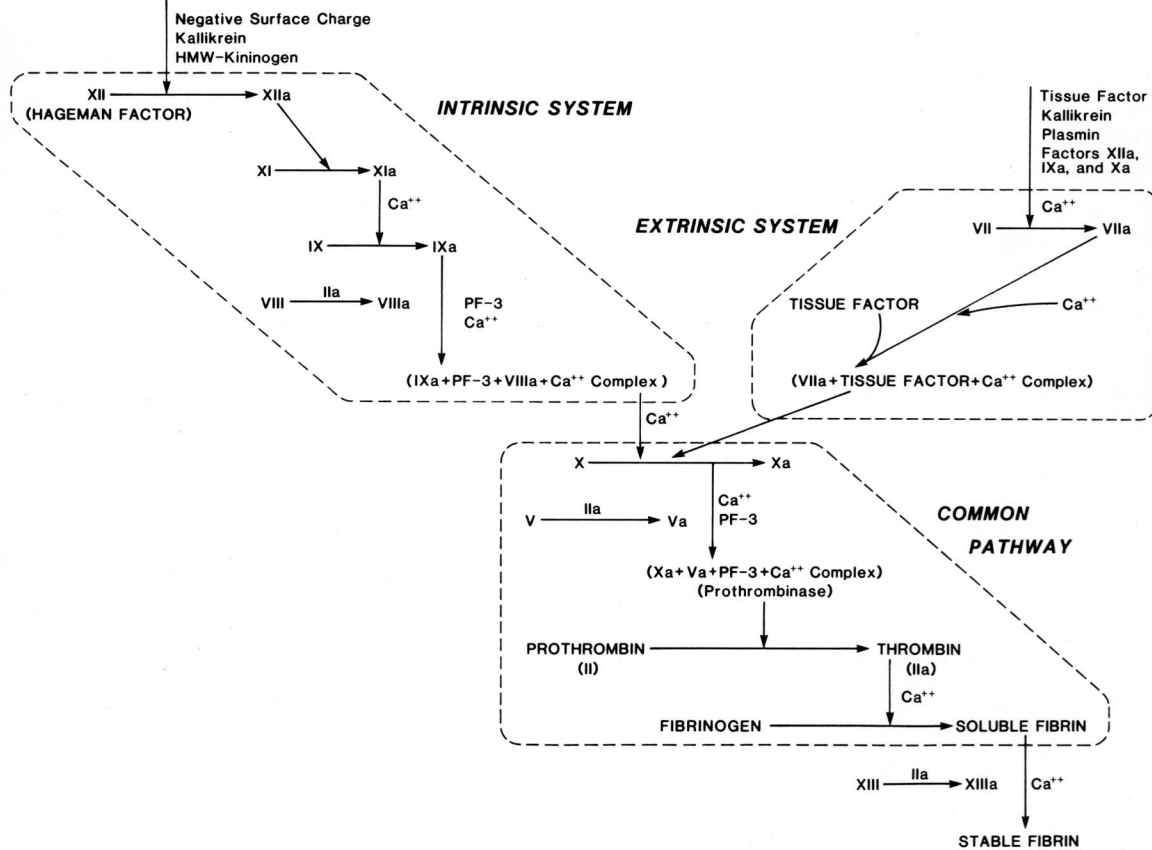

Fig. 14–3. Classic cascade mechanism of blood coagulation terminating in a stable fibrin clot formation. Factor XIIa plays a crucial role in the initiation of the intrinsic system, whereas factor VII and tissue factor complex initiate the extrinsic system. The two systems merge at the stage where factor X is activated to Xa, the first step of the common pathway. HMW-kininogen, high-molecular-weight kininogen; PF-3, platelet phospholipid. See Figure 14–4 for interactions of the activated Hageman factor with other biologic systems and Figure 14–5 for fibrin(ogen)olysis. See text for details.

reactions, sometimes called a "waterfall" or "cascade", provides a high net energy gain that allows for the explosive suddenness of the functionally important final step, the conversion of soluble fibrinogen to insoluble fibrin.

The nomenclature of various coagulation factors, established by an International Committe for the Nomenclature of Blood Clotting Factors, is given in Table 14–3 and a scheme for their interaction is given in Figure 14–3. In addition, Table 14–3 also lists the plasma levels, in vivo half-lives, turnover rates, and sites of biosynthesis of various coagulation factors. The factors are numbered (in Roman numerals) according to priority of discovery, not in order of their action. Note that the only nonprotein factor is calcium (factor IV), which is needed for most of the reactions. With the exception of tissue thromboplastin (factor III), each factor is present in normal plasma. Serum is deficient in factors I, II, V, and VIII and has diminished concentrations of factor XIII and increased concentrations of factor IX. Factors XII, XI, X, IX, VII, and II and prekallikrein possess serine at their active enzymatic sites, thus are classified as serine proteases (Thompson and Harker, 1983). Some of the coagulation proteins, e.g., factors II, VIII, IX, and X, have a sizable extravascular pool that can be mobilized into the circulation by physiologic and pathologic stimuli (Wintrobe et al., 1981).

Many schemes have been proposed to aid in understanding the clotting sequence, and one is outlined in Figure 14–3. Even with present knowledge, such schemes are still tentative. Clotting probably is not as orderly a step-by-step process as commonly diagrammed, nor are all the reactions truly proenzyme-enzyme transformations; and although the process is divided into steps or phases, parallel reactions in another "phase" are also occurring simultaneously. For example, coagulation factors VIII:vWF, V, and III, and HMW-kininogen act as cofactors rather than proteases (Davie et al., 1979; Thompson and Harker, 1983). Two phases can interact. Thrombin produced in later stages of clotting also is involved in activation of factor VIII, an earlier event. It is evident from Figure 14–3 that the coagulation process is probably one of four steps, namely, the *contact reaction, thromboplastinogenesis, thrombin formation*, and *fibrin formation*. Laboratory procedures have been developed to detect abnormalities of one or more of these steps (Table 14–4).

Coagulation Factors and Their Interactions

Factor XII (Hageman Factor)

The first step in the clotting sequence is the conversion of factor XII to its active state, XIIa,

Table 14–3. Nomenclature and Some Properties of Coagulation Factors*

Factor	Common Name	Molecular Weight	Plasma Level (μg/ml)	Half-life (hours)	Turnover Rate (μg/ml/day)	Biosynthesis
I	Fibrinogen	340,000	2500	123	500	Liver
II	Prothrombin	70,000	100	100	40	Liver; vitamin K-dependent
III	Tissue thromboplastin	45,000	0	—	—	Virtually all tissues
IV	Calcium ions	—	—	—	—	
V	Proaccelerin	330,000	5–12	25	10	Liver
VII	Proconvertin	63,000	1	5	2	Liver; vitamin K-dependent
VIII	Antihemophilic factor	1–2 million	7	10	25	FVIII:C, probably liver FVIII:vWF, endothelial cells and megakaryocytes
IX	Christmas factor	62,000	4	20	2	Liver; vitamin K-dependent
X	Stuart factor	59,000	5	65	6	Liver; vitamin K-dependent
XI	Plasma thromboplastin antecedent	200,000	4	65	<2	Liver
XII	Hageman factor	80,000	29	60	<2	?
XIII	Fibrin stabilizing factor	320,000	10	150	3	Liver?; megakaryocytes
—	Prekallikrein	85,000	—	—	—	Liver?
—	High-molecular-weight kininogen	120,000	—	—	—	Liver?

Data compiled from Giddings (1980), Thompson and Harker (1983), and Wintrobe et al. (1981).
*Factor designation is as recommended by an International Committee for the Nomenclature of Blood Clotting Factors. JAMA, *180*:733, 1962.

Table 14–4. Laboratory Diagnosis of Bleeding Disorders—Common Tests

Prothrombin Time (PT)
Assays extrinsic (factor VII) and common (factors X, V, II, and I) pathways

Activated Partial Thromboplastin Time (APTT)
Assays intrinsic (factors XII, XI, IX, and VIII) and (common factors X, V, II, and I) pathways

Thrombin Time (TT)
Assays fibrinogen (factor I)

Platelet Count
Examination of stained blood film for adequacy of platelet numbers.
Total platelet count is performed if smear indicates a decreased or markedly increased platelet number

an esterolytic enzyme. This is called the *contact reaction* because it occurs when blood comes in contact with glass or other agents such as asbestos, kaolin, or diatomaceous earth, which has a highly negative surface charge (Cochrane and Griffith, 1979) and is the basis for the measurement of clotting time (see Diagnostic Methods). Calcium is not utilized during contact activation of factor XII. Once activation occurs, factor XIIa successively converts factors XI and IX each to its activated form XIa and IXa; Ca^{++} is required to convert factor IX to its active form. Both factors XII and XI are adsorbed to glass or to a similar surface in the contact reaction. In vivo activation of factor XII occurs when collagen is exposed after tissue injury. Prekallikrein (also known as Fletcher factor) and HMW-kininogen (also known as Fitzgerald factor, Williams factor, Flaujeac factor) also participate in contact activation of factor XII. Kinin participation is needed for optimal activation of the intrinsic pathway; kallikrein can activate factors XII and XI. HMW-kininogen mainly enhances the action of factor XIIa during activation of factor XI. Although activities of each of these contact factors may be reduced by acquired or hereditary disorders, only low concentrations of factor XI are associated with abnormal bleeding.

Factor XII also may become activated in the fluid phase, i.e., in plasma, without surface activation, by a variety of proteolytic enzymes such as kallikrein, plasmin, and factor XIa and possibly by endothelial cells (Wintrobe et al., 1981).

In addition to the coagulation system, note that the kinin, complement, and plasminogen systems also merge at this initial step of the coagulation cascade (Fig. 14–4). The Hageman factor also is important in inflammation and disseminated intravascular coagulation (DIC). Factor XIIa, in reacting with exposed collagen, activates the plasma kinin system by the conversion of inactive prekallikrein to active kallikrein which in turn converts kininogen to active kinins (Zimmerman et al., 1977). Similarly, smaller proteolytic fragments of factor XII can activate prekallikrein, although they do not activate factor XI. Kinins are an important factor in inflammation because they cause edema, vasodilation, and increased capillary permeability and induce chemotaxis of leukocytes (see Chapter 26). Note that kallikrein also can be involved in the fibrinolytic system and has additional physiologic roles (Cochrane and Griffith, 1979; Heimark et al., 1980).

For a review of Hageman factor activity, see Kaplan et al. (1976).

Factor VIII (Antihemophilic Factor)

In the next sequence of the coagulation process, factor IXa forms a complex with factor VIII and PF-3 in the presence of Ca^{++}. This complex then activates factor X to Xa. Factor VIII first requires modification by a serine protease, such as thrombin, to exert its reactivity independently. The action of thrombin on factor VIII accelerates the generation of Xa.

Recent immunologic studies have revealed the heterogeneity of factor VIII (Bloom, 1980; Hoyer, 1981); this finding has clinical and diagnostic implications. It has been found that factor VIII is comprised of a major and a minor component, each having different biochemical and functional properties. The major component (MW about 1 million) called *factor VIII-related antigen* (FVIII:RAg) does not participate in the intrinsic pathway of coagulation, but is involved in formation of the hemostatic plug. FVIII:RAg is produced by endothelial cells and megakaryocytes. Factor VIII:vWF activity is associated with this component. The smaller moiety (MW 25,000–340,000) constitutes the factor VIII-coagulant (FVIII:C) activity and participates in coagulation. The FVIII:C site of biosynthesis is not known definitely, but studies in dogs (Webster et al.,

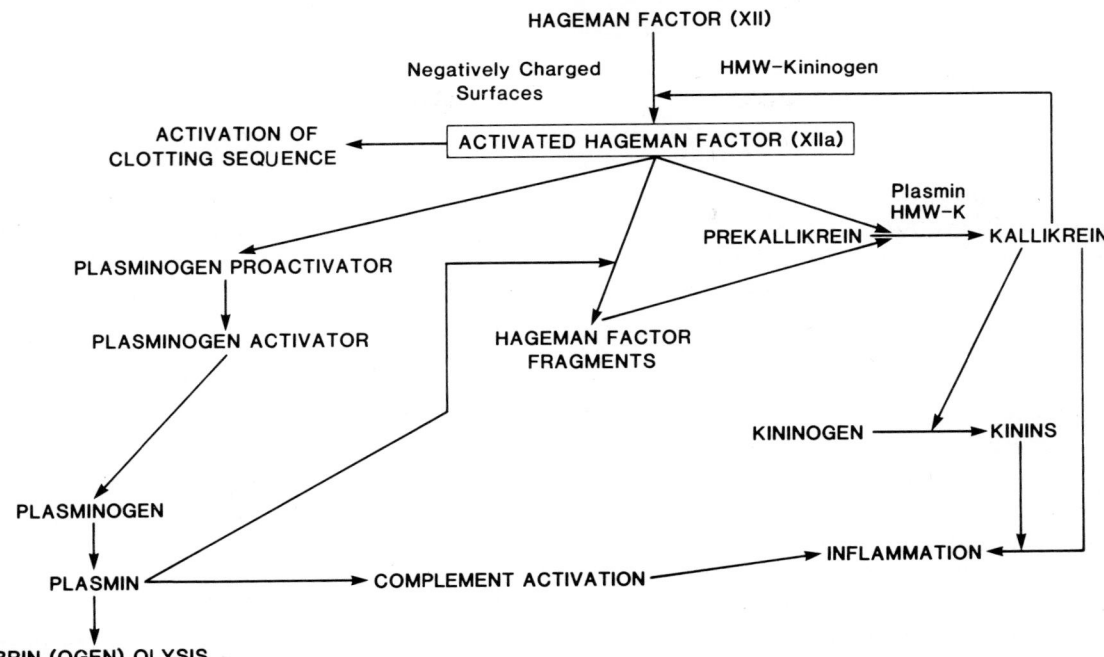

Fig. 14–4. Interactions between the coagulation, kinin, fibrinolytic, and complement systems. HMW-kininogen, high-molecular-weight kininogen. (Modified from Ruddy et al., 1972.)

1971) and pigs (Owen et al., 1979) indicate hepatic synthesis, probably by the mononuclear phagocyte system (MPS) (Jaffe, 1977; Jaffe et al., 1973). The half-life of FVIII:C is estimated at 8 to 12 hours and that of FVIII:RAg at 22 to 44 hours (Bennett and Ratnoff, 1972; Kernoff et al., 1974). Methods for their detection have been described (Feinstein et al., 1969; Hoyer, 1972, 1976, 1981; Stites et al., 1971; Zimmerman et al., 1977).

A significant extravascular pool of factor VIII exists, principally in the spleen (Weaver et al., 1964; Webster et al., 1971). Plasma concentrations of factor VIII can increase under a variety of circumstances, such as following vigorous exercise, infusion of epinephrine and 2–3 DPG, and death; in pregnancy; and in chronic thrombocytpenia. Factor VIII also acts as an acute phase protein.

Factor X (Stuart-Prower Factor)

Factor X is the meeting ground of the intrinsic and extrinsic systems (see Fig. 14–3). At this level and onward, the two systems share a common pathway. As mentioned, the intrinsic system is initiated by contact activation whereas in the extrinsic system, initi-

ation is via thromboplastin of tissue origin (factor III). In the intrinsic system, factor IXa, factor VIII, PF-3, and Ca^{++} form a complex to activate factor X. In the extrinsic system, thromboplastin released by tissue damage reacts with factor VII in the presence of Ca^{++} to form a complex for activation of factor X. Factor X can be activated in vitro by incubation with dilute trypsin or Russell's viper venom. Activated factor Xa is the prime activator of prothrombin (Dodds, 1980).

Prothrombin and Thrombin

Prothrombin is converted to thrombin in the presence of factor Xa, phospholipid (PF-3), Ca^{++}, and an accelerator (factor V). Although thrombin can be formed from prothrombin without the interaction of factors other than Ca^{++} and phospholipid, the reaction is slow. The reaction is accelerated by a labile factor called *proaccelerin* or *factor V*. In vitro activity of factor V is increased by action of proteolytic enzymes, e.g., thrombin, factor Xa, Russell's viper venom, and papain. Factor V is inactivated by EDTA.

Factors Xa and V react with platelet phospholipid in the presence of Ca^{++} to form a particulate complex with enzyme activity, also refered to as "prothrombin-converting activity" or "prothrombinase." Prothrombin is converted to thrombin by the action of prothrombinase. The phospholipid is thought to be organized in clusters or aggregates, and the action of prothrombinase takes place on the surface of these clusters. During activation of the coagulation cascade by the extrinsic system, tissue thromboplastin can substitute for the phospholipid from PF-3. Once formed, thrombin may activate its own production from prothrombin, but the reaction is slow.

Thrombin has both esterase and peptidase activity, and modifies or activates several reactions. Thrombin functions in the coagulation system at several stages, namely, conversion of fibrinogen to fibrin, promotion of platelet aggregation and release reaction, and activation of factors XIII, XII, VIII, and V. The enzymatic activity of thrombin is inhibited by heparin and natural antithrombins (see Regulation of the Clotting Process) present in plasma (Heimark, 1980). Thrombin also promotes conversion of plasminogen to plasmin and activation of the complement system.

Fibrinogen and Fibrin

Fibrinogen is a glycoprotein with a MW of 340,000. Its molecular structure is dimeric having several calcium binding sites. Each half of the fibrinogen molecule contains 3 pairs of polypeptide chains, alpha (α) or A, beta (β) or B, and gamma (γ) chains, having a MW of 73,000, 60,000, and 50,000, respectively (Doolittle, 1973; McKee et al., 1970). The chains are interconnected by disulfide bonds.

The proteolytic action of thrombin on fibrinogen results in conversion of fibrinogen to fibrin monomers and four fibrinopeptides (Lane, 1981). The reaction takes place in the absence of calcium. Two of the fibrinopeptides are derived from the alpha chain (fibrinopeptides A) and two from the beta chain (fibrinopeptides B). The rapid spontaneous polymerization of the fibrin monomers results in formation of the clot, a gelatinous mass of fibrin strands. Initially the clot is held together by weak noncovalent forces between the fibrin monomers; and so, the clot is sol-uble in urea. Within minutes, however, a stable clot is produced when the strands are joined covalently through the action of a cross-linking enzyme, factor XIIIa, in the presence of Ca^{++} (see Fig. 14–3). Factor XIIIa enables the clot to reach maturity and achieve its maximum strength (Babior and Stossel, 1984). Factor XIII (fibrin-stabilizing factor) exists in plasma as a proenzyme and also is supplied by platelets. Factor XIII is synthesized by megakaryocytes, liver, and placenta. It is activated by thrombin in the absence of calcium.

Fibrinopeptide B has other biologic activities such as potentiating the contraction of smooth muscle and the chemotactic action on human leukocytes (Collen, 1980; Francis et al., 1980).

Tissue Thromboplastin

Tissue thromboplastin (factor III) or tissue phospholipid provides a suitably charged surface to bind both Ca^{++} and factor VII to form an enzymatic complex that activates factor X to Xa. Factor VII activity can be enhanced by the action of kallikrein, plasmin, factor XIIa, factor IXa, and also by factor Xa. Factor VII has the shortest half-life of all the coagulation proteins (see Table 14–3).

Tissue thromboplastin is not present normally in blood but is released when tissue is damaged. It is present in large amounts in the brain, lungs, and placenta, and is also secreted by activated leukocytes (Zimmerman, 1977); it has been found in the intima of large vessels. Tissue thromboplastin is a protein-phospholipid complex associated with a microsomal fraction in cells. Lipid comprises one-third of the molecular weight of this factor and is essential for its activity (Bajaj et al., 1981). The action of tissue thromboplastin is species-specific attributable to its protein moiety.

SUMMARY OF COAGULATION AND PLATELET INTERACTIONS DURING HEMOSTASIS

Because of its complexity the overall clotting mechanism not only provides for many places where controls can be invoked but also provides for several places where defects can occur. Blood contains not only the clotting factors but also a series of safety devices to prevent clotting within the vessels and to dissolve any fibrin that may have formed.

It is evident from Figure 14–1 that the hemostatic response is mediated by the cell surfaces and collagen exposed at the wound site. Exposure to collagen initiates activation of the intrinsic coagulation system, beginning with conversion of factor XII to XIIa. Prekallikrein and HMW-kininogen at the injury site enhance the activation of the intrinsic pathway. Ruptured endothelial cells, smooth muscle cells, and other damaged cells exude tissue factor initiating the extrinsic pathway (beginning with factor VII). Simultaneously, platelets coming in contact with exposed collagen or thrombin (factor IIa) become activated, i.e., they become spherical and adherent. Platelets bind to collagen via their surface receptors for von Willebrand's factor complexed to factor VIII of endothelial cells. Activated platelets then undergo the release reaction. Platelets release a variety of substances including ADP and TxA_2, both of which cause more platelets to adhere and aggregate thus enlarging the platelet plug. Availability of PF-3 and factor V on the surface of activated platelets further potentiates the clotting process (Schrier, 1984).

Figure 14–2 illustrates continuation of the aforementioned processes. During the hemostatic phase, factor V molecules at the surface of platelets in the hemostatic plug serve as binding sites for factor Xa. The binding step localizes the clotting process and markedly enhances the speed of the reaction. In the fibrin-generation phase, the localized factor Xa molecules trigger formation of a path of cross-linked fibrin molecules in which red cells become trapped. The platelet surface membrane protects the attached factor Xa and possibly thrombin (factor IIa) from degradation by the antithrombin III-heparin complex or other serine protease inhibitors. Finally, in the wound repair phase, thrombosthenin, within clotted platelets, contracts, converting the bulky plug into a tidy patch.

Several regulatory mechanisms act concurrently to keep the clotting process localized. Thrombin bound to cell surface receptors triggers release of prostacyclin (PGI_2) from un-injured endothelial cells to limit the spread of platelet aggregation. The heparin-antithrombin III complex limits further activation of the clotting process in the fluid phase. Plasmin activated early in the process, begins to lyse the clot. Platelet growth factor stimulates formation of new endothelial cells and collagen-producing fibroblasts to colonize the wound area enabling repair to occur.

BIOSYNTHESIS OF CLOTTING FACTORS AND THE ROLE OF VITAMIN K

The liver is the site of the biosynthesis of most clotting factors. Those factors that are known or thought to be produced in the liver include fibrinogen (factor I), prothrombin (factor II), and factors V, VII, IX, X, XI, and XIII (Table 14–3). Factor VIII is believed to be synthesized in two parts, one portion (FVIII:vWF) coming from endothelial cells and megakaryocytes and the other (FVIII:C) coming from an unknown site, possibly the liver. Factor XIII is synthesized also by megakaryocytes. It is not known specifically where factor XII is made.

Lipid soluble vitamin K is essential for the synthesis of factors II, VII, IX, and X by the liver. These glycoproteins are synthesized initially as inactive precursors and require vitamin K for their activation. The N-terminal portions of peptide chains of all 4 of these clotting factors contain a series of glutamic acid residues, 19 of which must be carboxylated to gamma-carboxyglutamyl to bind calcium during the clotting process (Fernlund and Stenflo, 1975; Stenflo and Suttie, 1977; Stenflo, 1978). The enzymatic carboxylation of glutamic acid residues requires vitamin K as a cofactor. Most drugs commonly used as rodenticides with anticoagulation action and drugs used for long-term therapeutic anticoagulation act by interfering with this gamma-carboxylation.

Vitamin K also is required for the production of anticoagulant proteins known collectively as protein "C" (Gallop et al., 1980; Marder, 1984), and protein "M" (Seegers and Ghosh, 1980), which is present in bovine plasma. Protein "C" is a single chain glycoprotein having a MW of about 62,000. Protein "M" has not been characterized.

Vitamin K is available in the diet (vitamin K_1, phylloquinone) or is synthesized in the gut (vitamin K_2, menaquinone) where it is passed to the liver for action. Hence, a deficiency can arise owing to low dietary concentration, lack of bowel synthesis, lack of absorption, or lack of hepatic utilization. The effects of these conditions that lead to vitamin K deficiency are discussed in a later section of this chapter. More information is available in the reviews by Mount et al. (1982), Prydz (1974, 1977), Stenflo (1978), Suttie and Jackson (1977), and Vrins et al. (1983).

REGULATION OF THE CLOTTING PROCESS

The clotting process is regulated by two general mechanisms—the elimination of activated clotting factors and the destruction of the fibrin clot. Elimination of activated clotting factors from the circulation involves humoral and cellular processes. Several natural inhibitors of coagulation have been found in blood; these inhibitors function by inhibiting protease activity. Five of them, namely antithrombin III, C_1-inactivator, α_2-macroglobulin, α_1-antitrypsin, and α_2-antiplasmin act on one or more of the coagulation factors. Some clotting factors may be directly inactivated also in the plasma by protein "C" and other humoral inactivators (Babior and Stossel, 1984). Cellular removal of activated coagulation factors involves the MPS, the liver, the lungs, and the neutrophils. Constant flow of blood also tends to diminish the local concentration of activated coagulation factors, thereby regulating the extent of clot formation.

Antithrombin III is the principal physiologic inhibitor that is most studied. It is an α_2-glycoprotein (MW 67,000) produced by the liver and is found in plasma as well as at extravascular sites. Rabbit antithrombin III has a half-life of about 42 hours. Antithrombin III works by combining with a clotting factor to form a stable 1:1 complex. It acts against activated factors XII, XI, IX, X, and II. In other words, it acts against all proteolytic clotting factors except factor VIIa. Its importance in

vivo is demonstrated in patients with antithrombin III deficiencies that are at risk for thrombosis. Its action is greatly potentiated by heparin, a property that forms the basis for anticoagulant therapy. Antithrombin III is also active against plasmin and kallikrein. Methods for measuring antithrombin III concentrations are available and can be used to diagnose disorders of coagulation, particularly DIC and thrombosis (Green, 1984; Ødegård and Abildgaard, 1978; Raymond and Dodds, 1979). Feldman et al. (1981) found that 85% of dogs with DIC had decreased antithrombin III concentration in plasma.

C'$_1$inactivator is a neuraminoglycoprotein (MW 135,000) containing the highest amount (35%) of carbohydrate of any of the plasma protease inhibitors. In addition to inhibiting the action of the first component of complement, it is a protease inhibitor of factors XIIa and XIa, kallikrein, and plasmin.

α_2-macroglobulin is a glycoprotein of MW 725,000. It inhibits activities of thrombin, kallikrein, plasmin, and other proteolytic enzymes. Its site of production is unknown, but cultured fibroblasts have been found to produce it.

α_1-antitrypsin, present in plasma and on platelets, is an α-globulin with a MW of 40,000 to 50,000. It is the major trypsin inhibitor of plasma; it also inhibits chymotrypsin, urokinase, and plasmin as well as factor XIa.

α_2-antiplasmin is an α_2-glycoprotein with a MW of 65,000 to 70,000. It inactivates plasmin and urokinase, but does not inactivate other coagulation proteins. It is the major inactivator of plasmin.

Protein "C" is a vitamin K-dependent protein that neutralizes the thrombin-activated forms of factors V and VIII. Protein "C" functions only after it is activated by thrombin, therefore, its effect tends to be limited to regions where active clotting is taking place. It is complementary to antithrombin III, working on nonproteolytic clotting factors against which antithrombin III has no effect. Patients deficient in protein "C" have a greatly increased risk of venous thrombosis, which indicates that protein "C," like antithrombin III, plays an important role in the prohibition of coagulation in vivo (Marder, 1984).

Removal of activated coagulation factors by

the liver involves both hepatocytes and the MPS. Soluble forms of activated coagulation proteins are cleared by hepatocytes. The MPS mainly removes particulate coagulation products, e.g., prothrombinase, tissue thromboplastin, and certain fibrin degradation products (FDPs). Hence, MPS "blockade," as in the Shwartzman reaction, creates coagulation abnormalities. Particulate coagulation products (fibrin, fibrin monomers, and FDPs) also may be cleared by the lungs, macrophages in tissues, and blood leukocytes.

Destruction of the fibrin clot is discussed in the next section.

FIBRINOLYSIS

Fibrinolysis is the antithesis of blood coagulation. Fibrin is probably being laid down continuously and removed along blood vessel walls (Mosesson, 1974). Removal of the clot formed at the site of injury is a necessary step in wound healing and restoration of circulation through thrombosed vessels. The clot is removed by proteolytic action of plasmin bound to the clot, a process referred to as physiologic fibrinolysis, or simply fibrinolysis.

Recent interest in fibrinolysis stems from developments in the treatment of thromboembolic disorders, atherosclerosis, and cancer in humans. Fibrinolysis also plays a part in inflammation (since antifibrinolytic drugs have anti-inflammatory effects), repair of connective tissue, and promotion of healing. For general reviews on fibrinolysis, refer to Babior and Stossel (1984), Lijnen and Cullen (1982), and Wintrobe et al. (1981). Observations on various animal species have been made by Clifton and Downie (1950), Gajewski and Povar (1971), and Hawkey (1975).

Mechanisms

Blood clots in vitro can lyse spontaneously, thereby indicating that the mechanisms for clot lysis reside within the clot itself. Dissolution of the clot is accomplished by a regulated system of proteolytic enzymes and their activators and inactivators; these include plasminogen proactivators, plasminogen activators, plasminogen, plasmin, inhibitors of plasminogen proactivators and activators,

and antiplasmins (Fig. 14–5). *Plasminogen proactivator(s)* is a humoral precursor of plasminogen activator. It is converted to the activator form during contact activation of the clotting mechanism and also by prekallikrein, HMW-kininogen, thrombin, and coagulation factors XIIa and XIa. Plasminogen proactivators and activators are also present in tissues.

Plasminogen activators can be found in lysosomes of most cells, in red cells, in endothelium particularly of small vessels, and in body fluids such as saliva, tears, urine, milk, and semen. Their plasma concentration is normally low because of constant clearance by the liver. Lysosomal and endothelial plasminogen activators are released under a variety of stimuli such as exercise, emotional stress, surgery, epinephrine, histamine, bacterial pyrogens, and hypoxia (Fearnley, 1969; Meade et al., 1979; Wintrobe et al, 1981). Plasminogen activators in body fluids and tissues are sometimes called *cytofibrinolysokinases*. *Plasminogen* is a β-globulin (MW 81,000) probably synthesized by the liver. Eosinophils in the bone marrow may also be involved in its production or storage and transportation (Riddle and Barnhardt, 1965). Plasminogen is present also in extravascular locations and has a half-life of about 2.2 days.

Plasminogen forms complexes with fibrinogen and fibrin, and so during clot formation it is incorporated within the clot. Plasminogen activators released by endothelial damage, possibly gaining access to the clot by adsorption and diffusion activate plasminogen. The plasminogen activator, itself a highly active proteolytic enzyme, by limited proteolysis converts the proenzyme plasminogen to an active serine protease, plasmin, which proteolyses fibrin in an orderly manner into various fragments (Lijnen and Cullen, 1982). Thus, fibrinolysis is a reflection of activity of plasminogen activator located within the clot. Clot lysis probably proceeds slowly because the activator must enter by diffusion and also because of regulation by inhibitors. The concentration of activator at sites of injury, inflammation, or other trauma is raised by vasoactive stimuli (Lijnen and Cullen, 1982). Small amounts of plasminogen may be activated directly by factor XIIa or by kallikrein and factor XIa. The major pathway is ,

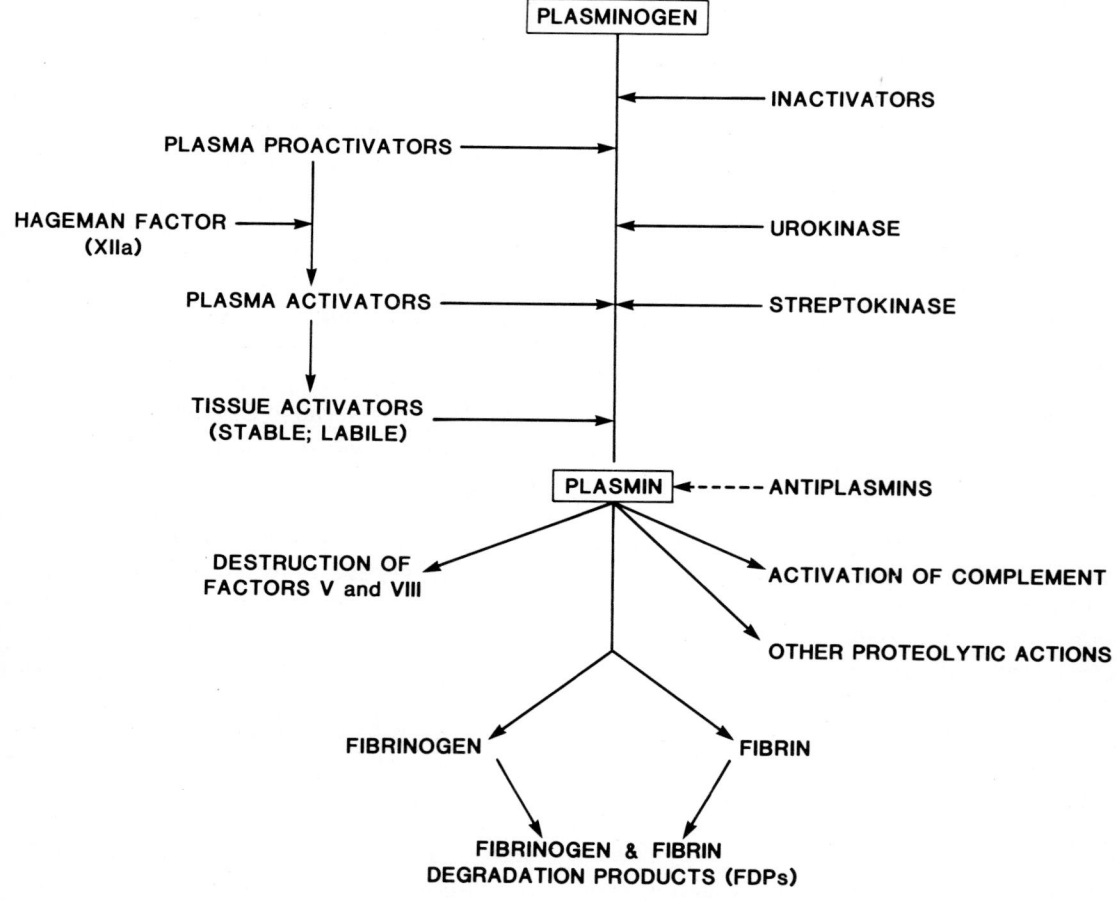

Fig. 14–5. The fibrinolytic system can be activated either intrinsically by factors present in the blood or extrinsically by tissue activators that are provided by damaged cells in the blood vessel wall. Both streptokinase and urokinase can convert plasminogen to plasmin to enhance fibrinolysis and can be used therapeutically as thrombolytic agents. Plasmin activity is regulated normally by antiplasmins in blood, but its excessive activity leads to increased fibrin(ogen)olysis with elevated concentrations of FDPs in blood. Other actions of plasmin are also shown. See text for details.

however, through the interaction of factor XIIa with a plasma proactivator to produce a plasminogen activator. Plasmin may also be produced by the action of other proteolytic enzymes such as thrombin and trypsin and by chemicals such as fatty acids, benzene, and chloroform.

This mechanism of fibrinolysis is responsible for the formation of circulating fragments of fibrin(ogen), called fibrin(ogen) degradation products (FDPs) or fibrin(ogen) split products (FSPs) in DIC, and for the lower concentrations of factors V and VIII in such patients (Feinstein, 1982). The molecular size of FDPs depends on the degree of plasmin activity. FDPs impair hemostasis because they have antiplasmin action, inhibit fibrin poly-

merization, and interfere with platelet function. FDPs are removed from the circulation by the liver, kidney, and MPS.

In addition to digesting fibrin(ogen) and coagulation factors V and VIII, plasmin also hydrolyzes complement components and certain hormones such as ACTH, growth hormone, and glucagon (Deykin, 1970). Plasmin is capable of hydrolyzing gelatin and casein, which is useful in the assay of its activity.

Plasma inhibitors of fibrinolysis include antiplasmins, antiactivators, and antiproactivators. There are at least five naturally occurring inhibitors of plasmin activity in plasma (see the preceding section); of these, α_2-antiplasmin is the most potent, α_2-macroglobulin is of major importance, and the slow-acting antiplasmin, α_1-antitrypsin, binds plasmin after the first two have become saturated (Wintrobe et al., 1981). Antiplasmin activity has been detected also in platelets and endothelium. Although both fibrin-bound plasmin and free plasmin can be destroyed by antiplasmins, physiologic proteolysis carried out by fibrin-bound plasmin generally is not inhibited by antiplasmins. Free plasmin is constantly inactivated by antiplasmins in blood at about a 10-fold higher concentration than plasmin. Hence, excessive production of plasmin must occur to effect pathologic proteolysis leading to formation of FDPs in abnormal amounts.

Filtrates from β-hemolytic streptococci also cause rapid liquefaction of fibrin clots (Christensen, 1945). This streptococcal fibrinolysin is called *streptokinase*. Its mechanism of action has not been clearly established, but one hypothesis is that streptokinase forms a complex with plasminogen (or plasmin) and the complex nonenzymatically activates plasminogen to plasmin, which then proteolyses the fibrin (Bajaj and Castellino, 1977). Species variations have been noted with regard to the fibrinolytic system activated by streptokinase. Urine also contains a powerful activator of the fibrinolytic system called *urokinase* or *urokase* (Williams, 1951), having a MW of 54,000 and trypsin-like protease action. It is synthesized by the kidney (Kucinski et al., 1968). See the section on Thrombosis for the use of these agents in promoting thrombolysis.

Measurements

The presence of plasmin in plasma indicates an advanced pathologic process, because its detection indicates that it is present in amounts sufficient to overcome the action of antiplasmins. Note, however, that plasma concentration of plasminogen activators, hence fibrinolytic activity, is increased following a variety of stimuli.

Although fibrinolysis in the normal state is so low it is often undetected, in certain diseases it is greatly enhanced. Accelerated fibrinolysis can be diagnosed by demonstrating FDPs in serum or by finding increased plasminogen activation (see "euglobulin lysis time" in the following paragraph) in plasma (Table 14–5). FDPs are potent inhibitors of

Table 14–5. Differences Between Primary Fibrin(ogen)olysis and Disseminated Intravascular Coagulation (DIC)

Parameter	Primary Fibrin(ogen)olysis	DIC
Platelet count	Normal	Low
Euglobulin lysis time	Shortened	Normal
Fibrin degradation products (FDPs)	Present	Present

coagulation and, like other anticoagulants, they cause abnormalities in the screening assays for prothrombin time (PT), activated partial prothrombin time (APTT), and especially thrombin time (TT) (Feldman, 1981b). Their presence may be suspected on that basis and confirmed by other tests (see Diagnostic Methods).

Most studies that measure fibrinolysis have had to do with conditions by which the system can be activated. What is usually measured is spontaneous clot lysis, euglobulin lysis time, hydrolysis of casein, or fibrinolysis using fibrin plates or ^{131}I-labeled fibrinogen. The euglobulin lysis method is frequently performed. The euglobulin fraction of plasma contains fibrinogen, all plasminogen activators, and plasminogen, but no antiplasmin. This fraction can be isolated and redissolved in neutral buffer containing a calcium-binding anticoagulant. When excess calcium is added to the euglobulin fraction, the clotting factors act on fibrinogen to produce a fibrin clot. This clot will dissolve after a few hours because of the unopposed action of newly formed plasmin generated by its activators during the period of incubation. The rate at which the clot dissolves is related closely to the quantity of circulating plasminogen activators present in the original plasma. The time required for the euglobulin fraction or precipitate to dissolve is referred to as the *"euglobulin lysis time"* and is a measurement of the fibrinolytic activity of the plasma. The shorter the euglobulin lysis time, the greater the fibrinolytic activity. The fibrinolytic activity in precipitated euglobulin was found to occur instantly in sera of guinea pigs but took about 1–5 hours in dogs and hamsters; 5–24 hours in the monkey, cat, mouse, and fish; and above 24 hours in humans, rabbits, cows, horses, pigs, sheep, rats, chickens, turkeys, ducks, and frogs (Irfan, 1968; Niewiarowski and Latollo, 1959; Ogston and Bennett, 1977).

Clinical Observations

Practical problems related to fibrinolysis in animals are rare except perhaps as they relate to DIC and to the management of thrombosis and thromboembolism. The clinician will find evidence of excessive fibrinolysis when spontaneous clot lysis occurs during clotting time or clot retraction tests. We have seen this occur in carcinoma of the dog (Schalm et al. 1975). Engen et al. (1974) reported a similar finding in a dog with a diaphragmatic hernia treated with epsilon aminocaproic acid (EACA). As mentioned previously, prolongation of clotting tests like PT, APTT, and TT would be another clue to increased fibrinolysis. Assays for coagulation factors V and VIII reveal reduced concentrations, and factor XIII also may be reduced in some patients. Hypofibrinogenemia may be modest to marked. Invariably the euglobulin lysis time is shortened.

Bleeding in patients with pathologic fibrinolysis is primarily a manifestation of antihemostatic effects of FDPs as in DIC. Treatment, therefore, involves the use of antifibrinolytic agents. Inhibition of fibrinolysis can be brought about by EACA; in low concentrations (10^{-4}M), EACA inhibits plasminogen activators but not free plasmin; in high concentrations (greater than 0.06M) it inhibits plasmin (Alkjaersig et al., 1959). Caution is recommended in treating patients with fibrinolysis with underlying DIC because of paradoxic pathogenesis. Use of EACA in conjunction with heparin or following heparin administration is suggested in such cases (see Wintrobe et al., 1981 for further discussion). Other drugs used therapeutically for systemic states of excessive fibrinolysis are aprotinin (Trasylol), p-aminocyclohexane carbolic acid, and p-aminomethyl benzoic acid.

DISORDERS OF COAGULATION

This area of veterinary medicine is expanding rapidly and so it is impossible to document every report. The extensive publications of Dodds are acknowledged (Dodds, 1970, 1974, 1975, 1977a, 1977b, 1977c, 1977d, 1980)

as are reviews by Feldman (1981b), Hall (1972), Jones (1979), Green (1981), Rebar and Boon (1980), and Troy (1984).

Hereditary Coagulopathies

Hereditary coagulation abnormalities are less common than acquired coagulation disorders. They are generally a manifestation of a single factor deficiency resulting from a deficient or defective biosynthesis. Regardless of the type of coagulation abnormality, patients with hereditary coagulopathies show similar clinical signs. Table 14–6 lists various hereditary coagulopathies in animals together with pertinent references.

Inheritance Patterns

The congenital coagulation disorders appear clinically as either spontaneous hemorrhage or extensive hemorrhage after trauma or surgery. The history usually indicates whether the disorder is congenital or acquired. The hereditary disorders appear in early life and are characterized by the presence of a single abnormality that can account for the entire clinical picture. With the exception of hemophilia A and B, all congenital coagulation defects have an autosomal inheritance pattern. Classic von Willebrand's disease (vWD) in humans is transmitted as an autosomal dominant disorder, i.e., a single autosomal gene (heterozygosity) causes the disease. The recessive form of vWD has been recognized in Poland-China swine, Scottish terriers and Chesapeake Bay retrievers. The incompletely dominant form is much more common and has been recognized in 28 breeds of dogs (Dodds, 1984). Other defects, such as factor X or V deficiency, are autosomal recessive disorders, i.e., two abnormal genes (homozygosity) must be present for bleeding signs to occur. In contrast, hemophilia A and B are X-chromosome-linked recessive disorders. Bleeding disorders occur in males who are hemizygous for the abnormal X chromosome, usually transmitted by a heterozygous asymptomatic mother.

In hemophilia A, factor VIII:C is deficient; in hemophilia B, factor IX activity is deficient. Each disorder results from a different defect in the X chromosome. In most female carriers, concentrations of factor VIII:C or factor IX are

Table 14–6.   Hereditary Coagulopathies in Animals

Disease	Species	Inheritance*	Reference
Congenital afibrinogenemia (hypofibrinogenemia)	Dogs	Autosomal incomplete dominance	Kammermann et al. (1971)
	Goats		Breukink et al. (1972)
Factor VII deficiency	Dogs	Autosomal incomplete dominance	Capel-Edwards and Hall (1968); Garner et al. (1967); Hall (1972); Mustard et al. (1962b); Poller et al. (1971); Spurling et al. (1972)
Hemophilia A (factor VIII deficiency)	Dogs	X-linked recessive	Dodds (1974, 1977c, 1980); Okin and Dodds (1980); Spurling et al. (1974); also see vWD and Hemophilia B
	Cats		Cotter et al. (1978)
	Horses		Archer (1961); Feldman and Giacopuzzi (1982); Hutchins et al. (1967); Nossel et al. (1962); Sanger et al. (1964)
	Swine		Muhrer et al. (1965)
Von Willebrand's disease	Dogs	Autosomal recessive; more commonly, incomplete dominance	Bouma et al. (1976); Brinkhous et al. (1973); Buckner and Hampton (1966); Dodds (1970, 1975, 1977a); Johnson et al. (1980)
	Poland China swine	Autosomal recessive	Bowie et al. (1968, 1973); Cornell and Muhrer (1964); Cornell et al. (1969); Fass et al. (1979); Hogan et al. (1941); Muhrer et al. (1965)
Hemophilia B (factor IX deficiency)	Dogs	X-linked recessive	Aronson et al. (1972); Dodds (1974, 1980); Mustard et al. (1960, 1962a); Peterson and Dodds (1979); Rowsell (1960), Sherding and DiBartola (1980); Slappendel (1975)
Factor X deficiency	Dogs	Autosomal incomplete dominance	Dodds (1974, 1980)
Factor XI deficiency	Dogs	Autosomal incomplete dominance	Dodds and Kull (1971)
	Cattle		Kociba et al. (1969); Gentry et al. (1975)
Factor XII (Hageman factor) deficiency†	Cats		Green and White (1977); Kaplan et al. (1976); Kier et al. (1980)

*X-linked recessive—carried by females and manifested in their sons; affected males produce normal sons but all daughters are carriers. Autosomal inheritance—seen in either sex.
†The Hageman factor is completely absent in marine mammals, fowl, and most reptiles.

about 40 to 60% of normal. Concentrations differ from one female carrier to another because of variable inactivation of the normal and abnormal X chromosomes in somatic cells during embryonic gene replication (Lyon phenomenon) (Bennett, 1977; Mammen, 1983). Genetic probability indicates that a female carrier of hemophilia mated to a normal male will transmit the defective X chromosome to half of her male offspring who will be hemophiliacs and to half of her female offspring who will be carriers. It is important to diagnose carriers since they should be removed from breeding programs. In rare situations both hemophilia A and B can be co-inherited.

Hemophilia A

Hemophilia A is the classic hemophilia. As previously stated, hemophilia A has a sex-linked recessive mode of inheritance carried by females and manifested in males. If hemophilic males are bred to carrier females, hemophilic females (homozygous) can also be produced. Hemophilia A is one of the most common inherited bleeding disorders in humans as well as in animals and appears in many dog and cat breeds and laboratory tests indicate that the disorder is similar in all species. As mentioned in the previous edition of this book, studies on hemophilia in animals have contributed significantly to knowledge regarding the disease in humans. Genetic variants of hemophilia A have been found in humans.

In the past it was believed that hemophilia A was due to the absence of factor VIII. Recent immunologic and functional studies have shown that basically three functions relating to the factor VIII complex can be measured. These are: factor VIII:C, factor VIII:RAg (the portion of factor VIII:vWF which has immunologic property), and factor VIII:vWF. Currently it is unknown whether factor VIII:C, factor VIII:RAg, and factor VIII:vWF represent the activity of a single multifunctional macromolecular complex or the physically separable activities of interrelated substances (Hoyer, 1976, 1981). Evidence indicates that the molecular structure is comprised of a small molecular weight subunit (factor VIII:C) and a larger molecular weight subunit (factor VIII:RAg in association with factor VIII:vWF). Synthesis or secretion of factor VIII:C is decreased in most patients with hemophilia A, although it is suspected that a defective form of factor VIII:C molecule is synthesized in others. Patients with hemophilia A have normal plasma and endothelial concentrations of factor VIII:vWF polymers and normal or even slightly elevated factor VIII:RAg levels. If a known amount of factor VIII:C is infused into a hemophilic patient deficient in that factor, factor VIII:C activity rises and decays in a predictable manner with a biologic half-life of 8 to 12 hours (Green, 1981). Similar infusion of normal or hemophilic plasma into a patient with vWD, however, results in an elevation of factor VIII:C 24 hours later or longer, and the concentration of factor VIII:C activity rises above the calculated infused rate.

The severity of the disease is correlated directly with the concentrations of factor VIII:C in the plasma. Hemophilic bleeding can be severe if factor VIII:C activity is less than 1 to 5% of normal, or mild with coagulant activity more than 5% but less than 20% of normal (Appendix Case 28). In severe (classic) hemophilia, spontaneous bleeding occurs in areas subject to mechanical stress such as joints and muscles. Hemarthroses, subcutaneous and intramuscular hematomas, and ecchymoses are frequent, and gastrointestinal and genitourinary bleeding may be present. Recurrent hemarthroses can cause permanent joint damage. Hematomas can cause neurologic or other tissue damage as a result of compression and diminished blood flow. Bleeding into any organ can follow trauma or surgery. In moderate and mild hemophilia, bleeding often is a problem only during or after surgery or in association with trauma (Dodds, 1974, 1977b, 1977d).

In both hemophilia A and B, the APTT is prolonged, whereas PT, thrombin time, bleeding time, fibrinogen concentration, and platelet count are normal or near-normal. Abnormal APTT is correctable by mixing the patient's plasma 1:1 with normal plasma. Platelet function is normal in hemophilia A. For proper therapy, specific assay of factor VIII:C, factor VIII:vWF, and factor IX activity must be accomplished to distinguish hemophilia A from vWD and hemophilia B. Schlink and Johnson (1983) have described an autoradiographic procedure to determine canine factor VIII:vWF. Factor VIII activity can fluctuate upon exercise and during epinephrine response, pregnancy, or CNS stimulation (Hoyer, 1981).

Bleeding episodes in patients with hemophilia A are treated by transfusing cryoprecipitate prepared from normal plasma. Cryoprecipitates contain both the factor VIII:vWF and the biologic portion of the factor VIII complex, factor VIII:C (Moake et al., 1982). Fibrinogen and fibronectin also are present (Feldman and Thomson, 1983). Following cryoprecipitate infusion, factor VIII:vWF polymers are deposited on subendothelial surfaces exposed in an injured blood vessel where they improve local platelet adherence, decrease bleeding time, and diminish blood loss. The therapeutic effect lasts for about a day or less, presumably because of the removal and catabolism of transfused circulating factor VIII:vWF as well as the catabolism of factor VIII:vWF polymers deposited on subendothelium. The half-life of cryoprecipitate in hemophilia A dogs was found to be 7.7 to 32.3 hours (Aufderheid et al., 1975).

Cryoprecipitate infusion must be repeated

to maintain normal hemostasis. Lyophilized (human) factor VIII concentrates contain relatively small quantities of factor VIII:vWF polymers and relatively large quantities of factor VIII:C and are therefore ideal for treating hemophilia A in humans. Factor VIII:C concentration of 10 to 20% of normal are usually adequate to effect hemostasis after minor trauma. For major injuries, factor VIII:C concentrations must be maintained at greater than 50% of normal. The half-life of transfused factor VIII:C is 8 to 12 hours (Moake et al., 1982; Moake and Funicella, 1983). Consequently, transfusions may have to be repeated 2 to 3 times daily. Since factor VIII is closely bound somehow to fibrinogen, the clotting defect is not corrected by normal serum but is corrected by normal plasma. See Dodds (1977b) for additional information on the management and treatment of hemophilia A.

It is possible that hepatic cells of patients with hemophilia A can produce a modest amount of functional factor VIII:C molecules. In these patients 1-diamino-8-D arginine-vasopressin (DDAVP), an analogue of vasopressin (antidiuretic hormone), has been used as an alternate to cryoprecipitate or lyophilized factor VIII concentrate. DDAVP causes the endothelial release of stored factor VIII:vWF polymers that circulate through the liver of patients with mild hemophilia A and carry additional functional factor VIII:C molecules into the circulation (Moake and Funicella, 1983). DDAVP also increases the endothelial release of plasminogen activator and thus the activation of plasminogen to plasmin.

Some human patients with severe hemophilia A develop antibodies to the factor VIII complex; a similar case in a dog is described in Appendix Case 28. Treatment of these patients has been unsatisfactory generally because the antibodies rapidly inactivate the transfused factor VIII protein. Occasionally, a patient with no history of transfusion or hemophilia A produces antibodies against factor VIII:C; this occurs perhaps because of an acquired defect in a suppressor T-lymphocyte population. Associated conditions include immunologic disorders such as systemic lupus erythematosus. Bleeding often is as severe in nonhemophilic patients with circulatory antibodies to factor VIII:C as in those with hemophilia A. The antibodies are usually IgG and are sometimes monoclonal (Kasper, 1981).

von Willebrand's Disease (vWD)

vWD is a deficiency of a plasma factor that affects normal platelet function. This disease occurs in many dog breeds and in Poland-China swine (see Table 14–6). Many variants (types I, IIa, and IIb) have been described in humans and many hypotheses have been proposed for their inheritance (Moake and Funicella, 1983). Two forms of the disease have been recognized in dogs (Slappendel, personal communication) and variant types have been produced in pigs by selective breeding (Fass et al., 1979).

vWD occurs in both sexes and is inherited as an autosomal incompletely dominant or autosomal recessive trait as mentioned previously. The disease clinically ranges from mild to severe in the same family or litter and can be confused with hemophilia A. Although vWD is usually less severe than hemophilia A, the clinical signs are the same. Special clotting tests and a thorough analysis of pedigree may be necessary to establish diagnosis. Bloody diarrhea; bleeding at estrus or postpartum; small surface hematomas as from vaccination procedures; excessive bleeding on nail clipping, ear cropping, or tail docking; and epistaxis and lameness are common signs as is poor survival of the newborn. Because most affected animals survive, it is important to identify and remove carrier animals to halt the spread of the disease.

In vWD, prolonged bleeding times are frequent as opposed to hemophilia A (Table 14–7). There is reduced platelet adhesiveness or retention in glass bead columns and abnormal platelet aggregation; these properties of platelets are a function of interaction of platelet surface receptors with factor VIII:vWF. There is usually slight to moderate prolongation of APTT and normal PT and TT. The definitive tests are the measurement of factor VIII:RAg and platelet function tests (Dodds, 1975, 1977a, 1977b; Feldman, 1981b).

Antibodies to the factor VIII complex have been produced. Their use has allowed the de-

Table 14–7. A Comparison of Hemophilia A and von Willebrand's Disease

Parameter	Hemophilia A	von Willebrand's Disease
FVIII:C	Decreased	Normal/decreased
FVIII:RAg	Normal/Increased	Decreased
APTT	Prolonged	Normal/Prolonged
Bleeding time	Normal	Prolonged
Platelet function	Normal	Abnormal

tection and quantitation of factor VIII:RAg. Factor VIII:RAg concentrations are normal in hemophilia A, whereas they are greatly reduced in classic vWD and may be normal to high in type II human patients (Wintrobe et al, 1981). Factor VIII antigen appears in plasma and some is attached also to the platelet membrane. The antigen is synthesized by endothelial cells and perhaps by megakaryocytes as well (Moake and Funicella, 1983). Therefore, vWD may represent a synthetic defect in one of these areas. Data are emerging, however, that indicate that an antibody directed against factor VIII:vWF may be involved in the pathogenesis of vWD (Ruggeri and Zimmerman, 1980).

Clinically, human patients with type I (classic) vWD have mucosal and petechial bleeding that is not usually of great consequence. Trauma or surgery, however, may invoke a previously undiagnosed disorder causing a hemophilic emergency. The diagnosis is made by finding reduced factors VIII:C and VIII:vWF (5 to 50% of normal), a prolonged bleeding time, and abnormal platelet functions. Factor VIII:C concentrations show a latent increase in patients with vWD but not in patients with hemophilia A following transfusion of normal or hemophilic plasma, as mentioned earlier.

Cryoprecipitate fractions of normal plasma are transfused to arrest bleeding in a patient with vWD or to prepare a vWD patient for surgery. In addition, because of the association of vWD with hypothyroidism in the Doberman Pinscher breed, thyroid extracts have been used to increase factor VIII:vWF temporarily in canine patients prior to surgery (Dodds, 1980). Note that lyophilized factor VIII concentrates contain relatively small quantities of factor VIII:vWF and are not effective in treating vWD in humans. In humans with type I vWD in whom factor

VIII:vWF synthesis is normal, the alternative therapeutic agent is DDAVP. DDAVP is not as effective in treating people with heterozygous type IIa or IIb vWD and is ineffective in homozygous type IIa vWD (Nachman, 1982).

Hemophilia B

Hemophilia B (Christmas disease) is an X chromosome-linked recessive deficiency of factor IX. It is characterized by decreased or defective synthesis or secretion of the factor IX molecule. Factor IX deficiency and hemophilia A are indistinguishable clinically, and the diagnostic and screening tests used are the same as for hemophilia A. Screening test results reveal abnormalities similar to those in hemophilia A except that in humans the PT is abnormal in some variants of hemophilia B. The thromboplastin generation test has been used to distinguish the two disorders; it was defective in people with hemophilia B (Wintrobe et al., 1981).

Hemophilia B has been reported in dogs (Table 14–6; Appendix Case 27) and the clinical signs are more severe in larger breeds (Dodds, 1974, 1980). The deficiency of factor IX usually is severe (frequently about 1% of normal factor activity). Carrier females can be identified by having 40 to 60% of normal concentrations of factor IX. Bleeding episodes in hemophilia B are treated with fresh plasma transfusions. Factor IX is stable in blood or plasma stored at 4°C (Feldman, 1981b). Transfused factor IX has a half-life of approximately 24 hours (Mustard et al., 1960).

Factor VII Deficiency

This rare autosomal recessive or incompletely dominant disease has been reported in dogs (Table 14–6). In dogs it is a benign condition that usually does not manifest itself by a bleeding diathesis like that in humans with factor VII deficiency. It is usually diagnosed only after a clinical work-up before surgery or in experimental animals before experimentation. In addition to the deficiency of factor VII, affected animals have prolonged prothrombin times.

Factor X, XI, and XII Deficiencies

These deficiencies are rare, but as noted in Table 14–6 they do occur in animals. Specific factor assays can be performed by immunologic and functional methods and a moderate deficiency generally can be found.

In factor X deficiency, mild to moderate prolongation of APTT, PT, Russell's viper venom time (RVVT), and whole blood clotting time have been noted.

Factor XI deficiency (sometimes called hemophilia C) in animals is similar to that of humans, generally manifesting as prolonged bleeding before surgery; spontaneous bleeding is rare. APTT is prolonged in deficient patients. Both sexes are affected and carrier heterozygotes can be detected by suitable laboratory procedures.

Hageman factor (factor XII) deficiency is manifested by a prolonged clotting time of whole blood or plasma and significantly prolonged APTT due to defective formation of thrombin via the intrinsic pathway. Patients usually are asymptomatic, although minor bleeding may occur. This disease has been well characterized in cats (Kier, A.B., et al., 1980).

Afibrinogenemia and Dysfibrinogenemia

Afibrinogenemia is rare in animals but some cases have been noted in dogs and goats (Table 14–6). A family history is necessary to establish the hereditary nature. It is transmitted in humans as an autosomal recessive trait often appearing at birth by bleeding from the umbilical cord. The deficiency in fibrinogen prevents completion of the final step of coagulation, namely the conversion of fibrinogen to fibrin; and so, PT, APTT, TT, and clotting time are prolonged. Bleeding time may be prolonged in about half of the patients.

Dysfibrinogenemia in humans is an autosomal dominant trait characterized by fibrinogen that is defective in its breakdown, polymerization, and stabilization (Wintrobe et al., 1981). Heat precipitation and immunologic methods for quantitation of fibrinogen give normal values, but TT is prolonged. PT may be variably prolonged, and patients are usually asymptomatic.

Multiple Deficiencies

Dodds (1974) described crossbreeding experiments in which dogs with hemophilia A have been bred to dogs with hemophilia B. Offspring with combined hemophilia A and B exhibited hemorrhagic episodes similar to animals with single hemophilia.

Acquired Coagulopathies

The acquired coagulation disorders are more common than the inherited disorders. Unlike the inherited disorders, the acquired disorders usually are associated with multiple coagulation abnormalities, less severe bleeding that correlates poorly with laboratory test results, and less effective factor replacement therapy. The diagnosis of these disorders is often indicated by associated clinical features and by results of screening tests such as PT, APTT, and TT.

Some conditions associated with acquired coagulopathies are described briefly. DIC and thrombosis, which are of major importance, are discussed separately. Coagulation abnormalities in dogs with neoplastic diseases have been reported (Madewell et al., 1980).

Platelet Disorders

Platelet disorders include thrombocytopenia, thrombasthenia, thrombocytopathy (abnormal platelet function), thrombocytosis, and thrombocythemia. Some of these disorders and associated clinical signs are outlined in Tables 14–1 and 14–2 and discussed in Chapter 17.

Vitamin K Deficiency and Antagonism

Vitamin K is essential in the formation of several coagulation proteins referred to as the vitamin K-dependent coagulation proteins, namely factors II, VII, IX, and X. The role of liver in synthesis of these coagulation factors has been discussed earlier in this chapter (Table 14–3).

A nutritional deficiency of vitamin K is rare

in animals, and so a deficiency due to lack of absorption is seldom found. Such a deficiency would have to exist for a long period to prevent absorption of the small amount of vitamin K needed to maintain hemostasis, and the animal probably would have had previous signs other than bleeding tendency. Vitamin K deficiencies develop with chronic gastrointestinal problems such as malabsorption and those brought about by long-term broad-spectrum antibiotic and sulfanilamide therapy. A lack of bile salts in the gut prevents absorption of the fat soluble vitamin, hence obstructive jaundice leads to a deficiency, and finally liver disease can promote a lack of utilization of the vitamin. Because of immaturity of the liver, human neonates have been found to exhibit a modest deficiency (20 to 50% of normal) of vitamin K-dependent coagulation factors (Wintrobe et al, 1981). Vitamin K administration did not correct the deficiency. Similar observations have been reported for sheep and cattle (Nockels et al., 1978). Neonatal vitamin K hypovitaminosis has been described in a foal (Jones, 1979).

Vitamin K antagonism is encountered in animals upon ingestion of rodenticides whose action depends on this antagonism (see Appendix Cases 21 and 22). Warfarin, indanediones (diphacinone and pindone), bromadialone, and brodifacoum are commonly involved in this toxicosis (Mount and Feldman, 1983). The biochemical lesion of major importance is the inhibition of the enzyme system (epoxide reductase enzyme) essential for recycling of vitamin K necessary for activation of precursor forms of coagulation factors produced by the liver. The degree of inhibition of the enzyme system by a rodenticide contributes to species and rodenticide toxicity differences. The coccidiostat sulfaquinoxaline also produces coagulopathies due to vitamin K antagonism.

Diagnosis of vitamin K deficiencies is based on history, clinical examination, laboratory evaluation of clotting abnormalities, and clinical and laboratory response to vitamin K_1 therapy. Clinical signs of warfarin intoxication include anemia, weakness, pallor, hypovolemia, dyspnea, hematemesis, epistaxis, hematuria, melena/bloody stool, external hematomas, hemarthroses, and neurolgic signs.

Acute death also may occur in such intoxications. Cases of vitamin K antagonism in the dog were discussed by Green et al. (1979) who noted that the spectrum of bleeding problems is broad and, in severe cases, involves frank bleeding from body orifices and shock that may require transfusion of fresh whole blood to modest cases with only vague signs that respond to vitamin K_1 therapy. Detection of a factor VII deficiency helped confirm the diagnosis as well as prolonged PT, APTT, and activated clotting time (ACT) tests. The ACT test was particularly helpful as a screening test. Assays for coagulation factors II, VII, IX, and X reveal subnormal values. Bleeding time and platelet counts are normal.

Vitamin K deficiency is treated with vitamin K_1 (phylloquinone series), K_2 (menaquinone derivatives), or the synthetic K_3 (menadione); remember that oral therapy is ineffective when an absorption problem exists. Menadione is converted to the vitamin K_2 series in vivo, but is poorly stored in the liver in comparison to K_1 so higher amounts are required to achieve the same physiologic effect. Providing menadione supplements to swine and poultry rations is a common practice to alleviate some forms of mycotoxin-induced bleeding syndrome (Green et al., 1979; Mount et al., 1982).

Treatment of vitamin K antagonism involves administratiion of vitamin K preparations and fresh plasma transfusions. When prompt control of bleeding is required, fresh plasma should be given every 6 hours and the volume infused should approximate about 5 to 10% of the patient's total blood volume. The method of vitamin K therapy varies with the incriminated toxic compound. Poisoning with warfarin-related compounds may be successfully treated in dogs with vitamin K_1 given in *divided* oral doses daily for a period of 4 to 6 days. A dose of 0.25 to 2.5 mg/kg body weight is recommended for use in small animals and 0.5 to 2.5 mg/kg body weight in large animals (Scott et al., 1978, 1979). Since diphacinone poisoning causes vitamin K antagonism for a much longer period (about 3 to 4 weeks) than warfarin because of differences in their half-lives (15–20 days for diphacinone versus 40 hours for warfarin), comparatively higher dose and longer therapy is indicated—5 mg/kg body weight in 3 divided daily doses for 3 weeks. Vitamin K_1 is given subcutaneously for the initial 2 or 3 treatments and then orally until no longer needed (Mount and Feldman, 1983). Intravenous injection is not recommended because of the potential danger of anaphylactic reactions. The half-life of vitamin K_1 is about 5 hours.

As discussed by Green (1981), half-lives of the functional forms of coagulation factors II, VII, IX, and X (see Table 14–3) should be kept in mind with relation to the time of ingestion of the antagonist and the appearance of clinical signs and clotting abnormalities. At least a week is needed for most antagonists to be catabolized and removed from the body. In the dog as little as 5 mg/kg of warfarin can induce a moderate coagulopathy.

Factors that influence the effect and duration of vitamin K therapy include total dosage and type of toxin ingested, presence of interacting drugs that may potentiate (e.g., salicylates) or antagonize (e.g., barbiturates) the effects of coumarin drugs, individual variation in biotransformation of toxin, and amount and type of vitamin K administered (Mount and Feldman, 1983; Wintrobe et al., 1981).

Liver Disease

The liver is the site of synthesis of coagulation proteins of significance in hemostasis (see Table 14–3), factors involved in fibrinolysis (plasminogen and plasminogen activator), and certain inhibitors of coagulation, namely antithrombin III, α_2-macroglobulin, and α_1-antitrypsin (Babior and Stossel, 1984). It is evident from Table 14–3 that the half-life of factor VII is the shortest (only 5 hours). Thus determination of factor VII activity would be the most useful measurement in both acute and chronic liver disease. The PT test also has a high prognostic value in acute liver disease. The new immunologic assays for clotting factors in human medicine have facilitated the diagnosis of changes in liver disease and even have given another dimension to the evaluation of liver function albeit these tests have limited value in the differential diagnosis of liver disease (Lechner et al., 1977).

In acute and chronic liver disease in hu-

Table 14–8. Causes of Hemorrhagic Diathesis in Liver Disease

Deficiency Biosynthesis
  Various coagulation proteins (see Table 14–1)
  Prekallikrein
  HMW-kininogen
  Plasminogen
  Antithrombin III
  Antiplasmins

Aberrant Biosynthesis
  Fibrinogen
  Factor VIII
  Inhibitors of coagulation

Inadequate Clearance
  Activated clotting factors
  Plasminogen activators
  Hemostatic "debris," e.g., fibrin monomers, fibrin degradation products (FDPs)

Accelerated Destruction of Coagulation Factors
  Disseminated intravascular coagulation (DIC)
  Primary fibrin(ogen)olysis

Thrombocytopenia
  Splenic sequestration
  Other causes

Others
  Abnormal platelet function
  Other poorly defined causes

mans, factor VII activity shows the greatest reduction, factor IX shows the least change, changes in factors II and X are intermediate, and factor VIII is often elevated (Strombeck et al., 1976; Wintrobe et al., 1981). Factor VIII is, however, qualitatively abnormal. Factor deficiencies in humans often correlate with hypoalbuminemia (Wintrobe et al., 1981) and similar observations have been made in dogs (Green, unpublished observations).

Bleeding in liver disease is usually mild to moderate but severe bleeding may occur in patients with cirrhosis, fulminating hepatitis, and the terminal phase of chronic liver disease. Severe canine infectious hepatitis with bleeding problems has been reported (Lindblad and Backgren, 1964). The routine screening tests of coagulation (PT, APTT, etc.) on peripheral blood are unreliable guides of the risk of bleeding after liver biopsy and, hence, have limited value in determining contraindications to this procedure (Ewe, 1981).

Many factors may contribute to the hemostatic defect in liver disease (Table 14–8). These include impaired or defective synthesis of several clotting factors and thrombocytopenia. In addition, increased fibrinolytic activity may occur when patients with chronic liver disease are exposed to surgery or trauma. This occurs because of impaired synthesis of antiplasmins by the diseased liver, and inadequate clearance of plasminogen activators released into the circulation following surgery or trauma.

Therapy of coagulopathies in liver disease varies with the cause and severity of the disease as do laboratory findings. It consists of administration of vitamin K, antifibrinolytic agents, anticoagulants, and factor replacement.

Dysproteinemias

In myeloma and other paraproteinemias (see Chapter 34), abnormal proteins may be adsorbed to fibrinogen and interfere with the fibrinogen-to-fibrin conversion and fibrin polymerization. Vascular wall damage, thrombocytopenia, abnormal platelet function, hypercoagulability, and abnormal fibrinolysis may also be found (Wintrobe et al., 1981). In a report on a dog with IgA myeloma, platelet adhesion was reduced markedly and bleeding time and APTT were prolonged. The APTT prolongation coincided with the peak in plasma protein concentration (Shepard et al., 1972).

Primary Pathologic Fibrinolysis

Primary pathologic fibrinolysis is a hemorrhagic state that may result from a marked increase in plasma fibrinolytic (plasmin) activity. It is, however, an uncommon cause of bleeding, and may occur when a large amount of tissue plasminogen activators are released into the circulation as a result of extensive trauma, such as that associated with a major operation or a breakdown of tumor tissue. Thus, bleeding due to primary pathologic fibrin(ogen)olysis may occur in some of the same disorders that also produce DIC (Cade and Robinson, 1975; Engen et al., 1974; Kaplan et al., 1976). The clinical picture in most of these cases is similar to DIC (Table 14–5). See previous section on Fibrinolysis for details.

Pathologic Inhibitors of Coagulation

Many abnormal anticoagulants that prevent normal coagulation have been found in blood of human patients with acquired coagulopathies. The following comments are based on observations reported by Wintrobe et al. (1981). Pathologic anticoagulants include antibodies to various coagulation proteins such as those against factors V, VIII, IX, XI, and XIII and "lupus inhibitors." Lupus inhibitors, originally found in patients with systemic lupus erythematosus, may be detected in a variety of unrelated disorders such as myeloma, myelofibrosis, and rheumatoid arthritis, and following therapy with certain drugs, e.g., chlorpromazine and penicillin. Lupus inhibitors are poorly defined. They appear to be IgG and IgM antibodies and probably act by interfering with the action of preformed prothrombinase by complexing with the lipid moiety of the enzyme complex. Patients with these anticoagulants exhibit prolonged APTT that is not corrected by mixing equal volumes of normal plasma with the patient's plasma. PT and TT are often prolonged. Clinical bleeding seldom occurs; however, it is associated with platelet abnormalities. Corticosteroids and other immunosuppressive drugs are effective, but therapy is seldom indicated. Similar observations on animals are being made (Feldman et al., 1983).

DISSEMINATED INTRAVASCULAR COAGULATION (DIC)

DIC or consumption coagulopathy is a disorder in which diffuse intravascular thrombosis causes a hemostatic defect due to the reduction of clotting factors and platelets as a result of their utilization in the thrombotic process and to anticoagulant properties of FDPs generated from activation of the fibrinolytic system. DIC may complicate a variety of clinical conditions. It was first described in dogs that had been given incompatible blood transfusions or the infusion of thrombin or thromboplastin. The dogs developed thrombocytopenia, prolonged PT, the appearance of fibrinolytic activity and shock, disseminated inflammatory reactions, and bleeding tendencies (McKay, 1956; McKay et al., 1955; Hardaway, 1961). A brief description of DIC is given here; additional information is available in recent reviews (Feldman, 1981a; Greene, 1975; Greene et al., 1977; Schiefer and

Table 14–9. Conditions in Veterinary Medicine Associated with Disseminated Intravascular Coagulation (DIC)

Malignancies
  Metastasizing carcinomas, hemangiosarcomas, leukemias
Severe hemolysis
Infections
  Bacterial, Viral, Protozoal, Mycotic, Metazoal (heartworm)
Endotoxins
Massive trauma
Heat stroke
Liver disease
Pancreatitis
Obstetric complications
Incompatible blood transfusion
Snake bites
Purpura hemorrhagica
Acidosis

Table 14–10. Distribution of 41 Cases of DIC in Dogs by Major Disease Categories*

Category	No.	%
Malignancy	16	39
Pancreatitis	12	30
Sepsis/hemolysis	1	2
Sepsis/shock	1	2
Chronic active hepatitis	6	15
Heat stroke	5	12
Total	41	100

*From Feldman, et al., 1981; courtesy of the American Journal of Veterinary Research.

Searcy, 1975) and in selected reports on dogs (Kociba, 1976; Owen and Bowie, 1977; Owen et al., 1973; Schalm, 1980; Slappendel et al., 1972; Strombeck et al., 1976; Wigton et al., 1976); cats (Weiss et al., 1980); cattle (Buntain, 1980; Dalgliesh et al., 1976; Ruehl et al., 1982); and pigs (Weiss et al., 1973).

Conditions Associated With DIC

DIC is rarely, if ever, a primary event. The majority of cases are traced to platelet activation and/or the release of thromboplastins into the circulation from tissue damage in a variety of conditions (Table 14–9). DIC can be acute, subacute, or chronic, and localized or generalized; its severity is related to the rate of release of thromboplastin, the duration of exposure to the etiologic agent, and the ability of the liver and bone marrow to replace consumed coagulation factors and platelets. Distribution of 41 cases of DIC in dogs with major disease categories is given in Table 14–10 and laboratory findings in these cases are given in Table 14–11.

Intravascular coagulation may be activated by relatively trivial stimuli such as mild trauma. The fact that fibrin is not being laid down continuously is because of a composite action of several inherent protective mechanisms. These mechanisms include antagonism by circulating inhibitors of activated clotting factors produced by the liver, localized activation of the fibrinolytic system, and the

rapid clearance of activated clotting factors and hemostatic "debris" by the MPS. Similarly, platelet aggregation is normally prevented by the instability of platelet aggregates and by the action of plasma adenosine diphosphatase (ADPase). Consequently, under normal circumstances significant microthrombosis does not occur.

Tissue necrosis and inflammation are common inciting causes of DIC through release of procoagulant or the thromboplastin-like substances and initiation of the coagulation sequence. Exposure of subendothelial collagen as a result of inflammation causes platelet activation, release of platelet factors, and subsequent initiation of coagulation. Red blood cells lysed at inflammatory sites release ADP, causing platelet activation. Intravascular hemolysis is a potential cause of DIC through contact activation of coagulation factors and platelets. In sepsis, contact activation of coagulation may be due to the presence of bacterial lipopolysaccharides. During viremia, antigen-antibody complexes may cause ADP release from platelets, contact activation of coagulation, or endothelial damage followed by a collagen-induced initiation of coagulation. Stagnant blood flow, acidosis, and hypoxia favor endothelial damage and DIC.

Pathophysiology

Tissue necrosis, inflammation, red cell or platelet damage, and antigen-antibody or endotoxin-induced endothelial damage initiates coagulation process, as stated, through thrombin generation (Fig. 14–6). Thrombin cleaves fibrinogen to fibrin monomers that polymerize to form a firm clot. Simultaneously, fibrinolytic and kinin systems are also activated. Plasmin, the active protease in fibrinolysis, degrades fibrinogen and fibrin

Table 14–11. Coagulation Abnormalities in 41 Dogs with DIC*

Parameter	Normal Range	Mean + 1 SD in All Cases	Percentage Abnormal	Mean + 1 SD in Abnormal Cases
Antithrombin III activity (%)	89–108	71 + 14	85	62 + 12
Prothrombin time (sec)	6.4–7.4	11.0 + 5.4	80	12.3 + 55
Activated partial thromboplastin time (sec)	9.5–10.5	16.7 + 6.7	87	18.3 + 61
Thrombin time (sec)	5.0–10.0	11.0 + 6.6	55	16.4 + 68
Platelet count ($\times 10^3/\mu l$)	200–500	147 + 98	80	111 + 45
FDPs ($\mu g/ml$)	<10	—	61	>10–40
Protamine sulfate test (fibrin monomer*)	0	+	55	+ + +
Fibrinogen (g/dl)	0.20–0.40	0.24 + 0.19	61	0.11 + 0.05
Burr cells and red cell fragments†	rare	+	71	+ +
Factor V activity (%)	80–120	81 + 27	46	58 + 18
Factor VIII:C activity (%)	75–125	88 + 26	29	66 + 13
Plasminogen activity (%)	88–120	82 + 23	49	63 + 17

Modified from Feldman et al., 1981; courtesy of the American Journal of Veterinary Research.
*Presence of gel or fibrin strand was considered abnormal; graded trace to 4+.
†Burr cells and fragmented red cells graded + = 5–10%; + + = 10–15%; + + + = >15%; greater than 5% was considered abnormal.

producing FDPs that have affinity for soluble fibrin monomers preventing polymerization. Plasmin is capable also of degrading coagulation factors (Hirsh and Brain, 1983). Thus bleeding tendency in DIC is a consequence of depletion of coagulation factors and platelets plus the anticoagulant properties of FDPs. FDPs are cleared by the MPS, hence MPS blockade augments DIC (Feldman, 1981a; Ruehl et al., 1982).

The resultant balance of coagulation and fibrinolysis is, thus, affected by the two proteases, thrombin and plasmin. If thrombin is dominant, thromboses occur, whereas if plasmin is dominant, hemorrhage will occur. Production of kinins, mediators of vascular permeability and pain, is associated with vasodilation and vascular stasis and a vicious cycle ensues with coagulation initiation, localized stasis, and organ ischemia. Kinins also activate the complement system causing granulocyte migration and cell lysis. Considering these multisystem phenomena, DIC might also be called acute disseminated intravascular proteolysis.

Diagnosis

The clinical aspects of DIC can be characterized by widespread formation of fibrin thrombi, multiple coagulation defects, bleeding tendency, and impaired organ function.

The syndrome is reported principally in dogs, although it has been described in other species as well. Presenting signs include shock of varying severity, generalized or localized bleeding, petechia and ecchymoses of skin and mucous membranes, evidence of intravascular hemolysis, and adrenocortical, pulmonary, renal, hepatic, pancreatic, or CNS involvement with their accompanying signs and clinical effects. See Appendix Case 25.

Laboratory diagnosis of DIC (Table 14–12) is usually based on the triad of prolonged PT, thrombocytopenia, and hypofibrinogenemia. The finding of FDPs, evidence of fragmented erythrocytes (schistocytes) in blood smears, and decreased concentrations of coagulation factors (usually factors V and VIII) and antithrombin III add additional weight to the diagnosis. APTT and TT are also prolonged. There is no single laboratory test pathognomic for the disease. Coagulation abnormalities in 41 dogs with DIC are presented in Table 14–11.

In chronic DIC, not all procoagulants are depleted since liver and bone marrow have varying capacities to increase production of coagulation factors and platelets. Although the bone marrow is capable of producing about 4 to 8 times the usual number of platelets, and the liver can generate coagulation factors at least 5 times the normal concentration (Owen and Bowie, 1977), continuous infusion of thromboplastin into dogs caused overcompensation of hepatic production leading to elevated concentrations of fibri-

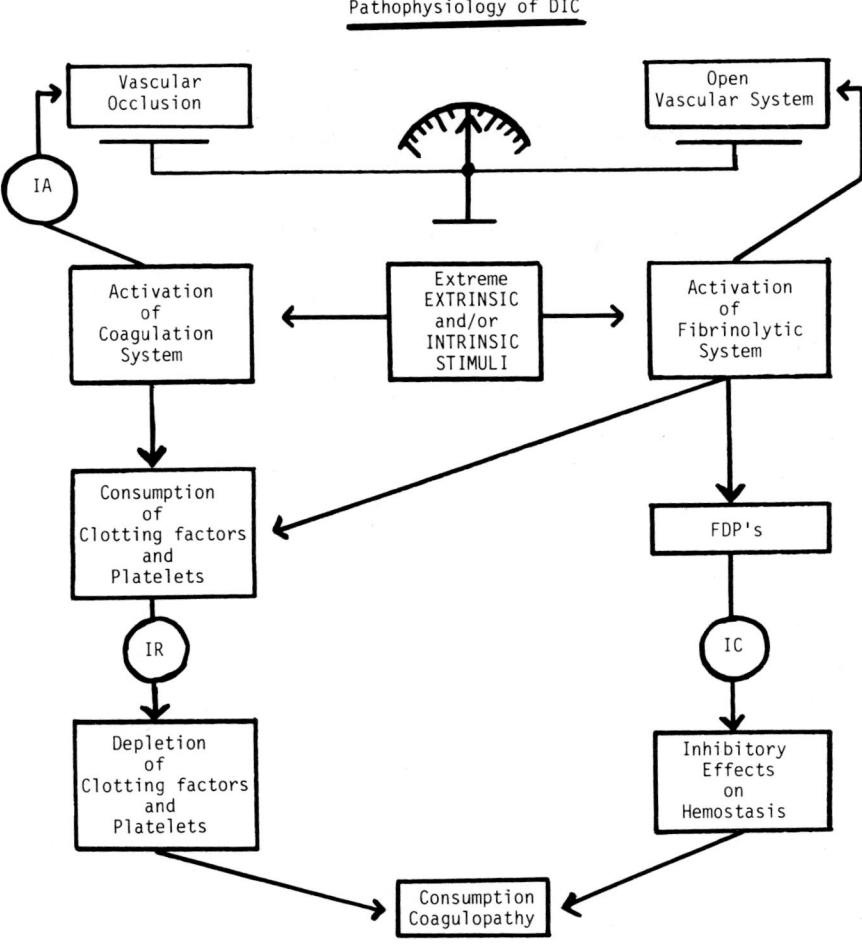

Pathophysiology of DIC

IA = Insufficient anticoagulation   IR = Insufficient repletion

IC = Insufficient clearance

Fig. 14–6. A schematic of various events associated with disseminated intravascular coagulation (DIC). (Prepared with the assistance of Dr. R. Slappendel.)

Table 14–12. Laboratory Findings in Disseminated Intravascular Coagulation (DIC)

Platelets	↓	Antithrombin III	↓
Schistocytes	+	Plasmin	↑
Fibrinogen	↓	Plasminogen	↓
FDPs	↑	Complement	↓
APTT	↑	Fibrin monomers	↑
PT	↑	Fibronectin	↓
TT	↑	Factors V and VIII	↓
Clotting time	↑	Protamine sulfate test	+
Clot lysis time	↓	BUN	↑

+ = present, ↑ = increased, ↓ = decreased.

nogen and factor V whereas the ability of the bone marrow to replace platelets was not as great (Owen et al., 1973).

Therapy

Treatment of acute DIC should be logical and sequential. The most important therapy is to remove the inciting cause. Such removal can be accomplished by appropriate antibiotic therapy for bacterial infections, surgical removal of neoplasms or necrotic tissue, normalizing body temperature in cases of heatstroke, or other measures capable of eliminating or mitigating the primary disease. When widespread metastatic disease exists, removal of the inciting cause is not possible. In such a situation specific treatment of DIC may be indicated.

Specific therapeutic measures may be separated into several categories including fluid therapy, administration of drugs such as heparin or aspirin to stop coagulation, and replacement of depleted blood constituents. Drugs that inhibit fibrinolysis are currently being investigated (Ruehl et al., 1982).

Fluid Therapy

Fluid therapy is indicated in animals with DIC. Specific goals are correction of hypovolemia, prevention or alleviation of vascular stasis, and dilution of thrombin, FDPs, and activators of fibrinolysis. Correction of hypovolemia and venous stasis decreases activation of the intrinsic system. Dilution of procoagulants aids in preventing coagulation protein activation, platelet activation, and fibrin polymerization (Ruehl et al., 1982).

The type of fluid administered is not critical in DIC and should be chosen on the basis of the primary disease and the acid-base, electrolyte, and hydration status of the patient. Total volume and rate of administration are determined by the status of the patient and monitored as in other cases of fluid therapy.

Inhibitors of Coagulation

Drugs to inhibit coagulation are indicated if the patient manifests direct evidence of bleeding, thrombosis, or organ dysfunction. Heparin is the most useful and most common choice at present. Heparin potentiates the action of plasma antithrombin III; its primary action is to inactivate thrombin and coagulation factors XIIa, XIa, Xa, and IXa.

Increased plasma concentration of thrombin is found in DIC, especially early in the process and in chronic situations. Provided that antithrombin III concentrations are adequate, administration of heparin to such patients would facilitate inactivation of thrombin and other coagulants, reducing the tendency for intravascular coagulation and thrombosis.

Heparin is injected usually by continuous intravenous (iv) infusion, but recent observations suggest that intermittent iv administration or subcutaneous administration is equally effective and produces fewer and less serious side effects (Feldman, 1981a). The recommended dosage of heparin for initial iv therapy is 10 units/kg body weight. The dose is then adjusted based on clinical response and changes in laboratory test results (ACT, PT, APTT, and fibrinogen level) used to monitor the patient's coagulation status. Normalizing test results indicates success of therapy. Heparin may be given subcutaneously in doses of 5 to 10 units/kg body weight every 8 to 12 hours. This method of heparin administration is safe, convenient, and does not interfere with in vitro tests used to monitor response (Ruehl et al., 1982). Heparinization in dogs (Green, 1980) and cats (Greene and Meriwether, 1982) can be monitored using the ACT test.

The most serious potential side effect of overzealous heparin therapy is bleeding resulting from too much anticoagulation and aided in some cases by thrombocytopenia. The mechanism of heparin-induced thrombocytopenia is poorly understood, but may, in part, involve an immune-mediated reaction (see Chapter 17).

Regardless of the method of administration, heparin requirements can vary widely among individuals. Patients with minimal activation of the coagulation system require relatively small doses; patients with extensive coagulation activation may need considerably larger doses. Furthermore, if excessive platelet activation is occurring, large quantities of PF-4 (heparin neutralizing factor) may be released, directly neutralizing heparin. Most importantly, if extensive DIC is occurring, plasma antithrombin III concentration will be reduced and even high-dose heparin therapy will be ineffective. In such patients, heparin therapy must be preceded or accompanied by fresh plasma administration to replenish antithrombin III necessary for heparin action (see Blood Component Therapy).

Inhibitors of platelet function such as aspirin may be used in DIC but are contraindicated in severely thrombocytopenic patients (platelet counts less than 50,000/μl of blood). One dose of aspirin carries with it the potential of impeding platelet function for 5 to 7 days (see Chapter 16). Other anticoagulants such as warfarin have not been effective.

Blood Component Therapy

When patients with DIC bleed, replacement of some or all blood constituents is indicated to replenish depleted coagulation factors and platelets. Some observers believe that replacement is contraindicated until after bleeding is controlled. Direct evidence that such replacement accelerates or maintains intravascular coagulation, however, is lacking. Plasma infusion is preferred, but whole blood can be given if red cell infusion is necessary. Infusion of red cells carries the risk of hemolysis and exacerbation of DIC (Hardaway et al., 1956; Rabiner and Friedman, 1968).

Plasma infusion to replenish antithrombin III is suggested when patients with DIC bleed and are unresponsive to heparin therapy. As mentioned earlier, heparin therapy must precede or accompany plasma infusion. Another approach has been to incubate fresh plasma with heparin (5 to 10 units/kg body weight) at room temperature for 30 minutes to activate antithrombin III and then infuse the plasma at 10 ml/kg every 3 hours as needed. An investigative approach to treat severe bleeding in humans with DIC has been the use of antithrombin III concentrates followed by administration of plasma and platelet suspensions (Abildgaard, 1979).

Plasma fibronectin concentration is reduced in DIC (Feldman and Thomson, 1983). Fibronectins are high molecular weight glycoproteins present on cell surfaces and in plasma. They mediate MPS clearance of bacteria and fibrin microaggregates. If the MPS is overwhelmed by fibrin microaggregates in DIC, clearance of activated coagulation factors will be inhibited with resultant ongoing activation of coagulation processes. Administration of fibronectin in the form of cryoprecipitates of plasma restores MPS function and will limit DIC. Cryoprecipitate is obtained by freezing fresh plasma and then allowing it to thaw at 4° to 10°C. The cryoprecipitate is aspirated. To restore MPS function, 10–20 ml of cryoprecipitate administered iv at 3-hour intervals will be sufficient. Overzealous cryoprecipitate therapy is contraindicated as the MPS may become suppressed. Cryoprecipitate is an investigational-type therapeutic agent (Ruehl et al., 1982).

Monitors of Effective Therapy

Various laboratory tests have been used to monitor anticoagulant therapy in DIC. These tests include ACT, PT, APTT, TT, quantitation of fibrinogen, assays for factors V and VIII, antithrombin III and FDPs, and platelet count (Gentry, 1977; Green, 1980; Greene and Meriwether, 1982; Ruehl et al., 1982). Normalization of the screening coagulogram (PT, APTT, and FDPs), usually denotes successful therapy. Return of normal fibrinogen concentration has proved to be a reliable and sensitive long-term indicator of effectiveness of heparin therapy, but fibrinogen concentrations may require 24 to 48 hours to normalize. Platelet counts often do not normalize for 7 to 14 days after cessation of bleeding (Feldman, 1981a; Ruehl et al., 1982).

THROMBOSIS

A thrombus is an intravascular deposit composed of fibrin and formed elements of blood. Thrombosis is the formation of this mass that completely or partially impedes the blood flow. Thrombi may form in arteries, veins, heart, and microcirculation. Thromboembolism results when a thrombus formed locally or one that dislodged from an upstream location occludes the vessel and shuts off the regional blood supply. DIC is a form of thrombosis in microcirculation. Thromboembolic complications have been reported in both humans and dogs in nephrotic syndromes (DeGaetano, 1981; Green and Kabel, 1982) and hypercorticism (Burns et al., 1981; Sjoberg et al., 1976). Increased thrombotic tendency is also noted in patients receiving treatment with glucocorticoids for prolonged periods (DeGaetano, 1981). Thromboembolism is of major importance in pathogenesis of heart attack and stroke in humans.

A brief description of pathogenesis, diagnosis, and therapy of thrombosis follows. For additional details excellent texts and reports may be seen (Dodds, 1977c; Feinstein, 1982; Hirsh, 1977; Migaki and Casey, 1975; Nemerson and Nossel, 1982; Verstraete, 1977).

Pathogenesis

The relative proportion of formed elements in thrombi differs from that in blood because their accumulation is partly selective. In addition, the relative proportion of different blood cells to each other and to fibrin is influenced by hemodynamics; therefore, the composition of arterial and venous thrombi is different (Hirsh and Brain, 1983).

Thrombi that form in the high-flow system (arteries) are composed mainly of platelet aggregates that are held together by a small amount of fibrin and are known as *platelet or white thrombi*. Red cells and leukocytes form a small component of these thrombi. Thrombi that form in areas of slow-to-moderate flow are composed of a mixture of red cells, platelets, and fibrin and are known as *mixed platelet thrombi*. Thrombi that form in areas of complete blood stasis are composed of red cells with a large amount of interspersed fibrin and are known as *coagulation or red thrombi*. Platelets and leukocytes are distributed randomly in these thrombi. Various thrombi may exhibit a lamellar arrangement of blood cells as they continue to grow gradually and may become organized as a fibrous plaque.

Thrombosis results from an imbalance between stimuli that initiate clot formation and protective mechanisms that inhibit or recede coagulation. Basically, thrombus formation involves the same sequence of events that leads to the formation of a hemostatic plug necessary to arrest escape of blood from an injured vessel wall (see section on Primary Hemostasis and Figs. 14–1 and 14–2). The only difference being that thrombus results when these processes continue unabated by mechanisms that ordinarily cause dissolution of the hemostatic plug after it has served its purpose (see sections on Regulation of the Clotting Process and Fibrinolysis). Hence the process of thrombogenesis is not described herein.

Thrombogenic factors include a variety of circumstances favoring localized platelet adhesion and aggregation and activation of the coagulation cascade. These factors include abnormalities of vessel wall, abnormalities of blood flow, hypercoagulable state of blood, and abnormalities of fibrinolysis (Table 14–13). Most of the probable thrombotic episodes recognized in animals are associated with infectious agents (bacteria, viruses, and fungi) that result in inflammation and damage to vascular endothelium (Migaki and Casey, 1975). Other causes of thrombosis in animals include infection with certain parasites, im-

Table 14–13.   Factors Implicated in the Pathogenesis of Thrombosis

Abnormalities of Vessel Wall
  Vascular injury—mechanical, chemical, immunologic, or infectious agents
  Diminished vascular tone
Abnormalities of Blood Flow
  Diminished or stagnant blood flow
  Turbulent or misdirected blood flow
  Hyperviscosity
Hypercoagulability of Blood
  Elevated levels of coagulation proteins—increased synthesis or reduced catabolism
  In vivo activation of coagulation cascade—entrance of tissue thrombplastins in blood
  Platelet abnormalities—decreased survival; increased adhesion, aggregation and release reaction; marked thrombocytosis; thrombocythemia
  Abnormalities of inhibitory mechanisms—deficiency of antithrombin III and protein "C," reduced levels of α-antiplasmin, defective clearance of activated coagulation factors by the liver or MPS
Abnormalities of Fibrinolysis
  Excessive α_1-antitrypsin inhibition of plasmin
  Deficiency of plasminogen activators
  Abnormal plasminogen

mune complex polyarthritis, neoplasia, vitamin E deficiency (in swine), and the use of indwelling catheters.

Diagnosis

The diagnosis of thrombosis includes angiography, impedence plethysmography, ^{125}I-fibrinogen scanning, and ultrasound (Hirsh, 1981). These studies are used in veterinary medicine but infrequently to diagnose thrombosis and are beyond the scope of this chapter. Generally the diagnosis is difficult, and in veterinary medicine thrombosis may not be recognized until it becomes a clinical emergency.

Laboratory findings associated with increased risks or the presence of thrombosis or thromboembolism include decreased antithrombin III concentration, deficient fibrinolysis, reduced platelet survival, increased platelet procoagulant activity (e.g., PF-4 and β-thromboglobulin), increased activity of clotting factors, and elevated levels of complexes of fibrin monomers, fibrinopeptide A, and FDPs in blood (Hirsh, 1977; Thompson and Harker, 1983).

A thrombus must be distinguished from postmortem clot found at necropsy. A thrombus is an antimortem clot that is generally partly or completely attached to the vascular endothelium. It is irregular in shape, varies in color, and has a dull appearance and roughened surface. It is friable and usually appears lamellar on cut surface. A postmortem clot, on the other hand, is entirely unattached to the vascular endothelium, dark red in color, molded to the vascular bed, and smooth and uniform in texture. A classic "chicken-fat" clot forms when rapid red cell settling occurs (as in the horse) prior to formation of a postmortem clot.

Therapy

Because of the important roles played by the coagulation system and the platelets in pathogenesis of thrombosis, therapeutic measures to control thrombosis or thromboembolism must be directed toward inhibiting abnormal activities of these blood constituents. Anticoagulants like heparin, coumarin, and indanediones and antiplatelet agents such as aspirin, sulfinpyrazone and dipyridamole are commonly used to dampen the "hypercoagulable state" and prevent formation of new thrombi. In addition, fibrinolytic agents such as streptokinase and urokinase have been used to effect dissolution of preformed thrombi, particularly during early stages of the disease. Mechanisms of actions of these drugs are summarized in Table 14–14.

Regardless of the therapeutic approach, if the patient is not selected and monitored carefully, serious bleeding complications can develop.

Anticoagulants

The major types of anticoagulants are heparin and vitamin K antagonists. See the discussion on heparin therapy in relation to DIC (p. 414) for the proper approach in treatment of thrombosis. Vitamin K antagonism was discussed previously as a cause of acquired coagulopathy (see p. 407).

Vitamin K antagonists reduce the blood concentration of functional (gammacarboxylated) forms of vitamin K-dependent coagulation factors II, VII, IX, and X by impairing their synthesis in the liver (Table 14–14). As blood concentrations of the factors able to be activated decline, their decarboxylated precursors accumulate in the blood, where they

not only perform poorly in coagulation but also act as weak anticoagulants. Thus, vitamin K antagonists such as warfarin have a different role in anticoagulant therapy than heparin and fibrinolytic agents. These latter substances are used to treat acute episodes of intravascular clotting and the courses of these agents are generally short—1 to 2 days (Bell and Meek, 1979). In contrast, vitamin K anticoagulants are used to prevent further clotting, not to treat immediate episodes of thrombosis. Therapy is monitored by performing the PT test. Dosage of the vitamin K antagonist is adjusted to prolong the PT to 2.5 times the baseline value. Once maintenance dosage is determined, the PT may be performed less frequently, at 1- to 3-week intervals. When selecting antithrombotic therapy with coumarin drugs, it is esential to recognize that many commonly used drugs may potentiate or inhibit the action of coumarin anticoagulants (Wintrobe et al., 1981).

The effect of warfarin in preventing coagulation in ponies (Scott et al., 1978, 1979) and in treating navicular disease (Vrins et al., 1983) has been studied.

Antiplatelet Drugs

Commonly used antiplatelet drugs include aspirin, sulfinpyrazone, and dipyridamole (Table 14–14). These agents are used mainly to prevent thrombosis at the arterial side of the circulation where clots are thought to originate as intravascular platelet aggregates as discussed previously (Thrombosis—Pathogenesis). These agents are less useful in combating thrombosis on the venous side because venous thrombosis appears to result mainly from inappropriate activation of the coagulation cascade. On an analogous basis, it should be obvious why heparin is beneficial in preventing venous thrombosis and less effective in preventing arterial thrombosis. Prophylactic or long-term therapeutic management of the thrombotic patient, however, often involves use of both anticoagulants and antiplatelet agents.

Aspirin blocks production of thromboxane and stable prostaglandins (see Fig. 16–6) by irreversibly inactivating platelet cyclo-oxygenase for the life of the affected platelet. Through its effect on thromboxane produc-

Table 14–14. **Mechanisms of Action of Selected Antithrombotic and Thrombolytic Agents**

Agent	Effect	Mechanism of Action
Heparin	Inhibition of serine proteases involved in clot formation	Potentiates the anticoagulant effects of antithrombin III by complexing with it
Coumarin-type drugs	Decreased supply of vitamin K-dependent functional clotting factors II, VII, IX, and X	Inhibition of the enzyme system necessary to recycle vitamin K for gammacarboxylation of the vitamin K-dependent clotting factors
Aspirin	Decreased thromboxane production, hence inhibition of platelet aggregation and release reaction	Inactivation of platelet cyclooxygenase (irreversible)
Sulfinpyrazone	Decreased thromboxane production, hence inhibition of platelet aggregation and release reaction	Inactivation of platelet cyclooxygenase (reversible)
Dipyridamole	Increased cAMP production, hence inhibition of platelet aggregation and release reaction	Inactivation of platelet phosphodiesterase: inhibition of intracellular CA^{++}
Streptokinase	Conversion of plasminogen to plasmin → thrombolysis	Formation of a nonenzymatic complex with plasminogen or plasmin
Urokinase	Activation of plasminogen to plasmin → thrombolysis	Enzymatic cleavage of plasminogen

tion, aspirin prevents the secondary wave of aggregation and release reaction undergone by platelets responding to weak stimuli. Its use as an antiplatelet agent is based on this effect. In very high dose, aspirin temporarily blocks the production of PGI_2, the natural inhibitor of platelet aggregation, by inactivating cyclo-oxygenase of the vascular endothelium. In the absence of PGI_2, platelet aggregation is efficient, enough to offset the antiaggregation effect of aspirin. Although the net effect of aspirin given in usual dosage is that of antithrombosis, a low-dose therapy may be desired to maintain this balance (Masotti et al., 1979).

Sulfinpyrazone inhibits platelet adhesion to collagen by blocking thromboxane production through reversible inhibition of platelet cyclo-oxygenase. Dipyridamole inhibits platelet adhesion and ADP-induced platelet aggregation as a result of increased production of cAMP within the platelets by impairing platelet phosphodiesterase activity. Clinical effectiveness of these drugs in veterinary medicine is being investigated.

Fibrinolytic Agents

The natural corollary to clot formation is activation of the fibrinolytic system (see Regulation of the Clotting Process). Hence, thrombolytic therapy involves activation of the endogenous fibrinolytic system. The most important fibrinolytic drugs are the plasminogen activators streptokinase and urokinase. As mentioned previously (Thrombosis—Therapy) and indicated in Table 14–14, streptokinase forms a complex with plasminogen (or plasmin) that nonenzymatically activates plasminogen precursors to plasmin. In contrast, urokinase (which is about 10 times more expensive than streptokinase) directly activates plasminogen to plasmin by an enzymatic process. Because urokinase is a natural product it is not inhibited as readily as streptokinase, which may be inactivated by antibodies present in blood (as a result of previous streptococcal infections), and is, therefore, given in higher doses or discontinued in "resistant" patients. Streptokinase is derived from streptococci; urokinase is a urine extract or derived from kidney cell cultures (Lijnen and Cullen, 1982).

Administration of either of these agents produces a systemic lytic state characterized by plasminogen depletion, presence of free plasmin in plasma, decrease in α_2-antiplasmin because of its binding to newly formed plasmin, decrease in fibrinogen concentration, increase in FDPs, and prolonged TT (Stampfer et al., 1982). Although the achievement of a systemic lytic state appears necessary for dissolving a pathologic clot, it increases the risk of uncontrolled bleeding. Note, the change in plasma coagulation proteins is not in itself a bleeding problem. The threat lies in the dissolution of a hemostatic plug or the prevention of plug formation. Experience with these drugs in veterinary medicine is limited (Albrechtsson et al., 1981; Sherry et al., 1955). Hence, discussion of therapy, patient selection, monitoring techniques, and success in therapy would be speculative. Statland and Ito (1984) give an excellent review of thrombolytic therapy.

DIAGNOSTIC METHODS

The veterinary clinician concerned with a bleeding problem has many techniques for adequate diagnosis. The information available must be carefully analyzed, however, and the problem approached systematically. This involves decision-making; that is, is the defect generalized or local, is it inherited or acquired, at what level is it (vascular, platelet, coagulation factor or a combination of these) and finally, what is the defect and how can it be corrected.

Acquired coagulation problems are more common than inherited problems in both humans and animals. Inherited problems are more common in animals, however, than in humans owing to inbreeding practices. A comprehensive medical history of the patient including current and previous bleeding problems, environmental and drug history, and the ancestry is a valuable adjunct to the clinical examination. Such a history should be reviewed for lameness, painful joints, anemia of unknown cause, or periodic weakness. A prolonged history of bleeding, especially in males with a family history of bleeding, should lead the clinician to suspect a congenital disorder.

The most obvious clinical signs in disorders of coagulation are spontaneous bleeding into the skin, mucous membranes, or internal tissues or excessive or prolonged bleeding after surgical procedures or trauma. Other signs to look for are petechiae, purpuras, ecchymoses, hematomas, hemarthroses, hematuria, and more obvious signs such as epistaxis or bleeding from the gums. During the physical examination, a tourniquet test can be performed—petechiae indicate possible thrombocytopenia or a defect in platelet function. The color of the mucous membranes is noted and capillary refill time determined (by pressing the gums and noting the time it takes for color to reappear). The blood smear can be helpful by noting the relative number and morphology of platelets and red cell abnormalities such as the presence of schistocytes.

Methods commonly used for testing the coagulation cascade are summarized in Table 14–4. Screening tests for the clotting cascade are carried out in plasma in which clotting has been prevented by a calcium sequestering agent such as sodium citrate. The cascade is initiated by adding calcium plus an activating agent, and the time required for the formation of a clot is measured. Three tests are used, each using a different activating agent and each examining a different portion of the cascade. These tests are PT, APTT, and TT, respectively measuring the intrinsic and extrinsic pathways and fibrinogen of the common pathway (Fig. 14–3). Selected references on tests of hemostasis in various species of animals are given (Abildgaard and Link, 1965; Benson et al., 1983; Bowie et al., 1973; Culbertson et al., 1979; Didisheim et al., 1959; Gajewski and Povar, 1971; Gentry et al., 1978; Johstone and Crane, 1980; Lewis, 1976; Lopocink et al., 1978; O'Rourke et al., 1982; Rowsell and Mustard, 1963; Seaman and Malinow, 1968).

Many tests are available for determining specific coagulation defects; these tests are useful in research on hemostasis but are not used routinely in clinical medicine. To assay for specific coagulation factor deficiencies, the clinician probably will need the services of an experienced coagulation laboratory. Reagents for diagnosis of human coagulation factor deficiencies are available commercially. Most of these reagents will work in animals. A pool of normal plasma should be used as a control. Results of factor assays are traditionally expressed as percentage of normal activity.

The screening tests PT and APTT differentiate between deficiencies of the intrinsic and extrinsic pathways. Coagulopathies with normal APTT and abnormal PT suggest factor

VII deficiency, whereas abnormal APTT and normal PT suggest factor VIII, IX, XI, XII, or Fletcher factor deficiency. To identify factor VIII deficiency, it is necessary to determine the concentrations of factor VIII:RAg and factor VIII:C. If factor VIII:C activity is low and factor VIII:RAg is normal or increased, hemophilia A is indicated. If factor VIII:C activity is low as well as factor VIII:RAg level, von Willebrand's disease is suspected.

A prolonged PT or APTT could be fully corrected by mixing the deficient plasma wih an equal volume of normal plasma or of a second plasma that lacked a different clotting factor (Feldman et al., 1983). The plasma in question would remain uncorrected. If the second plasma was deficient in the same factor that was missing from the plasma tested, the test results would not change. A clotting factor deficiency can therefore be diagnosed by showing that an abnormal PT or APTT is correctable by all but one of a panel of plasmas with known deficiencies; the unknown (patient's) plasma and the plasma that fails to correct the test are missing the same clotting factor.

The concentration of the deficient clotting factor, an important consideration in the treatment of clotting factor deficiency, can be determined from the PT or APTT using a standardized curve obtained with mixing normal plasma and plasma with a known deficiency. Clotting factor concentration as measured by immunologic testing in humans often agrees with concentrations measured functionally with the PT or APTT (Babior and Stossel, 1984).

Whenever an abnormal screening test is not corrected by mixing the defective plasma with an equal volume of normal plasma, the presence of an inhibitor is indicated. The potency of the inhibitor can be determined by measuring the effect of various concentrations of the inhibitor-containing plasma on the clotting properties of normal plasma. Identifying which factors the inhibitor acts against may be difficult because both the PT and APTT depend on the activation of many factors, and an inhibitor acting against any one of them will prolong clotting.

Screening Tests of Hemostasis

Bleeding Time

The bleeding time test, a crude but valuable screening test, is performed by measuring how long it takes for bleeding to stop from a fresh cut of determined size. A prolonged bleeding time usually indicates a platelet disorder (quantitative or qualitative) or probably an intrinsic blood vessel problem. In pure disorders of the clotting cascade the bleeding time is almost invariably normal.

Ivy Bleeding Time (Ivy et al., 1935; Mielke et al., 1969). This test can be performed on the skin of the abdomen near the umbilicus or in the flank. A moderately deep puncture is made with a No. 11 Bard Parker blade so that blood flows freely. A Mielke template device may be used to control the length and depth of the cut. Drops of blood are absorbed onto a circle of filter paper at 30-second intervals, and the time at which bleeding stops is noted. The paper should be moved each time so that each drop of blood falls on a fresh area. The normal bleeding time for most animals is 1 to 5 minutes.

Clotting Time

Clotting time is a measure of the overall functioning of the coagulation cascade. It is influenced by many factors such as the manner of blood withdrawal, the size and surface of the test tube, and the temperature of incubation. Care must be taken not to traumatize the veins during bleeding, and it is essential that the needle be inserted immediately into the vein to avoid inclusion of tissue thromboplastin in the test sample.

Lee-White Method. Blood in excess of 3.0 ml is drawn carefully from the best available vein avoiding tissue juices. If a glass syringe is used, timing is started immediately. Dispense the blood in 1.0-ml amounts down the sides of 3 tubes labeled 1 to 3 (10 × 75 mm each) starting with tube 3. If silicone-coated or plastic syringes are used, start timing now. Place tubes in a water bath or glass of water at 37°C. Tilt tube 1 at 30-second intervals until blood clots; then similarly tilt tube 2 and finally tube 3. The clotting time is the length of time required for the blood in tube 3 to clot. Normal clotting time by this method is 4 to

15 minutes in the horse, cow, and sheep; 3 to 13 minutes in the dog; and 8 minutes or so in the cat.

Activated Clotting Time (ACT). ACT is unique in that there is immediate contact activation of freshly drawn blood resulting in a shorter clotting time than obtained with the Lee-White method. Thus ACT is a more sensitive method to detect coagulation disorders of the intrinsic system. Contact activation of coagulation cascade occurs from mixing blood with diatomaceous earth in the collection tube (Byars et al., 1976; Hattersley, 1966, 1976). Following is the procedure for ACT:

Draw 2 ml of venous blood into a prewarmed (37°C) Vacutainer tube (Becton-Dickinson) containing purified siliceous earth; do not use this first tube for ACT determination. Leave the needle in the vein and exactly draw 2 ml of blood into a second prewarmed Vacutainer tube. Begin timing with a stop watch when blood first enters the tube. In the absence of ACT Vacutainer tubes, use glass tubes containing 12 mg of celite (Johns Manville Sales Co.). When blood ceases to enter the tube, remove the tube from the needle, invert 5 times to mix, and place it into a heating block or water bath at 37°C. After 1 minute, remove the tube at 5- to 10-second intervals and tilt it gently in front of a light source to watch for the first appearance of a visible clot. Continue to replace and remove the tube from the water bath to observe the clot. The end point is taken at the appearance of the first unmistakable, but not solid clot and should be timed to the nearest 5 seconds.

Inadequate mixing of blood and diatomaceous earth will cause the clotting time to be prolonged. The time for clot formation is temperature-dependent (Table 14–15; Middleton and Watson, 1978), therefore for standardiza-tion, it is customary to keep the tubes in a heating block or water bath before and during the test. Considerable time can elapse between the appearance of the first clot and a solid clot. Falsely increased times can result from failure to recognize the initial clot. Substances interfering with the ACT include salicylates, anticoagulants, certain antibiotics, and barbiturates.

In humans, the ACT is useful for monitoring anticoagulation therapy and deficiencies in factors VIII, IX, and XII, but not deficiencies in factor VII or defects due to platelet numbers or function. The ACT is a reliable, simple, and rapid test. Necessary materials are available commercially at low cost and the test can be done at the side of the animal; thus the test has many advantages for the practicing veterinarian. Results for the ACT test in normal animals are given in Table 14–15.

Routine Tests of Hemostasis

Activated Partial Thromboplastin Time (APTT)

The APTT measures the relative activity of factors in the intrinsic clotting sequence and the common pathway. It is a pivotal test for diagnosis and differentiation of hemophilias. The combination of an abnormal APTT with a normal PT establishes that a plasma coagulation disorder exists in the intrinsic pathway. The next step is the differentiation between a deficiency of factor VIII (hemophilia A) or factor IX (hemophilia B) by means of the *differential thromboplastin time*. In this test, suitably prepared reagents rich in either factor VIII or IX are added to the test plasma 1:1. The reagent correcting the APTT from abnormal to normal or near-normal level contains the deficient factor.

Table 14–15. Activated Coagulation Time (ACT) of Whole Blood in Some Animal Species

| Animal | Number | ACT in Seconds | | Reference |
		Range	Mean ± SD	
Dogs				
37°C	42	64–95	79 + 7.1	Middleton and Watson (1978)
Room temp.	42	83–129	102.6 + 10.7	Middleton and Watson (1978)
38°C	72	<60–125	77.5 + 14.7	Byars et al. (1976)
Ponies	37	115–280	152 + 35	Rawlings et al. (1975)
Horses	31	130–200	163 + 18	Rawlings et al. (1975)
Cows	10	120–180	145 + 18	Riley and Lasson (1979)

The APTT basically involves incubating platelet-poor plasma with a platelet substitute ("partial" thromboplastin) and a factor XII activator, and then measuring clotting time after recalcification (Hougie, 1972a). Plasma is activated by kaolin, diatomaceous silica (celite), or ellagic acid giving shorter clotting times and more reliable results than nonactivated plasma. A "complete" thromboplastin is prepared, for example, from dried brain, usually of rabbits. If this were to be used, hemophilic plasma would clot as rapidly as normal plasma. In the APTT, however, partial thromboplastins are used because they do not compensate for the lack of hemophilic factors. Partial thromboplastin is prepared by ether extraction of brain with the active material being crude cephalin, a phospholipid. Animal (cephalin) and vegetable (purified soy phosphatides) phospholipids available commercially can be used in the test in either manual or semiautomated formats using a fibrometer.

Collect plasma from blood anticoagulated with 3.8% sodium citrate in a ratio of 9 volumes of blood to 1 volume of the anticoagulant. Pipette 0.1 ml partial thromboplastin reagent into a 10 × 75 mm test tube and warm in a 37°C water bath for at least 1 minute. Add 0.1 ml of the test plasma into the tube and simultaneously start a stopwatch. Gently mix contents by twirling, and incubate at 37°C. After exactly 3 minutes, pipette 0.1 ml of prewarmed (37°C) 0.02 M calcium chloride solution into the tube, and simultaneously start a second stopwatch. Mix contents of the tube gently while holding it in the water bath. After 5 seconds, remove the tube from the water bath and gently tilt it back and forth. When fibrin strands appear or gel forms, stop the second stopwatch and record the clotting time. Repeat the test 2 or 3 times and average the results. Run a normal control with each patient of the same species if possible, although commercial human controls are available. Each laboratory should establish its own normal values. Our normal values are 9 to 11 seconds for the dog, 10 to 15 seconds for the cat, and 25 to 45 seconds for the horse. There may be variability at times due to the method of fibrin detection (Johnstone, 1984).

The APTT varies with animal species and source of partial thromboplastin. It is best to use pooled homologous plasma as a control. The test is affected by several other factors such as the anticoagulant, pH of the plasma, low fibrinogen levels, and FDPs. The presence of circulating inhibitors of coagulation (such as heparin and FDPs) in plasma is suspected when APTT is prolonged and remains prolonged after mixing equal amounts of normal plasma with the patient's plasma.

Prothrombin Time (PT)

Quick's one stage prothrombin time or simply PT offers a measure of the prothrombin complex, hence the extrinsic system and the common pathway, i.e., factors I, II, V, VII, and X. The end point involves the conversion of fibrinogen to fibrin, thus it is also a rough measure of fibrinogen (factor I) concentrations.

The principle of the test is based on the fact that plasma obtained from blood to which an anticoagulant (that binds Ca^{++}) has been added, will clot in a few seconds when recalcified in the presence of tissue thromboplastin (Hougie, 1972a, 1972b; Vollmer, 1976). The time recorded is the time elapsed between the addition of Ca^{++} and the appearance of a visible clot.

The procedure is as follows: collect 9 volumes of blood in a vial containing 1 volume of 3.8% sodium citrate solution, and remove the plasma by centrifugation. Add 0.1 ml of the citrated plasma to a small test tube (10 × 75 mm) and place it in a water bath at 37°C for 3 minutes. Thromboplastin solution (commercial rabbit brain thromboplastin) consists of equal volumes of thromboplastin and 0.02 M $CaCl_2$ solution (0.22 g of $CaCl_2$/dl distilled water). Warm the thromboplastin solution to 37°C for 5 minutes and add 0.2 ml by forcibly blowing out into the tube of plasma. Start timing by using a stopwatch. Maintain the tube at 37°C while shaking it gently. Remove the tube from the water bath and record the time when a visible clot forms. A nichrome loop (inserted and withdrawn until a clot forms) or a fibrometer with an automatic timer are alternative methods that can be used to time clot formation. Repeat until 2 or 3 PTs are within one second of each other. Run a normal control with each patient, preferably of the same species, although commercial human controls are available.

If semiautomatic test systems are used, the manufacturers' recommendations should be followed and each laboratory should establish its own normal values. Dodds (1980) recommends use of human brain thromboplastin because commercial rabbit brain thromboplastin does not detect minor deficiencies. The latter can be used, however, if diluted to give more prolonged clotting times. If homologous thromboplastin is used, values will differ from those obtained with rabbit or human reagents. Our normal values using rabbit thromboplastin are 6.4 to 7.4 seconds for the dog, 7.0 to 11.5 seconds for the cat, and 9.5 to 11.5 seconds for the horse.

The clinician without adequate facilities can use the local general hospital for this test provided the time between bleeding and testing is not prolonged. Transporting the blood on ice is recommended.

Abnormal PT can be found in DIC, liver disease, or deficiencies of factor VII and fibrinogen; and is a sensitive indicator of coagulation abnormality arising from vitamin K-deficiency or antagonism. PT can be used to monitor anticoagulant therapy and screen patients with severe liver disease.

Russell's Viper Venom Time (RVVT)

The RVVT is often performed when a need to differentiate between a deficiency of factor VII and factor X arises. Russell's viper venom (Stypven) in high dilutions is capable of activating factor X in recalcified normal plasma and plasma from patients with a deficiency of factors VII, VIII, and IX. The thromboplastic activity of the venom is dependent on the presence of platelet phospholipid, prothrombin, and factor V. Factor VII does not affect the reaction. A prolonged PT and normal RVVT are diagnostic of factor VII deficiency. The RVVT is prolonged in factor X deficiency and also in factor V deficiency.

Thrombin Time (TT)

The TT measures the time required and rate at which fibrin is formed, i.e., conversion of fibrinogen to fibrin monomers to initial clot. The test results are abnormal in patients with quantitative and qualitative abnormalities of fibrinogen, and when a patient's plasma contains inhibitors of the fibrinogen-to-fibrin conversion such as heparin and FDPs. A prolonged TT with a normal quantity of fibrinogen suggests dysfibrinogenemia or presence of inhibitors (Jim, 1957).

The TT is taken as the time it takes a standardized thrombin solution to clot plasma; this is a measure of the rate of conversion of fibrinogen to fibrin. All other steps in the coagulation sequence are bypassed.

The procedure for testing TT is as follows: obtain citrated blood as for the PT or APTT and remove the plasma. The plasma should be kept cold and used within 2 hours. Prepare concentrates of commercial thrombin (Parke Davis Co.) and store in small aliquots at -40°C until used. Just prior to performing the TT test, remove an aliquot of concentrated thrombin and make up to 10 units/ml of saline. Keep warm in a water bath at 37°C, and use within 30 minutes. Dispense 0.2 ml of fresh citrated patient plasma into 2 or 3 small (10 × 75 mm) test tubes. Warm the tubes at 37°C for 3 minutes. While holding a stopwatch in one hand, simultaneously blow 0.1 ml of thrombin into one tube and start the stopwatch. Remove the tube from the water bath and tilt and roll the tube back and forth under good light until a clot forms. Stop the watch when the clot forms and record the time. Repeat this procedure for the remaining tubes containing thrombin to obtain average TT. A control with homologous-pooled plasma should be run at the same time. Our normal values are 5 to 10 seconds for the dog, 10 to 19 seconds for the cat, and less than 30 seconds for the horse.

Hemostatic Tests for DIC and Fibrinolysis

Antithrombin III

A determination of inhibitors of blood clotting has diagnostic significance as in DIC. For determination of antithrombin III, the thrombin-agarose gel diffusion method can be used (Odegård and Abildgaard, 1978; Raymond and Dodds, 1979). Antithrombin III activity in normal dogs and dogs with DIC is given in Table 4–11. Stephens et al. (1984) have described a method for measuring antithrombin III in horses.

Fibrin Degradation Products (FDPs)

Fibrinogen and fibrin can be cleaved into several components, A, B, D, and E. Of these fragments, fragments D and E are quite antigenic. Commercially prepared antisera to fragments D and E adsorbed to latex particles in kit form are available (Thrombo Wellco Kit, Wellcome Reagents Ltd.). The sensitivity of the latex reagent is adjusted so that macroscopic agglutination of the latex particles occurs in the presence of FDP concentrations of 2 μg/ml or greater. The test is conducted as follows: collect 2 ml of blood into tubes containing a trypsin inhibitor (to inhibit plasmin) and bovine thrombin. Allow the blood to clot at room temperature or 37°C for 30 minutes or until a few drops of serum can be separated. Dilute serum to 1:5 and 1:20 with glycine buffer provided with the kit. Mix 1 drop of each serum dilution with 1 drop of the latex suspension on a glass slide and stir each mixture. Rock the slide gently to and fro for exactly 2 minutes while looking for macroscopic agglutination. Agglutination in 1:5 serum dilution indicates FDP concentration of greater than 10 μg/ml, while that in 1:20 dilution indicates a concentration of greater than 40 μg/ml. Normal concentration of FDPs in most species is generally less than 10 μg/ml.

The test is useful in detecting the occurrence of fibrinolysis. FDPs in plasma are short-lived but disruptive in that they impair thrombin mediated fibrin formation, fibrin polymerization, and platelet plug formation. Feldman et al. (1981) found elevated FDP levels in 61% of dogs with DIC (Table 14–11) indicating that intravascular coagulation and fibrinolysis were active.

Other tests for detection of FDPs include use of tanned erythrocyte hemagglutination inhibition assay (Mertens et al., 1969) and the staphylococcal clumping test based on the ability of FDPs to agglutinate *Staphylococcus aureus* (Allington, 1967; procedure #850, Sigma Chemical Co.). An indirect way to demonstrate FDPs is by paracoagulation tests (Mertens et al., 1969; Vollmer, 1976).

Fibrinogen Assays

Fibrinogen in coagulation studies usually is measured as a thrombin clottable protein. Enough thrombin is added to convert all the fibrinogen to fibrin, and the amount of protein in the resulting fibrin clot is determined by one of a variety of techniques. Fibrinogen can be determined also by an immunologic method or heat precipitation technique (see Chapter 2); these methods measure the fibrinogen by its structure, not by its function.

Fibrinolysis Tests

These tests are used to evaluate fibrinolysis as seen during intravascular coagulation or consumption coagulopathy. Fibrinolytic activity increases sharply during DIC or during treatment with streptokinase.

A simple test is the *clot lysis time* which can be done in conjunction with clot retraction time measurement. The blood will dissolve after clotting. Measurement at 37°C for times up to 48 hours is usually done although animal blood usually lyses in less than 24 hours.

Another test is the *euglobulin lysis time* (see section on Measurements under Fibrinolysis). Euglobulins are precipitated from plasma and redissolved by dilution and acidification. The redissolved precipitate, which contains fibrinogen, plasminogen, and plasminogen activator but not fibrinolytic inhibitors is then tested for lysis by endogenous plasmin (Vollmer, 1976). The test is not specific and is believed to reflect activator activity primarily. Kits such as DATA-FI by Dade are available for this test. The procedure for this test is as follows: Collect platelet-poor, citrated plasma as for other clotting tests. Place 0.5 ml of fresh plasma into a plastic centrifuge tube. Add 9 ml of cold distilled water and 0.1 ml of 1% acetic acid and mix gently by inversion. Keep the tube on ice or in the refrigerator for 10 minutes, and then gently centrifuge at 2000 G for 5 minutes. Gently discard the supernatant fluid and keep the tube inverted over an absorbent paper in a rack for 5 to 10 minutes. While keeping the tube in the inverted position, clean and dry the inside of the tube with cotton-tipped applicator sticks, being careful not to touch the precipitate. Add 0.5 ml of borate buffer, pH 9.0, to the tube and dissolve the precipitate by agitation at 37°C. Transfer the dissolved precipitate to a 12 × 75 mm plastic tube kept at 37°C. Add 0.1 ml of prewarmed 0.1 M $CaCl_2$ and 1 drop (50 μl) of concentrated thrombin (100 units/ml). Mix gently until a clot forms; then start a timer. Observe the clot at 10-minute inervals. The end point is at total lysis of the clot. Euglobulin lysis time is the interval of time between formation of the clot and its complete lysis.

Our normal values for euglobulin lysis time for some animals are: dogs, 60 to 120 minutes; horses, 3 to 6 hours; and monkeys, 2 to 6 hours. If fibrinogen is too low, the results may give a false impression of enhanced fibrinolytic activity.

Protamine Sulfate Test

The protamine sulfate test is used to detect fibrin monomers and early, clottable FDPs (Williams et al., 1972; Vollmer 1976). Kits are available to conduct the test (DATA-FI, Dade). The addition of protamine sulfate to citrated plasma causes a visible polymerization of monomer complexes and the test is usually positive in DIC. The test is performed as follows:

Obtain fresh citrated blood as for the APTT test and collect plasma. Use the plasma as soon as possible. Pipette 0.25 ml of plasma into a 10 × 75 mm test tube and warm at 37°C for 5 minutes. Place a small volume of reconstituted (1%) protamine sulfate solution (Eli Lilly or Upjohn) into a large test tube and warm to 37°C for 5 minutes. Add 0.025 ml of prewarmed 1% protamine sulfate solution to the plasma tube. Mix by gently tilting the tube once or twice and place in water bath at 37°C for 5 minutes. Examine for clot formation or fibrin strands. The test should be run in duplicate, and a positive control must be run simultaneously.

Hemostatic Tests for Fibrin Stabilization

Factor XIII Assay

Factor XIII deficiency can be found by determining clot solubility. The initial clot, held together only by weak noncovalent forces, is soluble in mild denaturing agents; a clot crosslinked by factor XIIIa is not. The solubility of a clot in a solution of a mild denaturant (urea or monochromatic acid) is used therefore to measure factor XIII (Giddings, 1980).

Platelet Tests

See Chapter 2 for methods to determine platelet counts, and Chapter 17 for comments on qualitative evaluation of platelets.

REFERENCES

(Titles in parentheses are English translations of foreign language titles.)

Abildgaard, U.: A Review of Antithrombin III. *In* Physiological Inhibitors of Coagulation and Fibrinolysis. Cullen, D. et al., eds. Elsevier North Holland, Biomedical Press, p. 63, 1979.

Abildgaard, C.F., and Link, R.P.: Blood Coagulation and Hemostasis in Thoroughbred Horses. Proc. Soc. Exp. Biol. Med., *119*:212, 1965.

Albrechtsson, U., et al.: Streptokinase Treatment of Dogs: Venous Thrombosis and Postthrombotic Syndrome. Arch. Surg., *116*:33, 1981.

Alkjaersig, N., et al.: ε-amino Caproic Acid, an Inhibitor of Plasminogen Activation. J. Biol. Chem., *234*:832, 1959.

Allington, M.J.: Fibrinogen and Fibrin Degradation Products and the Clumping of Staphylococci by Serum. Brit. J. Haematol., *13*:550, 1967.

Archer, R.K.: True Hemophilia (Hemophilia A) in a Thoroughbred Foal. Vet. Rec., *73*:338, 1961.

Aronson, D.L., et al.: A Quantitative Two-stage, Assay for Factor IX (Christmas Factor) using Plasma from Dogs with Christmas Disease. Thromb. Haemost., *27*:529, 1972.

Aufderheide, M., et al.: Clearance of Cryoprecipitated Factor VIII in Canine Hemophilia. A. Amer. J. Vet. Res., *36*:367, 1975.

Babior, B.M., and Stossel, T.P.: Hematology: A Pathophysiological Approach. Churchill Livingstone, New York, p. 171, 1984.

Bajaj, S.P., and Castellino, F.J.: Activation of Human Plasminogen by Equimolar Levels of Streptokinase. J. Biol. Chem., *252*:492, 1977.

Bajaj, S.P., et al.: Isolation and Characterization of Human Factor VII. J. Biol. Chem., *256*:253, 1981.

Bell, W.R., and Meek, A.G.: Guidelines for the Use of Thrombolytic Agents. New Eng. J. Med., *301*:1266, 1979.

Bennett, B.: Coagulation Pathways: Interrelationships and Control Mechanisms. Semin. Hematol., *14*:301, 1977.

Bennett, B., and Ratnoff, O.D.: Studies on the Response of Patients with Classic Hemophilia to Transfusion with Concentrates of an Antihemophilic Factor. A Difference in the Half-life of Antihemophilic Factor as Measured by Procoagulant and Immunologic Techniques. J. Clin. Invest., *51*:2593, 1972.

Benson, R.E., et al.: Efficiency and Precision of Electroimmunoassay for Canine Factor VIII-related Antigen. Amer. J. Vet. Res., *44*:399, 1983.

Bloom, A.L.: The von Willebrand Syndrome. Semin. Hematol., *17*:215, 1980.

Bouma, B.N., et al.: Infusion of Human and Canine Factor VIII in Dogs with von Willebrand's Disease: Studies of the von Willebrand and Factor VIII Synthesis Stimulating Factor. Scand. J. Haematol., *17*:263, 1976.

Bowie, E.J.W., et al.: Von Willebrand's Disease: A Critical Review. Hematol. Revs., *1*:1, 1968.

Bowie, E.J.W., et al.: Tests of Hemostasis in Swine: Normal Values and Values in Pigs Affected with von Willebrand's Disease. Amer. J. Vet. Res., *34*:1405, 1973.

Breukink, H.J., et al.: Congenital Afibrinogenemia in Goats. Zentralbl. Veterinaermed. A., *19*:661, 1972.

Brinkhous, K.M., et al.: Expression and Linkage of Genes for X-linked Hemophilias A and B in the Dog. Blood, *41*:577, 1973.

Buckner, R.G., and Hampton, J.W.: Canine Hemophilia. Blood, *27*:414, 1966.

Buntain, B.: Disseminated Intravascular Coagulopathy (DIC) in a Cow with Left Displaced Abomasum, Metritis, and Mastitis. Vet. Med. Small Anim. Clin., *75*:1023, 1980.

Burns, M.G., et al.: Pulmonary Artery Thrombosis in Three Dogs with Hyperadrenocorticism. J. Amer. Vet. Med. Ass., *178*:388, 1981.

Byars, T.D., et al.: Activated Coagulation Time (ACT) of Whole Blood in Normal Dogs. Amer. J. Vet. Res., *37*:1359, 1976.

Cade, J.F., and Robinson, T.F.: Coagulation and Fibrinolysis in the Dog. Can J. Comp. Med., *39*:296, 1975.

Capel-Edwards, K., and Hall, D.E.: Factor VII Deficiency in the Beagle Dog. Lab. Anim., *2*:105, 1968.

Christensen, L.R.: Streptococcal Fibrinolysis: A Proteolytic Reaction Due to a Serum Enzyme Activated by Streptococcal Fibrinolysin. J. Gen. Physiol., *28*:363, 1945.

Clifton, E.E., and Downie, G.R.: Variations in Proteolytic Activity of Serum of Animals Including Man. Proc. Soc. Exp. Biol. Med., *73*:559, 1950.

Cochrane, L.G., and Griffith, J.H.: Molecular Assembly in the Contact Phase of the Hageman Factor System. Amer. J. Med., *67*:657, 1979.

Collen, D.: On the Regulation and Control of Fibrinolysis. Thromb. Haemost., *43*:77, 1980.

Colman, R.W., et al.: Hemostasis and Thrombosis. J.B. Lippincott, Philadelphia, 1982.

Cornell, C.N., and Muhrer, M.E.: Coagulation Factors in Normal and Hemophiliac-type Swine. Amer. J. Physiol., *206*:926, 1964.

Cornell, C.N., et al.: Platelet Adhesiveness in Normal and Bleeder Swine as Measured in a Celite System. Amer. J. Physiol., *216*:1170, 1969.

Cotter, S.M., et al.: Hemophilia A in Three Unrelated Cats. J. Amer. Vet. Med. Ass., *172*:166, 1978.

Culbertson, R., Jr., et al.: Ontogeny of Bovine Hemostasis. Amer. J. Vet. Res., *40*:1402, 1979.

Dalgliesh, R.J., et al.: *Babesia argentina*: Disseminated Intravascular Coagulation in Acute Infection in Splenectomized Calves. Exp. Parasitol., *40*:124, 1976.

Davie, E.W., et al.: The Role of Serine Proteases in the Blood Coagulation Cascade. Adv. Enzymol., *48*:277, 1979.

DeGaetano, G.: Platelets, Prostaglandins and Thrombotic Disorders. *In* Clinics in Haematology. Prentice, C.R.M., ed. W.B. Saunders, Philadelphia, p. 297, 1981.

Deykin, D.: The Clinical Challenge of Disseminated Intravascular Coagulation. New Eng. J. Med., *283*:686, 1979.

Deykin, D., and Moake, K.: Acquired Platelet Function Disorders. Supplement to 1983 Amer. Soc. Hematol. Ann. Meeting, p. 37, 1983.

Didisheim, P., et al.: Hematologic and Coagulation Studies in Various Animal Species. J. Lab. Clin. Med.., *53*:866, 1959.

Dodds, W.J.: Canine von Willebrand's Disease. J. Lab. Clin. Med., *76*:713, 1970.

Dodds, W.J.: Hereditary and Acquired Hemorrhagic Disorders in Animals. *In* Progress in Hemostasis and Thrombosis. Vol. 2. Spaet, T.H., ed. Grune and Stratton, New York, pp. 215–247, 1974.

Dodds, W.J.: Further Studies on Canine von Willebrand's Disease. Blood, *45*:221, 1975.

Dodds, W.J.: Von Willebrand's Disease. Comp. Pathol. Bull., *9*:2, 1977a.

Dodds, W.J.: The Diagnosis, Management and Treatment of Bleeding Disorders. Mod. Vet. Pract., *58*:680, 756, 1977b.

Dodds, W.J.: First International Registry of Animal Models of Thrombosis and Hemorrhagic Diseases. Institute of Laboratory Animal Research News, *21*(1):A1–A23, 1977c.

Dodds, W.J.: Bleeding Disorders: Their Importance in Everyday Practice. Proc. Amer. Anim. Hosp. Ass., 44th Ann. Meet., pp. 147–154, 1977d.

Dodds, W.J.: Hemostasis and Coagulation. *In* Clinical Biochemistry of Domestic Animals. 3rd ed. Kaneko, J.J., ed. Academic Press, New York, p. 671, 1980.

Dodds, W.J.: Von Willebrand's Disease in Dogs. Mod. Vet. Pract., *65*:681, 1984.

Dodds, W.J., and Kull, J.E.: Canine Factor XI (Plasma Thromboplastin Antecedent) Deficiency. J. Lab. Clin. Med., *78*:746, 1971.

Doolittle, R.F.: Structural Aspects of the Fibrinogen to Fibrin Conversion. Adv. Protein Chem., *27*:1, 1973.

Engen, M.H., et al.: Fibrinolysis in a Dog with Diaphragmatic Hernia. J. Amer. Vet. Med. Ass., *164*:153, 1974.

Ewe, K.: Bleeding After Liver Biopsy Does Not Correlate with Indices of Peripheral Coagulation. Dig. Dis. Sci., *26*:388, 1981.

Fass, D.N., et al.: Inheritance of Porcine von Willebrand's Disease: Study of a Kindred of over 700 Pigs. Blood, *53*:712, 1979.

Fearnley, G.R.: Fibrinolysis. *In* Recent Advances in Blood Coagulation. Poller, L., ed. Little Brown, Boston, p. 229, 1969.

Feinstein, D.I.: Diagnosis and Management of Disseminated Intravascular Coagulation: The Role of Heparin Therapy. Blood, *60*:284, 1982.

Feinstein, D., et al.: Hemophilia A: Polymorphism Detectable by a Factor VIII Antibody. Science, *163*:1071, 1969.

Feldman, B.F.: Disseminated Intravascular Coagulation. Comp. Cont. Educ., *3*:46, 1981a.

Feldman, B.F.: Coagulopathies in Small Animals. J. Amer. Vet. Med. Ass., *179*:559, 1981b.

Feldman, B.F., and Giacopuzzi, R.L.: Hemophilia A (Factor VIII Deficiency) in a Colt. Equine Pract., *4*:24, 1982.

Feldman, B.F., and Thomson, D.B.: Fibronectin; Its Diagnostic and Therapeutic Implications. J. Amer. Anim. Hosp. Ass., *19*:1027, 1983.

Feldman, B.F., et al.: Disseminated Intravascular Coagulation: Antithrombin, Plasminogen, and Coagulation Abnormalities in 41 Dogs. Amer. J. Vet. Res., *179*:151, 1981.

Feldman, B.F., et al.: Hemorrhage in a Cat Caused by Inhibition of Factor XI (Plasma Thromboplastin Antecedent). J. Amer. Vet. Med. Ass., *182*:589, 1983.

Fernlund, P., and Stenflo, J.: Vitamin K and the Biosynthesis of Prothrombin. J. Biol. Chem., *250*:6125, 1975.

Fischbach, D.P., and Fogdall, R.P.: Coagulation. The Essentials. Williams & Wilkins, Baltimore, pp. 2–8, 1981.

Francis, C.W., et al.: Plasmic Degradation of Crosslinked Fibrin: Characterization of New Macromolecular

Complexes and a Model of Their Structure. J. Clin. Invest., 66:1033, 1980.

Gajewski, J., and Povar, M.L.: Blood Coagulation Values of Sheep. Amer. J. Vet. Res., 32:405, 1971.

Gallop, P.M., et al.: Carboxylated Calcium-binding Proteins and Vitamin K. New Eng. J. Med., 302:1460, 1980.

Garner, R., et al.: Factor VII Deficiency in Beagle Dog Plasma and Its Use in the Assay of Human Factor VII. Nature, 216:1130, 1967.

Gentry, P.A.: Interaction of Heparin with Canine Coagulation Proteins: In Vivo and In Vitro Studies. Can. J. Comp. Med., 41:396, 1977.

Gentry, P.A., et al.: Factor XI (Plasma Thromboplastin Antecedent) Deficiency in Cattle. Can. Vet. J., 16:160, 1975.

Gentry, P.A., et al.: Comparative Study of Blood Coagulation Test in the Horse and Pony. Amer. J. Vet. Res., 39:333, 1978.

Giddings, J.: The Investigation of Hereditary Coagulation Disorders. In Blood Coagulation and Haemostasis: A Practical Guide. 2nd ed. Thomson, J.M., ed. Churchill Livingstone, New York, p. 56, 1980.

Green, R.A.: Activated Coagulation Time in Monitoring Heparinized Dogs. Amer. J. Vet. Res., 41:1793, 1980.

Green, R.A.: Hemostasis and Disorders of Coagulation. Vet. Clin. North Amer. (Small Anim. Pract.), 11:289, 1981.

Green, R.A.: Clinical Implications of Antithrombin Deficiency. Comp. Cont. Educ., 6:537, 1984.

Green, R.A., and Kabel, A.L.: Hypercoagulable State in Three Dogs with Nephrotic Syndrome: Role of Acquired Antithrombin III Deficiency. J. Amer. Vet. Med. Ass., 181:914, 1982.

Green, R.A., and White, F.: Feline Factor XII (Hageman) Deficiency. Amer. J. Vet. Res., 38:893, 1977.

Green, R.A., et al.: Laboratory Evaluation of Coagulopathies due to Vitamin K Antagonism in the Dog: Three Case Reports. J. Amer. Anim. Hosp. Ass., 15:691, 1979.

Greene, C.E.: Disseminated Intravascular Coagulation in the Dog. A Review. J. Amer. Anim. Hosp. Ass., 11:674, 1975.

Greene, C.E., and Meriwether, E.: Activated Partial Thromboplastin Time and Activated Coagulation time in Monitoring Heparinized Cats. Amer. J. Vet. Res., 43:1437, 1982.

Greene, C.E., et al.: Disseminated Intravascular Coagulation Complicating Aflatoxicosis. Cornell Vet., 67:29, 1977.

Hall, D.E.: Blood Coagulation and Its Disorders in the Dog. Bailliere Tindall, Eastbourne, England, p. 188, 1972.

Hardaway, R.M.: Disseminated Intravascular Syndrome. Arch. Surg., 83:842, 1961.

Hardaway, R.M., III, et al.: Pathological Study of Intravascular Coagulation Following Incompatible Blood Transfusion in Dogs. Am. J. Surg., 91:24, 1956.

Hattersley, P.G.: Activated Coagulation Time of Whole Blood. JAMA, 196:436, 1966.

Hattersley, P.G.: Progress Report: The Activated Coagulation Time of Whole Blood (ACT). Amer. J. Clin. Path., 66:899, 1976.

Hawkey, C.M.: Comparative Mammalian Haematology. Whitefriars Press Ltd., London, 1975.

Heimark, R.L., et al.: Surface Activation of Blood Coagulation, Fibrinolysis and Kinin Formation. Nature, 286:456, 1980.

Hirsh, J.: Hypercoagulability. Semin. Hematol., 14:409, 1977.

Hirsh, J.: Blood Tests for the Diagnosis of Venous and Arterial Thrombosis. Blood, 57:1, 1981.

Hirsh, J., and Brain, E.A.: Hemostasis and Thrombosis. A Conceptual Approach. 2nd ed. Churchill Livingstone, New york, pp. 3–5, 1983.

Hogan, A.G.: A Hemophilia-like Disease in Swine. Proc. Soc. Exp. Biol. Med., 48:217, 1941.

Hougie, C.: Recalcification Time Test and Its Modifications (Partial Thromboplastin Time, Activated Partial Thromboplastin Time and Expanded Partial Thromboplastin Time). In Hematology. Willimas, W., et al., eds. McGraw-Hill, New York, p. 1400, 1972a.

Hougie, C.: The One Stage Prothrombin Time. In Hematology. Williams, W., et al., eds. McGraw-Hill, New York, p. 1403, 1972b.

Hoyer, L.W.: Immunologic Studies of Antihemophilic Factor (AHF, Factor VIII). IV. Radioimmuno Assay of AHF Antigen. J. Lab. Clin. Med., 80:822, 1972.

Hoyer, L.W.: von Willebrand's Disease. In Progress in Hemostasis and Thrombosis. Spaet, T.J., ed. Grune and Stratton, New York, p. 231, 1976.

Hoyer, L.W.: The Factor VIII Complex: Structure and Function. Blood, 58:1, 1981.

Hutchins, D.R., et al.: A Case of Equine Hemophilia. Aust. Vet. J., 43:83, 1967.

Irfan, M.: Fibrinolytic Activity in Animals of Different Species. Q. J. Exp. Physiol., 53:374, 1968.

Ivy, A.C., et al.: Bleeding Time as a Diagnostic Test. Surg. Gynecol. Obstet., 60:781, 1935.

Jaffe, E.A.: Endothelial Cells and the Biology of Factor VIII. New Eng. J. Med., 296:377, 1977.

Jaffe, E.A., et al.: Synthesis of Antihemophilic Factor Antigen by Cultured Human Endothelial Cells. J. Clin. Invest., 52:2757, 1973.

Jim, R.T.S.: Thrombin Time Test. J. Lab. Clin. Med., 50:45, 1957.

Johnson, G.S., et al.: A Bleeding Disease (von Willebrand's Disease) in a Chesapeake Bay Retriever. J. Amer. Vet. Med. Ass., 176:1261, 1980.

Johnstone, I.B., and Crane, S.: Determination of Canine Factor VIII-related Antigen Using Commercial Antihuman F VIII Serum. Vet. Clin. Path., 9(1):31, 1980.

Johnstone, I.B.: The Activated Partial Thromboplastin Time of Diluted Plasma (of Dog): Variability Due to the Method of Fibrin Detection. Can. J. Comp. Med., 48:198, 1984.

Jones, B.: [Diagnosis of Disorders of Haemostasis (Dog and Horse)]. Svensk Veterinärtiding, 31:423, 1979; Vet. Bull., Vol. 50, Ab #1009, 1980.

Kammermann, B., et al.: Afibrinogenamie beim Hund. Zentralbl. Veterinärmed. A., 18:192, 1971.

Kaplan, A.P., et al.: The Hageman Factor Dependent Pathways of Coagulation, Fibrinolysis and Kinin-Generation. Semin. Thromb. Hemostasis., 3:1, 1976.

Kasper, C.K.: Managment of Inhibitors of Factor VIII. Prog. Hematol., 12:143, 1981.

Kernoff, P.B.A., et al.: Transfusion and Gel Filtration Studies in von Willebrand's Disease. Brit. J. Haematol., 28:357, 1974.

Kier, A.B., et al.: The Inheritance Pattern of Factor XII (Hageman) Deficiency in Domestic Cats. Can. J. Comp. Med., 44:309, 1980.

Kociba, G.J.: Spontaneous Disseminated Intravascular Coagulation in Animals. In Animal Models of Thrombosis and Hemorrhagic Disorders, DHEW Pub No. 76–982, pp. 44–48, 1976. Nat'l. Inst. Health, U.S. Public Health Service, Washington, D.C.

Kociba, G.J., et al.: Bovine Plasma Thromboplastin Antecedent (Factor XI) Deficiency. J. Lab. Clin. Med., 74:37, 1969.

Kucinski, C.S., et al.: The Effect of Urokinase Antiserum on Plasminogen Activators. Demonstration of Immunologic Dissimilarity between Plasma Plasminogen Activation and Urokinase. J. Clin. Invest., 47:1238, 1968.

Lane, D.A.: Fibrinogen Derivatives in Plasma. Brit. J. Haematol., 47:329, 1981.

Lechner, K., et al.: Coagulation Abnormalities in Liver Disease. Semin. Thromb. Hemostas., 4:40, 1977.

Lewis, J.H.: Comparative Hematology Studies on Goats. Amer. J. Vet. Res., 37:601, 1976.

Lijnen, H.R., and Cullen, D.: Interaction of Plasminogen Activators and Inhibitors with Plasminogen and Fibrin. Semin. Thromb. Hemostas., 8:2, 1982.

Lindblad, G., and Bäckgren, A.W.: Megakaryocytes, Thrombocytes and Blood Clotting Times in Dogs with Experimental Hepatitis Contagiosa Canis. Acta Vet. Scand., 5:370, 1964.

Lopocink, S., et al.: Comparative Studies on Blood Coagulation Factor XIII. Proc. Soc. Exp. Biol. Med., 158:68, 1978.

Madewell, B.R., et al.: Coagulation Abnormalities in Dogs with Neoplastic Disease. Thromb. Haemost., 44:35, 1980.

Mammen, E.F.: Congenital Coagulation Disorders. Semin. Thromb. Hemostas., 9:1, 1983.

Marder, V.J.: Molecular Bad Actors and Thrombosis. New Eng. J. Med., 310:588, 1984.

Masotti, G., et al.: Differential Inhibition of Prostacyclin Production and Platelet Aggregation by Aspirin. Lancet, 2:1213, 1979.

McKay, D.G., et al.: Alterations in Blood Coagulation Mechanism after Incompatible Blood Transfusion. Am. J. Surg., 89:583, 1955.

McKay, D.G.: Pathologic Study of Intravascular Coagulation Following Incompatible Blood Transfusion in Dogs. II. Intra-aortic Injection of Incompatible Blood. Am. J. Surg., 91:32, 1956.

McKee, P.A., et al.: Subunit Structure of Human Fibrinogen, Soluble Fibrin, and Cross-linked Insoluble Fibrin. Proc. Natl. Acad. Sci. USA, 66:733, 1970.

Meade, T.W., et al.: Characteristics Affecting Fibrinolytic Activity and Plasma Fibrinogen Concentrations. Brit. Med. J., 1:153, 1979.

Mertens, B.F., et al.: Rapid Sensitive Method for Measuring Fibrinogen-Split Products in Human Serum. Mayo Clinic Proc., 44:114, 1969.

Middleton, D.J., and Watson, A.D.J.: Activated Coagulation Times of Whole Blood in Normal Dogs and Dogs with Coagulopathies. J. Small Anim. Pract., 19:417, 1978.

Mielke, C.H., et al.: Template Bleeding Time. Blood, 34:204, 1969.

Migaki, G., and Casey, H.W.: Conditions Associated with Thrombosis in Animals . *In* Animal Models of Thrombosis and Hemorrhagic Diseases. DHEW Publication No. (NIH) 76-982, pp. 55–65, 1975.

Moake, J.L., et al.: Unususally Large Factor VIII: von Willebrand Factor Multimers and Chronic Relapsing Thrombotic Thrombocytopenic Purpura. New Eng. J. Med., 307:1432, 1982.

Moake, J.L., and Funicella, T.: Common Bleeding Problems. Ciba Found. Symp., 35(3):2, 1983.

Mosesson, M.W.: Fibrinogen Catabolic Pathways. Semin. Thromb. Hemostas., 1:63, 1974.

Mount, M.E., and Feldman, B.F.: Mechanism of Dipha-cinone Rodenticide Toxicosis in the Dog and Its Therapeutic Implication. Amer. J. Vet. Res., 44:2009, 1983.

Mount, M.E., et al.: Vitamin K and Its Therapeutic Importance. J. Amer. Vet. Med. Ass., 180:1354, 1982.

Muhrer, M..E., et al.: Antihemophilic Factor Levels in Bleeder Swine following Infusions of Plasma and Serum. Amer. J. Physiol., 208:508, 1965.

Mustard, J.F., et al.: Canine Hemophilia B (Christmas Disease). Brit. J. Haematol., 6:259, 1960.

Mustard, J.F., et al.: A Comparison of the Effect of Serum and Plasma Transfusion on the Clotting Defect in Canine Haemophilia B. Brit. J. Haematol., 8:36, 1962a.

Mustard, J.F., et al.: Canine Factor-VII Deficiency. Brit. J. Haematol., 8:43, 1962b.

Nachman, R.L.: Von Willebrand's Disease, A Clinical and Molecular Enigma. West. J. Med., 136:318, 1982.

Nemerson, Y., and Nossel, H.L.: The Biology of Thrombosis. Annu. Rev. Med., 33:479, 1982.

Niewiarowski, S., and Latollo, Z.: Comparative Studies of the Fibrinolytic System of Sera of Various Vertebrates. Thromb. Haemost., 3:404, 1959.

Nockels, C.F., et al.: Factors Affecting Blood Clotting in Immature Sheep and Cattle. Brit. Vet. J., 134:286, 1978.

Nossel, H.L., et al.: Equine Hemophilia. Report of a Case and Its Response to Multiple Infusions of Heterospecific AHG. Brit. J. Haematol., 8:335, 1962.

O'Rourke, L., et al.: Coagulation, Fibrinolysis and Kinin Generatiion in Adult Cats. Amer. J. Vet. Res., 43:1478, 1982.

Ødegård, A.R., and Abildgaard, U.: Antithrombin III: Critical Review of Assay Methods: Significance of Variations in Health and Disease. Haemostasis, 7:127, 1978.

Ogston, D., and Bennett, B.: Haemostasis, Biochemistry, Physiology, Pathology. Wiley, New York, 202 p., 1977.

Okin, R., and Dodds, W.J.: Canine Hemophilia A and B. Canine Pract., 7(3):61, 1980.

Owen, C.A., Jr., and Bowie, E.J.: Chronic Intravascular Coagulation and Fibrinolysis (ICF) Syndrome (DIC). Semin. Thromb. Hemostas., 3:268, 1977.

Owen, C.A., Jr., et al.: Turnover of Fibrinogen and Platelets in Dogs Undergoing Induced Intravascular Coagulation. Thromb. Res., 2:251, 1973.

Owen, C.A., Jr., et al.: Generation of Factor VIII Coagulant Activity by Isolated, Perfused Neonatal Pig Livers and Adult Rat Livers. Brit. J. Haematol., 43:307, 1979.

Peterson, M.E., and Dodds, W.J.: Factor IX Deficiency in an Alaskan Malamute. J. Amer. Vet. Med. Ass., 74:1326, 1979.

Poller, L., et al.: Identification of a Congenital Defect of Factor VII in a Colony of Beagle Dogs. The Clinical Uses of the Plasma. J. Clin. Pathol., 24:636, 1971.

Prydz, H.: Biosynthesis of the Factors of the Prothrombin Complex. Thromb. Haemost., Suppl., 59:61, 1974.

Prydz, H.: Vitamin K-dependent Clotting Factors. Semin. Thromb. Hemostas., 4:1, 1977.

Rabiner, S.F., and Friedman, L.N.: The Role of Intravascular Hemolysis and the Reticuloendothelial System in the Production of a Hypercoagulable State. Brit. J. Haematol., 14:105, 1968.

Rawlings, C.A., et al.: Activated Coagulation Test in Normal and Heparinized Ponies and Horses. Amer. J. Vet. Res., 36:711, 1975.

Raymond, S.L., and Dodds, W.J.: Plasma Antithrombin Activity: A Comparative Study in Normal and Diseased Animals. Proc. Soc. Exp. Biol. Med., *161*:464, 1979.

Rebar, A.H., and Boon, G.D.: A Diagnostic Approach to Bleeding Disorders in the Dog. Proc. Amer. Anim. Hosp. Ass., 47th Annual Meeting, pp. 125–129, 1980.

Riddle, J.M., and Barnhart, M.I.: The Eosinophil as a Source of Profibrinolysin in Acute Inflammation. Blood, *25*:776, 1965.

Riley, J.H., and Lassen, E.D.: Activated Coagulation Times of Normal Cows. Vet. Clin. Path., *VIII*:31, 1979.

Rowsell, H.C., and Mustard, J.F.: Blood Coagulation in Some Common Laboratory Animals. Lab. Anim. Care, *13*:752, 1963.

Rowsell, H.C., et al.: A Disorder Resembling Hemophilia B (Christmas Disease) in Dogs. J. Amer. Vet. Med. Ass., *137*:247, 1960.

Ruddy, S., et al.: The Complement System of Man (First of Four Parts). New Eng. J. Med., *287*:489, 1972.

Ruehl, W., et al.: Rational Therapy in Disseminated Intravascular Coagulation. J. Amer. Vet. Med. Ass., *181*:76, 1982.

Ruggeri, Z.M., and Zimmerman, T.S.: Variant von Willebrand's Disease and Characterization of Two Subtypes by Analysis of Multimeric Composition of Factor VIII/von Willebrand Factor in Plasma and Platelets. J. Clin. Invest., *65*:1318, 1980.

Ruggeri, Z.M., et al.: Multimeric Composition of Factor VIII/von Willebrand Factor following Administration of DDAVP: Implications for Pathophysiology and Therapy of von Willebrand's Disease Subtypes. Blood, *59*:1272, 1982.

Sanger, V.L., et al.: Hemophilia in a Foal. J. Amer. Vet. Med. Ass., *144*:259, 1964.

Schalm, O.W.: Disseminated Intravascular Coagulation (DIC) in the Dog. Canine Pract., *7*:52, 1980.

Schalm, O.W., et al.:Veterinary Hematology. 3rd Ed. Lea & Febiger, Philadelphia, p. 297, 1975.

Schiefer, B., and Searcy, G.: Disseminated Intravascular Coagulation and Consumption Coagulopathy. Can. Vet. J., *16*:151, 1975.

Schlink, G.T., and Johnson, G.S.: A Sensitive Autoradiographic Procedure for Factor VIII-Related Antigen in Canine Plasma. Vet. Clin. Path., *12(3)*:21, 1983.

Schrier, S.L.: Disorders of Hemostasis and Coagulation. *In* Scientific American Medicine. Rubinstein, E., and Federman, D.D., eds. Scientific American, New York, *VI*:1, 1984.

Scott, E.A., et al.: Warfarin: Effects of Intravenous Loading Doses and Vitamin K on Warfarin Anticoagulation in the Pony. Amer. J. Vet. Res., *39*:1888, 1978.

Scott, E.A., et al.: Warfarin: Effects of Anticoagulant, Hematologic, and Blood Enzyme Values in Normal Ponies. Amer. J. Vet. Res., *40*:142, 1979.

Seaman, A.J., and Malinow, M.P.: Blood Clotting in Nonhuman Primates. Lab. Anim. Care, *18*:80, 1968.

Seegers, W.H., and Ghosh, A.: Activation of Prothrombin and Factor X: Function of Previously Unrecognized Plasma Protein. Thromb. Res., *17*:71, 1980.

Shepard, V.J., et al.: Gamma A Myeloma in a Dog with Defective Hemostasis. J. Amer. Vet. Med. Ass., *160*:1121, 1972.

Sherding, R.G., and DiBartola, S.P.: Hemophilia B (Factor IX Deficiency) in an Old English Sheepdog. J. Amer. Vet. Med. Ass., *176*:141, 1980.

Sherry, S., et al.: The Enzymatic Dissolution of Experimental Arterial Thrombi in the Dog by Trypsin, Chymotrypsin, and Plasminogen Activators. J. Clin. Invest., *33*:1303, 1955.

Sjoberg, H.E., et al.: Thromboembolic Complications, Heparin Treatment and Increase in Coagulation Factors in Cushing's Syndrome. Acta Med. Scand., *199*:95, 1976.

Slappendel, R.J.: Hemophilia A and Hemophilia B. in a Family of French Bulldogs. Tijdschr. Diergeneeskd., *100*:1075, 1975.

Slappendel, R.J., et al.: Response to Heparin of Spontaneous Disseminated Intravascular Coagulation in the Dog. Zentralbl. Veterinaermed. A., *19*:502, 1972.

Spurling, N.W., et al.: Hereditary Factor VII Deficiency in the Beagle. Brit. J. Haematol., *23*:59, 1972.

Spurling, N.W., et al.: Canine Factor VIII Deficiency. Experience with a Modified Thrombotest Method in Distinguishing between the Genotype. Res. Vet. Sci., *16*:228, 1974.

Stampfer, M.J., et al.: Effect of Intravenous Streptokinase on Acute Myocardial Infarction. New Eng. J. Med., *307*:1189, 1982.

Statland, B.E., and Ito, R.K.: Thrombocyte Therapy: Minimizing the Risks. Diagn. Med., *7*:25, 1984.

Stenflo, J.: Viamin K, Prothrombin and γ-carboxyglutamic Acid. Adv. Enzymol., *46*:, 1978.

Stephens, K.A., et al.: Measurement of Plasma Antithrombin III Activity in Healthy Horses. Amer. J. Vet. Res., *45*:351, 1984.

Stites, D.P., et al.: Factor VIII Detection by Hemagglutination Inhibition: Hemophilia A and von Willebrand's Disease. Science, *171*:196, 1971.

Strombeck, D.R., et al.: Coagulopathy and Encephalopathy in a Dog with Acute Hepatic Necrosis. J. Amer. Vet. Med. Ass., *169*:813, 1976.

Suttie, J.W., and Jackson, C.M.: Prothrombin Structure, Activation and Biosynthesis. Physiol. Rev., *57*:1, 1977.

Thompson, A.R., and Harker, L.A.: Manual of Hemostasis and Thrombosis. 3rd ed. F.A. Davis, Philadelphia, 1983.

Troy, G.C.: Clinical Approach to Hemostatic Disorders. Vet. Med. Small Anim. Clin., *79*:917, 1984.

Verstraete, N.: Haemostatic Drugs, A Critical Appraisal. Martinus Nijhoff Medical Division, The Hague, 1977.

Vollmer, K.: Protamine Sulfate Test for Fibrin Monomers in Plasma. Dade "Monographs," p. 18, 1972.

Vollmer, K.: Coagulation Procedures. In "Monograph." Dade Division American Hospital Supply Corp., Miami, Florida, pp. 18–19, 1976.

Vrins, A., et al.: Warfarin. A Review with Emphasis on Its Use in the Horse. Can. Vet. J., *24*:211, 1983.

Weaver, R.A., et al.: Antihemophilic Factor in Crosscirculated Normal and Hemophilic Dogs. Amer. J. Physiol., *206*:335, 1964.

Webster, W.P., et al.: Plasma Factor VIII Synthesis and Control as Revealed by Canine Organ Transplantation. Amer. J. Physiol., *220*:1147, 1971.

Weiss, R.C., et al.: Disseminated Intravascular Coagulation in Experimentally Induced Feline Infectious Peritonitis. Amer. J. Vet. Res., *41*:663, 1980.

Weiss, E., et al.: Volume Distribution and Ultrastructure of Platelets in Acute Hog Cholera. Thromb. Haemost., *30*:371, 1973.

White, J.G., and Gerrard, J.M.: Anatomy and Structural Organization of the Platelet. *In* Hemostasis and Thrombosis. Colman, R.W., et al., eds. J.B. Lippincott, Philadelphia, Chap. 21, 1982.

Wigton, D.H., et al.: Infectious Canine Hepatitis: Animal Model for Viral-Induced Disseminated Intravascular Coagulation. Blood, *47*:287, 1976.

Williams, J.R.B.: Fibrinolytic Activity of Urine. Brit. J. Exp. Path., *32*:530, 1951.

Williams, W.J., et al.: Hematology. McGraw-Hill, New York, pp. 1408–1409, 1972.

Wintrobe, M.M., et al.: Clinical Hematology. 8th ed. Chapters 16, 17, 45, 50, 51, and 52. Lea & Febiger, Philadelphia, 1981.

Zimmerman, T.S., et al.: Blood Coagulation and the Inflammation Response. Semin. Hematol., *14*:391, 1977.

Zucker, M.B.: The Functioning of Blood Platelets. Sci. Amer., *242*:86, 1980.

15

Megakaryocytopoiesis and Platelet Production, Survival, and Distribution

CYTOMORPHOLOGIC CHARACTERISTICS OF MEGAKARYOCYTOPOIESIS 432
Normal Features 432
Some Pathologic Findings 433

ULTRASTRUCTURE AND CYTOCHEMISTRY OF MEGAKARYOCYTES 433

PLATELET PRODUCTION FROM MEGAKARYOCYTES 437

REGULATION OF MEGAKARYOCYTOPOIESIS AND THROMBOPOIESIS 437

Stimulatory Factors 439
Inhibitory Factors 440
Thrombocyte Production in Iron Deficiency 440

PLATELET KINETICS AND DISTRIBUTION 441
Platelet Life Span 441
Distribution and Removal of Platelets 441
Abnormalities of Platelet Life Span and Distribution 442

In this and the subsequent two chapters, information from recent research on megakaryocytopoiesis; platelet production and kinetics; platelet structure, metabolism, and functions; and qualitative and quantitative disorders of platelets will be presented along with some of our own observations. Recent reviews on megakaryocytopoiesis and thrombopoiesis may be consulted for additional information (McDonald, 1981; Tavassoli, 1980;. Williams and Levine, 1982).

The terms *platelet* and *thrombocyte* are used interchangeably, although originally the term *thrombocyte* was introduced by Deckyusen in 1901 to describe the nucleated cell of lower vertebrates, the counterpart of the nonnucleated mammalian platelet first described by Bizzozero in 1882. In contrast to mammalian platelets, which represent cytoplasmic fragments of megakaryocytes, thrombocytes in lower vertebrates originate from a successive division of precursor cells (thromboblasts) within marrow sinusoids. The term *megakaryocyte* was introduced by Howell in 1890, and Wright in 1906 described the origin of platelets from the megakaryocytes.

Isotope labeling and electron microscopic studies have advanced knowledge regarding the development and maturation of megakaryocytes. Experimental evidence (Ebbe, 1976, 1979; Odell, 1974) suggests the existence in bone marrow of a self-replicating pluripotent stem cell (PPSC), which gives rise to a functionally recognizable megakaryocytic progenitor cell called the colony forming unit megakaryocyte, or CFU-Meg (Fig. 13–19). Progenitors of megakaryocytes have also been found in the peripheral blood (Burstein, 1980). The CFU-Meg is capable of dividing in such a manner that some of the progenies differentiate to become megakaryocytic precursors and some remain to self-perpetuate. This differentiation involves successive development through several intermediate cellular stages. These cells cannot be identified morphologically with Romanowsky stains, although cytochemical staining for acetylcholinesterase can be used as a marker for murine megakaryocytic cells. Division and differentiation of the PPSC into the CFU-Meg is influenced by hematopoietic microenvironment (HIM), cell-cell interactions and/or short-range humoral factors, whereas the differentiation of the CFU-Meg into megakaryoblast is regulated by a specific colony stimulating factor (Meg-CSF), and development of

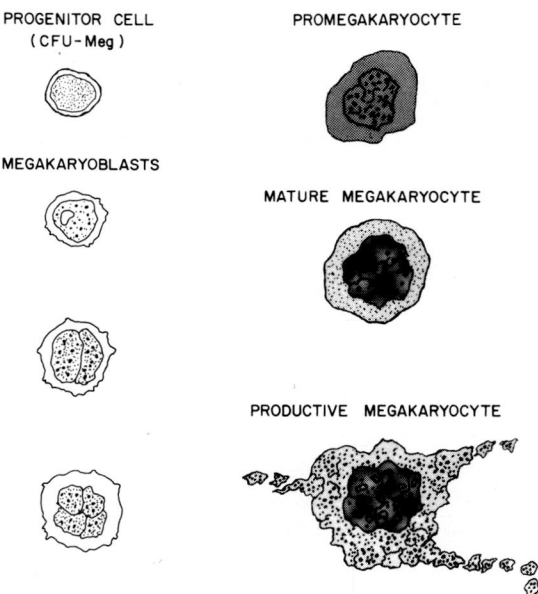

PROGENITOR CELL
(CFU-Meg)

MEGAKARYOBLASTS

PROMEGAKARYOCYTE

MATURE MEGAKARYOCYTE

PRODUCTIVE MEGAKARYOCYTE

Fig. 15–1. Megakaryocyte development and maturation. The megakaryocytic progenitor cell is a descendant of the pluripotential hematopoietic stem cell and an immediate precursor of the earliest morphologically recognizable cell of the series, the megakaryoblast. The megakaryoblast is initially a diploid cell with a single nucleus, but owing to endoreduplication (nuclear division without cytoplasmic division) it enlarges and becomes a polyploid cell with two to four nuclei. With progressive endoreduplication and maturation a megakaryoblast develops into a promegakaryocyte and then into a megakaryocyte. The nuclei of the promegakaryocyte and megakaryocyte appear multilobed rather than individually separated, and the cytoplasm of the latter cell shows prominent azurophilic granulation. Platelets are produced by cytoplasmic fragmentation of a mature productive megakaryocyte. (See also Fig. 15–5.)

megakaryocytes is influenced by thrombopoietin (Baldini and Ebbe, 1974; Williams and Levine, 1982). Development stages of a mature megakaryocyte leading to platelet production are shown in Figure 15–1. Megakaryocytopoiesis differs from erythropoiesis and granulocytopoiesis in that it involves polyploidization of the precursor cells owing to endoreduplication (nuclear division without cytoplasmic division).

CYTOMORPHOLOGIC CHARACTERISTICS OF MEGAKARYOCYTOPOIESIS

Normal Features

Megakaryocytes are the largest of the hematopoietic cells in the bone marrow. Their size

varies with the method of specimen preparation (Wickramasinghe, 1978; Levine et al., 1982). Megakaryocytes in a suspension of human bone marrow appear globular with a mean volume of about 4,700 ± 100 fl and a diameter of about 10 to 65 μm. In Wright-stained smears of marrow, cells of the megakaryocytic series measure more than 20 to about 160 μm in diameter, whereas in histologic sections of marrow fixed in Zenker's solution they appear much smaller (about 21 μm). Megakaryocytes in bone marrow specimens from various animal species also vary in size.

Megakaryocytic cells are generally classified into three types, stages, or groups according to their cytoplasmic and nuclear characteristics in Wright-stained marrow films. These are megakaryoblast, promegakaryocyte, and megakaryocyte, or, respectively, Stage I, II, and III cells, also called Group I, II, and III cells (Baldini and Ebbe, 1974; Bessis, 1973; Ebbe, 1979; Penington and Streatfield, 1975; Wickramasinghe, 1978; Wintrobe et al., 1981). Some have classified megakaryocytes as granular (Stage III) and mature or productive megakaryocytes (Stage IV) (Williams and Levine, 1982). *Megakaryoblast* is the most immature recognizable cell of the series. It has a highly basophilic, nongranular cytoplasm and a round nucleus with finely stippled chromatin and one or more nucleoli. The nucleus occupies most of the cell, giving a very high nucleus-to-cytoplasm ratio. Some megakaryoblasts have a few cytoplasmic vacuoles and small cytoplasmic twigs on the cell surface. The megakaryoblast does not undergo cell division and is, therefore, incapable of self-replication. Mitotic division of its nucleus without division of the cytoplasm (acytokinesis, endomitosis, or endoreduplication) leads to the production of a polyploid nucleus and an increase in cell size (Plate III–2). Repeated nuclear division produces cells having a polyploid DNA content of 4N, 8N, 16N, 32N, and sometimes 64N nuclear chromatin. Cells having two to four nuclei are also regarded as megakaryoblasts (Plates III–1, III–3).

Cells with more than four distinct nuclei are called *promegakaryocytes*. Cells with separate nuclei are extremely rare in normal marrow, but may be found when megakaryocytopoiesis is markedly stimulated in response to thrombocytopenia. More commonly, promegakaryocytes have a multilobed nucleus with indistinct separations, less basophilic cytoplasm, and a lower nucleus-to-cytoplasm ratio than megakaryoblasts (Plate III–4). Some promegakaryocytes may contain patches of fine azurophilic granules in the cytoplasm, particularly near the nucleus where granule formation begins. With maturation, the nucleus becomes more lobulated and the cytoplasm increases in amount, becomes less basophilic, and acquires increasing granularity. The *megakaryocyte* has a single multilobed nucleus, abundant pale-staining cytoplasm, and numerous small azurophilic granules (Plates III–4, III–5). An osteoclast, in contrast, has multiple separate nuclei and somewhat larger and fewer reddish purple cytoplasmic granules (Plate III–6).

Endoreduplication in megakaryoblasts and promegakaryocytes requires synthesis of DNA. Generally, endoreduplication precedes commencement of cytoplasmic maturation; both processes may occur simultaneously, however. Autoradiographic studies with tritiated thymidine (^{3}HTdR) have shown that DNA synthesis is largely restricted to the megakaryoblasts and promegakaryocytes (Wickramasinghe, 1978). DNA synthesis diminishes with increasing maturity and ceases at the 8N, 16N, or 32N stage, probably under the influence of a specific cytoplasmic regulator called thrombosthenin (Paulus, 1967). The predominant cell type is of the 8N ploidy (Levine et al., 1980). Cell size, nuclear volume, and cellular maturation are proportional to the DNA content of the nucleus (de Laval, 1968; Levine et al., 1982). Most of the low ploidy (4N–8N) megakaryocytes are immature, whereas those shedding platelets are of high ploidy (16N–32N). Thus, it is possible to observe mature megakaryocytes with differing cell size, nuclear mass, and cytoplasmic characteristics, depending on the degree of cytoplasmic maturation. Occasionally platelet-producing megakaryocytes are found to have pseudopod-like extensions of the cytoplasm (proplatelets) or individual platelets breaking away from the surface (Plate III–5). The entire process of megakaryocyte differ-

entiation and maturation takes about 6 days in humans, 3 days in dogs, and 2–3 days in rodents (Triplett, 1978; Wickramasinghe, 1978).

Some Pathologic Findings

Bleeding disorders due to intrinsic abnormalities of platelets may originate because of specific abnormalities in differentiation or proliferation of megakaryocytes and their precursors (Ebbe, 1979). Pathologic changes in megakaryocytes include changes in the proportion of various maturative stages, altered cell size, and nuclear and cytoplasmic abnormalities (Albrecht and Fulle, 1974; Bessis, 1973; Maldonado et al., 1975; Wickramasinghe, 1978). Increased ploidy and size of megakaryocytes accompany thrombocytosis, while decreased ploidy and cytoplasmic abnormalities may be seen in idiopathic thrombocytopenias. Degenerative morphologic changes such as cytoplasmic vacuolation and karyorrhexis may be seen in megakaryocytes in immune-mediated thrombocytopenia in dogs and humans (Fig. 15–2) (Joshi and Jain, 1977; McMillan et al., 1978). Reduced ploidy and micromegakaryocytes have been found in hematopoietic dysplasias. Megakaryoblasts are disproportionately increased in number in some cases of idiopathic thrombocytopenia, chronic lymphocytic leukemia, and myelometosis. Essential thrombocythemia is a neoplastic disorder of the hematopoietic stem cell.

Megakaryocytes exhibiting emperipolesis (transmigration) of neutrophils or other leukocytes may be seen as a nonspecific phenomenon under several unrelated circumstances (Parmley et al., 1982; Shamoto, 1981). We have seen such megakaryocytes in Wright-stained films of occasional bone marrow aspirates (Fig. 15–3).

ULTRASTRUCTURE AND CYTOCHEMISTRY OF MEGAKARYOCYTES

Megakaryocytopoiesis has been studied with the scanning (Aabo and Bendix-Hansen, 1982; Barnhart and Robinson, 1975; Djaldetti et al., 1979; Handagama et al., 1984; Ihzumi et al., 1977) and transmission (Behnke and

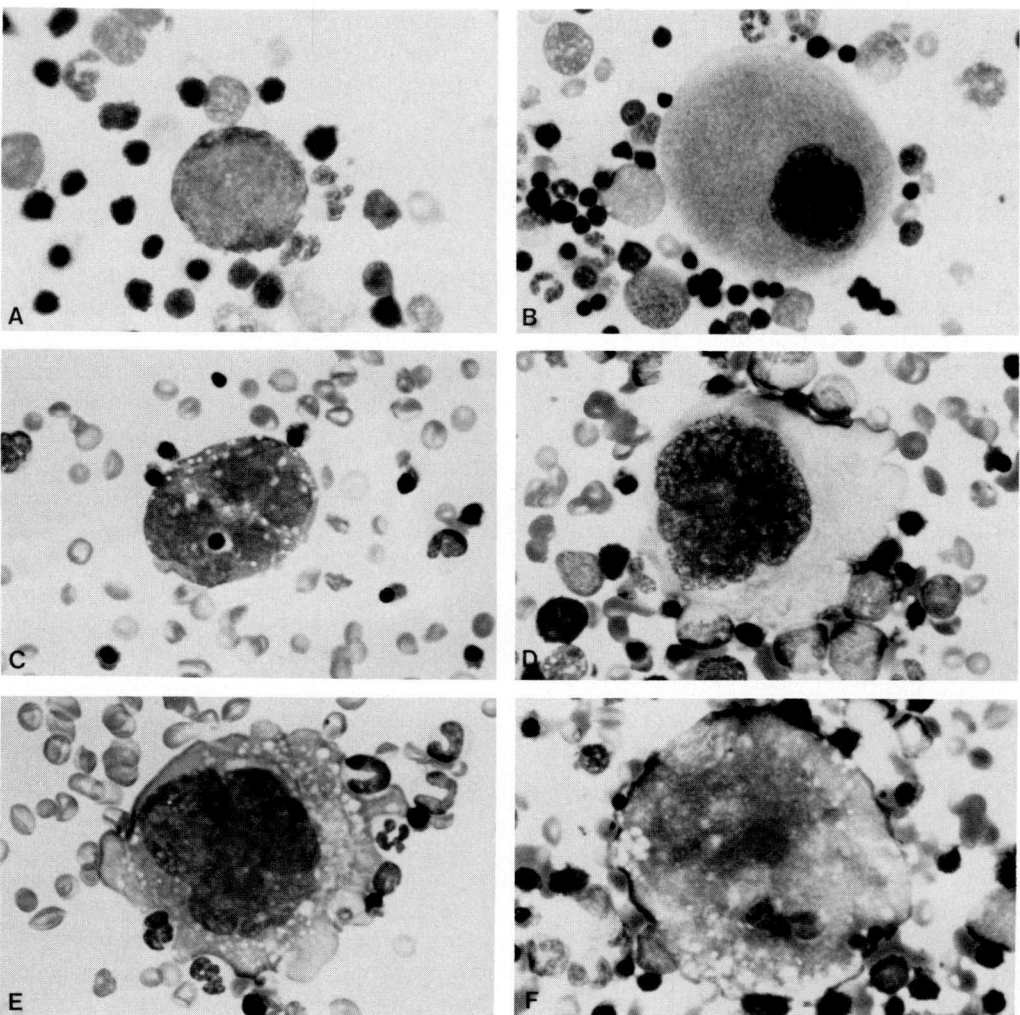

Fig. 15–2. Normal canine promegakaryocyte *(A)* and megakaryocyte *(B)* are compared with promegakaryocyte *(C)* and megakaryocytes *(D,E,F)* from dogs with autoimmune thrombocytopenia. Notice morphologic abnormalities such as karyolysis *(F)*, cytoplasmic vacuolation *(C,E,F)*, and deficiency in *(F)* or lack of *(D,E)* cytoplasmic granularity. Wright stain, ×700.

Pedersen, 1974; Kass et al., 1977; Penington and Streatfield, 1975; Wickramasinghe, 1978) electron microscopes, and cytochemical characteristics of megakaryocytes have been described (Bentfeld and Bainton, 1975; Kass et al., 1977). The megakaryocytes appear rather spherical and reveal varied surface morphology with the scanning electron microscope. Principal surface features include numerous ruffles and ridges, microprocesses of variable sizes and shape, and globular bud-like protuberances and scaly structures resembling platelets. Occasionally, several of these surface structures may be seen on the same cell. Some megakaryocytes may also have platelets

adhering to their surface. Internal structural details are visible with the transmission electron microscope (Figs. 15–4, 15–5).

The *megakaryoblast* contains a large round or indented nucleus with a small amount of condensed chromatin and several distinct nucleoli. The cytoplasm is relatively scanty and contains a prominent Golgi apparatus, many large mitochondria, a moderate number of polyribosomes and ribosomes, some segments of rough endoplasmic reticulum (RER), some strands of dense "demarcation membrane system," and a few alpha-granules.

Differentiation toward the *promegakaryocyte* is accompanied by increases in nuclear lob-

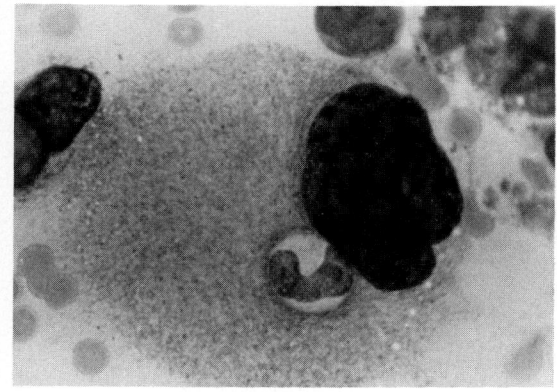

Fig. 15–3. Emperipolesis (transmigration) of a neutrophil metamyelocyte through the cytoplasm of a mature megakaryocyte. Wright-stained film of canine bone marrow.

ulation, cytoplasmic mass and contents, or activities of various organelles. The cytoplasm becomes packed with polyribosomes and ribosomes, the demarcation membrane system becomes more convoluted but less dense, and the granules and small mitochondria increase in number. Labeling with ^{35}S-sulfate has shown that formation of alpha-granules occurs in the Golgi apparatus, and the number of granules gradually increases from the vicinity of the nucleus toward the periphery of the cell (Behnke and Pedersen, 1974). Ultrastructural cytochemical studies demonstrated the presence of acid phosphatase–positive and aryl sulfatase–positive small vesicles (primary lysosomes) in immature and mature megakaryocytes from human and rat bone marrow (Bentfeld-Barker and Bainton, 1982). These lysosomes also originated from the Golgi complex, but were distinct from the alpha-granules. Formation of the demarcation membrane system begins near the cell membrane and extends through the cytoplasm toward the nucleus. It is formed by invagination of the megakaryocyte cell membrane (Tavassoli, 1980).

Maturation into a *megakaryocyte* (Figs. 15–4, 15–5) is characterized by a further increase in the cytoplasmic volume and progressive nuclear changes such as lobulation, chromatin condensation, and inactivity or disappearance of nucleoli. These changes are accompanied by development of an extensive demarcation membrane system with luminal openings to the cell surface, a decrease in the number of polyribosomes and large mitochondria, and an increase in small mitochondria, glycogen particles, and cytoplasmic granules. The ratio of granules to mitochondria gradually increases with ploidy stage and maturation. The external surface of the demarcation membrane system becomes coated with glycoprotein, which later constitutes the "exterior coat" of the platelets. Pseudopod formation and clearly defined platelet zones, wtih groups of granules separated by the demarcation membrane, may be seen in some larger and more mature megakaryocytes.

Additional ultrastructural and cytochemical features of megakaryocytes include the presence of: unpolymerized microtubule protein and scarce microtubules; thrombosthenin; primary lysosomes; aryl sulfatase and acid phosphatase in primary lysosomes, Golgi apparatus and RER; platelet antigens and pro-

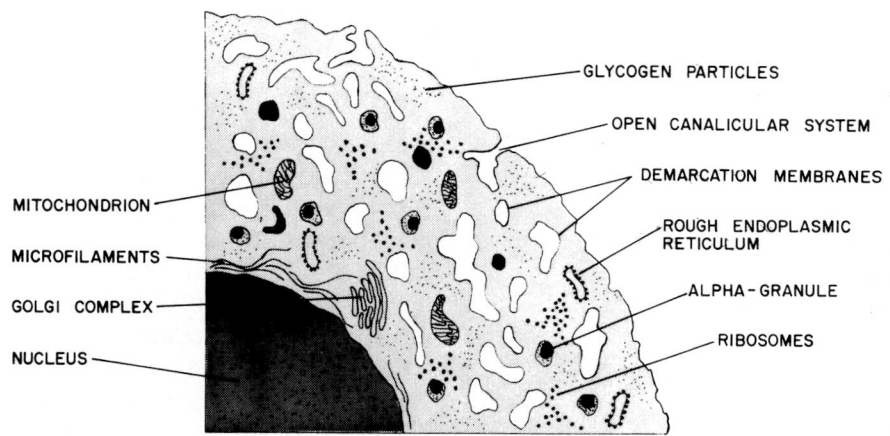

Fig. 15–4. A schematic drawing of morphologic features of a megakaryocyte. Only a portion is drawn.

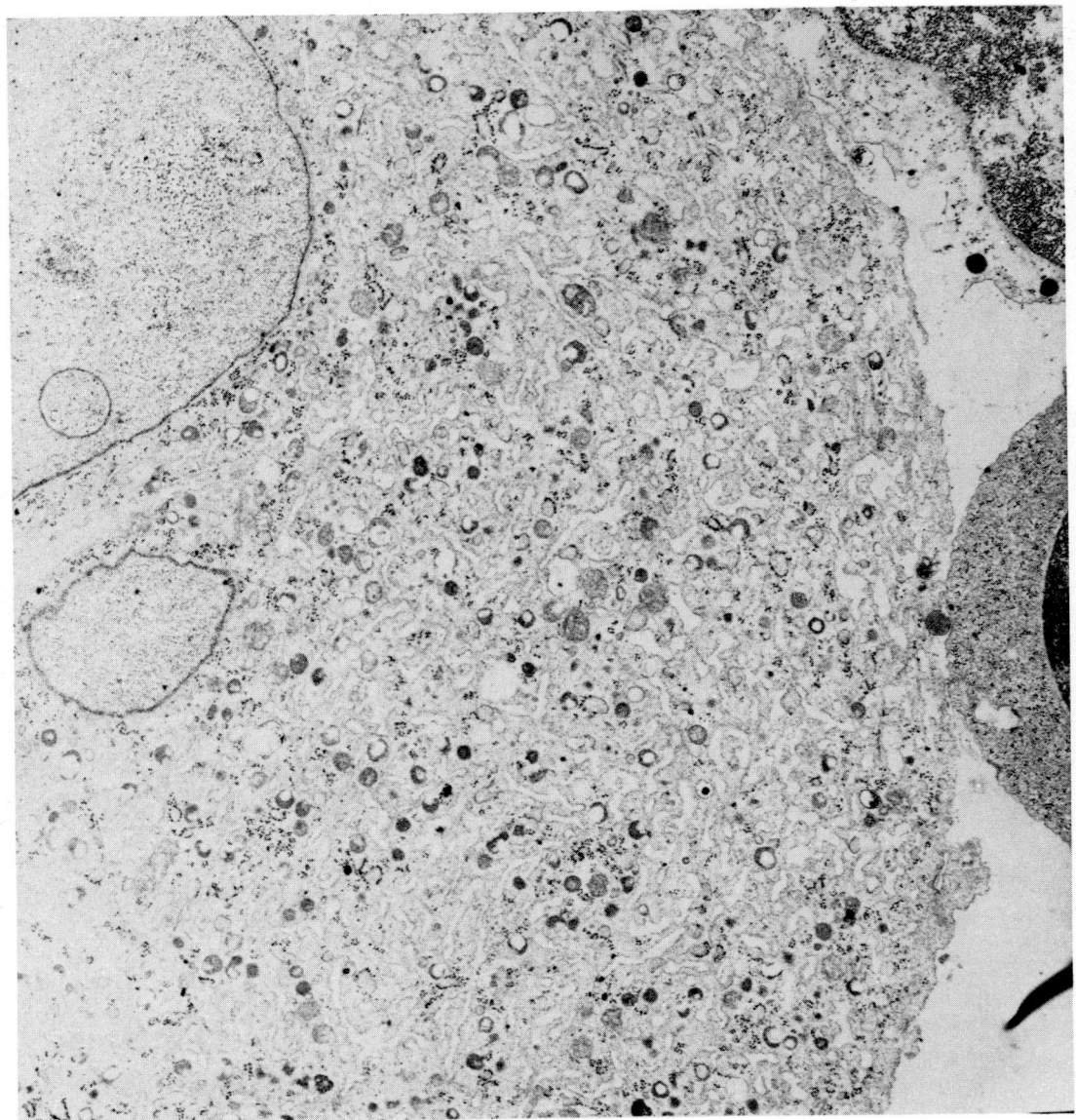

Fig. 15–5. A transmission electron photomicrograph of a portion of a canine megakaryocyte containing numerous granules, membranous tubules and vesicles, and ribosomes. Platelets are formed at the surface as a result of separation of cytoplasmic fragments by membranous channels. Parts of the nucleus are also seen at the upper left corner.

teins; antihemophilic factor; acetylcholinesterase in various membranous organelles of immature and mature megakaryocytes of the mouse and cat (Keyhani and Maigne, 1981; Tranum-Jensen and Behnke, 1981), but not human; a specific peroxidase in the nuclear envelope, RER, and dense tubular system; and the absence of dense bodies, characteristically found in circulating platelets. Isolated megakaryocytes possess the full complement of cyclooxygenase and lipoxygenase activities found in circulating platelets (Miller et al., 1982). The alpha-granules of megakaryocytes contain a variety of proteins of biologic significance including platelet factor 4, beta-thromboglobulin and the platelet-derived growth factor (Ryo et al., 1983). Myelofibrosis in acute megakaryocytic leukemia has been associated with local release of alpha-granule components from megakaryocytes in the bone marrow (Breton-Gorius et al., 1982; Castro-Malaspina and Moore, 1982).

PLATELET PRODUCTION FROM MEGAKARYOCYTES

The manner of platelet production from the megakaryocyte has been investigated both in vitro and in vivo. Wright in 1910 hypothesized that pseudopod-like projections arise from the surface of mature megakaryocytes and penetrate into the marrow sinusoids to shed platelets. This hypothesis has been confirmed in recent microcinematographic and electron microscopic studies of megakaryocytopoiesis in the bone marrow of several species (Becker and De Bruyn, 1976; Behnke and Pedersen, 1974; Bessis, 1973; Djaldetti et al., 1979; Lichtman et al., 1978; Radley and Scurfield, 1980; Scurfield and Radley, 1981; Theiry and Bessis, 1956; Tavassoli and Aoki, 1981; Weiss, 1981) and in the mouse spleen (Ihzumi et al., 1977). See reviews by De Bruyn (1981) and Tavassoli (1980). An alternate or additional mode of platelet formation through surface blebbing or budding has been described in recent years (Djaldetti et al., 1979; Handagama et al., 1984; Ihzumi et al., 1977; Lichtman et al., 1978). In studies on the mouse and rat bone marrow, megakaryocytes were seen to lie near the marrow sinusoidal wall, and in some places the wall structure of the sinus appeared to be completed by the megakaryocyte. In this position, platelets could be shed from cytoplasmic projections (Plate III–5) and surface blebs on the megakaryocyte, or the intact cell could enter the sinus to shed its platelets in the sinus lumen or elsewhere, particularly the pulmonary circulation. Platelet formation in such situations involves fragmentation of megakaryocyte cytoplasm, through fusion-fission reorganization of the dermarcation membranes (Tavassoli, 1980). The entry of intact megakaryocytes into the marrow sinus lumen and thence into the circulation entails transendothelial migration through apertures 6 µm in diameter located in the parajunctional areas of the sinus endothelium (Tavassoli and Aoki, 1981).

Megakaryocytes located in the subendothelial region of vascular sinusoids extend cytoplasmic extensions, villus processes or "proplatelets," through the endothelial cells into the sinusoidal lumen (Fig. 15–6). Proplatelets are elongated structures (circa 2.5 × 120 µm)

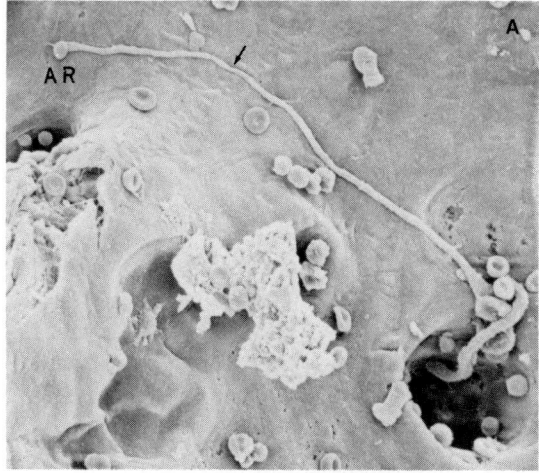

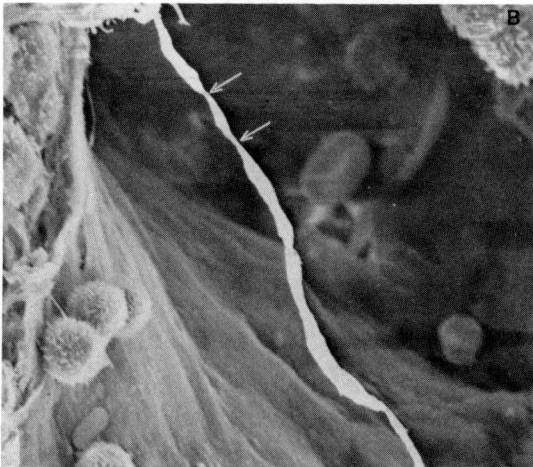

Fig. 15–6. Scanning electron photomicrographs of canine bone marrow depicting long slender extensions of proplatelets within sinusoidal lumen. Platelets may be shed by fragmentation of a proplatelet at the apical region (AR) or areas of intermittent constrictions (arrows). *A,* ×721; *B,* ×2,540. (Prepared with the assistance of Dr. Prem Handagama.)

and often occur in clusters. It is estimated that a mature megakaryocyte produces about 6 proplatelets per cell (Becker and De Bruyn, 1976), although this number seems to be a minimum. These proplatelets frequently present regional constrictions and beaded areas along their lengths, and it is envisioned that fragmentation at these locations by a pinching-off process leads to production of a heterogeneous population of platelets. It is conjectured that formation and fragmentation of proplatelets may involve fusion and fission of demarcation membrane system (Tavassoli and Yoffey, 1983), sol-gel transformation of megakaryocyte cytoplasm, and participation of microtubules and thrombosthenin, both of which are present in megakaryocytes as well as platelets (Behnke and Pedersen, 1974; Penington and Streatfield, 1975; White, 1979). In Wright-stained films of marrow aspirates, an occasional megakaryocyte may be seen at the verge of releasing platelets or may have a cluster of platelets adjacent to its surface. This may suggest extravascular release of platelets. Such platelets may gain entry to the circulation or be phagocytosed by marrow macrophages.

Some megakaryocytes are seen in extramedullary locations such as the lungs and occasionally in the spleen, liver, kidneys, and heart (Wickramasinghe, 1978). Pulmonary megakaryocytes have been investigated most and have been found to originate in the marrow. Several researchers have found that in health some intact mature megakaryocytes enter the circulation and shed their platelets in the lungs during passage through the pulmonary microcirculation (Crosby, 1975; Kaufman et al., 1965; Scheinin and Koivuniemi, 1963; Tavassoli, 1980; Wintrobe et al., 1981). Free nuclei are destroyed by pulmonary macrophages. Pulmonary and circulating megakaryocytes have been investigated in the dog (Warheit and Barnhart, 1980, 1981); about 7 megakaryocytes/ml of venous blood and 2/ml of arterial blood were found, and virtually all megakaryocytes were elongated (about 20–50 μm in length). Micromegakaryocytes and megakaryoblasts were found in the peripheral blood of three dogs with radiation-induced myelogenous leukemia (Tolle et al., 1983). Studies in mice indicate that the spleen contributes little to platelet production under normal conditions, but exhibits compensatory platelet production after bone marrow ablation (Layendecker and McDonald, 1982).

It has been estimated that there are about 150–500 megakaryocytes/10^6 nucleated cells in a suspension of normal canine marrow (Wickramasinghe, 1978). One to three megakaryocytes per low power microscopic field are found in smears of marrow aspirates from the ribs of a normal dog. In such smears there are about 70–84% mature and 16–30% immature megakaryocytes, with a ratio of 2.35–5.25:1 (Joshi and Jain, 1977).

A mature megakaryocyte normally produces about 2,000–8,000 platelets over a period of 3–12 hours (Bessis, 1973; Chernoff et al., 1980; Cronkite, 1958; Tavassoli, 1980; Triplett, 1978). The number produced is proportional to the cytoplasmic volume and ploidy value of the megakaryocyte. A rough correlation between platelet size and platelet number has been observed in various species (Lewis, 1975). Cyclic variations have been found to occur in platelet numbers, perhaps due to cyclic production and release (Morley, 1969; O'Neill and Firkin, 1964). Cyclic production of platelets at 11- to 14-day intervals was found to occur in gray collie dogs with congenital cyclic hematopoiesis (McDonald et al., 1976). The platelet size varied inversely with the platelet count, and significantly increased thrombopoietin levels were found at the beginning of active thrombopoiesis.

Young platelets are larger, denser, and metabolically and functionally more active than old platelets (Ebbe, 1976; Triplett, 1978). It has been suggested that the heterogeneity of circulating platelets, with regard to both size and density, stems from the origin of platelets from different populations of megakaryocytes (Penington et al., 1976). Small and young megakaryocytes produce large and dense platelets. That is, platelets from megakaryocytes with 8N nuclear ploidy appear larger and have a greater content of granules and mitochondria than those from 32N ploidy cells. The number and size of platelets produced vary considerably under pathologic conditions (see Chapter 17).

REGULATION OF MEGAKARYOCYTOPOIESIS AND THROMBOPOIESIS

The number of platelets in the circulation is remarkably constant in a healthy individual, although species variations occur in normal values for platelets, and the platelet number appears to be in excess of need. Platelet counts are lower in the newborn, and the normal adult level is reached in about 3 months. Experimental studies indicate that platelet number in blood is influenced by both positive and negative feedback mechanisms

(Ebbe, 1976; Wickramasinghe, 1978; Burstein and Harker, 1983).

Stimulatory Factors

Megakaryocytopoiesis is regulated by the number of circulating platelets. Thus experimental thrombocytopenia is followed by a rebound thrombocytosis, and, conversely, thrombocytopenia follows transfusion-induced thrombocytosis (Harker, 1968). Stimulation of megakaryocytopoiesis in thrombocytopenia is associated with an increase in the number of megakaryocytes and increases in their mitotic indexes, nuclear ploidy, and cell size. The maturation time of megakaryocytes is shortened, although a 2- to 3-day lag may be seen for the first evidence in blood of accelerated platelet production. In contrast, transfusion-induced thrombocytosis is associated with decreases in megakaryocyte number, size, and nuclear ploidy. The megakaryocyte maturation time remains normal or is prolonged.

The stimulatory influence of platelet number on megakaryocytopoiesis is mediated through a hormonal factor called thrombocytosis-stimulating factor (TSF) or thrombopoietin (Adams et al., 1978; Ebbe, 1976; Kawakita et al., 1981; McDonald, 1981; McDonald et al., 1976; Odell, 1974). The factor has been demonstrated in human urine and in blood of normal humans and animals. Partially purified thrombopoietin from the serum of thrombocytopenic rats was found to be a glycoprotein with a MW of about 48,000 (Dassin et al., 1983). The site of thrombopoietin production remains to be determined. Several studies have supported the concept that the kidney is at least one site of thrombopoietin production (see review by McDonald, 1981). Thrombocytopenia has been seen in up to 50% of human patients with kidney disease. Thrombopoietic activity is demonstrated in serum of mice experiencing "posthemorrhagic thrombocytopenia," in plasma of rats made thrombocytopenic by antiplatelet antibody, and in serum of vinblastine-treated rats, but not in nephrectomized control animals. A thrombocytopoietic factor from human kidney cell culture stimulates incorporation of ^{32}S and ^{75}Se-methionine into platelets, elevates platelet counts, and increases

platelet size in mice. This factor also stimulates megakaryocytopoiesis in vitro as evidenced by increases in the number of CFU-Meg, megakaryocytic colonies, and megakaryocytes, and in vivo as evidenced by increases in numbers of small acetylcholinesterase-positive cells (these are precursors of megakaryocytes in rodent bone marrow), megakaryocyte endomitosis, and megakaryocyte size and number. Immunologic, physical, and chemical similarities were found between TSF from kidney cell culture and TSF from human plasma and urine as well as from plasma of thrombocytopenic animals.

It is evident from the above and other studies that thrombopoietin seems to influence megakaryocyte production at least in three ways (Kawakita et al., 1981; McDonald, 1981; Odell, 1974): (a) by stimulating committed stem cells, i.e., increasing the rate of differentiation of unrecognizable megakaryocytic progenitors into megakaryocytic precursors, (b) by inducing additional endomitosis in immature megakaryocytes resulting in increased ploidy and cell volume, and (c) by shortening the megakaryocyte maturation time. The degree of stimulation of megakaryocytopoiesis is dose-dependent (Odell and Shelton, 1979). Recently, a two-level regulatory mechanism of megakaryocyte production has been proposed (see review by Williams and Levine, 1982). According to this hypothesis, proliferation of megakaryocyte progenitors into megakaryocytic colonies is stimulated by a megakaryocyte-colony stimulating factor (Meg-CSF), which is distinct from thrombopoietin, and megakaryocyte ploidy and possibly maturation are influenced primarily by thrombopoietin. It is not certain that both regulators are exclusive in their functional capacity, especially thrombopoietin, as evident from observations cited above. Experimental observations indicate that day-to-day requirements for thrombocytes are met not by modulation of CFU-Meg, but by modulation of more differentiated progenies, although CFU-Meg becomes involved in chronic thrombocytopenic states.

Meg-CSF is present in urine of patients with aplastic anemia and idiopathic thrombocytopenia (Kawakita et al., 1983), and its level in serum appears to be inversely related to marrow megakaryocyte number (Hoffmann et al., 1981). Thrombopoietin levels apparently vary inversely with the circulating platelet mass (Odell and Murphy, 1974). Although thrombopoietin levels in various conditions associated with altered platelet production remain to be determined, thrombocytopenia is presumably associated with increased levels and thrombocytosis with decreased levels. Regulatory mechanisms of thrombocytoses seen in myeloproliferative disorders and in many nonmalignant conditions remain unknown. The possibility of some nonspecific stimulation has been suggested in nonmalignant conditions (Burstein and Harker, 1983). Normal bone marrow has a capacity to undergo a fourfold to eightfold increase in platelet production (Wickramasinghe, 1978). A thrombocytosis-promoting factor, termed thrombocytosin, has been isolated from bovine bile and found to produce thrombocytosis in rats, dogs, sheep, and cattle (Begovic et al., 1973). Its physiologic and clinical significance remains to be determined. Vincristine, an antimitotic drug that has been used to promote thrombocyte production in dogs with immune-mediated thrombocytopenia (see Chapter 35), causes a dose-dependent thrombocytosis as well as thrombocytopenia in laboratory animals by mechanisms yet to be clearly defined (Choi et al., 1974).

Inhibitory Factors

Inhibitors of thrombopoiesis and thrombopoietin have also been investigated (Bessler et al., 1978; Wickramasinghe, 1978). Evidence has been presented to indicate that the spleen may produce an inhibitor of thrombopoiesis or thrombopoietin. This evidence is based on observations on splenectomized humans and laboratory animals. The magnitude of postsplenectomy thrombocytosis is much higher (twofold to sixfold) than accountable to the absence of splenic pooling. Because there is increased incorporation of ^{75}Se-methionine in platelets and the platelet life span remains normal after splenectomy, removal of an inhibitory factor is suspected. Postsplenectomy thrombocytosis in rats can be almost completely abolished by replanting as little as 10%

of the splenic tissue within the peritoneal cavity (Tarnuzi and Smiley, 1967). Furthermore, administration of splenic lymphocytes into splenectomized mice prevented thrombocytosis, and administration into normal mice caused thrombocytopenia (Bessler et al., 1978). An inhibitor of megakaryocytic colonies was found in normal human serum (Vainchenker et al., 1982). Suppression of megakaryocytopoiesis by suppressor T-cells was reported in eight patients with acute myelogenous leukemia (Worman et al., 1982).

Thrombocyte Production in Iron Deficiency

Thrombocytosis is often seen in iron deficiency anemia (Barnhart and Robinson, 1975; Table 12–2), and platelet counts increase at high altitude (Tocantins, 1938). It might be assumed that increased production of erythropoietin under such conditions may stimulate thrombopoiesis, but evidence to the contrary has been obtained. Erythropoietin does not stimulate thrombopoiesis, nor does thrombopoietin augment erythropoiesis (Evatt et al., 1976; O'Grady et al., 1968). Moreover, platelet production is diminished in severely anemic human patients and in mice exposed to severe hypoxia (McDonald et al., 1979) or given erythropoietin injections (Cooper and Cooper, 1977). This occurrence is explained on the basis of stem cell competition, leading to an increase in erythropoiesis with a concomitant decrease in megakaryocytopoiesis.

Thrombocytosis in severe iron deficiency anemia is associated with a twofold to threefold increase in megakaryocytopoiesis and platelet production. A few human patients with iron deficiency anemia exhibit thrombocytopenia associated with decreased megakaryocytopoiesis and platelet production. Platelet life span is normal in both types of responses. Based on experimental and clinical observations, a dual role of iron in thrombocyte production has been proposed (Karpatkin et al., 1974): (a) iron either directly or indirectly inhibits the increase in platelet count above steady-state levels via some inhibitory mechanisms, possibly against thrombopoietin; and (b) iron is also required for maximum platelet production under normal situations through an unknown mechanism.

Iron is required for the synthesis or production of an integral portion of the platelet. Further studies are needed to define the role of iron in thrombopoiesis.

PLATELET KINETICS AND DISTRIBUTION

Platelet Life Span

Several techniques have been used to determine intravascular distribution and life span of platelets (Finch et al., 1977; Harker, 1978; Mustard, 1978). Labeling with ^{51}Cr is considered a satisfactory method for platelet turnover and survival studies. ^{32}P-labeled orthophosphate is unsatisfactory, and DPF labeled with ^{32}P, ^{3}H, or ^{14}C and ^{14}C-serotonin are currently not recommended because of their elution and reutilization. ^{35}S-sulfate and ^{75}Se (selenomethionine) are incorporated into the cytoplasm of megakaryocytes and then into platelets. ^{111}In-oxine (^{111}indium-8-hydroxyquinoline) permits in vivo imaging of platelets in various organs and platelet localization at thrombogenic foci. ^{111}In-oxine is a cyclotron-produced, gamma-emitting isotope with a half-life of 2.8 days and is considered a "physiologic" platelet label (Heyns et al., 1980). A nonradioisotopic method, based on the measurement of malondialdehyde (MDA), an end product of platelet lipid peroxidation, has been developed to measure platelet life span (De Haas et al., 1979; Stuart et al., 1975). Oral ingestion of aspirin or in vitro exposure of platelets to aspirin inhibits cyclo-oxygenase enzyme needed for lipid-peroxidation. This defect persists for the remainder of the platelet life span. The emergence of newly formed, unaffected platelets is monitored by estimating the increase in MDA in serial blood samples taken over the next 10 days, and this increase in MDA constitutes a measure of time needed for platelet production.

The blood platelet has a finite life that is similar in humans and several domestic animals. Mean platelet survival time was found to be 10 days in calves (Mizuno et al., 1959), 9–11 days in sheep (Lander et al., 1965), and 9.9 ± 0.6 days in humans (Harker and Finch, 1969). Similar values were obtained for canine

platelets in early studies (Adelson et al., 1965), but shorter survival times were found in more recent studies. Mean survival of ^{111}In-oxine-labeled canine platelets was reported at 78.8 ± 2.0 hours (Rauls et al., 1982), 5.15 ± 0.3 days (Lotter et al., 1980), 5.9 ± 0.6 days (Sharefkin and Rich, 1982), and 6.6 ± 1.0 days (Badenhorst et al., 1982) and of ^{51}Cr-labeled canine platelets at 5.4 ± 0.3 days (O'Donnell et al., 1981). Platelet life span in rabbits (Morgan et al., 1955), mice (Odell and McDonald, 1961), and pigs (Robinson et al., 1961) is comparatively shorter. Platelet survival in 2- to 3-month-old calves was found to be about 5 days (Shaikh et al., 1978).

Distribution and Removal of Platelets

It has been observed that platelet numbers increase after epinephrine injection and after exercise (Aster, 1966; Bierman, 1962; Dawson and Ogston, 1969; Freedman et al., 1977). The increase due to the former is attributed to release of platelets from the spleen, whereas that due to the latter is associated with platelet release from the lungs. This is based on findings that epinephrine-induced platelet release is not seen in asplenic individuals, while exercise-induced change is not affected by splenectomy. Platelet counts in both cases return to normal levels within 30 minutes. These and other observations in normal and splenectomized persons and animals (Aster, 1966; Freedman et al., 1977) indicate existence of two rapidly mobilizable pools of platelets, one splenic and the other nonsplenic. About 30–40% of the total platelet mass in humans, dogs, and rabbits is sequestered in the spleen and can be rapidly mobilized. A disproportionately higher number of young platelets (megathrombocytes), besides senescent platelets, is sequestered in the spleen (Freedman and Karpatkin, 1975; Shulman et al., 1968). Normally, a dynamic exchange occurs between the splenic and the circulating platelets. Splenectomy is followed by a protracted thrombocytosis resulting largely from removal of the splenic reservoir and circulation of the total intravascular platelet mass and partly from increased thrombopoiesis (see Regulation of Megakaryocytopoiesis and Thrombopoiesis). In splenomegaly, as much as 90% of the platelet mass may be sequestered in the spleen.

The nonsplenic pool of platelets was investigated in splenectomized humans subjected to exercise and in splenectomized dogs and rabbits given epinephrine infusions (Freedman et al., 1977). The increase in platelet numbers in such subjects was transient, peaking at 3 minutes and returning to baseline at 5–7 minutes. In the dog and rabbit, the nonsplenic pool represented approximately half of the total rapidly mobilizable pool. Furthermore, in contrast to the splenic pool, the nonsplenic pool was not appreciably enriched with megathrombocytes. The site of this nonsplenic pool remained unknown. That such a nonsplenic pool of platelets may not be found in all species was evident from a study on normal and splenectomized ponies whose platelet counts and size were not significantly altered after exercise (Lepherd, 1977).

Physical and biochemical changes occur in platelets with aging (Harker, 1978), and normally platelets are cleared from the circulation by the spleen, liver, and bone marrow. Platelet turnover rate in humans was estimated to be 35,000 ± 4,300 platelets/μl of blood per day (Harker, 1968). Platelet destruction occurs in the mononuclear phagocyte (reticuloendothelial) system and is essentially age-dependent (linear disappearance), although some random destruction (exponential removal) is also observed (Harker, 1978; Hirsh and Dorey, 1972). Damaged and senescent platelets are sequestered mainly in the spleen or liver or both (Aster, 1969; Kaplan and Saba, 1978). Organ distribution of platelets was studied in humans (Heyns et al., 1980) and dogs (Lotter et al., 1980; Badenhorst et al., 1982; Sharefkin and Rich, 1982) through use of the newly introduced platelet label ^{111}In-oxine. In humans, platelet pooling in the spleen was 29.6%, which was in close agreement with previous studies. In addition, hepatic sequestration was found to be sizable, and some sequestration was found in the bone marrow. In the dog, platelet pooling was seen in the spleen (the major site), liver (an important site), and heart. The accumulation of labeled platelets in the various organs was rapid; in the spleen it was maximal after 15 minutes and comprised about 36.1% of the total platelet mass. Splenic size was found to vary from day to day among different dogs.

Abnormalities of Platelet Life Span and Distribution

Platelet distribution and life span in pathologic conditions are being investigated. In one study, three patterns of sequestration of ^{111}In-oxine-labeled platelets were found in eight human patients with idiopathic thrombocytopenic purpura; two patients had mainly splenic, two mainly hepatic, and three diffuse distribution, the major site being the bone marrow (Heyns et al., 1982). The pattern of sequestration was not predictive of response to glucocorticoid therapy or indicative of the necessity for splenectomy. However, information of this type on a larger number of patients is needed before a valid conclusion can be reached.

Platelet life span is reduced (<2 days) in a variety of pathologic conditions. These include immune-mediated thrombocytopenia (Burger et al., 1979; Heyns et al., 1982), acute promyelocytic leukemia (Uchida et al., 1979), and viral infections (Scott et al., 1978). Platelet survival is also decreased after administration of large doses of heparin (Bhattacharya, 1977). Platelet survival was shortened in 6 out of 15 dogs with localized tumors (4.4 ± 0.3 days versus normal mean of 5.4 ± 0.3 days) and in 30 out of 35 dogs with metastatic tumors (3.2 ± 0.2 days) (O'Donnell et al., 1981). Lifespan of ^{111}In-labeled platelets in hypomagnesemic lambs was 60 hours compared to 63 hours in control animals (Schneider et al., 1983). Platelet viability is diminished after storage at 4°C and after in vitro exposure to trypsin or neuraminidase (Harker, 1978). For additional information see Chapter 17.

REFERENCES

Aabo, K., and Bendix-Hansen, K.: Surface Structure of Intravascular Megakaryocytes: A Scanning Electron Microscopic Study. Acta. Pathol. Microbiol. Scand., 90A:85, 1982.

Adams, W.H., et al.: Humoral Regulation of Thrombopoiesis in Man. J. Lab. Clin. Med., 91:141, 1978.

Adelson, E., et al.: Platelet Tagging with Tritium Labeled Diisopropylfluorophosphate. Blood, 25:744, 1965.

Albrecht, M., and Fulle, H.H.: Morphologic der Megakaryozyten bei Blutkranke heiten. Blut, 28:109, 1974.

Aster, R.H.: Pooling of Platelets in the Spleen: Role in

the Pathogenesis of "Hypersplenic" Thrombocytopenia. J. Clin. Invest., *45*:645, 1966.

Aster, R.H.: Studies of the Fate of Platelets in Rats and Man. Blood, *34*:117, 1969.

Badenhorst, P.N., et al.: The Influence of the "Collection Injury" on the Survival and Distribution of Indium III-Labelled Canine Platelets. Brit. J. Haematol., *52*:233, 1982.

Baldini, M.G., and Ebbe, S. (eds.): Platelets: Production, Function, Transfusion and Storage. Grune & Stratton, New York, 1974.

Barnhart, M.I., and Robinson, J.A.: Structural Physiology of Platelets and Megakaryocytes. *In* Platelets: Recent Advances in Basic Research and Clinical Aspects. Ulutin O.N., ed. American Elsevier, New York, p. 57, 1975.

Becker, R.P., and De Bruyn, P.P.H.: The Transmural Passage of Blood Cells into Myeloid Sinusoids and the Entry of Platelets into Sinusoidal Circulation. Amer. J. Anat., *145*:183, 1976.

Begovic, S., et al.: Effect of Thrombopoietin Isolated from Bovine Bile on the Thrombocyte Count in Sheep. Veterinaria Yugoslavia, *22*:433, 1973.

Behnke, O., and Pedersen, N.T.: Ultrastructural Aspects of Megakaryocyte Maturation and Platelet Release. *In* Platelets: Production, Function, Transfusion and Storage. Baldini, M.G., and Ebbe, S., eds. Grune & Stratton, New York, Chap. 3, pp. 21–31, 1974.

Bentfeld, M.E., and Bainton, D.F.: Cytochemical Localization of Lysosomal Enzymes in Rat Megakaryocytes and Platelets. J. Clin. Invest., *56*:1635, 1975.

Bentfeld-Barker, M.E., and Bainton, D.F.: Identification of Primary Lysosomes in Human Megakaryocytes and Platelets. Blood, *59*:472, 1982.

Bessis, M.: The Living Blood Cell and Their Ultrastructure. Springer-Verlag, Berlin, 1973.

Bessler, H., et al.: Role of the Spleen and Lymphocytes in Regulation of the Circulating Platelet Number in Mice. J. Lab. Clin. Med., *91*:760, 1978.

Bhattacharya, D.K.: Survival and Rate of Utilization of Circulating Platelets following Administration of Heparin. Indian J. Exp. Biol., *15*:188, 1977.

Bierman, H.R.: Leucapheresis in Man. II. Changes in Circulating Granulocytes, Lymphocytes and Platelets in the Blood. Brit. J. Haematol., *8*:77, 1962.

Bizzozero, J.: Uber einen neuen Formbestandtheil de Blutes und die Rolle bei der Thrombose und der Blutgerinnung. Virchows Arch. (Pathol. Anat.), *90*:261, 1882.

Breton-Gorius, J., et al.: Myelofibrosis and Acute Megakaryocytic Leukemia in a Child: Topographic Relationship between Fibroblasts and Megakaryocytes with an α-Granule Defect. Leuk. Res., *9*:97, 1982.

Burger, T., et al.: Platelet Turnover and Megakaryocytopoiesis in ITP. Acta Med. Acad. Sci. Hung., *36*:45, 1979.

Burstein, S.A.: Studies of Marmoset Megakaryocytopoiesis in Vitro. Amer, J. Haematol., *8*:61, 1980.

Burstein, S.A., and Harker, L.A.: Control of Platelet Production. Clinics in Haematology, *12*:3, 1983.

Castro-Malaspina, H., and Moore, M.A.S.: Pathophysiological Mechanisms Operating in the Development of Myelofibrosis: Role of Megakaryocytes. Nouv. Rev. Fr. Hematol., *24*:221, 1982.

Chernoff, A., et al.: Origin of Platelet-Derived Growth Factor in Megakaryocytes in Guinea Pigs. J. Clin. Invest., *65*:926, 1980.

Choi, S., et al.: Effects of Vincristine on Platelet Production. *In* Platelets: Production, Function, Transfusion

and Storage. Baldini, M.G., and Ebbe, S., eds. Grune & Stratton, New York, Chap. 6, pp. 51–61, 1974.

Cooper, G.W., and Cooper, B.: Relationships between Blood Platelets and Erythrocyte Formation. Life Sciences, *20*:1517, 1977.

Cronkite, E.P.: Regulation of Platelet Production. *In* Homeostatic Mechanisms. Brookhaven Symp. Biol. (Upton, N.Y.), *10*:96, 1958.

Crosby, W.H.: Normal Platelet Numbers: Pulmonary Platelet Interactions. Ser. Haematol., *8(3)*:89, 1975.

Dassin, E., et al.: Partial Purification of a Thrombocytopoiesis Stimulating Factor Present in the Serum of Thrombocytopenic Rats. Acta Haematol., *69*:249, 1983.

Dawson, A.A., and Ogston, D.: Exercise-Induced Thrombocytosis. Acta Haematol. (Basel), *42*:241, 1969.

De Bruyn, P.P.H.: Structural Substrates of Bone Marrow Functions. Semin. Hematol., *18*:179, 1981.

De Haas, H.A., et al.: A Modified Non-Radioisotope Method for Measurement of Platelet Production Tissue. Brit. J. Haematol., *43*:737, 1979.

de Laval, M.: Contribution a l'etude de la Maturation de Megacaryocytes dans la moelle Ossense de Cobaye. Arch. Biol. Paris, *79*:597, 1968.

Djaldetti, M., et al.: SEM Observations on the Mechanism of Platelet Release from Megakaryocytes. Thromb. Haemost., *42*:611, 1979.

Ebbe, S.: Biology of Megakaryocytes. Prog. Hemost. Thromb., *3*:211, 1976.

Ebbe, S.: Experimental and Clinical Megakaryocytopoiesis. Clin. Haematol., *8*:371, 1979.

Evatt, B.L., et al.: Relationships between Thrombopoiesis and Erythropoiesis with Studies of the Effects of Preparation of Thrombopoietin and Erythropoietin. Blood, *48*:547, 1976.

Finch, C.A., et al.: Kinetics of the Formed Elements of Human Blood. Blood, *50*:699, 1977.

Freedman, M.L., and Karpatkin, S.: Heterogeneity of Rabbit Platelets v. Preferential Splenic Sequestration of Megathrombocytes. Brit. J. Haematol., *31*:255, 1975.

Freedman, M., et al.: Presence of a Non-Splenic Platelet Pool. Blood., *50*:419, 1977.

Handagama, P.J., et al.: Scanning Electron Microscopic Studies of Megakaryocytes and Platelet Formation in the Dog and Rat. (Unpublished Observations) 1984.

Harker, L.A.: Kinetics of Thrombopoiesis. J. Clin. Invest., *47*:458, 1968.

Harker, L.A.: Platelet Survival Tissue: Its Measurement and Use. Prog. Hemost. Thromb., *4*:321, 1978.

Harker, L.A., and Finch, C.A.: Thrombokinetics in Man. J. Clin. Invest., *48*:963, 1969.

Heyns, A.D., et al.: Kinetics, Distribution and Sites of Destruction of "Indium" Labelled Human Platelets. Brit. J. Haematol., *44*:269, 1980.

Heyns, A.D., et al.: Kinetics and Sites of Destruction of Indium-Oxine-Labelled Platelets in Idiopathic Thrombocytopenic Purpura: A Quantitative Study. Amer. J. Hematol., *12*:167, 1982.

Hirsh, J., and Dorey, J.C.G.: Platelet Function in Health and Disease. Prog. Hematol., *7*:185, 1972.

Hoffmann, R., et al.: Assay of an Activity in the Serum of Patients with Disorders of Thrombopoiesis that Stimulate Formation of Megakaryocytic Colonies. New Eng. J. Med., *305*:533, 1981.

Howell, W.W.: Observations upon the Occurrence, Structure and Formation of the Giant Cells of the Marrow. J. Morphol., *4*:117, 1890.

Ihzumi, T., et al.: Megakaryocyte and Platelet Formation: A Scanning Electron Microscope Study in Mouse Spleen. Arch. Histol. Jpn., 40:305, 1977.

Joshi, B.C., and Jain, N.C.: Experimental Immunologic Thrombocytopenia in Dogs: A Study of Thrombocytopenia and Megakaryocytopoiesis. Res. Vet. Sci., 22:11, 1977.

Kaplan, J.E., and Saba, T.M.: Platelet Removal from the Circulation by the Liver and Spleen. Amer. J. Physiol., 235:H314, 1978.

Karpatkin, S., et al.: Role of Iron as a Regulator of Thrombopoiesis. Amer. J. Med., 57:521, 1974.

Kass, L., et al.: Megakaryocytes in the Giant Platelet Syndrome. A Cytochemical and Ultrastructural Study. Thromb. Haemost., 38:652, 1977.

Kaufman, R.M., et al.: Circulating Megakaryocytes and Platelet Release in the Lung. Blood, 26:720, 1965.

Kawakita, M., et al.: Thrombopoiesis and Megakaryocyte Colony Stimulating Factors in the Urine of Patients with Idiopathic Thrombocytopenic Purpura. Brit. J. Haematol., 48:609, 1981.

Kawakita, M., et al.: Characterization of Human Megakaryocyte Colony Stimulating Factor in the Urinary Extracts from Patients with Aplastic Anemia and Idiopathic Thrombocytopenia Purpura. Blood, 61:556, 1983.

Kessel, R.G., and Kardon, R.H.: Tissues and Organs: A Text-Atlas of Scanning Electron Microscopy. W.H. Freeman, San Francisco, 1979.

Keyhani, E., and Maigne, J.: Acetylcholine Esterase in Cat Megakaryocyte: Evidence for Extracellular Secretion. Cell Biol. Int. Rep., 5:805, 1981.

Lander, H., et al.: Studies of Platelet Survival and Behavior in Sheep. J. Lab. Clin. Med., 66:887, 1965.

Layendecker, S.J., and McDonald, T.P.: The Relative Roles of the Spleen and Bone Marrow in Platelet Production in Mice. Exp. Hematol., 10:332, 1982.

Lepherd, E.E.: Effect of Exercise on Platelet Size and Number. Vet. Rec., 1012:488, 1977.

Levine, R.F., et al.: Flow Cytometric Analysis of Megakaryocyte Ploidy: Comparison with Feulgen Microdensitometry and Discovery that 8N is the Predominant Ploidy Class in Guinea Pig and Monkey Marrow. Blood, 56:210, 1980.

Levine, R., et al.: The Significance of Megakaryocyte Size. Blood, 60:1122, 1982.

Lewis, J.H.: Comparative Hematology: Mammalian Platelets. In Platelets, Recent Observations in Basic Research and Clinical Aspects. Ulutin, O.N., ed. American Elsevier, New York, pp. 18–23, 1975.

Lichtman, M.A., et al.: Parasinusoidal Location of Megakaryocytes in Marrow: A Determinant of Platelet Release. Amer. J. Hematol., 4:303, 1978.

Lotter, M.G., et al.: Kinetics, Distribution and Sites of Destruction of Canine Blood Platelets with In-111 Oxine. J. Nucl. Med., 21:36, 1980.

Maldonado, J., et al.: The Ultrastructure of the Platelet Line in Myeloproliferative Disease. In Platelets, Recent Advances in Basic Research and Clinical Aspects. Ulutin, O.N. ed. American Elsevier, New York, p. 472, 1975.

McDonald, T.P., et al.: Effects of Hypoxia on Thrombocytopoiesis and Thrombopoietin Production of Mice. Proc. Sco. Exp. Biol. Med., 160:335, 1979.

McDonald, T.P., et al.: Canine Cyclic Hematopoiesis: Platelet Size and Thrombopoietin Level in Relation to Platelet Count. Proc. Soc. Exp. Biol. Med., 153:424, 1976.

McDonald, T.P.: Array and Site of Production of Thrombopoietin. Brit. J. Haematol., 49:493, 1981.

McMillan, R., et al.: Antibody against Megakaryocytes in Idiopathic Thrombocytopenic Purpura. JAMA, 239(23):2460, 1978.

Miller, J.L., et al.: Arachidonic Acid Metabolism in Guinea Pig Megakaryocyte. Biochem. Biophys. Res. Commun., 107:752, 1982.

Mizuno, N.S., et al.: Life Span of Thrombocytes and Erythrocytes in Normal and Thrombocytopenic Calves. Blood, 14:708, 1959.

Morgan, M.C., et al.: Survival of Radiochromate-Labelled Platelets in Rabbits. J. Lab. Clin. Med., 45:521, 1955.

Morley, A.: A Platelet Cycle in Normal Individuals. Aust. Ann. Intern. Med., 18:127, 1969.

Mustard, J.F.: Platelet Survival. Thromb. Haemost., 40:154, 1978.

Odell, T.T., Jr.: Megakaryocytopoiesis and Its Response to Stimulated Suppression. In Platelets: Production, Function, Transfusion and Storage. Baldini, M.G., and Ebbe, S., eds. Grune & Stratton, New York, pp. 11–20. 1974.

Odell, T.T., Jr., and McDonald, T.P.: Life Span of Mouse Blood Platelets. Proc. Soc. Exp. Biol. Med., 106:107, 1961.

Odell, T.T., Jr., and Murphy, J.R.: Effects of Degree of Thrombocytopenia on Thrombocytopoietic Response. Blood, 44:147, 1974.

Odell, T.T., Jr., and Shelton, C.: Increasing Stimulation of Megakaryocytopoiesis with Decreasing Platelet Count. Proc. Soc. Exp. Biol. Med., 161:531, 1979.

O'Donnell, M.R., et al.: Platelet and Fibrinogen Kinetics in Canine Tumors. Cancer Res., 41:1379, 1981.

O'Grady, L.F., et al.: Effect of Erythropoietin on Transplanted Hematopoietic Tissue. Amer. J. Physiol., 215:176, 1968.

O'Neill, B., and Firkin, B.: Platelet Survival Studies in Coagulation Disorders, Thrombocythemia and Conditions Associated with Atherosclerosis. J. Lab. Clin. Med., 64:188, 1964.

Parmley, R.T., et al.: Emperipolesis of Neutrophils by Dysmorphic Megakaryocytes. Amer. J. Hematol., 13:303, 1982.

Paulus, J.M.: Multiple Differentiation in Megakaryocytes and Platelets. Blood, 29:407, 1967.

Penington, D.G., and Streatfield, K.: Heterogeneity of Megakaryocytes and Platelets. Ser. Haematol., 8:22, 1975.

Penington, D.G., et al.: Megakaryocytes and the Heterogeneity of Circulating Platelets. Brit. J. Haematol., 34:639, 1976.

Radley, J.M., and Scurfield, G.: The Mechanism of Platelet Release. Blood, 56:996, 1980.

Rauls, D.O., et al.: Evaluation of Platelet Kinetics in 47 Dogs Using Indium-111. J. Surg. Res., 33:362, 1982.

Robinson, G.A., et al.: Labeling of Blood Platelets of the Pig with 32S Sulphate. Brit. J. Haematol., 7:271, 1961.

Ryo, R., et al.: New Synthesis of a Platelet. Specific Protein: Platelet Factor 4 Synthesis in a Megakaryocyte Enriched Rabbit Bone Marrow Culture System. J. Cell Biol., 96:515, 1983.

Scheinin, T.M., and Koivuniemi, A.P.: Megakaryocytes in the Pulmonary Circulation. Blood, 22:82, 1963.

Schneider, M.D., et al.: Life Span and Tissue Distribution of [111]Indium Labeled Blood Platelets in Hypomagnesemic Lambs. Amer. J. Vet. Res., 44:806, 1983.

Scott, S., et al.: Effect of Viruses on Platelet Aggregation and Platelet Survival in Rabbits. Blood, 52:47, 1978.

Scurfield, G., and Radley, J.M.: Aspects of Platelet Formation and Release. Amer. J. Hematol., *10*:285, 1981.

Shaikh, B.S., et al.: A Technique to Assess Fibrinogen Platelet and Red Cell Kinetics in Calves with Artificial Hearts or Circulatory Assist Devices. Trans. Am. Soc. Artif. Intern. Organs, *24*:524, 1978.

Shamoto, M.: Emperipolesis of Hematopoietic Cells in Myelocytic Leukemia. Virchows Arch. (Cell Pathol.), *35*:283, 1981.

Sharefkin, J., and Rich, N.M.: Technical Considerations in the Study of Indium-111-Oxine Labelled Platelet Survival Patterns in Dogs. Lab. Anim. Sci., *32*:183, 1982.

Shulman, N.R., et al.: Evidence That the Spleen Will Change the Youngest and Hemostatically Most Effective Platelets. Amer. J. Physiol., *81*:302, 1968.

Stuart, M.J., et al.: A Simple Nonradioisotope Technique for the Determination of Platelet Lifespan. New Eng. J. Med., *292*:1310, 1975.

Tarnuzi, A., and Smiley, R.K.: Hematologic Effects of Splenic Implants. Blood, *29*:373, 1967.

Tavassoli, M.: Megakaryocyte-Platelet Axis and the Process of Platelet Formation and Release. Blood, *55*:537, 1980.

Tavassoli, M., and Aoki, M.: Migration of Entire Megakaryocytes through the Marrow-Blood Barrier. Brit. J. Haematol., *48*:25, 1981.

Tavassoli, M., and Yoffey, J.M.: Platelet Production and Release. *In* Bone Marrow Structure and Function. Alan R. Liss, New York, 1983.

Theiry, J.P., and Bessis, M.: Mechanisme de la Plagnettogenese: Etude in vitro par la Microcinematographie. Revue D'Hematologie, *11*:162, 1956.

Tocantins, L.M.: The Mammalian Blood Platelet in Health and Disease. Medicine, *17*:175, 1938.

Tolle, D.V., et al.: Circulating Micromegakaryocytes preceding Leukemia in Three Dogs Exposed to 2.5 R/Day Gamma Radiation. Vet. Pathol., *20*:111, 1983.

Tranum-Jensen, J., and Behnke, O.: Acetylcholinesterase in the Platelet Megakaryocyte System. I. Structural Localization in Platelets of the Rat, Mouse and Cat. II. Structural Localization in Megakaryocytes of the Rat, Mouse and Cat. Eur. J. Cell Biol., *24*:275, 1981.

Triplett, D.A.: The Platelet: A Review. *In* Platelet Function: Laboratory Evaluation and Clinical Application. Triplett, D.A., ed. Amer. Soc. Clin. Pathologists, Chicago, p. 1, 1978.

Uchida, T., et al.: Shortened Platelet Survival in Acute Promyelocytic Leukemia. Tohoku J. Exp. Med., *129*:205, 1979.

Vainchenker, W., et al.: Normal Human Serum Contains a Factor(s) Capable of Inhibiting Megakaryocyte Colony Formation. Exp. Hematol., *10*:650, 1982.

Warheit, D.B., and Barnhart, M.I.: Circulating Megakaryocytes and the Microvasculature of the Lung. Scan. Electron Microsc., *3*:225, 1980.

Warheit, D.B., and Barnhart, M.I.: Ultrastructure of Circulating and Platelet Forming Megakaryocytes: A Combined Correlative SEM-TEM and SEM Histochemical Study. Ann. N.Y. Acad. Sci., *370*:30, 1981.

Weiss, L.: Haemopoiesis in Mammalian Bone Marrow. Ciba Found. Symp., *84*:5, 1981.

White, J.G.: Current Concepts of Platelet Structure. Amer. J. Clin. Path., *71*:363, 1979.

Wickramasinghe, S.N.: The Megakaryocytes, chap. 8, pp. 260–292, and Megakaryocytes in Various Diseases, chap. 10, pp. 368–380. *In* Human Bone Marrow. Blackwell Scientific Publications, London, 1978.

Williams, N., and Levine, R.F.: The Origin, Development and Regulation of Megakaryocytes. Brit.J. Haematol., *52*:173, 1982.

Wintrobe, et al.: Clinical Hematology. 8th ed. Lea & Febiger, Philadelphia, 1981.

Worman, C.P., et al.: A Megakaryocytic Thrombocytopenia Associated with an Excess of Leu 2a$^+$ Suppressor Cells. Scand. J. Haematol., *28*:215, 1982.

Wright, J.H.: The Origin and Nature of Blood Platelets. Boston Med. Surg. J., *154*:643, 1906.

Wright, J.H.: The Histogenesis of the Blood Platelets. J. Morphol., *21*:263, 1910.

16

The Platelets: Structural, Biochemical, and Functional Aspects

MORPHOLOGIC FEATURES 446
  Light and Electron Microscopic
    Structure 446
  Structural and Functional Relationships 450
  Structural Abnormalities 453

PLATELET BIOCHEMISTRY AND
    METABOLISM 454
  General Biochemistry 454
  Arachidonic Acid Metabolism 455

FUNCTIONS OF PLATELETS 456
  Hemostasis 457
  Vascular Integrity 458

Blood Coagulation 458
Inflammation and Tissue Damage 458
Phagocytosis and Bactericidal Property 459
Thrombosis 459
Atherosclerosis 459
Role in Tumor Cell Metastasis 460

PLATELET AGGREGATION AND RELEASE
    REACTION 460

Understanding the structure and function of platelets is essential to understanding clinical conditions associated with qualitative abnormalities of platelets. Clues as to morphological alterations in platelets may be obtained from close examination of a well-stained blood film prepared from a carefully drawn blood sample. Functional abnormalities require special in vitro tests with patient's platelets and may not manifest morphologically. Over the last decade interest in platelets has grown beyond the realm of hemostasis. Important newer functions such as roles in tumor metastasis, atherosclerosis, and inflammation have been ascribed to these tiny cytoplasmic fragments of megakaryocytes as their biochemical aspects, particularly arachidonic acid metabolism, and cellular components are being studied. Following is a brief presentation of these aspects of the blood platelet. References cited in specific areas may be consulted for further details. A recent issue of *Clinics in Haematology* (volume 12, 1983) was completely devoted to platelet disorders.

MORPHOLOGIC FEATURES
Light and Electron Microscopic Structure

Platelets of various animal species present a heterogeneous morphology in stained blood films (Figs. 16–1, 16–2; Plate IX–1). Individual platelets appear as discoid, spheroid, or elongated flat objects with granular organelles dispersed throughout the cytoplasm or sometimes located centrally (granulomere). The platelet cytoplasm (hyalomere) is clear and bounded by a delicate membrane that appears smooth or sometimes bears a few fine, thread-like surface projections (Fig. 16–1A, B). Platelets may be distributed singly or found in small to large clumps. If venipuncture is performed carefully and EDTA is used as the anticoagulant, platelet clumping can be minimized. Infrequently a platelet may overlie an erythrocyte. One or two platelets may sometimes be found attached to a neutrophil (Fig. 16–1C); this is called "platelet satellitism." It is usually seen in films prepared from EDTA-blood and is generally nonspecific (Skinnider et al., 1978), although it has been found in some human patients with antiplatelet antibodies, lymphocytic leukemia, and myeloproliferative disorders (Cohen et al., 1980; White et al., 1978; Payne, 1981).

A study of platelet volumes in 11 mammalian species revealed that platelets of the dog, pig, and human are similar in volume (7.6–8.3 fl), whereas those of the ox, horse,

446

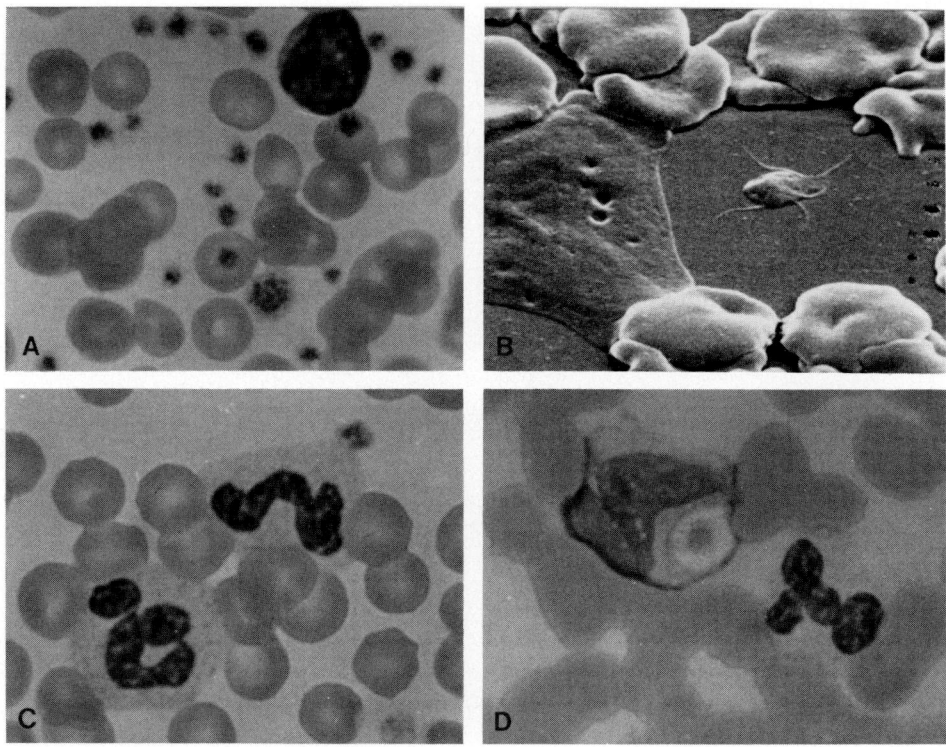

Fig. 16–1. *A,* Normal canine platelets exhibiting prominent granularity and some pleomorphism; an occasional one is as large as a red cell. *B,* Scanning electron photomicrograph of a blood film depicting a platelet with several distinctly visible fine dendritic processes; such processes are also seen in stained-blood films examined with the light microscope, but they are difficult to depict photographically as was the case with platelets shown in *A. C,* An example of platelet satellitism in which a canine platelet has adhered to a neutrophil. *D,* A rare example of platelet phagocytosis by a monocyte in peripheral blood of a thrombocytopenic dog (platelet count, 18,000/μl of blood). *A, C,* and *D* from Wright-stained blood films.

sheep, rat, guinea pig, and mouse are smaller (3.2–5.4 fl),and those of the cat larger (15.1 fl) (Prost-Dvojakovic et al., 1975). A recent study (Weiser and Kociba, 1984) reported mean platelet volume of 11.0–18.1 fl for 25 healthy cats. It is believed that in mammals platelet counts vary inversely, but nonlinearly, with platelet volume within and among species (von Behrens, 1972; Levin and Bessman, 1983). Larger platelets are considered metabolically and functionally more active than smaller platelets (Thompson et al., 1982).

Scanning electron microscopic studies have shown that platelets in carefully collected and well preserveed blood characteristically have a discoid or lentiform shape with a fairly smooth surface and slightly biconvex contour (Fig. 16–3). Shallow surface indentations and granularity may be seen on close examination of some platelets (Fig. 16–3*A, B, C*). Surface indentations are presumed to be external openings of the "open canalicular system" ramified within the body of the platelet, and surface granularity probably represents protractions of platelet granules. Surface features of platelets from the dog, cat, horse, cow, sheep, and goat are generally similar (Jain, 1975), although heterogeneity in shape and size is apparent between and within species (Fig. 16–3). Platelets in these species generally measure 1.3–4.7 μm in diameter or length and about 0.5 μm in thickness. A few transformed platelets (those with surface projections or pseudopods) may be found in blood samples of normal animals (Fig. 16–3*F*). Such dendritic platelets often develop within minutes of placing a drop of blood between a slide and coverslip. The surface projections vary in number and size; some may be several times the size of a platelet.

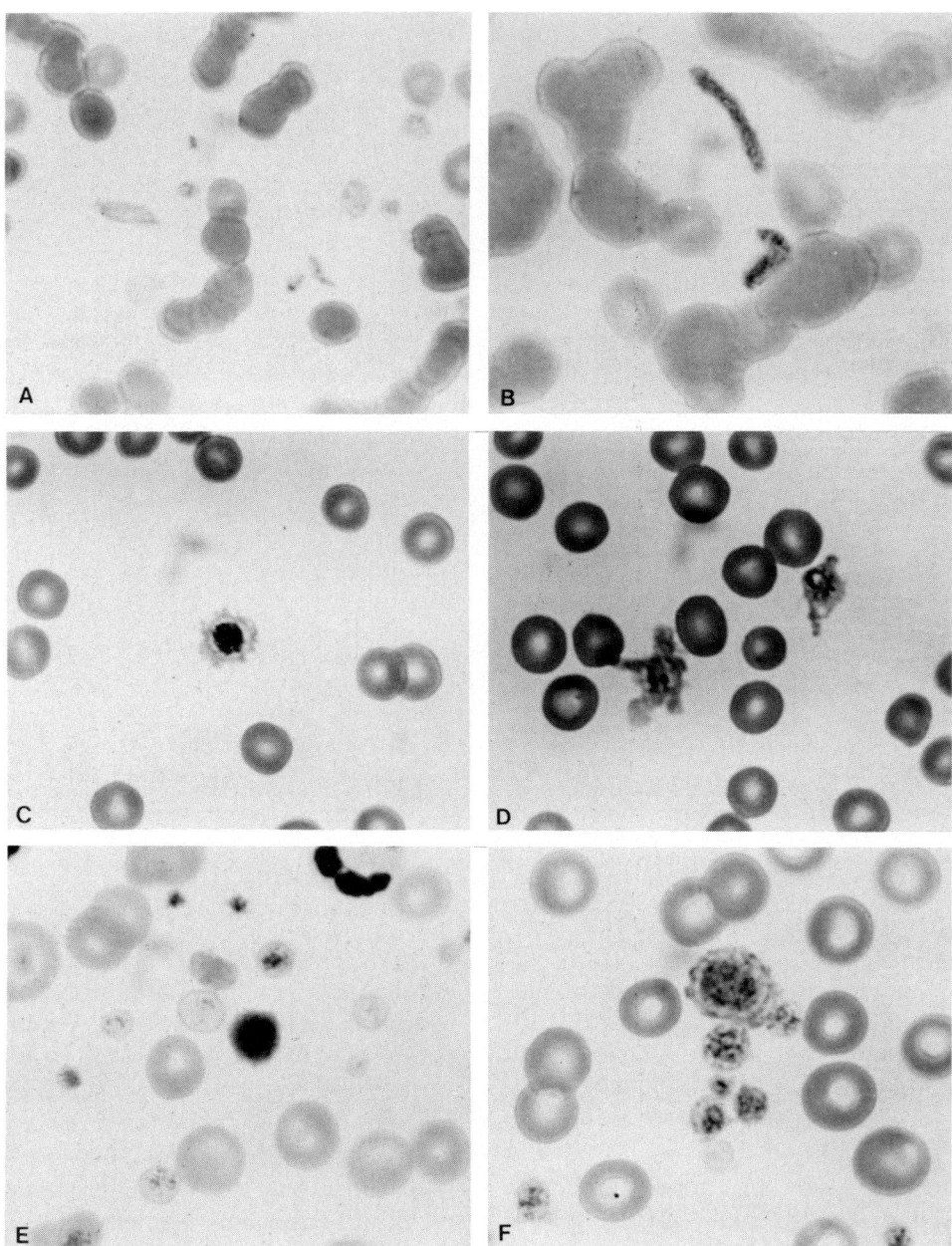

Fig. 16–2. *A,* Pleomorphic filamentous platelets in equine blood. *B,* Filamentous platelets in blood of a thrombocytopenic dog. *C,* A giant platelet with centripetal granularity. *D,* Abnormal giant platelets from a cat with lymphosarcoma. *E,* An excessively granular, several hypogranular, and few small granular platelets in a canine patient with thrombocytosis (platelet count, 824,000/μl of blood). *F,* A megathrombocyte in a canine patient. Wright-stained blood films.

The ultrastructure of platelets (Fig. 16–4) has been extensively investigated, particularly by White and associates (Gerrard and White, 1976; White, 1979, 1981; White and Clawson, 1980, 1981; White and Gerrard, 1976, 1978). The unit membrane of normal platelets is covered with some amorphous material forming a thin (20–50 nm) "external coat." Some fine filaments and a bundle of microtubules are found in the platelet matrix beneath the surface membrane. The internal structure is comprised of a heterogeneous

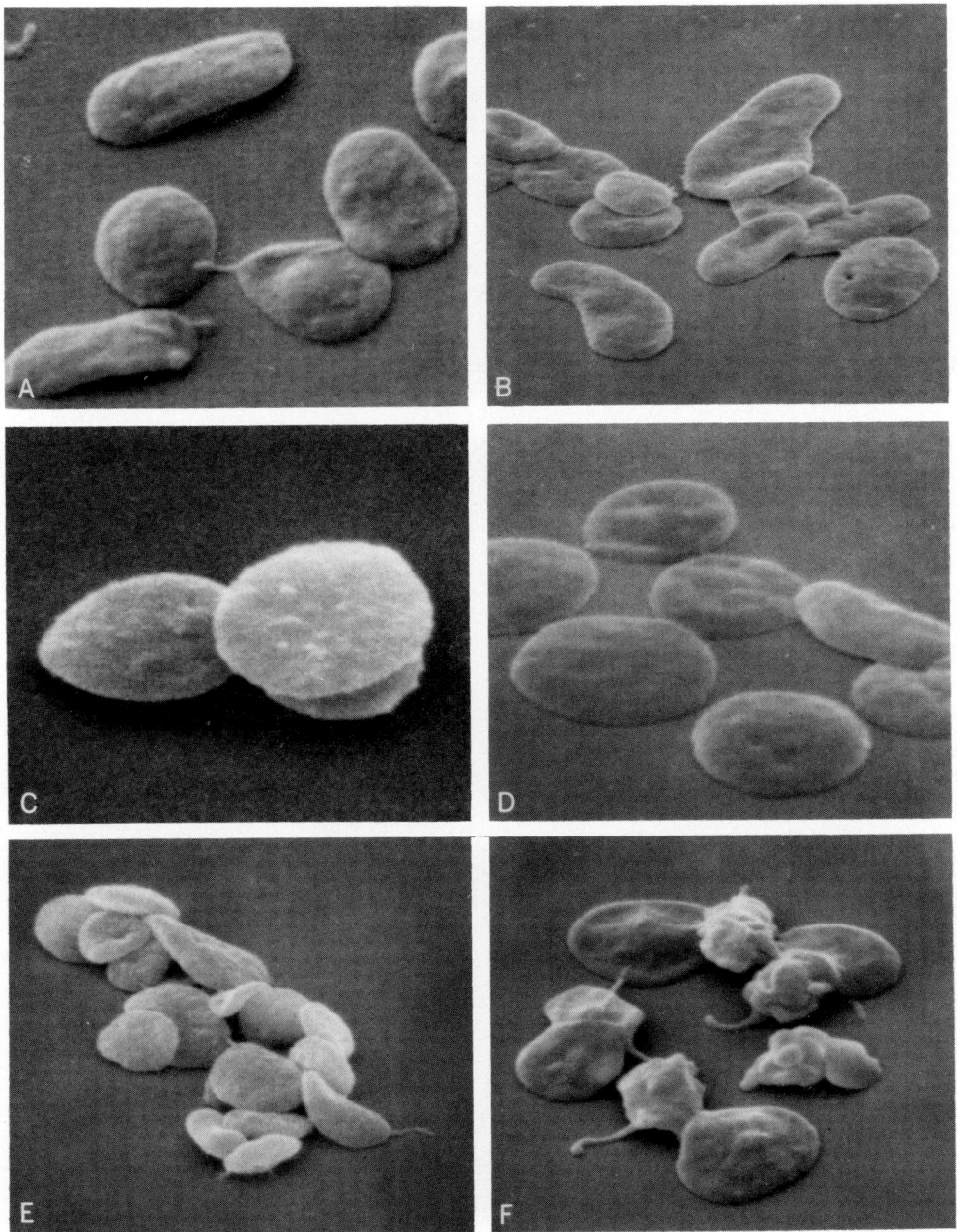

Fig. 16–3. Scanning electron photomicrographs of normal platelets from peripheral blood of various animal species. *A,* Canine platelets depicting discoid, oval and elongated morphology with or without surface projections. *B,* Equine platelets showing prominent pleomorphism, some with clearly visible surface pits. *C,* Uniformly discoid feline platelets with some surface roughness. *D,* Ovine platelets with relatively smooth surface except for some surface depressions. *E,* Bovine platelets of variable shapes and sizes, one having a short thin filament. *F,* Normal canine discoid platelets and activated platelets with centripetal aggregation of internal organelles *(upper left)* comparable to that seen with the light microscope (Fig. 16–2C), many surface buds and long pseudopods. (From Jain, 1975; courtesy of Thrombosis and Haemostasis [Stuttgart].)

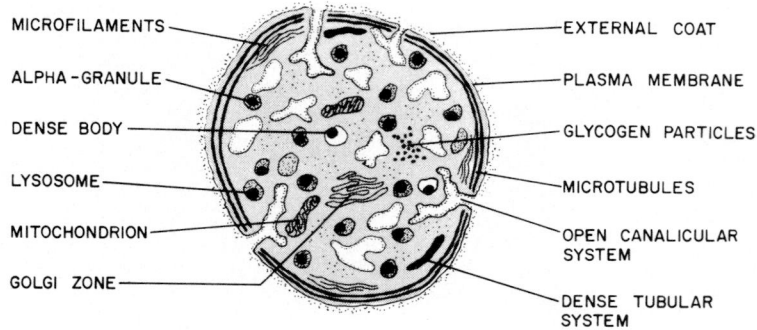

MICROFILAMENTS — EXTERNAL COAT

ALPHA-GRANULE — PLASMA MEMBRANE

DENSE BODY — GLYCOGEN PARTICLES

LYSOSOME — MICROTUBULES

MITOCHONDRION — OPEN CANALICULAR SYSTEM

GOLGI ZONE — DENSE TUBULAR SYSTEM

Fig. 16–4.   A schematic drawing of the ultrastructure of a platelet.

population of granules (alpha-granules), many glycogen particles, some electron-dense bodies (dense granules), and a few mitochondria, lysosomes, and peroxisomes. A poorly developed Golgi apparatus may be seen in a few platelets, while cisternae of smooth or rough endoplasmic reticulum and free ribosomes are rarely found. A sponge-like system of channels, called the "open canalicular system" (OCS) is randomly distributed in the platelet matrix. Channels of this system intercommunicate within the substance of the platelet and open on the platelet surface. Since it is formed by invagination of the platelet membrane, the OCS is lined by the same unit membrane and "exterior coat" that cover the platelet. Another series of channels, the "dense tubular system," is found just under the marginal band of microtubules; seemingly, it does not open on the platelet surface.

Platelets of various mammalian species present generally similar morphologic features (Fig. 16–5). The ultrastructure of equine, bovine, mink, and feline platelets has been described (Meyers et al., 1982b; White et al., 1975). The open canalicular system and dense tubular system were not readily identifiable in resting bovine platelets. The two types of granules, alpha- and dense granules, were found homogeneously distributed, but varied in electron density, number, and size.

Structural and Functional Relationships

The anatomic features of platelets have recently been divided into four structural regions by White (1979) in an attempt to correlate structural and functional aspects of

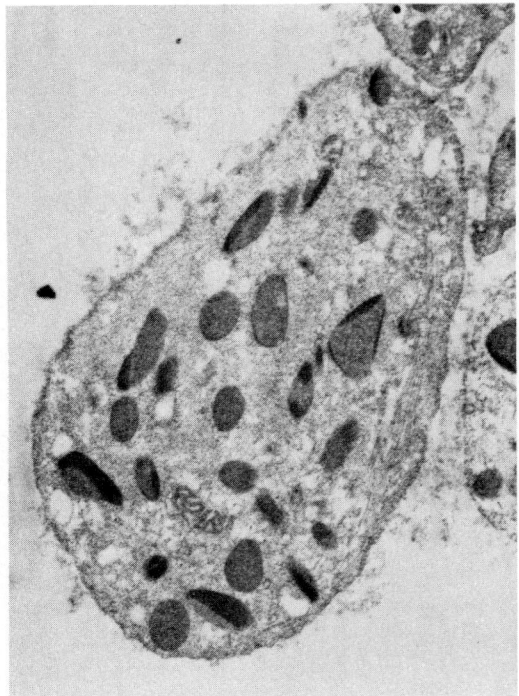

Fig. 16–5.   A transmission electron photomicrograph of a bovine platelet showing prominent granularity, some areas of the open canalicular system, a mitochondrion, and some profiles of microtubules near the surface membrane in the right area.

platelet physiology and pathology. These regions are briefly described below, and their constituents and possible functions are given in Table 16–1.

The *peripheral zone* is composed of the external or exterior coat, the unit membrane, and the submembranous area. This zone maintains platelet integrity and is concerned with reception and transmission of stimuli triggering platelet responses, particularly

Table 16–1.   Constituents and Possible Functions of Some Anatomic Units of Platelets

Anatomic Unit	Constituents	Possible Functions
Exterior coat	Fibrinogen	Platelet aggregation
	Glycoprotein	Platelet adhesion
Unit membrane	Arachidonic acid	Prostaglandin synthesis
	Platelet factor 3 (phospholipid)	Enhances coagulation
	cAMP	Inhibits release reaction
Microtubules	Tubulin	Provides cytoskeleton
		Forms contractile system
Microfilaments	Thrombosthenin	Shape change, clot retraction, release reaction
Alpha-granules	Beta-thromboglobulin	Impedes prostacyclin production by endothelial cells
	Catalase	Unknown
	Factor VIII–related antigen	Platelet adhesion to subendothelium
	Fibrinogen	Platelet aggregation and local coagulation
	Fibronectin	Adherence to extracellular matrix; promotes wound healing
	Growth factor(s)	Mitosis of endothelial and smooth muscle cells and fibroblasts
	High-molecular-weight kininogen	Blood coagulation
	Permeability factor	Increases vascular permeability
	Platelet factor 4	Antiheparin action
	Platelet factor 1	Acts as plasma coagulation factor V
	Thrombospondin	Unknown
Dense bodies	Adenine nucleotides	Platelet metabolism and hemostasis
	Histamine	Increases vascular permeability
	Serotonin	Vasoconstriction and enhancement of platelet aggregation
	Ca^{++}	Platelet stimulation
Lysosomal granules	Acid hydrolases, e.g., acid phosphatase and β-glucuronidase	Proteolysis
Dense tubular system	Ca^{++}	Platelet stimulation
	Enzymes for prostaglandin synthesis	Prostaglandin synthesis
Open canalicular system	Extensive surface area and canaliculi	Route for exocytosis, endocytosis, and phagocytosis
?	Antiplasmin	Inactivate plasmin
?	Epinephrine	Vasoconstriction

adhesion and aggregation reactions. The exterior coat is rich in glycoproteins and so is also known as the glycocalyx. It contains acid mucopolysaccharides and a Mg^{++}-dependent adenosine triphosphatase (ATPase). A number of plasma proteins (e.g., fibrinogen, IgG, and IgM) and coagulation factors (e.g., vitamin K–dependent factors and factors V and VIII) are found adsorbed onto the exterior coat. The glycoproteins provide receptors for agents causing platelet activation and furnish substrates for adhesion and aggregation reactions. At least seven glycoproteins have been identified in mammalian platelets, and some have been found to have functional significance. The glycoprotein Ib is the reaction site for the von Willebrand factor, a component of coagulation factor VIII necessary for platelet adherence to the endothelial surface of an injured vessel wall. Certain platelet defects have been related to a deficiency of one or more glycoproteins.

The unit membrane maintains platelet integrity and is rich in asymmetrically distributed phospholipids. Some platelet phospholipids participate in the coagulation process (e.g., platelet factor 3), and some supply a fatty acid substrate, arachidonic acid, for prostaglandin (PG) synthesis (Fig. 16–6).

The *sol-gel zone* is represented by the matrix of the platelet cytoplasm. Microfilaments in different states of polymerization and micro-

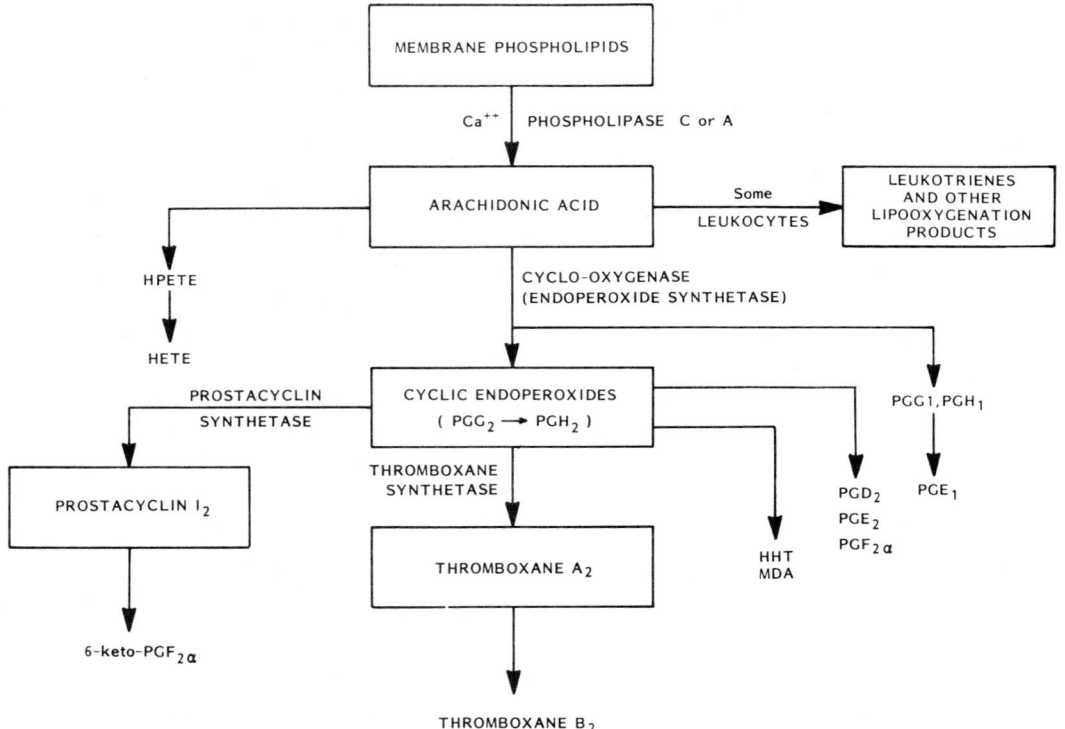

Fig. 16–6.   An outline of arachidonic acid metabolism leading to formation of various prostaglandins and thromboxane B_2. See text for details.

tubules are important structures of this zone. They provide the cytoskeleton for maintenance of normal discoid platelet shape and form a contractile system involved in shape change, pseudopod formation, internal contraction, and secretion of granule contents. Microfilaments are also involved in clot retraction. Thrombosthenin is associated with microfilaments and functions as a contractile protein owing to its actin- and myosin-like components. Microtubules are composed of tubulin and disappear in platelets kept at 4°C or exposed to colchicine and *Vinca* alkaloids, resulting in irregularities in platelet shape (Fig. 16–3F).

The *organelle zone* is composed of all internal structures except components of the sol-gel zone and the membrane system. Platelet granules form an important component of the organelle zone. They show morphologic and biochemical heterogeneity (Bogdanikowa et al., 1976; Kaplan et al., 1979; Giddings et al., 1982). The azurophilic granules seen in platelets in Wright-stained blood films correspond to the alpha-granules seen with the electron

microscope. The alpha-granules are membrane bound, oval or round, moderately electron dense structures. They contain platelet factor 4 (antiheparin), coagulation factor V, fibrinogen, beta-thromboglobulin (a thrombin-sensitive protein), fibronectin, factor VIII–related antigen, and a mitogenic or growth factor. Platelets in von Willebrand disease are deficient in factor VIII–related antigen (Giddings et al., 1982). Electron-dense granules, called delta-granules or dense bodies, contain a nonmetabolic pool of adenosine triphosphate (ATP) and adenosine diphosphate (ADP), Ca^{++}, and many monoamines such as serotonin and histamine. Serotonin is taken up from the plasma. Marked species differences have been reported for dense granule constituents (Meyers et al., 1982c). Lysosomal granules contain acid hydrolases such as acid phosphatase and β-glucoronidase. Specific locations of other platelet constituents remain to be determined (Table 16–1). Contraction of microtubules forces all internal organelles toward the center of the platelet with or without squeezing their contents to the exterior via the open canalicular system. Secretion of various constituents is triggered by platelet activation.

The *membrane system* is composed of the open canalicular system and the dense tubular system. The open canalicular system provides a passage for externalization of platelet secretory products and for internalization of substances from plasma into the platelets (White and Clawson, 1980). The dense tubular system provides a site for sequestration of Ca^{++} and localization of enzymes needed for prostaglandin synthesis. Release of Ca^{++} from this site into the platelet cytoplasm appears to be the key event in platelet aggregation.

Structural Abnormalities

Morphologic alterations such as sphering, budding, and pseudopod formation occur in platelets coming in contact with nonphysiologic surfaces (Fig. 16–1B) or after storage at low temperature (Fig. 16–3F). These alterations are attributed to disintegration and disappearance of microtubules. Exposure of platelets to aggregating agents causes extensive surface and ultrastructural changes. An excellent description of such morphologic changes with illustrations has been published (Allen et al., 1979).

Several hereditary disorders of platelet morphology with specific functional abnormalities have been described in humans (Biagini et al., 1982; Clemetson et al., 1980; White, 1979, 1982; White and Gerrard, 1976, 1978). These defects are associated with abnormal bleeding and are differentiated by various in vitro platelet function tests, by platelet contents, and by ultrastructural morphology. A brief description of features of some of the more common disorders follows. With few exceptions, similar studies on animals have not been reported.

Microthrombocytes are seen in *Wiskott-Aldrich syndrome*, a hereditary disorder of male children characterized by thrombocytopenia and increased susceptibility to infection. These platelets are also deficient in granules, dense bodies, mitochondria, adenine nucleotides, and serotonin; these deficiencies indicate that the defect may arise at the megakaryocyte level. Platelets of patients with

Glanzmann's thrombasthenia (see Hereditary Platelet Disorders in Chapter 17) show defective stickiness or aggregation due to a lack of glycoprotein IIIa and a markedly reduced amount of glycoprotein IIb. These platelets are also deficient in fibrinogen and another protein, α-actinin. Glanzmann's thrombasthenia has been described in dogs (see Chapter 17). The absence of glycoprotein Ib from platelets of patients with *Bernard-Soulier syndrome* has been related to a defective adhesion of platelets to subendothelial surfaces. Glycoprotein I is normal in von Willebrand's disease (discussed in Chapters 14 and 17) and Glanzmann's thrombasthenia. The Bernard-Soulier syndrome is an autosomal recessive bleeding disorder characterized by a mild thrombocytopenia, a prolonged bleeding time, and giant platelets that are not aggregated by ristocetin, human or bovine factor VIII, and bovine fibrinogen. The platelets also lack granules and contain disorganized microtubules. Platelets of patients with "*gray platelet syndrome*" (so named because of peculiar gray staining of their platelets in Wright-stained blood films) are devoid of alpha-granules, and a similar defect is seen in their megakaryocytes (Levy-Toledano et al., 1981). *Hermansky-Pudlak syndrome* is characterized by bleeding diathesis and impaired in vitro platelet function. There is a marked reduction in or an absence of dense bodies, and there are very low levels of serotonin and nonmetabolic pool of adenine nucleotides. In *Chédiak-Higashi syndrome*, platelets show a marked deficiency of storage pool of adenine nucleotides and serotonin. Rarely, platelets may reveal giant granules that are acid-phosphatase-positive (lysosomes) and an absence of dense bodies (White, 1982). In addition to the above, there is a miscellaneous group of hereditary platelet disorders of very rare occurrence.

Many acquired structural, metabolic, and functional defects of platelets have been found in humans with several hematologic abnormalities, particularly myeloproliferative disorders (Maldonado and Pierre, 1975; Pareti et al., 1982; Triplett, 1978; White and Gerrard, 1978; Zeigler et al., 1978). Platelet volume determination provides a means of detecting mega- and microthrombocytes in patient blood (Hunt, 1976; Roper et al., 1977). Megathrombocytes (giant platelets), about the size of a red cell or leukocyte, may be seen in human, canine, and feline blood (Fig. 16–2F). A transient megathrombocytosis was observed in a sick cow and is seen in piglets suffering from advanced neonatal isoimmune thrombocytopenic purpura (Dixon et al., 1980). Platelets age in the circulation by losing membrane fragments (Blajchman et al., 1981), and consequently senescent platelets appear small. Platelet fragmentation resulting in microthrombocytes has been seen in idiopathic autoimmune thrombocytopenia (Zucker-Franklin and Karpatkin, 1977). Platelets of pigs with von Willebrand's disease do not present unusual ultrastructural features (Lewis and Bowie, 1978). Morphologic abnormalities have been reported for platelets of cattle, mink, and cats with Chédiak-Higashi (CH) syndrome (Myers et al., 1982b, 1983; Prieur et al., 1976). Platelets of CH animals were found to be virtually devoid of dense granules and lacked giant granules that are characteristically present in leukocytes of CH animals and humans and considered diagnostic of the syndrome. Some in vitro functional differences in CH platelets were also found which seem to be related to a near absence of storage pool of adenine nucleotide and serotonin and a reduction in divalent cations in these platelets. Ultrastructural abnormalities (formation of vacuoles, pseudopods, and indentations and degranulation) were observed in platelets of cattle infected with East Coast fever (Kimeto, 1976).

PLATELET BIOCHEMISTRY AND METABOLISM

General Biochemistry

Proteins and carbohydrates constitute about 50% and 8.5%, respectively, of the platelet dry weight. The remainder is composed of mostly lipids and other constituents. The chief source of energy is anaerobic glycolysis, although enzymes of the hexose monophosphate pathway and oxidative phosphorylation in mitochondria are present (Reuter and Gross, 1978). The glycogen content of platelets is greater than that in granulocytes

and lymphocytes. A significant decrease in platelet glycogen occurs under the influence of substances that increase the intracellular content of cyclic adenosine monophosphate (cAMP) (Schneider, 1974). Discoid platelets contain a significant amount of cAMP, which regulates platelet activity probably through operation of the Ca^{++} pump. The ATP content of a platelet is about 150 times that of an erythrocyte (Wintrobe et al., 1981), and both ATP and ADP are distributed in metabolic (one-third) and nonmetabolic (two-thirds) pools, with a ratio of ATP:ADP of 3–5:1 and 0.9:1.0 in respective pools. Inducers of shape change and release reaction cause a profound increase in platelet metabolism, oxygen utilization, and glucose oxidation. About 10% of the total platelet protein is secreted during the release reaction. Platelets do not store endoperoxides, prostaglandins or thromboxanes; they are produced from the membrane phospholipids upon stimulation of platelets (Nossel, 1978). Platelets of various species differ in serotonin content (Dodds, 1978); relatively low levels are found in platelets of humans, nonhuman primates, rats, and guinea pigs, medium levels in platelets of dogs and horses, and high levels in platelets of cats. The serotonin content of equine platelets is about twice that of human platelets and their ATP:ADP ratio is greater, although the total content of adenine nucleotide is similar (White et al., 1975).

Glycoproteins of the platelet membrane have been separated by solubilization with the anionic detergent sodium dodecyl sulfate (SDS) and subsequent electrophoresis in polyacrylamide gels (Cierniewski et al., 1976; McMaster and Moelken, 1979; Nurden, 1977; Nurden et al., 1977). At least 7 glycoproteins have been identified and numbered I through VII. Species differences are found in relative rates of migration and abundance of various glycoproteins (Dodds, 1978; Lanillo and Cabezas, 1981; Taylor and Crawford, 1976; Toor et al., 1982). A basic SDS electrophoretic pattern consists of 2 to 4 high-molecular-weight (about 100,000 to 300,000) bands. Human, bovine, canine, porcine, and rabbit platelets contain 3 to 4 major glycoprotein bands, whereas feline platelets have only 2 such bands. Feline platelets lack glycoprotein I band (Nurden et al., 1977). Platelet membrane glycoproteins of dogs with thrombasthenic thrombopathia and von Willebrand's disease were studied, and an abnormality was detected in the former, but not in the latter condition (Raymond and Dodds, 1979). It has been suggested that differences in membrane protein and glycoprotein composition may help explain species differences of in vitro platelet aggregation (Toor et al., 1982). Two heparin-binding proteins have been purified from porcine platelets (Rucinski et al., 1983).

Platelet contractile proteins are actin, myosin, and an actin-binding protein filamin (Phillips et al., 1980; Pollard, 1979). These are located in the platelet membrane, and some myosin may be found in the interior of platelets. The arrangement of actin and myosin in activated platelets suggests that they may act like radially symmetric sarcomeres while pulling together fibrin strands during clot retraction.

Archidonic Acid Metabolism

In recent years arachidonate metabolites have been found to be of considerable significance in hemostasis and thrombosis involving platelet–vessel wall interactions. Several reviews are available concerning this aspect of platelet functions (Halushka et al., 1979; Harlan and Harker, 1981; Malmsten, 1979; Mustard and Kinlough-Rathbone, 1980; Weksler and Goldstein, 1980). Meyers et al. (1980) evaluated comparative aspects of arachidonic acid metabolism in animals and humans. The following brief discussion is derived from a review by Harlan and Harker (1981).

Prostaglandins and thromboxanes are not preformed but are newly synthesized and released from platelets, leukocytes, endothelial cells, and other body cells after appropriate stimulation (Fig. 16–6). Arachidonic acid is liberated from membrane phospholipids of stimulated cells by phospholipase C or phospholipase A. Platelet stimulation is achieved by thrombin, ADP, collagen, epinephrine, and calcium ionophores. Free arachidonic acid is rapidly oxygenated by cyclo-oxygenase to its cyclic endoperoxides, PGG_2 and its reduction product PGH_2, or by lipoxygenase to HPETE and HETE. Cyclo-oxygenase is also involved in conversion of di-homo linoleic

acid, a derivative of arachidonic acid, to PGG_1 and PGH_1, and the former is subsequently converted to PGE_1. Metabolism of arachidonic acid through another pathway in some leukocytes results in production of leukotrienes and lipoxygenation products having important biologic functions. PGG_2 and PGH_2 are nonenzymatically converted to HHT and malondialdehyde (MDA) or to the stable prostaglandins, PGD_2, PGE_2, and $PGF_2\alpha$; PGD_2 is the main product formed in the platelets. The major pathway of PGG_2 and PGH_2 in platelets is conversion to thromboxane A_2 by thromboxane synthetase. Thromboxane A_2 spontaneously hydrolyzes to thromboxane B_2.

The arachidonic acid pathway is characteristic of platelets in general, but considerable differences have been found between and within species (Meyers et al., 1980). Arachidonic acid metabolism is most prominent in human platelets, intermediate in those of the horse, and poorly developed in platelets of miniature pigs, cows, and mink. Individual variations are seen in the behavior of dog and cat platelets in this regard with low to high activity. There are also differences in platelet aggregation responses to arachidonic acid (see Platelet Aggregation and Release Reaction).

Arachidonic acid metabolism in vascular endothelium differs from that in platelets in certain respects. The lipoxygenase pathway is absent, nonenzymatic conversion of cyclic endoperoxidase primarily produces PGE_2, and the thromboxane synthetase pathway is less active, producing small amounts of thromboxane A_2 in some endothelial cells. The major pathway is conversion of cyclic endoperoxides to PGI_2 by prostacyclin synthetase. PGI_2 is very short-lived (half-life, 3 minutes at 37°C) and is hydrolyzed to an inactive stable product, 6-keto-$PGF_{1\alpha}$.

Various functions have been ascribed to arachidonate metabolites, and new roles are being defined. These include the following: HEPTE inhibits thromboxane synthetase, and both HEPTE and HETE are chemotactic for certain leukocytes. MDA cross-links proteins and inhibits certain enzyme activities. Thromboxane A_2 lowers platelet cAMP, causes vasoconstriction, and is the most potent platelet-aggregating agent described. PGG_2 and

PGH$_2$ also cause platelet aggregation. Platelet aggregation by ADP, epinephrine and low concentrations of collagen and thrombin is induced through production of thromboxane A$_2$ and is, therefore, blocked by inhibitors of cyclo-oxygenase and thromboxane synthetase. Aggregation by high concentrations of collagen and thrombin and calcium ionophores does not involve this mechanism. PGI$_2$ acts as a vasodilator and is the most potent platelet antiaggregating agent described. The relative concentration of PGI$_2$ needed to inhibit platelet aggregation varies among species; e.g., sheep and horse platelets are much less sensitive than human platelets (Dodds, 1978). PGI$_2$ acts primarily by increasing cellular levels of cAMP by stimulating adenylate cyclase. PGI$_2$ inhibits platelet adhesion to exposed subendothelium in vitro. The hypothesis that PGI$_2$ is a physiologic inhibitor of platelet adhesion and aggregation in vivo remains to be proven unequivocally.

Arachidonic acid metabolism is negatively influenced by some cellular components, and negative feedback control is also apparent. Increase in intracellular cAMP inhibits phospholipase activity. Blockage of the cyclo-oxygenase pathway by drugs leads to production of large quantities of HPETE and HETE. Oxygen radicals generated during bursts of oxygen consumption associated with endoperoxide production may inactivate cyclo-oxygenase and further substrate metabolism. This may be an important feedback regulator, especially in senescent or aggregated platelets.

A variety of drugs inhibit arachidonic acid metabolism and have proved effective or potentially important in controlling pathologic manifestations of platelet functions. For example, glucocorticoids and anti-inflammatory steroids inhibit phospholipase activity, but are not potent enough to exert antithrombotic action. Most clinically used inhibitors of prostaglandin or thromboxane synthesis inhibit cyclo-oxygenase activity. Aspirin irreversibly inactivates cyclo-oxygenase within minutes in platelets and probably also in bone marrow megakaryocytes. The defect persists for the life of the platelets, while newly formed platelets exhibit cyclo-oxygenase activity. Thus platelet life span can be determined by measurement of MDA activity after administration of aspirin (see Chapter 15). Cyclo-oxygenase active platelets return to the circulation in dogs more rapidly than in humans probably as a result of shorter platelet life span and more rapid turnover rate (Rao et al., 1981). In contrast to aspirin, indomethacin and sulfinpyrazone cause a transient and reversible inhibition of prostaglandin synthesis. Aspirin in low doses given intermittently has negligible action on prostacyclin synthetase activity of the blood vessel wall.

FUNCTIONS OF PLATELETS

The primary function of platelets is to maintain hemostasis. By interacting with endothelial cells, platelets help maintain vascular integrity. Platelets play an important role in blood coagulation by providing platelet phospholipid (platelet factor 3) and by carrying several coagulation factors on their surfaces. Platelets are essential for clot retraction, which is dependent upon their contractile protein system involving thrombosthenin. Other functions of platelets which have been delineated in recent years include their role in thrombosis and embolism, in inflammatory response through activation of chemotactic substances and release of cationic proteins and vasoactive amines, in phagocytosis of small particles and bacteria, and in atherosclerosis. Thus the platelet has come a long way in our understanding, from a mere fragment of megakaryocyte cytoplasm to a biologically important secretory cell that releases a number of proteins with procoagulant, antiheparin, inflammatory, and growth-promoting activities (Guzzo et al., 1980; Zucker, 1980). A brief description of various functions of the platelets follows. The reader is referred to other publications for details (Baldini and Ebbe, 1974; Day, 1976; Gaetano; 1981; Hardisty, 1981; Henry, 1977; Holmsen, 1974; Malmsten, 1979; Mustard and Kinlough-Rathbone, 1980; Salzman, 1976; Silver, 1981; Triplett, 1978; Vermylen et al., 1983; Zucker, 1980). Platelet functions in animals have been reviewed by Dodds (1978). Functional disorders of platelets are described in Chapter 17.

Hemostasis

The main function of platelets is in *hemostasis*. An adequate number of functionally normal platelets is essential to arrest hemorrhage after vascular injury and to prevent diapedesis of red cells from seemingly uninjured vessels. Larger and young platelets are more active in this respect (Blajchman et al., 1981; Harker and Ritchie, 1980; Haver and Gear, 1981; Smith et al., 1982; Thompson et al., 1982). An abnormality of the hemostatic function of platelets characteristically results in increased bleeding time and purpura.

Platelets do not adhere to each other or to capillary endothelium under normal conditions. This lack of adherence is partly attributed to thrombin-triggered production of prostacyclin (PGI$_2$), a powerful inhibitor of platelet adhesion and aggregation, by the normal endothelium, although unequivocal proof for this function of PGI$_2$ in vivo is awaiting. Denudation of capillary endothelium, with exposure of subendothelial collagen, immediately attracts platelets, and triggers them to undergo a series of complex physical and biochemical changes leading to the formation of a hemostatic plug (Fig. 16–7). At first,

platelets undergo a shape change to spiny spheres and then begin to adhere to the site of injury. Platelets also adhere to exposed basement membrane and elastic fibers. Adhesion to collagen in vitro requires Ca^{++} ions and von Willebrand factor (vWF), but Ca^{++} is not required for adhesion to noncollagenous surfaces (Triplett, 1978). Glycoprotein Ib on the platelet surface seems to be the reaction site for von Willebrand factor. Adhesion is followed by release of platelet granule contents. The release reaction promotes aggregation of assembled platelets as well as accumulation of more platelets, and thus a "chain reaction" sets in to form a covering mass to arrest bleeding. Platelet aggregation is a basic response to release of ADP in the presence of Ca^{++}. The ADP comes initially from the injured vessel wall and then from the platelets themselves (Born and Cross, 1963); ATP within the platelets is degraded to ADP by ATPase (Luscher, 1965). Activated platelets also synthesize and release several prostaglandins and thromboxane from arachidonic acid (Fig. 16–6). Thromboxane A$_2$ (TxA$_2$) is the most potent platelet-aggregating agent and inducer of release reaction. The hemostatic process is also assisted by several

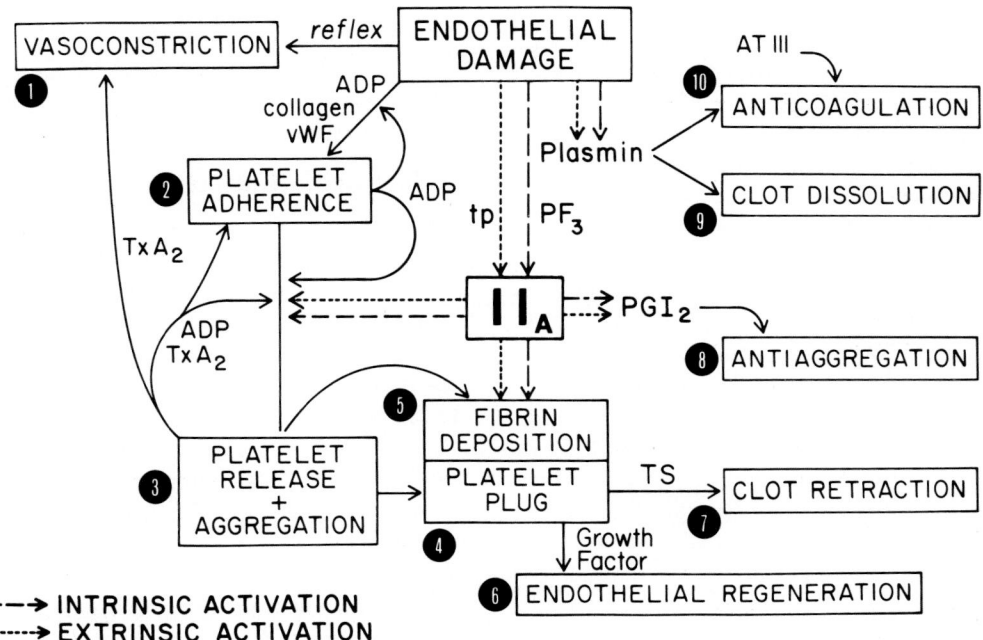

Fig. 16–7. A schematic presentation of a series of complex reactions associated with hemostasis at the site of a vascular injury. See text for details. (Prepared with assistance of Dr. R.J. Slappendel.)

other substances released from the interacting platelets (Day, 1976). Thus there exists a self-contained means of continuing platelet aggregation until an adequate mass has formed over the site of damage to the vessel wall.

Initially the hemostatic plug is of loose construction and incapable of arresting bleeding. Fusion of the platelet mass follows to form a solid plug through the process of viscous metamorphosis brought about by the action of thrombin. Injury to the vessel wall and availability of platelet factor 3 (PF-3) and other platelet coagulants activate the intrinsic system of coagulation at the site of injury. Thromboplastin (tp) released from the injured vessel triggers activation of the extrinsic system of coagulation leading to conversion of prothrombin (coagulation factor II) to thrombin (coagulation factor IIa). In addition to causing viscous fusion of the platelets, thrombin acts on fibrinogen, present on the platelet surfaces, converting it to a lattice of fibrin strands extending throughout the plug. The fibrin strands interconnect the platelet pseudopods. Thrombosthenin (TS) (Luscher, 1965), a contractile protein released from the platelets, further strengthens the hemostatic plug by pulling the fibrin strands taut, thereby producing clot retraction. This same action takes place in blood removed from the body, leading to shrinkage of the clot with separation of serum. Clot retraction requires viable platelets with intact energy metabolism and depends on reaction between ATP and thrombosthenin (Triplett, 1978). In the absence of thrombocytes, separation of serum from the clot does not take place in shed blood. Thus a simple test for thrombocytopenia is the "clot retraction test." Clot retraction is also dependent on fibrinogen concentration. In thrombocytopenia, the blood clot that forms at the site of an injury remains soft or gel-like and is less effective in sealing a damaged vessel. Thus bleeding time may also be prolonged in severe thrombocytopenia. Blood vessel wall abnormalities and functional defects of platelets are also associated with similar abnormalities in hemostasis. See Chapter 14 for further information.

Vascular Integrity

The integrity of capillary endothelium is dependent on an adequate supply of circulating platelets. Petechiae, ecchymoses, and bleeding from body orifices may accompany severe thrombocytopenia. Erythrocytes escape from intact vessels in thrombocytopenic individuals by squeezing through the weakened endothelial cells. A near straight-line relationship is noted between platelet count and bleeding time (Harker and Slichter, 1972). Transfusion of fresh, whole platelets prevents bleeding by contributing support to the endothelium of blood vessels. Incorporation of platelets or platelet material into capillary endothelium was demonstrated in ultrastructural (Johnson et al., 1966) and electron autoradiographic (Johnson, 1971) studies.

Blood Coagulation

Almost all plasma coagulation factors are found in association with platelets. More important, a variety of platelet proteins and lipoproteins, designated platelet factors 1 to 4, play a significant role in blood coagulation (Table 16–1). The best known is PF-3 which acts as an accelerator of the coagulation process. It participates during the interaction of coagulation factors IXa and VIII and of Xa and V to generate thrombin from prothrombin (Fig. 14–3). Platelets can promote proteolytic activation of factor XIII by kallikrein and of factor XI by both factor XII-dependent and factor XII-independent mechanisms (Walsh and Griffin, 1981). See Chapter 14 for additional information on roles of platelets in blood coagulation.

Inflammation and Tissue Damage

Platelets probably play a dual role in the inflammatory response. Release of platelet vasoactive amines and other substances, e.g., prostaglandins, cationic proteins, collagenase, elastase, histamine, serotonin, and a chemotactinogen, may initiate or contribute to an inflammatory response (Nachman and Palley, 1979; Vergaftig, 1976). Some of these factors are tissue damaging as well. For example, platelets have been implicated as mediators of tissue damage in many forms of renal disease (Jorgensen, 1981).

Neutrophils and macrophages at the inflammatory site may promote platelet release reaction (Clark and Klebanoff, 1979; Mencia-Huerta and Benveniste, 1979). The myeloperoxidase-H_2O_2-halide system of activated neutrophils can induce release of platelet constituents at the site of inflammation. A platelet-activating factor elaborated by neutrophils and macrophages has been found to induce platelet aggregation and release reaction.

Platelets were also found to exert some anti-inflammatory effect in studies of acute inflammation in the rat (Smith and Bolam, 1979). Platelets accumulated at the site of intradermal injection of zymosan and carrageen in normal rats, and the inflammatory response was significantly enhanced in thrombocytopenic rats.

Phagocytosis and Bactericidal Property

Chicken thrombocytes were found to phagocytize bacteria (Chang and Hamilton, 1976) and particulate matter (Awadhiya et al., 1980). Human platelets have been found to phagocytize bacteria and latex particles (Clawson and White, 1980; White and Clawson, 1981; Zucker-Franklin, 1981). These materials were found to be internalized through the pre-existing open canalicular system and not by pseudopod formation as in leukocytes. The process appears to be enzyme-dependent but is not accompanied by degranulation, although some release of granular material may occur. Platelets also bind endotoxin, possibly as an intermediate step in detoxification and clearance of endotoxin from plasma (Ausprunk and Das, 1978). Interaction of platelets with bacteria or their products may have serious consequences such as hemorrhage due to thrombocytopenia, disseminated intravascular coagulation (DIC), formation of septic emboli, occlusion of blood vessels, vasculitis, and endothelial necrosis (Clawson and White, 1980; Clawson et al., 1975). Platelets have been shown to play an important role in the pathophysiology of septic shock and in the development of shock-lung syndrome (Myrvold et al., 1977).

Beta-lysin, a thermostable bactericidal component of serum, has been localized in platelets and is secreted during blood coagulation, inflammation, antigen-antibody reactions, and bacteremia (Donaldson and Tew, 1977). It is conjectured that platelet beta-lysin plays a major role in maintaining sterile conditions in the body. Beta-lysin is bactericidal to certain bacteria *(Bacillus subtilis)* and damaging to others *(Escherichia coli)*. It is capable of amplifying the antibody and complement-mediated killing and lysis of gram-negative bacteria. Natural nonspecific immunity of rats to *Listeria monocytogenes* has been partly attributed to a platelet-dependent lysin (Davies et al., 1981).

Based on recently defined platelet functions in host defense, besides hemostasis, it has been suggested (Yankee, 1974) that thrombocytopenic patients may be given a prophylactic platelet transfusion therapy for the following reasons: (1) platelets aggregate bacteria and act as a means to clear bacteria from the circulation by the mononuclear phagocyte system, particularly in granulocytopenic patients; (2) platelets adsorb endotoxin and so are important in preventing and reducing shock in patients with gram-negative sepsis, and (3) platelets maintain tissue integrity of the gastrointestinal tract and thus may prevent entry of organisms into the general circulation.

Thrombosis

The role of platelets in thrombosis is receiving greater attention (Harker, 1976, 1978; Hardisty, 1981). Arterial or white thrombi are composed primarily of platelets because of high shear forces of circulating blood. There is a selective consumption of platelets, but the fibrinogen level remains normal. Such thrombi may be seen in cerebral vascular disease, diabetes mellitus, and renal vascular disease. Selective consumption of platelets can be prevented by inhibitors of platelet function such as dipyridamole and sulfinpyrazone, but not by heparin. Venous or red thrombi involve combined and equivalent consumption of both platelets and fibrinogen. The thrombus is composed of platelets, fibrin, and red cells owing to low shear flow. Such thrombi are found in pulmonary embolism and malignancy-induced deep venous thrombosis. Venous thrombosis may be prevented by heparin or warfarin, but not by drugs inhibiting platelet functions. See Chapter 14 for further information.

Atherosclerosis

Platelets contribute to the development of atherosclerosis by inflicting damage to the vascular endothelium by chemical mediators released after platelet activation and by initiating proliferation of smooth muscle cells in the arterial wall (Weksler and Nachman, 1981). A platelet-derived growth factor has been incriminated in the development of atherosclerotic lesions because of its mitogenic activity for smooth muscles and fibroblasts (reviewed by Harker and Ritchie, 1980; Zucker, 1980). Platelet-derived growth factor is also chemotactic for monocytes and neutrophils (Deuel et al., 1982). Macrophages also contain potent stimulators of mitogenesis for cells such as fibroblasts and smooth muscles (Ross et al., 1979).

Role in Tumor Cell Metastasis

Based on in vitro and in vivo experimental studies, it has been suggested that platelets play a role in the sequestration, adherence, and penetration of tumor cells through vascular endothelium; aggregated platelets prevent rapid clearance of tumor cells from the circulation and allow extravascular formation of nests of cells (Karpatkin and Pearlstein, 1981).

PLATELET AGGREGATION AND RELEASE REACTION

A series of biochemical and morphologic events occurs in platelets after contact with damaged vascular surface in vivo or after exposure to a variety of substances in vitro (Salzman, 1976; Triplett, 1978; White, 1974, 1979, 1981). Four such separable events have been recognized—adhesion, aggregation, contraction, and release reaction or secretion—one or more of which may occur simultaneously or independently depending on stimuli and environmental conditions. Derangement of any one process can lead to a bleeding disorder.

As described earlier, injury to the vascular endothelium initiates adherence of platelets to the site of injury. This stickiness of platelets to nonplatelet surfaces is termed *adhesion.* During this process platelets become spherical and develop dendritic processes as a result of changes in the organization of microtubules and release of intraplatelet Ca^{++}. Adherence of platelet to platelet is called *aggre-*

gation. Primary aggregation from initial activation of platelets is reversible, whereas secondary aggregation induced after the release reaction is irreversible. The *release reaction* (secretion) entails fusion of platelet granules with membranes of the open canalicular system and exocytosis of the granular contents into the canaliculi and thence to the outside. This process is aided by internal *contraction* of microtubules and microfilaments inducing central mobilization of platelet organelles.

A variety of conditions and substances make the platelet membrane stickier, induce platelet adherence to endothelial surface, and cause platelet aggregation and secretion (Day, 1976; Triplett, 1978; White, 1974). Endothelial damage promoting platelet adhesion may occur as a result of numerous factors, both physiologic (e.g., epinephrine) and pathologic (e.g., endotoxin, viral and bacterial infections). Platelet aggregation can be induced in vitro by ADP, epinephrine, collagen, thrombin, serotonin, calcium ionophores, TxA_2, immune complexes, endotoxin, ristocetin, viruses, and a variety of particulate matter. These agents are also capable of inducing platelet aggregation in vivo. In addition, platelet aggregation in vivo most often follows adhesion of platelets to ulcerated surfaces and skin, vascular grafts, and various artificial surfaces (Salzman, 1976). Platelet adhesiveness is increased in sheep with pasteurella infection (Sara et al., 1978). Dietary fats increase platelet aggregation (Renaud, 1975), and lipid phagocytosis by platelets may cause some degranulation (Ulutin, 1975). Azathioprine inhibits platelet aggregation, but not platelet adhesiveness (Bogdanikowa et al., 1976). Nonsteroidal anti-inflammatory agents such as phenylbutazone inhibit ADP-induced aggregation of equine platelets (Johnstone, 1983). Diethylcarbamazine, an anthelmintic, inhibited aggregation of equine platelets by ADP, collagen, and arachidonic acid, but caused a dose-dependent release of serotonin (Kowalski, 1983). A reduction in the intracellular level of cAMP in the platelets is associated with increased platelet aggregation, whereas an increase in the cAMP level has the reverse effect.

Platelet aggregation can be measured in

vitro with an aggregometer, which records the amount of light passing through a suspension of platelets. As platelets aggregate, the turbidity of the suspension decreases, permitting increased light transmittance. This provides a means of evaluating functional defects of platelets (Smith and Bolam, 1979). Platelet aggregation is influenced by the platelet state and by substances used. Two waves of aggregation—primary and secondary—are noticed with human platelets. Both primary and secondary aggregations are induced by ADP, thrombin, and epinephrine in different concentrations and conditions, whereas collagen causes only secondary aggregation. Species variations exist in aggregability of platelets to various agents (reviewed by Dodds, 1978; Manikeri et al., 1980; MacMillan and Sim, 1970; Murphy et al., 1980). Biphasic aggregation of human platelets is characteristically induced by ADP and epinephrine. However, such a response to ADP occurs irregularly in the dog and some monkeys, and high concentration of epinephrine is needed to elicit the effect in the dog. In contrast, most other animal species show monophasic, primary aggregation to ADP and no measurable response to epinephrine. Feline platelets exhibit biphasic aggregation with most aggregating agents. Equine platelets show biphasic response to ADP and serotonin. Platelets from all species respond to collagen. Bird and reptile thrombocytes respond only to thrombin. Responses to arachidonic acid also varied within and among species: platelets of mink, miniature pigs, horses, and cows did not aggregate, and those of dogs and cats showed variable aggregation in comparison to irreversible aggregation of human, guinea pig, and rabbit platelets (Harris et al., 1981; Meyers et al., 1980). Canine platelets are generally less sensitive to aggregation by TxA_2 and endoperoxides than those of other species, but they do undergo shape change (Chignard and Vargabtig, 1977; Harris et al., 1981) and produce TxA_2 upon stimulation (Harris et al., 1982). Breed differences have been reported in aggregability of canine platelets by arachidonic acid with a range of 0 to 100% aggregation (Clemmons and Meyers, 1984).

Abnormalities in platelet aggregation are believed to indicate functional defects of platelets and should be investigated in suspected cases in veterinary medicine. Response of platelets from a "bleeder" horse to collagen was delayed and less vigorous than that of platelets from a normal horse (White et al., 1975). An acquired absence of secondary aggregation wave was found in equine laminitis and positively correlated with severity of clinical signs of the disease (Bell et al., 1979). It has been suggested that the newborn foals may be at risk of platelet-associated hemorrhagic disorders because of less-developed ADP- and collagen-induced aggregability of their platelets, which progressively increases during the first week of life (Clemmons et al., 1984). Platelets of cats with Chédiak-Higashi syndrome showed no abnormality of response to arachidonic acid and serotonin (Meyers et al., 1980). See Chapter 17 for platelet functional defects in Glanzmann's thrombasthenia in pigs and dogs.

Most aggregating agents also induce shape changes in platelets (White and Clawson, 1980). Chilling causes platelets to become dendritic because of disappearance of or failure to form circumferential microtubules. However, platelets resume original shape on rewarming to 37°C. In contrast, shape changes induced by various substances at 37°C are associated with central shift of organelles and are generally irreversible. EDTA-induced spheroidal shape changes are related to alterations in the surface membrane and open canalicular system. Colchicine and Vinca alkaloids cause irreversible disruption of microtubules and result in failure of disc-sphere transformation. Vincristine inhibits platelet function through some mechanism other than disassembling of microtubules but not involving inhibition of prostaglandin synthesis (White and Rao, 1982).

The release reaction is a rapid and active process. Release of material from dense bodies is called release reaction I, while release reaction II is characterized by release of contents from the alpha-granules and lysosomes (Holmsen, 1974). Johnsen et al. (1966) reported that canine platelets are aggregated in vitro and in vivo by endotoxin without release of serotonin or PF-3, while aggregation followed by the release reaction was induced by collagen. Both processes were complement-dependent. Heparin can block the endotoxin-induced aggregation, but not the collagen-induced changes. Aggregation of canine platelets by endotoxin was confirmed in a recent study (Meyers et al., 1982a), but only slight and inconsistent clumping of bovine and equine platelets occurred, even at high endotoxin concentration.

The intracellular transmitter of aggregation and release reaction is Ca^{++}, and the basic reaction is cellular contraction requiring energy in the form of ATP (White, 1979). Aspirin ingestion inhibits the release reaction by blocking generation of thromboxane A_2 through inhibition of cyclo-oxygenase. This effect lasts for the life of the platelets. In comparison, indomethacin and most nonsteroidal anti-inflammatory substances similarly affect the platelet function, but the effect lasts only a few hours. Similarly, phenylbutazone was found to impair equine platelet functions for only 2 hours (Meyers et al., 1979). Dipyridamole interferes with platelet function by inhibiting the release of intracellular Ca^{++} needed for platelet aggregation. Sulfinpyrazone prevents the platelet release reaction by reversible inactivation of cyclo-oxygenase. The latter two drugs are useful in treatment of arterial thrombosis. Some studies on the effects of varous drugs on in vitro aggregation of animal platelets have been reported (Tippett, 1982). See Table 14–14 for additional information.

REFERENCES

Allen, R.D., et al.: Transformation and Motility of Human Platelets: Details of the Shape Change and Release Reaction Observed by Optical and Electron Microscopy. J. Cell. Biol., 83:126, 1979.

Ausprunk, D.H., and Das, J.: Endotoxin-induced Changes in Human Platelet Membranes: Morphologic Evidence. Blood, 51:487, 1978.

Awadhiya, R.P., et al.: Demonstration of the Phagocytic Activity of Chicken Thrombocytes Using Colloidal Carbon. Res. Vet. Sci., 29:120, 1980.

Baldini, M.G., and Ebbe, S.: Platelets: Production, Function, Transfusion and Storage. Grune & Stratton, New York, 1974.

Bell, T., et al.: Alteration of Platelet Function in Equine Laminitis. Fed. Proc., 38:1411, 1979.

Biagini, G., et al.: Platelets in Primary Thrombocythemia: Electron Microscopic Study. Nouv. Rev. Fr., Hematol., 24:19, 1982.

Blajchman, M.A., et al.: Hemostatic Function, Survival, and Membrane Glycoprotein Changes in Young versus Old Rabbit Platelets. J. Clin. Invest., 68:1289, 1981.

Bogdanikowa, B. et al.: The Influnce of Azathioprine on the Behaviour of Blood Platelets in Vitro. Folia Haematol., 103:248, 1976.

Born, G.V.R., and Cross, M.J.: The Aggregation of Blood Platelets. J. Physiol., 168:178, 1963.

Chang, C.F., and Hamilton, P.B.: Phagocytic Properties of Chicken Thrombocytes. Poultry Sci., 55:2018, 1976.

Chignard, M., and Vargabtig, B.B.: Synthesis of Thromboxane A_2 by Nonaggregating Dog Platelets Challenged with Arachidonic Acid or with Prostaglandin H_2. Prostaglandins, 14:222, 1977.

Cierniewski, C., et al.: Glycoproteins of Mammalian Platelet Membranes. Thromb. Haemost., 35:264, 1976.

Clark, R.A., and Klebanoff, S.J.: Myeloperoxidase-Mediated Platelet Release Reaction. J. Clin. Invest., 63:177, 1979.

Clawson, C.C., and White, J.G.: Platelet Interaction with Bacteria: Ultrastructure of Congenital Afibrinogenemic Platelets. Amer. J. Pathol., 98:197, 1980.

Clawson, C.C., et al.: Platelet Interaction with Bacteria. Amer. J. Pathol., 81:411, 1974.

Clemmons, R.M., and Meyers, K.M.: Acquisition and Aggregation of Canine Blood Platelets: Basic Mechanisms of Function and Differences Because of Breed Origin. Amer. J. Vet. Res., 45:137, 1984.

Clemmons, R.M., et al.: Haemostatic Mechanisms of the Newborn Foal: Reduced Platelet Responsiveness. Equine Vet. J., 16:353, 1984.

Clemetson, K.J., et al.: Additional Platelet Membrane Glycoprotein Abnormalities in Glanzmann's Thrombasthenia: A Comparison with Normals by High Resolution Two-Dimensional Polyacrylamide Gel Electrophoresis. Thromb. Res., 18:797, 1980.

Cohen, A.M., et al.: Satellitism of Platelets to Monocytes. Acta Haematol., 64:61, 1980.

Davies, W.A., et al.: Mechanisms for Nonspecific Immunity to Listeria monocytogenes in Rats Mediated by Platelets and the Clotting System. Infect. Immun., 33:477, 1981.

Day, H.J.: Role of Platelets in Hemostasis and Thrombosis. Ser. Haematol., 8:23, 1976.

Deuel, T.F., et al.: Chemotaxis of Monocytes and Neutrophils to Platelet Derived Growh Factor. J. Clin. Invest., 69:1046, 1982.

Dixon, P.M., et al.: Bovine Megathrombocytosis. Vet. Rec., 106:311, 1980.

Dodds, W.J.: Platelet Function in Animals: Species Specific. In Platelets: A Multidisciplinary Approach. G. de Gaetano and S. Garattini, eds. Raven Press, New York, p. 45, 1978.

Donaldson, D.M., and Tew, J.G.: Beta-Lysin of Platelet Origin. Bact. Review, 41:501, 1977.

Gaetano, G. de: Platelets, Prostaglandins and Thrombotic Disorders. Clin. Haematol., 10:297, 1981.

Gerrard, J.M., and White, J.G.: The Structure and Function of Platelets, with Emphasis on Their Contractile Nature. Pathobiol. Ann., 6:31, 1976.

Giddings, J.C., et al.: Immunohistochemical Comparison of Platelet Factor 4 (PF4), Fibronectin (Fn) and Factor VIII Related Antigen (VIIIR:Ag) in Human Platelet Granules. Brit. J. Haematol., 52:79, 1982.

Guzzo, J., et al.: Secreted Platelet Proteins with Antiheparin and Mitogenic Activities in Chronic Renal Failure. J. Lab. Clin. Med., 96:102, 1980.

Halushka, P.V., et al.: Prostaglandins, Thromboxanes,

and Platelet Function. Curr. Top. Hematol., 2:75, 1979.

Hardisty, R.M.: Disorder of Platelets. *In* Postgraduate Haematology, 2nd ed. Edited by A.V. Hoffbrand and S.M. Lewis. William Heinemann Medical Books, London, p. 635, 1981.

Harker, L.A.: Inhibitors of Platelet Function in the Prevention of Arterial Thrombosis. Ser. Haematol., 8:105, 1976.

Harker, L.A.: Platelet Survival Time: Its Measurement and Use. Prog. Hemost. Thromb., 4:321, 1978.

Harker, L.A., and Ritchie, J.L.: The Role of Platelets in Acute Vascular Events. Circulation, 62(suppl. V, pt. II):V13, 1980.

Harker, L.A., and Slichter, S.J.: The Bleeding Time as a Screening List for Evaluation of Platelet Function. New Eng. J. Med., 287:155, 1972.

Harlan, J.M., and Harker, L.A.: Hemostasis, Thrombosis, and Thromboembolic Disorders. The Role of Arachidonic Acid Metabolites in Platelet-Vessel Wall Interactions. Med. Clin. North Amer., 65:855, 1981.

Harris, R.H., et al.: Thromboxane A and the Endoperoxides Mediate Canine Platelet Activation. Thromb. Res., 23:521, 1981.

Harris, R.H., et al.: Endotoxin Interaction with Canine Platelets Fails to Stimulate Thromboxane Production. Proc. Soc. Exp. Biol. Med., 169:397, 1982.

Haver, V.M., and Gear, A.R.L.: Functional Fractionation of Platelets. J. Lab. Clin. Med., 97:187, 1981.

Henry, R.L.: Platelet Function. Semin. Thromb. Hemost., 4:93, 1977.

Holmsen, H.: Are Platelets Shape Change, Aggregation, and Release Reaction Tangible Manifestation of One Basic Platelet Function? Chap. 20. *In* Platelets: Production, Function, Transfusion and Storage. Baldini, M.G., and Ebbe, S., eds. Grune & Stratton, New York, pp. 207–220, 1974.

Hunt, F.A.: A Rapid Method for Assessing Megathrombocytes: Its Application to Thrombocytotic and Acquired Thrombocytopenic States. Pathology, 8:47, 1976.

Jain, N.C.: A Scanning Electron Microscopic Study of Platelets of Certain Animal Species. Thromb. Diath. Haemorr., 33:501, 1975.

Johnson, S.A.: Endothelial Supporting Function of Platelets. Chap. 10. *In* The Circulating Platelet. S.A. Johnson, ed. Academic Press, New York, p. 283, 1971.

Johnson, S.A., et al.: The Function of Platelets: A Review. Transfusion, 6:3, 1966.

Johnstone, I.B.: Comparative Effects of Phenylbutazone, Naproxen and Flunixin Meglumine on Equine Platelet Aggregation and Platelet Factor 3 Availability In Vitro. Can. J. Comp. Med., 46:172, 1983.

Jorgensen, K.A.: Platelets and Renal Disease. Dan. Med. Bull., 28:116, 1981.

Kaplan, K.L., et al.: Platelet and Granule Proteins: Studies on Release and Subcellular Localization. Blood, 53:604, 1979.

Karpatkin, S., and Pearlstein, E.: Role of Platelets in Tumor Cell Metastases. Ann. Intern. Med., 95:636, 1981.

Kimeto, B.A.: Ultrastructure of Blood Platelets in Cattle with East Coast Fever. Amer. J. Vet. Res., 37:443, 1976.

Kowalski, K.A.: Modulation of Equine Platelet Function by Diethylcarbamazine (DEC). Amer. J. Pathol., 113:1, 1983.

Lanillo, M., and Cabezas, J.A.: Isolation, Characterization and Chemical Composition of the Membrane from Sheep Platelets. Biochim. Biophys. Acta, 649:229, 1981.

Levin, J., and Bessman, J.D.: The Inverse Relation between Platelet Volume and Platelet Number: Abnormalities in Disease and Evidence that Platelet Size Does Not Correlate with Platelet Age. J. Lab. Med., 101:295, 1983.

Levy-Toledano, S., et al.: Gray Platelet Syndrome: Alpha-Granule Deficiency. J. Lab. Clin. Med., 98:831, 1981.

Lewis, J.C., and Bowie, F.J.: Ultrastructural Studies of Platelets of von Willebrand and Normal Swine. Lab. Invest., 53:179, 1978.

Luscher, E.F.: Biochemistry of Blood Platelets and Thrombus Formation. Ser. Haematol., 10:76, 1965.

MacMillan, D.C., and Sim, A.K.: A Comparative Study of Platelet Aggregation in Man and Laboratory Animals. Thromb. Diath. Haemorrh., 24:385, 1970.

Maldonado, J.E., and Pierre, R.V.: The Platelets in Preleukemia and Myelomonocytic Leukemia: Ultrastructural Cytochemistry and Cytogenetics. Mayo Clin. Proc., 50:573, 1975.

Malmsten, C.: Prostaglandins, Thromboxanes and Platelets. Brit. J. Haematol., 41:453, 1979.

Manikeri, S.R., et al.: Species Variation in Platelet Function and Blood Coagulation. Indian J. Med. Res., 71:44, 1980.

McMaster, J.F., and Moelken, M.E.: Studies on Human and Bovine Platelet Membrane Glycoproteins. Int. J. Biochem., 10:449, 1979.

Mencia-Huerta, J.M., and Benveniste, J.: Platelet-Activating Factor and Macrophages, I. Evidence for the Release from Rat and Mouse Peritoneal Macrophages and Not from Mastocytes. Eur. J. Immunol., 9:409, 1979.

Meyers, K.M., et al.: Phenylbutazone Inhibition of Equine Platelet Function. Amer. J. Vet. Res., 40:265, 1979.

Meyers, K.M., et al.: An Evaluation of the Arachidonate Pathway of Platelets from Companion and Food-Producing Animals, Mink, and Man. Thromb. Res., 20:13, 1980.

Meyers, K.M., et al.: Binding of ^{125}I-Labeled Endotoxin to Bovine, Canine and Equine Platelets and Endotoxin-Induced Agglutination of Canine Platelets. Amer. J. Vet. Res., 43:1721, 1982a.

Meyers, K.M., et al.: Ultrastructure of Resting and Activated Storage Pool Deficient Platelets from Animals with the Chédiak-Higashi Syndrome. Amer. J. Pathol., 106:364, 1982b.

Meyers, K.M., et al.: Comparative Study of Platelet Dense Granule Constituents. Amer. J. Physiol. Regul. Integr. Comp. Physiol., 12(2):R454, 1982c.

Meyers, K.M., et al.: Serotonin Accumulation in Granules of Storage Pool-Deficient Platelets of Chediak-Higashi Cattle. Amer. J. Physiol., 245:H150, 1983.

Murphy, T.L., et al.: Complement-Dependent Activation of Canine Platelets by Endotoxin and Collagen: In Vitro Studies. Clin. Immunol. Immunopathol., 16:57, 1980.

Mustard, J.F., and Kinlough-Rathbone, R.L.: Prostaglandins and Platelets. Ann. Rev. Med., 31:89, 1980.

Myrvold, H.E., et al.: The Role of Platelets and Fibrinogen in Experimental Septic Shock. Acta Chir. Scand., 143:131, 1977.

Nachman, R.L., and Palley, M.: The Platelet as an Inflammatory Cell. Adv. Inflam. Res., 1:169, 1979.

Nossel, H.L.: Secreted Platelet Proteins. Thromb. Haemost. 40:168, 1978.

Nurden, A.: A Different Organization of Bound Carbohydrate within Cat Platelet Membranes. Thromb. Haemost., 37:358, 1977.

Nurden, A.T., et al.: Comparative Studies on the Glycoprotein Composition of Mammalian Platelets. Comp. Bioch. Physiol., 56B:407, 1977.

Pareti, F.I., et al.: Biochemical and Metabolic Aspects of Platelet Dysfunction in Chronic Myeloproliferative Disorders. Thromb. Haemost., 47:84, 1982.

Payne, C.M.: Platelet Satellitism: An Ultrastructural Study, Amer. J. Pathol., 103:116, 1981.

Phillips, D.R., et al.: Identification of Membrane Proteins Mediating the Interaction of Human Platelets. J. Cell. Biol., 86:77, 1980.

Pollard, T.D.: Platelet Contractile Proteins. Thromb. Haemost., 42:1634, 1979.

Prieur, D.J., et al.: Ultrastructural and Morphometric Studies of Platelets from Cattle with the Chédiak-Higashi Syndrome. Lab. Invest., 35:197, 1976.

Prost-Dvojakovic, R.J, et al.: Study of Platelet Volumes and Diameter in 11 Mammals. In Platelets: Recent Advances in Basic Research and Clinical Aspects. Ulutin, O.N., ed. American Elsevier, New York, p. 30, 1975.

Rao, G.H.R., et al.: Rapid Return of Cyclo-Oxygenase Active Platelets in Dogs after A Single Oral Dose of Aspirin. Prostaglandins, 22:761, 1981.

Raymond, S.L., and Dodds, W.J.: Platelet Membrane Glycoproteins in Normal Dogs and Dogs with Hemostatic Defects. J. Lab. Clin. Med., 93:607, 1979.

Renaud, S.: Modifications of Platelet Functions by Dietary Fats. Adv. Exp. Med. and Biol., 63:264, 1975.

Reuter, H., and Gross, R.: Platelet Metabolism. Thromb. Hemost. Suppl., 63:87, 1978.

Roper, P.R., et al.: Profiles of Platelet Volume Distributions in Normal Individuals and in Patients with Acute Leukemia. Amer. J. Clin. Path., 68:449, 1977.

Ross, R., et al.: Cell Proliferation: Platelet and Macrophage Derived Growth Factor. Adv. Inflam. Res., 1:183, 1979.

Rucinski, B., et al.: Purification of Two Heparin-Binding Proteins from Porcine Platelets and Their Homology with Human Secreted Platelet Proteins. Blood, 61:1072, 1983.

Salzman, E.W.: Some Basic Mechanisms in Platelet Physiology. Ser. Haematol., 8:38, 1976.

Sara, I.S., et al.: Influence of Pasteurella Infection on Platelets, Platelet Adhesiveness, Plasma Clotting Time and Fibrinolysins in Sheep. Indian Vet. J., 55:282, 1978.

Schneider, W.H.G.: Regulation of Energy Metabolism in Human Blood Platelets by Cyclic AMP. Chap. 17. In Platelets: Production, Function, Transfusion and Storage. Baldini, M.G., and Ebbe, S., eds. Grune & Stratton, pp. 177–186, 1974.

Silver, M.J.: Mechanisms of Hemostasis and Therapy of Thrombosis: New Concepts Based On Metabolism of Arachidonic Acid by Platelets and Endothelial Cells. Adv. Pharmacol. Chemother., 18:1, 1981.

Skinnider, L.F., et al.: Platelet Satellitism: An Ultrastructural Study. Amer. J. Hematol., 4:179, 1978.

Smith, J.B., et al.: Platelet Physiology: Facts and Fiction. Prog. Lipid Res., 20:425, 1982.

Smith, M.J.H., and Bolam, J.P.: Anti-inflammatory Effects of Blood Platelets in the Rat. J. Pathol., 129:65, 1979.

Taylor, D.G., and Crawford, N.: Enzymatic and Chemical Analysis of Pig Platelet Membrane Subfractions Isolated by Zonal Centrifugation. Biochem. Biophys. Acta, 436:77, 1976.

Thompson, C.B., et al.: Size Dependent Platelet Subpopulations: Relationship of Platelet Volume to Ultrastructure Enzyme Activity and Function. Brit. J. Haematol., 50:509, 1982.

Tippett, F.E.: Reduction of Aspirin-Induced Inhibition of Collagen Stimulated Aggregation in Platelets of Malignant Hyperthermia Susceptible Pigs (abstract). Fed. Proc., 41:702, 1982.

Toor, B., et al.: Comparison of the Major Membrane Glycoproteins and Proteins of Human, Rabbit and Rat Blood Platelets. Thromb. Res., 26:317, 1982.

Triplett, D.A., ed.: Platelet Function: Laboratory Evaluation and Clinical Application. Amer. Soc. Clin. Pathologists, Chicago, 1978.

Ulutin, O.N.: Platelets: Recent Advances in Basic Research and Clinical Aspects. American Elsevier, New York, 1975.

Vergaftig, B.B.: Platelet and Inflammation. Agents Actions Suppl., 3:75, 1976.

Vermylen, J., et al.: Normal Mechanisms of Platelet Function. Clin. Haematol., 12:107, 1983.

von Behrens, W.E.: Evidence of Phylogenetic Canalization of the Circulating Platelet Mass in Man. Thromb. Diath. Haemorrh., 27:159, 1972.

Walsh, P.N., and Griffin, J.H.: Contribution of Human Platelets to the Protolytic Activation of Blood Coagulation Factors XII and XI. Blood, 57:106, 1981.

Weiser, M.G., and Kociba, G.J.: Platelet Concentration and Platelet Volume in Healthy Cats. Amer. J. Vet. Res., 45:518, 1984.

Weksler, B.B., and Goldstein, I.M.: Prostaglandins: Interactions with Platelets and Polymorphonuclear Leukocytes in Hemostasis and Inflammation. Amer. J. Med., 68:419, 1980.

Weksler, B.B., and Nachman, R.L.: Platelets and Atherosclerosis. Amer. J. Med., 71:331, 1981.

White, J.G.: Physiochemical Dissection of Platelet Structural Physiology. Chap. 22. In Platelets: Production, Function, Transfusion and Storage. Baldini, M.G., and Ebbe, S., eds. Grune & Stratton, New York, pp. 235–252, 1974.

White, J.G.: Current Concepts of Platelet Structure. Amer. J. Clin. Pathol., 71:363, 1979.

White, J.G.: Morphological Studies of Platelets and Platelet Reactions. Vox Sang., (Suppl. 1):8, 1981.

White, J.G.: Membrane Abnormalities in Congenital Disorders of Human Blood Platelets. Prog. Clin. Biol. Res., 97:351, 1982.

White, J.G., and Clawson, C.C.: The Surface Connected Canalicular System of Blood Platelets: A Fenestrated Membrane System. Amer. J. Pathol., 101:353, 1980.

White, J.G., and Clawson, C.C.: Effects of Large Latex Particle Uptake on the Surface Connected Canalicular System of Blood Platelets: A Freeze-Fracture and Cytochemical Study. Ultrastruct. Pathol., 2:277, 1981.

White, J.G., et al.: Platelet Studies in Normal and a Bleeder Horse. In Proc. First Int. Symp. Equine Hematol., Amer. Ass. Equine Pract., p. 209, 1975.

White, J.G., and Gerrard, J.M.: Ultrastructural Features of Abnormal Blood Platelets. Amer. J. Pathol., 83:590, 1976.

White, J.G., and Gerrard, J.M.: The Ultrastructure of Defective Human Platelets. Mol. Cell. Biochem., 21:109, 1978.

White, J.G., and Rao, G.H.R.: Effects of Microtubule Stabilizing Agent on the Response of Platelets to Vincristine. Blood, 60:474, 1982.

White, L.A., Jr., et al.: Platelet Satellitism and Phagocytosis by Neutrophils: Association with Antiplatelet

Antibodies and Lymphoma. Amer. J. Hematol., *4*:313, 1978.

Wintrobe, M.M., et al.: Clinical Hematology. 8th ed. Lea & Febiger, Philadelphia, 1981.

Yankee, R.A.: HL-A Antigens and Platelet Therapy. Chap. 28. *In* Platelets: Production, Function, Transfusion and Storage. Baldini, M.G., and Ebbe, S., eds. Grune & Stratton, New York, pp. 313–326, 1974.

Zeigler, Z., et al.: Microscopic Platelet Size and Morphology in Various Hematologic Disorders. Blood, *51*:479, 1978.

Zucker, M.B.: The Functioning of Blood Platelets. Sci. Amer. *242*:86, 1980.

Zucker-Franklin, D.: Endocytosis by Human Platelets: Metabolic and Freeze-Fracture Studies. J. Cell Biol., *91*:706, 1981.

Zucker-Franklin, D., and Karpatkin, S.: Red Cell and Platelet Fragmentation in Idiopathic Autoimmune Thrombocytopenia. New Eng. J. Med., *297*:517, 1977.

17

Qualitative and Quantitative Disorders of Platelets

QUALITATIVE OR FUNCTIONAL DEFECTS OF PLATELETS   466
Acquired Platelet Functional Disorders   467
Hereditary Platelet Disorders   468

VON WILLEBRAND'S DISEASE   468

QUANTITATIVE DISORDERS OF PLATELETS   469
Thrombocytosis   469
Thrombocythemia   471
Thrombocytopenia   472

Platelet disorders are broadly categorized as qualitative or quantitative. Qualitative or functional disorders include rare hereditary abnormalities like Glanzmann's thrombasthenia and more commonly occurring acquired defects seen in a number of pathologic conditions. Quantitative disorders include thrombocytopenia and thrombocytosis. Thrombocytopenia is by far the most common platelet abnormality encountered, and in fact is probably the most common cause of hemorrhagic diathesis in both humans and animals. Thrombocytosis, whether physiologic or reactive, occurs less freqently. A primary proliferative disorder of megakaryocytes in the bone marrow associated with tremendous thrombocytosis is termed thrombocythemia; it has been reported in humans, but not so far in animals. Abnormalities of platelet number and function may occur simultaneously as in cases of uremia, liver disease, and myeloproliferative disorders such as chronic myelogenous leukemia and thrombocythemia.

Both qualitative and quantitative platelet disorders may also be accompanied by abnormal platelet morphology (see Chapter 16). In some platelet dysfunctions bizarre platelet shape and size are common findings. The finding of such abnormalities in Wright-stained blood films may be the first clue to a disturbance of thrombopoiesis or platelet function. Megathrombocytes usually occur in reactive or compensatory thrombocytoses, and microthrombocytes are found in iron deficiency anemia and sometimes in acute leukemias (Roper et al., 1977). Structural abnormalities of platelets are frequently seen in

myeloproliferative disorders (Triplett, 1978). Giant platelets and platelet anisocytosis, however, may reflect increased thrombopoiesis in response to peripheral demands. Moreover, variations in platelet size and morphology may be found in a variety of diseases and are not necessarily associated with distinct functional abnormalities.

QUALITATIVE OR FUNCTIONAL DEFECTS OF PLATELETS

A number of hereditary and acquired defects of platelet function have been described in humans (Hardisty, 1977, 1983; Montiel, 1979; Morin, 1980; Triplett, 1978; Weinfeld et al., 1975), and some have been found to occur in animals. Such disorders vary in severity, often involve multiple functional abnormalities of platelets, and may stem from extrinsic abnormalities or defects in morphological and biochemical components of the platelets or megakaryocytes. Clinical manifestations referable to platelet dysfunction are generally similar in these disorders of diverse etiology, but pathogenetic mechanisms seem to be varied and largely poorly defined.

A functional platelet disorder may be suspected when an increased tendency to bleed and/or a prolonged bleeding time is observed in the presence of a normal or increased platelet count. Onset early in life and familial occurrence provide clues to a hereditary disorder. Initial evaluation of a patient with bleeding diathesis includes platelet count, examination of blood film for platelet distribution and morphology, bleeding time, prothrombin time, and partial prothrombin time. Further evaluation includes in vitro platelet aggregation tests using adrenalin, collagen, ADP, and ristocetin, and platelet retention tests in glass bead columns; and in vivo platelet adhesion tests. One or more of these platelet functions may be defective in the same patient. Most common demonstrable abnormalities in platelet function are those of aggregation, retention in glass bead column, and platelet factor 3 (PF–3) availability (Kasturi and Saraya, 1978; Morin, 1980).

Acquired Platelet Functional Disorders

Acquired functional disorders of platelets, with or without hemorrhagic manifestations, have been described in persons with a variety of diseases (Cowan, 1982; Malpass and Harker, 1980; Rao and Walsh, 1983). They are seen in renal disease with uremia; liver disease; myeloproliferative and lymphoproliferative disorders; Waldenström's macroglobulinemia and plasma cell myeloma; immunemediated disorders such as autoimmune thrombocytopenia, autoimmune hemolytic anemia, and systemic lupus erythematosus; conditions with circulating fibrin and fibrinogen-split products such as cirrhosis and disseminated intravascular coagulation (DIC); vitamin C deficiency; congenital heart disease; acquired storage pool disease (deficiency of contents of platelet dense bodies); and therapy with certain drugs, particularly nonsteroidal anti-inflammatory drugs, notably aspirin, Major findings in some of the disorders as reported in humans are described briefly below. Similar observations in animals are scarce. An acquired platelet defect, possibly related to defective adenine nucleotide storage pool or prostaglandin-mediated release, was associated with equine laminitis (Bell et al., 1979). Thrombocytosis associated with reduced platelet function was seen in a dog with amyloidosis (Ward, 1982).

Bleeding tendency in human patients with acute or chronic renal failure has long been known. In uremic patients it is ascribed largely to defects in platelet functions, although increased capillary fragility, decreased levels of plasma coagulation factors, and thrombocytopenia may occur (Hardisty, 1977; Jorgensen, 1981). Platelet abnormalities

in a number of patients include reduced in vivo adhesiveness to endothelium and in vitro defects of retention in glass bead columns, aggregation, PF-3 availability, and clot retraction. Abnormalities in bleeding time correlate well with clinical bleeding but not with various in vitro abnormalities of platelet function. These platelet abnormalities also do not seem to be related to the type of renal disease, but some relationship to the level of blood urea nitrogen and duration of uremia has been noted. Peritoneal dialysis or hemodialysis largely reverses these abnormalities within 24 to 48 hours. Urea per se does not seem to be directly detrimental, but its metabolites, guanidinosuccinic acid and phenolic acids, are believed to be involved. Decreased production of prostaglandin endoperoxides by platelets (Remuzzi et al., 1978b) and increased production of prostacyclin (PGI_2), an inhibitor of platelet adhesion and aggregation, by blood vessels (Remuzzi et al., 1978a) of uremic patients are thought to act synergistically and contribute to the bleeding tendency (Rao and Walsh, 1983).

Bleeding in chronic liver disease similarly appears to be multifactorial and poorly defined. The liver is the principal organ concerned with production of most of the procoagulants, and thus it is obvious that a bleeding diathesis would follow a significant decrease in this function of the liver. Additional contributory factors include thrombocytopenia, dysfibrinogenemia, enhanced fibrinolysis, and abnormalities of platelet functions (Rao and Walsh, 1983). Decreased platelet aggregation is seen in liver failure and with increases in fibrin and fibrinogen degradation products in circulation.

Patients with dysproteinemia may show a bleeding disorder as a result of thrombocytopenia as well as platelet dysfunction. Platelets show defective in vitro aggregation, adhesion, and PF-3 availability. It is believed that myeloma proteins and macromolecules such as dextran coat platelet surfaces and result in decreased platelet adhesiveness to connective tissues and defective in vitro aggregation. Both hemostatic and in vitro abnormalities of platelets in dysproteinemias are generally proportional to the amount of paraprotein in the circulation and are largely correctable by plasmapheresis. For further details see reviews by Lackner (1973) and Furie (1982).

Platelet abnormalities in myeloproliferative disorders include defective adhesiveness, aggregation, and availability of PF-3 as well as abnormal morphology (Boneu et al., 1980; Weinfeld et al., 1975; Weiss, 1977). Abnormalities of the coagulation system may also be present in some cases. It has been reported that some human patients, paradoxically, may develop both thrombotic and bleeding complications because of qualitative defects in platelets (Rao and Walsh, 1983).

Hereditary Platelet Disorders

Several hereditary disorders of platelet functions are described in humans (Hardisty, 1977, 1983; Montiel, 1979; Triplett, 1978). Two such disorders reported in animals are considered below. In addition, cats with Chédiak-Higashi (CH) syndrome have abnormal hemostasis with prolonged bleeding time and normal coagulation time. Their platelets show abnormal in vitro aggregation and storage pool deficiency as do platelets of CH mink and cattle (Meyers et al., 1981).

Glanzmann's Thrombasthenia

Glanzmann's thrombasthenia (Glanzmann, 1918) is a rare hemorrhagic disorder occurring in both sexes with autosomal recessive inheritance. It is characterized by greatly prolonged bleeding time in the presence of normal platelet numbers and coagulation factors. Patients show spontaneous purpuric mucosal and cutaneous bleeding, which starts in early life and decreases with advancing age. Bleeding can be controlled by platelet transfusion, while corticosteroids are ineffective.

The platelets appear round and individually distributed in peripheral blood smears. Their ultrastructure is normal. A characteristic finding is the absence of platelet aggregation with ADP, collagen, and thrombin, although shape changes do occur and there is aggregation with ristocetin. Clot retraction and PF-3 availability are also defective. Defective platelet aggregation is probably responsible for the prolonged bleeding time. The platelet dysfunction is attributed largely to absence of membrane glycoproteins IIb and IIIa and partly to lack of receptors for fibrinogen. Some metabolic abnormalities of platelets have also been found (Caen et al., 1977; Triplett, 1978), but their significance is unknown.

A hereditary disorder resembling Glanzmann's thrombasthenia has been described in dogs (Dodds, 1967, 1970). Platelet life span in these animals is reduced (4 days) or normal (7 days) (Dodds et al., 1972).

Hereditary Thrombopathia in the Basset Hound

A hereditary thrombopathia with autosomal inheritance pattern and markedly abnormal platelet function was described in basset hounds (Bell et al., 1982; Lotz et al., 1972). In 11 affected dogs studied recently (Bell et al., 1982), the rate and extent of ADP and collagen aggregation was significantly depressed. Plasma from affected dogs did not alter in vitro functions of normal platelets, whereas platelets of affected dogs behaved abnormally even in normal plasma. Bleeding time was variable (4.9 ± 4.9 minutes) and slightly prolonged compared to normal (1.5 ± 0.8 minutes). Clot retraction was normal, and there was no detectable platelet glycoprotein abnormality.

VON WILLEBRAND'S DISEASE

Von Willebrand's disease (vWD) is a hereditary bleeding disorder characterized by prolonged bleeding time but normal clot retraction time. It is a result of quantitative and qualitative abnormalities of von Willebrand's factor associated with factor VIII–related antigen (VIII:RAg), normally present in plasma. Although vWD is not a platelet defect per se, it is described here because it is similar to hereditary platelet defects. The VIII:RAg in plasma is believed to occur as a complex with factor VIII procoagulant protein and is essential for platelet-vessel wall interaction during normal hemostasis. Thus characteristic findings in vWD are decreased adherence of platelets to injured vessel walls and to glass beads, and defective ristocetin-induced platelet aggregation in patient's plasma. A number of variants or subtypes of vWD in humans

Table 17–1.   Normal Platelet Numbers in Various Animals

Animal Species	Platelet Count/μl of Blood	
	Range	Mean
Dog	200,000–500,000	300,000
Cat	300,000–800,000	450,000
Cow	100,000–800,000	500,000
Sheep	250,000–750,000	400,000
Goat	300,000–600,000	450,000
Horse	100,000–350,000	225,000
Pig	100,000–900,000	520,000

have been recognized in recent years (Triplett, 1978; Zimmerman and Ruggeri, 1983).

Von Willebrand's disease has been found to occur in Poland-China pigs (Hogan et al., 1941) and dogs (Dodds, 1970). Two forms of vWD have been recognized in the dog (R.J. Slappendal, personal communication). A colony of pigs with this disorder has been raised (Bowie et al., 1975a). The mode of inheritance is autosomal. Affected pigs develop purpuric lesions and bleed spontaneously from the nasopharynx and intestinal mucosa. The platelets show abnormalities of adhesiveness; other laboratory findings are similar to those found in human vWD, but also include abnormal viscous metamorphosis (Kahn et al., 1970). That the VIII:RAg may also contribute to pathogenesis of thrombosis and atherosclerosis was indicated by observations that pigs with vWD fail to develop atherosclerosis as rapidly as normal pigs and by the finding of significantly less platelet spreading and activation on injured vessel walls in vWD swine (Reddick et al., 1982). For additional comments on vWD see Chapter 14.

QUANTITATIVE DISORDERS OF PLATELETS

Platelet counts vary among species (Table 17–1). Platelet counts in small laboratory animals exceed 1 million/μl of blood, whereas in domestic animals they are generally below 1 million. For further details see information given on platelets of different species in Chapters 4 through 12 and in a report by Maupin (1978).

Thrombocytosis

An increase in platelet count beyond the normal range is referred to as thrombocytosis.

The increase is usually modest, transient, and asymptomatic, but in some cases substantially higher platelet counts may be encountered that may endanger life because of thromboembolism. *Physiologic thrombocytosis* results from increased mobilization of platelets from splenic as well as nonsplenic body pools. The nonsplenic (largely pulmonary) pool is mobilized during mild exercise, whereas epinephrine injection or release mobilizes the splenic pool. Platelets from both pools are mobilized during vigorous exercise. Species variations may be found in this regard. For example, a 10-minute exercise caused no significant changes in platelet counts in ponies (Lepherd, 1977). *"Reactive"* thrombocytosis is seen in association with a variety of conditions including hemorrhage (especially chronic), trauma, fractures, surgery, splenectomy and asplenic or hyposplenic state, acute or chronic infections, inflammatory conditions, malignancies, iron deficiency, Cushing's disease, and therapy with glucocorticoids and *Vinca* alkaloids (Tables 17–2, 17–3). It has been stated that the finding of an unexplained thrombocytosis should suggest the possibility of an occult malignancy (Triplett, 1978). In reactive thrombocytosis, megakaryocyte number is increased in the bone marrow, and the platelet count is directly proportional to the megakaryocytic mass and indirectly to the mean megakaryocyte volume (Wintrobe et al., 1981).

Thrombocytosis is also seen in primary diseases of the bone marrow, e.g., myeloproliferative disorders such as essential thrombocythemia (see below), polycythemia vera, and chronic myelogenous leukemia (Murphy, 1983).

Platelet counts following splenectomy in humans increase in 2–10 days, peak after 2 weeks, and gradually subside in 2–3 months (Triplett, 1978). A similar pattern, but with an earlier peak may be seen in the dog (Table 17–3). The increase in platelet number is attributed to the absence of a spleen-derived inhibitory factor in blood (see Chapter 15). Thrombocytosis following acute blood loss occurs after about 36 hours, and that following major surgery occurs between 3 and 10 days, with a return to normal platelet numbers in about 2 weeks. A "rebound" throm-

Table 17–2. Selected Examples of Thrombocytosis in the Dog, Cat, and Horse

Animal	Platelet Count/μl of Blood	Clinical Diagnosis or Finding
Dog	200,000–500,000	Normal range
	2,073,000	Vincristine and immunosuppressive therapy for autoimmune thrombocytopenia
	1,988,000	Suppurative bronchitis and enteritis
	1,148,000	Iron deficiency anemia
	828,000	Iron deficiency anemia
	755,000	Cushing's disease
	738,000	Squamous cell carcinoma
	737,000	Adenocarcinoma
	713,000	Prednisolone and immunosuppressive therapy for autoimmune hemolytic anemia
	673,000	Mastocytoma
	618,000	Nasal trauma
	613,000	Chronic inflammation/infection
Cat	300,000–800,000	Normal range
	2,046,000	Lymphocytic leukemia
	1,470,000	Anemia and bleeding disorder
	1,432,000	Mast cell sarcoma
	1,378,000	Myelogenous leukemia
	1,256,000	Myeloproliferative disorder
	1,163,000	Six days posttherapy for thrombocytopenia
	876,000	Erythremic myelosis
	872,000	Lymphocytic leukemia
Horse	100,000–350,000	Normal range
	632,000	Pleuritis
	611,000	Foal pneumonia
	510,000	Fluctuating temperature
	474,000	Combined immune deficiency
	472,000	CNS ataxia, abscess
	450,000	Strangles
	405,000	Pleuritis; heparin therapy for DIC

Table 17–3. An Example of Postsplenectomy Thrombocytosis in a Dog with an Idiopathic Anemia

Status	Platelet Count/μl of Blood
Presplenectomy	377,000
Postsplenectomy	
2 days	1,197,000
5 days	1,395,000
12 days	1,305,000
26 days	1,061,000
40 days	617,000

bocytosis also occurs during the recovery phase of thrombocytopenia. In humans, mild iron deficiency of short duration is associated with thrombocytosis, while a profound iron deficiency is accompanied by thrombocytopenia (see Chapter 15). The cause of this dichotomous relationship of iron with platelet numbers remains to be determined. Iron supplementation is associated with a quick (within 7–10 days) normalization of platelet counts (Murphy, 1983). Thrombocytosis, but not thrombocytopenia, has been observed in dogs with iron deficiency anemia. Therapy

with *Vinca* alkaloids such as vincristine is associated with increased thrombopoiesis (Jain and Switzer, 1981; Greene et al., 1982) and occasionally thrombocytosis of considerable magnitude. We have seen platelet counts of more than 1 million in several dogs and more than 2 million in two dogs treated with vincristine for immune-mediated thrombocytopenia. Thromboembolism may occur as a fatal complication in some such patients.

Selected examples of thrombocytosis are given for the dog, cat, and horse (Table 17–2). In these species, a mild thrombocytosis is more prevalent than marked increases in platelet numbers as shown in Figure 17–1 for the dog. Some canine patients receiving a combination of cytotoxic drugs and corticosteroids for control of neoplasia may develop thrombocytosis. A dog so treated for lymphosarcoma exhibited the following platelet numbers: August 28 (pretreatment), 320,000; September 24, 652,000; and October 8, 870,000. Such elevations of circulating platelet numbers may be a consequence of combined

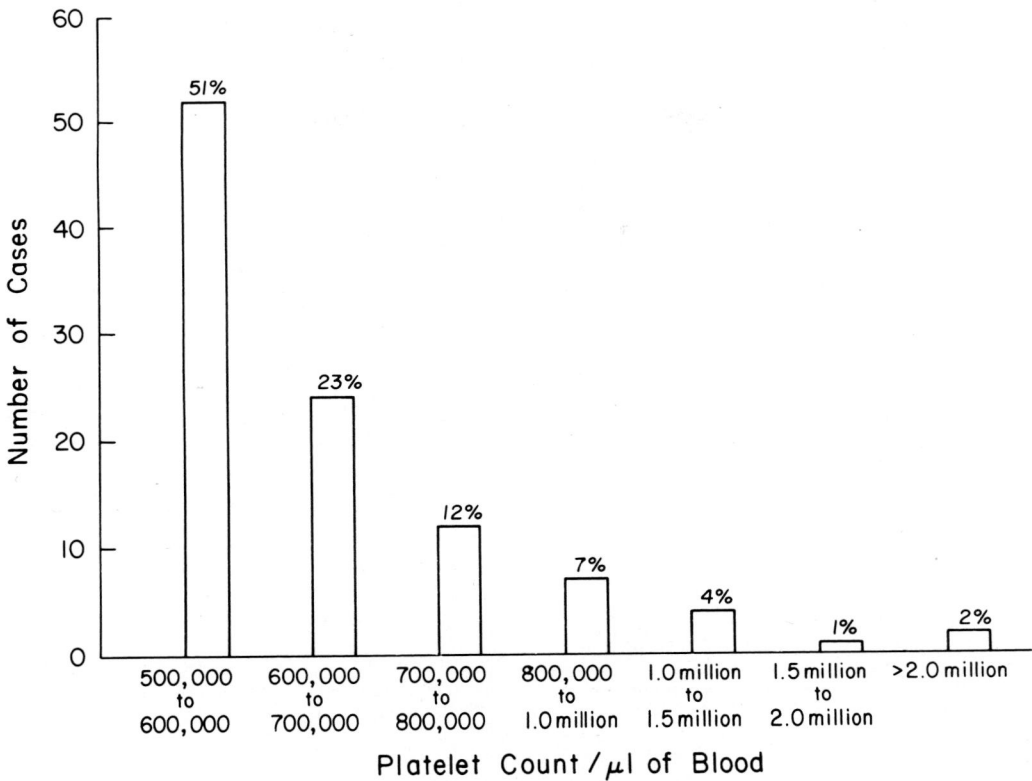

Fig. 17–1. Distribution of canine patients with various levels of thrombocytosis. Percentages of patients in each category are shown above the bar graphs.

effects of depression of splenic function (hyposplenism) and stimulation of megakaryocytopoiesis. Other signs of depressed splenic activity in some dogs on cytotoxic drugs and corticosteroids are the occurrence in the circulation of numerous Howell-Jolly bodies and, less frequently, of nucleated erythrocytes. The presence in peripheral blood of erythrocytes containing these nuclear structures, especially in the absence of anemia in remission, suggests loss of "pitting" function of the spleen. Accompanying this loss of function, there may be a reduction of potential of the spleen for retaining thrombocytes.

Thrombocythemia

A hemorrhagic syndrome associated with marked increase in circulating platelets resulting from "autonomous" overproduction of megakaryocytes is called thrombocythemia (Harker, 1970). The abnormal proliferation of marrow megakaryocytes categorizes the dis-

ease as a myeloproliferative disorder. The disorder has also been called essential thrombocythemia or megakaryocytic leukemia. Essential thrombocythemia is primarily seen in humans, although some cases of megakaryocytic leukemia have been reported in the cat and dog (see Chapter 32). Recently, thrombocythemia has been shown to be a clonal disorder originating from a pluripotent hematopoietic stem cell (Failkow et al., 1981). The disease is characterized in humans by recurrent spontaneous hemorrhages, purpura, epistaxis, gastrointestinal bleeding, splenomegaly, thromboembolic episodes, pseudohyperkalemia, and, at times, infarction atrophy of the spleen. Abnormalities of platelet morphology and function are also present. If anemia is present, it is microcytic hypochromic. Circulating platelet numbers are persistently elevated and exceed 1 million/μl of blood. The platelet count is unrelated to megakaryocyte volume, and megakaryocyte size is not decreased as in reactive thrombocytosis

Table 17–4.   Pathophysiologic Classification of Thrombocytopenia

A.   Decreased platelet production
   1.   Hereditary
   2.   Acquired: Drug toxicity; x-irradiation; mycotoxins; viral, rickettsial, and protozoan infections
   3.   Dysthrombopoiesis: Vitamin B_{12} or folate deficiency; uremia; myeloproliferative disorders; myelophthisis; aplastic anemia; severe iron deficiency; protozoan parasites
   4.   Defective thrombopoietin production
   5.   Miscellaneous

B.   Accelerated platelet destruction or utilization
   1.   Immune-mediated: Autoimmune, isoimmune, or neonatal; in association with other immune-mediated disorders; bacterial, viral, rickettsial, or protozoan infections; drug-induced; other causes
   2.   Nonimmune mechanisms: Anaphylaxis; DIC; microangiopathies; acute infections
   3.   Structural defects of platelets: Glanzmann's thrombasthenia; other hereditary or acquired defects

C.   Abnormal distribution
      Splenomegaly; hypothermia

D.   Excessive loss from blood
      Massive blood loss; exchange blood transfusion

(Wintrobe et al., 1981). The abnormal bleeding is associated with both increase in the platelet mass and functional defects of platelets. The bleeding may cease when platelet counts are reduced to normal (Triplett, 1978). Splenectomy is contraindicated; removal of the spleen leads to an even greater increase in platelet numbers and an intensification of bleeding episodes (Gunz, 1960). Therapy is directed toward reducing the platelet count by thrombocytopheresis, irradiation, and use of alkylating and antimitotic drugs. In a report of six human patients with primary thrombocythemia, erythrocyte and leukocyte numbers were elevated as well, and one of the patients died with acute myeloblastic leukemia (Ozer et al., 1960).

Thrombocytopenia

A reduction in the number of circulating platelets below the minimum normal level for the species is called thrombocytopenia. Pathophysiologic mechanisms of thrombocytopenia include decreased production, accelerated destruction or utilization, abnormal distribution, and excessive loss of platelets (Table 17–4). The first two are more common, and sometimes more than one mechanism

may be involved. Hence, in addition to platelet counts, bone marrow examination is important in diagnosis, particularly to distinguish between hypoproliferative and hyperdestructive causes of thrombocytopenia. In human studies such a distinction in some cases has also been made possible through correlations of platelet counts and mean platelet volumes (Gardner and Bessman, 1983). Low platelet counts may also be artifactual, resulting from in vitro clumping of platelets as reported for porcine (Ragan, 1972) and human (Baele et al., 1978) bloods anticoagulated with EDTA. Selected examples of thrombocytopenia are given for the dog, cat, and horse (Tables 17–5, 17–6, 17–7). Distribution of platelet counts in thrombocytopenia in the dog is shown in Figure 17–2. Specific instances and reports of thrombocytopenia in different species are summarized in the last section of this chapter.

Thrombocytopenia may be a primary or secondary abnormality depending on whether it is the principal finding (primary) or is associated with other conditions (secondary). It may have an acute onset or follow a chronic course. Idiopathic thrombocytopenic purpura (ITP) is defined as thrombocytopenia associated with purpuric lesions in the absence of a defined cause and with normal or increased numbers of megakaryocytes in the bone marrow. Acute ITP is common in children and usually resolves spontaneously, whereas chronic ITP predominates in adults and is rarely self-limiting. Such an age-related pattern of thrombocytopenia for young animals has not been observed. A compensated thrombocytopenic state exists when there is an increase in platelet destruction but platelet counts are within the normal range. This may be seen in cirrhosis, systemic lupus erythematosus (SLE), chronic DIC, and acute febrile illness.

Decreased platelet production may involve marrow hypoplasia, ineffective thrombopoiesis, and, very rarely, thrombopoietin deficiency. Platelet life span is usually normal or may be modestly decreased in such cases. Common causes of marrow hypoplasia are marrow damage by a variety of drugs, chemicals, or x-irradiation. Estrogen toxicity is a classical example in the dog (see Exogenous

Table 17-5. Selected Examples of Thrombocytopenia in the Dog, Cat, and Horse

Animal	Platelet Count/μl of Blood	Clinical Diagnosis or Finding
Dog	200,000–500,000	Normal range
	5,000	Estrogen toxicity
	6,000	Ehrlichiosis
	7,000	Autoimmune thrombocytopenia
	21,000	Myelogenous leukemia
	34,000	Autoimmune thrombocytopenia
	40,000	Splenomegaly
	47,000	Hemangiosarcoma
	64,000	Acute exacerbation of chronic hepatopathy
	102,000	Lymphosarcoma
	131,000	Addison's disease
	170,000	Autoimmune hemolytic anemia and thrombocytopenia
Cat	300,00–800,000	Normal range
	26,000	Feline leukemia virus infection
	51,000	Myelomonocytic leukemia
	101,000	Lymphosarcoma
	131,000	Autoimmune hemolytic anemia
	139,000	Squamous cell carcinoma
	160,000	Septicemia
	174,000	Erythremic myelosis
	188,000	DIC
Horse	100,000–350,000	Normal range
	11,000	Autoimmune hemolytic anemia
	12,000	Myelogenous leukemia
	19,000	Anemia associated with marrow hypoplasia
	31,000	DIC
	69,000	Salmonellosis with DIC
	53,000	Equine infectious anemia
	56,000	Ehrlichiosis
	61,000	Epistaxis
	88,000	Septicemia

Estrogen as a Cause of Thrombocytopenia). Marrow hypoplasia may also be seen in myelophthisis, aplastic anemia, and certain viral infections. Thrombocytopenia generally appears first and persists longer than the decrease in other hematopoietic cell lines. In thrombocytopenia due to ineffective thrombopoiesis, by contrast, there is increased megakaryocyte mass in the marrow, but decreased platelet production. This kind of thrombocytopenia is seen in humans in megaloblastic anemias of vitamin B_{12} and folate deficiencies, in myeloproliferative disorders, and sometimes in iron deficiency.

Increased platelet destruction or utilization as a mechanism of thrombocytopenia may involve an immunologic or nonimmunologic process. This subject was reviewed in the April and July 1982 issues of *Seminars in Thrombosis and Hemostasis*. Platelet survival is markedly reduced in such cases, while megakaryocytopoiesis is increased in some cases but diminished in others. Immune-mediated thrombocytopenia may be due to sensitiza-

tion of platelets by IgG, complement, or immune complexes and removal of such platelets by cells of the mononuclear phagocyte (reticuloendothelial) system (Karpatkin, 1983). Formation of autoantibody to platelets may occur for unknown reasons (idiopathic), or it may be secondary to a primary disease or drug therapy. In some situations, antiplatelet antibody may be detected without accompanying thrombocytopenia. Transfer of maternal antiplatelet antibodies to the fetus or newborn results in isoimmune thrombocytopenia. Nonimmunologic thrombocytopenia may be associated with bacterial or viral infections, uremia, transfusion of stored blood, cirrhosis, DIC, and various microangiopathic processes. Thrombocytopenia is an early manifestation of most septicemic bacterial and viral infections. Bacterial infection causes consumptive thrombocytopenia via induction of DIC, direct interaction with platelets, and platelet binding to vascular endothelium damaged by bacterial action (Wilson et al., 1982; Corrigan, 1977). It may also in-

Table 17–6.   Selected Data from Sequential Hemograms on a Dog with Autoimmune Hemolytic Anemia and Thrombocytopenia

Hemogram No.	Date	PCV (%)	MCV (fl)	Total Plasma Proteins (g/dl)	Reticulo- cytes (%)	WBC/μl	Thrombo- cytes/μl
1.	12-16-68[a]	23	117.0	6.5	36.0	25,550	38,000
2.	12-30-68	41	76.2	6.9	—	10,300	9,000
3.	1- 2-69	47	75.9	7.5	—	42,000	<1,000
4.	1- 6-69	44	70.9	7.5	—	18,700	13,000
5.	1- 8-69	42	69.3	7.1	—	20,400	<1,000
6.	1- 9-69	42	72.4	6.6	—	30,700	14,000
7.	1-13-69	38	70.0	7.5	—	16,500	5,000
8.	1-15-69	38	68.7	7.4	—	7,100	7,000
9.	1-17-69	38	67.4	7.4	—	14,200	10,000
10.	1-20-69	44	69.6	7.5	—	11,000	17,000
11.	1-24-69	43	67.8	6.9	—	10,800	2,000
12.	1-29-69	40	65.0	7.2	—	12,000	3,000
13.	2-22-69	33	60.3	7.0	6.0	14,100	5,000
14.	3-17-69[a]	10	113.6	4.5	30.5	42,200	4,000
15.	3-26-69	31	72.6	7.3	0.8	30,000	1,630,000
16.	4- 2-69	33	72.7	7.4	5.0	14,000	189,000
17.	4- 7-69	34	78.7	6.8	9.0	22,800	92,000
18.	4-14-69	35	75.3	7.5	rare	24,000	420,000
19.	4-22-69	35	75.0	8.0	rare	14,000	68,000
20.	4-28-69	36	72.6	8.0	0.8	13,700	78,000
21.	5- 6-69	41	73.5	8.3	0.8	14,600	24,000
22.	5-12-69	39	71.7	8.2	2.0	15,200	46,000
23.	9-23-69	48	75.5	8.0	6.0	9,400	9,000
24.	11-24-69	17	114.1	8.5	36.2	53,200	5,000
25.	12- 1-69	25	87.4	6.7	18.6	29,400	409,000
26.	2- 6-70	13	97.7	7.6	30.4	56,200	59,000
27.	2- 9-70	18	98.9	7.2	50.5	21,100	120,000
28.	2-12-70	23	83.3	7.7	15.8	22,300	125,000
29.	5-11-70	32	70.6	8.1	6.4	18,800	85,000

From Schalm and Ling, 1971; courtesy of *The California Veterinarian*.
[a]Period of no treatment December 16 to March 17, 1969.

Table 17–7.   Examples of Thrombocytopenia of Various Etiologies and Results of Therapy in the Dog

No.	Breed	Sex	Age (yr)	Clinical Complaint	Suspected Etiology	Treatment	Platelet No./μl of Blood (Elapsed time in days from first admission)				
1	Great Dane	M	2	Epistaxis	Sulfonamides, antibiotics	None	0 (0)	6,000 (1)	180,000 (3)	240,000 (5)	575,000 (7)
2	Shepherd type	F	6	Severe purpura	Overdose of es- tradiol cyclo- pentylpro- pionate	None	7,000 (0)	19,000 (2)	Died (2)		
3	Samoyed	F	1½	Anemia; large subcu- taneous hematoma	Consumption coagulopathy	Steroids	10,000 (0)	2,000 (2)	4,000 (3)	Rare (4)	Died (8)
4	Chihuahua	XF	11	Purpura and bleeding	Autoimmune	Steroids	10,000 (0)	31,000 (2)	102,000 (5)	251,000 (8)	410,000 (12)
5	Bull Mastiff	M	4	Generalized lymph- adenopathy; leuke- mia	Autoimmune	Steroids	46,000[a] (0)	107,000[a] (8)	288,000 (17)	424,000 (24)	210,000 (38)

From Schalm, 1971; courtesy of *The California Veterinarian*.
[a]Before beginning steroid therapy.

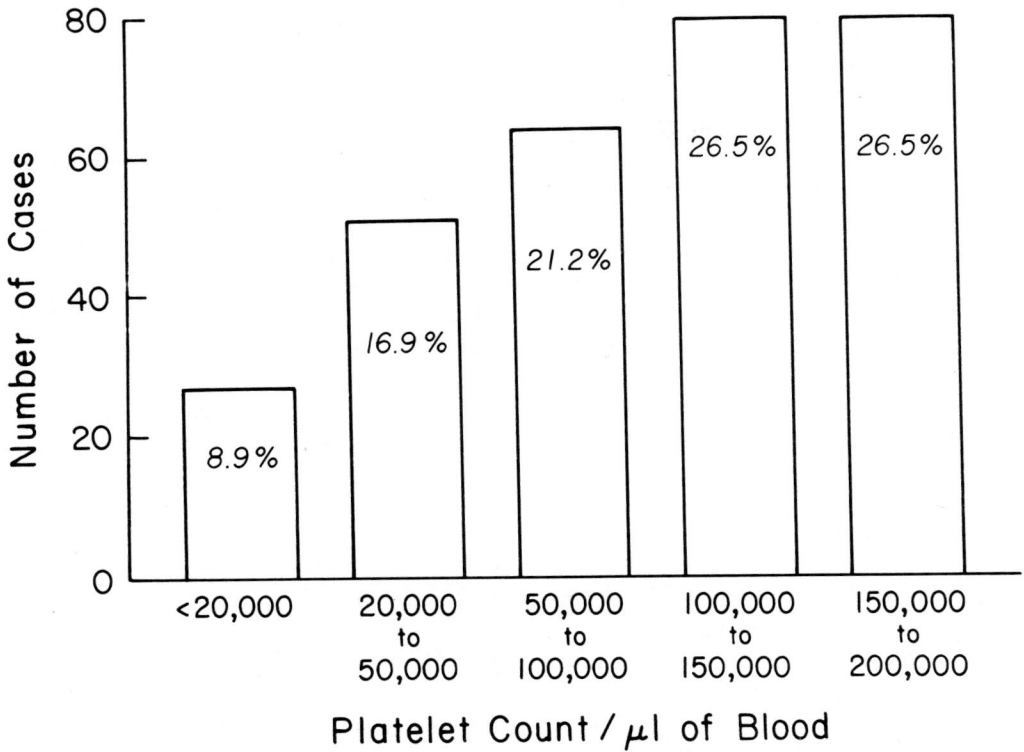

Fig. 17–2. Distribution of canine patients with various levels of thrombocytopenia. Percentages of patients in each category are shown in the bar graphs.

duce immune-mediated platelet destruction. Virus-induced thrombocytopenia may be due to decreased megakaryocytopoiesis from viral invasion of precursor cells in the bone marrow, or increased destruction of platelets by the virus or antigen-antibody complexes, or rarely it may be secondary to DIC. For additional information see recent reviews (Andrew and Kelton, 1984; Harlan, 1983; Kelton and Gibbons, 1982; Neame and Hirsh, 1982).

Abnormal distribution of platelets within the vasculature is a rare cause of thrombocytopenia. Normally about one-third of the circulating platelet mass is preferentially sequestered in the spleen. During splenomegaly or hypersplenism, abnormal platelet pooling occurs in the spleen and thrombocytopenia ensues. The degree of thrombocytopenia in such cases is related to the size of the spleen. In most cases, there is also a concomitant decrease in platelet life span. The liver is also an important site of platelet pooling in normal conditions, and abnormal portal sequestration may also lead to thrombocyto-

penia. Hypothermia causes morphologic changes in platelets, and thrombocytopenia occurs because of abnormal pooling.

Excessive loss of platelets to the level of thrombocytopenia may occur under unusual circumstances of extensive external hemorrhage.

Bleeding Tendency during Thrombocytopenic State

The normal range for circulating platelets is similar in humans and dogs—200,000–500,000/μl of blood. Platelet counts below 200,000 in the dog are representative of thrombocytopenia. However, danger of bleeding seldom exists until the count falls below 20,000/μl. Purpura, hemorrhage, prolonged bleeding time, and failure of clot retraction are commonly seen when circulating platelet numbers are below 10,000.

The relationship between the number of circulating platelets and the occurrence of hemorrhage was examined in 92 human patients with acute leukemia (Gaydos et al., 1962). It was reported that grossly visible hemorrhage rarely occurred when platelet counts were above 20,000/µl. Hemorrhage was observed 92% of the time when platelet counts were less than 10,000/µl, whereas at levels of 50,000–100,000/µl, hemorrhage occurred in only 8% of the cases. The inference is that as circulating platelet numbers decrease, blood vessel integrity diminishes proportionately, and the possibility of escape of erythrocytes through capillary walls increases.

Serious loss of blood in patients with hemostatic disorders is believed to result mainly from stress on blood vessels. Petechiation in thrombocytopenic patients is produced by application of either negative or positive pressure to the skin. Purpura and petechiation are observed most commonly in the dog in the skin of the ventral portion of the chest, abdomen, and inner thighs and in the oral mucous membranes. These areas of the body are most exposed to pressure stresses on surface capillaries. Bleeding into the gut is also a rather frequent event in thrombocytopenic dogs. Vessels close to the surface with little intervening tissue are at a disadvantage in resisting damage from comparatively light traumatic influences (Tocantins, 1947). Thus the small vessels running parallel to the surface of the upper respiratory, gastrointestinal, and urogenital tracts are commonly involved in hemorrhagic episodes associated with disorders of hemostasis.

Hemostasis in mammals is maintained by three interrelated mechanisms (Calaresu, 1960): platelet massing, formation of fibrin, and integrity of the blood vessel wall. Interference with one of these mechanisms is unassociated with death from spontaneous hemorrhage, but when more than one mechanism is interfered with, the incidence of death from hemorrhage increases. For example, thrombocytopenic rats displayed a 22% mortality rate that increased to 67% when stress was added in the form of intraperitoneal injections of 10% salt solution.

Bleeding episodes are much more common in the thrombocytopenic dog than in the thrombocytopenic cat. One might speculate that because cats are much less active than dogs when sick, they experience fewer bleeding episodes, probably as a result of less stress

being applied to their blood vessels. Schalm and Ling (1971) made long-term studies on the influence of physical stress on bleeding tendencies in a dog with autoimmune hemolytic anemia and thrombocytopenia. It was observed that during 54 days of confinement to a hospital cage, which limited stress on blood vessels, no serious bleeding occurred, although platelet counts were continuously less than 20,000 with 9 of 14 counts being under 10,000/µl (Table 17–6). During this same period, the PCV increased without any therapy from 23% to a peak of 47%. When the dog was at home and not confined, 6 episodes of serious bleeding occurred, the last event leading to death from exsanguination. The history of this canine patient supported the hypothesis that *stress on blood vessels plays a significant role in enhancing bleeding in the thrombocytopenic state.*

Exogenous Estrogen as a Cause of Thrombocytopenia

Clinical effects of large doses of natural or synthetic estrogens are hemorrhagic purpura, thrombocytopenia, profound leukocytosis followed by leukopenia, and progressive anemia. Bone marrow changes include depressed megakaryocytopoiesis and erythropoiesis and increased granulopoiesis followed by suppressed granulopoiesis.

The hematopoietic system of the dog seems to be more susceptible to estrogens than that of rhesus monkeys (Tyslowitz and Hartman, 1941), mice, rats, or guinea pigs (Tyslowitz and Dingemanse, 1941). Early experimental studies (Castrodale et al., 1941, Crafts, 1948) demonstrated that large doses of both stilbestrol and estradiol were toxic to the dog. Dogs of both sexes were affected, and the response was more rapid with estradiol than with stilbestrol. Profound changes occurred in the bone marrow and peripheral blood. Initially there was increased cellularity of the granulocytic cell series, followed by destruction of hematopoietic elements, at first of granulocytic cells and then of erythrocytic and megakaryocytic elements. Some dogs eventually developed general bone marrow hypoplasia and aplasia. These changes were reflected in the peripheral blood successively by leukocytosis, thrombocytopenia, anemia, and

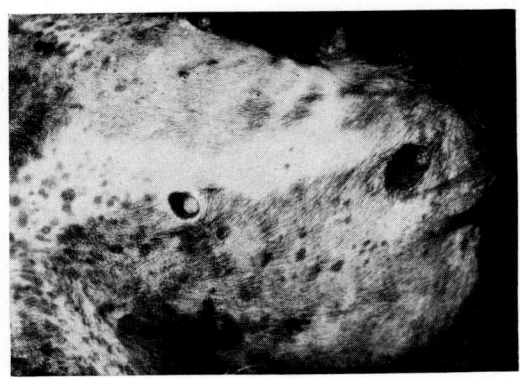

Fig. 17–3. Severe purpura on the ventral thorax and abdomen resulting from an overdose of estradiol cyclopentylpropionate for the prevention of pregnancy due to mismating.

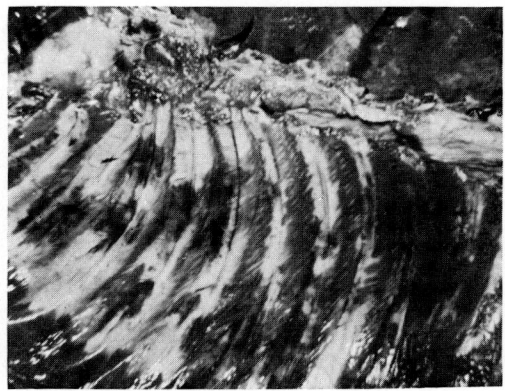

Fig. 17–4. Ecchymotic hemorrhages in the costal pleura of the same dog as presented in Figure 17–3.

leukopenia. Young dogs may be less susceptible to the toxic effects, and recovery may occur in the less severely affected animals. Death follows extensive bleeding and hemorrhage into vital organs and the cranial cavity.

An oil-soluble 17-β-cyclopentylpropionate ester of α-estradiol (Upjohn ECP) has a profound estrogenic effect and is employed therapeutically in female dogs for genitourinary disorders, including mismating, and in male dogs for treatment of prostatic hypertrophy and anal adenoma. Warning is given of the possible adverse effects of large doses on the hematopoietic system. Aplastic anemia occurred in a 6-year-old female fox terrier that had received two injections of ECP to correct false pregnancy (Steinberg, 1970).

Adverse effects of estrogen administration have been encountered in dogs admitted to our clinic (Schalm, 1971). For example, a female shepherd type dog (Table 17–7) had been mismated and was given a high dose (10 mg) of ECP. Two weeks later, the dog developed severe purpura involving the skin of the ventral thorax and abdomen (Fig. 17–3). The dog also had thrombocytopenia (7,000/µl), leukocytosis (56,000/µl) with neutrophilia accompanied by slight left shift to band cells and monocytosis, and a borderline anemia (PCV 36%). The dog became moribund and died on the second day after admission. Necropsy revealed diffuse hemorrhages of the costal pleura (Fig. 17–4) and petechiae in the stomach, urinary bladder, and lungs. Sub-

dural and parenchymatous hemorrhages were present in the brain. No megakaryocytes were observed in histologic sections of bone marrow taken at necropsy. Another dog given ECP at a dosage of 2 mg/week for 5 weeks, for the treatment of perianal adenoma, developed complete absence of thrombocytes, moderate anemia (PCV 25%), marked leukopenia (1,100/µl), and bleeding. Therapy with whole blood transfusions and prednisolone was ineffective. Hematologic changes in a Saint Bernard female dog treated for infertility with various preparations of estrogens are described in Appendix Case 11.

Experimental administration of 10 mg ECP to two 3-month-old female beagle dogs demonstrated a variable sensitivity to the drug (Table 17–8) with respect to changes in platelet and leukocyte numbers. Neither dog exhibited bleeding or other noticeable clinical signs during the observation period of 26 days. Perhaps the youth of the dogs played a significant role in modifying the effects of large doses of ECP. In another experimental study in dogs (Chiu, 1974), single intramuscular injections of 0.22 to 1.5 mg/kg of ECP produced an immediate increase in blood platelets with a peak between 5 and 7 days followed by a precipitous decrease to a level of 50,000/µl on day 13 and persistent thrombocytopenia thereafter. There was also leukocytosis (due to neutrophils and monocytes) with a peak between 17 and 23 days, followed by a rapid decline. The severity and duration of thrombocytopenia after day 13 and leukopenia after day 27 were age- and dose-

Table 17–8.   Effects of 10 mg of ECP[a] on Circulating Thrombocytes and Leukocytes in 3-Month-Old Female Beagle Dogs

| Elapsed Time (days) | Thrombocytes/μl | Total Leukocytes/μl | Absolute Leukocyte Numbers/μl | | | | |
| | | | Neutrophils | | Lymphocytes | Monocytes | Eosinophils |
			Bands	Segmenters			
Dog A							
0	194,000	8,300	0	4,358	2,324	1,618	0
5	386,000	26,700	134	18,230	4,005	3,872	400
10	82,000	39,000	0	27,300	3,510	7,995	0
13	16,000	24,300	486	15,674	2,308	5,589	122
18	10,000	54,400	2,720	41,344	4,352	5,712	272
20	45,000	73,900	6,651	53,578	8,129	4,434	1,108
26	212,000	40,500	202	30,780	7,086	2,228	202
Dog B							
0	392,000	8,600	0	4,472	2,021	1,935	175
5	390,000	18,000	0	10,260	4,230	2,520	990
10	205,000	18,700	0	10,659	2,338	5,516	187
13	81,000	12,300	62	6,519	2,030	3,382	123
18	481,000	31,500	0	20,318	5,985	4,252	945
20	486,000	28,700	0	19,085	5,310	3,300	1,004
26	517,000	24,400	0	16,348	5,368	1,830	854

[a]α-Estradiol (Upjohn).

dependent. The bone marrow exhibited suppression of erythropoiesis and megakaryocytopoiesis and stimulation of granulopoiesis on day 10. On day 20 and thereafter, young dogs exhibited regeneration of erythrocytes and megakaryocytes and cessation of granulopoiesis. Dogs receiving 0.9 mg/kg or more developed spontaneous hemorrhages between 11 and 22 days. Oral administration of ethinyl estradiol to female beagle dogs produced similar changes in blood and bone marrow cytology (Capel-Edwards et al., 1971).

Thrombocytopenia and Drug Sensitivity

Drug sensitivity leading to thrombocytopenia may develop within a few days of initiation of drug therapy. A number of drugs have been implicated (Hackett et al., 1982; Wintrobe et al., 1981). Discontinuance of the offending drug is rapidly accompanied by return of thrombocyte counts to the normal range. Mechanisms of drug-induced thrombocytopenia include direct bone marrow suppression and peripheral destruction of platelets via immune and nonimmune mechanisms.

Appendix Case 23 gives details of a possibly drug-induced thrombocytopenia and blood loss in a male Samoyed following postsurgical therapy with penicillin, streptomycin, and chlorpromazine. Hematomas, thrombocytopenia, and abnormalities of mature and im-

mature megakaryocytes were observed. The thrombocytopenia readily corrected itself when all therapy was stopped. Another instance of suspected drug sensitivity leading to thrombocytopenia was in a 2-year-old Great Dane (Table 17–7). The dog was given antibiotics and sulfamethazine for recurrent nodule formation over the entire body. Epistaxis associated with absolute thrombocytopenia developed on the eighth day. Termination of all therapy was accompanied by reappearance of platelets in the circulation in 24 hours, and a rapid increase followed, attaining levels in excess of 200,000/μl by the fifth day.

Immune-Mediated Thrombocytopenia

Immune-mediated or autoimmune thrombocytopenia (AITP) is frequent in the dog (Table 17–7) and infrequent in the cat and horse (reviewed by Jain and Switzer, 1981). The pathogenesis of autoantibody formation and its etiology remain unknown. In primary AITP, the principal finding is thrombocytopenia, whereas secondary AITP is often seen in association with other diseases or conditions or certain drug therapies and may occur along with autoimmune hemolytic anemia (AIHA) or other immune-mediated diseases such as systemic lupus erythematosus and rheumatoid arthritis. A number of drugs have been associated with thrombocytopenia in humans, including phenylbutazone, salicylates, sulfonamides, chlorothiazide, digitoxin, chloroquine, and hypoglycemic agents chlorpropamide and tolbutamide. Classical studies to elucidate the mechanisms of thrombocytopenia have been made with quinine, quinidine, and sedormid (see Chapter 35). Thrombocytopenia may develop within hours after injection of a drug, or it may develop slowly. Symptoms regress on discontinuation of the drug therapy as mentioned above. Thrombocytopenia is recognized as a complication of heparin therapy in about 5% of the human patients receiving this drug, occurring 3–16 days after the initial administration (Cimco et al, 1979; King and Kelton, 1984). The incidence is higher with bovine heparin than with porcine heparin. The mechanism is not clear, but may be partly immunologic.

Presenting clinical signs may be those of bleeding related to thrombocytopenia or the animal may be seen for another disorder and found to be thrombocytopenic. Definitive diagnosis requires demonstration of antiplatelet antibody either in serum or that associated with circulating platelets or marrow megakaryocytes of the patient. In cases in which antiplatelet antibody is not demonstrated, a presumptive diagnosis is made following succeessful management of thrombocytopenia with corticosteroids or other immunosuppressive drugs. Therapy consists of corticosteroids alone or in conjunction with cyclophosphamide and *Vinca* alkaloids. An increase in thrombocyte numbers occurs rapidly in those responding favorably to the drug therapy. Large or giant platelets believed to be young platelets are often found in the peripheral blood, indicating a compensatory increase in the thrombocyte production. AITP patients generally require continuous maintenance therapy with corticosteroids and a careful management and follow-up. See Chapter 35 for a detailed discussion of AITP.

Isoimmune or Neonatal Thrombocytopenia

Isoimmune or neonatal thrombocytopenia is a consequence of transfer of maternal antibodies to the newborn. Thrombocytopenia develops within a few days or 1 to 2 weeks after birth, but generally there is a sponta-

neous recovery. Affected animals develop prominent generalized petechial and ecchymotic hemorrhages, and death occurs in some cases, commonly due to intracranial hemorrhage. A hemorrhagic syndrome of piglets resulting from thrombocytopenia due to maternal isoimmunization was described by Stormorken et al. (1963). The sow was bred to the same boar for 4 litters. In the third litter, 6 of 11 piglets died of a hemorrhagic disease, while the remaining 5 piglets survived when raised artificially. The fourth litter consisted of 14 piglets. All were well until the fifth day, when the larger piglets became unthrifty and developed purpura; 1 developed epistaxis. Within 1 week, 8 piglets died. Autopsy revealed a widespread bleeding disorder. Two piglets having platelet counts of 28,000 and 37,000/μl of blood survived, as platelets increased over 12 days to 300,000 and 920,000/μl, respectively. Blood serum of the sow was found to agglutinate the platelets of the piglets. It was conjectured that isoantibodies against the platelets had been transferred through colostrum to the piglets. Subsequent transfer of thrombocyte agglutinating antibodies from sows to piglets after birth by colostrum consumption was found responsible for thrombocytopenia in blood and megakaryocytopenia in bone marrow, with clinical signs of a hemorrhagic diathesis in the skin and internal organs (Linklater, 1975; Schmidt et al., 1977). Isoimmune thrombocytopenia was produced experimentally by immunizing pregnant sows with boar's thrombocytes and allowing the piglets to suckle the dam.

Thrombocytopenia Due to Hypersplenism

This condition occurs rarely in animals. Enlargement of the spleen places demands on increasing numbers of circulating platelets to be retained within the organ. Perfusion of surgically removed human spleens with ^{51}Cr-labeled thrombocytes demonstrated a sizable pooling of the isotope that seemed to be dependent on the splenic size only (Penny et al., 1966). Increase in size of the splenic pool, which may be as high as 90%, rather than suppression of thrombopoiesis appears to be the main reason for thrombocytopenia in splenomegaly (Karpatkin, 1983). Splenectomy is indicated in such cases. Splenectomy

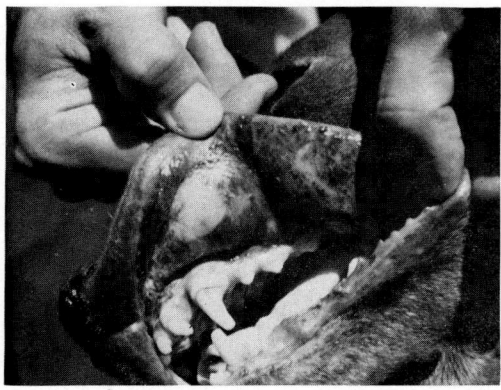

Fig. 17–5.   Edema and hemorrhagic foci in oral tissue of a dog with thrombotic thrombocytopenic purpura.

promoted complete recovery in 13 dogs that had had frequent and severe epistaxis with thrombocytopenia and enlarged spleens (Ascott, 1972).

Thrombocytopenia Due to Consumption Coagulopathy or Disseminated Intravascular Coagulation

Extensive intravascular clotting with disseminated thrombi is associated with significant consumption of blood clotting factors. This condition leads to thrombocytopenia and low levels of circulating fibrinogen, prothrombin, and coagulation factors V and VIII. Simultaneously, there is activation of the plasminogen system leading to the generation of fibrin and fibrinogen degradation products in the circulation. The development of an initial hypercoagulability of the blood thus can be followed by hypocoagulability. Clotting factors and platelets may be utilized to such a degree that hemostasis is no longer possible and hemorrhagic diathesis results (Case 3, Table 17–7, Fig. 17–5).

A variety of conditions may trigger the complex phenomenon of DIC. In humans and animals, DIC may be secondary to clinical conditions such as septicemia, transfusion reactions, surgery (especially of heart and lungs), snake bite (venoms), heat stroke, hypersensitivity reactions, certain viral infections, neoplasia (especially carcinoma and large hemangiomas), and leukemias (de Gruchy, 1970; Greene, 1975). Consumption coagulopathies in humans are commonly

acute disorders, but may be subacute or chronic.

DIC is being recognized increasingly in veterinary medicine, particularly in the dog (Slappendel et al., 1970) and less commonly in other species. DIC has been reported in dogs developing aflatoxicoses (Greene et al., 1977); calves with acute neonatal isoerythrolysis (Dimmoch et al., 1976); calves (Nagaraja et al., 1979), dogs (Fletcher and Ramwell, 1977; Garner et al., 1974), and pigs (Johannsen and Schoppmeyer, 1975) experimentally inoculated with endotoxin; gnotobiotic and specific pathogen–free piglets inoculated with *Erysipelothrix rhusiopathiae* (Schulz et al., 1971); and cats infected with feline infectious peritonitis virus (Weiss et al., 1980). For further details on DIC see Chapter 14.

Thrombocytopenia in Specific Diseases

Dogs. A modest thrombocytopenia (50,000–150,000/µl of blood) occasionally accompanies *canine lymphosarcoma*. Platelet numbers usually are not so low that bleeding occurs, although an infrequent patient may experience platelet reductions to levels at which hemorrhages may follow. Circulating platelet counts in 42 dogs with lymphosarcoma were: 21,000–89,000 (mean 49,000 ± 18,000) in 13 dogs; 101,000–173,000 (mean 123,000 ± 18,500) in 12 dogs; and 221,000–588,000 (mean 338,000 ± 88,000) in 17 dogs. Treatment with cytotoxic drugs and corticosteroids may correct thrombocytopenia in some patients. It is believed that the thrombocytopenia of chronic lymphocytic leukemia in humans is of autoimmune origin (Damshek, 1965), but such a relationship in the dog seems to be infrequent.

Tropical canine pancytopenia, in which epistaxis is a common clinical sign, is characterized by anemia, leukopenia, and thrombocytopenia. Coagulation and prothrombin times are normal, but bleeding time is prolonged, owing to the markedly low platelet number. The causative agent is *Ehrlichia canis* (Huxsoll et al., 1970). In experimental studies on *E. canis* infection in dogs (Pierce et al., 1977; Seamer and Snape, 1972; Smith et al., 1975), persistent thrombocytopenia developed 14 days after infection. Platelet life span was reduced to 4 days compared to the normal 9 days. Platelet destruction was found to occur primarily in the spleen. Megakaryocytopoiesis was increased, with an accelerated release of platelets, within 2–3 days compared to 5–6 days in normal dogs, leading to a marked increase in megathrombocytes. Recovery in clinical condition occurred in one study, but infection and thrombocytopenia persisted for months (Seamer and Snape, 1972). Oxytetracycline prevented experimental infection, while a thiosemicarbazone derivative delayed the onset of infection.

A *rickettsia-like* organism isolated from a dog was found to produce cyclic parasitemia and concurrent thrombocytopenia, but without hemorrhages, with a periodicity of 8–15 days (Harvey et al., 1978). The organism is very difficult to find in blood films, but careful search may reveal it in an occasional platelet in well-stained blood films (Fig. 17–6*A, B*) and by electron microscopy (Fig. 17–6*C*). The organism has recently been named *Ehrlichia platys,* and an indirect immunofluorescence test for its diagnosis has been developed (French and Harvey, 1983).

Thrombocytopenia has been observed in the dog in many other situations and experimental conditions. Dogs experimentally inoculated with the agent of *rocky mountain spotted fever* developed anemia, leukopenia proceeding to leukocytosis, thrombocytopenia, and characteristic cutaneous lesions including petechiae, ecchymoses, edema, and necrosis (Keenan et al., 1977). Clinical and pathologic manifestations of DIC including thrombocytopenia were seen in dogs inoculated intravenously with *hepatitis virus* (Wington, 1976). Other situations accompanied by thrombocytopenia include endotoxin injection (Fletcher and Ramwell, 1977), experimental peritonitis (Surgerman et al., 1982), dapsone administration (Lees et al., 1979), myasthenia gravis (Schutt and Kersten, 1977), and levamisole therapy for dirofilariasis (Atwell et al., 1981).

Cats. Moderate to marked thrombocytopenia is common in cats with various *myeloproliferative disorders*. Platelet morphology is often abnormal in such cases and megathrombocytes may be found. Experimental infection of kittens with the Kawakami-Theilen strain of feline leukemia virus induced erythroid hy-poplasia, transient thrombocytopenia followed by macrothrombocytosis, impaired in vitro platelet aggregation and release reaction, and decreased platelet life span (Boyce, 1984).

Ribavirin administration into cats exposed to calicivirus was associated with hemorrhages resulting from profound thrombocytopenia. Other abnormalities included reduced WBC and RBC counts, increased serum alanine aminotransferase activity, icterus, and loss of body weight (Povey, 1978). Toxic effects were largely reversed within a week of cessation of treatment.

Horses. Thrombocytopenia has been seen in cases of *equine ehrlichiosis* and *equine infectious anemia*. Isolated cases of idiopathic thrombocytopenia in the horse have been reported (Byars and Greene, 1982; Hammill and Helton, 1981; Morris and Whitlock, 1983; Valdez and Peyton, 1978).

In equine ehrlichiosis (Gribble, 1969), a transitory thrombocytopenia usually occurred on days 4 through 12 in experimentally produced disease. During this period, platelet counts were commonly less than 50,000/μl. A severe vasculitis, involving small arteries and veins, was a prominent histologic finding. It was suggested that the transitory thrombocytopenia was due to participation of platelets in the formation of the cellular thromboses characteristic of the disease. Platelet counts were lowest when vascular lesions were most severe. (See Plates XIV–1, XIV–2).

A 10-year-old quarter horse, in which the pathologic diagnosis at necropsy was equine infectious anemia, was observed over a period of 1 month. The horse progressively developed anemia, leukopenia, fever (105°F) and diarrhea (negative for *Salmonella* species). Epistaxis developed during the third week, and three platelet counts made during the final week, before the horse was destroyed, ranged from 2,000–14,000/μl. Bone marrow examination revealed only a rare megakaryocyte on the entire film.

Cattle. *Bracken fern poisoning* in cattle (Sippel, 1952) and poisoning of cattle fed soybean meal from which the oil had been extracted by *trichlorethylene* (Pritchard et al., 1956) produced aplasia of the bone marrow. Anemia, leukopenia, and thrombocytopenia devel-

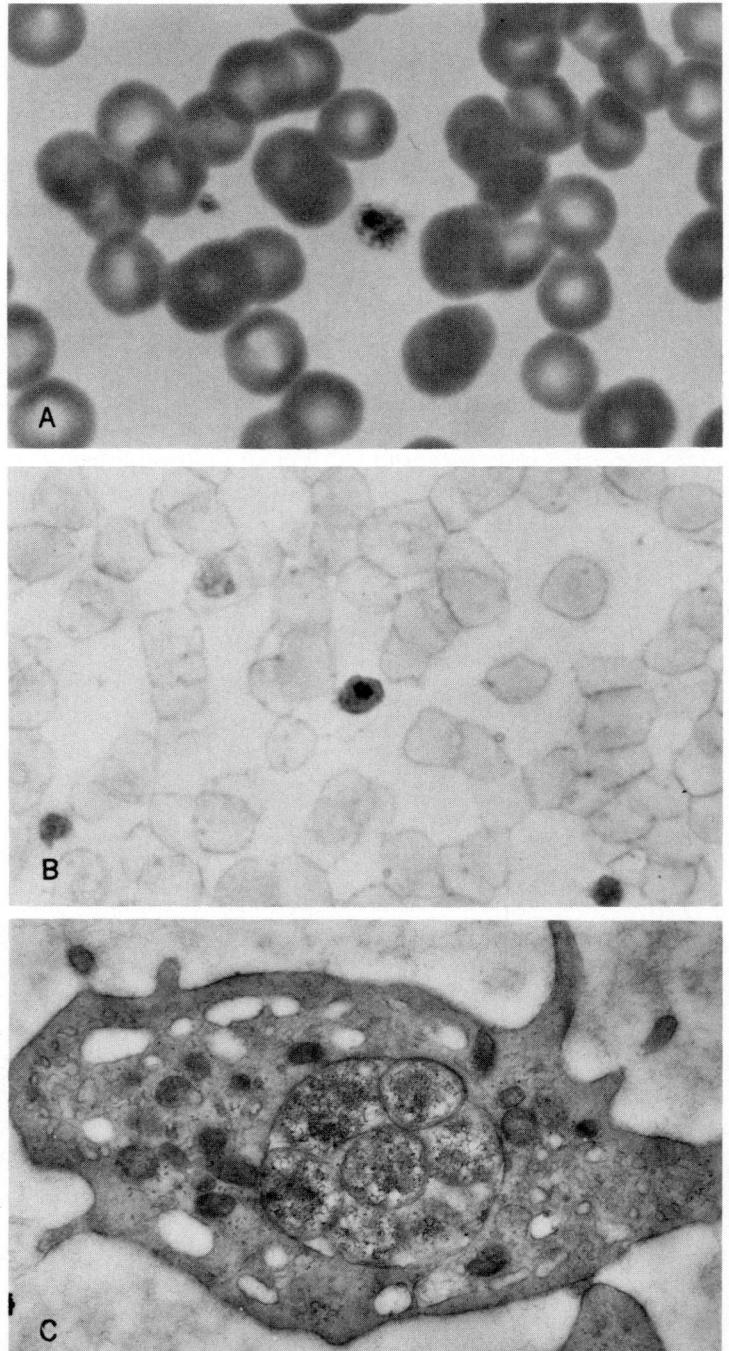

Fig. 17–6.   *Ehrlichia platys* in blood of a dog. *A,* Wright stain; *B,* New methylene blue stain; *C,* electron photomicrograph of a platelet containing a microorganism with seven subunits. (Courtesy of Dr. John Harvey).

oped. Bleeding from body openings was a characteristic finding in both diseases, and death was a common result.

Long-term administration of *furazolidone* to milk-fed calves was found to cause chronic poisoning in the form of a hemorrhagic syndrome with pancytopenia, hyperfibrinogenemia, prolonged clotting time, and bone marrow hypoplasia or aplasia (Hayashi et al., 1976; Hofmann, 1976). Beef calves fed on *reconstituted dried milk* developed a lethal hemorrhagic condition with thrombocytopenia as a characteristic finding (Espinasse et al., 1973). Food additives were suspected as the cause. Mycotoxic hemorrhagic syndrome with pancytopenia occurred in cattle fed on barley containing many potentially *toxic fungi* (Dyson and Reed, 1977).

Thrombocytopenia associated with petechial hemorrhages and pulmonary edema was seen in *East Coast Fever* (Kimeto, 1976). Thrombocytopenia has been observed repeatedly in cattle experimentally infected with *Trypanosoma congolense* and *T. vivax* (Forsberg et al., 1979; Maxie and Valli, 1978; Maxie et al., 1976, 1979; Preston et al., 1982; Wellde et al., 1978). Several mechanisms seem to be involved in its causation; these include reduced platelet life span, ineffective and/or reduced thrombopoiesis, and subacute to chronic DIC. Hereford cattle infected with *T. congolense* developed a thrombocytopenia that was most severe at peak parasitemia early in the course of infection (Wellde et al., 1978). DIC was also evident at 6–14 weeks of infection. As the disease progressed, parasite levels gradually decreased, and a corresponding increase in platelet numbers occurred. In chronically infected animals, platelet counts were reduced during and shortly after periods of patency. During extended remission, however, platelet numbers rose to normal or higher levels. Treatment of acutely ill, thrombocytopenic animals with Berenil resulted in thrombocytosis.

Thrombocytopenia accompanied by leukopenia was observed in the terminal stages of acute theileriasis in water buffaloes and cattle from experimental infection with *Theileria lawrencei* (Burridge and Odeke, 1973).

Sheep. Leukopenia, lymphopenia, and thrombocytopenia developed in sheep and cattle 1–3 weeks after *whole body gamma irradiation* (Sasser et al., 1973). In addition, agranulocytosis occurred in sheep exposed to *whole body x-irradiation* (Johannsen et al., 1978). Hemorrhagic diathesis due to thrombocytopenia and bacterial endotoxin occurred in these sheep shortly before death after 16–25 days of irradiation.

Sheep experimentally infected with the tick *Amblyomma variegatum* and *Hyalomma rufipes* developed anemia, thrombocytopenia, and leukocytosis (Dipeola and Ogunji, 1977). Sheep feeding on straw and hay contaminated with *Stachybotrys alternans* may develop toxicosis characterized by nasal hemorrhages and hemorrhagic enteritis, leukopenia, and thrombocytopenia (Danko, 1976). Production of thrombocytes and lymphocytes is inhibited. *Amporolium poisoning* in lambs caused hemorrhages associated with thrombocytopenia and anemia which were attributed to degenerative and hypoplastic changes in the bone marrow (Morgan et al., 1975).

Pigs. Infection of pigs with pathogenic strains of *swine fever virus* caused anemia, thrombocytopenia, and granulocytopenia (pancytopenia) and cellular necrobiosis of the spleen (Edwards, 1984; Popa, 1977). Viral antigen could be demonstrated by immunofluorescence in platelets and leukocytes, but not in erythrocytes (Leaniz et al., 1976). Morphologic changes of the release reaction occurred in platelets after viral pancytopenia. Observations on experimental infection with African swine fever virus suggested that thrombocytopenia was probably a consequence of increased platelet destruction associated with formation of immune complexes involving viral antigen and specific antiviral antibody (Edwards, 1984). Abnormal megakaryocytes indicating disturbed thrombopoiesis were seen in acute experimental *hog cholera* (Weiss et al., 1973). Marked thrombocytopenia developed, together with the virus-induced endothelial lesions and DIC, which was typical of the terminal state of the acute disease.

Thrombocytopenia and leukopenia developed in piglets experiencing *endotoxin shock* (Johannsen and Schoppmeyer, 1975) and in pigs experiencing *acute systemic shock* as a result of sensitization and subsequent challenge with ovalbumin (Wells et al., 1974).

REFERENCES

Andrew, M., and Kelton, J.: Neonatal Thrombocytopenia. Clin. Perinatol., *11*:359, 1984.

Ascott, E.W.: Epistaxis in the Dog: Treatment by Splenectomy. Rhodesian Vet. J., *3*:45, 1972.

Atwell, R.B., et al.: Suspected Drug-Induced Thrombocytopenia Associated with Levamisole Therapy in a Dog. Aust. Vet. J., *57*:91, 1981.

Baele, G., et al.: Pseudothrombocytopenia. Acta Clin. Belg., *33*:302, 1978.

Bell, T., et al.: Alteration of Platelet Function in Equine Laminitis. Fed. Proc., *38*:1411, 1979.

Bell, T.G., et al.: Platelet Function in Basset Hound Hereditary Thrombopathia (abstract). Fed. Proc., *41*:701, 1982.

Boneu, B., et al.: Platelets in Myeloproliferative Disorders. I. A Comparative Evaluation with Certain Platelets Function Tests. Scand. J. Haematol., *25*:214, 1980.

Bowie, E.J.W., et al.: Comparison of Abnormalities of Platelet Function in Human and Porcine von Willebrand's Disease. *In* Platelets: Recent Advances in Basic Research and Clinical Aspects. Ulutin, O.N., ed. American Elsevier, New York, pp. 420–423, 1975.

Boyce, J.T.: Erythroid Aplasia and Platelet Abnormalities in Cats Induced by the Kawakami-Theilen Strain of Feline Leukemia Virus. Diss. Abst. International B, *44*:3365, 1984.

Burridge, M.J., and Odeke, G.M.: Theileria lawrencei: Infection in the Indian Water Buffalo, Bubalus bubalis. Exp. Prasitol., *34*:257, 1973.

Byars, T.D., and Greene, C.E.: Idiopathic Thrombocytopenic Purpura in the Horse. J. Amer. Vet. Med. Ass., *180*:1422, 1982.

Caen, J.P., et al.: Adhesion and Aggregation of Human Platelets to Rabbit Subendothelium: A New Approach for Investigation: Specific Antibodies. Experientia, *33*:91, 1977.

Calaresu, F.R., and Jaques, L.B.: Thrombocytopenia in Experimental Production of Hemorrhagic Death by Multiple Factors. Can. J. Biochem. Physiol., *38*:1275, 1960.

Capel-Edwards, K., et al.: Hematological Changes Observed in Female Beagle Dogs Given Ethynylestradiol. Toxicol. Appl. Pharmacol., *20*:319, 1971.

Castrodale, D., et al.: Comparative Studies of the Effects of Estradiol and Stilbestrol upon the Blood, Liver and Bone Marrow. Endocrinology, *29*:363, 1941.

Chiu., T.: Studies on Estrogen-induced Proliferative Disorders of Hemopoietic Tissue in Dogs. Dissert. Abs. Int., *35B*:3104, 1974.

Cimco, P.L., et al.: Heparin-Induced Thrombocytopenia: Association with a Platelet Aggregating Factor and Arterial Thrombosis. Amer. J. Hematol., *6*:125, 1979.

Corrigan, J.J.: Heparin Therapy in Bacterial Septicemia. J. Pediatr., *91*:695, 1977.

Cowan, D.H.: Acquired Disorders of Platelet Function. *In* Hemostasis and Thrombosis: Basic Principles and Clinical Practice. Colman, R.W., et al., eds. J.B. Lippincott, Philadelphia, p. 516, 1982.

Crafts, R.C.: The Effects of Estrogens on the Bone Marrow of Adult Female Dogs. Blood, *3*:276, 1948.

Dameshek, W.: Idiopathic Thrombocytopenic Purpura. Ser. Haematol., *9*:61, 1965.

Danko, G.: On Stachybotryotoxicoses of Sheep. Magyar Allator Lapja, *31*:226, 1976.

de Gruchy, G.C.: Clinical Haematology in Medical Practice. 3rd ed. F.A. Davis, Philadelphia, p. 700, 1970.

Dimmoch, C.K., et al.: The Experimental Production of Haemolytic Disease of Newborn in Calves. Res. Vet. Sci., *20*:244, 1976.

Dipeola, O.O., and Ogunji, F.O.: Infested with the Ticks Amblyoma variegatum and Hyolomma rufipes. Bull. Amer. Health and Prod. Africa, *25*:25, 1977.

Dodds, W.J.: Familial Canine Thrombocytopathy. Thromb. Diath. Haemorrh. Suppl., *26*:241, 1967.

Dodds, W.J.: Canine von Willebrand's Diseae. J. Lab. Clin. Med., *76*:713, 1970.

Dodds, W.J., et al.: Platelet and Fibrinogen Survivals in Normal and Thrombopathic Dogs. 14th Int. Congr. Hematol., Sao Paulo, 1972, p. 234.

Dyson, D.A., and Reed, J.B.H.: Haemorrhagic Syndrome of Cattle of Suspected Mycotoxic Origin. Vet. Rec., *100*:400, 1977.

Edwards, J.F.: The Pathogenesis of Thrombocytopenia and Hemorrhage in African Swine Fever. Diss. Abst. International B, *44*:2675, 1984.

Espinasse, J., et al.: Observations and Comments on a Haemorrhagic Syndrome of Beef Calves Fed on Dried Milk. Rev. Med. Veterinaire, *124*:1503, 1973.

Failkow, P.J., et al.: Evidence That Essential Thrombocythemia Is a Clonal Disorder with Origin in a Multipotent Stem Cell. Blood, *58*:916, 1981.

Fletcher, J.R., and Ramwell, P.W.: Modification by Aspirin and Indomethacin of the Haemodynamic and Prostaglandin Releasing Effects of E. coli Endotoxin in the Dog. Brit. J. Pharmacol., *61*:175, 1977.

Forsberg, C.M., et al.: The Pathogenesis of Trypanosoma congolense Infection in Calves. IV. The Kinetics of Blood Coagulation. Vet. Pathol., *16*:229, 1979.

French, T.W., and Harvey, J.W.: Serologic Diagnosis of Infectious Cyclic Thrombocytopenia in Dogs, using an Indirect Fluorescent Antibody Test. Amer. J. Vet. Res., *44*:2407, 1983.

Furie, B.: Acquired Coagulation Disorders and Dysproteinemias. *In* Thrombosis and Hemostasis: Basic Principles and Clinical Practice. R.W. Colman, et al., eds. J.B. Lippincott, Philadelphia, p. 577, 1982.

Gardner, F.H., and Bessman, J.D.: Thrombocytopenia Due to Defective Platelet Production. Clin. Haematol., *12*:23, 1983.

Garner, R., et al.: The Role of Complement in Endotoxin Shock and Disseminated Intravascular Coagulation: Experimental Observations in the Dog. Brit. J. Haematol., *28*:393, 1974.

Gaydos, L.A., et al.: The Quantitative Relationship between Platelet Count and Hemorrhage in Patients with Acute Leukemia. New Eng. J. Med., *266*:905, 1962.

Glanzmann, E.: Hereditare hamorrhagische Thrombasthenic: Ein Beitray zur pathologic der Blutplatchen. Jahrbuch fur Kinderheilkrinde, *88*:113, 1918.

Greene, C.E.: Disseminated Intravascular Coagulation in the Dog. J. Amer. Anim. Hosp. Ass., *11*:674, 1975.

Greene, C.E., et al.: Disseminated Intravascular Coagulation Complicating Aflatoxicosis in Dogs. Cornell Vet., *67*:29, 1977.

Greene, C.E., et al.: Vincristine in the Treatment of Thrombocytopenia in Five Dogs. J. Amer. Vet. Med. Assoc., *180*:140, 1982.

Gribble, D.H.: Equine Ehrlichiosis. J. Amer. Vet. Med. Ass., *155*:462, 1969.

Gunz, F.W.: Hemorrhagic Thrombocythemia: A Critical Review. Blood, *15*:706, 1960.

Hackett, T., et al.: Drug-Induced Platelet Destruction. Semin. Thromb. Hemostas., *8*:116, 1982.

Hammill, D., and Helton, M.: Idiopathic Thrombocytopenia in a Mare. Mod. Vet. Pract., 62:392, 1981.

Hardisty, R.M. Disorders of Platelet Function. Brit. Med. Bull., 33:207, 1977.

Hardisty, R.M.: Hereditary Disorders of Platelet Function. Clin. Haematol., 12:153, 1983.

Harker, L.A.: Platelet Production. New Eng. J. Med., 282:492, 1970.

Harlan, J.M.: Thrombocytopenia Due to Non-Immune Platelet Destruction. Clin. Haematol., 12:39, 1983.

Harvey, J.W., et al.: Cyclic Thrombocytopenia Induced by a Rickettsia-Like Agent in Dogs. J. Inf. Dis., 137:182, 1978.

Hayashi, T., et al.: Hematological and Pathological Observations of Chronic Furazolidone Poisoning in Calves. Jpn. J. Vet. Res., 38:225, 1976.

Hofmann, W.: Chronic Furazolidone Poisoning in the Calf. Tierarztl. Prax., 4:453, 1976.

Hogan, A.G., et al.: A Hemophilia-Like Disease in Swine. Proc. Soc. Exp. Biol. Med., 48:217, 1941.

Huxsoll, D.L., et al.: Tropical Canine Pancytopenia. J. Amer. Vet. Med. Ass., 157:1627, 1970.

Jain, N.C., and Switzer, J.W.: Autoimmune Thrombocytopenia in Dogs and Cats. Vet. Clin. North Amer. (Small Anim. Pract.), 11:421, 1981.

Johannsen, U., et al.: Pathomorphology of Radiation Sickness in Sheep following Whole-body X-Irradiation. Arch. Exp. Vet. Med., 32:537, 1978.

Johannsen, U., and Schoppmeyer, K.: Experiments on the Pathogenesis of E. coli Enterotoxemia in Pigs. I. Comparison of the Action of Toxins from Two E. coli serotypes after Intestinal Injection. II. Intestinal Administration of E. coli Toxin. Arch. Exp. Vet. Med., 29:33, 1975.

Jorgensen, K.A.: Platelets and Renal Disease. Dan. Med. Bull., 28:116, 1981.

Kahn, R.A., et al.: Electron Microscopy of Bleeder Swine Platelets. Amer. J. Vet. Res., 31:679, 1970.

Karpatkin, S.: The Spleen and Thrombocytopenia. Clinics Haematol., 12:591, 1983.

Kasturi, J., and Saraya, A.K.: Platelet Functions in Dysproteinemia. Acta Haematol., 59:104, 1978.

Keenan, K.P., et al.: Studies on the Pathogenesis of Rickettsia rickettsii in the Dog: Clinical and Clinicopathologic Changes of Experimental Infection. Amer. J. Vet. Res., 38:851, 1977.

Kelton, J.G., and Gibbons, S.: Autoimmune Platelet Destruction: Idiopathic Thrombocytopenic Purpura. Semin. Thromb. Hemostas., 8:83, 1982.

Kimeto, B.A.: Ultrastructure of Blood Platelets in Cattle with East Coast Fever. Amer. J. Vet. Res., 37:443, 1976.

King, D.J., and Kelton, J.G.: Heparin-Induced thrombocytopenia. Ann. Int. Med., 100:535, 1984.

Lackner, H.: Hemostatic Abnormalities Associated with Dysproteinemias. Semin. Hematol., 10:125, 1973.

Leaniz, R., et al.: Swine Fever. II. Presence of Viral Antigen in the Platelets. Gaceta Vet., 38:100, 1976.

Lees, G.E., et al.: Fatal Thrombocytopenic Hemorrhagic Diathesis Associated with Dapsone Administration to a Dog. J. Amer. Vet. Med. Ass., 175:49, 1979.

Lepherd, E.E.: Effect of Exercise on Platelet Size and Number in Ponies. Vet. Rec., 101:488, 1977.

Linklater, K.A.: The Experimental Reproduction of Thrombocytopenic Purpura in Piglets. Res. Vet. Sci., 18:127, 1975.

Lotz, F., et al.: A Study of a Specific Congenital Platelet Functional Abnormality in Dogs. 3rd Congress

Thrombosis and Haemostasis, Washington, p. 220, 1972.

Malpass, T.W., and Harker, L.A.: Acquired Disorders of Platelet Function. Semin. Hematol., 17:242, 1980.

Maupin, B.: Bovinque de domias sur les plaquettes sanguines des animaux. Sciences et Techniques de l'Animal de Laboratoires, 3:766, 1978.

Maxie, M.G., et al.: A Comparative Study of the Hematological Aspects of the Diseases Caused by Trypanosoma vivax and Trypanosoma congolense in Cattle. In Pathophysiology of Parasitic Infection. Soubsby, E.J.L., ed. Academic Press, New York, pp. 183-198, 1976.

Maxie, M.G., Experimental Bovine Trypanosomiasis (Trypanosoma vivax and T. congolense). I. Symptomatology and Clinical Pathology. Tropenmed. Parasitol., 30:274, 1979.

Maxie, M.G., and Valli, V.E.O.: Pancytopenia in Bovine Trypanosomiasis. In Pathogenicity of Trypanosomes. Losos, G., and Chouinard, A., eds. International Dev. Res. Centre, Ottawa, pp. 135–136, 1978.

Meyers, K.M., et al.: Evaluation of the Platelet Storage Pool Deficiency in the Feline Counterpart of the Chédiak-Higashi syndrome. Amer. J. Physiol., 11:241, 1981.

Montiel, M.M.: The Role of Platelets in Hemostasis: Qualitative Defects of Platelets and Their Laboratory Evaluation. Tex. Med., 75(May):48, 1979.

Morgan, K.T., et al.: Amporolium Poisoning of Preruminant Lambs: An Investigation of the Encephalopathy and the Haemorrhagic and Diarrhoeic syndromes. J. Pathol., 116:73, 1975.

Morin, R.J.: The Role of Phospholipids in Platelet Function. Ann. Clin. Lab. Sci., 10:463, 1980.

Morris, D.D., and Whitlock, R.H.: Relapsing Idiopathic Thrombocytopenia in a Horse. Equine Vet. J., 15:73, 1983.

Murphy, S.: Thrombocytosis and Thrombocythaemia. Clin. Haematol., 12:89, 1983.

Nagaraja, T.G., et al.: Endotoxin Shock in Calves from Intravenous Injection of Rumen Bacterial Endotoxin. J. Anim. Sci., 49:567, 1979.

Neame, P.B., and Hirsh, J.: Increased Platelet Destruction. Semin. Thromb. Hemostas., 8:75, 1982.

Ozer, F.L., et al.: Primary Hemorrhagic Thrombocythemia. Amer. J. Med., 28:807, 1960.

Penny, R., et al.: The Splenic Platelet Pool. Blood, 27:1, 1966.

Pierce, K.R., et al.: Acute Canine Ehrlichiosis: Platelet Survival and Factor 3 Assay. Amer. J. Vet. Res., 38:1821, 1977.

Popa, M.: Some Properties and the Present Role of Lapinized Chinese Strain Virus in the Immunoprophylaxis of Swine Fever. Lucrar. Inst. de Cercet. Vet. se Biopra. "Pasteur," 13:49, 1977.

Povey, R.C.: Effect of Orally Administered Ribavirin on an Experimental Feline Calici Virus Infection in Cats. Amer. J. Vet. Res., 39:1337, 1978.

Preston, J.M., et al.: Trypanosoma congolense: Thrombocyte Survival in Infected Steers. Exp. Parasitol., 54:129, 1982.

Pritchard, W.R., et al.: Studies on Trichloroethylene-Extracted Feeds. I. Experimental Production of Acute Aplastic Anemia in Young Heifers. Amer. J. Vet. Res., 17:425, 1956.

Ragan, H.A.: Platelet Agglutination Induced by Ethylenediaminetetra-acetic Acid in Blood Samples from a Miniature Pig. Amer. J. Vet. Res., 33:2601, 1972.

Rao, A.K., and Walsh, P.N.: Acquired Qualitative Platelet Disorders. Clin. Haematol., *12*:201, 1983.

Reddick, R.L., et al.: Platelet Adhesion to Damaged Coronary Arteries: Comparison in Normal and Von Wilebrand Disease Swine. Proc. Natl. Acad. Sci., *79*:5076, 1982.

Remuzzi, G., et al.: Altered Platelet and Vascular Prostaglandin Generation in Patients with Renal Failure and Prolonged Bleeding Times. Thromb. Res., *13*:1007, 1978a.

Remuzzi, G., et al.: Bleeding in Renal Failure: Altered Platelet Function in Chronic Uremia Only Partially Corrected by Hemodialysis. Nephron, *22*:347, 1978b.

Roper, P.R., et al.: Profile of Platelet Volume Distribution in Normal Individuals and in Patients with Acute Leukemia. Amer. J. Clin. Pathol., *68*:449, 1977.

Sasser, L.B., et al.: Hematologic Response of Sheep and Cattle to Whole-Body Gamma Irradiation and Gastrointestinal and Skin Beta Irradiation. Amer. J. Vet. Res., *23*:1555, 1973.

Schalm, O.W.: The Blood Platelets (Thrombocytes). II. The Thrombocytopathics. Calif. Vet., *25*:6, June, 1971.

Schalm, O.W., and Ling, G.V.: The Blood Platelets (Thrombocytes). II. The Hemorrhagic Syndrome in Thrombocytopenia. Calif. Vet., *25*:10, August, 1971.

Schmidt, U., et al.: Thrombocytopenic Purpura in the Unweaned pig. Morphological, Haematological and Serological Studies. Zentralbl. Veterinarmed., *24B*:386, 1977.

Schulz, L.C., et al.: Microangiopathies Characterized by Blood Coagulation Disorder in Septicaemic Swine Erysipelas. Dtsch. Tierärztl. Wochenschr., *78*:563, 1971.

Schutt, I., and Kersten, U.: Myasthenia Gravis Pseudoparalytica in Three Female German Shepherd Dogs. Kleintierpraxis, *22*:45, 1977.

Seamer, J., and Snape, T.: Ehrlichia canis and Tropical Canine Pancytopaenia. Res. Vet. Sci., *13*:307, 1972.

Sippel, W.L.: Bracken Fern Poisoning. J. Amer. Vet. Med. Ass., *121*:9, 1952.

Slappendel, R.J., et al.: Spontaneous Consumption Coagulopathy in a Dog with Thyroid Cancer. Thromb. Diath. Haemorrh., *24*:129, 1970.

Smith, R.D., et al.: Platelet Kinetics in Canine Ehrlichiosis: Evidence for Increased Platelet Destrucion as the Cause of Thrombocytopenia. Infect. Immun., *11*:1216, 1975.

Steinberg, S.: Aplastic Anemia in a Dog. J. Amer. Vet. Med. Ass., *157*:966, 1970.

Stormorken, A., et al.: Thrombocytopenic Bleeding in Young Pigs Due to Maternal Iso-Immunization. Nature, *198*:1116, 1963.

Surgerman, H.J., et al.: Thrombocytopenia in Progressive Lethal Canine Peritonitis. Surg. Gynecol. Obstet., *154*:193, 1982.

Tocantins, L.M.: The Mechanism of Hemostasis. Ann. Surg., *125*:292, 1947.

Triplett, D.A.: Qualitative or Functional Disorders of Platelets. *In* Platelet Function: Laboratory Evaluation and Clinical Application. Chap. 5. Triplett, D.A., ed. Amer. Soc. Clin. Pathologists, Chicago, pp. 123–159, 1978.

Tyslowitz, R., and Dingemanse, E.: Effect of Large Doses of Estrogens on the Blood Picture of Dogs. Endocrinology, *29*:817, 1941.

Tyslowitz, R., and Harman, C.G.: Influence of Large Doses of Estrogens on the Blood Picture of Rhesus Monkeys (Macaca mulatta). Endocrinology, *29*:349, 1941.

Valdez, H., and Peyton, L.C.: Idiopathic Thrombocytopenia Associated with Hematoma of the Maxillary Sinus. J. Equine Med. Surg., *2*:379, 1978.

Ward, M.V.: Thrombocytosis, Reduced Platelet Function and Amyloidosis in a Dog. Calif. Vet., *36*:15, April, 1982.

Weinfeld, A., et al.: Platelets in the Myeloproliferative Syndrome. Clin. Haematol., *4*:373, 1975.

Weiss, E., et al.: Volume Distribution and Ultrastructure of Platelets in Acute Hog Cholera. Thromb. Diath. Haemorrh., *30*:371, 1973.

Weiss, R.C., et al.: Disseminated Intravascular Coagulation in Experimentally Induced Feline Infectious Peritonitis. Amer. J. Vet. Res., *41*:663, 1980.

Wellde, B.T., et al.: Trypanosoma congolense: Thrombocytopenia in Experimentally Infected Cattle. Exp. Parasitol., *45*:26, 1978.

Wells, P.W., et al.: Acute Systemic Immediate Hypersensitivity in the Pig. Res. Vet. Sci., *16*:347, 1974.

Wilson, J.J., et al.: Infection-induced Thrombocytopenia. Semin. Thromb. Hemostas., *8*:217, 1982.

Wington, D.H., et al.: Infectious Canine Hepatitis: Animal Model for Viral-induced Disseminated Intravascular Coagulation. Blood, *47*:287, 1976.

Wintrobe, M.M., et al.: Clinical Hematology. 8th ed. Lea & Febiger, Philadelphia, 1981.

Zimmerman, T.S., and Ruggeri, A.M.: Von Willebrand's Disease. Clin. Haematol., *12*:175, 1983.

18

Erythropoiesis and Its Regulation

ERYTHROCYTE PRODUCTION   487
    Nomenclature   487
    Light Microscopic Morphologic Features of
      Erythropoiesis   488
    Ultrastructural Features of
      Erythropoiesis   491
    The Birth of the Reticulocyte   495
    The Reticulocyte   499
    The Corrected Reticulocyte Count   501

ERYTHROKINETICS   501

REGULATION OF ERYTHROPOIESIS   503
    Erythropoietin   503
    Hormonal Influence on Erythropoiesis   507

MATERIALS ESSENTIAL FOR
    ERYTHROCYTE PRODUCTION   508
    Protein   508
    Minerals   509
    Vitamins   510

The mass of circulating red cells and the erythropoietic tissue in the bone marrow constitute a functional unit, the *erythron* (Boycott, 1929). Physiologic and pathologic states may affect the erythron, resulting in an absolute or relative change above or below the normal level. The erythron in health remains in delicate balance, for the daily production of erythrocytes equals the daily loss from destruction of senescent cells. The rate of erythrocyte replacement in a normal individual is incredibly fast; almost 1 million red cells are replaced every second in a healthy, 15-kg dog, for example. In response to anemia, normal hematopoietic tissues can undergo a six- to eightfold increase in erythrocyte production. An understanding of the process of erythropoiesis and exogenous and endogenous factors in its regulation is basic to effective treatment of the anemic patient.

ERYTHROCYTE PRODUCTION

It is postulated that primitive, undifferentiated pluripotential stem cells in the bone marrow give rise to unipotential cells, each committed to the erythrocytic, granulocytic-monocytic, or megakaryocytic series (see Chapter 13). The uncommitted and committed cell types have not been identified morphologically, although lymphocyte-like cells are considered to be the progenitor cells (Thomas et al., 1965). Functional existence of such cells has, however, been established by in vivo and in vitro experiments. Erythropoiesis in mammals begins with the differentiation of pluripotential stem cells into two erythroid progenitor cells, the burst forming unit–erythroid (BFU-E) and its progeny, the colony forming unit–erythroid (CFU-E) (Fig. 18–1, Table 18–1). The latter, under the influence of erythropoietin (Ep), subsequently gives rise to morphologically recognizable erythroid precursors, rubriblasts, which ultimately undergo at least four mitoses to produce mature erythrocytes.

Nomenclature

Different nomenclatures are in vogue for various morphologically identifiable cells of the erythroid series (Table 18–2). Recommendations of the Committee for Clarification of Nomenclature of Cells and Diseases of the Blood and Blood-Forming Organs (1950) have not been followed uniformly. Hence confusion regarding names of various immature erythroid cells flourishes, while hematologists continue to use a terminology under which even a nondividing cell is still given a "blast" suffix. *Veterinary Hematology* from its first edition adapted and continues to follow the terminology used in the reports of the committee.

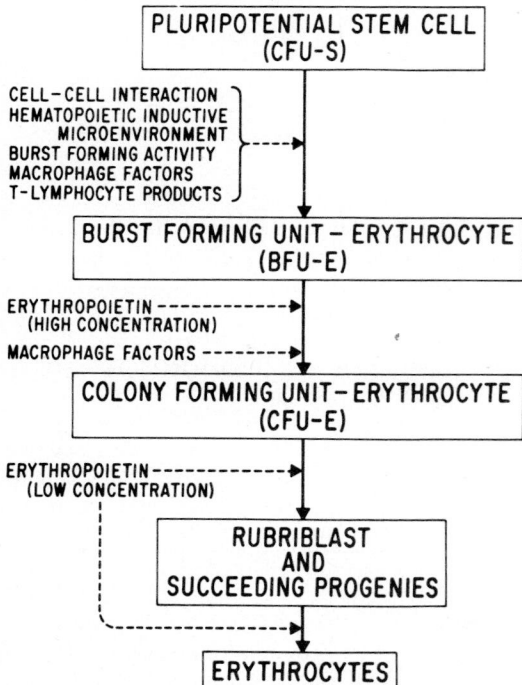

Fig. 18–1. Development of morphologically recognizable rubriblasts from morphologically unidentifiable but functionally recognizable progenitor cells. Also depicted are possible sites of interaction of various factors found to stimulate erythropoiesis in vitro and in vivo. See also Figure 18–12.

Light Microscopic Morphologic Features of Erythropoiesis

The earliest and most immature but recognizable cell of the erythrocytic series is the rubriblast. Erythrocytes are produced by mitotic division and maturation of rubriblasts in definite sequence (Table 18–2, Fig. 18–2). Cells in the mitotic compartment—from the rubriblast to the polychromatic rubricyte—normally undergo four mitotic divisions, one at each stage. Metarubricytes do not divide. Sequential maturation involves, besides loss of nucleoli and mitotic capacity, a progressive (a) decrease in size of both the cell and its nucleus, (b) increase in nuclear chromatin condensation, (c) decrease in cytoplasmic basophilia, and (d) increase in polychromasia followed by normochromasia in parallel with the amount of hemoglobin synthesized.

The developing erythroid cells in marrow are organized into small, discrete groups, *erythroblastic islands*, composed of a central reticulum cell surrounded by one ring or sometimes two rings of erythroid cells (Fig. 18–3) at various stages of differentiation and maturation (Bessis, 1973). The cytoplasm of the reticulum cell interdigitates between the erythroid cells. This arrangement of erythroid cells is readily seen in preparations of marrow carefully removed from a freshly opened bone and gently teased between a slide and a coverslip. Marrow aspiration disturbs the arrangement; hence it is not seen in smears of marrow aspirates. The reticulum cell hypothetically nourishes the developing erythroid cells, and so it is also called the nurse cell. It provides some ferritin to be used for heme synthesis and may be the immediate source of diffusible cellular substances needed for differentiation of erythroid progenitors into rubriblasts. Maturing erythroid cells move away from the nurse cell to become reticulocytes. The nurse cell also acts as a phagocytic cell to engulf free nuclei of the metarubricytes and aged red cells.

Table 18–1.   Some Features of Early and Late Erythroid Progenitor Cells

Burst Forming Unit–Erythrocyte (BFU-E)	Colony Forming Unit–Erythrocyte (CFU-E)
1. Originates from pluripotential stem cell.	Originates from BFU-E and is the immediate precursor of the rubriblast.
2. Relatively small and few in hematopoietic marrow tissue.	Relatively large and more abundant.
3. Forms large colonies, called "bursts," composed of many small subcolonies that mature in 7–8 days and contain several hundred to several thousand cells.	Forms small colonies of 8–128 nucleated cells in cultures of hematopoietic tissue in semisolid agar. The colonies mature in 2–7 days, and their number and size vary with concentration of erythropoietin in the culture.
4. Relatively erythropoietin-insensitive; hence requires higher (0.1–2.5 units) concentrations of erythropoietin for colony formation.	Erythropoietin-sensitive cell, responsive to fairly low (0.01–0.25 units) concentration of erythropoietin.
5. Their number changes very slightly after bleeding or hypertransfusion.	Their number increases markedly in blood loss anemia and decreases sharply after hypertransfusion.

Table 18–2.   Nomenclatures for Members of the Erythrocytic Series

Recommended Term	Other Terms
Rubriblast	Pronormoblast, Proerythroblast
Prorubricyte	Basophilic (or early) normoblast or erythroblast
Basophilic rubricyte	(included in the above category)
Polychromatic rubricyte	Early polychromatic normoblast or erythroblast
Metarubricyte	Late polychromatic normoblast or erythroblast, orthochromatic normoblast or erythroblast
Reticulocyte	Polychromatic erythrocyte
Erythrocyte	Red blood cell, Red cell

Light microscopic features of the erythroid series in a Wright-stained marrow film are given in Chapter 1 and are briefly described below.

The *rubriblast* is the largest cell of the erythrocytic series. It is round to oval and measures 15–20 μm in diameter. It has a nongranular, deep blue cytoplasm with or without a lightly stained peri- or paranuclear zone representing an active Golgi apparatus (Plate IV–1). The nucleus is round, occupies about three-fourths of the cell, and contains one or two

Patterns of Erythropoiesis

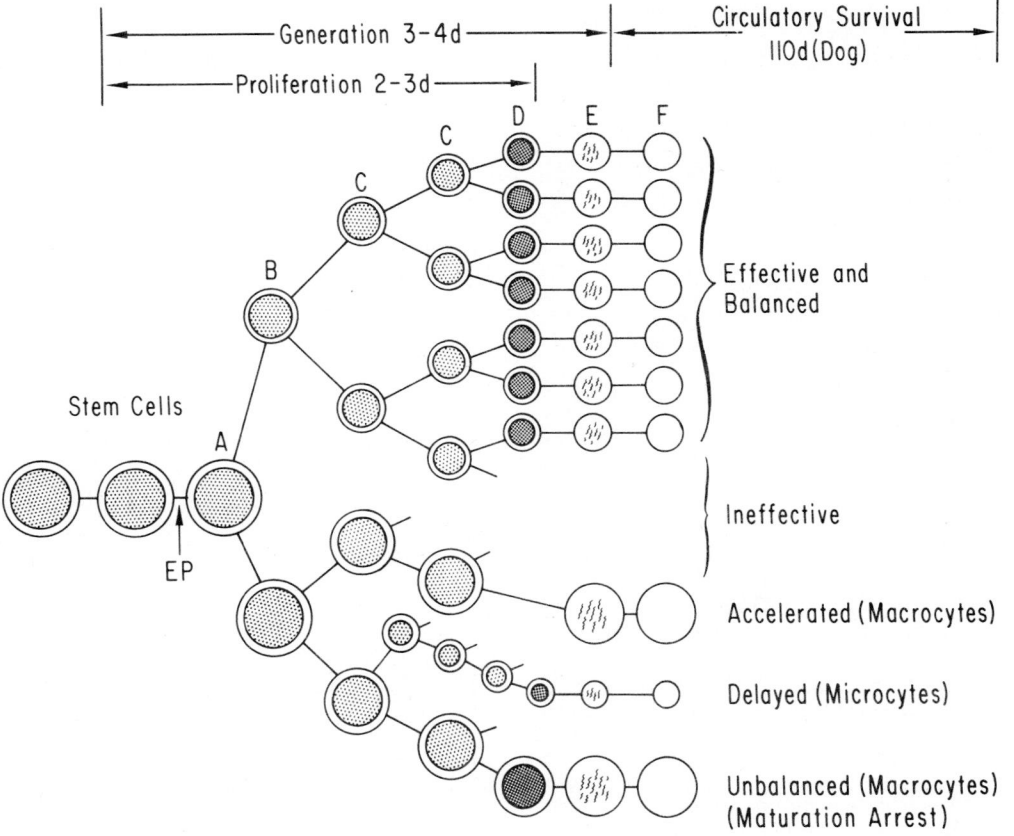

Fig. 18–2. Patterns of development and maturation of erythroid cells in health and disease. Erythropoiesis in health is mostly effective and balanced, although some ineffective erythropoiesis may occur. Examples of altered erythropoiesis shown are: accelerated erythropoiesis seen in responsive anemia, delayed erythropoiesis of iron deficiency, and unbalanced erythropoiesis of vitamin-B$_{12}$/folate deficiency. (A) rubriblast, (B) prorubricyte, (C) rubricyte, (D) metarubricyte, (E) reticulocyte, (F) erythrocyte. Average marrow proliferation and generation times of erythroid cells in days are given at the top along with life span of circulating red cells of the dog. (From Kaneko, 1980; courtesy of Academic Press.)

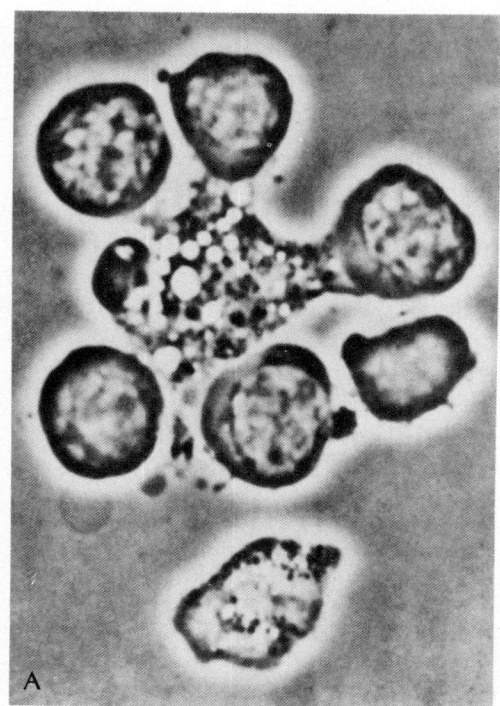

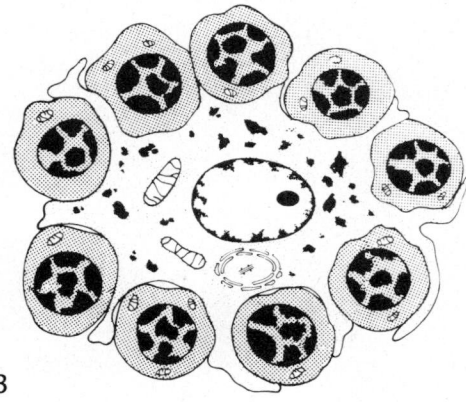

Fig. 18–3. *A,* An erythroblastic island examined in the living state by phase contrast microscopy; the cytoplasm of the reticulum cell can be identified by its many refractile inclusions. *B,* Schematic of an erythroblastic island; a corona of erythroid cells encircles the reticulum cell in which masses of hemosiderin can be seen. (From Bessis, 1973; courtesy of Springer-Verlag.)

nucleoli or nucleolar rings (Plates IV–1, IV–3). The nuclear chromatin is finely stippled and stains slightly more purple than in immature granulocytes. Rubriblasts are differentiated from myeloblasts and other similar-size blast cells by their more circular shape and deeper cytoplasmic and nuclear staining, the latter two characteristics reflecting, respectively, their slightly higher RNA and DNA contents. The *prorubricyte* has features identical to the rubriblast except for the absence of nucleoli (Plate IV–2). Some prorubricytes may be larger, have highly basophilic cytoplasm, and show slight chromatin condensation. The *basophilic rubricyte* is recognized by its condensed or coarsely granular nuclear chromatin, moderate to intense blue cytoplasm, and smaller size (Plates V–1, VI–6). Nucleoli are absent at this and subsequent stages. Sometimes it is difficult to distinguish between prorubricytes and basophilic rubricytes, particularly in the horse marrow. (Perhaps little would be compromised if these two cell series were combined into one category during routine evaluation of bone marrow films.) With increasing maturation, cytoplasmic color changes from blue to gray to orange owing to a reduction in the RNA and concomitant increase in the hemoglobin synthesis. Hence the *polychromatic rubricyte* has a grayish cytoplasm and increasingly prominent chromatin clumping (Plates IV–1, IV–5, VI–5). Cell size as well as nuclear size is reduced, and the nucleus occupies a relatively small area of the cytoplasm. The *metarubricyte* is the smallest of the nucleated erythrocytes and characteristically has a small, highly condensed nucleus that may stain homogeneously deep purple (pyknotic) or show a few light streaks or spots against a dark background (Plates IV–2, IV–5, VI–6). The cytoplasm of the metarubricyte is gray. Occasionally a metarubricyte and a late rubricyte may have normochromic cytoplasm. This is seen more often in equine and feline marrows. Cats with a myeloproliferative disorder involving the rubricytic series occasionally exhibit a higher frequency of normochromic metarubricytes in blood and bone marrow (Plate XIX–4). Extrusion of the metarubricyte nucleus gives rise to a polychromatic red cell, the *reticulocyte,* which later matures to become an erythrocyte. When a normochromic meta-rubricyte expels its nucleus, it skips the reticulocyte stage and gives rise to a giant red cell.

Ultrastructural Features of Erythropoiesis

Changes occurring in the cell structure during erythroid maturation have been studied with the electron microscope (Bessis, 1973; Fresco, 1974; Hertzberg and Orlic, 1981) and are shown in Figures 18–4 through 18–9. Ultrastructural abnormalities of the erythroid cells have also been described (Bessis, 1973; Fresco, 1981).

The rubriblast contains one or more prominent nucleoli and a nucleus having a predominantly loose chromatin (euchromatin) with little or no condensation (heterochromatin) near the nuclear envelope (Fig. 18–4).

The cytoplasm contains a well-developed Golgi apparatus, numerous ribosomes and polyribosomes, many mitochondria, a few strands of rough endoplasmic reticulum (RER), and scattered aggregates of ferritin molecules. The presence of ferritin helps identify the cell as belonging to the erythroid series. There is active DNA, RNA, and protein synthesis, but no hemoglobin synthesis. Deep basophilia seen in Wright-stained films is due to high RNA content.

The prorubricyte contains abundant free ribosomes and polyribosomes, many mitochondria, and traces of RER (Fig. 18–5). Its nucleus lacks or may have a small nucleolus and may show some evidence of beginning chromatin condensation. Globin synthesis begins at this stage and continues until the reticulocyte stage. Ribosomes are involved in

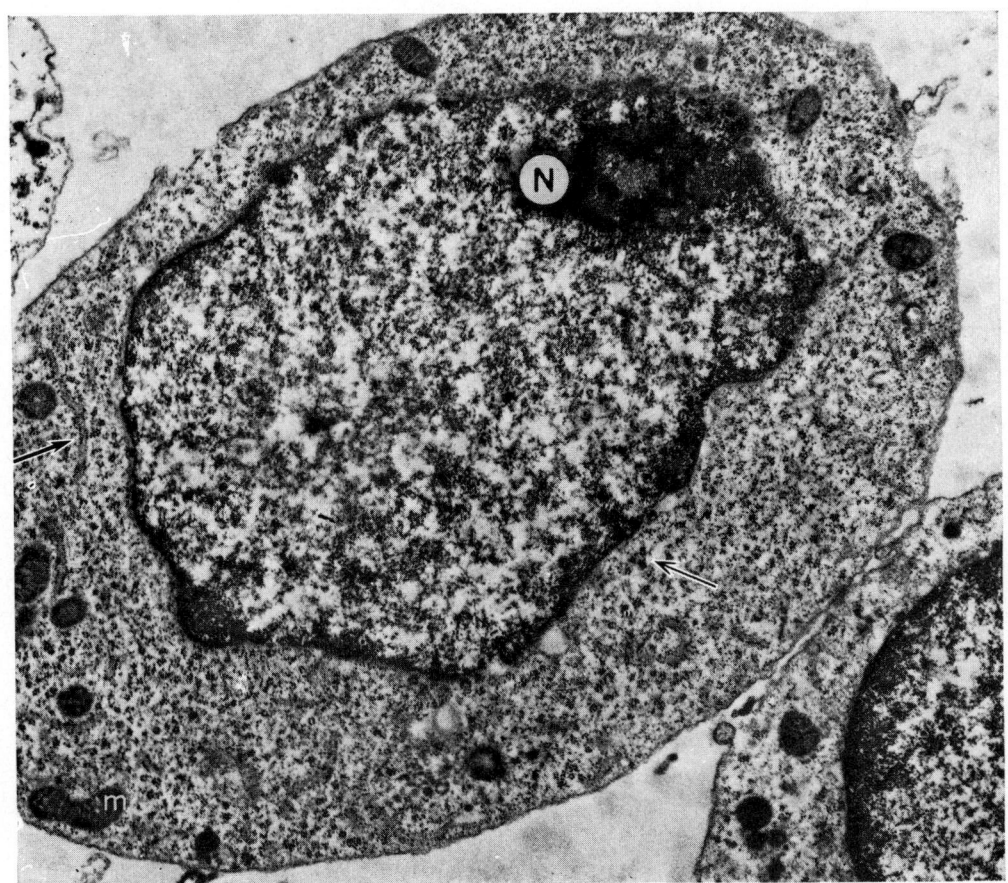

Fig. 18–4. An electron photomicrograph of a rubriblast from canine bone marrow. The nucleus has a nucleolus (N) and dispersed chromatin, some of which is marginated along the nuclear membrane. The cytoplasm is characteristically loaded with polyribosomes appearing as small black specks *(right arrow)*. Many mitochondria (m) and profiles of rough endoplasmic reticulum *(left arrow)* are also apparent. × 12,000.

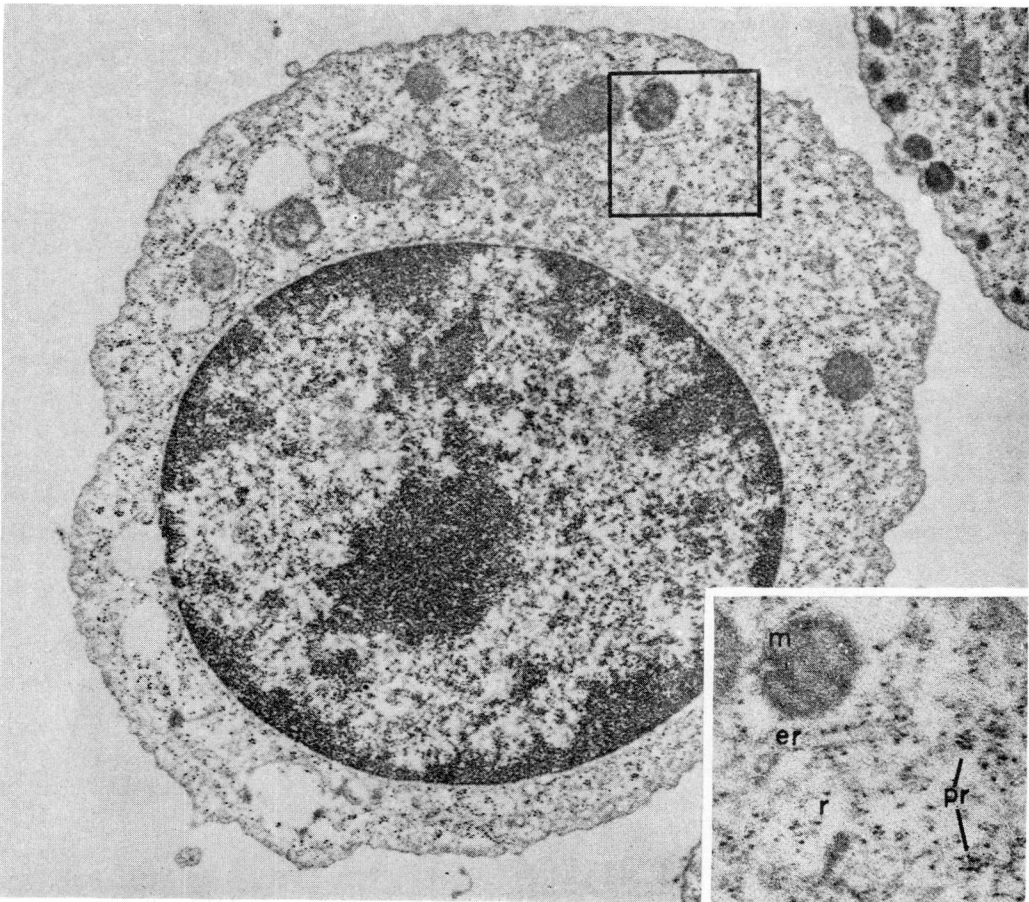

Fig. 18–5. A prorubricyte. The nucleus indicates incipient chromatin aggregation. The cytoplasm contains abundant polyribosomes and monoribosomes, many mitochondria, and traces of rough endoplasmic reticulum. ×16,000. Inset shows enlarged area in which a portion of the rough endoplasmic reticulum (er), a mitochondrion (m), ribosomes (r), and polyribosomes (pr) can be clearly seen. ×31,000.

the globin synthesis, while heme synthesis occurs in the mitochondria.

With maturation, the nucleoli disappear, and there is progressive condensation of the nuclear chromatin at first along the nuclear membrane and then centrally (Figs. 18–6, 18–7). Cytoplasmic structures such as ribosomes and mitochondria decrease in number, particularly after the basophilic rubricyte stage. There is a rapid loss of DNA and RNA synthesizing activity but an increase in the rate of heme synthesis. Thus the cytoplasm gradually loses its basophilic staining and becomes polychromatic. With accumulation of hemoglobin, cytoplasmic density increases.

In a condensed nucleus, a few small but well-defined areas of interchromatin material (Fig. 18–7) can be seen with the electron microscope, as is sometimes observed with the light microscope. These areas in rubricytes and metarubricytes consist of chromatin granules interspersed with hemoglobin (Fawcett and Witebsky, 1964), and they are contiguous with the cytoplasm at the nuclear pores (Fig. 18–7B, D). The number of nuclear pores decreases with cell maturation. No RNA of any form is synthesized after the basophilic stage of maturation and no DNA after the polychromatic stage. This cessation of RNA and DNA synthesis is thought to be due to interaction between intranuclear hemoglobin and nuclear histones (Stohlman, 1970). It is conjectured that an equilibrium exists between the intranuclear and cytoplasmic hemoglobin concentrations through the nuclear pores. Once a critical concentration of hemoglobin (circa 20%) is reached, a negative feedback presumably shuts off the nucleic acid synthe-

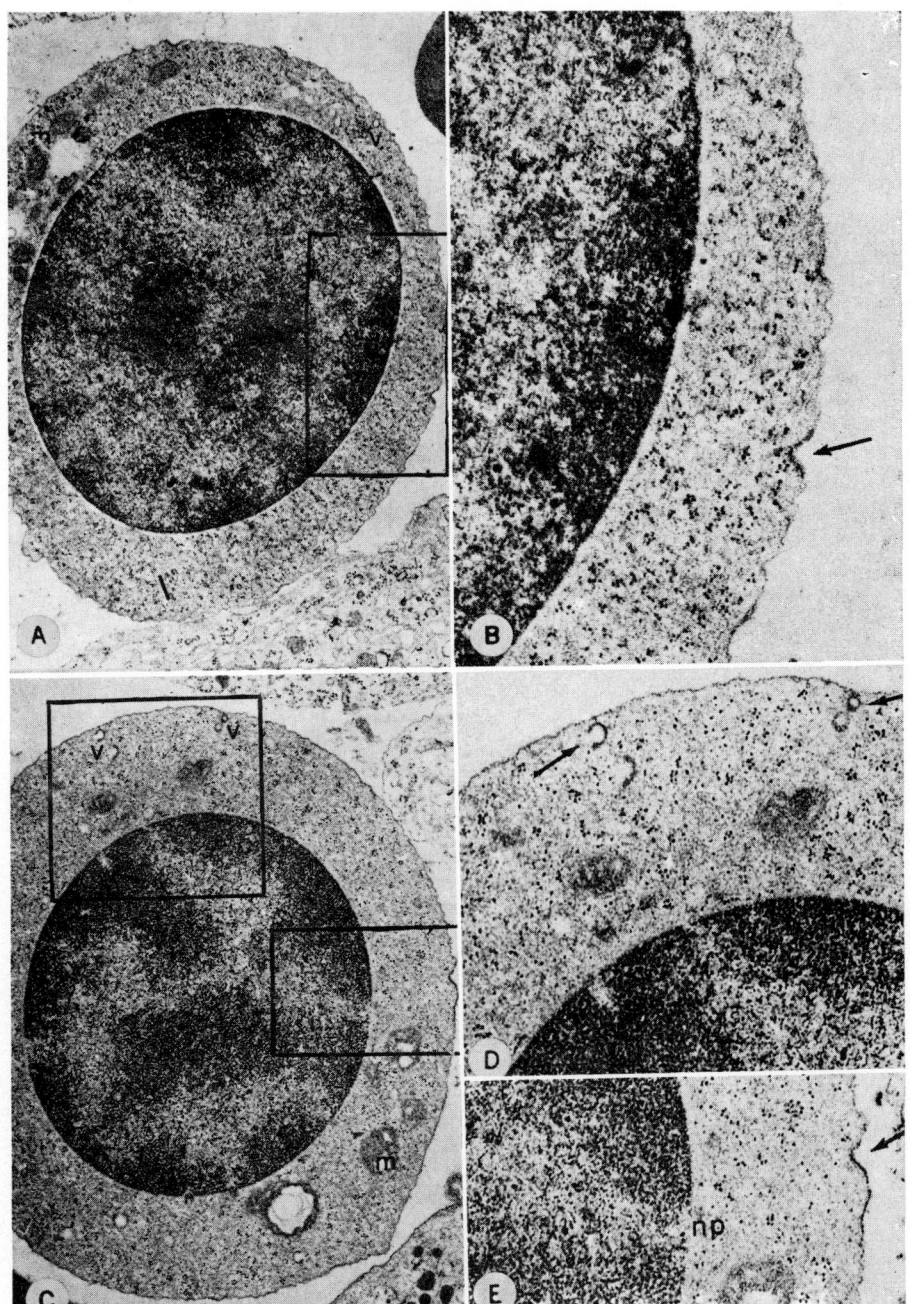

Fig. 18–6.   Early (*A*, ×10,560) and late (*C*, ×9,860) rubricytes. The nuclei in these cells are typically round and present areas of chromatin condensations having fuzzy demarcation zones that will become distinct with maturation. The cytoplasm contains fewer ribosomes and polyribosomes than the cell in Fig. 18–5. Some mitochondria (m), and pinocytotic vesicles (v) are in evidence. Insets show areas enlarged. *B* (×31,680) and *E* (×19,710) depict areas of surface membrane with fuzzy coating of ferritin granules and beginning of pinocytotic invaginations *(arrows)*; a nuclear pore (np) can be seen clearly in *E*. Pinocytotic vesicles *(arrows)* in the cytoplasm of the late rubricyte (*D*, ×19,710) are clearly visible at higher magnification.

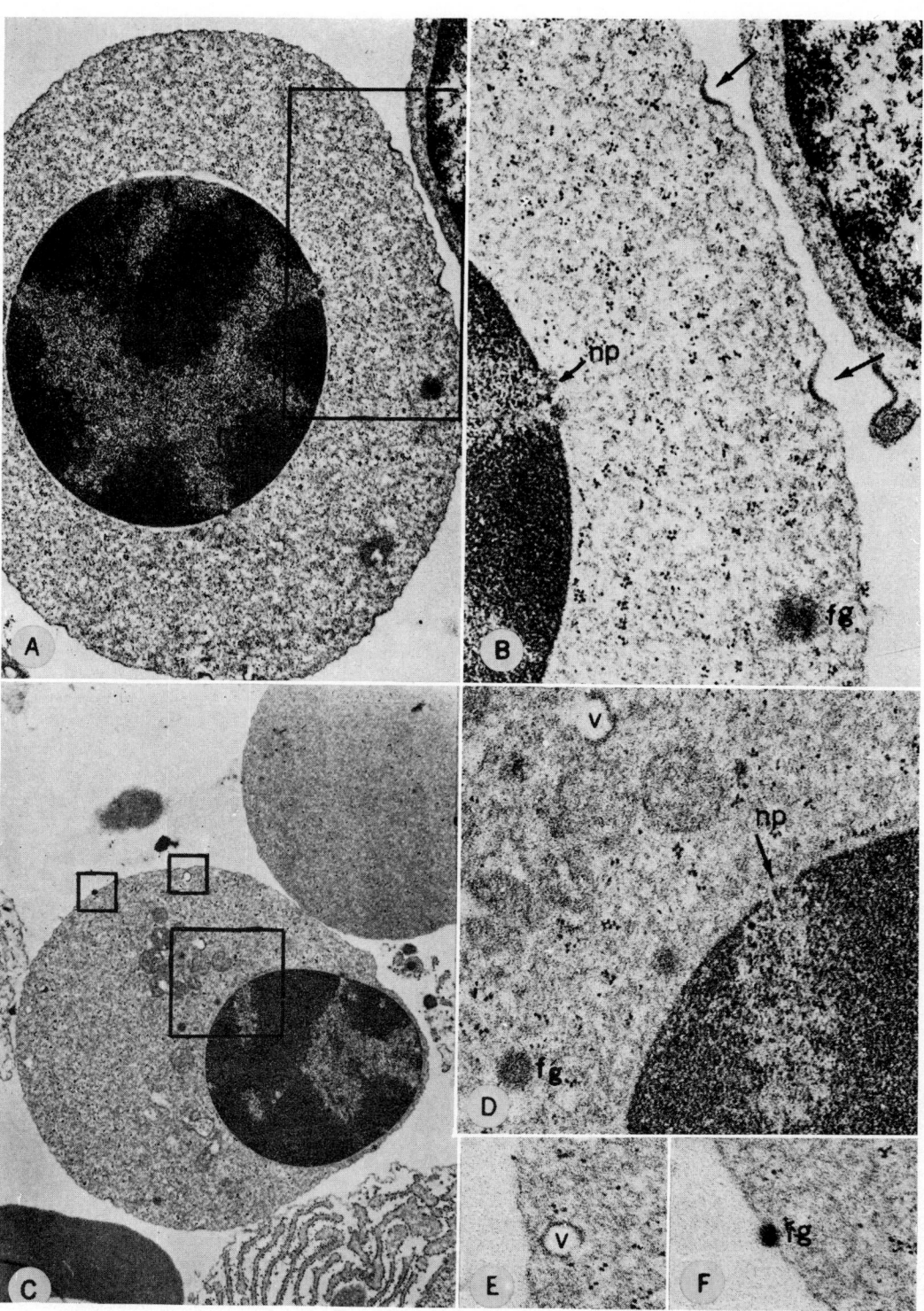

Fig. 18–7. Metarubricytes (*A*, ×11,900; *C*, ×8,000). The nuclei present marked chromatin condensations and some open areas. (These are hardly visible under the light microscope.) Insets show areas enlarged. Apparent also at this stage of maturation are pinocytotic invaginations of the surface membrane with coating of ferritin granules (*outer arrows* in *B*, ×25,000); pinocytotic vesicles, v (*D* and *E*, both ×36,000); and a dense accumulation of ferritin granules (fg) at the surface membrane (*F*, ×36,000) or in the cytoplasm (*B* and *D*). Nuclear pores (np) are more apparent at higher magnification (*B* and *D*); certain cytoplasmic and nuclear contents interchange through these regions. The metarubricyte in *C* has an eccentrically placed nucleus, which indicates that this cell is at a stage prior to denucleation.

sis. Thus the DNA synthesis, the number of mitotic divisions, and the cell size are controlled by the rate of hemoglobin synthesis. Asynchrony leads to pathologic changes in cell size and morphology. Delayed hemoglobin synthesis, as in iron deficiency, is associated with longer (continued) DNA synthesis, resulting in an extra mitosis and production of microcytes. In contrast, delayed DNA synthesis with a normal rate of hemoglobin synthesis, as in vitamin B_{12} and folate deficiencies, is associated with a reduction in mitotic division and production of macrocytes. Hemoglobin synthesis is slight at the basophilic rubricyte stage, moderate at the polychromic stage, and marked at the metarubricyte stage and continues after denucleation. About 15–20% of total hemoglobin is synthesized at the reticulocyte stage.

All erythroid precursors have characteristic small surface invaginations (Figs. 18–6, 18–7) at which ferritin granules may be seen. These invaginations, upon incorporation into the cell, form cytoplasmic vesicles containing aggregates of ferritin. Bessis (1973) called this process rhopheocytosis, which is akin to pinocytosis. Ferritin contains about 20% iron. Iron is also provided by transferrin through specific receptor sites present on the surface of immature erythroid cells, including the reticulocyte. Biochemically, the receptor sites are made up of glycoproteins with a MW of about 43,000–180,000 (Ecarot-Charrier et al., 1980; Steiner, 1980). Transferrin is a glycoprotein with a MW of about 83,000. It binds 2 atoms of iron in the ferric state. It attaches to the surface of the immature red cell, donates its iron at the receptor site, and detaches itself once again to be able to carry more iron. The iron receptor subsequently delivers the iron to the cytosol (Glass et al., 1980). Iron is taken up as early as the rubriblast stage, and the uptake decreases with increasing cell maturity. Excessive iron appears as hemosiderin and may be visualized as siderotic granules in the cytoplasm of nucleated red cells and mature erythrocytes stained with Prussian blue (Plates XII–10, XV–5). The number of such nucleated erythroid cells in normal human marrow may vary from 24–81% (Wintrobe et al., 1981). Cells containing hemosiderin—*sideroblasts* (nucleated erythrocytes) and *siderocytes* (erythrocytes)—increase in marrow in conditions associated with derangement of iron utilization by erythroid precursors.

Reticulocytes and young erythrocytes, as seen with the scanning electron microscope, display a variable degree of membrane folding and minute surface invaginations or pits (Fig. 18–10, *A–F*; Keeton and Jain, 1973). Transformation to mature erythrocytes is accompanied by a progressive decrease in the number of polyribosomes and mitochondria, loss of hemoglobin synthetic capacity, decrease in cell size, and change in cell shape to the biconcave form (Fig. 18–10, *G–J*).

The Birth of the Reticulocyte

The metarubricyte expels its nucleus within the marrow parenchyma by an active process. The process of denucleation has been studied in vitro (Bessis, 1973) and with the electron microscope (Skutelsky and Danon, 1970; Tavassoli, 1978). The metarubricyte has been observed to undergo violent cytoplasmic convulsions, pushing the nucleus to the periphery and suddenly expelling it (Bessis, 1973). Electron microscopic studies on dogs with hemolytic anemia indicate that the nucleus undergoes polarization, and many cytoplasmic vesicles accumulate in the vicinity of the deep surface of the nucleus prior to denucleation. These vesicles fuse with each other and with the cell membrane in such a way as to sever the nucleus from the main body (Simpson and Kling, 1968). Microfilaments have been observed for the first time in the cytoplasm of maturing erythroid cells in a position near the nucleus, suggesting an active role for these elements in the enucleation process (Repasky and Eckert, 1981). Nuclear expulsion usually occurs within the hematopoietic cords. The extruded nucleus, surrounded by a narrow rim of cytoplasm, is phagocytosed and digested by local macrophages (Fig. 18–8). Degradation of hemoglobin present in the cytoplasmic rim and also in the nucleus itself contributes to the "early peak" of bile excretion seen after administration of labeled hemoglobin components.

The newly formed reticulocytes display cytoplasmic characteristics of metarubricytes in that they retain polyribosomes, ribosomes,

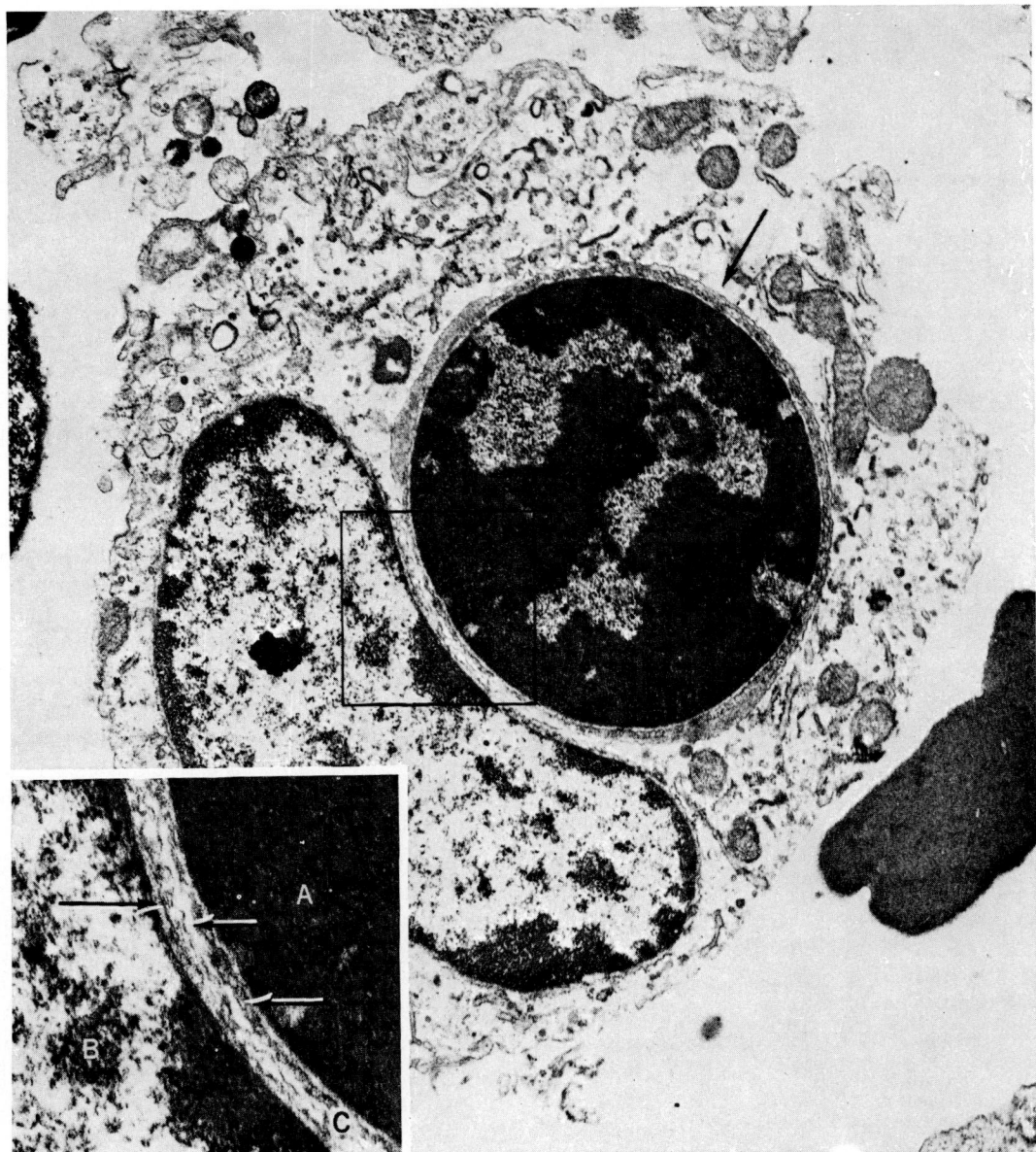

Fig. 18–8. An extruded metarubricyte nucleus *(arrow)* phagocytosed by a macrophage in the bone marrow. The metarubricyte nucleus is surrounded by a thin rim of cytoplasm (×11,200). The highly magnified inset (×25,200) presents portions of the metarubricyte nucleus (A) and phagocyte nucleus (B). The space (C) between the two nuclei contains three membranes: the membrane of the metarubricyte nucleus *(bottom arrow)*; the membrane of the phagosome, in which the extruded nucleus lies *(middle arrow)*; and the membrane around the macrophage nucleus *(top arrow)*.

and mitochondria (Fig. 18–9*A, B*) and continue to synthesize hemoglobin. Ribosomes and polyribosomes in a dispersed state contribute to the polychromatic appearance of reticulocytes with Wright stain. Vital stains such as new methylene blue and brilliant cresyl green produce aggregation of ribosomes and polyribosomes leading to the formation of a "reticulum" (Plate IV–6) (Rifkind et al., 1964). Under the electron microscope (Fig. 18–9*D)*, the reticulum is seen to be composed of both ribosomes and mitochondria or of ribosomes alone (Jensen, 1965; Orlic, 1970). The reticulocytes normally undergo a maturation process in the bone marrow for about 1–2 days, during which time there occurs a progressive decrease in polyribosomes (Rifkind et al., 1964), mitochondria (Simpson and

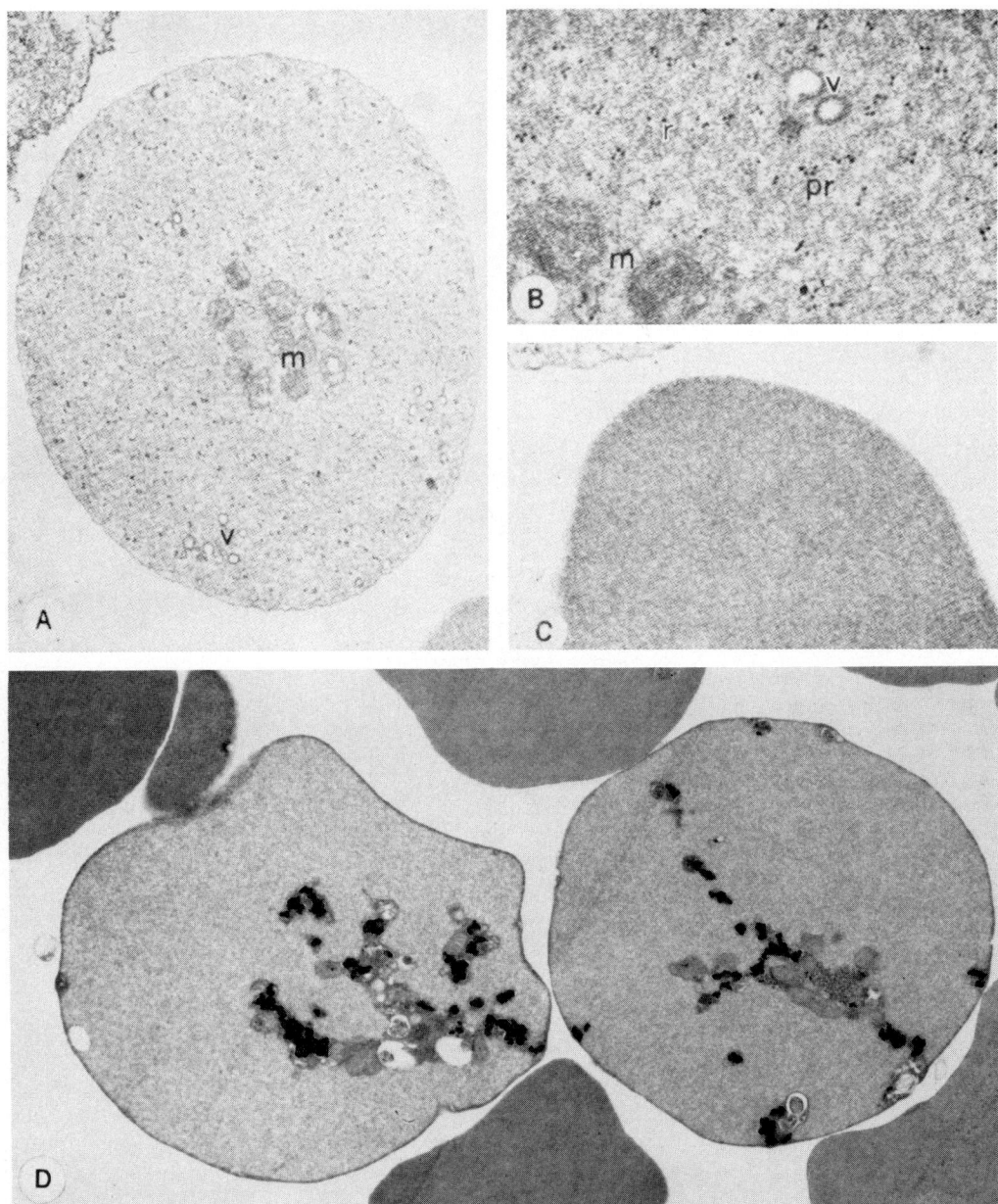

Fig. 18–9. A reticulocyte (*A*, ×12,740) and its enlarged portion (*B*, ×35,280) contain many ribosomes (r) and poly-ribosomes (pr). These form the characteristic reticulum when blood films are stained with new methylene blue vital stain (see Fig. 2–25;1). Mitochondria (m) and pinocytotic vesicles (v) are also present. Fuzzy, finely granular material in *B* is the hemoglobin. A portion of the mature erythrocyte shown in *C* exhibits homogeneous cytoplasm (×15,680). Two reticulocytes in *D* are from canine blood stained with new methylene blue to demonstrate their reticulum by electron microscopy. Cytoplasmic aggregates contain dense, stringy ribosomal material with entangled electron-light mitochondria (×11,500).

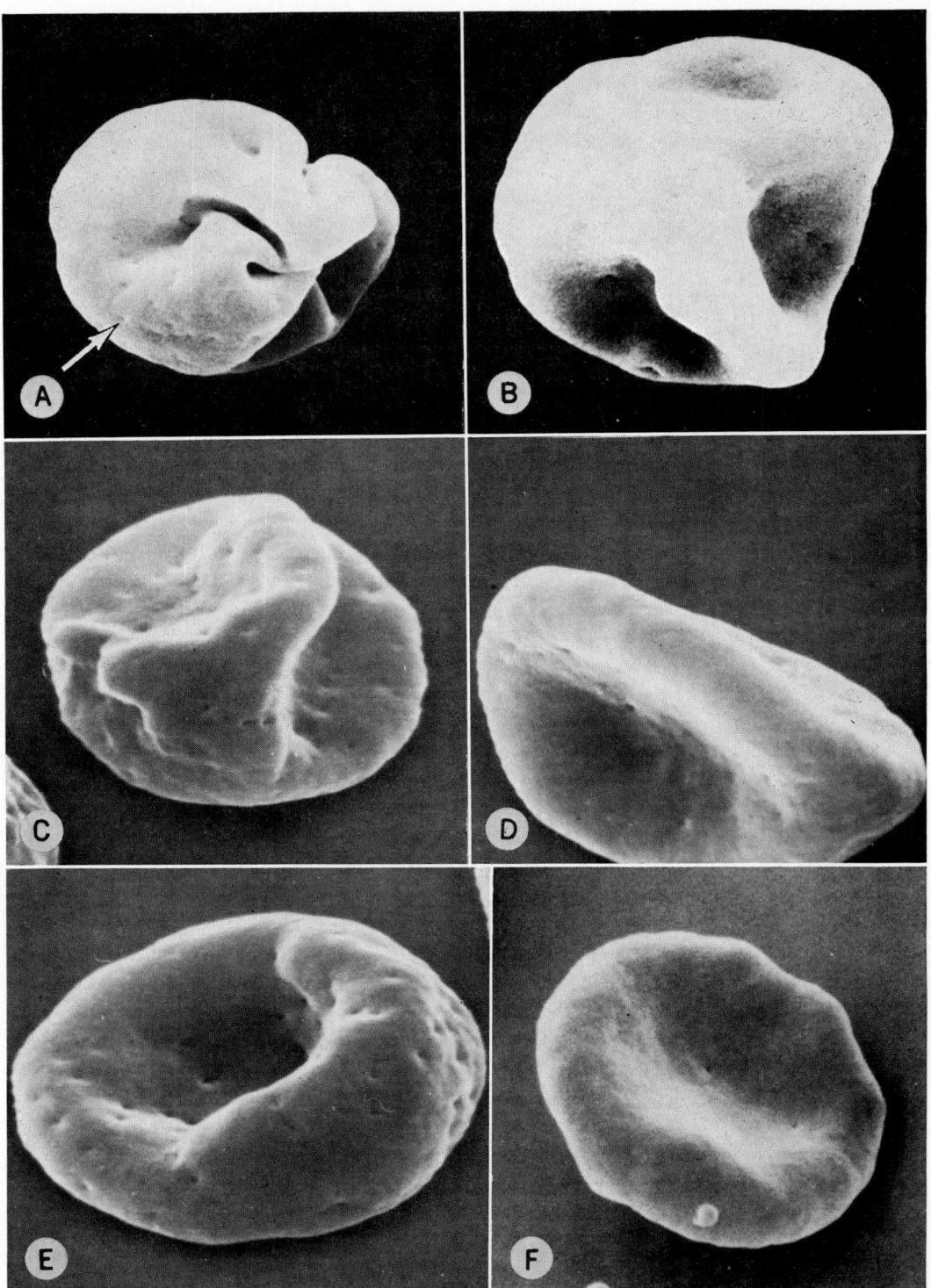

Fig. 18–10. (A–F). Scanning electron photomicrographs of maturing canine reticulocytes and erythrocytes. Such cells occur in the peripheral blood during remission following a severe blood loss or an episode of hemolytic anemia. *A* and *B,* Reticulocytes with characteristic irregular shape, membrane folding, invaginations of the surface, and many small shallow pits on the surface *(arrow).* The pits probably represent areas of pinocytotic activity. The reticulocyte in *A* is more immature than that in *B.* (*A,* ×7,700; *B,* ×8,200). *C* and *D,* Maturing reticulocytes possessing a transverse fold or a "bar" that indicates excessive surface area; the surface area is less than that of the cells shown in *A* and *B.* (*C,* ×10,300; *D,* ×9,700). *E,* An immature erythrocyte with a large concavity and highly thickened margins. (×9,700). *F,* An erythrocyte with the biconcave shape of maturity. The presence of a few surface pits as well as the slightly undulating margin indicate its young age. (×8,900). (Figs. *B–F* from Keeton and Jain, 1973; courtesy of *The California Veterinarian.*)

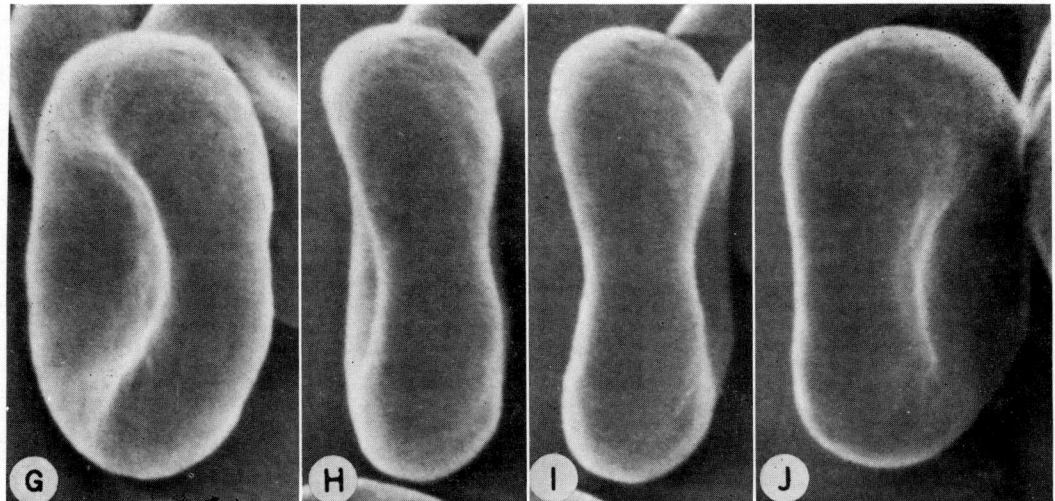

Fig. 18–10. (*G–J*). A canine erythrocyte photographed in succession at different angles of rotation to demonstrate the distinctive biconcave morphology as viewed with the scanning electron microscope. ×9,500.

Kling, 1968), membrane sialic acid and carbohydrate (Choy et al., 1979; Fukuda and Fukuda, 1981; Lutz and Fehr, 1979, and negative surface charge (Gattegno et al., 1979) and an increase in deformability (Leblond et al., 1971).

Reticulocytes enter the circulation by diapedesis (an active process) through endothelial cells lining the marrow sinusoids, probably through openings about 1–3 μm in diameter (Weiss, 1970; Orlic, 1970; also see Chapter 13). Reticulocytes have been found to exhibit ameboid movement in vitro (Walter, 1969). Normal release of maturing erythrocytes from the marrow is thought to be dependent upon cellular deformability and surface charge. The degree of reticulocyte release from the marrow into the peripheral blood varies among species (Leblond et al., 1971). After release into the circulation, the reticulocytes continue to mature for 24–30 hours before acquiring the uniformly homogeneous dense cytoplasm of the mature cell (Fig. 18–9C). This maturation may occur in the spleen since reticulocytes have been found to sequester preferentially in the spleen.

Normally, an occasional nucleated erythrocyte may cross the sinusoidal barrier and enter the general circulation. Nucleated erythrocytes are found in increasing numbers during intense erythropoietic response to anemia. Inappropriate release of nucleated erythrocytes is a pathologic consequence of marrow infiltration by leukemic cells, metastatic tumor, or granulomatous lesion; infection or septicemia; extramedullary hematopoiesis, and a variety of other situations such as lead poisoning and hemangiosarcoma.

The Reticulocyte

Reticulocytes are not found in health in the peripheral blood of the horse, cow, sheep, and goat. This means that the reticulocyte ripens in the bone marrow in these species. The dog and cat normally have an average of 0.5–1% reticulocytes in the peripheral blood, and the pig may have up to 2%. The rabbit, guinea pig, rat, and mouse normally exhibit 2–4% reticulocytes and are therefore good subjects for the demonstration of reticulocytes.

Reticulocytes increase in number in peripheral blood during response to blood loss, hemolytic diseases, or in remission of other types of anemia (Appendix Cases 20, 32, and 51). Reticulocytosis is not observed in peripheral blood of the horse in anemia in remission except under circumstances of continuous massive blood loss (Appendix Case 56). Reticulocytes were found to appear in bovine blood only after severe and sudden blood loss, and they disappeared during recovery even though macrocytosis persisted (Schnappauf et al., 1967). Marrow damage may be associated with release in blood of reticulocytes as well as nucleated red cells or of only the latter as mentioned above.

The time required for release of the newly formed reticulocytes in large numbers into the peripheral blood following a hypoxic stimulus is about 3–4 days, with the peak being attained by the seventh day (Appendix Case 69). When reticulocytes are released in large numbers, the mean corpuscular volume (MCV) generally increases in proportion to the number of immature cells present in the peripheral blood. In humans, the reticulocytes produced during normal conditions are about 20% larger than mature red cells (Kellman, 1964), and for every 10% increase in the reticulocyte count there is generally an increase of about 10 fl in the MCV (Harris and Kellermeyer, 1970). In the dog, the MCV increases about 8 fl for every 10% increase in the reticulocyte count (Fig. 18–11; Jain, 1980). However, a greater increase (two- to threefold) may be seen during intense erythropoiesis in other species (Appendix Case 69).

Reticulocytes are classified into 2 or 3 groups according to the amount of reticulum (see Chapter 5), which varies with the stage of maturation. In the normal animal, reticulocytes of the marrow are larger and less mature and contain more reticulum than those in the peripheral blood. Blood reticulocytes may contain a fully formed reticulum (aggregate reticulocytes) to a few specks or granules (punctate reticulocytes) in maturing cells. The former is usually seen in the dog, whereas the latter is often observed in the cat. The maturation time of reticulocytes in the peripheral blood of the dog was found to be 19–43 hours with the mean value of 31 hours (Nizet and Robscheit-Robbins, 1950). Longer values (range 26–54 hours, mean 39 hours) were obtained for human reticulocytes (Seip, 1953). In the cat, reticulocyte maturation time is slow, resulting in prolonged circulation of punctate reticulocytes (Alsakar et al., 1977; Cramer and Lewis, 1972; Fan et al., 1978). A maturation time of 12 hours for the heavily and moderately reticulated type and 3 days for the lightly reticulated type of feline reticulocytes has been reported (Fan et al., 1978).

In summary, the reticulocyte differs from the mature red cell in the following ways. It is a larger cell (macrocyte) that has not yet attained the typical biconcave shape. It has a great excess of membrane in relation to its contents, and so it may appear as a leptocyte. It is of lower specific gravity and does not participate in normal rouleau formation or pathologic agglutination (Stephens, 1940); hence it sediments slowly. It is more resistant to crenation (Key, 1921) (Fig. 2–24;1), to lysis by specific hemolytic serum (Cruz and Junaqueira, 1952), and to hypotonic lysis (Davis

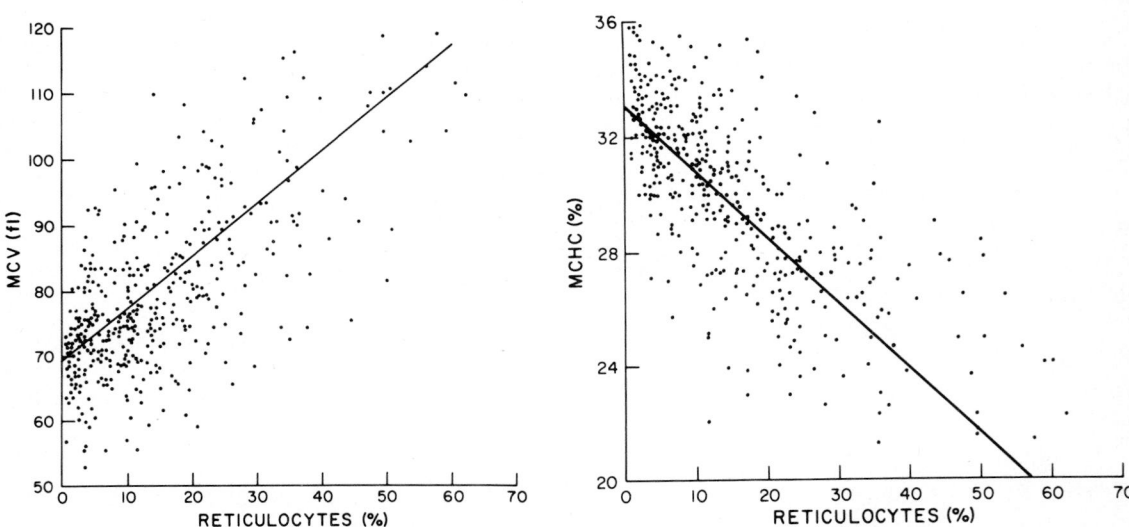

Fig. 18–11. Correlation of MCV *(left)* and MCHC *(right)* with reticulocyte count for anemic canine patients. (From Jain, 1979; courtesy of *The California Veterinarian.*)

et al., 1954; Johnson and Schwartz, 1971), and it is less susceptible to mechanical trauma in vitro (Stewart et al., 1950). It has greater negative surface charge (Skutelsky and Danon, 1970) and is sticky. It is able to synthesize hemoglobin. Many of these characteristics are protective in nature and give the cell a greater potential for survival in the circulation than the mature erythrocyte has. This inherent greater resistance to forces that may destroy the mature cell indicates existence of a natural mechanism whereby hemoglobin can be contributed to the circulation under conditions favoring destruction of mature erythrocytes. In anaplasmosis, the *Anaplasma marginale* is not seen in reticulocytes as these cells enter the circulation to replace the destroyed parasitized mature erythrocytes (Plate XVIII–7). Similarly, Heinz body formation and haemobartonellosis in cats rarely involve reticulocytes.

The Corrected Reticulocyte Count

The number of reticulocytes present in the peripheral blood can be considered indicative of effective erythropoiesis. In humans, there is a pool of reticulocytes in the bone marrow; its size is estimated to be approximately equal to the number of nucleated erythroid cells. The size of the marrow pool of reticulocytes in various animal species remains to be determined. There is also an oscillatory release of reticulocytes from the bone marrow into the peripheral blood. A measurement of the absolute number of circulating reticulocytes demonstrated that in some dogs there was a periodicity of release of reticulocytes, with peaks at about 14-day intervals (Morley and Stohlman, 1969).

A premature release of reticulocytes into the peripheral blood occurs under the influence of increased levels of erythropoietin (Ep). These cells, called "shift" or "stimulated" reticulocytes, are large and contain more reticulum. They require more time (about 1.5–3 days) to mature in the peripheral blood. Hence an increase in the reticulocyte count in peripheral blood may reflect increased production as well as increased accumulation. Therefore it is said that the reticulocyte count overestimates impression of enhanced erythropoiesis (Hillman, 1969) and

that the reticulocyte count will be more meaningful if it is corrected both for variations in the circulating red cell number and for changes in the maturation time (Hillman and Finch, 1969). Correction for the former variable can be made by determining the *absolute number* of circulating reticulocytes per μl of blood by multiplying the observed percentage of reticulocytes by the red cell count. Another approach is to obtain the *absolute percent* reticulocyte count by the formula:

> Absolute percentage = observed percent reticulocyte count × observed PCV ÷ mean normal PCV for the species

Hemoglobin concentration or RBC count may be substituted for PCV in the above formula for similar calculations of absolute percentage of reticulocytes. The second correction for prolonged maturation time is then introduced to obtain the "corrected reticulocyte count" or "reticulocyte production index."

> Corrected reticulocyte count = absolute percent reticulocyte ÷ reticulocyte maturation time for the degree of anemia

The alteration in the reticulocyte maturation time in the circulation is proportional to the increase in the Ep level and, therefore, usually to the degree of anemia. In humans, it is estimated that the maturation time of reticulocytes in the peripheral blood would be 1.5 days for a PCV of 35%, 2 days for a PCV of 25%, and 2.5 days for a PCV of 15% (Hillman and Finch, 1969). Similar figures for animal species are not available, except for limited observations on the dog and cat cited above.

ERYTHROKINETICS

The number of hematopoietic stem cells and erythropoietic progenitor cells in the bone marrow is small. These cells are self-replicating and normally have a slow regenerative cycle and a prolonged G_1 phase (the resting period following mitosis and preceding DNA synthesis). Increased concentration of Ep, as during anemia, shortens the G_1 phase of Ep-responsive cells and increases the number of late committed erythrocytic progenitor cells (CFU-E). Hence it is the recognizable erythroid compartment that usually undergoes expansion during increased erythropoietic response.

Isotope labeling has provided information on the time required for normal erythropoiesis. In the normal human bone marrow, at any one time about 2–5% rubriblasts, 5% prorubricytes and basophilic rubricytes combined, and 6% polychromic rubricytes are dividing. Each rubriblast on an average undergoes 4 mitotic divisions and gives rise to 16 mature erythrocytes. Proliferation and cellular maturation proceed simultaneously. The generation time for each maturative stage is approximately 24 hours. The turnover time (time taken for replacement of an entire population of cells) for metarubricytes is about 2 days, and for reticulocytes it is about 1–2 days. Thus in humans it may take as long as 8 days for a rubriblast to develop into a marrow reticulocyte. The bone marrow transit time for red cells in the dog has been estimated to be 7 days (Morley and Stohlman, 1969).

Turnover times for cells of the erythrocytic series have been estimated for a limited number of animal species. In the normal cow, turnover times for various cells are: prorubricytes, 10 hours; basophilic rubricytes, 17 hours; and polychromic rubricytes, 42–52 hours (Kaneko, 1970; Rudolph and Kaneko, 1971). Based on these estimates, the total transit time for erythroid cells from the proliferative through the maturative pools in the bovine marrow was estimated to be between 100 and 110 hours. This compared well with the observation of 72–96 hours required for the first appearance of ^{59}Fe-labeled red cells in normal calves after injection of the isotope and with the 8–10 days required for maximum labeling (Kaneko and Mattheeuws, 1966). Similar observations were made during acute experimental anaplasmosis (Appendix Case 69) in which the polychromic erythrocytes or reticulocytes appeared in peripheral blood on about the fourth day after massive removal of the parasitized erythrocytes, with the peak of activity being reached by the seventh day.

Because of cell death or skipping of a maturation stage, the normal sequence of maturation is not always followed. About 10% of cells die in the marrow at various stages of development. Such cell death is referred to as *ineffective erythropoiesis*, as opposed to effective erythropoiesis. An increase in ineffective erythropoiesis leads to anemia. In the normal dog, there is no ineffective erythropoiesis up to the metarubricyte stage, but about 20% of cell loss occurs between the process of enucleation and entry into the circulation (Lala et al., 1966). Ineffective erythropoiesis has been found in porphyric cattle (Kaneko, 1963). There is defective (delayed) maturation of reticulocytes (Smith and Kaneko, 1966) and metarubricytes (Rudolph, 1968) in porphyric cattle. This delay in maturation is associated with a marked decrease in heme synthesis and contributes to anemia.

In vitro studies on culture of bone marrow colonies indicated that bovine marrow cells have a very small proportion of pluripotent stem cells and that the hematopoietic progenitors do not exist in a wide spectrum of maturation as they do in mouse and human cells (Kaaya et al., 1979). These limitations may be responsible for slower recovery from a hematologic stress in the bovine than in other species. Also, directional competition of erythroid-granulocyte stem cells may occur in the bovine when there is increased need of a particular cell type (Kaaya and Maxie, 1980). See Chapter 13 for further information on this aspect of hematopoiesis.

Changes in the rate of hemoglobin synthesis are also reflected in the type of red cells produced. When erythropoiesis is stimulated, as in blood loss or hypoxemia, reticulocytes are released about a day earlier and the rate of erythropoiesis is accelerated, resulting in production of macrocytes. Acceleration of hemoglobin synthesis during erythroid stimulation results in a more rapid achievement of critical hemoglobin concentration, which in turn results in a skipped terminal division, early denucleation, and production of large cells (Stohlman, 1970). These macrocytes disappear from the circulation in a matter of days. This disappearance was attributed to their shortened life span (Brecher and Stohlman, 1962); however, other studies (Ganzoni et al., 1971; Shattil and Cooper, 1972) indicated that these macroreticulocytes mature in the circulation into normal long-lived erythrocytes, but only after loss of considerable hemoglobin, cell membrane, and intracellular organelles. The degree of macrocytosis within a species appears to be proportional to the degree of erythroid stimulation, but there are species differences in the magnitude of the erythroid response to a similar stimulus. When the rate of hemoglobin synthesis is reduced, as in iron deficiency, the marrow transit time is prolonged. Thus the time to reach the critical hemoglobin concentration in a developing rubricyte is lengthened in iron deficiency, permitting an additional cell division that produces microcytes (Stohlman, 1979).

REGULATION OF ERYTHROPOIESIS

Events associated with stem cell differentiation into erythrocytic progenitors and subsequent steps involved in erythrocyte production are depicted in Figures 18–1 and 18–2. Transformation of the pluripotential stem cell into BFU-E occurs under influences that remain to be fully defined. Hematopoietic inductive microenvironment (HIM), certain hormonal factors such as burst promoting activity (BPA), and some other substances may all be involved in the initial differentiation (Peschle, 1980; Fisher and Gross, 1977). Glycosaminoglycan may be an important part of HIM for erythropoiesis (Noordegraaf and Ploemoeher, 1980). Certain diffusible growth factors, including BPA produced by macrophages (Kurland et al., 1980; Gordon et al., 1980) and T-lymphocytes (Cline and Golde, 1979), were found to enhance differentiation of the pluripotential stem cell into the BFU-E. Macrophage factors were also associated with the transformation of BFU-E into CFU-E. Corticosteroids may also participate in the process of stem cell differentiation into BFU-E (Urabe et al., 1979). Prostaglandins (PG) of the E and A series stimulate erythropoiesis by acting on erythroid precursor cells and by increasing Ep production both from renal and extrarenal sources (Naughton et al., 1982). A variable direct effect of PG on erythroid differentiation has been observed; PGE has a stimulatory effect on BFU-E of humans, dogs, and sheep and an inhibitory effect on BFU-E of rats and guinea pigs (Peschle, 1980). Erythropoietin plays a minor role in the differentiation of

pluripotential stem cells into BFU-E, whereas differentiation of BFU-E into CFU-E is Ep-dependent. Ca^{++} may be necessary for this interaction (Misiti and Spivak, 1979) and may play a key role in terminal erythroid differentiation (Bridges et al., 1981). See also Chapter 13 for additional information.

Differentiation of CFU-E into rubriblasts and subsequent stages involves Ep. On the basis of in vitro observations, it has been suggested that enhanced erythropoiesis during hemolytic anemia may be due partly to the direct stimulatory effect of heme on terminal erythroid differentiation (Bonanou-Tzedaki et al., 1981). Endotoxin-induced marrow suppression of erythropoiesis is attributed to a reduction in the level of circulating erythropoietin (Udupa and Lipschitz, 1982).

Erythropoietin

The fundamental stimulus for erythropoiesis is tissue hypoxia, whether a consequence of changes in the size of the erythron (e.g., anemia) or a result of altered oxygen saturation of hemoglobin. In 1906, Carnot and Deflandre proposed that erythropoiesis was controlled not by direct oxygenation of the marrow, but by the concentration of a humoral factor, hematopoietin, elaborated outside the marrow in response to hypoxia. It was not until 1950, however, that the existence of a plasma hematopoietic factor was demonstrated. Chronic hypoxia in one partner of parabiotic rats was found to generate a plasma factor that stimulated erythropoiesis in the bone marrow of both rats of the pair (Reissmann, 1950; Erslev, 1953; Hodgson and Toha, 1954). Later, it was shown that plasma from anemic rabbits had a stimulatory effect on erythropoiesis in normal rabbits, while normal rabbit plasma was ineffective (Erslev, 1953; Hodgson and Toha, 1954). Subsequently, a plasma factor, increasingly elaborated under hypoxic conditions and capable of stimulating erythropoiesis, was found in many species including humans, dogs, cows, sheep, goats, pigs, guinea pigs, mice, birds, and fish (Krantz and Jacobson, 1970). This humoral factor is called erythropoietin. The present concepts of Ep production and regulation are depicted in Figure 18–12.

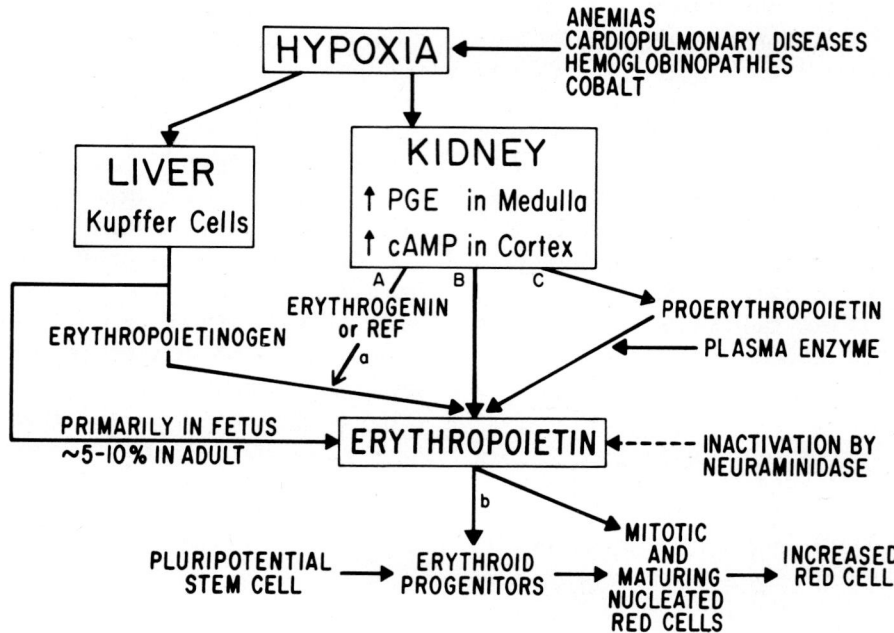

Fig. 18–12.   Current views (A, B, C) on synthesis of erythropoietin in response to various stimuli. Primary sites of stimulation of erythroid precursors by erythropoietin and sites of estrogen inhibition (a, large dose; b, small dose) of erythropoietin production or erythropoiesis are also shown. REF, renal erythropoietic factor.

Biologic Characteristics

Erythropoietin is the primary physiologic regulator of erythropoiesis in humans and animals in health as well as during anemia. It is normally found in small amounts in plasma and urine. The urine usually contains one-third to two-thirds the concentration found in plasma. It has also been found in the milk of lactating rats and mice (Grant, 1955). Highly purified Ep has been prepared from human urine and sheep plasma and is a glycoprotein containing 7.5–10% sialic acid (Graber and Krantz, 1978). The sialic acid residues are essential for biologic activity. The MW of human Ep is 27,000–60,000 and that of sheep Ep, 46,000–61,800. Ep is usually measured by bioassay because it is generally not species-specific, but other procedures, including a radioimmunoassay, have been developed. The amount of Ep in plasma and urine is inversely related to the hemoglobin level or tissue oxygenation. The oxygen affinity of hemoglobin also influences the production of Ep. Atmospheric, anemic, or cardiopulmonary hypoxia increases erythropoiesis by increasing Ep production, and hyperoxia and polycythemia,

created by transfusion of red cells, decrease erythropoiesis by decreasing Ep production. The Ep titer in the dog and in laboratory animals such as rabbits and rats can be raised by bleeding, by inducing hemolytic anemia or acute hypoxia, or by giving sublethal irradiation (Lowy, 1970). The plasma Ep titers increase in sheep and calves during anemic episodes associated with anaplasmosis (Jatkar and Kreier, 1967). During acute blood loss anemia in sheep, Ep levels increase precipitously to a maximum within 24 hours and subside rapidly after the third day and simultaneous with increases in the hematocrit value (Mohandas et al., 1980). In humans Ep production during acute hypoxia is increased within 12 hours, and maximum titer is reached at 3 days (Faura et al., 1969). The half-life of Ep is short; about 2–5 hours in rats (Reissmann et al., 1965), 7–10 hours in dogs (Bozzini, 1966; Weintraub et al., 1964), and 7–43 hours in humans (Rosse and Waldmann, 1964).

Site and Mechanism of Production

The kidney is the principal site of Ep production in the adult of many species, and it

Table 18–3. **Erythropoietin Production by Normal and Nephrectomized Dogs in Response to Bleeding, Cobalt Treatment, and Hypoxic Hypoxia**[a]

Treatment	24-hr Mean % RBC-^{59}Fe Uptake in Polycythemic Mice[b] ($\pm$ SEM)
Normal Dogs	
No treatment	0.61 $\pm$ 0.08
Bled to PCV 20%	8.85 $\pm$ 1.45
Cobalt (20 mg)	3.91 $\pm$ 0.57
Hypoxic hypoxia (10%)	11.14 $\pm$ 1.13
Nephrectomized Dogs	
No treatment	0.42 $\pm$ 0.01
Bled to PCV 20%	0.52 $\pm$ 0.02
Cobalt (20 mg)	0.37 $\pm$ 0.01
Hypoxic hypoxia (10%)	0.48 $\pm$ 0.03

[a]Modified from Mirand and Murphy, 1970, p. 497.

[b]Intravenously injected ^{59}Fe rapidly becomes incorporated in hemoglobin synthesized during erythrogenesis. Therefore, a determination of the amount of ^{59}Fe contained in newly formed erythrocytes can be taken as a direct measure of the rate of erythropoiesis (Plzak et al., 1955). Plasma from test animals (in this case, dogs) is injected by intravenous route into assay animals (in this case, polycythemic mice), which are then given a standard amount of ^{59}Fe. The degree of ^{59}Fe incorporation in red cells is determined at a suitable interval (in this case, after 24 hr). The presence of erythropoietin would be evidenced by an increase in the rate of ^{59}Fe incorporation. Thus erythropoietic activity of plasma from variously treated dogs shown in this table is proportional to the percent ^{59}Fe uptake and hence is an index of erythropoietin level.

is the sole source of Ep in the dog. A significant extrarenal production of Ep occurs in certain animals and anephric humans, but not in nephrectomized dogs. Erythropoiesis is almost completely depressed in dogs after nephrectomy and an amelioration of the developing azotemia by peritoneal dialysis does not restore red cell production. These animals do not respond to bleeding, hypoxic hypoxia, or cobalt treatment by demonstrable production of Ep (Naets, 1960; Mirand et al., 1968; Mirand and Murphy, 1970), as shown in Table 18–3. In contrast, significant quantities of Ep appear in dogs after renal transplants (Abbrect et al., 1968; Mirand et al., 1968).

Observations on laboratory animals, sheep, and humans (Fisher, 1979) indicate that extrarenal production of Ep during the fetal and neonatal periods, is primarily from the liver Kupffer cells. It is believed that in the adult extrarenal Ep normally plays an insignificant role in regulation of erythropoiesis, but it may be very important in an anephric patient. Extrarenal Ep probably helps in maintaining erythropoiesis during anemia of severe kid-

ney disease. Extrarenal Ep production is reduced following transfusion, while it is increased in response to bleeding or hypoxia but not by androgens.

Studies in rats have described a renal inhibitory factor reducing extrarenal (hepatic) Ep response to hypoxia (Naughton et al., 1981). Ep production has been detected in tissue cultures of normal adult kidney and fetal liver cell lines (Ogle et al., 1978). In vitro release of Ep from macrophages from various sources including the bone marrow, spleen, peritoneal exudate, lungs, and liver has been demonstrated (Rich and Kubanek, 1982). Administration of colloidal carbon or zymogen, which induces hyperplasia of liver mononuclear phagocytes (Kupffer cells), enhances EP production in nephrectomized rats exposed to hypoxia (Graber and Krantz, 1978).

The carotid body has been shown to control erythropoiesis in cats (Tramezzani et al., 1971), but not in humans (Lugliani et al., 1971).

The mechanism by which renal hypoxia is translated into chemical events leading to the production of Ep and the exact site of Ep production remain speculative. In vivo evidence favors the glomerulus as the site of Ep production, although other sites may also be involved (Ogle et al., 1978). Ep has been identified by fluorescent antibodies in the renal cortex (Busuttil et al., 1971). Two hypotheses exist with regard to the mode of Ep production (Fig. 18–12). According to one, the kidney regulates erythropoiesis by making an enzyme or principle called renal erythropoietic factor (REF) or erythrogenin. The latter can be extracted from the light mitochondrial or microsomal fraction of the kidney and is found in approximately equal quantities in the cortex and medulla (Gordon and Zanjani, 1970). Erythrogenin converts erythropoietinogen, an inactive plasma α-globulin produced by the liver, into active Ep. Another hypothesis is that Ep is synthesized in the renal medulla either in active form or in an inactive form (pro-Ep), which is activated by a serum factor at the time of release.

Stimulation of erythropoiesis by cobalt seems to be due to increased production of Ep resulting from histotoxic hypoxia induced by interference with certain enzymes concerned with the transport and utilization of oxygen (Goldwasser et al., 1958; Levy et al., 1950). It has been demonstrated recently that the kidney is capable of de novo synthesis of Ep and that cobalt potentiates the hypoxic stimulation of kidney Ep production (Katsuoka et al., 1983).

The formation and/or release of Ep by the kidney has recently been shown to be controlled by both hormonal and neural influences. Thus Ep production following hypoxia is abolished by cholinergic and β-adrenergic blockade or renal denervation. Activation of the β-adrenergic nervous system increases Ep production in normal or hypoxic animals. Albuterol, a $β_2$-adrenergic agonist, increased Ep production, while indomethacin decreased it (Jelkmann et al., 1979). Recent studies suggest that Ep production in response to renal hypoxia is modulated via the release of PG and/or prostacyclin and via activation of adenylate cyclase leading to elevation of renal cortical cyclic AMP levels (Fisher, 1980a, 1980b; Ghosal et al., 1980; Graber and Krantz, 1978). Evidence indicating that renal PGs trigger the production of Ep includes: (a) arachidonic acid as well as renal PGE_1 and PGE_2 are capable of increasing Ep production in the isolated perfused kidney; (b) renal hypoxia in the dog increases production of both PGE and Ep; (c) a prostaglandin synthetase inhibitor, indomethacin, blocks Ep production induced by perfusion of arachidonic acid or hypoxia; and (d) PGEs increase in vitro and in vivo erythroid colony formation in experiments with mice.

Effects of Erythropoietin

The primary target of Ep in the bone marrow is the committed erythropoietic progenitor cell, CFU-E, whose proliferation and maturation into rubriblasts is enhanced by a small amount of Ep. By comparison, BFU-E is relatively Ep-insensitive, requiring large amounts of Ep for differentiation into erythroid cells. Erythropoietin also exerts the following influences; (a) it stimulates proliferation of the rubriblasts and the developing rubricytes capable of mitosis; (b) it accelerates maturation of the rubricytic cells, thereby reducing the marrow transit time of erythroid

cells; and (c) it induces release of reticulocytes into the circulation (Gurney, 1970; Krantz and Jacobson, 1970). The primary molecular action of Ep is to stimulate RNA synthesis. This is followed by DNA synthesis, cell division, increased heme synthesis, and hemoglobin production in the responsive cells (Graber and Krantz, 1978).

Regulation of Fetal Erythropoiesis

Erythropoiesis in the fetus is not regulated by the maternal Ep but rather by its own Ep (Krantz and Jacobson, 1970; Scribner Seeley, 1970). The hormone has been demonstrated in the blood and urine of the human fetus at 32 weeks of gestation and also in the blood of sheep and goat fetuses. Maternal hypoxia stimulates fetal erythropoiesis through increased Ep production by the fetus and not by the mother (Zanjani et al., 1977). Fetal Ep does not cross the placental barrier to affect maternal erythropoiesis, nor does the exogenous or endogenous maternal Ep cross the placenta to influence fetal erythropoiesis (Krantz and Jacobson, 1970; Zanjani and Gordon, 1971). The primary site of production is the fetal liver and not the kidney. Studies with sheep fetuses indicate that the change in the site of Ep production from liver to kidney occurs gradually, beginning in utero during the last third of gestation (about 130 days) and reaching completion at about 40 days of postnatal life (McGlave and Zanjani, 1980; Zanjani, 1980).

Erythropoietin Production in Anemias and Polycythemias

It is obvious that anemia would ensue when there is insufficient production of Ep or inadequate bone marrow response, or both. Erythropoietin production in anemias of varied etiology has been determined (Erslev et al., 1980b; Ward et al., 1971). In anemias due to blood loss or hemolysis, there is an increase in both renal and extrarenal (Erslev et al., 1980a) production of Ep to stimulate erythropoiesis and reestablish the normal state. In secondary anemias (anemias secondary to nonhematologic diseases), there is either an inadequate Ep production or increased Ep production but inadequate bone marrow response, or both. The anemia of renal disease is due primarily to decreased production of Ep and is generally proportional to the degree of renal damage. About two-thirds of anemic human patients with rheumatoid arthritis, chronic infection, and some malignancie have inadequate Ep production, while one-third may show a mild increase (Ward et al., 1971). More recently it has been suggested that the diminished marrow response in malignancy and rheumatoid arthritis may be a result of one or more nonspecific erythropoietic inhibitors in circulation (Cavill and Bentley, 1982; Zucker et al., 1980). The anemia from protein deficiency partly involves inadequate Ep production since it can be corrected by Ep administration. Decreased Ep production as well as reduced stimulation of marrow cells may be found in endocrine deficiencies. The anemia of chronic respiratory disease is due primarily to decreased Ep production, although inadequate marrow response may be involved as well. Increased levels of Ep have been found in pernicious anemia, iron-deficiency anemia, sickle-cell anemia, leukemia, some cases of anemias associated with neoplasms, and various types of refractory anemias in humans. In these conditions, inadequate marrow response (erythropoiesis) may be the cause of anemia.

In humans, polycythemias secondary to renal tumors or cysts, hydronephrosis, tumors and hyperplasias of the endocrine organs, hepatomas, uterine leiomyomas, pulmonary disease, chronic heart disease, and the like are due to increased Ep production. It is conjectured that malignant or benign renal lesions induce Ep production, possibly through induction of local anoxia because of tissue compression from a space-occupying lesion. In primary polycythemia, however, Ep production is decreased. In addition, there are instances in which erythropoiesis is not Ep-dependent, e.g., polycythemia in mice induced by a strain of Friend leukemia virus (Mirand, 1970). Primary polycythemia is found in cattle, dogs, and cats, but observations with regard to Ep levels in such patients are scarce. The serum of a calf with familial primary polycythemia contained a factor probably similar to REF, which in itself was devoid of measurable erythropoietic activity but which when incubated with Ep, resulted in a fourfold enhancement of the activity (Van Dyke et al., 1968). Normal calf serum had no such effect. Polycythemia secondary to excessive production of Ep from a renal carcinoma was reported in a dog (Peterson and Zanjani, 1981).

Hormonal Influence on Erythropoiesis

A number of hormones play a physiologic role in controlling the size of the erythron (Gordon and Charipper, 1947; Krantz and Jacobson, 1970). This is shown by the fact that RBC counts tend to be slightly higher in males than in females in many mammalian species. In both humans and rats, removal of the gonads results in a change in the number of circulating erythrocytes. The RBC count increases in females following ovariectomy and decreases in males after castration. Parenteral administration of the respective sex hormone to the castrated individuals causes the RBC count to return to the normal level for the sex in question. Anemia may be associated with hypothyroidism (Appendix Case 6), adrenal cortical hypofunction (Addison's disease, Appendix Case 10), anterior pituitary insufficiency (Simmond's disease), and splenomegaly (Banti's disease, Appendix Case 24). On the other hand, evidence of intensified erythropoiesis may be observed in hyperfunction of the adrenal cortex (Cushing's disease, Appendix Case 9).

The pituitary, adrenals, thyroid, and gonads participate in the regulation of erythropoiesis largely through effects on metabolism and oxygen requirements, thereby increasing Ep production, and partly by altering the responsiveness of erythroid progenitors to other influences. Androgens, thyroid-stimulating hormone (TSH), adrenocorticotropic hormone (ACTH), growth hormone, prolactin, cortisone, thyroxine, epinephrine, norepinephrine, and angiotensin lead to increased Ep production, whereas estrogen and excessive glucagon exert an inhibitory action upon erythropoiesis (Krantz and Jacobson, 1970; Naets and Guns, 1980). In the presence of Ep, androgens, growth hormone, thyroxine, and corticosteroids also enhance the in vitro growth of erythroid precursor cells (How et al., 1979; Peschle, 1980).

Androgens have been used with variable

success in anemic patients to stimulate erythropoiesis. Androgens were found to produce an increase in Ep levels and the red cell mass in uremic human patients who had not undergone nephrectomy, but not in nephrectomized patients (Graber and Krantz, 1978). Testosterone increases renal Ep production in mice, rabbits, and dogs and stimulates erythropoiesis in rodents (Gurney, 1970). A greater increase in Ep is seen by the combination of testosterone and hypoxia than with either stimulus alone. Testosterone and thyroxine administration into intact and anephric sheep fetuses was found to stimulate erythropoiesis by stimulating hepatic Ep production (Zanjani and Banisadre, 1979).

Estrogen is thought to exert a dual role in the suppression of erythropoiesis depending on the dose administered. Small (physiologic) amounts directly affect the normal response of the committed stem cells to Ep. Larger (pharmacologic) amounts of estrogen depress Ep production by interfering with synthesis of the serum substrate erythropoietinogen by the liver (Fig. 18–12) (Siegal, 1970).

MATERIALS ESSENTIAL FOR ERYTHROCYTE PRODUCTION

The chemical composition of erythrocytes involves several factors: lipids, proteins, carbohydrates, minerals, vitamins, etc. Abnormal erythropoiesis results from insufficiency of those factors that are most critical for red cell production.

Protein

A dog maintained in an anemic state by repeated blood removal and fed a low-protein diet is unable to produce the usual amount of globin for hemoglobin synthesis even in the presence of a large excess of iron (Hahn and Whipple, 1939). The anemic dog kept on a protein-fasting diet was found to utilize protein from its own tissues to produce hemoglobin and plasma protein (Whipple et al., 1947). For every kilogram of weight loss, 50–140 g of blood protein was produced. Thus the body attempts to correct the anemia and hypoproteinemia by raiding its own tissues. Various proteins were found to differ in their biologic efficiency with respect to hemoglobin production. Casein, lactalbumin, whole egg protein, or liver protein in amounts of 150–250 g per week were able to maintain body weight and a strong positive nitrogen balance and produce considerable amounts of new hemoglobin and plasma proteins (Miller et al., 1947). In the rat, it was shown that protein intake is more essential than total caloric intake for maintenance of normal erythropoiesis (Bethard et al., 1958). Removal of protein from the diet was followed promptly by hemoconcentration, diminution of blood volume, and drastic reduction in erythropoiesis. These changes were reversible upon addition of protein to the diet. Protein deprivation in rats results in decreased Ep production in response to hypoxic stimulus. This can be corrected by feeding a single protein meal or amino acids such as methionine, leucine, or cystine (Anagnostou et al., 1978).

In sheep (Shutt and McDonald, 1965), the rate of hemoglobin synthesis was found to be independent of dietary protein, but the level of the circulating mass of hemoglobin after recovery from bleeding seemed to be influenced by the protein intake. Hemoglobin concentrations of lactating cows did not vary significantly with dietary protein levels of 13–17% (Esievo and Moore, 1979). These observations indicate some species differences with regard to influence of protein on erythropoiesis.

Although the above studies demonstrate the importance of protein in erythropoiesis under experimental conditions, a pure protein or specific amino acid deficiency in practice results in anemia only under exceptional circumstances. It has been suggested, however, that an absence of certain amino acids in the diet may affect the degree of megaloblastosis resulting from a deficiency of vitamin B_{12} or folate or both. Methionine and glycine appear to aggravate or provoke megaloblastosis, while homocysteine and serine may ameliorate the DNA defect in megaloblastosis in humans (Waxman et al., 1970).

Whipple and associates have made extensive studies on the value of various common dietary factors supporting hemoglobin production in dogs made anemic by bleeding

Table 18–4. Regeneration of Hemoglobin in Dogs Made Anemic by Bleeding and Fed Various Common Diet Factors[a]

Diet Factor (g/day)	Hb Produced over 2-wk Feeding Period (g)
Bread, 400	3
Milk, 450; bread, 400	3
Cream, 100; bread, 400	10
Butter, 100; bread 350	15
Asparagus, 200; bread 300	9
Spinach, 200; bread, 300	15
Raisins, 200; bread, 300	25
Apricots, 200; bread, 300	48
Eggs, 150; bread, 300	45
Whole fish, 250; bread, 300	13
Beef muscle, 250; bread, 300	17
Pig muscle, 250; bread, 300	30
Chicken gizzard, 250; bread, 200	80
Kidney, 250; bread, 300	70
Chicken liver, 250; bread, 300	80
Beef liver, 300; bread, 300	80
Beef liver, 450	95

[a]Data from Whipple and coworkers (Hahn and Whipple, 1939; Robscheit-Robbins et al., 1940; Miller et al., 1947; Whipple et al., 1947).

(Hahn and Whipple, 1939; Miller et al., 1947; Robscheit-Robbins et al., 1940; Whipple et al., 1947). Some results of their trials are summarized in Table 18–4. Dogs were observed to store ingredients for hemoglobin synthesis during periods of favorable diet. These carry-over materials rarely lasted more than 2 weeks under conditions of anemia from bleeding and an unfavorable diet. A dog in health and on an adequate diet readily replaces hemoglobin lost by hemorrhage. Haxhe (1967) demonstrated that the total red cell volume (mass) is closely related to the total body cell mass during experimental malnutrition and that erythropoiesis is blocked as soon as food restriction is induced. Dogs subjected to progressive malnutrition reduced their total red cell volume by 22% and body weight by 25%. The adaptive anemia of malnutrition required no transfusion but corrected itself as soon as refeeding began; blood tranfusion, when given, inhibited erythropoiesis.

Minerals

Iron, copper, and cobalt are the principal minerals required for red cell production. *Iron* is an integral part of the hemoglobin molecule and is therefore absolutely essential for hemoglobin synthesis. *Copper* is a cofactor for the enzyme ALA dehydrase required in the synthesis of heme (Fig. 19–1). *Cobalt* is essential to the diet of ruminants; vitamin B_{12} is synthesized in the rumen, and cobalt is required in the B_{12} molecule. Cobalt administered in excess to animals causes an increase in the red cell production and leads to polycythemia.

Vitamins

The essential vitamins for erythropoiesis are in the B series: riboflavin (B_2), pyridoxine (B_6), niacin or nicotinic acid, folate, thiamine, and B_{12}. All may not be required by every species of animal, but deficiencies may lead to development of anemia in one or more animal types. The ruminants are able to synthesize B_{12} in the rumen (Chapter 25), and the horse is capable of synthesizing it in the intesinal tract (Davies, 1971).

Vitamin A deficiency in humans is associated with anemia that precedes loss of night vision or decrease in serum vitamin A levels (Sauberlich and Hodges, 1979). The anemia is associated with decreased hemoglobin synthesis due to impaired mobilization of iron from the liver to the marrow. Vitamin E is a specific erythropoietic factor for nonhuman primates and swine and a potential erythropoietic factor for humans. Experimental vitamin E deficiency in nonhuman primates and swine causes a normocytic anemia, but it takes months to more than 2 years for the anemia to develop (Drake and Fitch, 1980). Bone marrow characteristically exhibits ineffective erythroid hyperplasia with numerous multinucleated cells (also see Chapter 25). Laboratory animals do not develop anemia from vitamin E deficiency.

REFERENCES

Abbrect, P.H., et al.: Plasma Erythropoietin and Renin Activity after Canine Renal Allotransplantation. J. Lab. Clin. Med., 71:766, 1968.

Alsaker, R.D. et al.: A Comparison of Polychromasia and Reticulocyte Counts in Assessing Erythrocytic Regenerative Response. J. Amer. Vet. Med. Ass., 170:39, 1977.

Anagnostou, A., et al.: Stimulation of Erythropoietin Secretion by Single Amino Acids. Proc. Soc. Exp. Biol. Med., 159:139, 1978.

Bessis, M.: Living Blood Cells and Their Ultrastructure. Springer-Verlag, New York, 1973.

Bethard, W.F., et al.: The Effect of Acute Protein Deprivation upon Erythropoiesis in Rats. Blood, *13:*216, 1958.

Bonanou-Tzedaki, S.A., et al.: Regulation of Erythroid Cell Differentiation by Haemin. Cell Differentiation, *10:*267, 1981.

Boycott, A.E.: The Blood as a Tissue: Hypertrophy and Atrophy of the Red Corpuscles. Proc. Roy. Soc., Med., *23:*15, 1929.

Bozzini, C.E.: Influence of the Erythroid Activity of the Bone Marrow on the Plasma Disappearance of Injected Erythropoietin in Dogs. Nature, *209:*1140, 1966.

Brecher, G., and Stohlman, F., Jr.: The Macrocytic Response to Erythropoietin Stimulation. *In* Erythropiesis. Jacobson, L.O., and Doyle, M., eds. Grune & Stratton, New York, 1962.

Bridges, K., et al.: Calcium Regulates the Commitment of Murine Erythroleukemia Cells to Terminal Erythroid Differentiation. J. Cell. Biol., *90:*542, 1981.

Busuttil, R.W., et al.: The Cytological Localization of Erythropoietin in the Human Kidney using the Fluorescent Antibody Technique. Proc. Soc. Exp. Biol. Med., *137:*327, 1971.

Carnot, P., and Deflandre, C.: Sur l'activite hemapoietique des differents organes au cours de la regeneration du sang. C.R. Acad. Sci., *143:*432, 1906.

Cavill, I., and Bentley, D.P.: Erythropoiesis in the Anemia of Rheumatoid Arthritis. Brit. J. Haematol., *50:*583, 1982.

Choy, Y.M., et al.: Changes in Surface Carbohydrates of Erythrocytes. Biochem. Biophys. Res. Commun., *410:*91, 1979.

Cline, M.J., and Golde, D.W.: Cellular Interactions in Haematopoiesis. Nature, *277:*177, 1979.

Committee for Clarification of Nomenclature of Cells and Diseases of the Blood and Blood-Forming Organs: First Report, Amer. J. Clin. Path., *18:*443, 1948. Second Report, *19:*56, 1949. Third, Fourth, and Fifth Reports, *20:*562, 1950.

Cramer, D.V., and Lewis, R.M.: Reticulocyte Response in the Cat. J. Amer. Vet. Med. Ass., *160:*61, 1972.

Cruz, W.O., and Junaqueira, P.C.: Resistance of Reticulocytes and Young Erythrocytes to the Action of Specific Hemolytic Serum. Blood, *7:*602, 1952.

Davies, M.E.: The Production of Vitamin B$_{12}$ in the Horse. Brit. Vet. J., *127:*34, 1971.

Davis, W.M., et al.: Changes in Red Cell Volume and Osmotic Fragility of Erythrocytes in the Rat following Acute Blood Loss. Amer. J. Physiol., *178:*17, 1954.

Drake, J.R., and Fitch, C.D.: Status of Vitamin E as an Erythropoietic Factor. Amer. J. Clin. Nutr., *33:*2386, 1980.

Ecarot-Charrier, B., et al.: Reticulocyte Membrane Transferrin Receptors. Can. J. Biochem., *58:*418, 1980.

Erslev, A.: Humoral Regulation of Red Cell Production. Blood, *8:*349, 1953.

Erslev, A.J., et al.: Renal and Extrarenal Erythropoietin Production in Anaemic Rats. Brit. J. Haematol., *45:*65, 1980a.

Erslev, A.J., et al.: Plasma Erythropoietin in Health and Disease. Ann. Clin. Lab. Med., *10:*250, 1980b.

Esievo, K.A.N., and Moore, W.E.: Effects of Dietary Protein and Stage of Lactation on the Haematology and Erythrocyte Enzymes Activities of High-Producing Dairy Cattle. Res. Vet. Sci., *26:*53, 1979.

Fan, L.C., et al.: Reticulocyte Responses and Maturation in Experimental Acute Blood Loss Anemia in the Cat. J. Amer. Hosp. Ass., *16:*219, 1978.

Faura, J., et al.: Effect of Altitude on Erythropoiesis. Blood, *33:*668, 1969.

Fawcett, D.W., and Witebsky, F.: Observations on the Ultrastructure of Nucleated Erythrocytes and Thrombocytes, with Particular Reference to the Structural Basis of Their Discoidal Shape. Z. Zellforsch., *62:*785, 1964.

Fisher, J.W.: Extrarenal Erythropoietin Production. J. Lab. Clin. Med., *93:*695, 1979.

Fisher, J.W.: Prostaglandins and Kidney Erythropoietin Production. Nephron, *25:*53, 1980a.

Fisher, J.W.: Mechanism of the Anemia of Chronic Renal Failure. Nephron, *25:*106, 1980b.

Fisher, J.W., and Gross, D.M.: Renal Prostaglandins and Kidney Production of Erythropoietin. *In* Kidney Hormones. Vol. 2. Fisher, J.W., ed. Academic Press, London, p. 354, 1977.

Fresco, R.: Ultrastructure of Blood Cells and Their Precursors. *In* Clinical Diagnosis by Laboratory Methods. 15th Ed. Davidson, I., and Henry, J.B., eds. Saunders, Philadelphia, p. 311, 1974.

Fresco, R.: Electron Microscopy in the Diagnosis of the Bone Marrow Disorders of the Erythroid Series. Semin. Hematol., *18:*279, 1981.

Fukuda, M., and Fukuda, M.N.: Changes in Cell Surface Glycoproteins and Carbohydrate Structures during the Development and Differentiation of Human Erythroid Cells. J. Supramol. Struct. Cell Biochem., *17:*313, 1981.

Ganzoni, A.M., et al.: Red Cell Aging in Vivo. J. Clin. Invest., *50:*1373, 1971.

Gattegno, L., et al.: Physiological Aging of Red Blood Cells and Changes in Membrane Carbohydrates. Biomedicine, *30:*194, 1979.

Ghosal, J., et al.: Effect of Different Prostaglandins and Methyl Testosterone on the Formation of Erythropoietin by Kidney. Indian J. Exp. Biol., *18:*377, 1980.

Glass, J., et al.: Transferrin-Binding and Iron-Binding Proteins of Rabbit Reticulocyte Plasma Membranes. Biochem. Biophys. Acta, *598:*293, 1980.

Goldwasser, E., et al.: Studies on Erythropoiesis. V. The Effect of Cobalt on the Production of Erythropoietin. Blood, *13:*55, 1958.

Gordon, A.S., and Charipper, H.A.: The Endocrine System and Hemopoiesis. Ann. N.Y. Acad. Sci., *48:*615, 1947.

Gordon, A.S., and Zanjani, E.D.: Some Aspects of Erythropoietin Physiology. *In* Regulation of Hematopoiesis. Vol. 1. Gordon, A.S., ed. Appleton-Century-Crofts, New York, 1970.

Gordon, L.I., et al.: Regulation of Erythroid Colony Formation by Bone Marrow Macrophages. Blood, *55:*1047, 1980.

Graber, S.E., and Krantz, S.B.: Erythropoietin and the Control of Red Cell Production. Ann. Rev. Med., *29:*51, 1978.

Grant, W.C.: The Influence of Anoxia of Lactating Rats and Mice on Blood of Their Normal Offspring. Blood, *10:*334, 1955.

Gurney, C.W.: The Control of Red Cell Production. *In* Blood Cells as a Tissue. Holmes, W.L., ed. Plenum Press, New York, 1970.

Hahn, P.F., and Whipple, G.H.: Hemoglobin Production in Anemia Limited by Low Protein Intake: Influence of Iron Intake, Protein Supplements and Fasting. J. Exp. Med., *69:*315, 1939.

Harris, J.W., and Kellermeyer, R.W.: The Red Cell, Production, Metabolism, Destruction: Normal and Abnormal. Harvard Univ. Press, Cambridge, Mass., 1970.

Haxhe, J.J.: Experimental Undernutrition. II. The Fate of Transfused Red Blood Cells. Metabolism, 16:1092, 1967.

Hertzberg, C., and Orlic, D.: An Electron Microscopic Study of Erythropoiesis in Fetal and Neonatal Rabbits. Acta Anat., 110:164, 1981.

Hillman, R.S.: Characteristics of Marrow Production and Reticulocyte Maturation In Normal Man in Response to Anemia. J. Clin. Invest., 48:443, 1969.

Hillman, R.S., and Finch, C.A.: The Misused Reticulocyte. Brit. J. Haematol., 17:313, 1969.

Hodgson, G., and Toha, J.: The Erythropoietic Effect of Urine and Plasma of Repeatedly Bled Rabbits. Blood, 9:299, 1954.

How, J., Davidson, R.J.L., and Bewsher, P.D.: Red Cell Changes in Hyperthyroidism. Scand. J. Haematol., 23:323, 1979.

Jain, N.C.: Hematologic Characteristics of Anemia. I. Pathophysiologic Features of the Erythrocyte. Calif. Vet., 33(5):9, 1979. II. Interpretive Aspects. Calif. Vet., 33(10):15, 1980.

Jatkar, P.R., and Kreier, J.P.: Relationship between Severity of Anemia and Plasma Erythropoietin Titer in Anaplasma-Infected Calves and Sheep. Amer. J. Vet. Res., 28:107, 1967.

Jelkmann, W., et al.: Indomethacin Blockade of Albuterol-Induced Erythropoietin Production in Isolated Perfused Dog Kidneys. Proc. Soc. Exp. Biol. Med., 162:65, 1979.

Jensen, W.N.: An Electron Microscopic Description of Basophilic Stippling in Red Cells. Blood, 25:933, 1965.

Johnson, L.W., and Schwartz, S.: Differential Lysis of Bovine and Canine Erythrocytes in Saline versus Saponin: Relation to Cell Age. Proc. Soc. Exp. Biol. Med., 138:871, 1971.

Kaaya, G.P., et al.: Bovine Granulocyte/Macrophage and Erythroid Colony Culture: Characteristics of the Colonies and the Assay System. Can. J. Comp. Med., 43:448, 1979.

Kaaya, G.P., and Maxie, M.G.: The Kinetics of Haemopoietic Differentiation Assessed by in Vitro Bone Marrow Culture in Endotoxin-Treated and in Anaemic Calves. Res. Vet. Sci., 29:63, 1980.

Kaneko, J.J.: Erythrokinetics and Iron Metabolism in Bovine Porphyria Erythropoietica. Ann. N.Y. Acad. Sci., 104:689, 1963.

Kaneko, J.J.: Porphyrin, Heme, and Erythrocyte Metabolism: The Prophyrias. In Clinical Biochemistry of Domestic Animals. Kaneko, J.J., and Cornelius, C.E., eds. Academic Press, New York, 1970.

Kaneko, J.J.: Clinical Biochemistry of Domestic Animals, 3rd Ed. Academic Press, New York, p. 121, 1980.

Kaneko, J.J., and Mattheeuws, D.R.G.: Iron Metabolism in Normal and Porphyric Calves. Amer. J. Vet. Res., 27:923, 1966.

Katsuoka, Y., et al.: Increased Levels of Erythropoietin in Kidney Extracts of Rats Treated with Cobalt and Hypoxia. Amer. J. Physiol., 244:F129, 1983.

Keeton, K.W., and Jain, N.C.: Erythrocyte Morphology During Response to Blood Loss, Calif. Vet., 27:13, Feb., 1973.

Kellman, S.-A.: On the Size of Normal Human Reticulocytes. Acta Med. Scand., 176:529, 1964.

Key, J.A.: Studies on Erythrocytes, with Special Reference to Reticulum, Polychromatophilia, and Mitochondria. Arch. Intern. Med., 28:511, 1921.

Krantz, S.B., and Jacobson, L.O.: Erythropoietin and the Regulation of Erythropoiesis. Univ. of Chicago Press, Chicago, 1970.

Kurland, J.I., et al.: Synthesis and Release of Erythroid Colony-Burst-Potentiating Activities by Purified Populations of Murine Peritoneal Macrophages. J. Exp. Med., 151:879, 1980.

Lala, P.K., et al.: An Evaluation of Erythropoiesis in Canine Marrow. Acta Haematol., 35:311, 1966.

Leblond, P.F., et al.: Cellular Deformability: A Possible Determinant of the Normal Release of Maturing Erythrocytes from the Bone Marrow. Blood, 37:40, 1971.

Levy, H., et al.: Effect of Cobalt on the Activity of Certain Enzymes in Homogenates of Rat Tissue. Arch. Biochem., 27:34, 1959.

Lowy, P.H.: Preparation and Chemistry of Erythropoietin. In Regulation of Hematopoiesis. Vol. 1, Gordon, A.S., ed. Appleton-Century-Crofts, New York, 1970.

Lugliani, R., et al.: The Role of the Carotid Body in Erythropoiesis in Man. New Eng. J. Med., 285:1112, 1971.

Lutz, H.U., and Fehr, J.: Total Sialic Acid Content of Glycophorins during Senescence of Human Red Blood Cells. J. Biol. Chem., 25:11177, 1979.

McGlave, P.B., and Zanjani, E.D.: Erythropoietin and Hemoglobin Switching. Tex. Biol. Med., 401:125, 1980.

Miller, L.L., et al.: Anemia and Hypoproteinemia: Weight Maintenance Effected by Food Proteins but Not by Mixtures of Pure Amino Acids. J. Exp. Med., 85:267, 1947.

Mirand, E.A.: Nonerythropoietin-dependent Erythropoiesis. In Regulation of Hematopoiesis. Vol. 1. Gordon, A.S., ed. Appleton-Century-Crofts, New York, 1970.

Mirand, E.A., et al.: Erythropoietin Response to Repeated Hemorrhage in Renal Allotransported, Nephrectomized or Intact dogs. Life Sci., 7:689, 1968.

Mirand, E.A., and Murphy, G.P.: Extrarenal Erythropoietin Activity in Man and Experimental Animals. In Regulation of Hematopoiesis, Vol. 1. Gordon, A.S., ed. Appleton-Century-Crofts, New York, 1970.

Misiti, J., and Spivak, J.L.: Erythropoiesis in Vitro: Role of Calcium. J. Clin. Invest., 64:1573, 1979.

Mohandas, N., et al.: Erythropoietic Stress, Macrocytosis, and Hemoglobin Switching in HbAA Sheep. Blood, 55:757, 1980.

Morley, A., and Stohlman, F., Jr.: Erythropoiesis in the Dog: The Periodic Nature of the Steady State. Science, 165:1025, 1969.

Naets, J.P.: The role of the Kidney in the Production of the Erythropoietic Factor. Blood, 16:1770, 1960.

Naets, J.P., and Guns, M.: Inhibitory Effect of Glucagon on Erythropoiesis. Blood, 55:997, 1980.

Naughton, B.A., et al.: A Renal Inhibitor to Hepatic Erythropoietin (Ep) Production. J. Med., 12:159, 1981.

Naughton, B.A., et al.: The Effects of Prostaglandins on Extrarenal Erythropoietic Production. Proc. Soc. Exp. Biol. Med., 170:231, 1982.

Nizet, A., and Robscheit-Robbins, F.S.: Reticulocyte Ripening in Experimental Anemia and Hypoproteinemia. Effect of Amino Acids in Vitro. Blood, 5:648, 1950.

Noordegraaf, E.M., and Ploemoeher, R.E.: Studies of the Haemopoietic Microenvironments. III. Glycosaminoglycan Levels in Relation to Phenylhydrazine-Induced Erythropoiesis in the Mouse Liver. Scand. J. Haematol., 24:152, 1980.

Ogle, J.W., et al.: Production of Erythropoietin in Vitro: A Review, In Vitro, 14:945, 1978.

Orlic, D.: Ultrastructural Analysis of Erythropoiesis. *In* Regulation of Hematopoiesis. Vol. 1, Gordon, A.S., ed. Appleton-Century-Crofts, New York, 1970.

Peschle, C.: Erythropoiesis. Ann. Rev. Med., 31:303, 1980.

Peterson, M.E., and Zanjani, E.D.: Inappropriate Erythropoietin Production from a Renal Carcinoma in a Dog with Polycythemia. J. Amer. Vet. Med. Ass., 179:995, 1981.

Plzak, L., et al.: Demonstration of Stimulation of Erythropoiesis by Plasma from Anemic Rats using Fe^{59}. J. Lab. Clin. Med., 46:671, 1955.

Reissmann, K.R.: Studies on the Mechanism of Erythropoietic Stimulation in Parabiotic Rats during Hypoxia. Blood, 5:372, 1950.

Reissmann, K.R., et al.: Influence of Disappearance Rate and Distribution Space on Plasma Concentration of Erythropoietin in Normal Rats. J. Lab. Clin. Med., 65:967, 1965.

Repasky, E.A., and Eckert, B.S.: A Reevaluation of the Process of Enucleation in Mammalian Erythroid Cells. Prog. Clin. Biol. Res., 55:679, 1981.

Rich, I.N., and Kubanek, B.: Release of Erythropoietin from Macrophages Mediated by Phagocytosis of Crystalline Silica. Res. J. Reticado. Soc., 31:17, 1982.

Rifkind, R.A., et al.: Alternations in Polyribosomes during Erythroid Cell Maturation. J. Cell. Biol., 22:599, 1964.

Robscheit-Robbins, F.S., et al.: Hemoglobin and Plasma Protein. Simultaneous Production during Continued Bleeding as Influenced by Diet Protein and Other Factors. J. Exp. Med., 72:479, 1940.

Rosse, W.F., and Waldmann, T.A.: The Metabolism of Erythropoietin in Patients with Anemia Due to Deficient Erythropoiesis. J. Clin. Invest., 43:1348, 1964.

Rudolph, W.G.: Autoradiographic Study of Erythroid Bone Marrow Cells in Normal and Porphyric Calves in Vitro. M.S. Thesis, Univ. of California, Davis, 1968.

Rudolph, W.G., and Kaneko, J.J.: Kinetics of Erythroid Bone Marrow Cells of Normal and Porphyric Calves in Vitro. Acta Haematol., 45:330, 1971.

Sauberlich, H.E., and Hodges, R.E.: Vitamin A Deficiency and Anemia. Nutr. Rev., 37:38, 1979.

Schnappauf, H., et al.: Erythropoietic Response in Calves following Blood Loss. Amer. J. Vet. Res., 28:275, 1967.

Scribner Seeley, V.A.: Renal Relations to Neonatal Erythropoiesis. *In* Regulation of Hematopoiesis. Vol. 1. Gordon, A.S., ed. Appleton-Century-Crofts, New York, 1970.

Seip, M.: Reticulocyte Studies: Liberation of Red Blood Corpuscles from Bone Marrow into Peripheral Blood and Production of Erythrocytes Elucidated by Reticulocyte Investigations. Acta Med. Scand. (Suppl. 282), 146:1, 1953.

Shattil, S.J., and Cooper, R.A.: Maturation of Macroreticulocyte Membranes in Vivo. J. Lab. Clin. Med., 79:215, 1972.

Shutt, D.A., and McDonald, I.W.: Rate of Haemoglobin Synthesis after Blood Loss in Sheep and the Influence of Dietary Protein. Aust. J. Exp. Biol. Med. Sci., 43:457, 1965.

Siegal, C.D.: Possible Hematopoietic Mechanisms in Nonmammalian Vertebrates. *In* Regulation of Hematopoiesis. Vol. 1. Gordon, A.S., ed. Appleton-Century-Crofts, New York, 1970.

Simpson, C.F., and Kling, J.M.: The Mechanism of Mitochondrial Extrusion from Phenylhydrazine-Induced Reticulocytes in the Circulating Blood. J. Cell. Biol., 36:103, 1968.

Skutelsky, E., and Danon, D.: Electron Microscopical Analysis of Surface Charge Labelling Density at Various Stages of the Erythroid Line. J. Membrane Biol., 2:173, 1970.

Smith, J.E., and Kaneko, J.J.: Rate of Heme and Porphyrin Synthesis by Bovine Porphyric Reticulocytes in Vitro. Amer. J. Vet. Res., 27:931, 1966.

Steiner, M.: Identification of the Binding Site for Transferrin in Human Reticulocytes. Biochem. Biophys. Res. Commun., 94:861, 1980.

Stephens, J.G.: Surface and Fragility Differences between Mature and Immature Red Cells. J. Physiol., 99:30, 1940.

Stewart, W.G., et al.: Age as Affecting the Osmotic and Mechanical Fragility of Dog Erythrocytes Tagged with Radioactive Iron. J. Exp. Med., 91:147, 1950.

Stohlman, F., Jr.: Kinetics of Erythropoiesis. *In* Regulation of Hematopoiesis. Vol. 1. Gordon, A.S., ed. Appleton-Century-Crofts, New York, 1970.

Tavassoli, M.: Red Cell Delivery and the Function of the Marrow-Blood Barrier: A Review. Exp. Hematol., 6:257, 1978.

Thomas, E.D., et al.: The Problem of the Stem Cell: Observations in Dogs following Nitrogen Mustard. J. Lab. Clin. Med., 65:794, 1965.

Tramezzani, J.H., et al.: The Carotid Body as a Neuroendocrine Organ Involved in Control of Erythropoiesis. Proc. Natl. Acad. Sci. U.S.A., 68:52, 1971.

Udupa, K.B., and Lispchitz, D.A.: Endotoxin-Induced Suppression of Erythropoiesis: The Role of Erythropoietin and a Heme Synthesis Stimulating Factor. Blood, 59:1267, 1982.

Urabe, A., et al.: The Influence of Steroid Hormone Metabolites on the in Vitro Development of Erythroid Colonies Derived from Human Bone Marrow. J. Exp. Med., 149:1314, 1979.

Van Dyke, D., et al.: Erythropoietin Enhancing Factor in Serum of a Calf with Primary Familial Polycythaemia. Nature, 217:1027, 1968.

Walter, H.: Factors in the Partition of Blood Cells in Aqueous Dextran-Polyethylene Two-Phase Systems. Prog. Separation Purification, 2:121, 1969.

Ward, H.P., et al.: Serum Level of Erythropoietin in Anemias Associated with Chronic Infection, Malignancy, and Primary Hematopoietic Disease. J. Clin. Invest., 50:332, 1971.

Waxman, S., et al.: Aggravation or Initiation of Megaloblastosis by Amino Acids in the Diet. JAMA, 214:101, 1970.

Weintraub, A.H., et al.: Plasma and Renal Clearance of Exogenous Erythropoietin in the Dog. Amer. J. Physiol., 207:523, 1964.

Weiss, L.: Transmural Cellular Passage in Vascular Sinuses of Rat Bone Marrow. Blood, 36:189, 1970.

Whipple, G.H., et al.: Raiding of Body Tissue Protein to Form Plasma Protein and Hemoglobin. What Is Premortal Rise of Urinary Nitrogen? J. Exp. Med., 85:277, 1947.

Wintrobe, M.M., et al.: Clinical Hematology. 8th ed. Lea & Febiger, Philadelphia, 1981.

Zanjani, E.D., et al.: Liver as the Primary Site of Erythropoietin Formation in the Fetus. J. Lab. Clin. Med., 89:640, 1977.

Zanjani, E.D., and Banisadre, M.: Hormonal Stimulation of Erythropoietin Production and Erythropoiesis in

Anephric Sheep Fetuses. J. Clin. Invest., *64*:1181, 1979.

Zanjani, E.D., and Gordon, A.S.: Erythropoietin Production and Utilization in Fetal Goats and Sheep. Israel J. Med. Sci., *7*:850, 1971.

Zanjani, E.D.: Liver to Kidney Switch of Erythropoietin Formation. Exp. Hematol. (Suppl.), *8*:29, 1980.

Zucker, S., et al.: Cancer Cell Inhibition of Erythropoiesis. J. Lab. Clin. Med., *96*:770, 1980.

19

Hemoglobin Synthesis and Destruction

HEMOGLOBIN SYNTHESIS   514
  Heme Synthesis   514
  Globin Synthesis   516

HEMOGLOBIN TYPES   516

HEMOGLOBINOPATHIES   519

HEMOGLOBIN DEGRADATION AND
  BILIRUBIN METABOLISM   520
  Intravascular Hemolysis   520
  Extravascular Hemolysis   521
  Bilirubin Formation and Excretion   521

Hemoglobin is essential to mammalian life because it carries and delivers oxygen necessary to cell survival. Hemoglobin production and destruction are balanced under physiologic conditions, and any deviation in either one is associated with a significant hematologic disorder. This chapter is concerned with some aspects of these processes.

HEMOGLOBIN SYNTHESIS

Hemoglobin is a conjugated protein consisting of heme and globin. There are some 400 million molecules of hemoglobin in the red cell, and these make up 95% of its dry weight. Each molecule consists of four heme units, each of which is associated with an individual polypeptide chain. The atomic model of horse hemoglobin has been constructed on the basis of x-ray crystallography studies and amino acid sequence analyses (Perutz et al., 1968) and subsequent events have been reviewed (Perutz, 1976). Comparative studies suggest unity of the hemoglobin model for different species. The hemoglobin molecule in three dimensions measures $65 \times 55 \times 50$ A° and can be regarded as a spheroid. Its molecular weight is 64,458.

Heme Synthesis

Heme consists of a protoporphyrin (type III) ring at the center of which is an iron atom in the ferrous state. The properties of hemoglobin are directly dependent upon maintaining this reduced state of the iron atoms. Heme is found not only in hemoglobin, but also in cytochromes, catalase, peroxidases, and myoglobin. The basic structure consists of four pyrrol rings linked together by four methene bridges to form the porphin nucleus common to all porphyrins (Dobriner and Rhoads, 1940; Shemin and Rittenberg, 1946).

Various steps involved in the biogenesis of heme are outlined in Figure 19–1. Succinyl-coenzyme A (CoA) and glycine formed in the tricarboxylic acid (TCA) cycle, react to form δ-aminolevulinic acid (ALA). The δ-ALA is synthesized only in mitochondria, and ALA synthetase is the rate-limiting enzyme in the entire sequence of heme synthesis. Pyridoxal phosphate (vitamin B_6) is necessary for the activation of glycine required for its initial condensation with succinyl-CoA. Deficiency of vitamin B_6 results in hypochromic anemia in some animals. Pantothenic acid is a component of coenzyme A; hence it is required for the formation of δ-ALA. Its deficiency is known to produce hypochromic anemia in birds and animals, but not in man. Two molecules of δ-ALA react to form, porphobilinogen (PBG). Four molecules of PBG react, ultimately forming the tetrapyrrolic ring component, uroporphyrinogen III. Both uroporphyrinogen I synthetase and uroporphyrinogen III cosynthetase are required for the formation of uroporphyrinogen III. Uroporphyrinogen III is converted to coproporphyrinogen III and then to protoporphyrinogen, which, upon oxidation yields protoporphyrin III. Protoporphyrin III subsequently combines with four moles of iron in ferrous state to form heme, four molecules of which finally

514

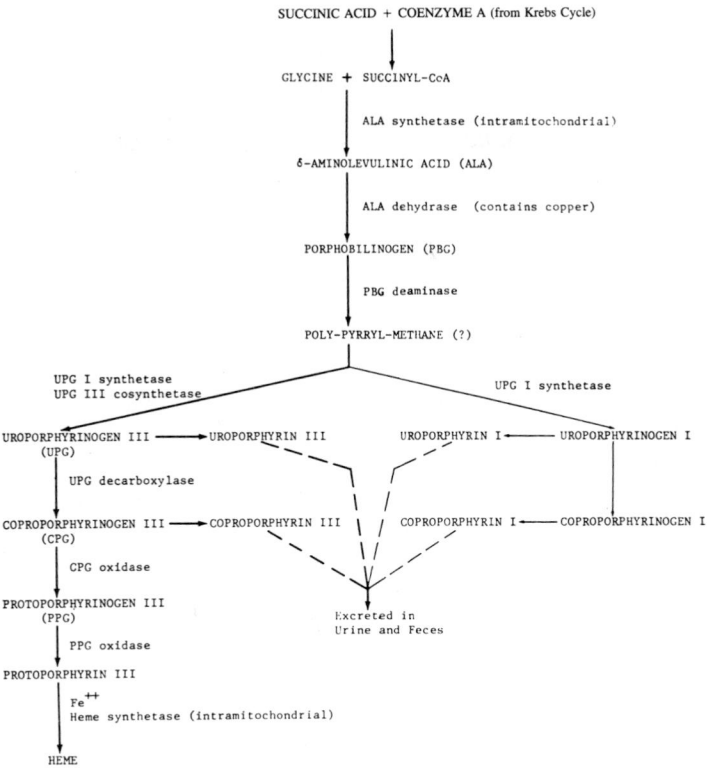

Fig. 19–1. A schematic presentation of steps involved in biogenesis of heme. Deficiency of certain vitamins required as cofactors at sites indicated may lead to anemia.

conjugate with four globin molecules to form one hemoglobin molecule.

Under normal conditions, most heme is synthesized before the erythrocyte nucleus is lost. Although the non-nucleated immature mammalian erythrocyte is capable of synthesizing heme in vitro, significant synthesis does not occur in mature erythrocytes (London et al., 1950). Thus, when immature erythrocytes enter the circulation, hemoglobin synthesis may continue bringing the cell to maturity. Heme is synthesized in the mitochondria. Mature mammalian erythrocytes are unable to synthesize heme de novo because they lack mitochondria. Both ALA-synthetase, involved in the first step of heme synthesis, and heme synthetase, involved in the last step of heme synthesis, are intramitochondrial enzymes and are therefore limited to erythroid precursors, including reticulocytes.

Protoporphyrin III accumulates to some extent in immature erythrocytes and is therefore present in increased concentration when re-

ticulocytosis occurs as in acute blood loss or hemolysis. Conditions associated with impairment of heme formation (e.g., iron deficiency anemia, the anemia of chronic infection, and lead poisoning) result in an increase in free erythrocyte protoporphyrin. Lead causes profound alterations in hemoglobin synthesis. It reduces heme synthesis by inhibiting ALA synthetase, ALA dehydrase, and heme synthetase, and it also retards biosynthesis of globin by inhibiting formation of polypeptide chains. The enzymes are inactivated because of blockade of SH-groups (White, 1975), and intermediates of heme and globin synthesis accumulate in red cells. Hence the anemia of lead poisoning is due partly to inadequate hemoglobin formation. Anemia is progressive and is characterized by the presence of many nucleated red cells in blood, prominent basophilic stippling in mature and/or somewhat polychromic erythrocytes, and abnormal ring sideroblasts. Reticulocytosis is absent or negligible. Iron deficiency potentiates the risk of developing lead toxicity (Freedman, 1979).

In addition to protoporphyrin of the hemoglobin molecule, two other natural porphyrins, coproporphyrin and uroporphyrin, are found in trace amounts in feces and urine; the former also occurs naturally in young erythrocytes (Schwartz and Wikoff, 1952). Coproporphyrin excretion is increased whenever erythropoiesis is intensified. Porphyrinuria is a term that is applied to increased excretion of porphyrins in the urine. An example, in addition to the increased formation following hemorrhage and hemolytic disease, is the occurrence of coproporphyrin III in abnormal amounts in the urine in lead poisoning.

Porphyria is a disease of porphyrin metabolism and is generally congenital. Both coproporphyrin and uroporphyrin are produced in excessive amounts, and since the latter has a predilection for the teeth and bones, these structures take on a brown or reddish color. Congenital porphyria of cattle is called "pink tooth" because of this discoloration of the teeth (Rhode and Cornelius, 1958; Appendix Case 72). The urine is brown to wine color because of the large amount of porphyrins present. The metabolic basis in bovine erythropoietic porphyria is a deficiency of uroporphyrinogen III-cosynthetase. The porphyrins have photosensitizing characteristics, and the white areas of the bodies of cattle affected with congenital porphyria may show lesions typical of photosensitization. For further details on porphyrias in animals, refer to Kaneko (1980).

Globin Synthesis

Globin required for the formation of hemoglobin is synthesized in the cytoplasm. The genetic information contained in the base sequence of DNA is carried from the nucleus to the cytoplasm by messenger RNA (mRNA). Through groups of three bases (a triplet or codon) acting as templates, mRNA translates the genetic information to the proteins that are assembled at the ribosomes (polyribosomes). Thus, specific peptide chains are formed on polyribosomes under the influence of mRNA from the nucleus. However, α and β chains are synthesized at an equal rate, but δ and γ chains are synthesized at a lower rate because of differences in the content of mRNA in erythroid cells. It takes about 90

seconds to form a complete alpha or beta chain, and about 800 hemoglobin molecules per second per cell are completed (Itano, 1966). Each of the polypeptide chains is controlled by a separate and distinct genetic locus. Mutations in these are reflected in the hemoglobin. The quantity and type of globin polypeptide chains synthesized appear to be influenced by genetic, ontogenetic, and environmental factors. Each heme group is attached to the corresponding peptide chain by a coordinate linkage from the iron of the heme to a specific histidine residue.

There are important interrelationships between the intracellular concentrations of heme and globin and their rates of synthesis. Excess heme inhibits the formation of more heme and stimulates the synthesis of globin. Excess globin synthesis, in turn, appears to stimulate heme synthesis and may inhibit further globin synthesis. The rates of heme and globin synthesis can be altered by various factors, such as starvation, ionizing radiations, and lead poisoning.

Investigations of the electrophoretic mobility of hemoglobin and fingerprinting of polypeptide chains have led to elucidation of the chemical and steric structure of the globin molecule. The human hemoglobin (HbA) molecule consists of two α and two β polypeptide chains (Rhinesmith et al., 1957). There are 141 amino acid residues in the α chain and 146 in the β chain. The chemical structure of normal human hemoglobins varies because of differences in one polypeptide chain and is written as $\alpha_2^A \beta_2^A$ (HbA), $\alpha_2^A \gamma_2^F$ (HbF), and $\alpha_2^A \delta_2^{A2}$ (HbA$_2$). Commitment to produce a particular hemoglobin type occurs at an early stage of erythroid differentiation (Mohandas et al., 1980; Nienhuis et al., 1980). Early erythroid progenitor cells (BFU-E) have been found to synthesize HbF, whereas late erythroid progenitor cells (CFU-E) synthesized only adult hemoglobin normally (Papayannopoulou et al., 1977). CFU-E can be induced to produce HbC in sheep (Nienhuis et al., 1980).

HEMOGLOBIN TYPES

Differences in the amino acid sequence of the globin moiety are responsible for phylogenetic and intraspecies differences in adult hemoglobins, differences between embryonic, fetal, and adult forms within a species, and heterogeneity within an individual (Kitchen, 1969; Kitchen and Brett, 1974). Many animal species exhibit hemoglobin polymorphism, wherein more than a single hemoglobin component exists within a species. The relative proportion of different types of hemoglobins is under genetic control and may vary in different individuals within a species. Electrophoretic techniques are used generally to demonstrate hemoglobin polymorphism, but they may not always reveal differences in hemoglobin components. In such cases, a structural comparison is essential to establish or determine the identity of the hemoglobins. Peptide chains of several animal species, including the horse, pig, sheep, goat, and cow, have been studied (Dayhoff, 1969). It has been shown that there are remarkable similarities between the α and γ chains of many species and that most of the polymorphism is due to β-chain variation. The length of both alpha and beta chains and the number of amino acid residues per chain appear to vary within a narrow range in different species. Differences in the number of various amino acids and their manner of sequential alignment account for species variation. Cat hemoglobin is unique in that it contains eight "reactive" cysteines, compared to two to four in normal hemoglobins of many other mammals (Taketa et al., 1967). The occurrence of Heinz bodies in feline erythrocytes does not seem to correlate with the type and amount of hemoglobin present in a particular cat (Jain, unpublished observations).

Embryonic, fetal, and adult types of hemoglobins have been found in many animal species (Table 19–1). One embryonic hemoglobin (HbE) has been found in the goat and rabbit, while two are found in the sheep and man, two to three in the cow, three in the cat and mouse, and two to four in the pig. One fetal hemoglobin (HbF) has been found in the cow, sheep, goat, rabbit, mouse, pig, rat, human, and subhuman primates; and one to two have been found in white-tailed deer. Embryonic or fetal hemoglobins in the dog and horse are indistinguishable electrophoretically from adult hemoglobins.

The quantity and type of hemoglobin synthesized vary during the growth in utero and after birth. In many mammalian species, HbF constitutes approximately 90–95% of the hemoglobin present at birth, compared to 30–80% concentration in human babies. It has been suggested that HbF may contribute to resistance of the human infant against malaria (Allison, 1957) and to resistance of neonatal calves against *Anaplasma marginale* (Williams and Jones, 1968). An association of hemoglobin type and resistance to helminthiasis has been described for sheep (Altaif and Dargie, 1978) and goats (Buvanendran et al., 1981). Erythrocyte osmotic fragility and alkaline denaturation of hemoglobin were correlated with hemoglobin types in cattle of various ages; both parameters were lower for calves having a higher proportion of HbF (Costea, 1979). Fetal hemoglobin is replaced by the adult type(s) in many animal species within 4–8 weeks after birth and in some it may take a few months. Bovine HbF disappears completely within 6–7 months after birth (Jelic et al., 1981). This is in sharp contrast to the more gradual decrease and replacement in humans, in which HbF is found in 1–2% concentration even in adults. In humans, 3 types of red cells are found; fetal red cells containing HbF exclusively or predominantly, most adult red cells containing HbA, and the so-called F cells containing 75–90% HbA and 10–25% HbF (Nienhuis et al., 1980). In the adult animal, different adult hemoglobins are found in the same cell, e.g., HbA and HbB, the two major hemoglobins of the cat are found within the same erythrocyte (Taketa et al., 1978).

Cellular and molecular mechanisms of hemoglobin switching are being investigated in humans and animals (Benz, 1980–1981; Nienhuis et al., 1980; Papayannopoulou and Stamatoyannopoulos, 1982; Testa et al., 1982). It has been determined that the change in globin expression during ontogeny is controlled at the level of progenitor cells by several rather undefined factors, and that the BFU-E has the potential to produce progenies forming fetal and adult hemoglobin (Papayannopoulou and Stamatoyannopoulos, 1982). Synthesis of HbF seems to be influenced by erythropoietin since its production increases

Table 19–1. Hemoglobin Types in Several Species[a]

Species	Hemoglobin Type			Comments
	Embryonic	Fetal	Adult	
Dog	0	[b]	1–2	No embryonic or fetal Hb distinguishable from adult Hb.
Cat	3	0	1–2	Three embryonic Hb present at 21 days after conception, but disappear between 30–35 days. Adult Hb is present between 20–30 days after conception and varies considerably in proportion.
Cow	2–3	1	1–5	Embryonic Hb clearly shown at 4 weeks after conception and disappears between 6–10 weeks. Fetal Hb appears at 6–8 weeks after conception and persists to 3–10 weeks after birth. Hb types vary in different breeds. Types A and B are most common.
Horse	0	[b]	1–2	No embryonic or fetal Hb component distinguishable from adult Hb. Majority of horses have 2 Hb in a ratio of approximately 70:30, but certain breeds may have only 1 component.
Sheep	2	1	1–4	Trace of embryonic Hb present only at early development. Fetal Hb present at 40 days, begins to decrease at birth, and disappears between 40–50 days of age. HbC appears soon after birth with a rise to about 15% followed by a gradual disappearance. HbC reappears in response to blood loss.
Goat	1	1	1–6	Embryonic and fetal Hb patterns same as in sheep. HbC appears soon after birth, approaching 100% at about 60 days with gradual disappearance and replacement with final adult Hb types. HbC reappears in response to blood loss.
Rabbit	1	1	1–4	At 12 days after conception, 3 Hb are present: 2 embryonic and 1 indistinguishable from the adult type; however, major component is embryonic. At 20 days of gestation, 2 components are present, the major one being the adult type. Near term, only the adult type is present.
Mouse	3	0	2–6	Embryonic Hb are present at the twelfth day and disappear by the fifteenth day after conception. Disappearance of embryonic components is followed by the appearance of the adult types.
Guinea Pig	0	0	1–2	No embryonic or fetal Hb was detected in blood studied approximately 20–25 days after conception.
Pig	2–4[c]	1	1	Fetal and embryonic Hb are present at 30 days after conception. Embryonic Hb disappears between 45 and 60 days and fetal Hb is present at birth. Fetal Hb is electrophoretically indistinguishable from the adult Hb. It can be identified only by peptide mapping.
Rat	0	1	4	Four Hb components are present at birth. One component disappears 8–12 days after birth; 4 Hb are present in the adult.
White-tailed Deer	0	1–2	1–8	At birth, 95% of the Hb present is of the fetal type. It is completely replaced by adult Hb 8–12 weeks after birth. The presence of high levels of fetal Hb precludes sickling in the young.

[a]Modified from Kitchen, 1972.
[b]Prenatal hemoglobins indistinguishable from adult types by electrophoresis or peptide-mapping techniques.
[c]From Bektas et al., 1981.

during recovery from anemia and in erythroid-colony cultures of bone marrow and blood cells in the presence of high levels of erythropoietin (Dover et al., 1979; Papayannopoulou, 1980). Some increase in HbF formation occurs during pregnancy, probably as a result of changes in maternal erythropoiesis (Chui et al., 1980). Development of an embryonic-type hemoglobin in extramedullary hematopoietic cells in the liver was demonstrated in adult rats during experimental hepatic carcinogenesis (Enomoto et al., 1980).

Environmental and hormonal factors may influence expression of the globin gene and in turn the type of hemoglobin synthesized in a given species (Benz, 1980–81). Two hemoglobins are found in normal adult sheep. Hemoglobin A ($\alpha_2\,\beta_2^A$) is electrophoretically fast and has a higher oxygen affinity than HbB ($\alpha_2\,\beta_2^B$). Sheep having the phenotype for HbA or HbAB but not HbB, when subjected to acute or prolonged anemia or hypoxia develop another hemoglobin component, HbC ($\alpha_2\,\beta_2^C$). With the advance of anemia, HbA is partially or completely replaced by the new hemoglobin, and the switch reverses after recovery from anemia. Naturally occurring HbC is seen in sheep during the growth period after birth, coincidental with loss of HbF($\alpha_2\,\gamma_2$), and in cases of severe parasitism. Such a switch has also been observed in the goat (Huisman et al., 1967; Jain et al., 1980), but not in the cat (Lessard and Taketa, 1969) or cow (Bell and Huisman, 1968).

The A to C switch appears to be mediated by selective globin gene expression rather than by a clonal or cellular selective mechanism, for both HbA and HbC are synthesized simultaneously (Nienhuis and Bunn, 1974). The inability of sheep homozygous for HbB to produce HbC in response to erythropoietic stimuli is due to the absence of a β^C globin gene from the non-α globin gene cluster of these animals (Benz et al., 1977).

The factor responsible for this A to C switch is thought to be erythropoietin (Boyer, 1969). Intravenous injection of erythropoietin in nonanemic sheep induces such a switch (Thurmon et al., 1970), and commitment to HbC production occurs within a few hours although its phenotypic expression is detected a few days later. Erythroid colonies from sheep and goat marrow have been found to produce HbC in vitro (Barker, 1980; Barker et al., 1980); the amount of HbC produced being roughly proportional to the concentration of erythropoietin incorporated in the culture (Nienhuis and Benz, 1977). Apparently, CFU-E at a certain stage of differentiation can be induced to produce HbC by exposure to high levels of erythropoietin (Nienhuis and Benz, 1977; Nienhuis et al., 1980). HbC production can also be induced by erythropoietin in cultures of fetal erythroid stem cells from bone marrow or liver (Barker et al., 1977, 1980). For additional comments on A to C switch in sheep see Chapter 8.

HEMOGLOBINOPATHIES

The production of abnormal hemoglobin molecules in humans has been associated with altered function and instability of the hemoglobin that produces hematologic disorders. The basic structure of heme appears to be fixed, and no variants have as yet been identified. The type and quantity of globin peptide chains that are synthesized appear to be influenced by genetic, ontogenetic, and environmental factors; the synthesis is stimulated by hypoxia. Each of the polypeptide chains is controlled by a separate and distinct genetic locus, and all loci may be on the same or different chromosomes. Mutations in one or more loci and other chromosomal abnormalities result in formation of abnormal peptide chains. In humans, amino acid substitutions have been found in the α, β, γ, and δ chains (especially in the β chain) leading to production of abnormal or different hemoglobin molecules. Hemoglobins S, C, and E are due to β-chain mutation, HbG$_{Philadelphia}$ is due to α-chain mutation and HbG/C is an example of mutation in both α and β chains.

More than a hundred structurally distinct hemoglobin variants have been reported in humans (Harris and Kellermeyer, 1970). Electrophoresis, chromatography, antigenic analysis, fingerprinting, and hybridization have been used to discover these variants. Some of the hemoglobin variants, e.g., HbS, HbC, and HbE, are associated with specific hematologic disorders and clinical abnormalities. Of these, HbS, responsible for sickle-cell anemia in the Negro race, is the best-known variant. Hemoglobin S is characterized by substitution of valine for a glutamic acid at position 6 in the β chain. This single amino acid substitution is the cause of the morphologic change of the red cells from biconcave to sickle shape during deoxygenation of the blood. The abnormal shape is due to a molecular aggregation of deoxygenated HbS into rods, which in turn deform the red cell membrane, producing the characteristic sickling (Pauling et al., 1949; Perutz and Mitchison, 1950). The change is reversible upon oxygenation. Sickling of erythrocytes in the white-tailed deer (Chapter 4) has been related to the presence of seven polymorphic hemoglobins in this species (Kitchen, 1969). It was shown that although sickling was not associated with any particular type of hemoglobin, it was not seen when hemoglobin V and VII were present. Fusiform and spindle-shaped erythrocytes in Angora goats result from intracellular polymerization of hemoglobin in the form of tubular fibers similar to those of hemoglobin S, but molecular aberrations remain unknown (chapter 9).

Amino acid substitutions leading to formation of abnormal hemoglobins in animals have not been identified. In contrast to the single amino acid substitutions found in the majority of human polymorphic hemoglobins, multiple amino acid substitutions are seen in most of the normal ruminant hemoglobins (Kitchen, 1969). Reduced exercise tolerance in a dog was associated with the finding of an abnormal hemoglobin having altered oxygen affinity; the new hemoglobin comprised 30% of the total hemoglobin (Jones et al., 1978).

Besides qualitative changes in hemoglobin production described above, variations in the quantity of different types of polypeptide chains would affect the proportion of respective types of hemoglobin formed, e.g., depression of α-chain formation in humans would lead to decreased production of HbA, HbA_2, and HbF, whereas depression of β chain would inhibit only HbA. Thalassemias in humans represent such defects in the synthesis of one or another of the globin polypeptide chains; α, β, and δ-thalassemias are due to depression of alpha, beta, and delta

polypeptide chains, respectively (Ingram and Stretton, 1959). The resulting imbalance of polypeptide chains leads to intracellular precipitation of the excessive, relatively unstable chains, resulting in cell damage and destruction of erythrocytes. The two abnormalities—type and number—in the polypeptide chain formation can coexist, e.g., sickle cell anemia and alpha-thalassemia. Mechanisms that control the concentration of one or another hemoglobin are not completely understood.

HEMOGLOBIN DEGRADATION AND BILIRUBIN METABOLISM

The stroma of the erythrocyte supports the hemoglobin and the two are bonded together. When an erythrocyte undergoes fragmentation, the hemoglobin does not escape but remains with the fragments. Hemoglobin is released in free form when hemolysis occurs and the bond between the hemoglobin and stroma is broken by a hemolytic agent. Free hemoglobin in blood plasma is quickly disposed of by oxidation to useless forms, is lost through the kidneys, or is destroyed by the mononuclear phagocyte (reticuloendothelial) system (MPS) (Crosby, 1957). Hemolyzed red cells can initiate disseminated intravascular coagulation and cause adverse effects on renal function (see Chapter 14).

Intravascular Hemolysis

Catabolism of circulating hemoglobin has been discussed thoroughly (Bunn, 1972; DeVenuto et al., 1979; Pimestone, 1972). Steps involved in catabolism of intravascular hemoglobin are outlined in Figure 19–2. Plasma clearance of hemoglobin is largely dependent upon the MPS and hepatocytic uptake of free and bound hemoglobin, and partly upon renal clearance. It is fast at low concentration and slow at high concentration, with a half disappearance time of about 1 hr and 7 hr, respectively (DeVenuto et al., 1979). It has been shown that free hemoglobin in plasma is first bound to haptoglobin, an α_2-macroglobulin formed in the liver, and the complex is then removed rapidly (T ½, 20–30 min) and degraded by the MPS, mainly in the liver and to some extent in the bone marrow and spleen. The haptoglobin-hemoglobin

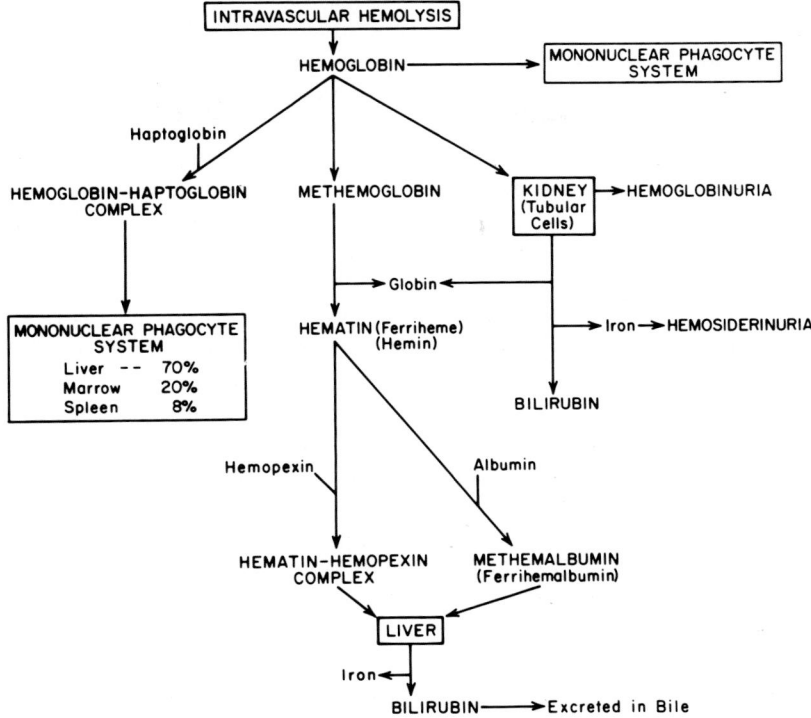

Fig. 19–2. An outline of steps involved in catabolism of free hemoglobin in the plasma.

complex, being a large molecule, does not clear through the kidney. Free hemoglobin may appear in plasma in sufficient concentration to impart a pink or red color when massive destruction of red cells occurs in the vascular bed. The condition is called *hemoglobinemia*. When more free hemoglobin is present than is required to saturate all the plasma haptoglobin, it is filtered by the renal glomeruli, probably in the form of dimers and possibly monomers of hemoglobin ($\alpha_2 \beta_2$ tetramer = 2 α or β dimers, each having a molecular weight of 32,000). This filtered hemoglobin is absorbed in the proximal tubular epithelium, where it is broken down to bilirubin, which is rapidly transported to the liver for excretion into the bile. The iron liberated at this site is mobilized slowly, and *hemosiderinuria* may result. Hemoglobin spills into the urine (*hemoglobinuria*) when the renal threshold for hemoglobin absorption is exceeded (Monke and Yuile, 1940). Excessive filtration of hemoglobin along with red cell membranes through the kidney may result in acute renal failure.

Free hemoglobin in the circulation is con-

verted to methemoglobin, which in turn dissociates liberating hematin (ferriheme). This hematin is bound first to hemopexin, a glycoprotein present in the plasma, and the hematin-hemopexin complex is removed slowly (T ½, 7–8 hr) from the plasma by the hepatocytes, in contrast to rapid (T ½, 20–30 min) removal of the hemoglobin-haptoglobin complex by the Kupffer cells (Bunn, 1972; DeVenuto et al., 1979). After saturation of the plasma hemopexin, any remaining unbound hematin is bound by albumin, with the formation of methemalbumin (ferrihemalbumin). Methemalbumin has a slow turnover rate and is last to disappear (DeVenuto et al., 1979). Hematin-hemopexin complex and methemalbumin are converted primarily to bilirubin in the liver.

When hemolysis is extreme, the plasma concentration of binding proteins decreases because of excessive utilization, e.g., during hemolytic crisis due to babesiasis in calves (Bremner, 1964). This may be taken as a useful indicator of hemolytic process. Plasma haptoglobin was found to be a sensitive indicator of hemolytic anemia in the horse (Allen and

Archer, 1971). Experimental studies in the dog (Thimel and Niepage, 1976), cat (Harvey and Gaskin, 1978), and cow (Richter, 1975), however, indicate that following a single episode of hemoglobinemia, haptoglobin levels are reduced rapidly and the decrease persists only for 12 to 24 hours. Haptoglobin is an acute phase protein. Increases in haptoglobin levels may occur in response to a variety of pathologic conditions and possibly also from some physiologic factors. Sex, age, pregnancy, and lactation were found to influence haptoglobin levels in pigs, but no such effects were observed for cattle (Richter, 1974). A considerable increase in haptoglobin levels occurred within 1.5 to 2.0 days in cattle and within 4 to 6 days in pigs after induction of a local sterile inflammatory lesion (Richter, 1975). Injection of adrenaline, corticotropin, corticosteroids, and bacterial products in both species also caused a rapid increase in haptoglobin. Plasma haptoglobin levels increased in cats in response to abscess formation, feline infectious peritonitis, upper respiratory infection, and splenectomy (Harvey and Gaskin, 1978). Increased haptoglobin levels were reported for horses with clinical and subclinical bacterial infections, and higher levels were also found 24 hours after surgery (Sheldrick et al., 1982). These observations indicate that haptoglobin concentration may not be as reliable an index of intravascular hemolysis as proclaimed, particularly in the presence of an inflammatory lesion. See Chapter 34 for further information on haptoglobin.

Extravascular (Intracellular) Hemolysis

Normally, hemoglobin is destroyed extravascularly by macrophages of the MPS. The hemoglobin molecule is split off, its iron and globin are reutilized and the protoporphyrin molecule is degraded (Fig. 19–3). Iron released from the hemoglobin is bound to transferrin, transported, and made available to the bone marrow for the synthesis of new hemoglobin. Some iron may also be stored as ferritin or hemosiderin. The porphyrin ring is first converted to biliverdin (green pigment) and then reduced to bilirubin (yellow pigment). Free bilirubin is released into the circulation, bound to albumin, and is transported to the parenchymatous cells of the

liver, where it is conjugated with glucuronic acid (Schmid, 1956), mainly as a diglucuronide. This conjugation takes place in the smooth endoplasmic reticulum of hepatocytes. Hereditary defects in the conjugation of bilirubin have been detected in man, rat, and sheep (Cornelius, 1980).

Bilirubin Formation and Excretion

The concentration of bilirubin in the plasma of the dog, cat, cow, sheep, and pig is very low, whereas a relatively large amount occurs in the plasma of the horse (Stone and Adams, 1950). Birds mainly excrete biliverdin into the bile; domestic animals primarily excrete bilirubin glucuronide. Liver tissue in birds is almost completely devoid of biliverdin reductase activity, which explains the formation of little or no bilirubin (Tenhunen, 1971). In sheep, cattle, and pigs, the bilirubin conjugate in the gall bladder is partly hydrolyzed to free bilirubin, some of which is reoxidized to biliverdin.

The origin of bile pigment from hemoglobin was suspected by Virchow (Rich, 1925). In 1847, he published the observation that a reddish-brown pigment, hematoidin (later shown to be identical to bilirubin), is found in tissues where hemorrhage had occurred. Virchow postulated that the pigment was derived from the hemoglobin of disintegrating erythrocytes. In 1889, Lowit (Rich, 1925) proclaimed that the phagocytic cells of the liver, spleen, bone marrow, and peripheral blood convert hemoglobin to bile pigments. The hypothesis is generally accepted that the catabolism of hemoglobin is a function of the MPS. By injecting ^{15}N-labeled hematin (heme) intravenously into the dog, it was demonstrated that hematin can be readily converted into bile pigment (London, 1950). One gram of hemoglobin gives rise to 35 mg of bilirubin in the dog (Hawkins and Johnson, 1939). The maximal capacity of dogs to catabolize hemoglobin has been studied (Couburn and Kane, 1968) by injecting varying quantities of damaged erythrocytes into the circulation. The maximum rate of hemoglobin catabolism in normal anesthetized dogs was found to average about 0.07 g/kg body wt/hr. It was also shown that hemoglobinemia can result from "overloading" the MPS with damaged eryth-

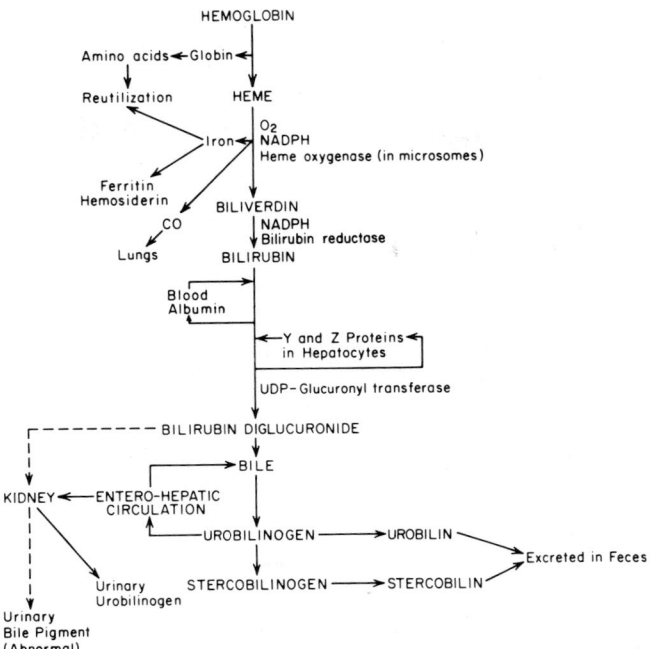

Fig. 19–3. An outline of steps involved in the normal catabolism of hemoglobin.

rocytes (>0.14 g of hemoglobin) and therefore may not always indicate intravascular hemolysis. Hemoglobin is cleared from plasma within a few hours. Renal threshold for hemoglobin in dogs was found to be 0.8–1.5 g/L of plasma (Allison and Rees, 1957).

Although hemoglobin is the main source of bile pigments, it has been shown that other porphyrins such as cytochrome pigments, myoglobin, and other unknown sources also contribute in small measure to the total bile pigment. Bilirubin from nonerythrocytic sources is primarily produced by the liver (Robinson, 1972). Increased ineffective erythropoiesis as well as stimulated effective erythropoiesis may contribute to increased levels of bilirubin in plasma, in the former case because of hemolysis and in the latter because of fragmentation (remodeling) of immature reticulocytes (Robinson, 1972). In a study of catabolism of Heinz bodies in rats (Goldstein et al., 1968), it was found that the heme moiety of solubilized Heinz bodies, in contrast to native hemoglobin, is not converted to bilirubin but is catabolized by an alternate pathway whose parameters remain to be fully determined.

In 1913, van den Bergh and Snapper (Rich, 1925) introduced a test for detecting bilirubin that involved the use of diazotized sulfanilic acid to form the reddish pigment azobilirubin. This technique has become widely known as the van den Bergh test for bilirubin. By 1916, van den Bergh recognized that bilirubin occurs in two forms; the methods to detect these are called the "direct" and "indirect" van den Bergh tests. Free bilirubin (i.e., bilirubin bound to albumin) present in plasma is insoluble in water (at physiologic pH), but soluble in alcohol hence it is also termed indirect-reacting bilirubin. In contrast, the bilirubin conjugate (i.e., bilirubin diglucuronide) is soluble in water and reacts with the diazo reagent without the addition of alcohol, hence the synonym direct-reacting bilirubin.

Prehepatic bilirubin in plasma is firmly bound to albumin, and therefore it does not filter through the kidney to enter the urine, but posthepatic bilirubin (conjugated form) is able to pass into the urine. In icterus or jaundice, the van den Bergh test is often used to aid in establishing the nature of the hyperbilirubinemia. In *hemolytic disease*, most of the bilirubin is prehepatic or indirect-reacting. In intrahepatic obstruction or extrahepatic occlusion of the bile duct, the interference with free flow of bile into the intestine leads to regurgitation of conjugated bilirubin into the bloodstream. Thus hyperbilirubinemia in *hepatic* or *obstructive* jaundice is due mainly to conjugated or direct-reacting bilirubin. In dogs, the kidney threshold for the conjugated bilirubin is low, permitting bile pigments to appear readily in the urine in many systemic diseases affecting the liver parenchymatous cells.

Generally, icterus and serum levels of bilirubin due to posthepatic obstruction are not as prominent as in hemolytic icterus, since bilirubin conjugate can escape into the urine. In severe hemolytic icterus, both forms of bilirubin are usually found in the plasma. The anemia results in a partial anoxia that may lead to swelling of liver cells and partial closing of the bile canaliculi.

The horse is somewhat unique in its bile pigment formation. Both in normal and in disease conditions, bilirubin in the plasma is primarily indirect-reacting (see Table 6–11). During anorexia or starvation, plasma levels of indirect bilirubin often increase significantly to raise icterus index to 50–100 units. This increase has been attributed to reduced excretion of the bilirubin from impaired uptake by the liver through some unknown mechanisms (see Chapter 6). Various factors possibly involved in fasting bilirubinemia (Bakken et al., 1971) and clinical aspects of hyperbilirubinemia due to unconjugated bilirubin (Powell, 1972) have been discussed extensively.

Hypobilirubinemia is commonly seen in chronic diseases such as infections, malignancies, and end stage kidney disease in the dog. This occurs because chronic diseases lead to depression of erythropoiesis and secondary anemia. As the number of erythrocytes available for removal by the MPS becomes reduced, the concentration of bilirubin in the plasma becomes lower and lower, and the plasma in turn becomes devoid of visible pigmentation.

Bilirubin glucuronide is normally excreted with the bile into the small intestine and is progressively reduced to urobilinogen by bacterial action in the terminal ileum and large intestine. A minute amount of conjugated bilirubin in the gut is also hydrolyzed to free bilirubin in the presence of intestinal and possible bacterial β-glucuronidase (Elder et al., 1972). Most of the urobilinogen passes out in the feces as stercobilin, which gives the color to normal feces. Some of the urobilinogen and a trivial amount of the free bilirubin that is formed are absorbed from the gut and reach the liver, through the portal circulation, to be excreted into the bile. The entire process is designated *enterohepatic circulation of bile pigments*. A small amount of absorbed urobilinogen enters the general circulation and is excreted in the urine to become the normal pigment of the urine. Determination of urinary urobilinogen concentration, in conjunction with the van den Bergh test on serum, is helpful in differentiating conditions affecting bilirubin excretion and catabolism. Urobilins and conjugated bilirubin are not absorbed from the intestinal tract. Diminished bowel movement (stasis of feces) increases urobilinogen absorption, while severe diarrhea is associated with increased excretion of unaltered bilirubin in the feces. Treatment with antibiotics may modify intestinal flora and alter production of the urobilinogen. Refer to Cornelius (1980) for a thorough discussion of bilirubin catabolism and excretion in various animal species.

In the newborn infant, bilirubin is the major pigment of meconium and feces, while urobilinogen is present only in minute quantities. In contrast to adults, the neonate has the ability to unconjugate a large amount of bilirubin conjugate excreted into the gut because of greater β-glucuronidase activity in the intestine. Free bilirubin is absorbed from the small intestine. It gains access into the general circulation, although some is excreted again into the bile after conjugation by the liver. This process may contribute significantly to the occurrence of physiologic neonatal hyperbilirubinemia due to other etiologic factors (Elder et al., 1972; Lester and Troxler, 1969). Hyperbilirubinemia or icterus in newborn calves (Cornelius, 1980) and elevated icterus index in newborn foals (see Table 6–5) have been recorded.

The genetic defects of bilirubin metabolism have been recognized in sheep. Defective uptake of bilirubin by hepatocytes in Southdown mutant sheep is associated with increased concentrations of indirect bilirubin in blood. A similar abnormality has been found in Gunn rats and in humans with Gilbert syndrome. Defective excretion of conjugated bilirubin by hepatocytes in Corriedale mutant sheep is associated with elevated concentrations of direct bilirubin in blood. Dubin-Johnson syndrome in humans is a similar disorder (Cornelius, 1980).

REFERENCES

(Titles in parentheses are English translations of foreign language titles.)

Allen, B., and Archer, R.K.: Haptoglobins in the Horse. Vet. Rec., 89:106, 1971.

Allison, A.C.: Malaria in Carriers of the Sickle-Cell Trait and in Newborn Children. Exp. Parasitol., 6:418, 1957.

Allison, A.C., and Rees, W.: The Binding of Haemoglobin by Plasma Proteins (Haptoglobins). Brit. Med. J., 2:1137, 1957.

Altaif, K.I., and Dargie, J.D.: Genetic Resistance to Helminths: Comparison of the Development of Ostertagia circumcincta Infections in Scottish Blackface Sheep of Different Haemoglobin Type. Res. Vet. Sci., 24:391, 1978.

Bakken, A.F., et al.: Stimulation of Hepatic Heme Oxygenase Activity by Fasting and by Hormones. Gastroenterology, 60:177, 1971.

Barker, J.E.: Hemoglobin Switching in Sheep: Characteristics of BFU-E Derived Colonies from Fetal Liver. Blood, 56:495, 1980.

Barker, J.E., et al.: Hemoglobin Switching in Sheep and Goats, Induction of Hemoglobin Synthesis in Cultures of Sheep Fetal Erythroid Cells. Proc. Natl. Acad. Sci., 74:5078, 1977.

Barker, J.E., et al.: Hemoglobin Switching in Sheep: A Comparison of the Erythropoietin-induced Switch to HbC and the Fetal to Adult Hemoglobin Switch. Blood, 56:488, 1980.

Bektas, M.S., et al.: The Embryonic Hemoglobins of Mammals. A New Hemoglobin, Hemoglobin Heide II (Hb He II: $\alpha_2 v_2$), and Demonstration of the Hemoglobin Structure of Gower I ($\delta_2 \epsilon_2$) in the Pig Embryo. Hoppe-Seyler's Z. Physiol. Chem., 362:991, 1981.

Bell, J.T., and Huisman, T.H.: Hemoglobin Types in an Anemic Cow. Amer. J. Vet. Res., 29:479, 1968.

Benz, E.J., Jr., et al.: Stability of the Individual Globin Genes during Erythroid Differentiation. Science, 196:1213, 1977.

Benz, E.J., Jr.: Hemoglobin Switching in Animals. Tex. Rep. Biol. Med., 40:111, 1980–1981.

Boyer, S.H.: Sheep Hemoglobins, Erythropoietin, and Genetic Regulation. In Hemopoietic Cellular Proliferation. Stohlman, F.J., ed. Grune and Stratton, New York, p. 141, 1969.

Bremner, K.C.: Studies on Haptoglobin and Haemopexin in the Plasma of Cattle. Anat. J. Exp. Biol. Med. Sci., 42:643, 1964.

Bunn, H.F.: Erythrocyte Destruction and Hemoglobin Catabolism. Semin. Hematol., 9:3, 1972.

Buvanendran, V., et al.: Haemoglobin Polymorphism and Resistance to Helminths in Red Sokoto Goats. Trop. Anim. Health. Prod., 13:217, 1981.

Chui, D.H.K., et al.: Proportion of Fetal Hemoglobin Synthesis Decreases during Erythroid Cell Maturation. Proc. Natl. Acad. Sci., 77:2757, 1980.

Cornelius, C.E.: Liver Function. In Clinical Biochemistry of Domestic Animals. Vol. 1. Kaneko, J.J., and Cornelius, C.E., eds. Academic Press, New York, 1980.

Costea, V.: Recherches sur la correlation entre les types d'hemoglobine et certains parametres sanguins chez les bovins. Archiva Veterinaria, 14:35, 1979.

Couburn, R.F., and Kane, P.B.: Maximal Erythrocyte and Hemoglobin Catabolism. J. Clin. Invest., 47:1435, 1968.

Crosby, W.H.: Diseases of the Reticuloendothelial System and Hematology: The Red Cell and Some of Its Problems. Annu. Rev. Med., 8:151, 1957.

Dayhoff, M.O.: Atlas of Protein Sequence and Structure. Vol. 4. National Biomedical Research Foundation, Silver Spring, Maryland, pp. D37–D63, 1969.

DeVenuto, F., et al.: Appraisal of Hemoglobin Solution as a Blood Substitute. Surg. Gynecol. Obstet., 149:417, 1979.

Dobriner, K., and Rhoads, C.P.: The Porphyrins in Health and Disease. Physiol. Rev., 20:416, 1940.

Dover, G.J., et al.: Production of Erythrocytes that Contain Fetal Hemoglobin in Anemia. J. Clin. Invest., 63:173, 1979.

Elder, G., et al.: Bile Pigment Fate in Gastrointestinal Tract. Semin. Hematol., 9:71, 1972.

Enomoto, K., et al.: Demonstration of Embryonic-Type Hemoglobin in Extramedullary Hematopoietic Cells in the Liver During Experimental Liver Carcinogenesis by 3'-methyl-4-dimethylaminoazobenzene. Cancer Res., 40:1769, 1980.

Freedman, M.L.: Ethanol, Lead and Benzene Inhibition of Reticulocyte Heme and Protein Synthesis: Increased in Vitro Toxicity in Iron-Deficient Cells. Environ. Res., 18:291, 1979.

Goldstein, G.W., et al.: The Catabolism of Heinz Bodies: An Experimental Model Demonstrating Conversion to Non-Bilirubin Catabolites. Blood, 31:388, 1968.

Harris, J.W., and Kellermeyer, R.W.: The Red Cell, Production, Metabolism, Destruction: Normal and Abnormal. Harvard Univ. Press, Cambridge, Mass., 1970.

Harvey, J.W., and Gaskin, J.M.: Feline Haptoglobin. Amer. J. Vet. Res., 39:549, 1978.

Hawkins, W.B., and Johnson, A.C.: Bile Pigment and Hemoglobin Interrelation in Anemic Dogs. Amer. J. Physiol., 126:326, 1939.

Huisman, T.H.J., et al.: The Structure of Goat Hemoglobins. I. Structural Studies of the Chains of the Hemoglobins of Normal and Anemic Goats. J. Biol. Chem., 262:2534, 1967.

Ingram, V.M., and Stretton, A.O.W.: Genetic Basis of the Thalassaemia Diseases. Nature, 184:1903, 1959.

Itano, H.A.: Genetic Regulation of Peptide Synthesis in Hemoglobins. J. Cell. Physiol., 67:65, 1966.

Jain, N.C., et al.: Fusiform Erythrocytes Resembling Sickle Cells in Angora Goats. Observations on Osmotic and Mechanical Fragilities and Reversal of Cell Shape During Anemia. Res. Vet. Sci., 28:25, 1980.

Jelic, Z., et al.: Use of Gel Electrofocusing in the Analysis of Bovine Haemoglobin. Acta Vet., Yugoslavia, 31:173, 1981.

Jones, D.R.E., et al.: Reduced Exercise Tolerance in a Dog Associated with an Abnormal Haemoglobin. Vet. Rec., 102:105, 1978.

Kaneko, J.J.: Clinical Biochemistry of Domestic Animals. 3rd Ed. Academic Press, New York, 1980.

Kitchen, H.: Heterogeneity of Animal Hemoglobins. Adv. Vet. Sci. Comp. Med., 13:247, 1969.

Kitchen, H.: Fetal Hemoglobins. Bull. Amer. Soc. Vet. Clin. Path., 1(3):25, 1972.

Kitchen, H., and Brett, I.: Embryonic and Fetal Hemoglobins in Animals. Ann. N.Y. Acad. Sci., *241*:653, 1974.

Lessard, J.L., and Taketa, F.: Multiple Hemoglobins in Fetal, Newborn, and Adult Cats. Biochem. Biophys. Acta, *175*:441, 1969.

Lester, R., and Troxler, R.F.: Recent Advances in Bile Pigment Metabolism. Gastroenterology, *56*:143, 1969.

London, I.M.: The Conversion of Hematin to Bile Pigment. J. Biol. Chem., *184*:373, 1950.

London, I.M., et al.: Synthesis of Heme in Vitro by the Immature Nonnucleated Mammalian Erythrocyte. J. Biol. Chem., *183*:749, 1950.

Mohandas, N., et al.: Erythropoietic Stress, Macrocytosis, and Hemoglobin Switching in HbAA Sheep. Blood, *55*:757, 1980.

Monke, J.V., and Yuile, C.L.: The Renal Clearance of Hemoglobin in the Dog. J. Exp. Med., *72*:149, 1940.

Nienhuis, A.W., and Benz, E.J.: Regulation of Hemoglobin Synthesis During the Development of the Red Cells. New Eng. J. Med., *297*:1430, 1977.

Nienhuis, A.W., and Bunn, H.F.: Hemoglobin Switching in Sheep and Goats: Occurrence of Hemoglobins A and C in Same Red Cell. Science, *185*:946, 1974.

Nienhuis, A.W., et al.: Overview: Mechanisms of the Regulation of Hemoglobin Synthesis at the Cellular Level. Ann. N.Y. Acad. Sci., *344*:189, 1980.

Papayannopoulou, T.H.: Fetal Hb Production During Acute Erythroid Expansion. I. Observation in Patients with Transient Erythroplastopenia and Post-Phlebotomy. Brit. J. Haematol., *44*:535, 1980.

Papayannopoulou, T.H., and Stamatoyannopoulos, G.: Human Hemoglobin Switching: Insights from Studies of Erythroid Cultures. J. Cell. Physiol. [Suppl.], *1*:145, 1982.

Papayannopoulou, T.H., et al.: Hemoglobin F Synthesis in Vitro: Evidence for Control at the Level of Primitive Erythroid Stem Cells. Proc. Natl. Acad. Sci. USA, *74*:2923, 1977.

Pauling, L., et al.: Sickle Cell Anemia, a Molecular Disease. Science, *110*:543, 1949.

Perutz, M.F.: Structure and Mechanism of Haemoglobin. Brit. Med. Bull., *32*:195, 1976.

Perutz, M.F., and Mitchison, J.M.: State of Haemoglobin in Sickle-Cell Anaemia. Nature, *166*:677, 1950.

Perutz, M.F., et al.: Three-Dimensional Fourier Synthesis of Horse Oxyhaemoglobin at 2.8 A Resolution: The Atomic Model. Nature, *219*:131, 1968.

Pimestone, N.F.: Renal Degradation of Hemoglobin. Semin. Hematol., *9*:31, 1972.

Powell, L.W.: Clinical Aspects of Unconjugated Hyperbilirubinemia. Semin. Hematol., *9*:91, 1972.

Rhinesmith, H.S., et al.: A Quantitative Study of the Hydrolysis of Human Dinitrophenyl (DNP) Globin: The Number and Kind of Polypeptide Chains in Normal Adult Human Hemoglobin. J. Amer. Chem. Soc., *79*:4682, 1957.

Rhode, E.A., and Cornelius, C.E.: Congenital Porphyria (Pink Tooth) in Holstein-Friesian Calves in California. J. Amer. Vet. Med. Ass., *132*:112, 1958.

Rich, A.R.: The Formation of Bile Pigment: Physiol. Rev., *5*:182, 1925.

Richter, H.: (Haptoglobin in Domestic Animals. III. Content in Plasma and Serum of Ruminants and Pigs under Various Physiological Conditions.) Arch. Exp. Veterinärmed., *28*(4):505, 1974.

Richter, H.: (Haptoglobin in Domesticated Mammals. IV. Experiments on Factors Affecting Haptoglobin Status.) Arch. Exp. Veterinärmed., *29*:217, 1975.

Robinson, S.H.: Formation of Bilirubin from Erythroid and Nonerythroid Sources. Semin. Hematol., *9*:43, 1972.

Schmid, R.: Direct-Reacting Bilirubin, Bilirubin Glucuronide, in Serum, Bile, and Urine. Science, *124*:76, 1956.

Schwartz, S., and Wikoff, H.M.: The Relation of Erythrocyte Coproporphyrin and Protoporphyrin to Erythropoiesis. J. Biol. Chem., *194*:563, 1952.

Sheldrick, R., et al.: Haemoglobin Binding Capacity of Serum as an Indicator of Infection in the Horse. Vet. Rec., *111*:128, 1982.

Shemin, D., and Rittenberg, D.: The Life Span of the Human Red Blood Cell. J. Biol. Chem., *166*:627, 1946.

Stone, E.C., and Adams, M.F.: Studies on Blood Plasma of Domestic Animals. I. Absorption Spectrums of Plasma of Some Individual Animals. Amer. J. Vet. Res., *11*:91, 1950.

Taketa, F., et al.: Studies on Cat Hemoglobin and Hybrids with Human Hemoglobin A. Biochemistry, *6*:3809, 1967.

Taketa, F., et al.: Hemoglobin A and B of the Cat: Occurrence in the Same Cell. Hemoglobin, *2*:371, 1978.

Tenhunen, R.: The Green Colour of Avian Bile: Biochemical Explanation. Scand. J. Clin. Lab. Invest., *27*:116, 1971.

Testa, U., et al.: Cellular and Molecular Mechanisms of Haemoglobin Switching in Man. Haematologica, *67*:64, 1982.

Thimel, H., and Niepage, H.: Die Hamoglobin—Bindungskapazitat in serum des unbehadelten Hundes und bei experimenteller Hamolyse. Fortschr. Veterinärmed., *25*:203, 1976.

Thurmon, T.F., et al.: Hemoglobin Switching in Non-Anemic Sheep. III. Evidence for Presumptive Identity Between A-C Factor and Erythropoietin. Blood, *36*:598, 1970.

White, J.M.: Lead and Haemoglobin Synthesis: A Review. Postgrad. Med. J., *51*:755, 1975.

Williams, E.I., and Jones, E.W.: Blood Transfusions During Patent Bovine Anaplasmosis. Amer. J. Vet. Res., *29*:703, 1968.

20

The Erythrocyte: Its Morphology, Metabolism, and Survival

SPECIES VARIATION IN ERYTHROCYTE MORPHOLOGY 527

RED CELL MEMBRANE 528
Membrane Lipids 531
Membrane Proteins 532

TRANSFORMATIONS AND ABNORMALITIES OF THE ERYTHROCYTE SHAPE 532
Descriptive Terminology 533
Abnormalities of Ionic Transport and Thermal Reactivity 543
Additional Comments 544

METABOLISM OF THE ERYTHROCYTES 545
Normal Erythrocyte Metabolism and Some Species Differences 545
Abnormalities of Erythrocyte Metabolism 546
Erythrocyte 2,3-Diphosphoglycerate (DPG) 546

ERYTHROCYTE LIFE SPAN 547
Normal Life Span 547
Shortened Intravascular Survival 548

DESTRUCTION OF ERYTHROCYTES 550
Erythrocyte Deformability 550
Modes of Erythrocyte Destruction 551

The primary function of the erythrocyte is to serve as a carrier of hemoglobin. The incorporation of hemoglobin in a special cell for circulation in the bloodstream makes possible the complex structure and specialized activities of the vertebrates. Hemoglobin in solution, in the concentration found in mammalian erythrocytes, does not increase viscosity of the blood, as thought previously (Schmidt-Nielsen and Taylor, 1968). At such a concentration, however, it exerts an osmotic pressure about three times as great as that caused by the plasma proteins alone. This pressure would have profound effects on the movement of fluids through capillary walls and particularly on filtration in the renal glomeruli. These effects are avoided by placing hemoglobin within a cell that is capable of passing through the bore of the smallest capillary. Another advantage is gained, for in the interior of the erythrocyte, the hemoglobin exists in an environment that is designed to take advantage of the pH, slightly more acid than plasma, at which hemoglobin is most efficient as a respiratory pigment (Barcroft, 1923, 1924). Other advantages of packaging

the hemoglobin in cellular units are: The hemoglobin is removed from the general metabolic pool, preventing its rapid turnover (the half-life of free hemoglobin in plasma is about three hours as opposed to weeks to months within red cells), and the hemoglobin is kept in close proximity to enzyme systems to maintain its chemical state required for oxygen transport. Each gram of hemoglobin carries 1.3 ml of oxygen at complete saturation.

SPECIES VARIATION IN ERYTHROCYTE MORPHOLOGY

The mammalian erythrocyte is anuclear; all other vertebrates have nucleated red cells. The shape of the erythrocyte can be studied readily in wet preparations under the light microscope. The morphology of erythrocytes in routinely stained blood films depends on the extent to which erythrocytes flatten and shrink during smear making. The mean corpuscular diameter of erythrocytes measured in a "dry" state is smaller than that measured in the "wet" state (Werre at al., 1970). The biconcave erythrocyte characteristically displays a distinct central pale area in modestly thick regions of the film. This central pallor is readily apparent in canine erythrocytes. Erythrocytes of the cat and horse generally stain diffusely or reveal limited evidence of central pallor; the red cells of the cow, sheep, goat, and pig may or may not present a pale central area. Thus, in stained blood films, except for the dog, the red cells of the common domestic animals do not appear distinctly biconcave, but tend to be shaped like flat discs with little or no central depression.

Stained blood films are not suitable for study of three-dimensional morphology. With the use of Nomarski differential interference-contrast microscopy, some depth of field is obtained, but scanning electron microscopy provides optimal definition of three-dimensional morphologic features. Erythrocytes of the common domestic animals (the dog, cat, cow, horse, sheep, and goat) have been examined with the scanning electron microscope (Jain and Kono, 1972, 1977a, b). Biconcave erythrocytes are found in health in each of these species, but the proportion of such cells and the degree of concavity vary. Typical biconcave erythrocytes are present in the dog (Fig. 20–1A), cow (Fig. 20–1C), and sheep (Fig. 20–1E and F); the erythrocytes of the horse (Fig. 20–1D) and cat (Fig. 20–1B) have a shallow concavity; and most of the erythrocytes of the goat may be rather flat or have a shallow surface depression (Fig. 20–2A). The cow and sheep also have a small number of uniconcave (bowl-shaped) erythrocytes (Fig. 20–1C). These cells may be present in different profiles. One or more wart-like protuberances (Fig. 20–1F) have been observed on the surface of a few erythrocytes of the sheep and goat and rarely on dog red cells. These structures may indicate the beginning of red cell senescence and represent gradual fragmentation that leads to complete red cell destruction (see Erythrocyte Fragmentation). The surface of mature erythrocytes in all species is smooth, whereas immature erythrocytes have a relatively rough surface and many small pits that correspond to sites of iron intake (see Fig. 18–10A; Keeton and Jain, 1973).

Species differences can be found in the erythrocyte shape. The family Camellidae,

which includes the camel, alpaca, and llama, is distinctive in having elliptical erythrocytes (Figs. 20–2E, F; Jain and Keeton, 1974). Erythrocytes of certain deer species can sickle after removal from the body. Sickle-shaped erythrocytes in deer are small, highly pliable, and nonfragile (normal mechanical fragility), unlike human sickle cells; hence, the presence of sickle cells in deer is innocuous (Whitten, 1967). Sickle-shaped erythrocytes were seen in three breeds of British sheep (Evans, 1968). Poikilocytosis (variation in cell shape) is prominent among erythrocytes of the goat—spindle-shaped, rod-like, pear-shaped, and triangular erythrocytes (Fig. 20–2B) can be found in some clinically normal goats. Poikilocytosis can be seen in newborn goats (Holman and Dew, 1964) and calves (Sato and Mizuno, 1982). Elliptical erythrocytes have been found in goat kids 1 to 3 months of age (Holman and Dew, 1964), and we have observed nearly all red cells to be perfectly discocytic in some goat kids from 1 day to about 2 months in age. Fusiform and match-stick form red cells, similar to those seen in deer blood and in humans with sickle cell anemia, have been found in goats of the Angora breed (Jain and Kono, 1977a,b). Light and electron microscopic observations (Figs. 9–3, 9–4) indicated that polymerization of hemoglobin in the form of longitudinal tubular fibers was responsible for conferring the fusiform and spindle shapes to erythrocytes. Microtubules and marginal bands were seen in camel red cells by electron microscopy, but they were thought nonessential for maintenance of the elliptical shape (Cohen, 1979). The ellipsoidal shape of nucleated red cells in nonmammalian vertebrates is attributed to marginal bands (Coiro et al., 1978) and/or transmarginal band material (Cohen et al., 1982). Prominent spherocytes (Fig. 20–2C) with no accompanying anemia were observed in 1 goat; it was probably an unusual case of hereditary spherocytosis (Jain, 1973). Acanthocytes (Fig. 20–2D) were found in blood from an apparently healthy cow (Jain, unpublished observations).

RED CELL MEMBRANE

The red cell membrane encloses the cellular components and is vital to the survival and

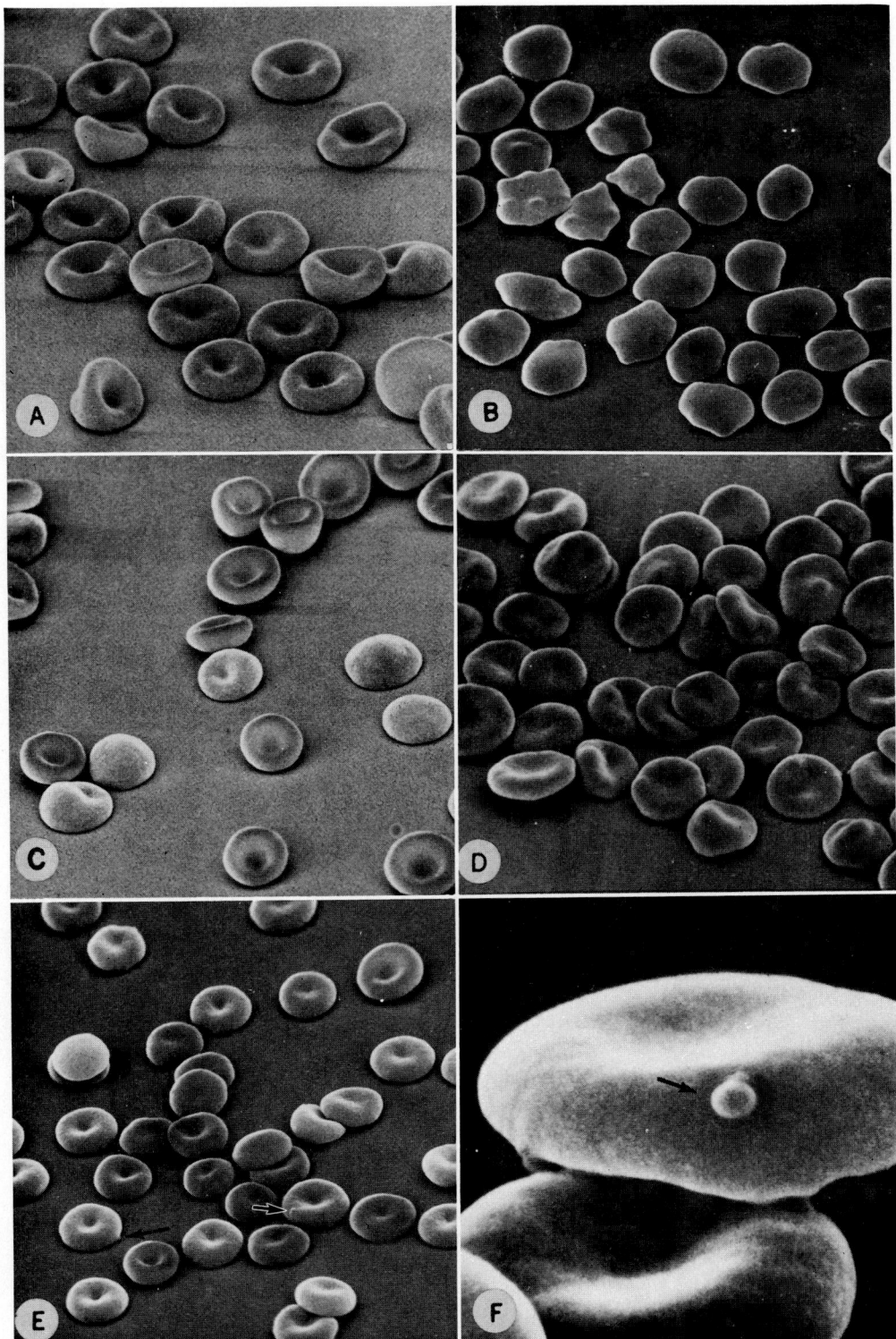

Fig. 20–1. Scanning electron photomicrographs of erythrocytes from a clinically normal dog (*A*, ×2,600), cat (*B*, ×2,500), cow (*C*, ×2,500), horse (*D*, ×2,550), and sheep (*E*, ×2,430; and *F*, ×12,000). Arrows in *E* and *F* point to small protuberances on the cell surface; such structures are often seen on sheep and goat erythrocytes and rarely on dog red cells. (*A,B,D,* and *E* from Jain and Kono, 1972; courtesy of *Research in Veterinary Science. C* from Jain, 1972b; courtesy of *The California Veterinarian.*)

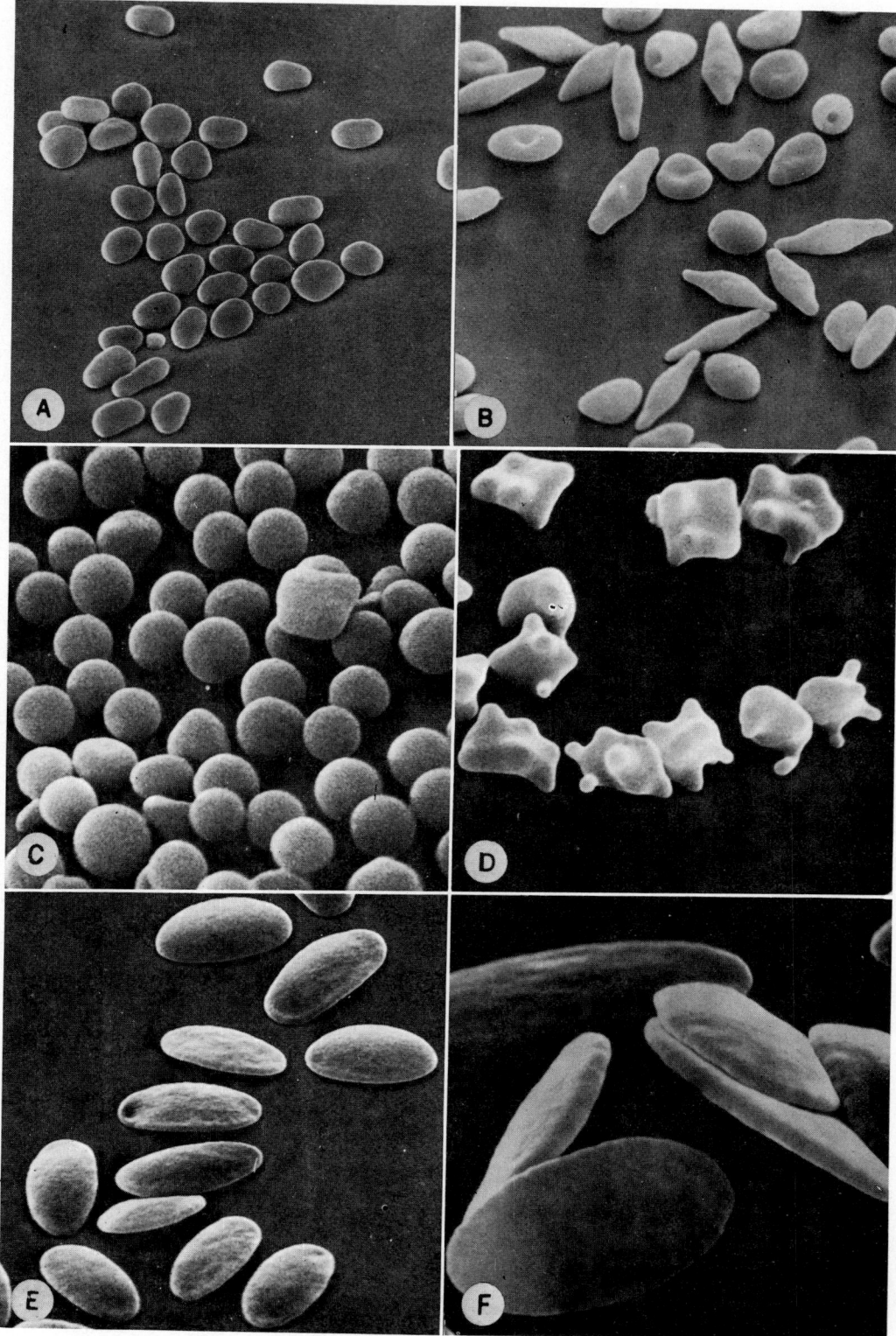

Fig. 20–2. Scanning electron photomicrographs of erythrocytes. *A* (×2,500), *B* (×3,150), and *C* (×3,275) are from clinically healthy goats. *D* (×3,000), acanthocytes from a normal cow. *E* (×2,400) and *F* (×6,500), erythrocytes from a camel; the side-view in *F* shows their waferlike thinness. (*A* from Jain and Kono, 1972; courtesy of *Research in Veterinary Science. F* from Jain and Keeton, 1974; courtesy of *British Veterinary Journal.*)

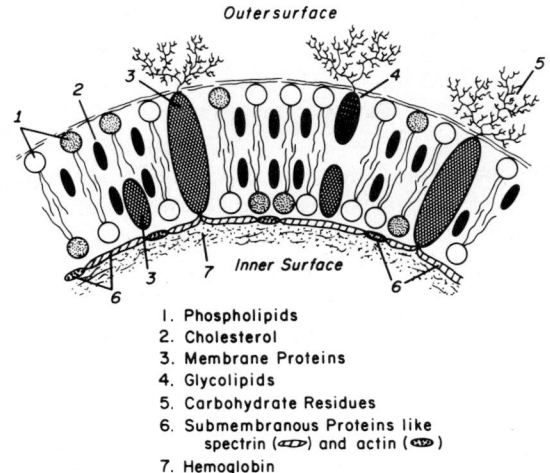

Outer surface

Inner Surface

1. Phospholipids
2. Cholesterol
3. Membrane Proteins
4. Glycolipids
5. Carbohydrate Residues
6. Submembranous Proteins like
     spectrin (⊂⊐) and actin (⊂▱)
7. Hemoglobin

Fig. 20–3. A schematic of erythrocyte membrane showing different structural components. (Modified from Zucker-Franklin et al.: Atlas of Blood Cells. Lea & Febiger, Philadelphia, 1981.)

function of the red cell. It bestows the red cell with deformability and resilience to survive circulation through minute capillaries of body tissues. Its unique transport functions and selective permeability to cations regulate the red cell contents and ionic gradient between the intracellular and extracellular environments. Membrane properties are important in regulating the interaction of the red cell with other cells (e.g., macrophages) or the surrounding medium. Several enzymes important to normal red cell function and survival are found in the membrane (Ballas and Krasnow, 1980; Delaunay, 1977).

Some knowledge of the structural and biochemical composition of the erythrocyte membrane is essential to understand aberrations in red cell shape. Several recent reviews are available on this aspect (Goodman and Shiffer, 1983; Gratzer, 1981; Lubin and Chin, 1982; Rice-Evans and Chapman, 1981). Morphologically, the red cell membrane consists of a bilayer structure composed of two electron-dense layers, each about 25Å thick, separated by a 20–30 Å electron-lucent zone. Biochemically, the membrane is composed of proteins (48%), lipids (44%), and carbohydrates (8%). The carbohydrate moiety is associated either with proteins or lipids in the membrane, forming glycoproteins or glycolipids, respectively. Protein and lipid components are asymmetrically distributed within the outer and inner portions of the erythrocyte membrane which consequently differ in protein and lipid composition. The biochemical structure of the red cell membrane is most satisfactorily represented by the fluid mosaic model (Fig. 20–3). It consists of a lipid bilayer comprised of phospholipid molecules arranged with their hydrophobic nonpolar groups directed inwardly toward each other and hydrophilic polar groups directed outwardly, forming the external and internal membrane surfaces. Cholesterol is interspersed between the phospholipid molecules. Protein molecules are asymmetrically distributed within the membrane (integral membrane proteins) and at submembranous locations (peripheral membrane proteins). Some membrane proteins remain intramembranous while others traverse the whole membrane, with their outer portion glycosylated and inner portion associated with submembranous structural proteins. Carbohydrate residues on the red cell membrane confer negative surface charge and serve as antigenic determinants (blood groups) and binding sites for viruses and lectins.

The membrane of the red cell has a negative surface charge that decreases with the age of the red cell and also when red cells are exposed to antibodies or proteolytic enzymes like trypsin. This charge is due largely to carboxyl groups of sialic acid residues localized in the glycoproteins of the external surface (Danon et al., 1971). An excellent correlation has been found between sialic acid molecules per unit surface area of red cells and red cell electrophoretic mobility for several species (Walter, 1969). This characteristic has been used to separate red cells of different ages.

Membrane Lipids

Membrane lipids are important determinants of red cell shape and surface area. The outer half of the red cell membrane is rich in phosphatidylcholine and sphingomyelin and has some phosphatidylethanolamine, whereas the inner half is rich in phosphatidylserine and phosphatidylethanolamine (Lubin and Chin, 1982).

Normal cholesterol to phospholipid ratio in human erythrocytes is about 0.9–1.0 (Cooper, 1980) and these molecules are in a dynamic state exchanging freely between membrane and plasma. A higher concentration of cholesterol is found in the membrane at the convex portion of the red cell than at the concavity. An optimal cholesterol to phospholipid ratio is essential to maintain normal red cell shape. Loss of cholesterol decreases the membrane surface area causing red cells to become osmotically more fragile, whereas an increase in cholesterol extends the surface area (giving the cell a folded contour), decreases red cell filtrability, and imparts resistance to osmotic lysis (Cooper, 1970, 1978; Cooper et al., 1980). Cholesterol and phospholipid contents and their ratios in the red cell membrane have been associated with altered red cell morphology in liver disease, "spur-cell anemia" and abetalipoproteinemia. "Stress-reticulocytes" of anemia and mature red cells derived from them have abnormal membrane lipid composition (Walter et al., 1978).

The lipid composition of red cell membrane varies considerably among species and can vary within the species (Atkinson et al., 1980; deGier and van Deenen, 1961; Luther et al., 1982; Nelson, 1967; O'Kelly, 1979). Erythrocytes of the neonate can also exhibit some differences (Thiele et al., 1979), and this can be due in part to the diet of the dam during pregnancy (Shand and Noble, 1981). De novo synthesis of phospholipid and cholesterol occurs in the reticulocyte, but not in the mature red cell. Furthermore, a decrease in lipid content of red cells occurs with increasing cell age (Krotlinger et al., 1980).

Membrane Proteins

Several proteins are delineated when red cell membrane is solubilized with sodium dodecyl sulfate and subjected to polyacrylamide gel electrophoresis (SDS-PAGE). These proteins from human red cells have been named according to their relative location from the place of migration besides certain specific names. Three classes of sialoproteins have been identified, namely, glycophorin A, B, and C. Glycophorin A and band 3 protein are the major integral membrane proteins. At least 4 of the peripheral membrane proteins are recognized to constitute the submembranous cytoskeleton; these are bands 1, 2,

4.1, and 5 (Bennett and Stenbuck, 1980; Goodman and Shiffer, 1983; Gratzer, 1981; Tsukita et al., 1980). Spectrin (bands 1 and 2) and actin (band 5) are the major cytoskeletal proteins, the former playing a key role in maintaining cell shape and cellular integrity (Marchesi, 1983). Spectrin is linked to the inner aspects of the red cell membrane by at least one other membrane protein called ankyrin or syndein. Changes in spectrin configuration (dephosphorylation) are associated with crenation (discocyte-echinocyte transformation). Abnormalities of spectrin have been implicated in altered red cell shape seen in certain disorders of humans, e.g., hereditary spherocytosis, hereditary elliptocytosis, and sickle cell anemia.

Some studies have been conducted on red cell membrane proteins of animal species. A complex mixture of proteins was obtained when acetic acid soluble proteins of bovine and sheep erythrocyte membrane were subjected to PAGE (Brandon, 1980; Maddy, 1970). At least 7 major polypeptide bands have been identified in goat red cell membranes by SDS-PAGE (Atkinson et al., 1980). Red cells of myotonic goats were found to have altered membrane-protein composition (decreased band A), increased membrane-bound calcium and sialic acid contents, and increased osmotic resistance (Atkinson et al., 1980). Five membrane glycoproteins were described for the horse, sheep, goat, and bovine erythrocytes (Klimas et al., 1982).

TRANSFORMATIONS AND ABNORMALITIES OF THE ERYTHROCYTE SHAPE

The normal shape of the red cell is one of equilibrium, determined by the structural properties of the cell membrane and hemoglobin, under the influence of intracellular and extracellular environments. The most common form is the biconcave shape. The erythrocyte is normally capable of regaining its shape after repeated alterations following passage through the microcirculation (Fig. 20–4). Ghosts of hemolyzed erythrocytes can also assume the biconcave shape in a proper environment. The red cell membrane is believed to be largely responsible for the bicon-

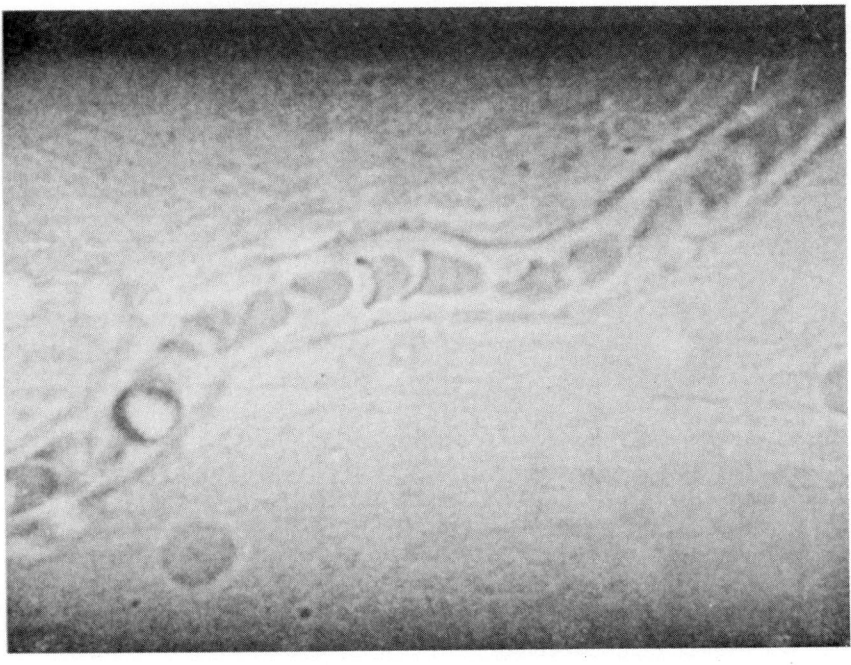

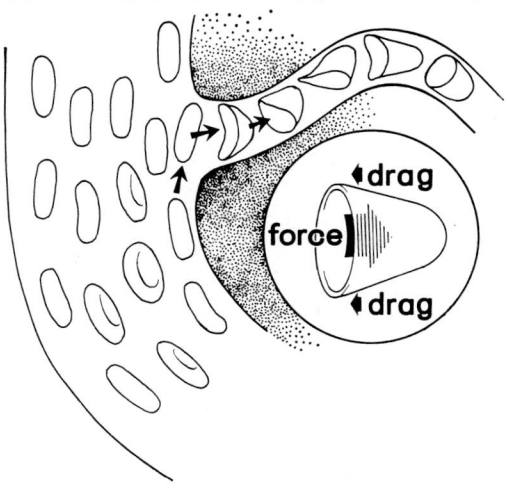

Fig. 20–4. *Top,* One frame of film taken at 3,200 frames per second showing red blood cells of the dog passing through a capillary. *Bottom,* Schematic representation of the predominant flow pattern in the arteriole and arteriolar end of a capillary. Circle inset shows the forces acting on the red blood cell during its passage through the capillary. (From Guest, et al., 1963; courtesy of *Science*.)

cave shape of the mature erythrocyte, but how the shape is maintained is still not completely understood. Membrane phospholipids, cholesterol, and proteins are important and ATP and Ca^{++} are essential for maintaining the normal shape. Metabolically depleted red cells are likely to exhibit artifactual alterations.

Descriptive Terminology

Abnormalities of red cell shape may be of diagnostic significance. In this regard, it is imperative that correct descriptive terminology (Table 20–1) is used for the observed red cell shape and that the artifactual form is distinguished from the true shape change.

Variations in red cell shape may occur under pathologic conditions as a result of intrinsic abnormalities of the red cell or because of changes in its environment. Many in vitro factors are also known to influence the red cell shape (Brecher and Bessis, 1972; Deuticke, 1968; Litchman et al., 1974; Quist, 1980; Szasz et al., 1978). Various abnormalities in

Table 20–1.   Terms Describing Erythrocyte Morphology and Their Greek or Latin Roots

Term	Greek or Latin Root	Meaning of Root
-cyte	Gr. kytos	Cell
Acanthocyte	Gr. akantha	Thorn, spicule, spine
Acuminocyte	L. acuminatus	Fusiform
Codocyte	Gr. kodea	Helmet, hat, cup-shaped
Cryohydrocyte	Gr. kryos + hydros	Frost
Dacryocyte	Gr. dakryon	Tear
Descicyte	L. de-siccus	Completely dry
Discocyte	Gr. diskoeites, diskos	Disc, round plate
Drepanocyte	Gr. drepano, drepanē	Sickle
Eccentrocyte	Gr. ekkentros	Out of the center
Echinocyte	Gr. echinos	Sea urchin
Elliptocyte	Gr. elleipsis	Defect
Fusocyte	L. fusus	Spindle
Hydrocyte	Gr. hydōr	Water
Keratocyte	Gr. keras, keratos	Horn
Knizocyte	Gr. knizo	Dimple
Leptocyte	Gr. leptos	Thin
Macrocyte	Gr. makros	Long
Megalocyte	Gr. megas	Large, great
Microcyte	Gr. mikros	Small
Ovalocyte	L. ovum, NL ovalis	Egg
Poikilocyte	Gr. poikilos	Variegated
Pyknocyte	Gr. pyknos	Compact
Pyropoikilocyte	Gr. pyr, pyros + poikilos	Fire + variegated
Schistocyte	Gr. schistos	Divided, divisible, split
Schizocyte	Gr. schizein	Cut, cleave, split
Selenocyte	Gr. selēnē	Moon
Siderocyte	Gr. siderōs	Iron
Spherocyte	Gr. sphaira	Sphere, ball
Stomatocyte	Gr. stoma, stomatos	Mouth
Torocyte	L. torus	Bulge, protuberance
Xerocyte	Gr. xeros	Dry

Note: The Greek root is preferred. The Latin root is substituted for lack of an appropriate Greek root.

the red cell shape are listed in the following sections along with a brief description of the cell morphology and conditions frequently associated with the particular cells in humans. The same terminology could be used to describe erythrocytes of various animal species, but conditions associated with a particular cell type need to be determined. A more varied erythrocyte morphology is found in animal bloods, however, which may require formulating new terms that conform with the Greek prefixes currently used to denote various forms of red cells in humans. Often more than one form of red cells are found in the same blood sample, and red cells of a particular shape may exhibit secondary shape changes. The latter event is described appropriately by combining relevant terms; e.g., spheroechinocyte, spherostomatocyte. In the following descriptions, our unpublished observations are given along with those from some literature reports on animal red cells (Jain, 1972b, 1975; Jain and Keeton, 1974; Jain and Kono,

1972, 1977a, 1977b; Perman and Schall, 1983; Pinkerton et al., 1974; Rebar et al., 1981; Shull et al., 1978; Smith et al., 1982, 1983). Interested readers should read the publications of Bessis (1972, 1973, 1977) and relevant reviews by Cooper (1978, 1980); Lessin et al., (1976); Rebar et al. (1981); and Weed (1975) for further information. Light and scanning electron photomicrographs of various forms of red cells are presented in Figures 20–5 through 20–9.

Acanthocytes are spiculated erythrocytes with several unevenly distributed surface projections that are irregular in length, thickness, and distribution (see Figs. 20–2*D*; 20–6*C*; 20–8*E*). The projections may be straight or curved and have knobby ends. The knobby end or the entire projection may fragment resulting in a spherocytic change prior to lysis, or the entire cell may be sequestered in the spleen and be removed prematurely. Acanthocytes are also called "spur" cells and have been confused with echinocytes. The

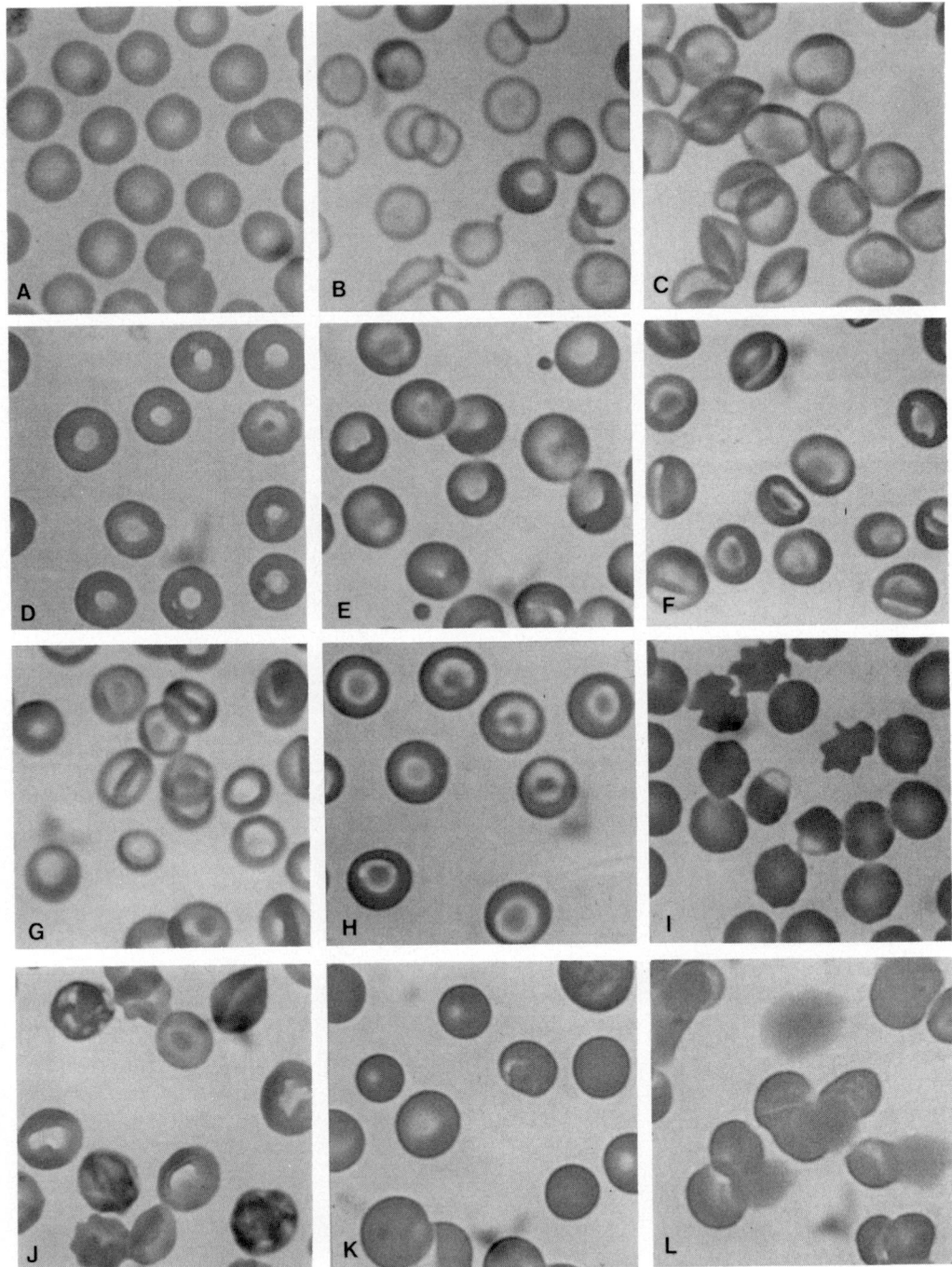

Fig. 20–5. Erythrocyte morphology in Wright-stained canine blood films examined with the light microscope. *A,* Normal discoid red cells with central pallor; *B,* hypochromic erythrocytes with a thin rim of hemoglobin and extended central pallor; *C,* thin leptocytes with variable foldings; *D,* punched-out red cells (torocytes); *E* and *F,* various forms of stomatocytes, a few small red cell fragments are also present in *E; G,* microcytic hypochromic red cells and a few leptocytic red cells with a central membranous fold (knizocytes); *H,* target cells (codocytes); *I,* hemoglobin crystallization in an occasional red cell; *J,* several polychromatic red cells with membranous folds typical of reticulocytes examined with the scanning electron microscope (see Fig. 20–8A); *K,* spherocytic red cells, those with a slight clear area are called spherostomatocytes; *L,* smudge cells.

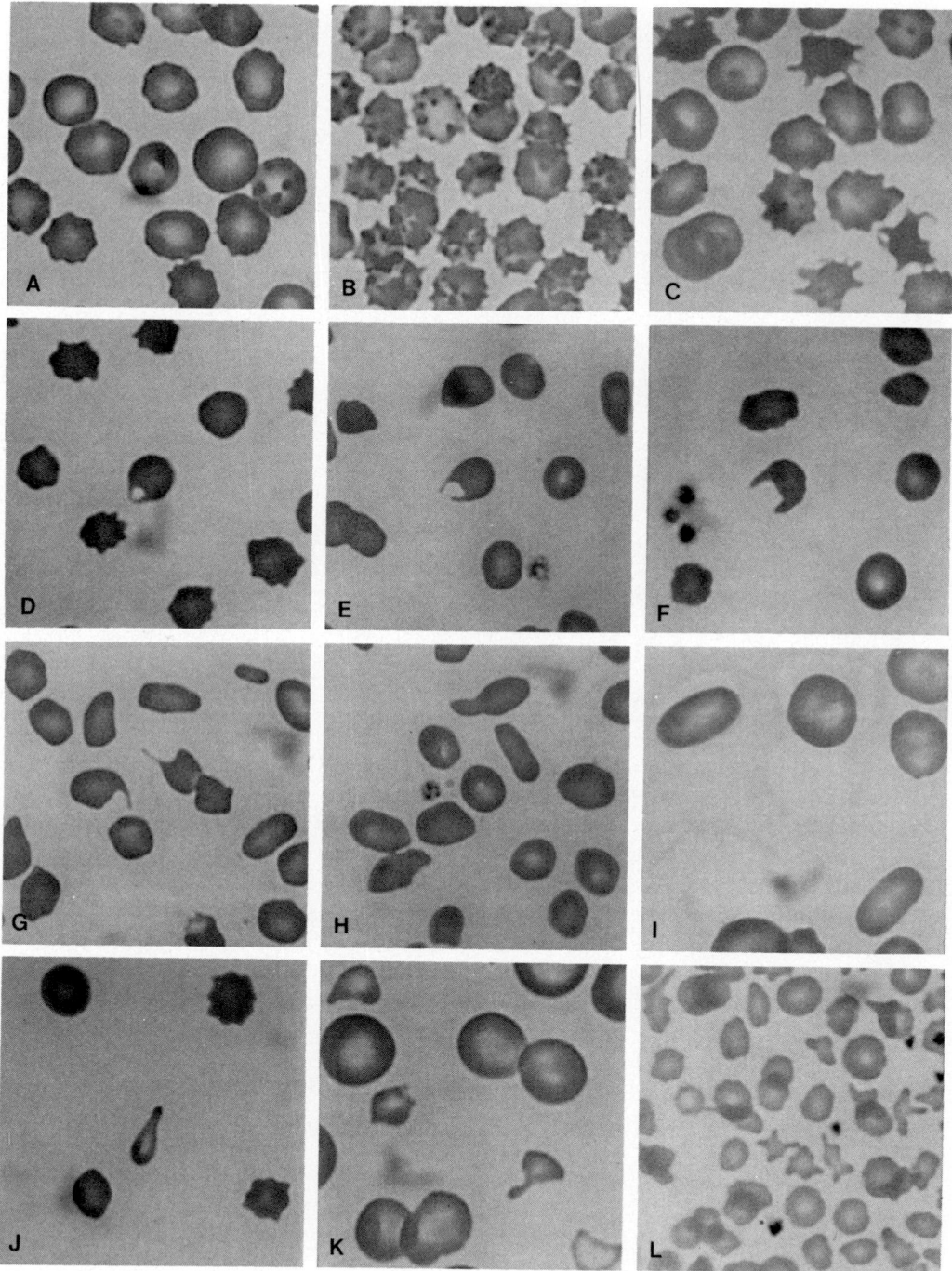

Fig. 20–6.   Erythrocyte morphology in Wright-stained blood films examined with the light microscope. *A,* discoid erythrocytes and slightly crenated canine red cells; *B,* highly crenated red cells and a few burr cells (echinocytes) in dog blood; *C,* acanthocytes in a dog blood; *D–G,* stages leading to formation of a keratocyte from a blister cell in cat blood; *H,* ovalocytic and match-stick forms of red cells in cat blood; *I,* ovalocytes in dog blood; *J,* a teardrop (dacryocyte) in cat blood; *K,* schistocytes in dog blood; *L,* poikilocytes in a calf with erythropoietic porphyria.

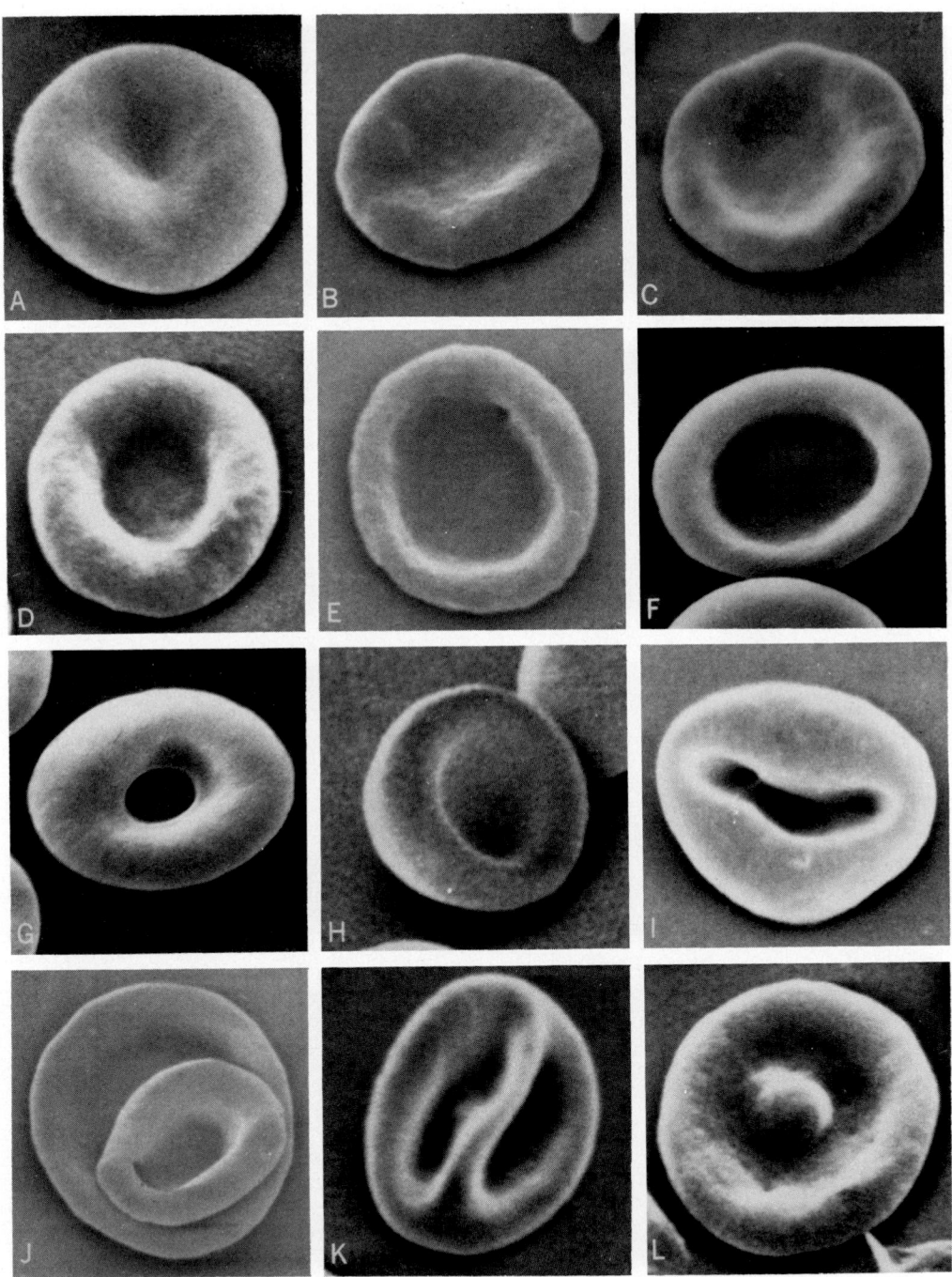

Fig. 20–7. Scanning electron photomicrographs of erythrocytes depicting various morphologic forms. *A–C,* normal discoid forms with varying degrees of concavity. *D,* a red cell with extreme concavity—such cells will appear as punched-out cells (torocytes) with light microscopy; *E,* and *F,* hypochromic red cells with a narrow rim of hemoglobin and extended central concavity; *G,* a torocyte; *H* and *I,* stomatocytes; *J,* a microcyte and a macrocyte; *K,* knizocyte; and *L,* codocyte.

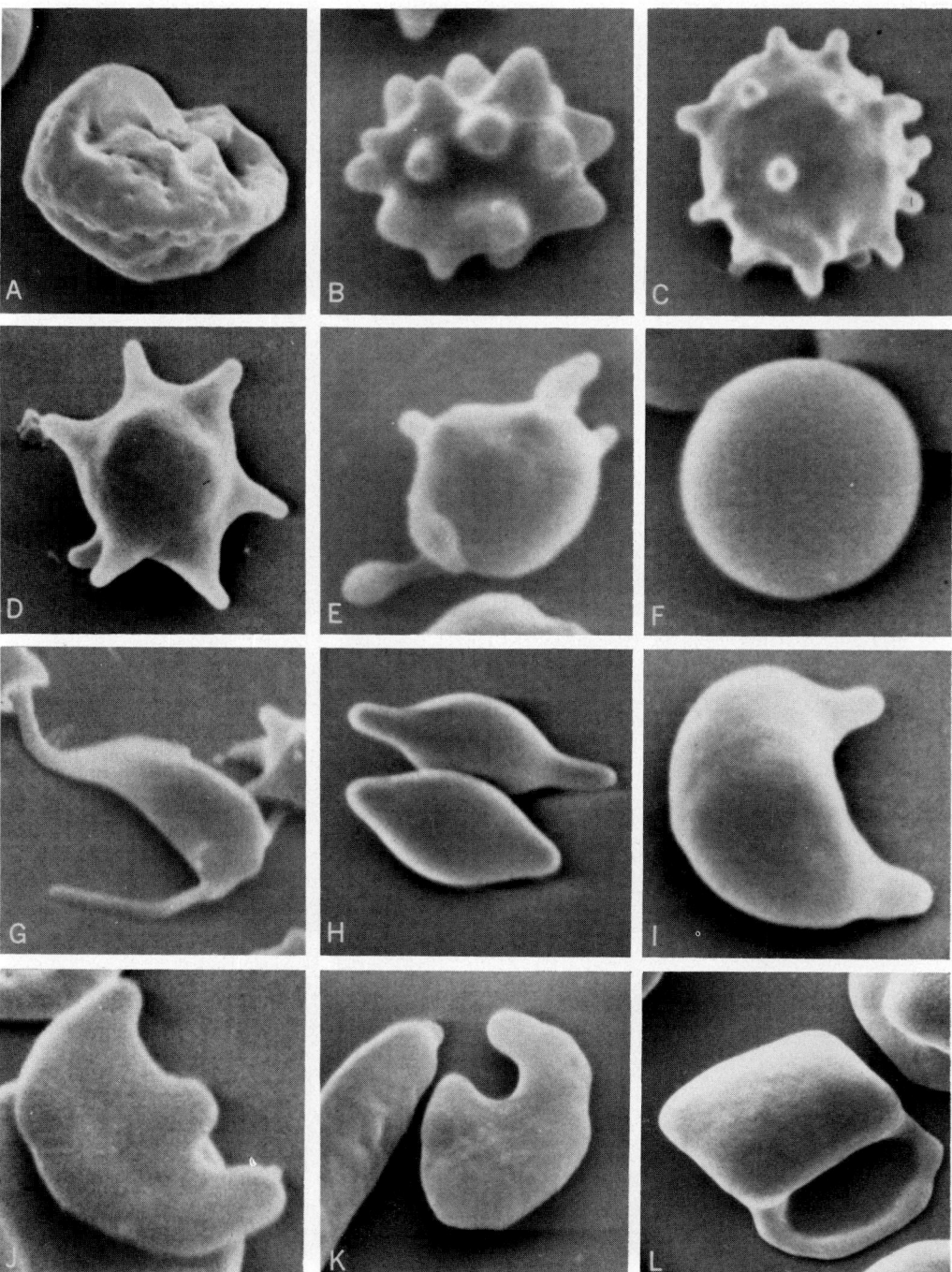

Fig. 20–8. Scanning electron photomicrographs of erythrocytes depicting various morphologic forms. *A*, reticulocyte; *B–D*, various forms of echinocytes, the cell in *D* may be called a burr cell; *E*, acanthocyte; *F*, spherocyte; *G*, drepanocyte; *H*, fusiform and spindle-shaped red cells; *I–K*, keratocytes; and *L*, a hemoglobin-crystal in a feline red cell.

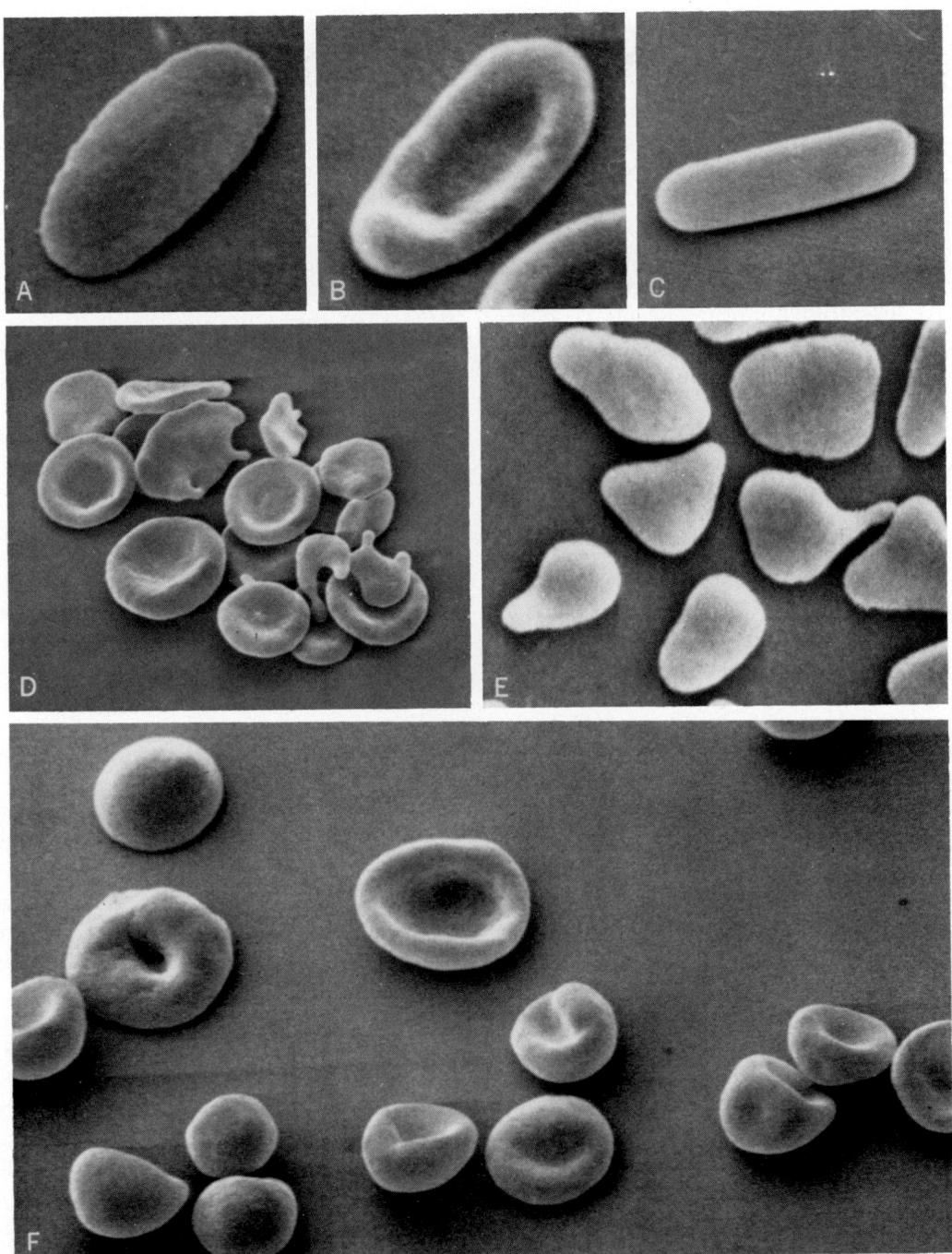

Fig. 20–9. Scanning electron photomicrographs of erythrocytes depicting various morphologic forms. *A* and *B*, ovalocytes; *C*, match-stick form; *D*, schistocytes admixed with normal-appearing red cells of varying sizes; *E*, dacryocytes and triangular cells; and *F*, leptocytes and stomatocytes in different profiles.

acanthocytes, in contrast to echinocytes, generally have a smaller cell size, fewer spicules and an irreversible cell shape. Acanthocytes, unlike echinocytes, can undergo echinocytic and stomatocytic changes. Their characteristic shape is attributed to an increase in membrane cholesterol (25–65%) unaccompanied by changes in membrane phospholipids, giving a cholesterol to phospholipid ratio of as high as 1.6. Acanthocytes are found in humans with congenital abetalipoproteinemia, liver disease, postsplenectomy state and after heparin therapy. Acanthocytes have been seen in dogs with splenic hemangioma or hemangiosarcoma (Gelberg and Stackhouse, 1977) and in dogs with a variety of diffuse liver diseases (Rebar et al., 1981; Shull et al., 1978). In addition to these conditions, we also have seen these cells in some dogs with portocaval shunts. Experimentally, acanthocytosis was produced in dogs fed a cholesterol-enriched, atherogenic diet (Cooper et al., 1980).

Acuminocytes and *fusocytes* are fusiform and spindle-shaped red cells. They are found in blood of certain normal goats, particularly of the Angora breed (Figs. 20–2B, 20–8H). Their biologic significance remains unknown.

Codocytes, commonly known as *target cells*, are thin, cup-shaped erythrocytes with a dense central area of hemoglobin that is separated partially or completely by a colorless or pale zone from the peripheral hemoglobinized region (Figs. 20–5H; 20–7L). This is a result of redistribution of hemoglobin within the cell probably as a result of excessive cell membrane, or a decrease in hemoglobin content, or both. These red cells may be hypochromic and appear as "Mexican hat" or "Greek helmet" cells. They may exhibit some echinocytic and stomatocytic change, and show increased osmotic resistance. Biochemical studies have shown that their membrane cholesterol is increased by 25 to 75% and lecithin is increased by 15 to 45%, resulting in an increase of about 15% in the ratio of the two lipids. Codocytes are found in humans with hypochromic anemias, liver disease with cholestasis, the rare deficiency of the enzyme lecithin-cholesterol acyltransferase (LCAT), certain hemoglobinopathies, and after splenectomy. In hypertonic plasma they may be seen as an artifact. Target cells have been found in dogs with conditions similar to humans except for hemoglobinopathies and LCAT-deficiency which have not been described in animal species.

Dacryocytes are erythrocytes shaped like a teardrop (see Figs. 20–6J; 20–9E). This shape is believed to be a result of the "pitting" function of the spleen on red cells containing inclusions or an impact of migration through the splenic or marrow sinusoids. It is believed that a change in the cytoskeleton proteins must occur as an associated event to make the normally highly deformable cell assume a distorted permanent shape. Such cells are found in humans with myelofibrosis, Heinz body anemias, bone marrow metastases, thalassemias, and aberrant hematopoiesis. We have seen such cells in dogs and cats with myeloproliferative disorders and in normal goat kids. Dacryocytic cells may appear as artifacts of smear making, particularly along the feather-edge of the blood film. In such areas most red cells show their tail-ends in the same direction, as opposed to chance orientation of true dacryocytes.

Discocytes are normal biconcave erythrocytes that are sometimes referred to as normocytes.

Drepanocytes are sickle-shaped erythrocytes produced as the result of polymerization of hemoglobin S or the like. They are found in humans in sickle cell anemia, hemoglobin C disease, and certain other hemoglobinopathies. Sickle-shaped erythrocytes have been found in normal deer (Figs. 12–7, 12–8), sheep, and goats. A cell of similar morphology may be found on rare occasions in blood films of other animal species (Fig. 20–8G). Drepanocytes may also exhibit echinocytic and stomatocytic changes. Hemoglobin crystallization seen in an occasional red cell in humans and animals with hemoglobin C disease (Figs. 20–5I; 20–8L) is a different phenomenon than hemoglobin polymerization leading to formation of drepanocytes.

Eccentrocytes are erythrocytes with condensed hemoglobin in one area of the cell. They have also been described as pyknocytes. Eccentrocytes have been observed in dogs with hemolytic anemia from acetylphenylhydrazine (Ham et al., 1973) and onion (Harvey and Rackear, 1985) toxicosis. They are thought to result from oxidative injury to the red cell membrane.

Echinocytes, in contrast to acanthocytes, have several blunt or pointed evenly spaced surface projections (Figs. 20–6A, B; 20–8B, C, D). These red cells are known commonly as crenated cells, and markedly echinocytic cells are often referred to as "burr" cells (Figs. 20–6B; 20–8D). Highly crenated cells have sometimes been erroneously called "spur" cells. The number, shape, and extent of surface projections vary with the nature and strength of the inciting agent as well as the species concerned. For example, the goat red cell may reveal only a few projections, while the dog red cell may show many. Red cells in the central part of a blood film appear more crenated than those along the featheredge. A variety of agents induce echinocyte formation in vitro, e.g., high pH and anionic agents, plasma heated at 37°C for 24 hr, lysolecithin, fatty acids, physiologic saline, and glass surface. The best way to confirm the phenomenon is to examine a drop of blood between plastic surfaces, thus eliminating artifactual occurrences of echinocytes. The echinocytic change is reversible to a certain extent, but not after transformation into a distinct spheroechinocytic form. Echinocytes are found in old blood as red cells become depleted of ATP. Highly echinocytic (burr) cells are seen often in kidney disease with uremia and in pyruvate kinase deficiency in humans.

Elliptocytes (ovalocytes) are red cells with an ellipsoid or oval shape and include other variants like the match-stick or cigar-shaped forms. They are seen in humans with hereditary elliptocytosis, megaloblastic anemia, thalassemia and iron deficiency, and in anemias of malignancy, leukemia, and enzyme deficiency. A few elliptocytes (less than 1%) may be found in normal human blood, and are said to increase in almost any type of anemia. Hereditary elliptocytosis resulting from band 4.1 deficiency occurs in the dog, presumably as an autosomal recessive trait (Smith et al., 1983). Elliptocytosis is characteristic of the family Camellidae (see Fig. 12–11). Elliptocytes in humans show some evidence of biconcavity, whereas those of the camel appear flat or have a slightly raised con-

tour (see Figs. 20–2E, F). Elliptical red cells are seen sometimes in cats with unexplained anemias, in dogs with lymphocytic leukemia or lymphoma, and in dogs and cats with myeloproliferative disorders (Figs. 20–6I; 20–9B). Cigar-shaped and match-stick form red cells may be seen in some normal deer and Angora goats (Fig. 20–9C), and may be found in dogs and cats with hematopoietic malignancies and unexplained anemias (Figs. 20–6G, H). These various cell types may appear crenated in some animals.

Gigantocytes are large (over $1\frac{1}{2}$ to 2 times the normal diameter) red cells, larger than macrocytes and megalocytes. They are occasionally seen in normal goats and rarely in other species in health or during erythropoietic response to severe anemia. It is believed that these cells arise from denucleation of occasional normochromic metarubricytes that may develop in the bone marrow during erythroid maturation.

Keratocytes have one or more pointed projections like horns and a slightly notched or somewhat flat surface between the projections (Figs. 20–6D through G; 20–8I through K). They are usually seen in conditions associated with formation of schizocytes. The spicules result from the rupture of a vacuole appearing near the cell surface (Figs. 20–6D through F) or from mechanical trauma to the red cell as it circulates passing fibrin strands or prosthetic devices within the cardiovascular system.

Knizocytes are erythrocytes with a central bar of hemoglobin and somewhat clear spaces on either side (Fig. 20–5G). They correspond to leptocytes with a central hemoglobinized-membranous fold and relatively lucent areas on both sides giving the appearance of a triconcave cell (Fig. 20–7K). They may be seen along with stomatocytosis and, more commonly, during response to anemia in humans and dogs.

Leptocytes are erythrocytes with increased diameter and decreased cell thickness. These cells are thin having a surface area that is greater than the contents; hence they tend to fold and may appear as target cells, folded bowl-shaped cells, or knizocytes (Figs. 20–5C, G; 20–7E, J through L; 20–9F) Leptocytes may vary in size and staining characteristics. They may appear orthochromic or polychromic in Wright-stained blood films. Orthochromic leptocytes are seen in liver disease, obstructive jaundice, and iron deficiency, whereas polychromic leptocytes are characteristic of responsive anemia and correspond to polychromic red cells or reticulocytes (Figs. 20–5J; 20–8A).

Macrocytes and *megalocytes*, are morphologically normal erythrocytes except for an MCV that is greater than normal for the species in question (Figs. 20–7J; 20–9F). They are found in blood during intensified erythropoiesis. Certain dogs of the poodle breed normally exhibit macrocytosis (see Chapter 25). Megalocytes are the hallmark of megaloblastic anemia due to vitamin B_{12} and folate deficiency in humans.

Microcytes are erythrocytes with an MCV smaller than normal for the species (Fig. 20–7J). Most of these cells have increased central pallor due to the reduced hemoglobin content. The clear area gradually merges with the peripheral hemoglobinized zone, as opposed to abrupt separation in punched-out cells (torocytes) (compare Fig. 20–5B and D with Fig. 20–7F and G). Their thickness:diameter ratio is normal, unlike that in spherocytes. Microcytic hypochromic red cells are the hallmark of iron deficiency anemia, and may be seen in anemias of inflammatory disease. Dogs of the Japanese Akita breed normally have smaller red cells with an MCV in the lower normal range or below that of the dogs of other breeds (at 60 fl), but their MCHC is similar and so they are not hypochromic.

Poikilocytes are erythrocytes having any morphology other than the normal. Thus, poikilocytosis is a general term encompassing any deviation of shape. With increased understanding of the behavior of red cells under in vitro conditions and factors affecting their shape in vivo, many of the abnormal morphologic forms have been assigned new names and so described, such as echinocytes, acanthocytes, and schizocytes. Hence, it is recommended that the term poikilocyte be used only for shapes that cannot be properly categorized (Figs. 20–6L; 20–9D, E) under the current terminology, or when a general description is desired.

Schizocytes or *schistocytes* are irregular fragments (triangular, rod, half-moon, spiculated, or other bizarre forms) of red cells (Figs. 20–6K; 20–9D) resulting from trauma in the circulation such as severing from fibrin filaments. These fragments are commonly seen in disseminated intravascular coagulation (DIC) and microangiopathic hemolytic anemias from abnormalities of vascular endothelium and insertion of prosthetic devices in humans. Normal blood may contain less than 0.5% schistocytes. Some schistocytes may appear spherical—spheroschistocytes or microspherocytes, e.g., those resulting from heat fragmentation in burn patients. Schistocytes have been observed in dogs with DIC; microangiopathic hemolytic anemia; congestive heart failure; glomerulonephritis; myelofibrosis; and neoplasms, particularly hemangiosarcoma (Madewell and Feldman, 1980; Rebar et al., 1981).

Selenocytes are crescent-shaped, poorly stained red cells. They are seen in diseases associated with hemolysis, e.g., toxemia, infections, and lipemia. Partial lysis of canine red cells in Wright-stained blood films of patients with lipemia or hemolytic anemia may sometimes be seen in the form of fuzzy areas of hemoglobin without a membranous outline (Fig. 20–5L).

Siderocytes are mature erythrocytes containing Prussian blue–positive iron granules visible with the light microscope (Plate XII–10). Reticulocytes may also present this feature. *Sideroblasts* are nucleated erythrocytes containing iron granules in the cytoplasm (Plate XV–5). These iron granules represent ferritin aggregates in the cytoplasm of normal rubricytes, whereas in abnormal cells they are made of crystallized ferritin aggregates, hemosiderin granules of variable shape, or iron-filled mitochondria. "Ringed-sideroblasts" contain iron-filled mitochondria arranged in a circular pattern around the nucleus. In normal human marrow, 30–50% of the nucleated erythrocytes may contain 1 or 2 and rarely 3 iron granules (Wintrobe et al., 1981). Siderocytes are decreased in iron-deficiency anemia. Increased numbers of siderocytes with abnormal iron granulation are found in sideroblastic anemias, refractory anemias, severe plumbism, and thalassemia major.

Spherocytes are intensely stained, small, spherical erythrocytes with reduced surface to volume ratio (Figs. 20–5K; 20–8F). Because of their smaller than normal size, they are also called "microspherocytes." Cells that appear typically spherical in blood films often appear to have a small depression or stomata when examined with the scanning electron microscope. Spherocytes are seen in humans in hereditary spherocytosis, in immune-mediated hemolytic anemias, and Heinz body anemias. Osmotic swelling of red cells produces macrospherocytes. Sphero-echinocytic and spherostomatocytic transformations (with normal volume) have been observed in vitro. Spherocytes are characteristically found in autoimmune hemolytic anemia (AIHA) in the dog (Plate XVII–4), but are difficult to recognize in blood films of other animal species, although they have been found occasionally in cats with AIHA. Their shape is distinctive also in specimens prepared for electron microscopy (Fig. 35–2B). A possible instance of hereditary spherocytosis was recorded in the goat (Fig. 20–2C). Hereditary spherocytosis as a result of spectrin deficiency occurs in the common house mouse (Bernstein, 1980).

Spiculated-erythrocytes are red cells with one or more surface spicules. Thus it is a general term encompassing several of the now well-recognized forms of red cells such as echinocytes, acanthocytes, dacryocytes, drepanocytes, keratocytes, and schizocytes. Therefore, it is recommended that this term be used for erythrocytes with surface spicules that cannot be categorized properly. For example, some red cells with one spicule (Fig. 20–6G), as seen in cats with nonresponsive anemias of varied etiologies, may be placed under this category.

Stomatocytes are erythrocytes that in Wright-stained films appear to have a slit- or mouth-like clear opening near the cell center (Figs. 20–5E, F). They present a uniconcave morphology in wet preparations and in specimens examined with the scanning electron microscope (Figs. 20–7H, I; 20–9F). This erythrocyte shape can be induced in vitro by lowering the pH and by cationic agents, e.g., chlorpromazine. Stomatocytes have been found in people with hereditary spherocytosis and hereditary hydrocytosis. Hereditary

stomatocytosis has been found in Alaskan malamutes as an autosomal recessive trait (Pinkerton et al., 1974). Stomatocytes have been found in dogs with chronic anemias. Sometimes a red cell may exhibit two stomata and infrequently a polychromatic erythrocyte may also appear stomatocytic. Thin leptocytes may also assume a stomatocytic appearance (Fig. 20–5C).

Torocytes are ring-shaped erythrocytes with a sharply defined clear central area and a thickened peripheral rim of hemoglobin; hence, they are commonly referred to as "punched-out" cells (Figs. 20–5D; 20–7D, G). They are believed to result from peripheral redistribution of hemoglobin. Torocytes are seen in hypochromic anemias (iron deficiency) and may occur as artifacts.

Abnormalities of Ionic Transport and Thermal Reactivity

Rare congenital abnormalities of ionic transport function and thermal reactivity of erythrocytes have been recognized in humans (Mentzer and Clark, 1983; Mohandas and Shohet, 1978). In the former, alterations in cell water are associated with changes in cell shape and deformability either because of reduction in surface area to volume ratio (hydrocytosis) or an increase in MCHC and thus internal viscosity (xerocytosis). In the latter, abnormalities of cell shape are associated with increased thermal reactivity of erythrocytes (pyropoikilocytosis). Salient features of these abnormalities in humans are given below; they have not been recognized as yet in animals. Defects of cytoskeletal protein, spectrin, have been identified in some of these disorders (Goodman and Shiffer, 1983; Gratzer, 1981).

Hydrocytosis is characterized by an accumulation of sodium in excess of potassium with an obligatory gain of cell water and an increase in the critical hemolytic volume of the red cells (Nathan and Shohet, 1970). This biochemical change in erythrocytes manifests as a hemolytic anemia. Red cells with increased water are designated hydrocytes. Morphologically they appear as stomatocytes. *Cryohydrocytes* are erythrocytes showing increased hemolysis in vitro at 4°C, without any in vivo relevance (Mentzer and Clark, 1983).

Xerocytosis (formerly called *desiccytosis*) is an autosomal dominant hemolytic anemia with osmotically resistant, low-potassium, high-sodium erythrocytes in which passive efflux of potassium and net potassium loss exceed passive sodium influx and net sodium gain (Glader et al., 1974; Platt et al., 1981). This leakage of potassium, with attendant water loss, produces an increase in MCHC. The red cells are called xerocytes (descicytes). They often appear as flattened cells, although a few echinocytic and stomatocytic forms may be present.

Pyropoikilocytosis is a congenital abnormality of red cells characterized by an apparent enhanced thermal reactivity (Zarkowsky et al., 1975) as a result of a defect in cell membrane (Mohandas et al., 1980). The red cells exhibit membrane budding and sphering at 44°C instead of 50°C, which is normal. They present marked anisocytosis, poikilocytosis, microspherocytosis, and bizarre morphology. Their osmotic fragility is increased and deformability is reduced.

Additional Comments

Certain shape changes are predictable. *Discocytic-echinocytic transformation* follows depletion of ATP and Mg^{++}, accumulation of Ca^{++}, increase in pH, exposure to anionic compounds, loss of fatty acid acylation capacity, and increase in lysolecithin content. *Discocytic-stomatocytic transformation* occurs at low pH and is induced by cationic compounds. Echinocytic and stomatocytic compounds act as antagonists (Sheetz and Singer, 1974). A "bilayer couple hypothesis" to explain abnormalities of the red cell shape was proposed by Sheetz and Singer (1974, 1976). Accordingly, electrostatic charge differences resulting from normal asymmetric distribution of phospholipids within the two leaflets of the red cell membrane form the basis for differences in transmembrane localization of various compounds, producing morphologic transformations. Thus, at equilibrium, anionic (echinocytic) agents intercalate preferentially into the outer half of the red cell membrane, whereas cationic (stomatocytic) agents preferentially partition into the inner half

(Hsu, 1980; Matayoshi, 1980). This results in asymmetric contraction or expansion of the surface areas of the two monolayers relative to one another and consequential observed outward (echinocytic) and inward (stomatocytic) curvature of the red cell membrane. Further observations indicate, however, that this hypothesis does not fully explain shape changes from some other factors, although the preferential distribution of a transforming agent could be demonstrated (Mohandas et al., 1978). Alterations in transmembrane potential (Glaser, 1979), alteration or rearrangement of membrane components (Alhanaty and Sheetz, 1981), and manipulations of the lipid bilayer (Fujii, 1981) may produce morphologic changes.

Changes in the membrane phospholipid and cholesterol composition have been related to abnormalities of the red cell shape in liver disease, whether hepatocellular or obstructive (see reviews by Cooper, 1978, 1980). Target cells are seen commonly in humans with obstructive jaundice, hepatitis, or cirrhosis. The lipid content as well as the cholesterol-to-phospholipid ratio is higher in target cells owing to a disproportionate increase in both cholesterol and phospholipids. In biliary obstruction, the increase in red cell cholesterol and phospholipid is proportional to the severity of the disease process (Okano et al., 1978, 1979). Severe hepatocellular disease is accompanied with "spur-cell anemia." Spur cells (acanthocytes) have a greatly increased membrane cholesterol with a normal or slightly elevated phospholipid content. Acanthocytosis is characteristic of abetalipoproteinemia; these red cells contain a normal or slightly elevated level of cholesterol, but there is a marked decrease in lecithin, producing a high cholesterol-to-phospholipid ratio. Cholesterol-laden red cells have a reduced deformability and life span that contribute to the anemia of liver disease.

Recently, it has been shown that the fluidity of the outer leaflet of the red cell membrane exceeds that of the inner leaflet, and that acanthocytosis and experimental cholesterol enrichment decrease the lipid fluidity of the outer but not the inner leaflet (Flamm and Schachter, 1982). Sphingomyelin-to-lecithin and cholesterol-to-phospholipid molar ratios are increased in acanthocytes. Sphingomyelin, which is localized primarily in the outer layer, decreases fluidity of the lipid bilayers. Exogenous cholesterol, which is incorporated preferentially into the outer layer, probably has a similar effect on membrane fluidity. Cooper (1978, 1980) suggested that formation of acanthocytes in vivo occurs in 2 phases: In the first phase, cholesterol loading causes membrane folding and scalloping of the cell margin resulting in formation of a regularly spiculated red cell. Such cells exhibit impaired flow properties. In the second phase, the altered red cells undergo "splenic conditioning," which is characterized by membrane loss and formation of irregularly spiculated cells—acanthocytes. Shape changes corresponding to the first phase may be apparent within 12–24 hours, whereas those of the second phase may occur over a period of 6–8 days after cholesterol enrichment of red cells.

Acanthocytes have been observed to develop in dogs fed a cholesterol-rich atherogenic diet (Cooper et al., 1980). Acanthocytosis was common in 2 cases of splenic hemangiosarcoma and in 1 case of splenic hemangioma in dogs (Gelberg and Stackhouse, 1977). Acanthocytosis in association with low red cell counts was found in some bovine calves (Gierber et al., 1975).

METABOLISM OF THE ERYTHROCYTES

Erythrocyte maturation through the polychromatophilic rubricyte stage is characterized by an active Krebs cycle, Embden-Meyerhof (EM) pathway, and pentose cycle or hexose monophosphate shunt. Their activities are reduced slightly at the metarubricyte stage and are limited in the reticulocyte. The mature erythrocyte derives its energy solely from glucose metabolism carried out predominantly (95%) via the anaerobic EM pathway and to some extent (5%) through the oxidative pentose cycle. It has only vestiges of the Krebs cycle and lacks capacity for oxidative phosphorylation because of the absence of intracellular organelles. In comparison, reticulocytes and young erythrocytes in general are metabolically more active (Agar et al., 1975a; Kaneko, 1974; Smith and Agar, 1975) and lev-

els of several key enzymes are reduced in senescent red cells. Erythrocyte metabolism of various animal species has been reviewed (Agar and Board, 1983; Kaneko, 1974).

Normal Erythrocyte Metabolism and Some Species Differences

Species and breed differences as well as individual variations exist in erythrocyte enzyme and metabolic activities, and erythrocytes of the neonate have higher enzyme activities (Agar et al., 1975b, 1976; Kaneko, 1974). Erythrocytes of the adult pig are peculiar in that they are impervious to glucose and do not metabolize it, yet they have a high concentration of adenosine triphosphate (ATP) and 2,3-diphosphoglyceric acid (DPG). Neonate pig red cells, however, can utilize glucose (Bartlett, 1970); this ability is lost within 3–4 weeks after birth (Imre and Sari, 1979; Kim, 1979; Thiele et al., 1979). Metabolic activities of bovine erythrocytes decrease with the age of the cell (Bartosz and Bartkowiak, 1981; Bartosz et al., 1981) and the age of the animal. For example, glucose consumption is reduced within 2–3 months after birth (Kim, 1979) and $Na^+K^+ATPase$ activity is markedly diminished in adult red cells (Thiele et al., 1979). Sheep have very low glucose-6-phosphate dehydrogenase, negligible 2,3-DPG and bimodal distribution of certain electrolytes and reduced glutathione (Agar and Suzuki, 1982).

The survival of erythrocytes depends on the functioning of existing enzyme systems. With aging, gradual attrition of its energy-generating metabolic activities occurs resulting ultimately in cell death and removal from the circulation. Physiologic significance of some important enzymes and coenzymes are briefly discussed.

Adenosine triphosphate, generated in the EM pathway, is a potential source of energy. It is utilized for maintenance of cell shape in most species by controlling the active movement of Na^+ out of and K^+ into the cell. Movement of Na^+ into and K^+ out of the cell are passive processes occurring by diffusion. A wide variation in the ATP content of red cells in different species exists (Bartlett, 1970; Harkness et al., 1969). *Reduced nicotinamide-adenine dinucleotide* (NADH) or reduced diphosphopyridine nucleotide (DPNH), also formed in the EM cycles is utilized for the enzymatic reduction of methemoglobin (having iron in the ferric form) to a functional hemoglobin (having iron in the ferrous form) capable of transporting oxygen. The enzyme NADH-methemoglobin reductase is involved in this conversion. *Reduced nicotinamide-adenine dinucleotide phosphate* (NADPH) or reduced triphosphopyridine nucleotide (TPNH) formed in the pentose cycle is utilized for the conversion of oxidized glutathione (GSSG) to reduced glutathione (GSH).

Reduced glutathione protects erythrocytes against hemolysis by oxidant drugs, and is utilized also for conversion of methemoglobin to functional hemoglobin. Inability to generate GSH may lead to precipitation of hemoglobin, in the form of Heinz bodies, upon auto-oxidation or oxidation by chemical oxidants (Allen and Jandl, 1961). Mature erythrocytes are able to synthesize GSH de novo. Glutathione reductase (GR) and glutathione peroxidase (GP) are involved in glutathione metabolism. Species differences were found in erythrocyte GR activity, being lowest in cats and highest in horses (Harvey and Kaneko, 1975). Glutathione peroxidase activity was found to be higher in calves than in adult cattle (Kursa et al., 1982). Glutathione peroxidase and superoxide dismutase activities are reduced in aging bovine erythrocytes (Bartosz and Bartkowiak, 1981). Glutathione peroxidase and selenium values were highly correlated in cows and sheep, but not in pigs (Thompson et al., 1976). A bimodal (low and high) distribution of GSH is found in the red cells of sheep and goats, but not in cattle (Agar, 1979; Agar et al., 1978; Smith, 1977). Red cell glutathione content may be increased during anemia (Roth et al., 1979) and a greater increase may occur in GSH-deficient sheep than in normal sheep (Agar et al., 1975a). Incorporation of GSH in blood to be used for transfusion in experimental hemorrhagic shock in the dog was found to increase the survival of animals considerably, perhaps by increasing the oxygen supply to the tissues (Horejsi, 1970).

Abnormalities of Erythrocyte Metabolism

In humans, several hematologic disorders have been uncovered that occur because of deficiencies of certain enzymes of the EM pathway, pentose cycle, or nonglycolytic metabolic pathway (Kahn et al., 1979; Valentine, 1970). The most common and well known are the deficiencies of glucose-6-phosphate dehydrogenase and pyruvate kinase. These enzyme deficiencies have an autosomal recessive mode of inheritance and are associated with chronic hemolytic anemias of mild to moderate degree. Similar enzyme deficiencies leading to hematologic disorders are being unveiled in animal species. A hereditary nonspherocytic hemolytic anemia due to pyruvate kinase deficiency has been found to occur in the Besenji dogs (Ewing, 1969; Searcy et al., 1979; Tasker et al., 1969) and Beagles (Harvey et al., 1977). Methemoglobinemia due to deficiency of NADH-methemoglobin reductase has been described in the dog (Atkins et al., 1981; Harvey et al., 1974; Letchworth et al., 1977). Methemoglobinemia in animals primarily results from exposure to oxidant drugs, e.g., nitrate, nitrite, phenacetin, acetaminophen, sulfonamides, benzocaine, aniline dyes, and dapsone (see Atkins et al., 1981 for references). An occasional cat has been observed at the Veterinary Medical Teaching Hospital, University of California, Davis, to develop methemoglobinemia during anesthesia with ketamine hydrochloride. A case of familial hemoglobinemia and hemolytic anemia in the horse was associated with decreased erythrocyte glutathione reductase and glutathione levels (Dixon et al., 1977).

Erythrocyte 2,3-Diphosphoglycerate (DPG)

Many mammalian erythrocytes contain 2,3-DPG in higher concentrations than do other tissue cells. In the red cell, 2,3-DPG not only acts as a potential regulator of energy metabolism through the EM pathway, but it also has an important function in regulating the release of oxygen from hemoglobin (Benesch and Benesch, 1967; Chanutin and Curnish, 1967). The latter property is essential in maintaining tissue normoxemic state under a variety of adverse clinical conditions. An increase in concentration of 2,3-DPG produces a corresponding decrease in intracellular pH that secondarily decreases oxygen affinity of human hemoglobin by Bohr effect. Thereby, more oxygen is released from hemoglobin to the tissues, as is seen in hypoxia, exercise, and anemia. The level of 2,3-DPG in human red cells is negatively correlated with the hemoglobin level in blood (Gerlach et al., 1970) in that it is higher in anemia and lower in polycythemia.

Species differences have been observed in the amount of 2,3-DPG and its influence on oxygen affinity of hemoglobin. The content of 2,3-DPG and ATP in red cells of several animal species has been determined (Bartlett, 1970; Bunn, 1971; Harkness et al., 1969) and the relationship of 2,3-DPG content to oxygen affinity of hemoglobin has been studied in several species (Bunn, 1971; Chiba and Sasaki, 1978; Taketa et al., 1971). Bunn (1971) reported that the hemoglobins of humans, horses, dogs, rabbits, guinea pigs, mice, rats, and pigs have relatively high (nonphysiologic) oxygen affinity and a strong reactivity with 2,3-DPG. The erythrocytes of these species also have high levels of 2,3-DPG. In contrast, sheep, goat, cow, and cat hemoglobins have low oxygen affinity and a weak reactivity with 2,3-DPG; the red cells of these species have low levels of 2,3-DPG. These observations indicate that 2,3-DPG plays a role in regulating blood oxygen in some animal species also. Red cells of newborn lambs and calves have a higher 2,3-DPG content (Agar et al., 1976; King and Mifsud, 1981; Noble et al., 1983) and more 2,3-DPG is found in red cells of sheep with low GSH than in sheep with high GSH (Agar and Roberts, 1977). A decrease in 2,3-DPG levels was observed in horses during training (Lewis and McLean, 1975). The response of the horse hemoglobin to 2,3-DPG is lower than that of human hemoglobin (McLean and Lewis, 1975), although a functional relationship between elevated 2,3-DPG levels and the oxygen dissociation curve has been found in equine red cells during anemia (Studzinski et al., 1978). Anemic cats have a two- to threefold higher content of 2,3-DPG (Norton and Smith, 1976). Phlebotomy-induced anemia in dogs did not alter 2,3-DPG content of red cells, although reticulocytosis and a concomitant increase in several erythrocytic enzymes were seen (Smith and Agar, 1975). In this regard, it is interesting to note that negligible quantities of 2,3-DPG were found in goat red cells both during the control periods and during anemia when the hemoglobin oxygen affinity curve had shifted to the right (Metcalfe and Dhindsa, 1970).

ERYTHROCYTE LIFE SPAN

Normal Life Span

Knowledge of the life span of the erythrocyte is of value in understanding the dynamics of red cell production and destruction. The erythrocyte of each species has a characteristic intravascular life span. Animal species having mean erythrocyte life spans of less than 100 days normally have some polychromatophilic erythrocytes or reticulocytes in peripheral blood, while no reticulocytes occur normally in the circulation in animal species with longer erythrocyte life spans (horse, cow, sheep, and goat).

Several methods for measuring red cell life span have been described. A serologic technique to ascertain the persistence of transfused compatible erythrocytes in the circulation was developed by Ashby in 1919. It involved treating the recipient's blood with specific immune serum to cause his red cells to agglutinate, leaving the donor or transfused cells unagglutinated for ease of detection. The post-transfusion survival time of canine erythrocytes was found to be 90–100 days when tested by such a differential agglutination technique using anti-A serum (Stohlman, 1956). A longer (112–133 days) erythrocyte survival time for canine erythrocytes was estimated using bilirubin production as a measure of the length of red cell life (Hawkins and Whipple, 1938).

Tagging or labeling erythrocytes with isotopes is considered a more accurate procedure. The isotopes commonly used for this purpose are ^{51}Cr, ^{55}Fe, ^{59}Fe, ^{15}N, ^{32}P, and ^{14}C. The methods for using these isotopes vary, and there are both advantages and disadvantages (Dagg et al., 1972; Eadie and Brown, 1953). An International Committee for Standardization in Hematology (1971) appointed to make recommendations on methods for radioisotope red cell survival studies in humans has outlined procedures to follow for using ^{51}Cr, $DF^{32}P$, and ^3H–DFP. The use of radiochromium represents a tagging method whereby the chromium becomes attached to the surface of the erythrocytes, while the other isotopes represent a labeling process in that the specific isotope is incorporated in the hemoglobin molecule as it is synthesized in new cells. In the labeling process, first the animal may be made anemic by bleeding or by producing hemolysis with phenylhydrazine. The isotope is then administered and becomes incorporated in the new generation of erythrocytes produced over a limited period of time. Another name for this process is "cohort labeling." Radioactivity of red cells is determined by serial sampling of blood over several weeks and the life span is calculated from data so obtained. Since red cell survival times may be expressed differently (mean red cell survival time, mean half-survival time, etc.), caution should be exercised when comparing results of different workers. Erythrocyte life span studies in various animals are summarized in Table 20–2.

Erythrocyte survival may be related to the age of the animal, but detailed studies in animals from birth onward have not been done. Rapid destruction of fetal erythrocytes was reported to occur in puppies between birth and 2 weeks of age (Lee et al., 1971). Erythrocyte survival in normal newborn humans is similar to that in adults (Berlin, 1964), although fetal red cells have a considerably shorter (70 days) life span (Harrison, 1979; Pearson, 1967).

The mean erythrocyte life span in Mongolian gerbils, cats, dogs, sheep, horses, and calves was inversely proportional to the pyrimidine 5' -nucleotidase activity of red cells and approximately proportional to the number of reticulocytes in these species (George et al., 1983).

In hibernating animals, the erythrocyte survival is extended (Brace, 1953). It was observed in the marmot (woodchuck) that during nonhibernation the mean life span of red cells was 36 ± 2 days, while during hibernation the life span was 112 ± 7 days.

Erythrocyte life span has been determined for some domestic birds. By the use of ^{14}C, the mean red cell survival time was found to be 20 days in the chicken and 39 days in the duck (Brace and Altland, 1956). Using ^{51}Cr,

the maximum erythrocyte life span was reported to be 35 days in the chicken, 35–45 days in the pigeon, and 42 days in the duck (Rodnan et al., 1957).

Erythrocyte survival studies (Cornelius et al., 1959) were made in the mule deer, aoudad sheep, and springbok antelope using glycine-2-^{14}C. For the mule deer and springbok the results were 95 and 80 days respectively. The aoudad sheep exhibited two distinctly separate populations of erythrocytes, one with survival time of 65 days and the other, 170 days.

Shortened Intravascular Survival

Erythrocyte survival time is reduced in hemolytic anemia caused by either an intracorpuscular or extracorpuscular defect or both. Erythrocytes produced during responsive phase of blood loss anemia may also have a shortened life span (Berlin and Lotz, 1951; Brecher and Stohlman, 1962). Other studies, however, do not support this contention (Shattil and Cooper, 1972). Nutritional deficiencies (vitamin B_{12}, folate, and iron) in humans are reported to result in defective red cells having shortened survival time (Harris and Kellermeyer, 1970). Erythrocyte life span studies have been made in swine with certain nutritional anemias (Bush et al., 1956a, b). In pyridoxine (vitamin B_6) deficiency, the erythrocyte survival time was normal, but in folate and copper deficiencies, it was decreased significantly.

In experimental molybdenosis of sheep (Kaneko et al., 1961a), two populations of erythrocytes were observed, one with a shortened life span of 20–28 days and the other with a life span of 80–84 days.

A potential life span of only 22–47 days was reported for erythrocytes in bovine congenital porphyria, compared to 160 days in normal cows (Kaneko, 1963). In a later study (Kaneko et al., 1971), erythrocyte survival time of 35.5–120 days was found in porphyric cows, in comparison to 135–162 days in normal cows. A significant correlation existed between the erythrocyte survival and the concentrations of erythrocyte coproporphyrin and protoporphyrin.

An eight- to tenfold decrease in red cell survival was found during hemolytic crisis in ex-

Table 20–2.   Erythrocyte Life Span in Various Animals as Determined by Use of Isotopes

Species	Mean Life Span (Days)	Isotope	Reference
Humans	127	^{15}N	Shemin and Rittenberg (1946)
Dog	119–122	^{55}Fe, ^{59}Fe	Stewart et al. (1950)
	110	^{55}Fe	Finch et al. (1949); Harrison et al. (1951)
	107	^{59}Fe	Brown and Eadie (1953)
	115	^{14}C	Bale et al. (1949)
	86–106	^{14}C	Cline and Berlin (1963)
Cat	77	^{15}N	Valentine et al. (1951)
	68	^{59}Fe	Brown and Eadie (1953)
	66–79	^{14}C	Kaneko et al. (1966)
	51 ± 15	^{59}Fe	Liddle et al. (1984)
Pig	62	^{14}C	Bush et al. (1955)
	63	^{59}Fe	Jensen et al. (1956)
	71	^{51}Cr	Hansard and Kincaid (1956)
Rabbit	45–50	^{55}Fe	Harrison et al. (1951); Burwell et al. (1953)
	65–70	^{15}N	Neuberger and Niven (1951)
	68	^{59}Fe	Brown and Eadie (1953)
Guinea pig	83	^{59}Fe	Everett and Yoffey (1959)
	80–90	^{51}Cr	Smith and McKinley (1962)
Hamster	60–70	^{51}Cr	Rigby et al. (1961)
Rat	45–50	^{55}Fe	Harrison et al. (1951); Burwell et al. (1953)
	68	^{14}C	Berlin et al. (1951)
	64	^{14}C	Berlin and Lotz (1951)
	65	^{51}Cr	Smith et al. (1959)
Mouse	20–30	^{55}Fe	Burwell et al. (1953); Harrison et al. (1951)
	41–45	^{32}P	Berlin et al. (1959)
Sheep			
Newborn lambs	75 ± 14.8	^{59}Fe	Tucker (1963)
Lambs, 3 months	46	^{59}Fe	Baker and Douglas (1957)
Lambs, 6 months	64	^{14}C	Kaneko et al. (1961b)
Lambs, 8 months	94 and 118	^{14}C	Kaneko et al. (1961b)
Lambs, 1 year	52	^{59}Fe	Baker and Douglas (1957)
Adult	76–133	Serological	Tucker (1963)
Adult	70–153	^{59}Fe	Tucker (1963)
Karakul ewe	130	^{14}C	Kaneko et al. (1961b)
Bighorn	147	^{14}C	Kaneko et al. (1961b)
Goat, adult			
Domestic	125	^{14}C	Kaneko and Cornelius (1962)
Himalayan tahr	160–165	^{14}C	Kaneko and Cornelius (1962)
Mixed breed	106 ± 13	^{51}Cr	Fitzsimmons et al. (1967)
Guanacos, mature			
(*Lama guanicoe*)	225	^{14}C	Cornelius and Kaneko (1962)
Cow			
Calf, 3 months	48–63	^{59}Fe	Baker and Douglas (1957)
Calf, 3–4 months	70–126	^{14}C	Johnson and Schwartz (1970)
Calf, 3 months	135–144	^{14}C	Kaneko et al. (1971)
Mature cows	160	^{14}C	Kaneko (1963)
Mature cows	157–162	^{14}C	Kaneko et al. (1971)
Horse	140–150	^{14}C	Cornelius et al. (1960)
	147 ± 8	^{32}P	Marcilese et al. (1966)

perimental anaplasmosis in splenectomized calves (Baker et al., 1961). In anemia of chronic fascioliasis in sheep, red cell survival was found to be curvilinear, compared to a linear disappearance in normal sheep (Sewell et al., 1968), thereby indicating some reduction in red cell life span. Half-time survival of ^{51}Cr-labeled red cells was reduced (128.8 and 168.8 hours) in 2 sheep infected with *Fasciola*

gigantica as compared to 2 control sheep (276 and 288 hours) (Ogunrinade and Anosa, 1981). A shortened red cell survival time (11 days) was reported in a steer suffering from chronic trichostrongyloidosis (Baker and Douglas, 1957).

Canine erythrocytes modified in vitro by influenza A virus have a significantly shortened life span (Stewart et al., 1955). Goats given homologous blood transfusion show about 5–7 times shorter red cell survival time for the transfused red cells than autologous red cells given by transfusion (Fitzsimmons et al., 1967).

One might expect a longer survival time in polycythemia vera. Red cell ^{51}Cr-half-survival time in a polycythemic cat (12 days), however, was found to be close to that in 2 normal cats (11.2 days) (Reed et al., 1970). Similarly, red cell survival was not significantly altered in a dog with polycythemia vera (Appendix Case 17). Erythrocytes of a cat with erythroleukemia were found to have a half-life of 5.4 days.

DESTRUCTION OF ERYTHROCYTES

The manner in which senescent red cells are removed from the circulation in the normal animal is a matter of conjecture. Biochemical and molecular changes resulting in cell death are not definitely known, even though billions of erythrocytes are destroyed every day. It is essential to be cognizant of the rheologic properties of blood to appreciate the stresses erythrocytes undergo in the circulation and yet escape destruction. This subject was discussed elegantly in a comprehensive publication (Weed, 1970). Blood flow through the microcirculation (capillaries) depends on such rheologic properties of whole blood as the intrinsic properties and number of red cells and the relative concentration of different plasma proteins. Proper flow through the microcirculation depends on the ability of the individual red cell to deform, especially when there is an increase in viscosity of the blood. The normal biconcave red cell has a remarkable ability to deform under little pressure and to pass through narrow capillaries whose diameters are as small as 3 μm. Species differences in the deformability of erythrocytes have been noted, with the smallest goat red cells being the most rigid and elliptical erythrocytes of camel and llama being markedly less deformable than their human counterpart (Gregersen et al., 1966; Smith, 1983; Smith et al., 1979, 1980). A decrease in deformability is associated with an increase in red cell rigidity, increase in blood viscosity, impeded blood flow, and cell frag-

mentation. Rigidity of the red cell seems to be more important than its shape in determining the rheologic property of the blood (Whitmore, 1981).

Erythrocyte Deformability

Erythrocyte deformability has been measured by several techniques including filtration through small pore filters, viscometry of cell suspensions, aspiration of cells into micropipettes, deformation of cells under fluid shear stress, and more recently by a laser diffraction technique using an instrument called ektacytometer (Groner et al., 1980; Mohandas et al., 1980; Smith, 1983).

The deformability of normal erythrocytes appears to depend on at least three main factors (Chien, 1977; Mentzer and Clark, 1983; Mohandas and Shohet, 1978; Weed, 1970): (a) maintenance of cell geometry or biconcave shape, (b) normal internal or hemoglobin fluidity, and (c) intrinsic membrane deformability or viscoelastic properties. Specific alterations of these factors have been uncovered in certain hereditary disorders of human red cells (Mohandas et al., 1980).

Maintenance of the biconcave shape depends on a high ratio of surface area to volume, i.e., relative amount of excess surface area. A decrease in this ratio either by osmotic swelling or by fragmentation results in progressive loss of the biconcave shape and a decrease in the ability of the cell to deform. Adequate energy in the form of ATP is critical to maintenance of ionic and osmotic equilibrium within the red cell. A decrease in blood pH and pO_2 can adversely affect the cell shape.

Normal internal fluidity of the cell depends primarily on the properties of normal hemoglobin. Abnormal hemoglobins that have a predisposition to undergo intracellular gelation or crystallization, as in sickle cell disease in humans, cause increased rigidity of red cells and predispose them to intravascular fragmentation. Similarly, Heinz-body formation is associated with increased rigidity. Decreased deformability of irreversibly- sickled human erythrocytes is related also to their markedly elevated membrane rigidity (Havell et al., 1978) and increased intracellular viscosity (Clark et al., 1980). Nucleated erythrocytes are less deformable (Gaehtgens et al., 1981).

Intrinsic membrane deformability is significantly affected by the relationship between intracellular ATP, Ca^{++}, and Mg^{++}. It is also influenced by cAMP and 2,3-DPG (Marcel, 1979). It may be affected by pH and oxygen tension in local regions of the microcirculation; both hypoxia and acidosis reduce red cell deformability. More importantly, physical properties of spectrin regulate the shape and deformability of the erythrocyte (Marchesi, 1983; Smith et al., 1980).

Membrane rigidity is increased in ATP-depleted red cells and in red cells with excess of Ca^{++}, but probably by different mechanisms (Clark et al., 1981). With intracellular accumulation of Ca^{++}, the red cell undergoes echinocytic shape transformation, becomes less deformable, and shows diminished survival (Kretchman and Rogers, 1981; Wiley and McCulloch, 1982). It is hypothesized that Ca^{++} interacts with the cytoskeletal proteins to alter their physical state or spatial arrangement such that there is a contractile response of the internal lipid layer which causes the echinocytic transformation (reviewed by Kretchman and Rogers, 1981). ATP can prevent or minimize the adverse effect of Ca^{++}, which is probably why lower ATP values in older red cells predispose them to accumulation of Ca^{++} and removal from the circulation. It was also shown that changes in cell water and cation content may be involved in Ca^{++}-induced red cell rigidity (Dreher et al., 1978) since red cells suspended in high K^+ buffers did not show shape changes even after an increase in Ca^{++} and a decrease in ATP. Ca^{++}-dependent morphologic and metabolic changes may vary in red cells of different species and of differing age, e.g., adult sheep red cells are unresponsive, although lamb red cells are responsive to sudden increases in intracellular Ca^{++} (Eaton et al., 1978).

Changes in one or more of the above factors may be involved in pathogenesis of certain hemolytic anemias. Aged red cells lose their deformability as a result of both decreased fluidity of hemoglobin and decreased filtrability (Tillman et al., 1980). The main modes of red cell destruction in health probably involve an alteration of erythrocyte deformability resulting largely from changes in the physiochemical properties of the surface membrane. Recent studies indicate that essential steps of red cell senescence occur in the cytosol leading to redistribution of membrane components, release of membrane vesicles, remodeling of the membrane, reduction in surface to volume ratio (spherocytosis), and reduced deformability (Bocci, 1981).

Modes of Erythrocyte Destruction

Destruction of affected red cells may occur by one or a combination of the following three processes: changes in membrane permeability, phagocytosis, and fragmentation (Jensen and Lessin, 1970; Weed and Reed, 1965, 1966). Red cell destruction through phagocytosis by macrophages of the mononuclear phagocyte system is known commonly as *extravascular hemolysis*. Lysis of erythrocytes within the circulation, as a consequence of membrane permeability changes or cellular fragmentation, is referred to as *intravascular hemolysis*. It should be remembered that the extravascular hemolysis is characterized by an elevated level of unconjugated bilirubin, whereas hemoglobinemia and hemoglobinuria are the hallmark of intravascular hemolysis.

Changes in Membrane Permeability, Increased Osmotic Fragility, and Hemolysis

Any derangement in the permeability of red cells to electrolytes (Na^+ and K^+) leads to osmotic swelling and lysis. It is generally accepted that the selectivity of the mammalian red cell membrane to cations and anions is due to the presence of water-filled "pores" with positive fixed charges (Passow, 1969). It has been shown that the normal human erythrocyte is able to maintain its biconcave shape by controlling the concentration of intracellular cations through ATPase-dependent active transport of Na^+ out and K^+ into the cell (Jandl, 1965). A similar mechanism has been shown to be active in sheep (Tosteson and Hoffman, 1960) and cattle (Keeton and Kaneko, 1972). Sheep and goats have been classified according to the ability of their red cells to transport Na^+ and K^+; high K^+ cells have higher active pump fluxes of Na^+

and K⁺ and more Na-K pumps per cell than low K⁺ cells (Dunham and Ellory, 1980; Lauf and Valet, 1980). The Na⁺-K⁺-ATPase and Ca⁺⁺-Mg⁺⁺-ATPase activities of bovine red cell membrane decrease with the age of the animal (Brown et al., 1978). Biochemical mechanisms involved in controlling the shape of erythrocytes having high Na⁺ and low K⁺ (e.g., in the dog and cat) are unknown. Anion transport in red cells of the dog and cat is similar to that in human red cells (Castranova et al., 1979). Red cells of the adult sheep, cattle, and goats lack the calcium-activated potassium channel present in human red cell membrane, but such channels are present in red cells of fetal and newborn lambs (Brown et al., 1978) and in canine erythrocytes (Richhardt and Fuhrmann, 1979). Thus, Ca⁺⁺ can induce an increase in K⁺ permeability of canine red cells (Richhardt and Fuhrmann, 1979).

The osmotic fragility of the red cell is related to its geometric configuration. In a hypotonic environment, an erythrocyte swells to its maximum (critical hemolytic volume) and becomes a sphere before hemolysis ensues. Any further increase in the cell volume by continuous stress stretches the red cell envelope and leads to the formation of holes (Baker, 1967; Seeman, 1967) large enough to permit hemoglobin leakage. Once started, the process of hemolysis is complete within a few seconds. The hemoglobin molecule is about 64 Å in diameter. Any break in the red cell membrane greater than 64 Å allows direct escape of hemoglobin without osmotic swelling. Red cells injured by the action of complement and antibody can hemolyse in this manner (Jandl, 1966).

Factors influencing erythrocyte osmotic fragility have been reviewed (Jain, 1972a). A linear relationship seems to exist between the red cell volume (MCV) of different species and the critical hemolytic volume that can be attained. Smaller red cells of the goat (average MCV 20 fl) were found to swell only about 25% compared to larger cells of the horse (average MCV 46 fl), which swell by 42% (Perk et al., 1964a, b). Therefore, erythrocytes of the horse can stand a lower concentration of NaCl before hemolysing completely than can the goat erythrocytes. The thin elliptical red cell

of the camel (Fig. 20–2F) is uniquely resistant to osmotic lysis; it can increase in volume by about 200% without undergoing lysis (Perk et al., 1964a, b). In this context, it has been observed also that elliptical erythrocytes of the camel have greater heat resistance than discocytic red cells of the horse, cow, goat, pig, and donkey (Germano and Barresic, 1976). The nucleated elliptical erythrocytes of birds also have lower osmotic fragility than discocytic mammalian red cells (Viscor and Palomeque, 1982).

It has been demonstrated that the osmotic fragility of human red cells is influenced by the cholesterol content of the membrane. A decrease in the membrane cholesterol is associated with sphering and increased osmotic fragility, while an increase in the membrane cholesterol, as in thalassemic red cells, is related to a decreased osmotic fragility (Cooper et al., 1980; Sagawa and Shiraki, 1980). The observations of spheroidal red cells in one clinically normal goat (Fig. 20–2C) and of highly acanthocytic erythrocytes in a normal cow (Fig. 20–2D) are interesting from this point of view. How such cells are able to survive circulatory dynamics and biochemical mechanisms involved in their formation remain to be determined. Erythrocytes that have been transformed into spheres in vitro by the action of surface-active agents such as bile and free fatty acids are more rigid than normal erythrocytes (Braasch, 1969; Coleman et al., 1980).

The determination of osmotic fragility of red cells in vitro is an attempt to correlate a possible similar behavior of these cells in vivo. The exact relationship between the in vitro measurement of red cell fragility and the ability of the cell to survive in vivo is unknown. A positive correlation exists, however, between abnormalities of osmotic and mechanical fragilities and shortened survival of red cells (Harris and Kellermeyer, 1970). The concentrations of hypotonic saline in which maximum and minimum hemolysis normally occurs have been determined for several animal species (Table 20–3), but much remains to be learned about changes occurring in disease. Increased osmotic fragility, preceded by a decrease in the erythrocytic acetylocholinesterase activity was observed in bovine an-

Table 20–3. Osmotic Fragility of Erythrocytes from Normal Adult Animals, as Indicated by Maximum and Minimum Resistance to Hypotonic Saline Solutions[a]

Animal	RBC Diameter (μm)[b]	% of Buffered NaCl Solution	
		(Max)	(Min)
Camel	7.5 × 4.4	0.21	0.30
Dog	7.0	0.29	0.50
Pig	6.0	0.29	0.52
Rat	6.3	0.30	0.42
Rabbit	6.7	0.30	0.50
Mouse	6.1	0.30	0.50
Guinea pig	7.5	0.30	0.52
Hamster	6.5	0.30	0.51
Horse	5.8	0.34	0.54
Donkey	6.2	0.35	0.54
Cat	5.8	0.36	0.60
Cow	5.8	0.38	0.59
Sheep	4.5	0.43	0.56
Goat	3.2	0.44	0.66

[a]From Perk et al., 1964a.
[b]Mean RBC sizes taken from Chapters 4 through 10 and 12.

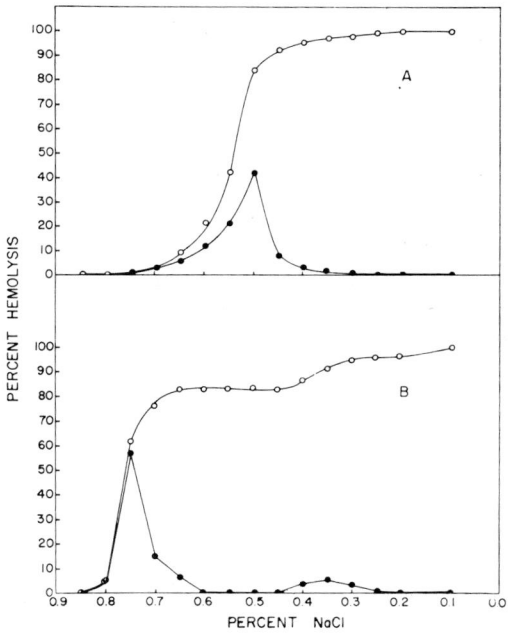

Fig. 20–10. *A*, Normal cumulative (—) and derivative (●–●) erythrocyte osmotic fragility curves drawn from mean values for 51 clinically healthy dogs. *B*, Cumulative (○–○) and derivative (●–●) curves for a dog with autoimmune hemolytic anemia. Three osmotically different populations of erythrocytes are apparent clearly from derivative curve (Chapter 2). (From Jain, 1973; courtesy of *The Cornell Veterinarian*.)

Fig. 20–11. *A*, Normal cumulative (○–○) and derivative (●–●) erythrocyte osmotic fragility curves drawn from mean values for 49 clinically healthy cats. *B*, Cumulative (○–○) and derivative (●–●) fragility curves for a feline patient with autoimmune hemolytic anemia. Two osmotically different populations of erythrocytes are evidenced clearly by the derivative curves.

aplasmosis (Wallace, 1967). Increased resistance to osmotic lysis of erythrocytes of porphyric cows was attributed to the presence of young erythrocytes (Kaneko and Mills, 1969). Mechanical fragility but not the osmotic fragility of canine erythrocytes was found to increase in the presence of postprandial li-

pemia (Jasper and Jain, 1965). Progressive increases in osmotic and mechanical fragilities of red cells occurred within a few hours in a dog given an intravenous injection of anticanine red cell immune serum (Castle, 1967). Marked increases in osmotic fragility were

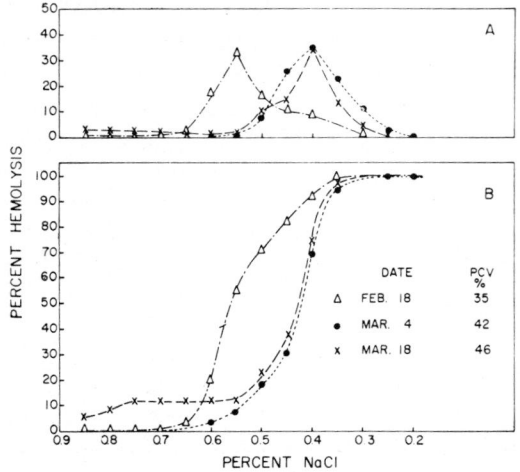

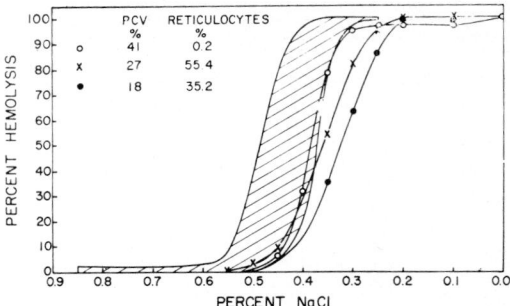

Fig. 20–14. Erythrocyte osmotic fragility curves of two anemic Basenji dogs are compared with a curve of a normal Basenji dog and a range of fragility for normal dogs of some other breeds (shaded area). The anemic Basenji dogs demonstrate increased resistance due to presence of large numbers of reticulocytes. (From Jain, 1973; courtesy of *The Cornell Veterinarian*.)

Fig. 20–12. Derivative (*A*) and cumulative (*B*) erythrocyte osmotic fragility curves for a canine patient with polyarthritis of possible autoimmune origin. Steroid therapy was started on February 18. Increased osmotic fragility was seen on February 18. On March 4, fragility was about normal, but on March 18, a slightly increased fragility was again apparent. (From Jain, 1973; courtesy of *The Cornell Veterinarian*.)

seen in a dog (Fig. 20–10*B*) and a cat (Fig. 20–11*B*) with autoimmune hemolytic anemia and also in a dog with polyarthritis of possible autoimmune origin (Fig. 20–12). An increase in the packed cell volume, in association with clinical improvement of such patients follow-

ing steroid therapy, was usually accompanied by a return of the osmotic fragility toward normal (Figs. 20–12 and 20–13). A marked increase in the osmotic fragility in autoimmune hemolytic anemia may produce erroneously high MCV and MCHC values because osmotically more fragile spherocytes may rupture in the diluting fluid used in obtaining RBC count by the Coulter electronic counter (see Chapter 2). An increase in osmotic fragility was also noted in a cat with haemobartonellosis (Jain, 1973). In familial nonspherocytic hemolytic anemia of Basenji dogs, the resistance of erythrocytes to osmotic lysis may be normal (Ewing, 1969) or slightly increased (Fig. 20–14) (Jain, 1973). Marked abnormalities in fragility of incubated red cells have been reported, however, in this condition (Searcy et al., 1971). Erythrocyte osmotic fragility is increased in chondrodysplastic pups (Terpin and Roach, 1981).

Phagocytosis of Damaged Erythrocytes

Rous and Robertson, in 1917, suggested that erythrophagocytosis plays a significant part in removal of red cells in the dog, rat, and guinea pig, but not in the cat. Current belief, however, is that erythrophagocytosis occurs in all animal species. Phagocytosis of the whole erythrocyte may be seen in peripheral blood in diseases involving the erythrocyte. In feline haemobartonellosis and in eperythrozoonosis in sheep, whole red cells have been observed on rare occasions within

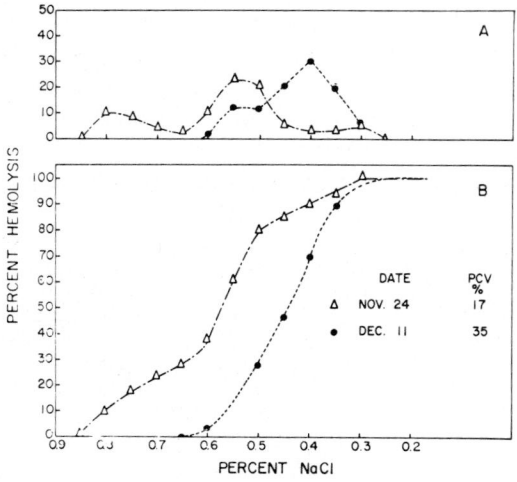

Fig. 20–13. Derivative (*A*) and cumulative (*B*) erythrocyte osmotic fragility curves for a canine patient with autoimmune hemolytic anemia. The derivative curves attest to the existence of two populations of erythrocytes having different osmotic fragility. Steroid therapy was initiated on November 24. (From Jain, 1973; courtesy of *The Cornell Veterinarian*.)

mononuclear cells in stained films of peripheral blood. Phagocytosis of erythrocytes by leukocytes in the peripheral blood is rare in comparison to phagocytosis by macrophages of the mononuclear phagocyte system (Plates XV–6, XVII–6). Macrophages destroy ingested erythrocytes through proteolytic and lipolytic enzymes, and subsequently hemoglobin is degraded with release of iron, globin, and bilirubin (see Chapter 19).

Erythrocytes damaged as a consequence of intrinsic defects or acquired abnormalities are prone to early sequestration by macrophages of the mononuclear phagocyte system particularly in the spleen and liver. One of the functions of the spleen is the removal of abnormal red cells from the circulation. It is generally agreed that the site of removal of abnormal erythrocytes depends on the degree of damage sustained (Rifkind, 1966). The spleen seems to remove minimally injured red cells preferentially, while the liver predominantly removes severely damaged red cells. On the basis of these findings, it has been postulated that the mononuclear phagocyte system plays a major role in the destruction of senescent erythrocytes. Splenic environment—principally low glucose concentration, mild hypoxia, hypercapnia, and relatively low pH—is deleterious to erythrocytes. The sites of major destruction, however, may vary in different species. Splenic sequestration is thought to be the major mode of normal red cell removal in mice and rats, while the bone marrow appears to be the chief site in rabbits (Ultmann and Gordon, 1965). In splenectomized rats, liver and bone marrow sequestration may increase about twofold, while in splenectomized mice, only hepatic sequestration may double. In humans, over a third of physiologic red cell destruction may occur in the bone marrow (Ehrenstein and Lockner, 1958). These observations also indicate that the long-term results of splenectomy in symptomatic treatment of certain anemias (e.g., AIHA) would depend on the extent to which the liver and bone marrow can expend their sequestrating capacities.

It has been demonstrated that erythrocytes containing Heinz bodies are either "pitted" (i.e., the Heinz body is removed from the red cell without destruction of the entire cell) or removed in toto ("culling") by phagocytic cells of the mononuclear phagocyte system (MPS) (Lawson et al., 1969). The pitted red cell may enter the general circulation, but it may not survive long because of acquired local membrane rigidity (Weed, 1970).

Factors involved in selective removal of erythrocytes by macrophages are poorly understood. An impressive in vitro demonstration by Bessis (1965) revealed that when a single red cell is shot with a laser beam of 1 μm, a minute lesion develops in the membrane and material released from the "dying" red cell stimulates macrophages to engulf the damaged cell immediately. It has been suggested that changes in the biophysical properties of the red cell membrane, especially the surface charge, can be detected by the macrophages (Danon et al., 1971). The zeta potential of the surface of both erythrocytes and leukocytes dictates a normal repulsive force that separates these cells by greater than 200 Å (Bangham, 1964). Any reduction in this force, e.g., by agglutinating antibody, would make the red cell prone to phagocytosis. Contrary to the belief, recent observations indicate that although the total sialic acid content is lower in old erythrocytes, there are no differences between young and senescent red cell surface charge densities relative to surface area (Luner et al., 1977; Seaman et al., 1977).

A role for anti-erythrocyte antibodies in removal of senescent red cells has been delineated in recent years. It has been shown that "physiologic" IgG autoantibodies selectively bind to an age-specific antigen on human senescent red cells in situ and initiate removal of such cells by phagocytosis (Kay, 1978; Lutz and Kay, 1981). It is hypothesized that a chemical modification within the red cell membrane may either form the age-specific antigen during aging or render it accessible during senescence. Upon binding a critical number of these autoantibody molecules (about 100 per cell) via their Fab region, mononuclear phagocytes attach to erythrocyte-bound IgG molecules by their Fc receptors and phagocytize the cells. The senescent antigen in human red cells was recently shown to be related immunologically to the band 3 membrane protein (Kay et al., 1983).

It is postulated also that senescent red cells

could be recognized owing to the presence of cytophilic antibodies on the surface of macrophages (Danon et al., 1977; Knyszynski et al., 1977). The antibodies are believed to be directed toward antigenic sites absent or shielded on young red cells but exposed on old red cells.

Erythrocyte Fragmentation

Erythrocytes may fragment because of extrinsic damage, intrinsic cellular abnormality, or partial phagocytosis (Weed and Reed, 1966). Early studies by Rous and coworkers (Rous, 1923; Rous and Robertson, 1917) suggested that fragmentation of erythrocytes is a major mechanism of normal red cell destruction and an important mechanism for removal of pathologic red cells. They proposed the hypothesis of fragmentation without loss of hemoglobin, the fragmenting portions continuing to become smaller and smaller until hemoglobin dust is produced and removed by the MPS. In support of this hypothesis, the authors stated that poikilocytes (Plate XVII–1) are not produced as such in the bone marrow but are found regularly in the spleen and only inconsistently in other organs. Doan and Sabin (1926) subsequently confirmed the concept of fragmentation of red cells in the circulation of the normal rabbit by studying films of fresh blood and observing the phenomenon. They considered the poikilocyte as the first stage in the process of fragmentation. How red cell fragments can seal spontaneously without loss of hemoglobin is unknown.

Scanning electron microscopic studies (Jain and Kono, 1972) of erythrocytes from apparently healthy animals have shown that a few erythrocytes in the sheep, goat, and dog have one or more wart-like protuberances on their surface (Fig. 20–1F). Protuberances of various forms were found on many erythrocytes of a canine patient. It is believed that these represent the beginning stage of red cell fragmentation and removal.

Fragmentation due to intrinsic abnormalities of red cells has been observed in anemias due to iron deficiency, sickle-cell disorder, Heinz bodies, and autoimmune disease (Weed and Reed, 1966). Fragmentation can be induced in vitro by exposing red cells to heat, urea, ammonium sulfate, or forced sieving (Weed and Reed, 1965). Erythrocyte fragmentation leading to formation of schistocytes occurs in microangiopathic anemias and conditions associated with intravascular fibrin deposition. It has been demonstrated that the red cell membrane is intolerant to stretching to more than 110% of its area (Rand, 1964). Stress on the cell beyond the tensile strength of the membrane, therefore, may result in tearing and formation of fragments. Fragmentation would contribute to a decrease in red cell enzyme activity and glycolysis, which will predispose to further fragmentation. Small spheroidal cells produced as the result of fragmentation (microspherocytes) have limited tolerance to both physical and metabolic stresses like spherocytes of autoimmune disease. They may be destroyed by osmotic hemolysis or by phagocytosis. Rebar et al., (1981) have recently reviewed erythrocyte fragmentation in disease.

REFERENCES

(Titles in parentheses are English translations of foreign language titles.)

Agar, N.S.: Red Cell Enzymes. V. Enzyme Activities in the Red Blood Cells of Saanen and Angora Goats. Comp. Biochem. Physiol., *64B*:239, 1979.

Agar, N.S., and Board, P.G.: Red Blood Cells of Domestic Mammals. Elsevier, Amsterdam, 1983.

Agar, N.S., and Roberts, J.: Biochemical Polymorphism and 2,3-Diphosphoglycerate in Sheep R.B.C. Experientia, *33*:300, 1977.

Agar, N.S., and Suzuki, T.: Red Cell Metabolism in Buffaloes and Camels. J. Exp. Zoo., *223*:25, 1982.

Agar, N.S., et al.: The Effect of Experimental Anaemia on the Levels of Glutathione and Glycolytic Enzymes of the Erythrocyte of Normal and Glutathione-Deficient Merino Sheep. Aust. J. Biol. Sci., *28*:233, 1975a.

Agar, N.S., et al.: Red Cell Enzymes. II. Enzyme Activities in the Red Blood Cell of High and Low K Sheep. III. Enzyme Activities in the Red Blood Cell of Different Breeds of Sheep. Comp. Biochem. Physiol., *51B*:467, 1975b.

Agar, N.S., et al.: Postnatal Changes in the Levels of 2,3 Diphosphoglycerate, Reduced Glutathione and Some Enzyme Activity in the Erythrocytes of Lambs. Res. Vet. Sci., *20*:223, 1976.

Agar, N.S., et al.: Glutathione Levels in the Red Blood Cells of Cattle. Comp. Biochem. Physiol., *59B*:141, 1978.

Alhanaty, E., and Sheetz, M.P.: Control of the Erythrocyte Membrane Shape: Recovery from the Effect of Crenating Agents. J. Cell. Biol., *91*:884, 1981.

Allen, D.W., and Jandl, J.H.: Oxidative Hemolysis and Precipitation of Hemoglobin. II. The Role of Thiols in Oxidant Drug Action. J. Clin. Invest., *40*:454, 1961.

Ashby, W.: The Determination of the Length of Transfused Blood Corpuscles in Man. J. Exp. Med., 29:267, 1919.

Atkins, C.E., et al.: Methemoglobin Reductase Deficiency and Methemoglobinemia in a Dog. J. Amer. Anim. Hos. Assoc., 17:829, 1981.

Atkinson, J.B., et al.: A Generalized Membrane Defect in Heritable Myotonia: U.S. Studies of Erythrocytes in an Animal Model and Patients. Proc. Soc. Exp. Biol. Med., 163:69, 1980.

Baker, N.F., and Douglas, J.R.: The Pathogenesis of Trichostrongyloid Parasites. II. Ferrokinetic Studies in Ruminants. Amer. J. Vet. Res., 18:295, 1957.

Baker, N.F., et al.: Erythrocyte Survival in Experimental Anaplasmosis. Amer. J. Vet. Res., 22:590, 1961.

Baker, R.F.: Ultrastructure of the Red Blood Cells. Fed. Proc., 26:1785, 1967.

Bale, W.F., et al.: Hemoglobin Labeled by Radioactive Lysine. Erythrocyte Life Cycle. J. Exp. Med., 90:315, 1949.

Ballas, S.K., and Krasnow, S.H.: Structure of Erythrocyte Membrane and Its Transport Functions. Ann. Clin. Lab. Sci., 10:209, 1980.

Bangham, A.D.: The Adhesiveness of Leukocytes with Special Reference to Zeta Potential. Ann. N.Y. Acad. Sci., 116:945, 1964.

Barcroft, J.: The Raison d'Etre of the Red Corpuscle. Harvey Lect., 1921–1922:146, 1923.

Barcroft, J.: The Significance of Hemoglobin. Physiol. Rev., 4:329, 1924.

Bartlett, G.: Patterns of Phosphate Compounds in Red Blood Cells of Man and Animals. Adv. Exp. Biol. Med., 6:245, 1970.

Bartosz, G., and Bartkowiak, A.: Aging of the Erythrocyte. II. Activities of Peroxide-Detoxifying Enzymes. Experientia, 37:722, 1981.

Bartosz, G., et al.: Aging of the Erythrocyte. III. Cation Content. Experientia, 37:723, 1981.

Benesch, R., and Benesch, R.E.: The effect of Organic Phosphates from Human Erythrocyte on the Allosteric Properties of Hemoglobin. Biochem. Biophys. Res. Commun., 26:162, 1967.

Bennett, V., and Stenbuck, P.J.: Human Erythrocyte Ankyrin. Purification and Properties. J. Biol. Chem., 255:2540, 1980.

Berlin, N.I.: Life Span of the Red Cell, *In* The Red Blood Cell. C. Bishop and D.M. Swigenor, eds. Academic Press, New York, pp. 423–450, 1964.

Berlin, N.I., and Lotz, C.I.: Life Span of the Red Blood Cell of the Rat Following Acute Hemorrhage. Proc. Soc. Exp. Biol. Med., 78:788, 1951.

Berlin, N.I., et al.: Life Span of the Rat Red Blood Cell as Determined by Glycine-2-C14. Amer. J. Physiol., 165:565, 1951.

Berlin, N.I., et al.: Life Span of Red Blood Cells. Physiol. Rev., 39:577, 1959.

Bernstein, S.E.: Inherited Hemolytic Disease in Mice: A Review and Update. Lab. Anim. Sci., 30:197, 1980.

Bessis, M.: Red Cell Shapes. An Illustrated Classification and Its Rationale. Nou. Rev. Franc. d'Hemat., 12:721, 1972.

Bessis, M.: Living Blood Cells and Their Ultrastructure. Springer-Verlag, New York, 1973.

Bessis, M.: Blood Smears Reinterpreted. Springer International, Springer-Verlag, Berlin Heidelberg, 1977.

Bessis, M.: Cellular Mechanisms for the Destruction of Erythrocytes. Haematologica, 2:59, 1965.

Bocci, V.: Determinants of Erythrocyte Aging: A Reappraisal. Brit. J. Haematol., 48:515, 1981.

Braasch, D.: The Relation Between Erythrocyte Deformability, Cell Shape and Membrane Surface Tension. Pflugers Arch., 313:316, 1969.

Brace, K.C.: Life Span of the Marmot Erythrocyte. Blood, 8:648, 1953.

Brace, K.C., and Altland, P.D.: The Life Span of the Duck and Chicken Erythrocyte as Determined with C14. Proc. Soc. Exp. Biol. Med., 92:615, 1956.

Brandon, D.L.: Studies of Sheep Red Blood Cell Membranes, Using Cleavable Crosslinking Reagents. Cell. Mol. Biol., 26:569, 1980.

Brecher, G., and Bessis, M.: Present Status of Spiculed Red Cells and Their Relationship to the Discocyte-Echinocyte Transformation: A Critical Review. Blood, 40:333, 1972.

Brecher, G., and Stohlman, F., Jr.: The Macrocytic Response to Erythropoietin Stimulation. *In* Erythropoiesis. L.O. Jacobson and M. Doyle, eds. Grune & Stratton, New York, 1962.

Brown, A.M., et al.: A Calcium Activated Potassium Channel Present in Foetal Red Cells of the Sheep but Absent from Reticulocytes and Mature Red Cells. Biochem. Biophys. Acta, 511:163, 1978.

Brown, I.W., Jr., and Eadie, G.S.: An Analytical Study of the in vivo Survival of Limited Populations of Animal Red Blood Cells Tagged with Radio-iron. J. Gen. Physiol., 36:327, 1953.

Bunn, H.F.: Differences in the Interaction of 2,3-Diphosphoglycerate with Certain Mammalian Hemoglobins. Science, 172:1049, 1971.

Burwell, E.L., et al.: Erythrocyte Life Span in Small Animals. Comparison of Two Methods Employing Radioiron. Amer. J. Physiol., 172:718, 1953.

Bush, J.A., et al.: Erythrocyte Life Span in Growing Swine as Determined by Glycine-2-C14. J. Exp. Med., 101:451, 1955.

Bush, J.A., et al.: Studies on Copper Metabolism. XIX. The Kinetics of Iron Metabolism and Erythrocyte Life-Span in Copper-Deficient Swine. J. Exp. Med., 103:701, 1956a.

Bush, J.A., et al.: The Kinetics of Iron Metabolism in Swine with Various Experimentally Induced Anemias. J. Exp. Med., 103:161, 1956b.

Castle, W.B.: Disorders of the Blood-Forming Tissues. *In* Pathologic Physiology: Mechanisms of Diseases, W.A. Sodeman and W.A. Sodeman, Jr., eds. 4th Ed. W.B. Saunders and Co., Philadelphia, 1967.

Castranova, V., et al.: Characteristics of Anion Transport in Cat and Dog Red Blood Cells. J. Membrane Biol., 49:57, 1979.

Chanutin, A., and Curnish, R.R.: Effect of Organic and Inorganic Phosphates on the Oxygen Equilibrium of Human Erythrocytes. Arch. Biochem. Biophys., 121:96, 1967.

Chiba, H., and Sasaki, R.: Functions of 2,3-bisphosphoglycerate and its Metabolism. Curr. Top. Cell. Regul., 14:75, 1978.

Chien, S.: Principles and Techniques for Assessing Erythrocyte Deformability. Blood Cells, 3:71, 1977.

Clark, M.R., et al.: Deformability of Oxygenated Irreversibly Sickled Cells. J. Clin. Invest., 65:189, 1980.

Clark, M.R., et al.: Separate Mechanisms of Deformability Loss in ATP-Depleted and Ca-Loaded Erythrocyte. J. Clin. Invest., 67:531, 1981.

Cline, M.J., and Berlin, N.I.: Erythropoiesis and Red Cell Survival in the Hypothyroid Dog. Amer. J. Physiol., 204:415, 1963.

Cohen, W.D.: Marginal Bands in Camel Erythrocytes. J. Cell. Sci., 36:97, 1979.

Cohen, W.D., et al.: The Cytoskeletal System of Nucleated Erythrocytes. I. Composition and Function of Major Elements. J. Cell. Biol., *93*:828, 1982.

Coiro, J.R.R., et al.: The Marginal Band and Its Role in the Ellipsoidal Shape of Geochelone Carbonaria Erythrocyte. Arch. d'Anato. Microscop., *67*:133, 1978.

Coleman, R., et al.: Membrane Lipid Composition and Susceptibility to Bile Salt Damage. Biochim. Biophys. Acta, *599*:294, 1980.

Cooper, R.A.: Lipids of Human Red Cell Membranes: Normal Composition and Variability in Disease. Gen. Hematol., *7*:314, 1970.

Cooper, R.A.: Influence of Increased Membrane Cholesterol on Membrane Fluidity and Cell Function in Human Red Blood Cells. J. Supramol. Struct., *8*:413, 1978.

Cooper, R.A.: Hemolytic Syndromes and Red Cell Membrane Abnormalities in Liver Disease. Sem. Hematol., *17*:103, 1980.

Cooper, R.A., et al.: Red Cell Cholesterol Enrichment and Spur Cell Anemia in Dog Fed a Cholesterol-Enriched, Atherogenic Diet. J. Lipid. Res., *21*:1082, 1980.

Cornelius, C.E., and Kaneko, J.J.: Erythrocyte Life Span in the Guanaco. Science, *137*:673, 1962.

Cornelius, C.E., et al.: Erythrocyte Survival Studies in the Mule Deer, Aoudad Sheep, and Springbok Antelope Using Glycine-2-C14. Amer. J. Vet. Res., *20*:917, 1959.

Cornelius, C.E., et al.: Erythrocyte Survival Studies in the Horse Using Glycine-2-C14. Amer. J. Vet. Res., *20*:1123, 1960.

Dagg, J.H., et al.: A Direct Method of Determining Red Cell Life Span Using Radioiron. An Application of the Occupancy Principle. Brit. J. Haematol., *22*:9, 1972.

Danon, D., et al.: The Sequestration of Old Red Cells and Extruded Erythroid Nuclei. *In* Red Cell Structure and Function, B. Ramot, ed. Academic Press, New York, 1971.

Danon, D., et al.: Phagocytosis of 'Old' Red Blood Cells by Macrophages from Syngeneic Mice in Vitro. Exp. Hematol., *5*:480, 1977.

deGier, J., and van Deenen, L.L.M.: Some Lipid Characteristics of Red Cell Membranes of Various Animal Species. Biochem. Biophys. Acta, *49*:286, 1961.

Delaunay, J.: The Enzymes of the Red Blood Cell Plasma Membrane. Biomedicine, *26*:357, 1977.

Deuticke, B.: Transformation and Restoration of Biconcave Shape of Human Erythrocytes Induced by Amphiphilic Agents and Changes of Ionic Environment. Biochem. Biophys. Acta, *163*:494, 1968.

Dixon, P.M., et al.: Familial Methaemoglobinaemia and Haemolytic Anaemia in the Horse Associated with Decreased Erythrocytic Glutathione Reductase and Glutathione. Equine Vet. J., *9*(4):198, 1977.

Doan, C.A., and Sabin, F.R.: Normal and Pathological Fragmentation of Red Blood Cell: The Phagocytosis of these Fragments by Desquamated Endothelial Cells of the Blood Stream: the Correlation of the Peroxidase Reaction with Phagocytosis in Mononuclear Cells. J. Exp. Med., *43*:839, 1926.

Dreher, K.L., et al.: Retention of Water and Potassium by Erythrocytes Prevents Calcium Induced Membrane Rigidity. Amer. J. Pathol., *92*:215, 1978.

Dunham, P.B., and Ellory, J.C.: Stimulation of the Sodium-Potassium Pump by Trypsin in Low Potassium Type Erythrocytes of Goats. J. Physiol., *301*:25, 1980.

Eadie, G.S., and Brown, I.W., Jr.: Red Blood Cell Survival Studies. Blood, *8*:1110, 1953.

Eaton, J.W., et al.: Intracellular Calcium: Lack of Effect on Ovine Red Cells. Proc. Soc. Exp. Biol. Med., *157*:506, 1978.

Ehrenstein, G.V., and Lockner, D.: Sites of the Physiological Breakdown of the Red Blood Corpuscles. Nature, *181*:911, 1958.

Evans, E.T.R.: Sickling Phenomenon in Sheep. Nature, *217*:74, 1968.

Everett, N.B., and Yoffey, J.M.: Life of Guinea Pig Circulating Erythrocyte and Its Relation to Erythrocyte Population of Bone Marrow. Proc. Soc. Exp. Biol. Med., *101*:318, 1959.

Ewing, G.O.: Familial Nonspherocytic Hemolytic Anemia of Basenji Dogs. J. Amer. Vet. Med. Ass., *154*:503, 1969.

Finch, C.A., et al.: Iron Metabolism. Erythrocyte Iron Turnover. J. Lab. Clin. Med., *34*:1480, 1949.

Fitzsimmons, W.M., et al.: Blood Transfusion and Red Cell Survival in the Goat. Brit. Vet. J., *123*:192, 1967.

Flamm, M., and Schachter, D.: Acanthocytosis and Cholesterol Enrichment Decrease Lipid Fluidity of Only the Outer Human Erythrocyte Membrane Leaflet. Nature, *298*:290, 1982.

Fujii, T.: Role of Membrane Lipids and Proteins in Discocyte, Echinocyte and Stomatocyte Transformation of Erythrocytes. Acta Biol. Med. Germ., *40*:361, 1981.

Gaehtgens, P., et al.: Comparative Rheology of Nucleated and Non-nucleated Red Blood Cells. I. Microrheology of Avian Erythrocytes During Capillary Flow. Pflugers Archiv., *390*:278, 1981.

Gelberg, H., and Stackhouse, L.L.: Three Cases of Canine Acanthocytosis Associated with Splenic Neoplasia. Vet. Med. Small Anim. Clin., *72*:1183, 1977.

George, J.W., et al.: Comparison of Pyrimidine 5'-Nucleotidase Activity in Erythrocytes of Sheep, Dogs, Cats, Horses, Calves, and Mongolian Gerbils. Amer. J. Vet. Res., *44*:1968, 1983.

Gerlach, E., et al.: Metabolism of 2,3-Diphosphoglycerate in Red Blood Cells under Various Experimental Conditions. Adv. Exp. Biol. Med., *6*:155, 1970.

Germano, D., and Barresi, C.: (Effects in vitro of Heat on Blood Cell Mammals, Horse, Donkey, Cattle, Goat, Swine, Dromedary.) Annuli della Facolta' di Medicina. Veterinaria Messina, *13*:143, 1976.

Gierber, H., et al.: (Severe Deformity of Erythrocytes in Calves.) Archiv. für Tierheilkunde, *117*:341, 1975.

Glader, B.E., et al.: Congenital Hemolytic Anemia Associated with Dehydrated Erythrocytes and Increased Potassium Loss. New Eng. J. Med., *291*:491, 1974.

Glaser, R.: The Shape of Red Blood Cells as a Function of Membrane Potential and Temperature. J. Membrane Biol., *51*:217, 1979.

Goodman, S.R., and Shiffer, K.: The Spectrin Membrane Skeleton of Normal and Abnormal Human Erythrocytes: A Review. Amer. J. Physiol., *244*:C121, 1983.

Gratzer, W.B.: The Red Cell Membrane and Its Cytoskeleton. Biochem. J., *198*:1, 1981.

Gregersen, M.I., et al.: Species Differences in the Flexibility and Deformation of Erythrocytes (RBC). 5th European Conference on Microcirculation, Gothenburg, 1966. Bibl. Anat., No. 10, 104–108.

Groner, W., et al.: New Optical Technique for Measuring Erythrocyte Deformability with the Ektacytometer. Clin. Chem., *26*:1435, 1980.

Guest, M.M., et al.: Red Blood Cells: Change in Shape in Capillaries. Science, *142*:1319, 1963.

Ham, T.H., et al.: Physical Properties of Red Cells as Related to Effects in Vivo. IV. Oxidant Drugs Producing Abnormal Intracellular Concentration of Hemoglobin (Eccentrocytes) with a Rigid-Red-Cell Hemolytic Syndrome. J. Lab. Clin. Med., 82:898, 1973.

Hansard, S.L., and Kincaid, E.: Red Cell Life Span of Farm Animals. J. Anim. Sci., 15:1300, 1956.

Harkness, D.R., et al.: A Comparative Study on the Phosphoglyceric Acid Cycle in Mammalian Erythrocytes. Comp. Biochem. Physiol., 28:129, 1969.

Harris, J.W., and Kellermeyer, R.W.: The Red Cell, Production, Metabolism, Destruction: Normal and Abnormal. Harvard University Press, Cambridge, Mass., 1970.

Harrison, B.A., et al.: Erythrocyte Life Span in Small Animals. Fed. Proc., 10:357, 1951.

Harrison, K.L.: Fetal Erythrocyte Life Span. Aust. Paediatr. J., 15:96, 1979.

Harvey, J.W., and Kaneko, J.J.: Mammalian Erythrocyte Glutathione Reductase: Kinetic Constants and Saturation with Cofactors. Amer. J. Vet. Res., 10:1511, 1975.

Harvey, J.W., and Rackear, D.: Experimental Onion-Induced Hemolytic Anemia in Dogs. Vet. Pathol., 22:387, 1985.

Harvey, J.W., et al.: Methemoglobin Reductase Deficiency in a Dog. J. Amer. Vet. Med. Ass., 164:1030, 1974.

Harvey, J.W., et al.:Erythrocyte Pyruvate Kinase Deficiency in a Beagle Dog. Vet. Clin. Pathol., 6:13, 1977.

Havell, T.C., et al.: Deformability Characteristics of Sickle Cells by Microelastimetry. Amer. J. Hematol., 4:9, 1978.

Hawkins, W.B., and Whipple, G.H.: The Life Cycle of the Red Blood Cell in the Dog. Amer. J. Physiol., 122:418, 1938.

Holman, H.H., and Dew, S.M.: The Blood Picture of the Goat. II. Changes in Erythrocytic Shape, Size and Number Associated with Age. Res. Vet. Sci., 5:274, 1964.

Horejsi, J.: Effect of Glutathione and Some Other Substances on the Oxygen Dissociation Curve of Hemoglobin and Experimental Therapy of Hemorrhagic Shock with Solutions Enriched with Glutathione. Adv. Exp. Med. Biol., 6:9, 1970.

Hsu, R.C.: The Formation of Echinocytes by the Insertion of Oxygenated Sterol Compounds into Red Cell Membranes. Blood, 56:109, 1980.

Imre, S., and Sari, B.: Comparative Study of the Metabolism and Filtrability of Red Blood Cells of the Calf and Adult Cattle. Acta Physiol. Acad. Sci. Hung., 53:23, 1979.

International Committee for Standardization in Hematology. Recommended Methods for Radioisotope Red Cell Survival Studies. Blood, 38:378, 1971.

Jain, N.C.: Measurement and Significance of Osmotic Fragility of Canine Erythrocytes. Bull. Amer. Soc. Vet. Clin. Pathol., 1(3):9, 1972a.

Jain, N.C.: Morphology of Blood Cells in Three Dimensions. Calif. Vet. 26(12):16, 1972b.

Jain, N.C.: Osmotic Fragility of Erythrocytes of Dogs and Cats in Health and in Certain Hematologic Disorders. Cornell Vet., 63:411, 1973.

Jain, N.C.: Echinocytic and Stomatocytic Transformations of Red Cells of the Goat. Blood Cells, 1:385, 1975.

Jain, N.C., and Keeton, K.S.: Morphology of Camel and Llama Erythrocytes as Viewed with the Scanning Electron Microscope. Brit. Vet. J., 130:288, 1974.

Jain, N.C., and Kono, C.S.: Scanning Electromicroscopy of Erythrocytes of Dog, Cat, Cow, Horse, Sheep and Goat. Res. Vet. Sci., 13:489, 1972.

Jain, N.C., and Kono, C.S.: Fusiform Erythrocytes Resembling Sickle Cells in Angora Goats: Light and Electron Microscopic Observations. Res. Vet. Sci., 22:169, 1977a.

Jain, N.C., and Kono, C.S.: Fusiform Erythrocytes in Angora Goats Resembling Sickle Cells: Influences of Temperature, pH and Oxygenations on Cell Shape. Amer. J. Vet. Res., 38:983, 1977b.

Jandl, J.H.: Leaky Red Cells. An Analytical Review. Blood, 26:367, 1965.

Jandl, J.H.: The Pathophysiology of Hemolytic Anemias. Amer. J. Med., 41:657, 1966.

Jasper, D.E., and Jain, N.C.: Effects of Lipemia upon Erythrocyte Fragility, Sedimentation Rate and Plasma Refractometer Indexes in the Dog. Amer. J. Vet. Res., 26:332, 1965.

Jensen, W.N., and Lessin, L.S.: Membrane Alterations Associated with Hemoglobinopathies. Semin. Hematol., 7:409, 1970.

Jensen, W.N., et al.: The Kinetics of Iron Metabolism in Normal Growing Swine. J. Exp. Med., 103:145, 1956.

Johnson, L.W., and Schwartz, S.: Isotopic Studies of Erythrocyte Survival in Normal and Porphyric Cattle. Influence of Light Exposure, Blood Withdrawal, and Splenectomy. Amer. J. Vet. Res., 31:2167, 1970.

Kahn, A., et al.: Advances in Hereditary Red Cell Enzyme Anomalies. Hum. Genet., 50:1, 1979.

Kaneko, J.J.: Erythrokinetics and Iron Metabolism in Bovine Porphyria Erythropoietica. Ann. N.Y. Acad. Sci., 104:689, 1963.

Kaneko, J.J.: Comparative Erythrocyte Metabolism. Adv. Vet. Sci. Comp. Med., 18:117, 1974.

Kaneko, J.J., and Cornelius, C.E.: Erythrocyte Survival Studies in the Himalayan Tahr and Domestic Goats. Amer. J. Vet. Res., 23:913, 1962.

Kaneko, J.J., and Mills, R.: Erythrocyte Enzyme Activity, Ion Concentrations, Osmotic Fragility, and Glutathione Stability in Bovine Erythropoietic Porphyria and Its Carrier State. Amer. J. Vet. Res., 30:1805, 1969.

Kaneko, J.J., et al.: Erythrocyte Survival Studies in Experimental Molybdenosis of Sheep. Proc. Soc. Exp. Biol. Med., 107:924, 1961a.

Keneko, J.J., et al.: Erythrocyte Survival Studies in Domestic and Bighorn Sheep, Using Glycine-2-C^{14}. Amer. J. Vet. Res., 22:683, 1961b.

Kaneko, J.J., et al.: Erythrocyte Survival in the Cat as Determined by Glycine-2-C^{14}. Proc. Soc. Exp. Biol. Med., 123:783, 1966.

Kaneko, J.J., et al.: Erythrocyte Porphyrin and Erythrocyte Survival in Bovine Erythropoietic Porphyria. Amer. J. Vet. Res., 32:1981, 1971.

Kay, M.M.B.: Role of Physiologic Autoantibody in the Removal of Senescent Human Red Cells. J. Supramol. Struct., 9:555, 1978.

Kay, M.M.B., et al.: Senescent Cell Antigen is Immunologically Related to Band 3. Proc. Natl. Acad. Sci., 80:1631, 1983.

Keeton, K.S., and Jain, N.C.: Erythrocyte Morphology during Response to Blood Loss. Calif. Vet., 27:13(Feb.) 1973.

Keeton, K.S., and Kaneko, J.J.: Characterization of Adenosine Triphosphatase in Erythrocyte Membranes of the Cow. Proc. Soc. Exp. Biol. Med., 140:30, 1972.

Kim, H.D.: Cow Red Blood Cells. III. Postnatal Adaptation of Energy Metabolism in the Calf Red Blood Cells. Biochim. Biophys. Acta, *588*:44, 1979.

King, M.E., and Mifsud, C.V.J.: Postnatal Changes in Erythrocyte 2,3-Diphosphoglycerate in Sheep and Cattle. Res. Vet. Sci., *31*:37, 1981.

Klimas, N.C., et al.: Comparison of Receptor Properties of Erythrocyte Membrane Glycoproteins. Dev. Comp. Immunol., *6*:765, 1982.

Knyszynski, A., et al.: Phagocytosis of "Old" Red Blood Cells by Macrophages from Syngeneic Mice in Vitro. Exp. Hematol., *5*:480, 1977.

Kretchman, J., and Rogers, B.S.: Erythrocyte Shape Transformation Associated with Calcium Accumulation. Amer. J. Med. Technol., *47*:561, 1981.

Krotlinger, F., et al.: Bovine J Blood Group Activity in the Lipids of Erythrocytes of Different Age. Blut, *40*:417, 1980.

Kursa, J., et al.: Glutathione Peroxidase Activity in the Blood of Cattle. Biologizace a Chemizace Zivocisne Vyroby-Veterinaria, *18*:89, 1982.

Lauf, P.K., and Valet, G.: Cation Transport in Different Volume Populations of Genetically Low K+ Lamb Red Cells. J. Cell. Physiol., *104*:283, 1980.

Lawson, N.S., et al.: Splenic Ultrastructure in Drug-Induced Heinz Body Hemolysis. Arch. Path., *87*:491, 1969.

Lee, P., et al.: Turnover of Red Blood Cell Mass in Newborn Puppies. Fed. Proc., *30*:195, 1971.

Lessin, et al.: Clinical Implications of Red Cell Shape. Adv. Intern. Med., *21*:451, 1976.

Letchworth, G.J., et al.: Cyanosis and Methemoglobinemia in Two Dogs Due to NADH-methemoglobin Reductase Deficiency. Amer. Anim. Hosp. Ass., *13*:75, 1977.

Lewis, I.M., and McLean, J.G.: Physiological Variation in Levels of 2-3 Diphosphoglycerate in Horse Erythrocytes. Res. Vet. Sci., *18*:186, 1975.

Liddle, C.G., et al.: A Comparison of Chromium-51 and Iron-59 for Estimating Erythrocyte Survival in the Cat. Lab. Anim. Sci., *34*:365, 1984.

Litchman, M.A., et al.: The Effect of Incubated Plasma and Lysolecithin on the Shape and Membrane Lipid Composition of Red Cells Studies "in vitro." Nouv. Rev. Fr. Hematol., *14*:5, 1974.

Lubin, B., and Chin, D.: Membrane Phospholipid Organization in Pathologic Human Erythrocytes. Prog. Clin. Biol. Res., *97*:137, 1982.

Luner, S.J., et al.: Red Cell Charge is Not a Function of Cell Age. Nature, *269*:719, 1977.

Luther, D.G., et al.: Fatty Acid Composition of Equine Erythrocytes. Amer. J. Vet. Res., *43*:1007, 1982.

Lutz, H.U., and Kay, M.M.B.: An Age-Specific Cell Antigen is Present on Senescent Human Red Blood Cell Membranes. A Brief Note. Mech. Ageing Dev., *15*:65, 1981.

Maddy, A.H.: Erythrocyte Membrane Proteins. Semin. Hematol., *7*:275, 1970.

Madewell, B.R., and Feldman, B.F.: Characterization of Anemias Associated with Neoplasia in Small Animals. J. Amer. Vet. Med. Ass., *176*:419, 1980.

Marcel, G.A.: Red Cell Deformability: Physiological, Clinical and Pharmocological Aspects. J. Med., *10*:409, 1979.

Marchesi, V.T.: The Red Cell Membrane Skeleton: Recent Progress. Blood, *61*:1, 1983.

Marcilese, N.A., et al.: Red Cell Survival Time in the Horse, Determined with Di-Isopropyl-Phosphorofluoridate-P[32]. Amer. J. Physiol., *211*:281, 1966.

Matayoshi, E.D.: Distribution of Shape-Changing Compounds Across the Red Cell Membrane. Biochemistry, *19*:3414, 1980.

McLean, J.G., and Lewis, I.M.: Oxygen Affinity Responses to 2,3-Diphosphoglycerate, and Methaemoglobin Formation in Horse and Human Haemoglobins. Res. Vet. Sci., *19*:259, 1975.

Mentzer, W.C., Jr., and Clark, M.R.: Disorders of Erythrocyte Cation Permeability and Water Content Associated with Hemolytic Anemia. Biomembranes, *11*:79, 1983.

Metcalfe, J., and Dhindsa, D.S.: A Comparison of Mechanisms of Oxygen Transport Among Several Mammalian Species. Adv. Exp. Med. Biol., *6*:229, 1970.

Mohandas, N., and Shohet, S.B.: Control of Red Cell Deformability and Shape. Curr. Top. Hematol., *1*:71, 1978.

Mohandas, N., et al.: Bilayer Balance and Regulation of Red Cell Shape Changes. J. Supramol. Struct., *9*:453, 1978.

Mohandas, N., et al.: Analysis of Factors Regulating Erythrocyte Deformability. J. Clin. Invest., *66*:563, 1980.

Nathan, D.G., and Shohet, S.B.: Erythrocyte Ion Transport Defects and Hemolytic Anemia: "Hydrocytosis" and "Desiccytosis." Semin. Hematol., *7*:381, 1970.

Nelson, G.J.: Lipid Composition of Erythrocytes in Various Mammalian Species. Biochim. Biophys. Acta, *144*:221, 1967.

Neuberger, A., and Niven, J.S.F.: Haemoglobin Formation in Rabbits. J. Physiol. (London), *112*:292, 1951.

Noble, N.A., et al.: Mechanisms of Red Cell 2,3-Diphosphoglycerate Increase in Neonatal Lambs. Blood, *61*:920, 1983.

Norton, J.M., and Smith, R.P.: Drugs Acting on Hemoglobin and the Oxygen Transport System. Pharmacol. Ther. B., *2*:523, 1976.

Ogunrinade, A.F., and Anosa, V.O.: Red Blood Cell Survival and Faecal Clearance in Sheep Infected with *Fasciola gigantica*. J. Comp. Path., *91*:381, 1981.

Okano, Y., et al.: Mechanisms for Lipid Abnormalities of Erythrocyte Membrane in Biliary Obstruction: Lecithin Content and Its Fatty Acyl Composition. Clin. Chim. Acta, *88*:237, 1978.

Okano, Y., et al.: Abnormalities of Erythrocyte Membranes in Biliary Atresia: Ultrastructural and Lipid Composition. Clin. Chim. Acta, *94*:317, 1979.

O'Kelly, J.C.: The Lipid Composition of Erythrocytes in European Cattle and Buffalo Steers. Lipids, *14*:983, 1979.

Passow, H.: Passive Ion Permeability of the Erythrocyte Membrane. Prog. Biophys. Mol. Biol., *19*:425, 1969.

Pearson, H.A.: Life-Span of the Fetal Red Blood Cell. J. Pediatr., *70*:166, 1967.

Perk, K., et al.: Osmotic Fragility of Red Blood Cells of Young and Mature Domestic and Laboratory Animals. Amer. J. Vet. Res., *25*:1241, 1964a.

Perk, K., et al.: The Degree of Swelling and Osmotic Resistance in Hypotonic Solutions of Erythrocytes from Various Domestic Animals. Refuah Vet., *20*:122, 1964b.

Perman, V., and Schall, W.D.: Diseases of the Red Blood Cells. *In* Textbook of Veterinary Internal Medicine. Diseases of the Dog and Cat. Vol. II. Ettinger, S.J., ed. W.B. Saunders Co., Philadelphia, p. 1938, 1983.

Pinkerton, P.H., et al.: Hereditary Spherocytosis with Hemolytic Anemia in the Dog. Blood, *44*:557, 1974.

Platt, O.S., et al.: Exercise-Induced Hemolysis in Xerocytosis. J. Clin. Invest., 68:631, 1981.

Quist, E.E.: Regulation of Erythrocyte Membrane Shape by Ca^{2+}. Biochem. Biophys. Res. Commun., 92:631, 1980.

Rand, R.P.: Mechanical Properties of the Red Cell Membrane. II. Viscoelastic Breakdown of the Membrane. Biophys. J., 4:303, 1964.

Rebar, A.H., et al.: Red Cell Fragmentation in the Dog: An Editorial Review. Vet. Path., 18:415, 1981.

Reed, C., et al.: Polycythemia Vera in a Cat. J. Amer. Vet. Med. Ass., 157:85, 1970.

Rice-Evans, C., and Chapman, D.: Red Blood Cell Biomembrane Structure and Deformability. Scand. J. Clin. Lab. Invest., 41(Suppl 156):99, 1981.

Richhardt, H.-W., and Fuhrmann, G.F.: Dog Red Blood Cells Exhibit a Ca-stimulated Increase in K Permeability in the Absence of (Na, K) ATPase Activity. Nature, 279:248, 1979.

Rifkind, R.A.: Destruction of Injured Red Cells in Vivo. Amer. J. Med., 41:711, 1966.

Rigby, P.G., et al.: Erythrocyte Survival in Hamsters Using Intra-peritoneal NA$_2$Cr^{57}O$_4$. Proc. Soc. Exp. Biol. Med., 106:313, 1961.

Rodnan, G.P., et al.: The Life Span of the Red Blood Cell and the Red Blood Cell Volume in the Chicken, Pigeon and Duck as Estimated by the Use of NA$_2$Cr^{57}O$_4$. With Observations on Red Cell Turnover Rate in the Mammal, Bird and Reptile. Blood, 12:355, 1957.

Roth, E.F., et al.: Reticulocytes Contain Increased Amounts of Reduced Glutathione Except when Produced by Acetylphenylhydrazine. Biochem. Med., 21:333, 1979.

Rous, P.: Destruction of the Red Blood Corpuscles in Health and Disease. Physiol. Rev., 3:75, 1923.

Rous, P., and Robertson, O.H.: The Normal Fate of the Erythrocytes. I. The Findings in Healthy Animals. J. Exp. Med., 25:651, 1917.

Sagawa, S., and Shiraki, K.: Changes of Osmotic Fragility of Red Blood Cells Due to Repletion or Depletion of Cholesterol in Human and Rat Red Cells in vitro. J. Nutr. Sci. Vitaminol., 26:161, 1980.

Sato, T., and Mizuno, M.: Poikilocytosis of Newborn Calves. Jpn. J. Vet. Sci., 44:801, 1982.

Schmidt-Nielsen, K., and Taylor, C.R.: Red Blood Cells: Why or Why Not? Science, 162:274, 1968.

Seaman, G.V.H., et al.: Red Cell Aging. Surface Charge Density and Sialic Acid Content of Density-fractionated Human Erythrocytes. Blood, 50:1001, 1977.

Searcy, G.P., et al.: Congenital Hemolytic Anemia in the Basenji Dog Due to Erythrocyte Pyruvate Kinase Deficiency. Can. J. Comp. Med., 35:67, 1971.

Searcy, G.P., et al.: Animal Model of Human Disease: Pyruvate Kinase Deficiency. Animal Model: Pyruvate Kinase Deficiency in Dogs. Amer. J. Pathol., 94:689, 1979.

Seeman, P.C.: Transient Holes in the Erythrocyte Membrane During Hypotonic Hemolysis and Stable Holes in the Membranes after Hemolysis by Saponin and Lysolecithin. J. Cell Biol., 32:55, 1967.

Sewell, M.M.H., et al.: Studies on the Aetiology of Anaemia in Chronic Fascioliasis in Sheep. Brit. Vet. J., 124:160, 1968.

Shand, J.H., and Noble, R.C.: The Maternal Diet and Its Effect on the Lipid Composition and Osmotic Fragility of Neonatal Ovine Erythrocytes. Biol. Neonate, 40:150, 1981.

Shattil, S.J., and Cooper, R.A.: Maturation of Macroreticulocyte Membranes in Vivo. J. Lab. Clin. Med., 79:215, 1972.

Sheetz, M.P., and Singer, S.J.: Biological Membranes as Bilayer Couples. A Molecular Mechanism of Drug-Erythrocyte Interactions. Proc. Natl. Acad. Sci., 71:4457, 1974.

Sheetz, M.P., and Singer, S.J.: Equilibrium and Kinetic Effects of Drugs on the Shapes of Human Erythrocytes. J. Cell Biol., 70:247, 1976.

Shemin, D., and Rittenberg, D.: The Life Span of the Human Red Blood Cell. J. Biol. Chem., 166:627, 1946.

Shull, R.M., et al.: Spur Cell Anemia in a Dog. J. Amer. Vet. Med. Ass., 173:978, 1978.

Smith, J.E.: Elevated Erythrocyte Glutathione Associated with Elevated Substrate in High- and Low-glutathione Sheep. Biochim. Biophys. Acta, 496:516, 1977.

Smith, J.E.: Erythrocyte Deformity. In Red Blood Cells of Domestic Mammals. Agar, N.S., and Board, P.G., eds. Elsevier, Amsterdam, p. 55, 1983.

Smith, J.E., and Agar, N.S.: The Effect of Phlebotomy on Canine Erythrocyte Metabolism. Res. Vet. Sci., 18:231, 1975.

Smith, J.E., et al.: Variability in Erythrocyte Deformability Among Various Mammals. Amer. J. Physiol., 236:H725, 1979.

Smith, J.E., et al.: Deformability and Spectrin Properties in Three Types of Elongated Red Cells. Amer. J. Hematol., 8:1, 1980.

Smith, J.E., et al.: Interaction of Amphipathic Drugs with Erythrocytes from Various Species. Amer. J. Vet. Res., 43:1041, 1982.

Smith, J.E., et al.: Hereditary Elliptocytosis with Protein Band 4.1 Deficiency in the Dog. Blood, 61:373, 1983.

Smith, L.H., and McKinley, T.W., Jr.: Erythrocyte Survival in Guinea Pigs. Proc. Soc. Exp. Biol. Med., 111:768, 1962.

Smith, L.H., et al.: Life Span of Rat Erythrocytes as Determined by Cr and Differential Agglutination Methods. Proc. Soc. Exp. Biol. Med., 100:29, 1959.

Stewart, W.B., et al.: Age as Affecting the Osmotic and Mechanical Fragility of Dog Erythrocytes Tagged with Radioactive Iron. J. Exp. Med., 91:147, 1950.

Stewart, W.B., et al.: The Survival Time of Canine Erythrocytes Modified by Influenza Virus. Blood, 10:228, 1955.

Stohlman, F., Jr.: Red Cell Survival in the Dog Determined by a Method of Differential Agglutination Employing Canine Anti-A Serum. J. Lab. Clin. Med., 47:83, 1956.

Studzinski, T., et al.: Effect of Anaemia on the 2,3 Diphosphoglycerate Content of Equine Erythrocytes. Acta Physiol. Pol., 29:335, 1978.

Szasz, I., et al.: Biconcave Shape and Its Transformations in Human Red Cells. Acta Biol. Acad. Sci. Hung., 29:1, 1978.

Taketa, F., et al.: B-Chain Amino Termini of the Cat Hemoglobins and the Response to 2,3-Diphosphoglycerate and Adenosine Triphosphate. J. Biol. Chem., 246:4471, 1971.

Tasker, J.B., et al.: Familial Anemia in the Basenji Dog. J. Amer. Vet. Med. Ass., 154:158, 1969.

Terpin, T., and Roach, M.R.: Chondrodysplasia in the Alaskan Malamute: Involvement of Arteries, as well as Bone and Blood. Amer. J. Vet. Res., 42:1865, 1981.

Thiele, O.W., et al.: Lipid Pattern of Erythrocyte Membrane of Calf and Adult Cattle. Zentralbl. Veterinärmed., 26:425, 1979.

Thompson, R.H., et al.: The Levels of Selenium and Glutathione Peroxidase Activity in Blood of Sheep, Cows, and Pigs. Res. Vet. Sci., *20*:229, 1976.

Tillmann, W., et al.: Rheological Properties of Young and Aged Human Erythrocytes. Klin. Wochenschr., *58*:569, 1980.

Tosteson, D.C., and Hoffman, J.F.: Regulation of Cell Volume by Active Cation Transport in High and Low Potassium Sheep Red Cells. J. Gen. Physiol., *44*:169, 1960.

Tsukita, S., et al.: Cytoskeletal Network Underlying the Human Erythrocyte Membrane. Thin Section Electron Microscopy. J. Cell Biol., *85*:567, 1980.

Tucker, E.M.: Red Cell Life Span in Young Adult Sheep. Res. Vet. Sci., *4*:11, 1963.

Ultmann, J.E., and Gordon, C.S.: Life Span and Sites of Sequestration of Normal Erythrocytes in Normal and Splenectomized Mice and Rats. Acta Haematol., *33*:118, 1965.

Valentine, W.H.: The Hereditary Hemolytic Anemias Associated with Erythrocyte Enzyme Deficiencies. Adv. Intern. Med., *16*:303, 1970.

Valentine, W.H., et al.: Heme Synthesis and Erythrocyte Life Span in the Cat. Proc. Soc. Exp. Biol. Med., *77*:244, 1951.

Viscor, G., and Palomeque, J.: Method for Determining the Osmotic Fragility Curves of Erythrocytes in Birds. Lab. Anim., *16(1)*:48, 1982.

Wallace, W.R.: Loss of Erythrocytic Acetylcholinesterase Activity and Its Relationship to Osmotic Fragility of Erythrocytes in Bovine Anaplasmosis. Amer. J. Vet. Res., *28*:55, 1967.

Walter, H.: Factors in the Partition of Blood Cells in Aqueous Dextran-Polyethylene Glycol Two-Phase Systems. Prog. Separation Purifi., *2*:121, 1969.

Walter, H., et al.: Abnormal Membrane Lipid-related Properties During Maturation of Reticulocytes from Severely Anaemic Rats as Measured by Partition in Two Polymer Aqueous Phases. Brit. J. Haematol., *39*:391, 1978.

Weed, R.I.: Membrane Structure and Its Relation to Haemolysis. Clin. Haematol., *4*:3, 1975.

Weed, R.I.: The Importance of Erythrocyte Deformability. Amer. J. Med., *49*:147, 1970.

Weed, R.I., and Reed, C.F.: The Relation of Erythrocyte Fragmentation to Cellular Destruction. Blood, *26*:894, 1965.

Weed, R.I., and Reed, C.F.: Membrane Alterations Leading to Red Cell Destruction. Amer. J. Med., *41*:681, 1966.

Werre, J.M., et al.: Cause of Macroplania of Erythrocytes in Diseases of the Liver and Biliary Tract with Special Reference to Leptocytosis. Brit. J. Haematol., *19*:223, 1970.

Whitmore, R.L.: The Influence of Erythrocyte Shape and Rigidity on the Viscosity of Blood. Biorheology, *18*:557, 1981.

Whitten, C.F.: Innocuous Nature of the Sickling (Pseudosickling) Phenomenon in Deer. Brit. J. Haematol., *13*:650, 1967.

Wiley, J.S., and McCulloch, K.E.: Calcium Ions, Drug Action and the Red Cell Membrane. Pharmacol., Ther., *18*:271, 1982.

Wintrobe, M.M., et al.: Clinical Hematology. 8th ed. Lea & Febiger, Philadelphia, 1981.

Zarkowsky, H.S., et al.: A Congenital Hemolytic Anemia with Thermal Sensitivity of the Erythrocyte Membrane. Brit. J. Haematol., *29*:537, 1975.

21

Clinical and Laboratory Evaluation of Anemias and Polycythemias

CLINICAL SIGNS OF ANEMIA 563

CLASSIFICATION OF ANEMIAS 564
    Pathophysiologic Classification 564
    Morphologic Classification 564
    Classification Based on Bone Marrow
       Response 566

**LABORATORY EVALUATION OF
      ANEMIAS 566**
    Red Cell Parameters 566
    The Reticulocyte Count 567

Red Cell Indices 568
Erythrocyte Morphology 569
Other Hematologic Findings 570
Bone Marrow Examination 570
Other Laboratory Tests 571

THERAPEUTIC ASPECTS OF ANEMIA 571

POLYCYTHEMIA 572
    Absolute Polycythemia 573
    Relative Polycythemia 575

Anemia may be suspected from clinical signs and presenting history of a patient. Hematologic findings of below normal red cell count, hemoglobin concentration, and/or packed cell volume establish the existence of anemia. Anemia is rarely a primary disease; rather, it generally reflects a secondary development, and, therefore, the unqualified term *anemia* is not a satisfactory diagnosis. Anemia is a sign and more commonly only one of the results of a generalized disease process. Once anemia has been detected, its pathogenesis or etiology should be thoroughly searched.

Accurate diagnosis of anemia in terms of the causative disease process(es) is often challenging and is necessary for proper therapeutic management of the patient. Anemias can be evaluated and classified on the basis of erythrocyte morphology, pathogenetic mechanisms, and bone marrow erythroid response. Although none of the approaches are completely satisfactory by themselves, they are complementary and, together, provide a logical means of analyzing the anemia. It is common practice to evaluate a hemogram (CBC) at first to classify the anemia morphologically on the basis of mean corpuscular volume (MCV) and mean corpuscular hemo-globin concentration (MCHC). Then evidence is searched for bone marrow response to anemia by finding reticulocytosis or increased polychromasia in the blood. These changes, together with other hematologic findings, patient history, and clinical observations may provide clues to pathogenesis or etiology of the anemia. There may be situations, however, when a bone marrow examination (as in nonresponsive or hypoproliferative anemias) or other laboratory tests (such as Coombs test, urinalysis, fecal examination, serum chemistries) need to be performed in conjunction with or following blood examination to determine the specific etiology. Treatment is not to be directed at the anemia per se except as an emergency measure, for such an approach will result in failure to diagnose and treat the primary disease, which must be defined and attended by all possible means.

CLINICAL SIGNS OF ANEMIA

The clinical signs referable to anemia are the result of reduced oxygen-carrying capacity of the blood as well as a consequence of certain physiologic adjustments designed to increase the efficiency of the reduced circulating red cell mass and reduce the work load of the heart. Development of various clinical signs and their magnitude depend on the rapidity of onset, the degree, and the cause of the anemia as well as the physical activity of the animal. Signs common to anemias of diverse etiology include reduced exercise tolerance, pallor of mucous membranes, increased heart rate sometimes with murmurs, increased respiratory rate, depression, and dementia. A mild anemia usually passes undetected unless the animal is allowed to exert or is brought to the clinic for other reasons. The patient may present other signs referable to a specific disease or pathogenesis of anemia (see below).

In hemorrhage, when one-third of the blood volume is lost in a short period, shock occurs and death may ensue. Tachycardia and dyspnea become prominent signs. When this occurs, blood transfusions or plasma expanders are indicated to prevent death. Animals with a large spleen, such as the horse, sheep, and goat, may be able to withstand large losses of blood, up to 25% of the circulating blood volume, without serious consequences (see Chapter 3). When blood is lost more slowly, as much as 50% may be lost over a 24-hour period without danger to life. The slower loss permits replacement of blood volume by movement of fluids into the circulation from the tissues.

Clinical signs resulting from acute hemolytic anemia may be icterus, hemoglobinemia, hemoglobinuria, and fever. Icterus without hemoglobinuria is observed when the accelerated destruction of the erythrocytes occurs within the mononuclear phagocyte (reticuloendothelial) system, whereas with massive hemolysis of red cells within the bloodstream, hemoglobinemia follows and hemoglobinuria may ensue (see Chapter 19). Nephrosis may develop from hemoglobinuria. The sudden release of hemoglobin and the end products of erythrocyte breakdown lead to pyrexia. Thus, in acute hemolytic disease, a temperature rise should be anticipated, and its occurrence does not necessarily reflect the existence of an infectious process. Significant intravascular hemolysis may induce disseminated intravascular coagulation.

In chronically developing anemia, the hemoglobin level may drop to below 50% of the normal minimum without the patient revealing signs of hypoxemia unless exerted. For example, exercise intolerance is an early sign observed in a working or racing animal. This sign occurs because the body makes certain adjustments to compensate for the lower oxygen-carrying capacity of the blood at rest but cannot quickly meet requirements imposed by increased physical activity.

Compensatory adjustments occur in chronic anemia. Heart rate and, later, heart size increase to reduce circulation time of the erythrocytes. Blood volume is reduced to bring about a greater concentration of the erythrocytes in the plasma, and constriction of peripheral capillaries takes place to reduce the total vascular space. As anemia progresses, plasma protein concentration may be decreased, thus reducing blood viscosity and work load on the heart. In chronic anemia, certain clinical signs may develop as a result of overcompensation—heart murmur associated with cardiac hypertrophy, extreme pallor of the mucous membranes from reduction of blood volume and capillary constriction, and edema as a result of reduction in plasma protein concentration.

CLASSIFICATION OF ANEMIAS

Anemias are classified in various ways to determine possible pathophysiologic mechanisms and narrow down probable causes in search of the etiologic diagnosis.

Pathophysiologic Classification

A broad categorization of various causes is presented in Table 21–1 and includes anemias from acute or chronic blood loss, intravascular or extravascular hemolysis, and selective or generalized hypoplasia or aplasia of the bone marrow including deficiency or defective utilization of nutrients essential for erythrocyte production. Anemia of a particular etiology may involve more than one pathogenetic mechanism such as a hemolytic component as well as suppression of erythropoiesis.

Morphologic Classification

Anemias may be classified on the basis of erythrocyte morphology employing the two

Table 21–1. Pathophysiologic Classification of Anemias

I. Blood Loss or Hemorrhagic Anemias (see Table 22–1)
 Acute and chronic blood loss from various causes

II. Hemolytic Anemias (see Table 23–1)
 Blood parasites, bacterial, viral, and rickettsial agents
 Chemicals and drugs
 Poisonous plants
 Metabolic diseases
 Intraerythrocytic defects
 Immune-mediated disorders
 Miscellaneous causes

III. Depression or Hypoproliferative Anemias (see Table 25–1)
 Nutritional deficiency anemias
 Anemia of inflammatory disease
 Organic or tissue disorders
 Parasitic diseases
 Aplastic or hypoplastic anemias
 Myeloproliferative disorders

red cell indices, MCV and MCHC. The MCH is not of direct practical value; its usefulness lies in the fact that it changes directly with the MCV, and any disproportionate change in its value should evoke suspicion of a laboratory error in determinations of RBC and hemoglobin values. In iron deficiency anemia, however, MCH may diminish far more than anticipated for the reduction in MCV. The size of the erythrocyte in the anemic state is designated macrocytic, normocytic, or microcytic, and the mean hemoglobin concentration is designated either normochromic or hypochromic (Table 21–2). A true hyperchromic state is said to be impossible because

hemoglobin would precipitate at a concentration of 37% or more. Morphologic categorization of anemia must be confirmed by microscopic examination of erythrocyte populations.

The morphologic classification of anemia is noncommittal as to etiology but is helpful in limiting possible causes and providing clues to probable pathophysiologic mechanisms. It also forms a basis for consideration and selection of a program of treatment. A predictable etiologic relationship can be found in certain typical cases, but more often additional information is needed to establish the pathophysiologic mechanisms.

The *macrocytic anemias* may be normochromic or hypochromic and may be divided into transitory or true macrocytic anemias. True macrocytic anemias have normochromic erythrocytes, whereas transitory or pseudomacrocytic anemias characteristically have a below normal MCHC value as a result of reticulocytosis.

Macrocytic normochromic anemia in humans is characteristic of vitamin B_{12} and folate deficiency. Other causes have been administration of certain antimitotic drugs, severe liver disease, splenectomy, myeloproliferative disorders involving red cells (erythremic myelosis), and some leukemias. Anemic cats with myeloproliferative disorders sometimes have such red cell indices. Such an anemia results from asynchrony of erythropoiesis whereby maturation arrest occurs at the prorubricyte-basophilic rubricyte stages, which leads to

Table 21–2. Morphologic Classification of Erythrocyte Populations

	Based on MCV	*Based on MCHC*	*Clinical Interpretation*
I.	Normocytic	Normochromic	Normal erythrocyte morphology Depression anemias (see Table 25–1) excluding certain nutritional deficiencies and some cases of myeloproliferative disorders in the cat (see below)
II.	Normocytic	Hypochromic	Early iron deficiency
III.	Macrocytic	Normochromic	Pernicious anemia in humans and primates Vitamin B_{12} and folate deficiencies Cobalt deficiency in ruminants Erythremic myelosis and erythroleukemia in cats Defective erythrogenesis as in Poodle macrocytosis
IV.	Macrocytic	Hypochromic	Anemia in remission, either blood loss (see Table 22–1) or hemolytic (see Table 23–1)
V.	Microcytic	Normochromic	Characteristic of the Japanese Akita dogs Iron deficiency in progression
VI.	Microcytic	Hypochromic	Iron and copper deficiencies and chronic blood loss (see Table 22–1); pyridoxine deficiency

megaloblastic erythroid cells in the bone marrow. Macrocytic normochromic erythrocytes unaccompanied by anemia have been observed in some dogs of the Poodle breed (Chapter 25). The possibility of a deficiency or defective utilization of vitamin B_{12} and folate has not been investigated in such dogs and cats. It has been reported that cattle on cobalt-deficient or molybdenum-rich pastures have developed macrocytic normochromic anemia, but this is rare (see Chapter 25).

Macrocytic hypochromic anemia is observed during remission in acute blood loss or acute hemolytic anemia. Reticulocytosis in response to the anemia contributes to an increase in the MCV and a decrease in the MCHC (Fig. 18–11). Several days must elapse from the onset of anemia before manifestation of such a red cell morphology. Recovery from anemia is accompanied by maturation of these cells into erythrocytes with normal indices.

The *normocytic-normochromic* anemias occur when there is selective depression of erythrogenesis in chronic diseases, e.g., infections, nephritis with uremia, malignancies, and certain endocrine disorders. In such cases, reticulocyte response is absent or insignificant. This may be due to a deficiency in erythropoietin elaboration, marrow depression, or defective iron utilization. Hematinics, B-vitamins, and liver-extract injections are not indicated, because the erythropoietic tissue is unable to utilize these substances. Efforts should be directed toward diagnosis of the primary disease rather than toward treatment of the anemia. In protracted depression anemia, the erythrocytes may become microcytic but remain normochromic.

The *microcytic hypochromic* anemias are specific for iron deficiency or failure to utilize iron. The degree of changes in erythrocyte morphology depends on the duration and severity of the anemia. Determination of serum iron, iron binding capacity, and bone marrow iron are helpful in evaluating iron supply and utilization. Chronic blood loss or iron, copper, and pyridoxine deficiencies must be considered. In severe iron-deficiency anemia, blood transfusions are indicated as an emergency measure and as a means of direct administration of iron (Appendix Cases 33 and 34). Microcytic normochromic and normocytic hypochromic red cells may occur during development of classic iron-deficiency that would manifest later as microcytic hypochromic anemia. Microcytic normochromic red cells are a normal finding in some Akitas.

Classification Based on Bone Marrow Response

Based on bone marrow erythropoietic response evident in the peripheral blood, anemias are classified as responsive or regenerative and nonresponsive or nonregenerative. This classification is helpful in differentiation of blood loss and hemolytic anemias (generally responsive) from depression anemias (nonresponsive). A valid interpretation may require calculation of a corrected reticulocyte count or reticulocyte production index (see The Reticulocyte Count).

LABORATORY EVALUATION OF ANEMIAS

In this section, brief general and comparative comments are made on anemias of various types. Details on specific anemias can be found in Chapters 22 through 25. Interested readers may consult some recent reviews on the subject (Bamidele, 1979; Harvey, 1980; Hathaway, 1976; Hinton and Jones, 1977; Sutton, 1977).

Red Cell Parameters

Anemia is indicated when one or more of the red cell parameters (PCV, hemoglobin, and RBC count) is below the normal level for the age, sex, and breed of the species concerned. Geographic location with regard to altitude and laboratory errors affecting red cell parameters should be considered. Of the three red cell parameters, the packed cell volume (PCV) provides a simple, quick, and accurate means of detecting anemia; however, the PCV should not be considered a reliable indicator of anemia if the animal is known to have an exceptionally high (Poodles) or low (Akitas) MCV in health. In such cases, hemoglobin concentration should be considered to establish the presence of anemia. Dehydration and splenic contraction may mask the anemia at the initial blood examination but may be found, respectively, after the patient is rehydrated and emotionally adjusted. Females during the latter half or last trimester of pregnancy may have lower red cell values ("spurious anemia") than nonpregnant females because of increased plasma volume, although iron deficiency may also be a factor (see Chapter 22). Similarly, hemodilution following fluid therapy would temporarily reduce red cell parameters. Determination of both PCV and total plasma protein concentration is generally helpful in differentiating these variables. The protein value increases during dehydration, whereas it decreases during hemodilution and remains essentially unchanged when splenic contraction is involved. The changes in plasma protein concentration and the PCV during dehydration may be disproportionate in that the former may undergo a greater increase than the latter (Boyd, 1981). The PCV is influenced by changes in the MCV that vary inversely with alterations in the plasma osmolarity.

An analysis of admission hemograms of 1,000 canine patients indicated that mild anemia is more prevalent than marked anemia (Table 21–3). About two-thirds of the dogs exhibited mild anemia (PVC between 31 and 36%), about one-fourth had moderate anemia (PCV between 21 and 30%), and less than one-tenth had marked to severe anemia (PCV < 20%). The degree of anemia seemed to vary with the nature, extent, and duration of the disease process (Table 21–4).

The Reticulocyte Count

The reticulocyte count (Chapter 18) can be considered as the best semiquantitative indicator of effective marrow erythropoietic activity. For this reason, anemias are broadly classified as regenerative (responsive) or nonregenerative (nonresponsive).

Interpretation of reticulocyte counts should be made in relation to species differences in erythropoiesis and release of young red cells into the circulation. A small number of reticulocytes are normally found in the blood of dogs and cats but are not found in cattle, sheep, goats, and horses. Dogs respond to increased erythroid stimulation as do humans. Varied morphology of reticulocytes in the cat (Chapter 5) poses difficulty in obtaining a valid reticulocyte count and its proper interpretation; "punctate" reticulocytes exceed "aggregate" reticulocytes and persist in blood longer. In ruminants, the magnitude of reticulocyte response is less, and the presence of even some reticulocytes is evidence of responsive anemia. Horses do not exhibit reticulocytosis even when the anemia is extreme. Sometimes, a horse may respond with a marked anisocytosis as a result of macrocytosis (see Appendix Case 55). Until another means of evaluating erythropoietic response to anemia is discovered, bone marrow examination must be performed in the anemic horse to find evidence of increased erythroid precursors and reticulocytes.

The reticulocyte count generally varies with the degree of anemia (Table 21–3); the greater the marrow stimulation, the greater the reticulocytosis, and, conversely, the greater the marrow suppression, the greater the reticulocytopenia. Individual variations in reticulocyte counts may be noted, however, depending on the nature, duration, and extent of the disease process. The degree of reticulocytosis must be viewed in concert with the

Table 21–3. Degree of Anemia and Its Relationship to Reticulocyte Counts in Peripheral Blood of Canine Patients at Initial Examination

PCV* (%)	Patients		Number of Patients†	Reticulocyte Count (%)	
	Number	%		Range	Mean
<10	10	1.0	10	0–48.6	12.66
11–15	25	2.5	23	0–35.4	11.06
16–20	39	3.9	36	0–29.5	5.45
21–25	74	7.4	73	0–27.0	5.44
26–30	189	18.9	176	0–21.6	2.29
31–36	663	66.3	455	0–15.6	1.48

*Degree of anemia determined by packed cell volume (PCV) evaluation, normal range being 37–55%. A total of 1,000 patients were evaluated.

†Reticulocyte counts were performed only for 773 patients.

From Jain, 1979; courtesy of *California Veterinarian*.

Table 21–4. Degree of Anemia in Relation to Clinical Signs and Diagnosis at Initial Examination of 1,000 Canine Patients

PCV (%)	Clinical Signs or Diagnosis
<10	Autoimmune hemolytic anemia, chronic blood loss, lymphosarcoma, idiopathic.
11–15	Autoimmune hemolytic anemia, renal disease, hepatic disease, splenic tumor, idiopathic.
15–20	Autoimmune hemolytic anemia, idiopathic or autoimmune thrombocytopenia, renal disease, bleeding disorder, hemorrhage, babesiasis.
20–25	Autoimmune hemolytic anemia, idiopathic or autoimmune thrombocytopenia, bleeding disorder, renal disease, liver disease, hemorrhage. Lymphocytic leukemia; chronic and suppurative lesions; bacterial, viral, and fungal infections, chronic weight loss; neurologic disturbance.
26–30	Similar to dogs with PCV of 20–25% with addition of disseminated intravascular coagulation, dirofilariasis, Cushing's syndrome, Addison's disease.
31–36	Similar to dogs with PCV of 20–25% with addition of ectoparasites; immune-mediated disorders such as systemic lupus erythematosus, rheumatoid arthritis, and gammopathy; endocrine disorders such as Addison's disease, diabetes mellitus, and hypothyroidism.

From Jain, 1979; courtesy of *California Veterinarian.*

degree of anemia. For example, a reticulocyte count of 4% at a PCV of 15% in the dog indicates an inadequate response, whereas it would be an adequate response at a PCV of 32%. Calculation of an absolute reticulocyte count or a corrected reticulocyte count or "reticulocyte production index" (Chapter 18) eliminates error in misinterpretation from the degree of anemia and premature release of reticulocytes from the bone marrow into the circulation. The magnitude of reticulocytosis generally is greater in hemolytic anemia than in blood loss anemia, and it is least in nonresponsive (depression) anemias. One must be cognizant, however, that it takes about 3 days for a significant reticulocytosis to be found in blood after an acute hemolytic or hemorrhagic episode. It takes about 5–7 days for a maximum response, provided the bone marrow is functioning optimally and required ingredients are plentiful. The response sub-

sequently diminishes and reticulocytosis disappears by 2 weeks. A particularly anemic patient may be seen when the erythropoietic response is not necessarily at the peak level. For example, a dog on the first day of blood loss or hemolytic episode may appear to have a nonresponsive, normocytic-normochromic anemia that can be mistaken for a hypoproliferative anemia. Repeat reticulocyte counts, at least 3 days apart, must be made to distinguish such situations, particularly when history and clinical signs are not helpful diagnostically.

Thus, reticulocytosis in an anemic patient indicates increased red cell destruction or blood loss. Reticulocytosis without evidence of anemia may indicate reduced oxygenation of blood causing an artificial hypoxic situation leading to increased erythropoietin production which in turn stimulates erythropoiesis and release of reticulocytes from the bone marrow. On the contrary, the absence of reticulocytosis in an anemic patient is suggestive of reduced erythropoietin production, marrow depression or failure, defective iron utilization, or increased ineffective erythropoiesis. Bone marrow examination is necessary to evaluate erythrogenesis in such patients.

Red Cell Indices

Red cell indices have been commented on in the previous section, Morphologic Classification. It is emphasized that erthrocyte morphology, noted on careful examination of blood film, must always be considered in conjunction with MCV and MCHC values for proper interpretation of the red cell indices. The red cell indices represent values for an average (mean) erythrocyte in a given population. Usually there is a good correlation between red cell indices and carefully gained microscopic impression of red cell size and hemoglobin content. Differences in a minority of red cell population or extreme changes in the opposite direction, however, may not be reflected in the red cell indices, but may be evident on smear examination. For example, the MCV may be within the normal range despite a marked reticulocytosis (Fig. 18–11). This may occur when reticulocytosis is accompanied with a significant number of spherocytes or microcytic red cells. The MCHC may be disproportionately reduced when reticulocytosis is accompanied with hypochromic red cells, whether they are normocytic or microcytic. One should also remember that a slight technical error or diurnal variation in red cell parameters can so alter the red cell indices that two hemograms on the same patient may appear inconsistent.

Erythrocyte Morphology

The diagnostic significance of erythrocyte morphology has not been explored as much in veterinary medicine as in human medicine. Important clues as to the specific cause(s) or pathophysiologic process(es) of anemia and bone marrow erythropoietic activity can be obtained from careful examination of erythrocyte morphology in a good, Wright-stained film (Figs. 20–5, 20–6). Canine red cells are normally uniformly biconcave with central pallor and measure about 7.0 µm in diameter; these cells offer more of an opportunity to witness morphologic changes than other animal species' red cells. The red cells should be examined for abnormalities of size, shape, and color, the degree of such abnormality, and the presence of inclusions. The following section gives a brief description, and Fig. 21–1 depicts red cell morphology in various anemias. For additional information on abnormal erythrocyte morphology and its interpretation see Chapter 20.

Comments regarding the significance of finding macrocytic and microcytic red cells, whether hypochromic or normochromic, have been made in the previous section. Hypochromic red cells show an increase in the area of central pallor and are fairly easy to detect. Experience is necessary to detect macrocytosis or microcytosis in blood films. A comparison with morphology of erythrocytes in a normal blood film may be helpful in such situations. Nucleated red cells or erythrocytes containing Howell-Jolly bodies appear in increasing numbers during responsive anemia, but may also reflect other causes such as reduced splenic function (see Chapter 18). Nucleated erythrocytes may occur in excessive numbers in dogs with lead poisoning and in cats with myeloproliferative disorders, e.g., erythremic myelosis and erythroleukemia.

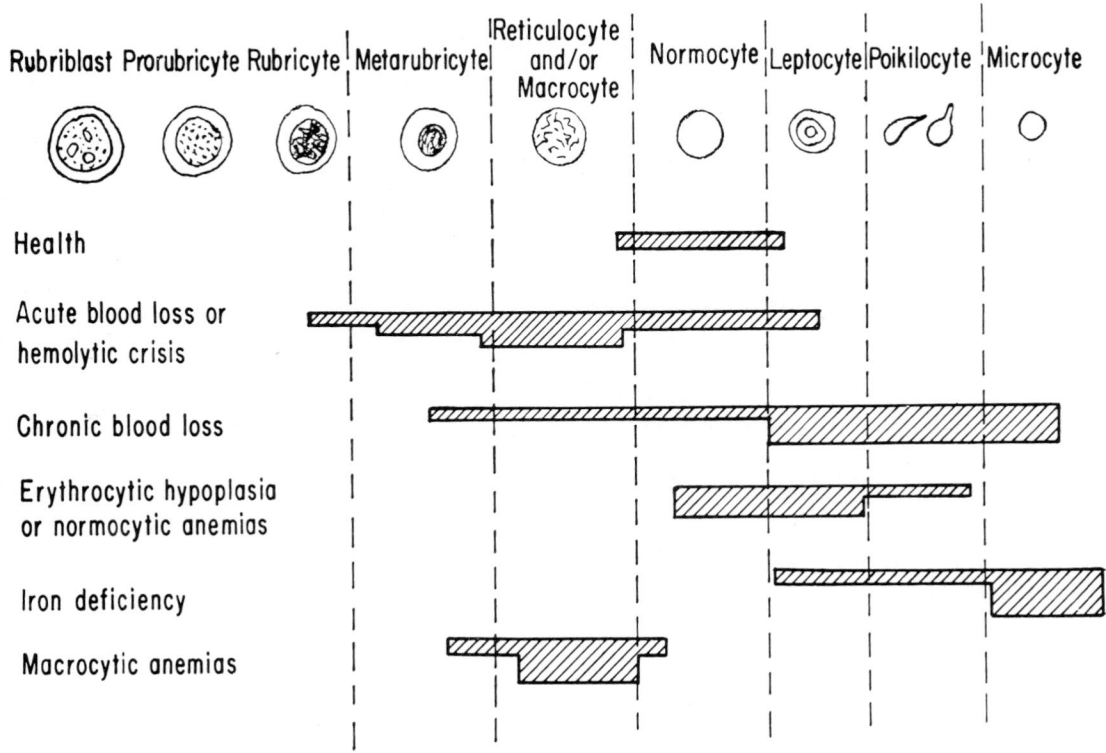

Fig. 21–1. Erythrocyte morphology in the various types of anemias.

The occurrence in peripheral blood of nucleated erythrocytes in conjunction with immature neutrophils (shift to the left) is termed *leukoerythroblastic reaction*. Such a blood picture may be observed in a variety of conditions such as during an intense hematopoietic response to acute blood loss or hemolytic anemia, disseminated hemangiosarcoma, and myeloproliferative disorders (Delsol et al., 1979; Shull, 1981b). Heinz bodies indicate oxidative denaturation of hemoglobin and are associated with causation of hemolytic anemia. Pappenheimer bodies (Plate XII–9), small bluish granules that stain positive for iron (Plate XII–10), are found in an occasional young red cell during responsive anemia (particularly hemolytic anemia). Basophilic stippling, representing aggregation of ribosomal material, is seen characteristically in dogs with lead poisoning, but it also may be seen in dogs and cats during an intense response to anemia. It is a normal occurrence in ruminants during responsive anemia.

Crenation is artifactual and is found to a variable extent in almost all blood films. Markedly crenated red cells known as "burr" cells are seen characteristically in humans who have renal disease with uremia; they have also been found in some canine patients with the same disease. Acanthocytes are typically seen in humans with abetalipoproteinemia and liver disease with hemolytic anemia. They have been seen in dogs with hemangiosarcoma and severe liver disease with hyperbilirubinemia. Spherocytes are characteristic of autoimmune hemolytic anemia, and agglutinated erythrocytes indicate the presence of cold agglutinins with or without concurrent anemia. Poikilocytes occur in anemias involving red cell fragmentation and are found in iron deficiency anemia. Schistocytes or other fragmented forms of red cells occur in a variety of conditions associated with hemolytic anemias from red cell trauma and suggest the possibility of disseminated intravascular coagulation (DIC) or hemolytic-uremic syndrome (Musgrave et al., 1978; Rebar et al., 1981). Target cells occur in anemias involving reduced hemoglobin synthesis, in liver disease with icterus, in obstructive jaundice, after splenectomy, and in marrow suppression. Leptocytes may be found along with target cells, particularly in chronic diseases and in liver disease. Leptocytosis may be seen in dogs with hypothyroidism. "Tear drop" red cells and ovalocytes are indicative of disordered erythropoiesis as in myeloproliferative disorders, myelofibrosis, or myelophthisis. For additional details of erythrocyte morphology see Chapter 20 and Figs. 20–5 through 20–9.

Other Hematologic Findings

Icterus index may be increased in hemolytic anemias, and it is normal in depression anemias and in anemias from blood loss except when hemorrhage occurs in body cavities. Hemoglobinemia is an early manifestation of a severe hemolytic anemia developing from intravascular lysis of red cells. Total plasma protein concentration is usually reduced in anemias from external blood loss and infestation with bloodsucking parasites; depression or hemolytic anemias do not show such changes in plasma protein levels. Total and differential leukocyte counts are variable, more so because of the primary disease responsible for the anemia than because of the anemia itself. During an intense response to anemia, however, reticulocytosis may be accompanied by a neutrophilia with left shift (see Chapter 18). This is particularly common in hemolytic anemias in the dog. Monocytosis often is encountered in autoimmune hemolytic anemia in the dog. Osmotic fragility is increased in hemolytic anemias from a variety of causes (see Chapter 20).

Bone Marrow Examination

Bone marrow examination in anemias is performed primarily to evaluate the erythropoietic response. Generally, during responsive phase hemolytic and blood loss anemias are accompanied with an increased erythropoiesis and a reduced myeloid:erythroid ratio (Table 6–13). This is often evident from reticulocytosis in the peripheral blood, and a bone marrow examination is usually unnecessary. Erythropoiesis is reduced in depression anemias yielding an elevated myeloid:erythroid ratio (Table 6–13). Erythropoiesis is disturbed in anemias of nutritional deficiencies such as those of iron (Chapter 22) and vitamin B_{12} (Chapter 25). Megaloblastic erythroid precursors are a remarkable finding in erythremic myelosis and erythroleukemia in the cat (Chapter 32).

Bone marrow of Poodles with macrocytosis simulating vitamin B_{12}-folate deficiency exhibits hypersegmented neutrophils, giant metamyelocytes, erythrocytes with multiple Howell-Jolly bodies, and aberrant nuclear mitosis and fragmentation in erythroid cells. Bone marrow iron, estimated after Prussian blue staining (Plate XII–11) is decreased in iron deficiency anemias, whereas it is increased in anemias of inflammatory disease. Both of these situations are associated with decreased numbers of marrow sideroblasts, although sideroblasts are increased in iron-overload situations and the so-called sideroblastic anemia (Cartwright and Deiss, 1975).

Bone marrow examination is essential to evaluate response to anemia in the horse (Schalm, 1975). In this species, reticulocytes normally mature in the bone marrow prior to their release as red cells into the circulation in health and during response to anemia, whether from blood loss or hemolytic process. In such instances, an increase in marrow reticulocyte numbers of over 5% is considered evidence for an effective erythropoiesis.

Other Laboratory Tests

The newly formed red cells released into the peripheral blood present certain biochemical attributes that could be measured to detect effective erythrogenesis. Those with promising application have included red cell adenosine-5-triphosphate (Smith and Agar, 1976), creatine (Fehr and Knob, 1979; Shull, 1981a; Wu et al., 1983), and glucose-6-phosphate dehydrogenase (Shull, 1981a). Measurement of red cell lactic dehydrogenase was considered a good measure of response to hemolytic anemia (Shull, 1981). These observations need to be extended to provide a routinely applicable laboratory procedure for evaluation of responsive anemia in the horse.

Fecal examination for occult blood is usually positive during bleeding into the gastrointestinal tract. Omnivores often have a positive fecal blood test because of hemoglobin in the meat diet. Excretion of urobilinogen in the urine increases during hemolytic anemias. Urinary excretion of bile also increases in hemolytic anemia as long as the liver is able to conjugate excessive hemoglobin released during the hemolytic process. See Chapter 19 for details of urinary excretion of bile and urobilinogen. Hemoglobinemia, methemoglobinemia, and hemoglobinuria may be evident in hemolytic anemia. Total serum bilirubin is normal in depression anemias and anemias from blood loss to external sites. A van den Bergh test may help differentiate hyperbilirubinemia of hemolytic anemia from hepatic disease and intrahepatic or posthepatic cholestasis, particularly in the dog (Chapter 19). Haptoglobin (Marchand et al., 1980), hemopexin, and methemalbumin determinations also may be helpful in defining hemolytic anemias (see Chapter 19). Radiologic examination and other necessary diagnostic tests may have to be performed to determine the primary cause of the anemia. Comments regarding a variety of specific tests performed in evaluating a particular type of anemia are made at appropriate places in Chapters 22 through 25.

THERAPEUTIC ASPECTS OF ANEMIA

After an anemia has been detected, it is important to determine its duration and significance in relation to the possible pathophysiology and effect on the patient. A mild anemia may be of little consequence to the patient, but it may have a serious cause such as a bleeding tumor. On the contrary, a moderate anemia affects the patient's well-being and marked anemia may undoubtedly be life-threatening, regardless of the cause. Similarly, acute anemia is more serious than chronic anemia in which physiologic adjustments have incurred. Massive blood loss within a short period requires immediate treatment for shock and restoration of blood volume for adequate oxygenation. Subsequently, materials essential for erythrocyte production must be provided to ensure a rapid and appropriate bone marrow response. This entails providing an adequate and nutritious diet and rational administration of hematinics that include various iron preparations, B-vitamins, and trace elements. Most important, the cause of anemia should be sought and appropriately managed or treated, if possible. Specific measures may vary from surgical intervention to treatment with antibiotics, specific drugs, and various immunosuppressive agents. Corticosteroids and androgens have been used to stimulate red cell production.

Blood transfusions are given: *(a)* to prevent shock from loss of blood volume in acute hemorrhage; *(b)* to improve the oxygen-carrying capacity of the blood, which permits the patient to function more normally; and *(c)* to attempt to restore a normal maturation of erythrocytes in certain "idiopathic" anemias by temporarily giving the erythropoietic tissue a rest.

The existence of anemia by itself is not justification for a blood transfusion. In chronically developing anemia, the physiologic adjustments are such that the hemoglobin may drop to 50% of the minimum normal without significant signs of anemia. We have seen dogs with a PCV of less than 10% still standing; such cases fall into category *(b)* of the reasons for giving blood transfusions as described above. In end stage kidney disease, depression of erythropoiesis occurs, and a progressive anemia develops. The PCV may fall below 20%, but this does not mean that a blood transfusion is required or will be helpful. In fact, these cases are terminal, and the administration of blood is a waste of the veterinarian's time and the client's financial resources (Appendix Case 5).

We commonly give blood transfusions to a dog with a PCV of 12% or less and to a cat with a PCV of 10% or less. The need for whole blood transfusion becomes less once evidence of active erythropoiesis makes its appearance in the circulation, provided there is no continuing blood loss through hemorrhage. Increased erythropoietic activity is immediately suppressed following blood transfusion (Fig. 35–1).

For more information on blood transfusion see Chapter 35.

POLYCYTHEMIA

An increase in erythrocyte number above normal in blood is generally referred to as polycythemia (Table 21–5). *Primary polycythemia,* a myeloproliferative disorder, is usu-

Table 21–5. Classification of Polycythemias in Humans and Animals

A. Absolute Polycythemia
   Primary Polycythemia
      Polycythemia vera, a malignant hematopoietic stem cell disorder

   Secondary Polycythemia
      Hypoxic increase in erythropoietin production
         Reduced atmospheric oxygen
         Pulmonary hypoxia
         Cardiovascular disease (right to left shunts)
         Reduced oxygen transport by hemoglobin
      Autonomous increase in erythropoietin production
         Nonneoplastic renal diseases, e.g., cysts and hydronephrosis
         Neoplastic diseases, e.g., renal tumors, hepatomas, uterine leiomyomas, cerebellar hemangioblastomas
      Familial erythrocytosis in humans
B. Relative Polycythemia
      Dehydration from various causes
      Splenic contraction

ally called polycythemia vera. It is characterized by abnormal proliferation of erythroid, granulocytic, and megakaryocytic cells leading to an absolute increase in red cell mass along with elevated total leukocyte and platelet counts. *Secondary polycythemia,* sometimes called erythrocytosis, accompanies a variety of conditions associated with increased erythropoietin production. Measuring the body red cell mass using ^{51}Cr-labeled red cells and the body plasma volume using ^{131}I-albumin or other suitable methods is indicated in patients with suspected polycythemia. An increase in total red cell mass without a significant decrease in plasma volume is suggestive of primary or secondary polycythemia, whereas *relative polycythemia* (erythrocytosis) is characterized by a normal red cell mass and a decreased plasma volume.

Differentiation of primary and secondary polycythemias requires a detailed history, thorough physical examination, chest roentgenogram, and laboratory tests necessary to establish the diagnosis. Determination of arterial PO_2 and serum or urinary erythropoietin concentration is essential. Arterial oxygen saturation is low and serum or urinary erythropoietin levels are high in secondary polycythemia, whereas in primary polycythemia the oxygen saturation is normal and erythropoietin levels are usually below normal. In relative polycythemia, oxygen saturation as well as erythropoietin levels are normal.

Therapeutic management is based on correct diagnosis. A mild erythrocytosis is inconsequential, but excessive red cell mass increases blood viscosity and pulmonary vascular resistance and decreases cardiac output. This leads to decreased blood flow and reduced tissue oxygenation (Murray, et al., 1963). In primary polycythemia, phlebotomy is done to reduce erythrocyte counts to a low-normal range and chemotherapy and radiation therapy (^{32}P) are given to diminish erythropoiesis. Death occurs from vascular complications or other undetermined causes.

Absolute Polycythemia

Primary Polycythemia

In human medicine, primary polycythemia is referred to by various names such as polycythemia rubra vera, polycythemia vera, erythremia, and Vaquez-Osler disease. Studies on the pathogenesis of polycythemia vera indicate that it is an acquired clonal disorder of the pluripotential stem cell resulting in expansion of committed stem cell pools, primarily of the erythrocytic lines (Golde and Cline, 1976). Thus, polycythemia vera is a myeloproliferative disorder mainly involving overproduction of red cells. Leukocytosis and thrombocytosis commonly accompany the disorder, and it may eventually terminate in myelofibrosis or acute granulocytic leukemia. Diagnosis of polycythemia vera requires the demonstration of an absolute increase in total erythrocyte volume associated with a normal arterial blood oxygen saturation of no less than 90%. In the absence of cardiopulmonary lesion, an intravenous pyelogram is done to rule out abnormalities of renal perfusion; this is followed by hemoglobin characterization and determination of oxygen dissociation curves. Most importantly, erythropoietin levels are measured in plasma or urine. Plasma erythropoietin level is either normal or subnormal. Red cell life span is normal and morphology is unchanged unless iron deficiency exists. Splenomegaly and hepatomegaly may be seen in some patients. Bone marrow findings include excessive hematopoiesis, increased magakaryocyte ploidy, and reduced iron stores.

Polycythemia vera is a rare disease in animals although it has been described in the dog, cat, and ox. Cole (1954) described polycythemia in a 2-year-old cocker spaniel, and Miller (1968) briefly described polycythemia vera in a 3-year-old boxer dog. Neither author performed blood volume and oxygen saturation studies for lack of facilities. Donovan and Loeb (1959) reported the first authentic case of canine polycythemia vera in a 5-year-old male English cocker spaniel. Their diagnosis was based on blood volume studies, with verification at necropsy of the absence of heart disease, pulmonary disease, and dehydration. Carb (1969) diagnosed polycythemia vera in a 2-year-old male terrier-type dog that had PCV values of 77–80%, hemoglobin levels of 21.5–24.5 g/dl, and RBC counts of 10.1–10.5 million/µl of blood. Erythrocyte morphology was normal. Total leukocyte count was elevated moderately initially (22,370/µl) but later diminished to normal. Platelet counts were below normal (82,000–136,000/µl) but increased to normal during therapy. Carb stated that the polycythemia vera was treated successfully by removing relatively large amounts of blood and administering uracil mustard to depress the production of erythrocytes. Polycythemia vera in a 5-year-old Labrador retriever bitch was treated using ^{32}P (Bush and Fankhouser, 1972). Polycythemia vera in a 14-month-old intact female Old English sheepdog is described in Appendix Case 17. McGrath (1974) and Peterson and Randolph (1982) reviewed literature on polycythemia vera in the dog and presented three additional cases each. In comparison to humans, canine patients appeared to be young to middle-age dogs without sex or breed distribution; rarely present splenomegaly and hepatomegaly; do not exhibit pruritus, peptic ulceration, hyperkaratosis, and hyperuricemia; and rarely have accompanied leukocytosis and thrombocytosis. Treatment of three dogs with hydroxyurea was found to manage the disease successfully for a mean period of 16.6 months (Peterson and Randolph, 1982).

Polycythemia vera in a 15-year-old altered male Maltese cat was reported by Reed et al. (1970).

A Hereford steer, approximately 8 months

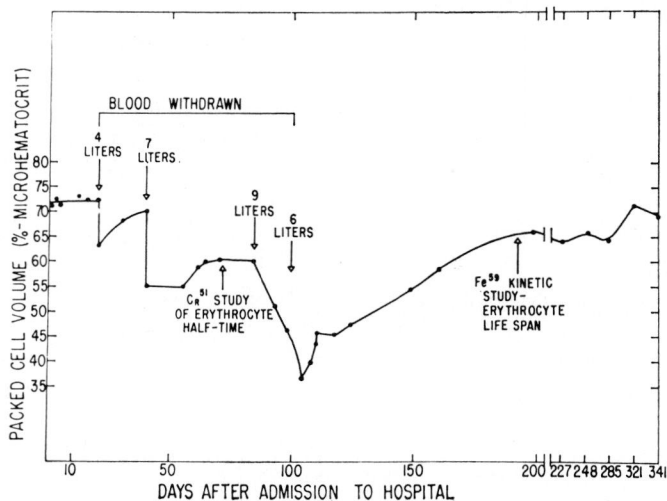

Fig. 21–2. Packed cell volumes of erythrocytes in a steer with polycythemia vera. Effects of blood withdrawal on the PCV and subsequent regeneration of erythrocytes are shown. (From Fowler et al., 1964; courtesy of *Cornell Veterinarian*.)

of age, was presented to our clinic with apparent blindness and nervous irritability. Physical examination revealed a steer in good flesh with an ulceration of the anterior border of the dental pad, a nasal discharge, and intensely red conjunctival mucous membrane. The PCV was 70–72% with the Wintrobe hematocrit method and 60–65% with the Drummond microhematocrit method, the difference being due to retention of a greater amount of trapped plasma in the red cell column by the former technique (see Chapter 2). The steer was maintained under observation for 1 year, and blood was withdrawn in amounts of 4–9 liters on 4 separate occasions. The series of phlebotomies, conducted over a period of 70 days, reduced the PCV from 71% to 35% (Fig. 21–2). The steer's vision improved, and weight gain averaged 0.8 lb/day. After the last bleeding, the PCV gradually increased again, reaching 48% at 1 month, 58% at 2 months, 63% at 3 months, and finally approached the admission level of 70%. When the PCV was at its maximum level, RBC counts were 20–24 million/µl and hemoglobin concentration was 20–23 g/dl. The erythrocytes were normocytic-normochromic and erythrokinetic studies with ^{51}Cr and ^{59}Fe indicated an overproduction of erythrocytes of normal life span. Total blood volume was calculated to be 18.5 liters, and red cell mass to be 10 liters. Total leukocyte counts were between 12,000 and 18,000/µl with normal differential distribution of various leukocytes. Central nervous system signs of circling and irritability were observed terminally. The steer was destroyed, and a detailed gross necropsy and histopathologic examination revealed no significant anatomic or pathologic deviations that could account for the polycythemia vera. Fowler et al. (1964) concluded that all laboratory studies confirmed the case to be primary polycythemia.

Familial polycythemia in 14 Jersey calves, all members of an inbred family of Jersey cattle maintained for genetic studies at the University of California, was described by Tennant et al. (1967). Polycythemia developed as early as the second month of life and persisted throughout the first year among 5 surviving calves. This development was followed by remission of signs of plethora by maturity. The genetic pattern was consistent with a simple recessive mode of inheritance. The polycythemic state was characterized by PCV values of 60–80%, RBC counts of 15.8–25.5 million/µl, hemoglobin concentrations of 19.2–27.2 g/dl, and WBC counts varying from normal to a high of 33,000/µl. Clinical signs were congested mucous membranes, dyspnea, and reduced weight gains. Arterial oxygen tension was within normal limits in 2 calves studied. Erythrocyte life span studies in one calf gave normal findings. Total erythrocyte and plasma volume studies on 4 calves indicated significantly elevated erythrocyte volumes, thereby establishing the primary nature of the polycythemia. Necropsy findings further substantiated the primary nature of the polycythemia, for no lesions were found that might have induced a polycythemia.

Secondary Polycythemia

Secondary polycythemia is a result of increased erythropoiesis mediated by an excessive production of erythropoietin. Erythropoietin levels are increased either as a compensatory physiologic response by the kidney to tissue hypoxia or as a result of autonomous production independent of tissue oxygen supply.

Secondary polycythemia in response to tissue hypoxia is seen in people and animals living at high altitudes. It may be anticipated in some cardiovascular diseases and chronic pulmonary diseases. Secondary polycythemia is seen in animals with tetralogy of Fallot, a congenital cardiac disorder leading to shunting of a portion of blood from the right to the left side of the heart, bypassing the lungs (Appendix Case 18). Tetralogy of Fallot has been described in the dog (Hamlin et al., 1962; Meredith and Clarkson, 1959), cat (Bolton et al., 1972; Bush et al., 1972), cow (Cordy and Ribelin, 1950; Fisher and Pirie, 1964), and horse (Prickett et al., 1973). Arterial oxygen saturation is below normal in such patients. Carboxyhemoglobinemia in cigarette smokers and rare hemoglobinopathies interfering with oxygenation have been found to cause mild polycythemia in humans.

Other forms of secondary polycythemia occur in humans more commonly in association with certain types of kidney disease (hydronephrosis, cysts, carcinoma, and adenoma) and less commonly in association with neoplasms of the liver, cerebellar hemangioblastoma, pheochromocytoma, adrenal adenoma, and uterine fibroid. Polycythemia associated with space-occupying lesions of the kidney and neoplasia of various organs appears to be the result of stimulation of erythrogenesis by lesion-related erythropoietin production (Penington, 1965). Arterial oxygen saturation is normal in these forms of polycythemia. Tumor-induced secondary polycythemia has been reported in canines with renal carcinoma (Peterson and Zanjani, 1981; Scott and Patnaik, 1972).

A familial erythrocytosis due to autonomous erythropoietin production has been described in a few human families (Wintrobe et al., 1981).

Erythrocytosis of rather undefined etiology was reported in a horse with normal serum erythropoietin levels (Beech et al., 1984).

Relative Polycythemia

Relative polycythemia is commonly encountered in animals as a result of reduction in plasma volume from dehydration. Water intake by sick animals commonly is inadequate to maintain normal body water content. Diseases accompanied with excessive loss of water (e.g., diarrhea, vomiting, and polyuria from electrolyte imbalance) can quickly produce dehydration. First body water is given up by the muscles and skin but finally the blood plasma also becomes involved in water loss, leading to concentration of the formed elements and some chemical constituents (hemoconcentration). Examples are Cushing's disease and pancreatitis. Profuse sweating in horses, as during endurance rides, can cause hemoconcentration (Fig. 6–4).

Another form of relative polycythemia occurs in excitable animals, such as certain breeds of dogs and horses, as the result of the injection of a mass of concentrated erythrocytes into the circulation on contraction of the spleen (see Chapter 6). Splenic contraction also may occur under conditions of severe pain, e.g., in horses with colic. Although splenic contraction does not ordinarily cause relative polycythemia in humans (Wintrobe et al., 1981), a form of relative polycythemia, termed "stress polycythemia" is described, most commonly in obese, chronically anxious, middle-aged males with a high incidence of hypertension (Lawrence and Berlin, 1952). Relative polycythemia reverts to normal as dehydration is relieved or when circumstances leading to splenic contraction no longer exist. Phlebotomy and chemotherapy are contraindicated.

REFERENCES

Bamidele, O.: Clinico-Pathological Studies of Anaemia in Domestic Ruminants. Bull. Anim. Health Prod. Africa, *27*:181, 1979.

Beech, J., et al.: Erythrocytosis in a Horse. J. Amer. Vet. Med. Ass., *184*:986, 1984.

Bolton, G.R., et al.: Tetralogy of Fallot in Three Cats. J. Amer. Vet. Med. Ass., *160*:1622, 1972.

Boyd, J.W.: The Relationship Between Blood Haemoglobin Concentration, Packed Cell Volume, and Plasma Protein Concentration in Dehydration. Brit. Vet. J., *137*:166, 1981.

Bush, B.M., and Fankhouser, R.: Polycythemia Vera in a Bitch. J. Small Anim. Pract., *13*:75, 1972.

Bush, M., et al.: Tetralogy of Fallot in a Cat. J. Amer. Vet. Med. Ass., *161*:1679, 1972.

Carb, A.V.: Polycythemia Vera in a Dog. J. Amer. Vet. Med. Ass., *151*:289, 1969.

Cartwright, G.E., and Deiss, A.: Sideroblasts, Siderocytes, and Sideroblastic Anemia. New Eng. J. Med., *292*:185, 1975.

Cole, N.: Polycythemia in a Dog. North Amer. Vet., *35*:601, 1954.

Cordy, D.R., and Ribelin, W.E.: Six Congenital Cardiac Anomalies in Animals. Cornell Vet., *40*:249, 1950.

Delsol, G., et al.: Leukoerythroblastosis and Cancer Frequency, Prognosis and Physiopathologic Significance. Cancer, *44*:1009, 1979.

Donovan, E.F., and Loeb, W.F.: Polycythemia Rubra Vera in the Dog. J. Amer. Vet. Med. Ass., *131*:36, 1959.

Fehr, J., and Knob, M.: Comparison of Red Cell Creatine Level and Reticulocyte Count in Appraising the Severity of Hemolytic Processes. Blood, *53*:966, 1979.

Fisher, E.W., and Pirie, H.M.: Tetralogy of Fallot in a Friesian Heifer. Brit. Heart J., *26*:97, 1964.

Fowler, M.E., et al.: Clinical and Erythrokinetic Studies on a Case of Bovine Polycythemia Vera. Cornell Vet., *54*:153, 1964.

Golde, D.W., and Cline, M.J.: Pathogenesis of Polycythemia Vera—New Concepts. Amer. J. Hematol., *1*:351, 1976.

Hamlin, R.L., et al.: Antemortem Diagnosis of Tetralogy of Fallot in a Dog. J. Amer. Vet. Med. Ass., *140*:948, 1962.

Harvey, J.W.: Canine Hemolytic Anemias. J. Amer. Vet. Med. Ass., *176*:970, 1980.

Hathaway, J.E.: Feline Anemia. Vet. Clin. North Amer., *6*:495, 1976.

Hinton, M., and Jones, D.R.E.: Anaemia in the Dog: An Analysis of Laboratory Data. J. Small Anim. Pract., *18*:701, 1977.

Jain, N.C.: Hematologic Characteristics of Anemia. II. Interpretive Aspects. Calif. Vet., *33*(10):15, 1979.

Lawrence, J.H., and Berlin, N.I.: Relative Polycythemia-The Polycythemia of Stress. Yale J. Biol. Med., *24*:498, 1952.

Marchand, A., et al.: The Predictive Value of Serum Haptoglobin in Hemolytic Disease. J. Amer. Vet. Med. Ass., *243*:1909, 1980.

McGrath, C.J.: Polycythemia Vera in Dogs. J. Amer. Vet. Med. Ass., *164*:1117, 1974.

Meredith, J.H., and Clarkson, T.B.: Tetralogy of Fallot in the Dog. J. Amer. Vet. Med. Ass., *135*:326, 1959.

Miller, R.M.: Polycythemia Vera in a Dog. Vet. Med. Small Anim. Clin., *63*:222, 1968.

Murray, J.F., et al.: The Circulatory Effects of Hematocrit Variations in Normovolemic and Hypervolemic Dogs. J. Clin. Invest., *42*:1150, 1963.

Musgrave, J.E., et al.: The Hemolytic Uremic Syndrome. Clin. Pediatr., *17*:218, 1978.

Penington, D.G.: Polycythaemia in Neoplastic Diseases. Proc. Roy. Soc. Med., *58*:488, 1965.

Peterson, M.E., and Randolph, J.F.: Diagnosis of Canine Primary Polycythemia and Management with Hydroxyurea. J. Amer. Vet. Med. Ass., *180*:415, 1982.

Peterson, M.E., and Zanjani, E.D.: Inappropriate Erythropoietin Production from a Renal Carcinoma in a Dog with Polycythemia. J. Amer. Vet. Med. Ass., *179*:995, 1981.

Prickett, M.E., et al.: Tetralogy of Fallot in the Thoroughbred Foal. J. Amer. Vet. Med. Ass., *162*:552, 1973.

Rebar, A.H., et al.: Red Cell Fragmentation in the Dog. An Editorial Review. Vet. Pathol., *18*(4):415, 1981.

Reed, C., et al.: Polycythemia Vera in a Cat. J. Amer. Vet. Med. Ass., *157*:85, 1970.

Schalm, O.W.: Equine Hematology: Part IV. Erythroid Marrow Cytology in Response to Anemia. Calif. Vet., *29*(10):8, 1975.

Scott, R.C., and Patnaik, A.K.: Renal Carcinoma Associated with Secondary Polycythemia in the Dog. J. Amer. Anim. Hosp. Ass., *8*:275, 1972.

Shull, R.M.: Biochemical Changes in Equine Erythrocytes During Experimental Regenerative Anemia. Cornell Vet., *71*:280, 1981a.

Shull, R.M.: Inappropriate Marrow Release of Hematopoietic Precursors in Three Dogs. Vet. Pathol., *18*:569, 1981b.

Smith, J.E., and Agar, N.S.: Studies on Erythrocyte Metabolism Following Acute Blood Loss in the Horse. Equine Vet. J., *8*:34, 1976.

Sutton, R.H.: Some Anaemias of Farm Livestock. N. Z. Vet. J., *25*:308, 1977.

Tennant, B., et al.: Familial Polycythemia in Cattle. J. Amer. Vet. Med. Ass., *150*:1493, 1967.

Wintrobe, M.M., et al.: Clinical Hematology. 8th Ed. Lea & Febiger, Philadelphia, 1981.

Wu, M.-J., et al.: Using Red Blood Cell Creatine Concentration to Evaluate the Equine Erythropoietic Response. Amer. J. Vet. Res., *44*:1427, 1983.

22

Blood Loss or Hemorrhagic Anemias

ACUTE BLOOD LOSS 577
    Changes in the Peripheral Blood 577
    Bone Marrow Response 580

CHRONIC BLOOD LOSS 581
    Iron Deficiency Anemia 581
    Blood Loss Anemia Associated with
      Parasitism 584

Hemodynamic effects and changes in total blood volume as well as plasma volume following acute and chronic blood losses have been described in Chapter 3. Additional information on acute blood loss in the horse is given in Chapter 6. This chapter is concerned primarily with hematologic changes in blood and bone marrow following such losses of blood.

ACUTE BLOOD LOSS

Changes in the Peripheral Blood

A significant loss of blood within a few minutes to over several hours constitutes acute blood loss. Such losses may occur owing to a variety of circumstances (Table 22–1). Hemodynamic, blood volume, and hematologic changes vary with the amount of blood loss and its location. Experimental studies on various animal species have provided information in this regard. Blood may be lost externally or internally into body cavities. A small amount of blood loss in relation to body weight is well tolerated, whereas a larger volume may have significant immediate effects and could be fatal (see Chapter 3). Manifestation of hemodynamic effects and circulatory adjustments begin immediately. Splenic reserve of erythrocytes is injected into the circulation of certain animal species, particularly the horse (see Chapter 6). Even though extravascular fluid begins to move into the vascular space within a few minutes of a significant blood loss, a blood sample taken within a few hours often yields normal values for RBC count, PCV, hemoglobin level, and total plasma protein concentration. Expansion of

Table 22–1. Causes of Blood Loss or Hemorrhagic Anemias

Acute Blood Loss
  Trauma and surgical procedures
  Bleeding lesions
  Coagulation disorders
    Bracken fern poisoning in cattle
    Sweet clover hay (dicumarol) poisoning in cattle
    Warfarin poisoning
    Disseminated intravascular coagulation from various causes
  Thrombocytopenia (see Table 17–4)
  Parasites
    Haemonchus; hookworms; coccidia

Chronic Blood Loss
  Gastrointestinal lesions
    Neoplasms particularly leiomyomas; ulcers, parasitism such as coccidiosis
  Neoplasms with bleeding into body cavities and tissues
    Hemangiosarcoma in the dog
  Coagulation disorders
    Vitamin K and prothrombin deficiencies
    Hemophilia A in dogs and foals
  Thrombocytopenia
  Parasites
    Ticks, bloodsucking lice, sticktight fleas; hookworms; haemonchus

plasma volume is indicated by a diminishing total plasma protein concentration, which precedes decreases in red cell parameters. Such a decrease in plasma protein concentration may be evident as early as 1 hour after blood loss and a significant diminution is seen by 4 hours (Table 22–2). A 100% restoration of blood volume may be accomplished within 24 hours (Torten and Schalm, 1964). The resulting hemodilution produces a fall in red cell parameters and plasma protein concentrations. Thus, a blood sample collected after a day or so of blood loss, remarkably reveals a normocytic-normochromic anemia accompanied by hypoproteinemia. Reticulocyte response is not evident for the first 3–4 days, hence blood loss anemia at this stage can be mistaken for a depression anemia. Information derived from patient history and physical examination should help differentiate this. Plasma protein concentration begins to increase by 2–3 days and is usually normal within 5–7 days, long before restoration of red cell parameters.

A persistently low level of plasma proteins suggests continuing blood loss. Also, a diminished plasma protein value in an anemic patient is suggestive of external blood loss wherein both red cells and plasma components are lost. In contrast, plasma protein levels are usually within the normal range in patients with internal blood loss and hemolytic anemias. In addition, internal blood loss may also elevate icterus index; external blood loss does not.

Platelet numbers increase immediately to shorten coagulation time and hasten hemostasis.

The leukocyte number increases within hours owing to an increase in neutrophils. Later, as reticulocytes are released from the bone marrow, immature leukocytes also appear in the blood. The magnitude of the "shift to the left" may be correlated with the intensity of the erythropoietic response. In acute hemolytic anemias, leukocytosis and a temperature rise are to be anticipated and should not be interpreted as evidence of an infectious process.

Immature erythrocytes begin to appear in the circulation 72–96 hours after the onset of the blood loss or red cell destruction. The peak of release of reticulocytes occurs usually between the fifth and seventh days, followed by a gradual decline as the emergency is met and red cell parameters return to normal. Persistent reticulocytosis without an increase in RBC counts suggests an uncompensated blood loss anemia requiring a search for the bleeding lesion. During the peak response the blood profile is characterized by polychromatic macrocytes, nucleated erythrocytes, and erythrocytes with nuclear remnants called Howell-Jolly bodies (Plates XII–9, XVII–3). Thus, a triad of anemia, hypoproteinemia, and reticulocytosis is considered a hallmark of responsive blood loss anemia.

The greater size of erythrocytes (MCV) and their reduced hemoglobin concentration (MCHC) characterize the anemia during this stage as macrocytic hypochromic. Macrocytic polychromatic erythrocytes (reticulocytes) often assume leptocytic forms and contribute to moderate to marked anisocytosis common to such a response. This should be contrasted with orthochromic leptocytes seen in chronic diseases.

The degree of reticulocytosis generally varies with the magnitude of blood loss, the period over which blood loss occurred, and the species. Dogs and cats exhibit the most commonly observed picture of a regenerative blood loss anemia, the type previously described. Even in these animals, peak erythropoietic responses to blood loss are usually less than those seen in hemolytic anemias from a variety of causes. Other species differences should also be remembered for they are significant. For example, in the cat, "aggregate" reticulocytes disappear earlier than "punctate" reticulocytes; thus the presence of many "punctate" reticulocytes suggests that a blood loss or hemolytic episode has occurred (see Chapter 5). Horses responding to acute blood loss may show no obvious changes in erythrocyte morphology or exhibit only anisocytosis owing to increases in MCV (Appendix Case 55).

Basophilic stippling (Plate XVIII–10) is an additional finding during vigorous erythrogenesis in ruminants, and may precede macrocytosis. Reticulocyte response and changes in red cell parameters and MCV have been described for goats (Tables 9–4 and 9–5) and water buffaloes (Table 12–30). Ruminants may display little or no reticulocytosis following acute blood loss, however, and there may be some age effect (see Chapter 7). For example, a maximal reticulocyte response of only 1.6% was seen in 4-month-old calves phlebotomized to reduce hemoglobin concentration by 40% over a period of 14 days (Bremmer, 1966). Calves experiencing a 60% reduction in PCV from blood loss over 24 hours, however, exhibited a maximal reticulocyte response of 14% (Schnappauf et al., 1967). The hematologic response of a 7-month-old Holstein-Friesian bull subjected to repeated massive blood withdrawal demonstrated impres-

Table 22–2. Erythrocyte Parameters and Plasma Protein Concentrations in Response to Repeated Blood Withdrawal from a 7-month-old Holstein-Friesian Bull

Day	Blood Withdrawn (l)	RBC ($\times 10^6/\mu l$)	PCV (%)	Hb (g/dl)	MCV (fl)	MCHC (%)	MCH (pg)	Reticulocytes (%)	Nucleated RBC/100 WBC	Plasma Proteins (g/dl)
1	7.5	9.15	37.0	12.8	40.4	34.6	14.0	0	0	7.3
2	6.5	6.05	24.0	8.1	39.0	33.8	13.4	0	0	6.2
3	3.0	3.19	14.0	5.0	43.9	35.7	15.7	rare	0	4.8
4	—	2.90	13.0	4.2	44.8	32.3	14.5	2.8	0.5	5.0
5	—	3.14	15.0	4.8	47.8	32.0	15.3	3.9	2.0	5.4
6	—	3.11	17.0	5.2	54.7	30.6	16.7	8.4	1.0	5.5
7	5.0	3.01	17.0	5.5	56.5	32.3	18.3	12.8	3.5	5.5
8	3.5	2.70	16.0	4.9	59.2	30.6	18.1	19.6	4.0	5.5
9	2.5	1.83	14.0	3.9	76.5	27.8	21.3	21.8	3.0	4.9
15	—	2.39	14.0	4.0	58.6	28.6	16.7	10.6	1.0	4.6
20	—	3.90	20.0	6.5	51.3	32.5	16.6	4.4	3.0	5.2
28	—	6.95	27.0	9.0	38.8	33.3	12.9	0	0	6.2
48	—	9.00	33.0	10.5	36.7	31.8	11.7	0	0	7.1

From Schalm, 1980; courtesy of *Bovine Practice.*

sive changes in various erythrocyte parameters, Wintrobe indexes, and plasma protein concentrations (Schalm, 1980; Table 22–2). A brief description is given below:

Six separate blood withdrawals, ranging from 7.5 liters down to 2.5 liters were made for a total removal of 28 liters over a period of 9 days. Using growth standards for Holstein-Friesian cattle, the bull's weight was estimated to be 225 kg. Blood volume was estimated to be 14.1 liters on a basis of 6.25% body weight (Chapter 3). The volume of blood withdrawn on day 1 (7.5 liters) was equal to slightly more than one-half the bull's estimated total blood volume. Total blood removed over the 9-day period was equal to 2 times the estimated prebleeding volume. Twelve samplings of jugular blood were made over the first 48-hour period of blood withdrawal. In Table 22–2, the data on blood composition on each day of blood withdrawal are representative of the blood prior to the removal of the stated volume of blood withdrawn on that day. For example, blood composition data on day 1 are representative of prebleeding (normal) values, while the data on day 2 represent the changes in blood composition resulting from the withdrawal of 7.5 liters of blood 24 hours previously.

Hemodilution was evidenced in blood values of day 2, but the magnitude of change was not proportional to the amount of blood removed (about one-half blood volume) and restoration of plasma volume (almost 100%) within 24 hours in that the data did not reveal a 50% reduction in RBC, PCV, hemoglobin concentration, and plasma protein values, rather a 33% reduction in erythrocytes and plasma protein concentration. Such observations are a common finding in blood loss anemia and are explained by an initial partial replacement of erythrocytes from the splenic reserve, and the movement of protein, particularly albumin, from extravascular stores into the circulation. As blood loss continued, plasma protein concentration somewhat stabilized by increased hepatic synthesis of albumin and decreased rate of destruction.

The first evidence of a real beginning release of newly formed erythrocytes (reticulocytes) from the bone marrow to blood appeared 72 hours (day 4) after the initial blood withdrawal. Reticulocytes increased steadily to 12.8% by day 7 at which time a new series of blood withdrawal was started. Erythropoiesis had been greatly intensified in response to the blood withdrawal of 17 liters of blood in the first series of phlebotomies so that the immediate response to the second series of blood withdrawal was an increase of reticulocytes in the circulation to 19.6% on day 8 and 21.8% on day 9.

Erythrocyte morphology during the period of intensified erythropoiesis was characterized first by the appearance of the erythrocytes exhibiting basophilic stippling followed by macrocytic polychromatic cells, nucleated erythrocytes, and erythrocytes with Howell-Jolly bodies.

Changes in red cell indexes were reflective of increases in the number of immature erythrocytes in blood. Between day 1 and day 9, MCV increased from 40.4 fl to 76.5 fl, MCH increased from 14.0 pg to 21.3 pg, and MCHC decreased from 34.6% to 27.8%. The relationship of RBC count and MCV to changing PCV values was nicely demonstrated from the data on days 8, 9, and 15. There was a 39% reduction in RBC count and only a 17.6% reduction in PCV between days 8 and 9. The difference in the response of these two erythrocyte parameters was due to the rapid increase in MCV between the two days, 59.2 fl to 76.5 fl, thereby causing the PCV to exhibit a smaller reduction in the face of a much greater fall in RBC counts. The RBC count increased from 1.83 million to 2.39 million between days 9 and 15 but the PCV values remained at 14% on both days. As the RBC count increased, MCV decreased to 58.6 fl so that the PCV values were temporarily stabilized at 14%.

After day 9, when no further blood withdrawal was made, there followed a gradual return of all erythrocyte parameters and plasma protein concentration to levels consistent with normal ranges, with the exception of MCV which was below the minimum normal of 40.0 fl. [Schalm, 1980].

Bone Marrow Response

Hematopoietic potential of the bone marrow can be stimulated 6–8 folds under appropriate circumstances. Hypoxic state created by acute blood loss increases erythropoietin production which then stimulates erythropoiesis (see Chapter 18 for details). Although erythropoietin production is enhanced within hours of the establishment of a hypoxic state, significant erythrogenesis in bone marrow is not evident until 2–3 days later, with maximal changes occurring about a day or two prior to peak reticulocytosis in the peripheral blood, and subsiding as recovery follows. During this period M:E ratio is anticipated to be below normal (Appendix Case 19). Prerequisites for an optimal response are that adequate supplies of nutrients essential to erythrogenesis, particularly iron, must be available and the functional ability of the marrow should not be compromised. Some stimulation of granulopoiesis may also be evident, depending on the magnitude of stimulus for overall hematopoietic stimulation. Thrombopoiesis may also be stimulated, particularly in blood loss situations demanding their excessive usage. When thrombocytopenia appears to be the cause of blood loss, platelet production may be reduced and morphologic abnormalities of platelets as well as magakaryocytes may be discernible.

CHRONIC BLOOD LOSS

Periodic removal of a small quantity of blood from an animal may be inconsequential, but unrestricted continuous loss can lead to an uncompensated blood loss anemia. For example, once a week withdrawal of up to 20 ml of blood from an average-sized cat and 60 ml from an average-sized Beagle dog for 3–4 weeks can be tolerated by the animal with no evident signs of anemia. In comparison, chronic loss of only a small quantity of blood from a bleeding gastrointestinal tumor can lead to anemia. This becomes evident from the fact that 1 ml of blood contains about 0.5 mg of iron, and normally about 1 mg of iron is absorbed and excreted daily. Thus, an iron-deficient state can manifest easily when iron balance is tilted in favor of increased loss. The anemia is typically recognized as that of iron deficiency.

Iron Deficiency Anemia

Iron deficiency is rare among domestic animals. The major portion (about two-thirds) of iron in the body is found as hemoglobin iron, but a substantial amount exists as non-hemoglobin iron in the form of ferritin, hemosiderin, myoglobin, iron-containing enzymes, and other undefined forms. Iron balance in an individual is maintained largely by the rate of iron absorption and to a lesser extent by the rate of iron loss. Physiologically, a small amount of iron is lost in feces owing to exfoliation of epithelial cells of the gastrointestinal tract and excretion of bile, and a minor portion is lost in the skin, nails, hair, and urine. Women and primates lose iron from blood loss during menstruation. Daily iron loss varies directly with the iron content of the body and inversely with the body weight; it is lower in humans, cows, sheep, and dogs than in laboratory animals (Finch et al., 1978). Normally, these losses are balanced by absorption of an equivalent amount of iron from the diet. Iron metabolism has been reviewed by Conrad and Barton, 1981; Jacobs and Worwood, 1980; Kaneko, 1980; Nimeh and Bishop, 1980; and Turnbull, 1974.

Iron deficiency from reduced intake of iron develops in baby pigs reared in a sanitary environment (concrete floors), pups and kittens raised on milk, and animals grazing on iron-deficient pastures. Neonates not provided with adequate iron supplement exhibit anemia within a few weeks of birth; e.g., pigs (see Chapter 10), lambs (Tait and Dubeski, 1980), and cats (Weiser and Kociba, 1983). A congenital iron deficiency anemia, probably as a result of impaired in utero transfer of iron from the dam to the fetus, was described in dairy calves (Tennant et al., 1975). More commonly, however, iron deficiency results from chronic blood loss (Table 22–1) as in animals with a bleeding ulcer, a tumor of the gastrointestinal or urinary tract, or heavy infestation with bloodsucking external parasites such as fleas and lice or internal parasites such as Haemonchus in sheep and hookworms in puppies (Appendix Case 34). Thrombocytopenia is another significant cause of chronic blood loss anemia. Certainly, dogs and cats in the United States, when not infested with bloodsucking parasites, generally will have adequate stores of iron from their diet. Chronic blood loss from a bleeding tumor of the gastrointestinal tract, e.g., leiomyoma of the duodenum, has been a cause of iron deficiency in the dog. In humans, these smooth-muscle tumors are known to bleed massively (Huntley et al., 1960). Menorrhea in primates leads to iron deficiency anemia. Frequent blood withdrawals from blood-donor dogs may lead to iron deficiency anemia. It should also be remembered that conditions influencing synthesis of protoporphyrin or availability of iron for heme synthesis may also mimic hematologic abnormalities of iron deficiency.

Absorption and Transport of Iron

Dietary sources of iron are varied; meat, eggs, legumes, and dirt have a high content of iron, while milk is a poor source. Iron is absorbed from the gut in bivalent or ferrous form, whereas it occurs in nature in organic complexes (phytates, oxalates, and phosphates) in the ferric form. Hydrochloric acid of the stomach releases the iron from the organic complex, and reducing substances (ascorbic acid) in the alkaline medium in duodenum aid in converting the ferric iron into the ferrous iron (see Chapter 13). In humans, faulty iron absorption results from achlorhydria (lack of HCl) in the stomach; apparently this condition rarely occurs in animals. A high phosphorus level in the diet ties up the iron, thus making it unavailable for absorption. Conversely, a low phosphorus intake may increase iron absorption (Hegsted et al., 1949). Iron absorption is promoted by protein in the diet.

Iron absorption by mucosal cells occurs mainly in the upper duodenum. It is an energy-dependent mechanism and involves binding of iron to specific receptors on the cell surface. It has been shown that iron at this location is bound by a "mucosal transferrin," a protein with properties similar to serum transferrin, prior to absorption (Morgan, 1980). The mucosal cell either releases the ferrous iron into the plasma for transport to other parts of the body or converts it back to the ferric form for storage as ferritin, which may be reused or lost into the gut when the cell exfoliates. The extent of each of these events regulates iron metabolism in the body. The rate of mucosal cell iron absorption varies inversely with the body's iron stores and directly with the rate of erythropoiesis as well as with the availability of iron in the diet. Normally the amount absorbed equals that which is lost through "excretion," although a larger amount is absorbed during body growth, pregnancy, and anemic state and a smaller amount is absorbed in iron overload. The "mucosal block" theory of iron absorption is further discussed in Chapter 13.

Transfer of iron from the mucosal cell to the plasma transport protein, transferrin, is promoted by ATP, citrate, and ceruloplasmin. Transferrin is a pink glycoprotein migrating in the β_1-globulin fraction of the serum. It is synthesized by the liver and to some extent by macrophages and other tissues. Normally transferrin is saturated one-third with iron, and each molecule carries two atoms of iron in the ferric form. Different polymorphic forms of transferrin (MW 75,000–83,000) are present in various species, but no functional differences have been found. The major function of transferrin is to transport iron, but by being an iron chelator it also acts as a bacteriostatic agent. For further details of transferrin, see recent reviews (Aisen and Brown, 1977; Jacobs and Worwood, 1980).

Iron needed for heme synthesis largely comes from reutilization of iron in the storage compartment which is replenished from iron conserved after degradation of hemoglobin molecules and from dietary sources. Iron is stored mainly in two forms, ferritin and hemosiderin, the latter being more stable and less reusable. The major storage organs are the liver, spleen, and bone marrow. Macrophages in the bone marrow serve as a great reservoir of recycled iron derived from hemoglobin of phagocytized red cells. Macrophages, however, primarily supply iron to the plasma transferrin; this process is aided by ceruloplasmin and ascorbate. Erythroid cells in the bone marrow can extract up to 85% of transferrin iron presented to them. Transferrin donates iron on the cell surface or after internalization through attachment to specific surface receptors. These sites in electron photomicrographs of erythroid cells are characterized by focal accumulations of ferritin (Figs. 18–6, 18–7). The process of iron intake by developing erythroid cells has been termed ropheocytosis. About 80–90% of iron taken in by the erythroid cell is utilized for heme synthesis and the remainder is largely converted to ferritin for temporary storage or ultimate excretion. Erythroid ferritin is recognized as "siderosomes" and forms the basis for recognition of "sideroblasts" and "siderocytes" in bone marrow and blood films stained with Prussian blue. Ferrokinetic measurements provide information regarding rates of iron utilization and erythropoiesis.

Species variations are noted in the dietary requirements of iron (Kolb, 1963; Kaneko, 1980). Generally, it is low in adults and high in growing children and animals. Iron need is increased during pregnancy, particularly in the last trimester. Iron requirements of cows, horses, and swine are higher than those for dogs, sheep, and cats. Women and female primates require more iron than males because of menstrual bleeding.

Clinical and Laboratory Findings in Iron Deficiency Anemia

Hematologic and serum iron studies have been made on dogs with chronic iron defi-

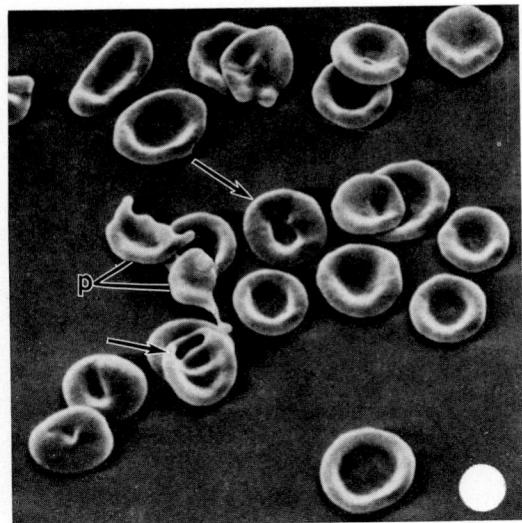

Fig. 22–1. Scanning electron photomicrographs of erythrocytes from a dog with microcytic hypochromic anemia. Hypochromic erythrocytes with markedly enlarged concavity, poikilocytes (*p*), and erythrocytes with membrane defects (*arrows*) are apparent. ×2,200. (Courtesy of N.C. Jain and K.S. Keeton.)

ciency anemia (Harvey et al., 1982; Weiser and O'Grady, 1983). Iron deficiency occurs gradually; hence, changes observed in blood depend on the extent of iron depletion. Changes in iron metabolism precede morphologic abnormalities (Dallman, 1977). The anemia in early stages is normocytic-normochromic, whereas a microcytic hypochromic anemia characterizes the blood picture of fully expressed iron deficiency. In iron deficiency, hemoglobin synthesis is more deficient than erythrocyte production. Thus, the RBC count is not as markedly reduced as the hemoglobin concentration with the result that microcytosis precedes hypochromasia. During early stages of iron deficiency, microcytosis is better appreciated from erythrocyte volume distribution curves than MCV determinations, and hypochromasia is readily apparent on careful examination of a good Wright-stained blood film than by MCHC (see Chapter 21). Microcytosis and hypochromasia manifest in Wintrobe indexes only when the majority of erythrocytes are so involved.

The anemia is usually nonresponsive in nature, although some reticulocytosis may be observed. The iron-deficient erythrocyte has a narrow rim of lightly stained hemoglobin with a variable but greater than normal area of central pallor (Plate XVII–1; Fig. 22–1). The poorly structured red cells break apart in circulation, producing often encountered poikilocytes (Fig. 22–1). Red cell life span is modestly shortened probably because of reduced red cell deformability (Tillmann and Schroter, 1980). Thrombocytosis of inexplicable origin is a common finding in iron deficiency anemia (see Chapter 17). Hypoproteinemia may be found in some animals, and leukocyte numbers are variable because of the primary disease.

In the bone marrow, a maturation arrest takes place in the late rubricyte stage so that while these cells are awaiting hemoglobin synthesis, further cell division may take place, with the production of some erythrocytes that are smaller than normal and deficient in hemoglobin (see Chapter 18); this gives rise to microcytic-hypochromic anemia. Thus, the bone marrow cytology is characterized by a predominance of late rubricytes and metarubricytes (Plate XVII–2 and Appendix Case 33). These nucleated red cells often exhibit scanty irregularly stained cytoplasm and ragged cellular boundaries. Marrow macrophage iron is depleted and sideroblasts are reduced in number (Table 22–3).

Iron status of a patient can be assessed by measuring serum iron (SI) and total iron binding capacity (TIBC, a measure of serum transferrin level) and calculating the percent saturation of transferrin (100 × SI/TIBC). Species variations occur in serum iron and transferrin values and percent saturation may vary from 20–60% (Jacobs and Worwood, 1980; Kaneko, 1980). Generally, normal animals and humans have an average serum iron level of about 100 μg/dl, a TIBC of 300 μg/dl, and a percent saturation of 33%. A comparison of changes in iron metabolism in iron deficiency anemia and anemia of chronic disorders is presented in Table 22–3. In human patients with iron deficiency, SI and transferrin saturation are generally reduced and TIBC is increased (Table 22–3). Recent studies on dogs, however, revealed decreased SI and transferrin saturation, but no significant changes in TIBC values (Harvey et al., 1982; Weiser and O'Grady, 1983).

A small amount of ferritin is found in blood in concentration proportional to iron stores in

Table 22–3.   Comparative Features of Iron Deficiency Anemia and Anemia of Chronic Disorders

Feature	Iron-Deficiency Anemia	Anemia of Inflammatory Disease
Iron Absorption		
Intestinal absorption of iron	Increased	Decreased
Serum Measurements		
Serum Iron	Normal to decreased	Normal to decreased
TIBC*	Normal to increased	Decreased
TIBC % saturation	Decreased	Decreased
Serum copper, zinc, and ceruloplasmin	—	Increased
Serum ferritin	Decreased	Normal or increased
Erythrocyte Measurements		
Erythrocyte parameters	Moderate to marked, nonresponsive anemia	Mild to moderate, nonresponsive anemia
Free RBC Protoporphyrin	Increased	Increased
RBC life span	Slightly decreased	Slightly decreased
Bone Marrow Measurements		
Erythropoiesis	Normal or impaired	Impaired
Marrow macrophage iron	Decreased	Normal or increased
Marrow sideroblasts	Decreased	Decreased
Hepatic Measurements		
Superoxide dismutase	?	Decreased

*TIBC, total iron binding capacity or transferrin concentration.

the body; hence measurement of serum ferritin levels is useful for detection of iron deficiency. In human patients, serum ferritin is decreased in iron deficiency, whereas it is normal or increased in liver disease, neoplasms, inflammatory diseases and β-thalassemia (Dallman, 1977; Hershko et al., 1979). Serum ferritin concentrations are markedly elevated in cows following parturition (Furugouri et al., 1982). In horses, serum ferritin is increased after iron therapy and decreased after phlebotomy (Smith et al., 1984a). Serum ferritin levels have been measured to estimate iron stores in neonatal pigs (Smith et al., 1984b).

Free erythrocytic protoporphyrin is increased severalfold, even before anemia becomes apparent (Dallman, 1977).

Treatment of iron deficiency varies with the primary etiology. Neonates should be provided sufficient dietary iron by iron supplementation or by administering iron compounds. Chronic blood loss as a cause of iron deficiency requires treating the condition responsible for blood loss first and then providing adequate iron supplementation. Iron supplementation in dogs and cats has been discussed (Dodds and Ward, 1980). In horses, iron dextran causes adverse reactions but iron

cacodylate appears to be safe. Acute iron intoxication leading to death from administration of a hematinic can occur not only in piglets, but also in ruminants (Nicholson et al., 1983).

Blood Loss Anemia Associated with Parasitism

Several blood sucking parasites produce blood loss anemia. A report of anemia in cattle caused by the bloodsucking louse *Haematopinus eurysternus* (Peterson et al., 1953) stated that the condition of the animals became critical when PCV decreased to 13% and that a PCV as low as 9% was observed. Removal of the lice was followed by a prompt recovery from the anemia. In the case of the dog, our clinic has encountered several instances of advanced anemia associated with heavy infestations with the sticktight flea, *Echidnophaga gallinacea* (Appendix Case 34). The hookworm *Ancylostoma caninum* is a prodigious bloodsucker, and it has been reported that a single worm may remove as much as 0.8 ml of blood in a 24-hour period (Landsberg, 1939). In acute hookworm disease, the blood picture is one of acute blood loss characterized by macrocytic-hypochromic anemia, whereas in the more chronic disease, the anemia may be microcytic-hypochromic.

Anemia and hypoproteinemia have been observed in acute and chronic helminthiasis in cattle and sheep. Although the pathogenesis of anemia has not been definitely established, blood loss is believed to be primarily responsible for anemia associated with bloodsucking stomach worms such as *Haemonchus contortus* in sheep and *H. placei* in cattle, whereas impaired erythropoiesis is thought to be involved in anemia from nonbloodsucking parasites such as *Trichostrongylus* spp., *Ostertagia* spp., and *Cooperia* spp. (Baker and Douglas, 1966; Greenwood, 1977; Jennings, 1976; Soulsby, 1982; Viana and Campos, 1975). Impaired erythropoiesis has been attributed to a variety of causes including increased ineffective erythropoiesis, copper deficiency, specific animo acid deficiency from disturbed protein metabolism, and toxic marrow suppression, all resulting from chronic parasitism. An interference with iron utilization, as in anemia of chronic disease (Chapter 25), may also be involved as indicated by normal to increased plasma iron and excessive iron stores in the liver (Baker and Douglas, 1966). In addition, a shortened red cell life span may contribute to the anemia from both chronic blood loss and impaired erythropoiesis. Hypoproteinemia in helminthiasis is primarily a result of hypoalbuminemia developing because of protein-losing gastroenteropathy, with anorexia and malabsorption accentuating the problem to some extent (Dargie, 1975; Greenwood, 1977). Edema of the lips and intermandibular space (bottle jaw) may develop in animals with severe hypoproteinemia (Appendix Case 71). Breed differences have been observed in susceptibility of sheep to develop anemia and hypoproteinemia from helminthiasis (Greenwood, 1977).

Heavy infestations with *H. contortus* in sheep present a blood picture of acute blood loss, i.e., macrocytic-hypochromic anemia with evidence of increased erythropoiesis in blood and bone marrow. In chronic haemonchosis, the anemia gradually becomes well advanced and may appear as normocytic-normochromic or microcytic-hypochromic with little or no evidence of reticulocytosis (Baker and Douglas, 1966). Normocytic normochromic anemia is common to trichostrongyloidosis in cattle (Baker and Douglas, 1966), but hypochromasia may sometimes be seen (Appendix Case 71). Acute helminthiasis in sheep (infections with *Haemonchus* spp., *Trichostrongylus* spp., and *Strongyloides* spp.) was characterized by a rapid increase in helminth egg output coupled with over a 50% decrease in erythrocyte parameters within 7 weeks. In comparison, chronic infection was associated with a slow and irregular increase in helminth egg output and a slow but steady decline of less than 40% in red cell parameters (Ogunsusi, 1978). It has been calculated that an adult *haemonchus* worm consumes about 0.05 ml of blood per day and that blood loss in feces is apparent first at 6 to 12 days postinfection and precedes appearance of eggs in feces (Clark et al., 1962). Experimental infection of lambs with *H. contortus* showed that a worm count of as low as 374 could cause severe anemia (Malviya et al., 1979).

Experimental studies by Dargie and Allonby (1975) in Merino sheep demonstrated that anemia from severe haemonchosis develops in 3 phases. During the first phase, between 7 and 25 days of infection (prepatent period), severe anemia results from blood loss. Erythropoietic response to anemia is absent due to a delay in adaptation, and serum iron levels remain within the normal range. During the second phase, prevailing for 6 to 14 weeks, a compensatory steady state anemia seems to persist because of increased erythropoiesis in face of continued blood loss. Iron deficiency gradually develops because of increased iron utilization accompanied by increased fecal iron loss and diminished iron absorption. This sets the stage for the third phase in which anemia becomes more pronounced as erythropoiesis wanes from iron depletion in blood and bone marrow and possibly inadequate globin synthesis ascribed to specific amino acid deficiency from disturbed protein metabolism (Baker and Douglas, 1966; Soulsby, 1982). Thus, in progressive haemonchosis, the regenerative anemia observed during the early stage of the disease gradually terminates into a nonregenerative anemia of iron deficiency (Appendix Case 73). Hence anthelminthic therapy must accompany prolonged adequate iron supplementation to replenish body stores of iron and insure recovery from anemia (Baker and Douglas, 1966).

Heavy infestations with coccidia will lead to bloody diarrhea and anemia. In 9 dogs experimentally infected with coccidia, the average RBC count fell from a normal of 6.3 million/µl to 3.4 million/µl in 6 days and then returned to the normal level over the next 11 days (Lee, 1934).

Experimental schistosomiasis (*Schistosoma matthei*) in sheep was found to cause blood loss anemia and hypoalbuminemia. In addition, decreased erythropoiesis, elevated plasma volume, and increased catabolism of albumin contributed to changes seen in blood values (Preston and Dargie, 1972).

The liver fluke, *Fasciola hepatica*, produces a blood loss anemia in cattle and sheep when large numbers of adult flukes are present in the liver (Sewell et al., 1968). The anemia is accompanied by hypoalbuminemia and hypergammaglobulinemia (Ross, 1967). Hemorrhage in the peritoneal cavity may be prominent during the migratory phase of immature flukes through the liver. The adult fluke was shown to be hematophagic on the evidence of the presence of degraded hemoglobin in the flukes' ceca (Todd and Ross, 1966). The primary cause of anemia in sheep infected with adult flukes was loss of blood into the gut via the bile (Holmes and MacLean, 1969); about 0.5 ml of red cells may be lost per day per fluke (Jennings, 1976). The degree of anemia seems to be related to the animal's erythropoietic capacity, which is substantially lower in poorly fed animals (Berry and Dargie, 1978). A shortening of erythrocyte survival time in blood may also occur and contribute to anemia (Furmaga and Gunlach, 1978; Holmes et al., 1971). Plasma iron level was found to fluctuate with duration of the disease. Early decrease in plasma iron was related to diminished iron mobilization associated with a defective function of the mononuclear phagocyte system resulting from ascorbic acid deficiency (Gameel, 1982).

An example of severe fascioliasis was observed in a California flock of 1,488 breeding ewes (Hjerpe et al., 1971). Clinical signs consisted of pallor, bottle jaw, ascites, and weight loss. Blood studies were conducted on 15 of the severely affected ewes to characterize the hematologic effects and responses. All 15 ewes were severely anemic, with RBC counts ranging between 1.86 and 6.15 million/µl (average, 3.48 million/µl) and PCV values of 8.0–22.0% (average, 15.0%). Intensification of erythropoiesis was indicated by the observation of moderate anisocytosis, polychromasia, and variable basophilic stippling of erythrocytes, as well as by reticulocyte counts ranging from 2.3–16.4% (average, 8.5%). MCV ranged from 33.0–64.5 fl (average, 43.0 fl), and MCHC ranged from 20.8–38.0% (average, 28.0%), indicating a trend toward macrocytic hypochromic erythrocytes. Serum iron levels ranged from 47–141 µg/dl (average, 81.9 µg/dl), compared with normal levels of 111–170 µg/dl. Icterus index was 2 to 5 units (normal) in 13 ewes and 10 and 20 units in the remaining two ewes, suggesting liver dysfunction in the latter two ewes. Hypoproteinemia was present in 12 of the 15 ewes, with total plasma protein ranging from 3.3–5.8 g/dl (average, 4.9 g/dl). As indicated by Ross (1967), the hypoproteinemia is due to a marked reduction in albumin, and this correlates with the edema characteristic of severe fascioliasis. Generally, there was a moderate leukocytosis due to neutrophilia and a moderate suppression of circulating lymphocyte numbers.

Experimental infection of sheep with *Fasciola gigantica* produced a marked anemia between 10 and 14 weeks of infection (Kadhim, 1976).

REFERENCES

Aisen, P., and Brown, E.B.: The Iron Binding Function of Transferrin in Iron Metabolism. Semin. Hematol., *14*:31, 1977.

Baker, N.F., and Douglas, J.R.: Blood Alterations in Helminth Infection. *In* Biology of Parasites. E.J.L. Soulsby, ed. Academic Press, New York, pp. 155–183, 1966.

Berry, C.I., and Dargie, J.D.: Pathophysiology of Ovine Fascioliasis: The Influence of Dietary Protein and Iron on the Erythrokinetics of Sheep Experimentally Infected with *Fasciola hepatica*. Vet. Parasitol., *4*:327, 1978.

Bremmer, K.C.: The Reticulocyte Response in Calves Made Anemic by Phlebotomy. Aust. J. Exp. Biol. Med. Sci., *44*:251, 1966.

Clark, C.H., et al.: Measurements of Blood Loss Caused by *Haemonchus contortus* Infection in Sheep. Amer. J. Vet. Res., *23*:977, 1962.

Conrad, M.E., and Barton, J.C.: Factors Affecting Iron Balance. Amer. J. Hematol., *10*:199, 1981.

Dallman, P.R.: New Approaches to Screening for Iron Deficiency. J. Pediatr., *90*:678, 1977.

Dargie, J.D.: Application of Radioisotopic Techniques to the Study of Red Cell and Plasma Protein Metabolism in Helminth Diseases of Sheep. Symp. Br. Soc. Parasitol., *13*:1, 1975.

Dargie, J.D., and Allonby, E.W.: Pathophysiology of Single and Challenge Infections of *Haemonchus contortus* in Merino Sheep: Studies of Red Cell Kinetics and "Self-Cure" Phenomenon. Int. J. Parasitol., *5*:147, 1975.

Dodds, W.J., and Ward, M.V.: Iron Supplementation in Dogs and Cats. Mod. Vet. Pract., *61*:496, 1980.

Finch, C.A., et al.: Body Iron Loss In Animals. Proc. Soc. Exp. Biol. Med., *159*:335, 1978.

Furmaga, S., and Gunlach, J.L.: Behaviour of Morphologic Blood Elements and Levels of Iron and Transferrin in the Blood Serum of Calves Experimentally Infected with *Fasciola hepatica* (Trematoda). Acta Parasitol. Polonica, *25*:179, 1978.

Furugouri, K., et al.: Ferritin in Blood Serum of Dairy Cows. J. Dairy Sci., *65*:1529, 1982.

Gameel, A.A.: *Fasciola hepatica*: Plasma Ascorbic Acid, Plasma Iron and Iron-Binding Capacity in Experimentally Infected Sheep. Z. Parasitenkd., *68*:185, 1982.

Greenwood, B.: Haematology of the Sheep and Goat. *In* Comparative Clinical Haematology. Archer, R.K., and Jeffcott, L.B., eds. Blackwell Scientific, Oxford, pp. 320–332, 1977.

Harvey, J.W., et al.: Chronic Iron Deficiency Anemia in Dogs. J. Amer. Anim. Hosp. Ass., *18*:946, 1982.

Hegsted, D.M., et al.: The Influence of Diet on Iron Absorption. II. The Interrelation of Iron and Phosphorus. J. Exp. Med., *90*:147, 1949.

Hershko, C., et al.: Serum Ferritin and Mean Corpuscular Volume Measurement in the Diagnosis of β-Thalassaemia Minor and Iron Deficiency. Acta Haematol., *62*:236, 1979.

Hjerpe, C.A., et al.: Ovine Fascioliasis in California. J. Amer. Vet. Med. Ass., *159*:1266, 1971.

Holmes, P.H., and MacLean, J.M.: Intestinal Loss of Iron and Its Possible Reabsorption in Chronic Ovine Fascioliasis. Res. Vet. Sci., *10*:488, 1969.

Holmes, P.H., et al.: A Study of the Onset and Development of the Anaemia and Hypoproteinaemia in Chronic Ovine Fascioliasis. *In* Pathology of Parasitic Diseases. Gaafar, S.M., et al., eds. Purdue University, Lafayette, p. 69, 1971.

Huntley, B.F., et al.: Hemorrhage from Leiomyomas of the Gastrointestinal Tract. Arch. Intern. Med., *106*:245, 1960.

Jacobs, A., and Worwood, M.: Iron in Biochemistry and Medicine, II. Academic Press, London, 1980.

Jennings, F.W.: The Anemias of Parasitic Infections. *In* Pathophysiology of Parasitic Infection. Soulsby, E.J.L., ed. Academic Press, New York, pp. 41–67, 1976.

Kadhim, J.K.: Haematological Changes During the Course of Experimental Infection with *Fasciola gigantica* in Sheep. *In* Pathophysiology of Parasitic Infection. Soulsby, E.J.L., ed. Academic Press, New York, p. 105, 1976.

Kaneko, J.J.: Iron Metabolism. *In* Clinical Biochemistry of Domestic Animals. 3rd Ed. Kaneko, J.J., ed. Academic Press, New York, p. 649, 1980.

Kolb, E.: The Metabolism of Iron in Farm Animals under Normal and Pathologic Conditions. Adv. Vet. Sci., *8*:49, 1963.

Landsberg, J.W.: Hookworm Disease in Dogs. J. Amer. Vet. Med. Ass., *94*:389, 1939.

Lee, C.D.: The Pathology of Coccidiosis in the Dog. J. Amer. Vet. Med. Ass., *85*:760, 1934.

Malviya, H.C., et al.: Measurement of the Blood Loss Caused by *Haemonchus contortus* Infection in Sheep. Indian Vet. J., *56*:709, 1979.

Morgan, E.H.: Comparative Iron Metabolism. *In* Iron in Biochemistry and Medicine II. Jacobs, A., and Worwood, M., eds. Academic Press, New York, pp. 641–687, 1980.

Nicholson, S.S., et al.: Acute Intoxication from a Hematinic in Calves. J. Amer. Vet. Med. Ass., *182*:616, 1983.

Nimeh, N., and Bishop, R.C.: Disorders of Iron Metabolism. Med. Clin. North Amer., *64*:631, 1980.

Ogunsusi, R.A.: Changes in Blood Values of Sheep Suffering from Acute and Chronic Helminthiasis. Res. Vet. Sci., *25*:298, 1978.

Peterson, H.O., et al.: Anemia in Cattle Caused by Heavy Infestations of the Blood-Sucking Louse, *Haematopinus eurysternus*. J. Amer. Vet. Med. Ass., *122*:373, 1953.

Preston, J.M., and Dargie, J.D.: The Anaemia of Ovine Schistosomiasis *(S. mattheei)*. Trans. R. Soc. Trop. Med. Hyg., *66*:530, 1972.

Ross, J.G.: An Epidemiological Study of Fascioliasis in Sheep. Vet. Rec., *80*:214, 1967.

Schalm, O.W.: Differential Diagnosis of Anemias in Cattle. Part I. Massive Blood Loss By Repeated Phlebotomies. Bovine Pract., *1*:10, 1980.

Schnappauf, H., et al.: Erythropoietic Response in Calves Following Blood Loss. Amer. J. Vet. Res., *28*:275, 1967.

Sewell, M.M.H., et al.: Studies on the Aetiology of Anaemia in Chronic Fascioliasis in Sheep. Brit. Vet. J., *124*:160, 1968.

Smith, J.E., et al.: Serum Ferritin as a Measure of Stored Iron in Horses. J. Nutr., *114*:677, 1984a.

Smith, J.E., et al.: Serum Ferritin and Total Iron-Binding Capacity to Estimate Iron Storage in Pigs. Vet. Pathol., *21*:597, 1984b.

Soulsby, E.J.L.: Helminths, Arthropods, and Protozoa of Domesticated Animals. 7th ed. Lea & Febiger, Philadelphia, pp. 234–235; 238–239, 1982.

Tait, R.M., and Dubeski, P.L.: Iron Deficiency Anemia in Young Lambs. J. Anim. Sci., *51*(Suppl. 1):454, 1980.

Tennant, B., et al.: Hematology of the Neonatal Calf. III. Frequency of Congenital Iron Deficiency Anemia. Cornell Vet., *65*:543, 1975.

Tillmann, W., and Schroter, W.: Deformability of Erythrocytes in Iron Deficiency Anemia. Blut, *40*:179, 1980.

Tobias, G.: Congenital Porphyria in a Cat. J. Amer. Vet. Med. Ass., *145*:462, 1964.

Todd, J.R., and Ross, J.G.: Origin of Hemoglobin in the Cecal Contents of *Fasciola hepatica*. Exp. Parasitol., *19*:151, 1966.

Torten, M., and Schalm, O.W.: Influence of the Equine Spleen on Rapid Changes in the Concentration of Erythrocytes in Peripheral Blood. Amer. J. Vet. Res., *25*:500, 1964.

Turnbull, A.: Iron Absorption. *In* Iron in Biochemistry and Medicine. Jacobs, A., and Worwood, M., eds. Academic Press, New York, p. 369, 1974.

Viana, E.S., and Campos, J.M. de: Haemogram of Calves

Free from Helminths and of Naturally Parasitized Calves. Vet. Bull., *45*:5344, 1975.

Weiser, M.G., and Kociba, G.J.: Sequential Changes in Erythrocyte Volume Distribution and Microcytosis Associated with Iron Deficiency in Kittens. Vet. Path., *20*:1, 1983.

Weiser, G., and O'Grady, M.: Erythrocyte Volume Distribution Analysis and Hematologic Changes in Dogs with Iron Deficiency Anemia. Vet. Path., *20*:230, 1983.

23

Hemolytic Anemias Associated with Some Infectious Agents

HEMOLYTIC ANEMIAS ASSOCIATED WITH BLOOD PARASITES AND RICKETTSIAL INFECTIONS   590
Anaplasmosis   590
Babesiosis   596
Haemobartonellosis   602
Eperythrozoonosis   608
Theileriasis   610
Trypanosomiasis   612
Cytauxzoonosis in Cats   615
Sarcocystosis in Cattle and Goats   616

HEMOLYTIC ANEMIAS ASSOCIATED WITH SOME BACTERIAL INFECTIONS   616
Leptospirosis   616
Bacillary Hemoglobinuria in Cattle and Sheep   617

HEMOLYTIC ANEMIAS ASSOCIATED WITH SOME VIRAL INFECTIONS   618
Equine Infectious Anemia   618

Hemolytic anemias result primarily from increased erythrocyte destruction, whether intravascular or extravascular. An *uncompensated hemolytic anemia* is said to exist when the rate of red cell destruction exceeds the capacity of bone marrow for enhanced erythropoiesis and delivery of young erythrocytes to the circulation. A *compensated hemolytic disorder* exists when both red cell destruction and marrow erythropoiesis are increased, and red cell values are within the normal range.

Hemolytic anemias have numerous causes (Table 23–1) and involve several pathophysiologic mechanisms, one or more of which may be operative in a particular instance. Although a particular disease may produce certain specific clinicopathologic changes, some of the clinical and laboratory findings are common to hemolytic anemias of various causes. Clinical signs may vary with the specific etiology and the degree of anemia. The onset may be sudden or progressive. Signs of anemia such as pale mucous membranes, weakness, fatigue, and tachycardia may be present depending on the severity of anemia. Rarely, mucous membranes may be discolored—reddened due to intense hemolytic process. Hemoglobinuria may occur in an occasional patient, and icterus may be evident in some cases. The former indicates an acute hemolytic episode, and the latter, significant persistent red cell destruction. Fever, constant or intermittent, of a variable degree may be present and is related partly to the hemolytic process. Disseminated intravascular coagulation (DIC) may occur as a sequel to lysis of a large number of erythrocytes.

A variety of abnormalities may be found in blood values, bone marrow cytology, serum chemistries, and urinalysis. The extent of changes depends on the severity and duration of the inciting etiology. One may find a variable degree of anemia (reduced red cell parameters); a variable hemoglobinemia; a normal or increased icterus index; a variable hyperbilirubinemia from increases in both conjugated (direct) and unconjugated (indirect) bilirubin, the latter usually exceeding the former; plasma protein concentration usually within the normal range; typical evidences of a regenerative anemia, i.e., increased anisocytosis, polychromasia, and reticulocyte numbers with or without marrow release of nucleated red cells in all species except the horse; a macrocytic hypochromic anemia during remission in most species but very rarely in the horse; abnormal erythrocyte morphology such as spherocytes, leptocytes, schis-

589

Table 23–1. Some Causes of Hemolytic Anemia in Various Animal Species

A. Blood Parasites and Rickettsial Agents
  Anaplasmosis in cattle, sheep, and goats
  Babesiosis in cattle, dogs, horses, sheep, and goats
  Haemobartonellosis in cats, dogs and cattle
  Eperythrozoonosis in cattle (splenectomized), sheep, and pigs
  Cytauxzoonosis in cats
  Trypanosomiasis in cattle
  Theileriasis in cattle
  Ehrlichiosis in dogs and horses

B. Bacterial Infections
  Leptospirosis in cattle, sheep, and dogs
  Bacillary hemoglobinuria in cattle and sheep
  Staphylococcus pyogenes infection (gangrenous mastitis in cows)

C. Viral Infections
  Equine infectious anemia

D. Chemicals and Drugs
  Copper poisoning in sheep, cattle, and pigs
  Lead poisoning in dogs, horses, and cattle
  Phenothiazine toxicosis in horses and sheep
  Methylene blue and Acetaminophen toxicosis in cats
  Nitrate and nitrite poisoning in cattle
  Phenol compounds, benzene and related compounds, naphthalene in moth balls

E. Poisonous Plants and Venoms
  Onion toxicity in cattle, sheep, horses, and dogs
  Rape and kale poisoning in cattle and sheep
  Castor bean toxicity in cattle
  Other miscellaneous toxic plants
  Snake venom

F. Intraerythrocytic Defects or Enzyme Deficiencies
  Congenital porphyria in cattle, cats, and pigs
  Pyruvate kinase deficiency in dogs
  Methemoglobinemia in dogs, cats, and horses

G. Immune-Mediated Hemolytic Anemias
  Autoimmune hemolytic anemia in dogs, cats, and horses
  Neonatal isoerythrolysis in cattle and horses
  Transfusion reactions

H. Metabolic Diseases
  Postparturient hemoglobinuria in cattle

I. Miscellaneous Causes
  Water intoxication in cattle

tocytes, and other forms of poikilocytes; leukocytosis due to neutrophilia with regenerative left shift, particularly during vigorous erythropoietic response; a decreased myeloid:erythroid ratio in bone marrow aspirates indicating an elevation of erythropoiesis; increased numbers of reticulocytes (>5%) in a responsive marrow from a horse; an infrequent hemoglobinuria; and increased serum lactic dehydrogenase and decreased serum haptoglobin levels during acute hemolytic crisis. Certain hematologic findings

(Heinz bodies, spherocytes, schistocytes) may provide clues to pathophysiologic processes that may be involved in hemolytic anemias, while others (hemoparasites) may be of etiologic significance or coincidental. For further general comments see Chapter 21.

Some important diseases or conditions associated with hemolytic anemia in various animal species are discussed briefly in this chapter. Additional information can be found in the references cited.

HEMOLYTIC ANEMIAS ASSOCIATED WITH BLOOD PARASITES AND RICKETTSIAL INFECTIONS

In the eighth edition of Bergey's Manual of Determinative Bacteriology, *Anaplasma, Paranaplasma, Haemobartonella,* and *Eperythrozoon* are classified as separate genera belonging to the family Anaplasmataceae in the order Rickettsiales (Ristic and Kreier, 1974). This classification is based on some structural and antigenic similarities between these hemoparasites and their resemblance to rickettsiae.

Anaplasmosis

Anaplasmosis is an infectious disease of cattle, sheep, goats, and some wild ruminants caused by *Anaplasma* species. The organism is an obligate, intraerythrocytic parasite and extremely host-specific. Causative agents of anaplasmosis in cattle are *Anaplasma marginale, A. centrale, Paranaplasma caudatum,* and *P. discoides* and in sheep and goats *A. ovis.* In cattle, *A. marginale* is the most pathogenic, while *A. centrale* causes a mild clinical disease and anemia (Kuttler, 1966). *A. ovis* is nonpathogenic. Anaplasmosis is enzootic in certain areas of California, the southern and western United States, and most tropical areas of the world. The disease may occur in acute, subacute, or chronic form. A marked parasitemia is present during the acute phase of the disease, while a low level of infection, lasting from months to years, may be detected during the carrier state. The disease has been reviewed (Ristic, 1968, 1980).

Clinical and Hematologic Findings

Anaplasmosis is characterized by fever, marked hemolytic anemia without hemoglo-

Table 23–2.   Ranges, Means, and Standard Deviations in Hemogram Data of 38 Cattle with Natural Infection Due to *Anaplasma marginale*

	Range	Mean ± 1 SD
Erythrocytes ($\times 10^6/\mu$l)	0.85–5.6	2.26 ± 1.18
Hemoglobin (g/dl)	2.30–8.2	4.42 ± 1.59
PCV (%)	7.0–25.0	14.86 ± 4.89
MCV (fl)	41.7–110.0	71.71 ± 17.25
MCHC (%)	23.1–35.8	29.73 ± 2.86
MCH (pg)	13.6–34.4	21.11 ± 4.71
Icterus index units	0–100	20 ± 24
Plasma proteins (g/dl)	6.0–9.4	7.71 ± 0.75
Fibrinogen (g/dl)	0.20–0.90	0.65 ± 0.17
Reticulocytes (%)	0–31.8	8.4 ± 7.6
WBC/μl	2,900–38,800	12,744 ± 6,743
Band neutrophils	0–1,900	319 ± 387
Mature neutrophils	377–20,370	4,520 ± 3,727
Lymphocytes	1,960–16,464	6,299 ± 3,102
Monocytes	0–2,910	924 ± 787
Eosinophils	0–2,000	288 ± 397
Basophils	0–194	21 ± 44
WBC (%)		
Band neutrophils	0–18.0	2.5 ± 3.2
Mature neutrophils	7.0–75.5	33.5 ± 15.1
Lymphocytes	15.0–83.0	52.9 ± 15.9
Monocytes	0.0–20.0	7.3 ± 5.2
Eosinophils	0.0–10.0	2.0 ± 2.3
Basophils	0.0–1.0	0.2 ± 0.3

binuria, icterus, and splenomegaly. The natural disease may be difficult to diagnose if blood studies are delayed many days beyond the hemolytic crisis. The *Anaplasma* bodies increase in number during the incubation period, which varies from 15–45 days, and during this time the animals are asymptomatic. Clinical signs of the disease appear suddenly within 2–21 days of establishment of parasitemia. The parasitized erythrocytes may be removed over a period of a few days, and the mass of circulating red cells may drop by 50–80%. At the time of greatest decrease in RBC count, the body temperature becomes elevated (105–106°F) and the animal shows anorexia, depression, dehydration, loss of milk production, icterus, and other signs of anemia. Some animals may develop abnormalities of the central nervous system and abort, and death may occur in certain cases. Within 4–5 days, *Anaplasma* bodies may be too few in number to permit a certain diagnosis. By this time, the anemia is in remission, and reticulocytosis, polychromasia, anisocytosis with macrocytosis, and basophilic stippling are evident (Plates XVIII–7, XVIII–10). The PCV may fall as low as 7%, which is generally unfavorable. However, a PCV of 11% with evidence of anemia in remission need

cause little concern. Such an animal has a good prognosis without blood transfusion if carefully nursed and kept from overexertion. Convalescence usually lasts 1–2 months, but it may take 3 or more months. It is followed by the carrier state, which may disappear later or become activated by another disease.

Table 23–2 summarizes the hematologic findings in 38 cattle with natural infection due to *A. marginale*. Some cattle were in the earliest stage of the disease when icterus was a prominent clinical sign (100 units) and evidence of remission of anemia was lacking (MCV 42 fl). Other individuals were well advanced in their response to the hemolytic crisis with MCV of 110 fl and a normal icterus index. Leukocytosis due primarily to neutrophilia was seen in some cattle. Erythrophagocytosis and evidence of increased erythropoiesis are found in the bone marrow (Kreier et al., 1964). Erythropoietin levels are increased during anemia; peak levels coincide with the maximal occurrence of anemia (Jatkar and Kreier, 1967). Serum chemistry values have also been determined for infected cows (Allen et al., 1981).

The changes in erythrocyte parameters that follow massive destruction of parasitized erythrocytes as seen in experimentally in-

Table 23–3.   Changes in RBC Number, Size, and Hemoglobin Concentration in Experimentally Induced Anaplasmosis

	Postinoculation Day							
	30	31	33	35	39	42	46	66
PCV (%)	13.0	12.0	12.0	12.0	14.0	17.0	18.9	24.0
RBC ($\times 10^6/\mu l$)	3.16	2.58	1.88	1.24	1.41	1.83	2.51	4.88
Hb (g/dl)	4.4	3.8	3.4	3.4	3.8	4.6	5.2	7.9
MCV (fl)	43.0	45.0	72.0	96.7	99.2	94.0	75.5	49.2
MCHC (%)	29.3	31.6	28.0	28.0	27.1	27.0	27.5	33.0
MCH (pg)	13.9	14.3	18.0	27.4	26.9	25.1	20.7	16.2

duced anaplasmosis are shown in Table 23–3 (see also Appendix Case 69). From the thirtieth to the thirty-fifth day postinoculation of blood from an *A. marginale* carrier cow, the PCV remained essentially stationary, but the RBC count fell an additional 60%, while hemoglobin fell only 22%. The PCV on the thirty-fifth day was maintained by the greatly increased size of the newly released erythrocytes (MCV 96.7 fl). The hemoglobin concentration in the average erythrocyte on a volume basis (MCHC 28%) was reduced, but on a weight basis (MCH 27.4 pg), it was twice as much as in the mature erythrocytes as recorded on day 30. The marked increase in MCV and MCH during the peak response to the hemolytic crisis rapidly regressed toward normal (day 66) as newly formed erythrocytes underwent splenic molding and maturation.

Pathogenesis

The anemia in anaplasmosis results largely from extravascular destruction of parasitized erythrocytes; phagocytosis of such erythrocytes can be demonstrated in the spleen and bone marrow. This erythrophagocytosis results in marked icterus without hemoglobinemia and hemoglobinuria. Hence, common necropsy findings include splenomegaly, an enlarged and friable liver, and a distended gall bladder. Under experimental situations, the prepatent (incubation) period is about 2–6 weeks, after which anemia begins to develop; maximum decline in red cell parameters is seen 1–6 days after the occurrence of peak parasitemia. See also Table 23–3.

The degree of anemia is often out of proportion to the prevailing parasitemia (Schroeder and Ristic, 1968). This situation is attributable to immune-mediated destruction of nonparasitized erythrocytes in addition to that of parasitized erythrocytes. Immunologic

studies (Ristic, 1961; Schroeder and Ristic, 1965a, 1965b, 1968) indicate that during anaplasmosis, the host produces antibodies directed against the *Anaplasma* organism as well as against its own red cells. Only the antierythrocyte antibodies are implicated in the causation of immune-mediated anemia. The antibody (IgG) can be eluted off the erythrocytes, and such an antibody can sensitize normal autologous and homologous red cells to undergo in vitro phagocytosis (Ristic, 1961; Ristic et al., 1972). Thus parasitized erythrocytes as well as nonparasitized erythrocytes coated with the autoantibody in vivo are phagocytized by cells of the monocyte macrophage (reticuloendothelial) system rather than undergoing intravascular hemolysis, although erythrocyte osmotic fragility is increased. A positive Coombs test has been demonstrated in anaplasmosis. Autoagglutinins can be found bound to erythrocytes and free in serum of cattle during the acute and convalescent stages of anaplasmosis (Mann and Ristic, 1963) and act as cold-reacting IgM antibody. Demonstration of their presence requires use of trypsinized-erythrocytes. Autoagglutinins are thought to be produced as a result of alteration in the red cell membrane by the *Anaplasma*. In this context it has been shown that phospholipid concentration of infected erythrocytes is decreased (Schroeder and Dimopoullis, 1963) and that *Anaplasma* produces neuraminidase (Rao and Ristic, 1963). In addition to the antibody-dependent mechanisms involved in anemia, red cell destruction in anaplasmosis may also occur through a T cell–mediated antibody-independent mechanism (Kakoma, 1978).

Morphology of the Organism

Morphology of *Anaplasma* organisms associated with the disease in the Pacific Coast

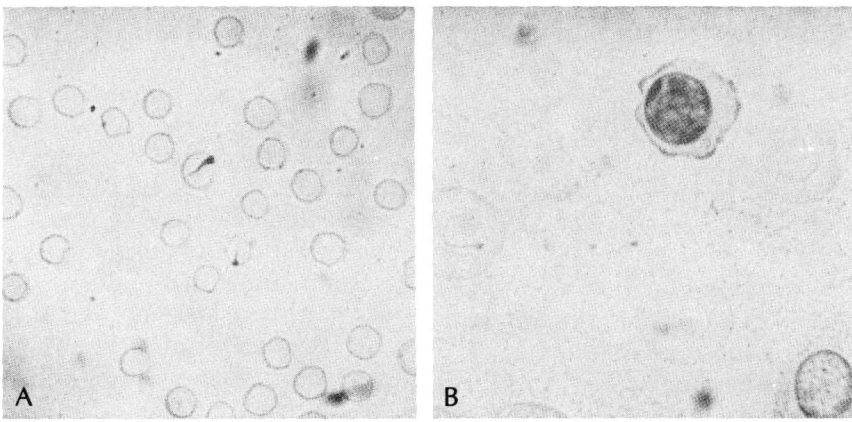

Fig. 23–1. Appendages associated with marginal bodies in anaplasmosis of cattle as demonstrated with new methylene blue vital staining technique.

states and in Mexico differs from the general conception of the organism seen in blood films stained by Romanowsky stains. Boynton (1932), in a study of anaplasmosis in California cattle, observed ring and tailed forms of *Anaplasma.* He considered the ring and tail-like structures associated with the typical marginal bodies of *Anaplasma* to be either erythrocytic substance or a portion of the parasite itself. Lotze and Yiengst (1942) and Franklin and Redmond (1958), using conventional staining, reported the presence of tails or appendages in association with their strains of *A. marginale.*

Espana and coworkers (1959, 1963) in Mexico employed phase contrast microscopy and the electron microscope to demonstrate ring, matchstick, comet, and dumbbell forms of the parasite. They also showed that the percentages of tailed and nontailed organisms varied markedly with the animal and the stage of the disease.

Pilcher et al. (1961), in Oregon, lysed erythrocytes containing *A. marginale* and described appendages not seen in the same blood stained by Giemsa method. The most common form consisted of a spherical head located at the periphery of the cell and a tail portion extending completely across the cell. Some spherical bodies without tails were observed, and a variant dumbbell form was described that consisted of two heads located at opposite edges of the cell connected by a thin band similar to the tails of the more common form. Madden (1962) investigated these pe-

culiar forms by fluorescent antibody technique. Schalm et al.(1962) reported that tails and loop-like appendages were readily demonstrable in unfixed blood films stained with new methylene blue (Figs. 23–1, 2–25). All these observations revealed the existence of two morphologically different forms of *Anaplasma:* the classical punctate structures, described by Theiler (1909) and observed in blood smears stained with Romanowsky stains, and the more complex tailed forms. The organism of *A. centrale* appears more frequently near the center of the erythrocyte whereas *A. marginale* appears near the cell margin.

Kreier and Ristic (1963a, b, c) made an extensive comparison of Florida and Oregon isolates of *Anaplasma.* The Florida isolate consisted of only one morphologic form, typical round marginal bodies. Three morphologic classes were identified for the Oregon isolate. The predominant form was the round marginal body. A second form had a marginally situated head with a body and a tail, and a third had a bipolar disc shape. The Oregon isolate was inoculated into calves, sheep, and deer. The authors concluded that the parasite forms with appendages were distinct from *A. marginale* and were present in blood in combination with *A. marginale.* They suggested the name *Paranaplasma caudata* (now *Paranaplasma caudatum*) for the tailed form and *Paranaplasma discoides* for the form with two heads at opposite sides of the erythrocyte connected by a band. These proposals were

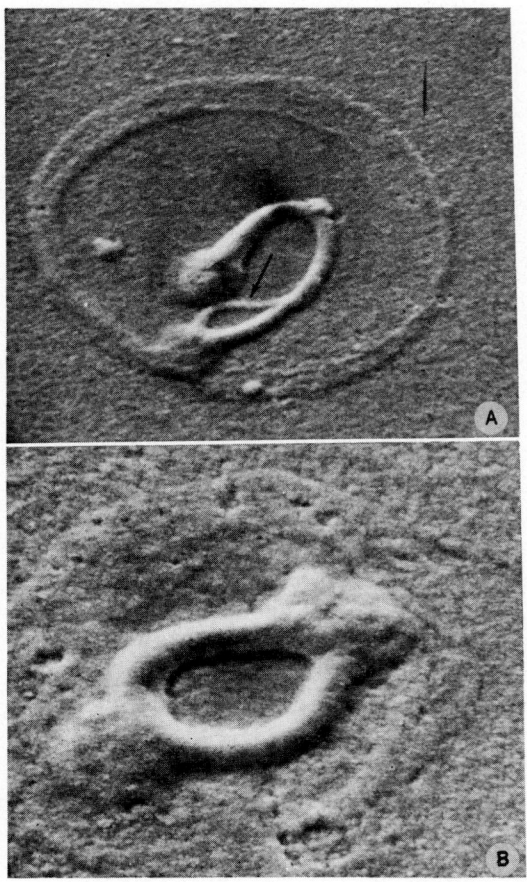

Fig. 23–2. Scanning electron micrographs of hemolyzed red cells parasitized with *Paranaplasma* organisms. *A,* Dumbbell form with two heads joined by a long, thin filament. Note the presence of a small, slender secondary filament *(arrow)* (×5,775). *B,* Discoid form, two heads doubly joined by tails (×10,625). (From Keeton and Jain, 1973; courtesy of the *Journal of Parasitology.*)

made on the basis that passage through sheep eliminated *P. caudatum* but permitted survival of *A. marginale* and *P. discoides*. In passage through the deer, only *A. marginale* survived. Fluorescein-labeled antibody and cross-immunity studies with premune cattle demonstrated the marginal body of the Oregon isolate to be antigenically identical to the Florida isolate, while the forms having appendages were antigenically and immunologically distinct from the Florida isolate. Keeton and Jain (1973), using the scanning electron microscope, have delineated more clearly the tailed organisms (Fig. 23–2).

The ultrastructure of *Anaplasma* has been studied by many workers (DeRobertis and Epstein, 1951; Foote et al., 1958; Gates et al., 1967; Ristic, 1967; Ristic and Watrach, 1961, 1963; Scott et al., 1961; Simpson et al., 1967; Summers and Padgett, 1970). The marginal body of *A. marginale* is a membrane-bound structure consisting of four to eight subunits or initial bodies, each of which is also membrane-bound. The initial bodies are round or oval structures measuring about 0.3 μm in diameter. It is believed that the initial body penetrates the erythrocyte membrane by invagination, resides within a vacuole, and divides by binary fission to form the marginal body. Thus various developmental stages of the organism can be observed in erythrocytes, smaller marginal bodies being evident during the early stage and larger ones during the peak of infection. It is believed that the cycle is completed by rupture of the marginal body and release of the initial bodies for penetration into additional erythrocytes. In vitro studies (Erp and Fahrney, 1975) indicate that the organism may leave the erythrocyte without lysing the cell, i.e., by exocytosis, and that red cell penetration can occur within 12–16 hours (Kreier and Ristic, 1961), probably by endocytosis. Histochemical staining of *A. marginale* demonstrated it to contain DNA, RNA, organic iron, and protein (Moulton and Christensen, 1955).

In comparison, ultrastructural studies of *Paranaplasma* have been limited (Espana et al., 1959; Keeton and Jain, 1973a; Ritchie, 1962; Simpson et al., 1965). Simpson et al. (1965) observed with the transmission electron microscope that the tailed portion of the organism did not appear membrane-limited and blended into the surrounding medium of the parasitized erythrocyte. The tailed structures appeared as elongated cylinders with a pattern of longitudinal and transverse striations indicating a periodicity of internal structure. It was concluded that the filaments and tails formed from organization of erythrocytic material and did not constitute part of the organism. In the scanning electron microscopic studies of Keeton and Jain (1973a), the filaments and tails seemed to be an integral part of the organism and continuous with the head structure. This finding was in accord with observations of Madden (1962), who by fluorescent antibody technique showed that the tail-like structures were an integral part of the organism.

Diagnosis

Diagnosis is based on history, clinical findings, and blood examination for evidence of anemia with or without remission and, most importantly, the presence of the organism. In Wright-stained blood films, *A. marginale* characteristically appears as a typical round, dark-staining inclusion along the margin of the mature erythrocytes (Plates XVIII–4, XVIII–5, XVIII–7). Immature erythrocytes seem to be resistant to penetration by *Anaplasma*, although rarely inclusion bodies may also be observed in polychromatic red cells. Usually one and infrequently two inclusion bodies are seen in a single erythrocyte. *Paranaplasma caudatum* and *P. discoides* present tail and loop forms evident only by special staining procedures including the new methylene blue stain. Only the marginal body is seen in Wright-stained films of blood infected with both of these organisms. It is stated that platelets may also become invaded by *A. marginale*, usually during the initial stage of parasitemia and less frequently when erythrocytes are heavily parasitized (Ristic and Watrach, 1962). This has not been our experience.

Detection of the carrier state may require inoculation of splenectomized calves, but it is costly and lengthy. Serologic tests such as indirect fluorescent antibody, complement-fixation, capillary agglutination, and card agglutination tests can be performed to detect the carrier state. The indirect fluorescent antibody and complement-fixation tests are highly sensitive and more accurate, the former being more sensitive (Gonzalez et al., 1978), while the card agglutination test is less accurate but is useful for a general herd survey. An ELISA test may be a better method of detection of infected animals in herds with *Anaplasma* infection (Thoen et al., 1980).

Therapy and Control

Acutely infected animals require rest and must avoid undue excitement. Treatment consists of administration of tetracycline and imidocarb. Effects of tetracycline therapy vary with the stage of the disease process, being most effective during the patent period. The carrier state can be eliminated by administration of tetracycline mixed in feed, but the animals become susceptible to reinfection. Blood transfusion may be given in severely anemic or nonresponsive animals.

Susceptibility of cattle to anaplasmosis seems to be age-related. Clinically the disease appears to be mild in calves up to 1 year of age, acute but rarely fatal in cattle up to 2 years of age, acute and occasionally fatal in cattle up to 3 years of age, and often peracute and fatal in cattle over 3 years of age. Calves for unknown reasons are naturally resistant to *Anaplasma* infection. The most susceptible animal is the splenectomized cow; splenectomized calves and intact cows are less susceptible. Immunization with an attenuated vaccine is possible, but the problem of vaccinated dams becoming sensitized to alloantigens in the vaccine has clouded the issue; calves born of such dams may exhibit neonatal isoerythrolysis (see Chapter 35). Vector control and elimination of natural reservoirs of infection are essential to limit spread of the disease, but seem impractical. In utero transmission of anaplasmosis has also been reported (Zaugg, 1985).

Infection can be transmitted readily between deer, from deer to cattle, and from cattle to deer. Several species of ticks, particularly *Boophilus*, have been found capable of transmitting anaplasmosis under experimental conditions (Ristic, 1968). The two most important ones are *Dermacentor occidentalis* and *Dermacentor andersoni*. The former is the most important vector of *Anaplasma* on the Pacific West Coast of the United States. Several species of *Tabanus* can also transmit the disease under experimental conditions. Mechanical transmission by surgical equipment may spread the disease. Flies and mosquitoes were not found to transmit *Anaplasma* in some experimental situations. Columbian black-tailed deer and the Rocky Mountain mule deer were found to serve as natural reservoirs for *A. marginale* infection of cattle occupying the same range (Boynton and Woods, 1933, 1940). The parasite was capable of biological transmission from deer to cattle by the tick *Dermacentor occidentalis*, and two additional species of ticks gave mechanical transfer (Boynton et al., 1936). These observations on the susceptibility of deer to *A. marginale* and the further demonstration of the actual presence of *A. marginale* carriers among the deer population of California were extended by Christensen et al. (1958, 1960) and Osebold et al. (1959). Wild elk also act as carriers of *Anaplasma* (Renshaw et al., 1976). White-tailed deer in southern Illinois were recently found to harbor *A. marginale* (Smith et al., 1982).

Anaplasmosis in Sheep and Goats

Intact or splenectomized sheep do not become infected with *A. marginale* (DeKock and Quinlan, 1926), although the organism may survive in such animals (Du Toit, 1934). DeKock and Quinlan (1926) found a distinct strain, *Anaplasma ovis*, in South African sheep which apparently produced only a mild subclinical disease in the intact animal. When carriers of *A. ovis* were splenectomized, "grave symptoms set in which in some instances proved to be fatal." *A. ovis* failed to infect either intact or splenectomized cattle but regularly became established in goats. In recent studies, splenectomy of asymptomatic, supposedly carrier sheep from endemic areas of Africa resulted in a serious infection with *A. ovis* and/or *Babesia ovis* within 21–70 days followed by a marked anemia within 7 days (Anosa et al., 1979).

The presence of *A. ovis* in the United States was first reported by Splitter et al. (1955, 1956). They recovered the parasite in Kansas from sheep originating from the Rocky Mountain region. Morphologically, *A. ovis* was identical to *A. marginale*, and cross antigenicity was observed in the complement-fixation test. Experimentally, the strain of *A. ovis* failed to infect splenectomized calves or cattle, and it did not produce any detectable immunity in cattle against *A. marginale*. Goats, however, developed a more severe reaction to *A. ovis* than sheep, and splenectomy increased susceptibility of both goats and sheep. While there are no reports of natural infection of deer with *A. ovis*, successful experimental infection was produced in two Virginia white-tailed deer (Kreier and Ristic, 1963d).

Recently, clinical observations, development of complement-fixing antibodies, and electron microscopic studies of *A. ovis* infection in Idaho sheep were described (Magonigle et al., 1981). *A. ovis* infection was experimentally transmitted to and recovered from splenectomized calves, although the organisms could not be found in circulating erythrocytes (Kuttler, 1981). Also, a transient infection of *A. marginale* into splenectomized goats was described (Maas and Buening, 1981).

Babesiosis (Piroplasmosis)

Protozoan parasites belonging to the family Babesiidae and the order Piroplasmoeda occur within erythrocytes of vertebrates and cause a hemolytic anemia. Reviews dealing with babesiosis in domestic animals have been published (Callow, 1977; Carmichael, 1956; Furie, 1982; Mahoney, 1977; Malherbe, 1956; Neitz, 1956; Purnell, 1981; Reik, 1968; Ristic, 1980, 1981; Ristic and Kreier, 1981). Levine (1971) enumerated 71 species of *Babesia* in various vertebrate hosts with 18 of the species causing disease in common domestic animals. Babesiosis in cattle is caused by *B. bigemina*, *B. bovis* (synonymous with *B. argentina*), *B. major*, and *B. divergens*; *B. bigemina* and *B. bovis* are economically more important. In sheep and goats babesiosis is caused by *B. ovis* and *B. motasi*; in horses by *B. equi* and *B. caballi*; in swine by *B. trautmanni* and *B. perroncitoi*; in dogs by *B. canis*, *B. gibsoni*, and *B.vogeli*; and in cats by *B. felis*.

Historically, *Babesia bigemina*, the cause of Texas fever of cattle, is of special interest. It was the first disease in which it was demonstrated that an arthropod could serve as an intermediate host and vector of the disease. Control of Texas fever through destruction of the intermediate host *(Boophilus annulatus)* by routine dipping of cattle in an insecticide led to discovery of the means to control malaria and yellow fever of humans through elimination of the breeding places of the mosquito vector.

Babesiosis is of great economic importance, particularly in the tropics and subtropics. The disease is transmitted by ixodid ticks. All domestic animal species are susceptible. Babesia are species-specific, and thus normally babesiosis does not spread between unrelated animal species. However, extremely rare

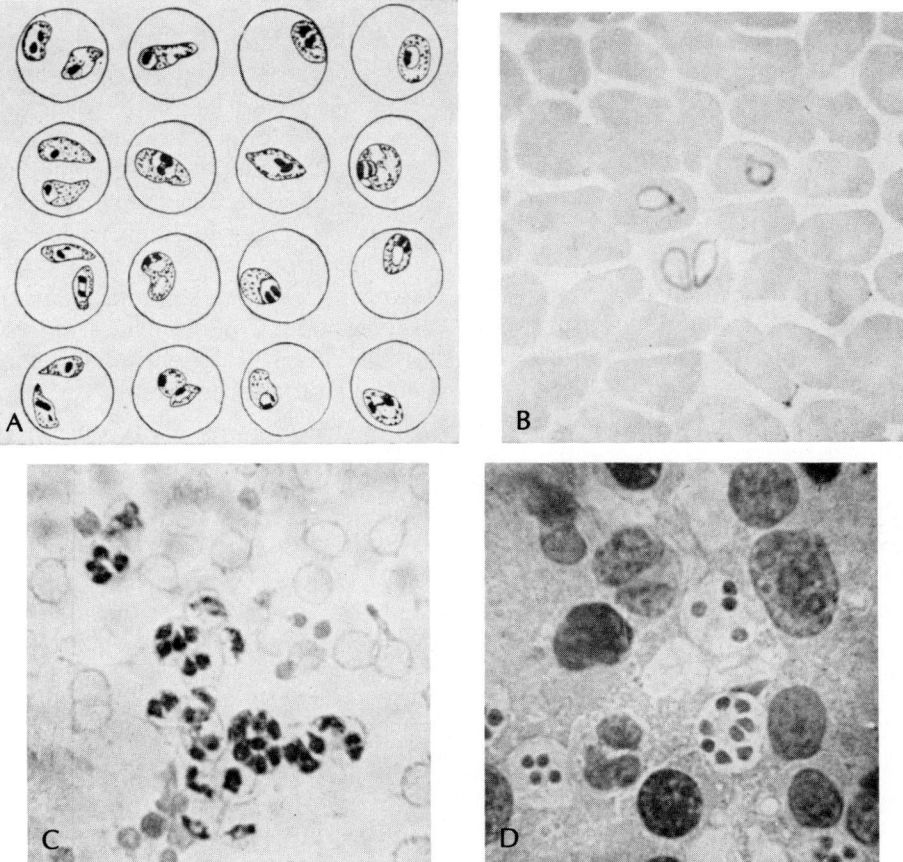

Fig. 23–3. Drawings and photographs of *Babesia canis.*

cases of human infection with *Babesia* species of animal origin have been reported (Jennings, 1976). In the United States, babesiosis has been known in the dog since 1934 (Sanders, 1937) and in the horse since 1961 (Sippel et al., 1962). Dikmans (1935) presented a series of sketches (Fig. 23–3A) depicting the morphology of the protozoon as observed in the first known case of canine babesiosis in the United States. Hematologic observations on experimental bovine babesiosis have been made (Lohr et al., 1977; Purnell et al., 1977; Wright, 1973).

Clinical Signs and Clinicopathologic Findings

The organisms (trophozoites) characteristically occur in the erythrocytes of the vertebrate host and present a round, ameboid, bizarre, rod-shaped, or typical pyriform morphology. *B. bigemina* is a large piroplasm

(4.0–5.0 × 2.0–3.0 μm), while *B. bovis* is small (2.4 × 1.5 μm). The pyriform organisms are connected at their narrow ends by a thin, filamentous structure and are arranged typically at an angle forming a morphologic basis for distinguishing *Babesia* species. The ultrastructure of *B. bovis* has been described (Todorovic, 1981). The organism divides by binary fission or a budding-like process within the erythrocyte and destroys the red cells intravascularly during escape from the cell (Callow and Pepper, 1974). Hence hemoglobinemia is often a prominent finding during the acute phase of the disease. The mechanism of red cell penetration is unknown, but studies with *B. rodhaini* in rats indicate that complement is critical in facilitating the infection (Ward and Jack, 1981). Surface proteins of *B. bovis*–infected erythrocytes of calves have been studied in this regard (Howard et al., 1980). Some *Babesia* species *(B. bovis, B. equi,* and *B. caballi)* also develop in other tissues of the host, e.g., the vascular endothelium.

The incubation period for babesiosis varies from 5–14 days depending on the species of *Babesia* involved. Prominent clinical signs of acute infection include fever, anorexia, dehydration, anemia, hemoglobinuria, terminal icterus, and death. The anemia is usually regenerative with erythrocyte indexes categorizing it as macrocytic and hypochromic. The degree of anemia is usually out of proportion to the degree of parasitemia—a finding that has been interpreted as indicating hemolysis not only of parasitized red cells but also of some unparasitized red cells, perhaps by an immune mechanism. Central nervous system signs may be seen in acutely ill cattle, and posterior paresis is common in sheep. Death is attributed to organic failure.

Prominent clinicopathologic findings of babesiosis include icterus, splenomegaly, reticuloendothelial cell hyperplasia with excessive hemosiderin, swollen and dark liver, distended urinary bladder with brownish-red urine, and enlarged and red kidneys. A unique finding with *B. bovis* and *B. canis* infections is that autoagglutination of both parasitized and nonparasitized erythrocytes blocks capillaries of the skin and brain (Ristic, 1981). *B. bovis* has a predilection for brain capillaries and can be detected in smears of gray matter of the cerebral cortex. DIC may occur as a complication of hemolytic anemia from babesiosis (Dalgliesh et al., 1976).

Diagnosis

Blood examination is essential to demonstrate babesiosis. However, the diagnosis of babesiosis, especially in chronic form, is often difficult without experimental animal inoculation. The erythrocytes containing the protozoa in the early acute stage are usually so numerous that there is little difficulty in finding infected cells. When the disease enters the chronic phase, however, the number of involved erythrocytes may be so small that diagnosis even from daily blood examination on numerous occasions may be impossible. Two helpful features should be kept in mind, both related to characteristics of erythrocytes harboring the parasite: (1) infected red cells are of lower specific gravity than noninfected mature erythrocytes, and (2) infected cells tend to be larger than noninfected cells. These features cause infected erythrocytes to concentrate to a greater extent in capillary blood; also the infected cells accumulate at the periphery of the blood film. Capillary blood from an ear should be tried, and the periphery of stained blood films should be given special attention in the search for the protozoon. *Babesia* organisms may also be found in erythrocytes in the bone marrow, spleen, and liver.

Watkins (1962) described a concentration and staining technique for equine blood that consisted of centrifuging blood at 1,500–2,000 rpm and collecting the erythrocytes from the top of the red cell column. Being of lower specific gravity, the infected cells tend to accumulate below the buffy coat. A thick film is prepared and placed in Giemsa stain that has been prepared in buffered, distilled water. The erythrocytes are lysed, leaving the protozoa intact. A second concentration technique consists of allowing blood to settle as in the erythrocyte sedimentation test and then transferring the plasma to a small centrifuge tube. The plasma is centrifuged at 2,500 rpm for 10 minutes and then decanted for preparation of films from the sediment. Staining is accomplished as mentioned.

Diagnosis in some cases may require transmission in a splenectomized animal. The effect of splenectomy varies with the species of *Babesia* involved; e.g., splenectomy rarely precipitates parasitemia in cattle infected with *B. bovis*, whereas a nonfatal parasitemia is a consistent finding with *B. bigemina* infection (Ristic, 1981).

Several serologic tests have been developed to detect carriers of infection; the complement fixation and the indirect immunofluorescence tests are used widely.

Treatment and Control

Control of the disease involves treatment, immunization, and vector control. Treatment involves administering a babesiacidal drug (Kuttler, 1981). Various drugs that have been used in treatment of babesiosis include derivatives of quinoline (e.g. acaprin), acridine, and diamidine (e.g. amicarbalide and diminazene aceturate). Imidocarb has also been used. In general, small babesiae are more refractory to treatment than large ones (Ristic, 1981). Eradication of tick vectors seems impractical and economically not feasible. Active immunization against babesiosis has been achieved with virulent strains, irradiated parasites, inactivated parasites in adjuvant, and more recently, in the case of *B. bovis*, with antigens derived from in vitro cell cultures (Ristic, 1981). The disease caused by *B. bovis* is more serious and difficult to control than that by *B. bigemina*. Cattle of certain breeds are more resistant to babesiosis, and calves of all breeds display a natural immunity and react minimally when infected up to the age of 7 months (Ristic, 1981), probably as a result of a serum factor (Levy et al., 1982). Newborn calves may develop the disease. Horses are highly resistant to infection, whereas puppies are very susceptible.

Recovery from an acute infection is followed by development of a carrier state. However, the carrier state in adult animals is generally created by premunition as a result of infection while young. Mild to marked relapses may occur following stress or splenectomy.

Canine Babesiosis

Both *B. canis* and *B. gibsoni* have been found in North America. *B. canis* is one of the largest *Babesia* species, measuring up to 5 μm in length and 2.5–3.0 μm in width. It is usually pyriform and sometimes may appear ameboid. As many as sixteen parasites can be found in a single erythrocyte. In comparison, *B. gibsoni* is usually much smaller and appears spherical, oval, elongate, ameboid, or rod-shaped; pyriform morphology is rare. An occasional Maltese cross form may be seen, as described for *B. equi* infection in horses. The ultrastructure of *B. canis* (Simpson et al., 1963) and *B. gibsoni* (Mimori et al., 1982) has been described. In a comparison of morphology of *B. canis* and *B. divergens*, the former organism appeared intracellular, forming surface bulges, and the latter was found partially epicellular (Gorenflot et al., 1979). Several reports describe clinicopathologic characteristics of babesiosis in the dog (Alperin and Bevins, 1963; Breitschwerdt, et al., 1983; Farwell et al., 1982; Groves and Yap, 1968; Mae-

graith et al., 1957; Malherbe, 1956; Moore, 1979a, 1979b; Moore and Williams, 1979).

Babesiosis in the dog may occur concurrently with other blood parasites, e.g., *Ehrlichia canis* and *Haemobartonella canis* (Ewing, 1969). Patients with dual infection become seriously ill and develop a severe normocytic-normochromic anemia. The anemia results from increased red cell destruction as well as from depressed erythropoiesis, the former being a result of *B. canis* and the latter of *E. canis* infection (Ewing and Buckner, 1965). A single intramuscular injection of imidocarb dipropionate, administered at a dose of 5 mg/kg, was found to result in successful recovery of 83.9% of dogs having babesiosis and 95.8% of dogs having ehrlichiosis (Adeyanju and Aliu, 1982).

The acute disease is characterized by fever, anorexia, depression, hemolytic anemia, hemoglobinuria, bilirubinuria, bilirubinemia, and icterus. Parasitemia is often detectable on blood examination (see experimental case described below). Dogs infected with *B. gibsoni* become listless and anorectic, develop an intermittent or constant fever, but rarely exhibit icterus and hemoglobinuria. DIC may occur as a complication during the acute phase of the disease (Moore, 1979a, 1979b; Moore and Williams, 1979). Splenomegaly and hepatomegaly are often seen (Seneviratna, 1965a, 1965b). As mentioned above, *B. canis*, like *B. bovis*, may be associated with agglutination of red cells in cerebral capillaries (Piercy, 1947; Purchase, 1947). In addition, dogs with *B. canis* infection develop metabolic acidosis (Button, 1979), in contrast to alkalosis seen in calves with *B. bovis* infection (Wright et al., 1982). Experimental babesiosis in dogs has been studied (Botros et al., 1975; Groves and Dennis, 1972).

Diagnosing the chronic form is a challenge and requires persistence. A low-grade or progressive anemia may be seen in such cases, but parasitemia is often undetectable. Serologic examination is particularly helpful in diagnosing such cases (Anderson et al., 1980; Popovic and Ristic, 1970; Ristic et al., 1971). The difficulty of diagnosis by blood examination facing the veterinarian in chronic babesiosis in the dog was dramatically demonstrated by the following case history:

A 2-year-old male German shepherd dog had wintered in Arizona and moved to the San Francisco Bay area. The dog was clinically normal on June 18, 1962, when first observed by the referring veterinarian. On July 3, the dog was depressed, the mucous membranes were pale, body temperature was 106°F, the PCV was 28%, and the WBC was 7,800/μl of blood. By July 9, the PCV had fallen to 18%. The dog was referred to the Veterinary School clinic on July 11. At that time, the hemogram revealed the following: PCV, 25%; WBC, 14,900; and lymphocytes, 38.5% (5,736/μl of blood). These findings indicated *anemia* associated with *lymphocytosis*. Erythrocyte morphology was typical of maturity, with slight anisocytosis, rare polychromasia, and a moderate number of leptocytes. The anemia was normocytic (MCV 65 fl) normochromic (MCHC 35.2%). The corrected erythrocyte sedimentation rate was -18 mm (observed rate of 17 mm minus anticipated rate of 35 mm for the PCV). The lymphocytosis was associated with normal-appearing lymphocytes. A bone marrow study revealed some late rubricytes with fragmenting nuclei and a few large phagocytic cells containing engulfed erythrocytes or red cell debris. The cause of the anemia and lymphocytosis was undiagnosed, and the dog was released to the owner on July 20th.

The dog was readmitted on August 8 for further study. A blood sample at this time revealed a few erythrocytes containing typical *B. canis* (Plate XVIII–6). This was a most fortunate occurrence, for although the dog was kept under close observation for 10 months, *B. canis* were never again observed in blood films prepared from either venous or capillary blood. During the first month, following the initial observation of *B. canis*, hemograms were taken almost daily and at various times of the day. The single most constant feature of the hemogram was a persistent lymphocytosis. Occasionally, the lymphocyte numbers dropped to within the high normal range (4,000–5,000), but more commonly lymphocytes comprised 35–60%, with values falling in the range of 40–46% after September 1962. The last hemogram, dated May 7, 1963, revealed PCV to be 46%, WBC 15,950, and lymphocytes 48% or 6,540/μl.

A mixed-female dog, 12 weeks old, was splenectomized on August 16. Ten ml of blood was taken from the German shepherd dog on August 27 and injected intravenously into the young splenectomized dog. The first temperature rise to 102.8°F occurred 96 hours later, and *B. canis* appeared in moderate numbers in peripheral blood at this time (Fig. 23–3*B*). Three days later, *B. canis* was found in blood with difficulty, and then it was not observed in venous blood collected during the next 7 days. The protozoon reappeared in venous blood on September 5 and rapidly increased in numbers (Fig. 23–3*C*). At this time the PCV dropped from the preinoculation level of 35% to 24%. From September 5 to September 15, the PCV fell to 6%. Despite the rapid fall in PCV, clinical icterus did not manifest until the day of death (September 15). Lymphocyte numbers did not exceed the normal range, like that seen in chronic disease of the German shepherd dog, but gradually diminished, as would be anticipated in stress-induced release of corticosteroids. The final leukogram on the day of death was typical of a degenerative left shift, falling lymphocyte numbers, eosinopenia, and monocytosis.

Examination of bone marrow, removed immediately after death, revealed erythrocytes containing multiple parasites (Fig. 23–3*D*). Search for an initial stage of development of the parasite within the red cell was unsuccessful.

Lymphoid hyperplasia was observed in dogs with chronic babesiosis, and the increased lymphocytic activity was directly correlated with the numbers of lymphocytes present in the peripheral blood (Dorner, 1969). Lymphocytosis, as observed in the German shepherd described above, seems to be a feature in the dog chronically infected with *B. canis*. Lymphokine-mediated activation of normal macrophages was observed during infection with *B. gibsoni* (Ishimine et al., 1979).

Anderson et al. (1979) recently described probably the first case of *B. gibsoni* infection in a standard poodle dog in the United States. Clinical signs included vomiting, anorexia, and rectal temperature of 40°C. A severe anemia was evident and 0.2–1.6% red cells were parasitized with one to many ring forms of *B. gibsoni*. Successful experimental transmission was achieved in an intact dog and a splenectomized dog, both of which exhibited parasitemia by the sixth day, and as many as 29% erythrocytes were parasitized shortly before death by the twenty-seventh day. A sensitive and reproducible indirect fluorescent antibody test for a North American isolate of *B. gibsoni* has been developed (Anderson et al., 1980). Comparative features of *B. canis* and *B. gibsoni* infections have been described recently (Farwell et al., 1982). A positive Coombs test was found in many of the infected dogs.

Feline Babesiosis

Futter and colleagues (1980a, 1980b, 1981) have described observations on natural and experimental babesiosis in domestic cats. Lethargy, anorexia, and anemia were seen in both situations. Red cell parameters in experimental cases decreased within 7–10 days, and a marked anemia developed within 3 weeks of infection. Icterus was present in only occasional cases; fever was absent. Death occurred in all untreated cases. Blood examination revealed increased polychromasia, Howell-Jolly bodies, nucleated erythrocytes, anisocytosis, macrocytosis (increased MCV), and hypochromasia (decreased MCHC) indicative of a regenerative anemia. Erythrophagocytosis by monocytes was also observed. A moderate increase occurred in serum bilirubin with indirect-reacting bilirubin being usually higher than the direct-reacting pigment. Total plasma protein concentration did not change, but γ-globulins were increased.

Equine Babesiosis

Babesia equi and *Babesia caballi* infect horses, mules, donkeys, and zebras (Knowles and Uniss-Floyd, 1983; Mahoney, 1977; Maurer, 1962a, 1962b; Purnell, 1981). The organisms divide by binary fission, giving rise to two or four daughter trophozoites. *B. caballi* are most readily recognized in erythrocytes as paired pyriform bodies with their pointed ends meeting at an acute angle. They are usually 2.5–4.0 μm in greatest dimension and resemble *B. bigemina*. The trophozoites of *B. equi* are quite pleomorphic with round, oval, and/or ring forms predominating. They are most readily distinguished when observed as small (2.0 μm in length), pyriform bodies in groups of four with pointed ends meeting to form a Maltese cross. The ultrastructure of *B. equi* has been described (Simpson and Neal, 1980; Simpson et al., 1963; Moltmann et al., 1983). Crystalline inclusions were found in a few red cells parasitized with *B. equi* following treatment of ponies with imidocarb (Simpson and Neal, 1980).

Presently, equine piroplasmosis from *B. caballi* is considered endemic in certain parts of the United States (Knowles et al., 1980). In early reports, *B. equi* was found to have a wider distribution and generally greater pathogenicity than *B. caballi* (Maurer, 1962a, 1962b). An acute case usually displays clinical signs of a progressive hemolytic anemia. Parasitemia is evident in such animals, particularly during febrile periods for 36–72 hours, and not in convalescing or carrier animals. Mortality may be as high as 20%. *Dermacentor nitens* is considered the principal vector of *B. caballi* (Roby and Anthony, 1963). Clinical disease develops in a susceptible horse 14–21 days after the horse is placed with infected horses in endemic areas of equine piroplasmosis. Transmission through contaminated instruments may occur. Experimental infection has been produced in intact and splenectomized horses and donkeys (Knowles et al., 1980; Nafie et al., 1982). The incubation period was 7 days in splenectomized horses and 11 days in intact horses. Infected animals developed fever, edema of limbs, anemia, icterus, and leukopenia or leukocytosis. Recent in vitro and in vivo studies (Moltmann et al., 1983; Schein et al., 1981) demonstrated that tick-borne *B. equi* sporozoites invade lymphocytes of the horse and develop into schizonts from which merozoites are produced that subsequently invade the erythrocytes.

In an attempt to control and eventually eradicate equine babesiosis from the United States, serologic methods for the diagnosis of carriers have been developed. These include a gel precipitation method, a one-step fluorescein-labeled antibody inhibition test, a complement fixation test, and an indirect fluorescein-antibody method to detect carrier horses experimentally infected with *B. caballi* (Knowles et al., 1980; Madden and Holbrook, 1968; Ristic and Sibinovic, 1964).

Haemobartonellosis

The blood parasites of the genus *Haemobartonella* are morphologically similar to *Eperythrozoa*. Seamer (1959) briefly described *Haemobartonella* as small cocci or beaded bacilli on the surface of the erythrocyte, and *Eperythrozoa* as cocci or rings on or between the red cells. Peters and Wigand (1955) questioned the justification for two generic names on trifling differences in morphology.

Haemobartonellosis in Cats

The blood parasite responsible for feline infectious anemia (FIA) of cats was first reported in the United States from Colorado by Flint and Moss (1953). The name *Haemobartonella felis* was given to the parasite by Flint and McKelvie (1955) and is currently in use. Seamer and Douglas (1959) observed the parasite in anemic cats in Great Britain and preferred the name *Eperythrozoon felis* because Clark (1942) of South Africa had already so named it.

The morphologic features of *H. felis* are well documented (Seamer and Douglas, 1959; Splitter et al., 1956). The organism is highly pleomorphic; it may appear as a coccoid body, a delicate ring, or a small rod. The predominant form seen may vary with the stage of the disease and the individual cat; small ringlike forms may be seen in large numbers on the surface of erythrocytes at the height of parasitemia (Plates XVIII–1, XVIII–2). The organisms may appear singly, in pairs, in a small group, or as short chains of coccoid bodies attached to the erythrocytes. Although both mature and immature erythrocytes may be parasitized, the former are more commonly involved. Rarely, organisms may be observed in the plasma (Seamer and Douglas, 1959; Small and Ristic, 1971). Our experience has been that the organism often detaches from erythrocytes in refrigerated anticoagulated blood, and so examination of fresh blood is essential for diagnostic evaluation.

Results of electron microscopic studies (Demaree and Nessmith, 1972; Simpson et al., 1978; Small and Ristic, 1971) of *H. felis* have confirmed and extended observations made with the light microscope which showed that the organism occupies an epicellular location.

The erythrocyte membrane at the site of parasitic attachment is usually indented and may be partially eroded. The organism is membrane-bound, and its internal contents include electron-dense granules, short fine filaments, and microtubules. It is anuclear, but both DNA and RNA can be demonstrated. Indications were that the organism reproduces by both binary fission and budding. Jain and Keeton (1973) used the scanning electron microscope to demonstrate the pleomorphic nature of the organism and a deep pitting of the erythrocyte surface by the parasite (Fig. 23–4).

Specific diagnosis of FIA presents a problem because infected cats may not be presented in the initial acute stage when the parasite is present in peripheral blood in large numbers. Great care must be taken to avoid confusing the parasite with the stain precipitate. When the disease is suspected but the parasite has not been observed in the stained blood film, it is advisable to examine the blood on at least four occasions, generally on consecutive days (see Appendix Case 52). Small and Ristic (1967) compared Giemsa, acridine orange, and fluorescent-labeled antibody staining methods for detection of *H. felis*. Close agreement was found between the acridine orange and fluorescent-labeled antibody methods, but Giemsa staining was less than 50% reliable.

Feline infectious anemia is a disease seen largely in male cats (Flint et al., 1958). Among 30 domestic cats developing a natural infection and presented to our clinic in various stages of disease, 27 were male and 3 were female. Data from admission hemograms of these 30 cats are summarized in Table 23–4. A common complaint was that the cat had been lethargic and anorectic for 2 or more days. Variable clinical signs included fever, dehydration, and enlarged lymph nodes and spleen. Frequently medical history included stress; sometimes the cat had been away from home for several days and had returned in an exhausted condition, or it had been in a fight several weeks before, suffering bite wounds resulting in abscess formation. Stress appeared with sufficient frequency in the medical history to suggest activation of a latent infection as the body's defenses became

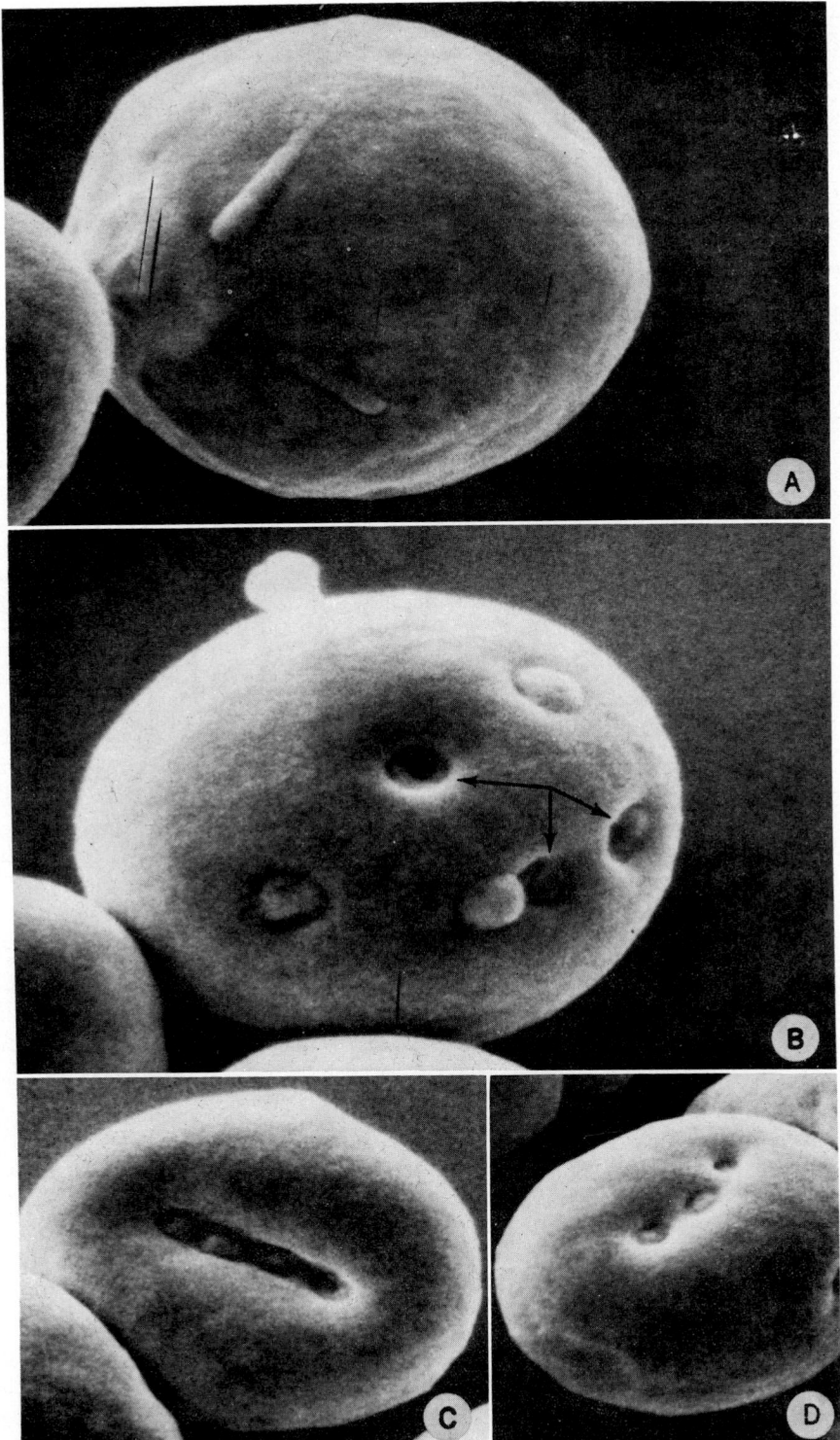

Fig. 23–4. Scanning electron photomicrographs of erythrocytes from a cat naturally infected with *Haemobartonella felis. A*, An erythrocyte with two rod-shaped organisms attached lengthwise (×16,600). *B*, An erythrocyte with coccoid bodies and surface lesions *(arrows)* apparently produced by parasitic adhesions and becoming evident after the parasite had become dislodged (×18,500). *C*, An erythrocyte with coccoid bodies and sites of parasitic attachment aligned in a rod-shaped groove that would appear as a short chain of *Haemobartonella* bodies under the light microscope (×12,500). *D*, An erythrocyte with three sites of parasitic attachment in the form of a short chain (×10,850). (From Jain and Keeton, 1973; courtesy of *The American Journal of Veterinary Research*).

Table 23–4. Ranges, Means, and Standard Deviations in Hemogram Data of 30 Cats with Natural Infection Due to *Haemobartonella felis*

	Range	Mean ± 1 SD
Erythrocytes ($\times 10^6/\mu$l)	0.63–5.60	2.32 ± 1.18
Hemoglobin (g/dl)	1.8–6.8	4.4 ± 1.5
PCV (%)	6.0–23.0	14.5 ± 4.6
MCV (fl)	33.9–109.9	70.8 ± 20.0
MCHC (%)	20.0–35.8	29.5 ± 4.0
MCH (pg)	12.1–28.8	20.8 ± 4.8
Plasma protein (g/dl)	5.7–10.9	7.9 ± 1.1
Icterus index units	0.0–75.0	8.0 ± 15.6
WBC/μl	2,300–49,000	12,660 ± 8,840
Band neutrophils	0–2,200	430 ± 490
Mature neutrophils	1,220–36,995	8,395 ± 7,365
Lymphocytes	560–5,984	2,828 ± 1,575
Monocytes	0–4,165	870 ± 869
Eosinophils	0–630	116 ± 179
Basophils	0–245	13 ± 47
WBC (%)		
Band neutrophils	0.0–8.0	3.0 ± 2.3
Mature neutrophils	35.0–93.0	61.9 ± 14.1
Lymphocytes	2.0–53.0	26.8 ± 12.3
Monocytes	0.0–22.0	7.0 ± 5.5
Eosinophils	0.0–5.0	1.0 ± 1.5
Basophils	0.0–1.0	0.1 ± 0.3

weakened. In addition, *H. felis* may reappear in peripheral blood of carrier cats afflicted with a severe terminal or systemic disease. It has been reported, however, that exogenous administration of corticosteroids failed to induce relapse in carrier cats; rather it helped erythropoietic recovery in the face of parasitemia (Harvey and Gaskin, 1977). Perhaps the nature and extent of stress under natural conditions is different than under experimental situations. Carrier cats appear to be immune to the parasite, since hemolytic destruction of erythrocytes does not take place. Occasionally, a cat with a past history of FIA has subsequently developed erythroleukemia or lymphosarcoma. Such occurrences may be coincidental. Haemobartonellosis is associated with an increased incidence of feline leukemia virus (FeLV) infection (Priester and Hayes, 1973).

The degree of anemia seen on presentation of the cat to the veterinarian will depend on the stage of the disease. Among 30 cats (Table 23–4), PCV values varied from 6–23% on admission, and the icterus index varied from 0–75 units. It is possible that cyclic bouts of parasitemia lead to the more advanced stages of anemia. Plasma protein concentration is generally increased somewhat above normal because of some hemoconcentration. Evidence of immaturity of erythrocytes in peripheral blood (polychromasia or reticulocytosis) is to be anticipated; its extent varies with the degree of recent erythrocyte destruction (Appendix Case 53). MCV varied from 33.9–109.9 fl with a mean of 70.8 fl. Thus, in a few cats, evidence of remission of the anemia was lacking, while in a few others the evidence was very marked at the time of admission.

Feline infectious anemia may affect cats of all ages; the majority of cases occur between 1 and 3 years of age (Flint et al., 1958). The range in our data was from 7 months to 12 years, with 50% of the cases falling within 1–3 years of age.

The mode of transmission of the parasite among cats under natural conditions is not known, although it can be demonstrated to be an infectious disease by inoculation of intact cats with blood from an infected cat (Appendix Case 53). Flint et al. (1959) found the effect of splenectomy to be minimal in experimental transmission of the parasite. It is possible, however, that removal of the spleen may favor reappearance of the parasite in the blood of cats with latent infection. For this reason, cats intended for use as blood donors in our clinic are splenectomized and monitored closely by blood film examination for freedom from latent infections.

Harvey and Gaskin (1977) produced exper-

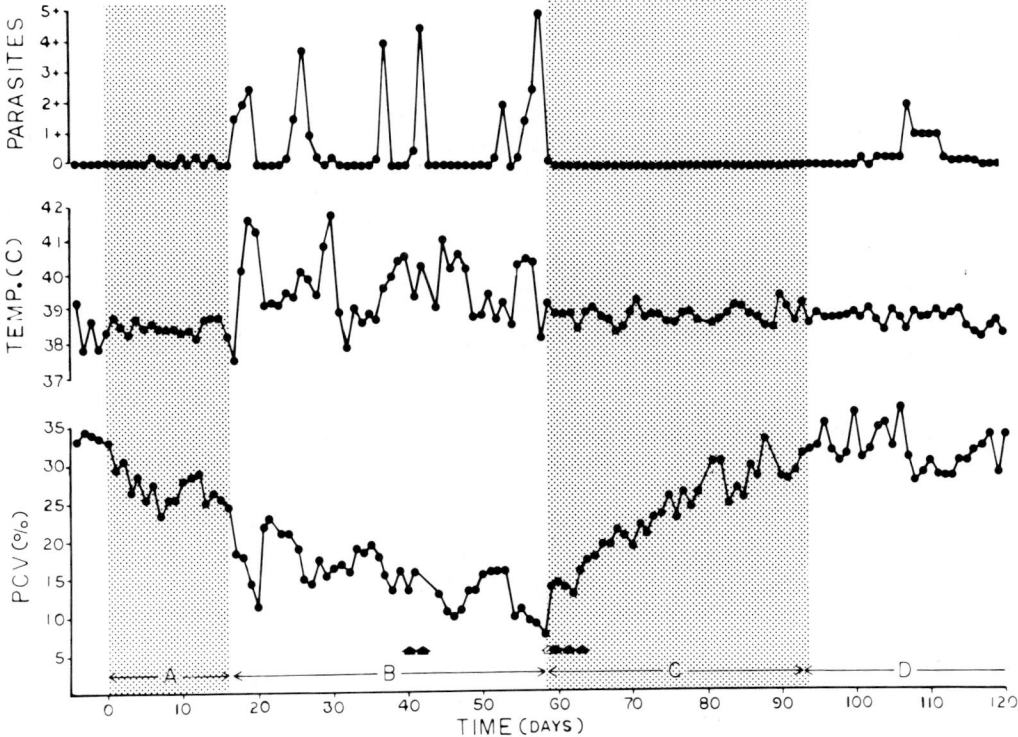

Fig. 23–5. Packed cell volume (PCV), rectal temperatures, and blood parasite values in a cat following intravenous inoculation with *Haemobartonella felis*–infected blood on day 0. Closed arrows indicate IV thiacetarsamide sodium (1 mg/kg) administration. Open arrow indicates a 25-ml IV whole blood transfusion. Phases of disease are indicated by letter and shading; A is the preparasitemic phase, B is the acute phase, C is the recovery phase, and D is the carrier phase. (From Harvey and Gaskin, 1977; courtesy of the *Journal of the American Animal Hospital Association.*)

imental haemobartonellosis in eight normal, nonsplenectomized cats by intravenous inoculation of 1.0 ml blood from a natural case of *H. felis* in Florida. All cats developed anemia following one or more bouts of parasitemia (Fig. 23–5). The first parasitemia was apparent within 2–17 (mean 8.4) days. A parasitemic episode rarely persisted beyond 4 days and usually lasted 1–2 days. Infrequently parasites were eliminated within a few hours so that 18.6% of the time very few parasites were demonstrable in blood films, and 35.5% of the time none were demonstrable. The PCV usually decreased as the parasitemia heightened, whereas the disappearance of parasites from the circulation was in many cases associated with a sudden increase in PCV. In general, anorexia and weight loss were constant findings, but fever and icterus were infrequent. Prominent laboratory findings during the acute phase included icterus, slight to marked increase in erythropoiesis, decreased myeloid:erythroid ratio, absence or

low levels of serum haptoglobin, and a moderate increase in total plasma protein concentration. Leukocyte numbers varied widely from leukopenia to leukocytosis with a regenerative left shift.

One cat died during the acute phase of the disease, one was treated, and the remaining spontaneously attained preinoculation levels of PCV by 2–4 months postinfection and became chronic carriers of *H. felis*. Three kittens were born of an infected pregnant cat. No parasites were found in the kittens at birth, but parasitemia was observed in one kitten at 3 days of age and in the other two at 3 months of age. The mode of transmission of infection to the kittens was unknown. The possibility that *H. felis* could be transmitted transplacentally or via the milk was suggested in a recent report (Fisher et al., 1983).

In other experimental studies with *H. felis*, it was found that erythrocyte osmotic fragility was increased with development of parasitemia and loss of red cell cholesterol and phospholipid (Maede, 1980), the direct Coombs test was positive for an average of 15 days after the first appearance of *H. felis*, and half-time survival of ^{51}Cr-labeled red cells was reduced by about 50% (Maede, 1975; Maede and Hato, 1975). Radioisotopic and electron microscopic studies indicated that parasitized red cells sequester mainly in the spleen, and that erythrophagocytosis occurs, or the parasite is removed by macrophages and the pitted red cells are returned to the circulation (Maede, 1978, 1979). In splenectomized cats, red cell destruction occurred in the lungs, liver, and bone marrow (Maede, 1978; Maede and Murata, 1978). Parasitemia was longer in splenectomized cats. Erythrophagocytosis was also seen in 11 of 15 cats for about 20 days after the first appearance of parasites in the blood (Maede and Hato, 1975).

Therapy of FIA varies with clinical condition of the patient. Blood transfusion is recommended when PCV is less than 12% and fluids are given to dehydrated animals. Tetracycline is administered specifically to combat the infection. Corticosteroids have been found beneficial (Harvey, 1980).

Haemobartonellosis in Dogs

Haemobartonella canis can be found in normal dogs, but it is seldom pathogenic for an intact (nonsplenectomized) dog. Isolated incidences of anemia in intact dogs from this infection have been reported (Austerman, 1979; Lumb, 1961; North, 1978; Pryor and Bradbury, 1975; Sonoda et al., 1978; West, 1979). Clinical anemia develops when a carrier dog is splenectomized for experimental or therapeutic purposes (Benjamin and Lumb, 1959; Brodey and Schalm, 1963; Carr and Essex, 1944; Knutti and Hawkins, 1925; McNaught et al., 1935; Middleton et al., 1982; Rhoads and Miller, 1935); or when a carrier dog develops another disease such as bacterial or parasitic infection (Oduye and Dipeolu, 1976; Sonoda et al., 1978); or when a splenectomized dog is transfused with blood from a donor that is a carrier of *H. canis* (Schalm and Theilen, 1972). The incubation period of canine haemobartonellosis is about 15 days.

Schalm and Theilen (1972) reported an unusual occurrence of haemobartonellosis fol-

lowing a blood transfusion to a dog with depressed splenic activity due to lymphosarcoma and corticosteroid therapy. The donor dog was subsequently shown to be a carrier of *H. canis*. The infection can be transmitted experimentally in splenectomized dogs by the dog tick *Rhipicephalus sanguineus* (Seneviratna et al., 1973).

Clinically affected dogs exhibit listlessness, episodes of fever, hemolytic anemia, icterus, and bilirubinemia. Hematologic findings are typical of a regenerative anemia. Leukocytosis from neutrophilia with left shift may be seen in an occasional patient.

H. canis differs in morphology from *H. felis* in that it more commonly forms chains extending across the surface of affected erythrocytes, although individual organisms appearing as small dots or rods are also seen (Plate XVIII–3). The degree of parasitemia is variable, staining is delicate, and a diligent search must be made to observe the organism when present in small numbers. The ultrastructure of *H. canis* and its relation to the erythrocyte has been investigated (Venable and Ewing, 1968; Sonoda et al., 1978). The organism adheres to, but does not penetrate, the erythrocyte membrane. Single organisms were found to dimple the surface of the erythrocyte, while aggregates (chains) produced grooves or deep infoldings in the erythrocyte surface.

We have recently made scanning and transmission electron microscopic studies of erythrocytes of an anemic dog with haemobartonellosis (Jain, unpublished observations, 1982). *H. canis* was found singly, in small groups, or in chains on the surface of erythrocytes (Fig. 23–6A, B, C). Indentation of the erythrocyte surface was observed by transmission electron microscopy, but erosion of the red cell membrane was not evident (Fig. 23–6D). It is conjectured that anemia in *H. canis* infection probably does not result from direct damage to the erythrocyte and may involve some other mechanisms such as immune-mediated red cell destruction. Bundza et al. (1976) have observed *H. canis* infection in a dog with Coombs-positive anemia.

Haemobartonellosis in Cattle

Haemobartonella bovis has been observed in cattle from some Asian, European, and Af-

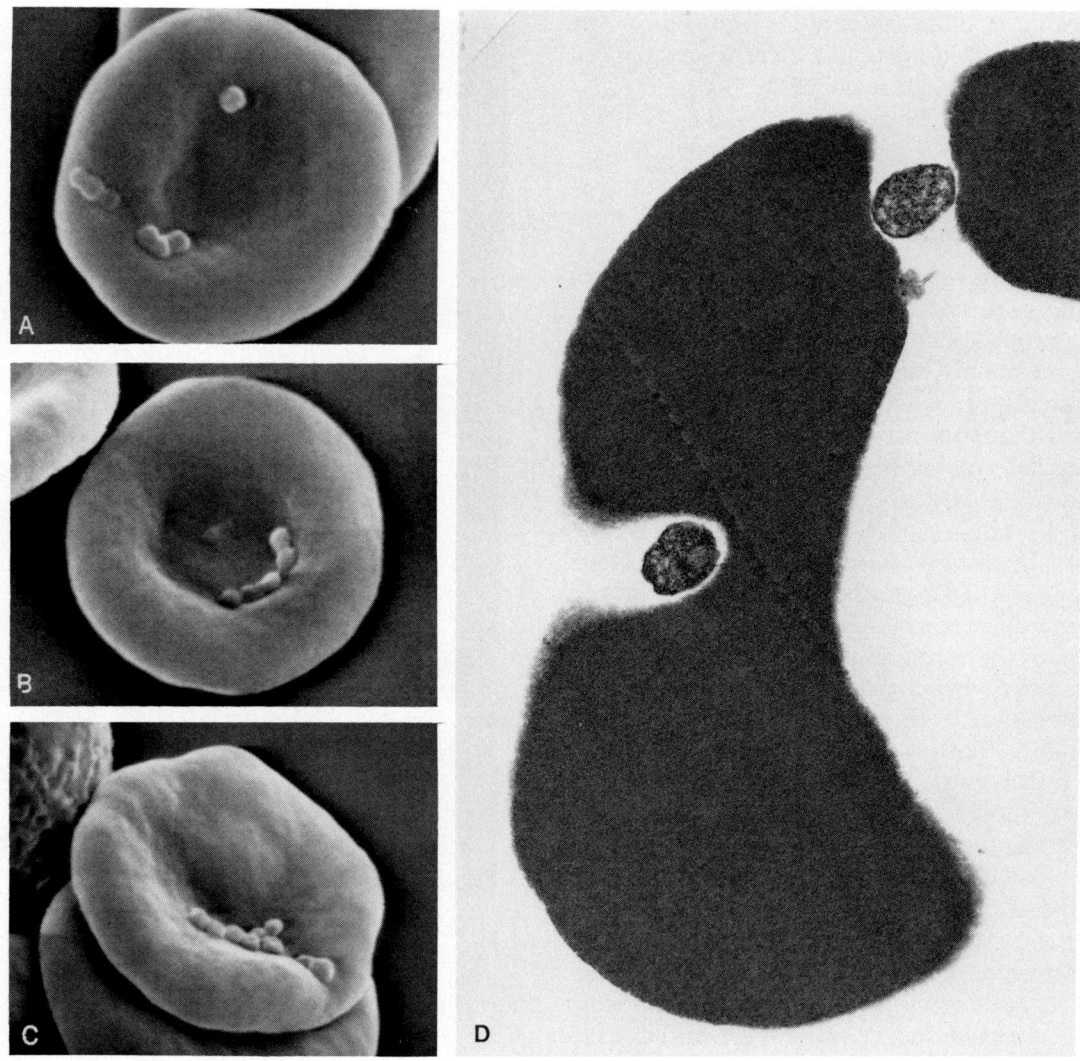

Fig. 23–6.   Scanning *(A–C)* and transmission *(D)* electron photomicrographs of *Haemobartonella canis*. Single organisms as well as small groups and short chains are seen epicellularly on the erythrocytes with surface indentations at some locations. A–C ×6,000, D ×10,000.

rican countries (see review by Kreier and Ristic, 1968), but is rarely considered to be the cause of anemia. It can also be found in association with other protozoan diseases (Barnett and Brocklesby, 1971; Brocklesby, 1970).

This organism was observed by Simpson and Love (1970) to be closely associated with the surface of the erythrocyte, but separated from the erythrocytic membrane by a narrow and definite space. The parasite was rod-shaped, ovoid, or chained. In the liver, erythrocyte-associated organisms were observed in

phagocytic vesicles of Kupffer cells. These authors concluded that erythrophagocytosis, and not hemolysis, appeared to be responsible for the anemia produced by *H. bovis* in splenectomized calves.

Love and McEwen (1972) observed the appearance of a *Haemobartonella*-like parasite in each of ten splenectomized calves. The mean incubation period was 18 days, and parasitemia persisted a mean of 8 days. The parasites were attached to the surface of the erythrocytes and were also found free in the plasma. A decrease in PCV occurred at the peak of parasitemia, and there was a marked fall in blood glucose concentration.

Eperythrozoonosis

Eperythrozoonosis in Cattle

Eperythrozoon wenyoni, a red cell parasite of cattle, was first described by Adler and Ellenbogen (1934) in a splenectomized calf. The organisms in Giemsa-stained films appeared coccoid and vesicular in nature, either scattered regularly on erythrocytes, arranged in irregular chains, or in tight groups of 50-60 parasites. The organisms measured about 0.2–1.5 μm in diameter and appeared to multiply by binary fission or budding. Neitz (1940) studied eperythrozoonosis in cattle and found delicate ring forms to be most common with ovoid, comma, rod, dumbbell, and tennis racket forms also present. The parasites were seen both epicellularly and in the plasma. Similar organisms were also observed in cattle used in studies on anaplasmosis (Lotze and Yiengst, 1941). These morphologic forms of *E. wenyoni* are readily seen in blood films stained with Wright (Plates XVIII–4, XVIII–5) or other Romanowsky stains.

Kreier and Ristic (1963) performed a detailed study of the morphologic characteristics of *E. wenyoni* and *E. ovis* using various techniques. Delicate basophilic rings, about 1 μm in diameter, were seen in the plasma and on erythrocytes in Giemsa-stained films, while spherical organisms were observed in wet preparations examined with the phase contrast microscope. Electron photomicrographs of shadow-cast preparations revealed the organisms to be oblong or circular in shape and attached to the erythrocyte surface, often in peripheral position or free in plasma.

Keeton and Jain (1973) studied morphologic characteristics of *E. wenyoni* with the scanning electron microscope. Coccoid and oval organisms were seen in epicellular locations as solitary bodies and arranged in chains, clusters, or pairs (Fig. 23–7). Budding seemed to be the primary mode of replication. The erythrocyte surface at the site of parasitic adherence in some instances seemed to be

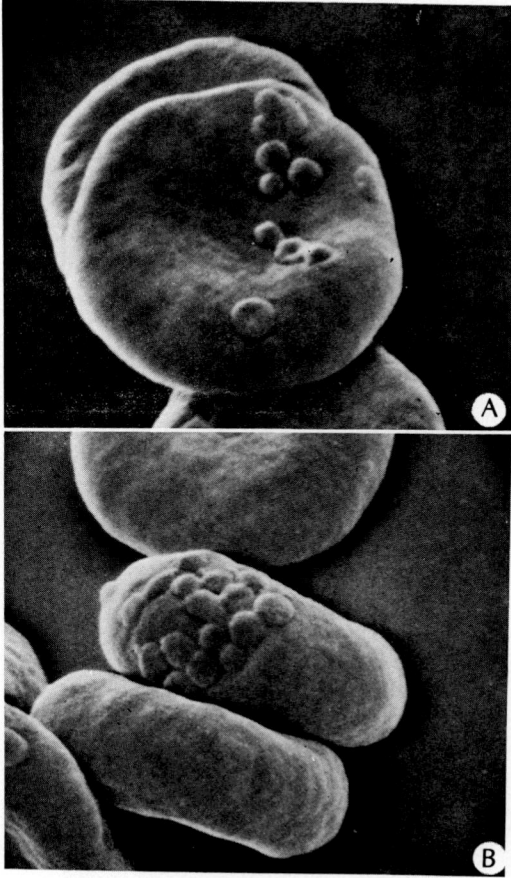

Fig. 23–7. Scanning electron micrographs of bovine erythrocytes parasitized with *Eperythrozoon wenyoni. A,* ×7,840. *B,* ×8,400. (From Keeton and Jain, 1973; courtesy of the *Journal of Parasitology.*)

slightly depressed, but surface erosions and altered red cell morphology, as seen with *Haemobartonella felis* (Fig. 23–4), were not found. The lack of notable erythrocyte membrane alterations was considered important in that anemia was not seen during or following parasitemia in the case studied.

The infection is typically latent in cattle, but is encountered clinically in splenectomized cattle or cattle severely ill from other causes. Numerous *Eperythrozoa* were observed in blood samples from three Hereford cattle and a Holstein cow, all exhibiting edema of the hind legs. These occurrences were unassociated with any evidence of anemia or increased icterus index. Hemolytic anemia is encountered most commonly as a clinical entity under experimental conditions when calves are splenectomized for transmission trials with anaplasmosis (Lotze and Yiengst, 1941), although in some splenectomized cattle only a slight reduction in RBC may be seen (Kreier and Ristic, 1963; Neitz, 1940). After splenectomy of calves harboring a latent infection, a period of mild depression and temperature elevation of 103–106°F may occur in a week to 10 days. During the febrile phase, myriads of tiny coccoid and rod-like organisms appear on the surface of the erythrocytes and in the plasma between the red cells. The calves may develop anemia as evidenced by a reduction in RBC, hemoglobin, and PCV of 25–50% and blood morphology typical of anemia in remission. This is followed by rapid recovery.

In experimental transmission of anaplasmosis to splenectomized calves, the donor blood may harbor infection with *Eperythrozoa* and *Anaplasma*. The incubation period of the former is shorter than that of the latter, so an initial illness due to eperythrozoonosis may precede by several days the more severe disease of anaplasmosis. Interference between anaplasmosis and eperythrozoonosis has been reported in experimentally infected splenectomized cattle (Foote et al., 1957).

Eperythrozoonosis in Sheep and Goats

Eperythrozoon ovis was described and named by Neitz et al. (1934). They encountered the parasite under experimental conditions in splenectomized sheep inoculated with blood from other animals. The organisms typically appeared as delicate vesicular rings, 0.5–1.0 μm in diameter, occurring both on the erythrocytes and in the plasma. In addition, ovoid forms, irregular triangles, and rod, dumbbell, and comma forms were seen. Eperythrozoonosis in sheep differs from the disease in cattle in that *E. ovis* is more pathogenic and may produce a clinical syndrome of anemia under natural conditions.

Eperythrozoonosis was reported in lambs on two adjacent properties in New South Wales (Littlejohns, 1960). Mortality was 10% among 390 unweaned lambs. Clinical signs were profound anemia and staggering, with apparent stiffness of the hindquarters. The parasite was readily found in the blood in early stages but disappeared when the anemia became advanced. Littlejohns com-

mented that "possibly the pathogenicity of *E. ovis* may to some extent be dependent on the presence of factors operating in a synergistic or simple additive manner."

It has been reported that *E. ovis* may induce a severe hemolytic anemia in heavily infected sheep, but usually only slight manifestations of disease are noted (Overas, 1969). Primary infection with *E. ovis* can induce anemia in lambs (Daddow, 1979b). The anemia is thought to result predominantly from intravascular hemolysis and partly from erythrophagocytosis (Sutton, 1978). *E. ovis* can be transmitted to goats, which develop a lower degree of parasitemia than sheep and become chronic carriers (Daddow, 1979a).

Sheep are not susceptible to *E. wenyoni* even when splenectomized (Neitz, 1940). A close serologic relationship was found between *E. wenyoni* and *E. ovis* by a fluorescein-labeled antibody technique (Kreier and Ristic, 1963).

Eperythrozoonosis in Pigs

Eperythrozoon suis and *Eperythrozoon parvum* were first described by Splitter (1950) as blood parasites of swine in the United States. The former is the more pathogenic, being capable of causing clinical anemia and icterus in young pigs under natural conditions. The latter is nonpathogenic for intact pigs but manifests in splenectomized swine. In reports from Great Britain, *E. parvum* has been described as appearing in the bloodstream within 9 days of splenectomy and capable of producing severe anemia in such pigs (Jennings and Seamer, 1956; Seamer, 1960).

The *Eperythrozoa* of swine are similar in morphology to *E. wenyoni* and *E. ovis* but may be somewhat larger. Rods, rings, and coccoid and budding forms averaging 0.8–1.0 μm in diameter, with an occasional form up to 2.5 μm have been described. The parasites are observed to be on the surface of the erythrocyte and in the plasma. An excellent photograph of *E. suis* was published by Savage and Isa (1958), and recent observations are summarized by Henry (1979).

The natural disease in swine was designated "ictero-anemia" by Brock et al. (1951) before the causative agent was identified as *E. suis*. The severity of clinical signs suggested that the disease may appear in peracute, acute, and subacute forms in young swine. Temperature elevations of 106–107.5°F, depression, anorexia, muscular weakness, and icterus were common clinical signs. Anemia may develop rapidly with RBC counts reduced to below 3 million/μl of blood. The bone marrow remains active, and signs of anemia in remission such as anisocytosis, polychromasia, Howell-Jolly bodies, and nucleated erythrocytes are observed (Adams et al., 1959). Anemia and mild icterus are also seen in newborn pigs (Henry, 1979).

Despite the natural occurrence of the disease in intact pigs, the disease is reproduced experimentally with regularity only in splenectomized swine. The mechanism of anemia and icterus in acute porcine eperythrozoonosis seems to be related to formation of cold-reacting IgM agglutinins preceding massive parasitemia (Zachary, 1983). Parasite-erythrocyte membrane interactions are presumed to play an important role in production of such antibodies (Zachary and Basgall, 1985). Rapid disappearance of the parasite from the blood is associated with the occurrence of regenerative changes in blood morphology (Splitter and Williamson, 1950). The parasite can be transmitted to susceptible pigs by the common hog louse, *Haematopinus suis*, and by the transplacental route (Henry, 1979). Subclinical eperythrozoonosis in pigs is not associated with anemia, but may compromise breeding performance and gain in body weight.

Theileriasis

Theileriasis is caused by a small protozoan parasite of the genus *Theileria* infecting the lymphocytes and erythrocytes of ruminants, especially cattle, sheep, and goats. The infection is spread by bloodsucking arthropods, particularly by ticks of the family Ixodidae. The subject has been reviewed (Barnett, 1968; Irvin and Cunningham, 1981; Uilenberg, 1981).

There are several species of *Theileria*, but *T. parva* is the most important species economically, for it is the cause of East Coast fever of cattle in East and Central Africa. The mortality rate is almost 100% in susceptible cattle, while some cattle have a high degree of innate resistance. Other species of *Theileria* are less pathogenic or even nonpathogenic. *T. annulata* causes tropical theileriasis in cattle in the Mediterranean area, Asia, and Africa. *T. Mutans* has a greater worldwide distribution, but is of lesser pathogenicity. *T. hirci* and *T. ovis* cause theileriasis in sheep and goats, the former having slight or no pathogenicity and the latter being moderately to highly pathogenic.

The life cycle of *T. parva* has been described (Schein et al., 1977). Sporozoites injected with tick saliva into the vertebrate host invade local lymphocytes in whose cytoplasm they multiply by a reproductive cycle resembling schizogony to produce macro- and micro-schizonts. The latter give rise to merozoites, which upon release from the infected lymphocytes invade erythrocytes to form piroplasms capable of infecting feeding ticks. This process takes about 2 weeks.

Theileria species are distinguished on the basis of virulence and nature of immunity. The morphology of pathogenic and nonpathogenic forms (piroplasms) in the erythrocyte is similar (Neitz, 1959). The organisms are pleomorphic and appear as rod-shaped, comma-shaped, oval, round, or *Anaplasma*-like. The nucleus at the wider end of the piroplasm appears as a deeply stained, minute, reddish-purple granule near the cell margin. The cytoplasm of the parasite stains a light blue, although with the *Anaplasma*-like forms it can hardly be seen. *T. parva* organisms are numerous in blood during the initial stage of infection, but not thereafter. *T. mutans* and *T. annulata* remain in blood in small numbers for a long time. *T. hirci* and *T. ovis* occur in sheep and goats in small numbers for a prolonged period. Schizonts (Koch bodies) are found in the cytoplasm of lymphocytes in the peripheral blood and lymph nodes. The schizonts usually have a blue cytoplasm containing numerous reddish-purple, dot-like granules. Infected lymphocytes often undergo blast transformation, and such cells can be cultured to establish cell lines harboring the parasite (Brown, 1979).

The incubation period of *T. parva* following tick transmission in susceptible animals is 8–25 (mean 13–14) days, and the duration of infection varies from 4–25 (mean 12–15) days (Barnett, 1968). Experimental inoculations may take 3–7 days (Saidu, 1982) or several weeks and occasionally months to produce the disease (Barnett, 1968). Clinicopathologic changes vary with the severity of the disease. The disease is characterized by fever of variable duration, swelling of superficial lymph nodes, anorexia, lacrimation and nasal discharge, depression, and diarrhea with bloody feces. Occasionally nervous system signs may be seen. Death may occur within 14 days but more commonly within 18–24 days. Surviving animals show a progressively poor condition. Adult cattle are more susceptible than calves, and surviving animals develop strong immunity but are susceptible to other antigenic strains of the organism. Both cell-mediated and humoral immunity have been demonstrated in theileriasis (Allison and Eugui, 1981). Complement activation and fibrinolysis have also been found to occur (Shitakha et al., 1983).

Anemia may or may not be significant in *T. parva* infection, but leukopenia is marked and slight bilirubinemia may be seen. In comparison, *T. mutans* usually produces only a slight anemia, but in severe cases anemia is marked and hemoglobinuria and icterus may be seen (Rogers and Callow, 1966). Anemia is inversely proportional to the degree of parasitemia and is regenerative in nature (Saidu, 1982). *T. annulata* induces a consistent anemia with bilirubinemia and bilirubinuria, occasional clinical icterus, rare hemoglobinuria, and leukocytosis. Experimental infection of sheep with *T. hirci* produced a variable degree of anemia, with hemoglobin levels as low as 4.4 g/dl, and icterus (Sisodia and Gautam, 1983). Red cell destruction in theileriasis may involve erythrophagocytosis from immune-mediated mechanisms (Uilenberg, 1981).

Prominent pathologic findings in *T. parva* infection include generalized lymphoid hyperplasia followed by necrosis, pulmonary edema, hyperemia and emphysema, splenomegaly, hepatomegaly, petechial hemorrhages on serosal and mucosal surfaces of various organs, and abomasal and intestinal ulceration. Because superficial lymph nodes are initial sites of *T. parva* infection, examination of needle aspirates of prominent lymph nodes for lymphocytes containing macroschizonts is of diagnostic significance.

Theileria mutans is the only protozoon of the family Theileridae to have been reported in the United States. Its presence in cattle and deer in the United States is mostly of academic interest, for the protozoon is encountered occasionally in blood of animals employed experimentally in transmission experiments with anaplasmosis. The first published report of *T. mutans* in the United States was by Splitter (1950b), who reported its presence in a splenectomized calf 12 days after inoculation of blood from a known carrier of anaplasmosis. Experimental transmission of the protozoon to susceptible animals was readily accomplished by intravenous injection of carrier blood. The incubation period was 12–18 days, and mild fever, anemia, and anorexia resulted in several splenectomized calves. The clinical signs were of short duration, and prompt recovery followed. The parasite was demonstrated consistently in one calf over a period of 8 months. *T. mutans* was observed in a splenectomized calf in California during experimental transmission trials with anaplasmosis.

Theileria species have been reported in the deer, *Dama virginiana*, native to Missouri (Kreier et al., 1962). The infection was detected in a deer 4 weeks after splenectomy. The parasite was transmitted by blood inoculation to a second splenectomized deer. Hematologic data indicated that a microcytic anemia developed. Schaeffler (1963) indentified the protozoon in the deer as *Theileria cervi*, and he applied serologic tests to 115 deer killed by hunters in southern Illinois; four were positive, and the protozoon was found in blood smears of two of these deer. Osebold et al. (1959), in their study of anaplasmosis in wild deer, reported observing parasites in the red cells of fawns which were tentatively classified as *Theileria* species. White-tailed deer (*Odocoileus virginianus*) in the southwestern United States were found to carry *Theileria cervi* and *Trypanosoma cervi*, both occurring in 49% of the animals (Davidson et al., 1983).

Detection of carrier animals involves use of various serologic tests among which the indirect fluorescent antibody test is the most widely used; an ELISA test seems to be equally promising. Control of the disease involves immunization, limiting transport of cattle, and vector control. Therapy consists of administration of oxytetracycline at the time of initial infection. Use of certain antimalarial and other drugs has been found highly effective against clinical theileriasis (MacHardy et al., 1976; Schein and Voigt, 1979; Uilenberg, 1981).

Trypanosomiasis

Trypanosomes are flagellated protozoa appearing in the blood of all classes of vertebrates; in some instances, they may invade the tissues. Most of the trypanosomes are nonpathogenic, but some are of great concern. Trypanosomes are the cause of African sleeping sickness of humans (*Trypanosoma gambiense* and *T. rhodesiense*), which is spread by the tsetse fly (*Glossina*); they are also implicated in Chagas disease of humans (*T. cruzi*).

Many species of trypanosomes infect animals without any host specificity. Thus a particular trypanosome may infect several animal species, and more than one species of trypanosome may be found in the same animal. Some important trypanosomes of animals include *T. congolense*, *T. vivax*, *T. brucei*, and *T. evansi* infecting cattle; *T. suis* infecting pigs; and *T. equiperdum* infecting horses. Trypanosomiasis in a 4-year-old German shepherd dog that had been to Africa with its owner was seen in our clinic (Schalm, 1979).

Trypanosomiasis in animals has been assigned various names: "Nagana" in cattle of Africa is caused primarily by *T. congolense*, although other species may be involved; "Surra" in cattle of India and other countries is caused by *T. evansi*; and "Dourine" in horses is caused by *T. equiperdum*. Wild animals serve as a reservoir. Many modes of transmission have been described, the most important being insect and other arthropod vectors. Certain breeds of cattle are relatively resistant to infection, e.g., N'Dama, a West African breed of cattle. An excellent review of the historic and economic importance of trypanosomes in livestock was published by Hornby (1949), and a later review provided further details (Lumsden and Wells, 1968).

In the United States and Canada, trypanosomiasis is of only academic interest; the nonpathogenic species *T. theileri* (*T. americanum*, Crawley, 1909, 1912) may be encountered in rare instances in small numbers in the stained blood films of cattle or in cultures of bovine fetal tissues and organs. Trypanosomes have been observed not more than a half dozen times among several thousand blood films originating from both normal and clinically sick California cows (Fig. 23–8). The distribution of this nonpathogenic trypanosome, *T. theileri*, is worldwide in cattle, and the organism apparently is more prevalent than observations of its occurrence in the bloodstream would indicate.

Trypanosomes are typically elongated organisms having a pointed, blunt, or round posterior end; a terminal, subterminal, or marginal kinetoplast; and a poorly or well-defined undulating membrane. Various species of *Trypanosoma* in cattle can be distinguished by their morphology and their behavior in wet preparations of fresh blood. Blood forms of *T. theileri* measure about 25–120 μm in length, while most other animal trypanosomes are relatively short. Although some overlap in size occurs, *T. congolense* is usually smaller, *T. vivax* intermediate, and *T. brucei* larger. The surface of the trypanosomes is coated with a thin (15 nm) layer of glycoproteins, which readily changes antigenicity and has been shown to be important in persistent infection of the host (Morrison et al., 1981).

Pathogenesis involves initial multiplication of the organism in local lymph nodes and then transport to blood via lymphatics. The organisms multiply in blood by binary fission and exhibit erratic parasitemia, which usually corresponds with febrile peaks. Destruction of trypanosomes is mediated by antigen-antibody reaction. Hemolytic crisis develops from erythrophagocytosis and shortened red cell survival and is attributed to enzymatic effects of the parasite (Esievo et al., 1982) and immune mechanisms (Jennings, 1976). The anemia is preceded by hemodilution from expansion of plasma volume as shown in studies with *T. congolense* infection in cattle and *T. vivax* infection in sheep (Clarkson, 1976). Clinicopathologic aspects of *T. congolense* infection in goats have been described (Kaaya ·et al., 1977).

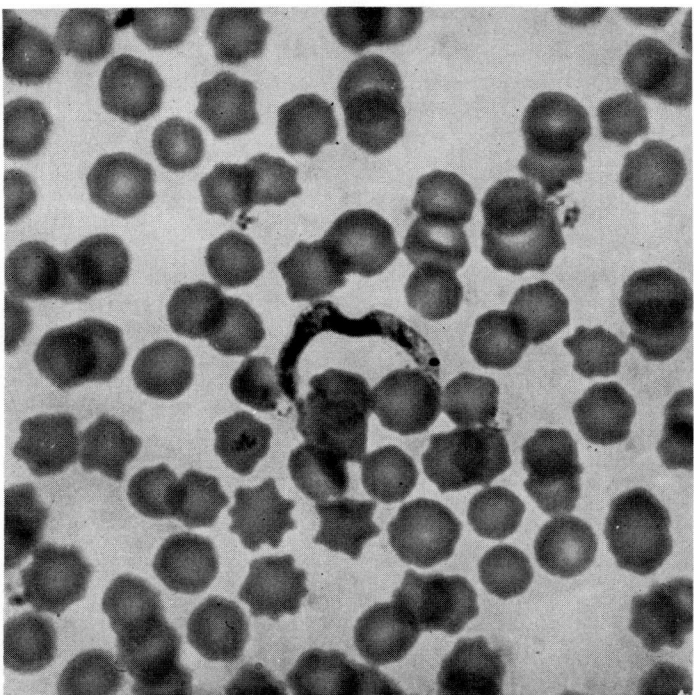

Fig. 23–8. *Trypanosoma theileri* (*T. americanum*, Crawley) in the blood of a cow in California.

Intrauterine transfer of the trypanosome from dam to fetus takes place in some instances, as indicated by isolation of trypanosomes from the stomach contents of an aborted fetus (Dikmans et al., 1957) and from a primary culture of fetal bovine kidney cells (Lundholm et al., 1959). At times it may be associated with abortion (Levine, et al., 1956).

Although *T. theileri* is ordinarily nonpathogenic, it may occasionally cause acute disease with fulminating parasitemia. Infected cattle show reduced milk production (Ristic and Trager, 1958) and may develop serious clinical signs and even die when conditions of stress lower the animal's resistance (Levine, 1961). Death may occur by trypanosomiasis itself, or it may be associated with other bacterial, viral, or parasitic diseases probably as a result of immune suppression by trypanosomiasis (Rurangirwa et al., 1978; Whitelaw et al., 1979). Death in trypanosomiasis usually follows a chronic relapsing infection with cachexia and infrequent presence of organisms in the circulation.

Clinical signs of trypanosomiasis include intermittent fever, enlarged superficial lymph nodes, anemia, tachycardia, progressively poor condition, stunted growth, and decreased fertility. The incubation period in cattle varies from 3–20 days or more, while clinical signs take about 2–4 weeks to appear. The disease may take an acute, subacute, or chronic form. An extremely acute infection, usually produced by *T. vivax*, may assume a septicemic form with fever, marked parasitemia, and massive hemorrhage (Morrison et al., 1981).

Diagnosis and control involve parasitological examination of blood, cerebrospinal fluid (CSF), lymph nodes, and material from lesions of living or dead animals. Blood can be examined in several ways (Leeflang et al., 1978; Toro et al., 1981). Thick blood films, lysed to destroy erythrocytes before staining with a Romanowsky stain, are satisfactory for finding the organism, but thin blood films are essential for identifying the species of trypanosome. Ear vein blood is said to be better than jugular blood for parasitologic examination (Greig et al., 1979).

Blood and CSF may be concentrated and buffy coat smears prepared to increase chances of finding the organism. During centrifugation of blood in a microhematocrit, trypanosomes settle at the interface of the buffy coat and the plasma layer. The microhematocrit tube can be examined directly under the light microscope, or the tube can be broken slightly above the buffy coat layer and contents poured on a clean glass slide for microscopic examination. Blood cultures can be performed in some cases. Inoculation of susceptible laboratory animals is a valuable procedure for detecting subclinical infections of some trypanosomes, e.g., *T. brucei.* Serologic diagnosis is by complement fixation and indirect immunofluorescence tests. A variety of drugs have been used to treat trypanosomiasis, and vector control has been attempted to prevent spread of infection.

Hematologic changes in trypanosomiasis in cattle have been investigated in detail (Dargie et al., 1979; Esievo, 1981; Jura and Losos, 1980; Kaaya et al., 1980; Maxie et al., 1976, 1979; Morrison et al., 1981; Naylor, 1971; Preston et al., 1979, 1982; Valli and Mills, 1980; Valli et al., 1978, 1979; Wellde et al., 1978). Anemia, in two phases, is the most prominent finding in natural infection (Morrison et al., 1981). The severity of the first phase, which lasts 3–4 months, is proportional to the degree of parasitemia. The anemia is hemolytic in nature and results primarily from erythrophagocytosis in the spleen, liver, lungs, hemal lymph nodes, bone marrow, and even the circulation and partly from intravascular hemolysis. Bone marrow response is typical of increased erythropoiesis but is inadequate. Petechiation and ecchymoses may be seen, but frank bleeding is absent. Treatment with trypanocidal drugs usually results in recovery. The second phase of anemia begins between 4 and 6 months after infection. Parasitemia progressively disappears or becomes difficult to discern, and response to therapy is poor. Necropsy findings suggest impaired erythropoiesis and continuous red cell destruction through erythrophagocytosis. Ferrokinetic studies indicate defective iron metabolism in both phases with retention of iron in macrophages (Dargie et al., 1979). Anemia in deer mice experimentally infected with *T. brucei* was associated with erythrophagocytosis, and iron supply did not seem to be a limiting factor (Anosa and Kaneko, 1983a, 1983b).

Although significant differences have been noted in the onset and duration of various blood and bone marrow abnormalities in infection with *T. vivax* and *T. congolense,* the general trend is similar. Evidence has been presented for a multiplicity of mechanisms of anemia; these have included hemodilution, increased red cell destruction from erythrophagocytosis, reduced erythropoiesis, and possibly blood loss as a complication of marked thrombocytopenia. In experimental infections, anemia is milder in neonatal calves than in calves 6 months in age or older. Reduction in red cell parameters is evident by 10–13 days of infection, and a severe anemia develops by 34–36 days (Maxie et al., 1976). The anemia is normocytic-normochromic in early stages and becomes macrocytic-normochromic as bone marrow response to anemia manifests by 4–6 weeks. This response is followed by a return of red cell values to normal in infection with *T. vivax* but not with *T. congolense,* in which case a normocytic-normochromic anemia persists. Microcytic-hypochromic anemia develops when there is a concomitant iron deficiency. Bone marrow cytology during the acute phase of the disease indicates a regenerative anemia, although a transient or mild continued erythroid depression may be present (Valli and Mills, 1980). Bone marrow response is much more marked for *T. congolense* than *T. vivax* (Maxie et al., 1976).

Half-survival time of ^{51}Cr-labeled erythrocytes is reduced by almost 50% in the acute phase, but hemoglobinuria is not seen. The liver seems to be the major site of red cell destruction. Red cell destruction in *T. vivax* infection seems to be by immunologic means as indicated by a positive direct Coombs test (Maxie et al., 1976) and other evidence (Banks, 1980). Both alternate and classic pathways of complement fixation are activated leading to decreased total circulating levels of complement (Nielsen et al., 1978b). In experimental infection of calves with *T. vivax,* red cells were found to be coated with complement, IgG, and IgM; the last two after elution from the red cells were shown to have antibody activity against antigens of the trypanosome (Facer et al., 1982). Infection with *T. vivax* and *T. congolense* is associated with marked increases in levels of serum IgM (Clarkson, 1976) and IgG (Nielsen et al., 1978a).

A transient leukopenia develops in trypanosomiasis owing to neutropenia and lymphopenia. Neutropenia is attributed to reduced myelopoiesis secondary to increased erythropoiesis (Valli et al., 1979) and production of a circulating factor inhibiting granulopoiesis (Kaaya et al., 1980). Other mechanisms of leukopenia have also been suggested (Esievo and Saror, 1983), but their significant contribution remains to be shown. The leukopenia is soon followed by leukocytosis. A marked thrombocytopenia also develops by 8–10 days postinfection, the degree being related to the level of parasitemia. Platelet survival time is reduced by one-third in calves infected with *T. congolense* (Preston et al., 1982). A natural or experimental infection with *T. vivax* may lead to a hemorrhagic diathesis with typical coagulation abnormalities (Wellde et al., 1983).

Prominent pathologic findings include cardiomyopathy, generalized lymphadenopathy, splenomegaly, plasmacytosis in lymphoid tissues and organs, and mononuclear phagocyte proliferation with some erythrophagocytosis.

Lymphocytosis in cattle has been associated with the presence of trypanosomes in the blood. In 920 blood samples examined in two herds, 20% of the trypanosome-positive samples had accompanying lymphocytosis (Cross et al., 1971). Among eight calves inoculated with blood containing *T. theileri*, lymphocyte numbers increased an average of 3,500/µl of blood above preinoculation levels in seven calves (Cross et al., 1971). Lymphocytosis was seen in chronic experimental infection of calves with *T. congolense* (Valli et al., 1978). Lymphocytosis unrelated to bovine lymphosarcoma has presented problems in detection of lymphosarcoma herds (see Chapter 32). On the other hand, in a survey of a leukosis-positive and a leukosis-negative herd for *T. theileri* by culture isolation, the trypanosome was found in 70.8% of cattle in the leukosis-positive herd and in 28.7% of cattle in the leukosis-negative herd (Hare et al., 1970). A positive correlation (p <0.05) was found between trypanosomiasis and lymphocytosis.

Cytauxzoonosis in Cats

A protozoan parasite resembling organisms of the genus *Cytauxzoon* was reported as a cause of fatal disease in domestic cats first from Missouri (Wagner, 1976) and subsequently from other parts of the United States (Ferris, 1979; Hauck et al., 1982; Kier et al., 1977; Wagner et al., 1979). Clinical signs of cytauxzoonosis in these cats included lethargy, anorexia, pale and icteric mucous membranes, fever, and dehydration. The cats usually died within a few days after clinical evidence of the disease. Pathologic findings included icterus, petechial and ecchymotic hemorrhages over the surface of the heart and lungs, excessive clear yellow fluid in the pericardial sac, engorged abdominal vessels, splenomegaly, and swollen and hyperemic lymph nodes. In addition, large numbers of schizonts characteristic of *Cytauxzoon* were found in mononuclear phagocytes of the liver, lungs, spleen, and lymph nodes. Hemolytic anemia was attributed to the protozoan parasites invading the erythrocytes; the degree of red cell parasitization varied from as low as 1% to as high as 25%.

The protozoon infecting cats has been named *Cytauxzoon felis* (Kier et al., 1982b). *Cytauxzoon* organisms have been described in ungulates in Africa. The source and mode of *Cytauxzoon* infection in domestic cats and its possible treatment remain to be described. The infection can be transmitted experimentally to healthy domestic cats (Ferris, 1979; Wagner et al., 1980) and some bobcats (Kier et al., 1982b; Wagner et al., 1980) by parenteral inoculation of blood from infected domestic cats. Experimentally infected domestic cats most frequently develop fever, anorexia, depression, and dehydration and usually die within 20 days. The ultrastructure of *C. felis* has been described (Simpson et al., 1985).

Cytauxzoon-like organisms were seen in two cheetahs examined at our clinic and found to have no clinical abnormality or anemia associated with the parasitic infection (Zinkl et al., 1981). In addition, *Cytauxzoon*-like piroplasms were found in 0.5–5.0% erythrocytes from 13 of 21 wild, trapped bobcats in Oklahoma

(Glenn et al., 1982). Responsive anemia was seen in only one of the infected bobcats. Experimental transmission of the infection from bobcats to domestic cats produced clinical signs of feline cytauxzoonosis with death occurring within 2 weeks (Kier et al., 1982a).

Sarcocystosis in Cattle and Goats

Anemia is seen in natural and experimental cases of sarcocystosis in cattle. In experimental infections in calves (Fayer and Prasse, 1981; Prasse and Fayer, 1981), about a 50% decline in hemoglobin levels occurred by 25–35 days postinfection. Anemia appeared during the period (also 25–35 days postinfection) of development of second generation schizonts in vascular endothelium and multiplication of merozoites in the circulation. Red cell morphology was suggestive of a normocytic-normochromic anemia, but its hemolytic origin was indicated by several findings such as rapidity of onset, the presence of hyperbilirubinemia, and marked iron deposition in the liver. Hemoglobinuria was not a feature, possibly because of extravascular red cell destruction. Abnormalities of coagulation and platelet function were also observed in infected calves. In similar studies with goats (Dubey et al., 1981), a mild to marked anemia was observed between 18 and 68 days after inoculation. The anemia was accompanied by hyperbilirubinemia, primarily due to increase in indirect bilirubin. The cause of anemia remained undetermined.

HEMOLYTIC ANEMIAS ASSOCIATED WITH SOME BACTERIAL INFECTIONS

Leptospirosis

Hemolytic anemia in calves and lambs may be caused by *Leptospira* organisms. Over 100 serotypes of leptospires are known, and more than one serotype may infect a particular animal species. The disease in cattle and swine is caused by *L. pomona*, *L. grippotyphosa*, *L. icterohaemorrhagiae*, and *L. canicola*. In sheep, it is caused by the first two and *L. hardjo*, which may also cause a mild infection in cattle. Leptospires are shed in urine and transmitted through contact with urine droplets.

The clinical signs are variable. Icterus and hemoglobinuria are sufficiently common in calves and cows to be listed among the more frequent signs of the disease (Reinhard, 1951, 1953) and occur at 4–8 days postinfection in conjunction with fever. Similar findings are reported for lambs with leptospirosis (Davidson and Hirsh, 1980). Leptospirosis in sheep has been found to produce cold-reacting IgM antibody–mediated hemolytic anemia (Bhasin et al., 1971). Anemia is accompanied by an erythropoietic response in blood 7–10 days postinfection with remission occurring 17–18 days postinfection. An increase in erythrocyte osmotic fragility and occurrence of erythrocyte sedimentation are sometimes found.

Leukopenia due to lymphopenia and/or neutropenia occurs at 7–12 days postinfection. Thrombocytopenia is a constant feature of leptospirosis and other spirochetal infections and is considered a useful diagnostic feature.

Hemorrhages are seen in infection due to *L. icterohaemorrhagiae* and *L. pomona*. Hemorrhagic diathesis is one of the most striking manifestations in acute leptospirosis (Higgins, 1981; Navarro and Kociba, 1982). In experimental infections with *L. icterohaemorrhagiae*, DIC was seen. The primary cause of DIC remains unknown, but evidence favors mediation through a toxic factor in leptospires.

Clinical signs of leptospirosis in the dog vary according to the form of the disease (mild to septicemic) and include fever (105–107°F), depression, anorexia, vomiting, and increased thirst. Hematologic and other laboratory findings vary with the severity of the disease. Moderate to marked anemia, icterus, and hemoglobinuria have been described, but in some cases anemia may not be evident (see Table 36–2). Infection with *L. canicola* is not commonly associated with a hemolytic process, but when the infection is due to *L. icterohaemorrhagiae*, hemolytic crisis with hemoglobinuria may be anticipated. Coinfection may occur.

Hemoconcentration may be suggested by high total plasma protein values. Fibrinogen and erythrocyte sedimentation rate are usually elevated. Modest leukocytosis due to neutrophilia with left shift may be evident, and other leukocyte numbers may reveal a corticosteroid effect. Blood urea nitrogen levels are generally increased, proteinuria may be a prominent finding, and glucosuria may occur.

Diagnosis of leptospirosis is based on demonstrating the organisms in urine and agglutinating antibody in serum. Fresh urine at body temperature is examined by dark-field microscopy; organisms are found about 1 week after infection and for weeks and months thereafter. Urine may be inoculated intraperitoneally into hamsters or guinea pigs to propagate and demonstrate the presence of leptospires. Serologic testing involves determination of increasing serum antibody titers between two samples taken 10–15 days apart during acute infection and of high titers in chronic infection. Agglutinating antibody appears in serum within 5–10 days, increases in titer for 1–3 weeks, and then persists for months to years. Hence, finding of a single positive serologic test result does not accurately reflect the stage of the disease. (See Chapter 36 for further discussion of leptospirosis in the dog.)

Bacillary Hemoglobinuria in Cattle and Sheep

Bacillary hemoglobinuria is a specific infectious disease caused by *Clostridium novyi* Type D (previously *C. hemolyticum*) and is characterized by sudden onset, high fever, anorexia, depression, rapid hemolysis, hemoglobinuria, reddish nasal discharge, and sometimes rapid death. The disease is endemic in certain areas of the western United States and is most likely to occur in pastures where drainage is poor (Records and Vawter, 1945). The RBC counts may fall to less than 2 million/μl of blood, and the hemoglobin may drop as low as 3.5 g/dl. If the animal lives long enough for the anemia to enter a stage of remission, the blood picture is typical of a marked response, with polychromatic macrocytes, basophilic stippling, and nucleated erythrocytes. Leukocytosis with neutrophilia may accompany erythrocytic changes.

The disease is spread by ingestion of spores with contaminated food and water. The spores migrate to the liver, where they germinate and produce toxins under favorable conditions, e.g., liver necrosis by migrating flukes, intoxicants, or severe hepatic congestion (Janzen et al., 1981). The organism produces a highly lethal beta toxin (phospholipase C), which degrades lecithin and causes marked intravascular destruction of erythrocytes and also exerts a hepatotoxic effect. The disease is often peracute or acute, but it may be protracted, and some animals may recover. Mortality rate is high, with deaths occurring within 18–36 hours as a result of respiratory failure due to a combination of hypoxia and toxemia. Necropsy findings are characteristic of anemia and icterus in addition to specific lesions in the liver. The disease can be produced experimentally in cattle, sheep, and rabbits (Erwin, 1977; Olander et al., 1966).

Diagnosis of bacillary hemoglobinuria requires a good history, necropsy, examination of blood, and impression smears of the liver lesions and spleen. A fluorescent antibody test can be performed to identify tentatively the causative organism. Treatment consists of administration of antibiotics, fluids, and blood transfusion. Vaccination can be performed to prevent future occurrences of bacillary hemoglobinuria.

A clinical record of a herd problem diagnosed as bacillary hemoglobinuria (red water disease) was as follows:

A rancher in central Nevada lost 30 head of cattle from a herd of 100 between October and early January. At first, the deaths occurred in calves only, but later some older cows died. The course of the disease varied from sudden deaths to cases that lasted as long as 10 days. Some recoveries were observed. Outstanding clinical signs were temperatures ranging up to 105°F, nasal discharge, shortness of breath, and bloat. Several animals had red-colored urine, and in some, the nasal discharge was red-tinged. Many cattle went off-feed, became depressed, and stood away from the herd. Others died with no premonitory clinical signs. On January 6, a 2-year-old Shorthorn heifer was presented for examination. The heifer was in fairly good condition, although quite small for her age. Clinical examination detected paleness of mucous membranes, slight serous nasal discharge, rapid heart rate, dry scanty feces, normal urine color, and a rectal tem-

Table 23–5. Hematologic Findings in a 2-Year-Old Shorthorn Heifer with Bacillary Hemoglobinuria

	Jan. 7, a.m.	Jan. 7, p.m.	Jan. 8, p.m.	Jan. 10, p.m.
RBC ($\times 10^6/\mu$l)	2.18	1.65	1.78	2.26
WBC ($\times 10^3/\mu$l)	27.7/19.9	22.4/14.9	16.8/12.0	17.7/11.3 (corrected for
Hb (g/dl)	3.6	3.6	4.3	4.6 nucleated RBC)
PCV (%)	10.0	8.0	13.0	16.0
MCV (fl)	46.0	48.0	73.0	71.0
MCHC (%)	36.0	45.0[a]	33.0	28.7
Icterus index	10.0	7.5	5.0	5.0
Reticulocytes (%)	0.8	2.4	0.1	0.1
Nucleated RBC/100 WBC	39.5	50.0	37.0	55.0

[a]Free hemoglobin in the plasma produced this elevated MCHC value.

perature of 105.5°F. Blood studies revealed a marked anemia (Table 23–5). Examination of stained blood films revealed moderate anisocytosis and polychromasia followed by marked basophilic stippling. This animal recovered and was returned to the owner. A week later, a second animal was submitted for necropsy, and a diagnosis of bacillary hemoglobinuria was made upon the finding of the typical liver infarct and demonstration of the bacilli in stained liver impression smears.

HEMOLYTIC ANEMIAS ASSOCIATED WITH SOME VIRAL INFECTIONS

Equine Infectious Anemia

Equine infectious anemia (EIA) is a viral disease of Equidae that expresses itself in acute and subacute forms in highly susceptible horses but more commonly assumes a chronic course. It has an incubation period of 14–21 days and is characterized by cyclic occurrences of pyrexia, weakness, and anemia. Horses making an apparent recovery may remain carriers of the virus for many months and years and in some instances for the remainder of life (Stein et al., 1955). Mechanical transmission through hematophagous insects, particularly tabanids, may occur (Foil et al., 1983; Issel and Foil, 1984). A severe relapse may occur in carrier horses as a result of intercurrent disease or conditions leading to stress.

Intermittent fever, debility, emaciation, pallor, icterus, and edema of dependent parts are signs suggestive of EIA (Hyslop, 1966). Additional clinical signs include petechial and ecchymotic hemorrhages in mucous membranes and lymphadenopathy. Comprehen-

sive reviews on EIA have been published in recent years (Issel and Coggins, 1979; Henson and McGuire, 1974; Ishii and Ishitani, 1975; Johnson, 1976; Coggins, 1981).

Until 1970, an antemortem diagnosis of EIA was dependent on a combination of clinical signs, liver biopsy, and the demonstration of sideroleukocytes (Plate XIV–11) in peripheral blood (Ishii, 1963; Rothenbacher et al., 1962). Decreased serum albumin and increased γ-globulin were considered to be additional diagnostic aids, when they accompanied other signs common to EIA (Henson et al., 1967). Both γ- and β-globulins are increased. Liver specific serum enzymes are increased slightly. Liver changes showing Kupffer cells laden with hemosiderin, occurrence of sideroleukocytes in blood, and changes in the albumin:globulin ratio are not specific for EIA since they occur in other diseases of the horse. The pathology of EIA in 100 experimentally inoculated horses has been discussed by Konno and Yamamoto (1970). A confirmed diagnosis of EIA was dependent upon reproducing the disease by inoculation of a susceptible horse with blood taken from a suspected case.

A breakthrough in the search for a reliable diagnostic test came when Coggins and Norcross (1970) developed an agar gel immunodiffusion test. The test was demonstrated to be 95% accurate for the diagnosis of EIA in acute, chronic, and inapparent forms (Coggins et al., 1972). False-positive reactions can occur with Coggin's test, and false-negative reactions may be obtained during early stages of an acute fulminating form. Foals of Coggins-positive mares may give positive tests during the first months of life because of passive transfer of antibody through colostrum ingestion. An immunofluorescence test to detect antibodies to EIA in infected horses has also been described (Weiland et al., 1982).

The nature of the anemia has been controversial. Part of the problem has been the failure of peripheral blood to reveal clearly that a horse is responding to an anemia. The horse rarely releases immature erythrocytes (reticulocytes and nucleated erythrocytes) to the circulation even in response to a severe hemolytic or blood-loss anemia. Thus in EIA the anemia is normocytic-normochromic, and without bone marrow examination, it may not be possible to determine how active the erythropoietic response is. The horse also has the peculiarity of a rapidly elevating icterus index in severe disease in the absence of erythrocyte destruction (see Chapter 6), and therefore bilirubinemia in conjunction with anemia is not necessarily a valid indication of a hemolytic process in the horse.

Evidence indicating that erythrocytes in this disease become coated with an autoantibody and complement supports the concept of an immune-mediated hemolytic anemia in EIA (Squire, 1968). Antibodies involved may be IgG or IgM type. Autoagglutination of erythrocytes may be present in an occasional case. Erythrocyte destruction is greater during febrile peaks. In EIA induced experimentally, bone marrow cellularity was increased (Yamamoto and Konno, 1967). Hematopoietic cells, however, were reduced, particularly in acute and subacute disease, as a result of an increase in reticular cells, blastoid cells, and small round cells.

Clinical and laboratory data from a horse exhibiting the subacute form of EIA are presented in Appendix Case 57. The diagnosis of EIA in this horse was verified by animal inoculation. Typical clinical and hematologic findings of acute EIA are illustrated by the following case:

A 5-year-old gelding quarter horse was presented with a history of partial anorexia and depression. Physical examination revealed a rectal temperature of 104.0°F, a heart rate of 100/min, and rapid respiration. The mucous membranes were pale, and there was extensive edema of the distal portion of all extremities, the ventral abdomen and the prepuce. The hemogram revealed an anemia (PCV, 14%), leukopenia (WBC, 2,000/μl), and bili-

rubinemia (icterus index >100 units). The MCV, MCHC, and MCH were 51.0 fl, 32.1%, and 16.4 pg, respectively, indicating that the anemia was normocytic-normochromic. The differential leukocyte count demonstrated the following distribution of leukocytes: band neutrophils, 3.0%; mature neutrophils, 28.0%; lymphocytes, 61.0%; and monocytes, 8.0%. Thus a severe neutropenia and a modest lymphopenia were in evidence. The van den Bergh test on blood serum revealed direct-acting bilirubin to be 1.4 mg/dl and indirect-acting (unconjugated) bilirubin to be 5.2 mg/dl. Total serum protein was 6.4 g/dl, with an A:G ratio of 0.56:1.0. The immunodiffusion test for EIA was positive.

The horse died on the third day of hospitalization. At necropsy, the most prominent gross finding was an enlarged liver estimated to be twice the normal size. There were epicardial petechiae and ecchymoses, and all lymph nodes examined were enlarged and moist and presented reddish mottling. Histopathologic studies revealed a distinctive mononuclear and siderocytic infiltration of connective tissues, liver, kidneys, and lungs, and similar cells appeared within the lumen of blood vessels. These findings were considered to be compatible with a diagnosis of EIA.

Biological transfer principally occurs through biting insects. Mechanical transmission from a carrier horse to a susceptible horse can occur through horseflies or use of contaminated needles, syringes, and surgical equipment (Hawkins et al., 1973, 1976; Williams et al., 1981). Infected horses may be isolated from normal horses to prevent spread of infection. At present no effective treatment is available for EIA; corticosteroids may exacerbate the disease.

REFERENCES

Anaplasmosis

Allen, P.C., et al.: Clinical Chemistry of Anaplasmosis: Blood Chemical Changes in Infected Cows. Amer. J. Res., 42:322, 1981.

Anosa, V.O., et al.: Splenectomy in Sheep: Techniques, Haematological Changes, and the Haematology of the Precipitated Anaplasmosis and Babesiosis. Zentralbl. Veterinärmed., A26:327, 1979.

Boynton, W.H.: Further Observations on Anaplasmosis. Cornell Vet., 22:10, 1932.

Boynton, W.H., and Woods, G.M.: Deer as Carriers of Anaplasmosis. Science, *78*:559, 1933.

Boynton, W.H., and Woods, G.M.: Anaplasmosis among Deer in the Natural State. Science, *91*:168, 1940.

Boynton, W.H., et al.: Anaplasmosis Transmission by Three Species of Ticks in California. J. Amer. Vet. Med. Ass., *88*:500, 1936.

Christensen, J.F., et al.: Infection and Antibody Response in Deer Experimentally Infected with Anaplasma marginale from Bovine Carriers. J. Amer. Vet. Med. Ass., *132*:289, 1958.

Christensen, J.F., et al.: Persistence of Latent Anaplasma marginale Infection in Deer. J. Amer. Vet. Med. Ass., *136*:426, 1960.

DeKock, C., and Quinlan, J.: Splenectomy in Domesticated Animals and Its Sequelae, with Special Reference to Anaplasmosis in Sheep. 11th and 12th Reports, Dir. Vet. Educ. Res., Union of South Africa, p. 369, 1926.

DeRobertis, E., and Epstein, B.: Electron Microscope Study of Anaplasmosis in Bovine Red Blood Cells. Proc. Soc. Exp. Biol. Med., *77*:254, 1951.

Du Toit, P.J.: Anaplasmosis. (Author's Summary of Paper 52, 12th International Veterinary Congress.) Vet. Rec., *14*:1266, 1934.

Erp, E., and Fahrney, D.: Exit of Anaplasma marginale from Bovine Red Blood Cells. Amer. J. Vet. Res., *36*:707, 1975.

Espana, C., et al.: Anaplasma marginale. I. Studies with Phase Contrast and Electron Microscopy. Amer. J. Vet. Res., *20*:795, 1959.

Espana, E.M., and Espana, C.: Anaplasma marginale. II. Further Studies of Morphologic Features with Phase Contrast and Light Microscopy. Amer. J. Vet. Res., *24*:713, 1963.

Foote, L.E., et al.: Electron Microscopy of the Anaplasma Body: Ultra Thin Sections of Bovine Erythrocytes. Science, *128*:147, 1958.

Franklin, T.E., and Redmond, H.E.: Observation on the Morphology of Anaplasma marginale with Reference to Projections or Tails. Amer. J. Vet. Res., *19*:252, 1958.

Gates, D.W., et al.: Ultrastructure of Anaplasma marginale Fixed with Glutaraldehyde and Osmiun Tetroxide. Amer. J. Vet. Res., *28*:1577, 1967.

Gonzalez, E.F., et al.: Comparisons of the Complement Fixation, Indirect Fluorescent Antibody, and Card Agglutination Tests for the Diagnosis of Bovine Anaplasmosis. Amer. J. Vet. Res., *39*:1538, 1978.

Jatkar, P.R., and Kreier, J.P.: Relationship between Severity of Anemia and Plasma Erythropoietin Titer in Anaplasma-Infected Calves and Sheep. Amer. J. Vet. Res., *28*:107, 1967.

Kakoma, I.: Immunologically Mediated Target Cell Injury in Canine Ehrlichiosis and Bovine Anaplasmosis. Diss. Abst. Int., B*38*:4676, 1978.

Keeton, K.S., and Jain, N.C.: Scanning Electron Microscopic Studies of Paranaplasma sp. in Erythrocytes of a Cow. J. Parasitol., *59*:331, 1973.

Kreier, J.P., and Ristic, M.: Studies in Anaplasmosis. IV. Development of the Causative Agent in Deer Erythrocytes Transfused into Calves. Amer. J. Vet. Res., *22*:790, 1961.

Kreier, J.P., and Ristic, M.: Anaplasmosis. X. Morphologic Characteristics of the Parasites Present in the Blood of Calves Infected with the Oregon Strain of Anaplasma marginale. Amer. J. Vet. Res., *24*:676, 1963a.

Kreier, J.P., and Ristic, M.: Anaplasmosis. XI. Immunoserologic Characteristics of the Parasite Present in the Blood of Calves Infected with the Oregon Strain

of Anaplasma marginale. Amer. J. Vet. Res., *24*:688, 1963b.

Kreier, J.P., and Ristic, M.: Anaplasmosis. XII. The Growth and Survival in Deer and Sheep of the Parasite Present in the Blood of Calves Infected with the Oregon Strain of Anaplasma marginale. Amer. J. Vet. Res., *24*:697, 1963c.

Kreier, J.P., and Ristic, M.: Anaplasmosis. VII. Experimental Anaplasma ovis in White-Tailed Deer (Dama virginiana). Amer. J. Vet. Res., *24*:567, 1963d.

Kreier, J.P., et al.: Anaplasmosis. XVI. The Pathogenesis of Anemia Produced by Infection with Anaplasma. Amer. J. Vet. Res., *25*:343, 1964.

Kuttler, K.L.: Clinical and Hematologic Comparison of Anaplasma marginale and Anaplasma centrale Infections in Cattle. Amer. J. Vet. Res., *27*:941, 1966.

Kuttler, K.L.: Infection of Splenectomized Calves with Anaplasma ovis. Amer. J. Vet. Res., *42*:2094, 1981.

Lotze, J.C., and Yiengst, M.J.: Studies on the Nature of Anaplasma. Amer. J. Vet. Res., *3*:312, 1942.

Maas, J., and Buening, G.M.: Characterization of Anaplasma marginale Infection in Splectomized Domestic Goats. Amer. J. Vet. Res., *42*:142, 1981.

Madden, P.A.: Structures of Anaplasma marginale Observed by Using Fluorescent Antibody Technique. Amer. J. Vet. Res., *23*:921, 1962.

Magonigle, R.A., et al.: Anaplasma ovis in Idaho Sheep. Amer. J. Vet. Res., *42*:199, 1981.

Mann, D.R., and Ristic, M.: Anaplasmosis. XVI. The Isolation and Characterization of an Autohemagglutinin. Amer. J. Vet. Res., *24*:709, 1963.

Moulton, J.E., and Christensen, J.F.: The Histochemical Nature of Anaplasma marginale. Amer. J. Vet. Res., *16*:377, 1955.

Osebold, J.W., et al.: Latent Anaplasma marginale Infection in Wild Deer Demonstrated by Calf Inoculation. Cornell Vet., *49*:97, 1959.

Pilcher, D.S., et al.: Studies on the Morphology and Respiration of Anaplasma marginale. Amer. J. Vet. Res., *22*:298, 1961.

Rao, P.J., and Ristic, M.: Serum Sialic Acid Levels in Experimental Anaplasmosis. Proc. Soc. Exp. Biol. Med., *114*:447, 1963.

Renshaw, H.W., et al.: Anaplasmosis: Prevalence, Treatment and Cattle to Elk Transmission Studies. Proc. 79th Annu. Meeting U.S. Anim. Health Ass., 1976.

Ristic, M.: Studies in Anaplasmosis. III. An Auto-Antibody and Symptomatic Macrocytic Anemia. Amer. J. Vet. Res., *22*:871, 1961.

Ristic, M.: Anaplasmosis. XX. Electron Microscopy of the Causative Agent Stained by the Negative Contrast Technique. Amer. J. Vet. Res., *28*:63, 1967.

Ristic, M.: Anaplasmosis. In Infectious Blood Diseases of Man and Animals. Weinman, D., and Ristic, M., eds. Academic Press, New York, pp. 473, 478–542, 1968.

Ristic, M.: Anaplasmosis. In Bovine Medicine and Surgery. 2nd ed. Amstutz, H.E., ed. American Veterinary Publications, Santa Barbara, p. 324, 1980.

Ristic, M., and Kreier, J.P.: Family Anaplasmataceae. In Bergey's Manual of Determinative Bacteriology. 8th Ed. Buchanan, R.E., and Gibbons, N.E., eds. Williams and Wilkins, Baltimore, p. 906, 1974.

Ristic, M., and Watrach, A.M.: Studies in Anaplasmosis. II. Electron Microscopy of Anaplasma marginale in Deer. Amer. J. Vet. Res., *22*:109, 1961.

Ristic, M., and Watrach, A.M.: Studies in Anaplasmosis. V. Occurrence of Anaplasma marginale in Bovine Blood Platelets. Amer. J. Vet. Res., *23*:626, 1962.

Ristic, M., and Watrach, A.M.: Anaplasmosis. VI. Studies and a Hypothesis Concerning the Cycle of Development of the Causative Agent. Amer. J. Vet. Res., *24*:267, 1963.

Ristic, M., et al.: Anaplasmosis: Opsonins and Hemagglutinins in Etiology of Anemia. Exp. Parasitol., *31*:2, 1972.

Ritchie, A.E.: Simplified Specimen Preparation for Electron Microscopic Studies of an Intra-Erythrocytic Parasite, Anaplasma marginale. Proc. Soc. Exp. Biol. Med., *110*:532, 1962.

Schalm, O.W., et al.: Observation with New Methylene Blue Stain as Applied to Anaplasma marginale. Calif. Vet., *17*:36, May–June, 1962.

Schroeder, W.F., and Dimopoullos, G.T.: Studies of Bovine Erythrocytes in Anaplasmosis. III. Partition of Erythrocytic Phospholipids. Amer. J. Vet. Res., *24*:283, 1963.

Schroeder, W.F., and Ristic, M.: Anaplasmosis. XVII. The Relation of Autoimmune Processes to Anemia. Amer. J. Vet. Res., *26*:239, 1965a.

Schroeder, W.F., and Ristic, M.: Anaplasmosis. XVIII. An Analysis of Autoantigens in Infected and Normal Bovine Erythrocytes. Amer. J. Vet. Res., *26*:679, 1965b.

Schroeder, W.F., and Ristic, M.: Blood Serum Factors Associated with Erythrophagocytosis in Calves with Anaplasmosis. Amer. J. Vet. Res., *29*:1991, 1968.

Scott, W.L., et al.: Electron Microscopy of A. marginale in the Bovine Erythrocyte. Amer. J. Vet. Res., *22*:877, 1961.

Simpson, C.F., et al.: The Nature of Bands in Parasitized Bovine Erythrocytes. J. Cell Biol., *27*:225, 1965.

Simpson, C.F., et al.: Morphologic and Histochemical Nature of Anaplasma marginale. Amer. J. Vet. Res., *28*:1055, 1967.

Smith, R.D., et al.: Serologic Evidence of Anaplasma marginale Infection in Illinois White-Tailed Deer. J. Amer. Vet. Med. Ass., *181*:1255, 1982.

Splitter, E.J., et al.: Anaplasmosis in Sheep in the United States. J. Amer. Vet. Med. Ass., *127*:244, 1955.

Splitter, E.J., et al.: Anaplasma ovis in the United States. Experimental Study in Sheep and Goats. Amer. J. Vet. Res., *17*:487, 1956.

Summers, W.A., and Padgett, F.: Electron Microscopy of Negatively Stained Anaplasma marginale Theiler, 1910. Amer. J. Vet. Res., *31*:1679, 1970.

Theiler, A.: Anaplasma marginale (Genus et spec. nov.): The Marginal Points in the Blood of Cattle Suffering from a Specific Disease. Rept. Govt. Vet. Bact. Transvaal U., South Africa, p. 7, 1909.

Thoen, C.O., et al.: Enzyme-Linked Immunosorbent Assay for Detecting Antibodies in Cattle in a Herd in Which Anaplasmosis Was Diagnosed. J. Clin. Microbiol., *11*:499, 1980.

Zaugg, J.L.: Bovine Anaplasmosis: Transplacental Transmission as It Relates to Stage of Gestation. Amer. J. Vet. Res., *46*:570, 1985.

Babesiosis

Adeyanju, B.J., and Aliu, Y.O.: Chemotherapy of Canine Ehrlichiosis and Babesiosis with Imidocarb Dipropionate. J. Amer. Anim. Hosp. Ass., *18*:827, 1982.

Alperin, A.L., and Bevins, N.F.: Babesiosis in a California Dog. J. Amer. Vet. Med. Ass., *143*:1328, 1963.

Anderson, J.F., et al.: Canine Babesia New to North America. Science, *204*:1431, 1979.

Anderson, J.F., et al.: Canine Babesiosis: Indirect Fluorescent Antibody Test for a North American Isolate of Babesia gibsoni. J. Amer. Vet. Med. Ass., *41*:2102, 1980.

Botros, B.A.M., et al.: Some Observations on Experimentally Induced Infection of Dogs with Babesia gibsoni. Amer. J. Vet. Res., *36*:293, 1975.

Breitschwerdt, E.B., et al.: Babesiosis in the Greyhound. J. Amer. Vet. Med. Ass., *182*:978, 1983.

Button, C.: Metabolic and Electrolyte Disturbances in Acute Canine Babesiosis. J. Amer. Vet. Med. Ass., *175*:475, 1979.

Callow, L.L.: Vaccination against Bovine Babesiosis. Adv. Exp. Med. Biol., *93*:121, 1977.

Callow, L.L., and Pepper, P.M.: Measurement of and Correlation between Fever, Changes in Packed Cell Volume and Parasitaemia in the Evaluation of the Susceptibility of Cattle to Infection with Babesia argentina. Aust. Vet. J., *50*:1, 1974.

Carmichael, J.: Treatment and Control of Babesiosis. Ann. N.Y. Acad. Sci., *64*(art. 2):147, 1956.

Dalgliesh, R.D., et al.: Disseminated Intravascular Coagulation in Acute Babesia argentina Infections in Splenectomized Calves. Exp. Parasitol., *40*:124, 1976.

Dikmans, G.: Canine Babesiosis in the United States. North Amer. Vet., *16*(1):45, 1935.

Dorner, J.L.: Clinical and Pathologic Features of Canine Babesiosis. J. Amer. Vet. Med. Ass., *154*:648, 1969.

Ewing, S.A., and Buckner, R.G.: Manifestations of Babesiosis, Ehrlichiosis and Combined Infections in the Dog. Amer. J. Vet. Res., *26*:815, 1965.

Ewing, S.A.: Canine Ehrlichiosis. Adv. Vet. Sci. Comp. Med., *13*:331, 1969.

Farwell, G.E., et al.: Clinical Observations on Babesia gibsoni and Babesia canis Infections in Dogs. J. Amer. Vet. Med. Ass., *180*:507, 1982.

Furie, W.S.: Bovine Babesiosis. Comp. Cont. Ed. Pract. Vet., *4*:S272, 1982.

Futter, G.J., et al.: Studies in Feline Babesiosis. 4. Chemical Pathology, Macroscopic and Microscopic Post Mortem Findings. J. S. Afr. Vet. Ass., *52*:5, 1981.

Futter, G.J., and Belonje, P.C.: Studies on Feline Babesiosis. I. Historical Review. J. S. Afr. Vet. Ass., *50*:105, 1980a.

Futter, G.J., et al.: Studies of Feline Babesiosis. 3. Haematological Findings. J. S. Afr. Vet. Ass., *51*:271, 1980b.

Gorenflot, A., et al.: Morphologic des hematies parasitees lors de Babesiosis bovine (B. divergens) et canine (B. canis). Annales Pharmaceutigens Françaises, *37*:443, 1979.

Groves, M.G., and Dennis, G.L.: Babesia gibsoni: Field and Laboratory Studies of Canine Infections. Exp. Parasitol., *31*:153, 1972.

Groves, M.G., and Yap, I.F.: Babesia gibsoni in a Dog. J. Amer. Vet. Med. Ass., *153*:689, 1968.

Howard, R.J., et al.: Comparison of the Surface Proteins and Glycoproteins on Erythrocytes of Calves before and during Infection with Babesia bovis. J. Protozool., *27*:241, 1980.

Ishimine, T., et al.: An in vitro Study of Monocyte Phagocytosis in the Peripheral Blood of Healthy and Babesia-Infected Beagles. Jap. J. Vet. Sci., *41*:487, 1979.

Jennings, F.W.: The Anaemias of Parasitic Infections. In Pathophysiology of Parasitic Infection. Soulsby, E.J.L., ed. Academic Press, New York, pp. 41–67, 1976.

Knowles, R.C., and Uniss-Floyd, R.: Equine Piroplasmosis (Babesiosis) of the Babesia caballi Type. Equine Pract., *5*(3):18, 1983.

Knowles, R.C., et al.: Equine Piroplasmosis. Equine Pract., 2:10, 1980.

Kuttler, K.L.: Chemotherapy of Babesiosis: A Review. *In* Babesiosis. Ristic, M., and Kreier, J.P., eds. Academic Press, New York, pp. 65–85, 1981.

Levine, N.D.: Taxonomy of the Piroplasmas. Trans. Amer. Microsc. Soc., 90:2, 1971.

Levy, M.G., et al.: Age Resistance in Bovine Babesiosis: Role of Blood Factors in Resistance to Babesia bovis. Infect. Immun., 37:1127, 1982.

Lohr, K.F., et al.: Haematological Reactions to Experimental Babesia bigemina Infection in Splenectomized and Nonsplenectomized Cattle. Abl. Vet. Med. B., 24:508, 1977.

Madden, P.A., and Holbrook, A.A.: Equine Piroplasmosis: Indirect Fluorescent Antibody Test for Babesia caballi. Amer. J. Vet. Res., 29:117 1968.

Maegraith, B.G., et al.: Pathological Processes in Babesia canis Infections. Z. Tropenmed. Parasitol., 8:485, 1957.

Mahoney, D.G.: Babesia of Domestic Animals. *In* Parasitic Protozoa. Vol 4. Kreier, J.P., ed. Academic Press, New York, pp. 1–52, 1977.

Malherbe, W.P.: The Manifestations and Diagnosis of Babesia Infections. Ann. N.Y. Acad. Sci., 69:129, 1956.

Maurer, F.D.: Equine Piroplasmosis: Another Emerging Disease. J. Amer. Vet. Med. Ass., 141:699, 1962a.

Maurer, F.D.: Equine Piroplasmosis: Another Emerging Disease. Proc. 8th Amer. Ass. Equine Pract. Conv., p. 241, 1962b.

Mimori, T., et al.: Morphological Studies of Multiplication of Babesia gibsoni in Canine Erythrocytes. Jap. J. Vet. Sci., 44:699, 1982.

Moltmann, U.G., et al.: Fine Structure of Babesia equi Laveran, 1901 within Lymphocytes and Erythrocytes of Horses: An in Vivo and in Vitro Study. J. Parasitol., 69(1):111, 1983.

Moore, D.J.: Disseminated Intravascular Coagulation: Treatment. J. S. Afr. Vet. Med. Ass., 50:259, 1979a.

Moore, D.J.: Therapeutic Implications of Babesia canis Infections in Dogs. J. S. Afr. Vet. Ass., 50:346, 1979b.

Moore, D.J., and Williams, M.C.: Disseminated Intravascular Coagulation: A Complication of Babesia canis Infection in the Dog. J. S. Afr. Vet. Med. Ass., 50:265, 1979.

Nafie, T., et al.: Effect of Induced Equine Piroplasmosis on Some Blood Constituents. Assiut Vet. Med. J., 9:123, 1982.

Neitz, W.O.: Classification, Transmission, and Biology of Piroplasms of Domestic Animals. Ann. N.Y. Acad. Sci., 64 (art. 2):56, 1956.

Piercy, S.E.: Hyperacute Canine Babesia (Tick Fever). Vet. Rec., 59:612, 1947.

Popovic, N.A., and Ristic, M.: Diagnosis of Canine Babesiosis by a Gel Precipitation Test. Amer. J. Vet. Res., 31:2201, 1970.

Purchase, H.S.: Cerebral Babesiosis in Dogs. Vet. Rec., 59:269, 1947.

Purnell, R.E.: Babesiosis in Various Hosts. *In* Babesiosis. Ristic, M., and Kreier, J.P., eds. Academic Press, New York, pp. 25–63, 1981.

Purnell, R.E., et al.: The Haematology of Experimentally Induced B. divergens and E. phagocytophilia Infections in Splenectomized Calves. Vet. Rec., 100:4, 1977.

Reik, R.F.: Babesiosis. *In* Infectious Blood Diseases of Man and Animals. Vol 2. Diseases Caused by Protista. Weinman, D., and Ristic, M., eds. Academic Press, New York, p. 219, 1968.

Ristic, M.: Babesiosis. *In* Bovine Medicine and Surgery. 2nd ed. Amstutz, H.E., ed. American Veterinary Publications, Santa Barbara, p. 355, 1980.

Ristic, M.: Babesiosis. Curr. Top. Vet. Med. Anim. Sci., 6:443, 1981.

Ristic, M., and Kreier, J.P., eds. Babesiosis. Academic Press, New York, 1981.

Ristic, M., and Sibinovic, S.: Equine Babesiosis: Diagnosis by a Precipitation in Gel and by a One-Step Fluorescent Antibody-Inhibition Test. Amer. J. Vet. Res., 25:1519, 1964.

Ristic, M., et al.: Babesia canis and Babesia gibsoni Soluble and Corpuscular Antigens Isolated from Blood of Dogs. Exp. Parasitol., 30:385, 1971.

Roby, T.O., and Anthony, D.W.: Transmission of Equine Piroplasmosis by *Dermacentor nitens* Neumann. J. Amer. Vet. Med. Ass., 142:768, 1963.

Sanders, D.A.: Observations on Canine Babesiosis (Piroplasmosis). J. Amer. Vet. Med. Ass., 90:27, 1937.

Schein, E., et al.: Babesia equi (Laveran 1901). I. Development in Horses and in Lymphocyte Culture. Tropenmed. Parasitol., 32:223, 1981.

Seneviratna, P.: Studies of Babesia gibsoni Infections of Dogs in Ceylon. Ceylon Vet. J., 13:1, 1965a.

Seneviratna, P.: The Pathology of Babesia gibsoni (Patton, 1910) Infection in the Dog. Ceylon Vet. J., 13:107, 1965b.

Simpson, C.F., and Neal, F.C.: Ultrastructure of Babesia equi in Ponies Treated with Imidocarb. Amer. J. Vet. Res., 41:267, 1980.

Simpson, C.F., et al.: Electron Microscopy of Canine and Equine Babesia. Amer. J. Vet. Res., 24:408, 1963.

Sippel, W.L., et al.: Equine Piroplasmosis in the United States. J. Amer. Vet. Med. Ass., 141:694, 1962.

Todorovic, R.A., et al.: Ultrastructure of Babesia bovis (Babes, 1888). Vet. Parasitol., 8:277, 1981.

Ward, P.A., and Jack, R.M.: The Entry Process of Babesia Merozoites into Red Cells. Amer. J. Pathol., 102:109, 1981.

Watkins, R.G.: A Concentration and Staining Technique for Diagnosing Equine Piroplasmosis. J. Amer. Vet. Med. Ass., 141:1330, 1962.

Wright, I.G.: Observations on the Hematology of Experimentally Induced Babesia argentina and B. bigemina Infections in Splenectomized Calves. Res. Vet. Sci., 14:29, 1973.

Wright, I.G., et al.: Acute Babesia bovis Infections: Metabolic and Blood Gas Changes during Infection. Brit. Vet. J., 138:61, 1982.

Haemobartonellosis

Austerman, J.W.: Haemobartonellosis in a Nonsplenectomized Dog. Vet. Med. Small Anim. Clin., 74:954, 1979.

Barnett, S.F., and Brocklesby, D.W.: The Isolation of a Large Babesia Species and Other Blood Parasites from British Cattle. Vet. Rec., 88:260, 1971.

Benjamin, M.M., and Lumb, W.V.: Haemobartonella canis Infection in a Dog. J. Amer. Vet. Med. Ass., 135:388, 1959.

Brocklesby, D.W.: Haemobartonella bovis Detected in the Blood of British Cattle. Vet. Rec., 87:761, 1970.

Brodey, R.S., and Schalm, O.W.: Hemobartonellosis and Thrombocytopenic Purpura in a Dog. J. Amer. Vet. Med. Ass., 143:1231, 1963.

Bundza, A., et al.: Haemobartonellosis in a Dog in Association with Coombs Positive Anemia. Can. Vet. J., *17*:267, 1976.

Carr, D.T., and Essex, H.E.: Bartonellosis: A Cause of Severe Anemia in Splenectomized Dogs. Proc. Soc. Exp. Biol. Med., *57*:44, 1944.

Clark, R.: Eperythrozoon felis (sp. Nov.) in a Cat. J. S. Afr. Vet. Med. Ass., *13(1)*:15, 1942.

Demaree, R.S., Jr., and Nessmith, W.B.: Ultrastructure of Haemobartonella felis from a Naturally Infected Cat. Amer. J. Vet. Res., *33*:1303, 1972.

Fisher, E.W., et al.: Anaemia in a Litter of Siamese Kittens. J. Small Anim. Pract., *24*:215, 1983.

Flint, J.C., and McKelvie, D.H.: Feline Infectious Anemia: Diagnosis and Treatment. Amer. Vet. Med. Ass., 92nd Annu. Meeting, p. 240, 1955.

Flint, J.C., and Moss, L.C.: Infectious Anemia in Cats. J. Amer. Vet. Med. Ass., *122*:45, 1953.

Flint, J.C., et al.: Feline Infectious Anemia. I. Clinical Aspects. Amer. J. Vet. Res., *19*:164, 1958.

Flint, J.C., et al.: Feline Infectious Anemia. II. Experimental Cases. Amer. J. Vet. Res., *20*:33, 1959.

Harvey, J.W.: Feline Hemobartonellosis. *In* Current Veterinary Therapy VII. Kirk, R.W., ed. W.B. Saunders, Philadelphia, 1980.

Harvey, J.W., and Gaskin, J.M.: Experimental Feline Haemobartonellosis. J. Amer. Anim. Hosp. Ass., *13*:28, 1977.

Jain, N.C., and Keeton, K.S.: Scanning Electron Microscopic Features of Haemobartonella felis. Amer. J. Vet. Res., *34*:697, 1973.

Knutti, R.E., and Hawkins, W.B.: I. Bartonella Incidence in Splenectomized Bile Fistula Dogs. J. Exp. Med., *61*:115, 1925.

Kreier, J.P., and Ristic, M.: Haemobartonellosis, Eperythrozoonosis, Grahamellosis and Ehrlichiosis. *In* Infectious Blood Diseases of Man and Animals. Vol. 2. Diseases Caused by Protista. Weinman, D., and Ristic, M., eds. Academic Press, New York, p. 387, 1968.

Love, J.N., and McEwen, E.G.: Hypoglycemia Associated with Haemobartonella-like Infection in Splenectomized Calves. Amer. J. Vet. Res., *33*:2087, 1972.

Lumb, W.V.: Canine Haemobartonellosis and Its Feline Counterpart. Calif. Vet., *14*:24, 1961.

Maede, Y.: Studies on Feline Haemobartonellosis. IV. Life Span of Erythrocytes of Cat Infected with Hemobartonella felis. Jap. J. Vet. Sci., *37*:269, 1975.

Maede, Y.: Studies on Feline Haemobartonellosis. V. Role of the Spleen in Cats Infected with Haemobartonella felis. Jap. J. Vet. Sci., *40*:141, 1978.

Maede, Y.: Sequestration and Phagocytosis of Hemobartonella felis in the Spleen. Amer. J. Vet. Res., *40*:691, 1979.

Maede, Y.: Studies on Feline Haemobartonellosis. VI. Changes of Erythrocyte Lipids Concentration and Their Relation to Osmotic Fragility. Jap. J. Vet. Sci., *42*:281, 1980.

Maede, Y., and Hato, R.: Studies on Feline Haemobartonellosis. II. The Mechanism of Anemia Produced by Infection with Haemobartonella felis. Jap. J. Vet. Sci., *37*:49, 1975.

Maede, Y., and Murata, H.: Ultrastructural Observation of the Removal of Haemobartonella felis from Erythrocytes in the Spleen of a Cat. Jap. J. Vet. Sci., *40*:203, 1978.

McNaught, J.B., et al.: Bartonella Bodies in the Blood of a Non-Splenectomized Dog. J. Exp. Med., *62*:353, 1935.

Middleton, D.J., et al.: Haemobartonellosis in a Dog. Aust. Vet. J., *59*:29, 1982.

North, D.C.: Fatal Haemobartonellosis in a Non-Splenectomized Dog: A Case Report. J. Small Anim. Pract., *19*:769, 1978.

Oduye, O.O., and Dipeolu, O.O.: Blood Parasites of Dogs in Ibadan. J. Small Anim. Pract., *17*:331, 1976.

Peters, D., and Wigand, R.: Bartonellaceae. Bact. Rev., *19*:150, 1955.

Priester, W.A., and Hayes, H.M.: Feline Leukemia after Feline Infectious Anemia. J. Natl. Cancer Inst., *51*:289, 1973.

Pryor, W.H., and Bradbury, R.P.: Haemobartonella canis Infection in Research Dogs. Lab. Anim. Sci., *25*:266, 1975.

Rhoads, C.P., and Miller, D.K.: The Association of Bartonella Bodies with Induced Anemia in the Dog. J. Exp. Med., *61*:139, 1935.

Schalm, O.W., and Theilen, G.H.: Lymphosarcoma and Hemobartonellosis in a Bassett Hound. Calif. Vet., *28*:22, April, 1972.

Seamer, J.: Eperythrozoon and Haemobartonella. Vet. Rec., *71*:437, 1959.

Seamer, J., and Douglas, S.W.: A New Blood Parasite of British Cats. Vet. Rec., *71*:405, 1959.

Seneviratna, et al.: Transmission of Haemobartonella canis by the Dog Tick, Rhipicephalus sanguineus. Res. Vet. Sci., *14*:112, 1973.

Simpson, C.F., and Love, J.N.: Fine Structure of Haemobartonella bovis in the Blood and Liver of Splenectomized Calves. Amer. J. Vet. Res., *31*:225, 1970.

Simpson, C.F., et al.: Ultrastructure of Erythrocytes Parasitized by Haemobartonella felis. J. Parasitol., *64*:505, 1978.

Small, E., and Ristic, M.: Morphologic Features of Haemobartonella felis. Amer. J. Vet. Res., *28*:845, 1967.

Small, E., and Ristic, M.: Haemobartonellosis. Vet. Clin. North Amer., *1*:225, 1971.

Sonoda, M., et al.: Studies on Canine. I. Haemobartonella canis Detected in the Blood of Dogs Inoculated with Babesia gibsoni. Jap. J. Vet. Sci., *40*:335, 1978.

Splitter, E.J., et al.: Feline Infectious Anemia. Vet. Med., *51*:17, 1956.

Venable, J.J., and Ewing, S.A.: Fine Structure of Haemobartonella canis (Rickettsiales:Bartonellaceae) and Its Relation to the Host Erythrocyte. J. Parasitol., *54*:259, 1968.

West, H.J.: Haemobartonellosis in the Dog. J. Small Anim. Pract., *20*:543, 1979.

Eperythrozoonosis

Adams, E.W., et al.: Eperythrozoonosis in a Herd of Purebred Landrace Pigs. J. Amer. Vet. Med. Ass., *135*:226, 1959.

Adler, S., and Ellenbogen, V.: A Note on Two New Blood Parasites of Cattle, Eperythrozoon and Bartonella. J. Comp. Path. Therap., *47*:219, 1934.

Brock, W.E., et al.: Studies on the Pathology of Virus Anemia or Ictero-Anemia of Swine. J. Amer. Vet. Med. Ass., Proc. 88th Annu. Meeting, p. 160, 1951.

Daddow, K.N.: The Transmission of Sheep Strain of Eperythrozoon ovis to Goats and the Development of a Carrier State in the Goats. Aust. Vet. J., *55*:605, 1979a.

Daddow, K.N.: Eperythrozoon ovis: A Cause of Anemia, Reduced Production and Decreased Exercise Tolerance in Sheep. Aust. Vet. J., *55*:433, 1979b.

Foote, L.E., et al.: Interference between Anaplasmosis

and Eperythrozoonosis in Splenectomized Cattle. Amer. J. Vet. Res., *18*:556, 1957.

Henry, S.C.: Clinical Observations of Eperythrozoonosis. J. Amer. Vet. Med. Ass., *174*:601, 1979.

Jennings, A.R., and Seamer, J.: A New Blood Parasite in British Pigs. Nature, *178*:153, 1956.

Keeton, K.S., and Jain, N.C.: Eperythrozoon wenyoni: A Scanning Electron Microscope Study. J. Parasitol., *59*:867, 1973.

Kreier, J.P., and Ristic, M.: Morphologic, Antigenic, and Pathogenic Characteristics of Eperythrozoon ovis and Eperythrozoon wenyonii. Amer. J. Vet. Res., *24*:488, 1963.

Littlejohns, I.R.: Eperythrozoonosis in Sheep. Aust. Vet. J., *36*:260, 1960.

Lotze, J.C., and Yiengst, M.J.: Eperythrozoonosis in Cattle in the United States. North Amer. Vet., *22*:345, 1941.

Neitz, W.O., et al.: Eperythrozoon ovis (sp. nov.) Infection in Sheep. Onderstepoort J. Vet. Sci. Anim. Ind., *3*:263, 1934.

Neitz, W.O.: Eperythrozoonosis in Cattle. Onderstepoort J. Vet. Sci. Anim. Ind., *14*:9, 1940.

Overas, J.: Studies on Eperythrozoon ovis Infection in Sheep. Acta Vet. Scand. Suppl., *28*, 1969.

Savage, A., and Isa, J.M.: A Picture of Eperythrozoon suis. Cornell Vet., *48*:10, 1958.

Seamer, J.: Studies on Eperythrozoon parvum Splitter, 1950. Parasitology, *50*:67, 1960.

Splitter, E.J.: Eperythrozoon suis: The Etiologic Agent of Ictero-Anemia of an Anaplasmosis-like Disease of Swine. Amer. J. Vet. Res., *11*:324, 1950.

Splitter, E.J., and Williamson, R.L.: Eperythrozoonosis in Swine: A Preliminary Report. J. Amer. Vet. Med. Ass., *116*:360, 1950.

Sutton, R.H.: Observations on the Pathology of Eperythrozoon ovis Infection in Sheep. N.Z. Vet. J., *26*:224, 1978.

Zachary, J.F.: Immune Responses and Hematologic Alterations in Splenectomized Pigs Experimentally Infected with Eperythrozoon suis. I. A Possible Animal Model for Cold Agglutinin Disease in Man. Diss. Abst. Sect. B., *49*:2823, 1983.

Zachary, J.F., and Basgall, E.J.: Erythrocyte Membrane Altration with the Attachment and Replication of *Eperythrozoon suis*: A Light and Electron Microscopy Study. Vet. Pathol., *22*:164, 1985.

Theileriasis

Allison, A.C., and Eugui, E.M.: Theilerosis: Cell-Mediated and Humoral Immunity. Amer. J. Pathol., *102*:114, 1981.

Barnett, S.F.: Theileriasis. *In* Infectious Blood Diseases of Man and Animals. Vol. 2. Diseases Caused by Protista. Weinman, D., and Ristic, M., eds. Academic Press, New York, p. 269, 1968.

Brown, C.G.D.: Propagation of Theileria. *In* Practical Applications of Tissue Culture. Marmorasch, K., and Hirumi, H., eds. Academic Press, New York, p. 223, 1979.

Davidson, W.R., et al.: Observations on Theileri cervi and Trypanosoma cervi in White-Tailed Deer (Odocoileus virginianus) from the South Eastern United States. Proc. Halminthol. Soc. Wash., *50*(1):165, 1983.

Irvin, A.D., and Cunningham, M.P.: East Coast Fever. Curr. Top. Vet. Med. Anim. Sci., *6*:393, 1981.

Kreier, J.P., et al.: Theileria sp. in a Deer in the United States. Amer. J. Vet. Res., *23*:657, 1962.

MacHardy, N., et al.: Chemotherapy of Theileria parva Infection. Nature, *261*:698, 1976.

Neitz, W.O.: Theileriosis. Adv. Vet. Sci., *5*:241, 1959.

Osebold et al.: Latent Anaplasma marginale Infection in Wild Deer Demonstrated by Calf Inoculation. Cornell Vet., *49*:97, 1959.

Rogers, R.J., and Callow, L.L.: Three Fatal Cases of Theileria mutans Infection. Aust. Vet. J., *42*:42, 1966.

Saidu, S.N.A.: Bovine Theileriasis Due to Theileria mutans: A Review. Vet. Bull., *52*:451, 1982.

Schaeffler, W.F.: Serologic Tests for Theileria cervi in White-Tailed Deer and Other Species of Theileria in Cattle and Sheep. Amer. J. Vet. Res., *24*:784, 1963.

Schein, E., and Voigt, W.P.: Chemotherapy of Bovine Theileriosis with Halofriginone. Acta Trop., *36*:391, 1979.

Schein, E., et al.: Development of Theileria parva (Theiler, 1904) in the Gut of Rhipicephalus appendiculus (Neumann, 1901). Parasitology, *75*:309, 1977.

Shitakha, V.M., et al.: Complement Activation and Fibrinolysis during Infection with Theileria parva (East Coast Fever) in Cattle. Vet. Immunol. Immunopathol., *4*:361, 1983.

Sisodia, R.S., and Gautam, O.P.: Experimental Cases of Theileria hirci Infection in Sheep and Goats. Indian J. Anim. Sci., *53*:162, 1983.

Splitter, E.J.: Theileria mutans Associated with Bovine Anaplasmosis in the United States. J. Amer. Vet. Med. Ass., *117*:134, 1950b.

Uilenberg, G.: Theileria Infections Other Than East Coast Fever. Curr. Top. Vet. Med. Anim. Sci., *6*:411, 1981.

Trypanosomiasis

Anosa, V.O., and Kaneko, J.J.: Pathogenesis of Trypanosoma brucei Infection in Deer Mice (Peromyscus maniculatus): Hematologic, Erythrocytes, Biochemical, and Iron Metabolic Aspects. Amer. J. Vet. Res., *44*:639, 1983a.

Anosa, V.O., and Kaneko, J.J.: Pathogenesis of Trypanosoma brucei Infection in Deer Mice (Peromyscus maniculatus): Light and Electron Microscopic Studies on Erythrocyte Pathologic Changes and Phagocytosis. Amer. J. Vet. Res., *44*:645, 1983b.

Banks, K.L.: Injury Induced by Trypanosoma congolense Adhesion to Cell Membranes. J. Parasitol. *66*:34, 1980.

Clarkson, M.J.: Immunoglobin M in Trypanosomiasis. *In* Pathophysiology of Parasitic Infection. Soulsby, E.J.L., ed. Academic Press, New York, p. 171, 1976.

Crawley, H.: Studies on Blood and Blood Parasites. III. Trypanosoma americanum N. Sp.: A Trypanosome Which Appears in Cultures Made from Blood of American Cattle (Preliminary Notice). USDA Bur. Anim. Ind. Bull., *119*:21, 1909.

Crawley, H.: Trypanosoma americanum: A Common Parasite of American Cattle. USDA Bur. Anim. Ind. Bull. 145, 1912.

Cross, R.F., et al.: Observations on Trypanosoma theileri Infection in Cattle. Can. J. Comp. Med., *35*:12, 1971.

Dargie, J.D., et al.: Bovine Trypanosomiasis: The Red Cell Kinetics of Ndama dn Zebu Cattle Infected with Trypanosoma congolense. Parasitology, *78*:271, 1979.

Dikmans, G., et al.: Demonstration of Trypanosoma theileri in the Stomach of an Aborted Bovine Fetus. Cornell Vet., *47*:344, 1957.

Esievo, K.A.N.: Studies on an Aspect of the Anaemia of Bovine Trypanosomiasis (Trypanosoma vivax). Diss. Abstr. Int., *42*:1686, 1981.

Esievo, K.A.N., and Saror, D.I.: Leukocyte Response in

Experimental Trypanosoma vivax Infection in Cattle. J. Comp. Path., *93*:165, 1983.

Esievo, K.A.N., et al.: Variation in Erythrocyte Surface and Free Serum Sialic Concentration During Experimental *Trypanosoma vivax*. Res. Vet. Sci., *32*:1, 1982.

Facer, C.A., et al.: Immune Haemolytic Anaemia in Bovine Trypanosomiasis. J. Comp. Path., *92*:393, 1982.

Greig, W.A., et al.: Factors Affecting Blood Sampling for Anaemia and Parsitaemia in Bovine Trypanosomiasis. Brit. Vet. J., *135*:130, 1979.

Hare, W.C.D., et al.: Bovine Trypanosomes and Lymphocytosis-Parallel Studies. Bibl. Haematologica, *36*:504, 1970.

Hornby, H.E.: The Development of Our Knowledge of Animal Trypanosomiases. Vet. Rec., *61*:375, 1949.

Jennings, F.W.: The Anaemias of Parasitic Infections. *In* Pathophysiology of Parasitic Infection. Soulsby, E.J.L., ed. Academic Press, New York, pp. 41–67, 1976.

Jura, W.G.Z., and Losos, G.J.: A Comparative Study of the Diseases in Cattle Caused by Theileria lawrencei and Theileria parva. I. Clinical Signs and Parasitological Observations. Vet. Parasitol., *7*:275, 1980.

Kaaya, G.P., et al.: Clinico-Pathologic Aspects of Trypanosoma congolense Infection in Goats. Bull. Anim. Health Prod. Africa, *25*:397, 1977.

Kaaya, G.P., et al.: Inhibition of Leukopoiesis by Sera from Trypanosoma congolense Infected Calves: Partial Characterization of the Inhibitory Factor. Tropenmed. Parasitol., *31*:232, 1980.

Leeflang, R., et al.: Studies on Trypanosoma vivax: Comparison of Parasitological Diagnostic Methods. Int. J. Parasitol., *8*:15, 1978.

Levine, N.D.: Protozoan Parasites of Domestic Animals and of Man. Burgess Publishing Co., Minneapolis, 1961.

Levine, N.D., et al.: A Case of Bovine Trypanosomiasis Due to Trypanosoma theileri in Illinois. J. Parasitol., *42*:553, 1956.

Lumsden, W.H.R., and Wells, E.A.: Trypanosomiasis. *In* Infectious Blood Diseases of Man and Animals. Vol. 2. Diseases Caused by Protista. Weinman, D., and Ristic, M., eds. Academic Press, New York, p. 329, 1968.

Lundholm, B.D., et al.: Trypanosoma theileri as a Contaminant of Tissue Origin in Cultures of Fetal Bovine Kidney Cells in Vitro. Virology, *8*:394, 1959.

Maxie, M.G., et al.: A Comparative Study of the Hematological Aspects of the Diseases Caused by Trypanosoma vivax and Trypanosoma congolense in Cattle. *In* Pathophysiology of Parasitic Infection. Soulsby, E.J.C., ed. Academic Press, New York, p. 183, 1976.

Maxie, M.G., et al.: Experimental Bovine Trypanosomiasis (Trypanosoma vivax and T. congolense). I. Symptomatology and Clinical Pathology. Tropenmed. Parasitol., *30*:274, 1979.

Morrison, W.I., et al.: Bovine Trypanosomiasis. Curr. Top. Vet. Med. Anim. Sci., *6*:469, 1981.

Naylor, D.C.: The Haematology and Histopathology of Trypanosoma congolense Infection in Cattle. Trop. Anim. Health Prod., *3*:159, 1971.

Nielsen, K., et al.: Experimental Bovine Trypanosomiasis: Changes in the Catabolism of Serum Immunoglobulins and Complement Components in Infected Cattle. Immunology, *35*:811, 1978a.

Nielsen, K., et al.: Experimental Bovine Trypanosomiasis: Changes in Serum Immunoglobulins, Com-

plement and Complement Components in Infected Animals. Immunology, *35*:817, 1978b.

Preston, J.M., et al.: Trypanosoma congolense: Calf Erythrocyte Survival. Exp. Parasitol., *48*:118, 1979.

Preston, J.M., et al.: Trypanosoma congolense: Thrombocyte Survival in Infected Steers. Exp. Parasitol., *54*:129, 1982.

Ristic, M., and Trager, W.: Cultivation at 37°C of a Trypanosome (Trypanosoma theileri) from cows with Depressed Milk Production. J. Protozool., *5*:146, 1958.

Rurangirwa, F.R., et al.: Immunosuppressive Effect of Trypanosoma congolense and Trypanosoma vivax on the Mycoplasma mycoides subsp. mycoides. Res. Vet. Sci., *25*:395, 1978.

Schalm, O.W.: Uncommon Hematologic Disorders: Spirochetosis, Trypanosomiasis, Leishmaniasis, Pelger-Huët Anomaly. Canine Pract., *6*(6):46, 1979.

Toro, M., et al.: Haematocrit Centrifugation Technique for the Diagnosis of Bovine Trypanosomiasis. Vet. Parasitol., *8*:23, 1981.

Valli, V.E.O., and Mills, J.N.: The Quantitation of Trypanosoma congolense in Calves. I. Hematological Changes. Tropenmed. Parasitol., *31*:215, 1980.

Valli, V.E.O., et al.: The Pathogenesis of Trypanosoma congolense Infection in Calves. II. Anemia and Erythroid Response. Vet. Path., *15*:732, 1978.

Valli, V.E.O., et al.: The Pathogenesis of Trypanosoma congolense Infection in Calves. III. Neutropenia and Myeloid Response. Vet. Path., *16*:96, 1979.

Wellde, B.T., et al.: Trypanosoma congolense: Thrombocytopenia in Experimentally Infected Cattle. Exp. Parasitol., *45*:26, 1978.

Wellde, B.T., et al.: Haemorrhagic Syndrome in Cattle Associated with Trypanosoma vivax Infection. Trop. Anim. Health Prod., *15*:95, 1983.

Whitelaw, D.D., et al.: Immunosuppression in Bovine Trypanosomiasis: Studies with Louping-Ill Vaccine. Res. Vet. Sci., *26*:102, 1979.

Cytauxzoonosis

Ferris, D.H.: A Progress Report on the Status of a New Disease of American Cats: Cytauxzoonosis. Comp. Immunol. Microbiol. Infect. Dis., *1*:269, 1979.

Glenn, B.L., et al.: Cytauxzan-like Piroplasms in Erythrocytes of Wild-Trapped Bobcats in Oklahoma. J. Amer. Vet. Med. Ass., *181*:1251, 1982.

Hauck, W.N., et al.: Cytauxzoonosis in a Native Louisiana Cat. J. Amer. Vet. Med. Ass., *180*(12):1472–1474, 1982.

Kier, A.B., et al.: Diagnostic Features of a Newly Described Blood Protozoan Disease in Domestic Cats—A Cytauxzoon Species. *In* Proc. 20th Annu. Meet., Am. Ass. Vet. Lab. Diagnosticians., p. 123, 1977.

Kier, A.B., et al.: Experimental Transmission of Cytauxzoon felis from Bobcats (Lynx rufus) to Domestic Cats (Felis domesticus). Amer. J. Vet. Res., *43*:97, 1982a.

Kier, A.B., et al.: Interspecies Transmission of Cytauxzoon felis. Amer. J. Vet. Res., *43*:102, 1982b.

Simpson, C.F., et al.: Ultrastructure of the Intraerythrocytic Stage of Cytauxzoon felis. Amer. J. Vet. Res., *46*:1178, 1985.

Wagner, J.E.: A Fatal Cytauxzoonosis-like Disease in Cats. J. Amer. Vet. Med. Ass., *168*:585, 1976.

Wagner, J.E., et al.: Experimentally Induced Cytauxzoonosis-like Disease in Domestic Cats. Vet. Parasitol., *6*:305, 1980.

Wagner, L.D., et al.: Feline Cytauxzoonosis: A Newly

Reported Blood Protozoan Disease from Southwestern Missouri. Mo. Vet., *25(2)*:12, 1979.

Zinkl, J.G., et al.: Cytauxzoon-like Organisms in Erythrocytes of Two Cheetahs. J. Amer. Vet. Med. Ass., *179*:1261, 1981.

Sarcocystosis

Dubey, J.P., et al.: Sarcocystosis in Goats: Clinical Signs and Pathologic and Hemotologic Findings. J. Amer. Vet. Med. Ass., *178*:683, 1981.

Fayer, R., and Prasse, K.W.: Hematology of Experimental Acute Sarcocystis bovicanis Infection in Calves. I. Cellular and Serologic Changes. Vet. Path., *18*:351, 1981.

Prasse, K.W., and Fayer, R.: Hematology of Experimental Acute Sarcocystis bovicanis Infections in Calves. II. Serum Biochemistry and Hemostasis Studies. Vet. Path., *18*:358, 1981.

Leptospirosis

Bhasin, J.L., et al.: Properties of a Cold Hemagglutinin Associated with Leptospiral Hemolytic Anemia of Sheep. Infect. Immun., *3*:398, 1971.

Davidson, J.N., and Hirsh, D.C.: Leptospirosis in Lambs. J. Amer. Vet. Med. Ass., *176(2)*:124, 1980.

Higgins, R.: A Minireview of the Pathogenesis of Acute Leptospirosis. Can. Vet. J., *22*:277, 1981.

Navarro, C.E.K., and Kociba, G.J.: Hemostatic Changes in Dogs with Experimental Leptospira interrogans serovar icterohaemorrhagiae Infection. Amer. J. Vet. Res., *43(5)*:904, 1982.

Reinhard, K.R.: A Clinical Pathological Study of Experimental Leptospirosis of Calves. Amer. J. Vet. Res., *12*:282, 1951.

Reinhard, K.R.: Present Knowledge and Concepts of Leptospirosis in Farm Animals. J. Amer. Vet. Med. Ass., *123*:487, 1953.

Bacillary Hemoglobinuria

Erwin, B.G.: Experimental Induction of Bacillary Hemoglobinuria in Cattle. Amer. J. Vet. Res., *38*:1625, 1977.

Janzen, E.D., et al.: Bacillary Hemoglobinuria Associated with Hepatic Necrobacillosis in a Yearling Feedlot Heifer. Can. Vet. J., *22*:393, 1981.

Olander, H.J., et al.: Bacillary Hemoglobinuria: Induction by Liver Biopsy in Naturally and Experimentally Infected Animals. Path. Vet., *3*:421, 1966.

Records, E., and Vawter, L.R.: Bacillary Hemoglobinuria of Cattle and Sheep (Red Water Disease). Univ. Nev. Agr. Exp. Sta. Bull., *173*, 1945.

Equine Infectious Anemia

Coggins, L.: Equine Infectious Anaemia. *In* Virus Diseases of Food Animals. Vol. 2. Gibbs, E.P.J., ed. Academic Press, London, pp. 719–730, 1981.

Coggins, L., and Norcross, N.L.: Immunodiffusion Reaction in Equine Infectious Anemia. Cornell Vet., *60*:330, 1970.

Coggins, L., et al.: Diagnosis of Equine Infectious Anemia by Immuno-Diffusion Test. Amer. J. Vet. Res., *33*:11, 1972.

Foil, L.D., et al.: Mechanical Transmission of Equine Infectious Anemia Virus by Deer Flies (Chrysops flavidus) and Stable Flies (Stomoxys calcitrans). Amer. J. Vet. Res., *44*:155, 1983.

Hawkins, J.A., et al.: Role of Horse Fly (Tabanus fuscucostatus) and Stable Fly (Stomoxys calcitrans) in Transmission of Equine Infectious Anemia to Ponies in Louisiana. Amer. J. Vet. Res., *34*:1583, 1973.

Hawkins, J.A., et al.: Transmission of Equine Infectious Anemia Virus by Tabanus fusciocostatus. J. Amer. Vet. Med. Ass., *168*:63, 1976.

Henson, J.B., and McGuire, T.C.: Equine Infectious Anemia. Prog. Med. Virol., *18*:143, 1974.

Henson, J.B., et al.: The Diagnosis of Equine Infectious Anemia Using the Complement-Fixation Test, Siderocyte Counts, Hepatic Biopsies, and Serum Alterations. J. Amer. Vet. Med. Ass., *151*:1830, 1967.

Hyslop, N.St.G.: Equine Infectious Anemia (Swamp Fever): A Review. Vet. Rec., *78*:858, 1966.

Ishii, S.: Equine Infectious Anemia or Swamp Fever. Adv. Vet. Sci., *8*:263, 1963.

Ishii, S., and Ishitani, R.: Equine Infectious Anemia. Adv. Vet. Sci. Comp. Med., *19*:195, 1975.

Issel, C.J., and Coggins, L.: Equine Infectious Anemia: Current Knowledge. J. Amer. Vet. Med. Ass., *174*:727, 1979.

Issel, C.J., and Foil, L.D.: Studies on Equine Infectious Anemia Virus Transmission by Insects. J. Amer. Vet. Med. Ass., *184*:293, 1984.

Johnson, A.W.: Equine Infectious Anemia: The Literature 1966–1975. Vet. Bull., *46*:559, 1976.

Konno, S., and Yamamoto, H.: Pathology of Equine Infectious Anemia: Proposed Classification of Pathologic Types of Disease. Cornell Vet., *60*:393, 1970.

Rothenbacher, H.J., et al.: Equine Infectious Anemia. II. The Sideroleukocyte Test as an Aid in the Clinical Diagnosis. Vet. Med., *57*:886, 1962.

Squire, R.A.: Equine Infectious Anemia: A Model of Immunoproliferative Disease: A Review. Blood, *32*:157, 1968.

Stein, C.D., et al.: Some Observations on Carriers of Equine Infectious Anemia. J. Amer. Vet. Med. Ass., *126*:277, 1955.

Weiland, F., et al.: Equine Infectious Anemia: Detection of Antibodies Using an Immunofluorescence Test. Res. Vet. Sci., *33*:347, 1982.

Williams, D.L., et al.: Studies with Equine Infectious Anemia Virus: Transmission Attempts by Mosquitoes and Survival of Virus on Vector Mouthparts and Hypodermic Needles, and in Mosquito Tissue Culture. Amer. J. Vet. Res., *42*:1469, 1981.

Yamamoto, H., and Konno, S.: Pathological Studies on Bone Marrow in Equine Infectious Anemia. II. Histopathology of Vertebral, Sternal and Femoral Bone Marrow. Natl. Inst. Anim. Health Quart. (Tokyo), *7*:84, 1967.

24

Hemolytic Anemias of Noninfectious Origin

HEMOYLTIC ANEMIAS ASSOCIATED WITH SOME CHEMICALS AND DRUGS 627
Copper Poisoning 627
Lead Poisoning 628

HEMOLYTIC ANEMIAS ASSOCIATED WITH HEINZ BODY FORMATION 632
Heinz Bodies and the Spleen 633
Heinz Bodies in Phenothiazine Toxicosis 633
Heinz Bodies Associated with Consumption of Kale or Onions 634
Heinz Bodies in Cattle 634
Heinz Bodies in Cats 634

HEMOLYTIC ANEMIAS ASSOCIATED WITH SOME POISONOUS PLANTS 640
Castor Beans, Brassica Species, Onions, and Red Maple Leaves 640
Nitrate and Nitrite Poisoning 642

HEMOLYTIC ANEMIAS ASSOCIATED WITH METABOLIC DISEASES 642
Postparturient Hemoglobinuria 642

HEMOLYTIC ANEMIAS ASSOCIATED WITH INTRAERYTHROCYTIC DEFECTS 643
Methemoglobinemia 643
Pyruvate Kinase Deficiency in the Dog 645
Congenital Erythropoietic Porphyria 646

IMMUNE-MEDIATED HEMOLYTIC ANEMIAS 647
Autoimmune Hemolytic Anemia 647
Neonatal Isoerythrolysis 650

HEMOLYTIC ANEMIAS OF MISCELLANEOUS ORIGIN 650
Water Intoxicosis 650

Various causes of hemolytic anemias are listed in Table 23–1, and hemolytic anemias associated with infectious agents are described in Chapter 23. Hemolytic anemias associated with causes other than infectious agents are described in this chapter. For general comments on various hematologic abnormalities encountered during a hemolytic anemia, see Chapter 21.

HEMOLYTIC ANEMIAS ASSOCIATED WITH SOME CHEMICALS AND DRUGS

The list of chemicals and drugs that can cause hemolytic anemia is long and includes copper, lead, phenothiazine, methylene blue, saponins, naphthalene, and certain drugs such as acetanilid, nitrofurantoin, neoarsphenamine, phenacetin, and some sulfanilamides. A brief description of hematologic abnormalities associated with copper and lead poisoning follows.

Copper Poisoning

Sheep are especially sensitive to development of hemolytic crisis under conditions of stress when the liver has a high content of copper. Growing lambs are most susceptible. Copper accumulates in the liver of animals receiving copper from drenches or feeding on copper-contaminated forage or certain plants having a high copper content. This accumulation of copper occurs over a prolonged period during which animals are usually asymptomatic, although evidence of liver damage can be found on histopathologic examination or in serum biochemistry. Under conditions of stress, copper is released to the bloodstream to bring about rapid erythrocyte destruction. Liver damage precedes increase in blood copper level. The strain of traveling is an important stress factor in promoting hemolytic crisis in sheep. Starvation after good feeding, exposure to cold, and sudden, unaccustomed exercise are other important predisposing stress factors leading to copper release from the liver (Pearson, 1956).

Acute hemolytic crisis with hemoglobinemia and hemoglobinuria is an outstanding finding. This is associated with respiratory distress, anorexia, and extreme weakness. The condition is usually fatal; death occurs within 24–48 hours. If the individual sheep lives long enough, the sclera becomes icteric, and the blood picture is one of marked bone marrow response to acute blood destruction. It has been stated that loss of body weight is one of the principal factors precipitating a hemolytic crisis in sheep that have large stores of copper in the liver. Thus deaths may increase when pastures dry up, unless the animals receive supplementary feeding to prevent the loss of body weight (Pierson and Aanes, 1958). Diagnosis is based on clinical signs and demonstration of high levels of copper in the liver and kidney specimens and forage.

Hemolytic anemia from copper poisoning has been reported also in swine (Gordon and Luke, 1957), calves (Shand and Lewis, 1957), and chickens (Goldberg et al., 1956). Pigs are relatively tolerant to dietary copper, but may develop a progressive, fatal anemia accompanied by icterus, stomach ulceration, and accumulation of copper in the liver and kidney (Higgins, 1981). Chronic copper toxicosis in growing pigs can manifest as iron deficiency anemia (Hatch et al., 1979), probably as a result of impaired iron absorption from the gastrointestinal tract (Gipp et al., 1974). Horses are relatively tolerant to copper accumulation in the liver (Smith et al., 1975).

Recently an inherited (autosomal recessive) copper toxicosis with progressive hepatopathy was described in Bedlington terriers, but acute hemolytic anemia was seen in only a small number of such dogs (Johnson et al., 1980; Owen and Ludwig, 1982; Twedt et al., 1979). Red cell survival was normal in three affected dogs studied (Su et al., 1982a). The disease resembles Wilson's disease of humans in many respects and was found to have a similar metabolic defect of impaired biliary excretion of copper (Su et al., 1982b).

In ruminants, the metabolism of copper, molybdenum, and sulfate ions is interrelated (Buck, 1981). Copper-molybdenum complex, in the presence of inorganic sulfate, is believed to inhibit urinary excretion and metabolism of copper in tissues, particularly in the liver, leading to impaired synthesis of ceruloplasmin. Copper toxicosis is common when the copper:molybdenum ratio in forage is greater than 10:1 either because of excessive copper or deficiency of molybdenum. Zinc and iron interact with copper in nonruminants, particularly in pigs, to exert a protective effect from copper toxicosis.

The mechanism of hemolysis from copper toxicity is under investigation (Asano et al., 1983; Hochstein et al., 1978; Kumar et al., 1978). It has been suggested that the primary cytotoxic effects of copper result from its interaction with the sulfhydryl groups of membrane proteins. Such an interaction leads not only to cross linking of membrane proteins, which affects cell viability, but also to the formation of cuprous ions, which then interact with oxygen to form superoxide. Hydrogen peroxide generated within the plasma membrane by the dismutation of superoxide so formed may participate in the initiation of lipid peroxidation, membrane damage, and hemolysis. Hemolysis in vitro is prevented in the presence of lipid antioxidants such as butylated hydroxyanisole. In addition to its interaction with membrane sulfhydryl groups, copper may also participate directly in the initiation of membrane lipid peroxidation. Copper may also exert some cytotoxic effect by inhibition of several important red cell enzymes such as glutathione reductase, glucose-6-phosphate dehydrogenase, and pyruvate kinase, (Boulard et al., 1972; Fairbanks, 1967), depletion of reduced glutathione (GSH), and increased methemoglobin formation (Asano et al., 1983).

Lead Poisoning

Lead poisoning may be acute or chronic, but anemia is evident only in the latter. Dogs seem to be highly sensitive, particularly young dogs, while cattle, horses, and sheep are less susceptible and pigs are relatively resistant to lead intoxication. Hematologic aspects of lead poisoning in humans and animals have been reviewed (George and Duncan, 1979; Schalm, 1980).

Canine Plumbism

Clinical signs of lead poisoning in the dog commonly mimic those of other diseases and may be confused with the distemper complex, infectious hapatitis, and gastrointestinal disorders. Although lead poisoning may occur in dogs at any age, it is particularly likely to develop in young dogs (less than 1 year of age) because of their habit of chewing on objects of all kinds (O'Brien, 1981), some of which may contain lead or be painted with lead-base paints. Dietary factors influence lead absorption: dogs on a high-fat, low-calcium diet were found to absorb more lead and have markedly elevated blood lead levels (Hamir et al., 1982). Also, lead accumulates more in young dogs than in older dogs.

The clinical signs of lead poisoning have been divided into abdominal or gastrointestinal and nervous responses (Dodd and Staples, 1956). Vomiting, diarrhea, colic, abdominal pain, and restlessness are frequent manifestations of plumbism in the dog. Body temperature is usually normal. The pain referable to the abdominal area may cause the dog to whine or cry constantly. The nervous system signs include irritability, hysterical barking, convulsions, muscular tremors, blindness, champing of the jaws and frothing due to excessive salivation, weakness, lethargy, and posterior ataxia. The nervous signs may follow the abdominal responses, but either group of clinical responses may occur without prior or subsequent appearance of the other. The dog usually loses weight and may fail to recognize its owner.

Lead poisoning in the dog should be suspected when a routine blood examination reveals a significant number of polychromatic erythrocytes and *nucleated erythrocytes* out of proportion to the PCV, which may be well within the normal range (Appendix Case 35). Although anemia is a common finding in chronic plumbism, it is generally not present in the more acute form. The finding of increased numbers of immature erythrocytes in the presence of a normal PCV calls for careful inspection of both nucleated and nonnucleated erythrocytes for evidence of *basophilic stippling* (Plate XVIII–11). The basophilic stippling may be in the form of distinct granules

(punctate) or more diffuse and web-like material (reticulated). The latter form is more common (Zook et al., 1970). The stippling effect is attributed to unusual clumping of ribosomes (Albahary, 1972; Jensen et al., 1965). Erythrocytes with basophilic stippling do not stain for iron by Prussian blue stain, whereas erythrocytes with Pappenheimer bodies (fine, bluish granules) do take up the stain and are then called siderocytes. Thus the stippled erythrocytes are immature cells whose ribosomal structure has been altered by the toxic effects of the lead.

It has been demonstrated (Valentine, et al., 1976) that lead poisoning in humans induces an acquired deficiency of erythrocyte pyrimidine-specific 5'-nucleotidase (P5N). Ribosomal RNA in normal reticulocytes is degraded to 5'-pyrimidine nucleotides, which are subsequently dephosphorylated by P5N. Deficiency of this enzyme is therefore associated with accumulation and aggregation of ribosomes, which assume the form of basophilic stippling in stained blood films. An autosomal recessive inherited deficiency of P5N associated with increased erythrocyte basophilic stippling has been reported in some human families (Beutler et al., 1980; Valentine et al., 1974). Among various animal species studied so far, erythrocytes of gerbils have the highest P5N activity, and in order of decreasing activity are feline, canine, ovine, equine, and bovine erythrocytes (George, 1981; George and Duncan, 1982). P5N was approximately proportional to the percentage of reticulocytes and inversely proportional to the mean red cell life span in these species.

The anemia of chronic lead poisoning varies in degree and appears to result from both impaired formation of heme (Chisolm, 1963) and accelerated removal of altered erythrocytes from the circulation (shortened survival). The latter forms the basis of hemolytic anemia. Evidence indicates that lead inhibits several enzymes of heme synthesis, e.g., δ-aminolevulinic acid (ALA) dehydrase, ALA synthetase, and heme synthetase. Hence elevations are found in levels of free erythrocyte protoporphyrins and urinary excretion of delta-ALA and coproporphyrin. There is also impaired globin synthesis. The anemia is usually normocytic-normochromic with a tendency to be slightly microcytic-hypochromic, and there may be some reticulocytosis. Erythrocyte osmotic fragility is reduced, but mechanical fragility is increased. Bone marrow shows erythroid hyperplasia along with some ineffective erythropoiesis. Increased formation of ring sideroblasts (iron accumulation in mitochondria) has been observed in experimental animals (Jensen, et al., 1965). Leukocytosis due to neutrophilia with a regenerative left shift is a common finding. This may be related to an increase in the bone marrow myeloid:erythroid ratio (Mitema et al., 1980).

The morphologic features of erythrocytes in lead poisoning as detected in peripheral blood films vary in degree from day to day in the same dog and among dogs. The nucleated erythrocytes varied between 1 and 163/100 WBC in nine dogs with lead poisoning (Bond and Kubin, 1949) and between 1 and 218/100 WBC in 60 dogs with lead poisoning (Zook et al., 1969). Defective hemoglobin synthesis leads to a buildup of metarubricytes in the bone marrow and provides the basis for their appearance in peripheral blood. Whether the inappropriate release of nucleated erythrocytes involves lead-induced alterations in the marrow sinusoidal-blood barrier remains to be established. The number of stippled erythrocytes also varies, and some authors have failed to observe any stippled cells in association with lead poisoning. Such failure may relate to the method of preparation of the blood film. Zook et al. (1970) have indicated that the number of stippled erythrocytes may decrease by 25–30% because of prolonged exposure to the anticoagulants EDTA and potassium oxalate or fixation of blood films with alcohol before staining. They also observed that acidic buffer solutions tend to reduce the stippling effect, although slow or rapid drying of the blood film did not significantly influence the development of stippled cells.

Stippled erythrocytes in the dog may occur in diseases other than lead poisoning, but to a much lesser extent (Zook et al., 1970). It was reported that more than 15 red cells with basophilic stippling per 10,000 erythrocytes was suggestive and more than 40/10,000 was almost pathognomonic of lead poisoning in the dog. We have observed some basophilic stippling in dogs and cats during intense erythropoietic response (e.g., polychromasia and reticulocytosis) to anemia from causes other than lead poisoning. Thus one should exercise caution in interpreting such a finding. Although erythrocytic stippling is often strongly suggestive of plumbism, a firm diagnosis must be based on the demonstration of an excessive lead concentration in the body. Blood and urine show increased lead levels when poisoning exists. The normal range for blood lead concentration in 40 dogs was found to be 0.01–0.05 mg/dl of whole oxalated blood (Zook et al., 1970). A lead concentration in blood in excess of 0.06 mg/dl was considered evidence of lead poisoning in the dog.

Therapy of lead poisoning is based on chelation with calcium EDTA. Satisfactory results in dogs have been obtained by administering EDTA daily for 5 days using a dosage of 110 mg/kg of body weight per day divided in four equal doses. The EDTA is added to 5% dextrose solution at the rate of 10 mg/ml and injected subcutaneously (Zook et al., 1969). Clinical signs of lead toxicosis begin to disappear within 2–3 days of the start of therapy. However, in dogs with particularly high blood lead concentrations, a second series of injections may be necessary. Chelation leads to an increase in excretion of the heavy metal in the urine. Lead concentration in urine collected in the morning before administration of EDTA and again in posttreatment urine collected in the afternoon have been measured (Pettit et al., 1956). In patients with lead objects found on radiologic examination of the gastrointestinal tract, surgery may be necessary to remove such objects.

Equine Plumbism

Chronic lead poisoning in horses pastured on areas adjacent to smelters has occurred periodically in California (Knight and Burau, 1973). Clinical signs are harsh hair coat, muscular weakness, stiffness of joints, dyspnea with roaring on exercise, and foreign body pneumonia as a sequel to pharyngeal paralysis. The major abnormalities result from disturbance of peripheral nerve functions, and in terminal cases loss of condition and severe incoordination are seen. Gastrointestinal signs or central nervous system disturbances are either absent or rarely seen. Fetal growth may be affected when mares during advanced pregnancy consume feed with high levels of lead. Some horses develop "lead line" on the gums. Blood lead levels of 0.35 ppm or more are considered significant, particularly in the presence of clinical signs.

A modest anemia with PCV values between 21 and 28% has occurred in some horses exhibiting chronic lead poisoning. Basophilic stippling of erythrocytes or the presence of large numbers of nucleated erythrocytes in peripheral blood has not been characteristic of plumbism in the horse. Only on careful search of the blood film have we found an occasional stippled erythrocyte or stippled metarubricyte (Plate XVIII–12). Even the bone marrow, with markedly increased numbers of metarubricytes, has lacked significant numbers of stippled cells. The reason for failure of a diagnostic blood picture in lead toxicosis in the horse may be the unique characteristic in the horse that nucleated and polychromatic erythrocytes are rarely released to blood even during anemia in remission. Perhaps such changes would manifest after a greater insult to the bone marrow. A recent report on experimental lead toxicosis in ponies fed smelter effluent–contaminated hay or given lead acetate stated that typical clinical signs developed along with anemia or marginal anemia, which was accompanied by the appearance of nucleated red cells and Howell-Jolly bodies in peripheral blood (Burrows and Borchard, 1982). Lead poisoning in the horse has been reviewed (Burrow, 1982).

Chronic lead poisoning in horses was reported to have been treated successfully with calcium EDTA (Holm et al., 1953).

Bovine Plumbism

Lead poisoning in calves and cows is most commonly an acute disease due to an apparent craving for lead and an uncanny ability of cattle to locate sources of lead (Fenstermacher et al., 1946). The literature contains contradictory reports regarding relative susceptibility of cattle and horses to lead toxicosis; early reports indicate that horses are much more tolerant than cattle, whereas later epizootologic studies suggest the opposite (Aronson, 1972; Hammond and Aronson, 1964). More recent observations indicate that the dose level required to produce chronic lead poisoning in horses is greater than that for cattle (Dollahite et al., 1978).

The effect of lead on blood morphology generally has not been discussed in papers on lead poisoning in cattle. Gross and microscopic changes in nine cattle affected with naturally occurring lead poisoning of 1 to 32 days' duration have been described (Christian and Tryphonas, 1971). Central nervous system involvement gave rise to the most common signs—blindness, grinding of teeth, and depression. Ruminal stasis was also a common finding. One steer and two pregnant heifers were given lead acetate orally. Hematologic values for the steer and one heifer remained within normal limits. The second heifer showed evidence of "blood-loss" anemia after more than 100 days of blood lead levels in excess of 0.5 ppm. Increased free erythrocytic porphyrin concentrations were noted at the time of necropsy. The authors concluded that the anemia was caused by increased destruction of erythrocytes as a result of increased osmotic fragility.

In a recent study, chronic lead poisoning in three calves was found to induce marked elevations of free erythrocyte protoporphyrins (George and Duncan, 1981). Lynch et al. (1976) reported finding basophilic stippling and nucleated erythrocytes in calves overdosed with lead for 6 weeks. Experimental observations indicated that increased basophilic stippling in lead-poisoned calves may be attributed to a decrease in erythrocyte P5N activity (George and Duncan, 1982).

Ovine Plumbism

Sheep may develop chronic lead poisoning. It can be detected by measurement of erythrocyte δ-ALA dehydrase activity, which was found to be strongly inhibited by relatively low doses of lead (Rolton et al., 1978). Urinary porphyrins and basophilic stippling were not sensitive indicators, whereas urinary lead and δ-ALA were too variable. Blood lead concentration paralleled the degree of lead exposure.

Porcine Plumbism

Pigs seem to be highly tolerant of lead. Blood lead concentrations of up to 290 μg/dl were associated with only mild clinical signs,

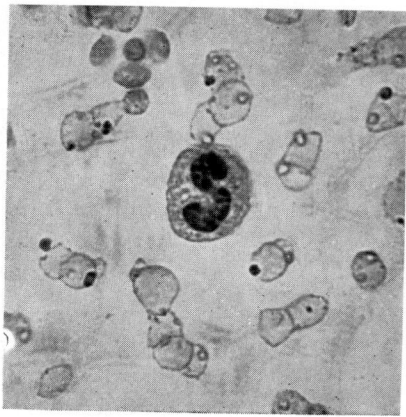

Fig. 24–1. Heinz bodies in phenothiazine toxicosis in the horse. New methylene blue stain applied to the dry, unfixed blood film.

but a marked decrease was seen in δ-ALA-dehydrase along with a moderate anemia (Lassen and Buck, 1979). Basophilic stippling was evident in erythrocytes of affected animals.

Feline Plumbism

Little is known about lead poisoning in cats. Lead poisoning in a cat from ingestion of food contaminated with lead-base paint has been reported (Jacobs, 1979). The cat had a PCV of 28.5%, reticulocyte count of 2.6%, and occasional basophilic stippling of erythrocytes. The latter prompted determination of serum lead, which was 0.7 ppm (normal <0.1 ppm), and of excretion of lead in urine, which was 0.2 ppm. Treatment with calcium-EDTA was successful.

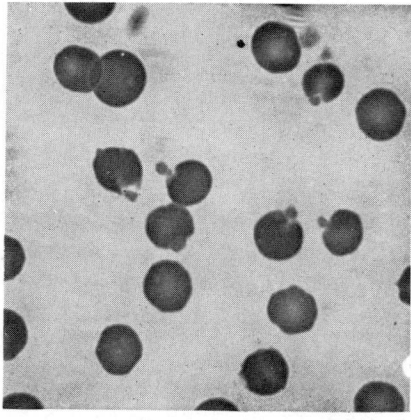

Fig. 24–2. Heinz bodies in phenothiazine toxicosis in the horse. Wright-Leishman stain.

HEMOLYTIC ANEMIAS ASSOCIATED WITH HEINZ BODY FORMATION

Heinz (1890) described the occurrence of inclusions within the erythrocytes of humans and animals, following exposure to certain coal-tar drugs, that resulted in hemolytic destruction of the involved cells. The inclusions, now referred to as Heinz bodies, were described as round, oval, or serrated, highly refractile granules commonly located near the margin of the cell or protruding from the cell. Size varied greatly, probably depending on the intensity of the causative factor.

During the early stages of formation of the Heinz body, several small, granular bodies are seen within the cell that subsequently coalesce to form a single larger body. Heinz bodies in all stages of development are best demonstrated with vital stains such as crystal violet, brilliant cresyl blue, or new methylene blue (NMB) applied to an unfixed blood film (Jain, 1973a; Figs. 2–25(5), and 24–1, 24–3). Heinz bodies are seen as bluish-green structures with the routinely employed stain for making reticulocyte counts (Plate XVIII–8).

Heinz bodies do not stain after a blood film has been fixed in methanol in preparation for staining with Wright stain. In such a preparation, a large Heinz body may occasionally appear as a whitish spot within the erythrocyte or near the cell margin. Detection requires careful examination of the stained blood film under an immersion oil lens. When the Heinz body projects from the surface of the cell, it is readily detected (Fig. 24–2). Small Heinz bodies escape detection, and areas of crenation or short spicules on the erythrocyte surface may be mistaken for Heinz bodies. Hence any suspicion of the presence of Heinz bodies in Wright-stained blood films should be confirmed by examination of an unfixed film stained with NMB.

The nature of the Heinz body has been debated for years, and there is a large body of literature on this subject (Beaven and White, 1954; Good, 1950; Harley and Mauer, 1961; Jacob, 1970; Jandl et al., 1960; Webster, 1949). It is generally agreed that Heinz bodies are formed by precipitation of oxidatively denatured hemoglobin. Hemoglobin is normally constantly oxidized at a slow rate by the oxygen it carries and by superoxide radical and hydrogen peroxide generated within the erythrocyte. This process of oxidation is reversed by a reducing system comprised of metabolically generated NADPH and glutathione present within the red cell. Administration of an oxidant such as methylene blue and acetaminophen to cats and phenothiazine to horses and sheep, or ingestion of materials containing an oxidant, e.g., onions and red maple leaves, can overwhelm the natural protective machinery of the red cells and result in Heinz body formation and hemolytic anemia.

Heinz body formation in humans also results from a deficiency of glutathione or enzymatic defects of glutathione metabolism and the pentose phosphate pathway. A deficiency of glucose-6-phosphate dehydrogenase (G6PD) has been associated with susceptibility to Heinz body formation (Carson et al., 1956). Heinz bodies in the newborn have been attributed to inactivity of erythrocyte enzymes important in protecting hemoglobin from oxidative denaturation (Brown, 1966). Furthermore, a congenital Heinz-body anemia has been attributed to the presence of an unstable hemoglobin fraction within the erythrocyte (Grimes and Meisler, 1962). The anemia is typically hemolytic and is followed by a compensatory increase in erythropoiesis and typical changes in blood and bone marrow cytology.

Heinz Bodies and the Spleen

The presence of Heinz bodies within the erythrocyte reduces deformability of the cell, thereby impeding passage of erythrocytes through the microcirculation of the spleen. Sequestration within the spleen leads to erythrophagocytosis or hemolysis of the more severely damaged erythrocytes within the splenic pulp (Rifkind, 1965; Jensen and Lessin, 1970).

Heinz bodies appeared in about 15% of erythrocytes of two horses following splenectomy. Heinz bodies were consistently found over a period of 5 years, after which the horses were sacrificed. The Heinz bodies were not of sufficient size to be detected in routinely stained blood films, but they were readily seen in dry, unfixed films stained with

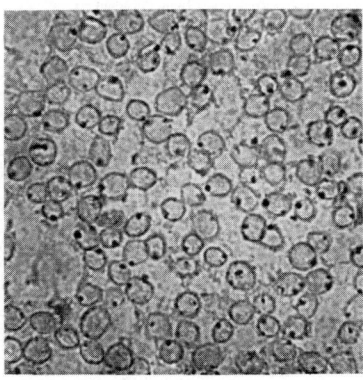

Fig. 24–3. Heinz bodies occurring under natural conditions of disease in a sheep. New methylene blue on dry, unfixed blood film.

NMB. Their occurrence in the circulation following splenectomy of these horses indicates that formation of small Heinz bodies probably takes place normally, as part of the aging process of the erythrocyte and that they are removed by the spleen, possibly through its pitting function (see Chapter 13).

Small Heinz bodies were found in 17 of 31 human patients who had undergone splenectomy (Selwyn, 1955). Heinz bodies increased in number in splenectomized patients taking the drug phenacetin, while intact persons taking the drug did not develop Heinz bodies. It was concluded that absence of the spleen or of splenic function was essential for the appearance of Heinz bodies when phenacetin was taken in normal doses. We have observed that the erythrocytes of dogs receiving daily doses of prednisolone may exhibit numerous small Heinz bodies. Suppression of splenic function by corticosteroid therapy may permit the formation of these small Heinz bodies. Their presence did not appear to lead to any dysfunction of the involved erythrocytes.

Heinz Bodies in Phenothiazine Toxicosis

Heinz body formation associated with hemolytic anemia has been observed in some horses receiving phenothiazine (McSherry et al., 1966; Schalm, 1962). Appendix Case 56 details a clinical instance of hemolytic anemia in a horse following administration of phenothiazine by the horse's owner (Fig. 24–2). The blood morphology of this clinical case was duplicated experimentally in another horse by administration of large doses of phenothiazine (Fig. 24–1). We have observed Heinz bodies occasionally in sheep (Fig. 24–3) in association with idiopathic hemolytic anemia. In one instance, Heinz bodies were observed by chance in blood of a sheep approximately one month after the flock had been treated with phenothiazine.

Heinz Bodies Associated with Consumption of Kale or Onions

Heinz bodies accompanied by hemolytic anemia and hemoglobinuria have been observed in cows fed kale. Hematologic findings were marked reduction in circulating erythrocytes after formation of Heinz bodies, followed by a marked reticulocytosis and recovery after kale was removed from the ration. Sheep and goats fed kale develop Heinz body–induced hemolytic anemia, but they are less affected than cattle. Excessive consumption of onions produces Heinz body–induced hemolytic anemia in cattle, sheep, horses, and dogs. See Hemolytic Anemias Associated with Some Poisonous Plants, below, for additional comments on kale toxicity and on onions as a cause of Heinz body–induced anemia.

Heinz Bodies in Cattle

Heinz body formation was induced in calves by a daily dose of 8 mg of phenylhydrazine/kg body weight for 6 weeks (Lynch et al., 1978). Heinz bodies were seen within the first week, and anemia followed by reticulocytosis was seen by the third week. Heinz body anemia was reported to occur in cattle grazing rye (*Secale cereale*) pastures (Simpson and Anderson, 1980).

A severe hemoglobinuria was found to develop 2–4 weeks postpartum in more than 40% of cows in some herds in New Zealand (Martinovich and Woodhouse, 1971). Heinz bodies were demonstrated in 3–50% of erythrocytes in clinically ill cattle, but they were also seen in up to 40% of erythrocytes in 20 clinically normal cows in the same herd. In addition to Heinz bodies, erythrocyte morphology in anemic cows was characterized by anisocytosis, microcytosis, polychromasia, and basophilic stippling. It was postulated

that Heinz bodies may have resulted from the production of hydroxylamine in the rumen.

Heinz Bodies in Cats

The routine application of NMB stain to dry, unfixed blood films led to the observation that nearly all normal domestic cats, as well as other members of the family Felidae, have a small but variable number of erythrocytes that contain a single small to medium-sized refractile body at the margin of the cell. Similar structures of much greater sizes were observed in some domestic cats admitted to the clinic with a variety of diseases (Fig. 2–25(3), Plate XVI). Because these structures occurred in cats without a history of treatment with oxidant drugs, they were initially referred to as erythrocyte refractile (ER) bodies (Schalm and Smith, 1963). In some instances, when the ER bodies were so large as to project from the margin of the erythrocyte, there was evidence of a hemolytic anemia in remission (Plate XVI–1).

Schmauch in 1899 described the natural occurrence of "endoglobulare Korperchen" in the erythrocytes of the domestic cat. The structures were found to vary in size, shape, and position in the cell. More commonly, however, the larger inclusions were irregular in shape and were located at the margin of the erythrocyte. The inclusions stained readily with 1% methyl violet in 0.85% saline solution, both in wet blood preparations and in dry, unfixed films. The number of involved erythrocytes varied among cats, and only 3 of 18 cats examined were free of the inclusion bodies. Beritic (1965) observed "Schmauch bodies" in 0.3–96.1% of the erythrocytes of 93 of 94 randomly chosen, clinically normal domestic cats. There was no relationship with age of cats, nor with disease or hemolytic anemia, even in cats in which the majority of erythrocytes contained the inclusions. Beritic concluded that the erythrocyte inclusions found physiologically in cats were similar morphologically and in staining characteristics to the Heinz bodies formed by toxic compounds in humans and animals.

Collins et al. (1968) investigated the ultrastructure of naturally occurring Heinz bodies in cats. The bodies were described as large, randomly distributed, irregular or round,

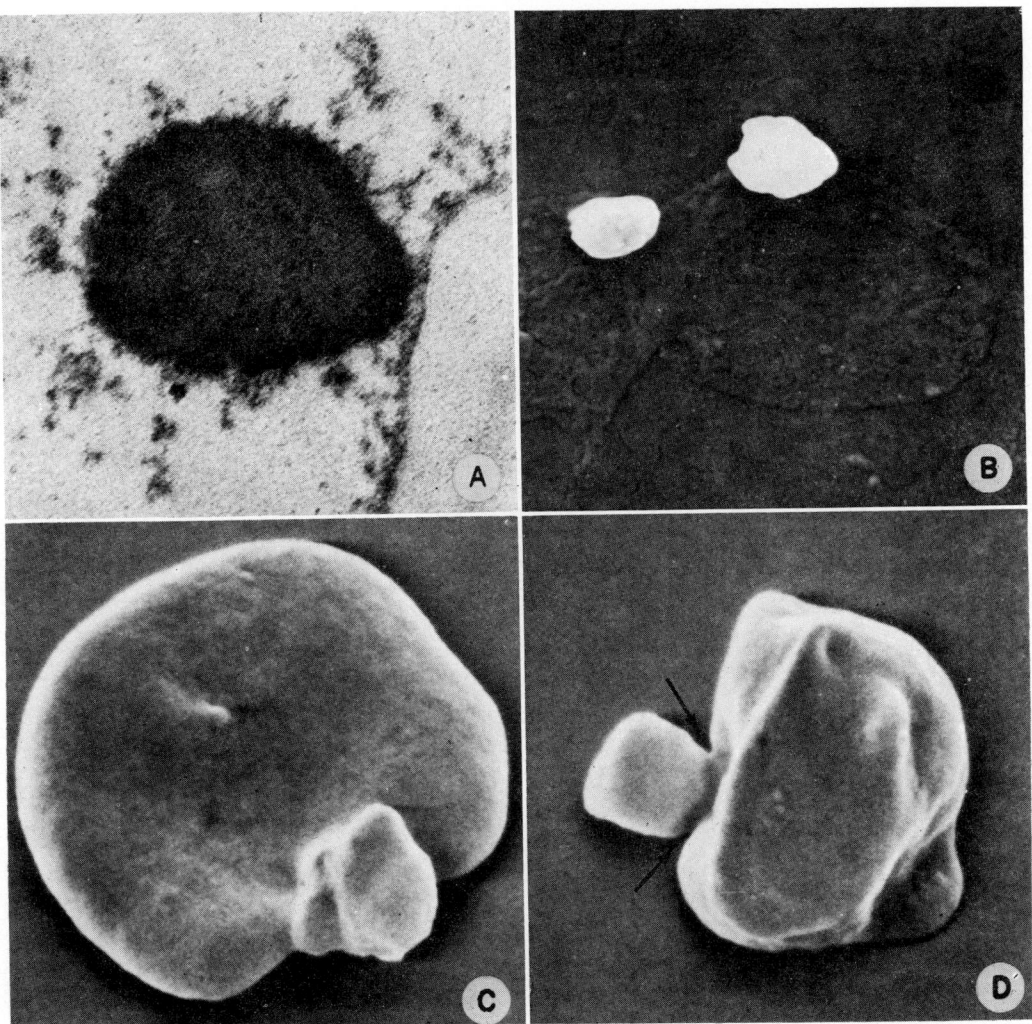

Fig. 24–4. Transmission (*A*) and scanning (*B–D*) electron micrographs of Heinz bodies in feline erythrocytes. *A,* An ultrathin section of a large Heinz body within a portion of an erythrocyte ghost. The Heinz body is composed of highly electron-dense mass; to the periphery are attached strands of reticular material of an electron density similar to that seen elsewhere within the plasma membrane of the empty ghost. ×42,000. (From Jain, 1973a; courtesy of *Bull Amer. Soc. Vet. Clin. Path.*) *B,* Erythrocyte ghosts containing Heinz bodies. ×6,800. *C,* An intact erythrocyte with marginal Heinz body. ×11,700. *D,* Side view of an erythrocyte showing a protruding Heinz body. Notice the constriction of cell membrane at the base of the Heinz body *(arrows).* ×11,700. (Courtesy of N.C. Jain and K.S. Keeton.)

finely granular masses of electron-dense material lacking a definite limiting membrane (Fig. 24–4*A*) and resembling mature Heinz bodies described by Rifkind and Danon (1965). Thus the ER or Schmauch bodies are nothing but Heinz bodies. These naturally occurring Heinz bodies in cats, when viewed with the scanning electron microscope after partial lysis of a blood film, appear as three-dimensional dense structures commonly located at the margin of the erythrocyte ghost (Jain and Keeton, 1975; Fig. 24–4*B*). Extrusion of Heinz bodies from intact erythrocytes is shown in Figs. 24–4*C* and *D*.

Jain (1973b) studied the role of the spleen in removal of Heinz bodies in the cat and concluded that the spleen plays a minor role in this species, unlike in the dog and the horse. This conclusion was based on the following findings: *(a)* splenectomy in a cat having a high but declining Heinz body count did not prevent further reduction in numbers of Heinz bodies (Fig. 24–5*A*); *(b)* splenectomy was not associated with a significant elevation

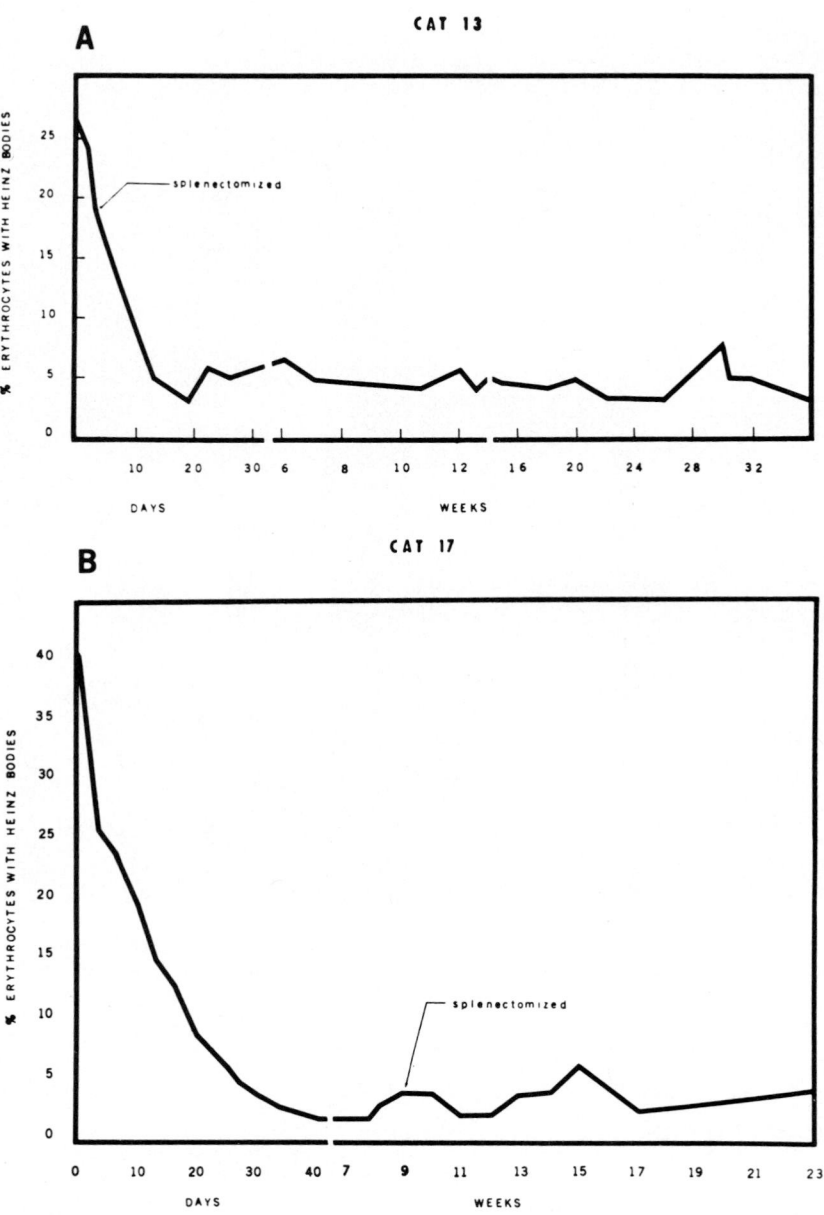

Fig. 24–5.   *A,* Cat 13 had 26% erythrocytes with Heinz bodies at first sampling; this declined to 18% in three days. It was splenectomized on the third day to determine if further spontaneous reduction of Heinz bodies would be delayed in the absence of the spleen. Regardless, Heinz body counts fell by half by the fourth day and were less than 5% by the tenth day, after which they remained at a 1–8% level over a period of 34 weeks. *B,* Naturally occurring Heinz bodies in this cat were seen in 40% of the erythrocytes at the first sampling. This level declined spontaneously to less than 5% in 30 days and ranged between 3% and 6% by the ninth week, when splenectomy was performed. Postsplenectomy counts in this cat did not increase beyond 9%.

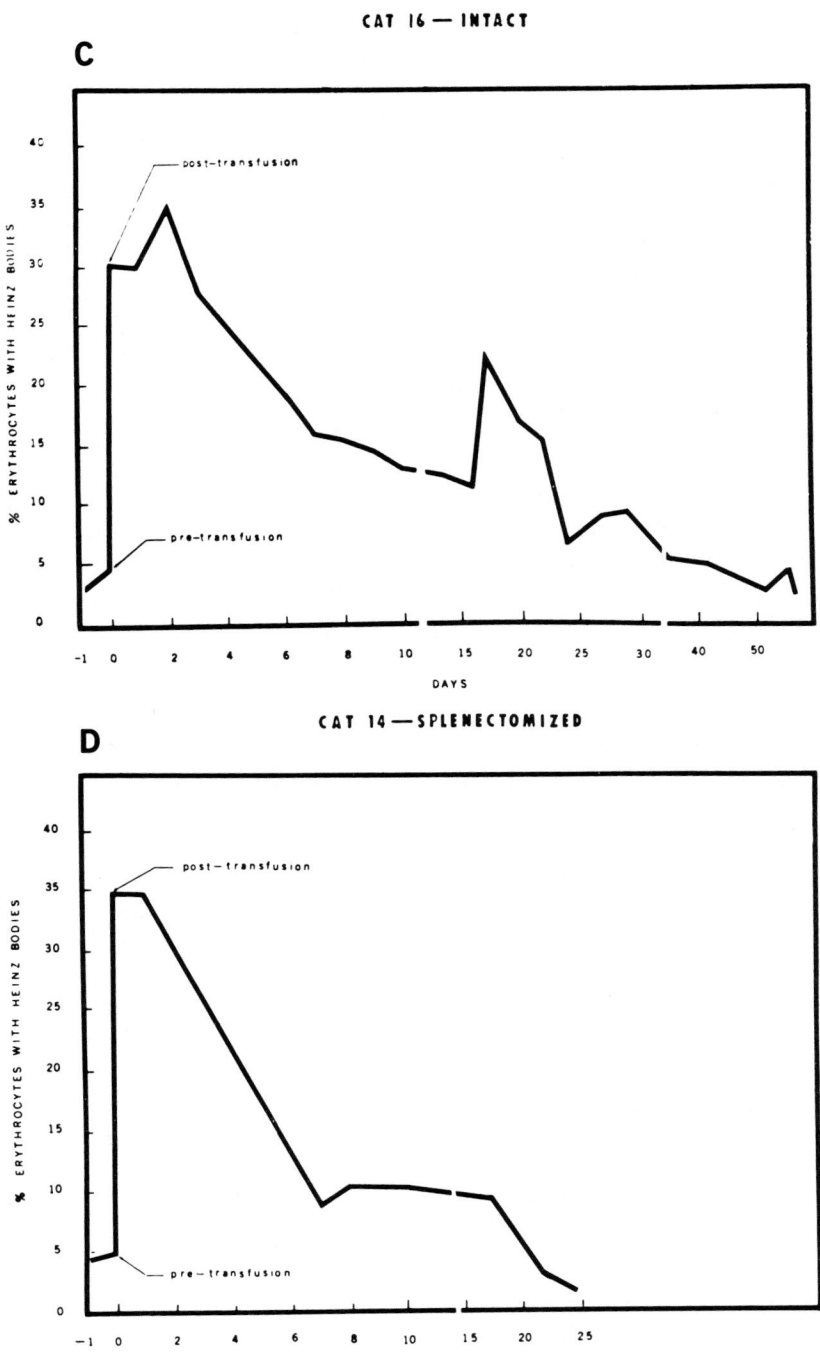

Fig. 24–5. *C*, Cat 16, an intact cat with a Heinz-body count of 5%, was transfused 100 ml of whole blood with 97% Heinz-body-containing erythrocytes. The donor cat was cross-matched and then given aniline to induce Heinz-body formation and bled 8 days later. Heinz body counts in Cat 16 increased to 30% after transfusion and decreased by half by the eighth day. On the sixteenth day, this cat had a Heinz-body count of 14%, but on the seventeenth day the count increased to 22.5% without any apparent changes in other hematologic parameters and clinical signs. On the next day, the count decreased to 17% and then gradually declined to less than 5% by the thirty-third day. *D*, Cat 14, a splenectomized cat with a Heinz-body count of 5%, was transfused 100 ml of whole blood (like Cat 16) with 84% Heinz-body-containing erythrocytes. Its Heinz-body count increased to 35% after transfusion, diminished by half by the fourth day, and was less than 5% by the twenty-first day after transfusion. (Drawn from results published by Jain, 1973b.)

in number of Heinz bodies over a period of several weeks (Fig. 24–5B); (c) transfused Heinz body–containing erythrocytes were removed from the blood of an intact or splenectomized cat at similar rates (Fig. 24–5C, D). Furthermore, it was interesting that in the splenectomized cat, transfused Heinz bodies were removed at the same rate recorded for her own erythrocytes containing Heinz bodies when the cat was intact.

The natural occurrence of Heinz bodies in the domestic cat is a unique phenomenon that remains to be explained. Indications are that the hemoglobin of the family Felidae is highly susceptible to oxidation because of its eight sulfhydryl (SH) reactive groups compared to two in most other species (Taketa et al., 1967). This makes the feline hemoglobin remarkably unstable and subject to denaturation by oxidation under a variety of circumstances not deleterious to other species' erythrocytes. Heinz body formation is also accelerated by the marked tendency of cats to form methemoglobin because of their low rate of methemoglobin reductase activity compared to that in other species (Stolk and Smith, 1966).

We have noted large Heinz bodies in cats in association with severe intestinal disturbances. It is interesting to note that Selwyn (1955) described a splenectomized human patient who exhibited a marked increase in Heinz bodies on two separate occasions in association with severe intestinal disturbances. Selwyn postulated that "it seems likely that these peaks were due to an autotoxic factor derived from the intestine."

A severe hemolytic anemia has been described in some cats receiving oral adminis-

tration of urinary antiseptics containing methylene blue (Schecter et al., 1973). Small Heinz bodies began to appear in erythrocytes within 24 hours and rapidly increased in number and size to involve up to 100% of the erythrocytes. By 7–10 days, the Heinz bodies were large enough to be seen projecting from the margin of the erythrocyte in routinely stained blood films. In blood from such cats, hemoglobin values determined with the spectrophotometer are spuriously elevated because the Heinz bodies remain suspended in the solution of hemolyzed erythrocytes, thereby decreasing light transmission. The MCHC values may exceed 40% because of erroneously high hemoglobin estimation. Proper hemoglobin values can be obtained by centrifugation of the hemolysate to remove the Heinz bodies before light transmission is measured. An occasional cat was found to be resistant to the action of methylene blue contained in the medication given. Cats developing a hemolytic anemia from treatment with drugs containing methylene blue will recover upon removal of the drug, although Heinz bodies may continue to be seen in gradually decreasing numbers over a period of several weeks.

That experimental administration of methylene blue in cats leads to hemolytic anemia from Heinz body formation is demonstrated by the following: Two cats were given by mouth 7 doses of 5.4 mg each of methylene blue (in gelatin capsules) at 8-hour intervals. The result was severe; each cat rapidly developed hemolytic anemia. Within 24 hours, Heinz bodies increased in size and number from small bodies involving fewer than 2% of red cells (Fig. 24–6A) to medium-sized struc-

Fig. 24–6. Erythrocyte morphology during development of Heinz-body hemolytic anemia in the cat resulting from oral administration of methylene blue. ×2,700. A, New methylene blue stain applied to unfixed blood film of a cat before administration of methylene blue. An eosinophil leukocyte is shown. Small Heinz bodies are present in less than 2% of the erythrocytes. B, Medium-sized Heinz bodies in nearly 100% of the erythrocytes 24 hours after the first oral dose of methylene blue. The Heinz body appears black when in focus and refractile when out of focus. New methlyene blue stain. C, Large Heinz bodies at 96 hours after the first dose of methylene blue. A neutrophil leukocyte is seen in the center. New methlyene blue stain. D, Same blood as in C stained by Wright-Leishman method. Note projection of large Heinz bodies from cell margins. Also, note a lysed erythrocyte in center field containing a Heinz body. E, Many reticulocytes (stippled cells) and few erythrocytes containing large Heinz bodies at the eighth day after initial administration of methylene blue. Two neutrophil leukocytes are also seen. New methylene blue stain. F, Blood taken on thirteenth day and stained by Wright-Leishman method. The anemia is in remission. A nucleated erythrocyte, an erythrocyte with a Howell-Jolly body, several macrocytes, and a few residual erythrocytes with large Heinz bodies are seen.

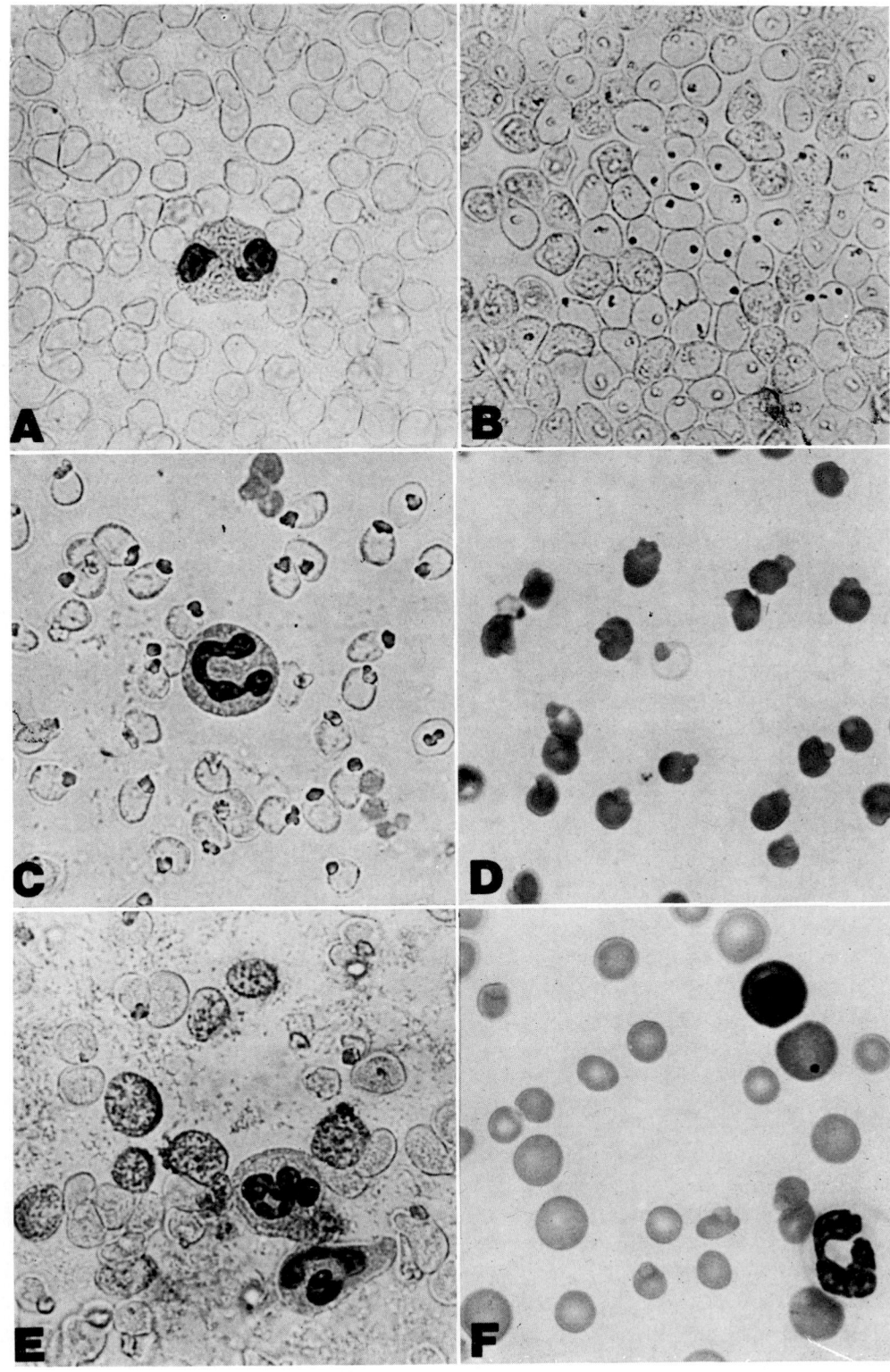

Fig. 24–6.

tures in 92–100% of the erythrocytes (Fig. 24–6B). By the forty-eighth hour after the initial dose all erythrocytes were involved, and by the ninety-sixth hour the Heinz bodies were very large (Fig. 24–6C) and readily observable as structures projecting from the red cell margin in the routinely stained blood films (Fig. 24–6D). In addition, some erythrocytes were lysed and appeared as ghost forms containing a Heinz body. The PCV dropped from around 43% to 13% within 6 days. The color of the plasma suggested the presence of both free hemoglobin and bilirubin. By the seventh day after the initial dose of methylene blue, the percentage of erythrocytes containing Heinz bodies started to decline as a result of their removal and replacement by newly formed erythrocytes (Fig. 24–6E, F). By the eighteenth day, only small Heinz bodies were seen in less than 5% of erythrocytes.

Heinz body hemolytic anemia was seen in a dog with chylothorax that was given methylene blue to locate thoracic lymph vessels for surgical correction (Schalm, 1978). A severe hemolytic anemia identical to that seen in the two cats receiving methlyene blue was observed in a feline patient receiving acetaminophen (325 mg once a day) for 6 days. In addition, 33% of the hemoglobin was methemoglobin. Others have observed Heinz body formation in cats given acetaminophen (Finco et al., 1975) and phenazopyridine (Harvey and Kornick, 1976). Heinz body formation with oxidant drugs has been observed in other species as mentioned above.

It is intriguing that natural Heinz body formation in cats is not associated with anemia, but anemia follows Heinz body formation from an oxidant drug. It is the author's opinion that anemia associated with administration of an oxidant drug such as methylene blue may not be due solely to formation of Heinz bodies. It may also involve oxidative damage to the erythrocyte membrane, with or without binding of intracellular Heinz bodies to the altered membranous sites. The change in red cell surface membrane may provide the key signal to the mononuclear phagocyte system for partial or complete erythrophagocytosis. It is possible that normal cats with naturally occurring Heinz bodies do not develop anemia because Heinz body formation in these cats is not accompanied by a significant oxidative damage to the erythrocyte membrane. Certainly research needs to be performed to delineate such a mechanism. Drug-induced membrane alterations have been associated with shortened intravascular survival of reticulocytes (Jain and Hochstein, 1980).

HEMOLYTIC ANEMIAS ASSOCIATED WITH SOME POISONOUS PLANTS

Excessive ingestion of a wide variety of plants or their products has been found on rare occasions to cause hemolytic anemia in animals. These include castor beans, oak shoots, frosted turnips, broom, ranunculus, convolvulus, colchicum, ash, privet, hornbeam, hazel, hellebore, wild onions, and plants of the Brassica family (e.g., rape and kale).

Castor Beans, Brassica Species, Onions, and Red Maple Leaves

Castor bean consumption in a 14-month-old, shorthorn heifer was found to cause marked respiratory distress, reddened mucous membranes and skin of teats, hemoglobinemia, severe anemia, and hemoglobinuria (Coles, 1980). Ricins from the beans were incriminated as the cause of erythrocyte destruction.

Kale causes Heinz body anemia in cattle, sheep, and goats (Dunbar and Chambers, 1963; Greenhalgh et al., 1969; Penny et al., 1961). Lactating cows, particularly after calving, are most susceptible. Sheep develop a relatively mild anemia, but sheep with low levels of glutathione (GSH) are more susceptible than those with high levels. There are two types of GSH deficiency in sheep. Some breeds (Corriedale and merino) have decreased activity of GSH synthetase enzyme and normal red cell life span; in some other breeds (Finnish Landrace) GSH content is low for unknown reasons and red cell life span is shortened (Smith, 1976). Sheep with GSH deficiency are more prone to anemia from ingesting kale but not from oxidants like primaquine. Heinz bodies become evident after the sheep feed on kale for 1–3 weeks, and anemia manifests after an additional 1–2 weeks. Recovery occurs over a period of 3–4 weeks after feeding on kale is stopped (Smith, 1980). Affected animals show retarded growth, hemoglobinuria, icterus, and hemosiderin deposits in the liver, spleen, and kidneys. Kale feeding in goats induced a hemolytic anemia, but recovery followed even though kale feeding was continued (Greenhalgh et al., 1969).

Senescent erythrocytes are more vulnerable to the effects of kale. Kale contains S-methyl cysteine and its sulfoxide (SO), which give rise to methanethiol and dimethyl disulfide in the rumen. It is believed that the latter product, after absorption, interacts with reduced glutathione in the erythrocytes to induce Heinz body formation and resultant anemia. Disulfides were found to produce hemolytic anemia experimentally in goats (Smith, 1980) and dogs.

Onions, wild and domestic, contain n-propyl disulfide, which produces Heinz body anemia in cattle (Hutchinson, 1977; Koger, 1956), sheep (Van Kampen et al., 1970),

horses (Pierce et al., 1972; Thorp and Harshfield, 1939), and dogs (Gruhzit, 1931; Harvey and Rackear, 1985; Lees et al., 1979; Schalm, 1978; Williams et al., 1941). We observed hemolytic anemia and some deaths among steers being fed cannery offal consisting of onions and tomato pulp and vines. Among 20 head, 2 died; at necropsy the tissues were icteric, and there was a distinct odor of onions. Losses ceased after the steers were moved to a pasture and the feeding of the cannery offal was stopped.

Hemograms of four affected steers in various stages of hemolytic anemia due to Heinz body formation are presented in Table 24–1. Steer 1 exhibited many Heinz bodies (Plate XVIII–8) but had not yet developed massive hemolytic destruction of its erythrocytes. This situation is indicated by the PCV value of 25% and the normal MCV and MCHC values. Steer 2 also had many erythrocytes containing Heinz bodies, but hemolytic destruction was under way, as was beginning remission of anemia. The PCV of 18% reflected the devel-

Table 24–1.   Hemograms in Onion Poisoning (Heinz-Body Hemolytic Anemia) in Cattle

	Steer Number and Breed			
	1 Holstein	2 Angus	3 Angus	4 Angus
RBC ($\times 10^6/\mu$l)	6.39	2.76	1.39	1.42
Hb (g/dl)	8.9	5.3	3.3	3.5
PCV (%)	25.0	18.0	11.0	13.0
MCV (fl)	39.1	65.2	79.0	91.5
MCHC (%)	35.6	29.4	30.0	27.1
MCH (pg)	13.9	19.2	23.7	25.7
Icterus index units	15	15	20	15
Plasma proteins (g/dl)	6.6	7.1	7.3	6.7
Fibrinogen (g/dl)	0.6	0.6	0.6	0.5
Reticulocytes (%)	0	10.2	20.0	26.8
Nucleated RBC/100 WBC	0	5	37	18
WBC/μl	9,300	7,200	17,000	8,700
WBC corrected for nucleated RBC	0	6,900	12,500	7,400
Band neutrophils	93 (1.0%)	0	1,000 (8.0%)	74 (1.0%)
Segmenters	1,488 (16.0%)	3,864 (56.0%)	4,812 (38.5%)	2,146 (29.0%)
Lymphocytes	7,440 (80.0%)	2,484 (36.0%)	6,062 (48.5%)	5,032 (68.0%)
Monocytes	279 (3.0%)	207 (3.0%)	62 (0.5%)	148 (2.0%)
Eosinophils	0	345 (5.0%)	500 (4.0%)	0
Basophils	0	0	62 (0.5%)	0
Anisocytosis	slight	moderate	marked	marked
Polychromasia	—	moderate	marked	marked
Basophilic stippling	—	few	—	moderate
Heinz bodies	many	many	few	few

oping anemia, and beginning remission was indicated by a reticulocytosis of 10.2% and an MCV of 65.2 fl. Steers 3 and 4 were well advanced in hemolytic destruction of damaged erythrocytes; only a few erythrocytes containing Heinz bodies remained in their blood. Marked anemia, macrocytosis, and reticulocytosis characterized their hemograms. Despite the serious nature of the hemolytic anemia, only Steer 3 presented a neutrophilia with modest left shift, and Steer 2 experienced a mild lymphopenia.

Horses ingesting *red maple (Acer rubrum) leaves* developed acute hemolytic anemia from an oxidant present in the leaves (Divers et al., 1982; King et al., 1981; Tennant et al., 1981). Clinical observations included weakness, polypnea, tachycardia, depression, icterus, cyanosis, and brownish discoloration of the blood and urine. Hematologic findings included methemoglobinemia, free plasma hemoglobin, decreased PCV, and Heinz bodies in erythrocytes. Pathologic findings were typical of acute hemolytic anemia and included generalized icterus, splenomegaly with erythrocyte sequestration in sinusoids, and swollen, black kidneys with tubular nephrosis and hemoglobin casts. The disease was reproduced in a pony fed dried, ground red maple leaves.

Nitrate and Nitrite Poisoning

Nitrate poisoning is a serious problem in ruminants, particularly cattle. It may result from drinking of contaminated water, but a more common cause is consumption of feeds containing abnormally high amounts of nitrates. Sudan grass (*Sorghum vulgare* var *sudanensis)* is involved in both nitrate poisoning and cyanide toxicity, but the former is more likely to manifest. Nitrate toxicity may be acute, subacute, or chronic, with clinical signs appearing within hours to one week. Poorly nourished animals are less tolerant. Acute toxicity results when the nitrate content of water is about 1,500 ppm (0.15%) and that of forage is about 1% or more (dry weight). Clinical signs of acute toxicity, e.g., dyspnea, cyanosis, weak pulse, and muscular weakness, appear within one-half to four hours and are attributable to lack of oxygen. Excessive salivation, diarrhea, and abdominal pain may be

seen. In terminal stages convulsions are seen and death occurs in 12–24 hours. Chronic nitrate poisoning has variable effects which are usually nonspecific. Animals show poor growth, abortion and infertility may occur, and vitamin A deficiency and goiter may develop. Goiter develops from inhibition of iodine uptake by the thyroid gland. The mechanism of vitamin A deficiency remains unknown, but administration of vitamin A seems to help.

The mechanism of nitrate toxicity resides in conversion of nitrate to its reduced form, nitrite, by the microorganisms in the rumen. The former is innocuous, while the latter is highly toxic because of its oxidative action. The nitrite is partly absorbed from the rumen and oxidizes hemoglobin in blood to produce methemoglobinemia. Blood appears chocolate brown when about 30–40% of the total hemoglobin is in the form of methemoglobin; death occurs when its level reaches about 80–90%.

Diagnosis of nitrate poisoning involves consideration of clinical signs, characteristic color of blood, increased levels of methemoglobin, and determination of nitrate and nitrite levels in feed, water, intestinal contents, plasma, serum, and urine. Nitrate and nitrite remain stable in plasma or serum samples up to 48 hours and for a much shorter time in whole blood; chronic poisoning is suggested by a nitrate level of <25 μg/ml and by a nitrite level of <0.75 μg/ml (Kaneko, 1983). Treatment consists of administration of methylene blue to induce reduction of methemoglobin (ferric iron) to deoxyhemoglobin (ferrous iron). This paradoxical action of methylene blue depends on activation of the NADPH-dependent methemoglobin reductase system. Methylene blue is given at the rate of 1–4.4 mg/kg body weight intravenously in the form of a 2–4% solution; one or more treatments may be required. The dosage of methylene blue is crucial, for an excess may induce a life-threatening methemoglobinemia. For details see Ruhr and Osweiler, 1981.

HEMOLYTIC ANEMIAS ASSOCIATED WITH METABOLIC DISEASES

Postparturient Hemoglobinuria

Postparturient hemoglobinuria in cattle is characterized by hemoglobinuria following intravascular hemolysis. The disease usually occurs within 2–3 weeks after calving but may manifest as many as 42 days after parturition. The visible mucous membranes first become pale and later very icteric, and the RBC count may drop below 2 million/µl of blood. The bone marrow responds in typical fashion to acute blood destruction. The MCV is greatly increased during remission of the anemia, and basophilic stippling of erythrocytes is common between the fifth and ninth days. The disease has been reported from New Zealand as a herd problem with up to 40% incidence, usually affecting first and second lactation cows. In North America it has been reported as a sporadic occurrence in high-producing cows in third to sixth lactations (see review by MacWilliams et al., 1982).

The mechanism of red cell destruction is not known definitely, although several possibilities have been suggested. In North America, the inorganic phosphorus values of the blood plasma were found to be low, suggesting a relationship of the disease to phosphorus deficiency (Madsen and Nielsen, 1939; Parkinson and Sutherland, 1954; Penny, 1956). Phosphorus deficiency may predispose to deleterious effects of a plant hemolysin, e.g., saponins from sugar beets or alfalfa (Parkinson and Sutherland, 1954). Copper deficiency and Heinz body formation as a result of feeding on poisonous plants have been associated with this condition in New Zealand (Black, 1981; Caple, 1981; Gardner et al., 1976; MacWilliams et al., 1982; Smith, 1973). Researchers have suggested that copper deficiency would lead to a diminished level of superoxide dismutase, a copper metalloenzyme, in the red cells and compromise their ability to withstand oxidative damage.

Treatment in North America consists of administering sodium acid phosphate (60 g in 300 ml of water) by intravenous infusion, 100 g of bone meal as a drench twice a day, fluids to restore hydration, and blood transfusion if necessary. Preventive measures include removal of factors causing hypophosphatemia such as dietary imbalance and poisonous plants. Investigators from New Zealand also recommend giving copper glycerate in cases associated with a copper deficiency. (See also Heinz bodies in Cattle, above.)

Postparturient hemoglobinuria is also seen in Indian water buffaloes (Kurundkar et al., 1981; Nagpal et al., 1968; Samad et al., 1979). Affected animals typically show hemoglobinuria, bilirubinemia, decreased serum inorganic phosphate (<2 mg/dl versus normal of 5.75 mg/dl), and anemia. Mortality rate varies from 20–70%. Necropsy findings are typical of anemia and icterus. Affected animals in most instances respond favorably to treatment with sodium acid phosphate. A similar disease has also been reported in sheep (Stamp and Stewart, 1953) and a goat (Setty and Narayana, 1975).

Jacob and Amsden (1971) reported on a severe but reversible hemolytic anemia in a human patient with profound hypophosphatemia that was corrected by parenteral phosphate supplementation. Serum phosphate is very low (<0.2 mg/dl) in human patients with hemolytic anemia due to hypophosphatemia. Erythrocyte ATP and 2,3-DPG levels are reduced, and this reduction is associated with decreased red cell deformability and hemolytic anemia. Additional findings include a bleeding diathesis with abnormal clot retraction and thrombocytopenia with reduced platelet survival. Hemolytic anemia has been reproduced in hyperalimented dogs (Jacob and Amsden, 1974).

HEMOLYTIC ANEMIAS ASSOCIATED WITH INTRAERYTHROCYTIC DEFECTS

Methemoglobinemia

During transport and delivery of oxygen to body tissues hemoglobin molecules in the erythrocyte constantly undergo reversible oxidation reduction reactions. Oxygen binding to the hemoglobin molecule results in formation of oxyhemoglobin with iron in the ferric state (Fe^{3+}) and generation of a heme-bound superoxide anion (Wintrobe et al., 1981). After the oxygen is delivered to the tissues, the process is normally reversed, and native (deoxy-) hemoglobin is formed. During the process of oxygen binding to the hemoglobin molecule, a small amount of methemoglobin (MetHb) is produced. The iron in the MetHb is in a nonfunctional ferric state, while that in the native hemoglobin is in the functional ferrous form (Fe^{2+}). Methemoglobin is also produced by direct action of superoxide anion and hydrogen peroxide, both of which are also generated within the red cells. Methemoglobinemia results when formation of MetHb exceeds the capacity of the erythrocyte to reduce it back to the native state. Oxidative damage by superoxide anion and hydrogen peroxide to erythrocytes also includes oxidation of membrane sulfhydryl groups and denaturation of globin moiety, resulting in Heinz body formation. These abnormalities of red cells not only create a serious functional disturbance of oxygen transport, but can be accompanied by hemolytic anemia.

Oxidative denaturation of hemoglobin is prevented by methemoglobin reductase, superoxide dismutase (SOD), glutathione peroxidase, and catalase. MetHb in erythrocytes is reduced nonenzymatically by ascorbic acid and reduced GSH and, most important, enzymatically by either NADH (generated by glucose metabolism via the Embden-Meyerhof pathway) or NADPH (generated via the pentose phosphate pathway) as electron donors. The predominant mechanism for MetHb reduction under normal conditions is a reaction involving NADH and the enzyme NADH-methemoglobin reductase. The enzyme system utilizing NADPH as an electron donor is of minor importance under normal conditions, but becomes highly functional in the presence of methylene blue. Thus it forms the basis of methylene blue therapy during methemoglobinemia from various causes. Care must be exercised, however, in use of methylene blue; in certain situations it may potentiate the oxidative denaturation of hemoglobin and aggravate hemolysis, as happened in a human patient with aniline-induced methemoglobinemia and in experiments with cats (Harvey and Keitt, 1983).

Superoxide dismutase, a copper-zinc enzyme, catalyzes the dismutation of superoxide to oxygen and H_2O_2. Hydrogen peroxide is degraded through a reaction involving glutathione peroxidase, a selenium-containing enzyme, and reduced GSH. During this process oxidized GSH (GSSG) is formed. The supply of reduced glutathione is maintained either by de novo synthesis of GSH by the erythrocytes or by rapid reduction of GSSG to GSH by a reaction involving glutathione reductase and NADPH (Fig. 24–7). GSH is essential not only to detoxify H_2O_2, but also to prevent oxidation of hemoglobin and sulfhydryl groups in the red cell membrane and in turn for erythrocyte survival. Thus inadequacies of GSH are usually associated with Heinz body formation. Catalase is of minor significance in degradation of H_2O_2 in the red cell.

Several situations are known to cause methemoglobinemia in humans and animals. Certain oxidants, perhaps those with a mild to moderate oxidative action, produce only methemoglobinemia, whereas strong oxidants also react with globin chains to induce denaturation and precipitation of hemoglobin in the form of Heinz bodies. For example, acetaminophen in cats produces both methemoglobinemia and Heinz body formation, while nitrite poisoning in cows and pigs produces only methemoglobinemia. We have observed development of significant methemoglobinemia in an occasional cat anesthetized with ketamine hydrochloride at the Veterinary Medical Teaching Hospital, University of California, Davis. Cats develop Heinz bodies without methemoglobinemia under natural conditions and after methylene blue administration. The latter may cause a serious hemolytic anemia in cats (see Heinz Bodies in Cats, above). Horses feeding on red maple (*Acer rubrum*) leaves developed acute hemolytic anemia from methemoglobinemia and Heinz body formation (Divers et al., 1982; Tennant et al., 1981). Methemoglobinemia and hemolytic anemia associated with diminished levels of red cell glutathione and decreased glutathione reductase were seen in a mare and her dam (Dixon et al., 1977). NADH-methemoglobin reductase deficiency has been observed in a dog and appears to be congenital in origin (Kaneko, 1983).

Animals with methemoglobinemia exhibit weakness, lethargy, anorexia, dyspnea, tachycardia, and, most important, dark, muddy brown mucous membranes and chocolate brown blood.

Quantitation of hemoglobin concentration by the cyanmethemoglobin method measures all forms of hemoglobin in blood, whereas the

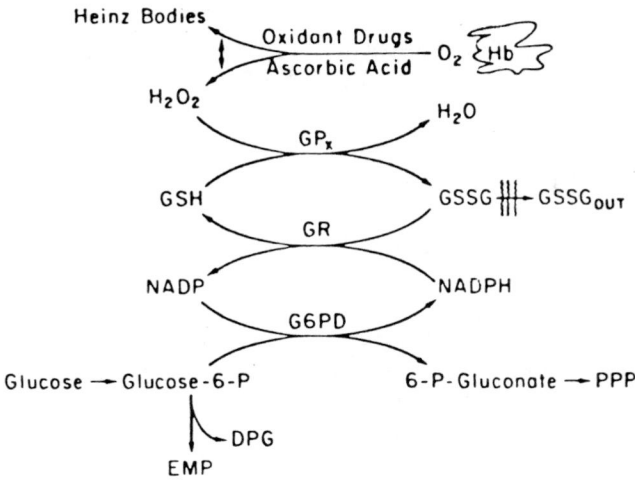

Fig. 24–7. Glutathione metabolism in the RBC. (From Kaneko, 1980; courtesy of Academic Press.)

oxyhemoglobin method measures oxyhemoglobin and not other forms including MetHb. Therefore hemoglobin values obtained by the two methods are incongruous for bloods containing excessive amounts of MetHb. In fact, using both methods provides a means of quantification of MetHb; the difference between the two values provides a good estimate of the MetHb present in that blood sample. Normal values of MetHb are 0–1.1% of normal hemoglobin concentration for dogs and 0–1.0% for cows (Kaneko, 1983).

Pyruvate Kinase Deficiency in the Dog

The occurrence of a familial hemolytic anemia within the basenji breed of dogs was reported simultaneously by Tasker et al. (1969) in New York and Ewing (1969a) in California. The defect was attributed to a deficiency of the erythrocytic enzyme pyruvate kinase (PK) (Searcy et al., 1971, 1979). Phosphoenol pyruvate, the substrate for PK, is significantly increased in erythrocytes of affected animals, and enzymes of the glycolytic cycle are also elevated. Additional reports of PK deficiency in the basenjis have been published (Andresen, 1977; Hogg et al., 1978). Pyruvate kinase deficiency has also been found in the beagle (Harvey et al., 1977; Prasse et al., 1975).

The mode of inheritance in the basenji is autosomal recessive, and age at detection of the anemia is often less than 6 months and usually less than 3 years. The PK deficiency leads to impaired erythrocyte energy metabolism (decreased glucose utilization and ATP formation) and a consequential premature red cell destruction. Half-life of ^{51}Cr-labeled red cells was found to be markedly reduced to 2.5 and 3 days in two affected basenji dogs compared to 20 days in normal dogs (Searcy et al., 1971). The erythrocyte osmotic fragility was found to be normal. The autohemolysis test is positive in that erythrocytes incubated with ATP do not hemolyze whereas those incubated with glucose hemolyze as a result of defective ATP generation. The erythrocyte osmotic fragility may be lower than normal in bloods with marked reticulocytosis (Fig. 20–14).

Ewing (1969a) reported that affected basenji dogs were normal in their general appearance, size, body weight, and growth pattern. They were less tolerant of exercise than normal littermates. Pale mucous membranes and splenomegaly were the usual findings on physical examination. The degree of anemia as reflected by mean values plus one standard deviation for the 22 basenji dogs in his study was as follows: RBC, 2.59 ± 1.8 million/μl; hemoglobin concentration, 6.07 ± 0.78 g/dl; and PCV, 22.5 ± 2.9%. The intensity of erythrogenesis, in response to the shortened erythrocyte life span, was mirrored in the following values: reticulocytes, 40.2 ± 11.0%; MCV, 85.9 ± 4.3 fl; MCHC, 27.2 ± 1.6%; and MCH, 23.4 ± 2.0 pg. Tasker et al. (1969) reported the M:E ratio of two affected basenji dogs to be 0.73:1 and 0.82:1, while Ewing (1969a) reported M:E ratios of 0.21–0.39:1.0. The latter values appear to be more representative of the intense erythrogenesis required to maintain a circulating reticulocyte population at the high levels characteristic of the disease. Myelofibrosis and osteosclerosis are common sequels (Searcy et al., 1979).

In an extension of the California study, 22 anemic basenji dogs (13 males and 9 females), 7 weeks to 30 months of age, some of which were littermates, were observed for varying lengths of time. Multiple hemograms were developed on individual dogs; data from five representative anemic basenji dogs are presented in Table 24–2. The anemia is characterized by macrocytic-hypochromic erythrocytes resulting from marked reticulocytosis. The degree of reticulocytosis varied among the dogs. Spherocytes were absent, and various tests for autoantibody to erythrocytes were negative.

Congenital Erythropoietic Porphyria

Several forms of porphyrias are known to occur in humans; these include hereditary or acquired erythropoietic and hepatic porphyrias. Congenital erythropoietic porphyria (porphyria erythropoietica or congenital porphyria), commonly called pink tooth, is an infrequently encountered inborn error of metabolism in cattle. Fourie (1936), in South Africa, made the first observations on the disease in grade shorthorn cattle. From results of breeding trials, he concluded that the disease had an autosomal recessive mode of inheritance. Rimington (1936) reported on the biochemistry of the defect and postulated that it was due to a failure or inhibition of a selectively catalyzed enzymatic reaction that normally results in the elaboration of adequate quantities of series III porphyrins, the precursors of heme (see Chapter 19 for a description of different types of porphyrins). Owing to failure to form adequate amounts of protoporphyrin III for hemoglobin synthesis, abnormal quantities of the useless uroporphyrin and coproporphyrin accumulate in the bones, teeth, tissues, and organs and produce the clinical syndrome.

Watson et al. (1959) found bovine and human porphyria congenita to be fundamentally similar and characterized by excessive formation of type I uroporphyrin and coproporphyrin in some of the developing rubricytes in the bone marrow. Bovine congenital erythropoietic porphyria has been identified as a hereditary deficiency of the enzyme uroporphyrinogen (UROgen) III cosynthetase (Levin, 1968; Romeo and Levin, 1969). Carrier animals show intermediate levels of the URO-

Table 24–2. Congenital Hemolytic Anemia (Pyruvate Kinase Deficiency) in the Basenji Dog (mean values and 1 SD)

	Dog Number				
	1	*2*	*3*	*4*	*5*
Number of Hemograms	17	14	14	13	8
Sex	F	M	M	M	F
Age range (mo)	18–24	5–30	5–11	5–26	10–18
RBC ($\times 10^6/\mu$l)	2.0±0.2	3.1±0.5	2.6±0.4	2.3±0.3	2.9±0.4
Hb (g/dl)	5.2±0.5	6.9±1.1	6.2±0.8	5.3±0.7	7.0±0.7
PCV (%)	18.5±1.9	24.7±3.7	22.4±2.7	19.6±2.6	24.5±3.5
MCV (fl)	92.5±6.5	80.2±5.4	86.0±5.8	85.1±6.5	85.0±2.9
MCH (pg)	26.1±1.6	22.1±1.5	23.8±1.7	23.2±1.4	24.3±1.4
MCHC (%)	27.4±2.9	27.7±1.8	27.7±1.8	27.5±2.3	28.6±1.3
Reticulocytes (%)	27.6±6.0	30.9±9.8	45.7±8.4	41.1±10.2	36.1±9.0
Icterus index units	2.7±1.3	4.6±2.2	5.3±1.7	2.5±1.1	2.8±1.3
Protein (g/dl)	6.7±0.4	6.6±0.3	6.7±0.2	6.7±0.4	6.7±0.4
Fibrinogen (g/dl)	0.17±0.07	0.245±0.13	0.211±0.08	0.2±0.08	0.188±0.08
WBC ($\times 10^3/\mu$l)	17.3±1.3	17.3±2.8	21.8±3.9	25.6±6.4	19.3±2.8
WBC (%)					
Bands	0.9±0.8	0.5±0.5	1.0±0.9	1.0±0.9	1.3±1.1
Segmenters	46.5±5.3	59.8±5.2	61.0±6.8	61.8±8.4	61.5±3.1
Lymphocytes	40.7±6.5	24.7±6.4	23.6±6.8	23.7±8.9	24.9±5.1
Monocytes	10.3±3.7	11.5±2.9	13.0±5.0	12.5±3.8	8.9±2.4
Eosinophils	1.5±1.2	3.4±1.8	1.2±1.1	0.8±1.1	3.3±2.5
Basophils	0.0	0.0	0.0	0.0	0.0

gen III cosynthetase. The disease occurs mainly in Holstein cattle, but some other breeds may also be involved. Congenital porphyria in cattle has been reported from Arkansas (Railsback, 1939), California (Rhode and Cornelius, 1958), Michigan (Madden et al., 1958), and Minnesota (Watson et al., 1959).

Calves with congenital porphyria (Appendix Case 72) fail to grow at a normal rate, and the white parts of their bodies are subjected to photosensitization when exposed to sunlight. The animals become weak, acquire poor condition, and develop photophobia and dermatitis. The urine is pigmented with the brownish red uroporphyrin. The teeth are reddish-brown; that is why the disease is called pink tooth. The teeth and bones produce a pink fluorescence when exposed to ultraviolet light. Bones become weak, and spontaneous fractures may occur. Definitive diagnosis entails demonstration of excessive porphyrins in various tissues and body fluids, e.g., bone marrow, urine, erythrocytes, and plasma. Various clinical and pathological findings are attributed to accumulation of porphyrins in different tissues and associated photodynamic effects. If protected from sunlight, cattle may mature, reproduce, and live for years (Fourie, 1953).

Kaneko and associates (1963, 1971, 1980) have performed studies on blood and bone marrow of porphyric cattle to delineate pathogenesis of anemia in this disorder. The principal defect is inability to produce normal amounts of hemoglobin. Thus, depending on the degree of defect, the anemia varies in intensity among individuals. Marrow erythropoiesis is intensified, as expressed by the presence of macrocytic erythrocytes, basophilic stippling, nucleated erythrocytes, and polychromasia in peripheral blood. Iron turnover and red cell survival studies in animals with congenital porphyria revealed markedly shortened erythrocyte life spans compared with those of normal cattle (Kaneko, 1963; Kaneko et al., 1971). A statistically significant correlation was found between erythrocyte coproporphyrin and protoporphyrin concentrations and survival time of the erythrocytes. Furthermore, porphyrins induced hemolysis

and delayed maturation of reticulocytes and metarubricytes.

Calves homozygous for porphyria erythropoietica have exhibited, at birth, 200–300 nucleated erythrocytes/100 WBC in peripheral blood. In addition, anisocytosis, poikilocytosis, polychromasia, and basophilic stippling characterized the erythrocyte morphology. The nucleated erythrocytes and basophilic stippling tended to disappear by the end of the first week, while moderate anisocytosis and slight to moderate poikilocytosis were characteristic features of subsequent hemograms (Appendix Case 72).

Congenital porphyria with an autosomal dominant inheritance pattern has been reported in both pigs (Clare and Stephens, 1944; Jorgensen, 1959) and cats (Glenn et al., 1968; Tobias, 1964). Affected pigs do not show photosensitization, but discoloration and fluorescence of teeth may be observed. Porphyrinuria is observed in most severely affected pigs. The disorder in cats produces fluorescence of teeth and urine, but anemia is not seen.

IMMUNE-MEDIATED HEMOLYTIC ANEMIAS

Autoimmune Hemolytic Anemia

Autoimmune hemolytic anemia (AIHA) is a consequence of accelerated red cell destruction by an autoantibody directed against mature erythrocytes. It occurs in humans and has been encountered frequently in the dog and infrequently in the cat. Rare instances of AIHA have been reported in the horse (Farrelly et al., 1966; Reef, 1983; Sutton et al., 1978). AIHA has been reported in a 6-month-old heifer (Dixon et al., 1978). A hereditary AIHA is known to occur in the NZB strain of mice. A brief description is given below, and additional details are presented in Chapter 35.

Miller et al. (1957) were the first to call attention to the natural occurrence of AIHA in the dog. Lewis et al. (1963) described in detail a clinical syndrome of AIHA in 19 dogs. The disorder was associated with thrombocytopenia in approximately half of the dogs. AIHA with thrombocytopenia can lead to double complications because erythrocytes are lost by diapedesis through the capillary endothelium, as well as being destroyed by the mononuclear phagocyte system (MPS). In addition to hemolytic anemia and thrombocytopenia, some dogs may present an associated glomerulonephritis of autoimmune origin. The disease is then similar to systemic lupus erythematosus of humans (Lewis, 1965; Lewis et al., 1965).

Autoimmune hemolytic anemia may occur as a primary (idiopathic) disorder, or it may be seen in association with other diseases or conditions such as bacterial, viral, rickettsial, or protozoan infections, hepatopathy, and other autoimmune disorders. In the dog, most cases of AIHA are idiopathic and can occur at any age. The disorder is slightly more common in females, and there may be some familial predisposition. Clinical signs are related to the primary disease and/or to the amount and nature of autoantibody in circulation. Clinical findings may be reflective of anemia, hemolysis, thrombocytopenia, and cyanosis of extremities (acrocyanosis) when cold agglutinins are involved. The hemolytic anemia may have a peracute or acute onset, or more commonly it may be chronic with one or more relapses occurring over weeks or months.

Antibodies associated with AIHA are generally categorized as warm reactive (mostly at 37°C) and cold reactive (usually at <30–32°C) antibodies and are, respectively, principally of the IgG and IgM type. Most cases of AIHA are due to warm IgG, and a few involve cold IgM, the latter usually occurring in association with the former. Low levels of cold agglutinins may occur in some normal dogs and horses as in people and are inconsequential. The basis of autoantibody formation remains speculative. It is hypothesized that AIHA may result from a change in the antigenic structure of the self-erythrocytes, formation of cross-reactive antibodies, and/or a change in the immune status of the patient. A case of AIHA was reported in a horse with cold agglutinins associated with *Clostridium perfringens* cellulitis (Reef, 1983).

The antierythrocyte autoantibody commonly encountered in AIHA has been in the past and is still sometimes referred to as an "incomplete antibody" because agglutination does not occur in saline suspensions of sensitized erythrocytes. To demonstrate the presence of the antibody coating of the erythrocytes, a species-specific antiglobulin reagent is added to a saline-washed suspension of the patient's erythrocytes. Agglutination results if the erythrocytes are coated with the autoantibody. This serologic procedure is called the direct Coombs test (Coombs et al., 1945; see Chapter 2). It is now known that the antibody associated with AIHA is complete, but it does not promote agglutination by itself because negative charges on the cell surface repel the erythrocytes. A broad spectrum Coombs reagent consists of anti-IgG and anti-complement, the latter to detect complement-coated erythrocytes as well. In the indirect Coombs test, patient's serum is tested against homologous erythrocytes to detect free autoantibody.

Mechanisms of red cell destruction in AIHA are depicted in Fig. 35–1. The primary mechanism involves erythrophagocytosis by macrophages of the MPS, particularly in the spleen, as a result of coating of the erythrocytes by autoantibody (IgG) and/or fixation of complement component C3. Partial erythrophagocytosis is believed to result in formation of spherocytes which exhibit increased osmotic fragility (Figs. 20–10, 20–11, 20–13). In a stained blood film, spherocytes typically are small, densely stained cells readily distinguishable from the larger, immature erythrocytes released to blood in response to the anemia (Plate XVII–4). Spherocytes are difficult to detect in the blood of species other than the dog, but careful examination has revealed their presence also in some feline and equine patients with AIHA. On rare occasions, erythrophagocytosis may also be detected in peripheral blood. Vigorous complement fixation by IgG or IgM autoantibody may result in direct intravascular hemolysis and frank hemoglobinemia and hemoglobinuria. Cold autoantibody is deleterious only if in very high titer and upon cold exposure of the patient.

Hematologic findings in AIHA vary with the stage of the disease. Table 24–3 lists data from six dogs with AIHA according to the duration of their illness. At the beginning of AIHA, spherocytosis is a prominent feature

Table 24–3.   Representative Hemograms of Autoimmune Hemolytic Anemia in the Dog

	Dog Number					
	1	2	3	4	5	6
Sex	XF	XF	XF	M	F	M
Age (yr)	7	6	8	2	1	7
Days sick to date of admission	2	4	12	77	96	180
PCV (%)	18	20	18	25	23	31
MCV (fl)	70.9	98.5[a]	125.9	109.6[a]	117.0	72.6
MCHC (%)	32.8	35.5	22.2	29.2	25.7	32.9
Icterus index units	50	Free hemoglobin	7.5	2	2	7.5
Reticulocytes (%)	4.0	7.6	39.4	54.0[b]	36.0	20.8
Erythrocyte fragility at 0.85% saline	—	35.0%	—	92.5%	—	10%
Anisocytosis[c]	+	+ +	+ + + +	+ +	+ + + +	+ +
Polychromasia[c]	+	+ +	+ + + +	+ +	+ + + +	+ +
Spherocytosis[c]	+ + + +	+ + + +	+	+ + + +	+	+ + + +
Agglutination of erythrocytes	+ + + +	+ + + +	None	+ +	None	None
Nucleated RBC/100 WBC	0	25.5	707	28.5	34	84
Thrombocytes/μl	245,000	55,000	519,000	461,000	38,000	18,000
WBC/μl (corrected)	15,000	21,600	15,800	34,000	25,400	25,800
Coombs test[c]	+ + +	+ + + +	+ + +	+	+	+ + + +

[a]Not valid. Greater than actual RBC size due to erythrocyte hemolysis, leading to error in MCV.
[b]Not valid because lysis of spherocytes left reticulocytes out of proportion to their actual number.
[c]+ = occasional, + + = slight, + + + = moderate, + + + + = marked.

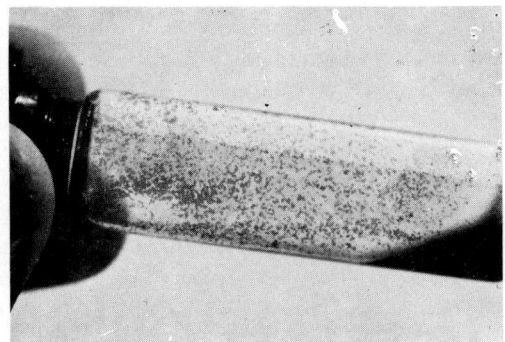

Fig. 24–8. Spontaneous agglutination of erythrocytes in drawn blood as seen in a dog with autoimmune hemolytic anemia.

and may be accompanied by spontaneous agglutination of the erythrocytes (Dog 1) due to formation of cold agglutinins (IgM). The agglutination may be so marked as to be visible grossly (Fig. 24–8).Physical examination of the patient may reveal icteric mucous membranes, and the icterus index may be 50 units or more (Dog 1). Hemoglobinemia and hemoglobinuria may be seen in some patients at this earliest stage of the disease because of the marked fragility of the spherocytes (Dog 2). As the first large mass of spherocytes is removed and replaced by polychromatic macrocytes, the icterus index rapidly decreases (Dog 3) and eventually attains normal values of 2 and 5 units during the less active phases of the disease (Dogs 4 and 5).

MCV and MCHC are ordinarily a measure of the intensity of release of immature erythrocytes to the blood in response to the anemia. In AIHA, however, the MCV may be spurious (Dogs 2 and 4) at times because of the fragile nature of spherocytes; agglutination of erythrocytes would have the same effect. A similar spurious result in the reticulocyte count was encountered at least once (Dog 4) when the more resistant reticulocytes remained to be counted while spherocytes were apparently hemolyzed by the staining solution. When large MCV values are valid, the MCHC is correspondingly reduced (Dogs 3 and 5), but when MCV is spurious, the MCHC either remains well within the normal range (Dog 2) or is only slightly reduced (Dog 4).

Total leukocyte counts are variable but tend to increase as the anemia enters a stage of remission. A neutrophilia with modest left shift is a common finding, as is a significant monocytosis. The mechanism of this regenerative left shift is unknown, but it may be due to concomitant release of a granulopoiesis-stimulating factor from the MPS engaged in active erythrophagocytosis.

Dogs 2, 5, and 6 had a variable thrombocytopenia. Dogs 5 and 6 had a history of periodic purpura and loss of blood, particularly into the gastrointestinal tract. These dogs could have had autoimmune thrombocytopenia.

Autoimmune hemolytic anemia occurs infrequently in the cat (Appendix Case 51). In stained films, cat erythrocytes normally exhibit little or no area of central pallor, and thus the typical spherocytic pattern is difficult to distinguish and requires a diligent search. The occurrence of irregular, small clumps of erythrocytes, sometimes including polychromatic red cells (Plate XVII–5), in blood films or agglutination of polychromatic red cells and rubricytes in bone marrow (Plate XIX–6) is considered indicative of the presence of an autoantibody. A familial occurrence of AIHA has been observed in two male sibling cats (Utroska, 1980).

Corticosteroid therapy is the treatment of choice in AIHA. Blood transfusions should be withheld as long as the PCV value exceeds 12% and there is evidence of remission. Blood transfusions should not be given except in life-threatening situations. Occasionally a dog fails to respond to corticosteroid therapy, as was the case with Dog 5. In such cases, chemotherapy with immunosuppressive drugs such as cyclophosphamide may be instituted in combination with prednisolone. See Chapter 35 for doses and other recommendations on therapy of AIHA in dogs and cats.

Neonatal Isoerythrolysis or Hemolytic Disease of the Newborn

Neonatal isoerythrolysis has been reported in mule foals, horse foals, and piglets (Cronin, 1950; Doll, 1952; Doll and Brown, 1954; Meyer et al., 1969). The young are normal at birth, but hemolysis begins within hours of ingestion of colostrum. At first the mucous membranes are pale, but later they become icteric. Hemoglobinuria may occur on the second or third day. If the animal does not die, the bone marrow response is typical of a hemolytic anemia.

The problem arises when the dam is bred more than once to the same stallion or boar so that antigens of the male's erythrocytes are transmitted to the erythrocytes of the fetus.

The dam develops antibodies against the fetal red cells when she becomes sensitized to them as a result of transfer across the placental membranes. The colostrum then contains the antibodies against the erythrocytes of the newborn. A technique for exchange blood transfusion for foals has been described (Farrelly et al., 1950).

Hemolytic disease in newborn pups has been encountered in rare instances. It may make its appearance when the bitch is blood group A-negative but has become sensitized to A-positive red blood cells and is mated to an A-positive male. Pups inheriting the A-positive factor experience hemolytic destruction of their red cells upon receiving anti-A antibody produced by the dam and passed into the colostrum. Young et al. (1951) have reproduced the condition experimentally. Bitches with A-negative erythrocytes were immunized with intravascular injections of A-positive dog red cells and mated with A-positive sires. All A-positive pups born to such dams developed hemolytic disease, provided they suckled the dam during the first day of life. There was no evidence of transfer of antibody across the placenta from mother to the pup. The degree of anemia in the A-positive pups varied widely, with PCV falling as low as 10%. Nucleated erythrocytes, reticulocytosis, and spherocytosis were present in the severely anemic groups. The erythrocyte osmotic fragility was substantially increased in all of the A-positive pups exposed to anti-A antibody.

Vaccination of females with tissue vaccines containing erythrocytes may sensitize the dam to red cell antigens that may later appear in erythrocytes of the newborn. On ingesting colostrum containing antibodies against red cell antigens, the newborn develops hemolytic anemia. An example is neonatal isoerythrolysis in calves born to cows vaccinated with an anaplasmosis vaccine of bovine blood origin (Dennis et al., 1970). For further details see Chapter 35.

HEMOLYTIC ANEMIAS OF MISCELLANEOUS ORIGIN

Water Intoxicosis

Cattle, particularly calves 2–10 months old, may develop hemoglobinuria from excessive intake of water. Calves raised on milk without water supplementation may drink excessive amounts of water when it becomes available in unlimited quantities. The amount of water consumed appears to be controlled only by physical limits of capacity (Kirkbride and Frey, 1967). Water-loaded calves have died within 2 hours (Laurance, 1965), although most such calves survive with no permanent ill effects and recover after 2 days (Wright, 1961).

Hematologic findings include hemolytic anemia, decreased total plasma protein concentration, and diminished serum sodium, chloride, and osmolality. Clinical signs of water intoxication are convulsions, coma, respiratory distress, hemoglobinuria, and death. Urine specific gravity is low. The most common necropsy lesion is edema of the lungs. It is believed that excessive water intake decreases blood electrolyte levels and induces osmotic destruction of erythrocytes. Hemolysis with attendant hemoglobinuria in some calves may be related to the fact that osmotic fragility of erythrocytes in calves is greatest at 4–5 months of age (see Chapter 7). Treatment consists of administering hypertonic fluids (2.5% NaCl and 10% dextran) and diuretics (mannitol) and other supportive therapy. A review of several literature reports on water intoxication in calves is available (Hannan, 1965). Experimental studies have been performed in dogs, sheep, and calves (Shimizu et al., 1979).

REFERENCES

Albahary, C.: Lead and Hemopoiesis. Amer. J. Med., 52:369, 1972.

Andresen, E.: Haemolytic Anaemia in Basenji Dogs. 2. Partial Deficiency of Erythrocyte Pyruvate Kinase (PK; EC 2.7.1.40) in Heterozygous Carriers. Anim. Blood Groups Biochem. Genet., 8:149, 1977.

Aronson, A.L.: Lead Poisoning in Cattle and Horses after Long-Term Exposure to Lead. Amer. J. Vet. Res., 33:627, 1972.

Asano, R., et al.: The Effect of Copper and Copper o-Phenanthroline Complex on Cattle Erythrocytes. Jap. J. Vet. Sci., 45:77, 1983.

Beaven, G.H., and White, J.C.: Oxidation of Phenylhydrazine in the Presence of Oxyhaemoglobin and the Origin of Heinz Bodies in Erythrocytes. Nature, 173:389, 1954.

Beritic, T.: Studies on Schmauch Bodies. I. The Incidence in Normal Cats (Felis domestica) and the Morphologic Relationship to Heinz Bodies. Blood, 25:999, 1965.

Beutler, E., et al.: Hemolytic Anemia Due to Pyrimidine-5'-nucleotidase Deficiency: Report of 8 Cases in 6 Families. Blood, 56:251, 1980.

Black, H.: Post-Parturient Haemoglobinuria in Northland. Proc. of the Society's 11th Seminar, Massey Univ., Palmerston North, New Zealand, May 22–23. Sheep and Beef Cattle Society of the N. Z. Vet. Ass., pp. 11–14, 1981.

Bond, E., and Kubin, R.: Lead Poisoning in Dogs. Vet. Med., 44:118, 1949.

Boulard, M., et al.: The Effect of Copper on Red Cell Enzyme Activities. J. Clin. Invest., 51:459, 1972.

Brown, A.K.: Erythrocyte Metabolism and Hemolysis in the Newborn. Pediatr. Clin. N. Amer., 13:879, 1966.

Buck, W.B.: Copper-Molybdenum. In Current Veterinary Therapy: Food Animal Practice. Howard, J.L., ed. W.B. Saunders, Philadelphia, p. 495, 1981.

Burrows, G.E.: Lead Poisoning in the Horse. Equine Pract., 4(6):30, 1982.

Burrows, G.E., and Borchard, R.E.: Experimental Lead Toxicosis in Ponies: Comparison of the Effects of Smelter Effluent-Contaminated Hay and Lead Acetate. Amer. J. Vet. Res., 43:2129, 1982.

Caple, I.W.: Post-Parturient Hemoglobinuria. In Current Veterinary Therapy: Food Animal Practice. Howard, J.L., ed. W.B. Saunders, Philadelphia, pp. 355–357, 1981.

Carson, P.E., et al.: Enzymatic Deficiency in Primaquine-Sensitive Erythrocytes. Science, 124:484, 1956.

Chisolm, J.J., Jr.: Disturbances in the Biosynthesis of Heme in Lead Intoxication. J. Pediatr., 64:174, 1963.

Christian, R.G., and Tryphonas, L.: Lead Poisoning in Cattle: Brain Lesions and Hematologic Changes. Amer. J. Vet. Res., 32:203, 1971.

Clare, N.T., and Stephens, E.H.: Congenital Porphyria in Pigs. Nature, 153:252, 1944.

Coles, E.H.: Veterinary Clinical Pathology. W.B. Saunders, Philadelphia, p. 106, 1980.

Collins, J.D., et al.: Ultrastructure of Erythrocyte Refractile Bodies in the Peripheral Blood of Cats. Amer. J. Vet. Clin. Path., 2:75, 1968.

Coombs, R.R.A., et al.: A New Test for the Detection of Weak or "Incomplete" Rh Agglutinins. Brit. J. Exp. Path., 26:255, 1945.

Cronin, M.T.I.: Haemolytic Disease in Foals. Irish Vet. J., 4:138, 1950.

Dennis, R.A., et al.: Neonatal Immunohemolytic Anemia and Icterus of Calves. J. Amer. Vet. Med. Ass., 155:1861, 1970.

Divers, T.J., et al.: Hemolytic Anemia in Horses after the Ingestion of Red Maple Leaves. J. Amer. Vet. Med. Ass., 180(3):300, 1982.

Dixon, P.M., et al.: Familial Methaemoglobinaemia and Haemolytic Anaemia in the Horse Associated with Decreased Erythrocytic Glutathione Reductase and Glutathione. Equine Vet. J., 9:198, 1977.

Dixon, P.M., et al.: Bovine Auto-Immune Haemolytic Anaemia. Vet. Rec., 103:155, 1978.

Dodd, D.C., and Staples, E.L.J.: Clinical Lead Poisoning in Dogs. N. Z. Vet. J., 4:1, 1956.

Doll, E.R.: Observations on the Clinical Features and Pathology of Hemolytic Icterus of Newborn Foals. Amer. J. Vet. Res., 13:504, 1952.

Doll, E.R., and Brown, R.G.: Isohemolytic Disease of Newborn Pigs. Cornell Vet., 44:86, 1954.

Dollahite, J.W., et al.: Chronic Lead Poisoning in Horses. Amer. J. Vet. Res., 39(6):961, 1978.

Dunbar, G.M., and Chambers, T.A.M.: Suspected Kale Poisoning in Dairy Cows. Vet. Rec., 75:566, 1963.

Ewing, G.O.: Familial Nonspherocytic Hemolytic Anemia of Basenji Dogs. J. Amer. Vet. Med. Ass., *154*:503, 1969.

Fairbanks, V.F.: Copper Sulfate–Induced Hemolytic Anemia. Arch. Intern. Med., *120*:428, 1967.

Farrelly, B.T., et al.: The Technique of Exchange Transfusion in the New-Born Foal. Vet. Rec., *62*:403, 1950.

Farrelly, B.T., et al.: Autoimmune Haemolytic Anaemia (AHA) in the Horse. Irish Vet. J., *20*:42, 1966.

Fenstermacher, R., et al.: Lead Poisoning in Cattle. J. Amer. Vet. Med. Ass., *108*:1, 1946.

Finco, D.R., et al.: Acetaaminophen Toxicosis in the Cat. J. Amer. Vet. Med. Ass., *166*:469, 1975.

Fourie, P.J.J.: The Occurrence of Congenital Porphyrinuria (Pink Tooth) in Cattle in South Africa (Swaziland). Onderstepoort J. Vet. Sci., *7*:535, 1936.

Fourie, P.J.J.: Does Bovine Congenital Porphyrinuria (Pink Tooth) Produce Clinical Disturbances in Animal Which is Protected from the Sun? Onderstepoort J. Vet. Res., *26*:231, 1953.

Gardner, D.E., et al.: Haematological and Biochemical Findings in Bovine Post-Parturient Haemoglobinuria and the Accompanying Heinz-Body Anaemia. N. Z. Vet. J., *24*:117, 1976.

George, J.W.: Hematology of Lead Poisoning in Cattle. Diss. Abstr. Int. B., *41*:3705, 1981.

George, J.W., and Duncan, J.R.: The Hematology of Lead Poisoning in Man and Animals. Vet. Clin. Path., *8*:23, 1979.

George, J.W., and Duncan, J.R.: Erythrocyte Protoporphyrin in Experimental Chronic Lead Poisoning in Calves. Amer. J. Vet. Res., *42(9)*:1630, 1981.

George, J.W., and Duncan, J.R.: Pyrimidine-Specific 5'-Nucleotidase Activity in Bovine Erythrocytes: Effect of Phlebotomy and Lead Poisoning. Amer. J. Vet. Res., *43(1)*:17, 1982.

Gipp, W.F., et al.: Effect of Dietary Copper, Iron and Ascorbic Acid Levels on Hematology, Blood and Tissue Copper, Iron and Zinc Concentrations and ^{64}Cu and ^{59}Fe Metabolism in Young Pigs. J. Nutr., *104*:532, 1974.

Glenn, B.L., et al.: Congenital Porphyria in the Domestic Cat (Felis catus): Preliminary Investigations on Inheritance Pattern. Amer. J. Vet. Res., *29*:1653, 1968.

Goldberg, A., et al.: Studies on Copper Metabolism. XXII. Hemolytic Anemia in Chickens Induced by the Administration of Copper. J. Lab. Clin. Med., *48*:442, 1956.

Good, M.G.: Heinz Body Phenomenon in Erythrocytes: Critical Remarks. Blood, *5*:885, 1950.

Gordon, W.A.M., and Luke, D.: Copper Poisoning in the Pig. Vet. Rec., *69*:37, 1957.

Greenhalgh, J.F.D., et al.: Kale Anemia. I. The Toxicity to Various Species of Animal of Three Types of Kale. Res. Vet. Sci., *10*:64, 1969.

Grimes, A.J., and Meisler, A.: Possible Cause of Heinz Bodies in Congenital Heinz-Body Anaemia. Nature, *194*:190, 1962.

Gruhzit, O.M.: I. Anemia in Dogs Produced by Feeding of Whole Onions and of Onion Fractions. Amer. J. Med. Sci., *181*:812, 1931.

Hamir, A.N., et al.: The Effects of Age and Diet on the Absorption of Lead from the Gastrointestinal Tract of Dogs. Aust. Vet. J., *58*:266, 1982.

Hammond, P.B., and Aronson, A.L.: Lead Poisoning in Cattle and Horses in the Vicinity of a Smelter. Ann. N.Y. Acad. Sci., III (art. 2):595, 1964.

Hannan, J.: Water Intoxication of Calves. Irish Vet. J., *19*:211, 1965.

Harley, J.D., and Mauer, A.M.: Studies on the Formation of Heinz Bodies. II. The Nature and Significance of Heinz Bodies. Blood, *17*:418, 1961.

Harvey, J.W., and Keitt, A.S.: Studies of the Efficiency and Potential Hazards of Methylene Blue Therapy in Aniline-Induced Methemoglobinaemia. Brit. J. Haematol., *54*:29, 1983.

Harvey, J.W., and Kornick, H.P.: Phenazopyridine Toxicosis in the Cat. J. Amer. Vet. Med. Ass., *169*:327, 1976.

Harvey, J.W. and Rackear, D.: Experimental Onion-Induced Hemolytic Anemia in Dogs. Vet. Pathol., *22*:387, 1985.

Harvey, J.W., et al.: Erythrocyte Pyruvate Kinase Deficiency in a Beagle Dog. Vet. Clin. Path., *6(3)*:13, 1977.

Hatch, R.C., et al.: Chronic Copper Toxicosis in Growing Swine. J. Amer. Vet. Med. Ass., *174(6)*:616, 1979.

Heinz, R.: Morphologische Veranderungen der rothen Blutkor-perchen durch Gifte. Virchows Arch. (Pathol. Anat.), *122*:112, 1980.

Higgins, R.J.: Chronic Copper Poisoning in Growing Pigs. Vet. Rec., *109*:134, 1981.

Hochstein, P., et al.: Mechanisms of Copper Toxicity in Red Cells. Prog. Clin. Biol. Res., *21*:669, 1978.

Hogg, G.G., et al.: Inherited Pyruvic Kinase Deficiency and Normal Haematological Values in Australian Basenji Dogs. Aust. Vet. J., *54*:367, 1978.

Holm, L.W., et al.: The Treatment of Chronic Lead Poisoning in Horses with Calcium Disodium Ethylenediamine-Tetraacetate. J. Amer. Vet. Med. Ass., *123*:383, 1953.

Hutchinson, T.W.S.: Onions as a Cause of Heinz Body Anemia and Death in Cattle. Can. Vet. J., *18*:358, 1977.

Jacob, H.S.: Mechanisms of Heinz Body Formation and Attachment to Red Cell Membrane. Semin. Hematol., *7*:341, 1970.

Jacob, H.S., and Amsden, T.: Acute Hemolytic Anemia with Rigid Red Cells in Hypophosphatemia. New Engl. J. Med., *285*:1446, 1971.

Jacob, H.S., and Amsden, T.: Acute Hemolytic Anemia with Rigid Red Cells in Hypophosphatemia. J. Lab. Clin. Med., *84*:643, 1974.

Jacobs, G.: Lead Poisoning in a Cat. J. Amer. Vet. Med. Ass., *179(12)*:1396, 1979.

Jain, N.C.: Demonstration of Heinz Bodies in Erythrocytes of the Cat. Bull. Amer. Soc. Vet. Clin. Path., *2*:13, 1973a.

Jain, N.C.: Studies on the Occurrence and Persistence of Heinz Bodies in Erythrocytes of the Cat. Folia Haematol., *99*:28, 1973b.

Jain, N.C., and Keeton, K.S.: Scanning Electron Microscopy of Heinz Bodies in Feline Erythrocytes. Amer. J. Vet. Res., *36(12)*:1691, 1975.

Jain, S.K., and Hochstein, P.: Membrane Alterations in Phenylhydrazine-Induced Reticulocytes. Arch. Biochem. Biophys., *201*:683, 1980.

Jandl, J.H., et al.: Oxidative Hemolysis and Precipitation of Hemoglobin. I. Heinz Body Anemias As an Acceleration of Red Cell Aging. J. Clin. Invest., *39*:1818, 1960.

Jensen, W.N., and Lessin, L.S.: Membrane Alterations Associated with Hemoglobinopathies. Semin. Hematol., *7*:409, 1970.

Jensen, W.N., et al.: An Electron Microscopic Description of Basophilic Stippling in Red Cells. Blood, *25*:933, 1965.

Johnson, G.F., et al.: Inheritance of Copper Toxicosis in

Bedlington Terriers. Amer. J. Vet. Res., *41(11)*:1865, 1980.

Jorgensen, S.K.: Congenital Porphyria in Pigs. Brit. Vet. J., *115*:160, 1959.

Kaneko, J.J.: Erythrokinetics and Iron Metabolism in Bovine Porphyria Erythropoietica. Ann. N.Y. Acad. Sci., *104*(art. 2):689, 1963.

Kaneko, J.J.: Porphyrins, Heme and Erythrocyte Metabolism: The Porphyrias. *In* Clinical Biochemistry of Domestic Animals. 2nd ed. Kaneko, J.J., ed. Academic Press, New York, p. 119, 1980.

Kaneko, J.J.: Personal communication. 1983.

Kaneko, J.J., et al.: Erythrocyte Porphyrin and Erythrocyte Survival in Bovine Erythropoietic Porphyria. Amer. J. Vet. Res., *32*:1981, 1971.

King, J.M., et al.: Acute Hemolytic Anemia, Methemoglobinemia, and Heinz Body Formation Associated with Ingestion of Red Maple Leaves by Horses. J. Amer. Vet. Med. Ass., *179*:143, 1981.

Kirkbride, C.A., and Frey, R.A.: Experimental Water Intoxication in Calves. J. Amer. Vet. Med. Ass., *15*:742, 1967.

Knight, H.K., and Burau, R.G.: Chronic Lead Poisoning in Horses. J. Amer. Vet. Med. Ass., *162*:781, 1973.

Koger, L.M.: Onion Poisoning in Cattle. J. Amer. Vet. Med. Ass., *129*:75, 1956.

Kumar, K.S., et al.: Copper-Induced Generation of Super Oxide in Human Red Cell Membrane. Biochem. Biophys. Res. Commun., *83*:587, 1978.

Kurundkar, V.D., et al.: Biochemical and Pathological Changes in Clinical Cases of Haemoglobinuria in Buffaloes. Indian J. Anim. Sci., *51*:35, 1981.

Lassen, E.D., and Buck, W.B.: Experimental Lead Toxicosis in Swine. Amer. J. Vet. Res., *40(10)*:1359, 1979.

Laurance, J.A.: Water Intoxication in Calves. J. S. Afr. Vet. Med. Ass., *36*:277, 1965.

Lees, G.E., et al.: Idiopathic Heinz Body Hemolytic Anemia in Three Dogs. J. Amer. Anim. Hosp. Ass., *15*:143, 1979.

Levin, E.Y.: Uroporphyrinogen III Cosynthetase in Bovine Erythropoietic Porphyria. Science, *161*:907, 1968.

Lewis, R.M.: Clinical Evaluation of the Lupus Erythematosus Cell Phenomenon in Dogs. J. Amer. Vet. Med. Ass., *147*:939, 1965.

Lewis, R.M., et al.: A Syndrome of Autoimmune Hemolytic Anemia and Thrombocytopenia in Dogs. Proc. 100th Annu. Meeting Amer. Vet. Med. Ass., p. 140, 1963.

Lewis, R.M., et al.: Canine Systemic Lupus Erythematosus. Blood, *25*:143, 1965.

Lynch, G.P., et al.: Physiological Responses of Calves to Cadmium and Lead. J. Anim. Sci., *42*:410, 1976.

Lynch, G.P., et al.: Heinz Body Formation in Calf Erythrocytes. J. Dairy Sci., *61*:1161, 1978.

MacWilliams, P.S., et al.: Bovine Postparturient Hemoglobinuria: A Review of the Literature. Can. Vet. J., *23*:309, 1982.

Madden, D.E., et al.: The Occurrence of Congenital Porphyria in Holstein-Friesian Cattle. J. Hered., *49*:125, 1958.

Madsen, D.E., and Nielsen, H.M.: Parturient Hemoglobinemia of Dairy Cows. J. Amer. Vet. Med. Ass., *94*:577, 1939.

Martinovich, D., and Woodhouse, D.A.: Post-Parturient Haemoglobinuria in Cattle: A Heinz Body Haemolytic Anemia. N. Z. Vet. J., *19*:259, 1971.

McSherry, B.J., et al.: The Hematology of Phenothiazine Poisoning in Horses. Can. Vet. J., *7*:3, 1966.

Meyer, R.C., et al.: A Hemolytic Neonatal Disease in Swine Associated with Blood Group Incompatibility. J. Amer. Vet. Med. Ass., *154*:531, 1969.

Miller, G., et al.: Studies on Destruction of Red Blood Cells by Canine Autoantibodies in Normal Dogs and in a Dog with Naturally Occurring Autoimmune Hemolytic Disease. Amer. J. Dis. Child., *93*:35, 1957.

Mitema, E.S., et al.: Effect of Chronic Lead Exposure on the Canine Bone Marrow. Amer. J. Vet. Res., *41(5)*:682, 1980.

Nagpal, M., et al.: Haemoglobinuria in Buffaloes. Indian Vet. J., *45*:1048, 1968.

O'Brien, D.P.: Lead Toxicity in a Dog. J. Amer. Anim. Hosp. Ass., *17*:845, 1981.

Owen, C.A., Jr., and Ludwig, J.: Inherited Copper Toxicosis in Bedlington Terriers: Wilson's Disease (Hepatocellular Degeneration). Amer. J. Pathol., *106*:432, 1982.

Parkinson, B., and Sutherland, A.K.: Post-Parturient Haemoglobinuria of Dairy Cows. Aust. Vet. J., *30*:232, 1954.

Pearson, J.K.L.: Copper Poisoning in Sheep Following the Feeding of a Copper-Supplemented Diet. Vet. Rec., *68*:766, 1956.

Penny, R.H.C.: Post-Parturient Haemoglobinuria (Haemoglobinaemia) in Cattle. Vet. Rec., *68*:238, 1956.

Penny, R.H.C., et al.: Heinz-Ehrlich Bodies Associated with Kale Feeding. Vet. Rec., *73*:747, 1961.

Pettit, G.D., et al.: Lead Poisoning in a Dog. J. Amer. Vet. Med. Ass., *128*:295, 1956.

Pierce, K.R., et al.: Acute Hemolytic Anemia Caused by Wild Onion Poisoning in Horses. J. Amer. Vet. Med. Ass., *160*:323, 1972.

Pierson, R.E., and Aanes, W.A.: Treatment of Chronic Copper Poisoning in Sheep. J. Amer. Vet. Med. Ass., *133*:307, 1958.

Prasse, K.W., et al.: Pyruvate Kinase Deficiency Anemia with Terminal Myelofibrosis and Osteosclerosis in a Beagle. J. Amer. Vet. Med. Ass., *166*:1170, 1975.

Railsback, L.T.: Porphyrinuria in a Yearling Hereford. Vet. Med., *34*:102, 1939.

Reef, V.B.: Clostridium perfringens Cellulitis and Immune-Mediated Hemolytic Anemia in a Horse. J. Amer. Vet. Med. Ass., *182*:251, 1983.

Rhode, E.A., and Cornelius, C.E.: Congenital Porphyria (Pink Tooth) in Holstein-Friesian Calves in California. J. Amer. Vet. Med. Ass., *132*:112, 1958.

Rifkind, R.A.: Heinz Body Anemia: An Ultrastructural Study. II. Red Cell Sequestration and Destruction. Blood, *26*:433, 1965.

Rifkind, R.A., and Danon, D.: Heinz Body Anemia: An Ultrastructural Study. I. Heinz Body Formation. Blood, *25*:885, 1965.

Rimington, C.: Some Cases of Congenital Porphyrinuria in Cattle: Chemical Studies upon the Living Animals and Post-Mortem Material. Onderstepoort J. Vet. Sci., *7*:567, 1936.

Rolton, C.E., et al.: Evaluation of Tests for the Diagnosis of Lead Exposure in Sheep. Aust. Vet. J., *54*:393, 1978.

Romeo, G., and Levin, E.Y.: Uroporphyrinogen III Cosynthetase in Human Congenital Erythropoietic Porphyria. Proc. Natl. Acad. Sci. USA, *63*:856, 1969.

Ruhr, L.P., and Osweiler, G.D.: Nitrate Accumulators. *In* Current Veterinary Therapy: Food Animal Practice. Howard, J.L., ed. W.B. Saunders, Philadelphia, pp. 433–435, 1981.

Samad, A., et al.: Some Biochemical and Clinical Aspects

of Haemoglobinuria in Buffaloes. Indian Vet. J., *56*:230, 1979.

Schalm, O.W.: Equine Clinical Hematology. Proc. 8th. Annu. Amer. Ass. Equine Pract. Conv., p. 107, 1962.

Schalm, O.W.: Methylene Blue Induced Heinz Body Hemolytic Anemia in a Dog. Canine Pract., *5(2)*:20, 1978.

Schalm, O.W.: Hematology of Lead Poisoning in the Dog. Canine Pract., *7(2)*:55, 1980.

Schalm, O.W., and Smith, R.: Some Unique Aspects of Feline Hematology in Disease. Small Anim. Clin., *3*:311, 1963.

Schecter, R.D., et al.: Heinz Body Hemolytic Anemia Associated with the Use of Urinary Antiseptics Containing Methylene Blue in the Cat. J. Amer. Vet. Med. Ass., *162*:37, 1973.

Schmauch, G.: Über Endoglobulare Korperchen in den Erythrocyten der Katze. Virchows Arch. (Pathol. Anat.), *157*:14, 1899.

Searcy, G.P., et al.: Congenital Hemolytic Anemia in the Basenji Dog Due to Erythrocyte Pyruvate Kinase Deficiency. Can. J. Comp. Med., *35*:67, 1971.

Searcy, G.P., et al.: Pyruvate Kinase Deficiency in Dogs. Amer. J. Pathol., *94*:689, 1979.

Selwyn, J.F.: Heinz Bodies in Red Cells after Splenectomy and after Phenacetin Administration. Brit. J. Haematol., *1*:173, 1955.

Setty, D., and Narayana, K.: A Case of Non-Febrile Haemoglobinuria in a She Goat. Indian Vet. J., *52*:149, 1975.

Shand, A., and Lewis, G.: Chronic Copper Poisoning in Young Calves. Vet. Rec., *69*:618, 1957.

Shimizu, Y., et al.: The Experimental Study on the Mechanism of Hemolysis on Paroxysmal Hemoglobinemia and Hemaglobinuria in Calves Due to Excessive Water Intake. Jap. J. Vet. Sci., *41*:583, 1979.

Simpson, C.F., and Anderson, B.: Heinz Body Anemia in Cattle Grazing Rye Pastures. Florida Vet. J., *9*:26, 1980.

Smith, B.: Copper and Molybdenum Imbalance in Relationship to Post-Parturient Haemoglobinuria in Cattle. N. Z. Vet. J., *21*:240, 1973.

Smith, J.D., et al.: Tolerance of Ponies to High Levels of Dietary Copper. J. Anim. Sci., *41*:1644, 1975.

Smith, J.E.: Inherited Erythrocyte Glutathione Deficiency. Amer. J. Pathol., *82*:233, 1976.

Smith, R.H.: Kale Poisoning: The Brassica Anaemia Factor. Vet. Rec., *107*:12, 1980.

Stamp, J.T., and Stewart, J.: Haemolytic Anaemia with Jaundice in Sheep. J. Comp. Pathol., *63*:48, 1953.

Stolk, J.M., and Smith, R.P.: Species Differences in Methemoglobin Reductase Activity. Biochem. Pharmacol., *15*:343, 1966.

Su, Le-Chu, et al.: A Comparison of Copper Loading Disease in Bedlington Terriers and Wilson's Disease in Humans. Amer. J. Physiol., *243(3)*:G226, 1982a.

Su, Le-Chu, et al.: A Defect of Biliary Excretion of Copper in Copper-Laden Bedlington Terriers. Amer. J. Physiol., *243*:G231, 1982b.

Sutton, R.H., et al.: Autoimmune Haemolytic Anaemia in a Horse. N. Z. Vet. J., *26*:311, 1978.

Taketa, F., et al.: Studies of Cat Hemoglobin and Hybrids with Human Hemoglobin A. Biochemistry, *6*:3809, 1967.

Tasker, J.B., et al.: Familial Anemia in the Basenji Dog. J. Amer. Vet. Med. Ass., *154*:158, 1969.

Tennant, B., et al.: Acute Hemolytic Anemia, Methemoglobinemia, and Heinz Body Formation Associated with Ingestion of Red Maple Leaves by Horses. J. Amer. Vet. Med. Ass., *179*:143, 1981.

Thorp, F., Jr., and Harshfield, G.S.: Onion Poisoning of Horses. J. Amer. Vet. Med. Ass., *94*:52, 1939.

Tobias, G.: Congenital Porphyria in a Cat. J. Amer. Vet. Med. Ass., *145*:462, 1964.

Twedt, D.C., et al.: Clinical, Morphologic, and Chemical Studies on Copper Toxicosis of Bedlington Terriers. J. Amer. Vet. Med. Ass., *175(3)*:269, 1979.

Utroska, B.: Auto-Immune Hemolytic Anemia in Sibling Cats. Vet. Med. Small Anim. Clin., *75*:1699, 1980.

Valentine, W.N., et al.: Hereditary Hemolytic Anemia with Human Erythrocyte Pyrimidine 5'-Nucleotidase Deficiency. J. Clin. Invest., *54*:866, 1974.

Valentine, W.N., et al.: Lead Poisoning: Association with Hemolytic Anemia, Basophilic Stippling, Erythrocyte Pyrimidine 5'-Nucleotidase Deficiency and Intraerythrocytic Accumulation of Pyrimidines. J. Clin. Invest., *58*:926, 1976.

Van Kampen, K.R., et al.: Hemolytic Anemia in Sheep Fed Wild Onion (Allium validum). J. Amer. Vet. Med. Ass., *156*:328, 1970.

Watson, C.J., et al.: Some Studies of the Comparative Biology of Human and Bovine Erythropoietic Porphyria. Amer. Med. Ass. Arch. Intern. Med., *103*:436, 1959.

Webster, S.H.: Heinz Body Phenomenon in Erythrocytes: A Review. Blood, *4*:479, 1949.

Williams, H.H., et al.: Biochemical Studies of the Blood of Dogs with N-propyl-disulfide Anemia. J. Lab. Clin. Med., *26*:996, 1941.

Wintrobe, M.M., et al.: Clinical Hematology. 8th ed. Lea & Febiger, Philadelphia, 1981.

Wright, M.A.: Haemoglobinuria from Excessive Water Drinking. Vet. Rec., *73*:129, 1961.

Young, L.E., et al.: Hemolytic Disease in Newborn Dogs. Blood, *6*:291, 1951.

Zook, B.C., et al.: Lead Poisoning in Dogs. J. Amer. Vet. Med. Ass., *155*:1329, 1969.

Zook, B.C., et al.: Basophilic Stippling of Erythrocytes in Dogs, with Special Reference to Lead Poisoning. J. Amer. Vet. Med. Ass., *157*:2092, 1970.

25
Depression or Hypoproliferative Anemias

NUTRITIONAL DEFICIENCY ANEMIAS   655
    Vitamin Deficiencies   656
    Poodle Macrocytosis Simulating Vitamin
      B_{12}–Folate Deficiency   661
    Mineral Deficiencies   662

APLASTIC ANEMIA   665
    Bracken Fern Poisoning   666
    Radiation Syndrome   666
    Other Causes   668

SECONDARY ANEMIAS FROM ERYTHROID
    HYPOPLASIA   668
    Anemia of Chronic Disorders or
      Inflammatory Disease   668
    Renal Disease with Uremia   669
    Liver Disease   670
    Neoplasia   671
    Endocrine Diseases   671
    Parasitism in Sheep and Cattle   671

Anemias associated primarily with reduced erythropoiesis are discussed in this chapter. Some causes of these anemias are listed in Table 25–1. Such anemias may result from limited supply or defective utilization of nutrients essential for red cell production or from anatomic disruption, functional impairment, or lack of stimulation of hematopoietic tissue.

There is an important distinction between anemias of nutritional deficiencies and anemias secondary to chemical or drug toxicity and organic diseases. In the former, erythropoiesis is suppressed and disturbed because of the lack of nutrients essential to red cell production, but bone marrow is fully capable of resuming normal erythropoietic activity as soon as adequate materials are supplied. By contrast, in the latter, the bone marrow's ability to produce red cells is often suppressed or destroyed by the insulting agent or disease so that anemia ensues in the face of adequate essential nutrients. Cellular damage in such cases may be mild and reversible upon removal of the primary cause, or it may be severe and permanent. In most cases of marrow suppression secondary to drugs, chemicals, or organic diseases, the anemia is normocytic-normochromic. However, a microcytic or macrocytic anemia may manifest following deficiency of iron or vitamin B_{12}–folate, respectively.

Table 25–1.   Depression or Hypoproliferative Anemias and Some of Their Causes in Various Animal Species

Nutritional deficiency anemias
  Protein deficiency
  Mineral deficiencies
    Iron, copper, cobalt, and selenium
  Vitamin deficiencies
    B_{12}, folic acid, niacin, pyridoxine, thiamine, pantothenic acid, riboflavin, ascorbic acid, and vitamins A and E

Anemia of inflammatory disease

Anemias associated with organic or tissue disorders
  Nephritis with uremia in the dog
  Malignancies
  Endocrine disorders such as hypothyroidism and hypoadrenocorticism in the dog
  Liver disease

Anemias associated with parasitic diseases
  Trichostrongylosis in sheep and cattle

Aplastic or hypoplastic anemias
  Irradiation
  Bracken fern
  Trichloroethylene-extracted soybean meal
  Estrogen toxicity in the dog

Anemias associated with myeloproliferative disorders

NUTRITIONAL DEFICIENCY ANEMIAS

Prolonged nutritional deficiencies of protein and several vitamins and minerals essential for erythrocyte production lead to anemia in humans and animals. The type of anemia varies with the nutrient lacking and the animal species involved. Most extensive experimental work in this regard has been done with pigs (Table 25–2). In this species, mild to modest normocytic anemia develops fol-

Table 25–2.   Hematologic Characteristics of Experimental Nutritional Deficiencies in Swine

| Deficiency | Anemia | | Leukopenia | Plasma Iron | Serum Copper | E.P. | Bone Marrow Morphology |
	Type	Severity					
Protein	N	+	None	Normal	Low	Normal	Normoblastic
Lysine	N	+	None	Normal	Normal	—	Normoblastic
Tryptophane	N	+ +	Present	Normal	—	Normal	Normoblastic
Iron	MH	+ + + +	None	Low	Normal	Normal	Normoblastic
Copper	MH	+ + + +	Present	Low	Low	Normal	Normoblastic
Pyridoxine	Mi	+ + + +	None	High	Normal	Low	Normoblastic
Niacin plus protein	N	+ +	None	Normal	Low	Normal	Normoblastic
Riboflavin	N	+	None	—	—	—	Normoblastic
Pantothenic acid	N	+ +	None	—	—	—	Normoblastic
Folate	Ma	+ + + +	Present	High	Normal	Low	Macronormoblastic
B_{12}	N	+	None	—	—	—	Normoblastic
Folate plus B_{12}	Ma	+ + + +	Present	—	—	—	Macronormoblastic with a few megaloblasts
Vitamin E	N	+ + + +	None	Normal	—	—	Abnormal*

From Wintrobe et al., 1981, p. 145.
Types of anemia: N = normocytic, MH = microcytic hypochromic, Mi = microcytic, and Ma = macrocytic.
E.P. refers to free erythrocyte protoporphyrin.
*Hyperplasia with multinucleated cells.

lowing deficiencies of protein and vitamins such as niacin, riboflavin, and pantothenic acid. A marked, normocytic anemia with bone marrow abnormalities develops in vitamin E deficiency. Severe microcytic anemia is characteristic of iron, copper and pyridoxine deficiencies. Vitamin B_{12} deficiency causes only a slight normocytic anemia, but macrocytic anemia results from deficiencies of folate or both folate and vitamin B_{12}.

Vitamin Deficiencies

Vitamin B_{12} and Folic Acid

Vitamin B_{12} and folic acid (folate) are essential for normal erythropoiesis (Vilter et al., 1950). Before vitamin B_{12} was discovered, it was common knowledge that an "animal protein factor" was required for adequate growth of some animals, e.g., chickens and swine. This factor is now defined as vitamin B_{12}. Baby pigs in which deficiency of vitamin B_{12} and folate was produced grew markedly and exhibited marked reticulocytosis upon injection of vitamin B_{12} (Johnson and Nesheim, 1949). After 3 weeks of vitamin B_{12} therapy, a second reticulocyte peak was obtained after folate supplementation by oral route.

Growth was retarded during the first weeks of life in pigs on a vitamin B_{12}–deficient diet (Cartwright et al., 1951). There was no macrocytic anemia, and the bone marrow was not megaloblastic. When anemia developed, it was normocytic and accompanied by a moderately severe neutropenia. This was in contrast to the production in swine of macrocytic anemia accompanied by neutropenia and slight thrombocytopenia when fed a folate-deficient ration (Cartwright et al., 1950). Studies by means of colon cannulas and ^{57}Co-labeled vitamin B_{12} introduced into the colon, determined that the vitamin can be absorbed from the colon of swine (Henderickx et al., 1964).

Macrocytic-normochromic anemia with leukopenia has also been produced experimentally in the rat with folate-deficient diets (Kodicek and Carpenter, 1950).

Characteristic hematologic findings with deficiency of vitamin B_{12} and folate in humans are: a macrocytic-normochromic anemia; the presence of hypersegmented neutrophils, ovalocytes, macrocytic red cells (megalocytes), and erythrocytes with multiple Howell-Jolly bodies in peripheral blood; and the presence of megaloblastic erythroid cells and giant metamyelocytes and neutrophils in the bone marrow. In addition, because of defective synthesis of myelin, neurologic signs are seen in vitamin B_{12} deficiency but not in folate deficiency. Expression of various abnormalities varies with the degree of deficiency and its cause. It takes several years for vitamin B_{12} deficiency caused by dietary lack to manifest because body stores of vitamin B_{12} are great, whereas folate deficiency appears within 2–4 months owing to a relatively smaller body reserve. By contrast, deficiency from impaired metabolism of these vitamins manifests early. The liver is the principal storage site.

Deficiency of B_{12} and folate may develop for several reasons, which include dietary lack, malabsorption, increased physiologic need (during pregnancy and the neonatal period), liver disease, therapy for malignant diseases, and administration of certain anticonvulsive drugs such as diphenylhydantoin, primidone, and phenobarbital. Vitamin B_{12} of dietary origin is prepared for absorption from the gut by an intrinsic factor produced in the stomach. When this factor is lacking, pernicious anemia develops in humans. True pernicious anemia, due to lack of the intrinsic factor, has not been demonstrated in animals. The removal of seven-eights of the stomach, the entire duodenum, and 30 cm of the jejunum in dogs failed to result in development of pernicious anemia or a macrocytic anemia (Bachrach and Fogelson, 1938).

Folates in nature occur as monoglutamates and principally (90%) in conjugated forms as polyglutamates. The latter are converted to monoglutamates either before or after absorption. Important natural sources of folates are green vegetables and dairy products. Vitamin B_{12}, thyroxine, and vitamin C have been credited with playing an important role in folate metabolism. It appears that the dog is able to obtain folate from intestinal bacterial action (Krehl and Elvehjem, 1945). However, when nicotinic acid was restricted, the degree of folate synthesis was greatly decreased. Spontaneous folate deficiency in the dog has been described (Afronsky, 1954). See Chapter 13 for additional comments on absorption of dietary vitamin B_{12} and folate.

Ruminants are the source of natural vitamin B_{12} for all meat-eating animals; the vitamin is produced by the rumen flora and stored in large quantities in the liver and other glandular organs. Herbivores with simple stomach and a large cecum such as the horse and rabbit produce some vitamin B_{12} in the cecum (Clifford et al., 1956). The feces of all animals develop a high level of vitamin B_{12} with aging as a result of bacterial action. Contamination of the pasture with feces could be a source of vitamin B_{12} for horses. The mature horse does not have a dietary requirement for vitamin B_{12} because the vitamin is produced by bacterial action and is absorbed from the lower gastrointestinal tract (Stillions et al., 1971). The concentration of vitamin B_{12} in alimentary tract contents of horses was found to increase from stomach to rectum (Davis, 1971). Rabbits may get their supply as a result of habitual coprophagy.

Vitamin B_{12} in the plasma is transported bound to transcobalamins, principally transcobalamin II (Allen, 1975). Transcobalamin I (TC I) is usually completely saturated with vitamin B_{12}, while transcobalamin II (TC II) is partially saturated, and transcobalamin III (TC III) is ordinarily free. TC II appears to function as a transport protein, while TC I and TC III do not. The origin of TC I is uncertain, but circumstantial evidence suggests it originates from immature granulocytes, while TC II is produced by the liver, granulocytes, and macrophages, and TC III by mature granulocytes. The transport process involves binding of TC II–cobalamin to a specific cell receptor, internalization of the complex via endocytosis, and degradation of the complex releasing cobalamin. A congenital deficiency of TC II in humans is associated with megaloblastic anemia.

Fig. 25–1 is a schematic of folic acid metabolism and its interaction with vitamin B_{12} in DNA synthesis. In the body, folic acid is first converted to dihydrofolate (DHF) and then to tetrahydrofolate (THF); the latter conversion occurs under the influence of the enzyme DHF-reductase in the presence of NADPH. Folate in plasma is found as free or protein-bound 5-methyl-THF, which is produced in the intestinal mucosal cells and the liver. THF serves as a source of 5,10-methylene-THF, a folate coenzyme involved in the conversion of deoxyuridylate to thymidylate under the influence of thymidylate synthetase. Thymidylate is subsequently utilized for DNA synthesis. It is presently conjectured that folate deficiency is expressed in lack of the folate coenzyme, resulting in deranged DNA synthesis. Folate antagonists such as methotrexate inhibit DHF-reductase and deprive the cell of reduced folate. Vitamin B_{12} deficiency also leads to the depletion of the folate coenzyme as a consequence of some interaction between

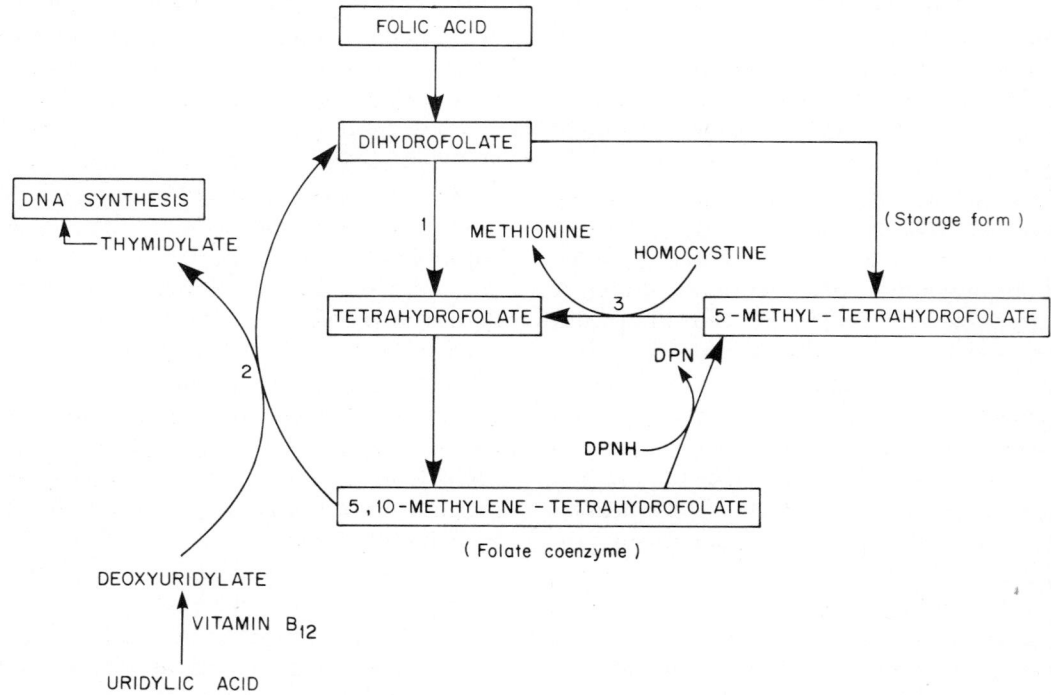

Fig. 25–1. Interaction of folic acid and vitamin B₁₂ in DNA synthesis. Sites of some enzyme interactions are also shown: 1, site of dihydrofolate reductase action + NADPH; 2, site of thymidylate synthetase action; 3, site of methyl B₁₂ (cobalamin), a vitamin B₁₂ coenzyme, action.

vitamin B_{12} and folate metabolism. According to the "methyl-tetrahydrofolate trap" hypothesis, vitamin B_{12} in the form of methyl cobalamin is needed as a coenzyme for the metabolic conversion of homocystine to methionine. During this process 5-methyl-THF, an inactive storage form of folate, is converted to THF. Most of the vitamin B_{12} in serum is in the form of methyl cobalamin. Vitamin B_{12} deficiency leads to impaired conversion of homocystine and trapping of folate as unusable 5-methyl-THF and consequently unavailability of 5,10-methylene-THF required for synthesis of DNA.

Whipple et al. (1955), using radioactive cobalt in the B_{12} molecule, were able to demonstrate in the dog the need for vitamin B_{12} in the first steps of stroma formation in the prorubricyte and basophilic rubricytes. In the absence of vitamin B_{12}, the S phase as well as the intermitotic period are prolonged, and maturation stops at the prorubricyte and basophilic rubricyte stages, causing these cells to be larger and more numerous in the bone marrow. A stained film from a dog or cat pre-

sumed to have vitamin B_{12} and/or folate deficiency presents an unusual number of large cells of varying sizes. The nuclei of these cells appear somewhat deficient in chromatin, for there seems to be more parachromatin separating clumps of chromatin (Plate XIX–1). Although mitosis is delayed or slowed for lack of synthesis of nucleoprotein, hemoglobin synthesis goes forward, leading to eventual extrusion of the nucleus and production of some larger than normal (macrocytic) erythrocytes. The large rubricytes are then called *megaloblasts*, and the marrow is said to be *megaloblastic*. Thus kinetic changes involve a slow rate of erythroid proliferation and an increase in the rate of ineffective erythropoiesis. A moderate reduction in red cell life span is seen. In humans, the resulting anemia is macrocytic-normochromic, but this has not been the case in the few instances of anemia of the dog and cat in which a vitamin B_{12}–folate deficiency was suspected. These animals had a normocytic-normochromic anemia, although a careful search of the blood film revealed an occasional macrocyte (Plate XI–8). Macrocytes were found to be more numerous, however, in the bone marrow in association with magaloblastoid rubricytes than in blood.

Defective nucleoprotein synthesis in vitamin B_{12}–folate deficiencies leads to reduced granulopoiesis and production of some giant metamyelocytes in the bone marrow. Maturation of the nucleus of the giant metamyelocytes leads to the development of large *hypersegmented neutrophils* that, when carefully searched for, can be found in small numbers in the bone marrow and blood (Plate XI–7). Megaloblastic changes disappear quickly after vitamin B_{12} therapy, but giant metamyelocytes may be found for several days. Care must be taken to distinguish between the megaloblastic marrow of vitamin B_{12}–folate deficiency and the primitive erythroid precursor cells that dominate the marrow in myeloproliferative disorders of the cat (Plates XV–4, XIX–2). The reader is referred to Chapter 32 for a discussion of myeloproliferative disorders in the cat.

Vitamin B_{12} deficiency develops in *cattle* and *sheep* on cobalt-deficient pastures (Maynard, 1954). A number of vitamin B_{12} analogues are produced in the rumen by bacterial fermentation. Cobalt is essential in the molecular structure of vitamin B_{12}, and so the term *cobalamins* has been given to this vitamin and its analogues. Cobalt-deficient areas have been reported in northern Michigan, northeastern Wisconsin, Florida, the British Isles, Australia, New Zealand, and Kenya. The condition produced in cattle and sheep has received various local names such as pine or pinning, salt sickness, brush sickness, enzootic marasmus, and nakuruitis. It has been reported that when horses, sheep, and rabbits grazed on a cobalt-deficient pasture, only the sheep exhibited signs of cobalt deficiency (Alexander and Davies, 1969). Clinical signs and hematologic changes in cobalt deficiency of cattle and sheep have been described (Marston, 1952). Prominent findings include unthriftiness, progressive wasting, marked macrocytic or normocytic anemia, and hemosiderosis. (Smith and Loosli, 1957; Marston, 1952). Neurologic abnormalities are not found. Excessive administration of cobalt is known to cause polycythemia (see Chapter 13).

The molecular structure of folate consists of three parts: pteridine, a yellow pigment; para-aminobenzoic acid, which is also found in the sulfonamide molecule; and glutamic acid. Its chemical name is pteroylglutamic acid or PGA. Because folate is required for cell multiplication, folate antimetabolites have been used in the treatment of leukemia to cause the malignant cells to accept a closely related chemical structure that cannot be utilized by the cell for growth and multiplication (Woolley, 1959). Such a chemical is 4-aminopteroylglutamic acid. In the treatment of bacterial infection with sulfanilamide, leukopenia sometimes develops. This can be explained on the basis of sulfanilamide acting as an antimetabolite for folate by virtue of its para-aminobenzoic acid.

Niacin

As discussed in the preceding section, in the dog the degree of folate synthesis was greatly decreased when niacin or nicotinic acid was restricted. Niacin is important to the dog; a deficiency of this vitamin in the presence of a low protein intake leads to development of a syndrome called *black-tongue*. The clinical signs are anorexia, marked dehydration, infection of the oral mucosa accompanied by buccal necrosis and ropy salivation, loss of body weight, and bloody diarrhea. Dogs on experimental nicotinic acid–deficient diets develop a severe macrocytic anemia with leukopenia (Handler and Dann, 1942; Handler and Featherston, 1943; Rhoads and Miller, 1933). Administration of niacin leads to an immediate reticulocytosis, and recovery ensues.

A relationship between tryptophan in the diet and the synthesis of nicotinic acid has been reported. Horses do not require nicotinic acid preformed because they are able to synthesize the vitamin from tryptophan (Schweigert et al., 1947). It has been shown that niacin is essential for normal erythropoiesis in pigs fed a low-protein diet (Cartwright et al., 1948). Lack of niacin was associated with development of a moderately severe normocytic anemia without leukopenia, but when tryptophan intake was adequate, niacin deficiency did not develop.

Vitamin B₆ or Pyridoxine

Experimental deficiency of vitamin B_6 causes microcytic-hypochromic anemia, iron overload, and neurological abnormalities in various animal species including the dog (Fouts et al., 1940), cat (Gershoff et al., 1959), mice (Keyhani et al., 1974), rats (Kornberg et al., 1945a), and pigs (Cartwright et al., 1944; Wintrobe et al., 1943a).

Vitamin B_6 was shown to be required by the dog for utilization of iron in the synthesis of hemoglobin (McKibbin et al., 1942). The blood plasma iron was abnormally high, and the copper values were at a low normal level during the anemia. The anemia was typically that of iron deficiency, namely microcytic-hypochromic. Oral administration of pyridoxine in doses of 60 μg/kg daily was followed in 4 days by reticulocytosis and a return of the erythron to normal. During the anemic phase, the MCV was reported to fall below 50 fl, and the MCHC varied from 24 to 28%.

Vitamin B_6 is needed for erythropoiesis chiefly because it serves as a cofactor for synthesis of δ-aminolevulinic acid. It is probably also required for optimal synthesis of heme from iron and protoporphyrin (Wintrobe et al., 1981).

Riboflavin

Although the precise role of riboflavin in erythrocyte metabolism remains to be defined, experimental dietary deficiency of riboflavin in rats (Kornberg et al., 1945b; Mookerjea and Hawkins, 1960), baboons (Foy et al., 1964, 1968), monkeys (Cooperman et al., 1945; Waisman, 1944), and pigs (Wintrobe et al., 1944) results in a normocytic-normochromic anemia from reduced erythropoiesis. The anemia is correctable by riboflavin administration.

In contrast, experimental riboflavin deficiency in dogs led to a microcytic-hypochromic anemia (Spector et al., 1943). Dogs that were on a riboflavin-deficient diet and were subjected to phlebotomy that removed up to 25% of the blood volume failed to regenerate hemoglobin. These dogs could not recover from the induced anemia unless riboflavin was given.

Riboflavin deficiency in growing pigs failed to produce anemia, but a marked increase in neutrophilic granulocytes was reported (Mitchell et al., 1950).

Vitamin C

Ascorbic acid or vitamin C is normally synthesized by all mammals, with the exception of primates and guinea pigs. The function of vitamin C is said to be the maintenance of intracellular substances of tissues derived from the mesenchyma. Severe deficiency in humans results in scurvy characterized by hemorrhagic manifestations, particularly bleeding in the gums and skin. A mild to moderate anemia that is usually normocytic-normochromic may be seen. Vitamin C also functions as a reducing agent for iron in the gut, thereby enhancing iron absorption, and as a participant in the conversion of folate to its active form. Thus the need for folate and iron is increased in ascorbic acid deficiency. It is interesting to note that high doses of vitamin C can destroy vitamin B_{12} (Herbert and Jacob, 1974) and may produce vitamin B_{12} deficiency (Hines, 1975). A megaloblastic anemia develops in monkeys fed milk diets deficient in ascorbic acid (Wallerstein and Wallerstein, 1976).

Pantothenic Acid

Experimental pantothenic acid deficiency in swine produced a moderate normocytic anemia, a severe sensory neuron degeneration, and an extensive colitis (Wintrobe et al., 1943b).

Vitamin E

Vitamin E deficiency rarely causes anemia in humans. In monkeys, it produces a normocytic-normochromic anemia after a prolonged period of 1–2 years depending on the breed involved (Ausman and Hayes, 1974; Brandy et al., 1982; Santiyanont et al., 1977). By contrast, growing pigs develop a severe anemia within 6–8 weeks (Lynch et al., 1977). The bone marrow in both species shows erythroid hyperplasia, ineffective erythropoiesis, and characteristically multinucleated rubricytes. The erythrocyte life span is reduced, and red cells are highly sensitive to hemolysis by H_2O_2 in vitro. Sheep on vitamin-E-deficient diet developed degenerative changes in bone marrow (Kimber and Allen, 1975).

Laboratory animals (Chou et al., 1978; Fitch, 1972) deficient in vitamin E ordinarily do not develop anemia, but their erythrocytes are sensitive to peroxide hemolysis (Smith and Mengel, 1968). Vitamin E functions as a lipid-soluble antioxidant. Hence it is conceivable that deficiency of this vitamin may be associated with oxidative damage to the erythrocytes. Erythrocyte deformability is reduced in rats deficient in vitamin E. Rats with combined vitamin E deficiency and lead toxicity develop an anemia that is more severe than that produced by either situation alone (Levander et al., 1977). See also Chapter 18.

Poodle Macrocytosis Simulating Vitamin B₁₂–Folate Deficiency

An unusual bone marrow dyscrasia, the cytology of which appears to simulate vitamin B₁₂–folate deficiency, is encountered infrequently in poodles, particularly in the miniature and toy breeds. The erythrocytes in the blood are distinctly macrocytic-normochromic (MCV, 85–95 fl; MCHC, 33–36%) and range in number from 4.5–6.0 million/μl of blood. Because of the large size of the erythrocytes, the hemoglobin concentration is near high normal and PCV is elevated (usually 50% or greater) out of proportion to the RBC count. Therefore anemia is not seen. At least two poodles of this type displayed oral mucous membrane defects that responded to parenteral vitamin B₁₂ injections, although morphology of erythrocytes and bone marrow cytology were not influenced significantly.

In addition to *macrocytic erythrocytes*, a search of the stained film may reveal an occasional erythrocyte with *multiple Howell-Jolly bodies* or other nuclear fragments (Fig. 25–2D). Furthermore, large *polychromatic erythrocytes* may be encountered in peripheral

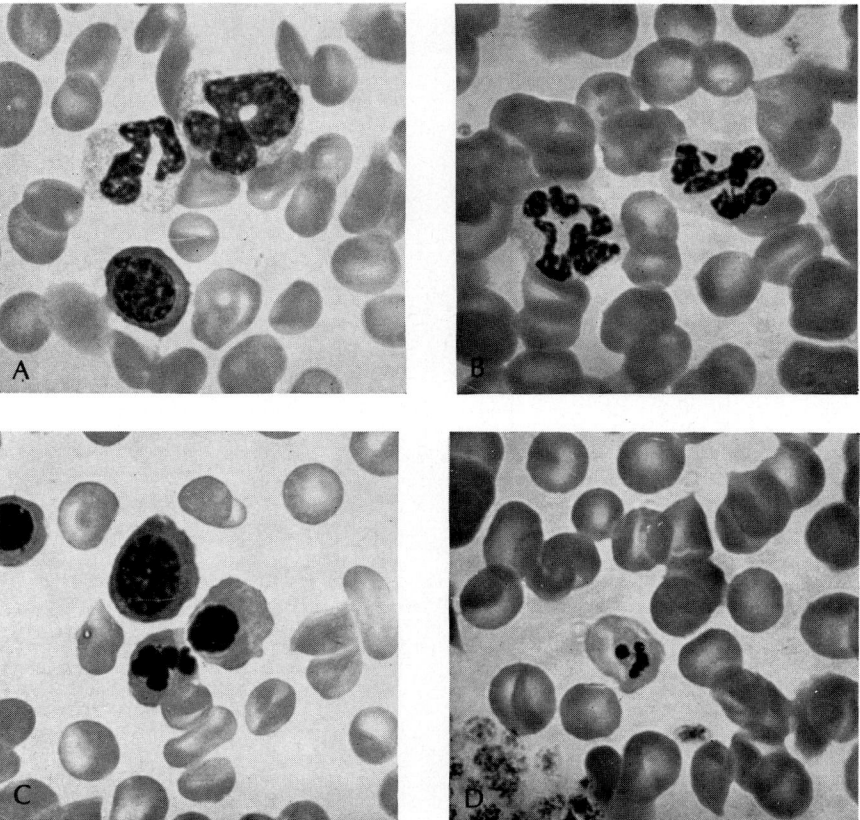

Fig. 25–2. Examples of abnormal maturation of erythrocytes and neutrophils in a poodle with a bone marrow dyscrasia simulating vitamin B₁₂ deficiency. A and C, bone marrow; B and D, peripheral blood.

blood in numbers apparently out of proportion to need for erythrocyte replacement when considered in relation to the elevated PCV and hemoglobin concentration. In some instances, an occasional *hypersegmented neutrophil* may be observed in the peripheral blood (Fig. 25–2B). Bone marrow examination will reveal *abnormal nucleated erythrocytes* characterized by incomplete separation of the two daughter cells in mitosis, larger than normal metarubricytes (megaloblasts) with fragmented nuclei (Fig. 25–2C), and an occasional giant metamyelocyte and hypersegmented or bizarre neutrophil (Fig. 25–2A). A few such nucleated erythrocytes may also be found in the peripheral blood in some cases.

Since the abnormality thus far has been limited to poodles, it would appear to be of genetic origin. The dyscrasia is discovered when blood studies are conducted on a poodle patient presented for complaints other than hematologic in nature. The abnormality is evident from the low normal RBC count associated with PCV and hemoglobin values approaching the maximum normal, which lead in turn to an MCV considerably in excess of normal and an MCHC within the normal range. If a regenerative anemia is seen in such a poodle, interpretation of macrocytosis should be made with caution.

Among 24 poodles with this bone marrow and blood dyscrasia, 15 were females and 9 were males. Their ages ranged from 3 months to 13 years, with a mean of 6.5 ± 4.2 years. Three poodles had no changes in red cell parameters over periods of 6, 7, and 13 months. It is conjectured that the aberration is present at birth and extends throughout life. Furthermore it appears that the abnormality does not seriously affect the well-being of the dog. Selected hematologic data on 9 poodles are presented in Table 25–3, which also lists means and standard deviations for the 24 poodles mentioned above (Schalm, 1976).

Mineral Deficiencies

Iron, copper, and cobalt are the minerals that become deficient most often in certain animals and whose deficiency leads to anemia. Trace mineral deficiencies in cattle have been reviewed (Smart et al., 1981).

Iron

Iron deficiency is discussed in Chapter 22.

Copper

Copper is one of the essential trace metals for humans and animals. It is a constituent of several important enzymes, e.g., superoxide dismutase, δ-aminolevulinic acid dehydrase, and oxidases such as cytochrome *c* oxidase. Many of the clinical abnormalities associated with copper deficiency in humans and animals can be traced to reduced activities of cupric enzymes (Danks, 1980; Demay et al., 1982).

Copper plays an important role in hematopoiesis. Copper deficiency interferes with iron metabolism and can cause impaired absorption, defective transfer from macrophages and hepatocytes to the plasma, and inability of rubricytes to utilize intracellular iron for hemoglobin synthesis (Goodman and Dallman, 1969; Lee et al., 1968, 1976; Williams et al., 1976, 1978; Wintrobe et al., 1981).

Thus in copper deficiency, a *microcytic-hypochromic anemia* very similar to that of iron deficiency is a prominent feature in some animals. Sideroblasts are found in increased numbers in the bone marrow as a result of intracytoplasmic accumulation of iron, probably because of defective mitochondrial uptake of iron consequential to reduced cytochrome *c* oxidase activity (Williams et al., 1976, 1978). The red cell life span is also reduced (Bush et al., 1956), probably as a result of deficiency of erythrocytic superoxide dismutase, a copper- and zinc-containing enzyme (Lynch et al., 1972).

In addition, in the absence of copper, growth rate is reduced, and the hair becomes rough and depigmented even before the anemia develops. Other prominent clinical findings include abnormal wool texture and growth in sheep, bone disorders such as osteoporosis and spontaneous fractures, infertility, cardiovascular defects, and gastrointestinal disturbances (McMurray, 1980). Copper-deficient lambs develop an extensive demyelinating neurologic disease known as "swayback" or "enzootic ataxia" (Underwood, 1977). Cattle and calves exhibit a cardiovascular disorder called "falling disease"; a pro-

Table 25-3. Hematologic Data of Poodles with an Erythrocytic Maturation Defect Leading to Macrocytosis

No.	Type*	Age	Sex	Clinical Complaint	PCV (%)	RBC (×10⁶/μl)	Hb (g/dl)	MCV (fl)	MCHC (%)	MCH (pg)	WBC/μl	Neutrophils/μl	
												Band	Mature
1	TP	3 mo	F	Vomiting	43	4.91	13.8	87.5	32.0	28.1	9,300	0	5,766
2	MP	1 yr	M	Diabetes insipidus	44	4.42	15.0	99.5	34.0	33.9	6,900	0	3,795
3	TP	15 mo	XF	Tracheitis	46	5.44	14.7	84.5	31.9	27.0	9,900	99	7,870
4	MP	3.5 Yr	F	Pharyngitis	53	6.20	18.4	85.5	34.7	29.6	7,600	0	5,244
5	MP	5 yr	M	Central nervous system signs	52	5.43	17.6	95.7	33.8	32.4	8,500	43	5,950
6	P	5 yr	M	Ulcerative colitis	47	4.40	15.7	106.8	33.4	35.7	5,800	29	3,625
7	TP	7 yr	F	Obesity	41	4.45	14.0	92.1	34.1	31.4	9,700	48	6,354
8	MP	11 yr	M	Glaucoma	48	4.93	16.6	97.4	34.6	33.7	7,700	38	4,505
9	P	11 yr	M	Myelitis	42	4.16	14.1	100.9	33.5	33.8	8,100	0	5,427
Means and 1 standard deviation					46.2 ± 4.2	4.99 ± 0.57	15.5 ± 1.6	94.4 ± 7.6	33.5 ± 1.0	31.7 ± 2.9	8,166 ± 1,346	28.6 ± 33.3	5,373 ± 1,322
Mean and 1 standard deviation for 24 poodles					45.5 ± 4.9	4.93 ± 0.66	15.1 ± 2.0	92.6 ± 6.9	33.2 ± 1.3	30.3 ± 3.9			

*TP = toy poodle, MP = miniature poodle, P = poodle.

gressive myocardial atrophy results in heart failure, usually after exercise or excitement. In New Zealand, copper deficiency has been implicated as a cause of postparturient hemoglobinuria in cattle because of copper's role in maintaining red cell integrity (Smith, 1975).

Copper is absorbed rapidly from the stomach and upper intestine. Copper absorption, transport, and distribution are thought to be regulated by metallothionein, a cysteine-rich, copper-binding protein (MW 6,000) present in the intestine, liver, and kidneys (Brimner, 1980). It provides a "mucosal block" for absorption of excessive copper, which induces its synthesis by mucosal cells.

Copper in plasma is largely (90–95%) found bound to ceruloplasmin, a blue glycoprotein (MW about 132,000) found in the α_2-globulin fraction of plasma, and to a lesser extent (5–10%) it is loosely bound to albumin and certain amino acids. It is conjectured that copper bound to albumin and amino acids is delivered from the mucosal cells to the liver for hepatocyte uptake and incorporation in ceruloplasmin or excretion into the bile. Ceruloplasmin is not involved in uptake of copper from the intestine, but it functions in transport of copper from the liver to other tissue sites. Ceruloplasmin binds 6–8 atoms of copper per mole. Ceruloplasmin regulates the rate at which ferrous iron is released from storage cells and is converted to ferric iron bound to transferrin. In addition, ceruloplasmin acts as an antioxidant, scavenges superoxide radicals, serves as an acute phase reactant, and may regulate plasma concentration of adrenaline and serotonin (Frieden, 1980). Neutrophil candidacidal activity is reduced in copper-deficient sheep and cattle (Jones and Suttle, 1981). Copper deficiency of the individual can be determined by measuring serum ceruloplasmin level, erythrocyte superoxide dismutase, and copper content of hair (McMurray, 1980). Reductions in serum ceruloplasmin occur rapidly, whereas those in superoxide dismutase occur slowly; thus these levels provide a means of determining the duration of copper deficiency (Mills, 1980).

In the body, the highest concentrations of copper are found in the liver, brain, and bone marrow. The liver plays the key role in copper metabolism; ruminants have a high hepatic storage capacity. Unlike iron, copper is said to be lost continuously in the excreta and must be replenished from dietary sources. Interaction of copper with certain other trace elements affects its metabolism (Mills, 1980). High levels of dietary zinc and cadmium inhibit copper absorption (through induction of metallothionein) and reduce serum levels of ceruloplasmin and cellular activity of cupric enzymes. Cadmium may be associated with enzootic ataxia of sheep. Interaction with zinc, iron, and cadmium is important in nonruminants, while interaction with molybdenum is much greater in ruminants (see below). Zinc and iron protect swine from adverse effects of copper, and conversely zinc and iron deficiencies accentuate the effects of copper deficiency (Buck, 1981). Studies on calves indicate that increased dietary iron intake can have a marked inhibitory effect on the utilization of dietary copper (Humphries et al., 1983). Molybdenum, at a much smaller dose level, produces the same effect, but clinical signs are different. It is hypothesized that a chemical reaction of dietary molybdate with sulphides in the rumen produces thiomolybdates, which interfere with copper absorption (see reviews by Mason, 1981, 1982).

Copper deficiency may be primary or secondary. Primary deficiency develops in animals fed on milk or on pastures deficient in copper. Copper-deficient areas are known in the United states and other parts of the world. A high mortality from severe anemia due to copper deficiency was reported in pigs 4–7 weeks old (Brooksbank, 1954). Observations have been made on experimentally induced copper and iron deficiencies in growing pigs (Cartwright et al., 1956; Lahey et al., 1952). It was concluded that copper deficiency anemia in swine is morphologically similar to iron deficiency anemia. However, it was reported that dogs made anemic as a result of iron deficiency developed microcytic-hypochromic anemia, but the anemia due to copper deficiency was characterized by normocytic-normochromic erythrocytes (Van Wyk et al., 1953).

Secondary copper deficiency in cattle and sheep occurs when such animals are pastured on soil having a high molybdenum content (Buck, 1981). Such soils have been found in the United States (in California, Oregon, Nevada, and Florida), England, Ireland, New Zealand, and Holland. Molybdenum in excessive amounts interferes with absorption of copper, and this effect is potentiated by dietary content of inorganic sulfate or sulfur amino acids. Studies in rats have shown that molybdenum exerts its effect through formation of tetrathiomolybdate (Mills, 1980). Cattle develop profuse diarrhea and become debilitated, and the pigmentation of their hair fades. Copper administration is used to control development of clinical signs of molybdenosis. Sheep are less susceptible than cattle to excess molybdenum, and horses are not susceptible at all (Marston, 1952). Investigation of the problem should include forage analysis for both copper and molybdenum. Treatment consists of adding copper sulfate to the diet or administration of copper glycinate subcutaneously.

In California, areas known to have high molybdenum content in the soil are Kern, Kings, Fresno, and Madera counties, principally on the west side in those areas that were formerly flooded by streams from the Sierra Nevada mountains. In these areas, cattle are most affected, with calves and young cattle showing the effects most noticeably. Hereford cattle become dirty yellow, and black animals turn mouse-gray. Hematologic findings of a Hereford calf about 6 months of age, one of a group of 20 calves affected with molybdenum poisoning, are presented in Table 25–4. The animal had profuse diarrhea, was dehydrated, and had a faded, dirty yellow hair color. Feces contained 15 ppm of molybdenum, and trichostrongyles were present. Moderate to marked anisocytosis and marked crenation of smaller cells was observed. Reticulocytes were absent. Dehydration masked the anemia, which was normocytic-normochromic.

Cobalt

The importance of cobalt to ruminants for synthesis of vitamin B_{12} by the rumen flora is discussed under Vitamin B_{12} and Folic Acid, above.

Selenium

Selenium is an essential component of the enzyme glutathione peroxidase (GSHPx), present in the erythrocytes. Hence erythrocyte-GSHPx content correlates directly with selenium deficiency in cattle, horses, pigs, sheep, goats, and humans, and measurement of GSHPx level can be used as a diagnostic tool to detect selenium deficiency (Wood and Smith, 1979; see Hussein and Jones, 1982, for references). The GSHPx is involved in the reduction of H_2O_2 and other hydroperoxides in the presence of reduced glutathione (GSH). In the erythrocyte this enzyme protects hemoglobin from oxidation by H_2O_2.

Neutrophil candidacidal activity is reduced in selenium-deficient cattle as in copper-deficient cattle (Boyne and Arthur, 1981).

APLASTIC ANEMIA

Aplastic anemia is characterized by pancytopenia and depressed hematopoiesis as a result of hypoplastic or aplastic marrow. Bone marrow depression may also be expressed as "unicytopenia" (reduction in a single component of the formed elements of blood), e.g., pure red cell aplasia or "bicytopenia" (reduction in two components), e.g., anemia and thrombocytopenia. Such changes usually signify an impending pancytopenia.

Aplastic anemia and pure red cell aplasia are usually acquired, and rarely they may be inherited. Two disorders of the latter type have been reported in children (Wintrobe et

Table 25–4. Hematologic Findings in a 6-Month-Old Female Hereford from a Herd Affected with Molybdenum Poisoning

RBC	6.8 million/μl	WBC	12,000/μl
Hemoglobin	7.8 g/dl	Bands	7%
PCV	23%	Neutrophils	43%
MCV	33.8 fl	Lymphocytes	45%
MCHC	33.9%	Monocytes	2%
		Unclassified cells	3%

al., 1981). The first, Fanconi's anemia, presents a variable clinical picture with pancytopenia, bone marrow hypoplasia, skeletal abnormalities, chromosomal aberrations, increased risks of leukemia and other tumors, and in rare cases pancreatic deficiency and defective uptake of folate. The second, congenital erythroid hypoplasia of Diamond-Blackfan, is a pure red cell aplasia characterized by severe anemia unassociated with leukocyte or platelet abnormalities.

Acquired hypoplasia or aplasia of the bone marrow may be produced by such agents as viral infections, bacterial toxins, radiation, chemicals (e.g., benzene), antimetabolites, and alkylating agents. Spontaneous hemorrhage due to thrombocytopenia and terminal infection as a result of granulocytopenia are common sequelae. Aplastic anemia from a variety of causes has been reported in the horse (Berggren, 1981), dog (Eldor et al., 1978; Glauberg and Beaumont, 1978), and cat. Estrogen toxicity in the dog has been associated with marrow hypoplasia (Legendre, 1976). Cases of transient erythroid hypoplasia have been reported in the dog (Weiss et al., 1982).

Sensitivity of the bone marrow to damage by drugs and chemicals varies among individuals, and bone marrow suppression may be reversible or irreversible. Even when it is reversible, the bone marrow defect may persist for weeks or months after discontinuation of the drug therapy. Some drugs may cause selective depression of a particular cell line, while others may induce a generalized hypoplasia or aplasia. For example, chloramphenicol produces a reversible marrow suppression primarily of the erythroid series in about 50% of human patients, whereas a severe, nonregenerative bone marrow depression occurs in the remainder. See Chapter 5 for observation on toxic effects of chloramphenicol on bone marrow of cats. Phenylbutazone causes more commonly a neutropenia than aplastic anemia.

Bone marrow failure in aplastic anemia can result from qualitative or quantitative abnormalities of hematopoietic stem cells, abnormal cellular or humoral control of hematopoiesis, and abnormalities of hematopoietic microenvironment (Fitchen and Cline, 1978). It has been suggested that drug-induced aplastic anemia may be due to the action of drugs on prostaglandin metabolism (Das, 1978).

Because of its general nonresponsiveness to various modes of therapy, aplastic anemia has also been referred to as refractory anemia. Several modes of therapy have been tried, but with limited success. These have included blood transfusions, splenectomy, administration of androgens and corticosteroids, and bone marrow transplantation. An immune-mediated aplastic anemia responsive to prednisone therapy has been reported (Bagby et al., 1979). Immunologic and hematologic concepts of marrow transplantation in cases of aplastic anemia have been reviewed (Storb, 1979; Thomas et al., 1975). Oral administration of an interferon-containing preparation produced remission of nonregenerative anemia associated with feline leukemia virus in four cats (Tompkins and Cummins, 1982).

Bracken Fern Poisoning

This is a disease of cattle that follows prolonged consumption of bracken fern when other forage is in short supply (Evans et al., 1958; Sippel, 1952). Under normal conditions, clinical signs appear after cattle have been feeding continuously on bracken fern for 1–3 months. High temperature, depression, anorexia, bleeding from body openings, and high mortality characterize the disease. The condition has been produced in sheep experimentally.

Bracken fern contains active carcinogens that are excreted in the urine of cattle feeding on bracken fern (McKenzie, 1978; Pamukcu et al., 1976). In natural and experimental situations, fern-fed cattle develop bladder and gastrointestinal tract tumors. Hematuria manifests as a prominent sign in such cattle, and so the syndrome has been called "chronic enzootic hematuria" or "bovine enzootic hematuria." Hematuria may develop as early as 2 months after commencement of fern feeding, and anemia and pancytopenia develop in later stages from severe damage to the bone marrow.

Radiation Syndrome

Clinical signs and other events in the dog following total-body x-radiation may be divided into several periods as follows:

	Peracute	
1–24 hours	Nausea	
1–7 days	Period of well-being	
7–21 days	Acute symptoms: anorexia, weight loss, depression, vomiting, and diarrhea followed by death or survival	
	Subacute	
25–40 days	Anemia and infertility	
	Chronic	
Over period of months	Obesity, lethargy, decreased efficiency	
	Latent	
Years later	Neoplasia, leukemia, cataract, shortened life span	

Lymphopenia develops within hours, while neutrophils tend to increase in the peripheral circulation during the first 24 hours followed by a gradual decline with marked granulocytopenia usually by the seventh day after exposure (Fig. 25–3). If the WBC count falls below 1,000/μl, few dogs survive.

Thrombocytopenia plus vascular fragility leads to occurrence of petechial and ecchymotic hemorrhages along the gastrointestinal tract in the musculature. If the dog survives, the radioresistant hematopoietic stem cells of the bone marrow and progenitor cells in the spleen and lymph nodes give rise to lymphocytes and granulocytes that begin to return to the peripheral blood around the fifteenth to twentieth day. At this time, because of the maturation arrest in erythropoiesis, a normocytic-normochromic anemia develops, from which the animal also later recovers.

Death is thought to be due to leukopenia and damage to the gastrointestinal tract that leads to septicemia. If bacterial infection is controlled, death can be delayed for several

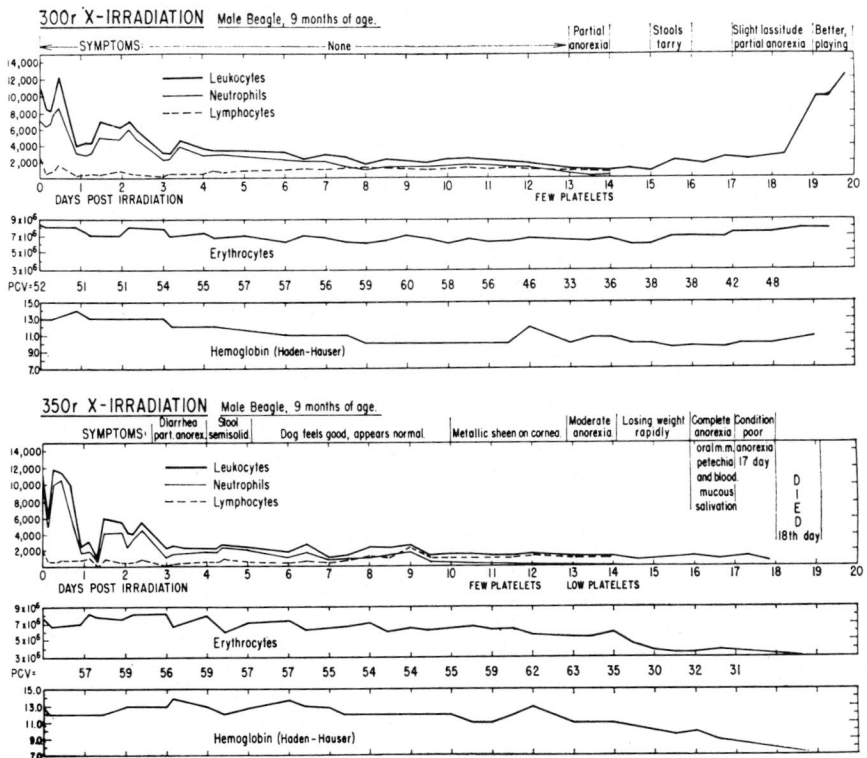

Fig. 25–3. Symptomatology and blood value changes in a beagle surviving a minimum lethal dose x-ray exposure, compared to values seen in a lethal exposure. (From Anderson, 1965; courtesy of the author.)

days. Animals surviving for 25 days have a good chance to recover from the acute radiation syndrome, but may develop tissue abnormalities later as a result of the exposure.

It is of interest that in hibernating animals, such as the marmot, exposed to whole-body irradiation, the destructive effects do not become apparent as long as the animal is hibernating (Brace, 1952; Smith and Grenan, 1951). Immediately upon termination of hibernation, the blood components rapidly diminish in number until death occurs 4–10 days later. This finding reveals that the rate of development of lethal process following radiation bears a close relationship to the metabolic rate.

Hematologic effects of whole-body gamma radiation in newborn Yorkshire pigs have been described (Case and Simon, 1972). Lymphopenia developed usually within 24 hours, while neutropenia and anemia appeared after 10–14 days.

Other Causes

Aplastic anemia has been reported in cattle fed extracted soybean meal (Rundles, 1958). It resulted from formation of a toxic factor (dichlorovinylcysteine) by the interaction of trichloroethylene used to extract the oil and cysteine in the beans (Strafuss and Sautter, 1967).

SECONDARY ANEMIAS FROM ERYTHROID HYPOPLASIA

A normocytic-normochromic anemia, usually unaccompanied by adequate reticulocyte response, is seen in a variety of conditions of diverse etiology. The finding of anemia in such patients is usually incidental and of secondary importance. Although a blood loss or hemolytic anemia, within the first three days of its occurrence, may manifest as a nonresponsive, normocytic-normochromic anemia, such anemias are to be excluded from consideration under secondary anemias from erythroid hypoplasia. Two broad categories of secondary anemias have been recognized (Wintrobe et al., 1981): (a) those without an obvious intrinsic marrow disease as in anemias associated with renal failure, liver disease, endocrine disorder, and deficiency or impaired utilization of iron; and (b) those with marrow abnormality as in anemias associated with marrow hypoplasia or aplasia, marrow infiltration by metastatic tumors or leukemic cells, and dyserythropoiesis.

Anemia of Chronic Disorders or Inflammatory Disease

A normocytic-normochromic, nonresponsive anemia is commonly found in association with chronic infections, chronic noninfectious inflammatory conditions, and some types of malignancies. These types of anemias are grouped under a common category presently referred to as anemia of inflammatory disease (AID). In natural cases in humans, anemia develops slowly, usually over a period of 1–2 months, and then becomes stabilized. The degree of anemia varies with the nature of the disease process but is usually mild to modest and without serious consequences. A variety of abnormalities have been found with regard to iron metabolism and erythropoiesis in such patients (Bierman, 1980; Cartwright et al., 1946; Douglas and Adamson, 1975; Erslev, 1972; Erslev and Gabuzda, 1979; Vaughan and Saifi, 1939). These are summarized in Table 22–3 and reviewed by Feldman and Kaneko (1981).

Although the anemia is usually normocytic-normochromic, in rare instances it may become microcytic-hypochromic, as in true iron deficiency. Early observations indicated that even a sterile abscess produced by injection of 1.0 ml of turpentine subcutaneously will diminish the production of new hemoglobin in the anemic dog (Robscheit-Robbins and Whipple, 1936). Similarly, anemia developed in cats injected with 0.75 ml of turpentine subcutaneously into the gluteal region (Mahaffey and Smith, 1978); PCV declined in all cats by as much as one third of basal value within 5 to 10 days.

Feldman (Feldman et al., 1981a, b, c, d) conducted a series of experiments in dogs to characterize the nature of AID and define its possible causes. A noninfectious local inflammation was induced in dogs by a single injection of 0.5 ml Freund's complete adjuvant subcutaneously in the flank region. Abscesses formed within 5–7 days and then began to open and drain. Formation of the abscesses was associated with reductions in red cell parameters by as much as 30% within 11–13 days, although a frank anemia (PCV <37%) was not evident. The red cell indexes and reticulocyte counts indicated red cell changes as normocytic, normochromic, and nonresponsive in nature. The depressed erythropoiesis was characterized by reduced levels of serum iron, decreased total iron binding capacity (serum transferrin), reduced percent saturation of transferrin, and decreased numbers of bone marrow sideroblasts. Free protoporphyrin concentration within red cells was increased, and similarly serum levels of copper, zinc, and ceruloplasmin were elevated. Bone marrow reticuloendothelial (macrophage) iron and hepatic nonheme iron were increased. Ferrokinetic studies indicated effective but inadequate erythropoietic response of the bone marrow limited mainly by the amount of iron available for this purpose. Iron stored in marrow macrophages seemed to be in a form that could not be readily mobilized by injection of deferoxamine, an iron-chelating agent.

Anemia of inflammatory disease has been attributed to a variety of causes such as shortened red cell survival, impaired marrow erythropoiesis, and defective iron metabolism (Cartwright, 1966; Zucker, 1974). Kinetic data indicate that anemia develops because bone marrow fails to compensate for a slight decrease in red cell life span (Cartwright, 1966; Cartwright and Lee, 1971; Cavill et al., 1977). This shortened red cell life span is probably the result of an extraerythrocytic factor of unknown character. The reason for impaired erythropoiesis seems to be the sequestration of iron in marrow macrophages so that it is unavailable for compensatory erythropoiesis. Lower levels of serum iron and transferrin saturation are primarily related to impaired mobilization of iron from storage sites in marrow macrophages and hepatocytes (Erslev, 1972; Feldman and Kaneko, 1981) and probably not to reduced iron absorption (Cartwright and Wintrobe, 1952). Cobalt is less effective in stimulating erythropoiesis in cats with AID than in normal cats. Administration of ferric citrate in cats with AID does not prevent occurrence of anemia, although serum iron may increase and some bone marrow response may be evident (Weiss et al., 1983). Thus administration of iron to treat anemia of this nature is uneventful; the cause of AID must be traced and alleviated to stimulate compensatory erythropoiesis. Iron deposits may be mobilized by administration of certain hormones, e.g., androgens and corticosteroids (Reeves et al., 1981).

Other abnormalities in AID include abnormalities of hemoglobin synthesis manifested as aberrant synthesis and excretion of porphyrins. For example, free erythrocyte porphyrin is elevated, and excretion of coproporphyrin I and III is increased. Hemoglobin synthesis by erythroid cells is also reduced in vitro (Kumar, 1979). Icterus index tends to be higher in AID than in anemia of iron deficiency (Nelson and Kehl, 1979).

Renal Disease with Uremia

End stage kidney disease (chronic interstitial nephritis) in the dog is generally associated with a normocytic-normochromic, nonresponsive anemia. A similar situation occurs in humans with chronic renal disease accompanied by uremia, the degree of anemia being directly related to the degree of nitrogen retention (Scarlett, 1929). Anemia may be masked by dehydration in which case it becomes prominent after hydration. An occasional human patient characteristically exhibits highly crenated red ("burr") cells and occasionally other red cell forms such as triangular and helmet cells (Wintrobe et al., 1981); the presence of burr cells is proportional to the degree of uremia (Fried, 1978). This has not been our experience with the dog. Appendix Case 5 is typical of the depression anemia associated with nephritis and uremia in the dog. See also Chapter 36.

The anemia of renal disease is due to inadequate erythrocyte production. Several pathogenic mechanisms have been proposed (Fried, 1978; Mansell and Grimes, 1979; Wallner and Vautrin, 1981) including decreased production of erythropoietin because of renal damage; production of a factor or factors inhibiting erythropoietic activity, e.g., guanidinosuccinic acid, phenols, and urea; and decreased erythrocyte survival because of extracellular and intracellular defects. Bone marrow studies in humans have revealed def-

inite evidence of hypoplasia of the erythrocytic tissues when the nonprotein nitrogen
level (BUN) of the blood was over 150 mg/dl
(Callen and Limarzi, 1950). Levin and
Gregory (1952) found normal or hypocellular
bone marrow in 50% of human cases of uremia and suggested hemolysis and functional
impairment of erythropoiesis as possible
causes of anemia.

Erslev (1958) experimentally reproduced
uremia in rabbits and made observations on
the erythropoietic factor. He concluded that
severe uremia is associated with significant
suppression of erythropoietic activity of
serum (erythropoietin) and depression of metabolism of erythropoietic cells. Recent studies with more sensitive methods to assay
erythropoietin have, however, indicated normal or even slightly increased levels (Radtke
et al., 1979). It is possible that a defective response of marrow to erythropoietin may be
involved in causation of anemia in such cases.
Red cells in chronic renal failure show several
metabolic abnormalities and appear to be in
hypermetabolic state (Mansell and Grimes,
1979; Rodriguez-Commes et al., 1979). Infusion of erythropoietin-rich plasma stimulated
erythropoiesis in subnephrectomized uremic
sheep regardless of the degree of uremia (Eschbach et al., 1984).

Neutrophil and immune functions may also
be compromised because patients with renal
disease are prone to infection (Fried, 1978).
Such patients also show functional abnormalities of platelets. Platelet count is either
normal or slightly increased, but platelet function is markedly impaired, resulting in hemostatic abnormality (see Chapter 17 for more
comments). Iron deficiency may develop as a
secondary complication of blood loss.

Therapeutic approaches to management of
anemia in human patients with kidney disease have been varied. Mild cases usually required no therapy. In severe cases, hemodialysis alleviated other symptoms of uremia
but did not improve the anemia. Kidney
transplantation is associated with increased
erythropoietin formation and red cell regeneration. Some stimulation of erythropoiesis
was observed after administration of androgens (Hendler et al., 1974).

Liver Disease

A normocytic-normochromic anemia is
seen in human patients with cirrhosis and
other uncomplicated liver diseases. Prominent findings include the presence of target
cells, "thin macrocytes," which are erythrocytes with increased diameter but normal
MCV, and acanthocytes (Figs. 20–6C, 20–8E).
The latter have been called "spur cells." Reticulocyte count is variable but may be elevated, and there is mild thrombocytopenia
and a variable leukocyte response. Bone marrow erythropoietic activity is reduced for the
degree of anemia. Anemia associated with
liver disease has been observed in animals,
but remains to be characterized fully.

Anemia is believed to result from either decreased erythrocyte survival (Felsher et al.,
1968; Hume et al., 1970) or impaired marrow
response (Kimber et al., 1965), the former
probably being the major cause. Other contributing mechanisms include chronic blood
loss from the gastrointestinal tract and iron
and folic acid deficiencies (Kimber et al.,
1965).

Although the precise mechanism of decreased erythrocyte survival remains to be defined, it may be a consequence of characteristic changes observed in erythrocyte
membrane lipids of such patients (see Chapter 20). Thin macrocytes have increased mem-
rane phospholipid and cholesterol, whereas
acanthocytes have increased cholesterol but
nearly normal phospholipids. Alterations in
red cell cholesterol:phospholipid ratios are attributed to a decrease in plasma LCAT (lysolecithin cholesterol acyltransferase) activity, increased plasma levels of bile salts, and
increased plasma free cholesterol:phospho-
lipid ratio (Cooper and Jandl, 1968, 1969,
1972). Increased rigidity promoting red cell
lysis was thought to result also from decreased intraerythrocytic ATP, probably secondary to hypophosphatemia common to hepatic disease (Wolf and Koett, 1980).
Inadequate erythroid response of the bone
marrow may be due to diminished erythropoietin production because of reduced hepatic function (see Chapter 13) or impaired
mobilization of hepatic iron.

Acute intravascular hemolysis, with hemoglobinemia and hemoglobinuria, has been observed in some horses with fulminating hepatic failure (Tennant et al., 1972; 1973). Although pathogenesis of the anemia remains unknown, it may be a consequence of altered structural integrity of the erythrocytes resulting from an acquired biochemical abnormality.

Neoplasia

Neoplasia, especially when malignant, causes a selective depression of erythrogenesis, although granulocytosis may be stimulated in some cases. Several mechanisms of anemia of malignancy have been proposed (DeGowin and Gibson, 1979; Madewell and Feldman, 1980; Zucker et al., 1980). These include more frequently marrow suppression, blood loss, autoantibody production, and hematopoietic dysplasia. Anemia may occur from a single pathophysiologic mechanism, but often more than one mechanism is involved. For example, when blood loss from the neoplasm is superimposed, the blood picture will show a combination of signs of depression of erythropoiesis, as well as a modest response to blood loss (reticulocytosis). Anemia may also occur from cancer chemotherapy.

Normocytic-normochromic, nonresponsive anemia associated with feline leukemia virus infection in cats is attributed to diminished erythropoiesis (Madewell et al., 1983). A case of tumor-associated chronic anemia in a cat is described in Appendix Case 46.

Endocrine Diseases

Hypothyroidism in the dog may be associated with anemia. The anemia is commonly borderline, with PCV ranging between 30 and 37%, although in some instances it may fall below 30%. The anemia is normocytic-normochromic, with leptocytosis commonly being a prominent feature (see Appendix Case 6 and Chapter 36). A mild, normocytic-normochromic anemia was reported in cattle afflicted with fluorosis and developing hypothyroidism (Hillman et al., 1979).

A mild to moderate anemia has been observed in humans with endocrine disorders of thyroid, adrenal, gonads, and pituitary, e.g., hypothyroidism, Addison's disease, hy-

pogonadism in males, hypopituitarism, and hyperparathyroidism. (See Chapter 18 for hormonal influences on erythropoiesis.) In hypothyroidism, erythrocyte morphology may be normocytic-normochromic, macrocytic-hypochromic, or macrocytic. The first two may be associated with decreased serum iron because of diminished iron absorption, while the last may be related to vitamin B_{12}–folate deficiency. Acanthocytes have been observed in about 20% of cases. Erythrocyte life span is normal or slightly increased in humans (Kiely et al., 1967; Tudhope and Wilson, 1960, 1969) as well as in dogs (Cline and Berlin, 1963). The anemia is considered "adaptive" in nature in that marrow erythropoietic activity is depressed in relation to diminished metabolic activity of the patient (Bomford, 1938; Kiely et al., 1967). Thyroid hormones were found to exert a direct effect on erythrogenesis (Malgor et al., 1975), but the in vivo response is very slow, taking 3–12 months to become evident (Tudhope and Wilson, 1960, 1969). A few patients with hyperthyroidism were also found to have anemia (Grenfell and Sheeler, 1979; Rivlin and Wagner, 1969).

Parasitism in Sheep and Cattle

The trichostrongyloid parasites of cattle and sheep (excluding *Haemonchus contortus*) may produce a severe normocytic-normochromic anemia that has all the appearances of selective depression of erythropoiesis (Appendix Case 71). The PCV may fall to 12%, and there is no evidence of reticulocytosis to compensate for the anemia. A PCV as low as 5% was observed in a lamb in association with a very heavy parasitism of this nature. See Chapter 22 for blood loss anemia associated with parasitism.

REFERENCES

Afronsky, D.: Folic Acid Deficiency in the Dog. Science, *120*:803, 1954.
Alexander, F., and Davies, M.E.: Studies on Vitamin B_{12} in the Horse. Brit. Vet. J., *125*:169, 1969.
Allen, R.H.: Human Vitamin B_{12} Transport Proteins. Prog. Hematol., *9*:57, 1975.
Andersen, A.C.: Effects of Ionizing Radiations on Blood. *In* Veterinary Hematology. 2nd ed. Schalm, O.W., ed. Lea and Febiger, Philadelphia, ch. 10, 1965.
Ausman, L.M., and Hayes, K.C.: Vitamin E Deficiency

Anemia in Old and New World Monkeys. Amer. J. Clin. Nutr., 27:1141, 1974.

Bachrach, W.H., and Fogelson, S.J.: The Role of the Upper Gastrointestinal Tract in the Etiology of Pernicious Anemia. J. Lab. Clin. Med., 24:249, 1938.

Bagby, G.G., et al.: Prednisone-Responsive Aplastic Anemia: A Mechanism of Glucocorticoid Action. Blood, 54:322, 1979.

Berggren, P.C.: Aplastic Anemia in a Horse. J. Amer. Vet. Med. Ass., 179:1400, 1981.

Bierman, A.H.: Recent Advances in the Clinical Hematology Laboratory: The Diagnosis of Anemia. J. Florida Med. Ass., 67:107, 1980.

Bomford, R.: Anemia in Myxoedema. Q. J. Med., 7:495, 1938.

Boyne, R., and Arthur, J.R.: Effects of Selenium and Copper Deficiency on Neutrophil Function in Cattle. J. Comp. Path., 91:271, 1981.

Brace, K.C.: Histological Changes in the Tissues of the Hibernating Marmot following Whole Body Irradiation. Science, 116:570, 1952.

Brandy, P.S., et al.: Erythrocyte Characteristics in Vitamin E-Responsive Anemia of the Owl Monkey (Aotus trivirgatus). Amer. J. Vet. Res., 43:1488, 1982.

Brimner, I.: Absorption, Transport, and Distribution of Copper. Ciba Found. Symp., 79:23, 1980.

Brooksbank, N.H.: Anaemia in Piglets Associated with a Copper Deficiency. Vet. Rec., 66:322, 1954.

Buck, W.B.: Copper-Molybdenum. *In* Current Veterinary Therapy: Food Animal Practice, Howard, J.L., ed. W.B. Saunders, Philadelphia, p. 495, 1981.

Bush, J.A., et al.: Studies on Copper Metabolism. J. Exp. Med., 103:701, 1956.

Callen, I.R., and Limarzi, L.R.: Blood and Bone Marrow Studies in Renal Disease. Amer. J. Clin. Path., 20:3, 1950.

Cartwright, G.E.: The Anemia of Chronic Disorders. Semin. Hematol., 3:351, 1966.

Cartwright, G.E., and Lee, G.R.: The Anemia of Chronic Disorders. Brit. J. Haematol., 21:147, 1971.

Cartwright, G.E., and Wintrobe, M.M.: The Anemia of Infection. *In* Advances in Internal Medicine. Dock, W., and Snapper, I., eds. Year Book Publishers, Chicago, p. 165, 1952.

Cartwright, G.E., et al.: Studies on Anemia in Swine Due to Pyridoxine Deficiency, Together with Data on Phenylhydrazine Anemia. J. Biol. Chem., 153:171, 1944.

Cartwright, G.E., et al.: The Anemia Associated with Chronic Infection. Science, 103:72, 1946.

Cartwright, G.E., et al.: Niacin Deficiency Anemia in Swine. Arch. Biochem., 19:109, 1948.

Cartwright, G.E., et al.: Experimental Production of Nutritional Macrocytic Anemia in Swine. III. Further Studies on Pteroylglutamic Acid Deficiency. J. Lab. Clin. Med., 36:675, 1950.

Cartwright, G.E., et al.: Hematologic Manifestations of Vitamin B12 Deficiency in Swine. Blood, 6:867, 1951.

Cartwright, G.E., et al.: Studies on Copper Metabolism. XVII. Further Observations on the Anemia of Copper Deficiency in Swine. Blood, 11:143, 1956.

Case, M.T., and Simon, J.: Whole-Body Gamma Irradiation of Newborn Pigs: Hematologic Changes. Amer. J. Vet. Res., 33:1217, 1972.

Cavill, I., et al.: Erythropoiesis in the Anemias of Chronic Disease. Scand. J. Haematol., 19:509, 1977.

Chou, S.C., et al.: Abnormalities of Iron Metabolism and Erythropoiesis in Vitamin E-Deficient Rabbits. Blood, 52:187, 1978.

Clifford, R.J., et al.: Effect of Feeding Penicillin and Vitamin B12 to Mature Debilitated Horses. Vet. Rec., 68:48, 1956.

Cline, M.J., and Berlin, N.I.: Erythropoiesis and Red Cell Survival in the Hypothyroid Dog. Amer. J. Physiol., 204:415, 1963.

Cooper, R.A., and Jandl, J.H.: Bile Salts and Cholesterol in the Pathogenesis of Target Cells in Obstructive Jaundice. J. Clin. Invest., 47:809, 1968; ibid., 48:906, 1969; ibid., 51:182, 1972.

Cooperman, J.M., et al.: Studies on the Requirements of the Monkey for Riboflavin and a New Factor in Liver. J. Nutr., 30:45, 1945.

Danks, D.M.: Copper Deficiency in Humans. Ciba Found. Symp., 79:209, 1980.

Das, U.N.: Drug-Induced Aplastic Anemia and Prostaglandins. Can. Med. Ass. J., 119:119, 1978.

Davies, E.: The Production of Vitamin B12 in the Horse. Brit. Vet. J., 127:34, 1971.

DeGowin, R.L., and Gibson, D.P.: Erythropoietin and the Anemia of Mice Bearing Extramedullary Tumor. J. Lab. Clin. Med., 94:303, 1979.

Demay, A., et al.: Effects of Copper on Humans, Laboratory and Farm Animals, Terrestrial Plants and Aquatic Life: Water Supply for Livestock. CRC Crit. Rev. Environmental Control, 12:229, 1982.

Douglas, S.W., and Adamson, J.W.: The Anemia of Chronic Disorders: Studies of Marrow Regulation and Iron Metabolism. Blood, 45:55, 1975.

Eldor, A., et al.: Androgen-Responsive Aplastic Anemia in a Dog. J. Amer. Vet. Med. Ass., 173:304, 1978.

Erslev, A.J.: Erythropoietic Function in Uremic Rabbits. Arch. Intern. Med., 101:407, 1958.

Erslev, A.J.: Anemia of Chronic Disorders. *In* Hematology. William, W.J., et al., eds. McGraw-Hill, New York, pp. 371–73, 1972.

Erslev, A.J., and Gabuzda, T.G.: Pathophysiology of Blood, W.B. Saunders, Philadelphia, pp. 23–113, 1979.

Eschbach, J.W., et al.: The Anemia of Chronic Renal Failure in Sheep. Response to Erythropoietin Rich Plasma in Vivo. J. Clin. Invest., 74:434, 1984.

Evans, I.A., et al.: Studies on Bracken Poisoning in Cattle. Part V. Brit. Vet. J., 114:253, 1958.

Feldman, B.F., and Kaneko, J.J.: The Anemia of Inflammatory Disease in the Dog. I. The Nature of the Problem. Vet. Res. Commun., 4:237, 1981.

Feldman, B.F., et al.: Anemia of Inflammatory Disease in the Dog: Ferrokinetics of Adjuvant-Induced Anemia. Amer. J. Vet. Res., 42:583, 1981a.

Feldman, B.F., et al.: Anemia of Inflammatory Disease in the Dog: Availability of Storage Iron in Inflammatory Disease. Amer. J. Vet. Res., 42:586, 1981b.

Feldman, B.F., et al.: Anemia of Inflammatory Disease in the Dog: Clinical Characterization. Amer. J. Vet. Res., 42:1109, 1981c.

Feldman, B.F., et al.: Anemia of Inflammatory Disease in the Dog: Measurement of Hepatic Superoxide Dismutase, Hepatic Nonheme Iron, Copper, Zinc, and

Ceruloplasmin and Serum Iron, Copper, and Zinc. Amer. J. Vet. Res., 42:1114, 1981d.

Felsher, B.F., et al.: Indirect Reacting Bilirubinemia in Cirrhosis: Its Relation to Red Cell Survival. Amer. J. Dig. Dis., 13:598, 1968.

Fitch, C.D.: The Red Blood Cell in the Vitamin E–Deficient Monkey. Amer. J. Clin. Nutr., 21:51, 1968; Ann. N.Y. Acad. Med., 203:172, 1972.

Fitchen, J.H., and Cline, M.J.: Recent Development in Understanding the Pathogenesis of Aplastic Anemia. Amer. J. Hematol., 5:365, 1978.

Fouts, P.J., et al.: Nutritional Microcytic Hypochromic Anemia in Dogs Cured with Crystalline Factor I. Amer. J. Med. Sci., 199:163, 1940.

Foy, H., et al.: Effect of Riboflavin Deficiency on Bone Marrow Function and Protein Metabolism in Baboons: Preliminary Report. Brit. J. Nutr., 18:307, 1964.

Foy, H., et al.: Isotopic and Cytologic Estimations of Marrow Erythroid Activity in Normal and Riboflavin Deficient Baboons. Acta Haematol., 39:118, 1968.

Fried, W.: Hematologic Complications of Chronic Renal Failure. Med. Clin. North Amer., 62:1363, 1978.

Frieden, E.: Ceruloplasmin: A Multi-Functional Metalloprotein of Vertebrate Plasma. Ciba Found. Symp., 79:93, 1980.

Gershoff, S.N., et al.: Vitamin B_6 Deficiency and Oxalate Nephrocalcinosis in the Cat. Amer. J. Med., 27:72, 1959.

Glauberg, A., and Beaumont, P.R.: Acquired Erythrocyte Aplasia in a Dog: A Case Report. J. Amer. Anim. Hosp. Ass., 14(5):635, 1978.

Goodman, J.R., and Dallman, P.R.: Role of Copper in Iron Localization in Developing Erythrocytes. Blood, 34:747, 1969.

Grenfell, R.F., and Sheeler, L.R.: Association of Thyroid Dysfunction and Anemia. J. Miss. State Med. Ass., 20:222, 1979.

Handler, P., and Dann, W.J.: The Biochemical Defects in Nicotinic Acid Deficiency. J. Biol. Chem., 145:145, 1942.

Handler, P., and Featherston, W.P.: The Biochemical Defect in Nicotinic Acid Deficiency. II. On the Nature of the Anemia. J. Biol. Chem., 151:395, 1943.

Hendler, E.D., et al.: Controlled Study of Androgen Therapy in Anemia of Patients on Maintenance Hemodialysis. New Eng. J. Med., 291:1046, 1974.

Hendrickx, H.K., et al.: Absorption of Vitamin B_{12} from the Colon of the Pig. J. Anim. Sci., 23:1036, 1964.

Herbert, V., and Jacob, E.: Destruction of Vitamin B_{12} by Ascorbic Acid. J. Amer. Med. Ass., 214:2035, 1974.

Hillman, D., et al.: Hypothyroidism and Anemia Related to Fluoride in Dairy Cattle. J. Dairy Sci., 62:416, 1979.

Hines, J.D.: Ascorbic Acid and Vitamin B_{12} Deficiency. J. Amer. Med. Ass., 234:24, 1975.

Hume, R., et al.: Red Cell Survival in Biliary Cirrhosis. J. Clin. Pathol., 23:397, 1970.

Humphries, W.R., et al.: The Influence of Dietary Iron and Molybdenum on Copper Metabolism in Calves. Brit. J. Nutr., 49:77, 1983.

Hussein, K.M., and Jones, B.-E.V.: Effects of Selenium Administration on Erythrocyte and Blood Plasma Glutathione Peroxidase Activity in Goats. Acta Vet. Scand., 23:559, 1982.

Johnson, B.C., and Nesheim, R.O.: Vitamin B_{12} and Pter-

oylglutamic Acid Deficiency in the Baby Pig, without Use of Antagonist. J. Anim. Sci., 8:622, 1949 (abstr.).

Jones, D.G., and Suttle, N.F.: Some Effects of Copper Deficiency on Leucocyte Function in Sheep and Cattle. Res. Vet. Sci., 31:151, 1981.

Keyhani, M., et al.: Erythropoiesis in Pyridoxine Deficient Mice. Proc. Soc. Exp. Biol. Med., 146:114, 1974.

Kiely, J.M., et al.: Erythrokinetics in Myxedema. Ann. Intern. Med., 67:533, 1967.

Kimber, R.J., and Allen, S.H.: An Abnormality of the Bone Marrow Associated with Vitamin E Deficiency in Sheep. Brit. J. Nutri., 33:357, 1975.

Kimber, C., et al.: The Mechanism of Anemia in Chronic Liver Disease. Q. J. Med., 34:33, 1965.

Kodicek, E., and Carpenter, K.J.: Experimental Anemias in the Rat. I. Macrocytic Anemia in Chronic Pteroylglutamic Acid Deficiency and after Splenectomy in Bartonella muris Infection. Blood, 5:522, 1950.

Kornberg, A., et al.: Blood Regeneration in Pyridoxine-Deficient Rats. Amer. J. Physiol., 143:434, 1945a.

Kornberg, A., et al.: Blood Regeneration in Rats Deficient in Biotin, Thiamin, or Riboflavin. Amer. J. Physiol., 145:54, 1945b.

Krehl, W.A., and Elvehjem, C.A.: The Importance of "Folic Acid" in Rations Low in Nicotinic Acid. J. Biol. Chem., 158:173, 1945.

Kumar, R.: Mechanism of Anaemia of Chronic Infection: Study of Haemoglobin Synthesis. Indian J. Med. Res., 70:463, 1979.

Lahey, M.E., et al.: Studies on Copper Metabolism. II. Hematologic Manifestations of Copper Deficiency in Swine. Blood, 7:1053, 1952.

Lee, G.R., et al.: Iron Metabolism in Copper-Deficient Swine. J. Clin. Invest., 47:2058, 1968.

Lee, G.R., et al.: Role of Copper in Iron Metabolism and Heme Biosynthesis. In Trace Elements in Human Health and Disease. Prasad, A., ed. Academic Press, New York, p. 373, 1976.

Legendre, A.M.: Estrogen-Induced Marrow Hypoplasia in a Dog. J. Amer. Anim. Hosp. Ass., 12(4):525, 1976.

Levander, O.A., et al.: Morphology of Erythrocytes from Vitamin E Deficient Lead-Poisoned Rats. J. Nutr., 107:1828, 1977.

Levin, W.C., and Gregory, L.: Hematological Effects of Uremia. Southern Med. J., 45:121, 1952.

Lynch, R.E., et al.: Copper and the Red Cell Membrane (abstr.). Blood, 40:963, 1972.

Lynch, R.E., et al.: The Anemia of Vitamin E Deficiency in Swine: An Experimental Model of the Human Congenital Dyserythropoietic Anemias. Amer. J. Hematol., 2:145, 1977.

Madewell, B.R., and Feldman, B.F.: Characterization of Anemias Associated with Neoplasia in Small Animals. J. Amer. Vet. Med. Ass., 176:419, 1980.

Madewell, B.R., et al.: Ferrokinetic and Erythrocyte Survival Studies in Healthy and Anemic Cats. Amer. J. Vet. Res., 44:424, 1983.

Mahaffey, E.A., and Smith, J.E.: Depression Anemia in Cats. Feline Pract., 8(5):19, 1978.

Malgor, L.A., et al.: Direct Effects of Thyroid Hormones on Bone Marrow Erythroid Cells of Rats. Blood, 45:671, 1975.

Mansell, M., and Grimes, A.J.: Red and White Cell Abnormalities in Chronic Renal Failure. Brit. J. Hematol., 42:169, 1979.

Marston, H.R.: Cobalt, Copper and Molybdenum in the Nutrition of Animals and Plants. Physiol. Rev., *32*:66, 1952.

Mason, J.: Molybdenum-Copper Antagonism in Ruminants: A Review of the Biochemical Basis. Irish Vet. Res., *35*:221, 1981.

Mason, J.: The Putative Role of Thiomolybdates in the Pathogenesis of Mo-Induced Hypocupraemia and Molybdenosis: Some Recent Developments. Irish Vet. J., *36*:164, 1982.

Maynard, L.A.: Animal Species That Feed Mankind: The Role of Nutrition. Science, *120*:164, 1954.

McKenzie, R.A.: Bovine Enzootic Haematuria in Queensland. Aust. Vet. J., *54*:61, 1978.

McKibbin, J.M., et al.: Studies on Anemia in Dogs Due to Pyridoxine Deficiency. J. Biol. Chem., *142*:77, 1942.

McMurray, C.H.: Copper Deficiency in Ruminants. Ciba Found. Symp., *79*:183, 1980.

Mills, C.F.: Metabolic Interactions of Copper with Other Trace Elements. Ciba Found. Symp., *79*:49, 325, 1980.

Mitchell, H.H., et al.: The Riboflavin Requirement of the Growing Pig at Two Environmental Temperatures. J. Nutr., *41*:317, 1950.

Mookerjea, S., and Hawkins, W.W.: Haematopoiesis in the Rat in Riboflavin Deficiency. Brit. J. Nutr., *14*:239, 1960.

Nelson, R.B., and Kehl, D.: Pale Plasma of Iron Deficiency: Meulengracht Test Revisited. Lancet, *1(8122)*:922, 1979.

Pamukcu, A.M., et al.: Naturally Occurring and Bracken-Fern-Induced Bovine Urinary Bladder Tumors. Vet. Path., *13*:110, 1976.

Radtke, H.W., et al.: Serum Erythropoietin Concentration in Chronic Renal Failure: Relationship of Degree of Anemia and Excretory Renal Function. Blood, *54*:877, 1979.

Reeves, W.B., et al.: Influence of Hormones on the Release of Iron by Macrophages. J. Reticuloendothel. Soc., *29*:173, 1981.

Rhoads, C.P., and Miller, D.K.: The Production in Dogs of Chronic Black Tongue with Anemia. J. Exp. Med., *58*:585, 1933.

Rivlin, R.S., and Wagner, H.N.: Anemia in Hyperthyroidism. Ann. Intern. Med., *79*:507, 1969.

Robscheit-Robbins, F.S., and Whipple, G.H.: Infection and Intoxication: Their Influence upon Hemoglobin Production in Experimental Anemia. J. Exp. Med., *63*:767, 1936.

Rodriguez-Commes, J.L., et al.: Metabolism of Red Blood Cells in Chronic Renal Failure. I. Glycolytic Enzyme Levels. Nephron, *24*:21, 1979.

Rundles, W.: Toxic Protein Derivatives Causing Aplastic Anemia: A Review. Blood, *13*:899, 1958.

Santiyanont, R., et al.: Accumulation of Orthochromatic Normoblasts in Bone Marrow of Vitamin E Deficient Monkey, Macaca fasicularis. J. Nutr., *107*:2026, 1977.

Scarlett, E.P.: The Significance of High-Grade Anemia in Chronic Nephritis. Amer. J. Med. Sci., *178*:215, 1929.

Schalm, O.W.: Erythrocyte Macrocytosis in Miniature and Toy Poodles. Canine Pract., *3(6)*:55, 1976.

Schweigert, B.S., et al.: The Metabolic Conversion of Tryptophan to Nicotinic Acid and to N-methylnicotinamide. Arch. Biochem., *12*:139, 1947.

Sippel, W.L.: Bracken Fern Poisoning. J. Amer. Vet. Med. Ass., *121*:9, 1952.

Smart, M.E., et al.: Trace Mineral Deficiencies in Cattle. A Review. Can. Vet. J., *22*:372, 1981.

Smith, B.: The Effects of Copper Supplementation on Stock Health and Production. N.Z. Vet., *23*:73, 1975.

Smith, F., and Grenan, M.M.: Circulating Blood Cells following Radiation in Hibernating Woodchuck. Fed. Proc., *10*:128, 1951.

Smith, K.A., and Mengel, C.E.: Association of Iron-Dextran Induced Hemolysis and Lipid Peroxidation in Mice. J. Lab. Clin. Med., *72*:505, 1968.

Smith, S.E., and Loosli, J.D.: Cobalt and Vitamin B$_{12}$ in Ruminant Nutrition. J. Dairy Sci., *40*:1215, 1957.

Spector, H., et al.: The Role of Riboflavin in Blood Regeneration. J. Biol. Chem., *150*:75, 1943.

Stillions, M.C., et al.: Utilization of Dietary Vitamin B$_{12}$ and Cobalt by Mature Horses. J. Anim. Sci., *32*:252, 1971.

Storb, R.: Immunologic and Hematologic Concepts in Marrow Transplantation as They Relate to Aplastic Anemia. Transplantation Proc., *11*:1916, 1979.

Strafuss, A.C., and Sautter, J.H.: Clinical and General Pathologic Finding of Aplastic Anemia Associated with S-(dichlorovinyl)-L-cysteine in Calves. Amer. J. Vet. Res., *28*:25, 1967.

Tennant, B.C., et al.: Intravascular Hemolysis Associated with Hepatic Failure in the Horse. Calif. Vet., *27*:15, 1972.

Tennant, B.C., et al.: Equine Hepatic Insufficiency. Vet. Clin. North Amer., *3(2)*:279, 1973.

Thomas, E.D., et al.: Bone Marrow Transplantation. New Eng. J. Med., *292*:832, 1975.

Tompkins, M.B., and Cummins, J.M.: Response of Feline Leukemia Virus–Induced Nonregenerative Anemia to Oral Administration of an Interferon-Containing Preparation. Feline Pract., *12(3)*:6, 1982.

Tudhope, G.R., and Wilson, G.M.: Anemia in Hypothyroidism. Q.J. Med., *29*:513, 1960.

Tudhope, G.R., and Wilson, G.M.: The Thyroid and the Blood. Charles C Thomas, Springfield, Ill., 1969.

Underwood, E.J.: Trace Elements in Human and Animal Nutrition. 3rd ed. Associated Press, New York, pp. 57–137, 1977.

Van Wyk, J.J., et al.: The Anemia of Copper Deficiency in Dogs Compared with That Produced by Iron Deficiency. Johns Hopkins Hosp. Bull., *93*:41, 1953.

Vaughan, J.M., and Saifi, M.F.: Haemoglobin Metabolism in Chronic Infections. J. Path. Bact., *49*:69, 1939.

Vilter, R.W., et al.: Studies on the Relationship of Vitamin B$_{12}$, Folic Acid, Thymine, Uracil, and Methyl Group Donors in Persons with Pernicious Anemia and Related Megaloblastic Anemias. Blood, *5*:695, 1950.

Waisman, H.A.: Production of Riboflavin Deficiency in the Monkey. Proc. Soc. Exp. Biol. Med., *55*:69, 1944.

Wallerstein, R.O., and Wallerstein, R.O., Jr.: Scurvy. Semin. Hematol., *13*:211, 1976.

Wallner, S.F., and Vautrin, R.M.: Evidence That Inhibition of Erythropoiesis Is Important in the Anemia of Chronic Renal Failure. J. Lab. Clin. Med., *97*:170, 1981.

Weiss, D.J., et al.: Transient Erythroid Hypoplasia in the Dog: Report of Five Cases. J. Amer. Anim. Hosp. Ass., *18(2)*:353, 1982.

Weiss, D.J., et al.: Studies on the Pathogenesis of Anemia of Inflammation: Mechanism of Impaired Erythrogenesis. Amer. J. Vet. Res., *44*:1832, 1983.

Whipple, G.H., et al.: Red Cell Stroma Protein Rich in Vitamin B_{12} during Active Regeneration: Anemia Studies Using Radioactive Cobalt-B_{12} in Dogs. J. Exp. Med., *102*:725, 1955.

Williams, D.M., et al.: Role of Copper in Mitochondrial Iron Metabolism. Blood, *48*:77, 1976.

Williams, D.M., et al.: Evidence for an Iron Carrier Substance in Copper Deficient Mitochondria. Prog. Clin. Biol. Res., *21*:539, 1978.

Wintrobe, M.M., et al.: Pyridoxine Deficiency in Swine. Bull. Johns Hopkins Hosp., *72*:1, 1943a.

Wintrobe, M.M., et al.: Pantothenic Acid Deficiency in Swine. Bull. Johns Hopkins Hosp., *73*:313, 1943b.

Wintrobe, M.M., et al.: Riboflavin Deficiency in Swine. Bull. Johns Hopkins Hosp., *75*:102, 1944.

Wintrobe, et al.: Clinical Hematology. 8th ed. Lea & Febiger, Philadelphia, 1981.

Wolf, P.L., and Koett, J.: Hemolytic Anemia in Hepatic Disease with Decreased Erythrocyte Adenosine Triphosphate. Amer. J. Clin. Path., *73*:785, 1980.

Wood, P.A., and Smith, J.E.: Pathogenesis and Diagnosis of Selenium Deficiency. Vet. Med. Small Anim. Clin., *74*:206, 1979.

Woolley, D.W.: Antimetabolites. Science, *129*:615, 1959.

Zucker, S.L.R.: Bone Marrow Erythropoiesis in Anemia of Inflammation. J. Lab. Clin. Med., *84*:620, 1974.

Zucker, S., et al.: Cancer Cell Inhibition of Erythropoiesis. J. Lab. Clin. Med., *96*:770, 1980.

26

The Neutrophils

MORPHOLOGY 676
    Light Microscopic Features 676
    Ultrastructure 677

LYSOSOMAL CONSTITUENTS AND THEIR
    POSSIBLE ROLES 683

METABOLISM AND CYTOCHEMISTRY 684

GRANULOPOIESIS AND
    GRANULOKINETICS 685
    Intramedullary Phase 686
    Intravascular Phase 689
    Tissue Phase 690
    Mechanisms of Neutrophilias 690
    Mechanisms of Neutropenias 695

REGULATION OF NEUTROPHIL
    HOMEOSTASIS 695
    Release of Marrow Neutrophils 695
    Control of Production 696

CHEMOTAXIS AND MIGRATION INTO
    TISSUES 698
    Techniques 698
    Factors Involved 699
    Mechanisms 700
    In Vivo Significance 700

FUNCTIONS 701
    Phagocytosis 701
    Microbicidal Activity 708
    Tissue Injury, Inflammation, and Neutrophil
        Lysosomes 712
    Antiviral Activity 714
    Parasite Destruction 714
    Cytotoxic Effect 714

MORPHOLOGIC AND FUNCTIONAL
    ABNORMALITIES 714
    Morphologic Abnormalities 715
    Functional Abnormalities 717

Neutrophils form the first line of cellular defense against microbial infection. This and other functions of neutrophils have become better defined during recent years, and more has become known about the pathophysiology of neutrophils. Subpopulations of neutrophils are being recognized based on differences in functional properties and cell surface antigens (Clement et al., 1983; Klempner and Gallin, 1978). A brief description of various aspects of neutrophils follows. Detailed information can be found in books (Cline, 1975; Gallin and Quie, 1978; Greenwalt and Jamieson, 1977; Klebanoff and Clark, 1978; Lisiewicz, 1980; Murphy, 1976; Snyderman, 1984; Wilkinson, 1982) and in specific reviews cited in the text.

MORPHOLOGY

Light Microscopic Features

Mature neutrophils characteristically have a polymorphic segmented nucleus with un-dulated nuclear membrane and clumped chromatin. Nuclear segmentation varies with the species from narrow nuclear constrictions to discernible short filaments separating the segments (Plates VII–8, VIII–8, IX–1, IX–4). Varying numbers of neutrophil leukocytes of the female of various species may show a nuclear appendage or extra chromatin lobe resembling a drumstick. The appendage is commonly referred to as the Barr body (Fig. 4–5; Plate XI–7).

The cytoplasm is clear and contains numerous granules that are typically neutral in reaction, staining pale pink with Wright or other Romanowsky stains. Staining is often so light that the cytoplasm may erroneously appear homogeneous and devoid of granules. Staining quality, however, varies with the species; granules of neutrophils from common domestic animals usually appear pale pink (Plate VIII–8). Neutrophils of the chicken and small laboratory animals such as rats, guinea pigs, and rabbits are pinkish red, and those of some primates such as the ring-tailed lemur stain highly azurophilic. The intense stainability of neutrophils in these species is probably related to their granule composition; such cells are often referred to as heterophils (from Greek *heteros*, "different").

A small number of band neutrophils may be found in blood in health. More immature neutrophils are normally found only in the bone marrow and appear in the circulation during granulocytic response to a disease process.

Sequential development of neutrophils occurs in the bone marrow as follows: myeloblast, promyelocyte or progranulocyte, myelocyte, metamyelocyte, band cell, and segmenter or mature neutrophil (Fig. 13–19; see also Chapter 1).

The myeloblast is the most immature, recognizable cell of the series (Plates V–3, V–5, VI–1). It has a round nucleus with stippled chromatin, one or more nucleoli or indistinct nucleolar rings, and distinct nuclear membrane. Rarely, a nucleolus or nucleolar ring is not visible. Its cytoplasm is fairly abundant and stains moderately blue in contrast to the deep blue cytoplasm of rubriblasts (Plates IV–1, VI–4).

The promyelocyte may be larger than its predecessor, but usually has similar nuclear features (Plates V–4, VI–2). The cytoplasm is more abundant, stains lighter blue, and characteristically contains distinct reddish purple, azurophilic granules. The number of azurophilic granules varies with the maturative stage of the cell, but their presence takes precedence over the nucleolus in classifying the cell as a promyelocyte.

The myelocyte may vary in size because it may divide twice before transforming into a metamyelocyte (Plate V–6). Its nucleus is round to slightly dented, lacks nucleolus, and displays some chromatin aggregation. Its cytoplasm stains faintly blue, particularly along the periphery, and contains numerous pale, "specific" granules. Azurophilic granules are normally not seen at this and subsequent stages. The presence of relatively abundant cytoplasm and the absence of conspicuously plaqued chromatin distinguishes myelocytes from lymphocytes present in the bone marrow.

The metamyelocyte may also vary in size, but its cytoplasmic features are similar to those of myelocytes (Plates V–3, V–6). Its nucleus is indented, akin to a kidney-bean, or is wide and elongated with fat ends.

The band neutrophil is about the size of the mature neutrophil, but has a slender, nonsegmented nucleus with less prominent chromatin clumping, smooth contour, and parallel-appearing sides (Plates V–6, VI–4, XII–3). It has clear cytoplasm and pale granules as in mature neutrophils.

Ultrastructure

Mature and developing neutrophils can be differentiated from eosinophils and basophils as early as the promyelocyte stage on the basis of granule structure. Observations on ultrastructure of neutrophils of different animal species, the dog in particular, are briefly described below. Readers interested in this subject are referred to excellent reports (Ackerman, 1968; Bainton and Farquhar, 1966, 1968, 1970; Wetzel et al., 1967) and reviews (Bainton, 1977; Poole, 1969; Spicer and Hardin, 1969; Wetzel 1970a, 1970b; Zucker-Franklin, 1968). Electron microscopic studies have been made on neutrophils of the dog (O'Donnell and Anderson, 1982; Shively et al., 1969; Sonoda and Kobayashi, 1970a), cat (Canfield, 1984; Grindem, 1985; Sonoda and Kobayashi, 1970b; Ward et al., 1972), horse (Bertram and Coignoul, 1982; Coignoul et al., 1984; Sonoda and Kobayashi, 1966), pig (Nafstad and Nafstad, 1968), sheep (Baggiolini et al., 1985; Rudolph and Schnabl, 1981; Yamada, 1970; Yamada and Sonoda, 1970), and cow (Baggiolini et al., 1985; Gennaro et al., 1983a), and goat (Baggiolini, et al., 1985).

The myeloblast is seldom seen in marrow specimens prepared for electron microscopy. It is characterized by a large, round nucleus with extremely dispersed chromatin, a prominent nucleolus, scattered rough endoplasmic reticulum (RER), abundant free ribosomes, and some mitochondria (Fig. 26–1). The nucleolus is thought to be involved in synthesis of protein necessary for biogenesis of cytoplasmic granules (Bernhard and Granboulan, 1968) or in directing cellular maturation and nuclear segmentation (Sainte-Marie and Sin, 1970). With maturation, the nucleus changes

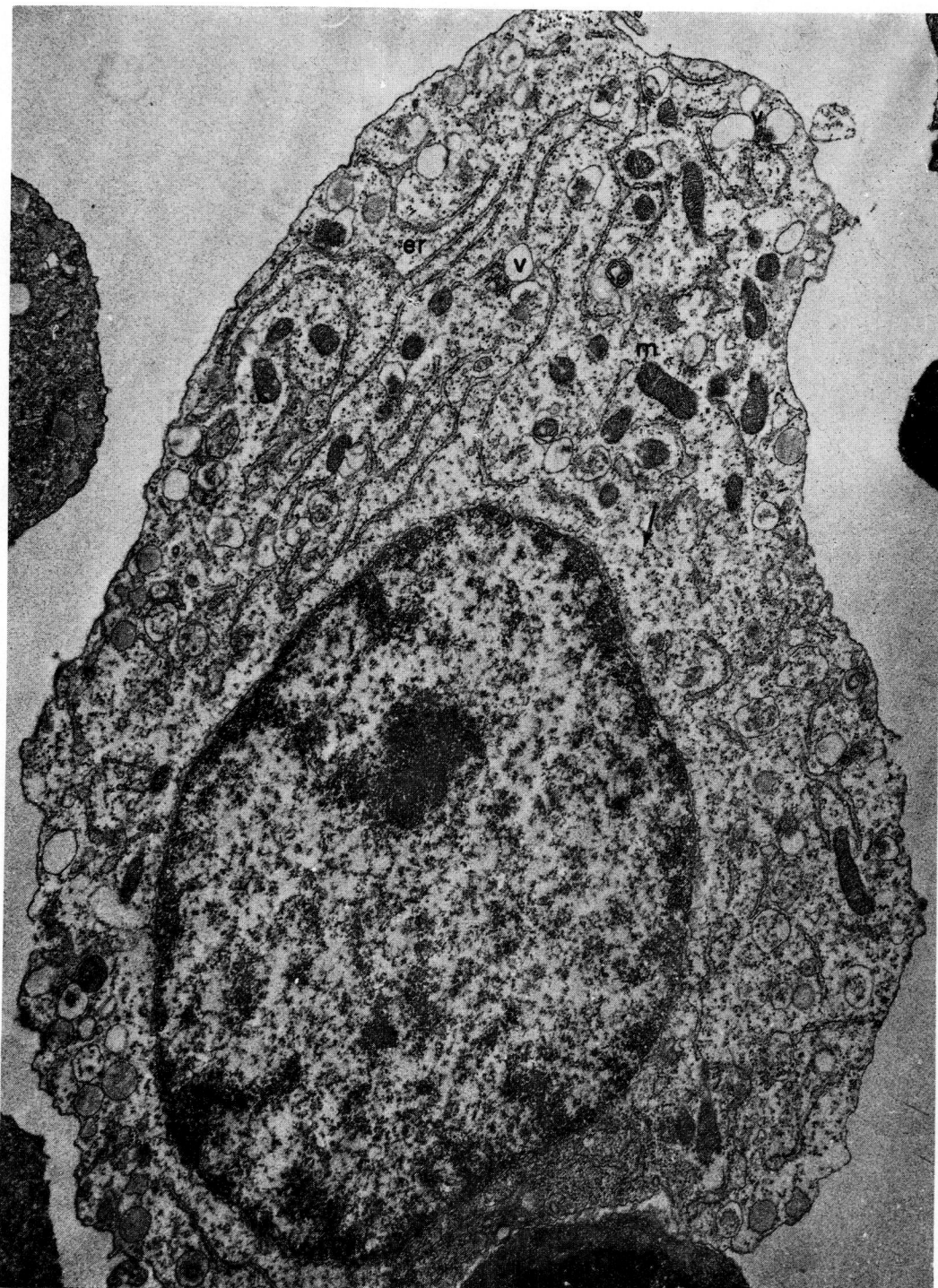

Fig. 26–1.   A late myeloblast from canine bone marrow. The oval nucleus exhibits minimal chromatin clumping with some margination along the inner aspects of the nuclear membrane. The cytoplasm contains prominent, long, and scattered cisternae of rough endoplasmic reticulum *(er)*, numerous ribosomes and polyribosomes *(arrow)*, many mitochondria *(m)*, and several vesicles *(v)*. The absence of cytoplasmic granules distinguishes this cell from the progranulocyte shown in Fig. 26–2. ×13,000.

shape, the nuclear outline undulates, the nuclear chromatin progressively condenses and marginates along inner aspects of the nuclear membrane, the nucleolus becomes inconspicuous, and mitochondria decrease in number. The RER and free ribosomes are prominent in the progranulocyte (Fig. 26–2A) and diminish in subsequent stages of cell maturation.

The most significant aspect of granulopoiesis is the formation of granules in the developing neutrophil. The presence of primary and secondary granules in developing and mature neutrophils can be demonstrated by electron microscopic, cytochemical staining techniques (Bainton and Farquhar, 1966) and immunochemical methods (Zucker-Franklin et al., 1981).

Neutrophilic promyelocytes in all species thus far studied seem to contain a single population of relatively large (about 0.4 μm), spherical, homogeneous, dense granules (Fig. 26–2A, B). Since these are the first granules to form, they are called primary granules and are analogous to the azurophilic granules seen with Romanowsky stains. Primary granules are peroxidase-positive; therefore this enzyme reaction can be used as a marker to study granule formation with the electron microscope. Primary granules develop by fusion of small, proteinaceous spherules secreted by the Golgi complex (Fig. 26–2B), mainly from its concave side. They predominate in promyelocytes and early myelocytes.

The myelocyte and the subsequent maturative stages are characterized by the appearance of relatively small (O.3 μm), less dense "secondary" granules that are peroxidase-negative (Fig. 26–3A). These secondary granules are analogous to the conventional specific granules of neutrophils. They are also formed by fusion of small vesicles secreted by the Golgi complex, in this instance from the convex side. Specific granules also appear homogeneous, and rarely they may appear crystalloid.

Formation of primary granules ceases with the appearance of secondary granules. Thus the number of primary granules is reduced by half with each cell division, while synthesis of secondary granules continues until the cell is no longer able to divide (past the mye-

locyte stage). Hence specific granules predominate in mature neutrophils. Although some primary granules are also present in mature neutrophils of common domestic animals, they no longer stain azurophilic because of loss of acid mucopolysaccharide during differentiation of the promyelocyte into the myelocyte. Their presence, however, continues to be demonstrable by peroxidase stain (Fig. 26–3B). The retention of azurophilia in primary granules in mature neutrophils is indicative of aberrant granulopoiesis and is called "toxic" granulation. Both primary and secondary granules are highly pleomorphic, and species differences in this regard have been noted (Fig. 26–4A through D).

The presence of very small, dense, pleomorphic, "tertiary" granules has been reported in neutrophils of some species (Wetzel et al., 1967). The so-called C-particles (Bretz and Baggiolini, 1974; Spitznagel et al., 1974) probably belong to this group of granules. A minor population of small, alkaline phosphatase–positive granules called "phosphasomes" was described in a recent study of human neutrophils (Wilson et al., 1981). In addition, catalase has been localized in "microperoxisomes" (Breton-Gorius et al., 1978) and gelatinase in particles smaller than the two conventional types of granules (Dewald et al., 1982, 1983) in human neutrophils. Neutrophils of cows, sheep, and goats were found to contain another granule type—large peroxidase-negative granules, larger than azurophilic and specific granules (Baggiolini et al., 1980).

Surface features of leukocytes have been studied with the scanning electron microscope (Newell, 1980; Lichtman et al., 1976; Michaelis et al., 1971). Proper fixation and processing of specimens are essential to prevent artifacts. Well-preserved leukocytes appear spherical and display a heterogeneous surface morphology comprised of many microvilli-like projections or random membranous folds (Fig. 26–5).

Despite the overlap in morphology of different kinds of leukocytes, suspensions of relatively pure preparations of leukocytes generally present distinguishing features (Newell, 1980). Normal lymphocytes generally present a villous surface, monocytes usu-

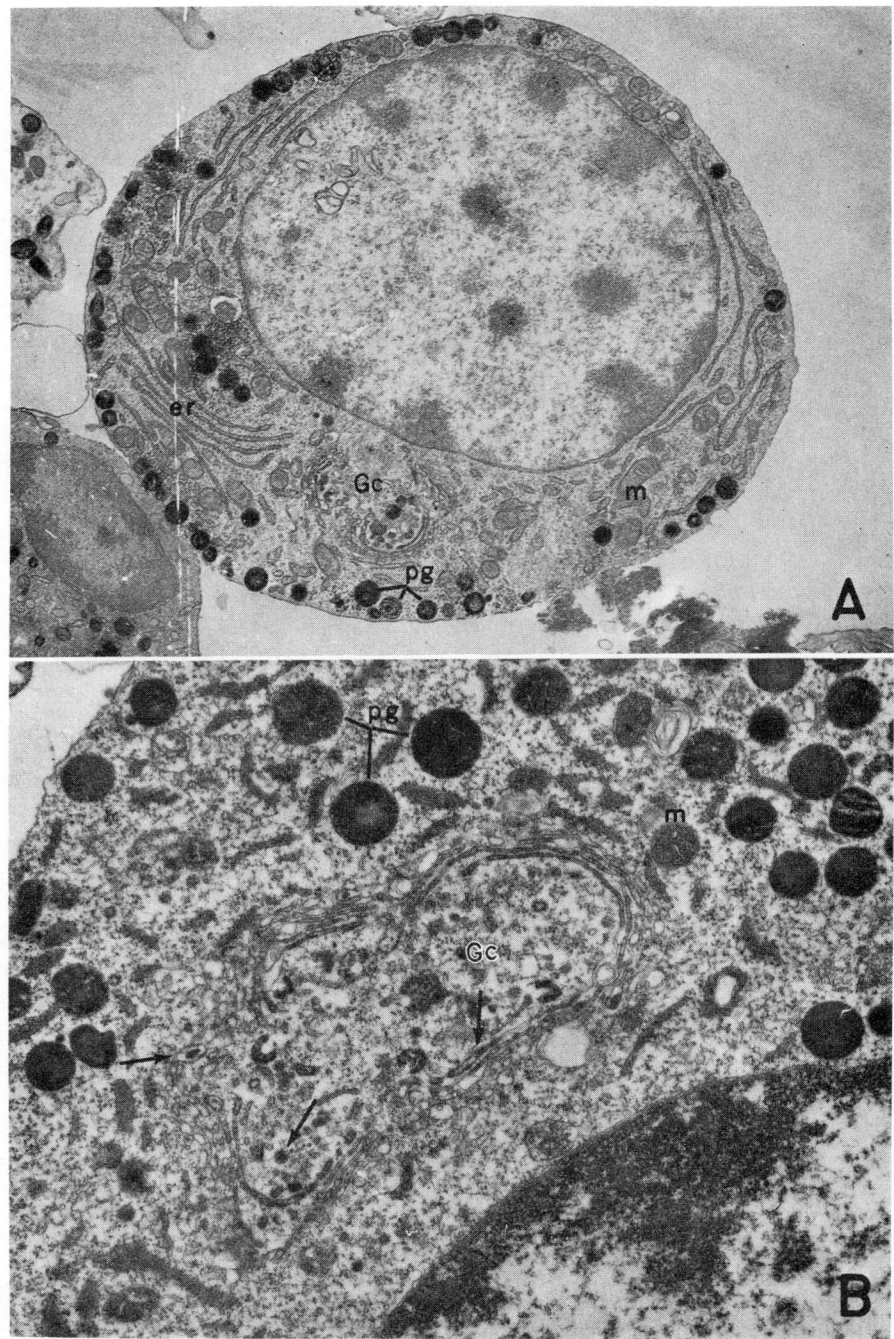

Fig. 26–2. Progranulocytes from canine bone marrow. These cells are characterized by the presence of numerous primary, or azurophilic, granules *(pg)*, which are peroxidase-positive; numerous mitochondria *(m)*; several profiles of prominent rough endoplasmic reticulum *(er)*; abundant ribosomes and polyribosomes. The nucleus shows slight chromatin clumping primarily along the nuclear membrane. The Golgi complex *(Gc)* is active and engaged in manufacturing primary granules. This is evident in *B*, in which tiny primary granules, vesicles containing condensing proteinaceous material, and cisternae containing condensing material can be seen in the Golgi complex area *(arrows)*. Peroxidase-stained specimen. *A*, ×6,300; *B*, ×21,600.

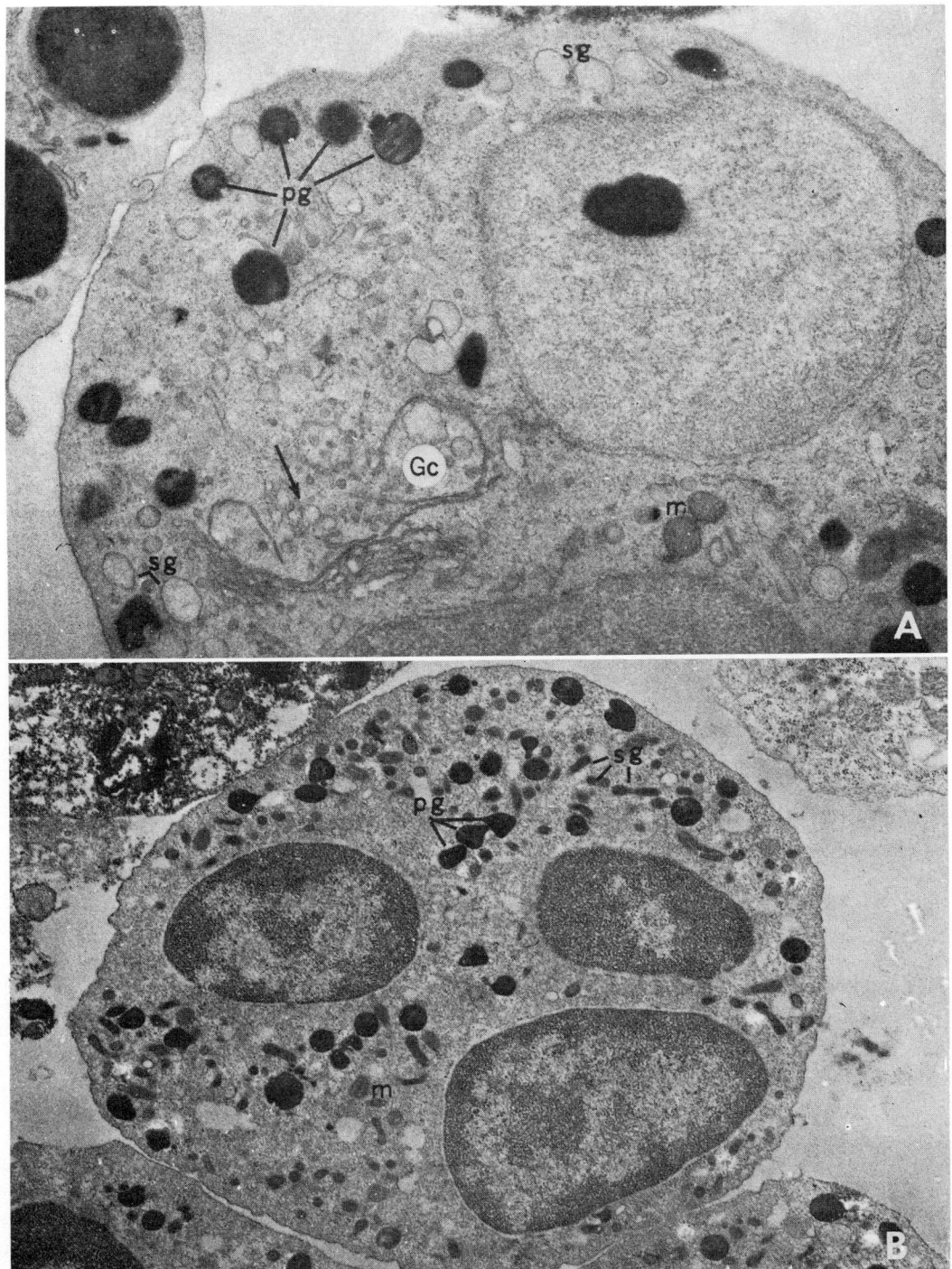

Fig. 26–3. A neutrophilic myelocyte *(A)* and a mature neutrophil *(B)* from canine bone marrow stained for peroxidase. These cells are characterized by the presence of both primary granules *(pg)*, which are peroxidase-positive, and secondary granules *(sg)*, which are peroxidase-negative. In the myelocyte *(A)*, notice the presence of an active Golgi complex *(Gc)* engaged in manufacturing secondary granules. Many clear saccules *(arrow)* of varying sizes can be seen in the vicinity of the Golgi complex, and similar large granules *(sg)* are apparent scattered in the cytoplasm. A few mitochondria *(m)* are also present. ×25,000. The mature neutrophil *(B)* distinctly contains larger, round, peroxidase-positive primary granules *(pg)* and smaller, pleomorphic, peroxidase-negative secondary granules *(sg)*. Romanowsky staining of blood films ordinarily demonstrates only one granule population because the primary granules by this stage have lost their acid mucopolysaccharide, which is responsible for their azurophilic staining at the progranulocyte stage. Some mitochondria *(m)* are also present. The nuclear lobes show condensation of chromatin. ×12,000.

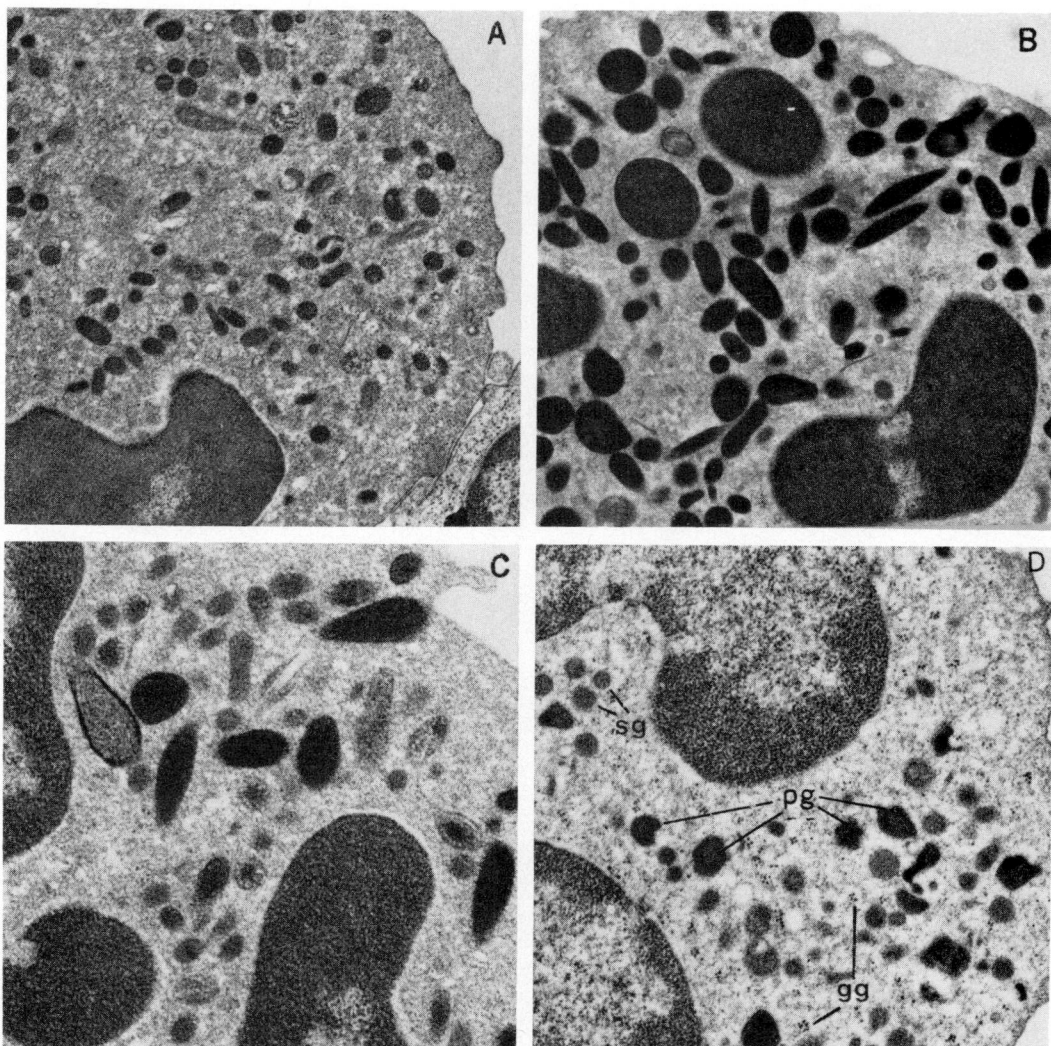

Fig. 26–4. *A,* Feline neutrophil with comparatively small, pleomorphic granules. ×11,200. *B,* Bovine neutrophil with highly pleomorphic, electron-dense granules. ×12,000. *C,* Equine neutrophil in which large, elongated, electron-dense primary granules contrast with smaller, pleomorphic, less dense secondary granules. ×20,800. *D,* Canine neutrophil with large, electron-dense granules *(pg)* and smaller, pleomorphic, less dense granules *(sg).* Compare the features of this cell with that stained for peroxidase (Fig. 26–3B), in which the two granule types can be more clearly distinguished. The neutrophil cytoplasm lacks rough endoplasmic reticulum and has scattered glycogen granules *(gg).* ×18,000.

ally display ruffles (broad-based, long, undulating, plate-like surface folds), and granulocytes have ridges (broad-based, narrow surface folds). Cell shape is altered during cellular locomotion, upon surface attachment, and by temperature, metabolic inhibitors, and agents influencing the surface membrane (Lichtman et al., 1976). Granulocytes in suspensions usually display an amoeboid shape characterized by a spherical, less rugose end and a multi-veiled end with broad

surface folds. Leukemic cells in general reflect the characteristic features of the cell of origin, but may appear abnormal or similar to immature leukocytes, in which surface features are absent or only partially developed. Bessis and Boisfleury (1970, 1971) have published excellent photomicrographs of living leukocytes during erythrophagocytosis. After extensive phagocytosis, neutrophils lose their surface foldings and appear rounded (Zakhireh et al., 1979).

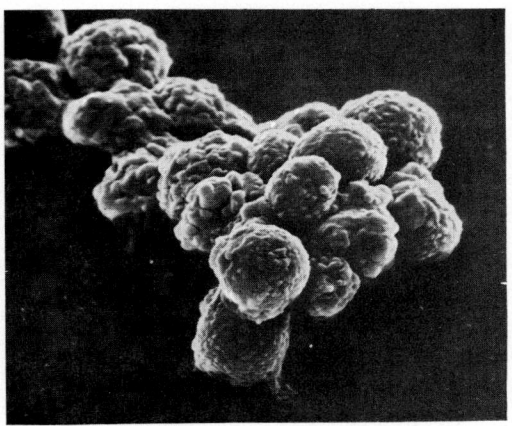

Fig. 26–5. A scanning electron photomicrograph of canine leukocytes from blood. The cells show numerous surface projections and cannot be identified as to their types on the basis of surface appearance. ×3,150.

LYSOSOMAL CONSTITUENTS AND THEIR POSSIBLE ROLES

The term *lysosome* was coined by de Duve et al. (1955) to describe intracellular membranous sacs (granules) containing acid hydrolytic enzymes. They also suggested that lysosomal components could be involved in causation of tissue injury. Cohn and Hirsch (1960) subsequently demonstrated that the granules of rabbit neutrophils are lysosomal in nature, for they contain several of the acid hydrolytic enzymes reported to be present in liver lysosomes. Strictly speaking, the primary granules of neutrophils which contain acid hydrolases can be regarded as lysosomes, whereas the secondary granules lacking such enzymes are not. Loosely, however, the term *lysosome* encompasses both types of granules, secondary granules being considered modified lysosomal granules. Bovine (Gennaro et al., 1983a, b), canine (O'Donnell and Andersen, 1982), and equine (Bertram and Coignoul, 1982) neutrophil granules have been characterized recently.

Neutrophil lysosomal granules exhibit a morphological as well as biochemical heterogeneity (reviewed by Shannon and Zellmer, 1982). Subpopulations of primary and secondary granules are being recognized. Neutrophil granules contain many enzymes and nonenzymatic substances (Table 26–1) that are compartmentalized from the cytoplasm by the unit membrane enclosing the granules

(Avila, 1979; Baggiolini, 1972; Olsson and Venge, 1980). Species differences in structure and biochemical constituents have been found. For example, bovine neutrophils have very little lysozyme (Rausch and Moore, 1975), and chicken heterophils lack myeloperoxidase (MPO) and catalase (Bellavite et al., 1977; Breton-Gorius et al., 1978). In the bovine, cationic proteins and lactoferrin are found in a large granule type that differs from both azurophilic and specific granules (Gennaro et al., 1983a). Alkaline phosphatase is believed to be present in specific granules; however, its ultrastructural location is being questioned. It has been associated with nongranular components—vesicular membranes, nuclear envelope, and irregular tubular structures (Borgers et al., 1978; Rustin et al., 1979; Wilson et al., 1981)—and is described as being present in separate organelles, called "phosphasomes" (Wilson et al., 1981). Similarly, catalase has been localized in the soluble fraction as well as in the particulate fraction comprised of small granules called "microperoxisomes" or "microbodies" (Breton-Gorius et al., 1978). The C-particles contain a minor portion of acid hydrolases.

Several functions have been suggested for the contents of specific and primary granules (Gallin and Fletcher, 1981; Gallin et al., 1982; Klebanoff and Clark, 1978). Specific granules contain factors regulating neutrophil adhesiveness and aggregation, hydroxyl radical formation, generation of complement-derived chemotactic factors, and myelopoiesis. Recently they have been shown to provide a source of new plasma membrane and receptors for neutrophils responding to chemoattractants. Substances from azurophilic granules are involved in modulation of inflammatory process through induction of capillary permeability, generation and inactivation of chemotactic factors, migration of neutrophils, and bactericidal effects.

Specific functions of several granular constituents have been delineated in recent years. For example, myeloperoxidase (MPO) and cationic proteins (including phagocytin and leukin) exert bactericidal effects, and some cationic proteins also induce an increase in vascular permeability. Lysozyme degrades bacterial cell walls and lyses certain bacterial

Table 26–1.   Some Enzymatic and Nonenzymatic Constituents of Mature Neutrophils

Primary or Azurophilic Granules	*Secondary or Specific Granules*	*Constituents of Uncertain Location*
Peroxidase	Alkaline phosphatase	Leukin
Sulfated mucopolysaccharides	Lysozyme (2/3)	Procoagulant activity
Cationic proteins	Lactoferrin	Endogenous pyrogen
Phagocytin	Aminopeptidase	Histamine
Lysozyme (1/3)	Specific collagenase	Kinin-forming and kinin-destroying enzymes
Acid proteases	C5-Inactivating factor	Aminopeptidase
Cathepsins B and D	Phospholipase A_2	
Neutral proteases	Transcobalamins	
Cathepsin G,		*"Microbodies"*
Elastase		Catalase
Nonspecific collagenase		
Proteinase 3		
Acid phosphatase		
Arylsulfatase	*Tertiary Granules*	
Acid hydrolytic enzymes	Acid phosphatase	
β-Galactosidase	Arylsulfatase	
β-Glucuronidase	β-Glycerophosphatase	
β-Glycerophosphatase	β-Glucuronidase	
5′-Nucleosidase	Acid mucosubstance	
α-Manosidase	Cathepsins B and D	

species. It increases phagocytic activity (Pruzanski and Saito, 1978); decreases chemotaxis, hexose monophosphate pathway activity, and superoxide generation (Gordon et al., 1979); and acts synergistically with cell extracts to kill certain bacteria (Neeman et al., 1974). The level of plasma lysozyme directly correlates with blood neutrophil turnover rate (Hansen, 1974; Hansen and Andersen, 1973). Lactoferrin is bacteriostatic and in some situations bactericidal (Bullen and Armstrong, 1979). Lactoferrin also increases adhesiveness of neutrophils (Oseas et al., 1981) and inhibits granulopoiesis (see Chapter 13). It may act synergistically with lysozyme in bactericidal action. Acid hydrolases are capable of degradation of carbohydrates, proteins, lipids, and nucleic acids at acidic pH. Neutral proteases and specific collagenase may be involved in tissue destruction during inflammation and abscess formation. The release of endogenous pyrogen contributes to increase in body temperature during infection. Phospholipase A_2 exerts a digestive rather than bactericidal effect (Elsbach, 1980).

METABOLISM AND CYTOCHEMISTRY

The major source of energy (about 90%) in neutrophils is anaerobic glycolysis, while a small amount (about 10%) is derived through the hexose monophosphate pathway. The former also supplies energy needed for neutrophil locomotion and phagocytosis. Glucose utilization and glycogen turnover rates are higher in neutrophils and monocytes than in lymphocytes. Glucose is freely permeable through the leukocyte membrane, but its utilization is decreased during diabetes mellitus. Glycogen is synthesized by neutrophils; it is evident in the form of periodic acid Schiff (PAS)–positive material in the cytoplasm at the myelocyte stage and increases with cell maturation (see Chapter 33).

It has been shown that neutrophils use different energy sources for movement and for phagocytosis (Borregaard and Herlin, 1982; Weisdorf et al., 1982a, b). Chemotaxis induces accelerated uptake of exogenous glucose, although stored glycogen may be catabolized for this purpose. By comparison, phagocytosis is associated with significantly enhanced glycogenolysis, even in the presence of extracellular glucose.

DNA, RNA, and protein synthesis and respiratory metabolism are higher in immature neutrophils and decrease with cell maturation. DNA synthesis is limited to cells capable of mitosis, i.e., up to the myelocyte stage. A decrease in RER, polyribosomes, and ribosomes is reflected in diminution in protein synthesis. A reduction in the number and size of mitochondria is associated with a decrease in the respiratory rate. Neutrophils are incapable of lipid synthesis, but can effect fatty acid chain elongation and synthesize lysolecithin from lecithin. Their membrane phospholipids and cholesterol exchange freely with those in the plasma. Neutrophils contain a significant amount of vitamin B_{12} and secrete transcobalamin II, which transports vitamin B_{12}.

Physiologic and pathologic variations occur in metabolic activities of neutrophils. Those associated with phagocytosis are described in a later section in this chapter (see Functions). In addition, neutrophils stimulated by phagocytosis or membrane perturbation can synthesize new protein as evidenced by production of endogenous pyrogen and plasminogen activator (Elsbach, 1980; Granellipiperno et al., 1977). Similarly, stimulated neutrophils metabolize phospholipids to generate prostaglandins, thromboxanes, and leukotrienes (Hansson and Radmark, 1980; Walsh et al., 1981). They can release various lysosomal substances and produce histaminase (Herman et al., 1979) and eosinophil chemotactic factor (Konig et al., 1978).

Glycolytic rate is higher in neutrophils from infants and in exudate neutrophils, and certain enzymatic activities are also higher in exudate neutrophils than in blood neutrophils (Takamori and Yamashita, 1980). An increase in plasma bilirubin level has an adverse effect on neutrophil hexose monophosphate pathway activity (Thong and Rencis, 1977). Glycogen content of neutrophils is increased during infection and in some glycogen storage diseases in humans, while it is decreased during chronic granulocytic leukemia. Metabolic activities such as DNA, RNA, and protein syntheses are higher in leukocytes of patients with granulocytic leukemia. Abnormalities of carbohydrate metabolism, lipid composition (Klock and Pieprzyk, 1979), and enzyme activities are also found in leukemic leukocytes (Eshelman et al., 1981). Abnormalities of protein metabolism have been reported in humans, e.g., cysteine crystals in neutrophils of patients with cysteinuria (Schneider et al., 1967).

Various constituents of neutrophils, and of their granules in particular, can be demonstrated by cytochemical methods. However, only some cytochemical reactions are commonly used for neutrophil identification (Jain, 1970; see Plate X). A distinctly positive staining is obtained for myeloperoxidase, Sudan black B, and naphthol AS-D chloroacetate esterase (Table 33–1). A faint to slight reactivity is seen for acid phosphatase. Alkaline phosphatase activity varies with the species. Equine, bovine, ovine, caprine, porcine, and human neutrophils exhibit a modest to strong positive reaction, whereas canine and feline neutrophils consistently give a negative reaction (see Table 33–1). Canine and feline eosinophils show positive alkaline phosphatase activity and should not be confused with neutrophils. PAS-positive material, in the form of fine to coarse granules, is present in the cytoplasm. Both alkaline phosphatase and PAS positivities of human neutrophils increase with cell maturation.

Changes in enzymatic activities of neutrophils may occur during disease states, but species variations may be found. For example, increases are seen in alkaline phosphatase, acid phosphatase, and naphthol AS-D chloroacetate esterase activities and nitro blue tetrazolium (NBT) reduction during infection in humans (Mackie et al., 1979). Alkaline phosphatase activity is markedly reduced during chronic myelogenous leukemia in humans. In contrast, canine and feline patients with myelogenous or myelomonocytic leukemias have increased alkaline phosphatase activity (Jain et al., 1981; Plates XXIII–6, XXIV–5). See Chapter 33 for further details on cytochemistry of animal leukocytes.

GRANULOPOIESIS AND GRANULOKINETICS

It is currently believed that in the microenvironment of the bone marrow, pluripotent hematopoietic stem cells give rise to bipotential committed stem cells, designated CFU-GM for colony forming unit granulocyte-monocyte. The latter under appropriate stimuli give rise to separate unipotential progenitors of neutrophils and monocytes. An orderly progression of multiplication and maturation of specifically committed progenitor cells, through various intermediate stages, results in the formation of mature neutrophils (Fig. 13–19). This concept of granulopoiesis is borne of in vivo and in vitro studies on bone marrow cells from normal and leukemic humans and laboratory animals by autoradiographic, tissue culture, cytogenetic, cytochemical, and electron microscopic techniques.

The life span of the granulocytes has three phases: the intramedullary, intravascular, and tissue phases. The first two have been investigated extensively, while the last phase remains to be studied adequately. Quantitative data regarding various phases of neutrophil life span are considered under granulokinetics.

A variety of techniques have been employed to study granulokinetics. Most accurate data are obtained with the use of radioisotopes, which include DNA labels—radiophosphate (^{32}P) and tritiated thymidine (^{3}HTdR)—and non-DNA labels—radioactive diisopropyl fluorophosphate (DF^{32}P), radioactive sulfate (^{35}S), radiochromate (^{59}Cr), and recently ^{111}In-oxine. The DNA labels are valuable for determining the life span of a cell from the time of DNA synthesis to its loss from the blood. The non-DNA labels are used primarily for determining intravascular distribution and life span of neutrophils. ^{3}HTdR is the most commonly used DNA label. Choice of a non-DNA label depends on the species and the purpose of the study. Labeling with ^{3}HTdR and DF^{32}P can be accomplished either in vitro or in vivo and is virtually complete within an hour (flash label). Migration of neutrophils into sites of inflammation can be followed by surface scanning of ^{111}In-oxine-labeled neutrophils (Thakur et al., 1976). Several reviews have been published on granulopoiesis and granulokinetics (Boggs, 1975; Carakostas et al., 1981a; Robinson and Mangalik, 1975; Vincent, 1977a, b).

Intramedullary Phase

Neutrophils and their precursors in the bone marrow can be divided into three pools based on cellular morphology and kinetic characteristics. The proliferative pool is comprised of myeloblasts, promyelocytes, and myelocytes; the maturative pool consists of metamyelocytes and band cells; and the storage or reserve pool consists of predominantly mature neutrophils. This division is not absolute and does not imply any anatomic separation; rather, it recognizes overlapping morphologic and functional boundaries.

The intramedullary phase of granulopoiesis is studied with DNA labels. Such studies have been conducted in humans and several animal species. The incorporation of a DNA label is limited to cells synthesizing DNA (S phase) at the time of injection. Cells of the proliferative pool become flash labeled after a single intravenous injection of ^{3}HTdR; cells of the maturative pool acquire the label with time only as progenies of labeled precursors. Metamyelocytes are generally considered non-mitotic, but mitosis was implied in studies on guinea pigs (Harris and Kugler, 1963) and calves (Valli et al., 1971) in which some labeled metamyelocytes were found within 1 hour after injection of ^{3}HTdR.

Because ^{3}HTdR is a weak beta particle emitter, it is ideal for microautoradiography. Marrow samples are obtained sequentially to follow the pattern of the label through various maturative stages. Because half of the labeled DNA remains in the daughter cells of a progenitor, several mitotic cycles must take place before the label is no longer detectable. Production rates of various granulocytes are determined by the "labeling index" (percentage of labeled cells), duration of the DNA synthetic phase (5 hours), and proportion of various types of cells. Compartment transit times (Table 26–2) are calculated by following the time it takes the label to appear in cells of various morphologically recognizable compartments.

Generally, granulopoiesis in different species involves three to seven (average 5) mitoses in vivo and as many as ten or eleven mitoses in vitro. For example, studies on granulopoietic islands in the thymus of the rat have shown that the granulocyte development involves seven successive mitoses: one at the myeloblast stage, two at the promyelocyte stage, three at the myelocyte stage, and one at the metamyelocyte stage (Sainte-Marie and Sin, 1970). Studies of granulopoiesis in human bone marrow indicated the occurrence of four consecutive mitoses, one each at the myeloblast and promyelocyte stages and two at the myelocyte stage (Boecker et al., 1978). Two mitoses at the myelocyte stage were associated with formation of large and small myelocytes, with small myelocytes predominating. About three to four mitoses are thought to occur during granulopoiesis in dogs and cats. Some diurnal variation in mitotic activity and oscillations in the production of neutrophils have been observed in human and canine studies (Robinson and Mangalik, 1975).

Maturation time of canine neutrophils was studied by autoradiographic analyses of marrow and blood cells from dogs given ^{3}HTdR (Patt and Maloney, 1959). In the marrow, about 15–20% of myelocytes became labeled within 2 hours; the label appeared in other cells as follows: metamyelocytes, 12–24 hours; bands, 24–36 hours; and segmented neutrophils, 2–3 days. Labeled segmenters appeared in the peripheral blood in 3–4 days and peaked (25–30%) at 4–5 days after the initial labeling of myelocytes in the marrow. Compartment transit times of cells of the neutrophilic series in canine bone marrow were calculated in subsequent studies (Table 26–2; Maloney et al., 1963; Maloney and Patt, 1968; Patt and Maloney, 1964). Considering the relative distribution of myelocyte to metamyelocyte of 1:0.75 in marrow smears and the rate of entry of metamyelocytes (5% per hour), it was estimated that for every 7.5 myelocytes, only 3.75 (0.75 × 5) myelocytes were transformed into metamyelocytes. This indicated a substantial "ineffective granulopoiesis" or the presence of a "myelocyte sink"; i.e., a large number of myelocytes do not undergo mitosis or mature to become metamyelocytes, but are lost in an unknown manner. Such a sink apparently also exists in humans.

A comparison of radioactivity of blood neutrophils in dogs injected with ^{32}P, ^{3}HTdR, ^{35}S, or DF^{32}P indicated that the time required for the last mitotic myelocyte to complete a generative cycle and traverse the postmitotic maturative and storage pools of the bone marrow is approximately 5 days (Boggs, 1967). Similar observations in humans provide estimates of longer marrow transit times and emergence time into the circulation (Table 26–2). Differences are also found in estimates obtained with different isotopes; the time taken for the development of mature neutrophils from myeloblasts in human bone marrow is estimated at 4–9 (mean 7) days with ^{3}HTdR and 8.5–14 (mean 11) days with DF^{32}P. Emergence time of 100–130 hours, with a peak at about 150 hours, was reported for calves (Vincent et al., 1974).

Myelopoiesis was studied by autoradiography in normal, anemic, and endotoxin-treated calves (Valli et al., 1971). The mean time of production of labeled neutrophils in such calves was, respectively, 5.77 ± 1.43, 5.75 ± 1.2, and 5.68 ± 1.37 days. The mean time of arrival of labeled neutrophils in the peripheral blood was 7.01, 6.19, and 6.91 days, respectively. These findings indicated that in the bovine, increased requirements for neutrophils, as during an infection, are met not by a shortening of the production time, but by an increase in the pool of proliferative cells.

Bone Marrow Reserve of Neutrophils

A functional storage compartment of neutrophils in the marrow was first demonstrated

Table 26–2. Estimates of Various Phases of Bone Marrow Granulokinetics in Dogs and Humans

Marrow Pools and Cellular Stages	Estimated Number of Mitoses	Dogs		Humans	
		Proportion of Cells (%)	Average Transit Time (hrs)	Proportion of Cells (%)	Average Transit Time (hrs)
Proliferative pool					
Myeloblast	1	1.0	10	0.9	24
Promyelocyte	1	1.3	8	3.3	47
Myelocyte	2	13.6	30	12.7	87
Maturative pool					
Metamyelocytes	0	8.8	20	15.9	33
Band cells	0	11.9	26	12.4	58
Storage pool					
Mature neutrophils	0	6.0	50	7.4	59
Emergence time in blood					
Myeloblast to mature neutrophils			144		308
Last myelocyte to mature neutrophils			106		179

with a technique called leukapheresis (Craddock et al., 1955, 1956; Perry et al., 1958). The size of the marrow reserve was found to be several times that of the number of circulating neutrophils. The method, as applied to the dog, consisted of removing the leukocytes from 1½ blood volumes every hour for 3 hours. This was accomplished by repeatedly removing 40–50 ml of blood, depleting it of leukocytes, and reinjecting it. Leukapheresis produced leukopenia in 15 of 17 dogs (2,000 or fewer leukocytes per/μl), but after a delay of 30–90 minutes, the leukocyte count began to increase, and in 4½ hours, the cells were back to normal value. The count continued to rise over the next 24–36 hours, when it was at 150–200% of normal level. Repeated leukapheresis after the leukocyte count had reached its maximum was accompanied by a progressive shortening of the delay period observed before leukocytosis began.

Both normal and irradiated dogs could rapidly replace the number of leukocytes circulating at any one time. However, the irradiated animal showed a more delayed replenishment, and if repeatedly leukapheresed, it was unable to respond because of depletion of leukocyte stores. In normal dogs, there was no change indicative of increasing immaturity of the marrow or circulating leukocytes until the third or fourth day. Thus the initial response did not depend upon an immediate production of cells by the bone marrow; rather, it involved release of preformed leukocytes from the storage compartment. Furthermore, increased production of leukocytes by an acceleration of granulopoiesis in the dog occurs only after a delay of 3–4 days.

A leukocyte reserve is necessary to prevent the occurrence of marrow depletion by the sudden imposition of a greatly increased rate of peripheral utilization. The marrow reserve affords a huge buffer between supply by growth, which is fixed within certain limits, and demand, which may vary widely. The storage pool is limited to segmented neutrophils and some bands, since cells less mature than bands are usually not found in blood initially upon increased demand for leukocytes (Thomas et al., 1965).

The marrow neutrophil reserve in the dog contains about a 5-day supply of cells at a normal rate of utilization (Boggs, 1967); there is about a 4- to 8-day reserve in normal human marrow (Rottini et al., 1979). Thus if the marrow granulocytic mitotic pool is severely damaged, as by x-radiation or disease, and if the rate of consumption is unaltered, neutropenia may not develop for 3–4 days. Reserves of similar or greater size have been demonstrated in the rabbit, mouse, and guinea pig (Boggs, 1967). A persistently low neutrophil count, despite an obviously stimulated granulopoiesis, indicates a depleted marrow reserve and/or ineffective granulopoiesis.

Techniques to assess marrow reserve of granulocytes have been described and include injection of a small dose of bacterial pyrogen or endotoxin, etiocholanolone, or corticosteroids (Dale et al., 1975; Korbitz et al., 1969; Robinson and Mangalik, 1975). Marrow reserve of granulocytes can be measured in cattle by subcutaneously injecting 5 μg/kg body weight of piromen, a polysaccharide complex of *Pseudomonas aeruginosa* (Lumsden et al., 1973), or intravenously injecting 5–10 μg *Escherichia coli* endotoxin (Jain and Lasmanis, 1978b) and in dogs by intravenously injecting 4 μg *Salmonella typhosa* endotoxin (Boggs et al., 1968b) or a smaller dose of endotoxin (Boggs et al., 1965a) or by giving 20 mg of prednisolone orally (see Chapter 4). Total and differential leukocyte counts are performed on preinjection and postinjection blood samples collected at 2-hour intervals for 12 hours. About a twofold increase in neutrophil numbers by 6–8 hours is considered indicative of an adequate marrow reserve. A similar approach may be followed for other animal species. In horses, prednisolone sodium succinate (200 mg, IV) mobilized marrow granulocyte reserve within three hours of injection, whereas etiocholanolone (0.3 mg/ kg, IM) failed to do so (Carakostas et al., 1981b).

Valli et al. (1969) carried out leukapheresis in calves and dogs by extracorporeal circulation of blood through siliconized glass wool. Continued leukapheresis for 5–7.6 hours produced granulocytopenia in blood and depletion of band and mature neutrophils in the bone marrow of both species. This was followed by a marked neutrophilia in dogs, noticeable on the first day after leukapheresis, whereas calves remained neutropenic for up to 1 week after leukapheresis. Since the marrow granulocyte reserve in dogs and calves was found to be similar (2×10^9 granulocytes/kg body weight), the faster recovery of dogs than of calves was attributed to a relatively larger pool of precursor cells in the marrow as well as to a shorter neutrophil generation time. Thus species differences in leukocyte response to acute infections appear to depend on the rapidity with which compensatory myeloid proliferation can occur.

Normally, mature neutrophils leave the marrow by a random process. Mechanisms controlling their release are insufficiently characterized, but involve changes in cellular deformability and adhesiveness, the more deformable and less sticky cells being the first to enter blood (see also Chapter 13). The peripheral blood neutrophil count may not necessarily reflect the rate of mobilization from marrow into the circulation and subsequently into the tissues. It has been shown that an enormous number of granulocytes can move from the bone marrow reserve into a site of acute inflammation, such as the peritoneal cavity, without a concomitant blood granulocytosis (Craddock et al., 1963). A typical clinical situation involving this pattern among animal species is acute peritonitis in a horse or dog.

Intravascular Phase

Neutrophils in circulation constitute the *circulating pool*, whereas those marginated along capillary walls constitute the *marginal pool* of granulocytes; the two together constitute the *total blood granulocyte pool*. Margination occurs throughout the microvasculature, but primarily in the lungs and to a lesser or negligible extent in the spleen and liver. Neutrophils in the two pools are in dynamic equilibrium and are generally considered to be a homogeneous population, although some doubts have been raised recently. On the basis of neutrophil alkaline phosphatase activity, it was found that the transfer of neutrophils from the circulating to the marginal pool is not random but selective, in favor of "older" cells (Fehr and Grossmann, 1979).

The distribution of neutrophils within the vascular system and their stay in the peripheral blood as well as their mode of disappearance have been studied using DNA and non-DNA labels. Estimates have been obtained for sizes of blood pools, intravascular half-time of disappearance ($T\frac{1}{2}$), and turnover rate of neutrophils. Under steady-state conditions, the marrow production rate, the marrow release rate, and the blood turnover rate of neutrophils should all be equal (Vincent, 1977b). Values may vary, however, between individuals and within the same individual at different times (Athens et al., 1961). On average, the marginal pool of granulocytes in humans, dogs, calves, and horses is approximately equal in size to the circulating pool, while that in cats is about twice as large (Table 26–3).

Different estimates of granulokinetics have been obtained in human and canine studies using different techniques and isotopes, although conclusions have not been different (Vincent, 1977a, b). Values obtained with ^{3}HTdR are presently considered most reliable, but DF^{32}P and ^{51}Cr provide a convenient and acceptable approach to clinical evaluation of granulokinetics. In comparison to ^{3}HTdR, DF^{32}P underestimates, while ^{51}Cr overestimates the $T\frac{1}{2}$ values in humans. Hence DF^{32}P overestimates and ^{51}Cr underestimates the granulocyte turnover rate, and both overestimate the marginal and total blood granulocyte pools.

Granulokinetic studies in developing calves, using ^{51}Cr-labeled neutrophils, indicated that young calves (8–16 days of age) have a significantly larger total blood granulocyte pool, shorter $T\frac{1}{2}$, and consequently a greater turnover rate than do older calves (187–380 days of age). The larger size of total blood granulocyte pool in the young calves is partly related to their greater blood volume (Carlson and Kaneko, 1975).

The $T\frac{1}{2}$ of circulating neutrophils in various species ranges between 6 and 14 hours, with a mean of about 6 hours (Table 26–3). Thus the total blood pool of neutrophils in most species is replaced about 2–2$\frac{1}{2}$ times a day. An exponential decrease of labeled neutrophils from the circulation in these studies indicated that neutrophils are lost from the pe-

Table 26–3. Blood Granulokinetic Data for Humans and Some Animals

Species	Label	TBGP	CGP	MGP	GTR	T½
Human[a, b]	DF[32]P	61	31	29	160	6.3
	[3]HTdR	40	22	17	87	7.6
Dog[c]	DF[32]P	90 ± 10	47 ± 8	43 ± 4	228 ± 40	5.2 ± 0.7
	[3]HTdR	75 ± 11	47 ± 8	23 ± 8	165 ± 22	7.6 ± 1.2
Cat[d]	^{3}H-DFP	228 ± 108	78 ± 24	210 ± 91	650 ± 186	7.4 ± 1.8
Calves[e] (age 187–380 days)	[51]Cr	63 ± 15	29 ± 9	34 ± 7	124 ± 3	8.9 ± 2.9
Horse[f]	[51]Cr	56 ± 15	27 ± 7	29 ± 9	88 ± 15	10.5 ± 1.3

Data from: a, Bishop et al., 1971; b, Dancey et al., 1976; c, Deubelbeiss et al., 1975; d, Prasse et al., 1973; e, Carlson and Kaneko, 1975; Carakostas et al., 1981a.

Mean values (± SD) are given for TBGP, total blood granulocyte pool ($\times 10^7$ cells/kg body weight); CGP, circulating granulocyte pool ($\times 10^7$ cells/kg body weight); MGP, marginal granulocyte pool ($\times 10^7$ cells/kg body weight); GTR, granulocyte turnover rate ($\times 10^7$ cells/kg/day), and T½, half-time of disappearance (hrs).

ripheral blood in a random manner, whereas loss of erythrocytes is age-dependent.

Neutrophils are normally lost in the lungs, saliva, gut, and urine. Some neutrophils may be lost because of senescence in the circulation (Fliedner et al., 1964). Once a neutrophil leaves the blood vessel, it does not normally return to recirculate. However, observations in patients with chronic granulocytic leukemia indicate that leukemic cells may return to the marrow (Moxley et al., 1965). This possibility was also suggested from observations on a calf given hydrocortisone 48 hours after being cross-transfused with [3]HTdR-labeled neutrophils from its chimeric, immunologically tolerant twin; both the labeling index and the number of labeled cells in blood increased after steroid injection (Vincent et al., 1974).

Tissue Phase

Normally neutrophils enter tissues by diapedesis through the intercellular junctions of vascular endothelium. Neutrophil migration into tissue has been studied by the skin window technique of Rebuck, in which a small area of the skin is abraded and sequential coverslips are applied to follow the pattern of leukocyte emigration (Rebuck and Crowley, 1955). Similar observations have also been made on leukocyte infiltrates in skin blisters or joint fluids after inducing a mild inflammatory reaction. More recently, ^{111}In-oxine has been used to tag neutrophils in vitro and follow their migration into various tissues after intravenous injection of labeled cells. ^{111}In-oxine is a gamma emitter and can be localized by surface imaging. Its short half-life

(2.5 days) makes it a very useful isotope for leukokinetic studies, particularly for localizing internal abscesses (Koblik et al., 1985; Thakur et al., 1976).

Neutrophil migration to sites of inflammation depends on the degree and duration of tissue injury (Boggs, 1975). In a mild lesion, neutrophil migration may be negligible by 24 hours, while in a moderate to severe lesion (e.g., acute mastitis, pyometra, or an abscess) it may continue for a long period. Neutrophil influx into the lesion is maintained by efflux from blood and bone marrow (Jain et al., 1978). Neutrophil efflux is decreased during neutropenic states, while neutrophilia does not necessarily mean an increased efflux, and immature neutrophils rarely egress (Boggs, 1975).

Granulokinetic studies in acute (Marsh et al., 1967; Rosenshein et al., 1979) and chronic (Athens et al., 1965; Galbraith et al., 1965) infection or inflammation have shown that increased margination and a shortened T½ occur in early acute infection because of increased egress into tissues. This increased margination is followed by an expansion of the total blood granulocyte pool and normalization or lengthening of T½ in established or chronic infection. Endotoxin markedly alters neutrophil behavior in that migration into inflammatory sites is markedly reduced (Rosenshein et al., 1979).

Mechanisms of Neutrophilias

Granulokinetic studies indicate that a change in the blood neutrophil count may be mediated by one or more of the following basic mechanisms: (1) the rate of granulopoiesis, (2) the extent of influx of granulocytes from the marrow, (3) a shift of cells between the circulating and the marginal pools, (4) the intravascular life span of cells, and (5) the rate of efflux from the blood (Boggs, 1967, 1975; Vincent, 1977a). An increase in the first, second, and fourth mechanisms and a decrease in the fifth mechanism will result in a neutrophilia, whereas the converse will induce a neutropenia (Table 26–4). One should be aware that redistribution of cells between the circulating and the marginal pools may occur rapidly and give an erroneous impression that a neutrophilia or neutropenia exists. It has been observed that because a considerable number of neutrophils are sequestered in the spleen, splenectomy in human patients may be associated with neutrophilia, and patients with diminished splenic function, as in sickle cell anemia, may also show neutrophilia (Walker and Willemze, 1980).

The regulation of peripheral blood leukocyte level has been investigated by means of transfusing labeled leukocytes into the dog (Ambrus and Ambrus, 1959). The transfused cells disappeared from the circulation in 2–3 hours, and, upon injection of epinephrine,

they reappeared in the blood. The main source of leukocyte release was said to be the pulmonary and splenic circulations and to a lesser degree, the splanchnic circulation. Transfused labeled granulocytes appeared to migrate to the capillaries in the pulmonary circulation and were either released again to circulate or marginated into the lung alveoli, subsequently appearing in the saliva. Transfused labeled lymphocytes migrated through the walls of the intestine and were eliminated. The investigators suggested that the continuously high level of elimination of leukocytes through the respiratory and gastrointestinal tracts may be a mechanism to protect these organs against infection.

There appears to be a constant ebb and flow of leukocytes moving into and out of the pulmonary circulation which is reflected peripherally as a fluctuating leukocyte count (Bierman et al., 1955). The liver is an important removal site, but is not as active as the lungs in this respect. The spleen is also said to be a potent leukocyte sequestration site (McMillan and Scott, 1968). However, splenectomy in the dog did not alter the blood gran-

Table 26–4. Neutrophil Kinetics in Certain Clinical and Experimental Situations

Cause	Blood Pools			Blood Half-life $(T\frac{1}{2})$	Marrow	
	CGP	MGP	TBGP		Production	Release
Epinephrine	I	D	NC	NC	NC	NC
Etiocholanolone	I	I	I	NC	NC	I
Corticosteroids						
Acute	I	I	I	I	NC	I
Sustained	I	I	I	I	NC/I	NC/I
Endotoxin						
Early phase	D	I	NC	NC	NC	NC
Intermediate phase	I	I	I	NC	NC	I
Late phase	I	I	I	NC	I	I
Infection						
Initial phase	NC/D	I	NC	D	NC	NC
Intermediate phase	NC	I/NC	I	NC/I	NC	I
Established	I	I	I	NC/I	I	I
Chronic granulocytic leukemia	I	I	I	I	I	I
Hypersplenism						
Shift neutropenia	D	I	NC/I	NC/I	NC	NC/I
True neutropenia	D	I	D	NC/D (rare)	D	D
Immune-mediated neutropenia	D	D	D	D	NC/I	I

Data compiled from: Athens, 1970; Athens et al., 1961; Bishop et al., 1968, 1971; Boggs et al., 1965a, 1968b; Carlson and Kaneko, 1976; Finch, 1972; Fruhman, 1972; Marsh et al., 1967; Vincent, 1977a, b.

CGP, circulating granulocyte pool; MGP, marginal granulocyte pool; TBGP, total blood granulocyte pool; I, increase; D, decrease; NC, no change.

Peripheral blood neutrophilia is indicated by I in CGP and neutropenia by D in CGP.

ulocyte pool sizes or the turnover rate (Raab et al., 1964).

The shift of neutrophils into and out of the marginal pool may involve changes in their surface property and adherence to vascular endothelium. Decreased adherence is probably associated with increased mobilization into the circulating pool. Within 5 minutes, epinephrine increases blood neutrophil counts by 80% and decreases adherence by less than 50%. These effects are abolished by the beta antagonist propanolol hydrochloride if given before injection of epinephrine (Boxer et al., 1980). Stimulation of beta receptors by epinephrine releases cAMP (cyclic adenosine monophosphate) from endothelial cells, which decreases neutrophil adherence. In vitro adhesiveness of neutrophils to nylon fibers correlates well with their adherence to vascular endothelium (Spagnuole et al., 1980). Endotoxin increases adherence of neutrophils to nylon fibers, probably via increased production of thromboxane A_2 since this effect is blocked by aspirin (Spagnuole et al., 1980). Neutrophils contain acidic proteins in their specific granules whose release may enhance surface adherence, and they also produce two low molecular weight (30,000) "neutrophil adherence factors" (Bockenstedt et al., 1980). For additional comments on neutrophil adherence to endothelial cells see Chapter 13.

Epinephrine-Induced Response

Increased release of epinephrine and norepinephrine during "fight-or-flight reaction" is associated with tachycardia, bronchodilation, peripheral vasoconstriction, neutrophilia, and lymphocytosis (Boxer et al., 1980). Neutrophilia also develops after stress, exercise, or epinephrine injection. This neutrophilia is attributed to an increase in the size of the circulating pool as a consequence of decrease in the marginal pool, and is called "stress," "shift," or "pseudo" neutrophilia because the size of the total blood granulocyte pool remains essentially unchanged. The $T\frac{1}{2}$ and the granulocyte turnover rate are unaltered (Athens et al., 1961). The increase in circulating granulocyte pool is generally rapid but transient, and its magnitude is usually two- to threefold. The many instances of transient neutrophilias seen in clinic patients may be stress neutrophilias. Conversely, neutropenia may develop as a result of a relative increase in the marginal pool (from shift of circulating neutrophils), e.g., after an intravenous injection of endotoxin.

Corticosteroid-Induced Response

Administration or excessive release of corticosteroids in vivo typically induces leukocytosis, neutrophilia, lymphopenia, eosinopenia, basopenia, and monocytosis or monocytopenia, depending on the species involved (Faucy et al., 1976; Jasper and Jain, 1965). Studies in humans, dogs, and calves indicate that neutrophilia from a single episode of release or injection of corticosteroids is due to a real increase in the total blood granulocyte pool (Athens et al., 1961; Bishop et al., 1968; Boggs, 1967; Carlson and Kaneko, 1976; Faucy et al., 1976). This increase is attributed to accelerated mobilization of mature neutrophils from the marrow storage pool and a decreased migration of cells out of the blood vasculature. Neutrophil $T\frac{1}{2}$ increases modestly, while granulocyte turnover rate remains normal because of the increased total blood granulocyte pool. Mobilization of neutrophils from the marginal pool is generally thought to be negligible (Bishop et al., 1968), but the suggestion (Carlson and Kaneko, 1976) that it may be a contributory factor requires exploration.

The blood level of corticosteroids after stress is proportional to the severity and duration of stress, but it returns to normal within 12–24 hours after the stress episode. The blood corticosteroid level increases immediately after stress-induced release of adrenocorticotropic hormone (ACTH) from the anterior pituitary. The biologic $T\frac{1}{2}$ of ACTH is 1–14 minutes and that of corticosteroids is 90 minutes; dexamethasone has a longer circulation time than cortisol (Nelson, 1980). Hence corticosteroid-induced neutrophilia typically lasts for only a few hours, with neutrophil counts becoming normal by 24 hours.

Neutrophilia of prolonged corticosteroid administration is associated with increased total blood granulocyte pool as a result of increased $T\frac{1}{2}$ from decreased egress with normal rates of production and release (Athens et al., 1961; Vincent, 1977a). Repeated administration is associated with a progressively diminished neutrophilia, probably due to depletion of marrow reserve by continuous accelerated drainage (Jasper and Jain, 1965). Corticosteroids have been found to either stimulate or inhibit myelopoiesis or to have no significant effect (Gorski, 1979).

Response to Infection and Inflammation

Neutrophil kinetics in infection or inflammation vary with the degree and duration of the disease process. The initial response is a reduction in neutrophil numbers due to increased margination and migration into tissues (Walker and Willemze, 1980). In the intermediate phase neutrophils from the marrow reserve are released into the vasculature causing an increase in the marginal granulocyte pool, but not in the circulating granulocyte pool (Boggs et al., 1965b; Craddock et al., 1963; Marsh et al., 1967; Vincent, 1977a; Walker and Willemze, 1980). This is called "masked granulocytosis" because the total blood granulocyte pool is increased. An increase in the size of the marginal pool in such instances may be beneficial to the host by providing more neutrophils for diapedesis into the tissues to combat infection or to modulate the inflammatory response.

As the inflammatory response progresses, a true neutrophilia develops from increases in both the marginal and the circulating granulocyte pools as a result of increased granulopoiesis and release of newly formed cells into the vasculature (Athens et al., 1965). The adjustment of granulopoietic activity in such cases involves increased stem cell input, decreased ineffective granulopoiesis, decreased generation time, additional mitoses, and decreased postmitotic time (Walker and Willemze, 1980).

Neutrophil T½ is reduced during the first few hours of infection, probably from increased egress of cells into the site of inflammation (Marsh et al., 1967), but in established infection it is normal or prolonged (Athens et al., 1965). The latter finding seems incongruous with the need for increased efflux of neutrophils into inflammatory sites; it has been suggested that this finding may be due to diminution of physiologic random loss of neutrophils into normal tissues (Cronkite and Vincent, 1969). In most instances of chronic neutrophilias, the turnover rate of granulocytes is normal or increased and the T½ value is longer than normal. This situation may persist for days or weeks. Human patients with immature granulocytes in the peripheral blood, as in chronic granulocytic leukemia, myelofibrosis, and myeloid metaplasia, have a relatively long neutrophil T½ (25–90 hours), compared with a T½ of less than 18 hours in neutrophilias mainly due to mature cells (Rottini et al., 1979). This long T½ is thought to reflect inability of immature cells to leave the blood rapidly and/or recirculation of immature cells through the bone marrow and spleen.

Endotoxin-Induced Response

Intravenous administration of endotoxin produces within minutes a marked neutropenia, followed by a rebound neutrophilia within a few hours. The former effect is attributed to shift of cells into the marginal pool and the latter to increased release of cells from the marrow reserve (Athens et al., 1961; Boggs et al., 1968a, b). The number of circulating platelets and lymphocytes also decreases following endotoxin administration. Such quantitative changes in blood cells have been found in humans (Boggs et al., 1968a; Dale et al., 1975; Mechanic et al., 1962; Quessenberry et al., 1972), dogs (Boggs et al., 1968b), cows (Jain and Lasmanis, 1978b; Lumsden et al., 1974), horses (Burrows, 1979), and water buffalo calves (Jain et al., 1980) given endotoxin intravenously and in cows inoculated with a large dose of endotoxin or viable coliform organisms into the mammary gland (Jain et al., 1978; Schalm and Lasmanis, 1976). It has been reported that subcutaneous injection of piromen, a polysaccharide of *Pseudomonas aeruginosa*, in the bovine produces a mild and transient neutropenia in comparison to a marked neutropenia of longer duration produced by intravenous administration (Lumsden et al., 1974). Intraperitoneal injection of endotoxin into horses results in neutropenia similar to that seen following intravenous administration (Burrows, 1979).

The bovine mammary gland is a convenient

and excellent model for studying migration of neutrophils into an inflammatory site and for assessing influence of inflammation on blood and bone marrow granulocytes. For example, blood neutrophil counts fell 4–6 hours after induction of acute bovine mastitis by intramammary injection of *E. coli* endotoxin (Jain et al., 1978). Simultaneously, neutrophils from bone marrow reserves began to mobilize so that the blood neutrophil count gradually increased. By 24–72 hours, there was a secondary decrease of blood neutrophils, probably due to redistribution of cells within the vascular granulocyte compartments. After 72 hours, a secondary increase in blood neutrophil numbers occurred, apparently from the continuous supply of newly formed cells as a result of increased granulopoiesis in the bone marrow. Granulopoietic activity returned to normal within 6–7 days.

The precise mechanisms of endotoxin-induced cytopenias are not known, although a variety of mechanisms have been proposed. These include participation of humoral factors, changes in cell surface properties, and generation of bioactive substances from activation of neutrophils, platelets, and vascular endothelial cells (Gimbrone and Buchanan, 1982). Endotoxin exerts a variety of effects on humoral and cellular components of blood (reviewed by Morrison and Ulevitch, 1978). For example, endotoxin can activate complement by both the classical and the alternate pathways, generate kallikrein through activation of Hageman factor (coagulation factor XII), stimulate arachidonic acid metabolism in platelets, neutrophils, and macrophages, and induce release of a variety of bioactive substances from platelets and leukocytes. Endotoxin-stimulated neutrophils also exhibit increased enzyme release and respiratory burst and decreased locomotion not inhibited by indomethacin (Dahinden et al., 1983). In all these reactions, the active portion of the endotoxin is the lipid A portion.

Studies in the cat and dog indicated that thrombocytopenia is dependent on activation of serum complement, while platelet injury and destruction were primarily involved in studies on piglets and baboons (reviewed by Hinshaw et al., 1982).

Endotoxin-induced neutropenia has been attributed to a number of factors. These include direct action of endotoxin and release or generation of chemotactic factors such as C5a (Gilbertsen et al., 1980; Hammerschmidt et al., 1981); thromboxane A_2 (Spagnuole et al., 1980); leukotriene B_4 (Bray, 1982; Ford-Hutchinson, 1983; Lindbom et al., 1982); platelet aggregating factor (Ford-Hutchinson, 1983); plasma kallikrein (Schapira et al., 1983); acidic proteins (Bockenstedt et al., 1980) and lactoferrin (Boxer et al., 1982; Lash et al., 1983; Oseas et al., 1981) from specific granules of neutrophils; and lymphokines (Badenoch-Jones, 1982). Prostaglandin E_2 was found to have no direct effect, but it potentiated the effect of C5 fragments (Tonnesen et al., 1982); C3 and C4 were not essential to development of neutropenia (see review by Morrison and Ulevitch, 1978).

In a recent study on neutrophils from a human patient deficient in specific granules, it was found that specific granule constituents are not required for adherence and aggregation in vitro or endotoxin-induced margination in vivo (Gallin et al., 1982). It is interesting that indomethacin inhibited endotoxin-induced neutrophil adherence (Spagnuole et al., 1980), but not granulocytopenia in rabbits (Howes et al., 1978). Factors promoting or inhibiting aggregation have been implicated to cause similar influences on neutrophil adherence (Ford-Hutchinson, 1983; Gilbertsen et al., 1980; Hammerschmidt et al., 1981; Schapira et al., 1983).

The role of endothelium in induction of thrombocytopenia and neutropenia has been investigated (reviewed by Gimbrone and Buchanan, 1982, and Tonnesen et al., 1982). Under in vitro conditions, platelets do not adhere to normal human and bovine endothelial cells, but neutrophils show some preferential adherence. There is marked platelet adherence to endothelium that has been "altered" as a result of virus infection, mechanical injury, and chemical or toxic modification (Gimbrone and Buchanan, 1982). Thus such a platelet-endothelium interaction in vivo may result in localized release of a variety of substances from platelets (see Table 16–1) and cause secondary accumulation of neutrophils at such sites.

The adherent properties of neutrophils

vary (Tonnesen et al., 1982); neutrophil–endothelial cell interaction requires divalent cations and is stimulated by action of chemotactic factors (such as FMLP, C5a, and bacterial filtrates) on either the endothelial cells or neutrophils (Hoover et al., 1978, 1980). Although basal neutrophil adherence to endothelial cells does not appear to involve cyclo-oxygenase derivatives of arachidonic acid or to be affected by prostacyclin, some lipo-oxygenase derivatives (e.g., leukotrienes) may be active in this process. In general, it has been shown that increased intracellular cyclic guanosine monophosphate (cGMP) is associated with increased granulocyte adherence, while increased intracellular cAMP is associated with decreased adherence (reviewed in Smith and Lumsden, 1983).

Neutrophilia is effected by generation of a "neutrophil releasing factor" and not by corticosteroids, although both are produced following endotoxin administration (Boggs et al., 1968a, 1968b). Subsequently, endotoxin triggers increased production of "colony stimulating factor," which then stimulates granulopoiesis (Quessenberry et al., 1972). Also see Release of Marrow Neutrophils section below.

Mechanisms of Neutropenias

Neutropenia has been studied less extensively. It may be caused by one or more of the following: (a) reduced total blood granulocyte pool with an equal or unequal distribution between the circulating and marginal pools (early endotoxin-induced response); (b) decreased survival (immune or nonimmune mediated change); (c) increased efflux (severe infection); (d) increased ineffective granulopoiesis (vitamin B_{12}–folate deficiency in humans); or (e) decreased granulopoiesis or release (iatrogenic) from the bone marrow. Neutropenia due to marrow retention of neutrophils is called "myelokathexis" (Zuelzer, 1964) and has been reported in certain dogs treated with nitrogen mustard (Boggs et al., 1966a). Neutropenia may result from a congenital defect in granulopoiesis as in gray collie dogs (see Chapter 4). Neutropenia of hypersplenism or that associated with enlarged spleen in humans is often due to excessive margination and sometimes due to shortened

survival time or a true reduction in the total blood granulocyte pool from decreased marrow production (Vincent, 1977a). Severe neutropenia results in increased susceptibility to infection.

REGULATION OF NEUTROPHIL HOMEOSTASIS

The number of neutrophils in circulation is normally maintained by a continuous process of random release of mature cells from the bone marrow. The rates of granulocyte production and release equal the rate of neutrophil egress from the circulation under steady state conditions. Several factors have been found to regulate granulopoiesis and egress of marrow granulocytes into the blood (Golde and Cline, 1974; Lichtman et al., 1977; Vogler and Winton, 1975). An interplay of these factors is involved at times of increased demand for neutrophils such as during infection and inflammation. The need may be met by: (a) increased release of mature neutrophils and some band cells from the marrow reserve; (b) shorter transit time of cells through the postmitotic maturative pool; (c) increase in mitosis at the myelocyte stage with a shorter cell cycle time (a decrease in ineffective granulopoiesis, which occurs at the myelocyte stage, may accomplish the same, particularly in the dog); and (d) increased stem cell input and differentiation of committed stem cells to form more granulocytes (van Furth and Willemze, 1979).

Release of Marrow Neutrophils

Release of marrow neutrophils is influenced by marrow microanatomy, geographic location of cells within the marrow, cellular age and properties, cell-releasing factors, and neurohormonal factors (reviewed by Lichtman et al., 1977). Granulopoiesis occurs at extravascular locations in the bone marrow, and mature neutrophils are found close to the sinusoidal wall. Electron microscopic studies of normal animal marrow have indicated that mature neutrophils traverse marrow vascular sinuses through narrow "migration pores" created in the sinusoidal endothelium by migrating cells. The cells pass through the endothelial cells and not through intercellular junctions, as is the case when granulocytes leave the microcirculation to enter tissues. At the migration sites, there may be interrupted basement membrane and fenestrated adventitial coat. Alterations in marrow microanatomy during disease may influence blood neutrophil counts; for example, endotoxin induces changes in the adventitial cells and marrow interstitium—basement membrane substance is decreased and lysosomal disruption occurs in endothelial cells—leading to enlargement of aperture and consequently neutrophilia (Weiss, 1970, 1976).

Cellular deformability and motility of neutrophils increase with maturation. These changes result partly from a decrease in the viscous property of the cytoplasm and partly from an increase in the nuclear flow property. Simultaneously, changes occur in surface composition (decrease in sialoproteins), causing a reduction in surface negative charge and diminution of surface adhesiveness. Hence mature cells are more deformable and less adhesive and are, therefore, the first to egress.

Blood flow in marrow sinusoids is influenced by neurohormonal mechanisms. For example, catecholamines affect marrow arteries, and ATP influences actomyosin in vascular endothelium. Hence neutrophil release is said to be directly proportional to the blood flow regulated by the intramedullary nerve supply and indirectly to the number of neutrophils in sinusoidal blood (Lichtman et al., 1977; Vincent, 1977a).

A humoral agent influencing release of neutrophils from the bone marrow was demonstrated in several species. This factor has been given different names such as leukocytosis promoting factor (LPF), leukocytosis inducing factor (LIF), neutrophil releasing factor (NRF), neutrophil releasing activity (NRA), granulocyte production factor (GPF), leukopoietin G, and renal granulopoiesis factor (RGF). It is found in serums of rats (Gordon et al., 1960; Handler et al., 1966) and rabbits (Fukuda and Matsumoto, 1959) and in plasma of dogs (Boggs et al., 1966b, 1966c) and humans (Dale et al., 1977). It is distinct from colony stimulating factor and is considered a physiologic regulator of neutrophil numbers in blood (Boggs, 1967). Its characteristics, site of origin, and mode of action remain to be

defined. It probably acts as a cytoattractant for mature neutrophils or alters sinusoidal wall structure, making cell egress possible. A C3 fragment was also found to enhance release of neutrophils from the bone marrow (Rother, 1972).

Control of Production

Regulation of granulocyte production is operative at various levels of granulopoiesis and involves participation of intramedullary and extramedullary factors. Marrow microenvironment plays an important role in early differentiation of pluripotent stem cells into committed progenitors. Humoral factors controlling development of granulocytic precursors and formation of mature neutrophils have been demonstrated in in vivo and in vitro studies (reviewed by Golde and Cline, 1974; Robinson and Mangalik, 1975; Vogler and Winton, 1975). These factors are broadly categorized as (a) colony stimulating factor (CSF) and colony inhibitory factor (CIF) and (b) chalone and antichalone. Both form a system of positive and negative feedback controls and are considered important regulators of granulopoiesis under physiologic and pathologic conditions. Abnormalities of such control mechanisms have been found in granulocytic leukemias and neutropenias from diminished production as in gray collie dogs (Golde and Cline, 1974).

Colony Stimulatory and Inhibitory Factors

Colony stimulating factor is found in small amounts in serum and urine and can be obtained from a variety of sources such as mature neutrophils, monocytes, macrophages, activated lymphocytes, embryonic kidney, spleen, lungs, and vascular endothelium (Rickard et al., 1971; Stanely and Metcalf, 1969). Three major types of CSF have been recognized, each being a glycoprotein and differing in molecular weight (23,000–60,000) and functional specificity. See Chapter 13 for details. The properties of CSF vary within and among species depending on its source and mode of action; e.g., patterns of differentiation of colonies depend on the type of CSF and its concentration. It acts on committed granulocyte precursors (CFU-GM) and must be continuously present for its in vitro effect to be accomplished (Rickard et al., 1971). It increases the number of dividing cells and decreases the cell cycle time.

Increased production of CSF is associated with an increase in granulopoiesis and blood neutrophil numbers. Hence CSF is considered a true granulopoietin. Neutrophilia associated with certain tumors may be due to increased secretion of CSF (Murphy, 1976). An inverse correlation has been found between blood neutrophil numbers and CSF in irradiated mice and in gray collie dogs with cyclic neutropenia (see Vogler and Winton, 1975). CSF and CIF have been detected in dogs made neutropenic by infusion of rabbit anticanine neutrophil serum (Rudolph and Kaneko, 1980).

Increased levels of CSF are found during the first 2–4 weeks after birth and are related to neutrophilia (Barak et al., 1980). Its production is increased during acute bacterial and viral infections and in response to neutropenias from a variety of causes. Endotoxin injection induces a 100-fold increase from secretion by macrophages. Lower levels of CSF are found in germfree mice, and higher levels are found during infection (Murphy, 1976). Increased levels appear in germfree mice after ureteral ligation (Foster and Mirand, 1970).

Colony inhibitory factor is also present in normal serum, urine, neutrophil extracts, monocytes, macrophages, and many other body cells. It is a glycoprotein with a molecular weight of 45,000, is dialyzable, and is heat labile (53–55°C for 30 minutes). It acts on CFU and on committed stem cells and blocks the action of CSF. Levels of CSF and CIF vary inversely in irradiated mice. Variable levels of CIF are found in acute and chronic granulocytic leukemias, and chronic granulocytic leukemia cells seem to be less suppressed by CIF (Broxmeyer et al., 1978).

Chalone and Antichalone

Chalones are tissue-specific, endogenous, nontoxic substances capable of inhibiting mitosis by negative feedback. They are present in many tissues and, importantly, are produced by the same cells whose function they regulate. Thus chalones are tissue- and cell-specific, but not species-specific.

Rytömaa and Kiviniemi (1968) demon-strated that granulocyte production in rats is controlled by a humoral feedback mechanism involving a specific inhibitor (chalone) and a specific stimulator (antichalone). Chalone is present in mature granulocytes, fresh serum, and splenic extracts. It is a polypeptide of low molecular weight (2,000–4,000) and is rapidly inactivated at 4°C. It decreases mitotic activity of the proliferative pool almost instantaneously, but its effect is transient.

Granulocyte antichalone is present only in the serum and has a molecular weight of 30,000–35,000. It causes a rapid, reversible, and short-term stimulation of cellular proliferation, affecting both DNA and RNA synthesis. In conditions of acute functional demand for granulocytes, antichalone appears in the serum and the content of chalone decreases markedly. Rytömaa suggested injecting chalone to control abnormal granulopoiesis as a therapeutic approach to leukemia (Rytömaa and Kiviniemi, 1970; Vogler and Winton, 1975). However, the use of this approach seems to be limited because neoplastic cells are relatively less sensitive to chalone's effect, and in certain cases such cells themselves produce increased amounts of chalone, which may suppress normal granulopoiesis.

Other Stimulators and Inhibitors of Granulopoiesis

Several other substances have been said to have a stimulatory or inhibitory effect on granulopoiesis. Stimulatory substances include PGI_2 (Miller et al., 1978), *Corynebacterium parvum* (Eliopoulos et al., 1980), *E. coli* endotoxin (Hammond et al., 1978), and lithium (Anonymous, 1980; Hammond and Dale, 1980). *C. parvum* increases granulopoiesis by increasing the number of CFU-GM and granulocytic series cells. Injection of *E. coli* endotoxin and lithium therapy ameliorate the cyclic pattern of granulopoiesis in gray collie dogs. Endotoxin increases production of CSF. Lithium augments production of CSF and directly stimulates pluripotent stem cells by inhibiting adenylate cyclase and thereby reducing the intracellular level of cAMP. For additional information see Chapter 13.

Inhibitory substances include PGE_1 and PGE_2, lactoferrin, and other cell products. PGEs make CFUs less responsive to CSF and modulate production of both granulocytes and monocytes (Miller et al., 1978). Macrophages produce both CSF and PGEs. CSF production is inhibited by lactoferrin, by a plasma factor from patients with chronic renal failure (Morris et al., 1980), and by a serum inhibitor found in certain neutropenic or marrow failure patients (Fitchen and Cline, 1980). Lactoferrin suppresses CSF production by mononuclear phagocytes, thereby decreasing granulopoiesis in vitro. Fully saturated lactoferrin is more inhibitory (Broxmeyer et al., 1980), and the polymerized molecule is inactive (Bagby and Bennett, 1982). Effects of endotoxin, testosterone, and corticosteroids may be mediated by lactoferrin (Broxmeyer et al., 1980). It is released by phagocytosing, but not resting neutrophils. CSF activity in chronic granulocytic leukemia is lower than normal (Szmitkowski et al., 1980). Neutrophils from chronic granulocytic leukemia patients contain lactoferrin, but about half of the cells fail to release it (Philip et al., 1981). Committed stem cells are also inhibited by products secreted by "null" lymphocytes (Broxmeyer 1979) and a high-molecular-weight substance in normal serum and leukemic cell extracts (Morris et al., 1980). A factor in plasma from patients with acute and chronic myeloid and lymphoid leukemias inhibits colony formation of normal bone marrow cells, but not of leukemic cells in vitro (Steinberg and Handler, 1979); the plasma factor is called "leukemia-associated inhibitory activity" (Broxmeyer et al., 1979). This factor is also present in normal bone marrow and blood cells and has been identified as an acidic isoferritin (Broxmeyer et al., 1982).

CHEMOTAXIS AND MIGRATION INTO TISSUES

Chemotaxis is a prerequisite for phagocytosis in tissues because the cells must sense and approach the site of infection before they can engulf the organism. *Chemotaxis* is defined as a directional movement of the leukocyte toward a concentration gradient of a chemotactic agent. Neutrophils can recognize a 1.0% gradient over a distance as small as one cell length, and can reverse polarity if a chemotactic agent is applied to the opposite end. *Chemokinesis* is defined as an enhanced nondirectional (random) movement. *Cytotaxin* (chemotaxin or leukotaxin) is a substance exerting direct chemotactic effect on the cells, while *cytotaxigen* is a substance inducing the formation of a cytotaxin. Neutrophils moving toward a chemoattractant constantly reorient and also show increased random movement (Cheung et al., 1982). Information on chemotaxis has been reviewed (Becker, 1977; Gallin and Quie, 1978; Smith and Lumsden, 1983; Walker and Willemze, 1980; Wilkinson, 1980, 1982).

Techniques

The ability of neutrophils to respond to chemoattractants can be measured in vitro by using the Boyden chamber (Cornely, 1966) or Harris tissue culture system (Kass and De Bruyn, 1967). Their ability to emigrate in tissues can be measured in vivo by the skin window technique of Rebuck (Rebuck and Crowley, 1955). These techniques have been modified to improve the method and obtain more reliable results.

The Boyden chamber consists of two compartments separated by a micropore filter. Leukocytes are placed in the upper compartment, and the chemotactic agent in the lower compartment. A concentration gradient is thus created between the compartments, and chemotaxis through the membrane ensues. After a specific interval at 37°C, the filter is removed and stained so that the cells that have passed through the filter and are located on the other side of the filter can be counted. In a modified procedure, two micropore filters are used, and the cells that have penetrated the upper filter and have reached the lower filter are counted. Zigmond and Hirsch (1973) have modified the Boyden chamber method to distinguish chemokinetic and chemotactic behaviors of neutrophils. A method has been described to study migration of neutrophils and monocytes through agarose (Nelson et al., 1975; Smith et al., 1985).

The skin window technique of Rebuck consists of applying a sterile coverslip to a slightly abraded area of the skin to allow for adhesion of emigrating neutrophils onto the glass surface. Sequential studies can be made by repeated application of additional coverslips.

These techniques have contributed a great deal to our understanding of neutrophil and monocyte mobilization in health and disease. A sluggish neutrophil response with any of these techniques is often correlated with lowered resistance to bacterial infection.

Factors Involved

A wide variety of factors influence chemotaxis (Becker, 1977; Fantone et al., 1982; Gallin, 1981; Keller et al., 1975; Wilkinson, 1980, 1982). Chemotaxis is temperature dependent, being optimal at 33–45°C; is independent of pH between 6.5 and 7.5; requires Ca^{++} and Mg^{++}; is energy dependent, being stimulated by glycolysis; and is depressed under hypoxic conditions (Casciato, 1978). Individual variations have been found in a quantitative evaluation of chemotactic response of neutrophils in studies on Beagle dogs (Latimer et al., 1981).

Since Menkin in 1956 first described "leukotaxin," numerous substances have been found to possess chemotactic properties (Table 26–5). The most important ones are those derived from the complement system, C5a being the most potent chemoattractant for neutrophils. Earlier studies had also suggested the chemotactic role of C3a and C567,

but recent observations with highly purified C3a did not support that claim (Hugli, 1978). Complement components are also chemotactic for eosinophils (see p. 741), basophils (see p. 761), and to a certain extent for monocytes (see p. 776; Fruhman, 1970). Neutrophil infiltration does not occur in complement-deficient animals.

Chemotactic complement fragments are generated more rapidly by the classical than by the alternate pathway of complement activation. Serum complement can be activated by immune complexes and by nonspecific proteases released from damaged tissues, neutrophils, and bacteria. C5 can be directly cleaved by lysosomal enzymes from neutrophils and by enzymes such as trypsin and plasmin. Fibroblasts can cleave C5 to C5a and also can elaborate chemotactic factors other than collagen in vitro (Sobel and Gallin, 1979). A heat-labile chemotactic factor for neutrophils is formed when *Staphylococcus aureus* is incubated in milk from endotoxin-infused mammary glands, but not in milk from normal glands (O'Gairbhidge et al., 1970). Generation of complement-derived chemotactic factors may be modulated by serum inhibitors of both the classical and alternate pathways of complement activation and by "chemotactic factor inactivators" in serum (Fantone et al., 1982).

Table 26–5. Neutrophil Chemoattractants and Inhibitors of Chemotaxis

Chemoattractants	Inactivators or Inhibitors
Activated complement components C5a, C567	Serum factors, e.g., chemotactic factor inactivator
Plasminogen activator	Cell-derived inhibitors
Kallikrein	Neutrophil immobilizing factor
Fibrin degradation products	Bacterial products
Collagen and its split products	Substances increasing cAMP levels
Factors from neutrophils, monocytes, macrophages, mast cells, and fibroblasts	Corticosteroids
Certain lymphokines	
Bacterial products—certain *N*-formyl methionyl peptides (FMP)	
Synthetic oligopeptides of FMP	
Viral products	
Casein and chemically altered proteins	
Tissue factors, e.g., lymph node permeability factor	
Fragments from IgG and IgM	
Arachidonic acid metabolites: PGFs, thromboxane B_2, leukotriene B_4, HHT. PGEs nd HETE have variable effects.	
Substances increasing cellular levels of cGMP	

Products of arachidonic acid metabolism exert a variable influence: PGFs, thromboxane B_2, leukotriene (LK) B_4, and HHT were found to exert a positive effect; PGEs and HETE had no or positive influence; and PGA and LK C_4 had no influence (Malnsten et al., 1980; Till et al., 1979). Chemokinesis was also increased by PGFs, HHT, and HETE, but not by PGEs and PGA. PGEs increase chemotaxis in the presence of serum albumin; hence they may be significant in inflamed areas where albumin accumulates as a result of increased capillary permeability (Till et al., 1979). Certain N-formyl methionyl peptides of bacterial origin and their synthetic analogues, particularly FMLP, have been found to exert chemotactic activity. The latter are being used increasingly to test this aspect of leukocyte function in vitro (Niedel and Cuatrecasas, 1980). Platelet aggregating factor, released from leukocytes, can act as a chemoattractant for neutrophils and also cause their aggregation, superoxide generation, and degranulation (Jouvin-Marche et al., 1982).

Mechanisms

A motile neutrophil has a broad leading edge of cytoplasm (lamellipodium) almost devoid of lysosomal granules, and a knob-like uropod having many long, retractile filaments at the posterior end. The nucleus is toward the posterior end, while most of the cytoplasm and granules are in front of the nucleus but behind the lamellipodium.

Locomotion of leukocytes is currently believed to involve their cytomusculoskeletal system, i.e., microfilaments and microtubules. Chemokinesis is presumably dependent on the microfilament system, whereas chemotactic orientation and movement of the cell depends largely on the organization of the microtubular system.

Agents affecting organization of microfilaments and microtubules interfere with various aspects of neutrophil functions (Goetzl and Gorman, 1978). For example, colchicine and vinblastine or vincristine, which cause disruption of microtubules, inhibit chemotaxis and degranulation, but have no effect on random movement and phagocytosis. Inhibition of chemokinesis by an inhibitor of microtubule assembly was reported in one study

(Valerius, 1979). Cytochalasin B, which alters microfilament assembly, inhibits random movement as well as chemotaxis and phagocytosis and promotes degranulation. Abnormalities of microtubules are associated with defective chemotaxis.

Studies with various synthetic peptides and complement-derived cytotaxins indicate that chemotaxis may involve interaction of the chemotactic factors with structurally specific receptors on the neutrophil surface (Becker, 1977; Gallin, 1980). Such an interaction leads to activation of a serine proesterase. This activation, along with participation of an already activated esterase, then may induce chemotaxis. Organophosphorus inhibitors such as DFP and phosphonate esters inhibit chemotaxis by inactivating esterases on the neutrophil surface (Ward and Becker, 1967).

Another mechanism of chemotaxis consists of an increase in the fluxes of monovalent (Na^+ and K^+) and divalent (Ca^{++} and Mg^{++}) cations, in part through activation of a membrane Na^+-K^+-dependent ATPase. An increase in intracellular level of ionized Ca^{++} is believed to induce breakdown and remodeling of membrane phospholipids and to sustain a series of unknown reactions leading to chemotactic factor–induced orientation and locomotion (Becker et al., 1983). Alterations in surface charge and degranulation or release of substances from specific granules have also been implicated (Gallin et al., 1978).

In Vivo Significance

Extravasation of neutrophils (diapedesis) begins shortly after microbial infection and is normally followed by chemotactic attraction toward the organism, its phagocytosis, and destruction. During the process of diapedesis, circulating neutrophils first adhere or marginate along the altered venular endothelial surface and then emigrate through intercellular junctions, cross the basement membrane, and enter the tissue.

Cyclic nucleotides, divalent cations, and probably prostacyclin may be involved in neutrophil adherence to the vascular endothelium. Adhesion of neutrophils is enhanced by exposure to C5a and by unidentified lysosomal substances released in the vicinity in response to the provoking agent such as

Gram-negative bacteria (An, 1980; Hoover et al., 1980).

Emigration may be facilitated by discharge of specific granules and plasmin activation at the site of migration (Baggiolini et al., 1980). Penetration of the basement membrane may involve partial destruction of the membrane by the proteolytic enzymes of the neutrophils in transit (Zakhireh et al., 1979).

The speed and magnitude of leukocyte mobilization varies with the tissues involved, with the physiologic state of the individual, and perhaps with the genetic makeup. The character of the exudate varies with the type of injury and changes during the course of an inflammatory response.

Experimental and clinical studies have established that an infection flares up when there are inadequate numbers of circulating neutrophils for mobilization into the tissues or when neutrophil mobilization is interfered with. In such situations, saprophytic organisms may proliferate, or uninhibited multiplication of pathogenic microorganisms occurs during the first few hours of entry into the tissue to produce a fatal disease.

For example, it has been shown that in the absence of neutrophil mobilization, an unrestricted growth of pneumococci occurs in tissues, even in the presence of humoral bactericidal factors (Rich and McKee, 1934). Severe neutropenias produced by use of antileukocyte serum, x-radiation, or nitrogen mustard result in increased susceptibility to exogenous and endogenous bacteria. It is stated that a reduction of more than 90% neutrophils is required to elicit such an effect (Fruhman, 1970); hence moderate neutropenias usually have little or no influence on susceptibility to infection.

In our studies on neutropenic cows (Jain et al., 1971; reviewed by Jain, 1976), it was demonstrated that severe coliform mastitis and permanent functional damage to the mammary glands occurred in the absence of adequate neutrophil mobilization into the experimentally infected mammary glands. Severe mastitis also developed in previously clinically normal mammary glands harboring micrococci (Schalm et al., 1976); in this instance, neutropenia curtailed neutrophil migration into the mammary glands and allowed unrestricted bacterial growth leading to mastitis.

In cyclic neutropenia of gray collie dogs, an increased susceptibility to infection develops during the neutropenic phase (Page and Good, 1958). It has been shown that about 200 cocci can be destroyed by as few as 10 neutrophils (Wilson et al., 1957). Theoretically, in the absence of neutrophils, 200 bacteria, by doubling their number every 30 minutes, would multiply to more than 3.2 million in just 7 hours, thus resulting in a serious infection.

FUNCTIONS

The best known and most investigated function of neutrophils is their role in the body's defense against pathogenic bacteria. Neutrophils also play an important role in the inflammatory process and can inflict tissue damage. Many new functional activities of neutrophils have been demonstrated in recent years, but the extent of their significance in vivo remains to be established. These include roles in coagulation and fibrinolysis, lymphocyte stimulation, iron absorption, and cytotoxicity for various body cells. Functional studies have been made on canine (Cook et al., 1978; Harvath et al., 1978), bovine (Beswick and Slater, 1977; Chambers et al., 1983; Nikolajczuk, 1978), and equine (Camp and Leid, 1982; Camp et al., 1979; Coigmoul et al., 1984; Jacobsen et al., 1982) neutrophils in addition to those from human and laboratory animals. Functional subpopulations of neutrophils have been recognized in human blood (Klempner and Gallin, 1978).

Phagocytosis

Phagocytosis, the ingestion of microscopically visible particles, and *pinocytosis*, the uptake of fluid vesicles by living cells, are considered essential phenomena of cell nutrition and self-defense among unicellular as well as multicellular organisms. The two processes together are called *endocytosis*. Phagocytosis on a surface is called "surface phagocytosis," and passive internalization of external medium along with the particle is called "piggyback phagocytosis."

Metchnikoff in 1893 introduced the term

phagocytosis (from the Greek *phagein*, "to eat") and conclusively demonstrated that phagocytic cells are of great importance for host defense against invading bacteria. It is now well established that resistance to infection depends principally upon an interaction of phagocytes, humoral factors (antibody and complement), and properties of the pathogen. Specific defects of the phagocytes and immunologic deficiencies in which susceptibility to certain bacterial diseases is increased have been demonstrated. Several reviews are available on these subjects (Austin and Cohn, 1963; Cohn and Austin, 1963; Rowley, 1962; Smith and Lumsden, 1983; Suter and Ramseier, 1964). Some observations have been made utilizing neutrophils from various animal species (Bertram et al., 1982; Jain, 1976; Jain and Lasmanis, 1978a; Mackie et al., 1982; Paape et al., 1979; Wakeyama et al., 1982).

Ingestion and Degranulation

Phagocytosis, whether in vivo or in vitro, is a two-step process involving at first "recognition" of the target and then its ingestion. The process of phagocytosis and post-phagocytic events have been studied by various means including electron microscopy and cytochemical and immunochemical methods (Klebanoff and Clark, 1978; MacRae et al., 1980; Pryzwanoky et al., 1979).

Chemotactically responsive neutrophils recognize bacteria through differences in surface properties and/or their opsonic receptors. They instantaneously undergo metabolic stimulation, advance pseudopods to entrap the bacterium, and then internalize it (Fig. 26–6). Pseudopod formation is a microfilament function. Fusion of the pseudopods around the bacterium results in formation of a membranous sac (phagocytic vacuole or "phagosome") containing the organism. The outer membrane of the phagocytic vacuole is made of the inner side of the plasma membrane, while its inner surface is made of the outer side of the plasma membrane.

Some rearrangement of membrane lipid and protein molecules is believed to occur during formation of phagocytic vacuoles which probably regulates their fusion with the cytoplasmic granules (lysosomes) (Rikihisa and Mizuno, 1978). Lysosomes in the vi-

cinity of the phagocytic vacuole fuse with the vacuolar membrane forming a "phagolysosome" or "secondary lysosome" and release their contents therein to kill and digest the bacterium (Fig. 26–7). It is believed, however, that the majority of the lysosomal hydrolytic enzymes discharged into the phagocytic vacuole serve a digestive function and are not directly involved in killing bacteria (Gobig, 1980). Various components of the bacteria are degraded at different rates, and the degradation products are excreted by the leukocyte into the surrounding medium (exocytosis), as shown by studies of the fate of radioactive organisms following phagocytosis (Ayoub and White, 1969).

The specific and azurophilic granules undergo degranulation sequentially or randomly as early as 5 seconds after the phagocytic event (Bainton, 1973; Segal et al., 1980; Pryzwanoky et al., 1979). Microfilaments and microtubules seem to be involved in this process (Zakhireh et al., 1979). The number of granules lost is proportional to the number and type of particles ingested. Granules not coming in contact with the phagocytic vacuole are not lysed. However, in contrast to such a selective, localized degranulation common to bacterial phagocytosis, generalized degranulation of the cells occurs after endocytosis of endotoxin or exotoxin (Zucker-Franklin, 1968). Polymyxin B sulfate inhibits endotoxin-mediated release of lysosomal enzymes from neutrophils (Bannatyne et al., 1977).

Degranulation leading to release of lysosomal enzymes into the surrounding milieu has also been observed (reviewed by Weissmann et al., 1979). It can occur in various ways:

(a) Bacterial toxins or detergents may cause cell death and induce passive release of cellular components.

(b) Phagocytosis of certain particles, such as urate crystals and silica, may be accompanied by formation of phagolysosomes and subsequent release of cellular components through perforation in the phagocytic vacuoles.

(c) Degranulation may occur during the process of phagocytosis of a larger particle such as zymosan, with release of

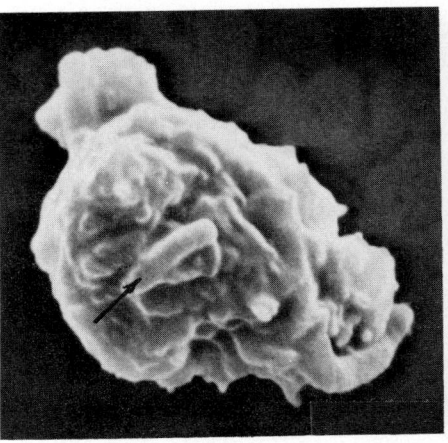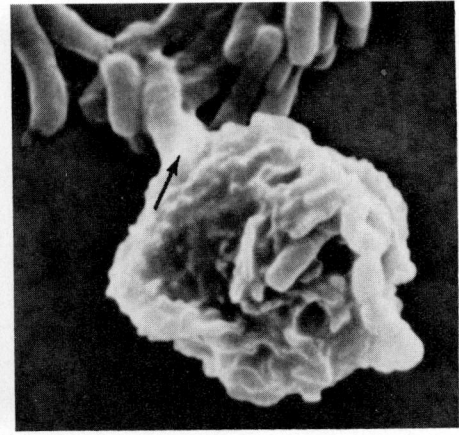

Fig. 26–6. Scanning electron photomicrographs of phagocytosis of opsonized *Escherichia coli* by bovine blood neutrophils after 1 minute. Partially ingested bacteria are clearly visible. Notice individual bacteria in the process of being ingested as evident from a veil of cell cytoplasm *(arrows)* over the bacterial surface. ×6,000. (Prepared with the assistance of Jan Vallinoti.)

contents to the outside, prior to closure of the phagocytic vacuole.

(d) Degranulation may follow unsuccessful attempts at phagocytosis of excessively large particles such as metazoan parasites coated with IgG and complement. This process is also referred to as "frustrated phagocytosis." It can also be induced by exposing neutrophils to cytochalasin B.

(e) Secretion of lysosomal components may be induced by certain substances without effect on the cellular viability.

Selective secretion of contents of specific granules is induced by certain substances such as concanavalin A, phorbol myristate acetate, FMLP, and C5a (Baggiolini et al., 1980; Dewald et al., 1982), while substances such as immune complexes and calcium ionophores induce secretion from both granule types (Smolen and Weissmann, 1981; Yurewucz and Zimmerman, 1977). Agents that cause disassembly of microtubules (e.g., colchicine) inhibit degranulation, whereas those promoting assembly of microtubules (e.g., deuterium oxide) enhance degranulation. Similarly, substances stimulating adenylate cylcase (e.g., β-adrenergic agents, PGE$_1$) inhibit degranulation, while those elevating cGMP promote degranulation. Lithium, in addition to its effect on granulopoiesis (see Chapter 13), can cause degranulation of both primary and specific granules in the absence

of phagocytic stimulus (Bloomfield and Young, 1982). C3a and C5a can also induce release of lysosomal enzymes (Herman et al., 1979; Menzel et al., 1978).

Contents of specific granules are released more easily and in higher amounts than those of azurophilic granules (Olsson and Venge, 1980); this may partly be related to the higher proportion of these granules in the mature neutrophils. Recent studies have shown that gelatinase present in an organelle other than primary and secondary granules may be secreted by neutrophils responding to chemotactic factors (Dewald et al., 1983). Under these conditions minor amounts of specific but not primary granule constituents are released.

Neutrophils may be destroyed in the process of killing bacteria. Furthermore, some bacteria, such as *Brucella abortus* and *Mycobacterium tuberculosis*, may escape destruction and survive within the leukocyte. In such cases, phagocytosis protects the bacteria from lethal effects of humoral factors and antibodies and helps in dissemination of the organisms to different tissues, thus accentuating the disease process.

Phagocytosis is best studied in test tubes. Suspensions of known numbers of bacteria and leukocytes in a suitable medium are mixed in test tubes. Bacteria and leukocytes may be exposed to various test substances such as opsonins and metabolic inhibitors, re-

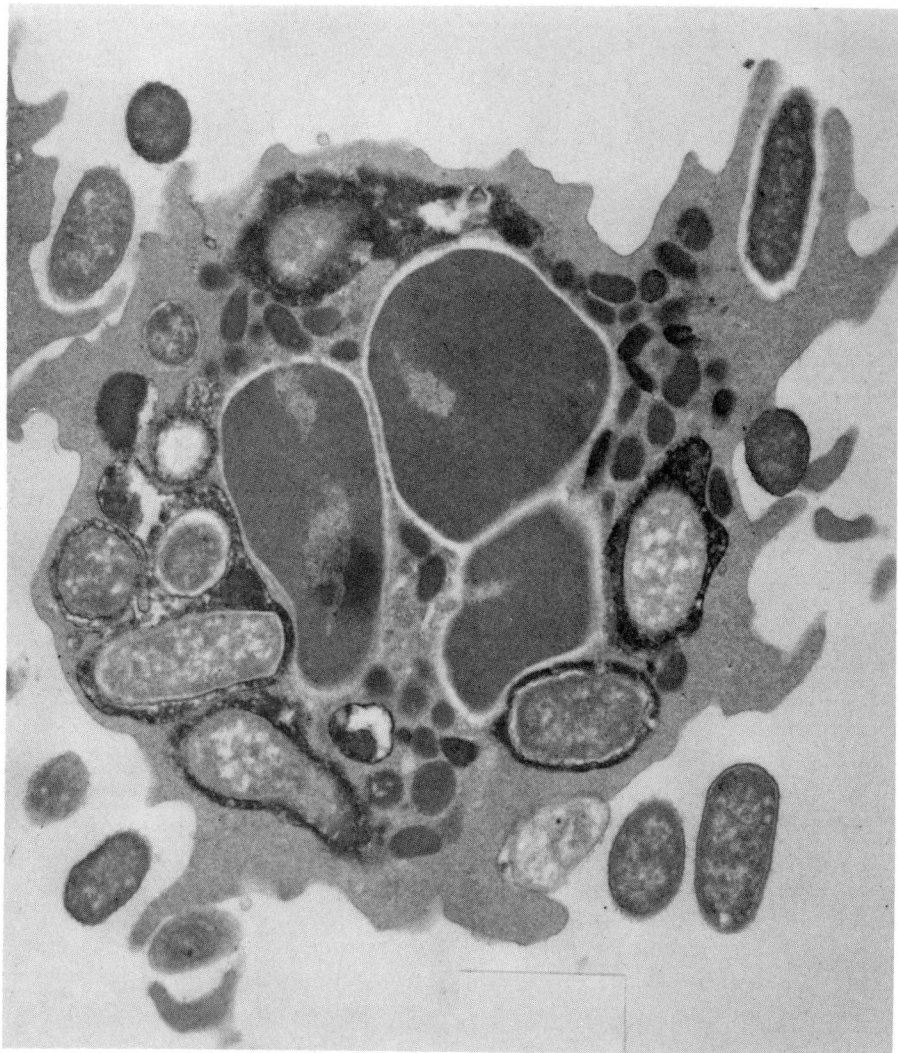

Fig. 26–7. Phagocytic and bactericidal activities of a bovine blood neutrophil that was allowed to interact with opsonized *Escherichia coli* for 1 minute. Active phagocytosis of extracellular bacteria as well as intracellular organisms is clearly evident. The cell was stained for peroxidase to delineate degranulation of peroxidase-positive primary (dark-stained) granules and peroxidase-negative specific (light-stained) granules. The presence of dark-stained material surrounding several bacteria indicates degranulation of primary granules within the confines of phagocytic vacuoles. × 16,800. (Prepared with the assistance of Jan Vallinoti.)

spectively, prior to mixing. The mixture is incubated at 37°C for a designed length of time, and then smears are prepared, stained with a Romanowsky stain, and examined. The number of active phagocytes (percentage of cells with ingested bacteria) and the phagocytic index (number of bacteria per cell) are determined to express the extent of phagocytosis. In addition, intracellular and extracellular bacteria counts may be made to evaluate bacterial killing. The number of active phagocytes, the phagocytic index, and the bacterial killing all vary with the bacte-

ria:leukocyte ratio, the type of test organism, and the length of incubation time.

Phagocytosis and bactericidal effects can also be assessed by measuring ingestion of ^{32}P-labeled bacteria and release of the label from phagocytic destruction of labeled bacteria incubated with viable leukocytes (Dulin et al., 1984). Inert particles or heat-killed bacteria can be used instead of viable bacteria to assess phagocytic function of neutrophils. Ingestion of labeled molecules can be measured to assess the degree of pinocytosis.

The nitro blue tetrazolium (NBT) reduction

test (conversion from yellow soluble form to insoluble blue-black deposits of formazan) provides a simultaneous measurement of phagocytic and postphagocytic metabolic burst. NBT reduction occurs on the cell surface and in phagosomes (Fig. 26–8). It is attributable almost exclusively to scavenging of superoxide anion and is inhibited by super-

oxide dismutase (Root and Cohen, 1981). NBT reduction is generally increased during bacterial infection.

Chemiluminescence (emission of light) measures metabolic changes occurring with or without phagocytosis (Harvath et al., 1978). Generation of chemiluminescence is dependent on availability of oxygen, forma-

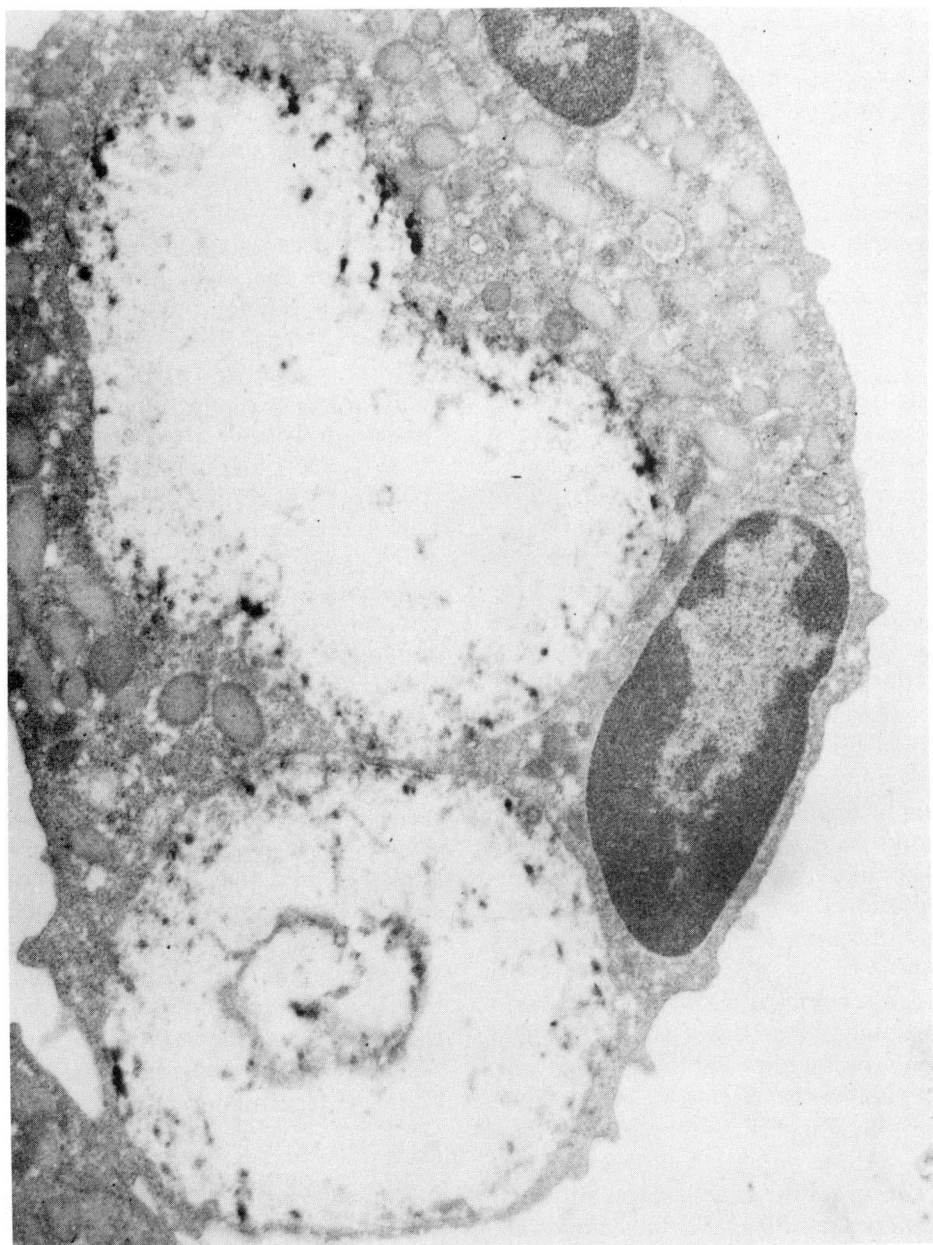

Fig. 26–8.   Nitro blue tetrazolium (NBT) reduction in a bovine blood neutrophil that has phagocytized two opsonized zymogen particles. The sites of NBT reduction are evident as electron dense, irregular specks, principally along the periphery of phagocytic vacuoles containing zymogen particles. Lysosomal granules are scattered throughout the cytoplasm of the cell.   ×24,000. (Prepared with the assistance of Jan Vallinoti.)

tion of superoxide anion, and myeloperoxidase (MPO) activity (Root and Cohen, 1981). Recent observations postulate that the metabolism of arachidonic acid via the lipo-oxygenase pathway, with generation of oxygen species, is the source of chemiluminescence (Cheung et al., 1983). A brief description of these and other phagocytosis-associated metabolic changes follows.

Metabolic Changes

Some elegant reviews are available on this subject (Karnovsky et al., 1981; Klebanoff, 1971; Root and Cohen, 1981; Sbarra et al., 1970; Zakhireh et al., 1979). Phagocytosis stimulates a coordinated series of changes in oxidative metabolism, collectively called the *metabolic burst*. These include increases in anaerobic glycolysis and lactate production, hexose monophosphate pathway (HMP) activity, oxygen consumption, production of superoxide and H_2O_2, lipid synthesis, and slight increases in RNA and protein syntheses. The intracellular concentration of ATP drops below the resting level (Borregaard and Herlin, 1982). Increases in the oxygen uptake, HMP shunt activity, and production of superoxide and H_2O_2 are called the *respiratory burst*. This event is reflected by increases in NBT reduction and chemiluminescence described in the preceding section. It has been established that phagocytosis is not essential for respiratory burst. It can be induced by perturbation of neutrophil plasma membrane by agents such as concanavalin A, phorbol myristate acetate, and C5a.

Increased anaerobic glycolysis supplies energy, in the form of ATP, required for chemotaxis and engulfment, while increased oxidative metabolic activities are related to intracellular bactericidal activity. Thus chemotaxis and phagocytosis, but not bactericidal activity, are inhibited by inhibitors of glycolysis, while neither is affected by inhibitors of respiration. Phagocytosis can occur under anaerobic as well as aerobic conditions, while bacterial killing is primarily aerobic, although oxygen-independent bactericidal systems are present in various leukocytes. Peritoneal macrophages behave like neutrophils, but in alveolar macrophages, oxidative phosphorylation provides energy for engulfment (Sbarra

et al., 1970); thus the process of phagocytosis by the alveolar macrophages is inhibited under anaerobic conditions. Intact RNA and protein synthesis are needed for expression of maximum bactericidal action. Lipid synthesis increases, probably to replace in part the portion of cell membrane utilized in formation of phagocytic vacuoles. Intracellular pH falls with increase in lactic acid formation.

Weissman and coworkers (1979, 1980) have proposed a sequence of events, called "the secretory code." that takes place in neutrophils following phagocytosis or ligand binding to specific surface receptors. Within 5–10 seconds, increases occur in membrane potential (hyperpolarization) and in the influx of Na^+ and Ca^{++}. Simultaneously, some Ca^{++} is lost from the plasma membrane subjacent to the area of ligand binding and membrane fluidity changes. These changes are followed by increases in oxidative metabolism and degranulation. Coupling of receptors to the membrane-bound adenylate cyclase is associated with some increase in cAMP (a level that does not inhibit degranulation), activation of a membrane NADPH oxidase, and generation of oxygen metabolites. Meanwhile membrane phospholipids, through arachidonic acid metabolism, generate various prostaglandins and thromboxanes. Intracellular events include condensation of subplasmalemmal microfilaments, microtubule assembly, and fusion of lysosomes (degranulation) with phagocytic vacuoles or portions of the plasma membrane. Degranulation leads to secretion of lysosomal enzymes into phagosomes or into the surrounding milieu. The extent of secretory activity or degranulation is believed to be regulated by prostaglandins via production of a four- to sixfold increase in cAMP. Hence compounds increasing intracellular levels of cAMP inhibit degranulation, whereas those increasing levels of cGMP enhance degranulation.

Factors Involved

Phagocytosis is affected by a variety of physical and chemical properties of both the phagocyte and the particle, and it is also affected by the environmental conditions (Braunsteiner and Zucker-Franklin, 1962). Neutrophils ingest rapidly dividing invasive or suppurative organisms, while mononuclear phagocytes ingest facultative or obligate intracellular organisms such as *Mycobacterium* and *Listeria*. Phagocytosis of viruses, certain protozoa, and other cells by neutrophils has also been described.

Factors influencing phagocytic properties of cells include cell age, energy, integrity of cellular components such as microfilaments and microtubules, chemotactic factors, Tuftsin and leukokinin, bacterial products and toxins, and viruses. Important properties of bacteria influencing phagocytosis are surface charge, cell wall composition, capsule, and toxins. Important environmental factors are temperature, pH, osmolarity, ionic composition, and interfacial tension. Phagocytosis is an active process requiring energy in the form of ATP. It occurs rapidly and most efficiently at pH 6–8 and at 37–40°C, but not at all at 4°C. A high concentration of salt and glucose (400–800 mg%) inhibits phagocytosis. Certain antibiotics (gentamicin, erythromycin, oxytetracycline, and chloramphenicol) in high concentration may depress phagocytic activity of neutrophils (Melby and Midtvedt, 1980).

Studies with bovine blood and milk neutrophils indicate that the phagocytic ability of neutrophils varies among cows, is reduced at parturition and following excessive release of corticosteroids in vivo, and is negatively influenced following phagocytosis of fat globules in milk and exposure to casein (Jain and Lasmanis, 1978a; Paape et al., 1979; Williams and Bunch, 1981). Neutrophils migrating into the mammary gland may ingest fat or cellular debris before entering alveolar lumen (Harmon and Heald, 1978). Normal skimmed milk promotes bacterial phagocytosis, and this property is enhanced in mastitic skimmed milk, whereas antibovine neutrophil serum is antiphagocytic (Jain and Lasmanis, 1978a). Cream reduces phagocytogenic oxygen uptake of bovine neutrophils and their bactericidal activity (Eshelman et al., 1981). Neutrophils from mastitic milk have considerably reduced myeloperoxidase activity (Gruner et al., 1982). Differences have been found in chemiluminescence of bovine neutrophils isolated from blood and milk of healthy cows (Weber et al., 1983).

Probably the most important and extensively studied promoters of phagocytosis are the humoral components known as *opsonins*. Opsonins are components of blood serum and are protein in nature. The process of opsonization involves adsorption of serum components to the surface of foreign particles, altering their surface properties and making them more liable to phagocytosis. Opsonization increases the rate and magnitude of ingestion for most organisms.

Neutrophils, monocytes, and macrophages have surface receptors for the Fc portion of IgG and for C3b; hence particles coated with these opsonic agents are easily phagocytosed. IgG antibodies bind to the surface of the organism via the Fab region, while the Fc region binds to the phagocyte surface. Chemotactic factors may enhance the expression of C3b and Fc receptors on neutrophils (Tauber, 1981). Cells may differ regarding the presence of these receptors. For example, bovine neutrophils have receptors for IgG_2 but not for IgG_1, while alveolar macrophages from gnotobiotic calves have receptors for IgG_1, and those from conventional calves also have receptors for IgG_2 (Howard et al., 1980). Bovine neutrophils, but not monocytes, have been shown to have Fc receptors for IgM (Grewal et al., 1978; Williams and Hill, 1982).

Opsonins can be specific or nonspecific (Miler, 1970). Specific opsonins are usually thermostable, specific antibodies that occur in high concentration after immunization; these are the most effective opsonins, but they have a restricted range. IgG is directly opsonic, while IgM exerts this effect largely through complement fixation. Phagocytosis of streptococci, smooth Gram-negative bacteria, and capsulated bacteria such as pneumococci is limited in the absence of specific antibodies. Precolostral calf serum is deficient in opsonic activity due to lack of immunoglobulins (Jain and Lasmanis, 1978a). Colostrum ingestion by the newborn calf increases opsonic activity of its serum within a few hours (Lombardo et al., 1979).

Nonspecific opsonins include α- and β-globulins, C-reactive protein, and complement components. They are usually thermolabile, are present in normal serum, and act on a wide range of bacteria as well as inert particles. Neutrophils themselves produce a "phagocytosis stimulating factor" from an intracellular precursor after phagocytosis and phagolysosome formation (Ishibashi and Yamashita, 1981). Certain lymphokines have been found to increase phagocytosis (Klostergaard et al., 1978). Low levels of staphylococcal alpha toxin have been found to enhance phagocytosis and killing of serum-opsonized staphylococci (Gemmell et al., 1982). Similarly, endotoxin stimulates both of these properties of neutrophils (Morrison and Ulevitch, 1978). Fimbriated *E. coli* are phagocytosed by neutrophils more readily than are nonfimbriated organisms, although neutrophil interaction with the former seems to be complex (Bjorksten and Wadstrom, 1982). Fibronectin has been found to increase chemotaxis, phagocytosis and NBT reduction of neutrophils (Jarstrand et al., 1982). Interferon has been found to promote phagocytosis of *E. coli* (Melby et al., 1982).

The participation of complement in phagocytosis is indicated by several studies employing anticomplement antibody and serums deficient in whole complement or various complement components (Jeter et al., 1961; Johnston et al., 1969; Miya and Marcus, 1961). Complement activation can occur by the classical pathway or via the alternate pathway. Fresh serum can opsonize particles by means of the properdin system in the absence of antibody. Ca^{++} is needed for complement fixation by the classical pathway, whereas Mg^{++} is needed for complement fixation by the alternate pathway. Both cations, however, promote phagocytosis. It is believed that the primary function of the C3b receptor is to facilitate particle recognition and adhesion, whereas that of the Fc receptor is to initiate phagocytosis. The former does not initiate ingestion, while the latter is inefficient in inducing adherence. However, a synergism exists between the two; e.g., the amount of IgG needed for phagocytosis is lower in the presence of complement. Both IgG and C3b participate in phagocytosis by neutrophils, while C3b binds particles to normal macrophages and induces phagocytosis by activated macrophages (Verhoef et al., 1977). The C3b receptor is susceptible to proteolysis and oxidative agents (Boxer et al., 1978).

Table 26–6.   Microbicidal Mechanisms in Neutrophils

Oxygen-dependent
  Myeloperoxidase-dependent
    Myeloperoxidase-H_2O_2-halide complex
  Myeloperoxidase-independent
    H_2O_2
    Superoxide anion
    Hydroxyl radical
    Singlet oxygen
Oxygen-independent
  Acidity in phagosomes
  Lysosomal constituents
    Cationic proteins
    Phagocytin and leukin
    Lysozyme
    Lactoferrin
    Proteases (cathepsins D, E, G)
    Phospholipase A_2
    "Bacterial permeability increasing protein"

Corticosteroids have been found to inhibit particle attachment or phagocytosis. In a recent study utilizing a new technique that enabled discrimination between attached and ingested particles, hydrocortisone was found to affect primarily the binding capacity of Fc and C3b receptors by human neutrophils (Forslid and Hed, 1982). Corticosteroids in high doses interfere with the binding of red cells coated with IgG or C3b to the corresponding receptors on monocytes (Schreiber et al., 1975). This mechanism makes corticosteroid therapy beneficial in treatment of immune-mediated hemolytic anemia and thrombocytopenia.

In contrast to classical opsonins, leukokinin and Tuftsin bind specifically to the surface of neutrophils in vitro and in vivo and stimulate both phagocytosis and bactericidal activities (Stabinsky et al., 1978). A similar effect is also recognized for macrophages. In addition, Tuftsin enhances random migration of monocytes, but not of neutrophils (Horsmanheimo et al., 1978). Tuftsin is a tetrapeptide fragment of leukokinin which is located in the Fc region of the IgG molecule. Its chemical structure is: L-threonyl-L-lysyl-L-prolyl-L-arginine. It is strongly basic; hence it binds to the sialic acid residues on cell surfaces.

Microbicidal Activity

Neutrophils phagocytize various organisms and kill them by different mechanisms that are broadly categorized as oxygen-dependent and oxygen-independent mecha-

Table 26–7. Microbial Resistance to Phagocytic Destruction

Process	Basis	Example
Avoidance of recognition	Surface antigens	Schistosomulae of *Schistosoma mansoni* are attacked, but not the adult worm.
Inhibition of chemotaxis	Bacterial products/toxins affecting neutrophils Failure to generate cytotaxin	*Staphylococcus aureus* mucopeptide; enterotoxin of *Echerichia coli*. *Pseudomonas aeruginosa* protease cleaves complement components.
Inhibition of ingestion after surface adherence	Increased membrane rigidity of the phagocyte	Viral attachment to neutrophils reduces their bacterial phagocytosis.
Suppression of metabolic burst	Unknown	*Brucella abortus* and vaccinia virus fail to stimulate hexose monophosphate pathway.
Inhibition of degranulation	Bacterial envelope composition	Acidic glycolipid from *Mycobacterium tuberculosis* inhibits degranulation. *Mycobacterium bovis* does this by increasing levels of cAMP.
Resistance to microbicidal activity	Enzymatic	Catalase-positive organisms destroy H_2O_2 generated in the phagocytes.
Destruction of the phagocyte	Bacterial products/toxins attacking cell membrane	Binding of staphylococcal leukocidin and streptolysin S to specific phospholipids; streptolysin O to cholesterol.

Abstracted from Densen and Mandell, 1980.

nisms (Table 26–6; reviewed by Karnovsky et al., 1981; Root and Cohen, 1981). Bacterial killing is assessed by culturing techniques to determine the number of bacteria killed or by release of the label from radio-labeled organisms.

Phagocytosis may or may not result in bacterial killing depending on microbial properties (Table 26–7). Bacterial killing is influenced by factors such as the presence of some exogenous substances, cell properties, and bacterial characteristics. Certain chemotactic (Issekutz, 1979) and phagocytosis-promoting factors (Menzel et al., 1978; Root and Cohen, 1981; Rottini et al., 1979) may enhance bactericidal activity of neutrophils as well. Immature neutrophils and neutrophils from milk and colostrum have reduced bactericidal activity (Jain and Lasmanis, 1978a; Paape et al., 1979; Pickering, 1980). In general, Gram-positive bacteria are destroyed more rapidly than are Gram-negative bacteria, and virulent organisms resist phagocytosis and postphagocytic destruction by various means (Densen and Mandell, 1980; Elsbach, 1980). For example, high molecular weight, negatively charged glycolipid sulfate of mycobacteria, lipopolysaccharide chain length of Gram-negative bacteria, and bacterial toxins adversely affect phagocytic and bactericidal properties of neutrophils.

Phagolysosome formation does not occur with organisms such as *Mycobacterium tuberculosis*, *Listeria monocytogenes*, and *Leishmania donovani*, although it occurs after exposure of the organisms to specific immune serums (Elsbach, 1980). *Brucella abortus* does not stimulate neutrophil HMP shunt activity (Kreutzer et al., 1979), and virulent salmonellae do not stimulate oxygen consumption by neutrophils (Densen and Mandell, 1980). Hence these organisms survive phagocytic destruction.

Species differences are found in various systems thought to be important for bactericidal action. For example, chicken neutrophils lack MPO, bovine neutrophils have a minute amount of lysozyme, and neutrophils of the rhesus monkey lack both lysozyme and lactoferrin (Rausch and Moore, 1975). Defective bactericidal activity has been found in many acquired and hereditary conditions in humans (see Functional Abnormalities later in this chapter) and is associated with increased susceptibility to infection.

Oxygen-Dependent Mechanisms

Increased glucose utilization via the hexose monophosphate pathway, enhanced respiratory activity, and activation of NADPH oxidase result in generation of superoxide anion. The major role of the superoxide anion is to serve as a precursor of H_2O_2 and to generate other oxygen metabolites—hydroxyl radicals and singlet oxygen. Among these, H_2O_2 seems to be the most important bactericidal agent, while hydroxyl radical and singlet oxygen are of lesser importance. The H_2O_2 complexes with MPO and a halide to form a potent bactericidal system—the MPO-H_2O_2-halide complex. This system kills a variety of bacteria, viruses, fungi, and mycoplasmata and destroys red cells (Root and Cohen, 1981).

Klebanoff et al. (1966) originally described a bacteriostatic system in milk consisting of lactoperoxidase, H_2O_2, and thiocyanate. It was later shown that thiocyanate could be replaced by a halide such as iodide, chloride, or bromide ion and that MPO from leukocytes was antibacterial in such a combination. Chloride is probably the physiologically important halide. Fusion of primary granules with the phagosomes releases MPO within the phagolysosomes, H_2O_2 is generated within the phagosomes and on the cell surface, and chloride is available intracellularly (Karnovsky et al., 1981).

The intracellular concentration of H_2O_2 has been estimated to range from 0.001 to 0.1 M, depending on the amount of phagocytosis and the intracellular pH (Iyer et al., 1961). It is noted that a concentration of 0.00005 M is enough for complete bacterial killing (Klebanoff, 1968). A two- to fourfold increase in H_2O_2 production occurs during phagocytosis (Paul et al., 1968). Phagocytosing alveolar macrophages produce less H_2O_2 than neutrophils (Sbarra et al., 1970). Although H_2O_2 by itself is bactericidal at high concentration, it exerts a similar effect at low concentration after complexing with MPO and a halide. Ascorbic acid and trace metals such as Cu^{++} potentiate the effect of H_2O_2.

Bacterial killing by the MPO-H_2O_2-halide system involves several mechanisms depending on the participating cofactor (halide) and is thought to occur via halogenation, deamination, and decarboxylation of the microbial wall (Karnovsky et al., 1981; Root and Cohen, 1981; Zakhireh et al., 1979). Singlet oxygen

and hydroxyl radicals kill bacteria via lipid peroxidation and oxidative damage to nucleic acid.

The amount of intracellular H_2O_2 may be regulated to a certain extent by cellular catalase. For example, animals treated with 3-amino-1, 2, 4-triazole, a catalase inhibitor, have about four times as much H_2O_2 in neutrophils as do untreated animals (Paul et al., 1968). Catalase-positive bacteria are resistant to the killing effect of the peroxide complex, while catalase-negative organisms are easily killed. Phagocytic cells escape toxic effects of various oxygen metabolites that diffuse in the cytosol by regulating their intracellular levels (Root and Cohen, 1981). The glutathione system and catalase regulate the level of intracellular H_2O_2 by reducing it to water. Superoxide dismutase (SOD) reduces superoxide anions to H_2O_2 at an accelerated rate and thus prevents their toxic effects. Similarly organisms containing SOD, e.g., *Staphylococcus aureus* and *E. coli*, are protected from the effect of superoxide anion.

Oxygen consumption and HMP shunt activity depend to some degree on the type of particle ingested. Strains of *E. coli* vary in this regard; their susceptibility to guinea pig neutrophils is proportional to the degree of oxygen consumption by neutrophils (Pickering, 1980). Similarly, decreased H_2O_2 production by neutrophils is associated with reduced bacterial killing. The best known example is chronic granulomatous disease (CGD) in humans, a sex-linked, recessive (in males) or autosomal recessive (in females) fatal disease of children, characterized by recurrent and chronic infections of the skin, bones, lungs, and liver. Neutrophils from these patients engulf bacteria normally but cannot kill them. Their glycolytic activity and concentration of lysozyme and phagocytin are normal. The basic defect in these children is that their neutrophils cannot mount a respiratory burst and form H_2O_2. Monocytes from such patients have a similar defect (Douglas and Fudenberg, 1969). This defect in the phagocytic cells is due to an absence of NADPH oxidase, presence of a mutant NADPH oxidase, or a defect in the activation of the oxidase (Gobig, 1980). Both the NBT reduction test and chemiluminescence are consequently markedly reduced. Catalase-negative bacteria that produce H_2O_2, such as streptococci, can be readily killed by these neutrophils, while catalase-positive bacteria that do not produce H_2O_2, such as *S. aureus* and *E. coli,* are not destroyed. The latter class of organisms therefore proliferate, causing premature death of such children. Fungal infections are frequent and extremely difficult to eradicate. In addition, defective pH of the phagocytic vacuoles was also found to contribute to the functional defect of neutrophils in Chédiak-Higashi syndrome (Segal et al., 1981).

Myeloperoxidase deficiency in neutrophils and monocytes leading to a unique susceptibility to *Candida albicans* has been detected in some human patients and has been shown to have an autosomal recessive mode of inheritance (Klebanoff, 1971). Studies on the bactericidal activity of peroxidase-deficient chicken heterophil leukocytes indicated that mechanisms other than MPO-H_2O_2-halide may exist for effective intracellular bacterial killing (Brune et al., 1972).

Oxygen-Independent Mechanisms

Oxygen-independent microbicidal mechanisms include acidic environment in the phagocytic vacuole and granule-associated substances such as cationic proteins, lysozyme, lactoferrin, phagocytin, and leukin (Table 26–6). The granule-associated substances are operative under anaerobic conditions and may also act synergistically with the oxygen-dependent mechanisms under aerobic conditions. Bovine neutrophil granules contain bactericidal substances active against both Gram-positive and Gram-negative bacteria (Gennaro et al., 1983b; Hakak-Berenji and Jain, 1983).

Increased *lactic acid* production from rise in anaerobic glycolysis following phagocytosis is believed to reduce the pH (to 3.0–6.0) inside the phagocytic vacuole within a few minutes and is believed to facilitate bacterial killing in several ways. The vacuolar acidity per se may be bactericidal for certain organisms (e.g., pneumococci); creates a favorable condition for certain antimicrobial systems to function, e.g., MPO; promotes the rate of superoxide reduction to H_2O_2; and facilitates digestion of killed organisms by the lysosomal acid pro-

teases and other hydrolytic enzymes (Jacques and Bainton, 1978).

Cationic proteins are active at pH near or greater than 7.0. They bind to acidic groups on bacterial surfaces and reduce microbial viability and growth by an unknown mechanism. They are also antifungal. Differences exist in microbicidal activity of various cationic proteins (Hakak-Berenji and Jain, 1983; Klebanoff and Clark, 1978; Spitznagel, 1977). Gram-positive bacteria are more susceptible to cationic proteins than are Gram-negative organisms. The sensitivity or resistance of Gram-negative organisms to purified cationic proteins varies with their membrane properties; rough organisms are killed quite readily, whereas smooth organisms are more resistant (Weiss et al., 1980). Cationic proteins may act synergistically with the MPO-H_2O_2-halide system (Root and Cohen, 1981).

Phagocytin, an antibacterial substance from rabbit neutrophils described by Hirsch, is a complex of arginine-rich cationic proteins each of which is bactericidal (Zeya and Spitznagel, 1966). *Leukin* (Skarnes and Watson, 1956) is a poorly characterized antibacterial protein present in neutrophils.

Lysozyme hydrolyzes bacterial cell wall components. It specifically attacks the β-1,4-glycosidic linkages in peptidoglycans. It acts on certain Gram-positive bacteria and fungi. Its action requires preexposure of the organism to antibody and complement, ascorbic acid and H_2O_2, or other "sensitizing" agents so that peptidoglycans become exposed or available for its action. Thus it is said that lysozyme may serve a digestive rather than microbicidal action (Elsbach, 1980). Lysozyme acts synergistically with other bactericidal systems and also enhances phagocytic activity of neutrophils (Neeman et al., 1974).

Lactoferrin exerts its bacteriostatic and possibly bactericidal effects by chelating iron needed for growth of certain bacteria. It is also associated with production of hypoferremia during infection. Lactoferrin acts synergistically with specific antibody to inhibit growth of *E. coli.* Its antimicrobial effect is probably extracellular because following phagocytosis most of the lactoferrin is secreted into the extracellular milieu rather than into the cytoplasm (Root and Cohen, 1981). Lactoferrin deficiency, as a consequence of the lack of specific granules, has been described in several human patients with recurrent infections (Breton-Gorius, 1980). Lactoferrin also seems to be important in neutrophil adhesion and aggregation and myelopoiesis (see Chapter 13). It also modulates hydroxyl radical production (Ambruso and Johnston, 1981).

Proteases—cathepsins D, E, and G—alter some Gram-negative bacteria for lysozyme action and are weakly bactericidal for staphylococci (Root and Cohen, 1981). Cathepsin G is also fungicidal. *Phospholipase A₂*, by increasing microbial envelope permeability, exerts a potent bactericidal effect on *E. coli* (Franson et al., 1977). In addition, a *"bacterial permeability increasing protein"* is described in rabbit neutrophils which increases permeability of the cell wall of *E. coli* and other Gram-negative bacteria (Olsson and Venge, 1980).

Tissue Injury, Inflammation, and Neutrophil Lysosomes

Studies of acute inflammation indicate that the early vascular response to a bacterial infection and other injuries is often biphasic (Hersh and Bodey, 1970; Vegad, 1979; Wilhelm, 1962; Willoughby, 1967). The initial increase in vascular permeability leading to edema is mainly due to the local release of one or more of the endogenous mediators, namely, histamine, serotonin, serum permeability factors, bradykinin, kallikrein, and leukotaxine, depending on the animal species. Serotonin has high vascular permeability-inducing potency in the rat, but it has a negligible effect in the rabbit and guinea pig. In the rat, histamine has a high level of activity (Miles and Wilhelm, 1960). Leakage of serum proteins and leukocyte diapedesis into the tissues occur after alteration of vascular permeability in venules, but the two events are often separate (Hurley and Spector, 1965).

In addition, a number of other plasma-derived and leukocyte-derived mediators are implicated in causation of inflammatory reaction (Pinckard, 1982). The former group includes complement components, particularly C5a, and factors resulting from activation of coagulation factors and the fibrinolytic system. The latter group includes factors from neutrophils (lysosomal constituents), lym-

phocytes (lymphokines), monocytes and macrophages (monokines), platelets (arachidonic acid metabolites), mast cells (platelet activating factor), and endothelial cells (arachidonic acid metabolites). Factors from eosinophils may also have some regulatory role (see Chapter 27).

Mechanisms responsible for the delayed phase of increase in vascular permeability and leukocyte emigration are complex and have not been clearly defined. These mechanisms may also involve some of the transiently acting stimuli incriminated in the initial phase of inflammation which are reformed after a lag period. Histamine, serotonin, leukotaxine, bradykinin, globulin permeability factor, compound 48/80, and kallikrein were shown to have very little effect in inducing leukocyte emigration, although they induced a marked vascular permeability to trypan blue (Spector and Willoughby, 1964). Tissue extracts, a permeability factor extracted from lymph node cells, and saline extracts of leukocytes induce significant leukocyte emigration in vitro as well as in vivo (Spector and Willoughby, 1970). Leukotrienes C4 and D4 have been found to cause increased vascular permeability (Malnsten et al., 1980). See p. 698 for more information on neutrophil migration in tissues.

The local accumulation of neutrophil leukocytes and release of leukocyte products play an important part in initiating vascular permeability and other forms of tissue injury in acute inflammation. Neutrophils are associated with development of severe tissue injury in certain instances such as Schwartzman and Arthus phenomena, as shown by neutropenic animals' failure to develop injury (Wasi et al., 1966). Furthermore, in rabbits made neutropenic by the use of antineutrophil serum or nitrogen mustard, the increase in vascular permeability was milder after heat injury or other forms of injury than in controls (Freedman et al., 1967; Taichman et al., 1966; Uriuhara and Movat, 1967). Intact or lysed neutrophil granules and an enzyme-free cationic protein or polypeptide from the neutrophil granules were shown to produce local leukocytosis and/or an increase in vascular permeability (Janoff and Schaefer, 1967;

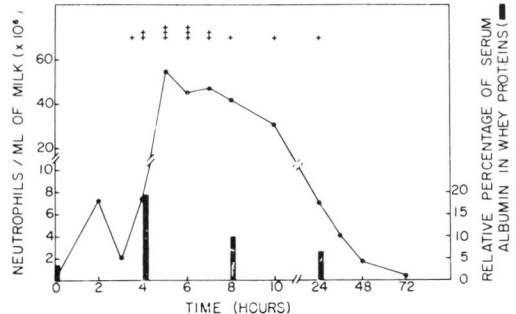

Fig. 26–9. Response of Cow 1547 to intramammary inoculation of 1.1 × 10⁹ intact leukocytes into a mammary gland. Plus signs indicate degree of swelling of the gland: +, slight swelling or firmness; + +, slight swelling and firmness; + + +, moderate swelling and firmness. (From Jain et al., 1972; courtesy of *The American Journal of Veterinary Research*.)

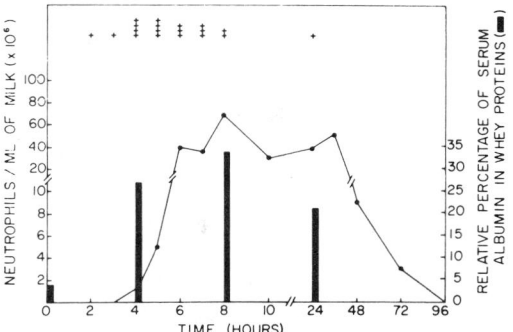

Fig. 26–10. Response of Cow 1556 to intramammary inoculation of a lysosomal preparation. Plus signs indicate degree of swelling of the gland: +, slight swelling or firmness; + +, slight swelling and firmness; + + +, moderate swelling and firmness; + + + +, marked swelling and firmness. (From Jain et al., 1972; courtesy of *The American Journal of Veterinary Research*.)

Golub and Spitznagel, 1966; Movat et al., 1964; Wasi et al., 1966).

Our studies in neutropenic and normal cows indicated that neutrophils influence the magnitude and duration of the cardinal signs of inflammation in the mammary gland during the early phase of acute coliform mastitis (Jain et al., 1968, 1969; Jain, 1976). Intramammary inoculation of intact (Fig. 26–9) or disrupted bovine neutrophils produced acute inflammatory changes (edema of the mammary gland and leukocytosis into the milk) in normal, lactating bovine mammary glands (Jain et al., 1972). The response varied with the number of leukocytes introduced into the gland cistern. Lysosomal preparations from neutrophils isolated from bovine mastitic milk also induced an inflammatory reaction in normal mammary glands (Fig. 26–10).

Neutrophils contain a variety of substances promoting or inhibiting inflammation and causing tissue injury (reviewed in Weissmann et al., 1979). Extracellular release of various preformed, granule-associated substances can be caused by a number of mechanisms, e.g., cell death, phagocytosis, chemotactic migration, secretion, and reversed endocytosis. Additional substances with similar activities are generated after metabolic stimulation of neutrophils by phagocytosis (Baggiolini et al., 1980; Muvat et al., 1964; Olsson and Venge, 1980; Weissmann et al., 1979). Substances promoting inflammation include cationic proteins, histamine, acid and neutral proteases, products of arachidonic acid metabolism, and oxygen metabolites. Substances regulating the inflammatory process include superoxide dismutase, catalase, ceruloplasmin, certain cationic proteins, lysozyme, PGI₂ and PGE₂, and kininase.

Neutrophil *proteases* can elicit mild to severe tissue injury, from inflammation to severe hemorrhagic necrosis, depending on the degree of enzyme release at the site of inflammation (Baggiolini et al., 1980; Movat, 1979; Olsson and Venge, 1980; Weissmann et al., 1980). They also have other effects. Species differences are found in the content and activity of neutral proteases. Neutral proteases are present primarily in azurophilic granules. They are released in larger amounts than acid proteases, and they function better in an extracellular environment.

Acid proteases *(cathepsins B and D)* are present in azurophilic granules. They generate leukokinin at acid pH, damage the vascular basement membrane, and function better in the phagocytic vacuole. A highly cationic protein (isoelectric point, pH greater than 11), termed "chymotrypsin-like protease" *(cathepsin G)* is present in azurophilic granules of human but not rabbit and guinea pig neutrophils. It is a serine protease and has four isozyme forms and a molecular weight of 25,500–28,500. It attacks substances like fibrinogen, casein, proteoglycan, complement components, and IgG.

Elastase occurs in three isozyme forms in specific granules. It has a molecular weight of 33,000–36,000 and an optimum pH of 8.5. It acts on elastin as well as on proteoglycans, complement components, and IgG. Because it acts on elastin, it has been implicated in causation of emphysema (Janoff et al., 1979).

A *specific collagenase* is present in specific granules; it forms a minor component of neutrophil collagenases and attacks only collagen. *Nonspecific collagenase* is a major constituent of azurophilic granules. It is a serine protease, has a molecular weight of 7,600, and is made of two nonidentical subcomponents. It attacks several substances in addition to collagen.

Gelatinase is a metalloproteinase that acts specifically on denatured collagen. In human neutrophils, it is localized in small, morphologically still unidentifiable organelles. It can be released rapidly from neutrophils independent of phagocytosis and stimulation of respiratory burst. It has been suggested that its secretion may be involved in the early events of neutrophil mobilization in response to chemotactic stimuli (Dewald et al., 1982).

Several protease inhibitors are present in plasma. These include α_1-antitrypsin, α_1-antichymotrypsin, σ_2-macroglobulin, and a "bronchial mucus inhibitor." These are active against chymotrypsin-like protease, and all except α_1-antichymotrypsin are active against elastase and nonspecific collagenase (Olsson and Venge, 1980). Ceruloplasmin, an acute phase protein, in extracellular location and superoxide dismutase in intracellular location scavenge oxygen-derived free radicals and lessen or obviate tissue damage (Weissmann et al., 1979).

Antiviral Activity

The role of phagocytic cells in viral infection is not well known. Viral defense is varied. Some viruses provoke almost exclusively humoral defense mechanisms, while others excite cellular antiviral mechanisms (Elsbach, 1980). Entry of viruses into phagocytic and nonphagocytic cells is by endocytosis. Macrophages play an important role in viral defense. Specific viral antibody promotes ingestion of viruses by macrophages and fusion of lysosomal granules with endocytotic vacuoles; postphagocytic events in macrophages probably prevent viral replication or promote intracellular degradation. B and T lymphocytes, through production of interferons, play an important role in viral immunity. Recent studies suggest a role for neutrophils in antiviral immunity (Grewal and Babiuk, 1980; Rouse, 1981; Rouse et al., 1978). Neutrophils were found to phagocytize opsonized herpes viruses and inflict antibody- or complement-dependent cell cytotoxicity.

Parasite Destruction

Participation of neutrophils in leukocyte-induced parasitic damage has been investigated. Although this is primarily a function of eosinophils, some neutrophil-induced damage has been demonstrated for *Trypanosoma cruzi* epimastigotes (Rimoldi et al., 1981), less virulent *Entamoeba histolytica* (Guerrant et al., 1981), schistosomulae of *Schistosoma mansoni* (Caulfield et al., 1980), and *Ascaris suum* larvae (Thompson et al., 1977). Bovine neutrophils were found to phagocytize *T. theileri* and mediate parasite killing by both intracellular and extracellular mechanisms (Townsend et al., 1982).

Cytotoxic Effect

Antibody-dependent cytotoxicity by neutrophils involves both oxidative and nonoxidative mechanisms (Conkling et al., 1982). Neutrophils bind to antibody-coated tumor cells and rapidly initiate lysis without phagocytosis, but increase in respiratory burst and superoxide generation are essential for this effect (Hafeman and Lucas, 1979). Studies with bovine leukocytes indicate that neutrophils are more active than eosinophils in antibody-dependent cytotoxicity (Roth and Kaeberle, 1981). Human neutrophils were found capable of destroying red cells in vitro by a mechanism involving formation of superoxide-mediated methemoglobin and subsequently a cytotoxic peroxide-ferriheme complex (Weiss, 1980).

MORPHOLOGIC AND FUNCTIONAL ABNORMALITIES

Investigations of functional aspects of human neutrophils over the past decade have shown that qualitative as well as quantitative changes in neutrophils may be associated with increased susceptibility to infection. Moreover, in-depth studies of the protective role of neutrophils have revealed that defective cellular activity may be found at various levels of functional execution. For example, interference with or defective adherence, migration, chemotaxis, ingestion, degranulation, metabolic activity, and microbicidal activity may occur and contribute to reduced resistance to infection, which may be fatal. Little is known about similar aspects of neutrophils of various domestic animals. A brief description of abnormalities encountered in human neutrophils follows to provide a basis for similar searches in veterinary medicine.

Morphologic Abnormalities

Morphologic abnormalities in neutrophils include aberrations of maturation, cell size, nuclear shape, granule characteristics, and cytoplasmic attributes (Table 26–8). Such changes may be acquired or hereditary and may be visible on light microscopy or demonstrable only by electron microscopy or cytochemical staining. For example, neutrophils of human patients with acute or chronic granulocytic leukemia may exhibit asynchronous cell maturation and abnormalities of granule formation (absence of azurophilic granules or specific granules), biochemical constituents (absence of peroxidase or alkaline phosphatase), or granule size and shape (Auer bodies) (Bainton, 1977). Selective deficiency of specific granules has been found in human patients (see Gallin et al., 1982 for references).

A brief description of some neutrophil abnormalities follows. Details can be found elsewhere (Cline, 1975; Wintrobe et al., 1981).

Neutrophils commonly display granular and cytoplasmic abnormalities referred to as *"toxic" changes.* These are encountered in conditions such as severe bacterial infections, septicemia, acute inflammatory conditions, and extensive burns. Cellular abnormalities include the presence of large, reddish purple "toxic" granules (Plate XI–12), Döhle bodies (Plates IX–2, XII–6), or cytoplasmic foaminess, vacuolation and/or increased diffuse basophilia (Plates XI–9, XI–10, XI–11). Ultrastructural studies have been made of human (McCall et al., 1969) and canine (Gossett and MacWilliams, 1982) toxic neutrophils. Toxic granules were shown to be analogous to the primary granules (McCall et al., 1969). They appear azurophilic in mature neutrophils because of retained acid mucopolysaccharide.

Döhle bodies are bluish cytoplasmic inclusions resulting from lamellar aggregation of rough endoplasmic reticulum (RER) (Fig. 26–11). They are more common in cats than in other animal species. Cytoplasmic foaminess and vacuolation reflect an "autolytic" change, probably due to lysosomal rupture or leakage of hydrolytic enzymes under the influence of bacterial toxins. Vacuolation is significantly greater in patients with bacteremia (Malcolm et al., 1979) and septicemia. The diffuse basophilic staining of the cytoplasm is due to retained ribosomes and RER, an indication of impaired cellular maturation. Sometimes, giant bizarre neutrophils (Plates IX–3, IX–4) may be seen, particularly in the cat, as a result of asynchronous granulopoiesis during acute or chronic active infection. Rarely, polyploid (binucleated) neutrophils may be seen during intense granulopoietic response. These toxic changes may occur singly or simultaneously, and sometimes immature neutrophils are also affected.

Auer rods are intracytoplasmic structures found in myeloid cells of some human pa-

Table 26–8. **Morphologic Abnormalities of Neutrophils**

Acquired	*Hereditary*
"Toxic" changes	Hypersegmentation
Cytoplasmic foaminess, vacuolation, and/or basophilia;	Macropolycytes
"toxic" granules; Döhle bodies; bizarre giant forms	Pelger-Huët anomaly
Hypersegmentation	May-Hegglin anomaly
Pseudo-Pelger-Huët anomaly	Alder-Reilly anomaly
Auer rods	Mucopolysaccharidosis
Asynchronous maturation	Chédiak-Higashi syndrome
Macropolycytes	Jordon's anomaly

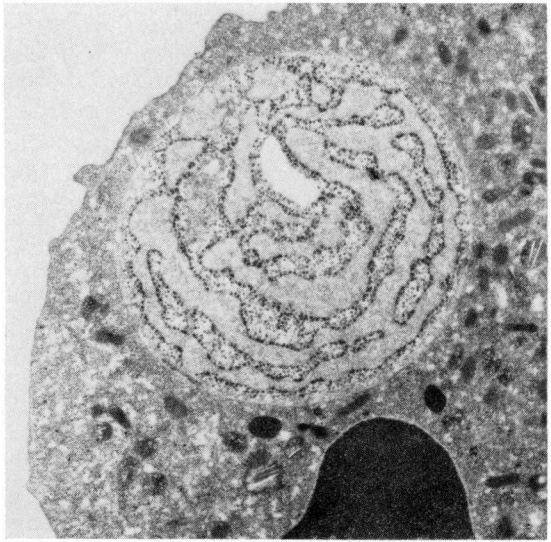

Fig. 26–11. Equine neutrophil with a whorl of rough endoplasmic reticulum. This structure would stain highly basophilic and appear as a Döhle body in blood films stained with a Romanowsky stain. ×14,400.

tients with acute myelogenous leukemia. They are found commonly in myeloblasts and promyelocytes and infrequently in other cells of the neutrophil series. They are derived from azurophilic granules and are best demonstrated in bone marrow films stained for myeloperoxidase. Auer rods have not been found so far in leukemic animals.

Pleokaryocytes and *macropolycytes* are, respectively, normal-size and giant neutrophils having a nucleus with or without increased nuclear lobes (more than 5). These cells have been seen in humans as a hereditary abnormality or as an acquired defect in vitamin B_{12} or folate deficiency; in iron deficiency; after prolonged therapy with corticosteroids; after treatment with antimetabolite drugs interfering with DNA synthesis, e.g., 6-mercaptopurine, cytosine arabinoside, and methotrexate; and in uremia. Nuclear segmentation is generally believed to be related to the cell age, but hypersegmented human neutrophils in vitamin B_{12} deficiency were not found to be older than normal (Cronkite and Vincent, 1969).

Hypersegmented neutrophils are found in poodles with macrocytic erythrocytes (Fig. 25–21B) and in dogs on long-term corticosteroid therapy. They were observed in a cat suspected of vitamin B_{12}–folate deficiency (Plate

XI–7). Idiopathic hypersegmentation of neutrophils was observed in a horse (Prasse et al., 1981). Animals with chronic neutrophilias, particularly the horse, may show occasional hypersegmented neutrophils in blood (Appendix Cases 42 and 60).

Pelger-Huët anomaly is a benign, autosomal dominant trait characterized by a reduced number of nuclear segments of granulocytes and coarseness of nuclear chromatin of lymphocytes and monocytes. Heterozygote humans have mature neutrophils with bilobed nuclei, while homozygotes have mature neutrophils with round nuclei and clumped chromatin. However, these cells are functionally normal (Johnson et al., 1980) or show minor defects of chemotaxis and phagocytosis which are inconsequential (Mills and Quie, 1980). Pseudo-Pelger-Huët anomaly may be found in myeloproliferative disorders and in other diseases such as severe infections and malignancies. Pelger-Huët anomaly has been found to occur in dogs as a hereditary (Fig. 4–8) or acquired (Shull and Powell, 1979) defect. In foxhounds with this anomaly, impaired neutrophil mobilization into skin and antibody response were found (Bowels et al., 1979). Pelger-Huët anomaly has been found in cats with a possible autosomal dominant mode of inheritance (Latimer et al., 1985). See Chapter 4 for additional information on dogs and Chapter 5 for cats.

Alder-Reilly anomaly is an autosomal recessive trait characterized by the presence of coarse (giant), intensely stained, azurophilic granules in mature neutrophils. Similar granules may also be present in other leukocytes and more commonly in bone marrow reticulum cells. Such cells are found in patients with *mucopolysaccharidosis* (MPS) and various bone and cartilage abnormalities. The basic defect is an abnormality of mucopolysaccharide (glycosaminoglycan) catabolism due to an enzyme deficiency so that it accumulates in leukocyte granules. Six genetic forms of enzyme deficiencies have been recognized in human mucopolysaccharidoses. Two genetic forms have been described in domestic cats: MPS I, associated with deficiency of α-L-iduronidase (Hurler's syndrome), and MPS VI, due to deficiency of arylsulfatase B activity (Maroteaux-Lamy syndrome) (Haskins et al., 1979a, b).

Abnormal granulation in leukocytes (Plates XIII–1 through XIII–4) was seen in three dachshund puppies affected with MPS (Schalm, 1977).

Chédiak-Higashi syndrome (CHS) is a lethal, autosomal recessive condition characterized in humans by partial ocular and cutaneous albinism, photophobia, a bleeding tendency, an increased susceptibility to pyogenic infections, and the presence of enlarged granules in most granule-containing cells such as granulocytes and melanocytes. Neutrophils often display single or multiple abnormal granules and sometimes whorls of unit membrane. Eosinophils and monocytes, but not lymphocytes, also show giant granules. The giant granules or structures result from aberrations of formation or fusion of primary and specific granules, as demonstrated by their reaction for cytochemical markers of both granule types (Rausch et al., 1978).

Formation of giant granules is attributed to defective microtubule assembly and inadequate production of cGMP (Oliver and Zurier, 1976; Oliver et al., 1976). Such neutrophils are also functionally abnormal. They display defective chemotaxis, degranulation, and bacterial killing. However, phagocytic ability seems to be unimpaired. A similar syndrome also occurs in Aleutian mink, Hereford cattle, cats, a strain of beige mice, and killer whales (see Kramer et al., 1977 for references). Three cats with the combination of yellow eye color and "blue smoke" hair color in a single line of 27 Persian cats were found to be affected with this anomaly (Kramer et al., 1977). Enlarged granules were found in neutrophils, eosinophils, basophils, and melanocytes. No susceptibility to infection was observed, but a bleeding tendency was noted. Monocytes may also contain enlarged granules and platelets are deficient in adenine nucleotides (Prieur and Collier, 1981). A pseudo-CHS may be seen in acute or chronic granulocytic leukemia and other myeloproliferative disorders as a manifestation of the underlying abnormal granule formation.

May-Hegglin anomaly is an autosomal dominant trait characterized by the presence of large (2–5 μm), basophilic inclusions similar to Döhle bodies in granulocytes and monocytes. Affected individuals also have megathrombocytes. Ultrastructurally, neutrophil inclusions appear as patches of particles and fibrils in a homogeneous background in the cytoplasm.

Jordon's anomaly is a recessive trait characterized by the presence of some large, lipid-containing vacuoles in the cytoplasm of granulocytes, monocytes, and occasionally lymphocytes and plasma cells. Such vacuoles may also occur in immature granulocytes in the bone marrow. Our observations are that the presence of fat-filled neutrophils is a common finding in milk from cows with inflamed mammary glands.

Table 26–9. Disorders of Neutrophil Functions Identified in Human Studies

Defects of locomotion and chemotaxis
  Intrinsic cellular defects of locomotion: differences due to age of the individual or of the cells; acquired or hereditary defects
  Defective or inadequate generation of cytotaxins
  Chemotactic "deactivation" of neutrophils
  Cytotaxin inactivation or inhibition by serum and cell-derived inhibitors
Defective phagocytosis
  Acquired or hereditary
    Cellular defects
    Humoral defects
Defective microbicidal activity
  Acquired or hereditary
    Abnormal degranulation or granular enzymes
    Defective metabolic activity

Functional Abnormalities

Specific defects of neutrophils and immunologic deficiencies in which susceptibility to infection is increased have been described in humans (Table 26–9), and similar abnormalities are being recognized in animals. Several reviews are available on this subject (Austin and Cohn, 1963; Baehner, 1975; Cohn and Austin, 1963; Gobig, 1980; Mills and Quie, 1980; Quie, 1983; Rowley, 1962; Smith and Lumsden, 1983; Suter and Ramseier, 1964; Tauber, 1981; Weston, 1976; Wolach et al., 1982), and observations on animal species have also been summarized (Smith and Lumsden, 1983).

Defects of Locomotion and Chemotaxis

Several factors have been found to interfere with neutrophil mobilization and hence to reduce resistance to infection even though the neutrophils may be capable of ingesting and killing the organisms. Inadequate emigration or inhibition of mobilization of the leukocytes may be a consequence of many intrinsic defects of phagocytes or of extracellular humoral defects (Table 26–9). A few examples follow.

Neutrophils of neonates exhibit decreased chemotactic responsiveness because of developmental immaturity of cells and humoral deficiency (Mease et al., 1981; Miller, 1969). Such neutrophils, particularly from stressed infants, also have reduced bactericidal activity (Shigeoka et al., 1979).

Immature neutrophils move slowly and respond poorly to chemotactic stimuli. Similarly, phagocytic ability of the neutrophils is related to their maturity (Hertzog, 1938); it develops between the myelocyte and metamyelocyte stage (Kass and De Bruyn, 1967).

Absence of some surface glycoproteins has been associated with defective adherence and chemotaxis or only chemotaxis (Gahmberg et al., 1979; Higgens et al., 1970).

Chédiak-Higashi neutrophils have an underlying defect of microtubule assembly, and so they exhibit defects of granule formation, locomotion, and degranulation. Agents increasing cGMP and decreasing cAMP, e.g., ascorbic acid and cholinergic agents, have been found to correct this defect in certain cases (Gallin et al., 1979; Wilkinson, 1977).

The leukocyte defect in "lazy leukocyte" syndrome is related to decreased membrane deformability resulting from an abnormality in interaction of membrane proteins and microfilaments (Gobig, 1980).

Neutrophils from patients with acute bacterial infections show a marked decrease in chemokinesis as well as chemotaxis due to impaired locomotion (Althaus et al., 1980).

Neutrophils infected with viruses or having surface-bound immunoglobulin or immune complexes show decreased chemotaxis (Starkebaum and Arend, 1979; Wilkinson, 1977).

Defective chemotaxis of neutrophils and monocytes is seen in human patients having eczematous and pustular dermatitis, markedly elevated serum IgE level, and recurrent "cold" staphylococcal skin abscesses and in burn patients (Weston, 1976).

Levamisole hydrochloride, an anthelmintic, consistently improved the chemotactic response of neutrophils from human patients with hyper-IgE syndrome and caused clinical improvement (Gallin, 1980).

Some observations have been made on leukocytes of common domestic animal species. Impaired chemotaxis was found in some dogs with bacterial pyodermas (Latimer et al., 1983) and Pelger-Huët anomaly (Bowles et al., 1979), but not in others (Krosse et al., 1981; Latimer and Prasse, 1982). Normal neutrophil migration was found in dogs with acquired hyposegmentation (Shull and Powell, 1979). Equine neutrophils normally exhibit either a weak (Zinkl and Brown, 1982) or no (Camp and Leid, 1982; Camp et al., 1979; Snyderman and Pike, 1980) chemotaxis to FMLP. Similarly, canine (Stickle et al., 1985) and porcine neutrophils have been found to lack receptors for FMLP (Chenoweth et al., 1980). Uterine neutrophils from mares susceptible to chronic endometritis were found defective in chemotaxis, deformability, and phagocytosis and killing of *Candida albicans* (Cheung et al., 1985; Liu et al., 1985).

Neutrophils from a Holstein heifer with a history of stunted growth, poor physical condition, and a chronic granulomatous lesion on the muzzle were found defective in their chemotactic and phagocytic abilities (Hagemoser et al., 1983).

Inadequate production of complement chemoattractants from acquired or hereditary deficiencies or defects is an obvious cause of poor chemotaxis. Decreased chemotactic response of neutrophils to a cytotaxin may occur as a result of preexposure of the cells to the same cytotaxin or to other chemotactic agents, phagocytable particles, or immune complexes (Dallegri et al., 1980; Kay et al., 1979; Lane et al., 1981; Ward and Becker, 1968). This phenomenon is called "chemotactic deactivation." It is a reversible process and is dependent on the functional state of the microtubular system (Dallegri et al., 1980). Bacterial toxins may immobilize cells in tissues or in vitro by attaching to specific sites on the cell membrane and exert an inhibitory effect (Wilkinson, 1980).

Inactivation of chemotactic factors is another cause of defective chemotaxis. Certain naturally occurring cytotaxin inactivators or chemotactic inhibitors may be found in serum (Keller et al., 1975). For example, an aminopeptidase called "chemotactic factor inactivator" inactivates complement-derived factors as well as other cytotaxins such as those derived from bacteria and lymphocytes. Its level is increased in many human cancer patients (Gobig, 1980).

A "neutrophil immobilizing factor" from human neutrophils and mononuclear leukocytes irreversibly inhibits chemotactic response of human neutrophils and eosinophils, but not of monocytes (Goetzl and Austen, 1972; Watt et al., 1983). Similarly, "migration inhibitory factor" from activated T-lymphocytes inhibits migration of monocytes.

Certain drugs, chemicals, hormones (e.g., corticosteroids), and bacterial products (e.g., endotoxin and streptolysin O) have been shown to depress chemotaxis. Substances that increase intracellular levels of cAMP decrease neutrophil mobility and chemotactic response, whereas those increasing cGMP levels have the opposite effect (Wilkinson, 1980). Heparin in high concentration and histamine have been found to inhibit chemotactic activity of neutrophils.

Phagocytic Defects

Phagocytic activity of neutrophils may be influenced by the age of the individual, the age of the neutrophils themselves, disease states, and drug therapy. Decreased phagocytic activity is exhibited by neutrophils of neonates and leukemic patients, neutrophils from exudate, milk, and colostrum, and neutrophils of patients with "cold abscesses" and diseases such as diabetes mellitus and acute bacterial infections. Certain antibiotics (gentamicin, erythromycin, oxytetracycline, and chloramphenicol) in high concentration may depress phagocytic activity of neutrophils (Melby and Midtvedt, 1980). Similar results were obtained when several antibiotics used in treatment of mastitis were tested in vitro for their effects on phagocytosis of ^{32}P-labeled *Staphylococcus aureus* by bovine neutrophils isolated from milk (Ziv et al., 1983).

Microbicidal Defects

Defective bactericidal activity may be related to cellular dysfunction of phagocytosis, postphagocytic events, and bactericidal action. Defective bactericidal activity of neutrophils has been found in various conditions (Table 26–9). These include iron deficiency (Prasad, 1979), vitamin E deficiency (Harris et al., 1980), folic acid deficiency (Youinou et al., 1982), pregnancy (El-Maaliem and Fletcher, 1980), severe bacterial infection (Hansen et al., 1976), viral infection (Faden et al., 1981), uremia (Wardle and Williams, 1980), and jaundice (Wardle and Williams, 1980). Drug therapy (e.g., amphotericin B, tetracyclines, certain sulfa drugs, corticosteroids, and some antineoplastic drugs such as methotrexate and *Vinca* alkaloids) may also affect this function of neutrophils (Mandell, 1982).

Changes in biochemical composition of neutrophils may be associated with defective functions. For example, reduced bactericidal activity of "toxic" neutrophils has been attributed to decreases in intracellular concentration of lysozyme and myeloperoxidase during acute bacterial infection (Hansen et al., 1976). Similarly, decreased H_2O_2 production, myeloperoxidase deficiency, and lactoferrin deficiency have been described in human patients with recurrent infections.

Impaired bactericidal activity has been reported for neutrophils from various animal species. Defective neutrophil bactericidal activity was found in a male Irish setter dog having a clinical history of recurrent, life-threatening bacterial infections with associated peaks of pyrexia and marked neutrophilia. This condition was called "canine granulocytopathy syndrome" (Renshaw et al., 1977). Defective bactericidal activity was found in the gray collie syndrome (Chusid et al., 1975), lead poisoning in dogs (Caldwell et al., 1979), dogs with severe inflammatory disease (Gossett et al., 1983), cattle infected with bovine virus diarrhea (Roth et al., 1981), Chédiak-Higashi cattle (Renshaw et al., 1974), and selenium and copper deficiencies in cattle (Boyne and Arthur, 1979, 1981).

REFERENCES

Ackerman, G.A.: Ultrastructure and Cytochemistry of the Developing Neutrophil. Lab. Invest., *19*:290, 1968.

Althaus, D., et al.: Impaired Neutrophil Locomotion during Acute Bacterial Infections. Int. Arch. Allergy Appl. Immunol., *61*:321, 1980.

Ambrus, C.M., and Ambrus, J.L.: Regulation of the Leukocyte Level. Ann. N.Y. Acad. Sci., *77*:445, 1959.

Ambruso, D.R., and Johnston, R.B.: Lactoferrin Enhances Hydroxyl Radical Production by Human Neutrophils, Neutrophil Particulate Fractions and an Enzyme Generating System. J. Clin. Invest., *67*:352, 1981.

An, T.: Fc Receptors on Human Neutrophils: Electron Microscopic Study of Natural Surface Distributors. Immunology, *40*:1, 1980.

Anonymous: Lithium in Haematology. Lancet, *2*(8195):626, 1980.

Athens, J.W.: Neutrophilic Granulocyte Kinetics and Granulocytopoiesis, *In* Regulation of Hematopoiesis. Vol. 2. Gordon, A.S., ed. Appleton-Century-Crofts, New York, p. 1143, 1970.

Athens, J.W., et al.: Leukokinetic Studies. IV. The Total Blood, Circulating and Marginal Granulocyte Pools and the Granulocyte Turnover Rate in Normal Subjects. J. Clin. Invest., *40*:989, 1961.

Athens, J.W., et al.: Leukokinetic Studies. XI. Blood Granulocyte Kinetics in Polycythemia Vera, Infection and Myelofibrosis. J. Clin. Invest., *44*:778, 1965.

Austin, K.F., and Cohn, Z.A.: Contribution of Serum and Cellular Factors in Host Defense Reactions. I. Serum Factors in Host Resistance. New Eng. J. Med., *268*:933, 1963.

Avila, J.L.: Comparative Biochemical Cytology of the Exoplasmic Apparatus in Polymorphonuclear Leukocytes. *In* Lysosomes in Applied Biology and Therapeutics. Dingle, J.T., et al., eds. North Holland, Amsterdam, pp. 235–266, 1979.

Ayoub, E.M., and White, J.G.: Intraphagocytic Degradation of Group A Streptococci: Electron Microscopic Studies. J. Bacteriol., *98*:728, 1969.

Badenoch-Jones, P.: Lymphokine-Induced Neutrophil Aggregation. Immunology, *47*:169, 1982.

Baehner, R.L.: Microbe Ingestion and Killing by Neutrophils: Normal Mechanisms and Abnormalities. Clin. Haematol., *4*:609, 1975.

Bagby, G.C., Jr., and Bennett, R.M.: Feedback Regulation of Granulopoiesis: Polymerization of Lactoferrin Abrogates Its Ability to Inhibit CSA Production. Blood, *60*:108, 1982.

Baggiolini, M.: The Enzymes of the Granules of Polymorphonuclear Leukocytes and Their Functions. Enzyme, *13*:132, 1972.

Baggiolini, M., et al.: Cellular Mechanisms of Proteinase Release from Inflammatory Cells and the Degradation of Extracellular Proteins. Ciba Found. Symp., *75*:105, 1980.

Baggiolini, M., et al.: Identification of Three Types of Granules in Neutrophils of Ruminants; Ultrastructures of Circulating and Maturing Cells. Lab. Invest., *52*:151, 1985.

Bainton, D.F.: Sequential Degranulation of the Two Types of Polymorphonuclear Leukocyte Granules during Phagocytosis of Microorganisms. J. Cell Biol., *58*:249, 1973.

Bainton, D.F.: Differentiation of Human Neutrophilic Granulocytes: Normal and Abnormal. *In* The Granulocyte: Function and Clinical Utilization. Alan R. Liss, New York, p. 1–27, 1977.

Bainton, D.F., and Farquhar, M.G.: Origin of Granules in Polymorphonuclear Leukocytes: Two Types Derived from Opposite Faces of the Golgi Complex in Developing Granulocytes. J. Cell Biol., *28*:277, 1966.

Bainton, D.F., and Farquhar, M.G.: Differences in Enzymes Content of Azurophil and Specific Granules of Polymorphonuclear Leukocytes. II. Cytochemistry and Electron Microscopy of Bone Marrow Cells. J. Cell Biol. *39*:299, 1968.

Bainton, D.F., and Farquhar, M.G.: Segregation and Packaging of Granule Enzymes in Eosinophilic Leukocytes. J. Cell Biol., *45*:54, 1970.

Bannatyne, R.M., et al.: Inhibition of the Biologic Effects of Endotoxin on Neutrophils by Polymyxin B Sulfate. J. Infect. Dis., *136*:469, 1977.

Barak, Y., et al.: Neonatal Neutrophilia: Possible Role of a Humoral Granulopoietic Factor. Pediatr. Res., *14*:1026, 1980.

Becker, E.L.: Stimulated Neutrophil Locomotion: Chemokinesis and Chemotaxis. Arch. Pathol. Lab. Med., *101*:509, 1977.

Becker, E.L., et al.: Some Early Ionic Events in Neutrophil Activation by Chemotactic Factors. Agents Actions Suppl., *12*:338, 1983.

Bellavite, P., et al.: Catalase Deficiency in Myeloperoxidase Deficient Polymorphonuclear Leucocytes from Chicken. FEBS Lett., *81*:73, 1977.

Bernhard, W., and Granboulan, N.: Electron Microscopy of the Nucleolus in Vertebrate Cells. *In* Ultrastructure in Biological Systems: The Nucleus. Vol. 3. Dalton, A.J., and Haguenan, J., eds. Academic Press, New York, p. 81, 1968.

Bertram, T.A., and Coignoul, F.L.: Morphometry of Equine Neutrophils Isolated at Different Temperatures. Vet. Pathol., *19*:534, 1982.

Bertram, T.A., et al.: Phagocytosis and Intracellular Killing of the Contagious Equine Metritis Organism by Equine Neutrophils in Serum. Infect. Immun., *37*:1241, 1982.

Bessis, M., and Boisfleury, A., de: Étude des Différentes Étapes de l'Erythro-Phagocytose par Microcinématographie et Microscopie Électronique à Balayage. Nouv. Rev. Fr. Hématol., *10*:223, 1970.

Bessis, M., and Boisfleury, A., de: Les Mouvements des Leucocytes Etudies au Microscope Electronique à Balayage. Nouv. Rev. Fr. Hematol., *11*:377, 1971.

Beswick, P.H., and Slater, T.F.: The "Metabolic Burst" in Bovine Blood Polymorphonuclear Leucocytes When Stimulated by Phagocytosis. Biochem. Soc. Trans., *5*:1299, 1977.

Bierman, H.R., et al.: The Sequestration and Visceral Circulation of Leukocytes in Man. Ann. N.Y. Acad. Sci., *59*:850, 1955.

Bishop, C.R., et al.: Leukokinetic Studies. XIII. A Non-Steady State Kinetic Evaluation of the Mechanism of Cortisone-Induced Granulocytosis. Jour. Clin. Invest., *47*:249, 1968.

Bishop, C.R., et al.: Leukokinetic Studies. XIV. Blood Neutrophil Kinetics in Chronic, Steady-State Neutropenia. J. Clin. Invest., *50*:1678, 1971.

Bjorksten, B., and Wadstrom, T.: Interaction of Escherichia coli with Different Fimbriae and Polymorphonuclear Leukocytes. Infect. Immun., *38*:298, 1982.

Bloomfield, F.J., and Young, M.M.: Influence of Lithium and Fluoride on Degranulation from Human Neutrophils in Vitro. Inflammation, *6*:257, 1982.

Bockenstedt, L.K., and Goetzl, E.J.: Constituents of Human Neutrophils That Mediate Enhanced Adherence to Surfaces: Purification and Identification as Acidic Proteins of the Specific Granules. J. Clin. Invest., *65*:1372, 1980.

Boecker, W.R., et al.: The Correlation of Human Myelocyte Size, DNA Content and Synthesis: Implication for Granulopoiesis Exp. Hematol., *6*:619, 1978.

Boggs, D.R.: The Kinetics of Neutrophilic Leukocytes in Health and Disease. Semin. Hematol., *4*:359, 1967.

Boggs, D.R.: Physiology of Neutrophil Proliferation, Maturation and Circulation. Clin. Haematol., *4*:535, 1975.

Boggs, D.R., et al.: Leukokinetic Studies. IX. Experimental Evaluation of a Model of Granulopoiesis. J. Clin. Invest., *44*:643, 1965a.

Boggs, D.R., et al.: Masked Granulocytosis. Proc. Soc. Exp. Biol. Med., *118*:753, 1965b.

Boggs, D.R., et al.: The Different Effects of Vinblastine Sulfate and Nitrogen Mustard upon Neutrophil Kinetics in the Dog. Proc. Soc. Exp. Biol. Med., *121*:1085, 1966a.

Boggs, D.R., et al.: Neutrophilia-Inducing Activity in Plasma of Dogs Recovering from Drug-Induced Myelotoxicity. Amer. J. Physiol., *211*:51, 1966b.

Boggs, D.R., et al.: Humoral Regulation of Neutrophil Release from Bone Marrow. J. Clin. Invest., *45*:988, 1966c.

Boggs, D.R., et al.: Neutrophil Releasing Activity in Plasma of Normal Human Subjects Injected with Endotoxin. Proc. Soc. Exp. Biol. Med., *127*:689, 1968a.

Boggs, D.R., et al.: Neutrophil-Releasing Activity in Plasma of Dogs Injected with Endotoxin. J. Lab. Clin. Med., *72*:177, 1968b.

Borgers, M., et al.: Alkaline Phosphatase Activity in Human Polymorphonuclear Leukocytes. Histochem. J., *10*:31, 1978.

Borregaard, N., and Herlin, T.: Energy Metabolism of Human Neutrophils during Phagocytosis. J. Clin. Invest., *70*:550, 1982.

Bowles, C.A., et al.: Studies of the Pelger-Huët Anomaly in Foxhounds. Amer. J. Pathol., *96*:237, 1979.

Boxer, L.A., et al.: Effects of Surface-Active Agents on Neutrophil Receptors. Infect. Immun., *21*:28, 1978.

Boxer, L.A., et al.: Diminished Polymorphonuclear Leukocyte Adherence: Functional Dependence on Release of Cyclic AMP by Endothelial Cells after Stimulation of β-Receptors by Epinephrine. J. Clin. Invest., *66*:268, 1980.

Boxer, L.A., et al.: Membrane-Bound Lactoferrin Alters the Surface Properties of Polymorphonuclear Leukocytes. J. Clin. Invest., *70*:1049, 1982.

Boyne, R., and Arthur, J.R.: Alterations of Neutrophil Function in Selenium-Deficient Cattle. J. Comp. Pathol., *89*:151, 1979.

Boyne, R., and Arthur, J.R.: Effects of Selenium and Copper Deficiency on Neutrophil Function in Cattle. J. Comp. Pathol., *91*:271, 1981.

Braunsteiner, H., and Zucker-Franklin, D.: The Physiology and Pathology of Leukocytes. Grune & Stratton, New York, 1962.

Bray, M.A.: Leukotrine B4: An Inflammatory Mediator with Vascular Actions in Vitro. Agents Actions Suppl., *11*:51, 1982.

Breton-Gorius, J.: Lactoferrin Deficiency as a Consequence of a Lack of Specific Granules in Neutrophils from a Patient with Recurrent Infections: Detection by Immunoperoxidase Staining for Lactoferrin and Cytochemical Electron Microscopy. Amer. J. Pathol., *99*:413, 1980.

Breton-Gorius, J., et al.: Cytochemical Distinction between Azurophils and Catalase-Containing Granules in Leukocytes. I. Studies in Developing Neutrophils and Monocytes from Patients with Myeloperoxidase

Deficiency: Comparison with Peroxidase Deficient Chicken Heterophils. Lab. Invest., *38*:21, 1978.

Bretz, U., and Baggiolini, M.: Biochemical and Morphological Characterization of Azurophil and Specific Granules of Human Neutrophilic Polymorphonuclear Leukocytes. J. Cell. Biol., *63*:251, 1974.

Broxmeyer, H.E.: Characteristics of Bone Marrow and Blood Cells in Human Leukemia That Produce Leukemia Inhibitory Activity (LIA). Leuk. Res., *3*:193, 1979.

Broxmeyer, H.E., et al.: Identification of Lactoferrin as the Granulocyte Derived Inhibitor of Colony-Stimulating Activity Production. J. Exp. Med., *148*:1052, 1978.

Broxmeyer, H.E., et al.: Persistence of Inhibitory Activity against Normal Bone Marrow Cells during Remission of Acute Leukemia. New Eng. J. Med., *301*:346, 1979.

Broxmeyer, H.E., et al.: Specificity and Modulation of the Action of Lactoferrin, a Negative Feedback Regulator of Myelopoiesis. Blood, *55*:324, 1980.

Broxmeyer, H.E., et al.: Monocyte-Macrophage-Derived Acidic Isoferritins: Normal Feedback Regulators of Granulocyte-Macrophage Progenitor Cells in Vitro. Blood, *60*:595, 1982.

Brune, K., et al.: Microbicidal Activity of Peroxidaseless Chicken Heterophil Leukocytes. Infect. Immun., *5*:283, 1972.

Bullen, J.J., and Armstrong, J.A.: The Role of Lactoferrin in the Bactericidal Function of Polymorphonuclear Leucocytes. Immunology, *36*:781, 1979.

Burrows, G.E.: Equine Escherichia coli Endotoxemia: Comparison of Intravenous and Intraperitoneal Endotoxin Administration. Amer. J. Vet. Res., *40*:991, 1979.

Caldwell, K.C., et al.: Induction of Myeloperoxidase Deficiency in Granulocytes in Lead Intoxicated Dogs. Blood, *53*:588, 1979.

Camp, C.J., and Leid, R.W.: Chemotaxis of Radiolabeled Equine Neutrophils. Amer. J. Vet. Res., *43*:397, 1982.

Camp, C.J., et al.: Chemotaxis (CT) and Chemokinesis (CK) of Isolated Equine Neutrophilic Leukocytes. Fed. Proc., *38*:1169, 1979.

Canfield, P.J.: An Ultrastructural Study of Granulocytic Development of Feline Bone Marrow. Anat. Histol. Embryol., *13*:97, 1984.

Carakostas, M.C., et al.: Intravascular Neutrophilic Granulocyte Kinetics in Horses. Amer. J. Vet. Res., *42*:623, 1981a.

Carakostas, M.C., et al.: Effects of Etiocholanolone and Prednisolone on Intravascular Granulocyte Kinetics in Horses. Amer. J. Vet. Res., *42*:626, 1981b.

Carlson, G.P., and Kaneko, J.J.: Intravascular Granulocyte Kinetics in Developing Calves. Amer. J. Vet. Res., *36*:421, 1975.

Carlson, G.P., and Kaneko, J.J.: Influence of Prednisolone on Intravascular Granulocyte Kinetics of Calves under Nonsteady State Conditions. Amer. J. Vet. Res., *37*:149, 1976.

Casciato, D.A.: Polymorphonuclear Neutrophil Chemotaxis under Aerobic and Anaerobic Conditions. Infect. Immun., *21*:381, 1978.

Caulfield, J.P., et al.: The Adherence of Human Neutrophil and Eosinophil to Schistosomula: Evidence for Membrane Fusion between Cells and Parasites. J. Cell Biol., *86*:46, 1980.

Chambers, W.H., et al.: Isolation of Bovine Polymorphonuclear Leukocytes by Density Gradient Centrifugation. Vet. Immunol. Immunopathol., *5*:197, 1983.

Chenoweth, D.E., et al.: Quantitative Comparisons of Neutrophil Chemotaxis in Four Animal Species. Clin. Immunol. Immunopathol., 15:525, 1980.

Cheung, A.T.W., et al.: Movement of Human Polymorphonuclear Leukocytes: A Videotape Analysis. J. Reticuloendothel. Soc., 31:193, 1982.

Cheung, A.T.W., et al.: Phagocytic and Killing Capacities of Uterine-Derived Polymorphonuclear Leukocytes from Mares Resistant and Susceptible to Chronic Endometritis. Amer. J. Vet. Res., 46:1938, 1985.

Cheung, K., et al.: The Origin of Chemoluminescence Produced by Neutrophils Stimulated by Opsonized Zymosan. J. Immunol., 130:2324, 1983.

Chusid, M.J., et al.: Defective Polymorphonuclear Leukocyte Metabolism and Function in Canine Cyclic Neutropenia. Blood, 46:921, 1975.

Clement, L.T., et al.: Identification of Neutrophil Subpopulations with Monoclonal Antibodies. Blood, 61:326, 1983.

Cline, M.J.: The White Cell. Harvard Univ. Press, Cambridge, Mass., 1975.

Cohn, Z.A., and Austin, K.F.: Contribution of Serum and Cellular Factors in Defense Reactions. II. Cellular Factors in Host Resistance. New Eng. J. Med., 268:1056, 1963.

Cohn, Z.A., and Hirsch, J.G.: The Influence of Phagocytosis on the Intracellular Distribution of Granule-Associated Components of PMN Leukocytes. J. Exp. Med., 112:1015. 1960.

Coignoul, F.L., et al.: Functional and Ultrastructural Evaluation of Neutrophils from Foals and Lactating and Nonlactating Mares. Amer. J. Vet. Res., 45:898, 1984.

Conkling, P., et al.: Comparison of Antibody-Dependent Cytotoxicity Mediated by Human Polymorphonuclear Cells, Monocytes, and Alveolar Macrophages. Blood, 60:1290, 1982.

Cook, L.O., et al.: In Vitro Functional Capabilities of Canine Polymorphonuclear Neutrophils Collected Simultaneously by Continuous-Flow Centrifugation and Continuous-Flow Filtration Leukapheresis. Amer. J. Hematol., 4:225, 1978.

Cornely, H.P.: Reversal of Chemotaxis in Vitro and Chemotactic Activity of Leukocyte Fractions. Proc. Soc. Exp. Biol. Med., 122:831, 1966.

Craddock, C.G., Jr., et al.: Studies on Leukopoiesis: The Technique of Leukapheresis and the Response of Myeloid Tissue in Normal and Irradiated Dogs. J. Lab. Clin. Med., 45:881, 1955.

Craddock, C.G., et al.: The Dynamics of Leukopoiesis and Leukocytosis, as Studied by Leukapheresis and Isotopic Techniques. J. Clin. Invest., 35:285, 1956.

Craddock, C.G., et al.: Control of the Steady State Proliferation of Leukocytes. In The Kinetics of Cellular Proliferation. Stohlman, F., ed. Grune & Stratton, New York, p. 242, 1963.

Cronkite, E.P. and Fliedner, T.M.: Granulopoiesis. New Engl. J. Med. 270:1347, 1403, 1964.

Cronkite, E.P., and Vincent, P.C.: Granulocytopoiesis. Ser. Hematol., 4:3, 1969.

Dahinden, C., and Fehr, J.: Granulocyte Activation by Endotoxin. II. Role of Granulocyte Adherence, Aggregation, and Effect of Cytochalasin B, and Comparison with Formylated Chemotactic Peptide-Induced Stimulation. J. Immunol., 130:863, 1983.

Dahinden, C., et al.: Granulocyte Activation by Endotoxin. I. Correlation between Adherence and Other Granulocyte Functions, and Role of Endotoxin Structure on Biologic Activity. J. Immunol., 130:857, 1983.

Dale, D.C., et al.: Comparison of Agents Producing a Neutrophilic Leukocytosis in Man: Hydrocortisone, Prednisolone, Endotoxin and Etiocholanolone. J. Clin. Invest., 56(4): 808, 1975.

Dale, D.C., et al.: Neutrophil-Releasing Activity in Plasma of Normal Human Subjects Injected with Etiocholanolone. Proc. Soc. Exp. Biol. Med., 156:192, 1977.

Dallegri, F., et al.: Evidence for a Reversible Functional State of Neutrophil Chemotactic Deactivation. Int. Arch. Allergy Appl. Immunol., 63:330, 1980.

Dancey, J.T., et al.: Neutrophil Kinetics in Man. J. Clin. Invest., 58:705, 1976.

de Duve, C., et al.: Tissue Fractionation Studies. 6. Intracellular Distribution Patterns of Enzymes in Rat-Liver Tissue. Biochem. J., 60:604, 1955.

Densen, P., and Mandell, G.L.: Phagocytic Strategy vs. Microbial Tactics. Rev. Infect. Dis., 2:817, 1980.

Deubelbeiss, K.A., et al.: Neutrophil Kinetics in the Dog. J. Clin. Invest., 55:833, 1975.

Dewald, B., et al.: Release of Gelatinase from a Novel Secretory Compartment of Human Neutrophils. J. Clin. Invest., 70:518, 1982.

Dewald, B., et al.: Exocytosis Induced in Neutrophils by Chemotactic Agents and Other Stimuli. Agents Actions Suppl., 12:371, 1983.

Douglas, S.D., and Fudenberg, H.H.: Host Defense Failure. The Role of Phagocyte Dysfunction. Hosp. Pract., 4:29, 1969.

Dulin, A.M., et al.: Determination of Phagocytosis of ^{32}P-labeled Staphylococcus aureus by Bovine Polymorphonuclear Leukocytes. Amer. J. Vet. Res., 45:786, 1984.

Eliopoulos, G., et al.: Effect of Corynebacterium parvum Stimulation on Granulopoiesis. Eur. J. Cancer, 16:1093, 1980.

El-Maaliem, H., and Fletcher, J.: Impaired Neutrophil Function and Myeloperoxidase Deficiency in Pregnancy. Brit. J. Haematol., 44:375, 1980.

Elsbach, P.: Degradation of Microorganisms by Phagocytic Cells. Rev. Infect. Dis., 2:106, 1980.

Eshelman, J.E., et al.: Effect of Cream on Bactericidal and Metabolic Function of Bovine Polymorphonuclear Neutrophils. Amer. J. Vet. Res., 42:738, 1981.

Faden, H., et al.: The in Vitro Effects of Newcastle Disease Virus on the Metabolic and Antibacterial Functions of Human Neutrophils. Blood, 58:221, 1981.

Fantone, J.C., et al.: Chemotactic Mediators in Neutrophil-Dependent Lung Injury. Ann. Rev. Physiol., 44:283, 1982.

Faucy, A.S., et al.: Glucocorticoid Therapy Mechanism of Action and Clinical Considerations. Ann. Intern. Med., 84:304, 1976.

Fehr, J., and Grossman, H.C.: Disparity between Circulating and Marginated Neutrophils: Evidence from Studies on the Granulocyte Alkaline Phosphatase, a Marker of Cell Maturity. Amer. J. Hematol., 7:369, 1979.

Finch, S.C.: Granulocytopenia (Ch. 75) and Granulocytosis (Ch. 76). In Hematology. Williams, W.J., et al., eds. McGraw-Hill. New York, 1972.

Fitchen, J.H., and Cline, M.J.: Serum Inhibitors of Myelopoiesis. Brit. J. Haematol., 44:7, 1980.

Fliedner, T.M., et al.: Granulopoiesis. I. Senescence and Random Loss in Neutrophilic Granulocytes in Human Beings. Blood, 24:402, 1964.

Ford-Hutchinson, A.W.: Neutrophil Aggregating Properties of PAF-Acether and Leukotriene B$_4$. Int. J. Immunopharmacol., 5:17, 1983.

Forslid, J., and Hed, J.: In Vitro Effect of Hydrocortisone on the Attachment and Ingestion Phase of Immunoglobulin G- and Complement Component C3b-Mediated Phagocytosis by Human Neutrophils. Infect. Immun., *38*:811, 1982.

Foster, R.S., and Mirand, E.A.: Bone Marrow Colony-Stimulating Factor following Ureteral Ligation in Germfree Mice. Proc. Soc. Exp. Biol. Med., *133*:1223, 1970.

Franson, R., et al.: Phospholipase A Activity Associated with the Membranes of Human Polymorphonuclear Leucocytes. Biochem. J. *167*:839, 1977.

Freedman, H.L., et al.: Inflammation and Tissue Injury. II. Local Release of Lysosomal Enzymes during Mixed Bacterial Infection in the Skin of Rabbits. Proc. Soc. Exp. Biol. Med., *125*:1209, 1967.

Fruhman, G.J.: Factors Influencing Neutrophil Mobilization. *In* Regulation of Hematopoiesis. Vol. 2. Gordon, A.S., ed. Appleton-Century-Crofts, New York, p. 873, 1970.

Fruhman, G.J.: Endotoxins and Leukocyte Mobilization. J. Reticuloendothel. Soc., *12*:62, 1972.

Fukuda, T., and Matsumoto, O.: Endogenous Factors Concerning the Febrile and the Leukocytic Response to Bacterial Endotoxin in Relation to the Adrenal Cortex. Jap. J. Physiol., *9*:274, 1959.

Gahmberg, C.G., et al.: Decrease of the Major High Molecular Weight Glycoprotein of Human Granulocytes in Monosomy-7 Associated with Defective Chemotaxis. Blood, *54*:401, 1979.

Galbraith, P., et al.: Patterns of Granulocyte Kinetics in Health, Infection and in Carcinoma. Blood, *25*:683, 1965.

Gallin, J.I.: Disorders of Phagocyte Chemotaxis. Ann. Intern. Med., *92*:520, 1980.

Gallin, J.I.: Abnormal Phagocyte Chemotaxis: Pathophysiology, Clinical Manifestations and Management of Patients. Rev. Infect. Dis., *3*:1196, 1981.

Gallin, J.I., and Fletcher, M.P.: Modulation of the Humoral and Cellular Components of the Inflammatory Process by Neutrophil Granules. *In* The Inflammatory Process. Venge, P., and Lindbom, A., eds. Almqvist & Wiksell International, Stockholm, pp. 183–201, 1981.

Gallin, J.I., and Quie, P.G.: Leukocyte Chemotaxis: Methods, Physiology and Clinical Implications. Raven Press, New York, 1978.

Gallin, J.I., et al.: Role of Secretory Events in Modulating Human Neutrophil Chemotaxis. J. Clin. Invest., *62*:1364, 1978.

Gallin, J.I., et al.: Efficacy of Ascorbic Acid in Chédiak-Higashi Syndrome: Studies in Humans and Mice. Blood, *53*:226, 1979.

Gallin, J.I., et al.: Human Neutrophil-Specific Granule Deficiency: A Model to Assess the Role of Neutrophil-Specific Granules in the Evolution of the Inflammatory Response. Blood, *59*:1317, 1982.

Gemmell, C.G., et al.: Effect of Staphylococcal α-Toxin on Phagocytosis of Staphylococci by Human Polymorphonuclear Leukocytes. Infect. Immun., *38*:975, 1982.

Gennaro, R., et al.: A Novel Type of Cytoplasmic Granule in Bovine Neutrophils. J. Cell Biol., *96*:1651, 1983a.

Gennaro, R., et al.: Potency of Bactericidal Proteins Purified from the Large Granules of Bovine Neutrophils. Infect. Immun., *40*:684, 1983b.

Gilbertsen, R.B., et al.: Effects of F-Met-Leu-Phe and Zymosan-Activated Serum on Rat Neutrophils in Vivo. J. Reticuloendothel. Soc., *27*:485, 1980.

Gimbrone, M.A., Jr., and Buchanan, M.R.: Interaction of Platelets and Leukocytes with Vascular Endothelium: In Vitro Studies. Ann. N.Y. Acad. Sci., *401*:171, 1982.

Gobig, T.G.: Leukocyte Abnormalities. Med. Clin. North Amer., *64*:647, 1980.

Goetzl, E.J., and Austen, K.F.: A Neutrophil-Immobilizing Factor Derived from Human Leukocytes. I. Generation and Partial Characterization. J. Exp. Med., *136*:1564, 1972.

Goetzl, E.J., and Gorman, R.R.: Chemotactic and Chemokinetic Stimulation of Human Eosinophil and Neutrophil Polymorphonuclear Leukocytes by 12-L-Hydroxy-5,8,10-Heptadecatrienoic Acid (HHT). J. Immunol., *120*:526, 1978.

Golde, D.W., and Cline, M.J.: Regulation of Granulopoiesis. New Eng. J. Med., *291*:1388, 1974.

Golub, E.S., and Spitznagel, J.K.: The Role of Lysosomes in Hypersensitivity Reactions: Tissue Damage by Polymorphonuclear Neutrophil Lysosomes. J. Immunol., *95*:1060, 1966.

Gordon, A.S., et al.: Evidence for a Circulating Leucocytosis-Inducing Factor (LIF). Acta Haematol., *23*:323, 1960.

Gordon, L.I., et al.: Modulation of Neutrophil Function by Lysozyme: Potential Negative Feedback System of Inflammation. J. Clin. Invest., *64*:226, 1979.

Gorski, A.: Corticosteroid-Dependent Alterations of Human Myelopoiesis in Vitro. Biomed., *30*:206, 1979.

Gossett, K.A., and MacWilliams, P.S.: Ultrastructure of Canine Toxic Neutrophils. Amer. J. Vet. Res., *43*:1634, 1982.

Gossett, K.A., et al.: In Vitro Function of Canine Neutrophils during Experimental Inflammatory Disease. Vet. Immunol. Immunopathol., *5*:151, 1983.

Granellipiperno, A., et al.: Secretion of Plasminogen Activator by Human Polymorphonuclear Leukocytes: Modulation by Glucocorticoids and Other Effectors. J. Exp. Med., *146*:1693, 1977.

Greenwalt, T.J., and Jamieson, G.A.: The Granulocyte: Function and Clinical Utilization. Alan R. Liss, New York, 1977.

Grewal, A.S., and Babiuk, L.A.: Complement-Dependent, Polymorphonuclear Neutrophil-Mediated Cytotoxicity of Herpesvirus-Infected Cells: Possible Mechanism(s) of Cytotoxicity. Immunology, *40*:151, 1980.

Grewal, A.S., et al.: Characterization of Surface Receptors on Bovine Leukocytes. Int. Arch. Allergy Appl. Immunol., *56*:289, 1978.

Grindem, C.B.: Ultrastructural Morphology of Leukemic Cells in the Cat. Vet. Pathol., *22*:147, 1985.

Gruner, E.R., et al.: A Comparison of Antibacterial Granule Components in Neutrophil Leukocytes from Bovine Blood and Milk after Endotoxin Infusion. J Dairy Sci., *65*(suppl. 1):164 (abstr.), 1982.

Guerrant, R.L., et al.: Interaction between Entamoeba histolytica and Human Polymorphonuclear Neutrophils. J. Infect. Dis., *143*:83, 1981.

Hafeman, D.G., and Lucas, Z.J.: Polymorphonuclear Leukocyte-Mediated, Antibody Dependent, Cellular Cytotoxicity against Tumor Cells: Dependence of Oxygen and the Respiratory Burst. J. Immunol., *123*:55, 1979.

Hagemoser, W.A., et al.: Granulocytopathy in a Holstein Heifer. J. Amer. Vet. Med. Ass., *183*:1093, 1983.

Hakak-Berenji, S.N., and Jain, N.C.: Antibacterial Activity of Bovine Blood Neutrophils and Their Cationic Proteins. J. Dairy Sci., *66*:1377, 1983.

Hammerschmidt, D.E., et al.: Complement-Induced

Granulocyte Aggregation in Vivo. Amer. J. Pathol., *102*:146, 1981.

Hammerschmidt, D.E., et al.: Synergy among Agents Inhibiting Granulocyte Aggregation. Inflammation, *6*:169, 1982.

Hammond, W.P., and Dale, D.C.: Lithium Therapy of Canine Cyclic Hematopoiesis. Blood, *55*:26, 1980.

Hammond, W.P., et al.: Canine Cyclic Hematopoiesis: Effects of Chronic Endotoxin Administration. Blood, *52*:1170, 1978.

Handler, E.S., et al.: Mechanisms of Leukocyte Production and Release. V. Studies on the Leukocytosis-Inducing Factor in the Plasma of Rats Treated with Typhoid-Paratyphoid Vaccine. J. Lab. Clin. Med., *67*:398, 1966.

Hansen, N.E.: Plasma Lysozyme, a Measure of Neutrophil Turnover: An Analytical Review. Munksgaard, Copenhagen, 1974.

Hansen, N.E., and Andersen, V.: Lysozyme Activity in Human Neutrophil Granulocytes. Brit. J. Haematol., *24*:613, 1973.

Hansen, N.E., et al.: Neutrophilic Granulocytes in Acute Bacterial Infection. Clin. Exp. Immunol., *26*:463, 1976.

Hansson, G., and Radmark, O.: Leukotriene C4: Isolation from Human Polymorphonuclear Leukocytes. FEBS Lett., *122*:87, 1980.

Harmon, R.J., and Heald, C.W.: Cytology of Bovine Neutrophil Migration in Mammary Tissue during Experimental Staphylococcus aureus Mastitis. J. Dairy Sci., *64*(suppl. 1):149, 1978.

Harris, P.F., and Kugler, J.H.: Mitosis in Metamyelocyte. Nature, *200*:712, 1963.

Harris, R.E., et al.: Consequences of Vitamin-E Deficiency on the Phagocytic and Oxidative Functions of the Rat Polymorphonuclear Leukocyte. Blood, *55*:338, 1980.

Harvath, L., et al.: Chemoluminescence of Human and Canine Polymorphonuclear Leukocytes in the Absence of Phagocytosis. J. Clin. Invest., *61*:1145, 1978.

Haskins, M.E., et al.: Mucopolysaccharidosis in a Domestic Short-Haired Cat: A Disease Distinct from That Seen in the Siamese Cat. J. Amer. Vet. Med. Ass., *175*:384, 1979a.

Haskins, M.E., et al.: Mucopolysaccharide Storage Disease in Three Families of Cats with Arylsulfatase B Deficiency: Leukocyte Studies and Carrier Identification. Pediatr. Res., *13*:1203, 1979b.

Haskins, M.E., et al.: Mucopolysaccharidosis VI Maroteaux-Lamy Syndrome: Arylsulfate B–Deficient Mucopolysaccharidosis in the Siamese Cat. Amer. J. Pathol., *105*:191, 1981.

Herman, J.J., et al.: Complement-Dependent Histaminase Release from Human Granulocytes. J. Clin. Invest., *63*:1195, 1979.

Hersh, E.M., and Bodey, G.P.: Leukocytic Mechanisms in Inflammation. Ann. Rev. Med., *21*:105, 1970.

Hertzog, A.J.: The Phagocytic Activity of Human Leukocytes, with Special Reference to Their Type and Maturity. Amer. J. Pathol., *14*:595, 1938.

Higgins, G.R., et al.: Granulocytasthenia: A Unique Leukocyte Dysfunction Associated with Decreased Resistance to Infection. Clin. Res., *18*:209A, 1970.

Hinshaw, L.B., et al.: Hematologic Disturbances during Sepsis: Platelets and Leukocytes. Adv. Shock Res., *7*:1, 1982.

Hoover, R.L., et al.: The Adhesive Interaction between Polymorphonuclear Leukocytes and Endothelial Cells in Vitro. Cell, *14*:423, 1978.

Hoover, R.L., et al.: Adhesion of Leukocytes to Endothelium: Roles of Divalent Cations, Surface Charge, Chemotactic Agents and Substrate. J. Cell. Sci., *45*:73, 1980.

Horsmanheimo, A., et al.: Effect of Tuftsin on Migration of Polymorphonuclear and Mononuclear Human Leukocytes in Leukocyte Migration Agarose Test. Clin. Immunol. Immunopathol., *11*:251, 1978.

Howard, C.J., et al.: Surface Receptors for Immunoglobulin on Bovine Polymorphonuclear Neutrophils and Macrophages. Res. Vet. Sci., *29*:128, 1980.

Howes, E.L., et al.: The Effect of Indomethacin on the Generalized Shwartzman Reaction. Amer. J. Pathol., *90*:7, 1978.

Hugli, T.E.: Chemical Aspects of the Serum Anaphylatoxins. Contemp. Top. Mol. Immunol., *7*:181, 1978.

Hurley, J.V., and Spector, W.G.: A Topographical Study of Increased Vascular Permeability in Acute Turpentine-Induced Pleurisy. J. Path. Bact., *89*:254, 1965.

Ishibashi, Y., and Yamashita, T.: Generation of a Phagocytosis-Stimulating Factor by Polymorphonuclear Neutrophils during Phagocytosis. Int. Arch. Allergy Appl. Immunol., *64*:181, 1981.

Issekutz, A.C.: Enhancement of Human Neutrophil Bactericidal Activity by Chemotactic Factors. Infect. Immunol., *24*:295, 1979.

Iyer, G.Y.N., et al.: Biochemical Aspects of Phagocytosis. Nature, *192*:535, 1961.

Jacobsen, K., et al.: Isolation of Equine Neutrophils and Analysis of Functional Characteristics by Chemiluminescence and Bactericidal Assays. Amer. J. Vet. Res., *43*:1912, 1982.

Jacques, Y.V., and Bainton, D.F.: Changes in pH within the Phagocytic Vacuoles of Human Neutrophils and Monocytes. Lab. Invest., *39*:179, 1978.

Jain, N.C.: A Comparative Cytochemical Study of Leukocytes of Some Animal Species. Folia Haematol., *94*:49, 1970.

Jain, N.C.: Neutrophil Leukocytes and Inflammation of the Bovine Mammary Gland. Theriogenology, *6*:153, 1976.

Jain, N.C., and Lasmanis, J.: Phagocytosis of Serum-Resistant and Serum-Sensitive Coliform Bacteria (Klebsiella) by Bovine Neutrophils from Blood and Mastitic Milk. Amer. J. Vet. Res., *39*:425, 1978a.

Jain, N.C., and Lasmanis, J.: Leukocyte Changes in Cows Given Intravenous Injection of Escherichia coli Endotoxin. Res. Vet. Sci., *24*:386, 1978b.

Jain, N.C., et al.: Experimental Mastitis in Leukopenic Cows: Immunologically Induced Neutropenia and Response to Intramammary Inoculation of Aerobacter aerogenes. Amer. J. Vet. Res., *29*:2089, 1968.

Jain, N.C., et al.: Comparison in Normal and Leukopenic Cows of Experimental Mastitis Due to Aerobacter aerogenes or Escherichia coli Endotoxin. Amer. J. Vet. Res., *30*:715, 1969.

Jain, N.C., et al.: Experimentally Induced Coliform (Aerobacter aerogenes) Mastitis in Normal Cows and in Cows Made Neutropenic by an Equine Anti-Bovine Leukocyte Serum. Amer. J. Vet. Res., *32*:1929, 1971.

Jain, N.C., et al.: Leukocytes and Tissue Factors in the Pathogenesis of Bovine Mastitis. Amer. J. Vet. Res., *33*:1137, 1972.

Jain, N.C., et al.: Neutrophil Kinetics in Endotoxin-Induced Mastitis. Amer. J. Vet. Res., *39*:1662, 1978.

Jain, N.C., et al.: Hematologic Changes in Buffalo Calves Inoculated with Escherichia coli Endotoxin and Corticosteroid. Unpublished observations, 1980.

Jain, N.C., et al.: Clinical Pathological Findings and Cytochemical Characterization of Myelomonocytic Leukaemia in 5 Dogs. J. Comp. Pathol., *91*:17, 1981.

Janoff, A., and Schaefer, S.: Mediators of Acute Inflammation in Leucocyte Lysosomes. Nature, *213*:144, 1967.

Janoff, A., et al.: Lung Injury Induced by Leukocytic Proteases. Amer. J. Pathol., *97*:111, 1979.

Jarstrand, C., et al.: Fibronectin Increases the Motility, Phagocytosis and NBT (Nitroblue Tetrazolium)-Reduction of Granulocytes. J. Clin. Lab. Immunol., *8*:59, 1982.

Jasper, D.E., and Jain, N.C.: The Influence of Adrenocorticotropic Hormone and Prednisolone upon Marrow and Circulating Leukocytes in the Dog. Amer. J. Vet. Res., *26*:844, 1965.

Jeter, W.S., et al.: Inhibition of Immune Phagocytosis of Diplococcus pneumoniae by Human Neutrophils with Antibody against Complement. J. Immunol., *86*:386, 1961.

Johnson, C.A., et al.: Functional and Metabolic Studies of Polymorphonuclear Leukocytes in the Congenital Pelger-Huët Anomaly. Blood, *55*:466, 1980.

Johnston, R.B., et al.: The Enhancement of Bacterial Phagocytosis by Serum: The Role of Complement Components and Two Cofactors. J. Exp. Med., *129*:1275, 1969.

Jouvin-Marche, E., et al.: Platelet-Activating Factor (PAF-Acether): An Activator of Neutrophil Functions. Agents Actions, *12*:716, 1982.

Karnovsky, M.J., et al.: Oxidative Cytochemistry in Phagocytosis: The Interface between Structure and Function. Histochem. J., *13*:1, 1981.

Kass, L., and De Bruyn, P.P.H.: Chemotaxis of Mature and Immature Blood Cells in Tissue Cultures. Anat. Rec., *159*:115, 1967.

Kay, N.E., et al.: Human Neutrophils Migratory Function: Modulating Effect of Interactions with Opsonized Particles. Infect. Immun., *26*:12, 1979.

Keller, H.U., et al.: Physiology of Chemotaxis and Random Motility. Semin. Hematol., *12*:47, 1975.

Klebanoff, S.J.: Myeloperoxidase-Halide-Hydrogen Peroxide Antibacterial System. J. Bacteriol., *95*:2131, 1968.

Klebanoff, S.J.: Intraleukocytic Microbicidal Defects. Ann. Rev. Med., *22*:39, 1971.

Klebanoff, S.J., and Clark, R.A.: The Neutrophil: Function and Clinical Disorders. North Holland, New York, 1978.

Klebanoff, S.J., et al.: The Peroxidase-Thiocyanate-Hydrogen Peroxide Antimicrobial System. Biochim. Biophys. Acta, *117*:63, 1966.

Klempner, M.S., and Gallin, J.I.: Separation and Functional Characterization of Human Neutrophil Subpopulations. Blood, *51*:659, 1978.

Klock, J.C., and Pieprzyk, J.K.: Cholesterol, Phospholipids, and Fatty Acids of Normal Immature Neutrophils: Comparison with Acute Myeloblastic Leukemia Cells and Normal Neutrophils. J. Lipid Res., *20*:908, 1979.

Klostergaard, J., et al.: Activation of Neutrophilic Granulocytes by Products of Human Lymphocytes. Int. Arch. Allergy Appl. Immunol., *57*:542, 1978.

Koblik, P.D., et al.: Use of ^{111}In-labeled Autologous Leukocytes to Image an Abdominal Abscess in a Horse. J. Amer. Vet. Med. Ass., *186*:1319, 1985.

Konig, W., et al.: Generation and Release of Eosinophil Chemotactic Factor from Human Polymorphonuclear Neutrophils by Arachidonic Acid. Eur. J. Immunol., *8*:434, 1978.

Korbitz, B.C., et al.: The Piromen Test: A Useful Assay of Bone Marrow Granulocyte Reserves. Curr. Ther. Res., *11*:491, 1969.

Kramer, J.W., et al.: The Chédiak-Higashi Syndrome of Cats. Lab. Invest., *36*:554, 1977.

Kreutzer, D.L., et al.: Interaction of Polymorphonuclear Leukocytes with Smooth and Rough Strains of Brucella abortus. Infect. Immun., *23*:737, 1979.

Krosse, F.G.M., et al.: Granulocyte Function Tests in Canine Infectious Diseases: Methods and Preliminary Clinical Results. Vet. Immunol. Immunopathol., *2*:455, 1981.

Lane, T.A., et al.: Phagocytosis-Induced Modulation of Human Neutrophil Chemotaxis Receptors. Blood, *58*:228, 1981.

Lash, J.A., et al.: Plasma Lactoferrin Reflects Granulocyte Activation in Vitro. Blood, *61*:885, 1983.

Latimer, K.S., and Prasse, K.W.: Neutrophilic Movement of a Basenji with Pelger-Huët Anomaly. Amer. J. Vet. Res., *43*:525, 1982.

Latimer, K.S., et al.: Quantitative Evaluation of Neutrophilic Chemotaxis in Beagles. Amer. J. Vet. Res., *42*:1254, 1981.

Latimer, K.S., et al.: Neutrophil Movement in Selected Canine Skin Diseases. Amer. J. Vet. Res., *44*:601, 1983.

Latimer, K.S., et al.: Pelger-Huët Anomaly in Cats. Vet. Pathol. *22*:370, 1985.

Lichtman, M.A., et al.: The Shape and Surface Morphology of Human Leukocytes in Vitro: Effect of Temperature, Metabolic Inhibitors and Agents That Influence Membrane Structure. Blood Cells, *2*:507, 1976.

Lichtman, M.A., et al., The Regulation of the Release of Granulocytes from Normal Marrow. *In* The Granulocyte: Function and Clinical Utilization. Alan R. Liss, New York, p. 53–75, 1977.

Lindbom, L., et al.: Leukotrine B4 Induces Extravasation and Migration of Polymorphonuclear Leukocytes in Vivo. Acta Physiol. Scand., *116*:105, 1982.

Lisiewicz, J.: Human Neutrophils. Charles Press Publishers, Bowie, Maryland, 1980.

Liu, I.K.: Comparison of Peripheral Blood and Uterine-Derived Polymorphonuclear Leukocytes from Mares Resistant and Susceptible to Chronic Endometritis: Chemotactic and Cell Elastimetry Analysis. Amer. J. Vet. Res., *46*:917, 1985.

LoBue, J.: Analysis of Normal Granulocyte Production and Release. *In* Regulation of Hematopoiesis, Vol. 2, Gordon, A.S. (ed.), Appleton-Century-Crofts, N.Y., Chapter 45, 1970.

Lombardo, P.S., et al.: Effect of Colostrum Ingestion on Indices of Neutrophil Phagocytosis and Metabolism in Newborn Calves. Amer. J. Vet. Res., *40*:362, 1979.

Lumsden, J.H., et al.: The Piromen Test as an Assay of Bone Marrow Granulocyte Reserves in the Calf. I. Studies on Bone Marrow and Peripheral Blood Leukocytes. Can. J. Comp. Path., *38*:56, 1974.

Mackie, D.P., et al.: Electron Microscopic Visualization of the in Vitro Phagocytosis of Group B Streptococci by Bovine Polymorphonuclear Leucocytes. Res. Vet. Sci., *33*:333, 1982.

Mackie, P.H., et al.: Neutrophil Cytochemistry in Bacterial Infections. J. Clin. Pathol., *32*:26, 1979.

MacRae, E.K., et al.: Scanning Electron Microscopic Observations of Early Stages of Phagocytosis of E. coli by Human Neutrophils. Cell Tissue Res., *209*:65, 1980.

Malcolm, I.D., et al.: Vacuolization of the Neutrophils in Bacteremia. Arch. Intern. Med., *139*:675, 1979.

Malnsten, C.L., et al.: Leukotriene B4: A Highly Potent and Sterospecific Factor Stimulating Migration of Polymorphonuclear Leukocytes. Acta Physiol. Scand., *110*:449, 1980.

Maloney, M.A., and Patt, H.M.: Granulocyte Transit from Bone Marrow to Blood. Blood, *13*:195, 1968.

Maloney, M.A., et al.: Myelocyte-Metamyelocyte Transition in the Bone Marrow of the Dog. Nature, *197*:150, 1963.

Mandell, L.A.: Effects of Antimicrobial and Antineoplastic Drugs on the Phagocytic and Microbicidal Function of the Polymorphonuclear Leukocyte. Rev. Infect. Dis., *4*:683, 1982.

Marsh, J.C., et al.: Neutrophil Kinetics in Acute Infection. J. Clin. Invest., *46*:1943, 1967.

McCall, C.E., et al.: Lysosomal and Ultrastructural Changes in Human "Toxic" Neutrophils during Bacterial Infection. J. Exp. Med., *129*:267, 1969.

McMillan, R., and Scott, J.L.: Leukocyte Labeling with Chromium. I. Technique and Results in Normal Subjects. Blood, *32*:738, 1968.

Mease, A.D., et al.: Irreversible Neutrophil Aggregation: A Mechanism of Decreased Newborn Neutrophil Chemotactic Response. Amer. J. Pathol., *104*:98, 1981.

Mechanic, R.C., et al.: Quantitative Studies of Human Leukocytic and Febrile Response to Single and Repeated Doses of Purified Bacterial Endotoxin. J. Clin. Invest., *41*:162, 1962.

Melby, K., and Midtvedt, T.: Effects of Some Antibacterial Agents on the Phagocytosis of 32p Labelled Escherichia coli by Human Polymorphonuclear Cells. Acta Pathol. Microbiol. Immunol. Scand. B, *88*:103, 1980.

Melby, K., et al.: Effect of Human Leukocyte Interaction on Phagocytic Activity of Polymorphonuclear Leukocytes. Acta Pathol. Microbiol. Immunol. Scand. B, *90*:181, 1982.

Menkin, V.: Biochemical Mechanisms in Inflammation. 2nd ed. Charles C Thomas, Springfield, Ill., 1956.

Menzel, J., et al.: Contribution of Immunoglobulins M and G, complement, and Properdin to the Intracellular Killing of Escherichia coli by Polymorphonuclear Leukocytes. Infect. Immun., *19*:659, 1978.

Michaelis, T.W., et al.: Surface Morphology of Human Leukocytes. Blood, *37*:23, 1971.

Miler, I.: Specific and Non-Specific Opsonins. Curr. Top. Microbiol. Immunol., *51*:63, 1970.

Miles, A.A., and Wilhelm, D.L.: The Activation of Endogenous Substances Inducing Pathological Increases of Capillary Permeability. In The Biochemical Response to Injury, Stoner, H.B., ed. Blackwell Scientific Publications, Oxford, 1960.

Miller, A.M., et al.: Modulation of Granulopoiesis: Opposing Roles of Prostaglandins F and E. J. Lab. Clin. Med., *92*:983, 1978.

Miller, M.E.: Deficiency of Chemotactic Function in the Human Neonate: A Previously Unrecognized Defect of the Inflammatory Response. Pediatr. Res., *3*:497, 1969.

Mills, E.L., and Quie, P.G.: Congenital Disorders of the Functions of Polymorphonuclear Neutrophils. Rev. Infect. Dis., *2*:505, 1980.

Miya, F., and Marcus, S.: Effect of Humoral Factors on in Vitro Phagocytic and Cytopeptic Activities of Normal and "Immune" Phagocytes. J. Immunol., *86*:652, 1961.

Morris, T.C.M., et al.: Inhibition of Normal Human Granulopoiesis in Vitro by Non-B, Non-T Lymphocytes. Brit. J. Haematol., *45*:541, 1980.

Morrison, D.C., and Ulevitch, R.J.: The Effects of Bacterial Endotoxins on Host Mediation Systems. Amer. J. Pathol., *93*:527, 1978.

Movat, H.Z.: Tissue Injury and Inflammation Induced by Immune Complexes: The Critical Role of the Neutrophil Leukocyte. Exp. Mol. Pathol., *31*:201, 1979.

Movat, H.Z., et al.: A Permeability Factor Released from Leukocytes after Phagocytosis of Immune Complexes and Its Possible Role in the Arthus Reaction. Life Sci., *3*:1025, 1964.

Moxley, J.H., et al.: Return of Leucocytes to the Bone Marrow in Chronic Myelogenous Leukaemia. Nature, *208*:1281, 1965.

Murphy, P.: The Neutrophil. Plenum Medical Book Co., New York, 1976.

Nafstad, H.J., and Nafstad, I.: An Electron Microscopic Study of Normal Blood and Bone Marrow in Pigs. Path. Vet., *5*:451, 1968.

Neeman, N., et al.: The Effect of Leukocyte Hydrolases on Bacteria. II. The Synergistic Action of Lysozyme and Extracts of PMN, Macrophages, Lymphocytes, and Platelets in Bacteriolysis. Proc. Soc. Exp. Biol. Med., *146*:1137, 1974.

Nelson, D.H.: The Adrenal Cortex: Physiological Function and Disease. W.B. Saunders, Philadelphia, 1980.

Nelson, R.D., et al.: Chemotaxis under Agarose: A New and Simple Method for Measuring Chemotaxis and Spontaneous Migration of Human Polymorphonuclear Leukocytes and Monocytes. J. Immunol., *115*:1650, 1975.

Newell, D.G.: Scanning Electron Microscopy of Normal and Leukaemic Human Leucocytes. Topical Rev. Hematol., *1*:87, 1980.

Niedel, J.E., and Cuatrecasas, P.: Formyl Peptide Chemotactic Receptors of Leukocytes and Macrophages. Curr. Top. Cell Regul., *17*:137, 1980.

Nikolajczuk, M.: Application of the NBT Test in Calves. Arch. Immunol. Ther. Exp., *26*:471, 1978.

O'Donnell, R.T., and Andersen, B.R.: Characterization of Canine Neutrophil Granules. Infect. Immun., *38*:351, 1982.

O'Gairbhidhe, C.P., et al.: Chemotactic Effect of Staphylococcus aureus on Neutrophils Isolated from the Bovine Mammary Gland. J. Dairy Sci., *53*:602, 1970.

Oliver, J.M., and Zurier, R.B.: Correction of Characteristic Abnormalities of Microtubule Function and Granule Morphology in Chédiak-Higashi Syndrome with Cholinergic Agonists: Studies in Vitro in Man and in Vivo in the Beige Mouse. J. Clin. Invest., *57*:1239, 1976.

Oliver, J.M., et al.: Carbamylcholine Prevents Giant Granule Formation in Cultured Fibroblasts from Beige (Chédiak-Higashi) Mice. J. Cell Biol., *69*:205, 1976.

Olsson, I., and Venge, P.: The Role of the Human Neutrophil in the Inflammatory Reaction. Allergy, *35*:1, 1980.

Oseas, R., et al.: Lactoferrin: A Promoter of Polymorphonuclear Adhesiveness. Blood, *57*:939, 1981.

Paape, M.J., et al.: Leukocytes: Second Line of Defense against Invading Mastitis Pathogens. Dairy Sci., *62*:135, 1979.

Page, A.R., and Good, R.A.: A Cinical and Experimental

Study of the Function of Neutrophils in the Inflammatory Response. Amer. J. Pathol., 34:645, 1958.

Patt, H.M., and Maloney, M.A.: Kinetics of Neutrophil Balance. In The Kinetics of Cellular Proliferation. Stohlman, F., Jr., ed. Grune & Stratton, New York, p. 201, 1959.

Patt, H.M., and Maloney, M.A.: A Model of Granulocyte Kinetics. Ann. N.Y. Acad. Sci., 113:515, 1964.

Paul, B., et al.: The Role of the Phagocyte in Host-Parasite Interactions. XVI. Effect of X-Irradiation on H_2O_2 Production in Guinea Pig Exudate Cells. J. Reticuloendothel. Soc., 5:538, 1968.

Perry, S., et al.: Rates of Appearance and Disappearance of White Blood Cells in Normal and in Various Disease States. J. Lab. Clin. Med., 51:501, 1958.

Philip, M.A., et al.: Failure of Chronic Granulocytic Leukaemia Leucocytes to Release an Inhibitor of Granulopoiesis. Lancet, 1(8225):866, 1981.

Pickering, L.K.: Polymorphonuclear Leukocytes of Human Colostrum. I. Oxidative Metabolism and Kinetics of Killing of Radiolabeled Staphylococcus aureus. J. Infect. Dis., 142:685, 1980.

Pinckard, R.N.: The "New" Chemical Mediators of Inflammation. In Current Topics in Inflammation and Infection. Majno, G., et al., eds. Williams & Wilkins, Baltimore, p. 38, 1982.

Poole, J.C.F.: Electron Microscopy of Polymorphonuclear Leucocytes. Brit. J. Derm., 81:11, 1969.

Prasad, J.S.: Leucocyte Function in Iron-Deficiency Anemia. Amer. J. Clin. Nutr., 32:550, 1979.

Prasse, K.W., et al.: Blood Neutrophilic Granulocyte Kinetics in Cats. Amer. J. Vet. Res., 34:1021, 1973.

Prasse, K.W., et al.: Idiopathic Hyposegmentation of Neutrophils in a Horse. J. Amer. Vet. Med. Ass., 178:303, 1981.

Prieur, D.J., and Collier, L.L.: Inheritance of the Chédiak-Higashi Syndrome in Cats. J. Heredity, 72:175, 1981.

Pruzanski, W., and Saito, S.: The Influence of Natural and Synthetic Cationic Substances on Phagocytic Activity of Human Polymorphonuclear Cells. Exp. Cell Res., 117:1, 1978.

Pryzwanoky, K.B., et al.: Early Degranulation of Human Neutrophils: Immunocytochemical Studies of Surface and Intracellular Phagocytic Events. Cell, 18:1025, 1979.

Quessenberry, P., et al.: Effect of Endotoxin on Granulopoiesis and Colony Stimulating Factor. New Eng. J. Med., 286:227, 1972.

Quie, P.G.: Clinical Disorders of Phagocyte Locomotion. Agents Actions Suppl., 12:398, 1983.

Raab, S.O., et al.: Granulokinetics in Normal Dogs. Amer. J. Physiol., 206:83, 1964.

Rausch, P.G., and Moore, T.G.: Granule Enzymes of Polymorphonuclear Neutrophils: A Phylogenetic Comparison. Blood, 46:913, 1975.

Rausch, P.G., et al.: Immunocytochemical Identification of Azurophilic and Specific Granule Markers in the Giant Granules of Chédiak-Higashi Neutrophils. New Eng. J. Med., 298:693, 1978.

Rebuck, J.W., and Crowley, J.H.: A Method for Studying Leukocytic Functions in Vivo. Ann. N.Y. Acad. Sci., 59:757, 1955.

Renshaw, H.W., et al.: Leukocyte Dysfunction in the Bovine Homologue of the Chédiak-Higashi Syndrome of Humans. Infect. Immun., 10:928, 1974.

Renshaw, H.W., et al.: Canine Granulocytopathy Syndrome: Defective Bactericidal Capacity of Neutrophils from a Dog with Recurrent Infections. Clin. Immunol. Immunopathol., 8:385, 1977.

Rich, A.R., and McKee, C.M.: A Study of the Character and Degree of Protection Afforded by the Immune State Independently of the Leucocytes. Bull. Johns Hopkins Hosp., 54:277, 1934.

Rickard, K.A., et al.: The in Vitro Colony-Forming Cell and the Response to Neutropenia. Blood, 37:6, 1971.

Rikihisa, Y., and Mizuno, D.: Different Arrangements of Phagolysosomes Membranes Which Depend upon the Particles Phagocytosed: Observations with Markers of the Two Sides of Plasma Membranes. Exp. Cell Res., 111:437, 1978.

Rimoldi, M.T., et al.: Trypanosoma cruzi: Sequence of Phagocytosis and Cytotoxicity by Human Polymorphonuclear Leucocytes. Immunology, 42:521, 1981.

Robinson, W.A., and Mangalik, A.: The Kinetics and Regulation of Granulopoiesis. Semin. Hematol., 12:7, 1975.

Root, R.K., and Cohen, M.S.: The Microbicidal Mechanisms of Human Neutrophils and Eosinophils. Rev. Infect. Dis., 3:565, 1981.

Rosenshein, M.S., et al.: Neutropenia, Inflammation, and the Kinetics of Transfused Neutrophils in Rabbits. J. Clin. Invest., 64:580, 1979.

Roth, J.A., and Kaeberle, M.L.: Isolation of Neutrophils and Eosinophils from the Peripheral Blood of Cattle and Comparison of Their Functional Activities. J. Immunol. Methods, 45:153, 1981.

Roth, J.A., et al.: Effects of Bovine Viral Diarrhea Virus Infection on Bovine Polymorphonuclear Leukocyte Function. Amer. J. Vet. Res., 42:244, 1981.

Rother, K.: Leucocyte Mobilizing Factor: A New Biological Activity Derived from the Third Component of Complement. Eur. J. Immunol., 2:550, 1972.

Rottini, G.D., et al.: Effect of Antibodies and Complement on the Interaction between Escherichia coli O 111:B4 and Polymorphonuclear Leukocytes. Infection, 7:160, 1979.

Rouse, B.T.: Role of Neutrophils in Antiviral Immunity. Adv. Exp. Med. Biol., 137:263, 1981.

Rouse, B.T., et al.: Neutrophils Are Mediators of Antiviral Immunity. Experientia, 34:346, 1978.

Rowley, D.: Phagocytosis. Adv. Immunol., 2:241, 1962.

Rudolph, R. and Schnabl, W.: (Fine Structure of Blood Leucocytes and Electron-Optical Demonstration of Peroxidase and Acid Phosphatase in Sheep Granulocytes). Zentralblat. Vet. Med., 28A:282, 1981.

Rudolph, W.G., and Kaneko, J.J.: Effect of Neutropenia on Colony Stimulating and Inhibiting Activity of Dog Serum. Proc. Soc. Exp. Biol. Med., 163:421, 1980.

Rustin, G.J.S., et al.: Studies on the Subcellular Localization of Human Neutrophil Alkaline Phosphatase. J. Cell Sci., 36:401, 1979.

Rytömaa, T., and Kiviniemi, K.: Control of Granulocyte Production. II. Mode of Action of Chalone and Antichalone. Cell Tissue Kinet., 1:341, 1968.

Rytömaa, T., and Kiviniemi, K.: Regression of Generalized Leukaemia in Rats Induced by the Granulocytic Chalone. Eur. J. Cancer, 6:401, 1970.

Sainte-Marie, G., and Sin, Y.M.: Morphologic Aspects and Kinetics of the Formation of Neutrophils and Eosinophils. In Regulation of Hematopoiesis. Vol. 2. Gordon, A.S., ed. Appleton-Century-Crofts, New York, p. 1109, 1970.

Sbarra, A.J., et al.: Metabolic and Bactericidal Activities of Phagocytizing Leukocytes. In Regulation of Hematopoiesis. Vol. 2. Gordon, A.S., ed. Appleton-Century-Crofts, New York, p. 1081, 1970.

Schalm, O.W.: Mucopolysaccharidosis. Canine Pract., 4(6):28, Dec., 1977.

Schalm, O.W., et al.: Conversion of Chronic Staphylococcal Mastitis to Acute Gangrenous Mastitis after Neutropenia in Blood and Bone Marrow Produced by an Equine Anti-Bovine Leukocyte Serum. Amer. J. Vet. Res., 37:885, 1976.

Schalm, O.W., and Lasmanis, J.: Cytologic Features of Bone Marrow in Normal and Mastitic Cows. Amer. J. Vet. Res., 37:359, 1976.

Schapira, M., et al.: Activation of Human Polymorphonuclear Leukocytes by Purified Human Plasma Kallikrein. Adv. Exp. Med. Biol., 156B:747, 1983.

Schneider, J.A., et al.: Increased Cystine in Leukocytes from Individuals Homozygous and Heterozygous for Cystinosis. Science, 157:1321, 1967.

Schreiber, A.D., et al.: Effect of Corticosteroids on the Human Monocyte IgG and Complement Receptors. J. Clin. Invest., 56:1189, 1975.

Segal, A.W., et al.: Kinetics of Fusion of the Cytoplasmic Granules with Phagocytic Vacuoles in Human Polymorphonuclear Leukocytes. J. Cell Biol., 85:42, 1980.

Segal, A.W., et al.: The Respiratory Burst of Phagocytic Cells Is Associated with a Rise in Vacuolar pH. Nature, 290:406, 1981.

Shannon, W.A., Jr., and Zellmer, D.M.: Heterogeneity in Polymorphonuclear Leukocyte Neutrophil Granules. Histochem. J.,14:847, 1982.

Shigeoka, A.O., et al.: Functional Analysis of Neutrophil Granulocytes from Healthy, Infected and Stressed Neonates. J. Pediatr., 95:454, 1979.

Shively, J.N., et al.: Fine Structure of Formed Elements in Canine Blood. Amer. J. Vet. Res., 30:893, 1969.

Shull, R.M., and Powell, D.: Acquired Hyposegmentation of Granulocyte (Pseudo-Pelger-Huët Anomaly) in a Dog. Cornell Vet., 69:241, 1979.

Skarnes, R.C., and Watson, D.W.: Characterization of Leukin: An Antibacterial Factor from Leucocytes Active against Gram-Positive Pathogens. J. Exp. Med., 104:829, 1956.

Smith, G.S., and Lumsden, J.H.: Review of Neutrophil Adherence, Chemotaxis, Phagocytosis and Killing. Vet. Immunol. Immunopathol., 4:177, 1983.

Smith, G.S., et al.: Chemotaxis of Porcine Neutrophil Under Agarose. Canad. J. Comp. Med., 49:43, 1985.

Smolen, J.E., and Weissmann, G.: Stimuli Which Provoke Secretion of Azurophil Enzymes from Human Neutrophils Induce Increments in Adenosine Cyclic 3', 5'-Monophosphate. Biochem. Biophys. Acta, 672:197, 1981.

Snyderman, R.: Regulation of Leukocyte Function. Plenum Press, N.Y., 1984.

Snyderman, R., and Pike, M.C.: N-formylmethionyl Peptide Receptors on Equine Leukocytes Initiate Secretion but Not Chemotaxis. Science, 209:493, 1980.

Sobel, J.D., and Gallin, J.I.: Polymorphonuclear Leukocyte and Monocyte Chemoattractants Produced by Human Fibroblasts. J. Clin. Invest., 63:609, 1979.

Sonoda, M., and Kobayashi, K.: Electron Microscopic Observations on the Blood of the Horse. I. Neutrophils in the Peripheral Blood of the Clinically Healthy Horse. Jap. J. Vet. Res., 14:71, 1966.

Sonoda, M., and Kobayashi, K.: Neutrophils of Canine Peripheral Blood in Electron Microscopy. Jap. J. Vet. Res., 18:37, 1970a.

Sonoda, M., and Kobayashi, K.: Feline Neutrophils in Electron Microscopy. Jap. J. Vet. Res., 18:63, 1970b.

Spagnuole, P.J., et al.: Thromboxane A2 Mediates Aug-

mented Polymorphonuclear Leukocyte Adhesiveness. J. Clin. Invest., 66:406, 1980.

Spector, W.G., and Willoughby, D.A.: The Effect of Vascular Permeability Factors on the Emigration of Leucocytes. J. Path. Bact., 87:341, 1964.

Spector, W.G., and Willoughby, D.A.: Mechanisms of Leukocyte Emigration in Inflammation. In Regulation of Hematopoiesis. Vol. 2. Gordon, A.S., ed. Appleton-Century-Crofts, New York, p. 959, 1970.

Spicer, S.S., and Hardin, J.H.: Ultrastructure, Cytochemistry, and Function of Neutrophil, Leucocyte Granules: A Review. J. Lab. Invest., 20(5):488, 1969.

Spitznagel, J.K.: Bactericidal Mechanisms of the Granulocyte. Prog. Clin. Biol. Res., 13:103, 1977.

Spitznagel, J.K., et al.: Character of Azurophil and Specific Granules Purified from Human Polymorphonuclear Leukocytes. Lab. Invest., 30:774, 1974.

Stabinsky, Y., et al.: Specific Binding Sites for the Phagocytosis Stimulating Peptide Tuftsin on Human Polymorphonuclear Leukocytes and Monocytes. Biochem. Biophys. Res. Commun., 83:599, 1978.

Stanley, E.R., and Metcalf, D.: Partial Purification and Some Properties of the Factor in Normal and Leukaemic Human Urine Stimulating Mouse Bone Marrow Colony Growth in Vitro. Aust. J. Exp. Biol. Med. Sci., 47:467, 1969.

Starkebaum, G., and Arend, W.P.: Neutrophil-Binding Immunoglobulin G in Systemic Lupus Erythematosus. J. Clin. Invest, 64:902, 1979.

Steinberg, H.N., and Handler, E.S.: Leukemic Host Influence on Normal Erythrocytic and Granulocytic Colony Formation in Vivo Plasma Clot Diffusion Chamber Cultures. Cancer Res., 39:1575, 1979.

Stickle, J.E., et al.: Neutrophil Function in the Dog: Shape Changes and Response to a Synthetic Tripeptide. Amer. J. Vet. Res., 46:225, 1985.

Suter, E., and Ramseier, H.: Cellular Reactions in Infection. Adv. Immunol., 4:117, 1964.

Szmitkowski, M., et al.: Granulopoietic Activity (GA) and Colony Stimulating Factor (CSF) in Myeloproliferative Diseases. Folia Haematol., 107:204, 1980.

Taichman, N.S., et al.: Inflammation and Tissue Injury. I. The Response to Intradermal Injections of Human Dentogingival Plaque in Normal and Leukopenic Rabbits. Arch. Oral Biol., 11:1385, 1966.

Takamori, K., and Yamashita, T.: Biochemical Properties of Polymorphonuclear Neutrophils from Venous Blood and Peritoneal Exudates of Rabbits. Infect. Immun., 29:395, 1980.

Tauber, A.I.: Current Views of Neutrophil Dysfunction. Amer. J. Med., 70:1237, 1981.

Thakur, M.L., et al.: Preparation and Evaluation of 111In-Labeled Leukocytes as an Abscess Imaging Agent in Dogs. Radiology, 119:731, 1976.

Thomas, E.D., et al.: Leukocyte Kinetics in the Dog Studied by Cross Circulation. J. Lab. Clin. Med., 67:64, 1965.

Thompson, J.M., et al.: An Ultrastructural Study of the Invasion of Ascaris suum Larvae by Neutrophils. J. Invertebr. Pathol., 30:181, 1977.

Thong, Y.H., and Rencis, V.: Bilirubin Inhibits Hexose-Monophosphate Shunt Activity of Phagocytosing Neutrophils. Acta Paediatr. Scand., 66:757, 1977.

Till, G., et al.: Chemokinetic and Chemotactic Activity of Various Prostaglandins for Neutrophil Granulocytes. Clin. Immunol. Immunopathol., 12:111, 1979.

Tonnesen, M.G., et al.: The Microvasculature in Inflammation: Interaction between Neutrophils and Vascular Endothelial Cells. Agents Actions Suppl., *11*:25, 1982.

Townsend, J., et al.: An Ultrastructural Study of the Interaction in Vitro between Trypanosoma theileri and Bovine Leukocytes. J. Cell Sci., *56*:389, 1982.

Uriuhara, T., and Movat, H.Z.: Role of PMN-Leukocyte Lysosomes in Tissue Injury, Inflammation and Hypersensitivity. V. Partial Suppression in Leukopenic Rabbits of Vascular Hyperpermeability Due to Thermal Injury. Proc. Soc. Exp. Biol. Med., *124*:279, 1967.

Valerius, N.H.: In Vitro Effect of R 17934, a New Drug with Antitubulin Activity, on Neutrophil Granulocyte Locomotion and Orientation. Acta Pathol. Microbiol. Scand. Sect. C Immunol., *87*:83, 1979.

Valli, V.E.O., et al.: Leukapheresis in Calves and Dogs by Extracorporeal Circulation of Blood through Siliconized Glass Wool. Res. Vet. Sci., *10*:267, 1969.

Valli, V.E.O., et al.: The Kinetics of Haematopoiesis in the Calf. I. An Autoradiographical Study of Myelopoiesis in Normal, Anemic, and Endotoxin Treated Calves. Res. Vet. Sci., *12*:535, 1971.

van Furth, R., and Willemze, R.: Phagocytic Cells during an Acute Inflammatory Reaction. Curr. Top. Pathol., *68*:179, 1979.

Vegad, J.L.: The Acute Inflammatory Response in the Sheep. Vet. Bull., *49*:555, 1979.

Verhoef, J., et al.: Human Polymorphonuclear Leucocyte Receptors for Staphylococcal Opsonins. Immunology, *33*:231, 1977.

Vincent, P.C.: Granulocyte Kinetics in Health and Disease. Clin. Haematol., *6*:695, 1977a.

Vincent, P.C.: The Measurement of Granulocyte Kinetics. Brit. J. Haematol., *36*:1, 1977b.

Vincent, P.C., et al.: The Intravascular Survival of Neutrophils Labeled in Vivo. Blood, *43*:371, 1974.

Vogler, W.R., and Winton, E.G.: Humoral Granulopoietic Inhibitors: A Review. Exp. Hematol., *3*:337, 1975.

Wakeyama, H., et al.: Superoxide-forming NADPH Oxidase Preparation of Pig Polymorphonuclear Leucocytes. Biochem. J., *205*:593, 1982.

Walker, R.I., and Willemze, R.: Neutrophil Kinetics and the Regulation of Granulopoiesis. Rev. Infect. Dis., *2*:282, 1980.

Walsh, C.E., et al.: Release and Metabolism of Arachidonic Acid in Human Neutrophils. J. Biol. Chem., *256*:7228, 1981.

Ward, J.W., et al.: Ultrastructure of Granulocytes in the Peripheral Blood of the Cat. J. Ultrastruct. Res., *39*:389, 1972.

Ward, P.A., and Becker, E.L.: Mechanisms of the Inhibition of Chemotaxis by Phosphonate Esters. J. Exp. Med., *125*:1001, 1967.

Ward, P.A., and Becker, E.L.: The Deactivation of Rabbit Neutrophils by Chemotactic Factor and the Nature of the Activable Esterase. J. Exp. Med., *127*:693, 1968.

Wardle, E.N., and Williams, R.: Polymorphonuclear Leucocyte Function in Uraemia and Jaundice. Acta Haematol., *64*:157, 1980.

Wasi, S., et al.: The Role of PMN-Leukocyte Lysosomes in Tissue Injury, Inflammation and Hypersensitivity. II. Studies on the Proteolytic Activity of PMN-Leukocyte Lysosomes of the Rabbit. Brit. J. Exp. Pathol., *47*:411, 1966.

Watt, K.W.K., et al.: Isolation of Two Polypeptides Comprising the Neutrophil-Immobilizing Factor of Human Leucocytes. Immunology, *48*:79, 1983.

Weber, L., et al.: The Chemiluminescent Response of Bovine Polymorphonuclear Leucocytes Isolated from Milk and Blood. Vet. Immunol. Immunopathol., *4*:397, 1983.

Weisdorf, D.J., et al.: Glycogenolysis versus Glucose Transport in Human Granulocytes: Differential Activation in Phagocytosis and Chemotaxis. Blood, *60*:888, 1982a.

Weisdorf, D.J., et al.: Granulocytes Utilize Different Energy Sources for Movement and Phagocytosis. Inflammation, *6*:245, 1982b.

Weiss, J., et al.: Resistance of Gram-Negative Bacteria to Purified Bactericidal Leukocyte Proteins. J. Clin. Invest., *65*:619, 1980.

Weiss, L.: Transmural Cellular Passage in Vascular Sinuses of Rat Bone Marrow. Blood, *36*:189, 1970.

Weiss, L.: The Hematopoietic Microenvironment of the Bone Marrow: An Ultrastructural Study of the Stroma in Rats. Anat. Rec., *186*:161, 1976.

Weiss, S.J.: The Role of Superoxide in the Destruction of Erythrocyte Targets by Human Neutrophils. J. Biol. Chem., *225*:9912, 1980.

Weissmann, G., et al.: The Secretory Code of the Neutrophil. J. Reticuloendothel. Soc., *26*:687, 1979.

Weissmann, G., et al.: Release of Inflammatory Mediators from Stimulated Neutrophils. New Eng. J. Med., *303*:27, 1980.

Weston, W.L.: Disorders of Phagocyte Function. Arch. Dermatol., *112*:1589, 1976.

Wetzel, B.K., et al.: Fine Structural Studies on the Development of Heterophil, Eosinophil, and Basophil Granulocytes in Rabbit. Lab. Invest., *16*:349, 1967.

Wetzel, B.K.: The Fine Structure and Cytochemistry of Developing Granulocytes with Special Reference to the Rabbit. In Regulation of Hematopoiesis. Vol. 2. Gordon, A.S., ed. Appleton-Century-Crofts, New York, p. 769, 1970a.

Wetzel, B.K.: The Comparative Fine Structure of Normal and Diseased Mammalian Granulocytes. In Regulation of Hematopoiesis. Vol. 2. Gordon, A.S., ed. Appleton-Century-Crofts, New York, p. 819, 1970b.

Wilhelm, D.L.: The Mediation of Increased Vascular Permeability in Inflammation. Pharmacol. Rev., *14*:251, 1962.

Wilkinson, P.C.: Physiology of Granulocyte Locomotion and Its Relation to Defects of Chemotaxis: A Review. Jour. Royal Soc. Med., *72*:606, 1977.

Wilkinson, P.C.: Leukocyte Locomotion and Chemotaxis: Effect of Bacteria and Viruses. Rev. Infect. Dis., *2*:293, 1980.

Wilkinson, P.C.: Chemotaxis and Inflammation. 2nd ed. Churchill Livingstone, London, 1982.

Williams, M.R., and Bunch, K.J.: Variation among Cows in the Ability of Their Blood Polymorphonuclear Leucocytes to Kill Escherichia coli and Staphylococcus aureus. Res. Vet. Sci., *30*:298, 1981.

Williams, M.R., and Hill, A.W.: A Role for IgM in the in Vitro Opsonisation of Staphylococcus aureus and Escherichia coli by Bovine Polymorphonuclear Leucocytes. Res. Vet. Sci., *33*:47, 1982.

Willoughby, D.A.: Mediators of the Inflammatory Response and Their Modification by Therapeutic Agents. Brit. Roy. Soc. Med., *60*:775, 1967.

Wilson, A.T., et al.: Fate of Non-Virulent Streptococci Phagocytized by Human and Mouse Neutrophils. J. Exp. Med., *106*:777, 1957.

Wilson, P.D., et al.: The Ultrastructural Localization of Human Neutrophil Alkaline Phosphatase in Normal Individuals during Pregnancy and in Patients with Chronic Granulocytic Leukaemia. Histochem. J., *13*:31, 1981.

Wintrobe, M.M., et al.: Clinical Hematology. 8th ed. Lea & Febiger, Philadelphia, 1981.

Wolach, B., et al.: Review: Clinical and Laboratory Approach to the Management of Neutrophil Dysfunction. Israel J. Med. Sci., 18:897, 1982.

Yamada, Y.: The Leukocytes of Ovine Peripheral Blood in Electron Microscopy. Jap. J. Vet. Res., 18(2):99, 1970.

Yamada, Y., and Sonoda, M.: Neutrophils of Ovine Peripheral Blood in Electron Microscopy. Jap. J. Vet. Res., 18(2):83, 1970.

Youinou, P.Y., et al.: Folic Acid Deficiency and Neutrophil Dysfunction. Amer. J. Med., 73:652, 1982.

Yurewucz, E., and Zimmerman, M.: Cytochalasin B–Dependent Release of Azurophil Granules Enzymes from Human Polymorphonuclear Leukocytes. Inflammation, 2:259, 1977.

Zakhireh, B., et al.: Neutrophil Function and Host Resistance. Infection, 7:88, 1979.

Zeya, H.I., and Spitznagel, J.K.: Antimicrobial Specificity of Leukocyte Lysosomal Cationic Proteins. Science, 154:1049, 1966.

Zigmond, S.H., and Hirsch, J.G.: Leukocyte Locomotion and Chemotaxis: New Methods for Evaluation and Demonstration of a Cell-Derived Chemotactic Factor. J. Exp. Med., 137:387, 1973.

Zinkl, J.G., and Brown, P.D.: Chemotaxis of Horse Polymorphonuclear Leukocytes to N-formyl-L-methionyl-L-leucyl-L-phenylalanine. Amer. J. Vet. Res., 43:613, 1982.

Ziv, G., et al.: Influence of Antibiotics and Intramammary Antibiotic Products on Phagocytosis of Staphylococcus aureus by Bovine Leukocytes. Amer. J. Vet. Res., 44:385, 1983.

Zucker-Franklin, D.: Electron Microscopic Studies of Human Granulocytes: Structural Variations Related to Function. Semin. Hematol., 5:109, 1968.

Zucker-Franklin, D., et al.: Atlas of Blood Cells: Function and Pathology. E.E. edi ermes Milano; Lea & Febiger, Philadelphia, 1981.

Zuelzer, W.W.: "Myelokathexis": A New Form of Chronic Granulocytopenia. New Eng. J. Med., 270:699, 1964.

27

The Eosinophils

MORPHOLOGY 731

BIOCHEMICAL COMPOSITION 737

METABOLISM 739

PRODUCTION AND RELEASE 739

SURFACE RECEPTORS AND
    CHEMOTAXIS 741

TISSUE DISTRIBUTION 742

FUNCTIONS 743
    Phagocytosis and Bactericidal Effect 743
    Parasiticidal Effect 743
    Regulation of Allergic and Inflammatory
      Reactions 746

Tissue Destruction 746
Other Functions 747

EOSINOPHILIAS 747
    Eosinophilia and Parasitism 748
    Pulmonary Infiltrates with Eosinophilia 749
    Hypereosinophilic Syndrome 749
    Eosinophilia and Estrus 750

EOSINOPENIAS 750
    Stress, Corticosteroids, and
      Eosinopenia 750
    Eosinopenia of Acute Infection and
      Inflammation 751

The last decade has witnessed extensive research on eosinophils to elucidate mechanisms of eosinophilia commonly associated with parasitic and allergic diseases, controls of eosinophil production, and eosinophil functions. This research has revealed a unifying concept of the genesis of eosinophilia seen in diverse diseases, a hormonal and T-lymphocyte-mediated control of eosinophil production, and an important role of eosinophils in controlling infection with helminthic parasites. Specific mechanisms, however, need to be further defined.

Eosinophil structure and composition have also been studied in detail. Most investigations have involved laboratory animals, but studies on humans are taking new dimensions as well. These findings may provide some basis for interpretation of abnormalities of the eosinophil leukocyte associated with various diseases in animal patients. The interested reader will find details on these topics in a monograph (Beeson and Bass, 1977), two books (Archer, 1963; Mahmoud and Austen, 1981), and numerous reviews (G.T. Archer, 1968; R.K. Archer, 1968; Bass, 1979; Bass and Szejda, 1979; Beeson, 1976; Butter-

field et al., 1983/84; Butterworth, 1977; Clark and Kaplan, 1975; Cline, 1975; Gleich, 1977; Kay, 1976, 1979; Mahmoud, 1977; Olsson and Venge, 1979; Sullivan, 1979; Valone, 1980; van Dallen, 1981; Weller and Goetzl, 1980; Zucker-Franklin et al., 1981).

MORPHOLOGY (Figs. 27–1 through 27–5)

Eosinophils characteristically have bright pinkish red, uniformly stained cytoplasmic granules and a polymorphic nucleus that is smoother and less segmented than that in mature neutrophils. The granules loosely pack the cell, and their size and shape vary among different animal species and sometimes within the same species. For example, granules in equine eosinophils are the largest among common domestic animals, and feline eosinophil granules are usually rod-shaped (Plates VII–6, VII–7). Canine eosinophils often display a few partially vacuolated granules (Plate XII–I); those of the greyhound particularly exhibit cytoplasmic vacuolation. A marked heterogeneity of eosinophil granules is seen in an occasional dog; a few granules

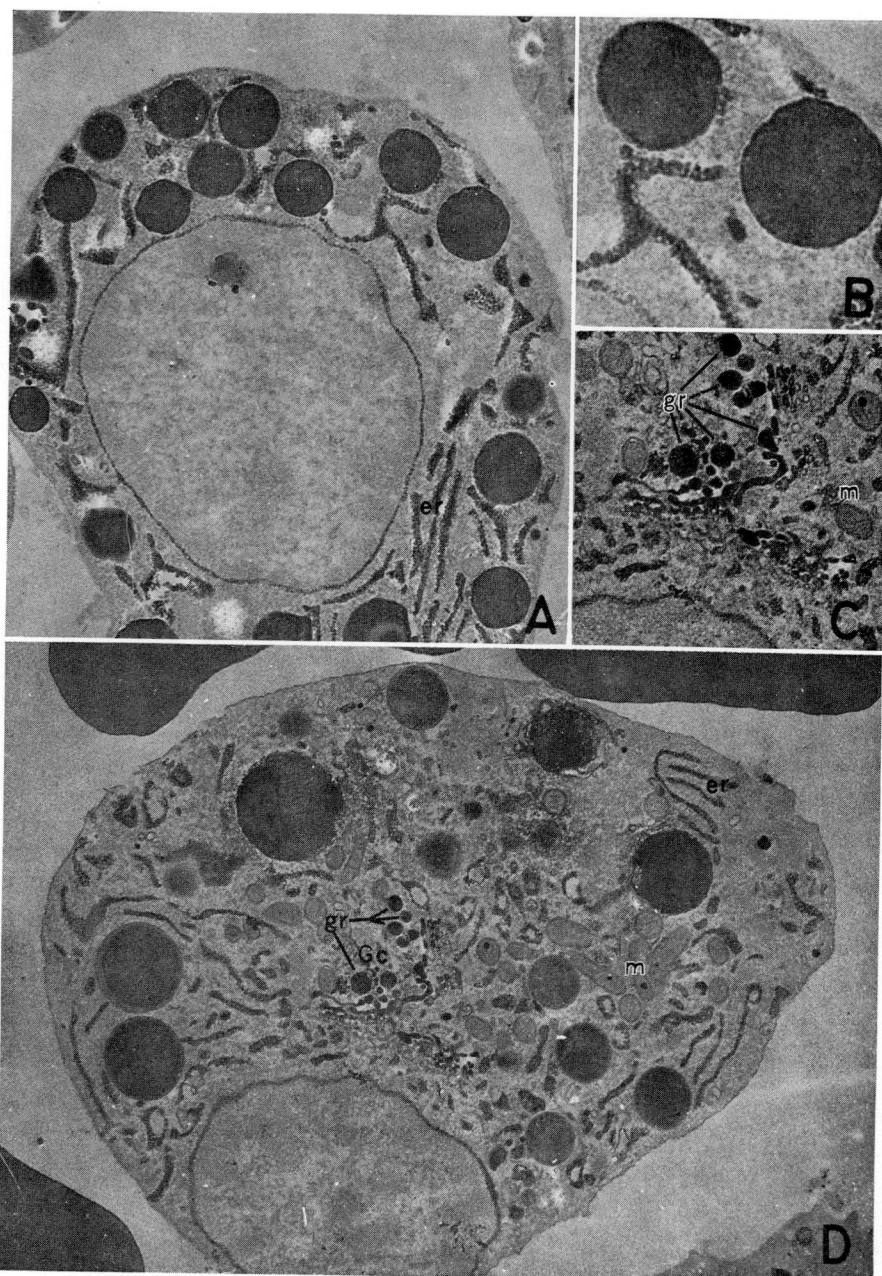

Fig. 27–1. Eosinophilic progranulocytes from canine bone marrow stained for peroxidase. An early progranulocyte *(A)* is characterized by the presence of many dense, homogeneous granules, while an intermediate or late progranulocyte *(D)* contains many condensing granules of varying morphology. *B* is an enlarged area of *A,* and *C* is an enlargement of the Golgi complex area of the cell in *D.* The Golgi complex *(C,D)* at this stage is very active in producing granules *(gr).* The cytoplasm at this stage contains elaborate cisternae of rough endoplasmic reticulum *(er)* and numerous mitochondria *(m).* In contrast to neutrophil progranulocytes, eosinophilic progranulocytes exhibit peroxidase activity in the rough endoplasmic reticulum, the Golgi complex, and along the outer nuclear membrane. *A,* ×10,080; *B,* ×18,900; *C,* ×14,280; *D,* ×10,080.

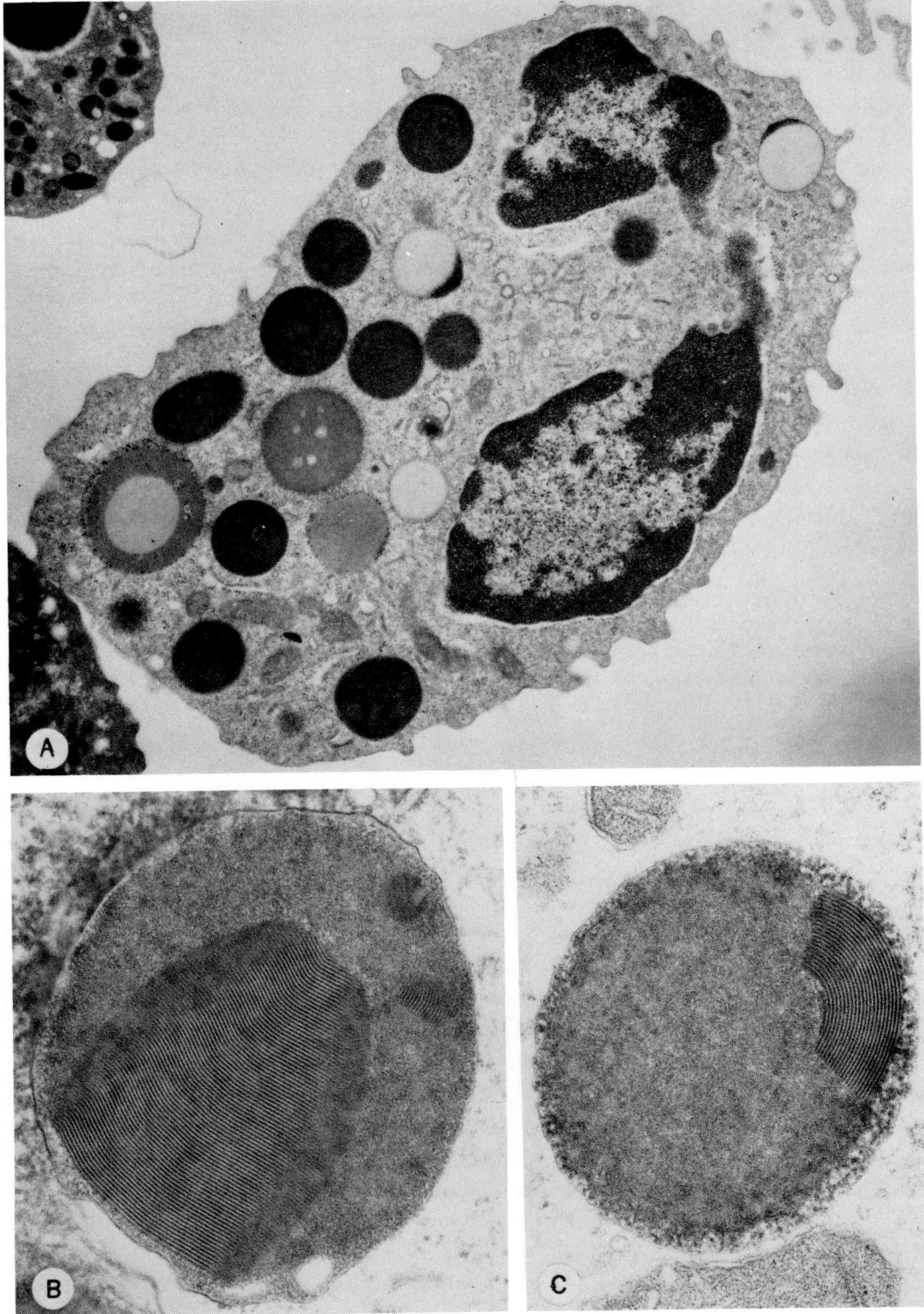

Fig. 27–2. *A,* A canine eosinophil containing granules of various morphologic types—dense homogeneous, dense amorphous mass surrounded by a narrow rim of somewhat light matrix, and clear vesicles with a cap and/or rim of dense material. A few mitochondria are present in the lower portion of the cell, a few remnants of rough endoplasmic reticulum are scattered throughout the cell, and some "microgranules" are visible in the cytoplasmic area between the nuclear lobes. ×32,000. *B* and *C,* Clearly defined "fingerprints" of portions of the crystalloid of two eosinophil granules. ×62,500

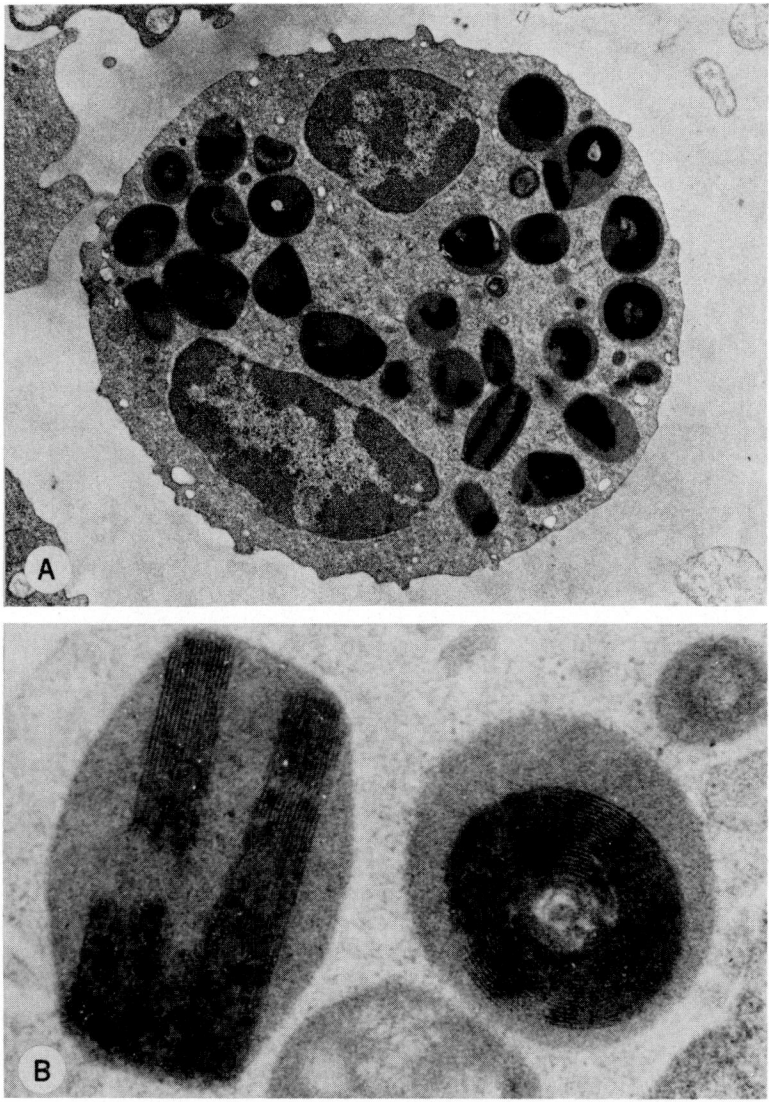

Fig. 27–3. *A,* A feline eosinophil with characteristic crystalloid granules and some "microgranules." ×11,200. *B,* Periodicity of lamellae in the crystalloid region of the granule is clearly visible at higher magnification. ×50,000.

may be as big as the red cell (Plate XII–2). A rare eosinophil may contain a few small, dark purplish-black granules, probably as a result of deranged eosinophil development under some toxic influence. Such azurophilic granules may also be found in an infrequent eosinophilic promyelocyte in the bone marrow (Plate XII–3).

Morphologic abnormalities in eosinophils have been observed in some hereditary and acquired disorders. For example, retarded nuclear segmentation is seen in eosinophils of humans (Kay et al., 1973) and dogs with Pel-

ger-Huët anomaly (see Fig. 4–8). Hypogranulation, vacuolation, and abnormally large granules have been observed in some human patients with hypereosinophilic syndrome and eosinophilia from other causes (Gleich, 1977; Olsen et al., 1980; Sullivan, 1979; Tai and Spry, 1981).

The surface topography of eosinophils, as observed with the scanning electron microscope, consists of sparse microvilli and some ridges, ruffles, and surface blebs. Granule contours are visible in cells with a partially collapsed surface membrane (Fig. 27–4A),

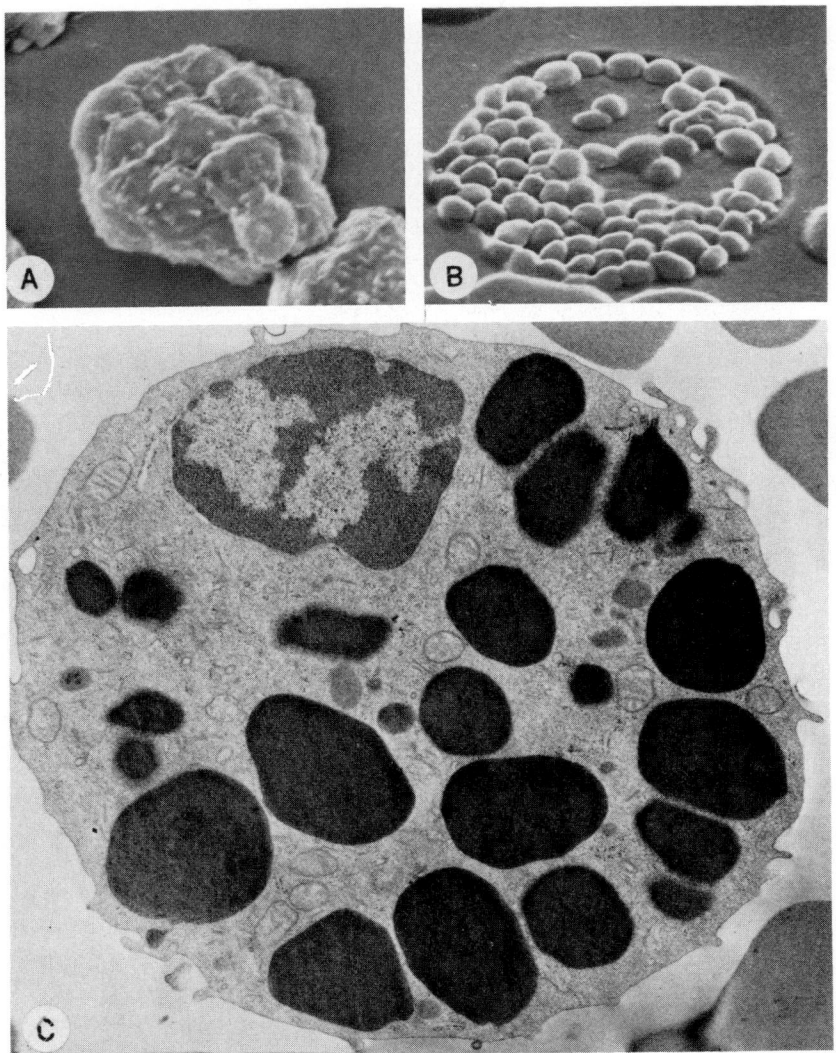

Fig. 27–4. Equine eosinophils. *A,* A scanning electron photomicrograph of a globular cell depicting some microvilli and granule contours. ×4,400. *B,* A scanning electron photomicrograph showing distinctly dispersed granules in a cell flattened from smear making. The nucleus (region devoid of granules) and cell membrane have collapsed. ×3,000. *C,* A transmission electron photomicrograph depicting characteristic large-round, homogeneous granules. Some mitochondria and rare profiles of rough endoplasmic reticulum are also present in the cytoplasm. A few microvillus-like projections are present on the cell surface. ×10,000.

and distinct granules are visible only in flattened eosinophils (Fig. 27–4*B*). Granules of unstained human eosinophils have been found to exhibit an unusual bright autofluorescence characteristic of the cell (Weil and Chused, 1981).

The ultrastructure of eosinophils and granule genesis have been described in various species (Ackerman, 1964; Atwal, 1976; Anteunis et al., 1977; Bainton and Farquhar, 1970; Cline, 1975; Fabiani et al., 1980; Maxwell, 1978; Nafstad and Nafstad, 1968; Presentey et

al., 1980). Two types of granules, homogeneous and crystalloid (0.60–1.0 μm), characterize these cells. A third type of small (0.1–0.5 μm) modestly homogeneous, round to elongated granule was found in some human eosinophils, particularly in hypereosinophilic patients (Parmley and Spicer, 1974). Mature eosinophils of 20 mammalian species including the dog, cat, and horse were found to contain pleomorphic "specific microgranules" about 0.02–0.2 μm in size (Schaefer et al., 1973). These resemble profiles

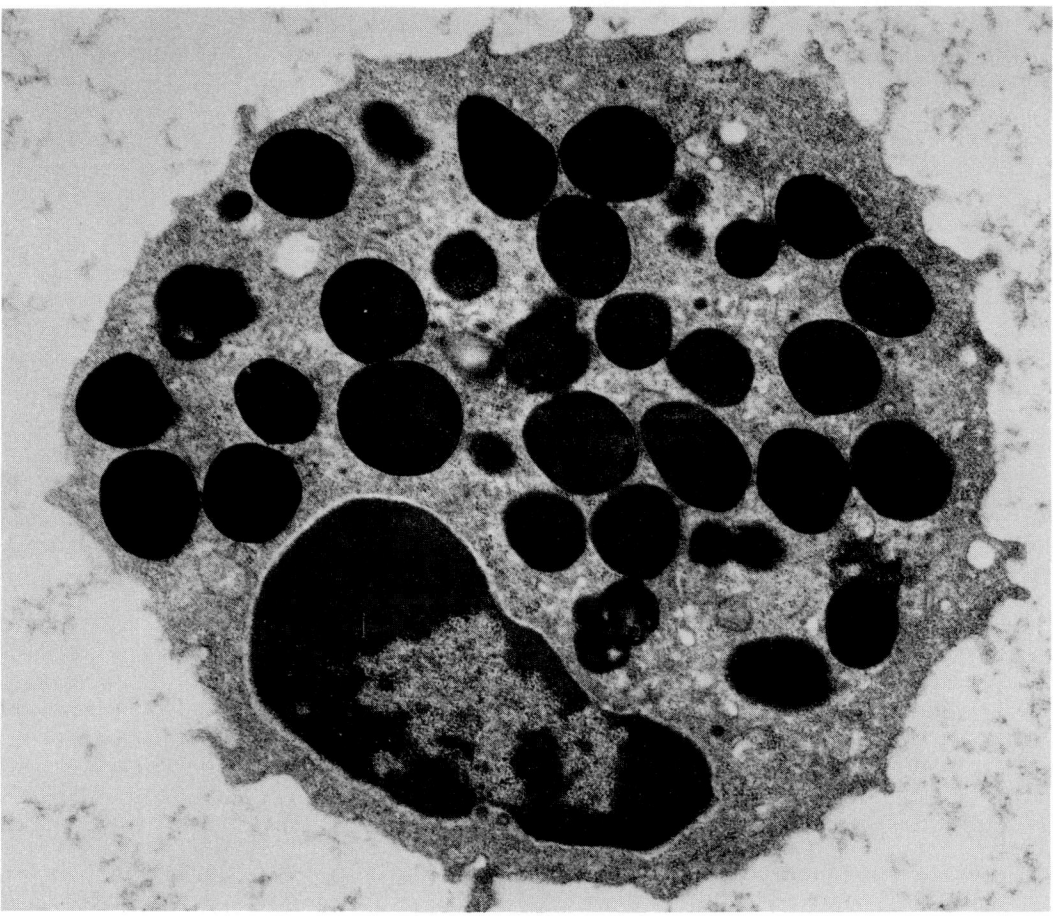

Fig. 27–5.   A bovine eosinophil with homogeneous, round granules of variable sizes. ×13,500.

of smooth endoplasmic reticulum and are more numerous in cells from patients with eosinophilias (Zucker-Franklin et al., 1981). We have also observed such structures in canine and feline eosinophils (Figs. 27–2, 27–3). Cytoplasmic organelles such as the Golgi complex, mitochondria, ribosomes, and rough endoplasmic reticulum (RER) are more prominent in mature eosinophils than in mature neutrophils (Clark and Kaplan, 1975; Sullivan, 1979).

The earliest morphologically identifiable precursor cell of the series (eosinophilic promyelocyte) contains large, spherical, electron-dense, homogeneous granules (Fig. 27–1A, B). These granules are formed by fusion and condensation of small saccules, vacuoles, or granular bodies elaborated by the Golgi complex (Fig. 27–1C, D). Their electron-dense, proteinaceous material is synthesized on po-

lyribosomes bound to the RER and is transported to the Golgi complex for packaging into granules (Bainton and Farquhar, 1970).

These granules exhibit azurophilic staining that disappears by the myelocyte stage (compare Plates V–5 and XII–3). It is believed that as the eosinophils mature, these homogeneous (primary) granules transform into the crystalloid (secondary) granules characteristic of mature eosinophils in most species, since transitional forms between the two granules can be seen in developing cells. Crystalloid granules are usually absent or rare at the promyelocyte stage (compare Figs. 27–1A and D with 27–2), become prominent at the myelocyte stage, and predominate at later stages in those animal species exhibiting such granules. This development of the secondary granules in eosinophils contrasts with that in neutrophils, in which primary and secondary granules are produced independently by the Golgi complex at the promyelocyte and myelocyte stage, respectively. The granule structure of pig eosinophils seems to be reversed in that homogeneous granules were seen in mature eosinophils, while granules with a specific internal structure were found in immature eosinophils (Nafstad and Nafstad, 1968).

The typical crystalloid granule in most species has an electron-dense core surrounded by a less electron-dense homogeneous matrix. The core shows longitudinal and cross-sectional periodicity (Gleich, 1977) and is resistant to dissolution by mechanical, osmotic, and certain enzymatic treatment. The appearance and density of the crystalloid granule vary with the species and the fixative used for electron microscopy (Zucker-Franklin, 1968). The size and shape of the granule are dependent on the size and rigidity of the crystalline core (Zucker-Franklin et al., 1981). Crystalloid granules are seen in the dog (Fig. 27–2), cat (Fig. 27–3), goat, guinea pig, mouse, rat, rhesus monkey, and human, while homogeneous granules are seen in the horse (Fig. 27–4), cow (Fig. 27–5), mink, and gorilla. Canine eosinophils (Fig. 27–2) often display a variety of granule morphology not encountered in other species, and only about 10% of the granules have distinct, lamellar, crystalloid cores surrounded by a thin rim of dense matrix (Hung, 1972). Almost all granules in mature feline eosinophils have electron-dense, tubular cores comprised of fibrillar periodicity resembling myelin figures and varying in location and shape (Fig. 27–3).

BIOCHEMICAL COMPOSITION

The eosinophil granules contain several cationic proteins and many lysosomal enzymes. Compared to neutrophils, human eosinophils have considerably higher peroxidase, β-glucuronidase, phospholipase, and arylsulfatase activities and lower hexokinase and alkaline phosphatase activities (Cline, 1965; Mahmoud and Austen, 1981). The small, homogeneous granules in human eosinophils react for acid phosphatase and arylsulfatase (Parmley and Spicer, 1974). Bovine and equine eosinophils stain for alkaline phosphatase as in-

tensely as neutrophils, while canine and feline eosinophils reveal a modest staining in contrast to the negative reaction of canine and feline neutrophils (Plate X–2). Rabbit eosinophils lack this enzyme activity.

A high content of zinc is present in the granule matrix in human, bovine, and murine eosinophils (Beeson and Bass, 1977, Cline, 1975). Plasminogen, activators of plasminogen and Hageman factor, kinin-producing activities and kininase, and thromboplastic activity have been described in eosinophils (Cline, 1975; Riddle and Barnhart, 1965). Eosinophils lack three important bactericidal substances found in neutrophils, namely lysozyme, lactoferrin, and phagocytin, and they also lack neutral proteases (Archer and Hirsch, 1963; Olsson and Venge, 1979). Morphologic, cytochemical, and electron microscopic studies of eosinophilic leukemia in humans have been published (Ackerman, 1964; Presentey at al., 1979).

Ultrastructural cytochemical studies have shown that eosinophilic promyelocytes reveal positive staining for peroxidase, acid phosphatase, and arylsulfatase in the RER, Golgi complex, and homogeneous granules, but only peroxidase activity is prominent in crystalloid granules of mature eosinophils (Bainton and Farquhar, 1970). Peroxidase (Bainton and Farquhar, 1970) and acid phosphatase (Seeman and Palade, 1967) are present in the matrix of the crystalloid granules, while phosphorylase, nonspecific esterase (naphthol AS-acetate substrate), and mucopolysaccharides are localized in the cytoplasm. Alkaline phosphatase is present in the plasma membrane and in intracytoplasmic locations other than the granules (Williams, et al., 1979).

The peroxidase in eosinophils differs from that in neutrophils with regard to spectral characteristics, antigenicity, genetic occurrence, and susceptibility to various inhibitors (Clark and Kaplan, 1975; Olsson and Venge, 1979; Wever et al., 1980). Recently it has been shown to have some antibacterial (DeChatelet et al., 1978; Jong et al., 1980; Migler et al., 1978), antiparasitic (Jong et al., 1979), and cytotoxic activities (Cline, 1975; Jong and Klebanoff, 1980). Eosinophil peroxidase is antibacterial when it forms a complex with H_2O_2 and iodide, chloride, or bromide as a halide, but the complex with iodide is particularly bactericidal (Jong et al., 1980). Such complexes can also degranulate mast cells releasing histamine (Henderson et al., 1980).

A hereditary (autosomal recessive) absence of peroxidase and phospholipid has been described in eosinophils of humans (Presentey, 1969); these eosinophils also have hypersegmented nuclei and sparse granules. Peroxidase is normally absent from eosinophils of the cat (Jain, 1967; Presentey et al., 1980).

The characteristic stainability of eosinophil granules is due to their highly basic (cationic) proteins (reviewed by Gleich, 1977, and Olsson and Venge, 1979). At least four such proteins are recognized in guinea pig eosinophils; the predominant one is referred to as the "major basic protein" (MBP). An analogous protein is found in human, bovine, and rat eosinophils. The predominant basic protein in human eosinophils is designated "eosinophilic cationic protein" (ECP).

The cationic proteins are located predominantly in the granule core, but some are also found in the granule matrix (Pimenta et al., 1980). The amount of MBP in eosinophils and its composition and molecular weight vary among species. The content of guinea pig MBP is about 3.5 μg/10^6 eosinophils and constitutes about 50% of the total granule protein. It is rich in arginine, has an isoelectric point of 10, and has at least two reactive sulfhydryl groups. Its molecular weight is 11,800, compared to 21,000 for human ECP and 16,000 for bovine MBP (Duffus et al., 1980).

The MBP differs from the Charcot-Leyden crystal protein of eosinophils (Gleich, 1977). Charcot-Leyden crystals are found in human tissues in various diseases associated with tissue eosinophilia, e.g., myeloid leukemia, asthma, allergy, and parasitic infections (Ackerman et al., 1981). The origin of Charcot-Leyden crystals from human basophils has also been described (Ackerman et al, 1982).

The eosinophilic MBP, unlike neutrophil cationic proteins, possesses a weak bactericidal activity and does not increase vascular permeability. It has little or no antihistaminic activity (Clark and Kaplan, 1975). However, it is highly cytotoxic in that it can damage larvae of *Schistosoma mansoni* and *Trichinella*

spiralis and various mammalian tissue cells including tracheal epithelium (Wassom et al, 1981). Bovine MBP was found to damage juvenile *Fasciola hepatica* (Duffus et al., 1980). In addition, human ECP has several dose- and time-dependent effects on the coagulation system and humoral mediators of inflammation (Mahmoud and Austen, 1981; Olsson and Venge, 1979); these include activation of factors XII and XI, generation of kallikrien and kinin, and activation of plasminogen. The MBP also neutralizes heparin (Olsson and Venge, 1979). An inhibitory effect on coagulation is also observed through interference with fibrinogen polymerization.

The ECP is released in serum and other body fluids such as saliva, where its concentration can be measured by a sensitive radioimmunoassay (Dahl and Venge, 1978; Frigas et al., 1981; Wassom et al., 1981). In persons with eosinophil numbers greater than 350/μl of blood, serum ECP levels correspond to blood eosinophil counts (Wassom et al., 1981). Increased levels are found in sputum of asthmatic patients (Frigas et al., 1981), although their serum levels may be low (Dahl and Venge, 1978). Many patients with skin diseases and normal eosinophil numbers may also have elevated serum ECP levels (Wassom et al., 1981). Such levels in serum and sputum may be in the range considered cytotoxic (Gleich et al., 1979a). The concentration of ECP may increase in serum in acute inflammation or acute infection despite a decrease in eosinophil numbers in blood. This increase is probably a result of degranulation of eosinophils infiltrating the site of inflammation or infection.

Eosinophil degranulation has been studied in vitro (Sher and Wadee, 1981; Tai and Spry, 1981). Substances that increase intracellular cyclic adenosine monophosphate (cAMP) prevent degranulation, whereas those that increase cyclic guanosine monophosphate (cGMP) have no effect. Eosinophils have been found to degranulate following ingestion of inert particles, antibody-coated erythrocytes or bacteria, and antigen-antibody complexes and after coming in contact with metazoan parasites.

METABOLISM

The major source of energy in eosinophils, as in neutrophils, is anaerobic glycolysis. The hexose monophosphate pathway (HMP) activity is somewhat more prominent in eosinophils than in neutrophils because of the presence of large and abundant mitochondria (Cline, 1975). Leukemic eosinophils and eosinophils from some patients with eosinophilias show increased metabolic activity (Bass et al., 1980b; Pincus et al., 1981; Winqvist et al., 1982).

Phagocytosis or perturbation of the plasma membrane stimulates metabolic activities of eosinophils; these include increases in HMP activity; oxygen consumption; generation of superoxide, hydroxyl radical, singlet oxygen, and H_2O_2; chemiluminescence; and reduction of nitro blue tetrazolium (Cline, 1975; De-Chatelet et al., 1977; Klebanoff et al., 1977; Pincus, 1980). It has been found that bovine neutrophils and eosinophils do not differ in their ability to reduce nitro blue tetrazolium (Roth and Kaeberle, 1981). Equine eosinophils have been found to generate in vitro about 4–5 times more slow-reacting substance than neutrophils (Jorg et al., 1982).

NADPH oxidase activity in eosinophils is about 3–6 times greater than that in neutrophils; oxidative burst and H_2O_2 production are greater as well (Bass, 1979; DeChatelet et al., 1977). Despite these phagocytosis-associated events, eosinophils have significantly lower phagocytic and bactericidal properties than neutrophils.

PRODUCTION AND RELEASE

The major site of eosinophilopoiesis is the bone marrow. Eosinophil production to a minor degree has been observed in the spleen, thymus, and cervical lymph nodes of laboratory animals (Hudson, 1968). The small intestine was considered another possible site of eosinophil formation in the dog (Godlowski, 1962), but these observations need confirmation. In general, eosinophils are produced in the bone marrow over a period of 2–6 days and enter the peripheral blood about 2 days later. Eosinophils circulate with a half-time of disappearance of a few hours and randomly enter tissues, where they may live for several days.

Eosinophils are produced in the bone marrow from a progenitor cell that is different from that for neutrophils and is designated colony forming unit–eosinophil (CFU-Eos) (Fig. 13–19). The CFU-Eos divides and differentiates into an eosinophilic myeloblast; both remain to be morphologically identified. The earliest precursor that can be morphologically and cytochemically recognized is the eosinophilic promyelocyte. It is infrequently encountered in marrow aspirates, but its progenies, eosinophilic myelocytes, are frequently encountered in a productive marrow. Eosinophilic promyelocytes and myelocytes are both capable of mitosis. Eventually eosinophilic myelocytes mature into metamyelocytes and band cells of the series and finally become mature eosinophils.

Kinetics of eosinophil production have been studied mostly in laboratory animals, although some data is available on humans. Mitotic, maturative, and storage compartments of eosinophils are recognized in the bone marrow. In the guinea pig, there are about 300 eosinophils in the bone marrow for every eosinophil in the circulation; about 75% of these are mature and constitute the storage compartment (Hudson, 1968). By contrast, the bone marrow to blood pool ratio of eosinophils in humans is about 3.4:1 (Walle and Parwaresch, 1979).

Studies in rats indicate normal cell cycle (generation) time of 30 hours, marrow transit time of 5.5 days, and minimum emergence time of eosinophils into blood of 41 hours (Spry, 1971a, 1971b). Shorter values were obtained in rats infected with *Trichinella spiralis*; the respective values were 9 hours, 3.6 days, and 18 hours. These observations indicate an accelerated production and release of eosinophils during parasitic infection. Production and release are probably accelerated in certain other infections as well. In rats, but not in humans, newly released eosinophils migrate into the spleen, where further maturation continues for 40 hours (Clark and Kaplan, 1975).

Some species differences are found in marrow kinetics of eosinophils. Observations in human studies provide the following estimates for normal eosinophilopoiesis: generation time, 1.5 days, postmitotic maturation time (in marrow), 2.5 days, and emergence time, 3.8 days.

Like neutrophils, eosinophils normally leave the circulation in a random manner. Their half-time of disappearance (T½) from blood varies with the species: about 30 minutes in the dog (Carper and Hoffman, 1966), 4.5–5 hours in humans (Herion et al., 1970), and 6–10 hours in the rat (Spry, 1971b). Eosinophils in human patients with benign eosinophilia have a markedly long blood half-life and appear to recirculate (Dale et al., 1976; Herion et al., 1970). In these patients, autologous ^{51}Cr-labeled eosinophils were found to leave the circulatory pool transiently within 3 hours of infusion and then reenter the circulatory pool to disappear from the circulation with a T½ of 44 hours.

Species differences may also exist in survival of eosinophils in tissues. Human eosinophils were found to survive in tissue culture for 8–12 days; neutrophils remained viable for 2–4 days, and basophils for 12–15 days (Osgood, 1937). In contrast, the tissue life span of rat eosinophils was estimated at 2–4 days (Cohen et al., 1967).

Separate controls for the production and release of eosinophils have been described in recent years. Experimental evidence indicated that eosinophilopoiesis in response to immune and nonimmune reactions is largely dependent on T-lymphocytes (Bartelmez et al., 1980b; Basten and Beeson, 1970; Beeson and Bass, 1977; Boyer et al., 1970; Mahmoud and Austen, 1981; Walls, 1977) and to some extent on other unknown factors (Pritchard and Eady, 1981; Tsuda et al., 1980).

In vitro studies of eosinophilopoiesis in semisolid (agar or methyl cellulose) or liquid cultures indicated humoral stimulation at the committed stem cell (CFU-Eos) level (Bartelmez et al., 1980a, 1980b). The factor responsible for the division and differentiation of these stem cells into colonies of recognizable eosinophils in semisolid agar is called eosinophil–colony stimulating factor (CSF-Eos). Antigen- or mitogen-stimulated lymphocytes are the major source of CSF-Eo, but cells of the mononuclear phagocyte system also produce it. CSF-Eo is distinct from neutrophil–or monocyte–colony stimulating factor. Murine CSF-Eo has a molecular weight of about 50,000 and acts slowly, producing maximum effect by 5–15 days. The factor stimulating growth of eosinophils in liquid cultures is called eosinophil growth stimulating factor (Eo-GSF). It is also released by antigen-stimulated lymphocytes, but is distinct from CSF-Eo and produces peak eosinophil production by the second day.

In vivo production of a factor stimulating eosinophilopoiesis was demonstrated in experiments with mice and rats made eosinopenic by an antieosinophil serum. Injection of the antieosinophil serum in normal mice is accompanied by increased numbers of newly formed eosinophils in the bone marrow. Serum from such eosinopenic mice also stimulates eosinophilopoiesis and induces eosinophilia in normal mice in 2–4 days.

The factor in serum is called "eosinophilopoietin" (EPP) and appears to be a low-molecular-weight (5,000) polypeptide, probably containing 5–10 amino acid residues. Its eosinophilopoietic effect is dose-dependent and lacks species specificity. The role of T-lymphocytes in secretion of EPP is suggested from studies on athymic nude mice, which do not elaborate EPP after receiving antieosinophil serum. However, injection of preformed EPP in nude mice induces increased production of eosinophils within 48 hours. In a recent study, EPP was also found to stimulate eosinophilopoiesis in liquid cultures of mouse bone marrow (Bartelmez et al., 1980b). Furthermore, on the basis of simlarities in kinetic patterns of eosinophil production by EPP and Eo-GSF they were considered identical substances. These factors are believed to stimulate eosinophil production by influencing myeloblasts and their progenies that are capable of mitosis.

Immune-mediated stimulation of eosinophilopoiesis in vivo also appears to be influenced by T-lymphocytes through elaboration of EPP. Intact thymus or T-lymphocyte function is essential for esoinophilia to develop in response to a variety of agents (Beeson and Bass, 1977; Jong and Klebanoff, 1980). For example mice depleted of T-lymphocytes fail to develop eosinophilia in response to *T. spiralis* infection, but develop neutrophilia in response to acute pyelonephritis. Similarly, nude mice fail to develop peripheral eosinophilia after *T. spiralis* infection compared to similarly infected control mice. In contrast, athymic nude mice that have received grafts of thymic tissue develop eosinophil responses to trichinosis. Cell-free media from cultures of splenic lymphocytes stimulated by a specific antigen induce eosinophilia in mice rendered eosinopenic by corticosteroids (Miller et al., 1976).

Eosinophilia associated with *T. spiralis* infection in rats was inhibited or reduced by neonatal thymectomy, antilymphocyte serum, or prolonged thoracic duct drainage, all of which are known to affect T cell responses (Basten and Beeson, 1970). Nude rats develop eosinophilia after intraperitoneal implantation of cell-tight diffusion chambers containing lymphocytes from *T. spiralis*–infected rats and *Trichinella* antigen. Similarly, animals depleted of T-lymphocytes fail to develop eosinophilia in response to *Ascaris lumbricoides, Schistosoma mansoni,* tetanus toxoid, and aluminium hydroxide (Pritchard and Eady, 1981). Passive transfer of sensitized thoracic duct lymphocytes results in an anamnestic eosinophilic response in previously sensitized syngeneic animals. Experiments with normal and nude rats infected with *Fasciola hepatica,* however, indicate that eosinophilia in such animals may develop irrespective of the thymic function (Doy and Hughes, 1982).

That the eosinophil response involved some cooperation of lymphocytes and bone marrow cells was shown in experiments in which rats were given whole body irradiation and then transfused with lymphocytes or bone marrow cells alone or in combination. The former group of animals failed to develop eosinophilia when challenged, whereas animals transfused with both lymphocytes and bone marrow cells responded with eosinophilia after a similar challenge (Beeson, 1976).

An "eosinophil releasing factor" (ERF) is found in plasma of rats infected with *T. spiralis* (Spry, 1971b). Intravenous injection of such plasma in normal rats produces a significant increase in eosinophil counts by the third hour, a peak at the sixth hour, and return to normal by 24 hours. Similar response

was seen in adrenalectomized or adrenalectomized-splenectomized rats. In studies with horses, continuous infusion of histamine for 2 hours was found to produce a transient eosinopenia followed by eosinophilia by 1½ hours which lasted for as long as histamine was injected (Archer, 1970). In both instances eosinophilia seems to be caused by mobilization of the marrow reserve of eosinophils.

SURFACE RECEPTORS AND CHEMOTAXIS

Eosinophils have surface receptors for IgE (Capron et al., 1981b; Weller and Goetzl, 1980), IgG (Kay, 1979; Sullivan, 1979; Weller and Goetzl, 1980), complement components C1, C3b, C3d, and C4 (Kay, 1979; Sullivan, 1979; Weller and Goetzl, 1980), glucocorticoids (Peterson et al., 1981), and histamine (Clark et al., 1978). The density of IgG and complement receptors on eosinophils is about 40% of that on neutrophils (Kay, 1979). This density may be one of the contributory factors for the low phagocytic activity of eosinophils. C3 receptors become better expressed as the cell matures. Expression of IgG, C3b, and C4 receptors is enhanced by "eosinophil chemotactic factor of anaphylaxis" (ECF-A), and expression of C3b and C4 receptors is enhanced by histamine and HETEs (hydroxyeicosatetraenoic acids, products of arachidonic acid metabolism) (Beeson and Bass, 1977; Capron et al., 1981a; Kay, 1979; Mahmoud and Austen, 1981).

The percentage of eosinophils with complement and IgG receptors and the number of such receptors per cell were found to increase during eosinophilias of diverse etiology (Zucker-Franklin et al., 1981). Eosinophils from human patients with eosinophilia due to parasitic infection form spontaneous rosettes with sheep red cells (De Simone et al., 1980).

Methods have been developed to separate highly pure populations of eosinophils of various species to study cell properties and functions. (Archer and Hirsch, 1963; Duffus et al., 1980; Gartner, 1980; Grewal and Babiuk, 1979; Jorg et al., 1978, 1982; Parrillo and Fauci, 1978). Eosinophils are as actively motile as neutrophils. A number of substances are chemotactic for eosinophils in vitro and produce local eosinophilia in vivo. These chemoattractants include antigen-antibody complexes, molecular aggregates of heterologous γ-globulin, fibrin, fibrinogen, products released from basophils, mast cells, and stimulated T-lymphocytes, and undefined tissue products (Archer, 1970; Butterworth, 1977; Honsinger et al., 1972; Sullivan, 1979; Ward, 1969).

The eosinophilotactic effect of antigen-antibody complexes is mediated through activation of complement components (C3a, C5a, and C567). Degranulation of mast cells and basophils through immunologic activation (interaction of surface IgE with specific antigen) or by nonimmune mechanisms is accompanied by release of several preformed or newly synthesized substances capable of attracting eosinophils (Butterworth and David, 1981; Olsson and Venge, 1979; Sullivan, 1979; also see Table 28–1). These include ECF-A, histamine, intermediate-molecular-weight peptides, and two products of arachidonic acid metabolism (HETEs and HHTs). Imidazole acetic acid, the oxidative deamination product of histamine, is also chemotactic for eosinophils (Turnbull and Kaur, 1976).

Stimulated lymphocytes release at least two inadequately characterized lymphokines that are chemotactic for eosinophils; one has a molecular weight of 24,000–56,000 and is called eosinophil stimulation promotor (ESP) (Green and Colley, 1974), and the other is a precursor substance which, after interaction with heterologous antigen-antibody complexes, gives rise to an active eosinophil chemotactic factor (ECF) (Cohen and Ward, 1971).

Histamine-induced release of an eosinophil-immobilizing factor from mononuclear cells was suggested to be partly responsible for accumulation of eosinophils in certain allergic diseases and nematode infections (Kowanatzki et al., 1977). In a paradoxical role, histamine itself in high concentration inhibits migration of eosinophils through H_2 receptors, increasing the intracellular concentration of AMP (Clark et al., 1978). A low-molecular-weight peptide chemotactic for eosinophils has been isolated from some carcinoma cells (Goetzl et al., 1978). A low-mo-

lecular-weight substance from severely affected muscles in three cases of bovine eosinophilic myositis was found chemotactic for eosinophils (Oghiso and Fijiwara, 1978).

Thus eosinophils are attracted into areas of immune-, complement-, and lymphocyte-mediated inflammation and tissue injury by a heterogeneous group of chemotactic stimuli (Sullivan, 1979). Some of these stimuli may exert synergistic effect; e.g., histamine may stimulate responsiveness to complement components (Clark et al., 1976). Some may also be released by other leukocytes, e.g., ECF from neutrophils (Frickhofen and Konig, 1979). However, histamine seems to play the key role in tissue localization of eosinophils, and thence in peripheral blood eosinophilia, as a consequence of its ability to stimulate eosinophil migration and to modulate eosinophil responsiveness to other chemotactic factors.

TISSUE DISTRIBUTION

Eosinophils are found in loose connective tissue, particularly beneath the epithelial surfaces at the portal of entry of foreign material, e.g., the gut, subcutis, and respiratory tract. Their distribution in tissues is quite extensive. The ratio of blood to tissue eosinophils has been estimated at 1:100 in humans (Osgood, 1954), 1:200 or 300 in the rat (Rytomaa, 1960), and 1:300 in the guinea pig (Hudson, 1968). Species differences in tissue distribution have been noted; e.g., many more eosinophils are found in the subcutaneous tissues of the rat than in those of humans. Furthermore, the number of eosinophils in some tissues may vary with the physiologic state of the animal. For example, the small number of eosinophils present in the uterus varies with the estrous cycle (Rytomaa, 1960). There are relatively few eosinophils in the intestinal submucosa of starved animals, and animals on a protein diet have many eosinophils in the thoracic duct lymph (Godlowski, 1962).

Tissue studies of eosinophils in rats revealed four main sites of concentration in the body: bone marrow, skin, intestinal tract, and lungs (Rytomaa, 1960). Eosinophils in 36 different organs of cows and pigs were found to range from 0–1,500/mm², with highest concentration in the intestinal tract, especially the small intestine, and modest concentration (50–200/mm²) in the stomach, lymph nodes, thymus, and conjunctiva (Vilpo et al., 1970). It is conjectured that the quantitative distribution of eosinophils in different organs may have a functional relationship to the organs' histamine content. For example, the intestine is rich in histamine, and it has been shown in rats that a large number of eosinophils are normally eliminated in the bowel (Sundell, 1958).

FUNCTIONS

Although functions of the eosinophils remain to be fully defined, it is becoming increasingly apparent that eosinophils are important in controlling infection with metazoan parasites. In addition, they seem to play an active role in regulating allergic and inflammatory reactions. The interested reader is encouraged to consult recent literature on these aspects of eosinophils for further information than is given below (Bass, 1979; Bartelmez at el., 1980b; Olsson and Venge, 1979; Sullivan, 1979; van Dallen, 1981). Regulatory functions of several eosinophil components are summarized in Table 27–1.

Phagocytosis and Bactericidal Effect

Eosinophils can phagocytize a wide variety of substances including bacteria (Fig. 27–6), mycoplasmata, yeasts, antibody-coated red cells, immune complexes, mast cell granules, and inert particles (Clark and Kaplan, 1975; Cline et al., 1968; Olsson and Venge, 1979; Sullivan, 1979). Eosinophils from allergic patients are inferior to normal eosinophils in phagocytic activity (Grover et al., 1978).

Phagocytosis is dependent on active glycolysis and is followed by an increase in oxidative metabolism and rapid degranulation (Fig. 27–6). Bactericidal effect is mediated through the peroxidase-H_2O_2-halide system, particularly with iodide as a halide, and through generation of oxygen metabolites such as superoxide anion and hydroxyl radicals.

Eosinophils, however, have a more limited phagocytic ability than neutrophils (Clark and Kaplan, 1975), and they are less efficient in killing bacteria despite a much higher content of peroxidase and a high metabolic activity in terms of oxidative response, H_2O_2 production, and iodination (Beahner and Johnston, 1971; Bass, 1979; DeChatelet et al., 1978; Mickenberg et al., 1972; Roth and Kaeberle, 1981). This more limited phagocytic and bactericidal ability may be due to differences in cellular properties and quantitative as well as qualitative differences in substances exerting bactericidal activity. Eosinophils lack lysozyme, lactoferrin, and phagocytin, and their cationic proteins are not or slightly bactericidal (Archer and Hirsch, 1963; DeChatelet et al., 1978; Jong et al., 1980; Mahmoud and Austen, 1981; Migler et al., 1978; Olsson and Venge, 1979). Thus eosinophils seem to be functionally limited in their capacity to provide host resistance to bacterial infection. However, eosinophil MBP, peroxidase, and oxygen radicals can effectively damage and kill various helminthic parasites as described below.

Parasiticidal Effect

It has been established in recent years that eosinophil-mediated destruction of parasites

Table 27–1. Regulatory and Other Functions of Eosinophil Components

Factor or Target	*Action by eosinophil component*
Histamine	Inactivated by histaminase; release inhibited by PGE and zinc, which also inhibits release of some other bioactive substances.
SRS-A (slow-reacting substance of anaphylaxis)	Inactivated by arylsulfatase B
Heparin	Neutralized by major basic protein
Platelet activating factor	Degraded by phospholipase D
Lysolecithin	Destroyed by lysolecithinase
IgE-antigen complexes, intact mast cell granules	Phagocytized
Helminthic parasite	Damaged by major basic protein, peroxidase, and superoxide radicals
Certain tissue cells	Damaged by major basic protein; injury potentiated by lysosomal hydrolases and superoxide radicals

For additional information see Schatz et al., 1981.

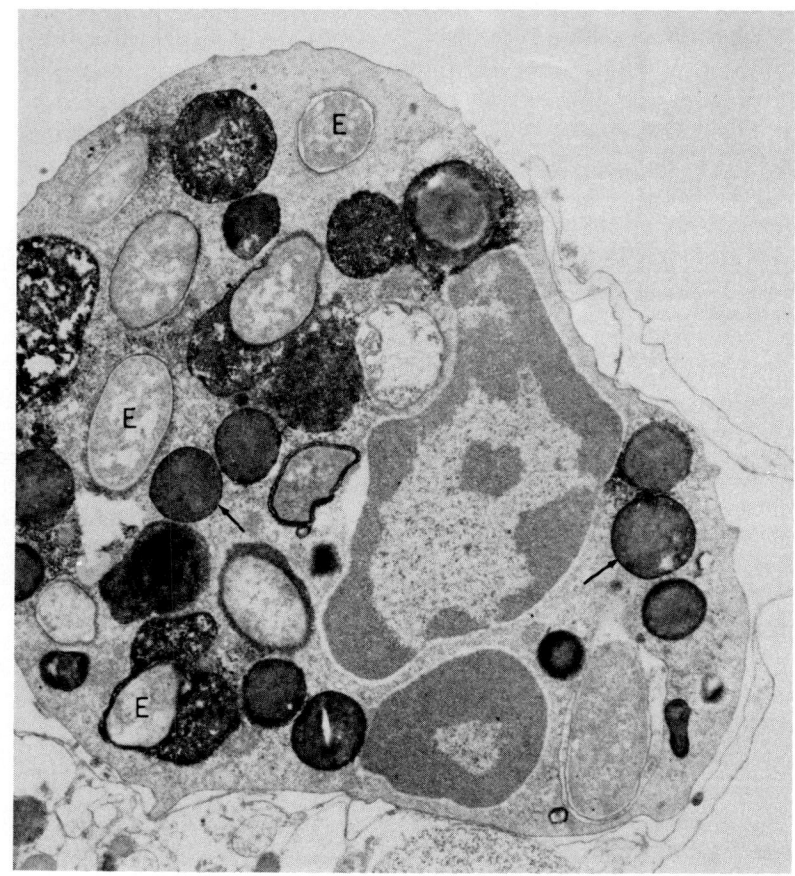

Fig. 27–6. Bovine eosinophil with intracellular *Escherichia coli* organisms *(E)* and intact peroxidase-positive eosinophil granules (arrows). Degranulation and accumulation of variable amounts of eosinophil granular material is evident in phagocytic vacuoles around some organisms. Peroxidase stain, ×14,700.

is an important mechanism of protective parasitic immunity. Such observations have been made from in vitro and in vivo studies on several parasites, e.g., the larvae (schistosomules) of *Schistosoma mansoni*, the larvae of *Trichinella spiralis*, microfilarae of *Onchocerca volvulus*, bloodstream forms of *Trypanosoma cruzi*, juvenile *Fasciola hepatica*, and *Trypanosoma theileri* (Duffus et al., 1980; Kipnis et al, 1981; Olsson and Venge, 1979; Sullivan, 1979; Townsend and Duffus, 1982; van Dallen, 1981). Butterworth (1977) has reviewed the role of eosinophils in immunity to helminthic infection, and Kay (1979) has summarized evidence supporting the concept that eosinophils and mast cell–derived mediators, acting together with complement, provide a highly effective mechanism for death of helminthic parasites. The interaction between IgE, mast

cells, eosinophils, and parasites is depicted in Fig. 27–7 and also discussed in Chapter 28.

Resistance to a helminthic infection is decreased by elimination of eosinophils. For example, treatment of mice with antieosinophil serum abolishes active or passive immunity to *S. mansoni* infection (Mahmoud and Austen, 1981; Mahmoud et al., 1975) and increases susceptibility of mice (Mahoud, 1977) and guinea pigs (Gleich et al., 1979b) to *T. spiralis* infection. In contrast, antilymphocyte, antineutrophil, and antimonocyte serums had no such effects (Mahmoud and Austen, 1981). Eosinophils were found to surround and kill schistosomules of *S. mansoni* in the skin of immune mice and primates (Sullivan, 1979). Such a reaction was not seen in non-immune animals and was markedly reduced in mice depleted of eosinophils by antieosin-

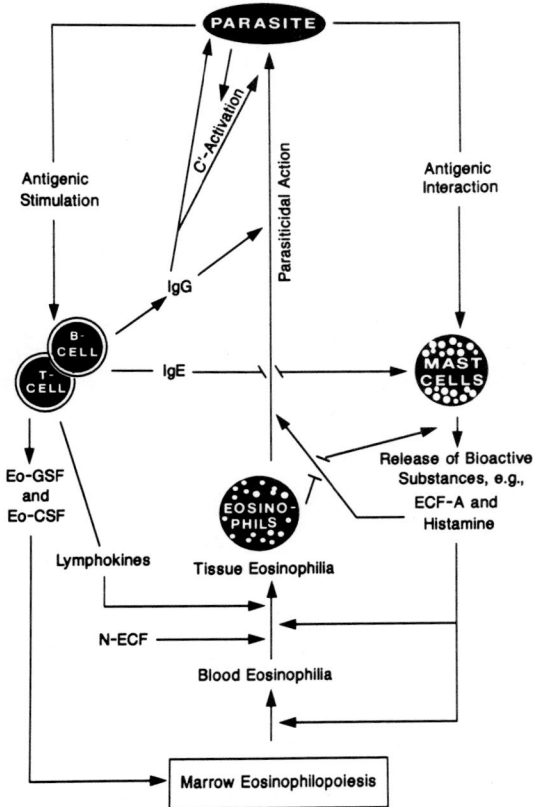

Fig. 27–7. Parasiticidal action of eosinophils via interaction with mast cells and lymphocytes. Parasitic antigens stimulate the lymphoid system. Stimulated T-lymphocytes produce eosinophil colony-stimulating factor (Eo-CSF) and eosinophil growth-stimulating factor (Eo-GSF), which promote bone marrow eosinophilopoiesis. IgE antibody, produced by certain subsets of stimulated B-lymphocytes, coats tissue mast cells. Interaction of parasitic antigen with specific IgE-coated mast cells induces release of bioactive substances, such as eosinophil chemotactic factor of anaphylaxis (ECF-A) and histamine, from the mast cells. These substances are highly chemotactic for eosinophils and thus promote blood and tissue eosinophilia. Lymphokines from stimulated T-lymphocytes and neutrophil-derived eosinophil chemotactic factor (N-ECF) also stimulate migration of eosinophils into tissues. Activation and degranulation of eosinophils are associated with parasiticidal action through eosinophil cationic proteins including major basic protein, the eosinophil peroxidase-hydrogen peroxide-halide complex, and phospholipases. Eosinophil attachment and killing of parasite is high in the presence of IgG antibody and complement (C), intermediate in the presence of C alone, and low when only IgG is present. C activation can be initiated indirectly by parasitic antigen or directly by IgG antibody. ECF-A and histamine increase expression of C receptors on eosinophils and also accelerate C-dependent parasiticidal action of eosinophils. Eosinophils also regulate release of bioactive substances from mast cells; the eosinophil peroxidase-hydrogen peroxide-halide complex promotes such a release, while eosinophil prostaglandins E_1, E_2, and zinc are inhibitory.

ophil serum. It is highly likely that eosinophils are also involved in killing other parasites because eosinophilic infiltrations in tissues are observed in association with other parasites, e.g., hepatic *F. hepatica*, intestinal *Oesophagostomum radiatum*, and lungworm *Dictyocaulus viviparus* infection in cattle (Butterworth, 1977).

Some observations have been made on the mechanisms of parasiticidal effect of eosinophils. In vitro and in vivo experiments indicate that direct phagocytosis of the parasite by eosinophils is not involved, but that after coming in close contact with an opsonized (antibody- and complement-coated) parasite, eosinophils undergo exocytosis to expel their granular constituents. This process is associated with release of label from ^{52}Cr-labeled parasites, ultrastructural surface changes in the parasite, and eventual death of the parasite (McLaren et al., 1978; Vadas et al., 1979). Damage to the various parasites is probably inflicted both by oxidative (peroxidase, H_2O_2 and superoxide radicals) and nonoxidative (eosinophil MBP) systems (Bass and Szejda, 1979; David et al., 1980; Jong et al., 1979). Experimental studies with schistosomules of *S. mansoni* indicated that the parasiticidal effect of eosinophils is higher in the presence of specific IgG antibody and complement and decreases progressively when only the complement or antibody is present (Kay, 1979; McKean et al., 1981). Complement can be activated by schistosomules and other parasites by both classical and alternate pathways resulting in the deposition of C3b on the parasite surface (Sullivan, 1979). This would promote their interaction with eosinophils and subsequent killing. ECF-A and histamine released from mast cells promote eosinophil-mediated, complement-dependent killing of schistosomules. This occurs probably through enhancement or unmasking of IgG and complement receptors on eosinophils (Capron et al., 1981a; Kay, 1979). Histamine has also been found to promote superoxide production by eosinophils (Pincus et al., 1982). Neutrophils also bind to schistosomules, but are relatively less effective in parasiticidal effect.

Eosinophils from different individuals may vary in their parsiticidal action. Circulating mature eosinophils can be activated by CSF to kill parasites by small amounts of antibody and complement (Dessein et al., 1982). Eosinophils from hypereosinophilic patients are less effective in parasiticidal effect, probably due to interference with cell surface receptors by immune complexes coating the surface of eosinophils in the peripheral blood of such patients (Kay, 1976).

Regulation of Allergic and Inflammatory Reactions

An allergic reaction is characterized by tissue and blood eosinophilia. Immune- and nonimmune-mediated degranulation of mast cells and basophils is followed by release of inflammatory mediators and release and generation of various chemoattractants for eosinophils as described (see Chapter 28). These observations, together with deleterious in vitro effects of various eosinophil constituents on certain mast cell mediators, form the basis of the hypothesis that eosinophils play a regulatory role in acute allergic and inflammatory processes. Eosinophils seem to modulate all stages of the allergic response, namely, release, inactivation, and replenishment of a mediator of inflammation such as histamine (Kay, 1976).

Eosinophils are believed to regulate allergic (immediate-type hypersensitivity reaction) and inflammatory reactions (Austen, 1978; Olsson and Venge, 1979; Sullivan, 1979) through a variety of mechanisms. Their ability to phagocytize immune complexes probably reduces availability of antigen for further immune response. Similarly, phagocytosis of intact mast cell granules would limit extracellular generation of inflammatory mediators. These phenomena also lead to exocytosis of eosinophil granules and/or their granular constituents (Olsson and Venge, 1979).

Earlier studies (Kovacs, 1950; Vercauteren, 1953) suggested that eosinophils contain an antihistamine and are specialized in detoxification of histamine. Studies on the horse and its eosinophils revealed that eosinophils are rapidly attracted into tissues by an increased concentration of free histamine and render histamine physiologically inactive by an unknown mechanism (Archer, 1963). More recently, eosinophils have been shown

to contain a histaminase that inactivates histamine (Zeiger et al., 1976), and factors inhibiting release and replenishment of histamine have also been identified in eosinophils (Gleich, 1977).

PGE_1 and PGE_2 inhibit mast cell degranulation and histamine release (Bass, 1979; Olsson and Venge, 1979). The high content of zinc released from eosinophils is thought to inhibit mast cell release of histamine and serotonin and to inhibit pletelet aggregation and macrophage migration (Beeson and Bass, 1977). In addition, eosinophil extracts inhibit edema-producing properties of serotonin and bradykinin (R.K. Archer, 1968, 1970). Slow reacting substance of anaphylaxis is inactivated by eosinophils by a more complex mechanism involving action of arylsulfatase, peroxidase, and peptidase (Bass, 1979; Wasserman et al., 1975). Phospholipase D from eosinophils causes inactivation of platelet aggregating factors released from basophils and mast cells (Kater et al., 1976). MBP binds heparin to neutralize it, and plasminogen reduces local thrombus formation (Bass, 1979).

Thus it would seem that eosinophils are armed with a variety of chemical substances that have antipholgistic properties. However, whether these substances occur in amounts sufficient to play a role in regulation of inflammation in vivo has been questioned. (Sullivan, 1979).

Tissue Destruction

An association between the accumulation of eosinophils beneath the tracheal epithelium and an increased mucous secretory activity of epithelial cells was suggested from studies on parasitized rats (G.T. Archer, 1968). Recent studies have shown that eosinophils may produce cell damage, through release of their MBP, during disease states associated with a prolonged, persistent hypereosinophilia (Gleich et al., 1979a; Mahmoud and Austen, 1981; Schatz et al., 1981). Purified eosinophils and MBP from their granules were found to exert antibody- and/or complement-dependent cytotoxicity for various types of cells (Frigas et al., 1980, 1981; Gleich et al., 1979a; Parrillo and Fauci, 1978) and neurotoxic effects (Durack et al., 1979). Damage induced by MBP could be augmented by other eosinophil cationic proteins, lysosomal hydrolases, or superoxide radicals (Schatz et al., 1981).

The eosinophil peroxidase-H_2O_2-halide system was found to have a potent cytotoxic effect on mouse ascites lymphoma cells (Jong and Klebanoff, 1980). Löffler's endomyocarditis in hypereosinophilia (Olsen et al., 1980; Olsson and Venge, 1979), central nervous system injury in certain diseases associated with eosinophilia (Durack et al., 1979), and tissue injury in eosinophilic gastroenteritis (Olsson and Venge, 1979) in human patients are ascribed to eosinophils. Clinical association of eosinophilia and cardiac disease in humans and in vitro observations of cardiac cell damage by eosinophilic basic protein are considered indicative of an active role of eosinophils in cardiotoxicity (Spry et al., 1983). A low-molecular-weight (18,400) polypeptide with neurotoxic properties has been isolated from human eosinophil granules (Durack et al., 1981).

Other Functions

There are other, less known functions of eosinophils as well. For instance, a high incidence of thrombosis in hypereosinophilic syndrome is associated with augmentation of coagulation through activation of Factor XII by ECP (Venge et al., 1979). A role in fibrinolysis is also suggested through activation of plasminogen. This may occur at a later stage than the procoagulant activation, but how the two processes interact remains unknown.

An inhibitory effect on granulopoiesis, probably mediated through PGE, was suggested from observations of an inverse relationship between eosinophilia and neutropenia in some human patients and an inhibitory effect of eosinophils on in vitro granulopoiesis (Tebbi et al., 1980).

Unlike neutrophil collagenase, which destroys connective tissue during the early stages of the inflammatory process, eosinophil collagenase is thought to play a role in remodeling connective tissue during late stages of the inflammatory process.

EOSINOPHILIAS

There are comparatively few eosinophils in the circulation in health, yet their numbers are sufficient to reflect significant changes in pathophysiology under certain conditions. A diurnal variation in the eosinophil count has been demonstrated, with the highest count at midnight and the lowest at noon. This is negatively related to variations in the endogenous corticosteroid level. An age relationship was seen in goats, the adults having twice as many eosinophils as the kids (Earl and Carranza, 1980).

Eosinophilia occurred in guinea pigs within 24 hours of severe hypoxia of high altitude (Grant and Hudson, 1969), in pigs after partial or complete hypophysectomy (Zintzsch, 1969), and in rats developing severe magnesium deficiency (Hungerford, 1964; Hungerford and Karson, 1960). Eosinophilia can be induced experimentally by injecting immune complexes, latex particles coated with γ-globulins, and parasitic infections (Butterworth, 1977). A genetic variation has been found in mice infected with parasites (Wakelin and Donachie, 1981).

Chronic eosinophilia is common to diseases of tissues and organs containing a high concentration of mast cells, e.g., the skin, lungs, gastrointestinal tract, and female genital organs. Eosinophilia is most often encountered in pathologic states associated with an interaction between antigen, IgE antibody, and mast cells or basophils (Olsson and Venge, 1979). These include certain parasitic infections, allergic respiratory diseases, and dermatoses. It is also seen in allergic reactions to drugs (Spry, 1980).

The release of histamine, ECF-A, and other chemotactic peptides from mast cells and activation of extravasated complement components in any organ or tissue, as a result of injury or an antigen-antibody (IgE) reaction, results in attraction of eosinophils into the area. Products released from T-lymphocytes during cell-mediated immune reactions provide additional stimuli. All these factors may initially produce a temporary eosinopenia as eosinophils are drained from the blood. However, as these factors, particularly histamine, are released from the injured tissue and enter the blood, eosinophils are attracted into the blood from the bone marrow leading to eosinophilia.

Eosinophilia from increased eosinophilopoiesis occurs within a few days after a sustained mast cell degranulation and after markedly high levels of serum histamine such as from daily injection of compound 48/80, a mast cell degranulator.

Thus eosinophilia is not an expression of a single disease entity such as parasitism or allergic reaction, but rather is an occurrence to be anticipated in a wide variety of chronic diseases involving continuous degranulation of mast cells. (Table 27–2).

Marked eosinophilia secondary to various inciting causes cannot be readily distinguished from malignant eosinophilia, although the latter occurs very rarely. Every effort should be made to determine the cause of a prolonged, persistent eosinophilia before considering the possibility of an eosinophilic granulocytic leukemia. The latter possibility is strongly suggested by the presence of a disordered differentiation and maturation of eosinophils in the bone marrow and by elimination of conditions commonly associated with an eosinophilia. A distinguishing feature may be that serum IgE levels are usually increased in eosinophilias from allergic causes, but not in patients with myeloproliferative disorders (Crowley and Myers, 1983).

Peripheral blood eosinophilia may result from increased eosinophilopoiesis, increased release of bone marrow reserve, preferential redistribution of cells from the marginal pool, or prolonged intravascular life span of eosinophils. Eosinophilia in most situations is probably due to increased production and enhanced release from the bone marrow as exemplified by the eosinophilia of parasitism (Beeson and Bass, 1977; Mahmoud et al., 1977, Mahmoud and Austen, 1981). Increased intravascular survival may also be a major contributory factor in certain hypereosinophilic patients (Dale et al.,1976; Olsen et al., 1980).

Several lines of evidence as discussed earlier in this chapter (see Production and Release) indicate that stimulus for eosinophilia is provided by substances released from T-lymphocytes, namely, CSF-Eo and Eo-GSF or EPP.

Eosinophilia and Parasitism

Eosinophilia in response to parasitism occurs when a sensitivity to the protein of the parasite has developed (allergic state) and the protein or secretory product of the parasite is released in the body. Helminthic antigens are potent inducers of reaginic or homocytotropic IgE antibody response. Thus high serum IgE levels and eosinophilia are characteristics of helminthic infections (Dessein et al., 1981; So-

Table 27–2.   Eosinophilia and Basophilia in the Dog and Cat

Number	Organ System or Disease Involvement	Eosinophils/μl		Basophils/μl	
		Mean ± 1 SD	Minimum-Maximum	Mean ± 1 SD	Minimum-Maximum
Dog					
143	Respiratory (lungs)	4,229 ± 3,786	1,330–15,958	356 ± 822	0–4,275
28	Skin	2,931 ± 1,931	1,536–12,627	91 ± 220	0–1,280
8	Ocular	2,841 ± 1,235	1,521– 5,785	74 ± 104	0– 292
20	GI tract	2,287 ± 1,447	1,424– 7,812	93 ± 155	0– 521
24	Bone and joint	2,649 ± 1,327	1,606– 6,700	80 ± 164	0– 750
24	Female genital	2,412 ± 1,337	1,379– 7,275	56 ± 117	0– 458
14	Urinary	2,250 ± 518	1,501– 3,182	52 ± 158	0– 612
22	Neurologic	2,294 ± 644	1,377– 3,625	45 ± 133	0– 522
7	Cardiac	1,918 ± 259	1,634– 2,431	92 ± 123	0– 344
28	Miscellaneous	3,931 ± 3,425	1,512–17,526	118 ± 211	0– 968
7	Suppurative	3,598 ± 2,695	1,609– 9,879	0	0
12	Neoplasia	2,149 ± 831	1,442– 4,446	56 ± 117	0– 458
Cat					
23	Skin	5,373 ± 4,408	1,500–22,230	111 ± 174	0– 537
11	Respiratory (lungs)	3,322 ± 1,539	1,522– 6,883	37 ± 41	0– 166
13	GI tract	2,706 ± 1,190	1,674– 6,341	114 ± 172	0– 564
12	Suppurative	2,964 ± 1,614	1,522– 7,375	156 ± 171	0– 486
13	Miscellaneous	3,147 ± 1,647	1,642– 7,832	132 ± 285	0–1,026

morin et al., 1978). Blood and tissue eosinophilia in such cases are proportional to the degree of antigenic stimulation or parasitic burden (Ackerman et al., 1981).

Filariasis in the dog is an excellent example of a parasitic state in which a dog may have a large number of viable microfilariae in its peripheral blood without a significant eosinophilia. Administration of chemotherapeutic agents to kill the microfilariae releases the specific protein to which the dog may be sensitive, in which case a marked but temporary eosinophilia is produced. Similarly eosinophilia and increased serum levels of MBP and Charcot-Leyden crystal protein were observed (with peaks at 1–2 weeks) after treatment of human patients infected with the helminth *Wuchereria bancrofti* (Ackerman et al., 1981).

Studies on the mechanisms of eosinophilia in parasitic infestations further indicate that it is a manifestation of immune response to parasitic antigens. For example, an intravenous inoculation of *T. spiralis* larvae into rats resulted in eosinophilia (primary response) with a peak on day 6 and a decline by day 10. Reinjection of the parasite 20 days later produced an enhanced eosinophilia (secondary response) with a higher peak and longer duration. Both primary and secondary eosinophil responses could be suppressed by agents known to modify the immune response (Boyer et al., 1970). Similarly, neonatal thymectomy, administration of antilymphocyte serum, and drainage of thoracic duct lymph significantly reduced the eosinophilic response to trichinosis (Basten and Beeson, 1970).

The key factor in genesis of eosinophilia in response to parasitism is the processing of parasite material by cells infiltrating the site of parasitic lodgment in tissues (Walls and Beeson, 1972). For example, intact *T. spiralis* larvae given intravascularly and larval extract in Freund's complete adjuvant given intramuscularly to normal rats produced eosinophilia, whereas injection of homogenized larvae and larval extract alone did not. However, the latter two effectively primed the animals to elicit eosinophilia on subsequent challenge and also elicited eosinophilia in previously sensitized rats. Thus eosinophilia is to be anticipated when parasitic larvae are migrating through tissues (Jenkins and Richard, 1984; Moncol and Batte, 1967). Reduction in parasitic burden by therapy is associated with diminution in eosinophil counts (Urch and Allen, 1980). Eosinophilia is least likely to accompany parasitism in which the parasite is free-living in the gut–remaining unattached to the gut wall (Chapter 6) and eosinophil counts in such cases are not influenced by anthelminthic treatment (Round, 1968).

Pulmonary Infiltrates with Eosinophilia

Pulmonary eosinophilias have been classified according to clinical characteristics of the syndromes and, more recently, their etiology (Schatz et al., 1981). The term *PIE* is applied to a clinical syndrome of pulmonary infiltrates (observed on radiologic examination) accompanied by peripheral blood eosinophilia. Pathologic conditions such as eosinophilic granuloma, in which blood eosinophilia is absent, are not included in this category.

PIEs have been divided into three groups (Schatz et al., 1981): (a) conditions in which PIE is a major part of the syndrome; these include allergic bronchopulmonary aspergillosis, chronic eosinophilic pneumonia, drug reaction, hypereosinophilic syndrome, parasitic infestation, and polyarteritis nodosa; (b) conditions in which PIE occurs infrequently and is a minor component; these include infections, neoplasms, and immunologic disorders; and (c) other conditions with PIE. In most diseases with PIE as a major component, serum IgE levels are elevated and treatment with corticosteroids is beneficial.

PIE occurs in the cat and, more commonly, in the dog (Grauer and Riedesel, 1977). Its causes in the dog include nonspecific allergic bronchitis, hypersensitivity to exogenous protein, heartworm disease, parasitic larval migration, and certain chronic infections.

Hypereosinophilic Syndrome

Hypereosinophilic syndrome (HES) is a heterogenous group of diseases characterized by persistent eosinophilia of undefined etiology and eosinophilic infiltration of tissues resulting in organ system dysfunction (Fauci et al., 1982; Hardy and Anderson, 1968). This syndrome in humans includes eosinophilic enteritis, Löeffler's syndrome, disseminated eosinophilic disease, and eosinophilic leukemia. The bone marrow is invariably hypereosinophilic and the heart and nervous system are most severely involved. Löeffler's syndrome is a condition of unknown etiology characterized by the presence of migratory pulmonary infiltrates, peripheral blood eosinophilia, and mild or no pulmonary symptoms lasting for 2–4 weeks.

A spectrum of HES, consisting of eosinophilic enteritis, disseminated eosinophilic infiltration of various organs and tissues, and eosinophilic leukemia, has been described in cats (Hendrick, 1981; Scott et al., 1985).

Eosinophilia and Estrus

We have observed eosinophilia in some dogs in estrus. The literature on this subject is limited. Estrogens injected into mice of both sexes were found to cause an increase in mast cells in various tissues (Arvy, 1955). In an investigation of the mast cell content of the uteri of 33 normal virgin heifers slaughtered at various times during the estrous cycle, the largest number of mast cells occurred in uteri in proestrus; the counts were lowest during estrus and on the first day proestrus (Weber et al., 1950). These findings indicate that degranulation of mast cells may take place during estrus and that eosinophilia may occur as a temporary and physiologic response to histamine release. Neoplasia of the ovary may be associated with eosinophilia in women (Wintrobe, 1981).

EOSINOPENIAS

The eosinophil count may be zero in some normal animals; hence eosinopenia is of limited significance. However, animals with circulating eosinophils characteristically develop eosinopenia after stress, endogenous release or administration of corticosteroids, and acute infection. Recent studies have demonstrated that these eosinopenic responses have independent mechanisms.

Stress, Corticosteroids, and Eosinopenia

Eosinopenia of physical and emotional stress is attributed to elevated levels of catecholamines, such as epinephrine, and adre-nocorticosteroids. Initial response to epinephrine injection is a mild eosinophilia, which peaks 1 hour postinjection, followed by eosinopenia by 4 hours (Beeson and Bass, 1977). The former effect is probably a result of mobilization of eosinophils from the spleen because it is not seen in splenectomized rats and guinea pigs. Epinephrine induces eosinopenia in intact animals, but was found to induce eosinophilia in adrenalectomized dogs (Henry et al., 1953) and rats (Thevathason and Gordon, 1958). However, eosinopenia ensued in the latter group of animals when both epinephrine and adrenocortical extracts were given. Such an effect was related to the dose of the epinephrine, but not to the dose of the adrenocortical extract.

The eosinopenic effect of catecholamines is purely a β-adrenergic effect, because (a) such a reaction was completely reversed by a pure β-adrenergic blocking agent, e.g., propanolol; and (b) isoproterenol, a pure β-adrenergic drug, produced eosinopenia as did epinephrine, while phenylepinephrine, a pure α-adrenergic drug, did not (Koch-Weser, 1968; Reed et al., 1970). Other studies revealed that the eosinopenic effect was a property of β_2-adrenergic stimulatory capacity (Dahl and Venge, 1978). PGE_1 and PGE_2 were found to produce eosinopenia in splenectomized rats; the effect did not seem to involve β-receptors, but was mediated through pituitary and adrenal activities (Kurosawa et al., 1978). Administration of adrenaline in sheep was found to decrease the number of eosinophils in the blood and lymph in 3 hours by about 70% and 50%, respectively, and insulin injection similarly produced a decrease of 72% and 43% (Mesipun and Kanarik, 1968).

The mechanism of ACTH- or corticosteroid-induced eosinopenia still remains to be unequivocally estalished. A variety of mechanisms have been proposed. Because corticosteroids have a neutralizing effect on histamine (Hicks and West, 1958) and histamine is chemotactic for eosinophils, decreased marrow release of eosinophils follows when the blood histamine level falls below normal after corticosteroid release or administration. Eosinophil release into the circulation is further diminished from inhibition of eosinophil adherence and chemotaxis by corticosteroids as demonstrated in in vitro and in vivo studies (Altman et al., 1981). Preexisting eosinophils in the blood disappear quickly because of corticosteroid-induced intravascular lysis (Navarrete and Petit, 1962), increased removal by the mononuclear phagocytes (Sundell, 1958), increased migration to the small intestine (Sundell, 1958), and/or reversible sequestration in organs rich in the mononuclear phagocyte system.

In a recent study, corticosteroid-induced eosinopenia was attributed to migration of eosinophils into lymphoid organs, namely the spleen, lymph nodes, and thymus, while eosinophilolysis or decreased production was not involved (Sabag et al., 1978). Migration into the lymphoid organs may be due to release of eosinophilotactic lymphokines from corticosteroid-induced lympholysis at such locations. The net result is an eosinopenia that persists until the blood histamine level rises again (convalescence). It has also been stated that continuous release of corticosteroids or prolonged steroid therapy causes decreased production of eosinophils (Beeson and Bass, 1977).

It is well known that administration of corticosteroids is beneficial in conditions associated with mast cell degranulation and release of histamine. Corticosteroids, besides neutralizing histamine, exert their beneficial effect by inhibiting degranulation of mast cells and basophils (Archer, 1970), perhaps by stabilizing lysosomal membranes (DeChatelet et al., 1977), thus reducing further histamine production and release.

The interrelationship of mast cell degranulation (release of histamine), the eosinotactic effect of histamine, and the neutralizing effect of glucocorticoids on histamine can serve as the basis for interpretation of the eosinophilia or eosinopenia seen in a variety of diseases of animals. One should realize, however, that the net result depends on the overwhelming effect of one or the other contributory factor.

Eosinopenia of Acute Infection and Inflammation

Eosinopenia characteristically accompanies acute infection and inflammatory reaction. It is often thought to be due to release of corticosteroids and catecholamines, but recent findings do not completely support this belief. Observations suggesting an independent mechanism have been summarized (Bass et al., 1980a; Beeson and Bass, 1977) and include the following: eosinopenia is found in some patients with adrenal insufficiency; acute infections suppress eosinophilia of trichinosis in guinea pigs and mice; acute pneumococcal infection in mice causes eosinopenia within 6 hours, but increase in corticosterone is not seen until 12 hours; bacterial and viral infections cause adrenal stimulation for only a brief period, while eosinopenia is seen for several days; adrenalectomized mice develop eosinopenia from acute infection or after injection of exudate from a pneumococcal abscess.

Several factors may be involved in causation of eosinopenia of acute infection and inflammation. Eosinophils seem to be actively involved in the inflammatory process (Olsson and Venge, 1979). Increased migration of eosinophils to the site of inflammation in response to locally-produced eosinophil chemotactic factors may partly reduce the blood eosinophil count (Bass et al., 1980a). Intravascular release of tissue products or activation of serum complement components may also be involved. For example, a nondialyzable glycoprotein (molecular weight >30,000) causing eosinopenia has been isolated from exudate (Bass, 1977; Beeson and Bass, 1977). Partially purified C5a given intravenously to rabbits was found to cause eosinopenia (Bass et al., 1980a). Decreased release of eosinophils from bone marrow during acute inflammation and decreased eosinophil production during chronic inflammation may also occur, the former through an unknown mechanism and the latter because of suppression of lymphocyte-mediated stimuli for eosinophil production (Mahmoud and Austen, 1981).

Although the above observations indicate a separate mechanism of initial eosinopenia of acute infection or inflammation, it is not unreasonable to think that a sustained eosinopenia during acute or chronic active inflammatory process may also be partly due to corticosteroids released under such situations.

Histamine was shown to be responsible for eosinopenia seen in stressed adrenalectomized dogs for pretreatment with antihistamines greatly reduced or in most cases abolished the eosinopenia from certain agents given in high doses (Swingle et al., 1955). Transient eosinopenia precedes eosinophilia from intravenous administration of histamine in horses and from injection of histamine liberator, compound 48/80 (Archer, 1970).

REFERENCES

Ackerman, G.A.: Eosinophilic Leukemia: A Morphologic and Histochemical Study. Blood, *24*:372, 1964.

Ackerman, S.J., et al.: Eosinophilia and Elevated Serum Levels of Eosinophil Major Basic Protein and Charcot-Leyden Crystal Protein (Lysophospholipase) after Treatment of Patients with Bancroft's Filariasis. J. Immunol., *127*:1093, 1981.

Ackerman, S.J., et al.: Formation of Charcot-Leyden Crystals by Human Basophils. J. Exp. Med., *155*:1597, 1982.

Altman, L.C., et al.: Effects of Corticosteroids on Eosinophil Chemotaxis and Adherence. J. Clin. Invest., *67*:28, 1981.

Anteunis, A., et al.: Ultrastructural Characteristics of Developing Eosinophil Leukocytes in Human Bone Marrow during Acute Leukemia. Inflammation, *2*:17, 1977.

Archer, G.T.: The Function of the Eosinophil. Proc. 11th Congr. Int. Soc. Blood Transf., Sydney, 1966. Bibl. Haematologica, 29, p. 1:71, 1968.

Archer, G. T., and Hirsch, J.G.: Isolation of Granules from Eosinophil Leukocytes and Study of Their Enzyme Content. J. Exp. Med., *118*:277, 1963.

Archer, R.K.: The Eosinophil Leucocytes. F.A. Davis, Philadelphia, 1963.

Archer, R.K.: The Eosinophil Leucocytes. Ser. Haematol. *1*:3, 1968.

Archer, R.K.: Regulatory Mechanisms in Eosinophil Leukocyte Production, Release, and Distribution. *In* Regulation of Hematopoiesis. Vol 2. Gordon, A.S., ed. Appleton-Century-Crofts, New York, p. 917, 1970.

Arvy, L.: Effect of Injections of Oestrogen on the Mast Cells of the White Mouse. Nature, *175*:506, 1955.

Atwal, O.S.: Ultrastructural Features of Eosinophil Leucocytes of Goat. I. Granule Development in the Bone Marrow. J. Comp. Path., *86*:183, 1976.

Austen, K.F.: Homeostasis of Effector Systems Which Can Also Be Recruited for Immunologic Reaction. J. Immunol., *121*:793, 1978.

Baehner, R.L., and Johnston, R.B., Jr.,: Metabolic and Bactericidal Activities of Human Eosinophils. Brit. J. Haematol., *20*:277, 1971.

Bainton, D.F., and Farquhar, M.G.: Segregation and Packaging of Granule Enzymes in Eosinophilic Leukocytes. J. Cell. Biol., *45*:54, 1970.

Bartelmez, S.H., et al.: Differential Regulation of Spleen Cell-Mediated Eosinophil and Neutrophil-Macrophage Production. Blood, *55*:489, 1980a.

Bartlemez, S.H., et al.: Stimulation of Eosinophil Production in Vitro by Eosinophilopoietin and Spleen-Cell-Derived Eosinophil Growth-Stimulating Factor. Blood, *56*:706, 1980b.

Bass, D.A.: Reproduction of the Eosinopenia of Acute Infection by Passive Transfer of a Material Obtained from Inflammatory Exudate. Infect. Immun., *15*:410, 1977.

Bass, D.A.: The Functions of Eosinophils. Ann. Intern. Med., *91*:120, 1979.

Bass, D.A., and Szejda, P.: Mechanisms of Killing of Newborn Larvae of Trichinella spiralis by Neutrophils and Eosinophils: Killing by Generators of Hydrogen Peroxide in Vitro. J. Clin. Invest., *64*:1558, 1979.

Bass, D.A., et al.: Eosinopenia of Acute Infection. Production of Eosinopenia by Chemotactic Factors of Acute Inflammation. J. Clin. Invest., *65*:1265, 1980a.

Bass, D.A., et al.: Comparison of Human Eosinophils from Normals and Patients with Eosinophilia. J. Clin. Invest., *66*:1265, 1980b.

Basten, A., and Beeson, P.B.: Mechanism of Eosinophilia. II. Role of the Lymphocyte. J. Exp. Med., *131*:1288, 1970.

Beeson, P.B.: Role of the Eosinophil. *In* Immunology of the Gut. Ciba Found. Symp., *92*:203, 1976.

Beeson, P.B., and Bass, D.A.: The Eosinophil. *In* Major Problems in Internal Medicine. Smith, L.H., Jr., ed. Vol. 14. W.B. Saunders, Philadelphia, 1977.

Boyer, M.H., et al.: Mechanism of Eosinophilia. III. Suppression of Eosinophilia by Agents Known to Modify Immune Responses. Blood, *36*:458, 1970.

Butterfield, J.H., et al.: The Eosinophil Leukocyte: Maturation and Function. Clin. Immunol. Rev., *2*:187, 1983/84.

Butterworth, A.E.: The Eosinophil and Its Role in Immunity to Helminth Infection. Curr. Top. Microbiol. Immunol., *77*:127, 1977.

Butterworth, A.E., and David, J.R.: Eosinophil Function. New Eng. J. Med., *304*:154, 1981.

Capron, M., et al.: Tetrapeptides of the Eosinophil Chemotactic Factor of Anaphylaxis (ECFA) Enhance Eosinophil Fc Receptors. Nature, *289*:71, 1981a.

Capron, M., et al.: Fc Receptors for IgE on Human and Rat Eosinophils. J. Immunol., *126*:2087, 1981b.

Carper, H.A., and Hoffman, P.L.: The Intravascular Survival of Transfused Canine Pelger-Hüet Neutrophils and Eosinophils. Blood, *27*:739, 1966.

Clark, R.A.F., and Kaplan, A.P.: Eosinophil Leucocytes: Structure and Function. Clin. Haematol., *4*:635, 1975.

Clark, R.A.F., et al.: Histamine-Dependent Inhibition and Enhancement of Eosinophil Migration to Chemotactic Agents. J. Allergy Clin. Immunol., *57*:191, 1976.

Clark, R.A.F., et al.: The Nature of Histamine Control of Eosinophil Localization. *In* Leukocyte Chemotaxis. Galli, J.I., and Quie, P.G., eds. Academic Press, New York, 1978.

Cline, M.J.: Metabolism of the Circulating Leukocyte. Physiol. Rev., *45*:674, 1965.

Cline, M.J.: The White Cell. Harvard Univ. Press, Cambridge, Mass., 1975.

Cline, M.J., et al.: Phagocytosis by Human Eosinophils. Blood, *32*:922, 1968.

Cohen, N.S., et al.: Mechanisms of Leukocyte Production and Release. VIII. Eosinophil and Neutrophil Kinetics in Rats. Scand. J. Haematol., *4*:339, 1967.

Cohen, S., and Ward, P.A.: In Vitro and in Vivo Activity of a Lymphocyte and Immune Complex-Dependent Chemotactic Factor for Eosinophils. J. Exp. Med., *133*:133, 1971.

Crowley, J.P., and Myers, T.J.: Humoral and Cellular Studies of Eosinophils in Reactive and Myeloproliferative Syndromes with Marked Eosinophilia. Amer. J. Clin. Pathol., *79*:301, 1983.

Dahl, R., and Venge, P.: Blood Eosinophil Leucocyte and Eosinophil Cationic Protein: In Vitro Study of the

Influence of β2 Adrenergic Drugs and Steroid Medication. Scand. J. Resp. Dis., *59*:319, 1978.

Dale, D.C., et al.: Eosinophil Kinetics in the Hypereosinophilic Syndrome. J. Lab. Clin. Med., *87*:487, 1976.

David, J.R., et al.: Mechanisms of the Interaction Mediating Killing of Schistosoma mansoni by Human Eosinophils. Amer. J. Trop. Med. Hyg., *29*:842, 1980.

DeChatelet, L.R., et al.: Oxidative Metabolism of the Human Eosinophil. Blood, *50*:525, 1977.

DeChatelet, L.R., et al.: Comparison of Intracellular Bactericidal Activities of Human Neutrophils and Eosinophils. Blood, *52*:609, 1978.

De Simone, C., et al.: Human Eosinophils and Parasitic Diseases: Light and Electron Microscopy Evidence of Interaction with Sheep Erythrocytes. Clin. Exp. Immunol., *39*:247, 1980.

Dessein, A.J., et al.: IgE Antibody and Resistance to Infection. I. Selective Suppression of the IgE Antibody Response in Rats Diminishes the Resistance and the Eosinophil Response to Trichinella spiralis Infection. J. Exp. Med., *153*:423, 1981.

Dessein, A.J., et al.: Enhancement of Human Blood Eosinophil Cytotoxicity by Semi-Purified Eosinophil Colony Stimulating Factor(s). J. Exp. Med., *156(1)*:90, 1982.

Doy, T.G., and Hughes, D.L.: The Role of the Thymus in the Eosinophil Response of Rats Infected with Fasciola hepatica. Clin. Exp. Immunol., *47*:74, 1982.

Duffus, W.P.H., et al.: Killing of Juvenile Fasciola hepatica by Purified Bovine Eosinophil Proteins. Clin. Exp. Immunol., *40*:336, 1980.

Durack, D.T., et al.: Neurotoxicity of Human Eosinophils. Proc. Natl. Acad. Sci., *76*:1443, 1979.

Durack, D.T., et al.: Purification of Human Eosinophil-Derived Neurotoxin. Proc. Natl. Acad. Sci., *78*:5165, 1981.

Earl, P.R., and Carranza, B.A.: Leukocyte Differential Counts of the Mexican Goat. Int. Goat Sheep Res., *1*:6, 1980.

Fabiani, O., et al.: Ultrastructural Observations on the Eosinophil Granulocytes in the Blood of the Horse. Annali della Facolta di Medicina Veterinaria di Pisa, *33*:347, 1980.

Fauci, A.S., et al.: The Idiopathic Hypereosinophilic Syndrome. Clinical, Pathophysiologic and Therapeutic Considerations. Ann. Int. Med., *97*:78, 1982.

Frickhofen, N., and Konig, W.: Subcellular Localization of the Eosinophil Chemotactic Factor (ECF) and its Inactivator in Human Polymorphonuclear Leucocytes (PMN). Immunology, *37*:111, 1979.

Frigas, E., et al.: Cytotoxic Effects of the Guinea Pig Eosinophil Major Basic Protein on Tracheal Epithelium. Lab Invest., *42*:35, 1980.

Frigas, E., et al.: Elevated Levels of the Eosinophil Granule Major Basic Protein in the Sputum of Patients with Broncheal Asthma. Mayo Clin. Proc., *56*:345, 1981.

Gartner, I.: Separation of Human Eosinophils in Density Gradients of Polyvinylpyrrolidone-Coated Silica Gel (Percol). Immunology, *40*:133, 1980.

Gleich, G.J.: The Eosinophil: New Aspects of Structure and Function. J. Allergy Clin. Immunol., *60*:73, 1977.

Gleich, G.J., et al.: Cytotoxic Properties of the Eosinophils Major Basic Protein. J. Immunol., *123*:2925, 1979a.

Gleich, G.J., et al.: The Effect of Antiserum to Eosinophils on Susceptibility and Acquired Immunity of the Guinea Pig to Trichostrongylus colubriformis. Immunology, *37*:873, 1979b.

Godlowski, Z.Z.: Allergy and Anaphylaxis as Metabolic Error. Vol 1. Dual Response to Antigenic Stimulation. Immuno-Metabolic Press, Chicago, 1962.

Goetzl, E.J., et al.: Production of a Low Molecular Weight Eosinophil Polymorphonuclear Leukocyte Chemotactic Factor by Anaplastic Squamous Cell Carcinoma of Human Lung. J. Clin. Invest., *61*:770, 1978.

Grant, J.B.F., and Hudson, G.: A Quantitative Study of Blood and Bone Marrow Eosinophils in Severe Hypoxia. Brit. J. Haematol., *17*:121, 1969.

Grauer, G.F., and Riedesel, D.H.: Pulmonary Infiltrates with Eosinophilia. Iowa State Univ. Vet., *39*:92, 1977.

Green, B.M., and Colley, D.G.: Eosinophils and Immune Mechanisms. II. Partial Characterization of the Lymphokine Eosinophil Stimulator Promoter. J. Immunol., *113*:910, 1974.

Grewal, A.S., and Babiuk, L.A.: Introduction: Isolation and Surface Marker Studies on Bovine Eosinophils. J. Immunol. Methods, *25*:65, 1979.

Grover, W.H., et al.: Phagocytic Properties of Isolated Human Eosinophils. J. Immunol., *121*:718, 1978.

Hardy, W., and Anderson, R.: Hypereosinophilic Syndromes. Ann. Int. Med., *68*:1220, 1968.

Henderson, W.R., et al.: Eosinophil Peroxidase-Induced Mast Cell Secretion. J. Exp. Med., *152*:265, 1980.

Hendrick, M.: A Spectrum of Hypereosinophilic Syndromes Exemplified by Six Cats with Eosinophilic Enteritis. Vet. Pathol., *18*:188, 1981.

Henry, W.L., et al.: Relationship between Actions of Adrenocortical Steroids and Adreno-Medullary Hormones in the Production of Eosinopenia. Amer. J. Physiol., *174*:455, 1953.

Herion, R.M., et al.: Eosinophil Kinetics in Two Patients with Eosinophilia. Blood, *36*:361, 1970.

Hicks, R., and West, G.B.: Adrenal Cortical Hormones and the Formation of Histamine and 5-Hydroxytryptamine. Nature, *181*:1342, 1958.

Honsinger, R.W., Jr., et al.: The Eosinophil and Allergy: Why? J. Allergy Clin. Immunol., *49*:142, 1972.

Hudson, G.: Quantitative Study of the Eosinophil Granulocytes. Semin. Hematol., *5*:166, 1968.

Hung, K.S.: Electron Microscopic Observations on Eosinophil Leukocyte Granules in Dog Blood. Anat. Rec., *174*:165, 1972.

Hungerford, G.F.: Role of Histamine in Producing the Eosinophilia of Magnesium Deficiency. Blood, *16*:1642, 1964.

Hungerford, G.F., and Karson, E.F.: The Eosinophilia of Magnesium Deficiency. Blood, *16*:1642, 1960.

Jain, N.C.: Peroxidase Activity in Leukocytes of Some Animal Species. Folia Haematol., *88*:297, 1967.

Jenkins, D.J., and Rickard, M.D.: Haematological and Serological Data from Dogs Raised Worm-free and Nonspecifically Infected with Helminths. Aust. Vet. J., *61*:309, 1984.

Jong, E.C., and Klebanoff, S.J.: Eosinophil-Mediated Mammalian Tumor Cell Cytotoxicity: Role of the Peroxidase System. J. Immunol., *124*:1949, 1980.

Jong, E.C., et al.: Toxic Effect of Eosinophil Peroxidase on Schistosomula of Schistosoma mansoni. Clin. Res., *27*:479A, 1979.

Jong, E.C., et al.: Bactericidal Activity of Eosinophil Peroxidase. J. Immunol., *124*:1378, 1980.

Jorg, A., et al.: A Rapid and Simple Method for the Isolation of Pure Eosinophilic Leukocytes from Horse Blood. Experientia, *34*:1654, 1978.

Jorg, A., et al.: Leukotriene Generation by Eosinophils. J. Exp. Med., *155*:392, 1982.

Kater, L.A., et al.: Isolation of Human Eosinophil Phospholipase D. J. Clin. Invest., *57*:1173, 1976.

Kay, A.B.: Functions of the Eosinophil Leucocyte. Brit. J. Haematol., *33*:313, 1976.

Kay, A.B.: The Role of the Eosinophil. J. Allergy Clin. Immunol., *64*:90, 1979.

Kay, N.E., et al.: Eosinophilic Pelger-Huët anomaly with Myeloproliferative Disorder. Amer. J. Clin. Pathol., *60*:663, 1973.

Kipnis, T.L., et al.: Cell-Mediated Cytotoxicity to Trypanosoma cruzi. II. Antibody-Dependent Killing of Bloodstream Forms by Mouse Eosinophils and Neutrophils. Amer. J. Trop. Med. Hyg., *30*:47, 1981.

Klebanoff, S.J., et al.: Functional Studies on Human Peritoneal Eosinophils. Infect. Immun. *17*:167, 1977.

Koch-Weser, J.: β-Adrenergic Blockade and Circulating Eosinophils. Arch. Intern. Med., *121*:255, 1968.

Kovacs, A.: Antihistamine Effect of Eosinophil Leukocytes. Experientia, *6*:349, 1950.

Kowanatzki, E., et al.: Histamine Induces Release of an Eosinophil Immobilizing Factor from Mononuclear Cells. Nature, *270*:67, 1977.

Kurosawa, M., et al.: Prostaglandin-Induced Eosinopenia in Splenectomized Rats. J. Allergy Clin. Immunol., *62*:33, 1978.

Mahmoud, A.A.F.: Antieosinophil Serum. Amer. J. Trop. Med. Hyg., *26:(Nov. suppl.)*:151, 1977.

Mahmoud, A.A.F., and Austen, K.F.: The Eosinophils in Health and Disease. New York, Grune & Stratton, 1981.

Mahmoud, A.A.F., et al.: A Role for the Eosinophil in Acquired Resistance to Schistosoma mansoni Infection as Determined by Antieosinophil Serum. J. Exp. Med., *142*:805, 1975.

Mahmoud, A.A.F., et al.: Eosinophilopoietin: A Circulating Low Molecular Weight Pepide-Like Substance Which Stimulates the Production of Eosinophils in Mice. J. Clin. Invest., *60*:675, 1977.

Maxwell, M.H.: Electron Microscopy of Developing and Mature Eosinophils in the Bone Marrow of the Fowl and the Duck. Histochem. J., *10(1)*:63, 1978.

McKean, J.R., et al.: Schistosoma mansoni: Complement and Antibody Damage, Mediated by Human Eosinophils and Neutrophils, in Killing Schistosomula in Vitro. Exp. Parasitol., *51*:307, 1981.

McLaren, D.J., et al.: Ultrastructural Evidence for Complement and Antibody-Dependent Damage to Schistosomula of Schistosoma manosoni by Rat Eosinophils in Vitro. Parasitology, *77*:313, 1978.

Mesipun, I., and Kanarik, V.: Changes in the Eosinophil Concentration in the Blood and Lymph of Sheep. Izv. Akad. Nauk. Eston. SSR. Biol., *17*:243, 1968.

Mickenberg, I.D., et al.: Bactericidal and Metabolic Properties of Human Eosinophils. Blood, *39*:67, 1972.

Migler, R., et al.: Human Eosinophilic Peroxidase: Role in Bactericidal Activity. Blood, *51*:445, 1978.

Miller, A.M., et al.: Spleen Cells from Schistosoma mansoni–Infected Mice Produce Diffusible Stimulator of Eosinophilopoiesis in Vivo. Nature, *262*:586, 1976.

Moncol, D.J., and Batte, E.G.: Peripheral Blood Eosinophilia in Porcine Ascariasis. Cornell Vet., *57*:96, 1967.

Nafstad, H.J., and Nafstad, I.: An Electron Microscopic Study of Normal Blood and Bone Marrow in Pigs. Path. Vet., *5*:451, 1968.

Navarrete, J.V., and Petit, D.W.: Induced Eosinopenia and Basophilopenia by "Free" Steroids in Vitro. Acta Endocrinol., *39*:135, 1962.

Oghiso Y., and Fujiwara, K.: Eosinophil Chemotactic Activity of Muscle Extracts from Bovine Eosinophil Myositis. Jap. J. Vet. Sci., *40*:41, 1978.

Olsen, E.G.J., et al.: The Pathogenesis of Löeffler's Endomyocardial Disease and Its Relationship to Endomyocardial Fibrosis. Prog. Cardiology, *8*:281, 1980.

Olsson, I., and Venge, P.: The Role of the Eosinophil Granulocyte in the Inflammatory Reaction. Allergy, *34*:353, 1979.

Osgood, E.E.: Culture of Human Marrow: Length of Life of Neutrophils, Eosinophils and Basophils of Normal Blood as Determined by Comparative Cultures of Blood and Sternal Marrow from Healthy Persons. J. Amer. Vet. Med. Ass., *109*:933, 1937.

Osgood, E.E.: The Number and Distribution of Human Hemic Cells. Blood, *9*:1141, 1954.

Parmley, R.T., and Spicer, S.S.: Cytochemical and Ultrastructural Identification of a Small Type Granule in Late Human Eosinophils. Lab. Invest., *30*:557, 1974.

Parrillo, J.E., and Fauci, A.S.: Human Eosinophils: Purification and Cytotoxic Capabilities of Eosinophils from Patients with Hypereosinophilic Syndrome. Blood, *51*:457, 1978.

Peterson, A.P., et al.: Glucocorticoid Receptors in Normal Human Eosinophils: Comparison with Neutrophils. J. Allergy and Clin. Immunol., *68*:212, 1981.

Pimenta, P.F.P., et al.: Ultrastructural Localization of Basic Proteins in Cytoplasmic Granules of Rat Eosinophils and Mast Cells. J. Histochem. Cytochem., *28*:238, 1980.

Pincus, S.H.: Comparative Metabolism of Guinea Pig Peritoneal Exudate Neutrophils and Eosinophils. Proc. Soc. Exp. Biol. Med., *163*:482, 1980.

Pincus, S.H., et al.: Metabolic Heterogeneity of Eosinophils from Normal to Hypereosinophilic Patients. Blood, *58(6)*:1175, 1981.

Pincus, S.H., et al.: Superoxide Production by Eosinophil: Activation by Histamine. J. Invest. Dermatol., *79(1)*:53, 1982.

Presentey, B.: Cytochemical Characterization of Eosinophils with Respect to Newly Discovered Anomaly. Amer. J. Clin. Pathol. *51*:451, 1969.

Presentey, B., et al.: Eosinophilic Leukemia: Morphological, Cytochemical, and Electron Microscopic Studies. J. Clin. Pathol., *32*:261, 1979.

Presentey, B., et al.: Genesis, Ultrastructure and Cytochemical Study of the Cat Eosinophil. Anat. Rec., *196*:119, 1980.

Pritchard, D.I., and Eady, R.P.: Eosinophilia in Athymic Nude (rnu/rnu) Rats: Thymus Independent Eosinophilia. Immunology, *43*:409, 1981.

Reed, C.E., et al.: Reduced Effect of Epinephrine on Circulating Eosinophils in Asthma and after β-Adrenergic Blockade or Bordetella pertussis vaccine. J. Allergy, *46*:90, 1970.

Riddle, J., and Barnhart, M.I.: Eosinophil as a Source for Profibrinolysin in Acute Inflammation. Blood, *25*:776, 1965.

Roth, J.A., and Kaeberle, M.L.: Isolation of Neutrophils and Eosinophils from the Peripheral Blood of Cattle and Comparison of Their Functional Activities. J. Immunol. Methods, *45*:153, 1981.

Round, M.C.: The Course of the Naturally Acquired Helminth Infections of Horses Given Regular Anthelminthic Treatment. Res. Vet. Sci., *9*:583, 1968.

Rytomaa, T.: Organ Distribution and Histochemical

Properties of Eosinophil Granulocytes in Rats. Acta Pathol. Scand., *50*:1, 1960.

Sabag, N., et al.: Cortisol-Induced Migration of Eosinophil Leukocytes to Lymphoid Organs. Experientia, *34*:666, 1978.

Schaefer, H.E., et al.: Spezifische Mikrogranula in Eosinophilen. Acta Haematol., *50*:92, 1973.

Schatz, M., et al.: Eosinophils and Immunologic Lung Disease. Med. Clin. North Amer., *65*:1055, 1981.

Scott, D.W., et al.: Hypereosinophilic Syndrome in a Cat. Feline Practice, *15*(1):22, 1985.

Seeman, P.M., and Palade, G.E.: Acid Phosphatase Localization in Rabbit Eosinophils. J. Cell Biol., *34*:745, 1967.

Sher, R., and Wadee, A.A.: Eosinophil Degranulation. Monitoring by Interference Contrast Microscopy. Inflammation, *5*:37, 1981.

Somorin, A.O., et al.: Correlation of Blood Eosinophils and Total Serum IgE. Cent. Afr. J. Med., *24*:255, 1978.

Spry, C.J.F.: Mechanism of Eosinophilia. V. Kinetics of Normal and Accelerated Eosinopoiesis. Cell Tissue Kinet., *4*:351, 1971a.

Spry, C.J.F.: Mechanism of Eosinophilia. VI. Eosinophil Mobilization. Cell Tissue Kinet., *4*:365, 1971b.

Spry, C.J.F.: Eosinophilia and Allergic Reactions to Drugs. Clin. Haematol., *9*:521, 1980.

Spry, C.J.F., et al.: The Cardiotoxicity of Eosinophils. Postgrad. Med. J., *59*:147, 1983.

Sullivan, T.J.: The Role of Eosinophils in Inflammatory Reactions. Prog. Hematol., *11*:65, 1979.

Sundell, B.: Variations in the Level of Eosinophils in the Wall of the Small Intestine of the Rat. Acta Endocrinol. *28(Suppl. 39)*, 1958.

Swingle, W.W., et al.: Prevention of Eosinopenia in Adrenalectomized Dogs by an Antihistaminic Drug. Amer. J. Physiol., *182*:256, 1955.

Tai, P.-C., and Spry, C.J.F.: The Mechanisms Which Produce Vacuolated and Degranulated Eosinophils. Brit. J. Haematol., *49*:219, 1981.

Tebbi, C.K., et al.: The Role of Eosinophils in Granulopoiesis. I. Eosinophilia in Neutropenic Patients. J. Pediatr., *96*:575, 1980.

Thevathason, O.I., and Gordon, A.S.: Adrenocortical-Medullary Interactions on the Blood Eosinophils. Acta Haematol., *19*:162, 1958.

Townsend, J., and Duffus, P.H.: Trypansoma theileri: Antibody Dependent Killing by Purified Populations of Bovine Leucocytes. Clin. Exp. Immunol., *48*:289, 1982.

Tsuda, S., et al.: Induction of T Cell–Independent Eosinophilia in Mice with Polymyxin B and Schistosoma Injection. Lab. Invest., *43*:495, 1980.

Turnbull, L.W., and Kaur, A.B.: Eosinophils and Mediators of Anaphylaxis: Histamine and Imidazole Acetic Acid as Chemotactic Agents for Human Eosinophil Leucocytes. Immunology., *31*:797, 1976.

Urch, D.L., and Allen, W.R.: Studies on Fenbendazole for Treating Lung and Intestinal Parasites in Horses and Donkeys. Equine Vet. Res., *12*:74, 1980.

Vadas, M.A., et al.: A New Method for the Purification of Human Eosinophils and Neutrophils, and a Comparison of the Ability of These Cells to Damage Schistosomula of Schistosoma mansoni. J. Immunol., *122*:1228, 1979.

Valone, F.H.: Modulation of Human Neutrophil and Eosinophil Polymorphonuclear Leukocyte Chemotaxis: An Analytical Review. Clin. Immunol. Immunopathol., *15*:52, 1980.

van Dallen, R.G.: The Eosinophil: Friend or Foe? Editorial. Mayo Clin. Proc., *56*:395, 1981.

Venge, P., et al.: Enhancement of Factor XII Dependent Reactions by Eosinophil Cationic Protein. Thromb. Res., *14*:641, 1979.

Vercauteren, R.: The Properties of the Isolated Granules from Blood Eosinophils. Enzymologia, *16*:1, 1953.

Vilpo, J.A., et al.: Distribution of Tissue Eosinophil Granulocytes in Cow and Pig Organs. Scand. J. Haematol., *7*:217, 1970.

Wakelin, D., and Donachie, A.M.: Genetic Control of Eosinophils: Mouse Strain Variation in Response to Antigens of Parasite Origin. Clin. Exp. Immunol., *51*:239, 1981.

Walle, A.J., and Parwaresch, M.R.: Estimation of Effective Eosinopoiesis and Bone Marrow Eosinophils Reserve Capacity in Normal Man. Cell Tissue Kinet., *12*:249, 1979.

Walls, R.S.: Eosinophil Response to Alum Adjuvants: Involvement of T Cell in Non-Antigen-Dependent Mechanisms. Proc. Soc. Exp. Biol. Med., *156*:431, 1977.

Walls, R.S., and Beeson, P.B.: Mechanism of Eosinophilia. VIII. Importance of Local Cellular Reactions in Stimulating Eosinophil Production. Clin. Exp. Immunol., *12*:111, 1972.

Ward, P.A.: Chemotaxis of Human Eosinophils. Amer. J. Pathol., *54*:121, 1969.

Wasserman, S.I., et al.: Inactivation of Slow Reacting Substance of Anaphylaxis by Human Eosinophil Arylsulfatase. J. Immunol., *114*:645, 1975.

Wassom, D.L., et al.: Elevated Serum Levels of the Eosinophil Granule: Major Basic Protein in Patients with Eosinophilia. J. Clin. Invest., *67*:651, 1981.

Weber, A.F., et al.: Tissue Mast Cells in the Virgin Bovine Uterus during the Estrous Cycle. Cornell Vet., *40*:34, 1950.

Weil, G.J., and Chused, T.M.: Eosinophil Autofluorescence and Its Use in Isolation and Analysis of Human Eosinophils Using Flow Microfluorometry. Blood, *57(6)*:1099, 1981.

Weller, P.F., and Goetzl, E.J.: The Human Eosinophil. Roles in Host Defense and Tissue Injury. Amer. J. Pathol., *100*:793, 1980.

Wever, R., et al.: Characterization of the Peroxidase in Human Eosinophils. Eur. J. Biochem., *108*:491, 1980.

Williams, D.M., et al.: Light Microscope and Electron Microscope Alkaline Phophatase Cytochemistry of Rat Bone Marrow Leukocytes. J. Histochem Cytochem., *27*:665, 1979.

Winqvist, I., et al.: Altered Density, Metabolism and Surface Receptors of Eosinophils in Eosinophilia. Immunology, *47(3)*:531, 1982.

Wintrobe, M.M., et al.: Clinical Hematology. 8th ed. Lea & Febiger, Philadelphia, 1981.

Zeiger, R.S., et al.: Histamine Metabolism. II. Cellular and Subcellular Localization of the Catabolic Enzymes, Histaminase and Histamine Methyl Transferase, in Human Leukocytes. J. Allergy Clin. Immunol., *58*:172, 1976.

Zintzsch, I.: Behaviour of Eosinophil Granulocytes in the Pig after Complete and Partial Hypophysectomy. Arch. Exp. Vet. Med., *23*:531, 1969.

Zucker-Franklin, D.: Electron Microscopic Studies of Human Granulocytes: Structural Variations Related to Function. Semin. Hematol., *5*:109, 1968.

Zucker-Franklin, D., et al.: Atlas of Blood Cells: Function and Pathology. E.E. edi ermes Milano, 1981.

28

The Basophil and the Mast Cell

PRODUCTION AND DISTRIBUTION   756

MORPHOLOGY   757

BIOCHEMICAL COMPOSITION   760

BIOLOGIC PROPERTIES   760

FUNCTIONS   762

BASOPHIL NUMBERS IN BLOOD   764

The basophil is a numerically insignificant but functionally important leukocyte. It has been studied less than other leukocytes, probably because of its scarcity in blood. In comparison, mast cells have been studied extensively. Recently, techniques have been developed to induce blood and bone marrow basophilia in laboratory animals, to isolate basophil-enriched cell preparations and their granules, and to maintain basophils in short-term cultures. These, together with newer methods of immunologic, cytochemical, and electron microscopic analyses, are increasing our understanding of basophil leukocytes and their functional significance in relation to mast cells. It is becoming apparent from these studies that the basophil is functionally not an end-stage cell; it is capable of resynthesizing its granules and perhaps has the potential to undergo blast transformation under appropriate conditions (Dvorak et al, 1982). Reviews on the basophil and the mast cell can be found (Denburg et al., 1980b; Dvorak and Dvorak, 1975, 1979; Dvorak et al, 1983; Galli, et al., 1984; Lichtenstein et al, 1978; MacGlashan et al., 1983; Metcalfe et al., 1981; Newball et al., 1980; Orr, 1977; Wasserman, 1979; Wintroub and Soter, 1981).

PRODUCTION AND DISTRIBUTION

The blood basophil bears some morphologic resemblance to the tissue mast cell and is believed to share a similar function. It is often debated whether basophils and mast cells share a common origin or whether they are one and the same cells, acquiring different morphology under the influence of local mi-croenvironment at different locations in the body. Some observations in this regard are mentioned below.

Mast cells are widely distributed in the connective tissues and are found in close association with blood vessels. The distribution of mast cells within the tissues and organs of the body varies among different species, but in general they are present in large numbers in the skin, subcutaneous tissues, lung parenchyma, the respiratory and digestive tracts, mammary glands, serosal membranes, particularly in pleural and peritoneal cavities, mesentery, scrotum, uterus, and thymus (Graham et al., 1955; West, 1959; Wintroub and Soter, 1981). The liver of the dog and the mesentery of the chicken are especially well supplied with mast cells.

The origin of basophils and mast cells from hematopoietic stem cells has been demonstrated. Basophils are produced in the bone marrow from mitosis of basophilic promyelocytes and myelocytes and maturation through the metamyelocyte and band stages. More immature precursors and the committed stem cell responsible for their production have not been clearly defined. It is assumed that basophil production follows a pattern similar to that delineated for the neutrophil and eosinophil (Fig. 13–19), although divergent evidence has been presented regarding the origin of basophils and mast cells. Basophil precursors have been found to circulate in humans (Denburg et al., 1980a) and rats (Zucker-Franklin et al., 1981).

It is generally believed that mast cells are produced from undifferentiated mesenchymal cells in the connective tissue, particularly near the blood vessels. Evidence has been obtained, however, that indicates that tissue mast cells also originate from a precursor in the bone marrow (Kitamura et al., 1979). Based on comparative cytochemical and immunologic studies, it has been hypothesized that rat mast cells and macrophages may originate from a common precursor (Zucker-Franklin et al., 1981). Also, ultrastructural evidence has been presented for the common origin of human mast cells and basophils: distinctive "intermediate" cells possessing electron microscopic features typical of both cell types were seen in three patients with myeloproliferative disorders (Zucker-Franklin, 1980).

In short-term cultures of guinea pig basophils, it was demonstrated that basophilopoiesis is antigen-specific and requires soluble factors, called "basophilopoietin(s)," derived from splenic T-lymphocytes (Denburg et al., 1980a). Basophil myelocytes have been identified in cultures of guinea pig bone marrow, and basophil growth and differentiation have been found to occur sequentially in 7 days (Denburg et al., 1981). In cultures of guinea pig peripheral blood basophils, basophiloblasts have been found to develop (Dvorak et al., 1982). They were thought to develop from blast transformation of mature basophils; confirmation of this observation would place basophils in line with lymphocytes, which are known to undergo blastogenesis under various stimuli. Basophilic promyelocytes were distinguished from other primitive cells in human patients with chronic myelogenous leukemia (Maine et al, 1979). Rabbit basophils have been found to possess T cell antigen on their surface, implicating an ontogenic relationship between T-lymphocytes and basophils (Denburg et al., 1980a).

Myeloid production of basophils in humans is similar to that of eosinophils and neutrophils. Tritiated thymidine labeling showed that it takes about 2.5 days for the newly formed basophils to appear in the peripheral blood, with a peak at about 7 days (Muraham, et al., 1969). The half-time of circulation is also similar to that of other granulocytes—about 6 hours—and is probably lengthened in leukemia (Parwaresch, 1976). Basophils migrate into tissues probably randomly and survive for about 10–12 days (Osgood et al., 1954) In contrast, mast cells have a much longer life span; their turnover time in mice was estimated at 9–18 months (Wintrobe et al., 1981).

MORPHOLOGY

Various morphologic and biochemical features of basophils and mast cells are summarized in Table 28-1. The basophil differs from the mast cell in having a smaller size, a regular round cell shape, a multilobed nucleus, and relatively evenly distributed, less numerous granules. The tissue mast cell is larger, has a stellate or round cellular outline, possesses a round nucleus, and contains numerous granules with somewhat eccentric distribution (Plate XII-4, XXII-6). Granule size and distribution in free mast cells, which may be found in the peripheral blood and bone marrow, vary and may be very similar to those in basophils. Immature mast cells usually have smaller granules.

A typical basophil in Wright-stained film is characterized by the presence of intense reddish violet granules that invariably fill the cytoplasm and mask the lobulated nucleus. The nuclear segmentation in basophils, as in eosinophils, is less pronounced (2–3 lobes) than in neutrophils. Basophil granules are soluble in water; hence some degranulation may be evident in stained films. The number, size, and stainability of granules vary among species. For example, canine basophils have larger and fewer granules than do bovine or equine basophils, and the feline basophil granules usually stain dull orange-gray against a grayish background, in contrast to the typical reddish violet staining in other species (Plates VII-5, VII-6, VII-7).

Basophil granules stain metachromatically at low pH with certain basic dyes such as Alcian blue, toluidine blue, and aldehyde fuchsin (Ackerman, 1963; Parwaresch, 1976). This characteristic metachromasia of basophil granules, by analogy to mast cell granules, has been attributed to their large content of proteoglycans (sulfated acid mucopolysaccharides [MPS]), particularly heparin. However, recent radioisotopic studies of guinea pig basophil granules have shown that they contain mostly (85%) chondroitin sulfate and

Table 28–1.   Comparison of Features of Basophils and Mast Cells

Criterion	Basophils	Mast cells
Location	Normally in blood and bone marrow; enter tissues during allergic and inflammatory processes	Normally in perivascular connective tissues; occasionally in bone marrow; very rare in blood (abnormal)
Origin	Bone marrow; committed stem cell not yet defined	Undifferentiated mesenchymal connective tissue cell; in bone marrow, pluripotential hematopoietic cell
Mitotic potential	Absent (?)	Present
Morphology in Wright-stained films	Small, round cell; bi- or trilobed nucleus; large, less numerous, loosely packed, intense reddish violet granules often masking the nucleus; species variation in granule size and staining	Relatively large, round to ovoid or stellate cell; round or oval nucleus; large, numeorus, darkly stained granules densely packing the cytoplasm, with some eccentric distribution and covering the nucleus
Surface morphology	Many short villi and some smooth folds; "uropod" in motile cells	Prominent microvilli and long, villous processes
Granule ultrastructure	Immature granules, homogeneous; mature granules, homogeneous, coarsely or finely particulate, fibrillar, or reticulated	In most species, homogeneous; in humans, characteristic scrolls, whorls, gratings, or lattices
Granule composition and cytochemistry		
Histamine	Relatively low	Relatively high
Serotonin	Present in rats and mice	Present in rats and mice
Dopamine	?	Present in ruminants
Heparin	Variable amounts	Relatively more; species variations
Other proteoglycans	Variable amounts	Variable amounts
Alkaline phosphatase	Present or absent	Present
Acid phosphatase	Absent	Present
Acid hydrolases	Absent	Present
Peroxidase	Present in humans and rabbits	Present
Degranulation process	Slow	Fast
Generation of arachidonate metabolites	Very small quantities of SRS-A and TxB$_2$	Comparatively larger amounts
Life span in tissues	Few days	Weeks to months

dermatan sulfate and only small amounts (about 15%) of heparin (Dvorak et al, 1979; Ornstein et al., 1977). Hence metachromasia of basophil granules in the guinea pig, and perhaps in other species, may be related to sulfated proteoglycans other than heparin. The absence of reddish violet granules in mature feline basophils is perhaps indicative of little or no MPS in such granules. An occasional basophil in the blood of some cats may contain a few reddish purple granules (Plate XII-5), which probably are indicative of disturbed basophilopoiesis of unknown cause. In Wright-stained films of feline bone marrow, basophil myelocytes and metamyelocytes often exhibit two granule types (Plates V–2, XII–4): large, darkly stained, reddish purple metachromatic granules and large, lightly stained, orange-gray granules common to mature basophils in this species (Plate VII-6). The former granule type probably corresponds to primary granules, and the latter to secondary granules similar to those seen in neutrophil precursors. Basophil precursors in other species lack metachromatic granules, and early immature cells have few such granules (Church and Holgate, 1980).

In preparations of resting cells examined with the scanning electron microscope, basophils appear spherical and display conspicuous, short villi and smooth folds on their surface (Galli et al., 1981). In addition, motile basophils exhibit a narrow, villi-covered cytoplasmic area, similar to the "uropod" seen in motile neutrophils and eosinophils. The surface morphology of mast cells is variable, but is characterized by prominent microvilli and long, villous extensions of plasma membranes (Wintroub and Soter, 1981).

The ultrastructure of basophil granules is

different from that of neutrophil and eosinophil granules, and some species differences have been found. The mature granules appear as homogenous, round, oval, or angular structures at low magnification (Fig. 28–1). Ovine basophil granules show a homogeneous and coarsely or finely granular ultrastructure (Yamada and Sonoda, 1972). At higher magnification, basophil granules present an array of dense particles (human and rabbit basophils) or fibrils or lamellae (guinea pig basophils) arranged in blocks or irregular bundles depending on the granule maturity (Terry et al., 1969; Wetzel, 1970a, b). A banded pattern is seen in mature granules, and an irregular arrangement of filaments is seen in immature ones. A second, relatively minor population of smaller granules has been described in human (Hastie and Chir, 1974) and feline (Ward et al., 1972) basophils. Granule formation occurs in the Golgi complex. Small granules coalesce to form large ones, and their contents condense with granule maturation.

In contrast, mast cell granules, in all species except humans, appear as electron-dense, spheroidal structures. Human mast cells contain characteristic crystalline inclusions in the

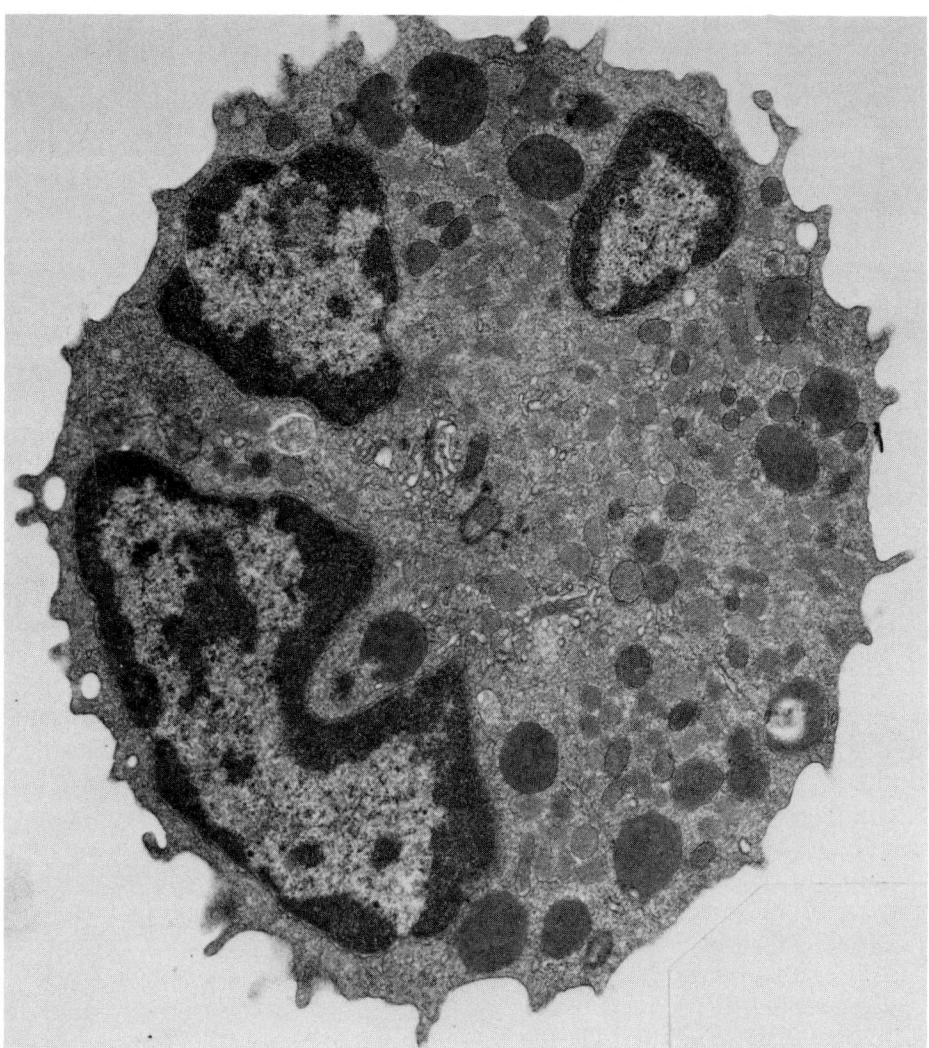

Fig. 28–1. A canine basophil containing numerous small to large, round granules of variable electron density. Central area of the cytoplasm contains profiles of the Golgi apparatus and centrioles. Some surface microvilli are also present. (×25,000).

form of scrolls, whorls, gratings, and lattices (Caulfield et al., 1980; Orr, 1977; Wintroub and Soter, 1981).

Other cytoplasmic organelles such as mitochondria, ribosomes, rough endoplasmic reticulum, and Golgi complex are poorly represented in mature basophils. Microtubules and microfilaments are present (Hastie and Chir, 1974). In some species, they characteristically display abundant cytoplasmic glycogen particles and a complex vesicular system concerned with endocytosis and exocytosis (Dvorak and Dvorak, 1975).

BIOCHEMICAL COMPOSITION

Mast cells and basophils contain a variety of preformed macro- and micro- molecular substances of biologic importance and are capable of generating several equally important substances upon immunologic and nonimmunologic stimulation (Table 28–2). These substances are released from the stimulated mast cell or basophil in a stepwise, secretory process and are important mediators of allergic, inflammatory, and cellular activities.

The composition of basophil and mast cell granules varies within and among species. Preformed histamine, heparin, hyaluronic acid, chondroitin sulfate, dermatan sulfate, serotonin, neutrophil chemotactic factor of anaphylaxis (NCF-A), and some other chemotactic factors and basophil kallikrein-like activities (BK-A) have been identified in basophil granules (Church and Holgate, 1980; Parwaresch, 1976; Wasserman, 1979; Wintroub and Soter, 1981). Histamine and heparin are probably bound to each other.

Antigen-stimulated (sensitized) basophils synthesize the slow reacting substance of anaphylaxis (SRA-A) (Austen et al., 1974), a platelet activating factor (PAF) (Austen et al., 1974; Benveniste, 1974; Benveniste et al., 1972; Parwaresch, 1976), and eosinophil chemotactic factor of anaphylaxis (ECF-A) (Czarnetzki et al., 1979). ECF-A is preformed in mast cells. Recent evidence indicates that different SRS-A represent products of arachidonic acid metabolism generated via the lipoxygenase pathway and are called leukotrienes C_1 and D (Wintroub and Soter, 1981). SRS-A, ECF, and PAF are also produced by neutrophils and monocytes. Human basophils produce much smaller amounts of arachidonic acid metabolites such as SRS-A and thromboxane B_2 than mast cells (MacGlashan et al., 1983).

Mast cells of ruminants contain histamine, serotonin, and dopamine, while avian mast cells are devoid of amines and contain only heparin (Chand and Eyre, 1978). Rat and mouse basophils contain serotonin, but human and rabbit basophils do not (Dvorak and Dvorak, 1975). The amount of histamine is estimated to be $1–2.4 \ \mu g/10^6$ cells in human basophils (Sampson and Archer, 1967), which is about 50-fold higher than that in neutrophils and eosinophils and about 20 times less than that in mast cells (Parwaresch, 1976). More recent estimates of histamine content of human mast cells are higher, $4–16 \ \mu g/10^6$ cells (MacGlashan et al., 1983). It is generally accepted that virtually all of the histamine in human blood is present in basophils, while in the rabbit about 25% is in basophils and 75% is in platelets (Dvorak and Dvorak, 1975) and in the guinea pig the respective proportion is 15% and 85% (Lett-Brown et al., 1981a). Basophils are equipped with an enzyme (histidine decarboxylase) necessary for histamine synthesis (Galli and Dvorak, 1975).

Species variations exist regarding certain enzymes demonstrable by cytochemical methods (Ackerman, 1963; Parwaresch, 1976). Mature basophil granules in humans and rabbits reveal positive staining for peroxidase but are negative for naphthol AS-D chloroacetate esterase (CAE), whereas the reverse is found in the cat (Plate X–10) and guinea pig. Mast cells are strongly positive for CAE. Basophils may reveal some alkaline phosphatase activity, but they do not stain for acid phosphatase and other acid hydrolytic enzymes. Dehydrogenases, diaphorases, and some glycogen can be demonstrated. Sudan black B reactivity is low in normal human basophils, but is high in basophils of patients with granulocytic leukemia, particularly basophilic leukemia.

BIOLOGIC PROPERTIES

Basophils and mast cells have receptors for IgE, IgG, β-adrenergic catecholamines, pros-

terium oxide) promotes histamine release (Church and Holgate, 1980). Interference with microfilament formation (by cytochalasin B) increases complement-mediated histamine release, but not that induced by allergen (Grant et al., 1977).

Some differences have been found between mast cells and basophils with regard to the process of mediator release. It is faster in mast cells than in basophils and probably involves a different mechanism. An increase in cyclic guanosine monophosphate (cGMP) increases histamine release from mast cells, while it has little or no effect on basophils (Church and Holgate, 1980). Furthermore, observations have been presented (Alm and Bloom, 1982) which imply that there is little or no correlation between histamine release from mast cells and intracellular levels of cAMP as described above.

Excellent electron microscopic studies of the degranulation phenomenon have been published in recent years (Dvorak et al., 1981a, 1981b, 1982, 1983). It has been shown that IgE-mediated degranulation of mast cells and basophils involves exocytosis and occurs in a stepwise manner. In the initial reaction, commencing within minutes, granules are stripped of their membranes and granular substances, rather than whole granules, are released to the exterior through formation of a single pore (guinea pig basophils) or multiple pores (human basophils and rat mast cells) in the plasma membrane. During this phase, the membrane bounding the granules fuses with the plasma membrane to form a degranulation sac or sacs. Next, the granules are extruded (Fig. 28–2) through the pore or pores, depending on the species.

Granule exocytosis may begin within minutes of the initial stimulation of basophils and continues for 6–36 hours and sometimes for as long as 72 hours. Subsequently, new granules are synthesized, and the cell morphology becomes normal within a few days. Species differences have been noted in this process; e.g., regranulation has not been demonstrated for human basophils. It has been shown that mouse mast cells may repeatedly undergo such cycles of degranulation and regranulation in vitro, and it is conjectured that the same may be true of basophils (Dvorak et

al., 1982). Granule lysis at the extracellular location may be rapid or slow, taking as long as three days (Dvorak et al., 1983). Slow granule lysis may contribute to the delayed phase of inflammatory reaction.

In most species, the major portion of histamine in the body is contained within mast cells and basophil leukocytes. Release of histamine and other potent vasoactive substances in the area of injury or in the target organ in the allergic response produces vasodilatation, blood stasis, and leakage of fluid into the tissues. In the sensitized animal, systemic reactions (such as urticaria, rhinitis, coughing, and dyspnea) differ, depending on the target organ, and an anaphylactic reaction ensues when massive, systemic mast cell degranulation occurs. Release of the platelet activating factor from basophils and mast cells causes aggregation of platelets and release of their vasoactive amines (Benveniste et al., 1972). Thus a chain reaction occurs which may have serious consequences. Mediator release can be modulated at various steps involving intensity of cellular stimulation, intracellular events associated with release and synthesis of various mediators, feedback control, and biodegradation of substances released (Church and Holgate, 1980). A simple, inexpensive in vitro test has been developed to determine allergic sensitivity of an individual on the basis of antigen-specific degranulation of basophils in whole blood (Benveniste, 1981; Benveniste et al., 1977).

Eosinophils are attracted chemotactically to the site of excess release of histamine in order to render the histamine inactive. The delicate balance between the functions of basophils/mast cells and eosinophils is intended first to initiate and then to modify the inflammatory response. The exudate in delayed immune reactions characteristically contains basophils and a low number of eosinophils (Wolf-Jurgensen, 1968).

It was postulated that the basophil, like the mast cell, releases its heparin in areas of inflammation in order to prevent clotting and stasis of blood and lymph (Fredericks and Moloney, 1959). The serosal linings of the body cavities contain many mast cells. Chronic bleeding into the chest or abdominal cavity is not followed by clotting of the blood.

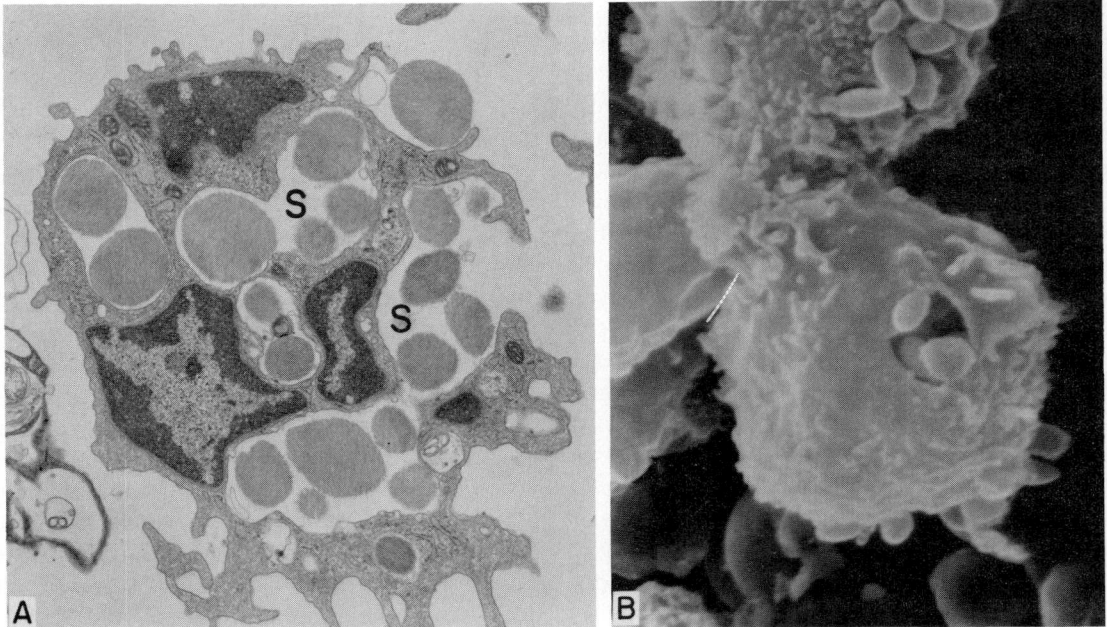

Fig. 28–2. In vitro anaphylactic degranulation of guinea pig basophils. *A,* Transmission electron photomicrograph, ×9,000. *B,* Scanning electron photomicrograph, ×10,000. (From Dvorak et al., 1981a; courtesy of *Laboratory Investigation.*)

This is no doubt a protective mechanism referable to the heparin in mast cells. Clotting of blood in body cavities would lead to formation of extensive adhesions.

Basophils facilitate triglyceride metabolism. Degranulation of basophils was observed upon feeding a meal high in fats to normal human subjects, while carbohydrates and proteins had no significant effects (Shelley and Juhlin, 1961). It was suggested that postprandial lipemia somehow acts upon the blood basophil to cause release of endogenous heparin, which then releases, and perhaps activates, lipoprotein lipase from the vascular endothelium to promote clearing of the lipemia. When heparin was injected intravenously at a level of 2 mg/kg into a dog with postprandial lipemia, the lactescence of the plasma disappeared within 15 minutes (Jasper and Jain, 1964). Lipoprotein lipase is normally found in plasma in negligible amounts.

BASOPHIL NUMBERS IN BLOOD

Basophils are rare in the peripheral blood and bone marrow. The normal range in various species is 0–300/μl of blood. They are encountered more frequently in ruminants and horses than in dogs and cats. Rabbits generally have as many as 10–15% basophils and so are a good species for research on these cells. An inverse relationship between the numbers of blood basophils and tissue mast cells is found in many species (Fulton et al., 1957). For example, the cat, mouse, hamster, rat, and fish have many mast cells, but few basophils. In contrast, the rabbit has few mast cells, but more basophils (Chapter 12). Mast cells are rare in the bone marrow and are normally absent in blood. An occasional mast cell may be seen in the peripheral blood of a severely stressed or injured animal or an animal in shock, and mastocytosis may occur in some dogs with malignant mast cell tumor. Mastocytemia (mast cells in venous blood), not associated with mast cell neoplasia, was found in 19 of 114 dogs—16 of 60 with suspected parvovirus infection, 2 with abdominal injuries, and 1 with renal insufficiency of unknown cause (Stockham et al., 1984).

The number of basophils in the blood seems to be influenced by the pituitary, adrenal, and thyroid grands and by sex hormones (Boseila, 1963), but the mechanism of the hormonal control has not been elucidated. Age and sex variations occur in humans, with slightly higher numbers in younger persons and women (Dvorak and Dvorak, 1975). A decrease in the basophil numbers is seen within 4 hours after an injection of adreno-corticotropic hormone (ACTH) into normal humans, rabbits, and pigs (Seidel et al., 1970; Wolf-Jurgensen, 1968). Injection of cortisone causes a rapid and prolonged reduction in basophil numbers, a decrease in blood histamine levels, and a time-dependent inhibition of histamine release from basophils (Dunsky et al., 1979; Saavedra-Delgado, et al., 1980; Schleimer et al., 1981). Corticosteroid-induced basopenia was seen in the cow (Table 7–12) and in physiologic stress in the horse (Fig. 6–4). A canine patient exhibiting a marked basophilia, with a long history of coughing and asthmatic attacks, responded with a 66% reduction in basophil count 7 hours after injection of ACTH (Table 28–3). The observation of a small number of basophils in some dogs with Cushing's syndrome (Appendix Cases 8 and 9) is not understandable in the light of the basopenic effect of glucocorticoids.

No significance is attached to basopenia in normal animals, while basophilia is considered significant. Basopenia has been observed during pregnancy in rabbits and in women (Selye, 1965). Basophilia has been observed in hypothyroidism, while basopenia is seen in thyrotoxicosis in humans (Boseila, 1963). Thyrotropin and L-thyroxine given to normal individuals cause a fall in circulating basophils, whereas D-thyroxine, which is metabolically inactive, causes an increase in basophils, possibly due to inhibition of the thyroid-stimulating hormone. Injection of es-trogen produces basophilia, while progesterone causes basopenia (Boseila and Uhrbrand, 1958).

Basophils have been investigated in various pathologic conditions of humans. A significantly higher number of basophils and higher blood histamine levels are found in chronic granulocytic leukemia (Jaranowski, 1972; Dvorak and Dvorak, 1975). Basophilia is also seen in humans in nephrosis, chronic liver disease, ulcerative colitis, hyperlipoproteinemia, and postprandial lipemia (Dvorak and Dvorak, 1975; Parwaresch, 1976). Increased numbers of basophils are usually seen in conditions associated with IgE production and release of lymphokines, such as allergic dermatitis, eczema, and delayed hypersensitivity reactions. In contrast, the basophil count is low in urticaria and immediately following anaphylaxis (Shelley, 1963). Anaphylactic shock in rabbits and guinea pigs results in a decrease in blood basophils. Basophils may infiltrate the skin or other organs in the absence of blood basophilia and are characteristically present in lesions of delayed type hypersensitivity (Dvorak and Dvorak, 1979).

Conditions associated with basophilia in dogs and cats are listed in Table 27–2.

Basophil numbers in blood increase following repeated intraperitoneal injection of certain antigens (heterologous serum) into guinea pigs and rabbits (Wolf-Jurgensen, 1968). This increase is preceded by substantial increases in basophil numbers in the bone marrow. Peak values occur in the bone marrow by 6–8 days and in the peripheral blood by 10–13 days (Dvorak and Dvorak, 1975). Experimental infection of guinea pigs with larvae of the tick *Dermacentor andersoni* produced basophilia in blood and bone marrow (Gordon and Allen, 1979).

Table 28–3. Effect of Natural Corticoids in Response to ACTH Administration upon the Hemogram of the Dog[a]

	Pretreatment Hemograms		ACTH Trial (Aug. 30)		30 hours Post-ACTH
	July 6	July 10	8:45 a.m.	3:45 p.m.	
WBC/μl	10,900	14,000	11,500	35,100	18,500
Neutrophils	6,540	7,700	7,360	31,064	13,135
Lymphocytes	1,800	2,450	1,725	1,228	925
Monocytes	381	1,260	805	2,457	1,850
Eosinophils	1,035	1,190	575	0	1,480
Basophils	1,144	1,330	1,035	351	1,110
Degenerated cells	—	70	—	—	—

[a]From Schalm, 1966; courtesty of *The California Veterinarian.*

REFERENCES

Ackerman, G.A.: Cytochemical Properties of the Blood Basophilic Granulocyte. Ann. N.Y. Acad. Sci., *103*:376, 1963.

Alm, P.E., and Bloom, G.D.: Cyclic Nucleotide Involvement in Histamine Release from Mast Cells: A Reevaluation. Life Sci., *30*:213, 1982.

Austen, K.F., et al.: Generation and Release of Chemical Mediators of Immediate Hypersensitivity. *In* Progress in Immunology. Vol. 2. Brent, L., and Holborow, E.J., eds. North Holland, Amsterdam, pp. 61–71, 1974.

Benveniste, J.: Platelet-Activating Factor: A New Mediator of Anaphylaxis and Immune Complex Deposition from Rabbit and Human Basophils. Nature, *249*:581, 1974.

Benveniste, J.: The Human Basophil Degranulation Test as an in vitro Method for the Diagnosis of Allergies. Clin. Allergy, *11*:1, 1981.

Benveniste, J., et al.: Leukocyte-Dependent Histamine Release from Rabbit Platelets: The Role of IgE, Basophils, and a Platelet-Activating Factor. J. Exp. Med., *136*:1356, 1972.

Benveniste, J., et al.: Detection of Immediate Hypersensitivity in Rabbits by Direct Basophil Degranulation. J. Allergy and Clin. Immunol., *59*:271, 1977.

Boseila, A.W.A.: Hormonal Influence on Blood and Tissue Basophilic Granulocytes. Ann. N.Y. Acad. Sci., *103*:394, 1963.

Boseila, A.W.A., and Uhrbrand, H.: Basophil-Eosinophil Relationship in Human Blood. Acta Endocrinol. (Copenh.), *28*:49, 1958.

Camussi, G., et al.: Release of Platelet-Activating Factor and Histamine .I. Effect of Immune Complexes, Complement and Neutrophils on Human and Rabbit Mastocytes and Basophils. Immunology., *33*:523, 1977.

Caulfield, J.P., et al.: Secretion of Dissociated Human Pulmonary Mast Cells: Evidence for Solubilization of Granule Contents before Discharge. J. Cell Biol., *85*:299, 1980.

Chand, N., and Eyre, P.: Rapid Method for Basophil Count in Domestic Fowl. Avian Dis., *22*:639, 1978.

Church, M.K., and Holgate, S.T.: The Basophil Leukocyte: Morphological, Immunological and Biochemical Considerations. Top. Rev. Haematol., *1*:65, 1980.

Czarnetzki, B., et al.: Comparison of Eosinophil Chemotactic Factor (ECF) in Basophils and Mast Cells. Monogr. Allergy, *14*:281, 1979.

Denburg, J.A., et al.: Chronic Myeloid Leukaemia: Evidence for Basophil Differentiation and Histamine Synthesis from Cultured Peripheral Blood Cells. Brit. J. Haematol., *45*:13, 1980a.

Denburg, J.A., et al.: Basophil Production. J. Clin. Invest., *65*:390, 1980b.

Denburg, J.A., et al.: Basophil Production. IV. Morphology of Basophils in Liquid Culture. Acta Haematol., *65*:114, 1981.

Dunsky, E.H., et al.: Early Effects of Corticosteroids on Basophils, Leukocyte Histamine, and Tissue Histamine. J. Allergy Clin. Immunol., *63*:426, 1979.

Dvorak, A.M., and Dvorak, H.F.: The Basophil: Its Morphology, Biochemistry, Motility, Release Reactions, Recovery, and Role in the Inflammatory Responses of IgE-Mediated and Cell-Mediated Origin. Arch. Pathol. Lab. Med., *103*:551, 1979.

Dvorak, A.M., et al.: Surface Membrane Alterations in Guinea Pig Basophils Undergoing Anaphylactic Degranulation: A Scanning Electron Microscope Study. Lab. Invest., *45*:58, 1981a.

Dvorak, A.M., et al.: Anaphylactic Degranulation of Basophilic Leukocytes. I. Fusion of Granular Membranes and Cytoplasmic Vesicles: Formation and Resolution of Degranulation Sacs. Lab. Invest., *44*:174, 1981b.

Dvorak, A.M., et al.: Anaphylactic Degranulation of Guinea Pig Basophilic Leukocytes. II. Evidence for Regranulation of Mature Basophils during Recovery from Degranulation in Vitro. Lab. Invest., *46*:461, 1982.

Dvorak, A.M., et al.: Basophil and Mast Cell Degranulation: Ultrastructural Analysis of Mechanisms of Mediator Release. Fed. Proc., *42*:2510, 1983.

Dvorak, H.F., and Dvorak, A.M.: Basophilic Leucocytes: Structure, Function and Role in Disease. Clin. Haematol., *4*:651, 1975.

Dvorak, H.F., et al.: Plasminogen Activator of Guinea Pig Basophils. Monogr. Allergy, *14*:249, 1979.

Fredericks, R.E., and Moloney, W.C.: The Basophilic Granulocyte. Blood, *14*:571, 1959.

Fulton, G.P., et al.: Humoral Aspects of Tissue Mast Cells. Physiol. Rev., *37*:221, 1957.

Galli, S.J., and Dvorak, H.F.: Histamine Synthesis by Guinea Pig Basophils in Short Term Tissue Culture. Fed. Proc., *34*:1045, 1975.

Galli, S.J., et al.: Guinea Pig Basophil Morphology in Vitro. I. Ultrastructure of Uropod-Bearing (Motile) Basophils and Modulation of Motile Structures by Serum and Substrate Effects. J. Immunol., *126*:1066, 1981.

Galli, S.J., et al.: A Cloned Cell with NK Function Resembles Basophils by Ultrastructure and Expresses IgE Receptors. Nature, *298*:5871, 1982.

Galli, S.J., et al.: Basophils and Mast Cells: Morphologic Insights into Their Biology, Secretory Patterns, and Functions. Prog. Allergy, *34*:1, 1984.

Gordon, J.R., and Allen, J.R.: The Basophil Response in Blood and Bone Marrow of Tick-Infested Guinea Pigs. Can. J. Comp. Med., *43*:380, 1979.

Graham, H.T., et al.: Mast Cells as Sources of Tissue Histamine. J. Exp. Med., *102*:307, 1955.

Grant, J.A., et al.: Complement-Mediated Release of Histamine from Human Basophils. III. Possible Regulatory Role of Microtubules and Microfilaments. J. Allergy Clin. Immunol., *60*:306, 1977.

Hastie, R., and Chir, B.: Study of the Ultrastructure of Human Basophil Leukocytes. Lab. Invest., *31*:223, 1974.

Henderson, W.R., and Kaliner, M.: Immunologic and Nonimmunologic Generation of Superoxide from Mast Cells and Basophils. J. Clin. Invest. *61*:187, 1978.

Ida, S., et al.: Enhancement of IgE-Mediated Histamine Release from Human Basophils by Immune-Specific Lymphokines. Clin. Exp. Immunol., *41*:380, 1980.

Jaranowski, J.: Basophil Leukocytes of Peripheral Blood in Various Pathological Conditions. Pol. Med. J., *11*:91, 1972.

Jasper, D.E., and Jain, N.C.: Postprandial Lipemia in Dogs. Calif. Vet., *18*:27, 1964.

Kitamura, Y., et al.: Distribution of Mast-Cell Precursors in Hematopoietic and Lymphopoietic Tissues of Mice. J. Exp. Med., *150*:482,1979.

Lett-Brown, M.A., et al.: Antigen-Induced Histamine Release from Guinea Pig Basophils. Int. Arch. Allergy Appl. Immunol., *64*-241, 1981a.

Lett-Brown, M.A., et al.: Modulation of Human Basophil

Migration in Vitro by a Soluble Factor from Virus-Stimulated Leukocytes. Clin. Immunol. Immunopathol., *20:*179, 1981b.

Lichtenstein, L.M., et al.: The Role of Basophils in Inflammatory Reactions. J. Invest. Dermatol., *71:*65, 1978.

MacGlashan, D.W., Jr., et al.: Comparative Studies of Human Basophils and Mast Cells. Fed. Proc., *42:*2504, 1983.

Magro, A.M.: Effect of Inhibitors of Arachidonic Acid Metabolism upon IgE and Non-IgE Mediated Histamine Release. J. Immunopharmacol., *4(1):*15, 1982.

Maine, J.P., et al.: Ultrastructural Localization of Peroxidase in Undifferentiated Blasts during the Blast Crisis of Chronic Granulocytic Leukemia. Brit. J. Haematol., *43:*539, 1979.

Malveaux, F.J., et al.: IgE Receptors on Human Basophils. Relationship to Serum IgE Concentration. J. Clin. Invest., *62:*176, 1978.

Marone, G., et al.: An Inhibitor of Lipooxygenase Inhibits Histamine Release from Human Basophils. Clin. Immunol. Immunopathol., *17:*117, 1980.

Marone, G., et al.: IgE-Mediated Histamine Release from Human Basophils: Differences between Antigen E- and Anti-IgE-Induced Secretion. Int. Arch. Allergy Appl. Immunol., *65:*339, 1981a.

Marone, G., et al.: Modulation of Histamine Release from Human Basophils in Vitro by Physiological Concentration of Zinc. J. Pharmacol. Exp. Ther., *217:*292, 1981b.

Metcalfe, D.D., et al.: The Mast Cell. CRC: Crit. Rev. Immunol., *3:*23, 1981.

Muraham, I, et al.: Studies on the Kinetics of Human Leukocytes in Vivo with 3H-Thymidine Autoradiography. II. Eosinophils and Basophils. Acta Haematol. Japan, *32:*384, 1969.

Newball, H.H., et al.: Basophil Mediators and Their Release, with Emphasis on BK-A. J. Invest. Dermatol., *74:*344, 1980.

Ornstein, N.S., et al.: Mucopolysaccharides Synthesized by Guinea Pig Basophil Leukocytes. Fed. Proc., *36:*1329, 1977.

Orr, T.S.C.: Fine Structure of the Mast Cell with Special Reference to Human Cells. Scand. J. Resp. Dis. Suppl., *98:*1, 1977.

Osgood, E.E., et al.: Duration of Life and the Different States of Maturation of Normal and Leukemic Leucocytes. Rev. Haematol., *9:*543, 1954.

Parwaresch, M.R.: The Human Blood Basophil: Morphology, Origin, Kinetics, Functions and Pathology. Springer-Verlag, New York, 1976.

Peters, S.P., et al.: Lipooxygenase Products Modulate Histamine Release in Human Basophils. Nature, *292:*455, 1981.

Saavedra-Delgado, A.M.P., et al.: Dose-Response Studies of the Suppression of Whole Blood Histamine and Basophil Counts by Prednisone. J. Allergy Clin. Immunol., *66:*464, 1980.

Sampson, D., and Archer, G.T.: Release of Histamine from Human Basophils. Blood, *29:*722, 1967.

Schleimer, R.P., et al.: Inhibition of Basophil Histamine Release by Anti-Inflammatory Steroids. Nature, *249:*581, 1981.

Seidel, H., et al.: Studies on Pigs. XXXIV. Determination of the Absolute Basophil Count as an Indicator of Adrenal Cortical Function. Arch. Exp. Vet. Med., *24:*349, 1970.

Selye, H.: The Mast Cells. Butterworths, Washington, D.C., 1965.

Shelley, W.B.: The Circulating Basophil as an Indicator of Hypersensitivity in Man: Experimental Novobiocin Sensitization. Arch. Dermatol., *88:*759, 1963.

Shelley, W.B., and Juhlin, L.: Degranulation of the Basophil in Man Induced by Alimentary Lipemia. Amer. J. Med. Sci., *242:*211, 1961.

Sinski, E., et al.: Immunological Investigations in Experimental Ostertagiosis in Sheep. V. Humoral Response Involving Homocytotropic Antibodies. Acta Parasitologica Polonica, *25:*373, 1978.

Stansworth, D.R.: Molecular Basis of Mast Cell Transferring Process. Monogr. Allergy, *14:*271, 1979.

Stockham, S.L., et al.: Idiopathic Mastocytemia in Dogs, Vet. Clin. Pathol., *13(1):*33, 1984.

Terry, R.W., et al.: Formation and Structure of Specific Granules in Basophilic Leukocytes of the Guinea Pig. Lab. Invest., *21:*65, 1969.

Ward, J.W., et al.: Ultrastructure of Granulocytes in the Peripheral Blood of the Cat. J. Ultrastruct. Res., *39:*389, 1972.

Wasserman, S.I.: The Mast Cell and the Inflammatory Response. *In* The Mast Cell: Its Role in Health and Disease. Pepys, J., and Edwards, A.M., eds. Pitman Medical, Turnbridge Wells, England, pp. 9–20, 1979.

West, G.B.: Tissue Mast Cells and Amines. Review article. J. Pharm. Pharmacol., *11:*513, 1959.

Wetzel, B.K.: The Fine Structure and Cytochemistry of Developing Granulocytes with Special Reference to the Rabbit. *In* Regulation of Hematopoiesis. Vol. 2. Gordon, A.S., ed. Appleton-Century-Crofts, New York, Ch. 33, p. 769, 1970a.

Wetzel, B.K.: The Comparative Fine Structure of Normal and Diseased Mammalian Granulocytes. *In* Regulation of Hematopoiesis. Vol. 2. Gordon, A.S., ed. Appleton-Century-Crofts, New York, Ch. 34, p. 819, 1970b.

Wintrobe, M.M., et al.: Clinical Hematology. 8th ed. Lea & Febiger, Philadelphia, pp. 203, 228–230, 1981.

Wintrobe, B.C., and Soter, N.A.: Biology of the Mast Cell and Its Role in Cutaneous Inflammation. Springer Semin. Immunopathol, *4:*55, 1981.

Wolf-Jurgensen, P.: The Basophilic Leukocyte. Ser. Haematol., *1(4):*45, 1968.

Yamada, Y., and Sonoda, M.: Basophils of Ovine Peripheral Blood in Electron Microscopy. Jpn. J. Vet. Sci., *34:*29, 1972.

Zucker-Franklin, D.: Eosinophil Function Related to Cutaneous Disorders. J. Invest. Dermatol., *71:*100, 1978.

Zucker-Franklin, D.: Ultrastructural Evidence for the Common Origin of Human Mast Cells and Basophils. Blood, *56:*534, 1980.

Zucker-Franklin, D. et al.: The Presence of Mast Cell Precursors in Rat Peripheral Blood. Blood, *58:*544, 1981.

29

The Monocytes and Macrophages

ORIGIN, DEVELOPMENT, AND
    KINETICS 769
  Monocytes 769
  Macrophages 770

MORPHOLOGY 771
  Monocytes and Their Precursors 771
  Macrophages, Epithelioid Cells, and Giant
    Cells 772

METABOLISM AND CYTOCHEMISTRY 775

SURFACE RECEPTORS AND
    CHEMOTAXIS 776

MONOCYTE NUMBERS IN BLOOD 777

FUNCTIONS 778
  Phagocytosis and Microbicidal Activity 779
  Scavenger Role 781
  Regulation of the Immune Response 782
  "Activated" or "Armed" Macrophages and
    Cytotoxicity 783
  Secretory Role 784

Knowledge of the origin, function, and fate of the blood monocyte and the tissue macrophage has advanced considerably during the past two decades. It has now been established that monocytes are derived from hematopoietic stem cells in the bone marrow, and shortly after entering the circulation, they migrate into various tissues and body cavities to become "fixed" or "free" macrophages.

The blood monocytes and tissue macrophages constituted important components of what until recently was called the reticuloendothelial system (RES). The term *reticuloendothelial system* was coined by Aschoff in 1924 to describe a collection of widely distributed cells capable of phagocytosis which, in addition to blood monocytes and tissue macrophages (histiocytes), included the reticular cells of the spleen and lymph nodes, reticuloendothelial cells of the lymph and blood sinuses, and the Kupffer cells of the liver.

The blood monocytes, the promonocytes and their precursors in the bone marrow, and the tissue macrophages are now considered to be components of the *mononuclear phagocyte system* (MPS). Members of the MPS include histiocytes in connective tissue; fixed and free macrophages in the lymph nodes, spleen, and bone marrow; pleural and peritoneal macrophages; Kupffer cells of the liver; alveolar macrophages; osteoclasts; and micro-

glial cells in the nervous system. Reticular cells, dendritic cells, fibroblasts and fibrocytes, and endothelial cells are excluded from the MPS.

The concept of the MPS evolved from morphologic, cytochemical, and functional similarities among various mononuclear phagocytes as well as from similarities in the origin and kinetics of these cells (van Furth et al., 1972; van Furth, 1980). However, mononuclear phagocytes at different stages of maturation have distinct morphologic features and different metabolic and functional characteristics (Territo and Cline, 1975). Furthermore, there is considerable heterogeneity with regard to these properties among macrophages from the same site, among macrophages from different sites, and between macrophages from normal animals and animals manipulated to yield "activated" macrophages (Bursuker and Goldman, 1983; Nelson, 1981). This heterogeneity is thought to originate, at least in part, from heterogeneity of monocytic precursors in the bone marrow (Bursuker and Goldman, 1983; Daems and De Bakker, 1982).

Functional aspects of the MPS have been discussed at length in a book (van Furth, 1980), and many reviews are available on various aspects of monocytes and macrophages (Davies and Bonney, 1979; Kay and Douglas, 1977; Kende, 1982; Lasser, 1983; Leder, 1967;

LoBuglio, 1970; Metcalf, 1985; Nathan, 1983; Nelson, 1981; Ogmundsottir and Weir, 1980; Roser, 1970; Shands, 1984; Sluiter et al, 1980; Takamura et al., 1984; Territo and Cline, 1975; van Furth et al., 1977; van Furth and Sluiter, 1983; Volkman, 1968, 1971; Wintrobe et al., 1981). One issue each of *Advances in Experimental Medicine and Biology* (vol. 155, 1982) and *Immunobiology* (vol. 161, nos. 3 and 4, 1982) have been devoted to topics related to the MPS.

ORIGIN, DEVELOPMENT, AND KINETICS

Monocytes

The myelogenous origin of monocytes has been amply demonstrated by in vitro and in vivo observations. These include: *(a)* studies in radiation chimeras transplanted with allogeneic bone marrow cells (Roser, 1970); *(b)* transfusion of tritiated thymidine (³HTdR)–labeled bone marrow cells into syngenic animals; *(c)* studies in x-radiated animals with partial shielding of the bone marrow; *(d)* in vitro studies with agar colonies (Bradley and Metcalf, 1966) and tissue culture transformation of bone marrow cells (Bennett and Cohn, 1966); and *(e)* cytochemical and ultrastructural studies of bone marrow cells (Leder, 1967; Nichols et al., 1971).

In vivo and in vitro studies (Metcalf, 1971; Volkman, 1971) have demonstrated that the pluripotential hematopoietic stem cell divides and gives rise to a bipotential committed stem cell, designated the colony forming unit–granulocyte, monocyte (CFU-GM), which serves as a progenitor for both neutrophils and monocytes (Fig. 13–19). The CFU-GM and its progenies, under appropriate stimulus, differentiate into either myeloblasts or monoblasts, the recognizable precursors of neutrophils and monocytes, respectively. The monoblast undergoes one mitosis and differentiates into a promonocyte, which continues to divide, at least once in the mouse and twice in humans, to produce monocytes. Monocytes and macrophages normally do not divide (van Furth and Cohn, 1968; van Furth et al., 1977), although they have been observed to proliferate in tissue culture (Greenwood, 1969).

Monocytopoiesis and monocyte kinetics have been studied in rats (Volkman and Gowans, 1965b; Whitelaw, 1966; Whitelaw et al., 1968), mice (van Furth and Cohn, 1968; van Furth et al.,1977; Volkman, 1971), and humans (Meuret et al., 1974a, 1974b; Meuret and Hoffmann, 1973) with generally similar results. A single injection of ³HTdR in rats was found to label 15–20% of promonocytes in the bone marrow and to give the following pattern of labeling in monocytes (Volkman and Gowans, 1965b): labeled monocytes started appearing in blood by the 16th hour, 18% were labeled at the 18th hour, 24% at the 36th hour, 19% at the 72nd hour, and 15% at the 120th hour. In similar experiments in mice (van Furth et al., 1970), 2 hours after a single injection of ³HTdR, about 69% of the promonocytes and 1% of the monocytes in the bone marrow and 2% of blood monocytes were labeled. The radioactivity in the promonocytes remained almost constant for 24 hours and then declined, while monocytes in marrow and blood became increasingly labeled, with peaks of 33.3% at 24 hours and 59% at 48 hours, respectively.

Kinetics of monocytopoiesis in humans were studied by observation of the appearance of labeled monocytes in blood after an injection of ³HTdR, which labeled promonocytes, and tritiated diisopropyl fluorophosphate (³HDFP), which labeled both promonocytes and monocytes (Meuret et al., 1974b). About 3% of the bone marrow cells were identified as promonocytes, with an average cell cycle time of 29 hours. Monocytes were produced over a period of 50–60 hours, from at least two mitotic divisions of promonocytes, and were released into the blood almost immediately. The minimum emergence time of monocytes from the bone marrow into the circulation is estimated at 5.7 hours in humans, 6 hours in the rat, and 2 hours in the mouse. These observations indicate that the newly formed monocytes leave the marrow rapidly and probably randomly. Thus the blood monocyte may be regarded as a relatively young cell (Volkman, 1968).

Species variations exist with regard to the bone marrow pool of monocytes. For example, in mice there are about two to three times more monocytes in the bone marrow than in the blood (Leder, 1967), while in humans there does not seem be a significant marrow reserve of monocytes (Meuret et al., 1974b).

Kinetics of blood monocytes were studied in humans after autotransfusion of blood cells labeled with ^{3}HDFP in vitro; their disappearance was followed in vivo by autoradiography of leukocyte concentrates obtained serially (Meuret and Hoffman, 1973). Monocytes were found distributed within the vascular system in the circulating and marginal pools with an average ratio of 1:3.5. Mean half-time of disappearance (T½) was 8.4 hours. The T½ reported for rodents was longer: 22 hours in mice (van Furth and Cohn, 1968) and 2 days in rats. The pattern of disappearance was exponential in humans and the mouse, but not in the rat. The turnover rate of blood monocytes was estimated at 168 million cells/day in humans and 3.6 million cells/day in rats (Whitelaw, 1966). Once in tissues, monocytes normally do not reenter blood to circulate.

The MPS of the bovine has been studied in recent years (Al-Izzi et al., 1982a, b, c). The bone marrow of healthy calves contains monoblasts, promonocytes, and monocytes in a ratio of 1:2.31:4.96. The mean production time of labeled monocytes in the bone marrow was found to be 36.4 ± 2.04 hours. The mean half-life of circulating monocytes varied between 19.5 and 22.5 hours, and their turnover rate was estimated at 5.4 ± 0.3% per hour. These values changed little in calves inoculated with *Corynebacterium parvum*.

Factors governing the rate of monocyte production in the bone marrow, release into the blood, migration into the tissues, and turnover in the tissues remain to be fully characterized. A monocytogenic factor was found in serums of rats injected with complete Freund's adjuvant into lymph nodes (Willoughby, 1967). A "factor increasing monocytopoiesis" (FIM) was demonstrated in serums of mice (van Waarde et al., 1977) and rabbits (Sluiter et al., 1980) during early phases of acute peritonitis, while a "monocytopoiesis inhibitor" (MPI), which reduced monocytopoiesis to normal level was found during the end of the inflammatory reaction (Sluiter et al., 1980; van Waarde et al., 1978). MPI also reduced the number of bone marrow

colonies and decreased the rate of macrophage proliferation in vitro.

FIM appears to be a protein with a molecular weight (MW) of 20,000 and is produced by macrophages at the site of inflammation (Sluiter et el., 1982). MPI has an MW of 50,000 or more and remains to be further characterized. FIM stimulates monoblasts to produce more promonocytes and decreases the cell cycle time of promonocytes, thereby increasing the rate of monocyte production (van Furth et al., 1977).

In vitro studies indicate that colony-stimulating factor (CSF), PGE$_2$, and lactoferrin affect mitotic activity of monocytic progenitor cells (Sluiter et al., 1982). A monocytopoietic CSF, distinct from the CSF stimulating granulocyte colonies, has been isolated from human urine (Stanley, 1975, 1976). It is a glycoprotein with an MW of 45,000–70,000 and acts at the level of committed stem cells (CFU-GM). PGE$_2$ produced by macrophages exerts inhibitory influence at this level. Lactoferrin may also affect monocytopoiesis through inhibition of PGE$_2$ production. Different subtypes of CSFs concerned with stimulation of granulopoiesis and monocytopoiesis are produced by a variety of cells including monocytes and macrophages, endothelial cells, and activated T-lymphocytes. For additional information see Chapter 13.

Macrophages

The myelogenous origin of macrophages was demonstrated in studies in which lethally irradiated rats were found to produce monocytes and macrophages after receiving ^{3}HTdR-labeled, syngenic bone marrow cells intravenously. Infusion of splenic cells in irradiated rats restored monocyte and macrophage production to a certain extent, but lymph node, thoracic duct, and thymic cells were ineffective in this regard (Volkman and Gowans, 1965a, b). In addition, mice that received whole body irradiation with hind limbs and pelvis shielded had a normal rate of macrophage production (van Furth et al., 1977). Current views on the ontogeny of macrophages have been reviewed (van Furth and Sluiter, 1983).

Tissue macrophages are far more numerous than circulating monocytes; a ratio of 50:1 is found in humans (Wintrobe et al., 1981). Such a high tissue localization of macrophages is perhaps related to their long life span, from several weeks to years (Cliff, 1966; Wintrobe et al., 1981).

Tissue macrophages are classified as fixed and free. For example, fixed macrophages are seen in the splenic sinusoids, liver (Kupffer cells), bone marrow (reticulum cells), lymph nodes, and lamina propria of the gastrointestinal tract. Free macrophages are found primarily in the pleural, peritoneal, and synovial cavities, alveolar spaces, and inflammatory sites.

The turnover of peritoneal macrophages is estimated to be low; in mice it is about 0.1%/hour which suggests a complete turnover time of nearly 6 weeks (van Furth and Cohn, 1968). Monocyte efflux into the peritoneal cavity is about 12% of the total blood monocyte influx from the bone marrow and is estimated at 1,250 cells/hour. This efflux may increase more than 10-fold during inflammatory conditions; about 50% of the circulating monocytes may leave blood to enter the peritoneal cavity (van Furth et al., 1977). Administration of corticosteroids or azathioprine in mice reduces release of monocytes from the bone marrow into the circulation and influx of monocytes into the peritoneal cavity.

Movement of macrophages from one tissue site to the other or peripheral localization to the organ of origin has been shown. For example, free macrophages of the peritoneal cavity were found to migrate via the draining lymphatics into other organs such as the spleen (Roser, 1970).

Mononuclear phagocytes accumulate at sites of acute and chronic inflammation, especially the latter. Lewis, in 1925, first clearly demonstrated that in tissue culture monocytes transform into macrophages, epithelioid cells, and multinucleated giant cells. Ebert and Florey, in 1939, reported that monocytes filled with carbon emigrated into tissues from vesicles in rabbit ear chambers and subsequently developed into active macrophages and eventually into sessile histiocytes. Cytochemical, ultrastructural, radiation chimera, and autoradiographic studies in recent years have confirmed such earlier observations (Bennett and Cohn, 1966; Cohn, 1965;

Leder, 1967; Sutton and Weiss, 1966). Formation of giant cells may involve participation of a lymphokine, "macrophage fusion factor" (Sone et al., 1981).

Thus tissue macrophages in acute and chronic inflammation are derived predominantly from the blood monocytes; the migration of circulating monocytes into tissues occurs through interendothelial regions of the venular wall (Marchesi and Florey, 1960). Although tissue macrophages normally do not divide, under certain circumstances some may arise from local proliferation (Blusse et al., 1981; Volkman, 1976).

MORPHOLOGY

Monocytes and Their Precursors

In Wright-stained blood films, monocytes are usually slightly larger than neutrophils. They characteristically display a highly pleomorphic nucleus that has been called "ameboid" because it may appear elongated or ovoid, irregularly contoured, folded, indented, horseshoe-shaped, and even slightly lobed, particularly in older cells (Plates VII–2, VII–4, VII–10). Some canine monocytes may have nuclei resembling those in young neutrophils—bands, metamyelocytes or myelocytes (see Plate VIII). The nuclear outline of a typical monocyte is usually indistinct, and nuclear chromatin is lacy or reticular and may exhibit some areas of condensation. The cytoplasm is relatively abundant, stains slightly gray blue, and appears like ground glass or foamy. A typical monocyte often contains some large vacuoles and many fine or indistinct, reddish purple (azurophilic) granules in the cytoplasm (Plate VIII–7).

Because of their nuclear shape and cytoplasmic granularity, monocytes may be confused with immature neutrophils, especially in the dog. A distinguishing feature in monocytes is that their cytoplasm always stains relatively blue with an overall darker background.

Supravital staining of monocytes with neutral red reveals numerous reddish bodies of varying sizes in the cytoplasm, often near the nucleus, and with Janus green, scattered spherical mitochondria become visible as greenish structures.

Monoblasts and promonocytes are found only in the bone marrow and are normally very rare and difficult to identify. They are found more frequently in cases of monocytic or myelomonocytic leukemia. Monoblasts may have some morphologic features of myeloblasts: a round or oval nucleus, with fine stringy chromatin and one or more nucleoli, and a small amount of moderate to deep blue cytoplasm. An undulated or clefted nuclear outline, when evident, is a distinguishing characteristic of monoblasts, although such a nucleus may be found, rarely, in a myeloblast (Plates VIII–1, VIII-2, XXIV–1 through XXIV–4).

Promonocytes typically have a large nucleus with moderate to deep indentations or undulations, fine chromatin, and a distinct or indistinct nucleolus. The cytoplasm is relatively abundant, less basophilic, and often agranular. The cytoplasmic outline may be uneven due to the presence of some pseudopods and vacuoles (Plate VIII–3).

Monocytes examined with the scanning electron microscope reveal many broad surface ruffles and irregular, ridge-like profiles, occasionally forming arch-shaped structures (Burkhardt, 1980). These structures correspond to broad and long filamentous surface projections seen on monocytes examined with the transmission electron microscope.

The ultrastructure of developing monocytes of the rabbit, guinea pig, and human has been described (Nichols et al., 1971). Canine monocytes have an ultrastructure similar to that of human monocytes (Sonoda and Kobayashi, 1970). Characteristics of bovine macrophage colonies (Al-Izzi et al., 1982c) and caprine monocytes (Liggitt, 1983) in culture have been described.

A brief description of electron microscopic features follows:

The *monoblast* is difficult to distinguish from the myeloblast. Its round to oval nucleus has dispersed chromatin and one or more nucleoli. The cytoplasm is scant and contains many ribosomes, polyribosomes, scattered profiles of rough endoplasmic reticulum (RER) many rod-shaped mitochondria, and a small Golgi complex.

The *promonocyte* has an irregular and indented nucleus. Its cytoplasm is abundant and contains numerous polyribosomes, a well-developed Golgi complex, and few cisternae of RER. A distinguishing feature of promonocytes and monocytes is the presence of some bundles of microfilaments near the nucleus. Many homogeneous and dense granules of varying size and shape are seen in the cytoplasm and appear to originate from the Golgi complex (Nichols et al., 1971). The RER, Golgi complex, and the granules are peroxidase-positive. The granules also react for arylsulfatase and acid phosphatase. Thus they appear to be primary granules or lysosomes. These granules are small and less numerous than those in promyelocytes.

The *monocyte* (Fig. 29–1) is smaller than the promonocyte and has a smaller nucleus and more abundant cytoplasm. The nucleus may be horseshoe shaped or lobed, shows dense chromatin condensation along the nuclear membrane, and may contain a small nucleolus. The cytoplasm contains a well-developed Golgi complex, many polyribosomes (but less than in promonocytes), many granules of varying size and shape, some vesicles, and a few cisternae of RER. Cessation of peroxidase-positive granule formation is indicated by the absence of peroxidase reaction in the RER and Golgi complex. However, formation of some peroxidase-negative granules has been observed in human monocytes (Bainton, 1976). Thus human monocytes contain both peroxidase-positive and peroxidase-negative granules.

Macrophages, Epithelioid Cells, and Giant Cells

Free macrophages are found primarily in body tissues and occasionally in bone marrow. They form a component of inflammatory exudates in body cavities, but are normally absent from blood. However, in certain diseases, e.g., subacute endocarditis, monocyte activation may occur in circulation, and cells resembling macrophages may be found in the peripheral blood (Wintrobe et al., 1981) (Plate VIII–10).

Morphologic, cytochemical, and metabolic characteristics of macrophages vary considerably depending on their maturity, site of origin, environmental conditions, and degree

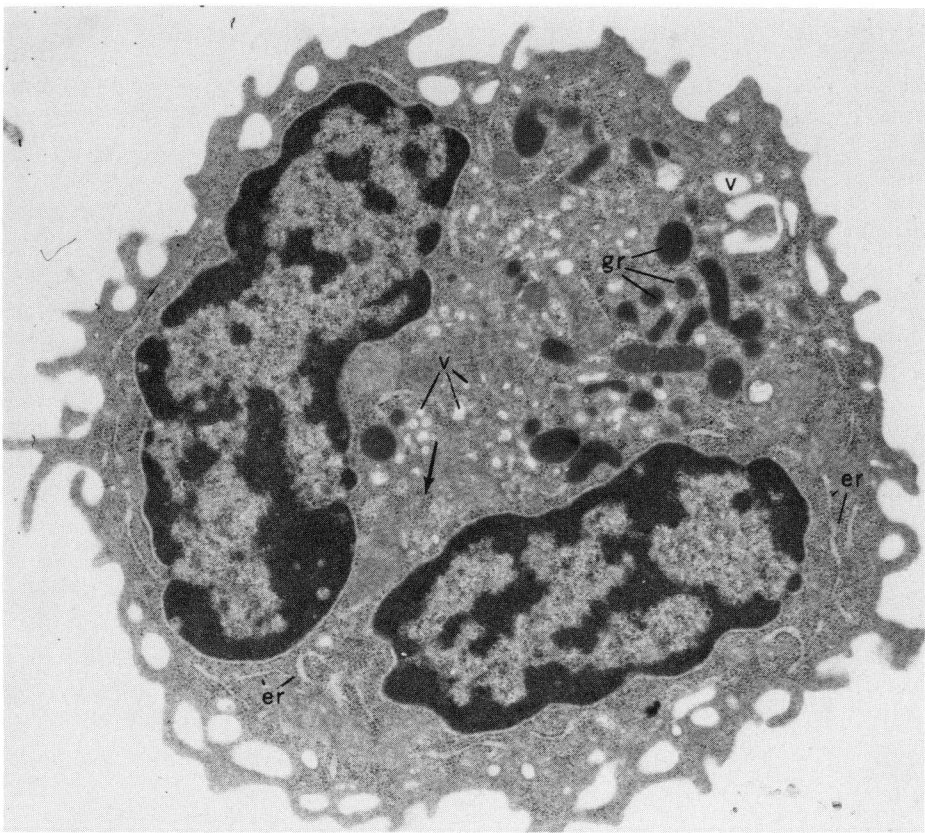

Fig. 29–1. Canine monocyte having many lysosomal granules *(gr)*, several small to large vesicles *(v)*, abundant ribosomes *(arrow)*, and prominent rough endoplasmic reticulum *(er)*, especially along the cell periphery. This cell also presents many microvillus-like projections along the cellular outline. The nucleus appears bilobed and shows heavy areas of chromatin condensation. ×17,500.

of stimulation (Cline, 1975). Generally macrophages have an oval, indented, or elongated nucleus with spongy chromatin, several prominent nucleoli, and a distinct nuclear membrane. Their cytoplasm is abundant, stains sky blue to pink to reddish, and contains many coarse, azurophilic granules or vacuoles of varying sizes, mitochondria, bundles of microfilaments and microtubules near the nucleus, scattered RER, and a well-developed Golgi complex. The presence of digestive cytoplasmic inclusions varies with the activity of the macrophage.

Macrophages in recently formed exudate resemble blood monocytes, while in older exudate they have a different structure (Nichols et al., 1971). Macrophages in peritoneal exudate collected 96 hours after induction of inflammation lack primary granules, but contain a more active Golgi complex, an increased amount of RER, many mitochon-

dria, and many digestive vacuoles of varying sizes (Fig. 29–2). The number and content of lysosomes is influenced by the stage of cellular maturation, location, and activity of the cell (Territo and Cline, 1975).

Alveolar macrophages are described to be of three distinct types and have unique biochemical properties such as high aerobic metabolism (Cohan and Cline, 1971). Ultrastructural differences have been found between macrophages of newborn and adult mice (Hardy et al., 1976) and between peritoneal and alveolar macrophages of germfree rats (Leake and Heise, 1967). Bovine alveolar macrophages are peroxidase-negative, stain strongly for nonspecific esterase, have receptors for IgG and complement, and are capable of mitosis in vitro (McGuire and Babiuk, 1982).

Macrophages have been defined according to their source or manner of procurement for

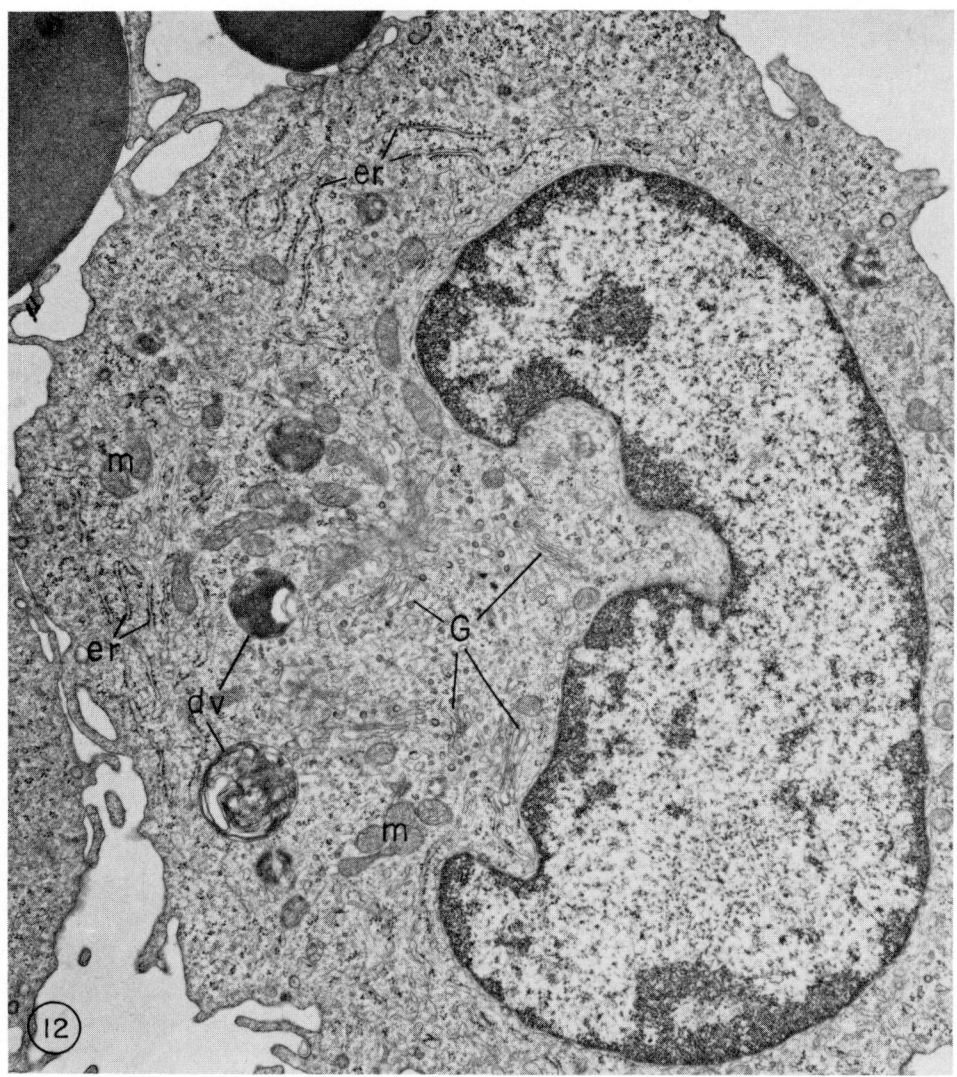

Fig. 29–2. Rabbit macrophage taken from a 96-hr peritoneal exudate. Numerous digestive vacuoles (dv) varying in size and content are present, but no secretory granules are evident. The Golgi complex (G) is large and contains numerous vesicles, many of which are coated. Rough ER (er) is moderately abundant, and mitochondria (m) are numerous. (×12,000). (From Bainton, 1980; courtesy of Elsevier/North-Holland.)

experimental work (Morahan, 1980; van Furth, 1980). *Resident (normal) macrophages* are cells obtained from a particular anatomic site in the absence of an exogenous or endogenous inflammatory stimulus. These cells show peroxidase-activity in the RER and the nuclear membrane. *Exudate macrophages* are cells present in an exudate. These originate from blood monocytes and have most of their characteristics, including peroxidase activity. *Exudate-resident (transitional) macrophages* are cells with characteristics in common with those of monocytes and resident macro-

phages. Peroxidase activity at the electron microscope level helps their identification. *Activated macrophages* are macrophages with enhanced (new or preexisting) functional activity that has been induced by any stimulus. *Elicited or evoked macrophages* are cells obtained after experimental procedures resulting in accumulation of macrophages at a particular anatomic site. This last term does not necessarily imply a morphologic or functional alteration in macrophages.

Epithelioid cells are larger than monocytes. They have an oval or indented nucleus with condensed chromatin and two to four nucleoli. The cytoplasm is abundant and contains microfilaments, numerous vacuoles, small vesicles in concentric rows, and relatively more organelles (free ribosomes, polyribosomes, mitochondria) than are present in macrophages. Epithelioid cells exhibit active protein synthesis and are highly phagocytic.

Giant cells are formed by fusion of macrophages or epithelioid cells or by amitotic division of monocytes. Differentiation of the mononuclear cells into macrophages, epithelioid cells, and giant cells has been observed in vitro and in vivo (see Wintrobe et al., 1981, for references). Monocytes have been observed to fuse and form giant cells in response to a soluble factor elaborated by antigen-stimulated T-lymphocytes (Postlelhwaite et al., 1982). Giant cells contain multiple nucleoli, multiple Golgi complexes, prominent mitochondria, numerous microfilaments, and large, clear cytoplasmic vacuoles. They have a few or no lysosomes, yet they are extremely rich in hydrolytic enzymes.

METABOLISM AND CYTOCHEMISTRY

The principal source of energy in monocytes and tissue macrophages is anaerobic glycolysis. However, metabolic activity of macrophages is dependent on several factors (Kay and Douglas, 1977), which include:

(a) Stage of cellular maturation. Glucose metabolism and protein synthesis increase with maturation through various stages, e.g., from promonocyte to monocyte to macrophage stage.

(b) Specific tissue location. Peritoneal macrophages utilize glucose primarily by anaerobic glycolysis, while alveolar macrophages use it primarily by oxidative metabolism because they have more mitochondria and higher succinic dehydrogenase and cytochrome oxidase activities (Simon et al., 1977). In addition, alveolar macrophages do not exhibit an increase in oxygen consumption following phagocytosis.

(c) Cellular activation. "Activated" macrophages have increased metabolic activities; both glycolysis and the hexose monophosphate pathways are increased.

(d) Endocytosis. Phagocytosis by peritoneal macrophages is followed by an increase in anaerobic glycolysis, while pinocytosis is dependent on aerobic glycolysis. Inhibitors of glycolysis depress phagocytosis by monocytes and tissue macrophages, inhibitors of oxidative metabolism decrease phagocytosis by alveolar macrophages, and inhibitors of oxidative metabolism or protein synthesis interfere with pinocytosis (Axline, 1970; Cline, 1975).

The differentiation of monocytes into macrophages in vivo and in vitro is accompanied by increases in the cell size, protein content, surface receptor expression, glucose utilization, lactate production, pinocytotic and phagocytic activities, enzyme synthesis, lysosome formation, number of mitochondria, activities of hydrolytic enzymes, and lipid droplets. However, there is an apparent reduction in the capacity to produce H_2O_2 and superoxide radicals (Nakagawara et al., 1981).

Cytochemical characteristics of blood monocytes have been compared with those of other leukocytes (Jain, 1970; Leder, 1967), and some species differences may be found (Table 33–1). Slight peroxidase, arylsulfatase, β-glucuronidase, and acid phosphatase activities are demonstrated in monocytes. With the light microscope, some monocytes appear peroxidase-positive (Plates X–5, X–6) and others peroxidase-negative, but both peroxidase-positive (primary) and peroxidase-negative (secondary) granules may be seen in monocytes examined with the electron microscope (van der Rhee et al., 1977). Monoblasts are usually negative or have a weak peroxidase activity in the RER and nuclear envelope, while promonocytes usually show a slightly positive peroxidase reaction in the RER, Golgi complex, and primary granules and catalase activity in secondary granules.

Macrophages are generally peroxidase-negative, but some may be peroxidase-positive depending on their stage of differentiation and environmental conditions. Resident and early exudate macrophages have peroxidase-positive nuclear envelope, RER, and granules, whereas macrophages from sites of chronic inflammation are peroxidase-negative and so are epithelioid cells and multinucleated giant cells. Giant cells are rich in microperoxisomes, which are highly catalase-positive; epithelioid cells have some microperoxisomes and slight catalase activity.

Monocytes characteristically reveal a positive cytoplasmic staining for nonspecific esterase (NSE), demonstrable with α-naphthyl acetate as a substrate, in contrast to negative staining for neutrophils. Monocytes and neutrophils contain an esterase that is demonstrable with naphthol AS-D acetate as substrate, but in monocytes this enzyme is significantly inhibited by sodium flouride treatment. In addition neutrophils contain an esterase demonstrable with naphthol AS-D chloroacetate as a substrate, while monocytes do not react for this enzyme. Staining for these esterases is helpful in characterizing myelogenous, myelomonocytic (Plate XXIV–6), and monocytic leukemias. A combined cytochemical method to demonstrate α-naphthyl acetate esterase in monocytes and chloracetate esterase in neutrophils has been developed for the differentiation of the respective cells in human blood and bone marrow preparations (Yam et al., 1971). This works well also for similar specimens from common domestic animals (Jain, 1981; see Plates X–8, X–9). This technique, in conjunction with peroxidase staining, may be useful in diagnosis of myelomonocytic and monocytic leukemias in the dog (Jain et al., 1981; Wilson and Shifrine, 1972). For additional information see Chapter 33.

Active protein metabolism directed toward production of lysosomal enzymes is present in monocytes and macrophages; the more mature the macrophage, the greater the protein synthesis (Kay and Douglas, 1977). Lysosomal enzyme synthesis and lysosome formation increase with enhanced endocytotic activity and are influenced by some other factors. Monocytes and macrophages can synthesize cholesterol as well as exchange it with that in serum. They can synthesize phospholipids and fatty acids and convert lysolecithin to lecithin for use in membrane synthesis needed after phagocytic and pinocytotic activities. DNA synthesis occurs in stimulated (immature) macrophages; ordinarily monocytes and mature macrophages do not synthesize DNA. Monocytes and macrophages synthesize RNA; interference with this synthesis diminishes pinocytosis.

SURFACE RECEPTORS AND CHEMOTAXIS

Studies on monocytes and macrophages of different species have demonstrated the presence of surface receptors for the Fc region of IgG on human (Kurlander, 1980; Morahan, 1980), canine (Lucas et al., 1980), and bovine (Birmingham and Jeska, 1980) monocytes and swine alveolar macrophages (Charley and Frenove, 1980); receptors for IgM on rabbit and human, but not on canine (Lucas et al., 1980) and bovine (Birmingham and Jeska, 1980) monocytes, and on rat and rabbit macrophages (Uher et al., 1981); receptors for IgA on human monocytes and neutrophils (Fanger et al., 1981); and receptors for IgE on human monocytes and human and murine macrophages (Melewicz et al., 1981). Receptors for complement components C3b and C3d have been found on human (Morahan, 1980), canine (Lucas et al., 1980), and bovine (Birmingham and Jeska, 1980) monocytes. Monoblasts and promonocytes also have IgG and C3 receptors (Kay and Douglas, 1977). Glucocorticoid receptors, more for dexamethasone than for cortisone, were demonstrated on human monocytes (Murakami et al., 1979) and were found to decrease with increasing maturation to the macrophage stage (van Furth, 1980). Macrophages also have receptors for other hormones, such as insulin, glucagon, and thyrotropin (van Furth, 1980).

Receptor activity may be altered by in vitro procedures, disease states (Rhodes et al., 1981), or therapy. Complement receptor activity is increased during monocyte cultures (Lucas et al., 1980) and macrophage activation by lymphokines (Griffin, 1981; Griffin and Mullinax, 1981). IgE receptors are better expressed on monocytes of patients with severe allergic states (Melewicz et al., 1981). Immune complexes were found to produce a reversible or irreversible reduction in Fc receptor activity (Kurlander, 1980). Corticosteroids may or may not inhibit binding of IgG-C3b-coated red cells to monocytes, but inhibit binding to neutrophils (Tolone et al., 1979).

Five antigens were identified on the surface of human monocytes by mouse monoclonal antibodies (Todd et al., 1981; Todd and Schlossman, 1982). The antigens Mo2 and Mo3 were specific for the monocyte-macrophage series, while Mo1 was also present on granulocytes and null cells but not on T- and B-lymphocytes, and Mo4 was also present on platelets. A platelet-specific antigen was also detected on monocytes as a result of platelet adherence to their membrane. Some monocytes and macrophages have Ia antigens on their surface membrane (Yamashita and Shevach, 1977).

Monocytes manifest active chemotaxis and particularly necrotaxis, i.e., attraction toward devitalized material (Lessin and Bessis, 1972). Complement components C3a and C5a are chemotactic for monocytes (Hausman et al., 1972; Wintrobe et al., 1981). A factor from neutrophils (Ward, 1968) and certain lymphokines are chemotactic for monocytes and macrophages (see Chapter 30). Kallikrien and a factor from corynebacteria are chemotactic for monocytes (Kay and Douglas, 1977). Levamisole increases the rate of migration of monocytes (Virolainen and Defendi, 1968).

Monocytes are highly chemotactic to lipid or lipid-rich material such as tubercle bacilli and lipopolysaccharide of Gram-negative bacteria, perhaps because of their high lipase activity compared to neutrophils and lymphocytes (Braunsteiner et al., 1964). Macrophages have been found to migrate into milk contained within the alveoli and ducts of involuting mammary glands of cows and ewes (Lee et al., 1969). There they are involved in phagocytosis of fat droplets. Macrophages can be obtained for in vitro studies from involuting mammary glands of cows or ewes a few days after intramammary inoculation of a minute amount of endotoxin (McDowell et al., 1969). Methods have been described to obtain monocyte-rich preparations from canine (Hart and Fidler, 1979; Shaw and Anderson 1984), bovine (Birmingham and Jeska, 1980; Matsson et al., 1985; Nagahata et al., 1985), caprine (Liggitt, 1983), ovine (Raghunathan et al., 1982), equine (Bruyninckx and Blancquaert, 1983), and human (Fluks, 1981; Norris, 1979) blood.

Chemotactic movement of monocytes involves solgel transformation of cytoplasm or intracellular alteration of microfilaments via contractile proteins (Kay and Douglas, 1977). Defective chemotaxis of monocytes was seen in neoplastic diseases, with reversal to normal level upon surgical removal of the tumor. Murine tumor cells were found to produce a low-MW macrophage chemotactic inhibitor factor which was active both in vitro and in vivo (Snyderman and Pike, 1976; van Furth, 1980). It was also present in blood of mice during tumor growth.

MONOCYTE NUMBERS IN BLOOD

The number of monocytes in blood is small. It depends on the number of actively dividing promonocytes and their cell cycle time in the bone marrow, positive and negative feedback regulations of monocytopoiesis, distribution of monocytes within the vascular pools, and tissue demands for monocytes. A 3–6 day periodicity is seen in the number of circulating monocytes in humans (Meuret et al., 1974a). Monocytosis and monocytopenia are seen in blood in many conditions, but the controlling mechanisms are not well known. Monocytosis is normal in the first two weeks of life of the infant (Territo and Cline, 1975).

Species differences have been observed in monocyte response to corticosteroids. For example, administration of a single dose of adrenocorticotropic hormone (ACTH) or corticosteroids characteristically produces monocytopenia in humans, mice, rats, and guinea pigs (Wintrobe et al., 1981), whereas monocytosis develops in the dog (Jasper and Jain, 1965) and a variable response is seen in the cat, horse, and cow (see Chapters 5, 6, and 7). These changes are evident within a few hours, and by the next day monocyte numbers return to normal. Monocytopenia is attributed to temporary sequestration of monocytes in the marginal pool (Fauci, 1979) and decreased release from the marrow (van Waarde et al., 1978). Monocyte production decreases with continued corticosteroid administration or endogenous release, resulting in a sustained monocytopenia. Glucocorticoids have been found to decrease production of monocyte and granulocyte colonies from committed bone marrow precursors in vitro (van Furth, 1980).

The exact mechanism of monocytosis in the dog remains to be investigated, but it is conjectured to involve shift of cells from the marginal pool or the bone marrow reserve, if present, or both. A bone marrow reserve seems to exists in the mouse, but not in humans. In species not consistently responding by monocytosis to corticosteroids, monocytopenia may develop in the initial stage of marked stress (cat, horse, and cow), but after the acute phase of the disease is over, it is followed by monocytosis. Recovery from endotoxin-induced monocytopenia is slower than that from granulocytopenia.

Acute experimental peritonitis in mice produced an increase in monocyte numbers in blood after 12 hours, with a peak at 48 hours and return to normal levels by 120 hours (van Furth et al., 1977). Administration of corticosteroids or azathioprine inhibited such a monocytosis in blood because these drugs decreased release of monocytes from the bone marrow and decreased monocytopoiesis.

During acute infection in humans half-time of disappearance of blood monocytes is slightly reduced, promonocytes in the bone marrow undergo additional mitosis with a shortened cell cycle time to increase monocyte production, and an increased number of immature cells are released into the peripheral blood (Meuret et al., 1974b). The net result is a monocytosis by 24–36 hours, probably preceded by a transient monocytopenia.

Monocytosis in subacute and chronic infection is strongly correlated with proportionate increases in total blood monocyte pool and monocyte turnover rate, while there is only a slight increase in the half-time of disappearance (maximum increase to 15 hours) and a moderate deviation in the ratio of circulating to marginal pool (Meuret and Hoffmann, 1973).

Monocytosis during inflammatory conditions is thought to result from increased elaboration of FIM from macrophages at the site of inflammation. The duration of monocytosis depends on the duration of the production of FIM. Monocytosis is seen in "high turnover" granulomas such as tuberculosis, in which marked elevation in monocytopoiesis and in-

Table 29–1. Functions of the Mononuclear Phagocyte Systems (MPS)

1. Transformation of monocytes into effector cells of the MPS, i.e., fixed and free macrophages in various tissues
2. Phagocytosis and microbicidal action, principally against intracellular bacteria, viruses, fungi, and protozoa
3. Regulation of the immune response, in both the afferent and efferent limbs of the immune response
4. Scavenger role: phagocytic removal of tissue debris, effete cells, antibody-coated cells, and other foreign material
5. Secretion of monokines, lysosomal enzymes, and other substances (see Table 29–2)
6. Cytotoxic effect against tumor cells and red cells
7. Regulation of hematopoiesis: control of granulopoiesis, monocytopoiesis, lymphopoiesis, and erythropoiesis
8. Other regulatory roles: in inflammation, tissue repair, and remodeling of embryonic tissues and bones
9. Coagulation and fibrinolysis: generation of several clotting factors and a plasminogen activator

creased release of monocytes are associated with high consumption and death of macrophages in tissues. In contrast monocytosis is not a consistent finding in "low turnover" granulomas such as sarcoidosis, in which monocytopoiesis is normal, monocyte turnover is low, and the tissue macrophage population is maintained because of the longevity of macrophages (Schmitt et al., 1977). Infections with intracellular parasites and hemolytic anemias may be associated with reactive hyperplasia of the MPS with clinically apparent increase in size of organs such as the spleen and liver.

Reactive or "toxic" monocytes have been found in humans with severe infection (Wintrobe et al., 1981). These cells may appear as macrophages (histiocytes) with highly vacuolated cytoplasm, a young-appearing nucleus with few indentations and folds, and more abundant and intensely stained cytoplasm. We have seen such cells in dogs with acute bacterial endocarditis, septicemia, and severe bacterial infections (Plate VIII–10).

FUNCTIONS

The monocyte exercises its function principally after transformation into a tissue macrophage, whether fixed or free. Several func-

Table 29–2. Secretory Products of the Mononuclear Phagocyte System[a]

Complement components
  C1 through C9, factors B and D, properdin
Antimicrobial or cytotoxic substances
  Interferons, a listericidal factor, oxygen metabolites (superoxide anion, hydroxyl radical, H_2O_2, and singlet oxygen), other cytotoxic factor(s)
Products of arachidonic acid metabolism
  Mostly PGE_2 and some PGI_2, $PGF_{2\alpha}$, thromboxane A_2, leukotrienes C_4 and D_4
Lysosomal enzymes
  Acid hydrolases (such as proteinases, esterases, lipases, sulfatases, ribonucleases, and cathepsins), neutral proteinases (such as collagenase, elastase, and plasminogen activator), arginase, and lysozyme
Factors modulating functions of other cells
  Factors enhancing growth of committed erythroid stem cells; colony stimulating factor enhancing granulopoiesis; lymphocyte activating factor for T and B cells; lymphocyte differentiation factor for T and B cells; lymphocyte proliferation inhibitor; mononuclear cell factor; angiogenic factor inducing microvascular proliferation; fibroblast cell proliferation factor; a factor enhancing collagen synthesis by fibroblasts; fibronectin as a chemotactic factor for monocytes, promoting phagocytosis, and with other activities; chemotactic factors for neutrophils and eosinophils; a platelet activating factor
Procoagulant and fibrinolytic factors
  Vitamin K–dependent clotting factors X, IX, VII, and prothrombin, factor V, and tissue thromboplastin-like activity; a plasminogen activator
Binding proteins
  Transferrin, ferritin, and transcobalamin II
Other factors
  Endogenous, pyrogen, haptoglobin, slow reacting substance, an α_2-macroglobulin (a plasma proteinase inhibitor), a growth factor promoting wound healing, a plasmin inhibitor

[a]Ascensao et al., 1981; Czarnetzki, 1980; Davies and Bonney, 1979; Feuerstein et al., 1981; Gordon, 1980; Hunninghake et al., 1980; Lasser, 1983; Morahan, 1980; Osterud et al., 1981; Rocklin et al., 1980.

tions have been well defined, while new ones are being discovered, particularly with regard to their secretory role (Tables 29–1 and 29–2).

The MPS plays important roles in defense against certain classes of mircoorganisms, especially intracellular organisms, in phagocytic removal of effete cells and cell debris, and in expression of the immune response.

Secretory activity of the MPS is associated with elaboration of monokines, endogenous pyrogen, lysosomal hydrolases, prostaglandins, and other substances of biologic importance. The MPS also plays a role in regulation of granulopoiesis through elaboration of colony-stimulating factor (CSF) and PGE (Bagby et al., 1981; Kurland et al., 1978; Metcalf, 1985; Verma et al., 1981) and in erythropoiesis by

providing a "nurse cell" in erythroblastic islands, by providing iron sequestered in macrophages, and by secreting erythroid proliferation factors (Ascensao et al., 1981; Zuckerman, 1981). Other roles are in defense against spontaneous tumors; wound repair; remodeling embryonic tissues and bones; clearing lipid from atherosclerosis lesions (Gerrity, 1981); and coagulation and fibrinolysis. Recently, macrophages were found to adhere in vitro to microfilariae of *Dipetalonema vitae* in the presence of IgE and to discharge lysosomal contents and exert lytic activity (Buaissi et al., 1981).

Phagocytosis and Microbicidal Activity

Cells of the MPS have great ability for phagocytosis and pinocytosis. The phagocytic capacity increases with progressive maturation from the promonocyte stage to the macrophage stage. Monocytes can rapidly engulf and destroy common pathogens, but at a slower rate than neutrophils (Matsson et al., 1985; Peterson et al., 1977; Verbrugh et al., 1978). They are usually called upon to handle the more difficult pathogens, especially intracellular organisms and those causing a granulomatous inflammatory response, e.g., fungi, protozoa, tubercle bacilli, and the *Listeria* and *Brucella* species. Some of these agents are capable of prolonged intracellular survival and multiplication. Infected animals may, however, display increased resistance in that the host's macrophages acquire enhanced capacity to kill the pathogen in the absence of humoral antibody. This ability was named "cellular immunity" by Mackaness (1964, 1968); see "Activated" or "Armed" Macrophages and Cytotoxicity, below.

Monocytes and fixed macrophages of the MPS may play an important role in host defense against viruses. This role is primarily attributed to production of interferon by the MPS (Acton and Myrvik, 1966). In addition, these cells have been found to remove and degrade antibody-virus complexes to low-MW metabolites (Silverstein, 1970). Macrophages have been linked to the natural resistance of cats to feline leukemia virus (FeLV) infection (Hoover et al., 1981). Macrophages from kittens were five times more susceptible to FeLV infection than those from adult cats, and temporary suppression of macrophage function markedly increased the susceptibility of adult cats to viral infection.

Current literature (see Birmingham and Jeska, 1980; Newman et al., 1980) indicates that C3 receptors enhance particle binding to blood monocytes and neutrophils, but not phagocytosis, oxidative metabolism, or degranulation. In comparison, Fc receptors induce binding as well as phagocytosis, while Fc and C3 receptors together have a synergistic action in promoting phagocytosis.

Macrophages may behave differently depending on their origin. For example, C3 receptors on "resident" peritoneal macrophages promote only particle attachment, but in "elicited" macrophages they induce phagocytosis, as do Fc receptors. Lectin-like receptors on macrophage membrane recognize sugars (glucose and galactose) in bacterial cell walls and in the membrane of tissue cells and promote binding of bacteria and tissue cells to macrophages (van Furth, 1980).

Fibronectin was found to enhance phagocytosis of inert particles by human monocytes in a dose-dependent manner (Czop et al., 1981) and phagocytic removal of blood-borne microaggregates such as immune complexes and certain activated coagulation factors by the MPS (Lanser and Saba, 1981). Fibronectin was also found to act as a chemoattractant for human monocytes, but not for neutrophils (Norris et al., 1982).

Mechanisms of bacterial killing by monocytes and macrophages are not well known, although they are thought to be generally similar to those in neutrophils. Microorganisms are ingested by active phagocytosis, but postphagocytic events differ with the organism. Within the cell, interaction of phagosomes and lysosomes also differs. For example, phagolysosome formation is not seen in *Toxoplasma gondi* and *Mycobacterium tuberculosis*, while *Leishmania donovani* survive and replicate within phagolysosomes protected from antiprotozoal lysosomal constituents because the organism secretes a polysaccharide protective factor (Jones, 1981; van Furth, 1980). Monocytes and macrophages, unlike neutrophils, can synthesize new proteins and replace expended lysosomes following active phagocytosis (Cohn, 1968). This ability arms them for a greater and continuous attack in combating infection. Various factors concerned with bactericidal, fungicidal, and cytotoxic activities of mononuclear phagocytes include peroxidase–H_2O_2–halide complex (Diamond et al., 1981), oxygen metabolites (Dyer et al., 1985; Koller and LoBuglio, 1981; Nathan, 1983; Sagone et al., 1981; van Furth, 1980), lysozyme (Lehrer, 1975), monocytin (Gershon and Olitzki, 1965), arginase (Farram and Nelson, 1980), and some other poorly defined substances (Nathan, 1983). Phagocytin and cationic proteins are absent, but lysozyme content in monocytes is higher than in neutrophils.

Products of oxygen metabolism such as superoxide anion, hydroxyl radical, singlet oxygen, and H_2O_2 are generated by mononuclear phagocytes less vigorously than in neutrophils (Reiss and Roos, 1978; van Furth, 1980), but enough to kill microorganisms, particularly in "activated" macrophages. These oxygen metabolites are produced by peritoneal macrophages, but not by alveolar macrophages whose basal oxygen consumption is high; hence it is possible that these products may not be of real functional consequence in alveolar macrophages.

The role of different oxygen metabolites in killing various intracellular bacteria and protozoa is summarized by Murray et al. (1980). This role in macrophages appears to depend on the interaction of several key factors including: *(a)* the effective triggering of the macrophage's respiratory burst, *(b)* the magnitude of the respiratory burst, *(c)* the generation of different oxygen metabolites, and *(d)* the activities of competitive intracellular mechanisms that scavenge superoxide anion and H_2O_2, e.g., superoxide dismutase (SOD), glutathione peroxidase (GP), and, more important, catalase present in macrophages and various pathogens.

A fair correlation between virulence and catalase activity, but not SOD levels, has been demonstrated for various bacteria including *Pasteurella, Brucella, Staphylococcus aureus,* and *M. tuberculosis.* Among intracellular protozoa, trypanosomes contain little or no catalase and are susceptible to H_2O_2. The related hemoflagellates, *Leishmania,* contain low levels of catalase and GP and are similarly susceptible to

H_2O_2. The extracellular protozoan *Entamoeba histolytica* has some GP, but virtually no catalase, and so is readily killed by exogenous H_2O_2. In contrast, *Toxoplasma* species are rich in catalase and GP and are, therefore, entirely resistant to concentrations of H_2O_2 that effectively kill *Trypanosoma cruzi, L. donovani,* and *E. histolytica. T. gondi* is susceptible to hydroxyl radicals and singlet oxygen, but not to superoxide anions and H_2O_2 because the last two can be degraded by its GP and catalase. Failure of monocytes and neutrophils to kill *Nocardia asteroides,* despite occurrence of the oxidative metabolic burst, was not related to SOD content of the nocardia since it was comparable to that of other bacteria (Filice et al., 1980), but catalase activity may well have been involved.

Genetic and acquired functional defects of monocytes and macrophages are associated with increased incidence of infections. Monocytes from patients with chronic granulomatous disease were found to have defective bactericidal and candidacidal activities as a result of impaired oxidative metabolism (Donowitz and Mandell, 1982; Douglas and Fundenberg, 1969; Lehrer, 1975). Heavy metals such as lead and cadmium reduce phagocytic and/or bactericidal activity of neutrophils and alveolar and peritoneal macrophages and increase susceptibility to endotoxin (Loose et al., 1978).

Corticosteroids depress bactericidal and fungicidal activities of monocytes (Thompson and van Furth, 1973). They affect functional competence of the MPS in a number of ways (reviewed by Kimberly and Ralph, 1983, and Lasser, 1983). They inhibit proliferation and maturation of monocytic precursors in the bone marrow, exudation of monocytes in inflammatory foci, and antibody- and complement-mediated phagocytosis by the MPS. In vitro, corticosteroids have been found to inhibit metabolic and cytotoxic properties of macrophages, block interaction in initiation of the immune response, and diminish expression of Fc receptors and production of neutral proteases and PGs. Corticosteroids inhibit activation of macrophages by rendering them unresponsive to lymphokines.

Scavenger Role

Macrophages normally phagocytize effete cells, undesirable cells or cellular debris, and foreign material. They phagocytize nuclei extruded from metarubricytes during erythrogenesis and defective erythrocytes in the bone marrow. Macrophages recognize changes in the red cell membrane induced by senescence, immunoglobulin coating, chemical injury, and disease states. Through their receptors for the Fc portion of IgG and complement component C3b and C3d, macrophages recognize and phagocytize antibody- and/or complement-coated red cells. This is an important mechanism for sequestration and removal of erythrocytes by the spleen in autiommune hemolytic anemia (AIHA). In addition, extracellular lysis by fixed macrophages of the spleen may also be involved in red cell destruction in AIHA (Hunt et al., 1980). Erythrophagocytosis is also a common feature in bone marrow in erythremic myelosis in cats.

After phagocytosis, the red cell membrane is digested by hydrolytic enzymes in the phagocytic vacuoles, and hemoglobin molecules are split so that globin is degraded into amino acids for reutilization, heme iron is complexed with apoferritin for storage as ferritin, and heme protoporphyrin is converted to bilirubin and transported to the liver for excretion into the bile.

Phagocytosed material may accumulate in tissue macrophages as a result of defective disposal because of genetic defects of enzyme functions, cellular overload, or other reasons (Cline, 1975). Such cells appear prominent in tissues because of their intracellular contents. In *Gaucher's disease,* glucocerebroside accumulates in macrophages due to deficiency of β-glucosidase or β-glucocerebrosidase, which catalyzes the hydrolysis of glucocerebroside. Gaucher's cells are seen in the bone marrow, spleen, and liver. These cells are large (20–60 μm) and have numerous vacuolar structures called Gaucher bodies in which tubular or fibrillar elements (aggregates of cerebroside) may be seen. These structures have high acid phosphatase activity and are probably secondary lysosomes. The principal source of cerebroside may be membranes of effete leukocytes and red cells. Gaucher's cells may be seen in other conditions, e.g., chronic myelogenous leukemia, in which the turnover rate of leukocytes is greater than normal.

In *Niemann-Pick disease*, sphingomyelin accumulates in macrophages due to deficiency of the catabolic enzyme, sphingomyelinase. Such cells are large (20-40 μm) and often vacuolated or foamy, but show no fibrils. They are also acid phosphatase–positive.

In *sea blue histiocyte syndrome*, macrophages are deficient in the enzyme sphingomyelinase; hence they accumulate cellular debris. Such pigmented sea-blue macrophages may be found in a variety of hematologic and nonhematologic conditions.

In *mucopolysaccharidosis* (Hurler's disease), macrophages, and sometimes lymphocytes in the peripheral blood, show large, reddish-purple granules known as Reilly bodies. For further description of storage diseases of the MPS, and for other references see Cline, 1975.

Regulation of the Immune Response

The MPS is intimately associated with many important pathways of immunity. Macrophages are involved in both phases of the immune response—in the afferent limb (induction of immunity to an antigen) and in the efferent limb (expression of cellular immunity). Macrophages interact with antigen through their membrane receptors. The antigen either remains bound to the macrophage membrane or is taken in, processed, and then presented by the macrophages to T- and B-lymphocytes in such a way that it stimulates them to mount an immune response. It is believed that a low-molecular-weight RNA from macrophages binds minute amounts of antigen and makes it highly immunogenic (Kay and Douglas, 1977). Such an antigen also remains bound to the macrophages for a longer period and elicits a greater immune response than soluble antigen.

Generally, a direct cell-to-cell contact is involved in macrophage-lymphocyte interaction. Lympocytes then produce antibodies or develop cell-mediated immunity specific to the paticular antigen. Certain antigens do not require macrophage participation. Particulate antigens, which are easliy phagocytosed by macrophages, act as good immunogens,

whereas soluble substances, which bypass macrophages, can induce a state of tolerance (Argyris, 1974).

The role of macrophages in humoral antibody production was initially suggested by observations that animals with readily phagocytosable particulate antigens gave a better immune response and that labeled antigen in intact animals could be found in association with macrophages and the dendritic processes of reticular cells for long periods (Territo and Cline, 1975). Further evidence was obtained in studies that revealed the following (Territo and Cline, 1975):

(a) Sublethal total body radiation inhibited the immune response of mice; this situation was reversed after administration of antigen containing macrophages and nonimmune lymphocytes.

(b) Overloading or destruction of the MPS prevented antibody synthesis.

(c) Antimacrophage serum inhibited phagocytosis by macrophages and produced an immunosuppressive effect.

(d) Pure populations of lymphocytes showed a reduced blastogenic and antibody response to specific antigens in vitro; addition of macrophages restored this response to the normal level.

(e) When substituted for intact macrophages, macrophage extract or RNA or supernatant from macrophage cultures stimulated antibody synthesis in vitro.

These findings form the basis of speculation that immunologic unresponsiveness of some newborn animals may be the result of immaturity of the MPS.

It has been shown that Ia antigens on the macrophages control in some way the recognition of antigens by the T cells (Unanue, 1980). Macrophages with Ia antigens are capable of presenting antigens to and interacting with T-lymphocytes, whereas macrophages lacking Ia antigens are incapable of doing so, although they can participate in the efferent limb of immune regulation and phagocytic activity.

The participation of macrophages in the efferent limb of immune response involves augmented phagocytosis and destruction of ingested pathogens or cells. In this respect, "activated" or "armed" macrophages exert a better phagocytic and cytotoxic effect than resting macrophages (Kay and Douglas, 1977; Ogmundsottir and Weir, 1980). See the following section for details.

In addition to these roles as antigen-presenting cells and secretors of lymphocyte activating factor in inducing immunity, macrophages also act as suppressors of cell-mediated immune responses (Bendixen et al., 1981; Nelson, 1981). Activated macrophages have been found to inhibit T cell responses, and they probably regulate suppressor T cells. These effects are probably mediated through soluble factors, especially prostaglandins (Stenson and Parker, 1980).

"Activated" or "Armed" Macrophages and Cytotoxicity

Macrophages participating in cytotoxicity have been divided into two categories of effector cells: *(a)* nonspecifically "activated" macrophages with a broader, less discriminatory cytotoxicity and *(b)* "armed" macrophages, which are actively cytotoxic against a specific target.

Metchnikoff proposed that phagocytic cells of actively immunized animals may be endowed with enhanced phagocytic and digestive activities independent of humoral antibody. This view is supported by several studies (Suter and Ramseier, 1964; Volkman, 1968). Characteristically, this state of "cellular immunity" (Mackaness 1964, 1968; Whitelaw, 1966; Whitelaw et al., 1968) or macrophage "activation" (Ogmundsottir and Weir, 1980) is induced by pathogens capable of prolonged association with the host, principally intracellular organisms, e.g., *Mycobacteria, Brucella, Listeria,* protozoa, and fungi. It has also been demonstrated that mononuclear phagocytes from mice and rabbits immunized against acute bacterial agents like *Salmonella typhimurium* and *Klebsiella pneumoniae* have enhanced functional capacity independent of measurable antibody (Miya and Marcus, 1961).

This activation of macrophages depends on the activity of T-lymphocytes (secretion of a lymphokine, macrophage activating factor; participation of a ribosomal self-duplicating RNA) as shown by studies on passive transfer of cellular response from immunized to normal animals by cells (Suter, 1961) and by in vitro exposure of macrophages to sensitized lymphocytes in the presence of the specific antigen or supernatants of such lymphocytes (Ogmundsottir and Weir, 1980; Suter and Ramseier, 1964). Several agents such as certain polyanions, endotoxin, immune complexes, and group A streptococcal cell wall material activate macrophages independent of T cell participation, probably through activation of complement by the alternate pathway. Interferons, complement, and colony-stimulating factors have also been found to activate or stimulate macrophages (Ghaffar, 1980; Kimberly and Ralph, 1983). Activation may also be influenced by disease states; e.g., monocytes from about 50% of human patients with cancer were found to have increased phagocytic activity (Ruco et al., 1980). Macrophage activation is facilitated by cyclooxgenase inhibitors and is inhibited by PGE_2 (Schnyder et al., 1981). Corticosteroids in high concentrations inhibit macrophage activation and accumulation in infective foci in the tissues (North, 1971).

Activated macrophages exhibit many morphologic, metabolic, and functional changes (Cline, 1975; Lasser, 1983; Ogmundsottir and Weir, 1980; Roubin et al., 1981). Such macrophages are larger and rich in intracellular organelles such as lysosomes and mitochondria and have an enlarged Golgi complex. Membrane ruffling is increased and pseudopods are more prominent. Metabolic activities such as protein synthesis, secretion and synthesis of lysosomal enzymes, and synthesis of monokines are increased. Activated macrophages have a greater frequency of surface receptors and exhibit increased chemotactic, pinocytotic, digestive, microbicidal, and cytotoxic activities.

Armed macrophages are actively cytotoxic against a specific target cell, e.g., tumor cells (Gordon, 1976). Macrophages from mice immunized with syngenic tumor cells show in vitro tumor cell destruction whereas, normal macrophages do not. This arming is independent of the presence of lymphocytes, but a "specific macrophage arming factor" (SMAF) produced from sensitized T cells is believed to be involved. SMAF consists of two components, a cytophilic site for macrophages and a recognition site for the target cell. The exact mechanism of cell destruction is unknown; cell to cell (macrophage to tumor cell) interaction is essential, although phagocytosis is not involved. Canine (Hart and Fidler, 1979) and bovine (Atluru and Johnson, 1982) monocytes, like human and murine monocytes, have been found to exert in vitro cytotoxicity for tumor cells.

Results of various in vivo and in vitro studies indicate that several extracellular soluble factors elaborated by activated macrophages may be involved in the tumoricidal activity. A tumor necrosis factor of 55,000 MW has been found in serums of mice and rabbits infected with *Mycobacterium bovis* BCG and given endotoxin. A neutral serine protease and H_2O_2 released by activated macrophages act synergistically to promote lysis of tumor cells. Cultured human monocytes have been found to release two cytostatic factors (MW 40,000 and 55,000) upon in vitro activation with lymphokines and endotoxin (Nissen-Meyer and Hammerstrom, 1982). Interestingly, in vitro tumoricidal activity of monocytes and macrophages was enhanced by lysozyme (LeMarbre et al., 1981) and fibronectin (Perri et al., 1982).

Secretory Role

Monocytes and macrophages have been found to secrete numerous low-MW substances after stimulation by a variety of agents such as bacteria, endotoxin, mitogens, or ionophores (Davies and Bonney, 1979; Gordon, 1980; Morahan, 1980; Nathan et al., 1980; Rocklin et al., 1980; Takamura et al., 1984). Some of these substances are referred to as "monokines" (Rocklin et al., 1980). These substances exhibit diverse biologic activities, playing roles in host defense, the inflammatory process, regulation of activities of other cells, and tissue destruction. Generally these substances are defined by their cellular functions; hence it is possible that a single factor may be given different names because of its multiplicity of functions. For example, lymphocyte activating factor (interleukin 1), an endogenous pyrogen, and serum amyloid A–inducing factor seem to be identical (Nelson, 1981).

The capacity of different populations of macrophages varies with regard to elaboration of various secretory products. For example, mouse resident macrophages release larger amounts of lysosomal hydrolases and synthesize more PGE_2 after stimulation by zymosan than elicited macrophages (Bonney et al., 1978). Agents known to increase the intracellular level of cyclic adenosine monophosphate inhibit secretory activity, while those increasing the intracellular level of cyclic guanosine monophosphate promote secretion (Foster, 1980; van Furth, 1980).

Various secretory products of the mononuclear cells are listed in Table 29–2. Histamine inhibits production of C2, C3, C4, and factor B and provides an important mechanism of controlling complement activation during the inflammatory process (Lappin et al., 1980). Oxygen metabolites are not only bactericidal, but may also damage tissue cells. Release of arginase into the environment of tumor cells may inhibit their growth. Release of some lysosomal enzymes (acid hydrolases) helps digest phagocytosed material, while others (proteinases) may break down tissue components and inflict tissue damage. Neutral proteinases are thought to play a key role in the pathogenesis of chronic inflammatory process (Gordon, 1976). Release of proteolytic enzymes from alveolar macrophages and inflammatory cells (both neutrophils and monocytes) is thought to initiate reorganization of the lung parenchyma leading to emphysema (Pierce and Senior, 1981).

Large quantities of lysosomal hydrolases are secreted in vitro by both normal and elicited macrophages independent of phagocytic stimulation (Schnyder and Baggiolini, 1978). Lysozyme is secreted in large amounts by leukemic monocytes, and determination of its level may be of diagnostic importance in monocytic and myelomonocytic leukemias (Stjernholm et al., 1972).

Mouse peritoneal macrophages have been found to produce several clotting factors, namely, the vitamin K–dependent factors VII, IX, X and prothrombin, factor V, and thromboplastin (Osterud et al., 1981). Generation of thromboplastin-like activity from human monocytes is stumulated by endotoxin, immune complexes, and C3b (van Furth, 1980).

Observations on macrophage procoagulants have been reviewed (Shands, 1984).

Plasminogen activator is secreted by activated macrophages, but not by resident macrophages, and its secretion is inhibited by corticosteroids treatment (van Furth, 1980). α_2-Macroglobulin, a plasma proteinase inhibitor, inhibits plasminogen activator.

A monocyte/macrophage-derived growth factor, similar in activity to that from platelets, may be of functional significance in wound repair during response to injury (Ross et al., 1982).

REFERENCES

Acton, J.D., and Myrvik, Q.N.: Production of Interferon by Alveolar Macrophages. J. Bacteriol., 91:2300, 1966.

Al-Izzi, S.A., et al.: Morphology and Cytochemistry of Bovine Bone Marrow Mononuclear Phagocytes. Can. J. Comp. Med., 46(2):130, 1982a.

Al-Izzi, S.A., et al.: The Kinetics of Mononuclear Phagocytes in Normal Calves and in Calves Given Corynebacterium parvum. Can. J. Comp. Med., 46(2):138, 1982b.

Al-Izzi, S.A., et al.: Proliferative, Morphologic, and Cytochemical Characteristics of Bovine Bone Marrow Macrophage Colonies in Liquid Culture. Amer. J. Vet. Res., 43:1869, 1982c.

Argyris, B.F.: Role of Macrophages in the Immune Response. In Developments in Lymphoid Cell Biology. Gottlieb, A.A., ed. CRC Press, Cleveland, ch. 2, 1974.

Ascensao, J.L., et al.: Production of Erythroid Potentiating Factor(s) by a Human Monocyte Cell Line. Blood, 57:170, 1981.

Atluru, D., and Johnson, D.W.: Bovine Monocyte-Induced Tumor Cell Cytotoxicosis. Amer. J. Vet. Res., 43:989, 1982.

Axline, S.G.: Functional Biochemistry of the Macrophage. Semin. Hematol., 7:142, 1970.

Bagby, G.C., et al.: Interaction of Lactoferrin, Monocytes and T Lymphocyte Subsets in the Regulation of Steady-State Granulopoiesis in Vitro. J. Clin. Invest., 68:56, 1981.

Bainton, D.F.: Primary Lysosomes of Blood Leukocytes. In Lysosomes in Biology and Pathology. Vol. 4. Dingle, J.T., and Dean, R.T., eds. Elsevier-North Holland, New York, 1976.

Bainton, D.F.: The Cell of Inflammation: A General View. In Handbook of Inflammation. Vol. 2. Glynn, L.E., et al., eds. Elsevier-North-Holland, New York, 1980, p. 1.

Bendixen, P.H., et al.: Inhibition of the Blastogenic Response of Peripheral Blood Mononuclear Cells to Mitogens and Antigens by Bovine Pulmonary Macrophages and Their Culture Supernatants. Res. Vet. Sci., 31:272, 1981.

Bennett, W.E., and Cohn, Z.A.: The Isolation and Selected Properties of Blood Monocytes. J. Exp. Med., 123:145, 1966.

Birmingham, J.R., and Jeska, E.L.: The Isolation, Long-Term Cultivation and Characterization of Bovine Peripheral Blood Monocytes. Immunology, 41:807, 1980.

Blusse, A., et al.: Origin and Kinetics of Pulmonary Macrophages during an Inflammatory Reaction Induced by Intravenous Administration of Heat-Killed Bacillus Calmette-Guérin. J. Exp. Med., 154:235, 1981.

Bonney, R.J., et al.: Regulation of Prostaglandin Synthesis and of Selective Release of Lysosomal Hydrolases by Mouse Peritoneal Macrophages. Biochem. J., 176:433, 1978.

Bradley, T.R., and Metcalf, D.: The Growth of Mouse Bone Marrow Cells in Vitro. Aust. J. Exp. Biol. Med. Sci., 44:287, 1966.

Braunsteiner, H., et al.: Lipase Activity in Leukocytes and Macrophages. Blood, 24:607, 1964.

Bruyninckx, W.J., and Blancquaert, A.-M.: Isolation of Horse Mononuclear Cells, Especially of Monocytes, on Isopaque-Ficoll Neutral Density Gradient. Vet. Immunol. Immunopathol., 4:493, 1983.

Buaissi, M.A., et al.: Dipetalonema vitae: Ultrastructural Study of the in Vitro Interaction between Rat Macrophages and Microfilariae in the Presence of IgE Antibody. Parasitology, 82:55, 1981.

Burkhardt, E.: Scanning and Transmission Electron Microscopy of Glass Blood Column-separated Monocytes from Mononuclear Leukocyte Suspensions of Peripheral Blood of the Chicken. J. Reticuloendothel. Soc., 28:103, 1980.

Bursuker, I., and Goldman, R.: On the Origin of Macrophages Heterogeneity: A Hypothesis. J. Reticuloendothel. Soc., 33:207, 1983.

Charley, B., and Frenove, B.: Fc and C3 Receptors on Swine Alveolar Macrophages. Res. Vet. Sci., 28:380, 1980.

Cliff, W.J.: The Behavior of Macrophages Labelled with Colloidal Carbon during Wound Healing in Rabbit Ear Chambers. J. Exp. Physiol., 51:112, 1966.

Cline, M.J.: The White Cell. Harvard Univ. Press, Cambridge, Mass., 1975.

Cohen, A.B., and Cline, M.J.: The Human Alveolar Macrophage: Isolation, Cultivation in Vitro, and Studies of Morphologic and Functional Characteristics. J. Clin. Invest., 15:1390, 1971.

Cohn, Z.A.: The Metabolism and Physiology of the Mononuclear Phagocytes. In The Inflammatory Process. Zweifach, B.J., et al., eds. Academic Press, New York, ch. 8, p. 337, 1965.

Cohn, Z.A.: The Structure and Function of Monocytes and Macrophages. Adv. Immunol., 9:163, 1968.

Czarnetzki, B.M.: Low Molecular Weight Eosinophil Chemotactic Factor (ECF) Production by Rat Peritoneal Mononuclear Phagocytes. Immunobiology, 157:62, 1980.

Czop, J.K., et al.: Augmentation of Human Monocyte Opsonin-Independent Phagocytosis by Fragments of Human Plasma Fibronectin. Proc. Natl. Acad. Sci., 78:3649, 1981.

Daems, W.T., and De Bakker, J.M.: Do Resident Macrophages Proliferate? Immunobiology, 161:204, 1982.

Davies, P., and Bonney, R.J.: Secretory Products of Mononuclear Phagocytes: A Brief Review. J. Reticuloendothel. Soc., 26:37, 1979.

Diamond, R.D., et al.: Monocyte-Mediated Serum: Independent Damage to Hyphal and Psuedohyphal Forms of Candida albicans in Vitro. J. Clin. Invest., 67:132, 1981.

Donowitz, G.R., and Mandell, G.L.: Monocyte Function in Patients with Chronic Granulomatous Disease of Childhood. Blood, 60:1151, 1982.

Douglas, S.D., and Fundenberg, H.H.: Host Defense Failure: The Role of Phagocyte Dysfunction. Hosp. Pract., 4:29, 1969.

Dyer, R.M., et al.: Production of Superoxide Anion by Bovine Pulmonary Macrophages Challenged with Soluble and Particulate Stimuli. Amer. J. Vet. Res., 46:336, 1985.

Ebert, R.H., and Florey, H.W.: The Extravascular Development of the Monocyte Observed in Vitro. Brit. J. Exp. Pathol., 20:342, 1939.

Fanger, M.W., et al.: The Specificity of Receptors for IgA on Human Peripheral Polymorphonuclear Cells and Monocytes. Cell. Immun., 60:324, 1981.

Farram, E., and Nelson, D.S.: Mechanism of Action of Mouse Macrophages as Antitumor Effector Cells: Role of Arginase. Cell. Immunol., 55:283, 1980.

Fauci, A.S.: Glucocorticoid Effects on Circulating Human Mononuclear Cells. J. Reticuloendothel. Soc., 26:727, 1979.

Feuerstein, N., et al.: Leukotrienes C4 and D4 Induce Prostaglandin and Thromboxane Release from Rat Peritoneal Macrophages. Brit. J. Pharmacol., 72:389, 1981.

Filice, G.A., et al.: Effects of Human Neutrophils and Monocytes on Nocardia asteroides: Failure of Killing despite Occurrence of the Oxidative Metabolic Burst. J. Infect. Dis., 142:432, 1980.

Fluks, A.J.: Three-Step Isolation of Human Blood Monocytes Using Discontinuous Density Gradients of Percoll. J. Immunol. Methods, 41:225, 1981.

Foster, S.J.: Cyclic Nucleotides and Cellular Secretion: Cyclic Nucleotides, Possible Intracellular Mediators of Macrophage Activation and Secretory Processes. Agents Actions, 10:556, 1980.

Gerrity, R.S.: The Role of the Monocyte in Atherosclerosis. I. Transition of Blood-Borne Monocyte into Foam Cells in Fatty Lesions. Amer. J.. Pathol., 103:181, 1981.

Gershon, Z., and Olitzki, A.L.: Monocytin: A Protecting Substance Produced by Murine Monocytes. Proc. Soc. Exp. Biol. Med., 119:32, 1965.

Ghaffar, A.: The Activation of Macrophages by Corynebacterium parvum: Effect of Anti-Complementary Agents Cobra Venum Factor and Sodium Cyanate. J. Reticuloendothel. Soc., 27:327, 1980.

Gordon, S.: Macrophage Neutral Proteinases and Chronic Inflammation. Ann. N.Y. Acad. Sci., 278:176, 1976.

Gordon, S.: Lysozyme and Plasminogen Activator: Constitutive and Induced Secretory Products of Mononuclear Phagocytes. *In* Mononuclear Phagocytes. Part 2. van Furth, R., ed. Martinus Nijhoff Publishers, The Hague, p. 1273. 1980.

Greenwood, B.: The Mitosis of Cultured Blood Monocytes from the Sheep. J. Physiol., 202:92P, 1969.

Griffin, F.M., Jr.: Role of Macrophage Fc and C3b Receptors in Phagocytosis of Immunologically Coated Cryptococcus neoformans. Proc. Natl. Acad. Sci., 78:3853, 1981.

Griffin, F.M., and Mullinax, P.J.: Augmentation of Macrophage Complement Receptor Function in Vitro. III. C3b Receptors That Promote Phagocytosis Migrate within the Phase of the Macrophage Plasma Membrane. J. Exp. Med., 154:291, 1981.

Hardy, B., et al.: Ultrastructural Differences between Macrophages of Newborn and Adult Mice. Jour. Reticuloendothel. Soc., 19:291, 1976.

Hart, I.R., and Fidler, I.J..: The Collection, Purification

and Characterization of Canine Peripheral Blood Monocytes. J. Reticuloendothel. Soc., 26:121, 1979.

Hausman, M.S., et al.: Humoral Mediators of Chemotaxis of Mononuclear Leukocytes. J. Infect. Dis., 125:595, 1972.

Hoover, E.A., et al.: Determinants of Susceptibility and Resistance to Feline Leukemia Virus Infection. I. Role of Macrophages. J. Natl. Cancer Inst., 67:889, 1981.

Hunninghake, G.W., et al.: Human Alveolar Macrophage-Derived Chemotactic Factor for Neutrophil. J. Clin. Invest., 66:473, 1980.

Hunt, J.S., et al.: Characterization of Human Erythrocyte Alloantibodies by IgG Subclass and Monocyte Interaction. Amer. J. Clin. Pathol., 74:259, 1980.

Jain, N.C.: A Comparative Cytochemical Study of Leukocytes of Some Animal Species. Folia Haematol., 94:49, 1970.

Jain, N.C.: Unpublished observations, 1981.

Jain, N.C., et al.: Clinico-Pathological Findings and Cytochemical Characterization of Myelomonocytic Leukemia in 5 Dogs. J. Comp. Pathol., 91:17, 1981.

Jasper, D.E., and Jain, N.C.: The Influence of Adrenocorticotropic Hormone and Prednisolone upon Marrow and Circulating Leukocytes in the Dog. Amer. J. Vet. Res., 26:844, 1965.

Jones, T.C.: Interactions between Macrophages and Obligate Intracellular Protozoa. Amer. J. Pathol., 102:127, 1981.

Kay, N.E., and Douglas, S.D.: Mononuclear Phagocyte: Development, Structure, Function, and Involvement in Immune Response. N.Y. State J. Med., 77:327, 1977.

Kende, M.: Role of Macrophages in the Expression of Immune Responses. J. Amer. Vet. Med. Ass., 181:1037, 1982.

Kimberly, R.P., and Ralph, P.: Endocytosis by the Mononuclear Phagocyte System and Autoimmune Disease. Amer. J. Med., 74:481, 1983.

Koller, C.A., and LoBuglio, A.F.: Monocyte-Mediated Antibody-Dependent Cell-Mediated Cytotoxicity: The Role of the Metabolic Burst. Blood, 58:293, 1981.

Kurland, J.I., et al.: Role for Monocyte-Macrophage-Derived Colony-Stimulating Factor and Prostaglandin E in the Positive and Negative Feedback Control of Myeloid Stem Cell Proliferation. Blood, 52:388, 1978.

Kurlander, R.J.: Reversible and Irreversible Loss of Fc Receptor Function of Human Monocytes as a Consequence of Interaction with Immunoglobulin G. J. Clin. Invest., 66:773, 1980.

Lanser, M.E., and Saba, T.M.: Fibronectin as a Co-Factor Necessary for Optimal Granulocyte Phagocytosis of Staphylcoccus aureus. J. Reticuloendothel. Soc., 30:415, 1981.

Lappin, D., et al.: Effect of Histamine on Monocyte Complement Production. II. Modulation of Protein Secretion, Degradation and Synthesis. Clin. Exp. Immunol., 42:515, 1980.

Lasser, A.: The Mononuclear Phagocytic System: A Review. Hum. Pathol., 14:108, 1983.

Leake, E.S., and Heise, E.R.: Comparative Cytology of Alveolar and Peritoneal Macrophages from Germfree Rats. Adv. Exp. Med. Biol., 1:133, 1967.

Leder, L.D.: The Origin of Blood Monocytes and Macrophages: A Review. Blut, 16:86, 1967.

Lee, C.S., et al.: The Importance of Macrophages in the Removal of Fat from the Involuting Mammary Gland. Res. Vet. Sci., 10:34, 1969.

Lehrer, R.I.: The Fungicidal Mechanism of Human Monocytes. I. Evidence for Myeloperoxidase-Linked and

Myeloperoxidase-Independent Candidacidal Mechanisms. J. Clin. Invest., *55*:338, 1975.

LeMarbre, P., et al.: Lysozyme Enhances Monocyte-Mediated Tumoricidal Activity: A Potential Amplifying Mechanism of Tumor Killing. Blood, *58*:994, 1981.

Lessin, L.S., and Bessis, M.: Morphology of Monocytes and Macrophages. *In* Hematology. Williams, W.J., et al., eds. McGraw-Hill, New York, ch. 86, p. 731, 1972.

Lewis, M.R.: The Formation of Macrophages, Epithelioid Cells and Giant Cells from Leukocytes in Incubated Blood. Amer. J. Pathol., *1*:91, 1925.

Liggitt, H.D.: Characterization of Short- and Long-Term Cultured Goat Peripheral Blood Monocytes. Amer. J. Vet. Res., *44*:919, 1983.

LoBuglio, A.: Factors Influencing Monocyte Development and Function. *In* Regulation of Hematopoiesis. Vol. 2. Gordon, A.S., ed. Appleton-Century-Crofts, New York, p. 983, 1970.

Loose, L.D., et al.: Influence of Cadmium on the Phagocytic and Microbicidal Activity of Murine Peritoneal Macrophages, Pulmonary Macrophages, and Polymorphonuclear Neutrophils. Infect. Immun., *22*:378, 1978.

Lucas, D.L., et al.: Characterization of Canine Monocytes in Vitro: Increased Receptor Activities for Fc, C3, and Heterologous Erythrocytes. Transplantation, *29*:133, 1980.

Mackaness, G.B.: The Immunological Basis of Acquired Cellular Resistance. J. Exp. Med., *120*:105, 1964.

Mackaness, G.B.: The Immunology of Antituberculosis Immunity. Amer. Rev. Resp. Dis., *97*:337, 1968.

Marchesi, V.T., and Florey, H.W.: Electron Micrographic Observations on the Emigration of Leucocytes. Q. J. Exp. Physiol., *45*:343, 1960.

Matsson, P., et al.: Evaluation of Flow Cytometry and Fluorescence Microscopy for the Estimation of Bovine Mononuclear Phagocytes. J. Immunol. Methods, *78*:13, 1985.

McDowell, G.H., et al.: Collection of Polymorphs and Macrophages from the Involuted Mammary Gland of the Ewe. Res. Vet. Sci., *10*:13, 1969.

McGuire, R.L., and Babiuk, L.A.: In Vitro Culture Characteristics of Bovine Alveolar Macrophages. J. Reticuloendothel. Soc., *31*:251, 1982.

Melewicz, F.M., et al.: Increased Peripheral Blood Monocytes with Fc Receptors for IgE in Patients with Severe Allergic Disorders. J. Immunol., *126*:1592, 1981.

Metcalf, D.: Transformation of Granulocytes to Macrophages in the Bone Marrow Colonies in Vitro. J. Cell. Physiol., *77*:277, 1971.

Metcalf, D.: The Granulocyte-Macrophage Colony-Stimulating Factors. Science, *229*:16, 1985.

Meuret, G., and Hoffmann, G.: Monocyte Kinetic Studies in Normal and Disease States. Brit. J. Haematol., *24*:275, 1973.

Meuret, G., et al.: Oscillation of Blood Monocyte Counts in Healthy Individuals. Cell Tissue Kinet., *7*:223, 1974.

Meuret, G., et al.: Kinetics of Human Monocytopoiesis. Blood, *44*:801, 1974.

Miya, F., and Marcus, S.: Effect of Humoral Factors on in Vitro Phagocytic and Cytopeptic Activities of Normal and "Immune" Phagocytes. J. Immunol., *86*:652, 1961.

Morahan, P.S.: Macrophage Nomenclature: Where Are We Going? J. Reticuloendothel. Soc., *27*:223, 1980.

Murakami, T., et al.: Glucocorticoid Receptor in Circulating Mononuclear Leukocytes. Endocrinology, *104*:500, 1979.

Murray, H.W., et al.: Macrophage Oxygen-Dependent Antimicrobial Activity. IV. Role of Endogenous Scavengers of Oxygen Intermediates. J. Exp. Med., *152*:1610, 1980.

Nagahata, H., et al.: Identification and Quantification of Monocytes in Bovine Cells. Jpn. J. Vet. Sci., *47*:325, 1985.

Nakagawara, A., et al.: Hydrogen Peroxide Metabolism in Human Monocytes during Differentiation in Vitro. J. Clin. Invest., *68*:1243, 1981.

Nathan, C.F.: Mechanisms of Macrophage Antimicrobial Activity. Trans. A. Soc. Trop. Med. Hyg., *77*:620, 1983.

Nathan, C.F., et al.: The Macrophage as an Effector Cell. New Eng. J. Med., *303*:622, 1980.

Nelson, D.S.: Macrophages: Progress and Problems. Clin. Exp. Immunol., *45*:225, 1981.

Newman, S.L., et al.: Development of Functional Complement Receptors during in Vitro Maturation of Human Monocytes into Macrophages. J. Immunol., *125*:2236, 1980.

Nichols, B.A., et al.: Differentiation of Monocytes, Origin, Nature, and Fate of Their Azurophil Granules. J. Cell Biol., *50*:498, 1971.

Nissen-Meyer, J., and Hammerstrom, J.: Physiochemical Characterization of Cytostatic Factors Released from Human Monocytes. Infect. Immun., *38*:67, 1982.

Norris, D.A.: Isolation of Functional Subsets of Human Peripheral Blood Monocytes. J. Immunol., *123*:166, 1979.

Norris, D.A., et al.: Fibronectin Fragment(s) Are Chemotactic for Human Peripheral Blood Monocytes. J. Immunol., *129*:1612, 1982.

North, R.J.: The Action of Cortisone Acetate on Cell-Mediated Immunity to Infection. J. Exp. Med., *134*:1485, 1971.

Ogmundsottir, H.M., and Weir, D.M.: Mechanisms of Macrophage Activation. Clin. Exp. Immunol., *40*:223, 1980.

Osterud, B., et al.: Production of Blood Coagulation Factor V and Tissue Thromboplastin by Macrophages in Vitro. FEBS Lett., *127*:154, 1981.

Perri, R.T., et al.: Fibronectin Enhances in Vitro Monocyte-Macrophage-Mediated Tumoricidal Activity. Blood, *60*:430, 1982.

Peterson, P.K., et al.: Kinetics of Phagocytosis and Bacterial Killing by Human Polymorphonuclear Leukocytes and Monocytes. J. Infect. Dis., *136*:502, 1977.

Pierce, J.A., and Senior, R.M.: Alveolar Macrophages' Secrets. J. Lab. Clin. Med., *97*:463, 1981.

Postlelhwaite, A.E., et al.: Formation of Multinucleated Giant Cells from Human Monocyte Precursors: Mediation by a Soluble Protein from Antigen and Mitogen Stimulated Lymphocytes. J. Exp. Med., *155*:168, 1982.

Raghunathan, R., et al.: Isolation of Ovine Lymphocytes, Granulocytes, and Monocytes by Counterflow Centrifugation Elutriation. Amer. J. Vet. Res., *43*:1467, 1982.

Reiss, M., and Roos, D.: Differences in Oxygen Metabolism of Phagocytosing Monocytes and Neutrophils. J. Clin. Invest., *61*:480, 1978.

Rhodes, J. et al.: Human Macrophage Function in Cancer: Systemic and Local Changes Detected by an Array for Fc Receptor Expression. J. Natl. Cancer Inst., *66*:423, 1981.

Rocklin, R.E., et al.: Mediators of Immunity: Lympho-kines and Monokines. Adv. Immunol., *29*:55, 1980.

Roser, B.: The Origin, Kinetics, and Fate of Macrophages Populations. J. Reticuloendothel. Soc., *8*:139, 1970.

Ross, R., et al.: Growth Factors from Platelets, Mono-cytes, and Endothelium: Their Role in Cell Prolifer-ation. Ann. N.Y. Acad. Sci., *397*:18, 1982.

Roubin, R., et al.: Markers of Macrophage Heterogenity: Altered Frequency of Macrophage Subpopulation after Various Pathologic Stimuli. J. Reticuloendothel. Soc., *29*:423, 1981.

Ruco, L.P., et al.: Increase Monocyte Phagocytosis in Cancer Patients. Eur. J. Cancer, *16*:1315, 1980.

Sagone, A.L., Jr., et al.: Characteristics of the Metabolic Response of Human Monocytes to Red Cells Sensi-tized with Anti-D Alloantibodies. J. Lab. Clin. Med., *98*:382, 1981.

Schmitt, E., et al.: Monocyte Recruitment in Tuberculosis and Sarcoidosis. Brit. J. Haematol., *35*:11, 1977.

Schnyder, J., and Baggiolini, M.: Secretion of Lysosomal Hydrolases by Stimulated and Non-Stimulated Mac-rophages. J. Exp. Med., *148*:435, 1978.

Schnyder, J., et al.: Effects of Cyclooxygenase Inhibitors and Prostaglandin E$_2$ on Macrophage Activation in Vitro. Prostaglandins, *22*:411, 1981.

Shands, J.W., Jr.: Macrophage Procoagulants. Haemos-tasis, *14*:373, 1984.

Shaw, S.E., and Anderson, N.V.: Isolation and Func-tional Analysis of Normal Canine Blood Monocytes and Resident Alveolar Macrophages. Amer. J. Vet. Res., *45*:87, 1984.

Silverstein, S.: Macrophages and Viral Immunity. Semin. Hematol., *7*:185, 1970.

Simon, L.M., et al.: Enzymatic Basis for Bioenergetic Dif-ferences of Alveolar versus Peritoneal Macrophages and Enzyme Regulation by Molecular O$_2$. J. Clin. Invest., *59*:443, 1977.

Sluiter, W., et al.: Humoral Control of Monocyte Pro-duction during Inflammation. *In* Mononuclear Phag-ocytes. Part 1. van Furth, R., ed. Martinus Nijhoff Publishers, The Hague, p. 325, 1980.

Sluiter, W., et al.: Regulation of Monocyte Precursor Cell Proliferation by Two Endogenous Factors. Immu-nobiology, *161*:219, 1982.

Sone, S., et al.: Kinetics and Ultrastructural Studies of the Indicator of Rat Alveolar Macrophage Fusion by Mediators Released from Mitogen-Stimulated Lym-phocytes. Amer. J. Pathol., *103*:234, 1981.

Sonoda, M., and Kobayashi, K.: Monocytes of Canine Peripheral Blood in Electron Microscopy. Jap. J. Vet. Res., *18*:67, 1970.

Stanley, E.R.: Colony-Stimulating Factor and the Regu-lation of Granulopoiesis and Macrophage Produc-tion. Fed. Proc., *34*:2272, 1975.

Stanley, E.R., et al.: Factors Regulating Macrophage Pro-duction and Growth: Identity of Colony-Stimulating Factor and Macrophage Growth Factor. J. Exp. Med., *143*:631, 1976.

Stenson, W.F., and Parker, C.W.: Prostaglandins, Mac-rophages, and Immunity. J. Immunol., *125*:1, 1980.

Stjernholm, R.L., et al.: Carbohydrate Metabolism by Leukocytes. Enzyme, *13*:7, 1972.

Suter, E.: Passive Transfer of Acquired Resistance to In-jection with Mycobacterium tuberculosis by Means of Cells. Amer. Rev. Resp. Dis., *83*:535, 1961.

Suter, E., and Ramseier, H.: Cellular Reactions in Infec-tion. Adv. Immunol., *4*:117, 1964.

Sutton, J.S., and Weiss, L.: Transformation of Monocytes in Tissue Culture into Macrophages, Epithelioid Cells and Multinucleated Giant Cells. J. Cell Biol., *28*:303, 1966.

Synderman, R., and Pike, M.C.: An Inhibitor of Mac-rophage Chemotaxis Produced by Neoplasm. Sci-ence, *192*:370, 1976.

Takamura, R., et al.: Secretory Products of Macrophages and Their Physiological Functions. Amer. J. Physiol., *246*:C1, 1984.

Territo, M.C., and Cline, M.J.: Mononuclear Phagocyte Proliferation, Maturation and Function. Clin. Hae-matol., *4*:685, 1975.

Thompson, J., and van Furth, R.: The Effect of Gluco-corticosteroids on the Kinetics of Promonocytes of the Bone Marrow. J. Exp. Med., *137*:10, 1973.

Todd, R.F., and Schlossman, S.F.: Analysis of Antigenic Determinants on Human Monocytes and Macro-phages. Blood, *59*:775, 1982.

Todd, R.F., et al.: Antigens on Human Monocytes Iden-tified by Monoclonal Antibodies. J. Immunol., *126*:1435, 1981.

Tolone, G., et al.: Effects of Hydrocortisone on Binding of IgG and C3b-Coated Erythrocytes to Human Mon-ocytes and Polymorphonuclear Leucocytes. J. Pharm. Pharmacol., *31*:563, 1979.

Uher, F., et al.: IgM-Fc Receptor-Mediated Phagocytosis of Rat Macrophages. Immunology, *42*:419, 1981.

Unanue, E.R.: Cooperation between Mononuclear Phag-ocytes and Lymphocytes in Immunity. New Eng. J. Med., *303*:977, 1980.

van der Rhee, H.J., et al.: Fine Structure and Peroxidatic Activity of Rat Blood Monocytes. Cell Tissue Res., *185*:1, 1977.

van Furth, R., ed.: Mononuclear Phagocytes: Functional Aspects. Parts 1 and 2. Martinus Nijhoff Publishers, The Hague, 1980.

van Furth, R., and Cohn, Z.A.: The Origin and Kinetics of Mononuclear Phagocytes. J. Exp. Med., *128*:415, 1968.

van Furth, R., and Sluiter, W.: Current Views on the Ontogeny of Macrophages and the Humoral Regu-lation of Monocytopoiesis. Trans. R. Soc. Trop. Med. Hyg., *77*:614, 1983.

van Furth, R., et al.: The Kinetics of Promonocytes and Monocytes in the Bone Marrow. J. Exp. Med., *132*:813, 1970.

van Furth, R., et al.: The Mononuclear Phagocyte System: A New Classification of Macrophages, Monocytes and Their Precursor Cells. Bull. WHO, *46*:845, 1972.

van Furth, R., et al.: The Regulation of the Participation of Mononuclear Phagocytes in Inflammatory Proc-ess. *In* Experimental Models of Chronic Inflamma-tory Diseases. Glynn, L.E., and Schlumberger, H.D., eds. Springer-Verlag, New York, p. 302, 1977.

van Waarde, D., et al.: Humoral Regulation of Mono-cytopoiesis during the Early Phase of an Inflamma-tory Reaction Caused by Particulate Substances. Blood, *50*:141, 1977.

van Waarde, D., et al.: Humoral Control of Monocyto-poiesis by an Activator and an Inhibitor. Agents Ac-tions, *8*:432, 1978.

Verbrugh, H.A., et al.: Phagocytosis and Killing of Staph-ylococci by Human Polymorphonuclear and Mono-nuclear Leucocytes. J. Clin. Pathol., *31*:539, 1978.

Verma, D.S., et al.: Prostaglandin E$_1$-Mediated Augmen-tation of Human Granulocyte-Macrophage Progeni-tor Cell Growth in Vitro. Leuk. Res., *5*:65, 1981.

Virolainen, M., and Defendi, V.: Ability of Hematopoietic Spleen Colonies to Form Macrophages in Vitro. Na-ture, *217*:1069, 1968.

Volkman, A.: The Function of the Monocyte. Bibl. Haematologica, 29(Pt. 1):86, 1968.

Volkman, A.: A Current Perspective of Monocytopoiesis. Curr. Top. Pathol., 54:76, 1971.

Volkman, A.: Disparity in Origin of Mononuclear Phagocyte Populations. J. Reticuloendothel. Soc., 19:249, 1976.

Volkman, A., and Gowans, J.L.: The Origin of Macrophages from Bone Marrow in the Rat. Brit. J. Exp. Pathol., 46:50, 1965a.

Volkman, A., and Gowans, J.L.: The Production of Macrophages in the Rat. Brit. J. Exp. Pathol., 46:62, 1965b.

Ward, P.A.: Chemotaxis of Mononuclear Cells. J. Exp. Med., 128:1201, 1968.

Whitelaw, D.M.: The Intravascular Lifespan of Monocytes. Blood, 28:455, 1966.

Whitelaw, D.M., et al.: Monocyte Kinetics: Observations after Pulse Labeling. J. Cell. Physiol., 72:65, 1968.

Willoughby, D.A.: A Monocytogenic Humoral Factor Released after Lymph Node Stimulation. Immunology, 12:165, 1967.

Wilson, F.D., and Shifrine, M.: Radiation-Induced Transplantable Myelomonocytic Leukemia in Beagles: Hematologic Parameters. Exp. Hematol., 22:41, 1972.

Wintrobe, M.M., et al.: Mononuclear Phagocytes (Monocytes and Macrophages). In Clinical Hematology 8th ed. Ch. 9. Lea & Febiger, Philadelphia, 1981.

Yam, L.T., et al.: Cytochemical Identification of Monocytes and Granulocytes. Amer. J. Clin. Pathol., 55:283, 1971.

Yamashita, U., and Shevach, E.M.: The Expression of Ia Antigens on Immunocompetent Cells in the Guinea Pig. II. Ia Antigens on Macrophages. J. Immunol., 119:1584, 1977.

Zuckerman, K.S.: Human Erythroid Burst-Forming Units. Growth in Vitro Is Dependent on Monocytes, but Not T Lymphocytes. J. Clin. Invest., 67:702, 1981.

30

The Lymphocytes and Plasma Cells

THE LYMPHOCYTES 790
    Morphology and Cytochemistry 791
    Characterization of B and T Cells and Their
      Subpopulations 795
    Lymphopoiesis 798
    Lymphokinetics 802

Recirculation 803
Functions of Lymphocytes 807
Lymphocyte Numbers in Peripheral
    Blood 811

THE PLASMA CELLS 812

The discipline of immunology is expanding by leaps and bounds. The lymphocytes play a pivotal role in the initiation and execution of the immune response. The increasing recognition of acquired and hereditary immunologic disorders in humans and animals has prompted in-depth studies of lymphocyte and plasma cell physiopathology. Lymphocytes from the peripheral blood and various lymphoid tissues are being characterized with new tools of research such as immunogenetic, immunologic, electron microscopic, radioisotopic, and cytochemical techniques. Methods are being developed to obtain highly pure preparations of lymphocyte subpopulations for specific structural and functional characterizations. Human and murine lymphocytes have been most studied to date, but information on lymphocytes of various domestic animals is being rapidly accumulated.

THE LYMPHOCYTES

Lymphocytes are a heterogeneous group of cells both morphologically and functionally. Morphologically similar lymphocytes may have different functions, and functionally identical cells may show morphologic diversity.

Morphologically, lymphocytes are generally classified as small, medium, and large, or simply as small (6-9 μm) and large (9-15 μm). The proportion of small and large lymphocytes varies in different species in health. The cell size, the degree of cytoplasmic basophilia, and, to a certain extent, the nuclear chromatin

pattern are thought to indicate relative age or maturity. The larger cell size, basophilic cytoplasm, or smooth chromatin are characteristics of relatively immature lymphocytes. Maturation has been correlated with decreases in the nuclear volume, cytoplasmic basophilia, DNA content, and histone dye–binding capacity and increases in chromatin clumping and the nucleus-to-cytoplasm ratio (Garcia and Iorio, 1968). These characteristics reverse when the small lymphocyte is stimulated to undergo blastogenesis in vitro and probably under similar conditions in vivo.

Functionally, lymphocytes are grouped on the basis of their involvement in the immune response. Lymphocytes concerned with cell-mediated immunity and immunoregulatory functions are variedly referred to as thymus-dependent, thymus-derived, thymus-processed, or T cells, while those concerned with the formation of humoral antibody are referred to as thymus-independent, bursa-derived in birds and bursa-equivalent or bone marrow–derived in mammals, or B cells. Increasingly precise characterization of these cells has been made possible in recent years through advances in techniques for isolation of pure populations of lymphocytes and production of highly specific monoclonal antibodies. Lymphocytes, and to a certain extent their subpopulations in various species, can now be distinguished by a variety of criteria (Table 30–1).

In most species, 80–95% of the peripheral blood lymphocytes are classified as T and B

Table 30–1. Criteria for Characterization of Lymphocyte Subpopulations in Various Species

B Cells	T Cells
Specific surface antigens	Specific surface antigens
Ia antigens	Brain-associated antigens
Surface immunoglobulin (sIg)	Reaction with antithymocyte serum
Cytoplasmic Ig (in pre-B cells)	Subsets with Fc receptors for various immunoglobulins
Receptors for Fc portion of various immunoglobulins	Spontaneous E-rosettes with erythrocytes of heterologous species
Erythrocyte-antibody rosettes	Stimulation by phytomitogens: phytohemagglutinin, concanavalin A, PWM, wax bean, and bovine serum albumin.
Receptors for C3: erythrocyte-antibody-complement-rosettes	
Receptors for Epstein-Barr virus	Receptors for *Helix pometia* antigen, peanut agglutinin, and C-reactive protein
Stimulation by pokeweed mitogen (PWM), antiglobulin serum, dextran, protein A, trypsin, and lipopolysaccharides	Receptors for measles virus
Adherence to nylon wool	Positive staining for Tdt in precursor cells and acid phosphatase, β-glucuronidase and α-naphthyl acetate esterase in mature T cells
Positive staining for terminal deoxyribonucleotidase (Tdt) in pre-B cells and 5'-nucleotidase in mature B cells (see Chapter 33)	

cells (Table 30–2). A minor, third population of mononuclear cells, referred to as "non-T, non-B" or "null" cells, is comprised of a variety of cell types whose markers, relative proportions, and functions are not yet clearly defined (Ferrarini et al., 1980; Grossi and Greaves, 1981).

Various subpopulations of lymphocytes are found in the peripheral blood as a result of production, release, and recirculation of lymphocytes at different stages of maturation and immunocompetence. Similarly, there are differences in the proportion of various lymphocytes in different lymphoid organs. Organ distribution and proportion of different subpopulations of lymphocytes change during disease. The reader is referred to recent reviews (Grossi and Greaves, 1981; Janossy, 1982; Kristensen et al., 1982; Moretta et al., 1984) on lymphocyte biology for further details on the topics disussed below.

Morphology and Cytochemistry

In Wright-stained blood films, lymphocytes appear as round to oval cells with scanty or moderately abundant cytoplasm of varying basophilia and a spherical or ovoid nucleus with distinct nuclear membrane and coarsely clumped chromatin. The nucleus may be indented or cleaved in some cells. Lymphocytes examined with the scanning electron microscope appear as globular cells with a smooth or villous surface exhibiting a variable number of stubby or finger-like microvilli. The surface morphology of lymphocytes is influenced by preparatory procedures and the stage of cel-

lular activation or maturation and is not indicative of their immunologic identity (Abugaber et al., 1981; Renau-Pigneres et al., 1980; Vos et al., 1980). Viable lymphocytes show a slow, ameboid movement, and motile cells assume a characteristic hand-mirror profile.

The ultrastructure of lymphocytes in various species is remarkably similar (Ackerman, 1970; Douglas, 1983a; Grossi and Greaves, 1981; Sonoda, 1971; Sonoda and Kobayashi, 1970; Sonoda and Marshak, 1970). However, there are some differences depending on size and age (Figs. 30–1, 30–2).

The nucleus presents patchy, dense clumps of heterochromatin in small lymphocytes, modestly dispersed chromatin in medium and large lymphocytes, and fairly dispersed chromatin in lymphoblasts. The nuclear membrane is distinct, and some nuclear pores are visible. Nucleoli are not seen in normal lymphocytes in Wright-stained blood films of various species except for an occasional cell in bovine blood. However, the presence of a small nucleolus is demonstrable by special procedures such as staining with methylene blue at pH 4.9 (Elves, 1967) or toluidine blue at pH 5.4 (Beran and Pospisil, 1967) and by electron microscopy (Fig. 30–1). The number of nucleoli within a lymphocyte varies among species; e.g., multiple nucleoli have been found in lymphocytes of cows, goats, pigs, guinea pigs, and mice (Beran and Pospisil, 1967).

Nuclear pockets have been observed on rare occasions in normal bovine lymphocytes from blood and lymph nodes and more fre-

Table 30–2.   Distribution of Lymphocyte Subpopulations in Peripheral Blood of Various Species from Selected Literature Reports

	B cell		T cell		
	% Lymphocytes*	Method**	% Lymphocytes	Method	Reference
Human	5–15 (10)	sIg	60–80 (75)	Sheep E-R	Grossi and Greaves (1981)
Rhesus Monkey					
Fetus, 60 days	12.5	EAC-R	13.5	Sheep E-R	Osburn et al. (1982)
Fetus, 120 days	16	EAC-R	38.7	Sheep E-R	Osburn et al. (1982)
Fetus, 165 days	16.8	EAC-R	71.8	Sheep E-R	Osburn et al. (1982)
Adult	20	EAC-R	63	Sheep E-R	Osburn et al. (1982)
	22	sIg			Osburn et al. (1982)
Dog	18	sIg	13	Human E-R	Chandler and Yang (1981)
			74	Antithymus Ab	Chandler and Yang (1981)
	30.5	sIg	38	Human E-R	Zander et al. (1975)
			68	Human E-R	Zander et al. (1975)
Cat	30	sIg	50	Guinea pig E-R	Rojko et al. (1982)
	34	EAC-R	23	Antithymus Ab	Rojko et al. (1982)
	36.5	EAC-R	28	Guinea pig E-R	Taylor and Siddiqui (1977)
	43	sIg	21	Guinea pig E-R	Mackey (1977)
Horse					
Foal	12–15	sIg	5–16	Guinea pig E-R	Frymus and Schollenberger (1979)
Adult	27	sIg			Banks and Henson (1973)
			38	Guinea pig E-R	Tarr et al. (1977)
Bovine					
Calf	Few	EAC-R	15	Sheep E-R	Wilkie et al. (1979)
Adult	17	sIg	83	Sheep E-R	Outteridge and Dufty (1981)
	23	EAC-R	26	Sheep E-R	Wilkie et al. (1979)
	25	sIg	60	Sheep E-R	Beldon et al. (1981)
	27	sIg	60	Sheep E-R	Grewal and Babiuk (1978)
	27	sIg	73	Antithymus Ab	Yang (1981)
Sheep					
Fetus	8	sIg	82	Antithymus Ab	Chandra et al. (1980)
Adult	16	sIg	79	Antithymus Ab	Chandra et al. (1980)
	16.6	sIg	28	Sheep E-R	Outteridge et al. (1981)
	36	EAC-R			Outteridge et al. (1981)
Goat	17	EAC-R	69	PNA	Banks and Greenlee (1982)
	19	sIg			Banks and Greenlee (1982)
Pig					
Piglet	15	EAC-R	47	Sheep E-R	Salmon (1979)
	15.6	sIg	30	Sheep E-R	Jaroskova and Kovaru (1978)
Adult			55–70	Antithymus Ab	Johnson et al. (1980)
	9	EAC-R	55	Sheep E-R	Salmon (1979)
	23.8	sIg			Reyero et al. (1978)
Buffalo	5–18	sIg	18	Sheep E-R	Kaura et al. (1979)

*mean and/or range.

**sIg, surface immunoglobulin; E-R, erythrocyte rosettes; EAC-R, erythrocyte-antibody-complement rosettes; Ab, antibody; PNA, peanut agglutinin.

quently in lymphocytes from leukemic cattle (Miller et al., 1969; Weber et al., 1969). A typical nuclear pocket is an invagination of the nuclear membrane in the form of a ring or loop extending from the usual nuclear contour and enclosing some cytoplasmic substance. Some thoracic duct lymphocytes of calves contain a "nuclear body" proximal to the nucleolus (Weber and Joel, 1966). A typical nuclear body is about the size of a nucleolus or slightly smaller and consists of a small, electron-dense central area surrounded by some fibrillar material.

Small lymphocytes present scanty cyto-plasm in which some free ribosomes, a few small mitochondria, a small Golgi complex, and little or no rough endoplasmic reticulum (RER) may be seen (Fig. 30–1). The amount of cytoplasm is more abundant in medium to large lymphocytes, and various organelles are more prominent in these cells. The centrioles are said to be more conspicuous in lymphocytes than in any other leukocytes (Grossi and Greaves, 1981). A few pinocytotic vesicles may be present in the cytoplasm near the plasma membrane. Glycogen granules may be seen in some lymphocytes as scattered particles or in small clumps somewhat indistin-

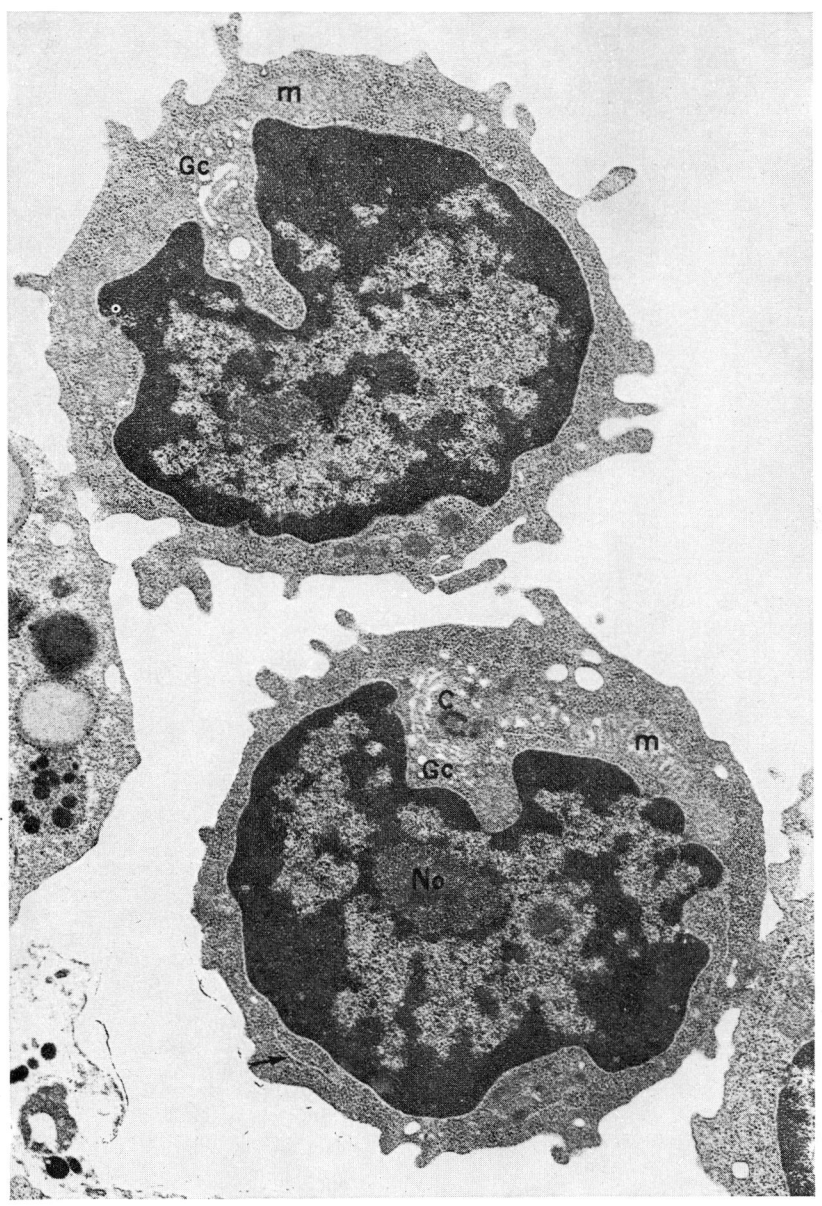

Fig. 30–1. Two canine lymphocytes from blood. The cytoplasm of both lymphocytes contains numerous ribosomes (dense particles), some indistinct mitochondria *(m)*, and an inconspicuous inactive area of the Golgi complex *(Gc)* represented by smooth, small, round vesicles or elongated tubules. The nuclei appear irregular in outline and contain areas of chromatin condensation, principally along the nuclear membrane. The lower lymphocyte also has a centriole *(C)*, a few profiles of rough endoplasmic reticulum in the cytoplasm along the periphery *(arrow)*, and a distinct nucleolus *(No)* with areas of chromatin condensation along the margin. A few cytoplasmic projections are also present on these cells. ×19,000.

guishable from ribosomes. Microfilaments and microtubules are seen in uropods of motile lymphocytes. Lysosomes are rare. A small proportion (5–15%) of T cells contain a few granules of variable electron density which correspond (Grossi and Greaves, 1981) to azurophilic granules seen in some lympho-

cytes in Wright-stained blood films (Plate VI–3). These granules are peroxidase negative. A large, spherical refractile structure called a Gall body may be seen in an occasional lymphocyte, and some lymphocytes in the guinea pig show an aggregate of reddish-purple granules known as a Kurloff body

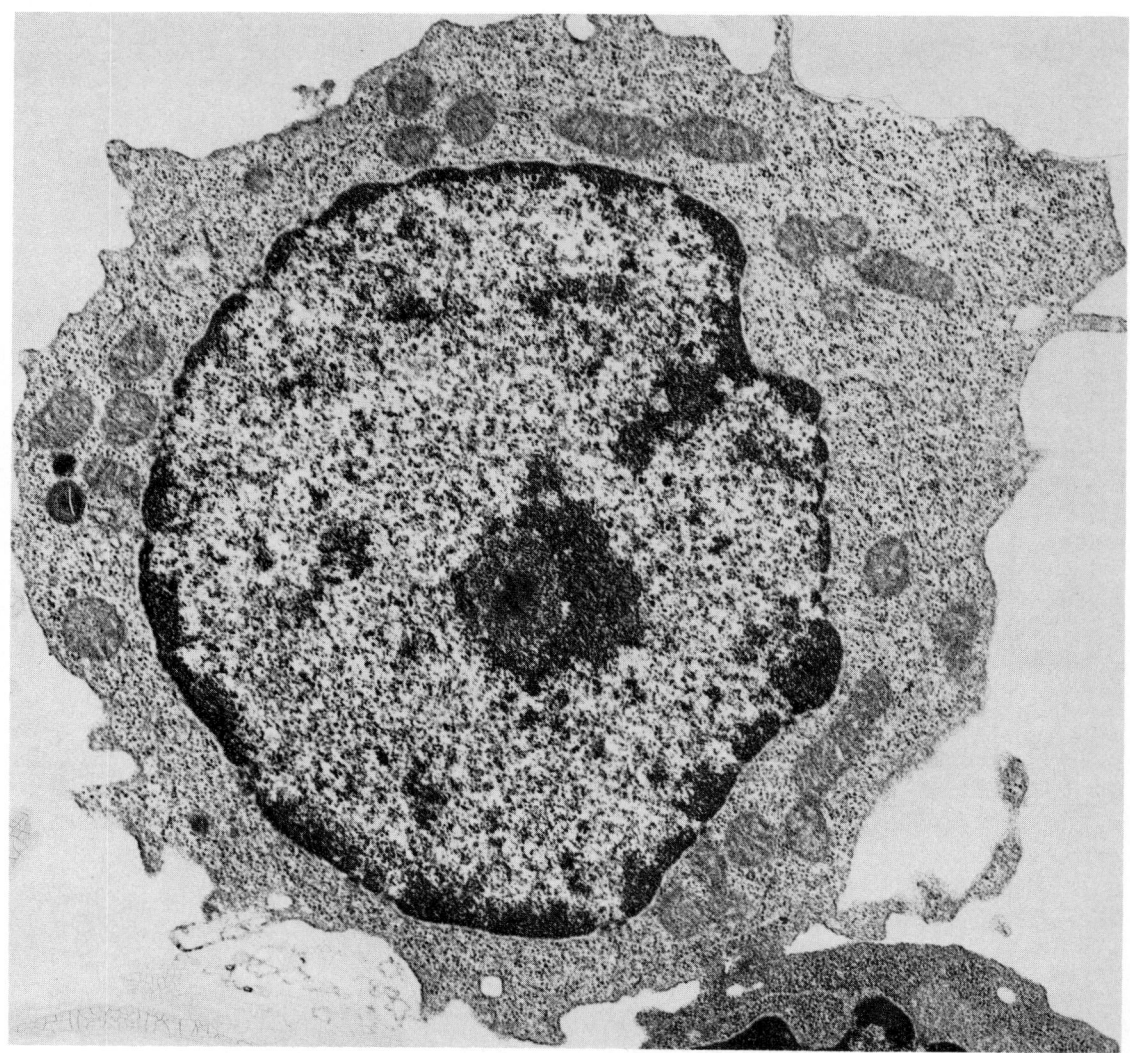

Fig. 30–2. A lymphocyte with a moderate amount of cytoplasm and a vesicular nucleus with a nucleolus. Nuclear pores and some chromatin condensation are evident along the nuclear membrane. The cytoplasm is rich in free ribosomes, has some profiles of rough endoplasmic reticulum and scattered mitochondria, and has a couple of dense granular structures. ×26,000.

(Fig. 12–4). The significance of these structures is unknown.

The number of ribosomes and polyribosomes varies among lymphocytes depending on the stage of cellular maturity and activity. Their number and distribution can be related to the degree and distribution of cytoplasmic basophilia seen in films stained with Wright stain (Plates IX–1, IX–3). The majority of peripheral blood lymphocytes reveal free ribosomes and appear unengaged in protein synthesis (Fig. 30–1). A small number may have some RER and polyribosomes, which are characteristic of cells engaged in protein syn-

thesis (e.g., antibody formation by B cells or lymphokine production by T cells), and a rare cell may even resemble a plasma cell (Fig. 30–3). Based on ribosomal pattern, two varieties of lymphocytes were described in the thoracic duct lymph of calves previously depleted of lymphocytes (Johnson et al, 1966).

Many acid hydrolytic and oxidative enzymes have been found in lymphocytes by biochemical or cytochemical methods (Grossi and Greaves, 1981; Gross et al., 1978). Pre-B and pre-T cells (immediate precursors of B and T cells) typically contain terminal deoxyribonucleotidase (Tdt). B-lymphocytes, plas-

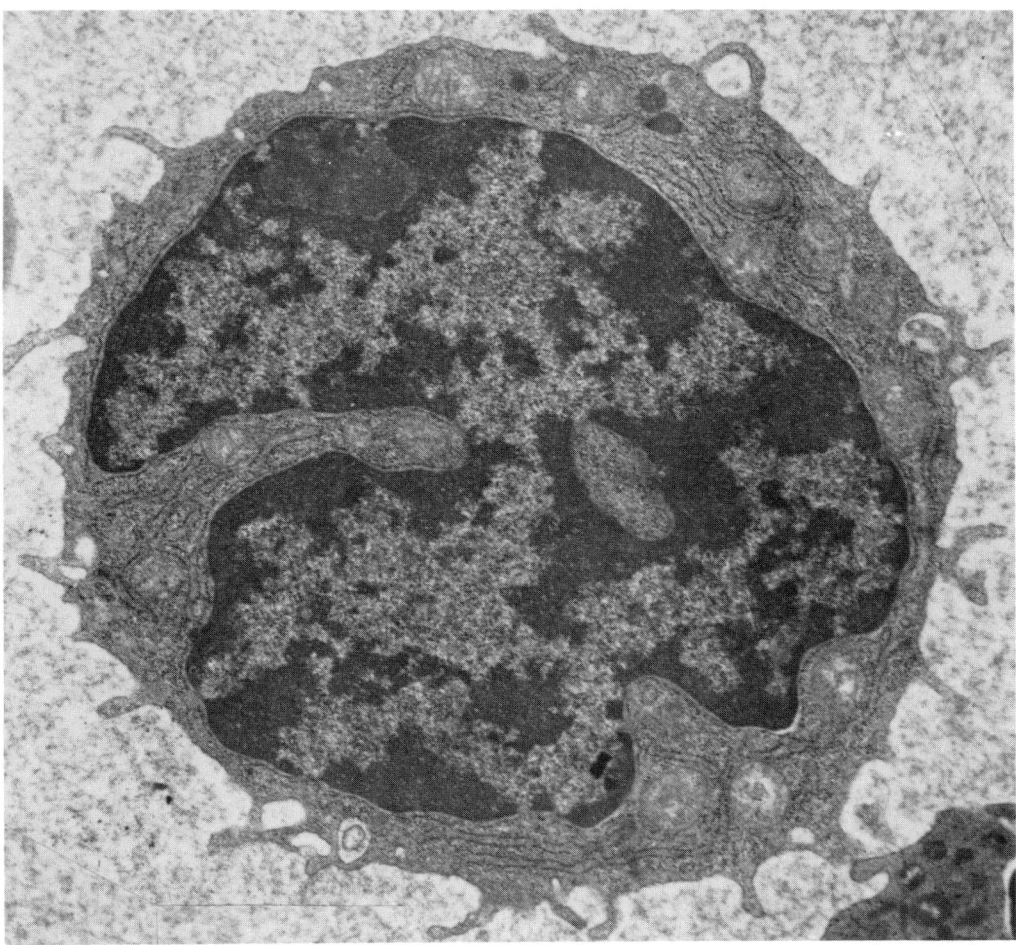

Fig. 30–3. A lymphocyte with a small amount of cytoplasm, rich in rough endoplasmic reticulum, and with an indented nucleus with condensed chromatin. This cell would appear blue in Wright-stained blood film and may be referred to as an "immunocyte." Some mitochondria and surface microvilli are also evident. ×25,000.

mablasts, and plasma cells stain for 5'-nucleotidase. Lysosomal enzymes such as acid phosphatase, β-glucuronidase, and acid α-naphthyl acetate esterase are present in T cells and activated B cells, but not in resting B cells. Staining intensities and patterns of these enzymes differ from those in other leukocytes; only one or two positive granular deposits are seen. Lymphocytes lack cytoplasmic alkaline phosphatase, peroxidase, sudan black B reactivity, and lysozyme.

Lymphocytes derive energy through glucose metabolism primarily via the glycolytic pathway (Cline, 1975). The pentose phosphate pathway is normally only of minor importance, but it may be stimulated under anaerobic conditions. Lymphocytes can synthesize protein, glycogen, and fatty acids.

Characterization of B and T Cells and Their Subpopulations

Several criteria are used to characterize lymphocytes and their subpopulations in different species (Table 30–1). To characterize lymphocyte populations it is necessary to have cell preparations enriched in T- and B-lymphocytes (Banks and Greenlee, 1981; Buschmann and Pawlas, 1980; Taylor and Siddiqui, 1977; Wysocki and Sato, 1978). Commonly used criteria include detection of specific surface membrane antigens, various immunologic and nonimmunologic surface receptors, surface or cytoplasmic immunoglobulins, and cytochemical reactions (Gross et al., 1978; Grossi and Greaves, 1981; Lydyard and Fanger, 1982; MacDonald, 1982; Morett et al., 1982; Sharon, 1983).

Different surface antigens are distinguished using monoclonal antibodies. Surface or cytoplasmic immunoglobulins (Ig) are demonstrated by fluorescent or autoradiographic techniques. The presence of receptors for heterologous erythrocytes has been demonstrated by detection of spontaneous rosette (E-rosettes) formation with red cells of various species. The presence of receptors for the Fc portion of Ig or the complement components (C3b and C3d receptors) is demonstrated, respectively, by rosette formation with antibody-coated erythrocytes (EA-rosettes) or antibody-complement-coated erythrocytes (EAC-rosettes); fluorescent and autoradiographic techniques have also been used for this purpose. Bacterial adherence to lymphocytes has been used in conjunction with the fluorescent antibody technique to identify bovine lymphocyte subpopulations (Canning et al., 1983). *Helix pometia* antigen has been used to characterize bovine (Johansson and Morein, 1983) and equine (Broström et al., 1985) T-lymphocytes.

All of these methods have proved useful in identification of functional subpopulations of lymphocytes in peripheral blood and lymphoid tissues in health and disease (reviewed by Kristensen et al., 1982). Such information is useful in clinical situations, particularly for patients with immunodeficiency disorders and lymphoid malignancies. These techniques have also provided new insights into characterization of leukemic lymphocytes and immunologic classification of leukemias in humans (Blatt et al., 1980; Bloomfield and Gajl-Peczalska, 1980; Lowenthal, 1982; Machin et al., 1980; Safai and Good, 1980) and animals (Cockerell et al., 1976a; Dutta et al., 1978; Holmberg et al., 1977; Kumar et al., 1978; Muscoplat et al., 1974a,b; Raich et al., 1983). Lymphoblasts and immature (partially differentiated) lymphocytes show phenotypic characteristics of their lineage.

The number of T- and B-lymphocytes in lymphoid tissues and peripheral blood varies in different species. In general, T cells predominate in the thymus, lymph nodes, thoracic duct lymph, and peripheral blood, while B cells predominate in the bone marrow and spleen (Douglas, 1983a; Grossi and Greaves, 1981; Kristensen et al., 1982). In peripheral blood, on an average, there are about 70% T cells and 20% B cells, and the remaining 10% probably constitute the null cells, although wide variations have been reported among and within species (Table 30–2). Such variations are attributed partly to technical factors and criteria used for characterization of lymphocyte subpopulations.

For example, E-rosetting for identification of T cells requires the use of particular species' red cells; otherwise negative or poor results are obtained. Sheep erythrocytes, commonly used for E-rosetting in various species, do not rosette with equine (Tarr et al., 1977) and feline (Mackey and Jarrett, 1975) lymphocytes. E-rosettes with neuraminidase-treated (Buschmann and Pawlas, 1980; Grewal and Babiuk, 1978; Wilkie et al., 1979) or trypsinized (Binns et al., 1979) erythrocytes give higher values than those with untreated red cells. In the dog, E-rosetting is considered nonspecific or highly variable and low in sensitivity (Chandler and Yang, 1981; Krakowka, 1980).

Fluorescent antibody techniques using antithymocyte antibody demonstrate a markedly higher percentage of T cells than the rosetting method in the dog (Chandler and Yang, 1981), cow (Yang, 1981), sheep (Chandra et al, 1980), and pig (Johnson et al., 1980). Peanut agglutinin (PNA) receptor is of special interest because it is recognized as a marker for cells in the thymic cortex (immature thymocytes) in mice and humans. It is also a specific marker for bovine, ovine, caprine, and equine T-lymphocytes (Banks and Greenlee, 1982; Sharon, 1983).

Surface Ig is considered the most reliable marker for identification of B cells (Chandler and Yang, 1981). It is a labile marker, however, and may be lost during cell washing (Kelly, 1980). Some surface Ig is also detected on T cells (Grossi and Greaves, 1981). Care must be taken not to confuse sIg^+ B cells with macrophages and other leukocytes (T_S and T_H) that bind sIg via Fc receptors, especially in fluorescent studies. Identification of B cells by EA- and EAC-rosettes generally yields higher values than those obtained through detection of surface markers.

The number of T and B cells in the peripheral blood and lymphoid tissues varies with age and the health of the individual. B cells are few during fetal life and steadily increase after birth until adult values are attained (Table 30–2). In the adult, age-related declines have been seen in B cells (Symons and Binns, 1975), T cells, and null cells (Outteridge et al., 1981).

Observations in the cow indicate that increased numbers of B cells and decreased numbers of T cells may be found in diseased cows (Giriunas et al., 1980). B-lymphocytes decrease during bovine mastitis (Ishikawa and Shimizu, 1983; Yang et al., 1980) and are very low or absent in agammaglobulinemia (Muscoplat et al., 1974a). Leukemic cows and cows with persistent lymphocytosis exhibit increased B cells (Kumar et al., 1978; Wilkie et al., 1979), comprising up to 97% of lymphocytes; and both T and B cells are reduced in acute lymphocytic leukemia (Muscoplat et al., 1974b). Compared to peripheral blood, secretions from dry bovine mammary glands contain a large proportion of T lymphocytes (Schore et al., 1981).

B Cells

In various species, about 20% of circulating lymphocytes are B cells. In most species, these are identified by the presence of surface immunoglobulins and receptors for C3b, C3d, and various immunoglobulins (Morett et al., 1982). Complement receptors are absent on plasma cells. Species differences and age-related changes are seen in the number of lymphocytes bearing various surface Igs. For example, most human lymphocytes have surface IgM (monomeric) and IgD, and some have IgG and IgA (monomeric), whereas about two-thirds of the canine B-lymphocytes have surface IgG and about one-third have IgM (Reif et al., 1975).

Human B-lymphocytes also exhibit some B-cell-specific and Ia-like antigens on their surface membrane (Grossi and Greaves, 1981). Ia antigens are glycoproteins, linked genetically to the major histocompatibility complex, with limited tissue distribution (Rifkind et al., 1980). They are found also in macrophages and early erythroid and myeloid precursors. Human B cells also form rosettes with mouse red cells and stain for 5'-nucleotidase (only in plasma membrane), but not for acid hydrolytic enzymes (Grossi and Greaves, 1981).

Ia-like antigens have been recognized on horse, cow, sheep, and pig lymphocytes in tests using monoclonal antibodies.

T Cells

About 21–85% of lymphocytes in the peripheral blood of various species have been identified as T cells by E-rosetting with heterologous erythrocytes (Kristensen et al., 1982); however, by antithymocyte antibodies, close to 70% of lymphocytes are classified as T-lymphocytes in most species (Table 30–2). Mature T-lymphocytes of humans, mice, rabbits, sheep, cattle, pigs, and monkeys form rosettes with sheep erythrocytes (Outteridge et al., 1981; Reeves and Renshaw, 1978; Salmon, 1979; Terrell et al., 1977; Vos et al., 1980). Similarly, canine T-lymphocytes form rosettes with guinea pig and human type O erythrocytes (Bowles et al., 1975); feline T-lymphocytes form rosettes with guinea pig, rat, and mouse red cells (Cockerell et al., 1976a; Mackey, 1977; Taylor et al., 1975); porcine T-lymphocytes also form rosettes with rabbit erythrocytes (Shimizu et al., 1976); and equine T-lymphocytes form rosettes with guinea pig erythrocytes (Frymus and Schollenberger, 1979; Tarr et al., 1977).

Specific surface antigens have been recognized as markers of T-lymphocytes during various developmental stages. Such antigenic differences were reported initially for the mouse, but have since been recognized for lymphocytes of humans and several animal species.

In addition, T-lymphocytes of humans and various animal species have receptors for the Fc portion of some immunoglobulins. Subsets of human T-lymphocytes with surface receptors for IgG, IgM, and IgA are referred to, respectively, as T_G, T_M, and T_A cells. Up to 85% of T cells are T_M cells; they are typically small to medium-sized cells having a relatively smooth surface, poorly developed cytoplasmic organelles, and no cytoplasmic granules. These cells constitute helper T cells. T_G cells account for about 5–15% of all T cells; these are large, contain azurophilic granules, show a villous surface, and have abundant cytoplasm (low nucleus-to-cytoplasm ratio) and well-developed organelles. This group of cells constitutes suppressor T cells.

Another important criterion for identification of T cells has been their mitogenic responses to nonspecific stimulatory agents such as the plant lectins phytohemagglutinin (PHA) and concanavalin (Con A) (Kristensen et al., 1982). Related observations are described under Blastogenesis in this chapter.

Cytochemical markers have also been studied. T cells stain for acid hydrolytic enzymes—acid phosphatase and β-glucuronidase. Acid α-naphthyl acetate esterase is also a useful marker (Bozdech and Bainton, 1981; Gross et al., 1978; Grossi and Greaves, 1981; Muller et al., 1981); it shows paranuclear staining in T_G cells, while a positive reaction in the form of one or two dots is seen in T_M cells.

These and other cytomorphologic and immunologic properties have been found helpful in differentiating subpopulations of T cells in various species (Gross et al., 1978; Grossi and Greaves, 1981; animal data reviewed in Kristensen et al., 1982).

Pre-T, Pre-B, and Null Cells

Pre-T and pre-B cells characteristically have Tdt activity. Pre-B cells show cytoplasmic IgM, but not surface Ig and complement receptors as do mature B-lymphocytes. Null cells are morphologically and cytochemically indistinguishable from T_G cells (Ferrarini et al., 1980). They lack specific markers of T and B cells, respond poorly to mitogens, do not produce immunoglobulins in vitro, and are nonadherent and nonphagocytic (Despont et al., 1981). Null cells have been assigned several roles such as being precursors of T and B cells as well as of myeloid and erythroid cells (Barr, 1979; Lipton and Nathan, 1980). Null cells have been described in the dog (Chandler and Yang, 1981), pig (Salmon, 1979), and sheep (Outteridge et al., 1981).

Lymphopoiesis

Lymphocytes are produced in the bone marrow; in the lymphoid organs, which include the thymus, lymph nodes, and spleen; and in gut-associated lymphoid tissues (GALT), which include the Peyer's patches, tonsils, and appendix. Quantitative studies indicate that the bone marrow is the body's largest lymphopoietic tissue (Douglas, 1983a).

Ontogeny

Studies on the ontogeny of hematopoiesis and lymphopoiesis have shown that pluripotent stem cells originate first from the embryonic yolk sac and later from the fetal liver, spleen, and bone marrow. The first step in differentiation of the pluripotent stem cell is the generation of committed myeloid and lymphoid stem cells (Fig. 30–4, Fig. 13–19). These committed stem cells produce various hematopoietic cells under the influence of undefined local microenvironmental factors and separate hormonal control mechanisms.

During the prenatal and postnatal periods, committed lymphoid stem cells from the bone marrow continually seed the thymus and the bursa of Fabricius in birds. (The bursa is a pouch-like structure formed from the epithelium of the cloaca.) At these locations, at least two functionally and phenotypically different populations of lymphoid precursors develop. These are known, respectively, as T cell precursors and B cell precursors. In mammals, the bone marrow serves as the bursa equivalent; hence B cell precursors develop in the bone marrow.

The thymus, the bursa of Fabricius, and the bone marrow are collectively referred to as *primary* or *central lymphoid organs*. They continually supply immunologically immature lymphoid precursors to the *peripheral* or *secondary lymphoid organs* (lymph nodes, spleen, and Peyer's patches), where immunocompetent subsets of T and B cells develop in response to antigenic stimulation. Evidence has been presented to indicate that at least some of the lymphoid precursors from the bone marrow may be committed to the T cell lineage before entering the thymus. Mechanisms involved in the preferential migration of stem cells to the primary lymphoid organs and of B and T cell precursors to specific areas in the secondary lymphoid organs are unknown. Ontogeny of the bovine immune system has been reviewed (Osburn et al., 1982).

The small lymphocytes produced in the lymph nodes and spleen are morphologically

DEVELOPMENT OF LYMPHOCYTES

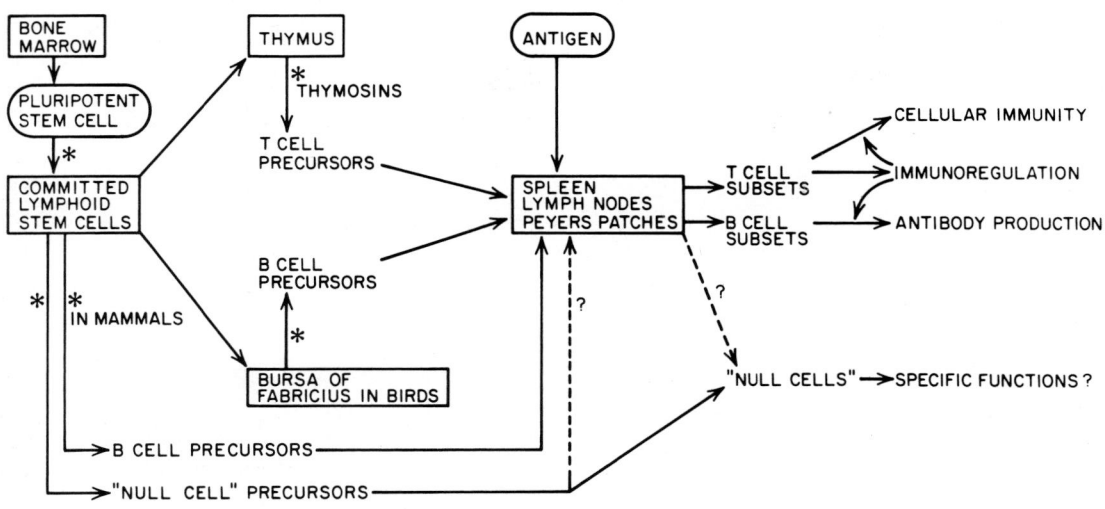

＊*Local Microenvironment*

Fig. 30–4. Sequential development of lymphocytes and their functional differentiation at various primary and secondary sites of lymphopoiesis. See text for details.

similar, but differ in histologic distribution and, more important, in functions. T cells are localized in the paracortical areas of lymph nodes, along the periarteriolar sheaths of the white pulp of the spleen, and in Peyer's patches. They or their progenies form the long-lived circulating lymphocytes concerned with immunoregulatory functions and cell-mediated immunity. B cells are localized in lymphoid follicles and medullary regions of the lymph nodes, in red pulp of the spleen, and in submucosal regions of the gut and respiratory tract. These cells are responsible for the synthesis of humoral antibodies.

Long and Short Production Pathways

The development of lymphocytes is thought to occur in the following order: stem cell, early precursor, lymphoblast, large lymphocyte, medium lymphocyte, small lymphocyte. The first two stages in the series have not been definitely identified morphologically. Two distinct types of pathways, one long and the other short, leading to the formation of small lymphocytes have been recognized. The long production pathway, associated with the production of T cells, involves six to eight mitoses and takes place

in the lymph nodes (Grundmann, 1958) and thymus (Leblond and Sainte-Marie, 1960). The short production pathway, associated with the production of B cells, involves two to three mitoses and takes place in the bone marrow (Osmond and Everett, 1964). Some lymphocytes may be produced by an intermediate pathway. Studies in dogs have shown that lymphocytes in DNA synthesis may enter the blood almost immediately after being labeled with tritiated thymidine (^{3}HTdR) (Cronkite et al., 1959).

Blastogenesis

Small lymphocytes rarely divide or incorporate ^{3}HTdR under normal conditions, but have the potential to proliferate if given a proper stimulus in a suitable environment. They transform into blast cells and divide in response to specific antigens and a variety of nonspecific stimuli. T and B cells vary with regard to their in vitro responses to various mitogens. Lymphocyte responses to various mitogens also vary among species (review by Kristensen et al., 1982). In humans and most animal species, PHA and Con A stimulate T cells. Pokeweed mitogen (PWM) stimulates both T and B cells to undergo blastogenesis, in some cases particularly the latter cells. Many other substances have been found to induce lymphocyte blastogenesis; these include lipopolysaccharides, dextran, trypsin, and anti-Ig antibody. Equine lymphocytes are also stimulated by M protein of *Streptococcus equi* (Srivastava and Barnum, 1982). In comparison to peripheral blood lymphocytes, lymphocytes from bovine milk may show a relatively lower proliferative response (Concha et al., 1978, 1980; Smith and Schultz, 1977). Proliferative response of T cells to mitogens is enhanced by exposure to proteases (Ahmed and Zweygarth, 1983) and indomethacin (Felsberg et al., 1983).

Many morphologic and metabolic changes accompany blast transformation, which may be optimal in 3–5 days. In the initial stages lectin or antigen binding to specific receptors on lymphocytes leads to changes in membrane permeability and transport of various nutrients and cations, particularly calcium (Segel, 1981). Cells enlarge, begin to synthesize DNA, and undergo mitosis. Nuclear chromatin becomes loose, nucleoli appear and become prominent, the cytoplasm becomes abundant and basophilic and acquires increased organelles, and the Golgi complex becomes more elaborate. RNA synthesis increases and so also the activities of lysosomal enzymes, glucose metabolism, and synthesis of glycogen, fatty acid, and protein. T cell lymphoblasts appear less basophilic than B cells because of their paucity of RER and may show large accumulations of glycogen.

Lymphocyte stimulation in different species is influenced by a variety of factors such as stress, hormones, diet, age, pregnancy, fetal proteins, certain serum components, disease, drug therapy, and season (Barta, 1983; Burrells et al., 1979; Kristensen et al., 1982; Lanweiler et al., 1983; Soper et al., 1978; Splitter and Everlith, 1982; Staples et al., 1983). Various bacterial, viral, mycotic, parasitic, and autoimmune diseases and lymphoid and nonlymphoid malignancies may transiently reduce the mitogenic response of lymphocytes (Barta, 1983; Kristensen et al., 1982), thereby impairing cell-mediated immunity. Factors inhibiting such a response may be found in serums of diseased animals (review by Barta, 1983), e.g., in dogs with generalized demodectic mange (Hirsh et al., 1975) and in cattle with lymphocytic leukemia (Jacobs et al., 1980) and squamous cell carcinoma (Dhingra et al., 1982). It was shown that serum-mediated immunosuppression in demodicosis in dogs is due to secondary bacterial infection because it was absent in animals with uncomplicated demodectic mange (Barta et al., 1983). Macrophages may also inhibit blastogenic response of peripheral blood lymphocytes (Bendixen et al., 1981).

Bone Marrow

Bone marrow is recognized as the body's major site of lymphocyte production and release (Douglas, 1983a). It contains a variable number of morphologically recognizable lymphocytes, depending on the species and age of the individual. In mice, 20–25% and in guinea pigs up to 50% of all nucleated marrow cells are lymphocytes. In humans, 16–21% of marrow cells constitute lymphocytes during adult life, while about 50% are present at birth and many more during fetal life (Williams et al., 1983). Among the common domestic animals, the cat has the largest number (5–15% of marrow cells) of lymphocytes in the bone marrow. Lymphocytes are diffusely distributed in the parenchyma of normal marrow, or they may appear as perivascular aggregates and rarely as nodules (in chickens).

Bone marrow lymphocytes have been classified according to morphology, immunologic attributes, origin, and cell age. In the following description, the proportions of various lymphocytes given in parentheses are for murine bone marrow, which has been extensively investigated (Osmond, 1980; Osmond et al., 1981; Wintrobe et al., 1981). Morphologically, most (80%) of the marrow lymphocytes are small, while some (20%) are large. The majority (60%) of the large lymphocytes have characteristics of pre-B cells, and most (80%) of the small lymphocytes are B cells. Some (8%) small lymphocytes are identified as T cells, and the remaining (12%) are classified as "non-T, non-B" or null cells. All of the T cells and about an equal proportion of the small B-lymphocytes are recirculating, long-lived, blood-borne lymphocytes. Studies with isotope labeling indicate that most of the small lymphocytes do not synthesize DNA and are nondividing, short-lived cells that originate locally from mitoses of large lymphocytes.

It takes about 30–36 hours for the newly formed marrow lymphocytes to mature and develop specific cell markers of B-lymphocytes. Labeled cells may appear in blood within 8 hours, and many of the newly formed small lymphocytes leave the bone marrow to seed the peripheral lymphoid organs, but most die in situ with a turnover time of 2–4 days. Thus bone marrow lymphopoiesis is largely ineffective, except in the guinea pig in which the majority of the marrow lymphocytes enter the blood (Yoffey, 1975).

In most species a decrease in marrow lymphopoiesis has little or no effect on blood lymphocyte numbers (Yoffey and Courtice, 1970). Conversely, production of lymphocytes in the bone marrow is not influenced by incoming, recirculating, blood-borne lymphocytes, thoracic duct drainage, or splenic or extracorporeal irradiation (Williams et al., 1983). In neonatally thymectomized or congenitally athymic mice, marrow lymphopoiesis is unaffected (Osmond et al., 1981). A basal level of lymphocyte production in the bone marrow is maintained by local microenvironmental factors and can be stimulated by nonspecific stimuli (Osmond et al., 1981).

Thymus

The thymus processes bone marrow-derived, committed lymphoid stem cells into cells destined to become immunocompetent T-lymphocytes. Lymphopoiesis occurs primarily in the cortex, and the newly formed lymphocytes continually move into the medulla, where little or no mitotic activity is observed (Wintrobe et al., 1981). The rate of mitotic activity in the thymus is about 5 to 10 times that in the peripheral lymphoid tissues, but the cell output is much less. The majority (about 95%) of the thymic lymphocytes have a short life span and die in situ. Only 5% of the thymic lymphocytes from the medulla and probably cortex enter the circulation via blood vessels or lymphatic channels. These cells are long-lived and migrate to T-dependent areas in the peripheral lymphoid organs where they further differentiate and mature

into subsets of T cells. Some differentiation is apparent in the thymus as evidenced by differences in cell surface antigens and steroid sensitivity; cells of the thymic cortex are corticosteroid-sensitive, while those in the medulla are relatively corticosteroid-resistant. In the thymus, only about 1% of the cells are recirculating lymphocytes, while the rest are locally produced.

Lymphoid differentiation toward T cell lineage in the thymus is influenced by several factors. These include thymic microenvironment, direct cellular contact between the stromal elements and lymphoid cells, thymic hormones, particularly thymosin and thymopoietin, lymphokines produced by medullary cells, and thymic macrophages (Bach and Papiernik, 1981; Janossy et al., 1981; Sell and Miller, 1980). Thymic hormones and interleukin-2 also influence T cell lymphopoiesis in the peripheral lymphoid organs (Bach and Papiernik, 1981). Recently it has been shown that the thymic medulla may contribute predominantly to the generation of helper T-lymphocytes (Janossy et al., 1981).

Peripheral Lymphoid Organs

Lymphopoiesis in the peripheral lymphoid organs such as the *spleen, lymph nodes,* and *Peyer's patches* occurs mainly in the germinal centers of lymphoid follicles, which play an important role in generation and differentiation of B-lymphocytes (Opstelten et al., 1981). Some B cell differentiation at these locations can occur independent of antigenic stimulation, but formation of germinal centers is induced by antigenic exposure and lymphokines. Most of the newly formed cells, however, die in situ, while some contribute to the pool of follicular B cells and migrate into the surrounding lymphoid tissue to develop into antibody-producing plasma cells and memory cells (Nieuwenhis et al., 1981; Opstelten et al., 1981). Memory cells are lymphocytes capable of eliciting a secondary immune response on contact with specific antigen at a later time—months to years. The localization of antigen to germinal centers is a highly C3-dependent process, and it is possible that C receptors on B cells may be involved in this process (Klaus and Humphrey, 1977). A minor degree of lymphopoietic activity leading to formation of T cells occurs in the paracortical areas of the lymph node and in the periarteriolar sheaths of the spleen (T-dependent areas).

Regulation of Lymphopoiesis

Lymphopoiesis in the lymph nodes and spleen is regulated primarily by an antigenic stimulus. In contrast, thymic lymphopoiesis and formation of pre-B cells in the bone marrow are independent of antigenic stimulus. B cell differentiation and plasma cell formation in the bone marrow are antigen-dependent, however. Thus in germfree rats and mice, lymphoid follicles in the lymph nodes and spleen are vestigial and B cell production in the marrow is reduced, while the thymus is near normal in size. Similarly, gnotobiotic dogs are deficient in B cells, although they have an unimpaired capacity to develop humoral immune response (Krakowka et al., 1978).

It has been estimated that about 0.5 million lymphocytes are formed each hour in a single axillary lymph node in health and about 2.6 million upon antigenic stimulation (Pierce, 1967). Lymphopoiesis varies greatly in different lymph nodes throughout the body (Mitchell et al., 1963), and existence of oligosynthetic lymph nodes has been recognized, a typical example being the popliteal lymph node in the guinea pig (Olson and Yoffey, 1967), mouse (Cottier et al., 1967), and sheep (Hall and Morris, 1965a).

Thymectomy leads to lymphopenia and impaired immune responses, but its effects vary with the species depending on the degree of cellularity of the peripheral lymphoid organs at birth (Cline, 1975). In the dog, the peripheral lymphoid organs are well developed at birth; hence little adverse effect is observed. In contrast, newborn mice, rats, and hamsters have poorly populated peripheral lymphoid organs, and so thymectomy results in serious immunologic impairment. Thymectomy of sheep fetuses between 55 and 77 days of gestation was associated with lymphopenia and decreased numbers of T cells for 8 months after birth (Fahey et al., 1980). In those species in which a significant amount of lymphopoiesis occurs in the bone marrow, e.g., the guinea pig, any factor influencing marrow ac-

tivity also affects the peripheral blood lymphocyte counts (Jones et al., 1967; Yoffey et al., 1968).

Lymphokinetics

Lymphokinetic studies have been difficult to perform and evaluate mainly because of the phenomenon of recirculation of lymphocytes and partly because of the lack of an end point in lymphocyte differentiation (Yoffey and Courtice, 1970). Injection of lymphocytes labeled in vitro, using ^{32}P, ^{51}Cr, ^{3}HTdR, and more recently ^{111}In-oxine (Wagstaff et al., 1981), and in vivo injection of ^{3}HTdR as a pulse label or continuous infusion have provided some information about the production and distribution of various lymphocyte populations. Unstimulated small lymphocytes have little or no DNA synthetic activity and so they do not incorporate ^{3}HTdR, while antigen- or phytomitogen-stimulated lymphocytes express this property. The generation time of large and medium-sized lymphocytes in the thymus of the adult mouse was reported to be 6–8 hours (Metcalf and Wiadrowski, 1966). Similar estimates have been obtained for lymphocytes in the germinal centers of lymph nodes and the spleen (Fliedner et al., 1964; Hanna, 1964). The turnover time of small lymphocytes in the thymus and the bone marrow of humans and some laboratory animals is reported to be 2–4 days (Matsuyama et al., 1966; Osmond and Everett, 1964).

Lymphopoiesis in external lymph nodes of two normal calves and two cows with lymphosarcoma was studied after injection of ^{3}HTdR in situ and measurement of grain counts of the labeled cells appearing in the efferent lymph (Kaneko et al., 1963). In normal calves, highest labeling occurred in large lymphocytes followed by medium and small lymphocytes. The generation time was estimated as 1–1.5 hours, T½ as 2 hours, and turnover time as 3 hours. At least two generations for the large and one for the medium lymphocytes were thought to occur.

Results in cows with lymphosarcoma indicated a marked increase in the rate of proliferation of large lymphocytes and an impairment in the generation of small lymphocytes. Labeling of large lymphocytes was greatly increased, but labeling of small lymphocytes was insignificant. The turnover of lymphocytes from the tumorous nodes was considerably increased. Other studies on bovine leukosis have reported similar findings (Chander and Gilman, 1974; Weiland and Straub, 1976). It has been reported that DNA synthesis and generation times are different in cytologically different populations of lymphocytes in the thoracic duct of the calf (Safier et al., 1967).

Quantitative studies on the rate of production of lymphocytes have been made in some species. In calves, about 200 million cells per minute enter the blood via the thoracic duct; of these, about 10% are new, while the rest are in the recirculation cycle (Cronkite et al., 1964). In sheep, about 300 million lymphocytes per hour are discharged per gram of lymph node tissue (Hall, 1967).

Qualitative and quantitative differences are found in lymphocytes from different regions of the body; for example, efferent lymph from the intestine contains a larger number of lymphocytes than that from other tissues and has IgA-bearing large lymphoid cells not present elsewhere. The cell population in lymph draining a particular tissue may change considerably due to physiologic and pathologic alterations in the tissue (Fahey et al., 1980; Issekutz et al., 1981). Lymphocyte production is increased after antigenic stimulation as described above.

The life span of lymphocytes is hard to estimate because, unlike neutrophils, they are not end stage cells. Subpopulations of lymphocytes are capable of undergoing blastic transformation and mitosis after an extended intermitotic interval. In early studies using ^{32}P as a DNA label (Ottesen, 1954), human lymphocytes were divided into two groups on the basis of life span: a small (11–22%) population with a short survival time of 2–4 days and the majority (78–89%) with a long survival time of 100–200 days. The existence of two populations of lymphocytes has been confirmed in other studies using different isotopes (Cronkite and Schiffer, 1970; Everett et al., 1964; Fitzgerald, 1964).

It is now believed that in the peripheral blood and various tissues, T cells are generally long-lived, B cells are short-lived, and memory T and B cells are very long-lived. In mice, almost all thoracic duct lymphocytes are long-lived; T cells have a life span of about 120–180 days and B cells of 35–50 days (Sprent and Basten 1973). Virtually all small lymphocytes in the bone marrow and thymus are short-lived, having a turnover time of about 2–4 days. In humans, the majority of lymphocytes in blood are long-lived; the average life span of human lymphocytes is estimated to be 4.3 years, and about 1% may live for at least 20 years (Buckton et al., 1967). No such information is available for common domestic animals, but a similar situation is believed to exist.

Recirculation

Gowans and colleagues (Gowans, 1959; Gowans and Knight, 1964) in a series of elegant studies with rats conclusively demonstrated that lymphocytes recirculate from blood to lymph nodes and back to blood. Hall and Morris (1962, 1965a,b) performed similar studies in fetal and adult sheep and provided further information. Recirculation has been studied by intravenously injecting lymphocytes labeled with ^{51}Cr, ^{3}HTdR, ^{111}indium oxine, and fluorescein isothiocyanate and tracking their appearance in various lymphoid organs and in efferent or thoracic duct lymph. Recirculation has been observed during fetal life, as early as 96 days of gestation in sheep (Pearson et al., 1976).

Significance

The recirculation phenomenon is significant in that it allows (a) a generalized distribution of immunocompetent cells, (b) exposure of a greater number of lymphocytes to an antigen deposited locally in the tissue, (c) a generalized relocation of antigenically primed cells and (d) immune surveillance. Thus it plays an extremely important role in establishing conditions for the generalized immune response to a local antigenic stimulus and protecting the body from development of undesirable clones of cells under normal circumstances. Recent observations on lymphocyte circulation in patients with lymphoproliferative disorders have introduced exciting new possibilities for therapy, including the use of labeled cells to home a source of ra-

RECIRCULATION OF LYMPHOCYTES

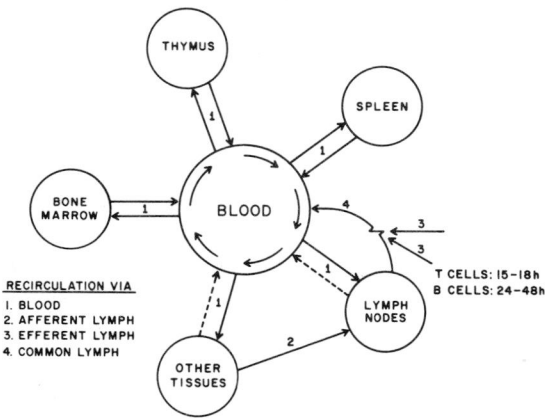

Fig. 30–5. Recirculation of lymphocytes through blood, bone marrow, lymphoid organs, and other body tissues. (Modified from Cline, 1975.)

diation preferentially to affected tissue (Crowther and Wagstaff, 1983).

Migration through Different Lymphoid Organs

It has been established that lymphocytes recirculate freely among the lymph nodes, spleen, GALT, and bone marrow and to a limited extent through the thymus (Brumby and Metcalf, 1967; Gowans and Knight, 1964; Keiser et al., 1967). Some lymphocyte migration also occurs into other tissues and body fluids, but cells from only the tissues and not the body fluids reenter the circulation through lymph. Migration of lymphocytes through various organs is depicted in Fig. 30–5. The migratory pathways of T-lymphocytes have been defined more clearly than those of B-lymphocytes.

The recirculation pattern of lymphocytes varies with the tissue and properties of the lymphocytes. Both T and B cells have been found to recirculate, but at different rates and following different pathways (Crowther and Wagstaff, 1983; Ford, 1979; Parrott and Wilkinson, 1981).

In rats, 90% of T-lymphocytes leaving the blood enter one of the three major sites of lymphocyte recirculation—the spleen (55%), the bone marrow (15%), and the lymph nodes (20%). The remaining (10%) migrate through the nonlymphoid tissues and enter blood through the peripheral lymph. Studies with

[111]indium oxine–labeled lymphocytes in humans indicate that these cells migrate initially to the liver, then reenter blood to circulate at first through the spleen and then through the lymph nodes (Wagstaff et al., 1981).

Most of the B cells in the peripheral blood are considered nonrecirculating; they represent freshly released, marrow-derived, virgin B cells on their way to the peripheral lymphoid organs. Recirculating B cells are primarily memory cells. In general, B cells move much more slowly than T cells; suppressor T cells circulate less than helper T cells; and lymphoblasts are usually noncirculating (Parrott and Wilkinson, 1981).

Transit time of lymphocytes also varies with the age of the animal, being longer in adult sheep and shorter during fetal life. Most of the circulation time is spent in the organs, where "homing" (returning to the site of production) occurs, while only a few hours are spent in the peripheral blood.

T and B cells distribute randomly, but some evidence in sheep indicates a preferential recirculation of T cell subpopulations through lymphoid and nonlymphoid tissues (Ford, 1979) and of B cells through GALT or peripheral lymph nodes, depending on their site of origin (Cahill et al., 1977; Hall et al., 1972). On this basis it was suggested that in adult sheep there may be two migratory pathways for lymphoid cells: one through the GALT and the other through the "somatic-splenic lymphoid tissues" (Hall et al., 1977). Such separation was not seen in the fetal lamb (Cahill et al., 1979).

Lymphocytes enter various tissues primarily at the region of postcapillary venules. The peripheral lymphoid organs have peculiar postcapillary venules with cuboidal or cylindrical endothelial cells. These so-called high endothelial venules (HEV) are located mainly in the deep cortex or paracortex and sometimes in the medullary cords of the lymph nodes and in the asinusoidal areas of the hemolymph nodes (Olah and Gliek, 1980). In the tonsils and Peyer's patches, they occur in the interfollicular areas.

Schoefl (1972), in an excellent electron microscopic study of single and serial tissue sections, demonstrated that lymphocytes migrate across the vascular endothelium *between* the endothelial cells and not *through* these cells as was believed earlier (Marchesi and Gowans, 1964). In lymph nodes, lymphocytes enter also through the afferent lymphatics. Reentry into the circulation from the lymph nodes in most species is essentially through efferent lymphatics, although a few cells may return via the vascular endothelium. The latter is the primary mode in the pig. Lymphocytes from the spleen, bone marrow, and thymus enter the blood predominantly through vascular endothelium (Osmond, 1980) and from Peyer's patches via lymph (Reynolds and Pabst, 1984).

Lymph Nodes. T-lymphocytes take longer to traverse the lymph nodes (15–18 hours in rats) than the spleen (5–6 hours in rats), but they migrate through both tissues much faster than B-lymphocytes do. In most species, T-lymphocytes enter the lymph nodes from the blood through HEV within 10–20 minutes and follow an ill-defined route within the paracortex to reach the medullary sinuses and the efferent lymphatics (Gowans and Knight, 1964; Opstelten et al., 1981; Parrott and Wilkinson, 1981). B-lymphocytes migrate through the HEV at a similar rate, but take a longer, devious route passing through follicular areas, particularly the coronas surrounding the germinal centers. Germinal centers are generally spared, although a certain subpopulation of B cells has been found to migrate into these areas (Opstelten et al., 1981). These lymphocytes subsequently find their way into the cortical and medullary sinuses and leave the node by way of the efferent lymph. Lymphocytes entering the lymph node via the afferent lymph show a different distribution; they become distributed throughout the superficial and deep cortex.

The relative proportion of lymphocytes entering a lymph node via the afferent lymph or directly from blood varies depending on the location of the lymph node in the lymphatic chain. Entry from the blood is also influenced to some extent by the number of lymphocytes entering via the lymph. In the peripheral lymph nodes, about 5–10% of the lymphocytes enter through the lymph, while 90% arrive by way of the blood (Hall and Morris, 1962, 1965b). This traffic pattern may be much different in centrally located nodes, and

the central lymph may differ in the number and types of cells, e.g., lymphocytes with surface immunoglobulins are four to five times more frequent in the central lymph than in the peripheral lymph (Miller and Adams, 1977).

Lymphocytes may leave a node to enter the blood either directly by traversing the postcapillary venules ("direct entry" lymphocytes) or indirectly by first entering efferent lymphatics and then appearing in the peripheral blood via the thoracic duct ("indirect entry" lymphocytes) (Yoffey, 1960). In the smaller laboratory animals, the direct entry lymphocytes consist mainly of newly formed cells, while the indirect entry lymphocytes are mainly recirculating (Yoffey, 1970). Direct entry lymphocytes represent a minor proportion of the total population leaving the lymph node because lymphatic blockage is followed by a decrease to almost zero in the number of circulating lymphocytes. Indirect entry lymphocytes may pass through one or several nodes before entering the blood.

Lymphocytes entering the blood through routes other than the thoracic duct, as from the right and cervical lymphatic ducts, are referred to as the "supplementary" lymphocytes (Yoffey and Courtice, 1956). The number of supplementary lymphocytes gaining access to the blood is about 4–12 times greater than that contributed by the thoracic duct (Yoffey, 1970).

Thoracic duct lymphocytes are derived mainly from mesenteric and intestinal lymphoid tissues (Cunningham et al., 1967). In most species they are comprised primarily (about 90%) of small lymphocytes and few (5–10%) medium to large lymphocytes. In the dog, 25–30% may be of the latter type (Elves, 1967). The majority of small lymphocytes (about 90%) in the thoracic duct are long-lived T cells, while the remaining (10%) are newly formed cells having a short life span (Everett and Tyler, 1967). Hence chronic drainage of the thoracic duct is associated with a significant decrease of T cells, but not of B cells in blood (Bohs et al., 1976).

Recirculation of lymphocytes in pigs is interesting. Pigs have large lymph nodes and a high lymphocyte count in the blood, but a considerably lower lymphocyte number

($<$10–250/μl) in the efferent lymph than that of other species (10^3–10^4/μl). These findings led Binns and Hall (1966) to suggest that lymphocytes in the pig recirculate into and out of the lymph nodes via the blood vascular system. Subsequent studies using labeled lymphocytes and other investigations have confirmed this mode of lymphocyte recirculation in the pig (review in Binns, 1982, and Bennel and Husband, 1981). It is related to the unique architecture of the lymph node in the pig—the conventional arrangement of the cortex and medulla is inverted. However, migration of lymphocytes from blood into the lymph node and spleen is comparable to that in other species (Pabst and Geisler, 1981).

Spleen. Studies in mice and rats indicate that both T and B cells enter the white pulp via the marginal zone, which functions as the HEV present in lymph nodes. Subsequently T cells move into the periarteriolar sheaths and then into the splenic venous blood to enter the circulation within 5–6 hours. B cells move into nodular areas, remain distributed in the parafollicular areas, and leave the spleen by 24 hours. More B cells recirculate through the spleen than through the lymph nodes (Ford, 1979).

Bone Marrow. Recirculating lymphocytes constitute only a small proportion of the total population of lymphocytes in the bone marrow (Ford, 1979; Osmond, 1980). Thoracic duct lymphocytes, comprised mainly of T cells, were found to have a short intramyeloid time (4–6 hours in mice and 2–3 hours in rats), similar to that in the spleen. Cells entering the marrow show a nonrandom distribution in the parenchyma, but a higher congregation is found along the periphery. The circulatory pattern for B cells remains unknown.

Mechanisms

Mechanisms involved in lymphocyte recirculation and its regulation are not definitely known, but various factors are considered important (Parrott and Wilkinson, 1981). Ecotaxis, i.e., separation of lymphocytes into T- and B-dependent areas of the lymphoid tissues, has been attributed to specific membrane properties of lymphocytes that are acquired during differentiation and is probably also related to the local microenvironment

and characteristics of the resident cells such as the reticulum cells.

It is conjectured that various populations of lymphocytes recirculate differently, probably because of variations in their surface characteristics, locomotion, and adherence to endothelial cells. Subsets within the T and B populations may show predilection for migration to certain lymphoid tissues, and cell age may also be important. For example, lymphoblasts are generally noncirculating or move very slowly through the lymph nodes.

Blood flow to the lymphoid organs was also found to affect recirculation, particularly after antigenic stimulation (Hay and Hobbs, 1977). Subcutaneous injection of antigen stimulates lymphocyte migration and trapping of lymphocytes within the lymph nodes, while intravenous or intraperitoneal injection of antigen increases lymphocyte migration to the spleen.

Antigenic, inflammatory, and cancerous processes in the drainage areas of regional lymph nodes may affect the traffic of lymphocytes through these nodes. The factors involved include vasoactive modulators of inflammation such as prostaglandins, histamine, bradykinin, and serotonin. These agents probably exert this effect through changes in cyclic nucleotide concentrations of the vascular tree and also of lymphocytes. Lymphocyte migration through popliteal lymph nodes of sheep was reduced by acute and chronic in vivo infusion of cyclic adenosine monophosphate (cAMP) and increased by similar infusions of cyclic guanosine monophosphate (cGMP) (Moore and Lachmann, 1982).

A variety of exogenous factors can influence lymphocyte migration. Pretreatment of lymphocytes with agents such as neuraminidase, trypsin, phospholipases A and C, plant lectins, and dextran has been found to affect lymphocyte surface charges, membrane properties, adhesion to vascular endothelium, and consequently recirculation (Parrott and Wilkinson, 1981). For example, small lymphocytes treated with plant lectins take more time to traverse the lymph nodes. Trypsinized lymphocytes do not migrate into the lymph nodes, GALT, and adjuvant-induced granulomas, but are capable of migrating into the spleen (Ford, 1979). Influenza and New-castle disease viruses attach to rat lymphocytes and inhibit their migration into the lymphoid organs (Woodruff and Woodruff, 1976). The effect is mediated through the viral neuraminidase, which digests sialic acid residues from the surface membranes of lymphocytes; both T- and B-lymphocytes are affected. Such lymphocytes do not attach to HEV of lymphoid organs, but can migrate to the liver. Similarly, heparin modifies the lymphocyte surface and induces lymphocytosis (Bradfield and Born, 1969; Jansen et al., 1962; see Lymphocyte Numbers in Peripheral Blood, below). Heat-damaged lymphocytes are retained preferentially by the lungs and liver.

Lymphoma, lymphocytic leukemia, and multiple myeloma are clonal lymphoproliferative disorders. The distribution of malignant lymphocytes in blood, bone marrow, and various lymphoid tissues in these disorders is extremely varied. Elucidation of migratory properties of such cells would be helpful in correlating varied laboratory findings of lymphocyte distribution and improved clinical management of the patient. Migration of malignant lymphocytes has been studied in humans (reviewed by Crowther and Wagstaff, 1983).

Functions of Lymphocytes

The primary role of lymphocytes is in humoral antibody formation and cell-mediated immunity. The immune response is age-dependent, the young and the old being less competent. Studies in various species have shown that immune competence is acquired gradually during fetal life, is fair (dog) to substantial (pig) at birth, and attains full expression during the first few months after birth (Bohs et al., 1976; Kristensen et al., 1982; Perryman et al., 1980). It declines with aging in association with thymic involution and lymphoid atrophy. Deficiency in one or both types of immune response has been found in humans and animals—for example, agammaglobulinemia from B cell deficiency (Banks et al., 1976; McGuire et al., 1976) and combined immune deficiency in the horse (McGuire et al., 1974). The reader is referred to a current immunology text for more information about the immune functions of lymphocytes than is given below.

Antibody Production

Although it has long been well accepted that the plasma cells are engaged in antibody synthesis, a similar role for the lymphocytes was debated until it was shown that pure populations of lymphocytes can synthesize antibodies both in vivo and in vitro (van Furth, 1969). Antibody formation occurs predominantly in the lymph nodes, to a lesser extent in the spleen and bone marrow, and to a variable extent locally in various tissues, including the Peyer's patches.

Antibody production generally involves interaction of the antigen with macrophages, T cells, and B cells and interactions among these cells (Bell, 1982; Hahn and Kaufmann, 1982; Melchers et al., 1982; Unanue, 1981; Wieczorek, 1980). However, antibody formation from certain antigens (e.g., lipopolysaccharides) may not require macrophage or T cell participation. Macrophages phagocytize and process the antigen for presentation in immunogenic form or hold the antigen on their surface for resting T and B cells to respond. Follicular dendritic cells in the germinal centers serve a similar function. Interaction of lymphocytes with macrophages is necessary for full expression of the immune response (Cline, 1975).

Various studies have shown that antigen-reactive T cells (helper or inducer T cells) and B cells through their surface receptors recognize the antigens and react specifically to them. To become activated, T helper cells through their specific surface immunoglobulins recognize the foreign antigen (carrier portion) and Ia antigen present on the macrophages. Similarly, activation of B cells involves recognition of the antigen (hapten portion) by specific immunoglobulin molecules (IgM) on their surface and also recognition of their surface Ia antigen by activated T helper cells. This double-signal recognition stimulates T and B cells to produce progenies specific for that particular antigen. This clonal proliferation is aided by lymphokines produced by antigen-stimulated T cells and is regulated by T suppressor cells and stimulatory (interleukin-1) and inhibitory (PGE) substances produced by macrophages (Kristensen et al., 1982; Ptak and Gershon, 1975). The antigen-specific progeny recognize the same antigen upon subsequent presentation and undergo a similar secondary proliferation. Some of the progeny become memory cells, while most express the specific immune response, whether humoral or cellular, depending mainly on the type of antigenic stimulation.

Transformation of B cells into antibody-producing immunocytes or plasma cells is the basis of humoral antibody response. Clonal proliferation results in the production of increasing amounts of antibody. Following antigenic stimulation, the different antibody classes appear in the blood in the order IgM, IgG, and IgA (Freedman and Gold, 1976). There is some evidence that this switching from one class of antibody to another requires T helper cells. For example, in T cell-deprived animals, there is usually some IgM response, but little or no IgG or IgA. Similarly, antibody response to T-independent antigens is predominantly IgM (Wieczorek, 1980). Individual plasma cells secrete only one type of antibody and of a single subclass (Cline, 1975; Grossi and Greaves, 1981). Plasma cells in the intestine specifically secrete IgA. Primary immune response takes about a week for peak expression, while secondary response is evident in less time, usually within 3–5 days.

The immunosuppressive effect of corticosteroids is mediated through various phases associated with the immune response. It has been suggested that a major mechanism involves lympholysis in "steroid-sensitive" animals (see Lymphocyte Numbers in Peripheral Blood, below), while in "steroid-resistant" species it is probably mediated through reduction in the number of Fc receptors on antigen-responsive cells and decreased production of lymphokines (Crabtree et al., 1980). Steroid-induced immunosuppression is more effective with respect to the primary immune response than the secondary response.

Cell-Mediated Immune Responses

The role of lymphocytes in mediation of such manifestations of cellular immunity as delayed type of hypersensitivity, homograft rejection, graft-versus-host reaction, tumor rejection, autoimmunity, and resistance to certain pathogens are being increasingly defined. T-lymphocytes are involved in these types of immune responses. Subpopulations of T cells are assigned different functions, some of which are seemingly opposite (Cantor, 1979; Gupta and Good, 1981). Cell-mediated immunity is measured by various in vitro tests such as macrophage migration inhibition, leukocyte migration inhibition, lymphocyte-mediated cytotoxicity, and lymphocyte transformation assays.

Immunoregulatory Role. T-lymphocytes exert an immunoregulatory influence on humoral antibody response (as discussed above) as well as cell-mediated immunity. T helper cells are involved in antigen recognition and stimulate B cells to produce antibody. T suppressor cells regulate activity of T helper cells and also regulate antibody production by B cells. T-lymphocytes from an animal unresponsive to a given antigen, when transferred to a normal animal, render the recipient specifically unresponsive. Such a suppressor function is probably involved in homeostatic control of the immune system and in preventing untoward autoimmune reactions and oncogenesis. T memory cells retain a capacity to respond upon stimulation by specific antigen at a later time.

Any disturbance in this immunoregulatory function of T cells may be expected to cause autoimmune disease. For example, it has been shown that serums of children with rheumatoid arthritis contain antibodies reactive with suppressor T cells, and a decreased number or selective dysfunction of suppressor T cells is seen in patients with systemic lupus erythematosus. This dysfunction of suppressor T cells could explain, at least in part, the exaggerated autoimmune responses seen in such patients (Giacco, 1980). It has been suggested that virus-induced depression of the host's immune protective mechanisms may be a necessary antecedent for the expression of oncogenic potential of feline leukemia virus in cats (Cockerell et al., 1976b).

Cytotoxic Function. Another function of T cells is the production of progeny capable of injuring or destroying cells that are recognized as antigenically foreign, e.g., tumor cells and cells infected with a virus. This is called the cytotoxic or killer function of T cells. Lymphocyte-mediated cytotoxicity has been found to involve three biologic activities of effector lymphocytes (Grossi and Greaves, 1981; Herberman, 1980):

1. Expression of T cell cytotoxic activity (cytotoxic T cells or immune cytotoxic T cells) requires previous antigenic exposure; hence, the phenomenon is antigen-specific.

2. Expression of K (killer) cell activity involves null cells and requires coating of the target cell by specific antibody. It is therefore also referred to as antibody-dependent cellular cytotoxicity (ADCC). K cells have Fc receptors and can be found in normal animals.

3. NK (natural killer) cell activity is expressed by a subpopulation of null cells against a wide spectrum of target cells. Killing by NK cells does not require antibody because these cells have receptors interacting with antigens on various target cells. Almost all human and rat NK cells have been morphologically identified as large lymphocytes with prominent azurophilic granules (Reynolds et al., 1981; Timonen et al., 1981).

In each of these cytotoxic activities, the target cell and the effector lymphocyte must come in contact for expression of the cytotoxic effect. The exact mechanism of killing is unknown (Sanderson, 1981). It should be remembered that ADCC is also exhibited by other leukocytes, namely, neutrophils, eosinophils, and monocytes and macrophages. Various characteristics of these cytotoxic lymphocytes have been reviewed (Djeu, 1982).

There is increasing evidence that NK cells are important in immune surveillance (Herberman, 1982; Herberman and Ortaldo, 1981). For example, these cells mediate natural resistance against tumors, certain bacterial and viral diseases, and bone marrow transplants. NK activity is affected by a variety of factors including interferons, lectins, and PGE (Herberman and Ortaldo, 1981); bacterial, viral, or protozoan infection (Campos et al., 1982; Hauser et al., 1982; Norley and Wardley,

1983); and immunosuppressive drugs and immunodeficiency disorders (Herberman, 1980). NK activity has been detected in normal humans and several species of animals (Herberman and Ortaldo, 1981; Huh et al., 1981; Krakowka, 1983; Leibold et al., 1980; Magnuson et al., 1985; Pinto, 1985).

This function is also age-dependent; e.g., fetal lambs at 70–138 days of gestation exhibited no cell-mediated lympholysis, and a markedly reduced level was seen at birth (Granberg and Hirvonen, 1980). Gnotobiotic young pigs are devoid of NK activity (Huh et al., 1981), but adult gnotobiotic dogs possess levels of NK activity comparable to those in conventional dogs (Krakowka, 1983).

Secretion of Lymphokines. Stimulated T-lymphocytes produce in vitro and also in vivo several soluble substances that have immense biologic significance, particularly in immunologic and inflammatory responses. These substances are called lymphokines (Dumonde et al., 1969). Activated B cells also produce some lymphokines. Nearly 100 different lymphokines have been described (review by Altman and Katz, 1982; Klesius, 1982; Rocklin et al., 1980), but some of these may be the same molecular species with different activities. Most of these are released upon antigenic stimulation, and some may be produced in response to nonspecific stimuli such as phytomitogens. Lymphokine synthesis is inhibited by agents inhibiting protein synthesis, affecting organization of microtubules and microfilaments, and increasing cellular levels of cAMP. Lymphokines can be found in circulation during an immune response.

Lymphokines have been classified functionally according to their effects on target cells: inhibitory or cytotoxic, stimulatory or proliferative, and inflammatory (review by Rocklin et al., 1980). The inhibitory lymphokines include substances that lyse (lymphotoxin) or inhibit proliferation (immune interferon) of their target cells. The stimulatory lymphokines include mitogenic factors that act upon lymphocytes or monocytes, colony stimulating factors, and lymphokines mediating T–B and T–T cell interactions. The role of T-lymphocytes in regulation of hematopoiesis is mediated principally through production of cell lineage–specific lymphokines

(Ascensao et al., 1981; Bagby et al., 1981; see also Chapter 13). The inflammatory lymphokines include factors related to the expression of cell-mediated immunity including migration inhibition factor (MIF), macrophage activating factor (MAF), chemotactic factors, as well as factors influencing vascular permeability and the clotting system. Lymphokines are also classified as antigen-specific or antigen-nonspecific (Altman and Katz, 1982). Brief descriptions of some lymphokines are given below.

Transfer factor is an antigen-specific, low-molecular-weight (less than 10,000) substance released within 1 hour of stimulation. It is capable of sensitizing a normal individual to initiate a cellular immune response upon contact with the antigen (delayed type hypersensitivity). It is species-specific.

Migration inhibition factor (MIF) inhibits the migration of monocytes and macrophages. It is produced within a few hours of interaction of a specific antigen with lymphocytes from a donor with delayed hypersensitivity (George and Vaughan, 1962). Lymphocytes stimulated by Con A and PHA also produce MIF. MIFs from different species appear to be proteins or glycoproteins with molecular weights between 23,000 and 65,000. Significant interspecies differences in the molecular structure of MIF seem to exist, although MIFs from different species affect heterologous macrophages. MIF reacts with surface receptors on monocytes and macrophages and makes the cells "sticky," thereby inhibiting cellular migration. It also increases their phagocytic and oxidative activities. Its production in vivo is thought to explain immobilization and accumulation of macrophages in lesions of delayed hypersensitivity and in granulomas. A similar factor capable of inhibiting the migration of neutrophils is called *leukocyte inhibiting factor* (LIF).

Macrophage activating factor (MAF) induces a variety of morphologic and functional changes typical of cellular activation. These include increased metabolic and functional activities such as augmented protein synthesis, lysosome formation, pinocytosis, phagocytosis, and bactericidal and tumoricidal capacities. It may initiate transformation of macrophages into epithelioid and giant cells.

MAF-induced activation of macrophages generally occurs after 1–3 days of interaction.

Mitosis stimulating factor (lymphocyte mitogenic factor or blastogenic factor) is released within 18–24 hours of T cell stimulation. It is a protein with a molecular weight of 15,000–50,000. It promotes blastogenesis of lymphocytes themselves; B-lymphocytes are particularly sensitive to its effect; hence it may be equally significant in humoral antibody response.

Lymphotoxin is a proteinaceous substance produced by reactive lymphocytes 2–5 days after exposure to a specific antigen or to nonspecific stimuli such as mitogens (Williams and Granger, 1969). Its molecular weight varies from 35,000–150,000 depending on the animal species, and three molecular subcomponents have been described. It is capable of destroying a wide variety of cells in tissue culture and is suspected of playing a similar role in vivo.

Interferons are newly synthesized glycoproteins (molecular weight 20,000–160,000) produced by a variety of cells including B cells after viral infection ("classical" or type I interferon) or by T-lymphocytes after mitogenic or antigenic stimulation ("immune" or type II interferon). Interferon production is suppressed following leukemic transformation of lymphocytes. Type I interferons include both α and β interferons, while type II is identical to γ interferon (Friedman and Vogel, 1983). Interferons have a wide range of antiviral activity and other biologic activities such as inhibition of tumor growth and regulation of cellular and humoral immune responses and macrophage function (De Maeyer-Guignard, 1981; Friedman and Vogel, 1983). Recent experimental studies in mice suggest that lymphopenia associated with viral infections in many cases may be due to virus-induced interferon rather than the virus itself (Schattner et al., 1983).

Interleukin-2 is a low-molecular-weight glycoprotein (murine, MW 30,000–35,000) or protein (human, MW 13,000–16,000) elaborated by T helper cells (Bendtzen, 1983). The latter are stimulated in the presence of appropriate antigen by interleukin-1 secreted from activated macrophages. Interleukin-2 is closely related, if not identical, to T cell growth factor, lymphocyte (thymocyte) mitogenic factor, thymocyte stimulating factor, and killer cell helper factor. It binds to specific receptors on activated T-lymphocytes and promotes their proliferation, thereby acting as a lymphocytic growth factor and modulator of immune response. It is thought that interleukin-2 promotes in vivo production of lymphokines and cytotoxic T-lymphocytes. Its use as a therapeutic agent in aberrant immune responses is being investigated (Gillis, 1983).

Production of interleukin-2 by bovine (Namen and Magnuson, 1984), ovine (English and Whitehurst, 1984), and canine (Cerruti-Sola et al., 1984) lymphocytes has been reported.

Lymphocyte Numbers in Peripheral Blood

The number of lymphocytes in the peripheral blood reflects a balance between cells leaving and entering the circulation; hence lymphocytosis or lymphopenia does not necessarily mean an altered lymphopoiesis (Yoffey et al., 1964). Changes in the rate of recirculation, production, destruction and/or elimination may or may not be reflected in the lymphocyte counts. For example, chronic drainage of lymph from calves produces a marked reduction in lymphocyte numbers in the lymph, but only a slight to moderate decrease is seen in the peripheral blood (Fish et al., 1969; Schnappauf and Schnappauf, 1968).

Similarly, a decrease in the size of lymphoid organs is not necessarily associated with a corresponding reduction in blood lymphocyte levels. For example, an increase in lymphocyte numbers in the blood was seen in humans with chronic lymphocytic leukemia when the palpable nodes were shrinking in response to cortisone therapy (Shaw et al., 1961).

A decrease in lymphopoiesis is usually associated with lymphopenia such as after thymectomy, corticosteroid administration, or irradiation, whereas a stimulation of lymphopoiesis may not result in lymphocytosis. Stimulation of lymphopoiesis during an immune response does not cause a significant increase in the number of circulating lymphocytes, although morphologic changes indicative of active protein synthesis may be seen in the cytoplasm of some lymphocytes (Crowther et al., 1969). Such lymphocytes (immunocytes) may be seen in blood of various animal species responding to a strong antigenic stimulus.

An intravenous injection of heparin produces a transient lymphocytosis in calves (Jansen et al., 1962) and rats (Bradfield and Born, 1969). In calves, this effect was attributed to increased mobilization of cells from lymphoid tissues, while in rats it was thought to be due to inhibition of lymphocyte emigration into the tissues. The duration of lymphocytosis depends on a critical concentration of heparin in the blood. An intravenous injection of *Bordetella pertussis* provokes a striking lymphocytosis in mice (Taub et al., 1972). This involves a reversible attachment of the pertussis factor onto the surface of lymphocytes, which prevents their homing back to lymphoid organs.

Results of studies with ^{3}HTdR-labeled lymphocytes and with extracorporeal irradiation indicate that there is a "rapidly accessible pool" of lymphocytes that can mix rapidly with the circulating lymphocytes (Cronkite and Schiffer, 1970). Its exact anatomic location is unknown, but it is thought to be analogous to the marginal pool of granulocytes. This pool of small lymphocytes numbers 2.5–3.4 $\times$ 10^9 lymphocytes/kg body weight for calves and sheep and 1.5–2.8 $\times$ 10^9 for dogs (Schnappauf and Schnappauf, 1968). In sheep and calves, this pool contains about 10 times and in dogs about 7 times the number of lymphocytes in the total circulating blood volume. In calves, this supply increased by 50% during the first 3 weeks of life. The existence of such a pool of lymphocytes may explain the physiologic lymphocytosis seen in some dogs (Table 4–5), cats (Table 5–3), and horses (Table 6–15).

Corticosteroids and sex hormones in physiologic concentrations affect lymphopoiesis (Mathur et al., 1979; Thomson et al., 1980), and increased concentrations of the former are known to cause lymphoid and thymic atrophy. Lymphoid atrophy also occurs in old age, malnutrition, and vitamin B deficiency (Esteban, 1968). Various species have been grouped according to the sensitivity of their lymphocytes to corticosteroids: rabbits, rats, and mice, are "steroid-sensitive" species and humans, monkeys, and guinea pigs are "steroid-resistant" species (Claman, 1972; Fauci et al., 1976). Glucocorticoid-sensitive populations of lymphocytes occur in various domestic animals (Kristensen et al., 1982).

Corticosteroid-induced lymphopenia is associated with lympholysis in blood and lymphoid tissues (rabbit) or altered distribution of lymphocytes out of the vascular pool into other body compartments such as the bone marrow (guinea pig), or both (mice and rats) (Cohen, 1972; Claman, 1972; Fauci, 1979; Fauci et al., 1976). Lymphopenia in different species involves various subpopulations of lymphocytes, but T cells are highly sensitive, particularly subsets of T cells with Fc receptors for IgM (T_M) (Fauci, 1979; Fauci et al., 1976; Hedman et al., 1980).

Several mechanisms of lympholysis have been proposed including inhibition of RNA and protein syntheses via inhibition of RNA polymerase, blockage of glucose transport and/or phosphorylation, and increase in protein degradation (Baxter and Forsman, 1972; McDonald et al., 1980). Redistribution of lymphocytes may be due to a direct effect of corticosteroids on the lymphocytes (alterations of surface charge) or on microvasculature (influencing adherence of lymphocytes to endothelial surface), or both (Fauci, 1979). It is generally believed that the lymphocyte functions are influenced by the number of glucocorticoid receptors present in the cell and the nature of the receptor interaction (Baxter and Forshan, 1972). Lymphopenia may be similarly influenced by glucocorticoid receptor interactions (Bloom et al., 1980).

Lymphopenia seen early in viral infection is attributed to changes in surface properties of the circulating lymphocytes and their increased sequestration in lymphoid tissues. Studies in mice indicate that viral neuraminidase (Woodruff and Woodruff, 1976) and interferon (Schattner et al., 1983) may alter the cell surface of lymphocytes and their pattern of circulation leading to lymphopenia. Corticosteroids produced as a result of viral infection did not seem to be involved because similar changes occurred in adrenalectomized mice and no evidence of lympholysis was found.

THE PLASMA CELLS

Plasma cells are identified by their characteristic morphologic features. These are (a) an abundant, highly basophilic cytoplasm that is frequently mottled or stippled, (b) a small clear area often seen in the cytoplasm near the nucleus, and (c) a small, usually eccentric nucleus with chromatin clumps somewhat more exaggerated than in lymphocytes and typically in the form of a cartwheel (Plate XI–4). The ultrastructure of plasma cells varies with the stage of maturity; e.g., a nucleolus is seen in the plasmablast. Plasma cells uniquely display a complex rough endoplasmic reticulum (RER) that occupies most of the cytoplasm (Fig. 30–6). The clear area in the cytoplasm, seen with the light microscope, is occupied by the Golgi complex. Mitochondria are few. Cytochemically, some glycogen and acid phosphatase can be demonstrated in plasma cells, but peroxidase and alkaline phosphatase are absent. The well-known pyroninophilic staining of the plasma cells (Plate X–12) is due to their elaborate RER rich in RNA.

Morphologic abnormalities are found in plasma cells, infrequently during an immune response and more frequently in myelomas and other pathologic conditions associated with plasmacytosis (Douglas, 1983b). A plasma cell engorged with antibody protein in its cytoplasm in the form of pinkish or bluish globules (Russell bodies) is occasionally seen in the bone marrow or lymph node aspirate and very rarely in the peripheral blood (Plate XI–5; Fig. 30–7). It is called a Mott cell. Plasma cells with reddish peripheral cytoplasmic staining, called "flame cells" (Plates XIII–7, XIII–8, XIII–9) have been found in IgA myelomas (Zinkl et al., 1983). Plasma cells with multiple nuclei are rare, but may be seen in the bone marrow and lymph nodes of patients with a vigorous immune response or gammopathy. Multinucleated plasma cells were frequently seen in the bone marrow of an unusual case of IgA myeloma in the dog (Zinkl et al., 1983). Such cells have been found rarely in normal human bone marrow (Douglas, 1983b), but not in domestic animal species.

Plasma cells are derived from B-lympho-

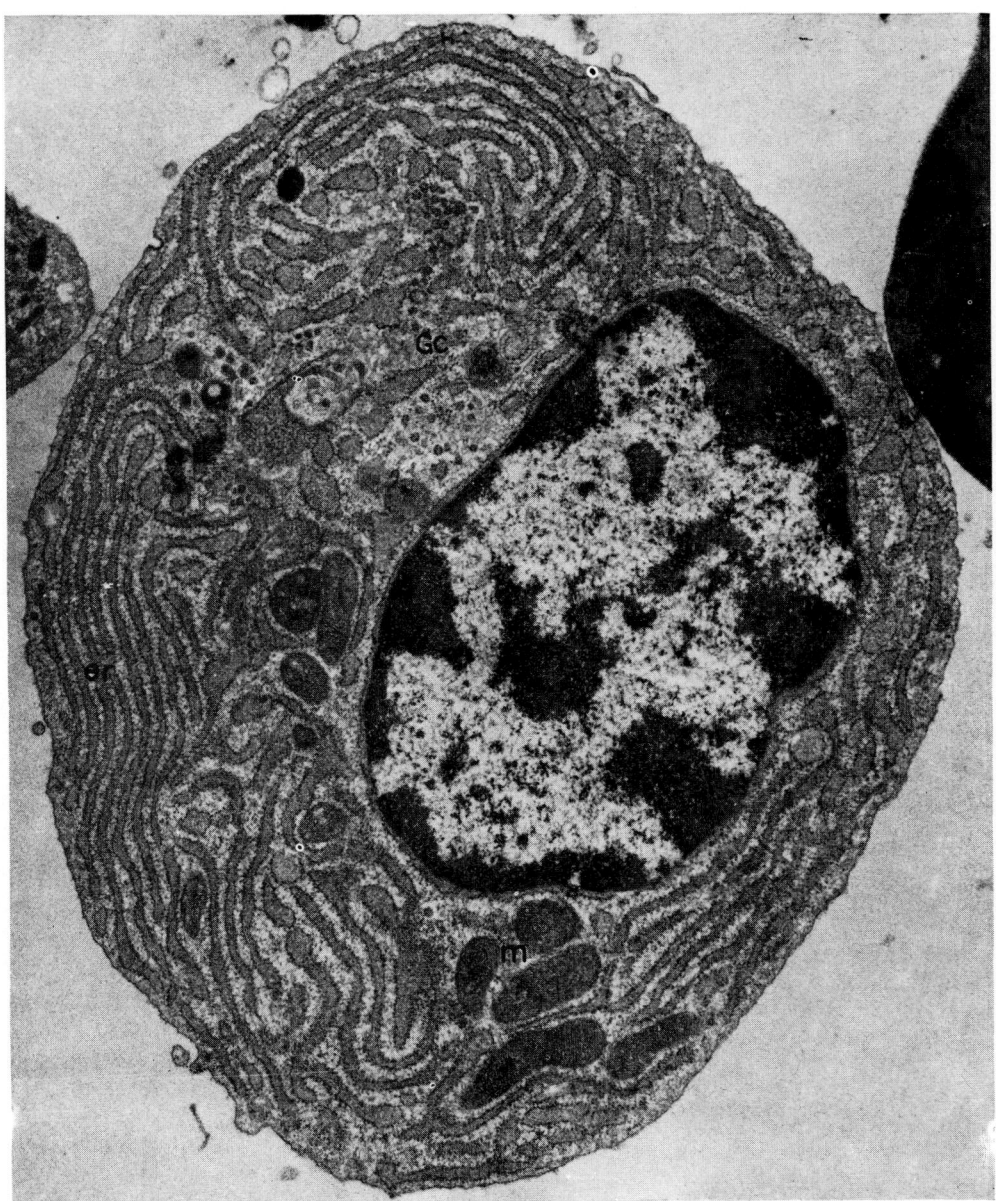

Fig. 30–6. A plasma cell from canine bone marrow. This cell characteristically displays patchy areas of chromatin condensation, in the form of a cartwheel, in the round eccentric nucleus and numerous elongated cisternae of endoplasmic reticulum *(er)* that almost fill the cytoplasm. Some mitochondria *(m)* are distributed among the cisternae of the rough endoplasmic reticulum. In the upper cytoplasmic portion near the nucleus, remnants of the Golgi complex *(Gc)*, cut transversely and represented as small round saccules, seem to be present. This area appears as a clear zone in the plasma cells in bone marrow smears stained with a Romanowsky stain (see Plate X). The rough endoplasmic reticulum contains flocculent proteinaceous material representing immunoglobulin molecules. ×18,000.

cytes after blastic transformation, mitoses, differentiation, and maturation in response to an antigen. Labeled lymphocytes from the efferent lymph of a sheep, when injected into the afferent lymphatics of a lymph node of an identical twin, were found to change into plasma cells (Birbeck and Hall, 1967). On average, 4–5 days are required for the generation of mature plasma cells. Plasmablasts and transitional (immature) plasma cells along with mature plasma cells are often seen in antigen-stimulated lymph nodes and other

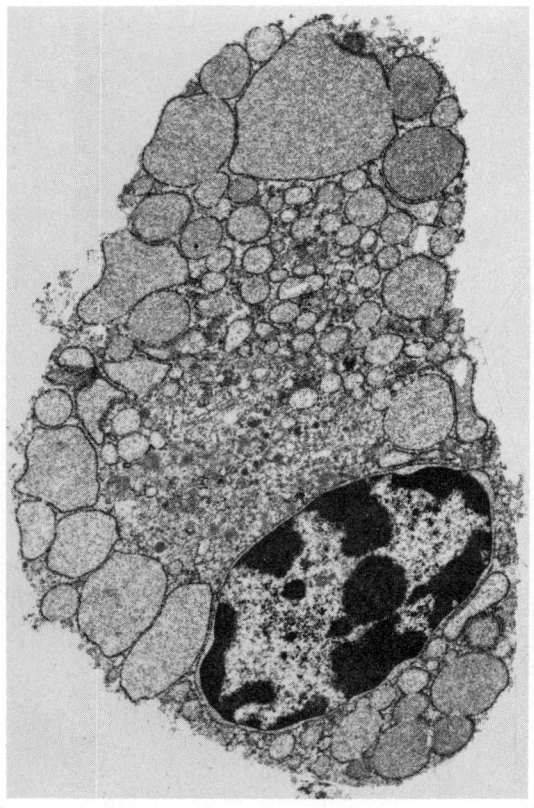

Fig. 30–7. A plasma cell with Russell bodies, which in this transmission electron photomicrograph appear as dilated vesicular structures (endoplasmic reticulum) containing amorphous material (immunoglobulin molecules). The eccentrically placed nucleus shows the characteristic cartwheel pattern of condensed chromatin. Although the cell membrane appears discontinuous or lost, cellular integrity is remarkably intact. ×22,000.

active lymphoid tissues such as the spleen and bone marrow. The terms "immunoblast" and "immunocyte" refer to antibody-producing lymphocytes without commitment to their specific cellular origin (Dameshek, 1963).

Plasma cells are concerned with the synthesis, storage, and release of immunoglobulins. They can be found in any tissue in the body, but are most numerous in tissues engaged in antibody formation. They are common in the medullary cords and germinal centers of lymph nodes, in the splenic white pulp and perivascular sheaths, and in connective tissues. Small numbers are found in the bone marrow, and a few are seen in the thymus of the guinea pig. They are rare in the thoracic duct. When the antigenic stimulus is local, plasma cells are found in the area of antigenic

deposition and in the draining lymph nodes. If the antigenic stimulus is systemic, they are found in greater numbers in various lymphoid organs, especially the spleen. Plasma cells are rare in the peripheral blood, even in plasma cell myeloma.

Some information about the genesis of the antibody molecule, has become available (Douglas, 1983b). The cisternae of the RER contain amorphous material representing immunoglobulins. Heavy and light chains of the immunoglobulin molecules are synthesized separately on polyribosomes attached to the RER. Light chains become detached and combine with heavy chains still bound to the polyribosomes. Antibody molecules are subsequently formed by disulfide linkages and are released free into the cisternae of the RER and move into the Golgi area. Carbohydrate is added to the antibody molecule in two stages: glucosamine is incorporated both in the RER and the Golgi complex, while galactose is added primarily in the latter (Douglas, 1983b).

One plasma cell synthesizes one type of antibody. How antibodies are released from the plasma cells is not known; their release may involve secretion (reverse pinocytosis), diffusion, or even cell death. The production of immunoglobulin is very rapid, taking about 1 or 2 minutes, and its appearance outside the cell takes about 15 minutes (Uhr and Finkelstein, 1967). The plasma cell secretes immunoglobulins at the rate of 2,000 molecules per second and probably dies after a few days or weeks (Freedman and Gold, 1976). Abnormalities in the secretion or synthesis of immunoglobulins have been found during bovine leukemia (Altura et al., 1979) and myelomas in various species (see Chapter 32).

REFERENCES

Abugaber, A.A., et al.: The Use of Various Buffers in the Preparation of Human Lymphocytes for SEM Observation. J. Microsc., 122(pt. 1):59, 1981.

Ackerman, G.A.: Structural Studies of the Lymphocyte and Lymphocyte Development. *In* Regulation of Hematopoiesis. Vol. 2. Gordon, A.S., ed. Appleton-Century-Crofts, New York, p. 1297, 1970.

Ahmed, J.S., and Zweygarth, E.: Potentiation of Proliferative Responses of Bovine Peripheral Blood Lymphocytes to Mitogens by Pronase. Zentralbl. Veterinärmed., 30:48, 1983.

Altman, A., and Katz, D.H.: The Biology of Monoclonal

Lymphokines Secreted by T Cell Lines and Hybridomas. Adv. Immunol., *33*:73, 1982.

Altura, D., et al.: B-Lymphocytes Differentiation Using Pokeweed Mitogen Stimulation: In Vitro Studies in Leukemic and Normal Cattle. Amer. J. Vet. Res., *40*:515, 1979.

Ascensao, J.L., et al.: Cell-Cell Interaction in Human Granulopoiesis: Role of T Lymphocytes. Exp. Hematol., *9*:473, 1981.

Bach, J.F.: Immunology. Wiley, New York, 1976.

Bach, J.F., and Papiernik, M.: Cellular and Molecular Signals in T Cell Differentiation. *In* Microenvironment in Haematopoietic and Lymphoid Differentiation. Porter, R., and Whelan, J., eds. Ciba Found. Symp. 84. Pitman Book Ltd., London, p. 215, 1981.

Bagby, G.C., Jr., et al.: Interaction of Lactoferrin, Monocytes and T Lymphocyte Subsets in the Regulation of Steady State Granulopoiesis in Vitro. J. Clin. Invest., *68*:56, 1981.

Banks, K.L., and Greenlee, A.: Isolation and Identification of Equine Lymphocytes and Monocytes. Amer. J. Vet. Res., *42*:1651, 1981.

Banks, K.L., and Greenlee, A.: Lymphocyte Subpopulations of the Goat: Isolation and Identification. Amer. J. Vet. Res., *43*:315, 1982.

Banks, K.L., and Henson, J.B.: Quantitation of Immunoglobulin-Bearing Lymphocytes and Lymphocyte Response to Mitogens in Horses Persistently Infected by Equine Infectious Anemia Virus. Immunology, *8*:679, 1973.

Banks, K.L., et al.: Absence of B Lymphocytes in a Horse with Primary Agammaglobulinemia. Clin. Immunol. Immunopathol., *5*:282, 1976.

Barr, R.D.: The Role of the Lymphocyte in Haemopoiesis. Scot. Med. J., *24*:267, 1979.

Barta, O.: Serum's Lymphocyte Immunoregulatory Factors (SLIF). Vet. Immunol. Immunopathol., *4*:279, 1983.

Barta, O., et al.: Lymphocyte Transformation Suppression Caused by Pyoderma: Failure to Demonstrate It in Uncomplicated Demodectic Mange. Comp. Immunol. Microbiol. Infect. Dis., *6*:9, 1983.

Baxter, J.D., and Forsham, P.H.: Tissue Effects of Glucocorticoids. Amer. J. Med., *53*:573, 1972.

Beldon, E.L., and Strelkauskas, A.J.: Mitogen and Mixed Lymphocyte Culture Responses of Isolated Bovine Lymphocyte Subpopulations. Amer. J. Vet. Res., *42*:934, 1981.

Beldon, E.L., et al.: Subpopulations of Bovine Lymphocytes Separated by Rosetting Techniques. Vet. Immunol. Immunopathol., *2*:467, 1981.

Bell, R.G.: Cell Interactions in Antibody Formation. J. Amer. Vet. Med. Ass., *181*:1011, 1982.

Bendixen, P.H., et al.: Inhibition of the Blastogenic Response of Peripheral Blood Mononuclear Cells to Mitogen and Antigens by Bovine Pulmonary Macrophages and Their Culture Supernatants. Res. Vet. Sci., *31*:272, 1981.

Bendtzen, K.: Biological Properties of Interleukins. Allergy, *38*:219, 1983.

Bennell, M.A., and Husband, A.J.: Route of Lymphocyte Migration in Pigs. I. Lymphocyte Circulation in Gut-Associated Lymphoid Tissue. Immunology, *42*:469, 1981.

Beran, M., and Pospisil, J.: A Contribution to the Comparative Morphology of Nucleolar Apparatus of Lymphocytes in the Peripheral Blood of Man and Some Animals. Folia Haematol., *88*(4):287, 1967.

Binns, R.M.: Organization of the Lymphoreticular System and Lymphocyte Markers in the Pig. Vet. Immunol. Immunopathol., *3*:95, 1982.

Binns, R.M., and Hall, J.G.: The Paucity of Lymphocytes in the Lymph of Unanaesthetised Pigs. Brit. J. Exp. Pathol., *47*:275, 1966.

Binns, R.M., et al.: Comparison of the Direct Antiglobulin Rosetting Reaction (DARR) and Direct Immunofluorescence (DIF) for Demonstration of sIg-Bearing Lymphocytes in Pigs, Sheep and Cattle. Immunology, *36*:549, 1979.

Birbeck, M.S.C., and Hall, J.G.: Transformation, in Vivo, of Basophilic Lymph Cells into Plasma Cells. Nature, *214*:183, 1967.

Blatt, J., et al.: Biochemical Markers in Lymphoid Malignancy. New Eng. J. Med., *303*:918, 1980.

Bloom, J.C., et al.: Glucocorticoid Receptors in Peripheral Blood Lymphocytes from Bovine Leukemia Virus–Infected Cows with Persistent Lymphocytosis. Cancer Res., *40*:2240, 1980.

Bloomfield, C.D., and Gajl-Peczalska, K.J.: The Clinical Relevance of Lymphocyte Surface Markers in Leukemia and Lymphoma. Curr. Top. Hematol., *3*:175, 1980.

Bohs, C.T., et al.: T Lymphocyte Depletion in Peripheral Blood of Sheep Undergoing Chronic Thoracic Duct Drainage. J. Reticuloendothel. Soc., *19*:383, 1976.

Bowles, C.A., et al.: Rosette Formation by Canine Peripheral Blood Lymphocytes. J. Immunol., *114*:399, 1975.

Bozdech, M.J., and Bainton, D.F.: Identification of α-Naphthyl Butyrate Esterase as a Plasma Membrane Ectoenzyme of Monocytes and a Discrete Intracellular Membrane-Bound Organelle in Lymphocytes. J. Exp. Med., *153*:182, 1981.

Bradfield, J.W.B., and Born, G.V.R.: Inhibition of Lymphocyte Recirculation by Heparin. Nature, *222*:1183, 1969.

Broström, H., et al.: A New Surface Marker on Equine Lymphocytes. II. Characterization and Separation of Purified Blood Lymphocytes with Receptors for Helix pomatia A Hemagglutin (HP). Vet. Immunol. Immunopathol., *8*:47, 1985.

Brumby, M., and Metcalf, D.: Migration of Cells to the Thymus Demonstrated by Parabiosis. Proc. Soc. Exp. Biol. Med., *124*:99, 1967.

Buckton, K.E., et al.: Lymphocyte Survival in Men Treated with X-rays for Ankylosing Spondylitis. Nature, *214*:470, 1967.

Burrells, C., et al.: Reactivity of Ovine Lymphocytes to Phytohaemagglutinin and Pokeweed Mitogen during Pregnancy and in the Immediate Post-Parturient Period. Clin. Exp. Immunol., *33*:410, 1978.

Buschmann, H., and Pawlas, S.: Characterization and Separation of Bovine Lymphocyte Populations. Comp. Immunol. Microbiol. Infect. Dis., *3*:299, 1980.

Cahill, R.N.P., et al.: Two Distinct Pools of Recirculating T Lymphocytes: Migratory Characteristics of Nodal and Intestinal T Lymphocytes. J. Exp. Med., *145*:420, 1977.

Cahill, R.N.P., et al.: The Migration of Lymphocytes in the Fetal Lamb. Eur. J. Immunol., *9*:251, 1979.

Campos, M., et al.: Natural Cell-Mediated Cytotoxicity of Bovine Mononuclear Cells against Virus-Infected Cells. Inf. Immun., *36*:1054, 1982.

Canning, P.C., et al.: Identification of Bovine Lymphocyte Subpopulations by a Combined Bacterial Adherence and Fluorescent Antibody Technique. Amer. J. Vet. Res., *44*:297, 1983.

Cantor, H.: Control of the Immune System by Inhibitors

and Inducer T Lymphocytes. Ann. Rev. Med., 30:269, 1979.

Cerruti-Sola, S., et al.: Interleukin- 1 and 2-like Activities in the Dog. Vet. Immunol. Immunopathol., 6:261, 1984.

Chander, S., and Gilman, J.P.W.: Bovine Leukosis. III. Relationship between Lymphocytosis and DNA Synthetic Lymphocytes. Can. J. Comp. Med., 38:430, 1974.

Chandler, J.P., and Yang, T.J.: Identification of Canine Lymphocyte Populations by Immunofluorescence Surface Marker Analysis. Int. Arch. Allergy Appl. Immunol., 65:62, 1981.

Chandra, P., et al.: Distribution of T and B Lymphocytes in Blood and Lymphoid Tissues of Fetal and Adult Sheep. Amer. J. Vet. Res., 41:2092, 1980.

Claman, H.N.: Corticosteroids and Lymphoid Cells. New Eng. J. Med., 287:388, 1972.

Cline, M.J.: The White Cell. Harvard Univ. Press, 1975.

Cockerell, G.L., et al.: Phytomitogen- and Antigen-Induced Blast Transformation of Feline Lymphocytes. Amer. J. Vet. Res., 36:1489, 1975.

Cockerell, G.L., et al.: Characterization of Feline T- and B-Lymphocytes and Identification of an Experimentally Induced T-Cell Neoplasm in the Cat. J. Natl. Cancer Inst., 57:907, 1976a.

Cockerell, G.L., et al.: Lymphocyte Mitogen Reactivity and Enumeration of Circulating B- and T-Cells during Feline Leukemia Virus Infection in the Cat. J. Natl. Cancer Inst., 57:1095, 1976b.

Cohen, J.J.: Thymus-Derived Lymphocytes Sequestered in the Bone Marrow of Hydrocortisone-Treated Mice. J. Immunol., 108:841, 1972.

Concha, C., et al.: Proportion of B and T Lymphocytes in Normal Bovine Milk. J. Dairy Res., 45:287, 1978.

Concha, C., et al.: Characterization and Response to Mitogens of Mammary Lymphocytes from the Bovine Dry-Period Secretion. J. Dairy Res., 47:305, 1980.

Cottier, H., et al., eds.: Germinal Centers in Immune Responses: Proceedings of a Symposium Held at the University of Bern, Switzerland, June, 1966. Springer, New York, 1967.

Crabtree, G., et al.: Mechanisms of Glucocorticoid Induced Immunosuppression: Inhibitory Effects on Expression of Fc Receptors and Production of T-Cell Growth Factor. J. Steroid Biochem., 12:445, 1980.

Cronkite, E.P., and Schiffer, L.M.: Kinetics of Normal Lymphopoiesis and Chronic Lymphocytic Leukemia. In Regulation of Hematopoiesis. Vol. 2. Gordon, A.S., ed. Appleton-Century-Crofts, New York, p. 1455, 1970.

Cronkite, E.P., et al.: The Use of Tritiated Thymidine in the Study of DNA Synthesis in Cell Turnover in Hemopoietic Tissues. Lab. Invest., 8:263, 1959.

Cronkite, E.P., et al.: Lymphocyte Production Measured by Extracorporeal Irradiation: Cannulation and Labeling Techniques. Ann. N.Y. Acad. Sci., 113:566, 1964.

Crowther, D., and Wagstaff, J.: Lymphocyte Migration in Malignant Disease. Clin. Exp. Immunol., 51:413, 1983.

Crowther, D., et al.: Lymphoid Cellular Responses in the Blood after Immunization in Man. J. Exp. Med., 129:849, 1969.

Cunningham, L., et al.: Studies on Lymphocytes. VIII. Short in Vivo Mitotic Time of Basophilic Lymphoid Cells in the Thoracic Duct of Calves after Simulated or Effective Extracorporeal Irradiation of Circulating Blood. Exp. Cell Res., 47:479, 1967.

Dameshek, W.: "Immunoblasts and Immunocytes": An Attempt at a Functional Nomenclature. Blood, 21:243, 1963.

De Maeyer, E., and De Maeyer-Guignard, J.: Interferons As Regulatory Agents of the Immune System. CRC Crit. Rev. Immunol., 2:167, 1981.

Despont, J.P., et al.: Functional and Biochemical Characteristics of Human "Null" Lymphoid Cells. Transplantation, 31:251, 1981.

Dhingra, V.K., et al.: Effect of Bovine Horn Cancer Serum on E-Rosetting Capacity of Peripheral Blood Lymphocytes from Normal Unaffected Animals. Res. Vet. Sci., 33:138, 1982.

Djeu, J.Y.: Antibody-Dependent Cell-Mediated Cytotoxicity and Natural Killer-Cell Phenomenon. J. Amer. Vet. Med. Ass., 181:1043, 1982.

Douglas, S.D.: Morphology of Lymphocytes. In Hematology. 3rd ed. Williams, W.J., et al., eds. McGraw-Hill, New York, Ch. 101, p. 883, 1983a.

Douglas, S.D.: Morphology of Plasma Cells. In Hematology. 3rd ed. Williams, W.J., et al., eds. McGraw-Hill, New York, ch. 102, p. 895, 1983b.

Dumonde, D.C., et al.: "Lymphokines": Non-Antibody Mediators of Cellular Immunity Generated by Lymphocyte Activation. Nature, 224:38, 1969.

Dutta, S.K., et al.: Lymphocyte Responsiveness to Mitogens and Quantitation of T and B Lymphocytes in Canine Malignant Lymphoma. Amer. J. Vet. Res., 39:455, 1978.

Elves, M.W.: The Lymphocytes. Yearbook Medical Publishers, Chicago, 1967.

English, L.S., and Whitehurst, M.: The Production of T-Cell Growth Factor (TCGF) in Vivo in Sheep. Cell. Immunol., 85:364, 1984.

Esteban, J.N.: The Differential Effect of Hydrocortisone on the Short-Lived Small Lymphocyte. Anat. Rec., 162:349, 1968.

Everett, N.B., and Tyler, R.W.: Lymphopoiesis in the Thymus and Other Tissues: Functional Implication. Int. Rev. Cytol., 22:205, 1967.

Everett, N.B., et al.: Recirculation of Lymphocytes. Ann. N.Y. Acad. Sci., 113:887, 1964.

Fahey, K.J., et al.: The Effect of Pre-Natal Thymectomy on Lymphocyte Sub-Populations in the Sheep. Aust. J. Exp. Biol. Med. Sci., 58:571, 1980.

Fauci, A.S.: Glucocorticoid Effects on Circulating Human Mononuclear Cells. J. Reticuloendothel. Soc., 26:727, 1979.

Fauci, A.S., et al.: Glucocorticosteroid Therapy: Mechanisms of Action and Clinical Considerations. Ann. Intern. Med., 84:304, 1976.

Felbserg, P.J., et al.: Potentiation of the Canine Lymphocyte Blastogenic Response by Indomethacin. Vet. Immunol. Immunopathol., 4:533, 1983.

Ferrarini, M., et al.: Ultrastructure and Cytochemistry of Human Peripheral Blood Lymphocytes: Similarities between the Cells of the Third Population and TG Lymphocytes. Eur. J. Immunol., 10:562, 1980.

Fish, J.C., et al.: Circulating Lymphocyte Depletion in the Calf. Effect on Blood and Lymph Lymphocytes. Arch. Surg., 99:664, 1969.

Fitzgerald, P.H.: The Immunological Role and Long Life Span of the Small Lymphocytes. J. Theor. Biol., 6:13, 1964.

Fliedner, T.M., et al.: Cell Proliferation in Germinal Centers of the Rat Spleen. Ann. N.Y. Acad. Sci., 113:578, 1964.

Ford, W.L.: Distribution of Lymphocytes in Health. J. Clin. Pathol., 32(13):63, 1979.

Freedman, S.O., and Gold, P., eds.: Clinical Immunology. 2nd ed. Harper & Row, Hagerstown, Md., 1976.

Friedman, R.M., and Vogel, S.N.: Interferons with Special Emphasis on the Immune System. Adv. Immunol., 34:97, 1983.

Frymus, T., and Schollenberger, A.: Circulating B and T Lymphocytes in Foals during First Five Months of Life. Zentralbl. Veterinärmed., 26:722, 1979.

Garcia, A.M., and Iorio, R.: Studies on DNA in Leukocytes and Related Cells of Mammals. V. The Fast Green-Histone and the Feulgen-DNA Content of Rat Leukocytes. Acta Cytol., 12:46, 1968.

George, M., and Vaughan, J.H.: In Vitro Cell Migration as a Model for Delayed Hypersensitivity. Proc. Soc. Exp. Biol. Med., 111:514, 1962.

Giacco, G.S.D.: T Cell Subpopulations and Diseases. Haematologica, 65:652, 1980.

Gillis, S.: Interleukin 2: Biology and Biochemistry. J. Clin. Chem., 3:1, 1983.

Giriunas, V.J., et al.: T and B Rosette-Forming Lymphocytes in the Peripheral Blood of Healthy Cows and Those Ill with Chronic Lympholeukosis. Proc. 2nd Int. Symp. Vet. Lab. Diagnosticians, June 24–26, 1980.

Gowans, J.L.: The Recirculation of Lymphocytes from Blood to Lymph in the Rat. J. Physiol., 146:54, 1959.

Gowans, J.L., and Knight, E.J.: The Route of Recirculation of Lymphocytes in the Rat. Proc. R. Soc. Lond. Ser. B., 159:257, 1964.

Granberg, C., and Hirvonen, T.: Cell-Mediated Lymphocytosis by Fetal and Neonatal Lymphocytes in Sheep and Man. Cell. Immunol., 51:13, 1980.

Grewal, A.S., and Babiuk, L.A.: Bovine T Lymphocytes: An Improved Technique of E Rosette Formation. J. Immunol. Methods, 24:355, 1978.

Gross, C.E., et al.: Morphological and Histochemical Analyses of Two Human T-Cell Subpopulation Bearing Receptors for IgM or IgG. J. Exp. Med., 147:1405, 1978.

Grossi, C.E., and Greaves, M.F.: Normal Lymphocytes. *In* Atlas of Blood Cells: Function and Pathology. Vol. 2. Zucker-Franklin, D., et al., eds. E.E. edi ermes Milano/Lea & Febiger, Philadelphia, p. 347, 1981.

Grundmann, E.: Die Bildung der Lymphocyten und Plasmazellen im Lymphatischen Gewebe der Ratte. Beitr. Path. Anat., 119:217, 1958.

Gupta, S., and Good, R.A.: Subpopulations of Human T Lymphocytes: Laboratory and Clinical Studies. Immunol. Rev., 56:89, 1981.

Hahn, H., and Kaufmann, S.H.E.: T Lymphocyte–Macrophage Interaction in Cellular Antibacterial Immunity. Immunobiology, 161:361, 1982.

Hall, J.G.: Quantitative Aspects of the Recirculation of Lymphocytes: An Analysis of Data from Experiments on Sheep. Q. J. Exp. Physiol., 52:76, 1967.

Hall, J.G., and Morris, B.: The Output of the Cells in Lymph from the Popliteal Node of the Sheep. Q. Exp. Physiol., 47:360, 1962.

Hall, J.G., and Morris, B.: The Immediate Effect of Antigens on the Cell Output of a Lymph Node. Brit. J. Exp. Pathol., 46:450, 1965a.

Hall, J.G., and Morris, B.: The Origin of the Cells in the Efferent Lymph from a Single Lymph Node. J. Exp. Med., 121:901, 1965b.

Hall, J.G., et al.: The Distribution and Differentiation of Lymph-Borne Immunoblasts after Intravenous Injection into Syngeneic Recipients. Cell Tissue Kinet., 5:269, 1972.

Hall, J.G., et al.: Studies on the Lymphocytes of Sheep.

III. Destination of Lymph-Borne Immunoblasts in Relation to Their Tissue of Origin. Eur. J. Immunol., 7:30, 1977.

Hanna, M.G.: An Autoradiographic Study of the Germinal Center in Spleen White Pulp during Early Intervals of the Immune Response. Lab. Invest., 13:95, 1964.

Hauser, W., Jr., et al.: Natural Killer Cells Induced by Acute and Chronic Toxoplasma Infection. Cell. Immunol., 69:330, 1982.

Hay, J.B., and Hobbs, B.B.: The Flow of Blood to Lymph Nodes and Its Relation to Lymphocyte Traffic and the Immune Response. J. Exp. Med., 145:31, 1977.

Hedman, L.A., et al.: Effect of Corticosteroids on Circulating Lymphocytes. Scand. J. Urol. Nephrol. Suppl., 54:120, 1980.

Herberman, R.B.: Natural Killer Cells and Cells Mediating Antibody-Dependent Cytotoxicity against Tumors. Clin. Immunobiol., 4:73, 1980.

Herberman, R.B.: Natural Killer Cells and Their Possible Relevance to Transplantation. Transplantation, 34:1, 1982.

Herberman, R.B., and Ortaldo, J.R.: Natural Killer Cells: Their Role in Defenses against Disease. Science, 214:24, 1981.

Hirsh, D.C., et al.: Suppression of in Vitro Lymphocyte Transformation by Serum from Dogs with Generalized Demodicosis. Amer. J. Vet. Res., 36:1591, 1975.

Holmberg, C.A., et al.: Malignant Lymphoma with B-Lymphocyte Characteristics in Dogs. Amer. J. Vet. Res., 38:1877, 1977.

Huh, N.D., et al.: Natural Killing and Antibody-Dependent Cellular Cytotoxicity in Specific-Pathogen-Free Miniature Swine and Germ-Free Piglets. II. Ontogenic Development of NK and ADCC. Int. J. Cancer, 28:175, 1981.

Ishikawa, H., and Shimizu, T.: Depression of B-Lymphocytes by Mastitis and Treatment with Levamisole. J. Dairy Sci., 66:556, 1983.

Issekutz, T.B., et al.: Lymphocyte Traffic through Chronic Inflammatory Lesions: Differential Migration versus Differential Retention. Clin. Exp. Immunol., 45:604, 1981.

Jacobs, R.M., et al.: Inhibition of Lymphocyte Blastogenesis by Sera from Cows with Lymphoma. Amer. J. Vet. Res., 41:372, 1980.

Janossy, G.: The Lymphocytes. Clin. Haematol., 11(3):487, 1982.

Janossy, G., et al.: The Human Thymic Microenvironment. *In* Microenvironment in Haematopoietic and Lymphoid Differentiation. Porter, R., and Whelan, J., eds. Ciba Found. Symp. 84. Pitman Book Ltd., London, p. 193, 1981.

Jansen, C.R., et al.: Studies on Lymphocytes. II. The Production of Leukocytosis by Intravenous Heparin in Calves. Blood, 20:443, 1962.

Jaroskova, L., and Kovaru, F.: Identification of T and B Lymphocytes in Pigs by Combined E-Rosette Test and Surface Ig Labelling. J. Immunol. Methods, 22:253, 1978.

Johansson, C., and Morein, B.: Evaluation of Labelling Methods for Bovine T and B Lymphocytes. Vet. Immunopathol., 4:345, 1983.

Johnson, H.A., et al.: Cytology-Variability of Ribosomal Aggregation in Lymphocytes. Nature, 211:420, 1966.

Johnson, H., Jr., et al.: Preparation and Characterization of an Antiserum Specific for T Cells of Pigs. Transplantation, 29:477, 1980.

Jones, H.B., et al.: Studies on Hypoxia. VII. Changes in

Lymphocytes and Transitional Cells in the Bone Marrow during Prolonged Rebound. Brit. J. Haematol., *13*:934, 1967.

Kaneko, J.J., et al.: Lymphocyte Proliferation by Normal and Tumorous Bovine Lymph Nodes. Ann. N.Y. Acad. Sci., *108*:1302, 1963.

Kaura, Y.K., et al.: Rosette Formation by Buffalos (Bos bubalis) T and B Lymphocytes. Vet. Res., *104*:386, 1979.

Keiser, G., et al.: Origin and Fate of Bone Marrow Lymphoid Cells of Dog. *In* The Lymphocyte in Immunology and Haemopoiesis. Yoffey, J.M., ed. Edward Arnold, London, p. 149, 1967.

Kelly, G.E.: Studies of Surface Markers on Canine Lymphocytes. Aust. J. Exp. Biol. Med. Sci., *58*:471, 1980.

Klaus, G.G.B., and Humphrey, J.H.: The Generation of Memory Cells. I. The Role of C3 in the Generation of B Memory Cells. Immunology, *33*:31, 1977.

Klesius, P.: Intercellular Communication: Role of Soluble Factors in Cellular Immune Responses. J. Amer. Vet. Med. Ass., *181*:1015, 1982.

Krakowka, S.: Mechanisms of E-Rosette Formation by Mitogen-Stimulated Canine Lymphocytes. Immunology, *39*:255, 1980.

Krakowka, S.: Natural Killer Cell Activity in Adult Gnotobiotic Dogs. Amer. J. Vet. Res., *44*:635, 1983.

Krakowka, S., et al.: Evaluation of B Lymphocyte Levels and Functions in Gnotobiotic Dogs. Amer. J. Vet. Res., *39*:1881, 1978.

Kristensen, F., et al.: The Lymphocyte Stimulation Test in Veterinary Immunology. Vet. Immunol. Immunopathol., *3*:203, 1982.

Kumar, S.P., et al.: Frequency of Lymphocytes Bearing Fc Receptors and Surface Membrane Immunoglobulins in Normal, Persistent Lymphocytotic and Leukemic Cows. Amer. J. Vet. Res., *39*:45, 1978.

Lanweiler, M., et al.: Effect of Antioxidant on the Proliferative Response of Canine Lymphocytes in Serum from Dogs with Vitamin E Deficiency. Amer. J. Vet. Res., *44*:5, 1983.

Leblond, C.P., and Sainte-Marie, G.: Models for Lymphocyte and Plasmocyte Formation. *In* Haemopoieses: Cell Production and Its Regulation. Wolstenholme, G.E., and O'Conner, M., eds. Ciba Found. Symp. Churchill, London, p. 152, 1960.

Leibold, W., et al.: Spontaneous Cell-Mediated Cytotoxicity (SCMC) in Various Mammalian Species and Chickens: Selective Reaction Pattern and Different Mechanisms. Scand. J. Immunol., *11*:203, 1980.

Lipton, J.M., and Nathan, D.G.: Cell–Cell Interaction in in Vitro Erythropoeisis. Blood Cells, *6*:645, 1980.

Lowenthal, R.M.: Lymphocyte Surface Marker Studies in Lymphoma and Leukemia. Pathology, *14*:283, 1982.

Lydyard, P.M., and Fanger, M.W.: Characteristics and Function of Fc Receptors on Human Lymphocytes. Immunology, *47*:1, 1982.

MacDonald, D.M.: Lymphocyte Receptors. Brit. J. Dermatol., *107*(suppl. 23):69, 1982.

Machin, G.A., et al.: Cytochemically Demonstrable β-Glucuronidase Activity in Normal and Neoplastic Human Lymphoid Cells. Blood, *56*:1111, 1980.

Mackey, L.J.: Distribution of T and B Cells in Thymus, Blood, and Lymph Nodes of the Cat. Res. Vet. Sci., *22*:225, 1977.

Mackey, L.J., and Jarrett, W.F.H.: Two Populations of Lymphocytes in a Cat. Vet. Rec., *96*:41, 1975.

Magnuson, N.S., et al.: Studies of Lymphocytes in Natural Killer Cell. Morphology from Horses with Hereditary Severe combined Immunodeficiency (SCID). Fed. Proc., *44*:594, 1985.

Marchesi, V.T., and Gowans, J.L.: The Migration of Lymphocytes through the Endothelium of Venules in Lymph Nodes: An Electron Microscopic Study. Proc. R. Soc. Lond. Ser. B., *159*:283, 1964.

Mathur, S., et al.: Cyclic Variations in White Cell Subpopulations in the Human Menstrual Cycle: Correlation with Progesterone and Estradiol. Clin. Immunol. Immunopathol., *13*:246, 1979.

Matsuyama, M., et al.: Autoradiographic Analysis of Lymphopoiesis and Lymphocyte Migration in Mice Bearing Multiple Thymus Grafts. J. Exp. Med., *123*:559, 1966.

McDonald, R.G., et al.: Glucocorticoids Stimulate Protein Degradation in Lymphocytes: A Possible Mechanism of Steroid-Induced Cell Death. Endocrinology, *107*:1512, 1980.

McGuire, T.C., et al.: Combined (B- and T-Lymphocyte) Immunodeficiency: A Fatal Genetic Disease in Arabian Foals. J. Amer. Vet. Med. Ass., *164*:70, 1974.

McGuire, T.C., et al.: Agamma-globulinemia in a Horse with Evidence of Functional T Lymphocytes. Amer. J. Vet. Res., *37*:41, 1976.

Melchers, F., et al.: Regulation of B Lymphocyte Replication and Maturation. J. Cellular Biochem., *19*:315, 1982.

Metcalf, D., and Wiadrowski, M.: Autoradiographic Analysis of Lymphocyte Proliferation in the Thymus and in Thymic Lymphoma Tissue. Cancer Res., *26*:483, 1966.

Miller, H.R.P., and Adams, E.P.: Reassortment of Lymphocytes in Lymph from Normal and Allografted Sheep. Amer. J. Pathol., *87*:59, 1977.

Miller, J.M., et al.: Incidence of Lymphocytic Nuclear Projections in Bovine Lymphosarcoma. J. Natl. Cancer Res. Inst., *43*:719, 1969.

Mitchell, J., et al.: Autoradiographic Studies on the Immune Response. 3. Differential Lymphopoiesis in Various Organs. Aust. J. Exp. Biol. Med. Sci., *41*:411, 1963.

Moore, T.C., and Lachmann, P.J.: Cyclic AMP Reduces and Cyclic GMP Increases the Traffic of Lymphocytes through Peripheral Lymph Nodes of Sheep in Vivo. Immunology, *47*:423, 1982.

Morett, L., et al.: Human Lymphocyte Surface Markers. Semin. Hematol., *19*:273, 1982.

Morreta, A., et al.: Recent Advances in the Phenotype and Functional Analysis of Human T Lymphocytes. Semin. Hematol., *21*:257, 1984.

Muller, J., et al.: Nonspecific Esterase in Human Lymphocytes. Int. Arch. Allergy Appl. Immunol., *64*:410, 1981.

Muscoplat, C.C., et al.: Lymphocyte Surface Immunoglobulin: Frequency in Normal and Lymphocytotic Cattle. Amer. J. Vet. Res., *35*:593, 1974a.

Muscopolat, C.C., et al.: Lymphocyte Subpopulations and Immunodeficiency in Calves with Acute Lymphocytic Leukemia. Amer. J. Vet. Res., *35*:1571, 1974b.

Namen, A.E., and Magnuson, J.A.: Production and Characterization of Bovine Interleukin-2. Immunology, *52*:469, 1984.

Nieuwenhuis, P., et al.: Histophysiology of Follicular Structures and Germinal Centres in Relation to B Cell Differentiation. *In* Microenvironment in Haematopoietic and Lymphoid Differentiation. Porter, R., and Whelan, J., eds. Ciba Found. Symp. 84. Pitman Book Ltd., London, p. 246, 1981.

Norley, S.G., and Wardley, R.C.: Investigation of Porcine Natural-Killer Cell Activity with Reference to African Swinefever Virus Infection. Immunology, *49*:593, 1983.

Olah, I., and Gliek, B.: Re-evaluation of the Lymphocyte Migration through the High-Endothelial Venules: Light and Electron Microscopic Studies on the Opposum's Lymph Node. Acta Biol. Acad. Sci. Hung., *31*:207, 1980.

Olson, I.A., and Yoffey, J.M.: Oligosynthetic and Polysynthetic Lymph Nodes. *In* The Lymphocytes in Immunology and Haemopoiesis: Symposium Held at Bristol, April, 1966. Yoffey, J.M., ed. Edward Arnold, London, p. 358, 1967.

Opstelten, D., et al.: Germinal Centers and the B-Cell System. VI. Migration Pattern of Germinal-Center Cells of the Rabbit Appendix. Cell Tissue Res. *218*:59, 1981.

Osburn, B.I., et al.: Ontogeny of the Immune System. J. Amer. Vet. Med. Ass., *181*:1049, 1982.

Osmond, D.G.: The Contribution of Bone Marrow to the Economy of the Lymphoid System. Monogr. Allergy, *16*:157, 1980.

Osmond, D.G., and Everett, N. B.: Radioautographic Studies of Bone Marrow Lymphocytes in Vivo and in Diffusion Chamber Cultures. Blood, *23*:1, 1964.

Osmond, D.G., et al.: Regulation and Localization of Lymphocyte Production in the Bone Marrow. *In* Microenvironments in Haemopoietic and Lymphoid Differentiation. Porter, R., and Whelan, J., eds. Ciba Found. Symp. 84. Pitman Books Ltd., London, pp. 68–86, 1981.

Ottesen, J.: On the Age of Human White Cells in Peripheral Blood. Acta Physiol. Scand., *32*:75, 1954.

Outteridge, P.M., and Dufty, J.H.: Surface Markers for Characterization of Bovine Blood Lymphocyte Populations and Changes in These from Birth to Maturity. Res. Vet. Sci., *31*:315, 1981.

Outteridge, P.M., et al.: Characterization of Lymphocyte Subpopulations in Sheep by Rosette Formation, Adherence to Nylon Wool and Mitogen Responsiveness. Vet. Immunol. Immunopathol., *2*:3, 1981.

Pabst, R., and Geisler, R.: The Route of Migration of Lymphocytes from Blood to Spleen and Mesenteric Lymph Nodes in the Pig. Cell Tissue Res., *221*:361, 1981.

Parrott, D.M.V., and Wilkinson, P.C.: Lymphocyte Locomotion and Migration. Prog. Allergy, *28*:193, 1981.

Pearson, L.D., et al.: Lymphopoiesis and Lymphocyte Recirculation in the Sheep Fetus. J. Exp. Med., *143*:167, 1976.

Perryman, L.E., et al.: Ontogeny of Lymphocyte Function in the Equine Fetus. Amer. J. Vet. Res., *41*:1197,1980.

Pierce, J.C.: Quantitation of Lymphocyte Production in Normal and Stimulated Lymph Nodes. Transplantation, *5*:967, 1967.

Pinto, A.J.: Natural Killer Cells in Yorkshire Swine: Properties, Specificity, and Regulation. Dissertation Abstracts International B, *46*:111, 1985.

Ptak, W., and Gershon, R.K.: Immunosuppression Effect by Macrophage Surfaces. J. Immunol., *115*:1346, 1975.

Raich, P.C., et al.: Cytochemical Reactions in Bovine and Ovine Lymphosarcoma. Vet. Pathol., *20*:322, 1983.

Reeves, J.H., and Renshaw, H.W.: Surface Membrane Markers on Bovine Peripheral Blood Lymphocytes. Amer. J. Vet. Res., *39*:917, 1978.

Reif, J.S., et al.: Local and Systemic Cell-Mediated Immunity in Viral Infection of the Canine Respiratory Tract. Transplant. Proc., *7*:561, 1975.

Renau-Pigneres, J., et al.: Effects of Preparatory Techniques on the Fine Structure of Human Peripheral Blood Lymphocytes. II. Effect of Glutaraldehyde Osmolarity. Mikroskopie, *36*:65, 1980.

Reyero, C., et al.: Development of Peripheral B and T Lymphocytes in Piglets. Z. Immun. Forsch., *154*:409, 1978.

Reynolds, C.W., et al.: Natural Killer (NK) Cell Activity in the Rat. I. Isolation and Characterization of the Effector Cell. J. Immunol., *127*:282, 1981.

Reynolds, J.D., and Pabst, R.: The Emigration of Lymphoyctes from Peyer's Patches in Sheep. Eur. J. Immunol., *14*:7, 1984.

Rifkind, R.A., et al.: Fundamentals of Hematology. 2nd ed. Year Book, Chicago, 1980.

Rocklin, R.E., et al.: Mediators of Immunity: Lymphokines and Monokines. Adv. Immunol., *29*:55, 1980.

Rojko, J.L., et al.: Characterization and Mitogenesis of Feline Lymphocyte Populations. Int. Arch. Allergy Appl. Immunol., *68*:226, 1982.

Safai, B., and Good, R.A.: Lymphoproliferative Disorders of the T-Cell Series: A Review. Medicine, *59*:335, 1980.

Safier, S., et al.: Studies on Lymphocytes. VI. Evidence Showing Different Generation Times for Cytologically Different Lymphoid Cell Lines in the Thoracic Duct of the Calf. Blood, *30*:301, 1967.

Salmon, H.: Surface Markers of Porcine Lymphocytes and Distribution in Various Lymphoid Organs. Int. Arch. Allergy Suppl. Immunol. *60*:262, 1979.

Sanderson, C.J.: The Mechanisms of Lymphocyte-Mediated Cytotoxicity. Biol. Rev., *56*:153, 1981.

Schattner, A., et al.: Involvement of Interferon in Virus-Induced Lymphopenia. Cell. Immunol., *79*:11, 1983.

Schnappauf, H., and Schnappauf, U.: Drainage des Ductus Thoracicus und Grösse der "Leicht mobilisierbaren" Lymphozyten bei Kälbern, Schafen und Hunden. Blut, *16*(4):209, 1968.

Schoefl, G.L.: The Migration of Lymphocytes across the Vascular Endothelium in Lymphoid Tissue. J. Exp. Med., *136*:568, 1972.

Schore, E.C., et al.: B and T Lymphocytes in the Bovine Mammary Gland: Rosette Formation and Mitogen Response. Vet. Immunol. Immunopathol. *2*:561, 1981.

Segel, G.B.: Membrane Alterations in Lymphocyte Proliferation. Amer. J. Pediatr. Hematol. Oncol., *3*(4):433, 1981.

Sell, K.W., and Miller, W.V.: The Lymphokines. Prog. Clin. Res., *58*:8, 1980.

Sharon, N.: Lectin Receptors as Lymphocyte Surface Markers. Adv. Immunol., *34*:213, 1983.

Shaw, R.K., et al.: A Study of Prednisone Therapy in Chronic Lymphocytic Leukemia. Blood, *17*:182, 1961.

Shimizu, M., et al.: T- and B-Lymphocytes in Porcine Blood. Amer. J. Vet. Res., *37*:309, 1976.

Smith, J.W., and Schultz, R.D.: Mitogen- and Antigen-Responsive Milk Lymphocytes. Cell. Immunol., *29*:165, 1977.

Sonoda, M.: Electron Microscopy of Lymphocytes in the Peripheral Blood of Clinically Healthy Horses. Jap. J. Vet. Sci., *33*:291, 1971.

Sonoda, M., and Kobayashi, K.: Lymphocytes of Canine Peripheral Blood in Electron Microscopy. Jap. J. Vet. Res., *18*:71, 1970.

Sonoda, M., and Marshak, R.R.: Electron Microscopic Observations on the Mononuclear Cells in the Peripheral Blood of the Clinically Normal and Lymphosarcoma Cows. Jap. J. Vet. Res., 18:9, 1970.

Soper, F.F., et al.: In Vitro Stimulation of Bovine Peripheral Blood Lymphocytes: Analysis of Variation of Lymphocyte Blastogenic Response in Normal Dairy Cattle. Amer. J. Vet. Res., 39:1039, 1978.

Splitter, G.A., and Everlith, K.M.: Suppression of Bovine T- and B-Lymphocyte Responses by Fetuin, a Bovine Glycoprotein. Cell. Immunol., 70:205, 1982.

Sprent, J., and Basten, A.: Circulating T and B Lymphocytes in the Mouse. II. Lifespan. Cell. Immunol., 7:40, 1973.

Srivastava, S.K., and Barnum, D.A.: Lymphocyte Stimulation Response in Horses against Phytohaemagglutinin and M Protein of Streptococcus equi Using Whole Blood. Can. J. Comp. Med., 46:51, 1982.

Staples, L.D., et al.: Influence of Certain Steroids on Lymphocyte Transformation in Sheep and Goats Studied in Vitro. J. Endocrinol., 98:55, 1983.

Symons, D.B.A., and Binns, R.M.: Immunoglobulin-Bearing Lymphocytes: Their Demonstration in Adult Sheep and Ontogeny in the Sheep Fetus. Int. Arch. Allergy Immunol., 49:658, 1975.

Tarr, M.J., et al.: Erythrocyte Rosette Formation of Equine Peripheral Blood Lymphocyte. Amer. J. Vet. Res., 38:1775, 1977.

Taub, R.N., et al.: Distribution of Labeled Lymph Node Cells in Mice during the Lymphocytosis Induced by Bordetella pertussis. J. Exp. Med., 136:1581, 1972.

Taylor, D.W., and Siddiqui, W.A.: Response of Enriched Population of Feline T and B Lymphocytes to Mitogen Stimulation. Amer. J. Vet. Res., 38:1969, 1977.

Taylor, D., et al.: Differentiating Feline T and B Lymphocytes by Rosette Formation. J. Immunol., 115:862, 1975.

Terrell, T.G., et al.: Immunologic Surface Markers on Nonhuman Primate Lymphocytes. Amer. J. Vet. Res., 38:503, 1977.

Thomson, S.P., et al.: Endogenous Cortisol: A Regulator of the Number of Lymphocytes in Peripheral Blood. Clin. Immunol. Immunopathol., 17:506, 1980.

Timonen, T., et al.: Characteristics of Human Large Granular Lymphocytes and Relationship to Natural Killer and K Cells. J. Exp. Med., 153:569, 1981.

Uhr, J.W., and Finkelstein, M.S.: The Kinetics of Antibody Formation. Prog. Allergy., 10:37, 1967.

Unanue, E.R.: The Regulatory Role of Macrophages in Antigenic Stimulation. Part Two: Symbiotic Relationship between Lymphocytes and Macrophages. Adv. Immunol., 31:1, 1981.

Van Furth, R.: The Formation of Immunoglobulins by Circulating Lymphocytes. Semin. Hematol., 6:84, 1969.

Vos, J.G., et al.: Ultrastructural Studies of Peripheral Blood Lymphocytes in T Cell–Depleted Rabbits. Cell Tissue Res., 213:221, 1980.

Wagstaff, J., et al.: A Method for Following Human Lymphocyte Traffic Using Indium-III Oxine Labelling. Clin. Exp. Immunol., 43:435, 1981.

Weber, A.F., and Joel, D.: Tabular and Ultrastructural Studies of Agranulocytes of the Thoracic Duct of Calves. Blood, 28:266, 1966.

Weber, A., et al.: Occurrence of Nuclear Pockets in Lymphocytes of Normal, Persistent Lymphocytotic and Leukemic Adult Cattle. J. Natl. Cancer Res. Inst., 43:1307, 1969.

Weiland, F., and Straub, O.C.: Biological Properties of Lymphocytes from Leukotic Cattle. Vet. Microbiol., 1:387, 1976.

Wieczorek, Z.: Cellular Mechanisms of Antibody Production. Acta Histochem. Suppl., 22:19–26, 1980.

Wilkie, B.N., et al.: Bovine Lymphocytes: Erythrocyte Rosettes in Normal Lymphomatous and Corticosteroid-Treated Cattle. Can. J. Comp. Med., 43:22, 1979.

Williams, T.W., and Granger, G.A.: Lymphocyte in Vitro Cytotoxicity: Mechanism of Lymphotoxin-Induced Target Cell Destruction. J. Immunol., 102:911, 1969.

Williams, W.J., et al.: Hematology. 3rd ed. McGraw-Hill, New York, 1983.

Wintrobe, M.M., et al.: Clinical Hematology. 8th ed. Lea & Febiger, Philadelphia, 1981.

Woodruff, J.J., and Woodruff, J.F.: Influenza A Virus Interaction with Murine Lymphocytes. I. The Influence of Influenza Virus A/Japan 305 (H2N2) on the Pattern of Migration of Recirculatory Lymphocytes. J. Immunol., 117:852, 1976.

Wysocki, L.J., and Sato, V.L.: "Panning" for Lymphocytes: A Method for Cell Selection. Proc. Natl. Acad. Sci., 75:2844, 1978.

Yang, T.J.: Identification of Bovine T- and B-Lymphocyte Subpopulations by Immunofluorescence Surface Marker Analysis. Amer. J. Vet. Res., 42:755, 1981.

Yang, T.J., et al.: Depression of B Lymphocyte Levels in the Peripheral Blood of Cows with Mastitis. Infect. Immun., 27:90, 1980.

Yoffey, J.M.: Quantitative Cellular Hematology. Charles C Thomas, Springfield, Ill., 1960.

Yoffey, J.M.: Lymphocyte Production in the Lymphomyeloid Complex. In Regulation of Hematopoiesis. Vol. 2. Gordon, A.S., ed. Appleton-Century-Crofts, New York, p. 1421, 1970.

Yoffey, J.M.: Bone Marrow Lymphocytes. Lymphology, 8:154, 1975.

Yoffey, J.M., and Courtice, F.C.: Lymphatics, Lymph and Lymphoid Tissue. Edward Arnold, London, 1956.

Yoffey, J.M., and Courtice, F.C.: Lymphatics, Lymph and the Lymphomyeloid Complex. Academic Press, New York, 1970.

Yoffey, J.M., et al.: The Source of the Lymphocytes in Thoracic Duct Lymph during Prolonged Drainage. Ann. N.Y. Acad. Sci. 113:1053, 1964.

Yoffey, J.M., et al.: Studies on Hypoxia. VI. Changes in Lymphocytes and Transitional Cells during the Intensification of Primary Hypoxia and Rebound. Ann. N.Y. Acad. Sci., 149:179, 1968.

Zander, A.R., et al.: Surface Markers on Canine Lymphocytes. Transplant. Proc. 7:369, 1975.

Zinkl, J.G., et al.: "Flaming" Plasma Cells in a Dog with IgA Multiple Myeloma. Vet. Clin. Pathol., 12(3):15, 1983.

31

Clinical Interpretation of Changes in Leukocyte Numbers and Morphology

SPECIES VARIATIONS IN TOTAL
    LEUKOCYTE RESPONSE IN
    DISEASE 821
  The Dog 823
  The Cat 823
  The Horse 823
  The Cow 823

CLASSIFICATION OF THE TOTAL AND
    DIFFERENTIAL LEUKOCYTE
    RESPONSES IN DISEASE 823
  Absolute and Relative Leukocyte
    Counts 824
  Regenerative Left Shift 824
  Degenerative Left Shift 824

Leukemoid Blood Picture 824
Leukoerythroblastic Reaction 825
Physiologic Leukocytosis 825

LEUKOCYTE RESPONSE IN RELATION TO
    THE TYPE OF DISEASE PROCESS 826

INTERPRETATION OF THE LEUKOCYTE
    PICTURE 827

THE LEUKOPENIAS 829
  Viral Diseases 829
  Rickettsial Infection 830
  Bacterial Endotoxins 831
  Bacterial Toxemia and Septicemia 836
  Anaphylaxis 836

Basic principles affecting leukocyte responses in disease are similar in all species. However, a single standard for interpreting the leukocyte pattern in disease in all domestic animals is not possible because the normal differential leukocyte count is not the same in all animals, and the leukocyte pattern in health significantly affects the pattern of leukocyte response to disease.

In the differential leukocyte count of domestic animals, the most significant species characteristic is the neutrophil:lymphocyte (N:L) ratio. Using mean percentages for neutrophils and lymphocytes in health, the N:L ratios are 3.5 for the dog, 1.8 for the cat, 1.1 for the young "hot-blooded" horse, and 0.5 for cattle (Schalm, 1962). The N:L ratio in humans is 1.5. Lymphocyte numbers are at their peak in young, growing animals, but gradually decrease with age. In comparison, neutrophil numbers remain stable. Thus the N:L ratio gradually, but slightly, increases with age (Table 4-1).

The reason for differences in the normal blood level of lymphocytes among the domestic animals is unknown. Selye (1937), in his studies on adaptation, observed that the adrenal cortical hormones depress and cause involution of lymphocytic tissues. In animals with a high proportion of lymphocytes, such as the mouse, rat, and rabbit, Dougherty and White (1944) found that an injection of ACTH produced leukopenia, lymphopenia, and neutrophilia. This is the case also in the cow (see below). On the other hand, animals with a high proportion of neutrophils respond to corticosteroids with leukocytosis, neutrophilia, and lymphopenia, although the extent may vary among species. In both types of animals, an eosinopenia is seen. Similarly, the magnitude of the total leukocyte count in response to disease correlates directly with the N:L ratio characteristic of the animal species in health (Table 31–1).

SPECIES VARIATIONS IN TOTAL LEUKOCYTE RESPONSE IN DISEASE

Different animal species vary not only in their normal total and differential leukocyte counts (Tables 1-3 and 1-41) but also in their leukocytic response to disease.

821

Table 31-1. Leukocyte Counts in Animal Patients and Their Relationship to the Neutrophil:Lymphocyte Ratio in Health[a]

Number of Leukocytes (/μl of blood) and Percentage of Patients within Designated Categories for Use in Clinical Interpretation[b]

| | | | | | | | | | | Leukocytosis | | | | | Range of Counts | |
| | | | | Leukopenia | | Normal Range | | Moderate | | Marked | | Extreme | | | | |
Animal	Number of Patients	Observation Period (yr)	N:L Ratio in Health	No.	%	No.	%	No.	%	No.	%	No.	%	Lowest	Highest
Dog	683	1½	3.5	<6,000	2.20	6,000–18,000	63.83	18,000–30,000	23.57	30,000–50,000	7.17	>50,000	3.22	1,300	174,000
Cat	273	3½	1.8	<8,000	22.30	8,000–20,000	51.00	20,000–30,000	16.50	30,000–50,000	8.00	>50,000	2.20	100	76,000
Horse	871	6	1.1	<7,000	2.00	7,000–14,000	71.93	14,000–20,000	16.88	20,000–30,000	7.58	>30,000	1.60	1,450	65,600
Cow	1,451	6	0.5	<4,000	6.88	4,000–12,000	61.54	12,000–20,000	24.60	20,000–30,000	5.72	>30,000	1.24	650	61,000

[a]Modified from Schalm, 1962; courtesy of the *Journal of the American Veterinary Medical Association.*

[b]Leukemia complex excluded from these data.

The Dog

The dog responds dramatically to microbial infections and stressful disease (Schalm, 1963). Total leukocyte counts of 30,000–50,000/μl of blood are common, and counts in excess of 50,000 are not rare. These counts are understandable when it is realized that both neutrophils and monocytes increase significantly in this species in response to the release of adrenocortical hormones in stress (Fig. 4-2).

The Cat

The cat, with a somewhat smaller N:L ratio than that of the dog, does not as a rule attain total leukocyte counts as high as the dog. Counts of 30,000 to 50,000 are not unusual in the cat, but maximum counts level off at about 75,000. Leukocyte numbers exeeding 100,000 (exclusive of the leukemia complex) are extremely rare. On the other hand, physiologic leukocytosis, in which lymphocytes often equal or even exceed neutrophil numbers, is common in frightened young cats (Table 5–3). This responsiveness of the cat to fear and excitement must be taken into consideration in viewing the hemogram (Appendix Case 53). Leukopenia is also a common finding in the cat. In young cats, it is usually due to infection with the panleukopenia virus, but in older cats a variety of toxemic diseases may depress granulopoiesis (Schalm, 1969). Bizarre young granulocytes are seen in the peripheral blood of these cats during the early stage of recovery from such an effect (Plate XV-10).

The Horse

In the horse, the general level of leukocyte response to infection is in the range of 15,000 to 25,000. Marked leukocytosis in the horse is 25,000 to 30,000 and extreme counts are in the range of 35,000 (Appendix Case 62).

The Cow

The cow is even less responsive than the horse. Very often, the total count remains within the normal range of 4,000 to 12,000, but there is neutrophilia of >50% and a left shift. A marked leukocytosis would be represented by counts of 20,000 to 30,000 and extreme leukocytosis by counts above 30,000. Total counts of 40,000 to 50,000 have been recorded but are rare. The dynamics of early leukocyte response to inflammatory disease in the cow are depicted in Fig. 7-3.

CLASSIFICATION OF THE TOTAL AND DIFFERENTIAL LEUKOCYTE RESPONSES IN DISEASE

Variations in leukocyte numbers may occur because of physiologic or pathologic influences. The suffix "-osis" or "-philia" is used to denote an increase above the normal maximum level, while the suffix "-penia" is used for a decrease below the normal minimum number of various cells. A leukocytosis may be physiologic such as that mediated by endogenous release of epinephrine and/or corticosteroids, or it may be pathologic in response to a disease process (reactive leukocytosis) or a result of a neoplastic change in hematopoiesis (proliferative leukocytosis). Leukopenia is always a pathologic event. Quantitative and qualitative changes in a particular leukocyte type indirectly reflect the nature of the disease process and the body's response to it.

Since neutrophils are the first line of defense against microbial infection and are important participants in inflammatory reactions, it is obvious why abnormalities of this leukocyte type attract the most attention. The term *right shift* was proposed by Arneth in 1904 and *left shift* by Shilling in 1929 to describe changes in blood neutrophil differential counts (Haden, 1935). Right shift indicates excessive numbers of neutrophils with increased nuclear segmentation (lobes) as in vitamin B_{12}–folate deficiency in humans, and left shift suggests prominence of immature neutrophils in blood as in an inflammatory response. A true right shift is not seen in blood of common domestic animals because their neutrophils are normally less segmented than those of humans, although an occasional hypersegmented neutrophil may be found during neutrophilic leukocytosis. Schilling further classified the left shift as a *regenerative* reaction associated with increased granulopoiesis or a *degenerative* reaction reflecting inhibited production and delayed maturation of neutrophilic cells.

Absolute and Relative Leukocyte Counts

A differential leukocyte count performed manually should be based on identification of a minimum of 200 cells, except in cases of advanced leukopenia, for which as many cells as possible should be counted. If nucleated red cells are found in a stained blood film, as part of a differential count, their number is recorded so that an appropriate correction can be made in the WBC count (see Chapter 2, for formula).

From the differential leukocyte count expressed in percentage (relative count) and the total leukocyte count per μl of blood, the number of each leukocyte type per μl of blood (absolute count) is calculated to determine whether an absolute increase or decrease has occurred. Errors of interpretation are less likely with absolute values than with percentages. When nucleated erythrocytes are encountered in a stained blood film, absolute numbers of the leukocyte types should be calculated from the corrected WBC count.

Regenerative Left Shift

Regenerative left shift is characterized by a leukocytosis due to neutrophilia and by the appearance of immature neutrophilic granulocytes in the peripheral blood. A slight shift to the left is limited to the occurrence of band neutrophils. A moderate left shift includes both band and metamyelocyte neutrophils, while in a marked left shift myelocytes and progranulocytes appear in the peripheral blood (Appendix Case 12). Rare instances of extreme left shift may also reveal myeloblasts.

In a typical regenerative left shift, the proportion of various immature neutrophils is orderly and follows a pyramidal distribution, with the most immature cell being the least numerous. Usually the mature neutrophils outnumber the immature cells.

It should be noted that leukocytoses involving eosinophils often show little or no left shift.

Degenerative Left Shift

The main feature of degenerative left shift is the occurrence of young neutrophilic granulocytes in the circulation in numbers exceeding mature neutrophils. The WBC count is often suggestive of leukopenia, but it may sometimes be within the normal range or, rarely, elevated. A degenerative left shift reflects the inability of the bone marrow to rise to the occasion and put forth a large number of mature cells. It is common in septicemia (Appendix Case 13). In rare situations of enhanced granulopoiesis, an extreme leukocytosis may have a left shift reflecting a degenerative pattern (Appendix Case 15). This is thought to be a reflection of continued excessive demand for neutrophils in tissue lesions above and beyond that met by mature cells.

In view of the current concept that separate mechanisms control production and release of neutrophils, it can be rationalized that a severe infection may provoke an extensive release into blood of mature as well as immature neutrophils from various marrow pools, viz., the reserve, maturative, and mitotic pools (see Chapter 26, pp. 685–696). With the overwhelming demand to combat infection, mature neutrophils are depleted from blood, and consequently immature neutrophils predominate, resulting in a degenerative left shift with leukopenia or normal WBC count. If the bone marrow has time to undergo granulopoiesis to meet increasing demands, events promoting inappropriate release of marrow neutrophils may produce a degenerative left shift pattern but, in this case, accompanied by leukocytosis (Appendix Cases 13 and 15). The prognosis in this situation is not as bad as when there is leukopenia, but still it is a matter of serious concern and could have fatal consequences.

Leukemoid Blood Picture

Krumbhaar, in 1926, introduced the concept of the leukemoid blood picture. It is characterized by an abnormality of total or differential leukocyte count that indicates leukemia but has been found to be otherwise. A leukemoid picture involving neutrophils is generally similar to a regenerative left shift. The leukogram suggests granulocytic leukemia in that there is a significantly elevated WBC count with left shift to include myelocytes and, at times, progranulocytes or even myeloblasts. The process stimulating the leukocytosis and the left shift is not leukemia, however.

Several criteria have been described to distinguish a leukemoid reaction from a granulocytic leukemia in humans (Goldman, 1981; Miale, 1982); these may be useful for animal species as well. Distinguishing features in the hemogram of a leukemoid reaction include the presence of toxic changes in neutrophils and the absence of marked anemia and thrombocytopenia. A thorough clinical and laboratory examination may provide essential clues to differentiate the two processes. Sequential hemograms may establish the temporary nature of a leukemoid reaction and a bone marrow examination may reveal myeloid hyperplasia with regular distribution of neutrophil granulocytes. Splenomegaly is common in granulocytic leukemia, and splenic aspirate often shows predominance of myeloid cells as opposed to lymphoid cells.

A leukemoid blood picture may also involve lymphocytes. Examples in animal species include lymphocytosis in young kittens, foals, and piglets; persistent lymphocytosis in cattle; and salmon poisoning in dogs wherein aberrant and immature lymphoid and monocytoid cells are present in blood (Plate XI–6, Appendix Case 36).

A leukemoid picture involving eosinophils may result from an extreme response to an allergic or parasitic disease or other causes. For example, eosinophil counts of over 60,000/μl of blood, initially suggestive of eosinophilic leukemia, were seen in two cats with intestinal lymphosarcoma (Prasse, 1983) as had been reported in humans.

Leukoerythroblastic Reaction

The leukoerythroblastic reaction is characterized by prominence of nucleated erythrocytes and immature neutrophil granulocytes in the peripheral blood. The WBC count may vary from leukopenia to slight leukocytosis. If anemia is a concomitant finding, then it is referred to as a leukoerythroblastic anemia. Generally, there is no reticulocyte response or the nucleated erythrocytes in blood are out of proportion to reticulocytes.

This type of blood picture is attributed to abnormalities of bone marrow architecture involving inappropriate release of immature erythroid and granulocytic cells. The mechanism involved remains unknown. Although a leukoerythroblastic reaction may be found in association with myeloproliferative disorders, it may occur as a nonspecific response to a severe disease process. It is not a specific disease entity. Causes of leukoerythroblastic reaction in humans include hematopoietic malignancies, myelophthisis, tumor metastasis in the bone marrow, myelosclerosis, multiple myeloma, and tuberculosis (Miale, 1982; Goldman, 1981; Wintrobe et al., 1981). Leukoerythroblastic reaction has been observed in dogs and cats with myeloproliferative disorders as well as some nonneoplastic diseases involving blood and bone marrow.

Physiologic Leukocytosis

An elevated WBC count as a result of muscular exercise, excitement, apprehension, or emotional disturbance constitutes physiologic leukocytosis. Wide variations are seen in the extent of leukocytosis and changes in differential leukocyte numbers, perhaps reflecting the intensity of the stress involved. The WBC count may increase by as much as 100 to 200%, primarily as a result of elevations in mature neutrophils; hence the condition is also called "pseudo" neutrophilia. Leukocytosis may also be a result of lymphocytosis, especially in young and growing animals, particularly the cat (Table 5–3) and the horse (Table 6–15). However, in some cases there may be an overall increase in various leukocyte types. Physiologic leukocytosis due to increases in neutrophils and lymphocyte numbers is generally considered an epinephrine effect.

Exogenous administration or endogenous release of corticosteroids is associated with predictable changes in total and differential leukocyte counts. A typical response consists of neutrophilia, lymphopenia, and eosinopenia. The neutrophilia is primarily made of mature neutrophils, although a slight increase in band neutrophils may be seen. Monocytopenia is a consistent feature in humans, whereas monocytosis is characteristic of the dog, and a variable response is seen in other animal species.

The overall effect is a leukocytosis in species with normal N:L ratios greater than one; WBC counts may reach as high as 30,000/μl in the cat and 40,000/μl in the dog (Prasse,

1983). Some species variations have been observed in these trends (see Table 4-4, and Fig. 4–2 for the dog; Fig. 5–3 for the cat; Table 6–14 for the horse; and Table 7–12 for the cow). These changes in leukocyte numbers are temporary and return to normal within 24 hours of an injection or release of endogenous corticosteroids. A continuous elevation in blood corticosteroid level, as from daily treatment, causes prolonged but diminishing elevations in leukocyte numbers (see p. 693).

LEUKOCYTE RESPONSE IN RELATION TO THE TYPE OF DISEASE PROCESS

The ability of the bone marrow to respond to a bacterial infection is measured by the total leukocyte count (particularly neutrophils), and the intensity of the response is gauged by the extent of the left shift. The degree of the left shift is generally proportional to the severity of infection or toxemia. The severity of the infection may also be assessed by the occurrence of toxic changes in the neutrophils; other leukocytes rarely show toxic changes (Appendix Cases 12, 13, 40, 63, and 66). The following are common manifestations of toxicity or qualitative changes in leukocytes in response to disease. See p. 715 for additional comments.

1. Diffuse basophilia of the cytoplasm or foamy blue cytoplasm of neutrophils. This may be seen in all domestic animals under conditions of extreme toxicity. A common manifestation of toxicity in neutrophils of the dog is the occurrence of moderate to many vacuoles so located along the periphery of the cell as to suggest a moth-eaten appearance (Plates VIII–11, VIII–12). Slight foamy vacuolation may appear as an artifact in canine neutrophils in EDTA blood more than 1 hour old (Gossett and Carakostas, 1984).

2. Occurrence of blue-black or reddish (azurophilic) granules, from few to many, in the cytoplasm of neutrophils. This is referred to as toxic granulation. This form of toxic manifestation has been seen in sheep, cattle, and horses (Plate XI-12). Hereditary abnormalities of neutrophil granulation are described in Chapter 26. The reddish purple granules of mucopolysaccharidosis are large,

are usually surrounded by a halo, and are present in a cell with cytoplasm more mature than that with toxic granules. Such granules are found in lymphocytes more often than in neutrophils.

3. Besides diffuse basophilia, bizarre giant neutrophils and Döhle bodies in the cytoplasm of neutrophils are common to cats in toxemic diseases (Plates IX–2, XI–10, XV–8, XV–9).

4. Polyploid neutrophils and acquired hyposegmentation of the neutrophil nucleus (pseudo-Pelger-Huët anomaly) reflect aberrant granulopoiesis. An occasional cell of this type may be encountered during reactive leukocytosis.

5. Hypersegmentation of the neutrophil nucleus results from longer intravascular survival, or it may be an in vitro artifact of degeneration.

6. Some cytoplasmic vacuolation is common in canine eosinophils, and it is much more extensive in eosinophils of the greyhound (see Chapter 4, p. 119). Rarely, a mature eosinophil may also show a few small reddish purple toxic granules.

7. Mature basophils of the cat normally lack metachromasia, but basophils with some reddish granulation are sometimes found in cat blood. It is perhaps a reflection of toxic effect on marrow basophil production or a response to agents stimulating IgE antibody production.

Various infectious and noninfectious disease processes in general may elicit the following responses. The degree of changes observed vary with the intensity and duration of the disease process, as well as with the cause, virulence of the organism, species and individual hematopoietic reactivity, location of the inflammatory process, and therapy (Miale, 1982). Species variations are also apparent.

1. The general response to *bacterial infections* is neutrophilia with or without left shift and toxic changes.

2. In bacterial infection with *septicemia,* there is often no leukocytosis; a degenerative left shift is more common. Toxic

changes in the form of cytoplasmic vacuolation and basophilia are prominent in neutrophils. Convalescence is accompanied by a regenerative left shift with diminution of toxic changes.

3. *Bacterial infection with localization and pus formation,* e.g., pyometra in a bitch, stimulates a marked neutrophilia in comparison to a generalized infection. Before the abscess becomes encapsulated, the total leukocyte count may be extremely high.

4. A variety of *noninfectious conditions* that stimulate release of endogenous corticosteroids and/or cause tissue destruction lead to neutrophilia. Examples are malignancy, chemical intoxication, metabolic intoxication such as uremia, and the postoperative state.

5. During *intense erythropoietic response* to hemolysis or significant blood loss, concomitant leukopoiesis often occurs resulting in neutrophilia with a variable left shift. Hemolytic anemia may also be accompanied by monocytosis reflecting increased disposal of antibody-coated erythrocytes. This is seen particularly in autoimmune hemolytic anemia. In rare cases, erythrophagocytosis by an occasional monocyte may be found in circulation.

6. *Antigen-antibody reactions, decomposition of tissue,* or a wide variety of *chronic diseases involving continuous degranulation of mast cells* and causing release of histamine commonly induce eosinophilia (Table 27–2). *Parasitism* results in eosinophilia only when sensitivity to a protein of the parasite has developed. Eosinophilia is common in dogs infected with *Dirofilaria immitis,* and increased basophil numbers may be found in some such cases.

7. A *chronic infection or inflammatory process* stimulates monocytosis. An increase in monocytes is a response to the body's need for destruction of pathogens too difficult for the neutrophils to handle and/or the need for the removal of tissue debris in the chronic inflammatory process. In the dog, monocytosis is also an

expression of response to the release of corticosteroids in stress.

8. *Toxins,* either endogenous (as in uremia), bacterial, or exogenous, may cause leukopenia by suppressing granulocytopoiesis or lymphopoiesis.

9. Most *diseases caused by viruses* produce leukopenia.

10. *Drug therapy* may alter leukocyte responses. There are many drugs of various classes that decrease leukocyte production and cause leukopenia. A good drug history is important in evaluating an animal's leukocyte response to disease. Comments about corticosteroids have been made earlier.

11. Certain *viral, rickettsial,* and *protozoal infections* may be found intracellularly in leukocyte cytoplasm. Distemper inclusions may occur in lymphocytes and neutrophils in addition to erythrocytes. Morulae of *Ehrlichia canis* are found primarily in lymphocytes, while those of *E. equi* are seen in neutrophils. *Leishmania* and *Histoplasma* organisms may be found in macrophages in the bone marrow and other tissues. *Leishmania* may rarely be found also in blood monocytes. On rare occasions, intracellular bacteria may be found in circulating neutrophils (Plate XIV–10).

INTERPRETATION OF THE LEUKOCYTE PICTURE

Any interpretation of a leukogram must take into consideration normal values for the species in question, age of the animal, and characteristic species-specific responses. Young animals have greater lymphocyte numbers and WBC counts than do adults. Hence lymphocytopenia is defined at a higher level of lymphocyte numbers in the young than in the adult, e.g., at $<2,000/\mu l$ of blood in a dog under 6 months in age, $<1,500$ in a dog under 2 years of age, and $<1,000$ in an adult dog. Breed may also be a consideration, particularly in cattle (see Chapter 7).

Differentiation of physiologic leukocytosis from reactive leukocytosis requires consideration of several other factors in the hemogram and is difficult at times. Sequential hemograms obtained daily on such patients are a valuable aid in this regard because physiologic leukocytosis is transient. In some situations, however, stress of the disease may override the effects of the disease per se and produce a classic stress leukogram.

A change in the WBC count may involve abnormalities of production, release, intravascular distribution, life span, and tissue egress of various leukocytes. For example, circulating neutrophils are in a dynamic equilibrium with neutrophils in the marginal pool (in capillary beds) and in the bone marrow reserve (see Chapter 26). An immediate functional demand for neutrophils is met *first* by mobilization of cells from the marginal and circulating pools, *then* from the marrow reserve, and *finally* by increased granulopoiesis and accelerated release. The latter is reflected in blood by a left shift. Thus the size of the marginal and circulating pools, the size of the marrow reserve, and the proliferative capacity of marrow are important determinants of the response to disease and the net level of circulating neutrophils. See Chapter 26 for comments on factors leading to neutrophilia and neutropenia. Conditions associated with changes in numbers of various leukocytes have been described at other places: neutrophilia (p. 691), neutropenia (p. 695), eosinophilia (p. 747), eosinopenia (p. 750), lymphocytosis and lymphopenia (p. 811), monocytosis and monocytopenia (p. 777) and basophilia and basopenia (p. 764).

Interpretations of certain trends in leukocyte numbers and abnormalities are given briefly below:

1. Neutrophilia with a slight left shift and with persistence of eosinophils suggests a mild infection or stress.
2. Neutrophilia with a modest lymphopenia and an absolute eosinopenia indicates a moderately severe to severe infection or other disease leading to severe stress.
3. Eosinopenia is usually a corticosteroid effect, but it may also be a direct result of disease process (see Chapter 27).
4. A marked absolute reduction in the lymphocyte count that persists despite therapy is not a favorable sign. Increasing numbers of lymphocytes indicate that recovery is taking place.
5. The occurrence of more immature than mature neutrophils (degenerative left shift) is an unfavorable sign. This interpretation does not apply to the cow in the initial response to infection.
6. A severe infection is indicated when toxic changes in neutrophils are a prominent feature. Prognosis should be guarded.
7. A diminishing leukocytosis with a reduction in numbers of neutrophils and a return of lymphocytes and eosinophils represent convalescence.
8. A leukopenia is common to viral diseases, but it is also present in overwhelming bacterial infections. Leukopenia is commonly observed in the early stages of acute mastitis and other similarly acute bacterial infections in the cow.
9. Eosinophilia is a response to histamine. It is common to antigen–antibody reactions involving IgE antibodies (allergy). These include those instances of parasitism wherein the animal has become sensitized to the protein or products of the parasite, as well as diseases leading to decomposition of body protein. The return of eosinophils to the blood in numbers indicative of eosinophilia in the face of neutrophilia and lymphopenia is to be viewed as a sign of worsening of the disease process. Eosinophilia is not uncommon in chronic suppurative diseases and certain malignancies when decomposition of tissue protein is taking place. Some association of eosinophilia with basophilia has been noted in the dog, especially in chronic respiratory diseases (Table 27–2).
10. Monocytosis generally reflects chronicity. Monocytosis is a characteristic feature of chronic suppurative and granulomatous diseases, and it also develops when there is escape of erythrocytes into the tissues and body cavities. In the dog, monocytosis is also seen in the acute phase of disease as an expression of the response to the corticosteroids of stress. Monocytosis accompanied by some im-

mature-looking monocytes in blood is indicative of a chronic inflammatory response rather than a corticosteroid effect. Monocytopenia is common in early phases of acute disease in the cat, cow, and horse.

11. Monocytosis accompanied by hyperfibrinogenemia and/or left shift indicates a chronic, active inflammatory response.

12. The presence of macrophages in blood indicates monocyte–macrophage transformation in circulation, probably due to a subacute or chronic bacterial infection, such as bacterial endocarditis.

13. The presence of an occasional polyploid or pseudo-Pelger-Huët neutrophil in circulation is indicative of aberrant granulopoiesis. The finding of an occasional hypersegmented neutrophil suggests that the neutrophilia is probably associated with increased circulating levels of corticosteroids. These aberrations of neutrophil morphology usually manifest during moderate to marked neutrophilia.

14. The presence of cytoplasmic basophilia in small to large lymphocytes and of cells resembling immunocytes or plasma cells indicates chronic antigenic stimulus and enhanced immunoglobulin synthesis as in a systemic disease or a local suppurative process.

15. Lymphoma in the dog and cat manifests as leukemia only in about 50% of the cases and in cats only in about 25% of the cases. In comparison, myeloproliferative disorders more often show immature and aberrant cells in the blood film. Bone marrow examination is essential to diagnosis of myeloproliferative disorders, while it is occasionally helpful in lymphoma.

16. Persistent lymphocytosis may be observed in cattle without any evidence of lymphocytic leukemia or lymphoma. An occasional lymphocyte with one or two nucleoli and aberrant morphology may be found in normal cattle, but it is an abnormal finding suggestive of lymphocytic leukemia in other animal species.

17. Fibrinogen elevation is a better indicator that a cow is responding to a disease than are the WBC count and neutrophil numbers.

18. Reversal of the N:L ratio in ruminants is generally indicative of a neutrophil response to an inflammatory process. A frank leukocytosis or neutrophilia may or may not be evident in such cases.

19. Mastocytemia, the presence of mast cells in the peripheral blood, is seen in about 10% of dogs with mastocytoma. It is also seen in dogs experiencing severe trauma and in some canine patients with acute inflammatory reaction, particularly of the gastrointestinal tract (Stockham et al., 1986).

THE LEUKOPENIAS

Leukopenia exists when the total leukocyte count in the peripheral blood falls below the normal minimum for the species concerned. Leukopenia may result from one or more of the following mechanisms: decreased production as in marrow damage or necrosis of lymphoid tissues; ineffective granulopoiesis or decreased release into the circulation; increased peripheral destruction or utilization as in sepsis; and shift of cells in the marginal pool as in early endotoxic effect or hypersplenism.

Some common causes of leukopenia are viral diseases; bacterial septicemia and toxemia; bacterial endotoxin; some instances of the leukemia complex; anaphylaxis; x-radiation; toxic substances of plant origin, such as bracken fern; certain drugs, such as the sulfonamides and similar chemicals, that compete with folic acid for utilization in cell growth and metabolism; nutritional deficiencies, such as deficiencies of protein, vitamin B_{12}, folic acid, and niacin; and some instances of hypersplenism in the autoimmune disease complex. Selected examples of the leukopenic state are discussed below.

Viral Diseases

A classic example of leukopenia in viral disease was the observation by Lewis and Shope (1929) that the demonstration of leukopenia in a herd of swine suspected of disease would add support to a diagnosis of *hog cholera*. They stated, "It is believed by us that for the present and until contradictory evidence appears, a leukocyte count of 8,000 per cu mm or less on three sick animals in a suspected herd indicates clearly that the condition is hog cholera." Many investigators have supported this original observation with respect to hog cholera. Dunne (1963) reported observations on more than 2,500 leukocyte counts taken at various times during the course of hog cholera produced experimentally. Leukopenia or WBC counts of less than 10,000/µl were found in approximately 50% of the pigs in the terminal stage of the disease.

Panleukopenia, a common viral disease of young cats, derives its name from the rapid and extreme reduction of all leukocyte types. Appendix Case 54 demonstrates the rapid fall in circulating leukocyte numbers in two cats infected experimentally with the virus of panleukopenia. Additional data are presented in Table 36–13. The leukopenia is attributed to decreased production. Neutrophilic leukocytosis often manifests in cats infected with *feline infectious peritonitis virus.*

Distemper and *canine infectious hepatitis* are two classic viral diseases of the dog in which leukopenia occurs in uncomplicated situations, but leukocytosis manifests following secondary bacterial infections. The diseases are discussed in Chapter 36. *Canine parvovirus* infection results in leukopenia due to neutropenia and lymphopenia, while *canine coronavirus* infection may produce lymphopenia but not neutropenia (Appel et al., 1979a, 1979b).

The development of leukopenia is commonly observed in experimentally produced *viral diseases* of domestic livestock. Luedke and coworkers (1964) found neutropenia, eosinopenia, and lymphopenia in 86% of lambs and ewes inoculated with the *bluetongue virus.* Heuschele and Barber (1963) observed a 67% reduction in total leukocyte counts of pigs 3 days after inoculation with the *rinderpest virus.* The leukocyte counts ranged from 6,500 to 7,500/µl, compared with counts of 18,000 to 27,000 in control pigs.

Easterday at al. (1962) exposed lambs and goat kids to the agent of *Rift Valley fever* and observed a leukopenia of short duration. Similarly, Storz et al. (1962) exposed cows to an agent of the *psittacosis-lymphogranuloma group* and found a leukopenia on the third and fourth days postinoculation, with a return to normal by the seventh day. The leukocytic response was said to be similar to the marked leukopenia observed in *virus diarrhea* of cattle (Baker et al., 1954). In contrast, infection of young calves resulted in leukocytosis. A word of caution is appropriate with regard to assigning as a cause of leukopenia in cattle the direct action of an infectious agent on the leukocytes. As indicated in Chapter 7, leukopenia may develop in the initial phases of any severe, acute inflammatory process in the cow. In fact, in all animals that normally present a low neutrophil:lymphocyte ratio, a localized severe inflammatory process may lead to draining off of neutrophils from the blood at a greater rate than they are replaced from the bone marrow, resulting in a temporary neutropenia; this, augmented by the lymphopenia and eosinopenia of stress, results in a frank leukopenia.

It is of interest that Maurer and Jones (1943) observed a leukocytosis, mainly due to neutrophilia, in uncomplicated cases of *equine influenza* developing from contact exposure. The total leukocyte count was usually normal or subnormal at the time of the first temperature rise, but shortly thereafter, the number of neutrophils increased, and neutrophil numbers as high as 17,000/µl were not uncommon.

Bryans et al. (1957) isolated the agent of "*viral arteritis*" and experimentally reproduced the disease in horses. Temperature elevations of 104 to 106.5° F persisted up to 9 days in some horses. The pyrexia was accompanied by a panleukopenia, with the lymphocyte number markedly depressed. In most horses, the leukopenia occurred 24 to 72 hours after the temperature elevation appeared, but in others the leukopenia was present at the onset of the fever.

Rickettsial Infection

Gribble (1969) and Stannard and coworkers (1969) described equine ehrlichiosis as a distinct disease in the horse characterized by panleukopenia, thrombocytopenia, and moderate anemia. A similar disease in the dog, caused by *Ehrlichia canis,* is characterized by pancytopenia. See Chapter 36 for further comments on ehrlichiosis in the horse and dog.

Bacterial Endotoxins

The endotoxins are high-molecular-weight, heat-stable complexes of phospholipid, polysaccharide, and a small amount of protein. They form an integral part of the outer cell wall of Gram-negative bacteria and are released on lysis of the bacteria. The lipid moiety is responsible for most of the endotoxic effects.

Endotoxemia from Gram-negative sepsis or experimental intravenous injection of endotoxin evokes a wide variety of biologic responses affecting almost all organs of the host (Majde and Person, 1981; Morrison and Ulevitch, 1978). These responses are characterized by generalized arteriolar constriction, fever, hypoglycemia, and hematologic abnormalities. Animals given lethal doses become anorectic, progressively weaker, and ataxic, and they generally develop a high fever. This is followed by respiratory distress, usually leading to the appearance of blood-tinged foam at the nostrils. Vomiting, fluid diarrhea, convulsions, and death within 24 hours represent a terminal pattern of clinical signs. Clinical signs of endotoxemia may vary with the amount of endotoxin injected.

Biochemical events associated with endotoxemia include activation of complement, generation of kallikrein and formation of procoagulants through activation of the Hageman factor, activation of the plasminogen system, and release of a number of bioactive substances including arachidonic acid metabolites from platelets and various other body cells (Morrison and Ulevitch, 1978).

Prominent hematologic changes include marked leukopenia (neutropenia and lymphopenia) and thrombocytopenia followed by a rebound neutrophilia. Leukocytes and platelets have been found to aggregate and sequester in the lungs, liver, and spleen (Hartman and Gordon, 1958). Kinetic studies indicate that the neutropenia is due to shift of cells from the circulating pool into the marginal pool and the neutrophilia is due to increased mobilization of cells from the marrow reserve into the circulation. Because of the latter effect, injection of a minute amount of a purified endotoxin has been found useful in assessing the marrow granulocyte reserve.

These quantitative changes have been observed in humans and a number of animal species including the dog, cow, horse, and water buffalo. However, it should be understood that hematologic effects of endotoxin vary with the amount of endotoxin injected (Fruhman, 1970; Jain and Lasmanis, 1978; Mechanic et al. 1962), and species vary in their sensitivity to endotoxin (Carrol et al., 1965). Leukopenia may be absent or minimal when smaller amounts are injected, whereas larger amounts may produce a leukopenia with degenerative left shift (see Table 31–2) and a rebound leukocytosis with left shift that may persist for a few days (Carroll et al., 1964). See p. 693 for additional comments and references on this topic.

Single intravenous injections of *Escherichia coli* endotoxin into normal cows produced dose-dependent leukocytic and febrile responses (Jain and Lasmanis, 1978). Injection of 5–20 μg induced a slight reduction in neutrophil and lymphocyte numbers within 1 hour followed by a neutrophilia 4–8 hours postinjection (Table 31–2). Injection of 50–500 μg produced a severe neutropenia for 4–6 hours followed by a gradual increase in neutrophil numbers along with slight to moderate left shift (Table 31–2). Higher doses caused progressively severe lymphopenia and greater increases in fever than the lower doses; rectal temperatures increased by 1.2–2.4°F, 2.2–2.4°F, and 2.8–6.4°F within 2 to 4 hours of injections of 5–20μg, 50μg, and 100–500 μg endotoxin, respectively, with a return to normal level by the eighth hour.

Similar hematologic changes have been observed in cows with severe endotoxin-induced or coliform mastitis (Carroll et al., 1964; Jain et al., 1978; Paape et al., 1974; Schalm and Lasmanis, 1976). As a result of massive leukocytosis in milk, these cows develop marked neutropenia and depletion of marrow reserve within 2–12 hours of the onset of acute mastitis. Thus it is conjectured that blood leukocytic changes during the early stage of endotoxin-induced mastitis are associated with both development of local inflammatory reaction as well as with systemic absorption of endotoxin. A similar analogy

Table 31–2. Changes in Peripheral Blood Leukocyte Numbers of Cows Given an Intravenous Injection of *Escherichia coli* **Endotoxin**

Endotoxin (μg)	Time (h)	Leukocyte count	Cells/μl blood		
			Immature neutrophils*	Mature neutrophils	Lymphocytes
5	0	7,200	0	2,376	3,924
	1	6,300	0	1,922	3,348
	2	5,500	0	2,117	3,080
	4	10,500	0	6,247	3,150
	6	10,500	0	5,652	3,780
	8	10,500	0	5,774	3,622
	10	8,100	0	3,888	3,280
	24	7,600	0	2,584	3,914
20	0	7,100	71 B	2,023	4,012
	1	6,000	0	1,920	3,600
	2	5,600	0	2,352	2,968
	4	7,600	0	3,876	2,850
	6	8,500	0	3,995	3,570
	8	8,600	0	3,569	4,042
	10	8,000	40 B	2,920	4,120
	24	6,800	0	1,530	4,352
50	0	8,100	0	3,078	4,212
	1	4,000	0	1,480	2,420
	2	2,300	58 B	402	1,610
	4	2,400	24 B	588	1,584
	6	3,500	70 B	1,015	2,152
	8	4,700	47 B	1,692	2,585
	10	5,300	26 B	1,404	3,418
	24	5,800	29 B	1,218	3,973
100	0	8,900	0	1,691	5,295
	1	1,700	0	68	1,496
	2	2,300	80 Mt	69	1,898
	4	1,600	16 B	80	1,336
	6	1,700	17 B	153	1,317
	8	3,900	468 Mt	643	2,281
	10	6,800	1,632 Mt	1,088	3,366
	24	11,600	2,088 Mt	3,422	5,104

From Jain and Lasmanis, 1978; courtesty of *Research in Veterinary Science*.
*Left shift up to: B, band cells; Mt, metamyelocytes

may be drawn for other diseases associated with Gram-negative infection.

Bryans and coworkers (Bryans, 1963; Rooney et al., 1963) described a fatal condition of horses of unknown etiology and named the disease colitis "X." The suddenness of occurrence of colitis X in apparently healthy horses and the violent clinical signs resemble those produced by endotoxin.

Hemograms on a 12-year-old gelding given 17 mg of endotoxin intraperitoneally are shown in Table 31–3 (Carroll et al., 1965). The horse collapsed within an hour after endotoxin administration, and a marked leukopenia (1,700 leukocytes/μl) was evident. Contraction of the spleen was indicated by an increase of PCV from 45% to 57% at the first hour. Subsequently, the PCV fell to 49% by

the fifth hour and then increased again, reaching 58% at the eighth hour, when the horse died (hemoconcentration from terminal fluid loss). Plasma protein concentration paralleled the pattern established by the PCV. Similar trials in other horses did not terminate in death. Burrows (1981) has reviewed endotoxemia in the horse.

Hemograms on a female cat, 18 months old, given 0.4 mg of endotoxin intraperitoneally are given in Table 31–4. It can be seen that, although a marked leukopenia was evident, there was no significant change in the PCV.

Davis and Smibert (1963) injected endotoxin into young swine. A marked decrease in leukocytes was seen as early as 4 minutes after injection. After 22 to 24 hours, there were increases in the erythrocyte sedimen-

Table 31–3.   Hemogram of the Horse after Intraperitoneal Administration of 17 mg of Enterobacter aerogenes Endotoxin[a]

Sample	PCV (%)	Plasma Protein (g/dl)	WBC/μl	Differential Leukocyte Count in Absolute Numbers/μl					
				Band Cells	Neutrophils	Lymphocytes	Monocytes	Eosinophils
Preinjection	45	8.2	10,100	151	6,060	2,727	555	555
1 hr postinjection	57	8.7	1,700	0	34	1,530	34	68
2 hr postinjection	56	8.8	1,800	0	72	1,674	0	36
3 hr postinjection	55	8.5	1,600	0	144	1,392	0	64
4 hr postinjection	51	7.8	1,900	19	285	1,520	0	76
5 hr postinjection	49	7.2	2,400	0	576	1,752	0	24
6 hr postinjection	51	8.1	2,800	56	728	1,820	0	168
7 hr postinjection	57	7.7	3,000	240	690	1,950	0	120
8 hr postinjection	58	8.7	4,800	528	2,016	1,920	48	96

[a]From Carroll et al., 1965; courtesy of the Journal of the American Veterinary Medical Association.

Table 31–4. Demonstration of the Leukocyte Responses in the Cat to the Intraperitoneal Injection of 0.4 mg of *Enterobacter aerogenes* Endotoxin in 1.0 ml of Saline

Time	Elapsed Time in Hours from Toxin Exposure (9 a.m.)	Temp. (°F)	PCV (%)	Nucleated RBC[a]/100 WBC	WBC/μl	WBC Corrected	Myelocytes	Meta-myelocytes	Band	Neutrophils	Lymphocytes	Monocytes	Eosinophils	Basophils	U.C.[b]	Degenerated Cells
8:30 a.m.	0	101.4	29	1	22,600	22,370	0	0	112	9,283	10,740	671	1,454	112	0	0
10 a.m.	1	101.6	27	5.5	4,100	3,886	0	0	78	1,185	2,234	0	350	0	0	38
11 a.m.	2	103.0	25	16	1,500	1,290	0	0	52	284	851	0	90	0	0	13
Noon	3	103.6	26	17	1,700	1,450	0	0	58	797	493	29	72	0	0	0
1 p.m.	4	104.4	26	10	5,300	4,770	0	0	858	2,766	954	0	190	0	0	0
2 p.m.	5	104.8	28	9	4,900	4,490	0	0	763	2,918	628	45	135	0	0	0
3 p.m.	6	104.0	28	3	11,500	11,155	0	223	2,007[c]	7,920[c]	836	0	111	0	56	0
4 p.m.	7	103.6	27	1	22,000	21,700	108	108	4,557[c]	16,275[c]	325	0	325	0	0	0
5 p.m.	8	103.8	26	0	26,000	—	0	131	2,882	21,877	917	131	262	0	0	0
9 a.m.	24[c]	102.6	29	1	36,100	35,740	0	0	179	29,664	5,003	357	536	0	0	0

[a]The increase in nucleated erythrocytes is relative rather than absolute, since the number remained essentially at the same level but appeared to increase in relation to the rapid decline in circulating leukocytes, i.e., 1 nucleated RBC/100 WBC at a level of 22,600 leukocytes/μl is essentially the same in real numbers as 16/100 WBC at a leukocyte level of 1,500/μl.

[b]Unclassified cells.

[c]Basophilia of cytoplasm.

Table 31–5. Total and Differential Absolute Leukocyte Numbers/µl of Blood in Experimental Anaphylaxis in a Young Hereford Steer

Elapsed Time	PCV (%)	Nucleated RBC/100 WBC	WBC	Metamyelo-cytes	Neutrophils		Lymphocytes	Monocytes	Eosinophils	Basophils
					Band	Mature				
0	35	0	7,650	0	0	1,645	5,049	421	536	0
5 min	40	0	2,150	0	0	43	2,064	43	0	0
15 min	38	3	3,200	32	160	352	2,400	64	192	0
30 min	36	0.5	4,500	0	158	652	3,082	68	518	0
1 hr	36	0	4,600	0	92	460	3,565	0	437	0
6 hr	32	0	4,500	0	22	968	2,970	158	382	0
24 hr	34	0	6,400	0	0	352	4,800	352	869	0
48 hr	34	0	9,500	0	0	1,282	6,270	902	902	142

Data obtained in cooperation with Dr. D.L. Dungworth.

tation rate, the total leukocyte count, and the percentage of immature neutrophils, but lymphocyte numbers remained below the preinoculation levels.

Bacterial Toxemia and Septicemia

Cats of all ages may develop leukopenia and signs of "toxic" interference with maturation of neutrophil granulocytes (Appendix Case 41). The horse is prone to acute accidents involving the intestinal tract and leading to volvulus, intussusception, and perforations. Characteristic findings in the hemogram (Appendix Case 63) are a markedly elevated PCV from splenic contraction and dehydration, increased icteric index, and a frank leukopenia in which all leukocyte types are depressed (Table 6–17). An additional finding, pointing to an unfavorable outcome, is the existence of a significant left shift in which the immature neutrophils are large and toxic (Plate XI–11). Leukopenia in a variety of clinical conditions in the cow has been discussed by Anderson (1970) (see also Chapter 7).

Anaphylaxis

Leukopenia and thrombocytopenia are characteristic hematologic findings in anaphylaxis. This is exemplified by an animal sensitized to egg albumin and subjected to an intravenous challenge of the antigen. A presensitized 16-month-old Hereford steer was given 20 ml of a 1 in 50 concentration of egg albumin intravenously. An immediate leukopenia and sudden increase in the PCV occurred (Table 31–5). The appearance of nucleated erythrocytes and immature neutrophils in the circulation within 15 minutes indicated an ill-defined effect on the bone marrow architecture whereby immature cells were released into the circulation under conditions of extreme stress. The rapid disappearance of neutrophils from large-vessel blood in anaphylaxis was similar to that produced by endotoxin.

REFERENCES

Andersen, H.A.: Evaluation of Leukopenia in Cattle. J. Amer. Vet. Med. Ass., *156*:858, 1970.

Appel, M.J.G., et al.: Canine Viral Enteritis. I. Status Report on Corona- and Parvo-like Viral Enteritides. Cornell Vet., *69*:123, 1979a.

Appel, M.J.G., et al.: Enteric Viral Infections of Dogs. 29th Gaine Vet. Symp., Gainesville, Florida, Oct. 17, 1979b.

Baker, J.A., et al.: Virus Diarrhea in Cattle. Amer. J. Vet. Res., *15*:525, 1954.

Bryans, J.T., et al.: The Blood Picture and Thermal Reaction in Experimental Viral Arteritis of Horses. Cornell Vet. *47*:42, 1957.

Bryans, J.T.: The Colitis Syndrome. Proc. 9th Annu. Meeting Assn. Amer. Equine Practitioners, 25, Dec., 1963.

Burrows, G.E.: Endotoxaemia in the Horse. Equine Vet. J., *13*(2):89, 1981.

Carroll, E.J., et al.: Experimental Coliform (*Aerobacter aerogenes*) Mastitis: Characteristics of the Endotoxin and Its Role in Pathogenesis. Amer. J. Vet. Res., *25*(106):720, 1964.

Carroll, E.J., et al.: Endotoxemia in a Horse. J. Amer. Vet. Med. Ass., *146*:1300, 1965.

Davis, J.W., and Smibert, R.M.: Studies on Hemolytic Escherichia coli Associated with Edema Disease of Swine. III. The Effect of Hemolytic and Nonhemolytic Escherichia coli Endotoxin on the Blood of Swine. Amer. J. Vet. Res., *24*:324, 1963.

Dougherty, T.F., and White, A.: Influence of Hormones on Lymphoid Tissue Structure and Function: The Role of the Pituitary Adrenotrophic Hormone in the Regulation of Lymphocytes and Other Cellular Elements of the Blood. Endocrinology, *35*:1, 1944.

Dunne, H.W.: Field and Laboratory Diagnosis of Hog Cholera. Vet. Med., *58*:222, 1963.

Easterday, B.C., et al.: Experimental Rift Valley Fever in Lambs and Sheep. Amer. J. Vet. Res., *23*:1224, 1962.

Fruhman, G.J.: Factors Influencing Neutrophil Mobilization. *In* Gordon, A.S., ed. Regulation of Hematopoiesis. Vol. 2. Appleton-Century-Crofts, New York, p. 873, 1970.

Goldman, J.M.: Normal Leucocytes. *In* Hoffbraud, A.V., and Lewis, S.M., eds. Postgraduate Haematology. 2nd ed. William Heinmann Medical Books, p. 381, 1981.

Gossett, K.A., and Carakostas, M.C.: Effect of EDTA on Morphology of Neutrophils of Healthy Dogs and Dogs with Inflammation. Vet. Clin. Pathol., *13*(2):22, 1984.

Gribble, D.H.: Equine Ehrlichiosis. J. Amer. Vet. Med. Ass., *155*:462, 1969.

Haden, R.L.: Qualitative Changes in Neutrophilic Leukocytes. Amer. J. Clin. Pathol., *5*:354, 1935.

Hartman, J.D., and Gordon, W.F.: Leucocyte Agglutinating Systems. Amer. J. Physiol., *195*:487, 1958.

Heuschele, W.P., and Barber, T.L.: Hematologic Studies of Rinderpest-Infected Swine. Can. J. Comp. Med. Vet. Sci., *27*:56, 1963.

Jain, N.C., and Lasmanis, J.: Leucocytic Changes in Cows Given Intravenous Injections of Escherichia coli Endotoxin. Res. Vet. Sci., *24*:386, 1978.

Jain, N.C., et al.: Experimentally Induced Coliform (*Aerobacter aerogenes*) Mastitis in Normal Cows and in Cows Made Neutropenic by an Equine Anti-Bovine Leukocyte Serum. Amer. J. Vet. Res., *32*:1929, 1971.

Jain, N.C., et al.: Neutrophil Kinetics in Endotoxin-Induced Mastitis. Amer. J. Vet. Res., *39*:1662, 1978.

Lewis, P.A., and Shope, R.E.: The Study of the Cells of the Blood as an Aid to the Diagnosis of Hog Cholera. J. Amer. Vet. Med. Ass., *74*:145, 1929.

Luedke, A.J., et al.: Clinical and Pathologic Features of Bluetongue in Sheep. Amer. J. Vet. Res., *25*:963, 1964.

Majde, J.A., and Person, R.J.: Pathophysiological Effects

of Endotoxins at the Cellular Level. Alan R. Liss, New York, 1981.

Maurer, F.D., and Jones, T.C.: The Blood Picture in Equine Influenza. Amer. J. Vet. Res., 4:257, 1943.

Mechanic, R.C., et al.: Quantitative Studies of Human Leukocytic and Febrile Responses to Single and Repeated Doses of Purified Bacterial Endotoxin. J. Clin. Invest., 41:162, 1962.

Miale, J.B.: Laboratory Medicine, Hematology. 6th ed. C.V. Mosby, St. Louis, 1982.

Morrison, D.C., and Ulevitch, R.J.: The Effects of Bacterial Endotoxins on Host Medication Systems: A Review. Amer. J. Pathol., 93:526, 1978.

Paape, M.J., et al.: Plasma Corticosteroid, Circulating Leukocyte and Milk Somatic Cell Responses to Escherichia coli Endotoxin Induced Mastitis. Proc. Soc. Exp. Biol. Med., 145:553, 1974.

Prasse, K.W.: White Blood Cell Disorders. *In* Textbook of Veterinary Internal Medicine: Diseases of the Dog and Cat. Vol. 2, 2nd ed. Ettinger, S.J., ed. W.B. Saunders, Philadelphia, ch. 78, p. 2001, 1983.

Rooney, J.R., et al.: Colitis "X" of Horses. J. Amer. Vet. Med. Ass., 142:510, 1963.

Schalm, O.W.: Leukocyte Responses to Disease in Various Domestic Animals. J. Amer. Vet. Med. Ass., 140:557, 1962.

Schalm, O.W.: Interpretation of Leukocyte Responses in the Dog. J. Amer. Vet. Med. Ass., 142:147, 1963.

Schalm, O.W.: Leukopenia and Resurgence of Granulopoiesis in the Cat. Calif. Vet., 23:16, (Feb.), 1969.

Schalm, O.W., and Lasmanis, J.: Cytologic Features of Bone Marrow in Normal and Mastitic Cows. Amer. J. Vet. Res., 37:359, 1976.

Schwartz, S.O., and Stansbury, F.: Significance of Nucleated Red Blood Cells in Peripheral Blood. J. Amer. Med. Ass., 154:1339, 1954.

Selye, H.: Studies on Adaptation. Endocrinology, 21:169, 1937.

Stannard, A.A., et al.: Equine Ehrlichiosis: A Disease with Similarities to Tick-Borne Fever and Bovine Petechial Fever. Vet. Rec., 84:149, 1969.

Stockham, S.L., et al.: Mastocytemia in Dogs with Acute Inflammatory Diseases. Vet. Clin. Pathol., 15:16, 1986.

Stoez, J., et al.: The Leukocytic Response of Cows and Calves to Acute Infection with an Agent of the Psittacosis-Lymphogranuloma Group. Amer. J. Vet. Res., 23:1200, 1962.

Teichman, I.-R.: Micro-Electrophoretic Investigations of Bovine Serum Proteins in Different Internal Disorders. Acta Vet. Scand., 18:335, 1977.

Weik, J.K., et al.: Leukoerythroblastosis: Diagnosis and Prognostic Significance. Mayo Clin. Proc., 49:110, 1974.

Wintrobe, M.M., et al.: Clinical Hematology. 8th ed. Lea & Febiger, Philadelphia, 1981.

32

The Leukemia Complex

GENERAL COMMENTS 838
  Laboratory Characterization of
    Leukemias 838
  Subclassification of Hematopoietic
    Malignancies 840
  Some Properties of Leukemic Cells 842
  Clonal Origin of Leukemias 842
  Incidence and Etiology of Leukemia 843

THE FELINE LEUKEMIA COMPLEX 844
  The Feline Leukemia Virus 844
  Lymphoproliferative Disorders 847
  Myeloproliferative Disorders 852

**THE LEUKEMIA COMPLEX IN THE
    DOG 869**
  Lymphoproliferative Disorders 869
  Myeloproliferative Disorders 876

THE BOVINE LEUKEMIA COMPLEX 884
  The Bovine Leukemia Virus 884
  Lymphoproliferative Disorders 886

**THE LEUKEMIA COMPLEX IN THE
    HORSE 890**
  Lymphoproliferative Disorders 890
  Myeloproliferative Disorders 894

**THE LEUKEMIA COMPLEX IN OTHER
    SPECIES 894**
  Goat 894
  Sheep 895
  Pig 896

**THERAPY OF LYMPHOPROLIFERATIVE AND
    MYELOPROLIFERATIVE
    DISORDERS 897**

Neoplastic processes involving hematopoietic cells can be grouped broadly as myeloproliferative disorders and lymphoproliferative disorders. The myeloproliferative disorders encompass disorders of hematopoietic stem cells as well as of granulocytic, monocytic, erythrocytic, and megakaryocytic series, whereas the lymphoproliferative disorders are restricted to the lymphoid series including plasma cells (Table 32–1). Such a categorization of hematopoietic neoplasias, although proposed many years ago (Dameshek, 1951), has found support in current concepts of hematopoietic differentiation.

GENERAL COMMENTS

Leukemia is a neoplastic disease involving one or more of the cell types of the hematopoietic tissues. The name implies white blood and was first used in 1845 by Virchow to distinguish *Weisses Blut* from the leukocytosis of infection. Neoplastic proliferation of hematopoietic precursor cells is not always associated with an above normal number of white cells in peripheral blood. In fact, in some instances, leukopenia may exist, as is common in lymphoma. Ellermann and Bang, in 1908, introduced "leukosis" as a more appropriate term to include both leukemic and nonleukemic forms of hematopoietic neoplasia.

Laboratory Characterization of Leukemias

To characterize the level of neoplastic cells in blood some have suggested using a combination of descriptive terms such as leukemic leukemia, subleukemic leukemia, and aleukemic leukemia (Dameshek and Gunz, 1964). In leukemic leukemia, the WBC count is extremely elevated or above normal and the abnormal or primitive cells are present in blood to permit diagnosis. This is the typical anticipated blood picture of a leukemic patient. The WBC count may be normal or decreased in both subleukemic leukemia and aleukemic leukemia, but in the former the primitive cells are present in blood in sufficient numbers to suggest a diagnosis of leukemia, whereas in the latter the primitive cells are either absent or present in such low numbers as to defy diagnosis.

Table 32–1. Classification of Hematopoietic Malignancies

MYELOPROLIFERATIVE DISORDERS
  Granulocytic
    Acute myeloid leukemias
      Acute myeloblastic leukemia
      Acute promyelocytic leukemia
      Acute eosinophilic leukemia
      Acute basophilic leukemia
    Chronic myeloid leukemias
      Chronic myelogenous leukemia
      Chronic eosinophilic leukemia
      Chronic basophilic leukemia
  Monocytic
    Acute monoblastic leukemia
    Acute monocytic leukemia
    Chronic monocytic leukemia
  Erythroid
    Acute erythremic myelosis
    Chronic erythremic myelosis
    Polycythemia rubra vera
  Megakaryocytic
    Acute megakaryocytic leukemia
  Mixed types
    Acute myelomonocytic leukemia
    Chronic myelomonocytic leukemia
    Erythroleukemia
    Acute lymphoblastic and myeloblastic leukemia
  Fibroblastic
    Acute myelofibrosis
    Chronic or idiopathic myelofibrosis
  Others
    Undifferentiated myeloproliferative disorder
    Mast cell leukemia
    Histiocytic medullary reticulosis ("malignant histiocytosis")
LYMPHOPROLIFERATIVE DISORDERS
  Lymphocytic
    Lymphoma
    Acute lymphoblastic leukemia
    Prolymphocytic leukemia
    Chronic lymphocytic leukemia
    "Histiocytic" lymphoma or "reticulum cell sarcoma"
    Hodgkin's or "Hodgkin's-like" disease
    Burkitt's lymphoma
  Plasma cells
    Multiple myeloma
    Waldenström's macroglobulinemia

Although this terminology appears paradoxical and may be confusing, it reflects the problem often encountered in diagnosing leukemia on the basis of blood examination only. Diagnosis of subleukemic and aleukemic leukemias may require making buffy coat smears and several sequential blood examinations as well as cytologic examination of other hematopoietic tissues such as bone marrow, lymph nodes, and spleen. Sometimes hematologic abnormalities of an undefined nature may precede development of a recognizable leukemia; the condition then in retrospect is referred to as "preleukemia."

The diagnosis of leukemia should also include categorization of the cell types involved, e.g., lymphocytic, granulocytic, monocytic, or myelomonocytic (Table 32–1). The leukemias involving the neutrophil and its precursors are traditionally called granulocytic, myelogenous, or myeloid leukemias, although the prefix "granulo-" commonly implies any of the three granular leukocytes (neutrophil, eosinophil, basophil) and the prefix "myelo" refers to the bone marrow or various marrow leukocytes except lymphocytes. Leukemias involving the eosinophils and basophils are specifically designated as eosinophilic leukemia and basophilic leukemia, respectively. The term nonlymphoid leukemia encompasses leukemias involving all cell lines except lymphocytic.

The leukemias may be categorized further as acute or chronic, based on cellular maturity, apparent onset, and clinical course. Acute leukemias are characterized by the presence of predominantly immature (blast) cells and a relatively shorter clinical course. Chronic leukemias characteristically reveal the presence of predominantly mature cells in blood and bone marrow and have a relatively longer clinical course. Except for typical cases, hematologic differentiation of acute and chronic leukemias in veterinary literature has been generally arbitrary. Precise criteria remain to be established. The FAB cooperative group (See Subclassification of Hematopoietic Malignancies, below) proposed that in humans over 30% of bone marrow blasts will suffice for the diagnosis of acute myeloid leukemia in any of its forms (Bennett et al., 1982).

Experience is necessary to recognize abnormal cells in Romanowsky-stained blood and bone marrow films of leukemic patients. A number of cytomorphologic features have been found helpful in distinguishing lymphocytic, granulocytic, and monocytic cell lines (Table 32–2). Although lymphocytic and granulocytic leukemias can be distinguished in most cases, acute leukemias comprised essentially of blast cells with little differentiation toward classic cell types are often difficult to classify. In such cases, certain cytochemical staining procedures can be performed and have been found useful (see Chapter 33). Electron microscopic studies may also reveal cellular differences. Clinical signs and other hematologic manifestations in such cases may be similar or not particularly distinctive.

Subclassification of Hematopoietic Malignancies

An accurate diagnosis of leukemia is essential for proper therapeutic management of the patient. Different modes of therapy are being instituted for different types of leukemias. In order to correlate success of therapeutic trials by a group of investigators or to compare results of different investigators in therapeutic management of similar leukemic patients, a systematic approach to nomenclature, classification, and characterization of acute leu-

kemias in humans was initiated and applied based on cytologic and some cytochemical properties of various leukocytes (Bennett et al., 1976). This led to what has become known as the FAB (French American British) classification of leukemias. It entails classification of acute leukemias into myeloid and lymphoid leukemias. Myeloid leukemias are subclassified into six categories (M1 through M6) and lymphoid leukemias into three categories (L1, L2, and L3) according to the direction and degree of cellular differentiation. The subgroup nomenclature of myeloid malignancies was: M1, myeloblastic leukemia without maturation; M2, myeloblastic leukemia with maturation; M3, hypergranular progranulocytic leukemia; M4, myelomonocytic leukemia; M5a, poorly differentiated monocytic (monoblastic) leukemia; M5b, differentiated monocytic leukemia; M6, erythroleukemia. Subsequently, more precise criteria were described to distinguish various subtypes of myeloid leukemias, and new categories were added (Bennett et al, 1980, 1985; Catovsky, 1982; Mertelsmann et al., 1980). These include an "M3 variant" in which leukemic blood cells have a bilobed, multilobed, or reniform nucleus and no or only a few fine cytoplasmic azurophilic granules; and M7, for acute megakaryoblastic leukemia. Criteria for subclassification of lymphoid leukemias have also been refined and correlated with incidence and prognosis of the disease (Bennett et al. 1981). Catovsky (1982) has briefly reviewed these findings.

Additional criteria that have been used to classify leukemias include isoenzyme determinations, chromosomal analysis, characterization of leukocyte specific membrane antigens by monoclonal antibodies, and patterns of in vitro growth of leukemic marrow cells. It has been shown that myelogenous leukemias may present a spectrum from a pure myelogenous leukemia to a pure monocytic leukemia, with the predominant form being a mixture of the two, namely, myelomonocytic leukemia. Pure acute monoblastic leukemia is rare in humans and animals in comparison to pure myelogenous leukemia. Cytochemical staining offers considerable help in distinguishing various subtypes of

Table 32–2. Cytologic and Cytochemical Features of Blood and Bone Marrow Cells in Leukemia

Characteristic	Lymphocytic	Granulocytic	Monocytic
Cell size	Usually small	Usually large	Usually large
Nuclear shape	Round to oval, smooth contour, rare clefting or slight indentation	Round to oval, smooth contour	Irregular, smooth or clefted contour; nuclear folds may be present
Nuclear chromatin	Fine to coarsely granular (gravel-like) or clumped	Finely stippled (sand-like)	Finely stippled or reticular (linearly fibrillar)
Nucleoli	One or more, distinct or inconspicuous	One or more, distinct or inconspicuous	One or more, distinct or inconspicuous
Amount of cytoplasm	Scant to moderately abundant	Moderately abundant	Moderately abundant
Nuclear : cytoplasmic ratio	High	Low to high	Low to high
Cytoplasmic basophilia	Slight to marked	Moderate	Moderate
Cytoplasm	Smooth, featureless, rarely vacuolated	Ground glass–like, no vacuoles unless toxic	Grayish blue, foamy or vacuolated
Azurophilic granules	Generally absent; rarely few and large	Many, small but distinct	Usually absent, sometimes fine and indistinct
Specific granules	−	+	−
Cytochemical markers:			
Peroxidase	−	+, usually strong	+, usually weak
Alkaline phosphatase	−	+, some cells	−
Lipase	−	−	+
Nonspecific esterase	−	−	+
Cell rafts	−	+	+
Proliferative cell line	Recognizable lymphocytic	Maturation toward neutrophilic series	Maturation toward monocytic cells

Note: Cell morphology varies with the patient and with time in the same patients. All cytologic criteria do not manifest in every case; mixed leukemias are sometimes encountered.

−, absent; +, present.

myelogenous leukemias (Table 32–2; see also Chapter 33).

The lymphoproliferative malignancies are classified in various ways employing a multitude of criteria (Kass, 1982; Lukes, 1979; Rappaport, 1966; Squire et al., 1973; Theilen and Madewell, 1979; Wintrobe et al., 1981). A simplistic traditional approach has been to label the tumor forming disease as malignant lymphoma, lymphoma, or lymphosarcoma. Lymphosarcoma has been preferred in describing lymphoid tumors of animals, while lymphoma has been commonly used in human medicine. The current trend in veterinary medicine, however, is also to use the term lymphoma. The disease in blood and/or bone marrow is labeled acute lymphoblastic (lymphocytic) leukemia or chronic lymphocytic leukemia. The diagnosis of leukemia can be made only when the total body burden exceeds 10^9 leukemic cells (Harmon, 1985). Thus, a patient with lymphoma may exhibit an overt leukemia or have only a few or no detectable leukemic cells in blood or bone marrow. Similarly, a patient with acute or chronic lymphocytic leukemia may or may not show tumor masses in other tissues and organs. The spectrum of distribution of leukemic cells in blood, bone marrow, lymph nodes, and other tissues and organs may be a reflection of abnormal biologic behavior of leukemic lymphocytes and the progressive nature of the disease. Strict compartmentalization of the disease as to its hemic or nonhemic location is a fallacy.

Anatomic categorization of lymphoma is based on major locations of tumor masses or neoplastic cells in various organs or tissues, e.g., thymic, alimentary, multicentric, cutaneous, or leukemic form. Histologic classification of lymphoma entails microscopic distribution of neoplastic cells, e.g., diffuse and nodular or their variants, and histocytologic categorization is based on the cell types involved, e.g., poorly differentiated, well differentiated, and "histiocytic" lymphoma. A National Cancer Institute–sponsored study of non-Hodgkin's lymphomas in humans has proposed a unified formulation of classification based on histologic criteria (Anonymous, 1982). A histocytologic appraisal has been done for lymphoid tumors of the dog, cat, and cow (Valli et al., 1981).

The current trend is to characterize various lymphoid malignancies also with regard to their immunologic cell surface markers, e.g., B, T, pre-B, pre-T, common (both B and T), and non-B non-T cell types or their subtypes. For various markers used in classification of subpopulations of lymphocytes see Chapter 30.

The usefulness of these various types of classification in prognosis and treatment of patients with lymphoid malignancies is a subject of deep interest and current investigation.

Some Properties of Leukemic Cells

Leukemic leukocytes exhibit morphologic as well as kinetic, biochemical, and functional abnormalities (Wintrobe et al, 1981). Leukemic blast cells may reveal nuclear and cytoplasmic features unlike those seen in normal blast cells. Abnormalities of DNA, RNA, and protein syntheses and defective enzyme activities have been found. Kinetic studies have shown that increased numbers of leukocytes in blood may be due to increased production and release of cells into the circulation, increased intravascular life span, or both. Abnormalities of cell distribution within the vascular system as well as rates of egress and ingress may also be involved. Extramedullary hematopoiesis, often apparent in myelogenous leukemia, may also be a contributory factor.

In lymphocytic leukemia, a somewhat different situation may be involved. Although there is increased production of lymphocytes in neoplastic lymph nodes, the rates of output and recirculation of lymphocytes may be decreased. The presence of leukemic lymphocytes in peripheral blood may be related to changes in their surface properties. A change in surface property increasing cellular cohesiveness may allow neoplastic lymphocytes to remain localized in the lymphoid tissue, cre-

ating an aleukemic leukemia, whereas surface changes decreasing adherence would allow such cells to increase in number in the circulation.

Functional abnormalities of neutrophils may manifest as reduced chemotaxis, phagocytosis, and bactericidal activity and those of lymphocytes as reduced cellular and humoral immunity so that leukemic patients having a tremendous leukocytosis are paradoxically prone to recurrent bacterial infections. Platelet abnormalities may also be present which manifest as defects of hemostasis.

Clonal Origin of Leukemias

Current concepts of hematopoietic differentiation are summarized in Fig. 13-19. In human studies, it has been shown that most hematopoietic neoplasms have a clonal origin (Wintrobe et al., 1981). For example, chromosomal analyses and determination of glucose-6 phosphate dehydrogenase (G6PD) isozymes of human patients with myelogenous leukemias have shown that chronic myelogenous leukemia originates at the level of the pluripotential stem cell so that such abnormalities are expressed not only in mature neutrophils, but also in erythroid and megakaryocytic series. In comparison, acute myelogenous leukemia originates primarily at the committed myeloid stem cell level and lymphocytic leukemias from committed lymphoid stem cells.

Although most hematopoietic neoplasms, being clonal in origin, are characterized by predominance of a single cell line, sometimes the disease may appear to involve two cell lines and rarely more. It is also accepted that hematopoietic malignancies are progressive. Thus the disease involving a single cell line may progress or change to involve other cell lines; e.g., myelogenous leukemia may transform into myelomonocytic leukemia and erythremic myelosis into erythroleukemia and in turn into myelogenous leukemia. In some cases transformations may occur within the same cell line so that different patterns of cellular differentiation become apparent, e.g., "blast crisis" of chronic myelogenous leukemia. Such changes may occur rapidly within weeks or slowly over a period of months or years. Progressions or conversions are more common in the myeloproliferative disorders than in the lymphoproliferative disorders.

A neoplastic change of a pluripotential stem cell preceding the level of bifurcation into myeloid and lymphoid stages could manifest in both of these cell lines; such an occurrence, although extremely rare, has been reported (Barr and Watt, 1978). In this context, it should be realized that between the well-defined maturative stages of various stem cells there may exist several subpopulations of cells whose neoplastic proliferation may manifest differently as mixed, atypical, or unclassifiable leukemias.

Incidence and Etiology of Leukemia

The incidence of leukemia varies with the type of leukemia, the species involved, and geographic location. The influence of age, sex, and breed on susceptibility to some leukemias has been described. In human leukemias, the incidence is higher in males, and granulocytic leukemias are more common during procreative periods of life. Although leukemia in animals can occur at any age, granulocytic leukemias are common in young animals and some age differences have been recognized in dogs, cats, and cattle with acute and chronic lymphocytic leukemia and different anatomic forms of lymphoma. A recent report (Schneider, 1983) gave adjusted annual incidence rates for all leukemias per 100,000 cats or dogs as 224.3 and 30.5, respectively. The cat had 6.1 times more lymphoma and 15.7 times more myeloproliferative disorder than the dog. In the cat, a bimodal age pattern was seen for all leukemias and for lymphoma alone, and a single early peak was seen for myeloproliferative disorder. In the dog, all age-specific patterns increased with age and peaked later in life. The neutered female cat and neutered male dog were at lowest risk. Neutering decreased the risk of leukemia in the female cat by approximately one-half, but not in the female dog. The age and sex preferences resembled those in humans. For additional comments, see the descriptions of leukemias in different species.

The etiology of leukemia is being extensively investigated. Although the molecular mechanisms associated with neoplastic transformation of the cell are unknown, cellular abnormalities leading to leukemia may develop as a result of certain viral infections, exposures to certain chemicals and physical agents, or from undefined causes. Ellermann and Bang, in 1908, reported the transmission of avian leukemia to two of five chickens receiving injections of material passed through a filter candle. The filtrate was clear and cell-free. This was the first indication that leukemia might possibly have a viral etiology. Rous, in 1911, reported successful transmission by cell-free filtrate of a spindle-cell sarcoma of chickens. The Rous sarcoma played a significant role in establishing the claim for viral etiology of oncogenesis.

Success in the search for viruses as etiologic agents of mammalian leukemia was reported by Gross, in 1951 (Gross, 1951a). Filtered AK mouse leukemic tissue extracts inoculated into infant mice resulted in development of leukemia at 6½ to 9 months of age in 7 of 25 exposed mice. Genetic or vertical transmission (Gross, 1951b) was demonstrated by the occurrence, at 14 to 20 months of age, of leukemia in 50% of offspring of matings of the originally inoculated mice. The Gross leukemogenic virus required particular strains of mice for successful transmission, thereby indicating a genetic influence on individual susceptibility to development of leukemia. In recent years leukemias and lymphomas of seemingly viral origin have been reported in a wide variety of species such as chickens, rodents, cats, cattle, sheep, and nonhuman primates (Hardy, 1978). In addition, some evidence has been forthcoming regarding possible association of RNA viruses with T-cell lymphomas and leukemias in humans (Gallo and Meyskens, 1978; Gallo and Wong-Staal, 1982; Weiss, 1981, 1982).

The avian and murine leukemogenic viruses are capable of causing different forms of leukemia and tumors, depending to some extent on dose, route of infection, and genetic makeup of the host (Burnester et al., 1959, Gross, 1964). Avian leukemia viruses (Graf and Stehelin, 1982) and viral lymphomagenesis in the domestic fowl (Payne, 1977) have been reviewed. Both avian and murine viruses may cause erythroblastosis, myeloblastosis, and lymphocytic leukemia or lymphoma. Leukemogenic viruses were present in some mice throughout life without producing leukemia. However, a high incidence of leukemia was induced in these virus-infected mice by exposure to x-radiation (Lieberman and Kaplan, 1959).

Viruses are classified by ultrastructure as A, B, and C types (Bernhard, 1960) and by their nucleic acid content as RNA or DNA viruses. The avian, murine, and feline leukemia viruses are C-type RNA viruses and further classified as oncornaviruses. Although most RNA viruses are retroviruses (i.e., they contain RNA-dependent DNA polymerase—reverse transcriptase), only a few are oncogenic. Reverse transcriptase activity and particles of retroviral density were demonstrated in short-term cultures of lymphoid tissue from a case of ovine lymphoblastic leukemia (Tomley et al, 1983b) and canine lymphoma (Tomley et al, 1983a). A few DNA viruses have been associated with tumor formation, e.g., Epstein-Barr virus with Burkitt's lymphoma and nasopharyngeal carcinoma in humans, Marek's disease virus with Marek's lymphoma of T cells in chickens, and *Herpes sylvilagus* with lymphoma in cottontail rabbits (Essex, 1982; Wintrobe et al., 1981).

Mechanisms involved in viral leukemogenesis are being investigated. A major role of the immune response in murine leukemogenesis has been demonstrated, but other possibilities also exist (Ihle et al., 1982). The molecular basis of lymphoid neoplasias has been reviewed (Croce et al., 1985; Gallo and Wong-Staal, 1982).

THE FELINE LEUKEMIA COMPLEX

It has been estimated that hematopoietic neoplasms represent about one-third of all cat tumors and the majority are lymphoid tumors (Dorn et al., 1968; Nielsen, 1983). The demonstration of virus particles in transmissible lymphoma in neonatal kittens by Jarrett, in 1964, (Jarrett et al., 1964a,b) was followed by extensive investigations on the nature of the virus, incidence of natural infection, immune responses, and associated clinical diseases. The virus became known as the feline leukemia virus (FeLV) even though the incidence of leukemia is low in the presence of a high

natural infection rate (Jarrett, 1973). A brief description of FeLV infection and related malignant hematopoietic diseases in cats is given here. Further details can be found in recent reviews (Essex, 1982; Hardy, 1981a, b, c; Jarrett, 1983; Neil and Onions, 1985).

The Feline Leukemia Virus

FeLV is a C-type oncornavirus (retrovirus) similar to the avian and murine leukemia viruses. In fact, immunological relationships between FeLV and endogenous rodent C-type viruses led some researchers to propose that the FeLV-related genes were transmitted from a rodent to a cat ancestor millions of years ago and afterwards perpetuated in the germ line of cats (Beneveniste et al., 1975). Virus particles budding from cell membranes can be demonstrated by electron microscopy (Fig. 32–1) in bone marrow and in a variety of other tissues and organs of the body (Anderson et al., 1971; Herz et al., 1970; Hoover and Kociba, 1974). The FeLV has several structural proteins (Hardy, 1981c), all of which are immunogenic (Essex, 1982). Some of the viral proteins and specific antibodies to them have been found extremely useful in seroepidemiologic studies of FeLV infection.

Diagnosis of FeLV Infection

The FeLV infection in cats can be demonstrated by virus isolation in tissue cultures and by serologic procedures such as immunofluorescence and enzyme-linked immunosorbent assay (ELISA).

Oncornaviruses have in common a group-specific antigen, p30 (p27 in case of FeLV), which is of great practical value because it is detectable by immunofluorescence (Hardy, 1981c; Jarrett, 1973). Antibody to this antigen has no protective significance (Cotter, 1979a). Development of an indirect immunofluorescent antibody (IFA) test by Hardy and co-workers for application to dry films of peripheral blood or bone marrow has proven to be a sensitive and practical method for the detection of FeLV-infected cats (Hardy et al., 1973a, b). A positive test means the cat is viremic; it does not indicate the presence of leukemia or lymphoma. In blood, the group-specific antigen occurs in leukocytes and platelets. In bone marrow it is also found in

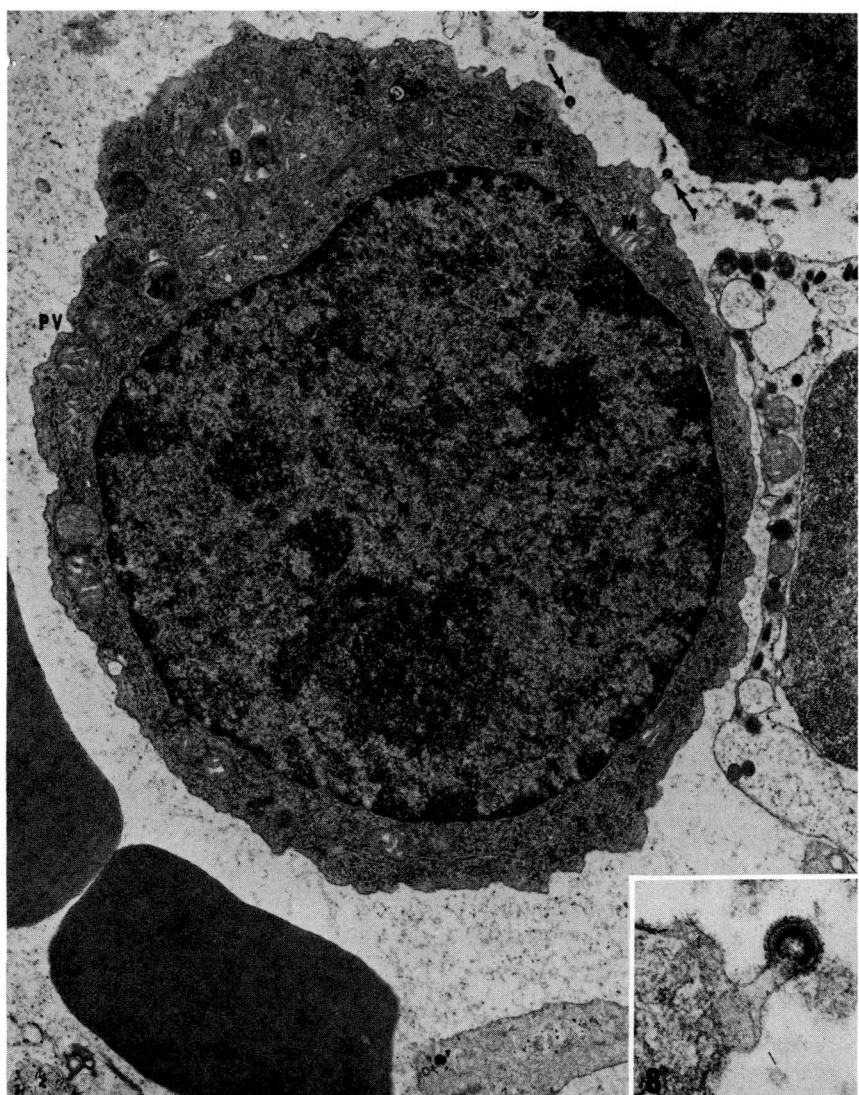

Fig. 32–1. Electron micrograph of a prominent atypical cell from the bone marrow of a cat with a myeloproliferative disorder. Arrows indicate two virus particles budding from the cell membrane ($\times$ 11,040). Inset is a higher magnification ($\times$ 64,560) of one of the virus particles. Ultrastructure of the cell reveals pinocytotic vesicles *(PV)* along the cell membrane. The nucleus *(N)* is round and eccentrically located and presents a large nucleolus *(Nu)*. A small amount of chromatin *(C)* is visible along the nuclear membrane. Numerous round mitochondria *(M)* and a well-developed Golgi apparatus *(G)* are evident. Free ribosomes and polysomes *(R)* are present in large numbers in the cytoplasm. The endoplasmic reticulum *(ER)* is limited to moderate numbers of long cisternae having numerous ribosomes along their surfaces. The cytoplasmic matrix is characteristically quite electron-dense, resembling that of a polychromatophilic rubricyte. (From Herz, et al., 1969a; courtesy of *California Veterinarian*.)

hematopoietic precursor cells of granulocytic, erythrocytic, and megakaryocytic series.

An ELISA (Leukassay-F; Pitman-Moore) test has been developed to detect soluble viral antigens in serum and plasma. It is a simple, sensitive test available for in-hospital use, but it usually gives more positive test results than those with the virus isolation or IFA proce-

dures. In a comparison (Hardy, 1981c) of studies of six groups of investigators the overall agreement of IFA and virus isolation with the ELISA test was 73.6% (range 38–93%); when ELISA-negative test results were compared with negative IFA or virus isolation tests, the overall agreement was 89.6% (range 87–100%); and when ELISA-positive test results were compared with positive IFA or virus isolation tests, the overall agreement was 58.6% (range 38–75%). Reasons for higher positivity of the ELISA test have been discussed (Lutz et al., 1980b; Jarrett et al., 1982b), but the issue still remains unsettled. In another comparative study, the majority of cats tested positive by the ELISA method alone were found to have hematologic or pathologic evidence of FeLV-related disease (Hirsch et al;, 1982).

Subgroups of FeLV

There are three FeLV subgroups designated A, B, and C (Sarma and Log, 1973) based on the presence of a type-specific envelope glycoprotein antigen, gp70. The antibody to gp70 is virus neutralizing, and a significant titer renders the cat immune to FeLV infection (Cotter, 1979a; Hardy, 1981c). Viruses of subgroup A usually infect only feline cells, whereas subgroup B and C viruses can grow in cells of several species (Hardy, 1981c; Sarma et al., 1975). Subgroups A and B were commonly present in cats with lymphoma as well as in FeLV-positive but clinically normal cats (Jarrett et al., 1978). Cats have age-related variations in their susceptibility to various subgroups of FeLV (Neil and Onions, 1985).

In experimentally inoculated kittens, a macrocytic anemia, associated with active erythropoiesis in the bone marrow and extramedullary hematopoiesis in the spleen, occurred in cats infected with subgroup A or A and B, although B alone was not accompanied by anemia, while cats infected with subgroup C developed a fatal aplastic or nonregenerative normocytic-normochromic anemia (Mackey et al., 1975). Persistent nonregenerative anemia is a relatively common development both in the absence of and in association with neoplasia induced by FeLV (Cotter, 1979b; Hoover et al., 1974). Anemia is rarely seen in FeLV-negative, lymphomatous cats (Hardy, 1981a).

Diseases Caused by or Associated with FeLV Infection

A host of neoplastic and non-neoplastic diseases are caused by or associated with FeLV infection in cats, the latter group of diseases occurring much more frequently than the former (Hardy, 1981a, b). These diseases include lymphoid and myeloid malignancies, regenerative and nonregenerative or aplastic anemia, thrombocytopenia, pancytopenia, panleukopenia-like syndrome, thymic atrophy, glomerulonephritis, abortion and fetal resorption, and neurologic syndrome.

A characteristic of FeLV infection is the development of immunosuppression, which places the cat in jeopardy of developing intercurrent infections and other associated diseases (Anderson et al., 1971; Cotter et al., 1975). A 15,000-molecular-weight polypeptide, p15, was found to be the mediator of immunosuppression through impairment of normal lymphocyte function in vitro and to abrogate immunity to FeLV in vivo (Mathes et al., 1979). A variety of viral, bacterial, and parasitic diseases have been found in association with FeLV-induced immunosuppression.

FOCMA Antigen and Antibody

An antigen distinct from the virus structure is produced on the membrane of altered host cells through action of the virus. This antigen is called FOCMA for feline oncornavirus cell membrane antigen. Host cells are induced to produce FOCMA by both FeLV and the feline sarcoma virus, FeSV (Essex et al., 1976). This tumor-specific antigen was found to be present on the membranes of naturally occurring feline lymphoma, myelogenous leukemia, and multicentric fibrosarcoma cells (Hardy et al, 1977a). High FOCMA antibody titers commonly protect against tumor development and leukemia, and about 25–38% of cats exposed to FeLV develop such titers of FOCMA antibodies (Hardy, 1981c). Cats infected with FeLV and exhibiting leukemia or lymphoma, as well as cats with FeLV-associated diseases, commonly have low or undetectable FOCMA titers, whereas those exposed to FeLV but remaining healthy develop high FOCMA titers. A strong correlation was found between antibody levels against FeLV and FOCMA antigen in serums of cats recovered from FeLV infection (Lutz et al., 1980a). FOCMA antibody has been found to lyse lymphoma cells in vitro and in vivo (Hardy, 1981a).

Incidence and Spread of FeLV Infection

Healthy cats in the natural environment generally do not show persistent FeLV infection. Little evidence of viremia (0–<1%) is found in stray cats, cats in single-cat households, and cats in multiple-cat households with no history of FeLV-related diseases, whereas cats in multiple-cat households with history of lymphoma or exposure to FeLV show a higher level (about 30%) of persistent FeLV infection (Hardy, 1981c). Thus natural infection with FeLV occurs commonly among cats in close contact, as in multiple-cat households or catteries (Hardy et al, 1973b; Pedersen et al., 1977).

In viremic cats large quantities of the virus are present in saliva, but rarely in urine, feces, and milk or in fleas recovered from such cats (Francis et al., 1977; Hinshaw and Blank, 1977). Healthy viremic cats excrete about 5–10 times more virus than leukemic cats and are 10–20 times more common than are sick cats (Essex, 1982). Horizontal spread of the virus between cats, by contact with the infected cats or their secretions and excretions, is the major means of propagation of the disease (Essex et al., 1977; Pedersen et al., 1977). Infection spreads through skin, oral, or respiratory routes, although the FeLV survives in the environment of the cat only for a few hours.

Pathogenetic studies (Jarrett et al., 1982a; Rojko et al., 1979) indicated that after initial exposure of the host to the virus, cats either become persistently infected and immunosuppressed or develop a self-limiting infection and immunity. Subsequently, leukemogenesis or induction of fatal non-neoplastic FeLV-related disease occurs in persistently infected cats.

Seroepidemiologic studies (Hardy, 1981c) suggested that about 30% of FeLV-exposed cats do not mount an adequate immune response to FeLV and become persistently infected; about 40% of FeLV-exposed cats produce high titers of antibody to FeLV envelope antigens (virus-neutralizing antibodies) and become immune to infection (some of these cats also develop FOCMA antibodies); and about 30% of cats become neither infected nor immune to FeLV and thus remain susceptible to infection. Nonviremic cats may develop a latent infection; virus can be demonstrated on bone marrow cultures of some of these cats (Madewell and Jarrett, 1983). The induction period for development of lymphoma or leukemia in naturally infected cats is prolonged; in a study of 18 cats the mean was 17.6 months and the range was 3–41 months (Francis et al., 1979).

Spread of FeLV among cats can be prevented by detection of viremic cats by the IFA test followed by removal of such cats from the environment (Hardy et al., 1976, 1977b). Occurrence of lymphoma, various types of leukemias, and myeloproliferative disorders, as well as the host of FeLV-associated diseases (Cotter, 1979a; Essex et al., 1975a.; Jarrett, 1975; Hardy, 1980) can be prevented by eliminating FeLV from the environment of pet domestic cats. In addition to test and removal of viremic cats, a vaccination program may become possible (Hardy et al., 1976; Jarrett et al., 1975; Olsen et al., 1980; Pedersen et al., 1979). Protocols of chemotherapy to prolong survival of cats with lymphoma have been developed (Cotter, 1983b), but treatment is not recommended in most cases because of the nature of FeLV infection (Hardy, 1981a).

Lymphoproliferative Disorders

The combined incidence of lymphoma and lymphocytic leukemia in cats is approximately 200/100,000 per year (Essex and Francis, 1976) and accounts for 80–90% of all feline hematopoietic neoplasms (Nielson, 1983). Lymphoma is the most frequently occurring form within the feline leukemia complex. About 70% of the cases of lymphoma are found in FeLV-positive cats, and about 30% of the cases occur in cats that are recognized as nonviremic or FeLV-negative (Essex, 1982). However, serologic studies indicate that FeLV is also the cause of lymphoma in cats in which the presence of virus cannot be demonstrated (Hardy, 1981a). Most of the FeLV-negative lymphomatous cats are over 7 years of age, and most such cases involve alimentary or unclassified forms of the tumor (Essex et al., 1975b; Hardy et al., 1981a; Niman et al., 1977; Theilen and Madewell, 1979).

Two morphologically similar C-type viruses have been described in association with feline lymphoma; the first, FeLV, is the etiologic agent of lymphoma (Jarrett et al., 1964b; Theilen and Madewell, 1979), and the second, feline C-type virus (RD-114) is an endogenous virus of the cat not known to cause disease (Livingston and Todaro, 1973; Mandel et al., 1979; Niman et al., 1977, 1979).

Anatomic Forms of Lymphoma

Clinical manifestations of lymphoma are so varied that several somewhat distinct anatomic patterns are now recognized. These are designated thymic or mediastinal, alimentary or abdominal, multicentric, and unclassified forms. The first two are for the most part limited to neoplastic involvement of the viscera and their associated lymph nodes. The multicentric form generally includes enlargement of some or all peripheral lymph nodes as well as variable involvement of internal organs. In the rare unclassified form, lymphoma may be located in the skin, eye, central nervous system, or any other nonlymphoid tissue. The thymic and alimentary forms taken together occur most frequently so that generalized superficial lymph node enlargement is not the most common finding in lymphoma of the cat, as is the case in the dog. Variations have been noted in geographical distribution of various forms of lymphoma and FeLV-associated hematologic diseases (Essex et al., 1975b).

The *thymic form* of lymphoma is characterized by a rapidly developing, space-occupying mass in the anterior ventral portion of the thorax. The mass may extend into the thoracic inlet, where it becomes palpable. Displacement of the trachea, esophagus, and regional lung lobes produces coughing, gagging, vomiting, and eventually dyspnea of varying degrees. Open-mouth breathing is sometimes seen. Respiratory distress is intensified as hydrothorax develops. A radiograph of the chest with the cat in standing position will reveal a fluid line, and after withdrawal of the fluid, the mass can be visualized radiographically. Radiologic features of 30 cases of thymic lymphoma have been described (Gruffydd-Jones et al., 1979).

Clinical signs similar to those of thymic lymphoma may be produced by pyothorax, chylothorax, diaphragmatic hernia, and chronic heart failure. Stained films of centri-fuged sediment of pleural effusions are generally diagnostic. Neutrophils and bacteria are present in large numbers in pyothorax. Chylothorax is characterized by a fluid that remains milky after centrifugation, and although lymphocytes are present in fair numbers, they are of the small mature type (Schalm, 1980a).

The chest fluid of nine cats with the thymic form of lymphoproliferative disease had white cells numbering from 5,000–295,000/µl, with a median of 40,000 and mean of 71,000 cells. Lymphoblasts or prolymphocytes were usually present, and 74–98% of cells were of lymphoid origin; mitotic figures were often present (Fig. 32–2).

The *alimentary or abdominal form* of lymphoma involves primarily the terminal ileum, mesenteric lymph nodes, liver, kidneys, and spleen. It is the most frequent form of lymphoma encountered in nonviremic (FeLV-negative) cats (Hardy, 1981a). The onset of clinical signs may be sudden and referable to the main lesion. Annular thickening of the ileum may lead to occlusion and vomiting, or there may be diarrhea from dilation and ulceration of the mucosal surface. Depression, anorexia, and rapid weight loss are frequent accompanying signs. Palpation reveals a firm mass in the mid-abdomen or, when the kidneys are grossly involved, bilateral firm masses in the region of the kidneys.

The *multicentric form* includes peripheral lymphadenopathy as well as internal lymph node and organ involvement. The spleen may be enlarged several times, and the liver may present a distinctly lobular pattern or numerous small foci of tumor cell infiltrations. The mesenteric nodes, kidneys, and mediastinal nodes may be involved. Clinical signs are referable to the extent and degree of tissue and organ involvement.

General clinical signs applicable to all forms of lymphoma are: depression, rapid wasting, fluctuating temperature elevations (with some cats remaining afebrile and others experiencing continuous pyrexia), vomiting and/or diarrhea, and progressive refractory anemia.

Age and sex data reveal equal susceptibility of the sexes, with distribution throughout the entire life span of the cat. Cats as young as 6

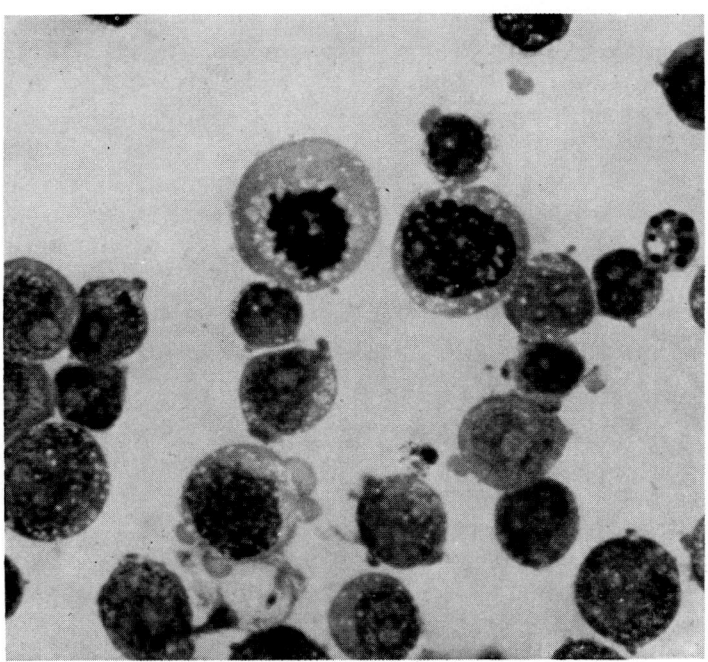

Fig. 32–2.   Cells in a sediment film of fluid from the chest cavity in feline lymphoma. This film was stained by Wright-Leishman method; however, new methylene blue stain (Chapter 2) is also suitable.

months of age have had lymphoma, most commonly the thymic form. Of 47 lymphomatous cats of known age, 46% were less than 3 years old, while 38% were 5 years of age and over. The oldest cat in the series was 13 years of age. In other studies it has been found that the thymic form is common in younger cats (mean age 2.5 years), the multicentric form in relatively older cats (mean age 4 years), and the alimentary form at a much higher age (mean age 8 years) (Hardy, 1981a). The average age of FeLV-infected cats with lymphoma was 3 years, while that of FeLV-negative cats with lymphoma was 7 years. No breed susceptibility has been reported.

Hematology of Lymphoid Malignancies

Hematologic changes in lymphoid malignancies are commonly not characteristic of a leukemia. Data on 49 cats with histologically proven lymphoid neoplasia are summarized in Table 32–3. Nineteen cats with the thymic type, 22 cats with the alimentary or multicentric type, and 8 cats with "histiocytic" lymphoma (reticulum cell sarcoma) are summarized separately.

PCV values obtained on all cats ranged from 4–46% with a mean of 27.4±9.3%. PCV of 33 (67.3%) of the cats fell within the broad normal range of 24–45%. Thus while anemia was present in about one-third of the cats, it was not a major feature in this group of cats. In another report, a mild to severe anemia was seen in 34 of 50 cats (68%) with FeLV-positive lymphoma in contrast to 2 out of 23 cats (9%) with FeLV-negative lymphoma (Hardy, 1981a). Anemia was common in the thymic or multicentric form but not in the alimentary form (Essex, 1982; Hardy, 1981a). The anemic cats usually display a persistent, nonregenerative, normocytic-normochromic anemia (Cotter, 1979b; Hathway, 1976).

Total plasma protein concentration of 25 cats ranged from 4.8 to 10.0 g/dl. A mean value of 7.4±1.1 g/dl suggests the possibility of elevation in some cats due to hemoconcentration. Only two cats were hypoproteinemic (4.8 and 5.3 g), and both were in the group diagnosed as having histiocytic lymphoma. In general, plasma fibrinogen values were within the normal range.

Total leukocyte counts varied from leukopenia (<5,500/μl) in seven cats to leukocytosis

Table 32–3. Hematology of Lymphoreticular Neoplasia in the Cat

	Form of Disease		
	Thymic	*Alimentary and Multicentric*	*Reticulum Cell Sarcoma*
No. of Cats	19	22	8
PCV (%)			
Range	9–46	4–39	20–37
Mean ± 1 SD	32.7 ± 8.3	23.5 ± 8.9	25.6 ± 6.8
No. cats tested	19	22	8
Plasma protein (g/dl)			
Range	6.9–8.8	6.1–8.2	4.8–10.0
Mean ± 1 SD	7.7 ± 0.7	7.3 ± 0.7	7.3 ± 1.8
No. cats tested	6	11	8
Fibrinogen (g/dl)			
Range	0.10–0.40	0.10–0.50	0.10–0.40
Mean ± 1 SD	0.26 ± 0.11	0.30 ± 0.15	0.24 ± 1.00
No. cats tested	5	11	7
Total WBC/μl			
Range	3,200–33,600	1,600–30,800	800–25,500
Mean ± 1 SD	15,605 ± 9,791	11,614 ± 8,149	11,468 ± 8,927
No. cats tested	18[a]	17[b]	8
Absolute lymphocyte count			
Range	56–6,200	500–9,009	240–2,719
Mean ± 1 SD	1,692 ± 1,441	2,935 ± 2,724	1,000 ± 757
No. cats tested	18[a]	17[b]	8

[a]One cat showed leukemia: WBC, 118,000; absolute lymphocytic count, 116,200.

[b]Five leukemic cats showed a WBC range of 65,000–693,000, with a mean of 210,000; six leukemic cats showed absolute lymphocyte counts ranging between 19,559 and 693,000; the mean was 56,221 ± 43,576.

(>19,500/μl) due to neutrophilia in 11 cats. A significant finding was that 25 cats (51%) had frank lymphopenia (<1,500 lymphocytes) at the time of admission (Appendix Case 48). Only 6 of 49 cats (12%) presented leukemic blood pictures with total counts ranging from 65,000 to 693,000/μl and absolute lymphocyte counts ranging from 19,559 to 693,000/μl. The cat with the highest count was 6 months old. One cat in the alimentary-multicentric group had a total leukocyte count of 22,000 of which 19,559 were lymphocytes, including lymphoblasts.

It is important to realize that although there was neoplastic involvement of lymphocytic tissues with tumor formation, the peripheral blood was lymphocytopenic in half of the cats. Similar observations have been made by others, although the proportions of cats with leukemic or leukopenic profiles have varied (Hardy, 1981a). Immunosuppression characteristic of FeLV infection may lead to lymphocytopenia resulting from thymic atrophy and depletion of other lymphoid tissues (Anderson et al., 1971; Mathes et al., 1979).

Lymphoblasts and prolymphocytes are larger than normal mature lymphocytes. Al-

though finely stippled chromatin pattern is the hallmark of immaturity (Fig. 32–3), the chromatin may sometimes be coarsely granular (compare Plates XXI–1 and XXI-3). When a nucleolar ring or rings are present (not to be confused with a condensed circular chromatin mass), the cell is identified as a lym-

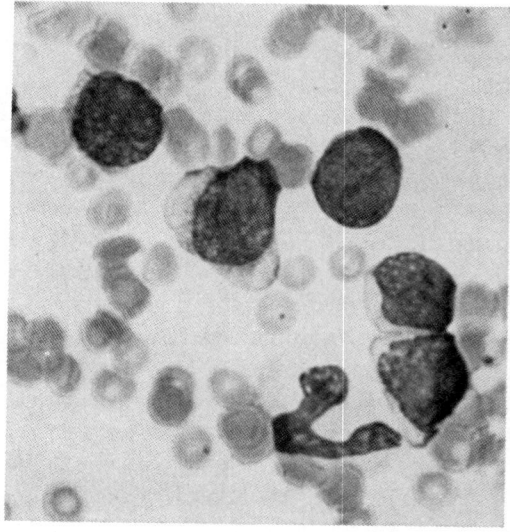

Fig. 32–3. Lymphoblasts and prolymphocytes in the bone marrow of a cat with lymphoma. ×2,700.

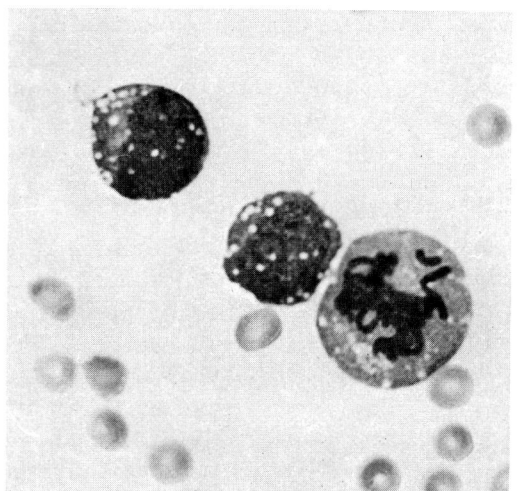

Fig. 32–4. Reticulum cells in pleural effusion in reticulum cell sarcoma of the cat. ×2,700.

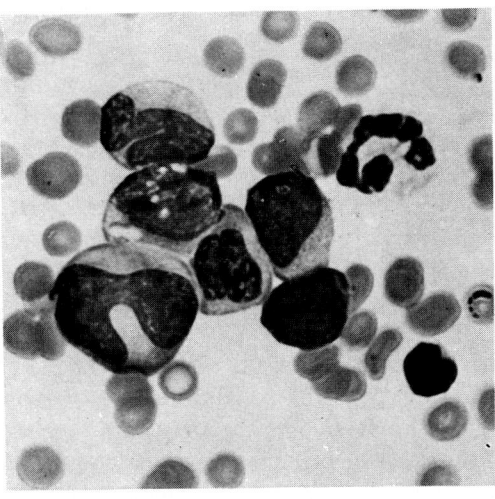

Fig. 32–6. Bone marrow from a cat with lymphoma. Center cluster of cells consists of two prolymphocytes and four granulocytes. Of particular interest is the giant metamyelocyte. ×2,700.

phoblast (Fig. 32-34). The cytoplasm of lymphoblasts and prolymphocytes is sparse and stains a deeper blue than that of the mature lymphocyte. Vacuoles may be present in the cytoplasm and sometimes in the nucleus. In histiocytic lymphoma, the neoplastic cells tend to be larger than typical lymphoblasts and prolymphocytes, the cytoplasm tends to stain a darker blue, and many round, discrete vacuoles commonly appear in both the cytoplasm and nucleus (Figs. 32-4, 32-7 and Plates XXI–5, XXI–6).

The *bone marrow* in lymphoid malignancies of cats may be moderately to massively infil-

trated by neoplastic lymphoid cells (Plate XXI–4). It should be recalled that normal feline marrow may present 5–15% small mature lymphocytes. Neoplastic infiltration of bone marrow is characterized by cells of varying size and maturity, ranging from mature lymphocytes to lymphoblasts (Fig. 32-5). Erythropoiesis is depressed, and granulopoiesis is sometimes abnormal; both are commonly manifestations of the FeLV infection rather than an effect of lymphoid infiltration since such changes could occur in the absence of

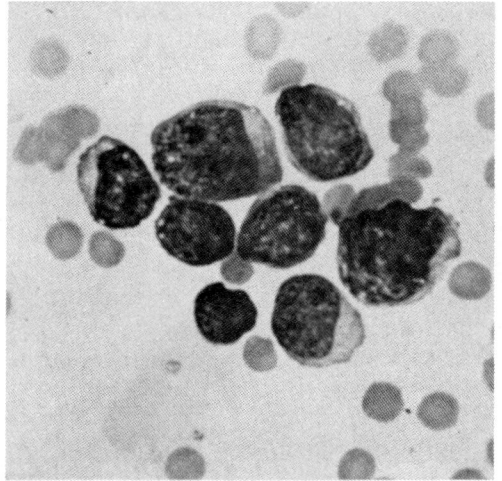

Fig. 32–5. Lymphocytes varying from normal to prolymphocytes in bone marrow of a cat with lymphoma. ×2,700.

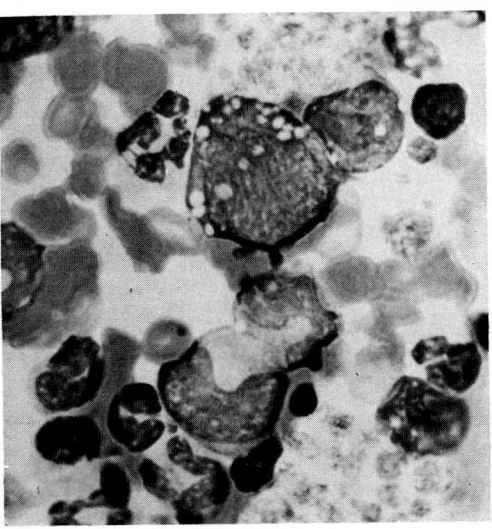

Fig. 32–7. Vacuolated reticulum cell in the bone marrow of a cat with reticulum cell sarcoma. ×2,700.

bone marrow involvement from FeLV infection. Large and bizarre granulocytic cells may be seen (Fig. 32–6). Cells typical of histiocytic lymphoma are also found in the bone marrow of affected cats (Fig. 32–7 and Plates XXI–5, XXI–6). Bone marrow was examined from 19 of the 49 cats in this series. Lymphocytic infiltration characteristic of lymphoid neoplasia was present in 12 cats (63%), while lymphoblasts or prolymphocytes were observed in peripheral blood of only 7 of the 12 cats.

Diagnosis of lymphoid neoplasia in the cat commonly requires a combination of blood studies, bone marrow aspiration, cytologic examination of pleural effusions, and lymph node aspirate or impression smears. In only a few instances, blood examination will by itself confirm the diagnosis. When a pleural effusion is present, it may support or exclude a diagnosis of neoplasia. Considerable experience is required for accurate interpretation of lymph node cytology, while bone marrow, when massively infiltrated by immature lymphocytes, presents no problem of diagnosis.

Other Laboratory Findings

Hypercalcemia associated with lymphoma was reported in a cat (Chew et al., 1975) as it has been in the dog, horse, and human. Chromosomal abnormalities in the form of marked aneuploidies were detected in two cats with acute lymphocytic leukemia (Goh et al., 1981). Serum complement levels are reduced in about 50% of viremic, apparently healthy cats and in all viremic cats with lymphoma (Kobilinsky et al., 1979). In the latter animals this reduction may be due to activation of complement through the classical pathway by circulating viral antigen-antibody complexes (O'Reilly-Felice et al., 1980). Complement depletion may also occur because of deposition with FeLV antigen-antibody complexes in the glomeruli of some viremic cats (Weksler et al., 1975).

Immunologic cell surface markers revealed that thymic lymphomas are composed of T cells, whereas alimentary lymphomas are composed of B cells and multicentric lymphomas either lacked B or T cell surface markers or were composed of T cells (Hardy, 1981a; Holmberg et al., 1976a; Mackey and Jarrett, 1975). All histologic types of lymphoma,

namely, undifferentiated lymphocytic, poorly differentiated lymphocytic, well differentiated lymphocytic, and "histiocytic," may occur in any of the various anatomic forms (Hardy, 1981a).

Acute Lymphoblastic Leukemia

Cats can develop acute lymphoblastic leukemia unassociated with solid tumor masses. In reports of cases of spontaneous feline lymphoid malignancies from the Angell Memorial Animal Hospital in Boston, 66 of 144 cases (46%) recorded between 1972 and 1975 were characterized as true leukemias with primary involvement of blood and bone marrow without clinically detectable tumor masses (Cotter and Essex, 1977). We, as well as others (Hardy, 1981a), have found it to be rare.

Clinical signs are vague and include pallor, lethargy, weakness, anorexia, weight loss, and fever. Hepatomegaly and lymphadenopathy may be found. Hematologic findings invariably show anemia, and total leukocyte count varies from leukopenia to extreme leukocytosis. The diagnosis is made by demonstrating the presence of abnormal lymphocytes in blood and/or bone marrow, and most of the lymphocytes appear to have immunologic features of T cells. The bone marrow is usually hypercellular, being infiltrated with lymphoblasts or prolymphocytes. Thrombocytopenia and bleeding tendencies are infrequent, unlike the findings in human patients with acute lymphoblastic leukemia.

Hodgkin's Disease

A case of Hodgkin's disease in a 9-year-old female tabby cat was reported recently (Roperto et al., 1983). Splenomegaly was evident on palpation and at necropsy. The presence of numerous cells having characteristics of Reed-Sternberg cells prompted the diagnosis of Hodgkin's disease.

Multiple Myeloma

This is described in Chapter 34.

Myeloproliferative Disorders

The term "myeloproliferative disorder" (MPD) was used by Dameshek (1951) to cover a clinical syndrome in humans resulting from abnormal proliferation of a variety of bone marrow cells that leads to profound anemia and commonly terminates in granulocytic leukemia. The foundation for the concept was laid by Di Guglielmo, in 1917, who proposed that the erythrocytic maturation series could proliferate abnormally, producing diseases he described as "erythremic myelosis" and "erythroleukemia" (Dameshek, 1969). Acute and chronic forms of erythremic myelosis have been recognized.

Myeloproliferative disorders may involve any one or a combination of the different cell lines comprising the cytology of bone marrow (Table 32–1). In the cat, all variants of MPD except the eosinophilic leukemia were found to be associated with FeLV infection (Hardy, 1981a). The feline leukemia virus has been demonstrated in various forms of MPD by electron microscopy (Herz et al., 1970; Schalm and Theilen, 1970) and immunologic tests (Crow et al., 1977a; Hardy et al., 1977a; Henness et al., 1977; Hoover and Kociba, 1974; Pedersen et al., 1977).

A schema, modified from one proposed by Nalbandian and coworkers (1968) is presented in Fig. 32-8 to explain the variety of cytologic patterns that may occur in MPD. Proliferation of the pluripotential stem cells may lead to the accumulation of primitive cells showing no clear-cut differentiation toward a recognizable cell line. The term "reticuloendotheliosis" was proposed by Gilmore et al. (1964) for this primitive cell form of MPD to distinguish it from lymphoma involving the bone marrow. While the name "reticuloendotheliosis" has served to call attention to the primitive nature of the abnormally proliferating bone marrow cell, it is not entirely appropriate. Acute erythremic myelosis has been suggested as more descriptive because cells with primitive erythroid characteristics are always present (Harvey, 1981). In my opinion, until more becomes known, the disease may best be described as an undifferentiated or poorly differentiated MPD since the bone marrow of such cats often shows predominance of primitive cells that cannot be properly classified, although occasional cells may exhibit restricted erythroid, myeloid, or mixed (both myeloid and erythroid features) differentiation.

Differentiation of the abnormally proliferating cells primarily into recognizable erythroid cells without significant participation of granulocytes may be termed "erythremic myelosis." An admixture of erythrocytic and granulocytic precursor cells suggests "erythroleukemia," and predominance of immature granulocytes is indicative of myelogenous leukemia.

The problem in nomenclature of MPD in cats stems largely from lack of well-defined criteria to categorize various forms of MPD in animal species and partly from limited opportunity to follow the natural progression of the disease because of death from secondary infections or elective euthanasia. Thus at present a simple diagnosis of MPD may be considered sufficient to formulate patient

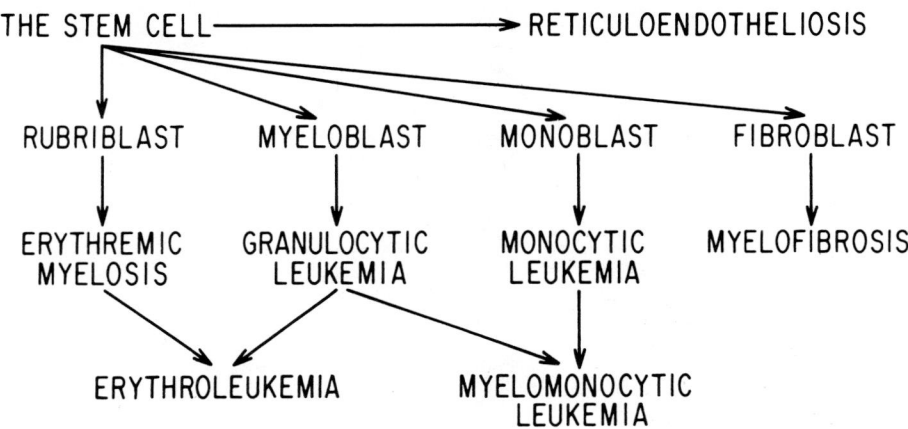

Fig. 32–8. A scheme indicating the origin of several different cell lines within the bone marrow from a pluripotential stem cell and the potential for development of different cytologic variation in myeloproliferative disorder.

management. It should also be mentioned that a broad diagnosis of MPD in cats may imply presence of erythroleukemia, erythremic myelosis, or undifferentiated or poorly differentiated MPD (reticuloendotheliosis).

Myelofibrosis (Plate XX–6) may develop in some cats with MPD as a terminal event, while bizarre proliferation of hematopoietic cells continues within the vascular spaces of the liver (Plate XX–5), spleen, and lymph nodes. Massive proliferation of hematopoietic cells in these extramedullary sites is a common event leading to splenomegaly, hepatomegaly, and, to a lesser extent, lymphadenopathy. Icterus becomes part of the syndrome when massive accumulation of hematopoietic cells within liver sinusoids (Fig. 32–9, Plate XX–5) leads to atrophy of the parenchyma. Icterus may also be due in part to hemolytic anemia from extensive erythrophagocytosis within the spleen and lymph nodes (Plate XVII–6). The existence of extramedullary hematopoiesis associated with advanced refractory anemia has been interpreted in the past as a response to the anemia rather than as the result of an erythroid myeloproliferative process.

Examples of significant findings in blood, bone marrow, and visceral organs of some of these forms of MPD in the cat are presented in Table 32–4. A brief description of the more commonly encountered forms follows.

Undifferentiated or Poorly Differentiated Myeloproliferative Disorder (Reticuloendotheliosis)

Typical cells have a reddish purple nucleus and blue cytoplasm, and they vary somewhat in size (Plates XV-1, XV-2). The nucleus occupies most of the cell and assumes an eccentric position. The nucleus may contain one or more nucleoli (Plate XV-1), but, more commonly, nucleoli are absent. The chromatin pattern (Fig. 32–10) and the ultrastructure of some of these primitive cells give an impression that they are closely related to an early erythroid precursor cell (Hurvitz, 1970). The cytoplasm of some cells contains a few to many reddish azurophilic granules (Plate XV-2), which is suggestive of the progranulocyte of the granulocytic cell series (Fig. 32–11).

Thus features of both erythroid and granulocytic precursor cells appear among the primitive undifferentiated cells. In some instances, particularly in blood, the cells may have a lighter cytoplasm, similar to that of the lymphocyte, but the nucleus retains a perfectly round shape and is eccentrically placed

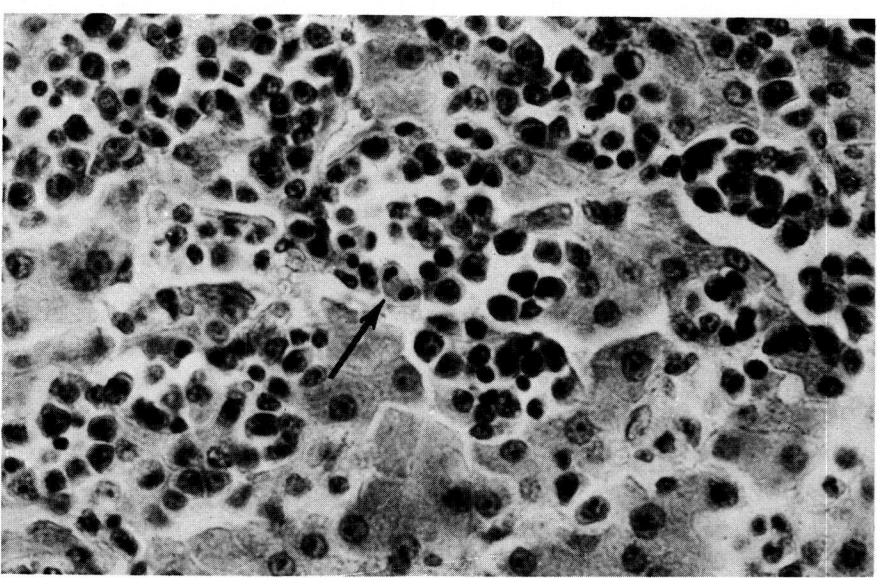

Fig. 32–9.   Liver section from a cat with undifferentiated myeloproliferative disorder reticuloendotheliosis. The liver sinusoids are packed with primitive cells. Arrow points to a cell in mitosis. H & E stain, ×400.

Table 32–4. Significant Findings in the Blood, Bone Marrow, and Visceral Organs in Myeloproliferative Disorders (MPD) of the Cat

Cat No.	Sex	Age	Cytologic Classification	PCV (%)	MCV (fl)	Icterus Index Units	Reticulocytes	Nucleated RBC/µl	WBC/µl	Left Shift to Include	Unclassified and Blast Cells (%)	Visceral Involvement[a]
1	XM	6 yr	Undifferentiated MPD	13	63.4	2	Rare	148	14,800	Bands	34.0	LN ++ LV ++ SP +++ BM +++
2	F	3 yr	Undifferentiated MPD	7	43.5	30	Rare	1,460	13,900	Bands	15.5	LN + LV + SP + BM +++[b]
3	M	7 yr	Erythremic myelosis	8	50.0	2	None	16,530	11,400	Progranulocytes	10.0	LN +++ LV + SP +++ BM +++[b]
4	M	2 yr	Erythremic myelosis	14	73.6	75	Moderate	435,000	45,100	Myelocytes	Few	LN ++ LV ++ SP +++ BM +++,LE[b]
5	XF	5 yr	Erythroleukemia	12	88.9	2	Rare	110,000	48,300	Myeloblasts	Rare	LN − LV + SP − BM ++,F,LE[b]
6	XM	mature	Erythroleukemia	12	61.5	2	Moderate	26	3,500	Myelocytes	4.0	LN ++ LV ++ SP +++ BM +++[b]
7	XM	2 yr	Hypoplastic anemia and leukopenia	8	69.6	7.5	Few	6,500	150	Bands	None	LN − LV − SP + BM +[c]
8	F	3 yr	Granulocytic leukemia	23	57.5	2	—	None	213,000	Blasts	1.0	LN − LV + SP + BM +++
9	F	7 mo	Granulocytic leukemia	22	44.0	2	None	None	4,000	Myelocytes	None	LN + LV + SP + BM +++

[a] —, not involved; +, slight; ++, moderate; +++, marked enlargement or infiltration; F, myelofibrosis; LE, lupus erythematosus cells seen; LN, lymph node; LV, liver; SP, spleen; BM, bone marrow.

[b] C-type virus demonstrated in bone marrow cells.

[c] C-type virus in megakaryocytes.

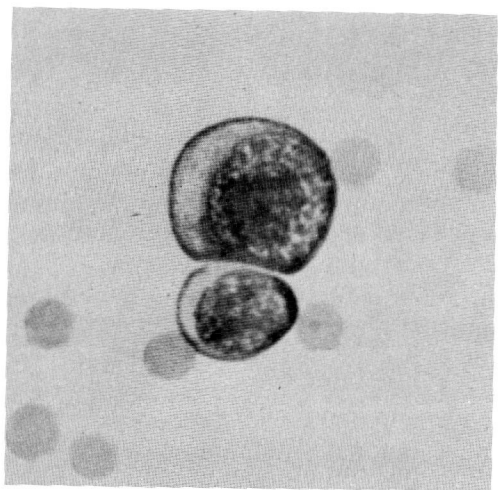

Fig. 32–10. Primitive cells in the blood of a cat with undifferentiated myeloproliferative disorder (reticuloendotheliosis). Nuclear chromatin pattern is suggestive of erythroid precursor cells. ×3,200.

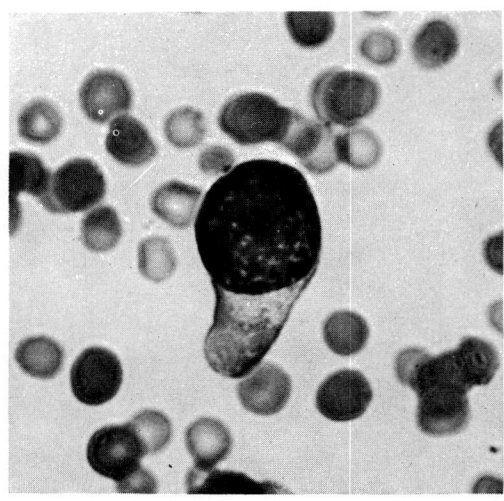

Fig. 32–12. Primitive cell with cytoplasmic pseudopod in the bone marrow of a cat with erythroleukemia. ×2,300.

so that generally more cytoplasm is evident than in the lymphocyte.

In the bone marrow, a monotonous pattern of round, deep blue cells is presented with almost complete absence of recognizable maturation forms (Plate XIX–2). There may be reduction in granulopoiesis, vacuolation of granulocytic cells, and an occasional giant metamyelocyte.

Care must be taken to distinguish the bone marrow cytology of this form of MPD from

that of deficiencies of vitamin B_{12} (Jarrett, 1973) and folic acid. These vitamin deficiencies result in a maturation arrest at the prorubricyte and basophilic rubricyte stages leading to an accumulation of deep blue–staining cells in the marrow. (Compare Plates XIX-1 and XIX-2.) Occurrence of large metamyelocytes in the bone marrow is also to be anticipated in these vitamin deficiencies.

An interesting feature that may accompany bone marrow cytology in this form of MPD is the occurrence of a pseudopod-like projection in some cells (Fig. 32-12). The cytoplasmic projection may contain azurophilic granules (Plate XV-3) or vacuoles, and there is a tendency for it to pinch off, forming anuclear cytoplasmic structures (Schalm, 1980b) of varying sizes in bone marrow and blood. When the pinched-off portion contains azurophilic granules, it may suggest an enormous blood platelet. When it is without granules and is deep blue in color, it may be confused with a giant polychromatic erythrocyte.

Erythremic Myelosis

This form of MPD may be suspected when, in the presence of a severe anemia, peripheral blood morphology is characterized by marked anisocytosis without an accompanying polychromasia (Plate XIX-3). There may be an occasional nucleated erythrocyte exhibiting asynchronism between cytoplasm and nu-

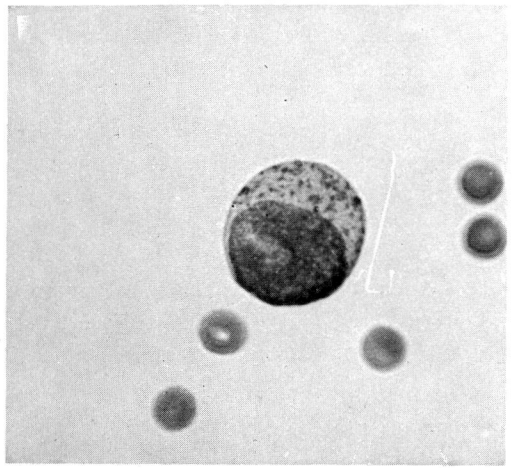

Fig. 32–11. Blast cell with large azurophilic granules in the blood of a cat with undifferentiated myeloproliferative disorder (reticuloendotheliosis). ×2,000.

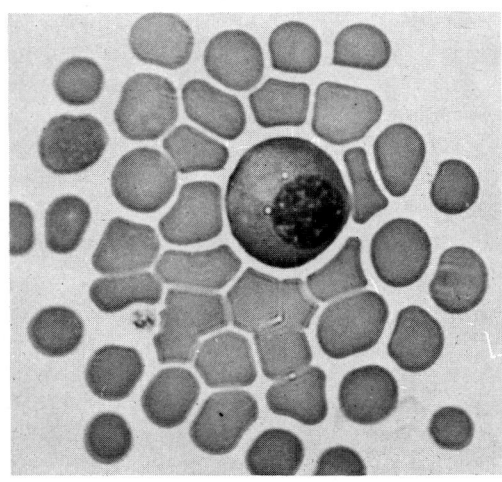

Fig. 32–13. A megaloblastoid nucleated erythrocyte in the blood of a cat as seen in erythremic myelosis or erythroleukemia. ×2,700.

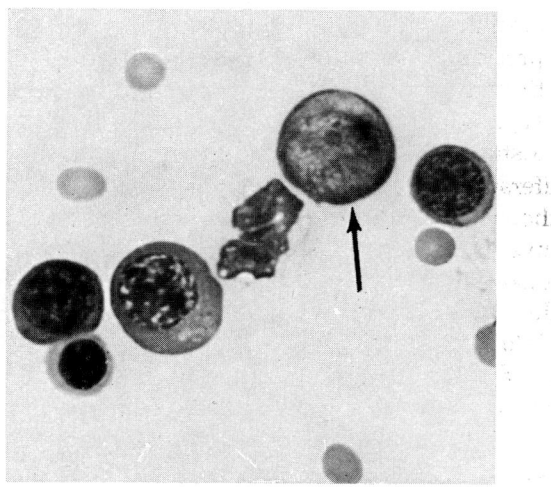

Fig. 32–14. Blood of a cat with erythroleukemia. A myeloblast *(arrow)* is shown together with four nucleated erythrocytes in various stages of maturation. ×2,700.

cleus (Fig. 32-13). In other patients, the blood may be characterized by a profusion of abnormal or relatively normal-appearing nucleated erythrocytes in all stages of development unaccompanied by polychromic erythrocytes (Cat 4, Table 32-4). These cells may have been derived in part from the sinusoids of the liver and spleen, from which they are probably released by pressure upon the cell-engorged organs (Plate XX-5). This situation was suspected in Cat 5 (Table 32–4) because the cells in the bone marrow were too primitive (Plate XIX-5) to have supplied the more mature nucleated cells in the circulation (Plate XIX-4).

Sequential examination of blood taken over a period of several days may reveal marked variations in the number and morphology of nucleated erythrocytes. A blood transfusion is commonly followed by a significant reduction in the number of circulating nucleated erythrocytes.

The bone marrow generally is characterized by a profusion of rubricytes in all stages of maturation (Schalm, 1980c). The majority of rubricytes may be of normal appearance but will be present in excessive number (Plate XIX-6), or megaloblastic rubricytes resulting from asynchronism between cytoplasm and nucleus may be a prominent feature (Plate XV-4). In rare instances, multiple nuclei (polyploidy) may be present in a large polychro-

matic cell (Plate XX-1). More commonly, metarubricytes with double nuclei have been encountered (Plate XIX-6). When the bone marrow is characterized by excessive proliferation of cells of the erythrocytic series, granulopoiesis is depressed and vacuolation of granulocytic precursor cells may be seen. Erythrophagocytosis by abnormally proliferating erythroid cells is seen on occasion (Schalm, 1980c) (Plate XX-2).

Erythremic myelosis in the cat was compared to the Di Guglielmo syndrome in humans (Zawidzka et al., 1964). In human patients with erythremic myelosis and erythroleukemia, abnormal erythroid cells in blood and bone marrow exhibit PAS-positive reaction (see Chapter 33). Similar PAS-positivity has been reported in two reports on erythremic myelosis in cats (Falconer et al., 1980; Zawidzka, 1964), but our findings on cats with erythremic myelosis and erythroleukemia have been negative.

Erythroleukemia

A clear separation between erythremic myelosis and erythroleukemia does not exist. In fact, the distinction is mostly arbitrary and is based on the finding of myeloblasts admixed with abnormal nucleated erythrocytes in peripheral blood (Fig. 32-14). Dameshek (1965) stressed the existence of three successive stages of MPD, initially involving the erythrocytic series and later the granulocytic precursors as follows: (1) a period of erythremic myelosis characterized by a striking erythroid hyperplasia of the bone marrow, (2) a stage of mixed erythroid and myeloid proliferation, namely, erythroleukemia, and (3) the eventual termination of some cases in myeloblastic leukemia. In some cases a preleukemic erythroid disorder may precede the development of an acute myelomonocytic leukemia (Kass, 1978). We observed a cat (Cat 6, Table 32-4) that seemed to be in the stage of progression from erythroleukemia to granulocytic leukemia (Herz et al., 1969a,b). The cat was observed over a period of 16 days. Four hemograms (Table 32-5) and two bone marrow aspirations were prepared. The PCV values ranged between 10 and 14%, and MCV varied between 61.5 and 88.0 fl. The blood was leukopenic on the initial hemogram, but leukocyte counts increased to between 8,000 and 12, 900/μl on other occasions.

The two bone marrow samples taken 10 days apart presented distinctly different cytologic patterns (Schalm, 1980d). In the first sample, the principal cellular abnormality was referable to the erythrocytic maturation series. Rubriblasts with a single large nucleolus (Figs. 32-15, 32-16) and megaloblastic rubricytes with normal or abnormal hemoglobinization were a prominent feature. The cytoplasmic color of megaloblastic rubricytes varied from dusky gray through light brown to the yellowish color of the normochromic erythrocyte (Plate XX-3). Granulocytic-series cells had vacuolated cytoplasm, and some cells were large with bizarre nuclei. The M:E ratio was 1.26:1.0. The M:E ratio in bone marrow sampled 10 days later had increased to 14.5:1.0. This reflected the change to a predominance of atypical granulocytic precursor cells with only an occasional megaloblastic rubricyte seen (Plate XX-4). *Haemobartonella felis* was observed in one microscopic field, and *Toxoplasma gondii* was found both intracellularly and extracellularly in several fields (Plates XIV-8, XIV-9). These parasites were not found in the first bone marrow sample. It was conjectured that the cat was a carrier of both parasites and that because of its debilitated condition and FeLV-mediated immunosuppression, the parasites were beginning to multiply.

At necropsy, multiple reddish white nod-

Table 32–5. Four Hemograms in a Cat with Bone Marrow Cytology Suggesting a Change from Erythroleukemia to Granulocytic Leukemia between December 3 and December 13

Date	Nov. 27	Dec. 3[a]	Dec. 12	Dec. 13
RBC ($\times 10^6$/μl)	1.95	1.89	1.30	1.25
PCV (%)	12.0	14.0	10.0	11.0
Hemoglobin (g/dl)	3.8	4.6	3.0	3.0
MCV (fl)	61.5	74.1	76.9	88.0
MCHC (%)	31.7	32.1	33.3	27.3
Icterus index units	2	2	—	10
Plasma proteins (g/dl)	7.6	6.9	—	6.9
Fibrinogen (g/dl)	0.20	0.20	—	0.20
Reticulocytes	moderate	moderate	—	few
Polychromasia	moderate	moderate	rare	rare
Anisocytosis	moderate	moderate	slight	slight
Nucleated RBC/100 WBC	26	29	5	1
WBC/μl (corrected)	3,500	8,000	12,900	12,000
Myelocytes	175 (5.0%)	0	0	0
Metamyelocytes	35 (1.0%)	0	0	420 (3.5%)
Band neutrophils	70 (2.0%)	0	580 (4.5%)	1,920 (16.0%)
Neutrophils (mature)	2,415 (69.0%)	6,320 (79.0%)	9,739 (75.5%)	5,340 (44.5%)
Lymphocytes	420 (12.0%)	1,040 (13.0%)	516 (4.0%)	720 (6.0%)
Monocytes	245 (7.0%)	640 (8.0%)	2,064 (16.0%)	3,360[b] (28.0%)
Eosinophils	0	0	0	0
Basophils	0	0	0	0
Unclassified cells	140 (4.0%)	0	0	240 (2.0%)
Parasites	—	—	few *H. felis*	few *H. felis* rare *T. gondii*

From Herz *et al.* 1969b; courtesy of *California Veterinarian*.
[a]Capillary blood from the ear; other three hemograms represent large-vessel blood.
[b]Although these cells were classified as monocytes, they may have been vacuolated myelocytes and metamyelocytes.

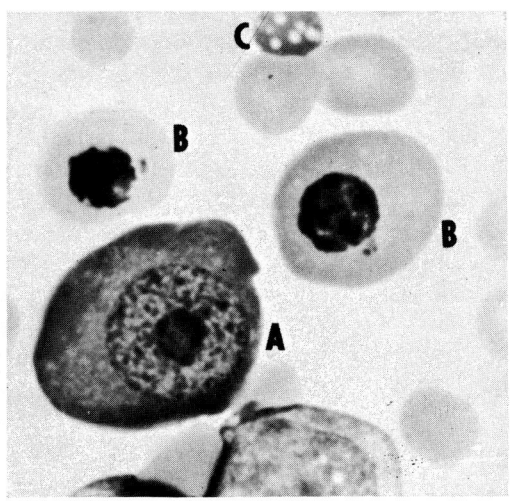

Fig. 32–15. Megaloblastoid rubriblast *(A)* and normochromic megaloblastoid rubricytes *(B)* in the bone marrow of a cat with erythremic myelosis or erythroleukemia. A vacuolated cytoplasmic fragment *(C)* is also shown. From Cat 6, Table 32–4. ×3,600.

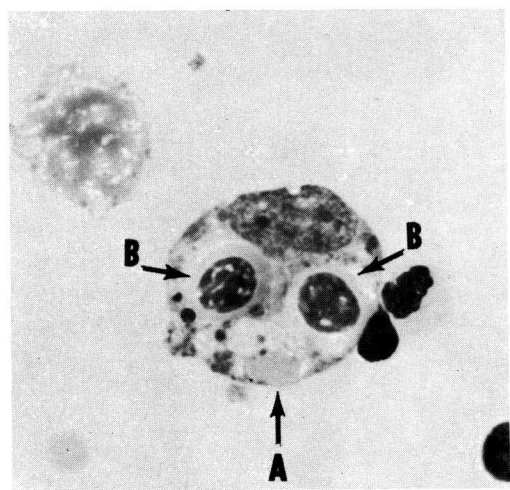

Fig. 32–17. Phagocytosis of an erythrocyte *(A)* and nucleated erythrocytes *(B)* by a macrophage in the bone marrow in erythremic myelosis of the cat. ×2,300.

ules of a type sometimes associated with granulocytic leukemia were scattered throughout the subcutaneous tissues. Lymph nodes were moderately enlarged and reddish and presented yellowish foci throughout. Both the liver and spleen were enlarged. The normal tissues of the spleen and lymph nodes were replaced by foci of undifferentiated cells as well as of cells classified as belonging to both the erythrocytic and granulocytic series.

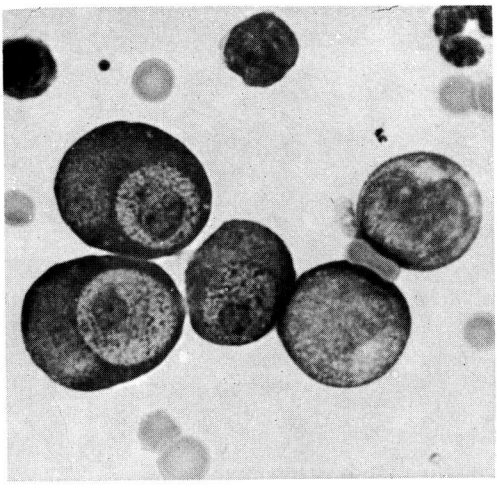

Fig. 32–16. Bone marrow from a cat with erythroleukemia. Three abnormal rubricytes and two myelocytes are seen. The rubricytes are deficient in nuclear chromatin, and each nucleus presents a large nucleolus. From Cat 6, Table 32–4. ×2,700.

Microscopically, the bone marrow contained mainly undifferentiated cells of the granulocytic series.

A bone marrow biopsy sample obtained at the time of the second marrow sampling was prepared for ultrastructural examination. The cells were of two types, megaloblastic erythroid cells showing maturation arrest and immature mononuclear cells with cytoplasmic vacuoles. C-type virus particles were found budding from the plasma membrane of this latter type of cell (Fig. 32-1). Virus particles were also found in intercellular spaces. No virus particles were seen associated with erythrocytic cells.

Such a changing pattern of MPD in cats has also been observed by others (Harvey et al., 1978). The fine structure of primitive erythroid cells in the blood of a cat with erythroleukemia was recently described (Maede and Murata, 1980). Cytologic (Roggli and Saleem, 1982) and cytochemical (Kass, 1978) observations on human cases of erythroleukemia have been summarized.

Additional Cytologic Features in Myeloproliferative Disorders

Phagocytosis of nucleated and mature erythrocytes by macrophages within the bone marrow (Fig. 32-17) is a common finding. Lupus erythematosus (LE) cells (Fig. 32-18) have been observed in fresh bone marrow of

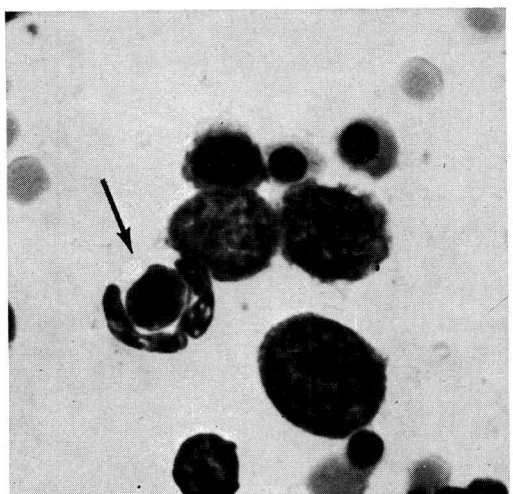

Fig. 32–18. Lupus erythematosus cell *(arrow)* in a film of freshly aspirated bone marrow from a cat with erythroleukemia. From Cat 4, Table 32–4. ×3,200.

three cats with MPD, suggesting the presence of an antinuclear antibody. Additional evidence of the action of antibody in MPD was seen in the bone marrow of two cats in which agglutination of polychromatic erythrocytes and metarubricytes was a prominent feature (Plate XIX-6). (See also Appendix Case 50).

Staining bone marrow films for iron has revealed the occurrence of iron particles within the cytoplasm of some megaloblastic rubricytes (Plate XV-5) and in some macrocytic erythrocytes. Terms commonly applied to such iron-containing cells are sideroblast and siderocyte, respectively. Dameshek (1965) equated sideroblastic (sideroachrestic) anemia of humans with erythremic myelosis in which a defect in heme synthesis exists, with apparent inability of nucleated erythrocytes to metabolize iron.

In a study on a 3-year old female domestic shorthair cat with erythroleukemia, it was found that the erythrocyte half-life was reduced by nearly 50%, total erythrocyte volume was reduced by 64%, and plasma volume was increased by 40%, compared with mean values for two control cats (Kaneko, unpublished observations).

Gross and Histopathologic Features of Myeloproliferative Disorders

Organ alterations characteristic of MPD are limited to the bone marrow, spleen, liver, and lymph nodes (Table 32–4). The proliferating hematopoietic cells infiltrate the vascular system and sinusoids of these organs to a varying degree. In the mildest form, the abnormally proliferating cells are limited to the bone marrow and blood. Little enlargement of the spleen, liver, or lymph nodes is noted. At the other extreme, the liver and spleen are enlarged three to four times, and all lymph nodes increase in size. Icterus may be seen when the liver is massively involved (Plate XX-5) or when there is aggressive erythrophagocytosis by the cells of the mononuclear phagocyte system (Plate XVII-6). Myelofibrosis (Plate XX-6) and osteoid metaplasia have been described as bone marrow alterations in some cats with FeLV infections (Flecknell et al., 1978; Schalm and Theilen, 1970; Ward et al., 1969). Varying degrees of medullary osteosclerosis were seen in 12 of 13 cats with nonregenerative anemia induced by intraperitoneal inoculation of FeLV into neonatal kittens (Hoover and Kociba, 1974).

Myelogenous or Granulocytic Leukemia

Neoplasia originating in the granulocytic cell series in the bone marrow is designated granulocytic or myelogenous leukemia. One thinks of typical granulocytic leukemia as being characterized by a leukocytosis with myelocytes, progranulocytes, and myeloblasts in peripheral blood in significant numbers. Several case reports have appeared in the literature on this disease in cats (Eyestone, 1951; Fraser et al., 1974; Grindem et al., 1985a,b; Holzworth, 1960; Meier and Patterson, 1956). Examples of a leukemic and a leukopenic form of granulocytic leukemia are included in Table 32-4.

Among 14 cats diagnosed as having granulocytic leukemia, three had total leukocyte counts of 65,000, 213,000 and 389,000/μl; in five cats, the leukocyte counts were between 26,000 and 45,000; in the remaining six cats, the leukocyte numbers were either within or below the normal range.

Cat 8, Table 32-4, with a leukocyte count of 213,000/μl, had 60% granulocytes, 34% monocytoid cells, and 6% lymphocytes. Among the granulocytes, only 4% consisted of myeloblasts, progranulocytes, and myelocytes, while mature neutrophils contributed 51%.

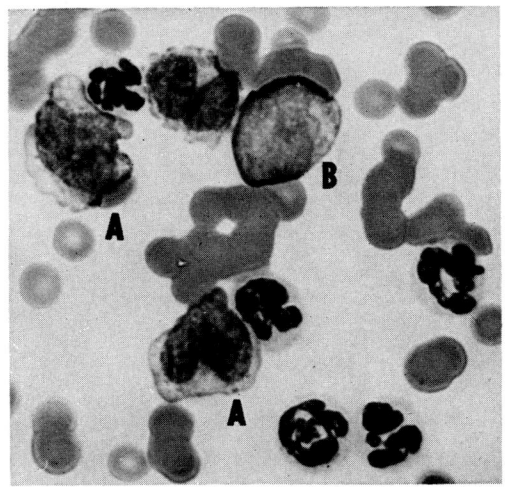

Fig. 32–19. Blood of a cat in myelomonocytic leukemia. *A,* monocytoid cells; *B,* a neutrophilic myelocyte. ×2,700.

The monocytoid cells (Fig. 32-19) were peroxidase-negative. It was concluded that this was best classified as a myelomonocytic leukemia. A leukemic process characterized by abnormal proliferation of both granulocytic and monocytic cells is classified as myelomonocytic leukemia. The monocyte is derived from a stem cell in common with the myeloblasts; therefore, neoplastic proliferation of the monocyte is classified as a myeloproliferative disorder. Diagnosis of monocytic leukemia is based on a characteristic folding of the nucleus of the primitive cells seen in blood and bone marrow (Schalm, 1980e).

A second cat with a leukocyte count of 389,000 of which 89.5% consisted of myelocytes, progranulocytes, and myeloblasts (Plate XXII) was a 1½-year-old male domestic shorthair. Illness extended over 2 months and started with watery and bloody diarrhea, anorexia, vomiting, and a rectal temperature of 105°F. Upon admission to our clinic 2 months later, the cat was weak, depressed, markedly dehydrated, and severely anemic (PCV 11%). The leukemia was classified as granulocytic on the basis of a predominance of progranulocytes in bone marrow cells (Plate XXII-2). Furthermore, cytochemical staining of bone marrow cells revealed the majority of large primitive cells to be peroxidase-positive.

Diagnosis may present a problem in the cat that has a normal or leukopenic leukocyte count with left shift to include at times myelocytes, progranulocytes, and occasionally myeloblasts. Cat 9, Table 32–4, is a case in point when all hemograms are considered. It was a 7-month-old female domestic shorthair cat that was admitted with the history of anorexia of 2 days' duration. The rectal temperature was 107.2°F, and although there was no vomiting or diarrhea, a diagnosis of panleukopenia was given consideration, since the cat had not been vaccinated. Thirty hemograms were obtained over a period of three months, of which nine were selected as representative of the changing total and differential leukocyte counts (Table 32-6).

A bone marrow aspiration on May 18 supported a diagnosis of granulocytic leukemia (Plate XX11-3). Many cells of the granulocytic series were abnormally large, with bizarre nuclear patterns, and erythropoiesis was almost absent. Necropsy revealed only minimal involvement of the liver, spleen, and lymph nodes. The spleen contained hemopoietic activity in the red pulp and presented many prominent megakaryocytes, but neoplastic cells were few. The liver exhibited small periportal foci of granulocytic cells, neoplastic blast cells, occasional mature granulocytes, and some erythropoietic elements. The degree of infiltration by obvious neoplastic cells varied among nodes and was never very great.

An interesting aspect concerning the technique of handling blood samples in granulocytic leukemia came to our attention with the case just described. After analysis of one of the blood samples, we decided to prepare a series of slides for teaching purposes. It was estimated that 1 hour had elapsed between preparation of the blood film for the original differential leukocyte count and preparation of the films for teaching purposes. Upon examining the latter films, we found that a major portion of the granulocytes had become vacuolated, giving the appearance of monocytes (compare Figs. 32–20 and 32–21). Leukemic granulocytic cells may be susceptible to rapid deterioration once the blood is withdrawn from the body. The anticoagulant was the disodium salt of EDTA. A similar vacuolation of leukemic granulocytes in old blood has been recorded for the dog (Fig. 32-28).

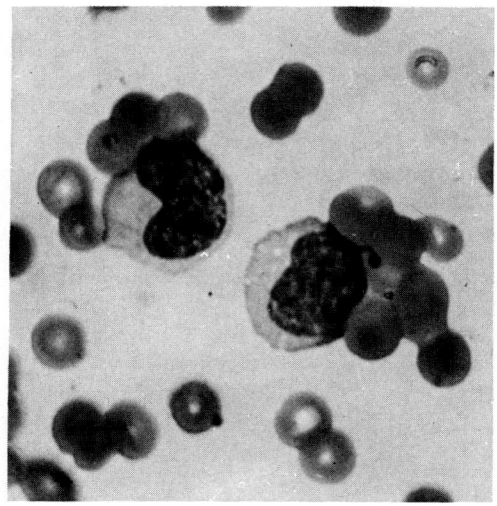

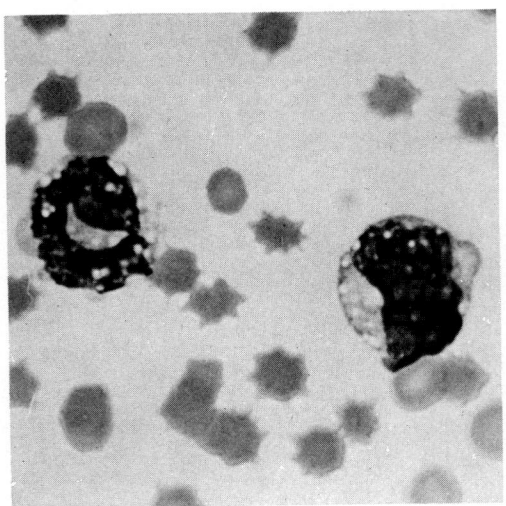

Fig. 32–20. Two metamyelocytes in freshly collected blood from the same cat as in Figure 32–21. From a case of subleukemic granulocytic leukemia. ×2,700.

Fig. 32–21. Two vacuolated granulocytes in the same blood as in Fig. 32–20. The blood stood for 1 hour in EDTA anticoagulant before the film was prepared. Leukemic granulocytes appear to be subject to degeneration upon aging of the blood. ×2,700.

The problem of diagnosis of subleukemic granulocytic leukemia in the cat is complicated by the fact that leukopenia with left shift to progranulocytes and/or myeloblasts occurs rather frequently in association with toxemic diseases. The bone marrow may be hypercellular, with many immature granulocytes with bizarre nuclei (Plates XV–8, XV–11). When the bone marrow is hypercellular with maturation arrest at the myelocyte stage, granulocytic leukemia may be suspected. Such maturation arrest forms the basis for the leukopenia and intermittent left shift to myeloblasts in peripheral blood. The erythrocytic maturation series may be complete but significantly reduced in relation to the prominent granulocytic precursor cells. In cats with

Table 32–6. Selected Hemograms Demonstrating the Marked Variation in Total and Differential Leukocyte Counts in Subleukemic Granulocytic Leukemia in a Young Cat (Cat 9, Table 32–4)

	March 15[a]	March 22	March 28	March 31	April 14	April 21	April 26	May 18[b]	June 22
Temperature (°F)	107.2	101.3	101.9	104.0	101.0	100.4	106.0	—	—
PCV (%)	22	22	18	15	22	24	20	15	6
Reticulocytes	—	—	0	0	many	0	—	mod.	0
Nucleated RBC/100 WBC	0	2	0	3	12	0	0	60	rare
WBC/μl	4,000[c]	2,800	7,700	9,900[c]	5,000	7,000[c]	5,500[c]	34,700[c]	4,000
Myeloblasts	0	0	0	rare	0	105	110	694	0
Progranulocytes	0	0	0	rare	0	140	275	694	0
Myelocytes (neut.)	160	0	0	792	0	945	825	3,470	0
Metamyelocytes (neut.)	480	0	0	1,485	0	1,540	825	3,644	160
Band neutrophils	1,560	0	308	1,782	50	385	275	1,388	240
Neutrophils (mature)	600	504	4,543	990	500	280	330	11,624	600
Lymphocytes	1,120	1,820	1,925	2,574	3,500	2,275	2,695	9,542	1,560
Monocytes	40	140	231	396	250	280	0	0	0
Eosinophils	40	336	539	495	700	210	110	1,041	240
Basophils	0	0	0	297	0	840	55	0	40
Unclassified cells	0	0	0	396	0	0	0	0	1,040
Degenerated cells	0	0	154	693	0	0	0	2,602	120

From Schalm and Switzer, 1968; courtesy of *California Veterinarian*.
[a]On antibiotics from March 15 through April 16; steroids between March 28 and April 16; no treatment from April 17 through April 19; returned to antibiotic therapy from April 28 to May 6, then all therapy stopped.
[b]Developed infected toe. On necropsy an abscessed lower molar was found.
[c]Immature neutrophils exhibited giant forms with bizarre nuclear patterns and basophilic cytoplasm.

an accompanying advanced anemia (PCV 10%), the erythrocytic maturation series is usually absent. The bone marrow film may reveal an occasional megaloblastic rubricyte. A finding of this type suggests the possibility of MPD in which the erythrocytic phase has given place to terminal granulocytic leukemia (Plate XXII–4).

Monocytic and Myelomonocytic Leukemias

Feline cases of monocytic leukemia (Henness et al., 1977; Holzworth, 1960; Tsujimoto et al., 1981) and myelomonocytic leukemia (Loeb et al., 1975; Madewell et al., 1979; Raskin and Krehbiel, 1985; Stann, 1979) have been described. Both sexes were involved and ages varied from 3 to 13 years. Many of these cats were FeLV-positive. Clinical findings were generally nonspecific. History consisted of anorexia, depression, vomiting, and lethargy of days' to weeks' duration. Physical findings included fever, pale mucous membranes, mild dehydration, diarrhea, emaciation, bilateral ocular and nasal discharges, dyspnea or hyperpnea, enlarged submandibular and axillary lymph nodes, splenomegaly, and mitral valve murmur.

Hematologic findings generally consisted of mild to severe anemia with macrocytic or normocytic red cell morphology, thrombocytopenia with abnormal platelet morphology, moderate to marked leukocytosis with left shift to promyelocytes and myeloblasts, and monocytosis with many immature cells. One cat initially had leukopenia but 4 months later had leukocytosis with 95–100% blast cells. Immature or abnormal monocytes predominated in cats with monocytic leukemia. In some cats, neutrophil cytoplasm was basophilic and contained Döhle bodies. Macropolycytes (giant, hypersegmented neutrophils) and erythrophagocytosis were seen in one case (Raskin and Krehbiel, 1985). Cytochemical findings supported the diagnosis of myelomonocytic or monocytic leukemia, and ultrastructure of leukemic cells confirmed the light microscopic diagnosis.

Bone marrow was usually hypercellular from increased myelopoiesis and monocytopoiesis. Erythropoiesis was diminished. The myeloid:erythroid ratio was increased significantly. Morphologic abnormalities in myeloid, erythroid, and megakaryocytic cells in an occasional cat indicated dyshematopoiesis. Erythrophagocytosis by monocytes and neutrophils was seen in one cat (Raskin and Krehbiel, 1985).

Significant necropsy findings were splenomegaly, hepatomegaly, and lymphadenopathy. Histopathologic examination revealed diffuse infiltration with leukemic blast cells of many organs including lymph nodes, liver, spleen, and bone marrow. In addition, extensive perivascular hemorrhagic infarcts were seen in the brain in two cats with monocytic leukemia, and one cat with similar diagnosis had hemorrhagic foci in lungs, urinary bladder, and gastrointestinal tract.

Eosinophilic Leukemia

This form of granulocytic leukemia is rare in the cat. Simon and Holzworth (1967) presented a well-documented case in a 4-year-old spayed female domestic shorthair cat. The total leukocyte count was 136,000/μl with 35% eosinophils and a PCV of 31%. Differential features between eosinophilic leukemia and eosinophilic enteritis were discussed. Hardy (1981a) found four cats with eosinophilic leukemia to be FeLV-negative.

We encountered one case of eosinophilic leukemia in a 2-year-old castrated male Maltese cat. The cat was presented with the history of vomiting and diarrhea for 3 weeks. The rectal temperature was 102.8° F, the pulse rate was 160/minute, and respiratory rate was 50/minute. The feces were not formed and presented a mucoid covering. Microscopic examination of the mucous revealed a profusion of eosinophils. The feces gave a strong (4+) occult blood test, but no parasitic ova were seen. A mass could be palpated in the midabdomen, and there was evidence of weight loss. The blood urea nitrogen was within the normal range.

The cat was kept under observation in the hospital and at home between April 26 and August 8, when it died. A total of 17 blood examinations and one bone marrow aspiration were made. Five hemograms depicting the course of events and the bone marrow cytology are presented in Table 32-7. Initially, daily treatment with prednisolone did not reduce the blood eosinophil count, which was

Table 32–7. Eosinophilic Leukemia in a 2-Year-Old Castrated Male Maltese Cat

	April 28	May 10[a]	May 24[b]	June 19	August 4[c]
RBC ($\times10^6$/μl)	6.01	5.75	4.71	3.87	5.66
Hemoglobin (g/dl)	9.9	8.4	7.2	6.9	8.7
PCV (%)	27.0	24.0	22.0	19.0	26.0
MCV (fl)	44.9	41.7	46.7	49.0	45.9
MCH (pg)	36.7	35.0	32.7	36.3	33.5
MCHC (%)	16.5	14.6	15.3	17.8	15.3
WBC/μl	244,000	242,000	50,000	184,000	186,000
Band neutrophils	1,220 (0.5%)	0	0	2,760 (1.5%)	1,860 (1.0%)
Mature neutrophils	21,960 (9.0%)	22,990 (9.5%)	7,750 (15.0%)	36,800 (20.0%)	42,780 (4.0%)
Lymphocytes	12,200 (5.0%)	19,360 (8.0%)	1,750 (3.5%)	5,520 (3.0%)	7,440 (4.0%)
Monocytes	2,440 (1.0%)	2,420 (1.0%)	750 (1.5%)	2,760 (1.5%)	9,300 (5.0%)
Metamyelocyte eosinophils	2,440 (1.0%)	4,840 (2.0%)	3,000 (6.0%)	1,840 (1.0%)	1,860 (1.0%)
Band eosinophils	34,160 (14.0%)	41,140 (17.0%)	11,000 (22.0%)	55,200 (30.0%)	11,160 (6.0%)
Eosinophils	169,580 (69.5%)	151,250 (62.5%)	25,750 (51.5%)	79,120 (43.0%)	111,600 (60.0%)
Basophils	0	0	0	0	0
Platelets/μl	62,000	—	271,000	352,000	160,000
Plasma proteins (g/dl)	6.5	—	7.6	8.1	8.0
Fibrinogen (g/dl)	0.10	—	0.10	0.10	0.20
Icterus index units	2	—	2	5 lipemic	5

Bone Marrow Cytology (Plate XXII–5)[c]	
Eosinophilic myelocytes	2.4%
Eosinophilic metamyelocytes	6.8
Eosinophilic bands	14.8
Eosinophils	58.0
Neutrophilic granulocytes	9.2
Rubricytes	4.0
Lymphocytes	4.8
M:E ratio 23.8:1.0	

[a]After treatment with prednisolone 5.0 mg b.i.d. for one week.
[b]After cyclophosphamide and prednisolone therapy.
[c]Samples taken at euthanasia.

about 200,000/µl. Therapy was then changed to a combination of cyclophosphamide and prednisolone, which resulted in a temporary reduction of the blood eosinophil number to nearly 40,000/µl (Table 32-7, May 24). Within 10 days, the blood eosinophil number increased again to >100,000, at which level it remained even though further therapy with cyclophosphamide and prednisolone was administered.

Hemograms before the beginning of therapy were characterized by neutrophilia, lymphocytosis, monocytosis, and eosinophilia, with the latter cells making up 80-85% of the total leukocyte count. No eosinophilic myelocytes appeared in peripheral blood, although a few metamyelocytes were constantly seen. Eosinophilic bands contributed 14-20% of the total leukocyte count, and later under therapy they contributed up to 30%. Mature eosinophils were the major cell both in peripheral blood and in the aspirated bone marrow. In the bone marrow, some eosinophilic myelocytes were considerably larger than normal and retained a deep blue cytoplasm (Plate XXII–5). The marrow was hypercellular, with 82% of cells in the eosinophilic series (Table 32-7). Nucleated erythrocytes contributed only 4.0% to marrow cytology and mature lymphocytes constituted 4.8% of marrow cells. Erythrocyte parameters in blood were at minimum normal levels on admission and fell during therapy so that a state of anemia developed. Blood platelet numbers were low on admission and again near termination but increased to normal levels during therapy, possibly in response to the administration of prednisolone.

At necropsy, all visceral lymph nodes of the thoracic and peritoneal cavities were found to be markedly enlarged. The liver and spleen were markedly enlarged. The liver had a reticulated pattern, and the spleen was dark red and of meaty consistency. Impression smears of lymph nodes, liver, spleen, and bone marrow revealed many eosinophils and granulocytic precursor cells, including progranulocytes and myelocytes. No evidence of virus was found in specimens of liver, spleen, lymph nodes, and bone marrow submitted for electron microscopy.

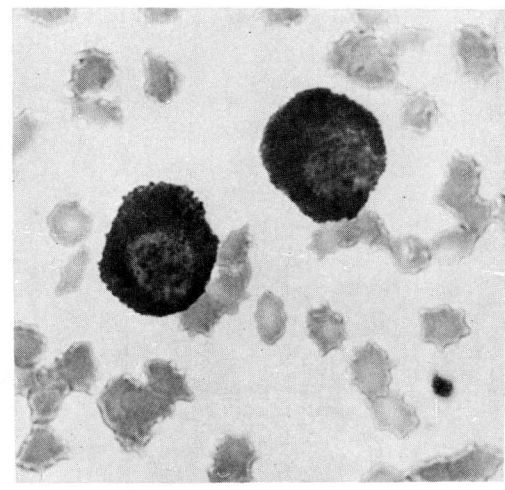

Fig. 32–22. Mast cells in the blood of a cat with mast cell leukemia ×2,700.

Basophilic and Mast Cell Leukemias

A possible instance of atypical basophilic subleukemic leukemia was encountered in a 4-year-old spayed cat (Henness and Crow, 1977). The leukocyte count was 15,700/µl with all stages of granulocytes from myeloblasts to mature neutrophils in the blood. Many primitive cells (44%) presented varying numbers of large purple cytoplasmic granules (Schalm, 1980f) somewhat similar to the granules of the immature basophil leukocyte of the cat. Attempts to obtain bone marrow were unsuccessful due to an existing myelofibrosis.

The mast cell is a tissue cell normally lying outside the vascular system. Due to some similarities to the basophil leukocyte, as encountered in some mammals other than the cat, a mast cell leukemia has at times been erroneously called basophilic leukemia. Occurrence of the mast cell in peripheral blood in large numbers in the cat in association with a greatly enlarged spleen has been reported several times in the literature (Garner and Lingeman, 1970; Lillie, 1931; Lucke, 1964; Meier and Gourley, 1957; Ohshima and Miura, 1965; Seawright and Grono, 1964). Mast cell leukemia in the cat has been encountered at the Angell Memorial Animal Hospital, Boston, almost as frequently as the undifferentiated form of MPD (reticuloendotheliosis)(Gilmore and Holzworth, 1971). However, it has been exceedingly rare at the VMTH, Davis, California.

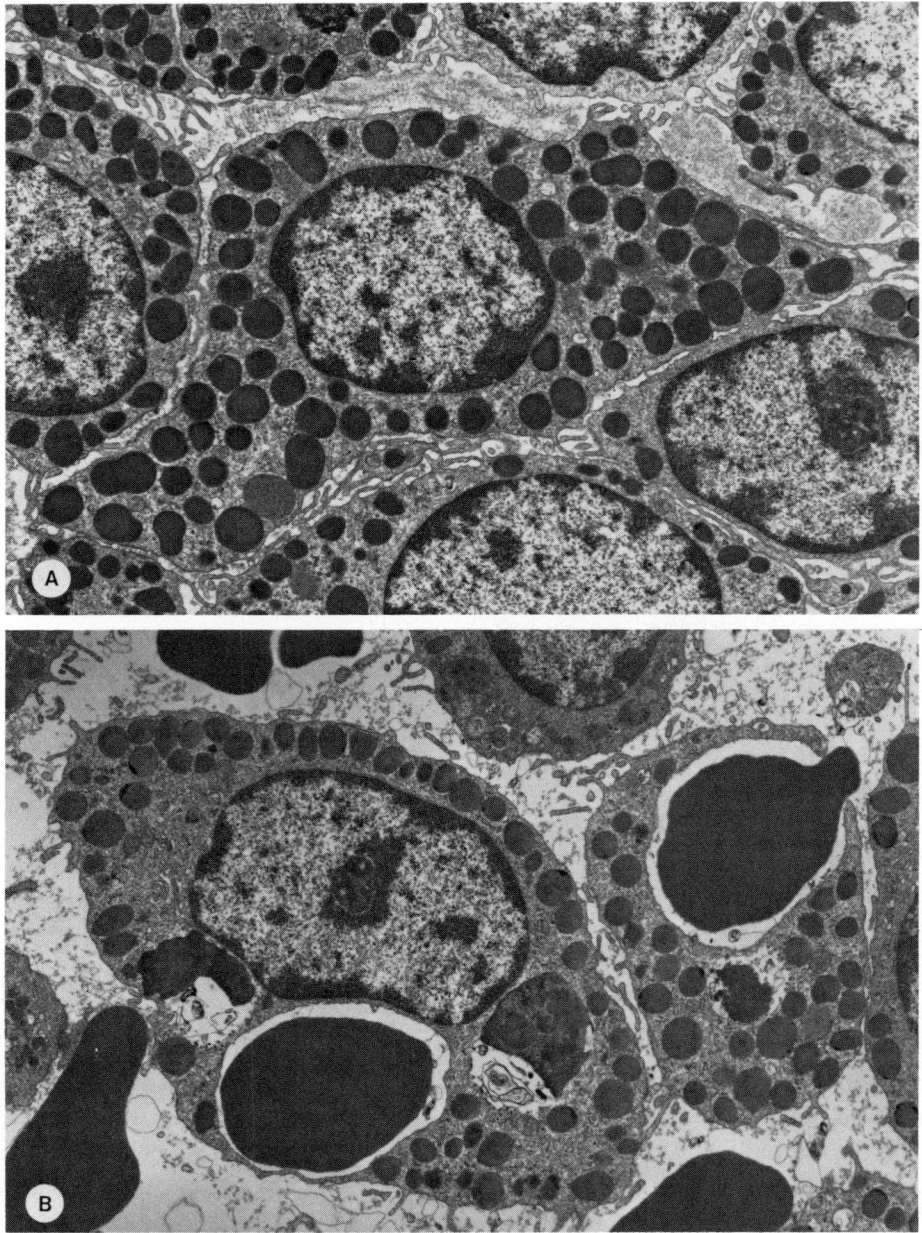

Fig. 32–23. Transmission electron photomicrographs of mast cells from splenic tissue of a cat with mast cell leukemia. Numerous small to large, homogeneously dense granules fill the cytoplasm of the mast cells in *A*; erythrophagocytosis is evident in cells in *B*. The large cell in *B* also shows two residual bodies originating from intracellular digestion of red cell stroma within the phagocytic vacuoles. Cell immaturity is evident from presence of a nucleolus and nuclei with poorly condensed chromatin in some of the cells. Short surface microvilli are also evident in some places. ×12,000. (Prepared with the assistance of Dr. Laurie O'Rourke.)

The most common gross lesion in mast cell leukemia is a marked enlargement of the spleen (Schalm, 1980g). There may be ulceration of the stomach and duodenum, sometimes leading to perforation and peritonitis, due to the high level of histamine in mast cells. A modest leukocytosis (25,000–30,000/ μl of blood) is characterized by the conspicuous presence of mast cells in the blood (Fig. 32-22), bone marrow (Plate XXII–6), spleen (Fig. 32-23), and liver, and with small foci of mast cells in other organs and tissues. Anemia and leukopenia may sometimes be seen.

Erythrophagocytosis by mast cells (Fig.

32–23) has been observed in a few cases of mast cell leukemia (Madewell et al., 1983; O'Rourke and Jain, 1982). Erythrophagocytosis by primitive malignant cells in the bone marrow and rarely in peripheral blood has been observed in myeloproliferative disorders in the cat (Plate XX-2) and by well-differentiated histiocytes in the bone marrow and other organs in a case of histiocytic medullary reticulosis ("malignant histiocytosis") in the dog (Schalm, 1978).

Megakaryocytic Leukemia

Megakaryocytic myelosis (leukemia) has been described in five cats (Hardy et al., 1981a; Michel et al., 1976; Schmidt et al., 1984; Sutton et al., 1978). It was characterized by a marked increase in circulating thrombocytes, with many giant and bizarre forms, and severe nonregenerative anemia. Hepatomegaly was present in two cases and splenomegaly in three cases. Megakaryocytes of abnormal morphology were present in the bone marrow, liver, and spleen. The megakaryocytes were tested to be FOCMA-positive in one case. A case of granulocytic leukemia with some evidence of megakaryocytic myelosis was reported in a cat (Sutton et al., 1978). The blood was characterized by numerous platelets, many of which were large and appeared immature, and many abnormal cells of the granulocytic series. Megakaryocytic proliferation was seen in the spleen. A role of megakaryocytes in development of myelofibrosis has been recently proposed (Castro-Malaspina and Moore, 1982).

Preleukemia and "Smoldering" Leukemia

Preleukemia, myelodysplastic syndrome, and hematopoietic dysplasia are terms used to describe a group of hypoproliferative hematologic abnormalities that precede development of an overt leukemia, usually acute myeloid leukemia (Bernard, 1976; Dreyfus, 1976; Fisher et al., 1973; Knospe and Gregory, 1971; Ricci et al., 1978; Sanal et al., 1979; Wintrobe et al., 1981). Prominent hematologic findings in preleukemic patients are anemia, neutropenia, and thrombocytopenia occurring singly or in combination. Morphologic abnormalities may also be seen in all three hematopoietic cell lines in blood and bone marrow.

In none of these disorders is there an excess of leukemic blast cells in the blood or bone marrow at the onset, and that the condition was preleukemic can be determined only in retrospect when the hematologic picture has progressed to an acute myeloid leukemia. The disease progresses very slowly, however, over a period of several months to years before terminating in an overt leukemia. In contrast to the preleukemic group, the "smoldering" or aleukemic leukemia shows more blast cells in marrow from the onset, while the blood shows cytopenias without blast cells (Fisher et al., 1973; Knospe and Gregory, 1971). The distinction may be subtle, however. New diagnostic criteria for the diagnosis of the various myelodysplastic syndromes in humans were proposed recently by the FAB cooperative group (Bennett et al., 1982). It has been suggested that patients considered to have smoldering leukemia already have a malignant clone established (Greenberg, 1983).

We have recognized such a syndrome of preleukemia in three cats (Table 32-8) with FeLV-associated hematopoietic disturbances preceding acute myeloid leukemia (Madewell et al., 1979). In all cats, blood picture was dominated by cytopenias and abnormal platelet morphology. In Cat 1, initial hematologic findings reflected anemia, macrocytosis, and leukopenia due both to neutropenia and lymphopenia. No blast cells were found in blood. However, bone marrow revealed predominance of poorly differentiated cells with some showing differentiation toward promyelocytes and some others toward monocytes. The disease progressed slowly for 3½ months before terminating in acute myelomonocytic leukemia recognized as blast crisis in blood. Cytochemical findings on blood and bone marrow leukocytes revealed distinct populations of cells with monocytic markers (α-naphthyl acetate esterase and α-naphthyl butyrate esterase) and with granulocytic markers (peroxidase and alkaline phosphatase).

In Cat 2, the initial hematologic abnormality included thrombocytopenia and leukopenia, primarily due to neutropenia. About 1 year later, it terminated in pancytopenia with left

Table 32–8.   Hematologic Findings in Three Preleukemic Cats

Factor	Cat 1		Cat 2		Cat 3	
	Day 0	Day 103	Day 0	Day 347	Day 0	Day 159
RBC ($\times 10^6/\mu l$)	1.99	2.59	5.19	1.68	7.36	4.26
Hemoglobin (g/dl)	3.7	5.4	8.7	3.1	10.2	6.7
PCV (%)	11	15	27	10	30	17
MCV (fl)	55.2	57.9	52.0	59.5	40.7	39.9
MCHC (%)	33.6	36.0	32.2	31.0	34.0	39.4
MCH (pg)	18.5	20.8	16.7	18.4	13.8	15.7
Plasma protein (g/dl)	8.0	8.0	7.5	7.8	7.0	6.1
Plasma fibrinogen (g/dl)	0.1	<0.1	0.4	0.2	<0.1	0.1
Reticulocytes (%)	rare	0	0	few	0	rare
Nucleated RBC (/100 WBC)	0	0	0	3	7	2
WBC[1]	1,900	178,400	3,400	2,700[2]	3,400[2]	40,700[2]
Blast cells	0	0	0	52% (1,404)	rare	72% (29,304)
Progranulocytes	0	0	0	6% (162)	rare	13% (5,291)
Myelocytes	0	0	0	4% (108)	rare	6% (2,442)
Metamyelocytes	0	0	0	2% (54)	1% (34)	2% (814)
Neutrophils	1,026	1,784	1,156	27	1,360	1,221
Segmented	52% (988)	1% (1,784)	34% (1,156)	0	39% (1,326)	2% (814)
Nonsegmented	2% (38)	0	0	1% (27)	1% (34)	1% (407)
Lymphocytes	42% (798)	4% (7,136)	49% (1,666)	35% (945)	48% (1,632)	4% (1,628)
Monocytes	2% (38)	0	17% (578)	0	3% (102)	0
Eosinophils	2% (38)	0	0	0	8% (272)	0
Basophils	0	0	0	0	0	0
Unclassified cells	0	95% (169,480)	0	0	0	0
Thrombocytes	Present	139,000	172,000	18,000	408,000	236,000
Platelet morphology	Pleomorphic; some very large	Pleomorphic;	Occasional; very large	Occasional; very large	Pleomorphic; many large	Many large

From Madewell et al., 1979; courtesy of *Veterinary Pathology*.
[1]Absolute values are expressed as cells/μl of blood.
[2]Leukocyte counts corrected for nucleated red blood cells.

shift to blast cells. A diagnosis of granulocytic (acute myeloblastic) leukemia was made on the basis of finding increased numbers of immature myeloid cells in blood and a predominance of myeloblasts and promyelocytes in bone marrow.

In Cat 3, the initial hematologic examination showed neutropenia and a leukoerythroblastic reaction (left shift with some immature cells to myeloblasts and nucleated erythrocytes). Bone marrow cytology showed a preponderance of myeloblasts and promyelocytes with complete myeloid and erythroid maturation. The blood and bone marrow findings were suggestive of subleukemic leukemia, but 5 months later, an overt granulocytic (acute myeloblastic) leukemia manifested in blood and bone marrow.

THE LEUKEMIA COMPLEX IN THE DOG

Lymphoma is the most common form of the leukemia complex in the dog. Primary lymphocytic leukemia is less common, and various forms of myelogenous leukemia have been described.

Lymphoproliferative Disorders

The annual incidence of lymphoma in the dog has been estimated at 24/100,000 (Dorn et al., 1967) and constitutes about 5–7% of all canine tumors seen (MacEwen et al., 1977b). Epidemiologic aspects of canine lymphoma have been summarized (Rosenthal, 1982; Schneider, 1983).

Viral Etiology and Pathogenesis

Etiology of canine lymphoma is being investigated. A canine leukemia virus has not been demonstrated unequivocally to be involved, although virus particles with retrovirus properties and reverse transcriptase activity have been found in lymphoid cells of dogs with lymphoma and lymphocytic leukemia (Onions, 1980; Tomley et., 1982, 1983a).

Pathogenesis of lymphocytic leukemia was studied in neonatal beagles inoculated with a cell line derived from a dog with lymphocytic leukemia and maintained in serial passages in neonates (Cohen et al., 1974). In subcutaneously inoculated dogs a local tumor mass developed, and leukemic cells were found to spread initially via the lymphatics to lymph nodes and subsequently by the blood stream to bone marrow and spleen; spread to the liver was considered secondary to the spleen via the portal venous system. The peripheral blood did not contain large numbers of neoplastic lymphocytes until after bone marrow and spleen were considerably infiltrated.

Clinical Findings

The most characteristic feature of canine lymphoma is bilateral painless swelling of superficial nodes. In fact, the owner often detects the disease while fondling the dog about the head and neck. Less frequently, the tonsils may be the cause of initial concern. Fleshy, nonulcerated enlargement of the tonsils may produce signs of choking and coughing. Although a low-grade fever may accompany lymphoma, the disease is more commonly afebrile. Edema of the face, throat, or limbs may be present in late stages of the disease. The edema may be more pronounced at one time than another.

Jarrett et al. (1966) divided the clinical manifestations of lymphoma into multicentric and alimentary types. Less common types may be classified as cutaneous, mediastinal (thymic), and miscellaneous forms (Theilen and Madewell, 1979). In addition, acute lymphoblastic and chronic lymphocytic leukemias may be encountered without solid tumor masses, although slight hepatosplenomegaly may be present (MacEwen et al., 1977b).

The *multicentric type* is by far the most common form and is characterized by bilateral lymphadenopathy of most superficial nodes, hepatosplenomegaly, and involvement of almost any other tissue or organ. It may develop in stages somewhat as follows: (1) initial lymphadenopathy in an active and relatively normal dog, (2) weight loss and mild alimentary disturbances, and (3) sudden change characterized by anorexia, listlessness, emaciation, dehydration, and death. About three-fourths of the dogs with this form of lymphoma show abnormal thoracic radiographs, and nearly half show abnormal abdominal radiographs (Ackerman and Madewell, 1980). Most multicentric lymphomas in the dog are of B-cell type (Holmberg et al., 1976b; Onions, 1977).

The *alimentary form* rarely involves superficial lymph nodes or the spleen, but the gut and mesenteric nodes are regularly involved. The alimentary type is characterized by progressive loss of condition, diarrhea, and a palpable mass in the mid-abdomen.

Although aforementioned clinical findings are common in dogs with lymphoma, they are not diagnostic. A definitive diagnosis requires laboratory finding of neoplastic cells in blood, bone marrow, and cytologic aspirates or biopsy specimens of lymph nodes or other tissues.

Age, Sex, and Breed Predilection

Among 75 dogs with lymphoma, age distribution was as follows: 2 to 4 years, 20%; 5 to 9 years, 61.3%; and 10 to 17 years, 18.6%. This age distribution is in agreement with many other reports stating that lymphoma occurs primarily in dogs 5 years of age and over. There were 37 females, of which 15 had been spayed, and 38 males, of which 3 had been castrated, thereby indicating no sex predilection.

Breed distribution was as follows: Four dogs were mongrels and dogs of thirty-eight different breeds were represented (eight German shepherd dogs, six boxer dogs, five beagles, four Labradors, and three each of cocker spaniels, collies, and English bulldogs). One dog each represented 31 additional breeds. It would appear *a priori* that incidence paralleled breed distribution in the general dog population of the community with the exception of boxer dogs and dachshunds. The incidence among boxers would appear to have been greater than could be attributed to breed popularity, and the incidence was less among dachshunds than might have been anticipated on the frequency of admissions of that breed to our hospital. Similar observations were reported in a larger survey in which breeds at relatively high risk included the boxer and Scottish terrier, whereas those at low risk included the dachshund (Rosenthal, 1982).

Blood Profile in Lymphoma

Means and standard deviations of various components for 72 dogs with lymphoma are presented in Table 32-9. Three dogs with total leukocyte counts of 120,000, 246,000, and 335,800/µl were excluded from the data (see Table 32-12). The oldest dogs (10–17 years) had a mean value of 35.1% for the packed cell volume (PCV), indicating presence of a borderline anemia. Among all 72 dogs, 37.5% of them had PCV values falling between 24 and 26%. Thus severe anemia was not a prominent feature in this group of lymphomatous dogs. The mild to modest anemia is often normocytic-normochromic and is generally believed to represent anemia of chronic disease. However, dogs with lymphoma may exhibit other types of anemias, e.g., immune-mediated, blood loss, diserythropoietic, microangiopathic, and aregenerative from therapy-induced marrow hypoplasia (Madewell and Feldman, 1980).

Mean values for total plasma proteins were similar for the three age groups (6.6-7.0 g/dl). However, 43% of the dogs had plasma protein concentrations falling below (4.5–6.5 g/dl) the anticipated normal values for their ages. Hepatosplenomegaly and generalized lymphadenopathy could be expected to result in decreased synthesis of plasma proteins, thus giving lower total values (Table 32-10). Elevated mean serum IgM levels have been reported in dogs with lymphoma (Madewell et al., 1980).

The mean total leukocyte counts among the 72 dogs were in the high normal range (15,500–16,500/µl) with a slight left shift, a modest monocytosis, and mean lymphocyte values within the normal range (Table 32-9). Table 32-11 summarizes the frequency of occurrence of leukocytosis (38.9%), neutrophilia (41.7%), lymphocytosis (20.8%), leukopenia (12.5%), and lymphopenia (25%). It is noteworthy that only 20.8% of the dogs with lymphoma exhibited a lymphocytosis (exclusive of the three dogs with extremely high counts referred to above) and 25.0% revealed frank lymphopenia. These findings are in agreement with those of other investigators in that *peripheral blood examination commonly is not diagnostic for canine lymphoma.* In other studies a frank leukemia was seen in 10% or less of the dogs with lymphoma (Cohen et al., 1974).

Careful examination of the stained blood film for lymphoblasts, prolymphocytes, or

Table 32–9. Blood Composition and Cytology in Canine Lymphoma in Three Age Groupings (means and 1 SD)

	14 Dogs 2–4 yr	45 Dogs 5–9 yr	13 Dogs 10–17 yr
PCV (%)	39.9 ± 8.3	39.9 ± 5.5	35.1 ± 5.3
RBC (× 10⁶/μl)	5.7 ± 1.3	5.7 ± 0.8	5.2 ± 0.8
Hb (g/dl)	13.2 ± 3.0	13.4 ± 2.0	11.7 ± 2.3
MCV (fl)	70.3 ± 3.8	69.5 ± 3.3	67.3 ± 3.0
MCHC (%)	32.9 ± 1.8	33.4 ± 1.6	32.8 ± 1.9
MCH (pg)	23.0 ± 1.2	23.3 ± 1.4	22.5 ± 2.3
Icterus index units	4.6 ± 4.4	5.4 ± 11.1	4.0 ± 4.8
Protein (g/dl)	6.9 ± 0.9	6.6 ± 1.1	7.0 ± 0.9
Fibrinogen (g/dl)	0.25 ± 0.10	0.223 ± 0.16	0.36 ± 0.13
WBC/μl	15,630 ± 10,570	16,547 ± 10,076	15,443 ± 8,333
Band neutrophils	363 ± 612	322 ± 630	520 ± 911
Neutrophils	9,510 ± 5,490	10,861 ± 6,994	12,678 ± 10,319
Lymphocytes	4,021 ± 4,831	3,436 ± 2,931	3,089 ± 3,538
Monocytes	1,481 ± 1,281	1,443 ± 2,219	1,168 ± 1,036
Eosinophils	93 ± 199	285 ± 550	181 ± 223
Basophils	142 ± 379	196 ± 843	3 ± 12
WBC (%)			
Band neutrophils	1.8 ± 2.6	1.1 ± 1.2	2.0 ± 2.6
Neutrophils	64.4 ± 16.9	66.3 ± 13.4	69.5 ± 16.7
Lymphocytes	21.5 ± 13.1	21.9 ± 12.9	20.5 ± 16.9
Monocytes	8.9 ± 3.9	7.8 ± 5.8	6.4 ± 3.6
Eosinophils	0.7 ± 1.3	1.8 ± 2.2	1.4 ± 2.1
Basophils	2.6 ± 8.2	0.8 ± 2.7	0.03 ± 0.12

large lymphocytes with diffuse nuclear chromatin revealed few to many lymphoblasts in 54% of the 72 dogs. An additional ten blood films contained some lymphocytes that were classified as immature. Significant cytologic features are lymphocytes of greater than normal size, a darker blue color of the cytoplasm than normal, and diffuse, coarsely clumped nuclear chromatin with or without nucleolar rings (Fig. 32-24). Presence of nucleoli or nucleolar rings permits classification of the cell as a lymphoblast (Plate XXI-1). Neoplastic lymphocytes may appear irregularly in small numbers in peripheral blood; therefore, their absence at initial examination does not exclude the possibility of finding lymphocytes of diagnostic significance in the blood at another time. It is generally believed that animals in advanced stages or terminal phases of lymphoma often exhibit neoplastic lymphocytes in blood and bone marrow. The fine structure of leukemic cells from such cases has been studied (Torres et al., 1976; Chapman et al., 1981).

Lymph node impression smears and films of aspirated fluid from an enlarged lymph node are generally more reliable than blood as a means of diagnosis (Plate XXI-2). Aspirated bone marrow may also be helpful, although the bone marrow is not regularly invaded in canine lymphoma (Schalm, 1980h). Cytologic specimens from other organs or tissues may also be helpful. In such cases finding excessive numbers of lymphoblasts or abnormal lymphocytes constitutes the diagnosis of lymphoma.

Blood platelet counts were made on 34 of the 72 dogs: normal range (200,000–500,000/ μl of blood); platelets numbered 221,000–588,000 in 16 dogs; 101,000–135,000 in 9 dogs, and 21,000–89,000 in the remaining 9 dogs. Thus 18 dogs (53%) exhibited some degree of thrombocytopenia, although none experienced bleeding problems.

Other Abnormalities

Hypercalcemia is frequently observed in dogs with lymphoma with a somewhat higher frequency in Saint Bernards and in males than in females (about 3:2). The hypercalcemia is attributed to bone-resorbing factors (e.g., osteoclast activating factor) released from tumor cells and not to "ectopic" secretion of parathormone (Heath et al., 1980; Weller et al., 1982a). Similar observations have been reported in humans (Grossman et al., 1981). Chromosomal abnormalities were found in a case of disseminated lymphoma (Idowu, 1976). An immune deficiency involving T cells has been described in dogs with lymphoma

Table 32-10. Representative Hemograms in Canine Lymphoma Characterized by Generalized Lymphadenopathy, Associated with Hepatomegaly in Four Dogs and Splenomegaly in Seven Dogs[a] (Selected cases from those summarized in Table 32-9)

Case No.	Breed	Sex	Age (yr)	PCV (%)	ESR[b]	Plasma Proteins (g/dl) Total	Fibrinogen	WBC/μl	Differential Leukocyte Count—Absolute Numbers/μl Band	Segmenters	Lymphocytes[c]	Monocytes	Eosinophils	Basophils	Unclassified	Degenerated
101186 G 8729	Cocker	M	6	32 (S)	13+	6.3	0.3 (H)	24,000	960	10,440	9,840++	1,080	240	0	0	1,440
67 S 1479 G 7331	Bulldog	F	5	46 (S)	2−	8.5	0.3	12,500	63	7,563	3,437+	1,125	250	63	0	0
100517 G 7888	Doberman	M	6	36 (S)	13+	5.6	0.0 (H)	15,400	0	3,619	11,550++	154	77	0	0	0
101497 G 9137	Collie	F	2	32	35+	9.6	0.3	8,500	510	6,035	255	510	0	0	935[d]	255
101509 G 9157	Border collie	M	9	38 (S)	14+	6.9	0.2	22,300	0	14,272	5,575++	2,119	335	0	0	0
102267 H 0379	Hound	M	7	33 (S)	16+	6.5	0.2 (H)	11,000	55	7,425	1,980+	990	495	55	0	0
100296 G 7643	Vizsla	M	8	39 (S)	—	5.7	0.35 (H)	17,800	0	12,913	3,827+	979	623	0	0	178
103132 H 1087	Chihuahua	M	7	33	—	6.6	0.3	12,300	61	7,381	2,783+	1,149	726	0	0	0
103792 H 3077	Cocker	F	9	26	14+	7.0	0.3	22,700	341	15,095	5,561+	1,703	0	0	0	0
66 S 2032 G 6040	German shepherd	F	10	40	9+	7.0	—	16,600	0	11,703	2,324	1,411	1,079	83	0	0
100379 G 7734	Boxer	M	7	44 (S)	4−	7.3	0.1	3,900	0	2,535	897+	195	156	117	0	0

[a]All dogs exhibited lymph node enlargement, in most cases generalized. Hepatomegaly is indicated by (H) following fibrinogen value; splenomegaly is indicated by (S) following PCV value.

[b]Corrected erythrocyte sedimentation rate at 1 hour.

[c]+, Occasional immature lymphocyte; ++, moderate number of immature lymphocytes.

[d]Large, dark neoplastic cells.

Table 32–11.   Number and Percentage of Dogs with Lymphoma in Three Age Groups with Leukocytosis, Lymphocytosis, Neutrophilia, Leukopenia, and/or Lymphophenia

Condition	14 Dogs 2–4 Yr Old	45 Dogs 5–9 Yr Old	13 Dogs 10–17 Yr Old	Total 72 Dogs
Leukocytosis (>17,000)				
No. of Dogs	5	16	7	28
% of All Dogs	35.7	35.5	53.8	38.9
Range per μl	17,800–47,200	17,800–47,200	18,300–52,800	17,800–52,800
Mean ± 1 SD per μl	28,600 ± 13,000	28,343 ± 8,995	28,542 ± 11,750	28,439 ± 10,037
Lymphocytosis (>5,000)				
No. of Dogs	3	9	3	15
% of All Dogs	21.4	20.0	23.1	20.8
Range per μl	8,036–17,382	5,005–12,600	7,164–14,892	5,005–17,382
Mean ± 1 SD per μl	13,750 ± 5,008	7,958 ± 3,285	9,826 ± 4,388	9,490 ± 4,234
Neutrophilia (>11,500)				
No. of Dogs	5	19	6	30
% of All Dogs	35.7	42.2	46.1	41.7
Range per μl	12,382–26,091	12,193–34,456	15,640–46,992	12,193–46,992
Mean ± 1 SD per μl	17,375 ± 5,300	18,103 ± 7,345	24,990 ± 11,858	18,379 ± 8,926
Leukopenia (<6,000)				
No. of Dogs	2	4	3	9
% of All Dogs	14.3	8.8	23.1	12.5
Range per μl	4,000–4,100	3,900–5,400	3,700–5,800	3,700–5,800
Mean ± 1 SD per μl	4,050 ± 70	4,650 ± 810	4,566 ± 1,097	4,488 ± 781
Lymphopenia (<1,200)				
No. of Dogs	5	10	3	18
% of All Dogs	35.7	22.2	23.1	25.0
Range per μl	255–1,066	378–1,060	440–823	255–1,066
Mean ± 1 SD per μl	840 ± 377	782 ± 275	634 ± 192	774 ± 275

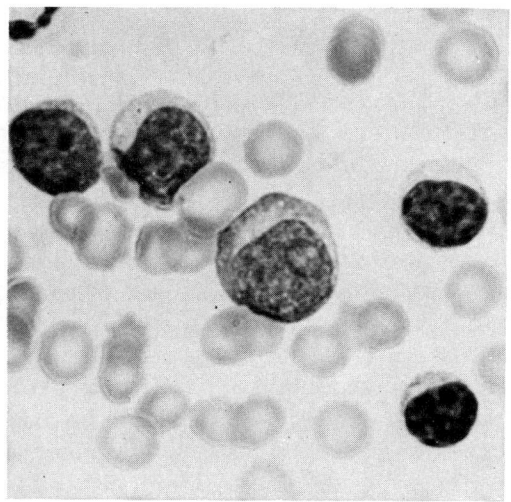

Fig. 32–24.   Blood in canine lymphoma with a total leukocyte count of 200,000/μl with 84% lymphocytes. The two smallest cells are normal lymphocytes, the center cell is a lymphoblast with a single large nucleolus, and the two medium-sized cells are prolymphocytes. ×2,700.

(Weiden et al., 1974). Paraneoplastic disorders in dogs with hematopoietic tumors have been reviewed (Weller, 1985).

Histopathologic and Immunologic Characterization

Morphologic and immunologic properties of 23 cases of canine lymphoma were studied by Holmberg et al., (1976b). Results indicated that (a) three distinct groups of histologic cell types were evident, namely, lymphocytic, poorly differentiated; "histiocytic"; and lymphocytic, well differentiated; (b) cells from "histiocytic" lymphoma were lymphocytes rather than histiocytes or macrophages; and (c) most lymphomas had a multicentric distribution and were of B-cell type. Histologic classification of lymphoma in 72 dogs was attempted according to the Rappaport classification of human lymphomas (Rappaport, 1966) with the following results (Weller et al., 1980b): nodular lymphoma was seen in 7 (9.7%) and diffuse in 65 (90.3%) cases. It was concluded that histologic classification of canine lymphomas according to the Rappaport schema cannot be used as a prognostic criterion in predicting therapeutic response, remission, or survival, although dogs with diffuse "histiocytic" lymphoma were found to have longer remission durations.

Acute and Chronic Lymphocytic Leukemias

In recent years acute lymphocytic leukemia (ALL) and chronic lymphocytic leukemia (CLL) have been recognized as distinct entities in the dog (Leifer and Matus, 1985; Matus et al., 1983). CLL is a disease of middle-aged to older dogs (mean age 9.4 years), while ALL is seen in relatively younger dogs (mean age 6.2 years). Both diseases seem to be more common in males than in females with a ratio of 3:2 for ALL and 2:1 for CLL. Breed distribution revealed German shepherd dogs to comprise 27% of the 30 cases of ALL reported by Matus (1983). The clinical course in CLL is more protracted and the physical signs (except for lymphadenopathy) are less pronounced in CLL and lymphoma than in ALL. The prognosis is said to be more favorable for CLL than for ALL (Leifer and Matus, 1985).

Acute lymphocytic leukemia is a rapidly progressive disease of sudden onset. It is characterized by high numbers of poorly differentiated lymphocytes (lymphoblasts) in the peripheral blood and bone marrow, usually unassociated with solid tumor masses. Chief complaints include lethargy, anorexia, vomiting, and diarrhea of a few weeks' duration. Clinical signs include anemia, splenomegaly, and hepatomegaly. Laboratory findings are, in addition to abnormal lymphocytes in blood and bone marrow, a nonregenerative normocytic-normochromic anemia and thrombocytopenia. Bone marrow shows myelosuppression with diminished megakaryocytopoiesis and erythropoiesis. Central nervous system involvement with leukemic cells may be seen (Rosin, 1982). Diminished B and T cell reactivity and mononuclear phagocytic function have been found (Leifer and Matus, 1985).

Chronic lymphocytic leukemia is a disease of long course manifesting over a period of several months or years and characterized by excessive numbers of well-differentiated (ma-

ture) lymphocytes in the peripheral blood and bone marrow. Bone marrow infiltration is patchy in early cases and diffuse in later cases. Clinical and laboratory findings may include lethargy, partial anorexia, anemia, ascites, azotemia, and proteinuria. Peripheral lymphadenopathy is generally absent, but internal lymph nodes may be slightly to moderately enlarged and hepatosplenomegaly may be seen.

Chronic lymphocytic leukemia is considered a disease of B-lymphocytes. Serum concentrations of IgM, IgG, and IgA may be increased, although hypogammaglobulinemia may be seen in about 10% of the cases (Hodgkins et al., 1980; Leifer and Matus, 1985). Over 50% of the cases show a monoclonal peak (usually IgM), and Bence Jones protein may be found in about half of the cases with monoclonal gammopathy. Hyperviscosity syndrome associated with monoclonal increase in IgA or IgM was observed in four dogs with lymphocytic leukemia (Braund et al., 1978; MacEwen et al., 1977a). Pathologic findings in chronic lymphocytic leukemia are generally similar to lymphoma.

Leukemia with peripheral leukocyte counts in excess of 100,000/μl, of which 85 to 97.5% of cells were of lymphoid origin, was seen in seven intact male dogs, 9 months to 13 years of age (Table 32-12). These seven dogs represented about 3% of all the dogs presented with the leukemia complex over a period of several years. Depression of several weeks' duration, periodic vomiting, occasional bouts of diarrhea, loss of appetite, increased thirst, weight loss, and occasionally elevated body temperatures were the most common clinical signs. Five of the dogs had bilateral peripheral lymphadenopathy, while no enlargement of external lymph nodes was detectable in two of the dogs. Aspiration of bone marrow from three of the dogs revealed massive displacement of marrow by neoplastic lymphocytes. Splenomegaly was present in four of five dogs on which necropsy was permitted. With the one exception of the 9-month-old collie dog, all dogs experienced anemia (PCV 16–31%), and two dogs had thrombocytopenia unaccompanied by bleeding. Hypoproteinemia was present in two of three dogs tested. The fact that three of seven dogs were boxers is

Table 32–12. Hemograms in Lymphocytic Leukemic Leukemia in the Dog

Breed	Age (yr)	Sex	Lymphadenopathy and Organ Involvement	PCV (%)	Plasma Proteins (g/dl)	WBC/μl	Differential Leukocyte Count (%)									
							Neutrophils			Lymphocytes			Mono-cytes	Eosino-phils	Baso-phils	Degener-ated
							Meta.	Band	Seg.	Blast	Pro	Mature				
Doberman	3	M	All nodes, spleno-megaly, kidneys, and bone marrow	21	—	575,000	0	0	2.0	0	2.0	95.0	1.0	0	0	0
Boxer	8	M	No external node involved. Spleen, bone marrow, and few internal nodes	24	—	580,000	0	0	0.2	0.6	6.8	89.6	0.2	0	0	2.6
Cairn terrier	10	M	Generalized with splenomegaly	23	—	120,000	0	0	12.0	+[b]	85.0	0	3.0	0	0	0
Boxer	6	M	Several peripheral nodes[a]	16	4.9	335,800	0	0.5	2.0	+[b]	97.5	0	0	0	0	0
Sealyham terrier	3	M	Generalized with bone marrow in-vasion	31	5.2	246,000	0	0	8.0	0	+[b]	88.5	3.0	0.5	0	0
Collie	¾	M	No peripheral node enlargement	42	7.9	131,000	0	0	4.5	0	94.5[c]	0	0	0	0	1.0
Boxer	13	M	Generalized, with hepatopathy and splenomegaly	28	—	216,000	0	0.5	0	0.05	1.5	82.0 (atypical)	0	0	0	7.0

[a]Necropsy not authorized.
[b]Seen on scanning only.
[c]All cells large atypical, in clusters.

of interest in view of the opinion expressed by others that boxers are more susceptible to lymphoma than other purebred dogs.

The two dogs having no enlargement of peripheral lymph nodes are of interest in that diagnosis was dependent entirely on blood studies. The 8-year-old boxer was observed for 18 months. During the first 6 months, the leukocyte count varied between 340,000 and 580,000. During the second 6 months, leukocyte counts were 106,000 to 393,000. In the final 6 months, 9-α-fluoro-hydrocortisone was administered daily by oral route. Leukocyte counts gradually decreased and were within the normal range during the last 3 months of life. However, the general condition of the dog deteriorated rapidly, with excessive weight loss. The dog was killed for humane reasons, and at necropsy, the spleen was found to be enlarged, as were the anterior cervical, renal, and hepatic lymph nodes. Histologically, the spleen and nodes were not diffusely involved with neoplastic lymphocytes, as is common to terminal lymphoma. This may have been a result in part of the protracted steroid therapy. The 9-month-old collie had exhibited depression, anorexia, polydipsia, and polyuria for 3 weeks and a loss of approximately 20 pounds of body weight. Blood examination revealed a leukocyte count of 131,000/μl, with 94.5% of cells described as large, atypical, vacuolated lymphoid cells with dark cytoplasm arranged in groups or clusters. The owner requested that the dog be destroyed, but necropsy was not permitted.

Burkitt's Lymphoma

Burkitt's lymphoma was initially considered a specific lymphoid tumor of children in Africa. It is a nonleukemic lymphoid tumor involving the visceral organs and bone marrow, particularly of the jaw. A characteristic feature is the scattering of phagocytic histiocytes among densely packed neoplastic lymphocytes, a pattern that gave rise to the term "starry sky" effect (O'Connor et al., 1965). The lymphoid cells involved have been invariably B-lymphocytes (Berard et al., 1978). A herpes-like virus, the Epstein-Barr virus, has been isolated from cells of many patients with Burkitt's lymphoma and is thought to be the etiologic agent of this disease. Although Lukes and coworkers (1966), in a histologic study of a large number of canine lymphomas, found many to present the starry sky pattern, true Burkitt's lymphoma has not been described in animals.

Hodgkin's Disease

Hodgkin's disease in humans is a lymphoid neoplasm recognized by its characteristic histology. The tumor in the lymph nodes begins with lymphocytic hyperplasia, followed by a gradual loss of normal architecture with replacement of the lymphocytes as the disease progresses. Binuclear or multinuclear giant cells, called Reed-Sternberg cells, are pathognomonic, and their presence is essential for diagnosis. In addition, lymph node histology consists of a mixed infiltrate of lymphocytes, histiocytes, eosinophils, plasma cells, and neutrophils. Typical Hodgkin's disease has not been found in animals, although several cases of possible Hodgkin's disease in the dog have been reported (Meier, 1957; Moulton and Bostick, 1958; Simon et al., 1964; Strandstrom and Rimaila-Parnanen, 1979) and reviewed (Hoerni et al., 1970; Wells, 1974).

Multiple Myeloma

This is described in Chapter 34.

Myeloproliferative Disorders

Myelogenous (Granulocytic) Leukemia

Acute and chronic granulocytic leukemias have been described in the dog (Barthel, 1974; Cooper and Watson, 1975; Green and Barton, 1977; Grindem, 1985; Grindem et al., 1977; Joiner et al., 1976; Leifer et al., 1983; Linnabary et al., 1978; Medway and Rapp, 1962; Meier, 1957; Roscher et al., 1960; Skelley, 1963; Weller et al., 1980c), and blast crisis in a case of granulocytic leukemia has been reported (Pollet et al., 1978). Six dogs with histologically verified granulocytic leukemia are briefly described in Table 32-12; Appendix Case 16 provides details of one of these cases. Four dogs were 16 months to 4 years of age, one dog was 5 years old, and the other was 7 years of age. These observations as well as reports of others seem to indicate that myelogenous leukemia is more common in young

Table 32–13. Hematologic and Other Data on Dogs Proven to be Histologically Positive for Granulocytic Leukemia

Breed, Sex, and Age	Clinical History and Clinical Signs	PCV (%)	WBC/μl	Differential Neutrophil Count (%)						Necropsy Findings and Other Comments
				Blast	Pro.	Myelo.	Meta.	Band	Segs.	
Walker hound, male, 16 mo	Progressive weakness and depression last few months; temp. normal	7.0	37,300–132,000	6.0	1.5	0.5	4.5	4.0	73.5	Hypersegmented mature neutrophils, platelets low. Spleen, liver, kidneys, and nodes enlarged.
German shepherd, XF, 17 mo (Plate XXIII–3)	Left eye corneal opacity, prescapular node enlarged; temp. 104°F	26.0	86,000–127,000	25.5	0.0	0.0	0.5	6.5	8.0	In blood, 57.0% large vacuolated monocytes. Bone marrow, many bizarre cell forms. Gross involvement of heart, spleen, liver, and kidneys.
German shepherd, XF, 2½ yr (Appendix Case 16)	Depression and anemia at 6 mo of age; last mo, anorexia, weakness, emaciation; temp. 103–105°F	9.0	116,000	3.3	2.4	2.4	1.0	0.7	64.5	In blood, 19.7% lymphocytes and 22.6% monocytes. M:E 36:1.0. Spleen 30 × 13 cm, wt. 400 gm, slight swelling of lymph nodes (Plate XXIII–4).
German shorthair pointer, XF, 5 yr	Gradual weight loss and anorexia for 1 week; temp. 102°F; hepatosplenomegaly	26.0	10,800	0.0	0.0	0.0	3.0	7.0	70.5	Liver 2½ times and spleen 3–4 times normal size, massively infiltrated by blasts to mature neutrophils. M:E 2.4:1.0.
Irish setter, female, 7 yr (Plate XXIII–2)	Less active for 1 year; extreme weight loss last 3 mo	26.0	29,900	3.0	3.0	55.0	3.0	5.0	20.0	Platelets 107,000/μl. Spleen enlarged. Kidneys 2 times normal size, mottled red. Liver mottled; greenish cast to both liver and bone marrow.[a] Slight swelling of lymph nodes.
Doberman pinscher, male, 4 yr (est.) (Figs. 32–25, 32–26, 32–28)	Sudden onset of conjunctivitis, vomiting, and depression. Jaw paralysis one week later.	16.0	124,000	1.0	1.5	7.5	20.0	15.0	49.0	Gross neoplastic involvement of all major organs, including trigeminal and vagus nerves. Greenish cast to neoplastic tissue.[a]

[a]Greenish color is said to be due to myeloperoxidase; the condition is referred to as chloroma.

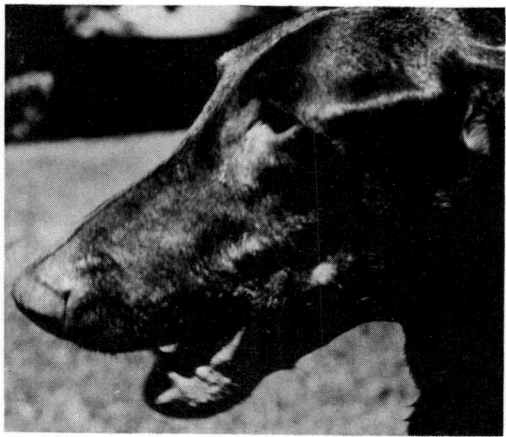

Fig. 32–25. Jaw paralysis in a dog with granulocytic leukemia involving the fifth, seventh, and ninth cranial nerve sheaths. See also Table 32–13.

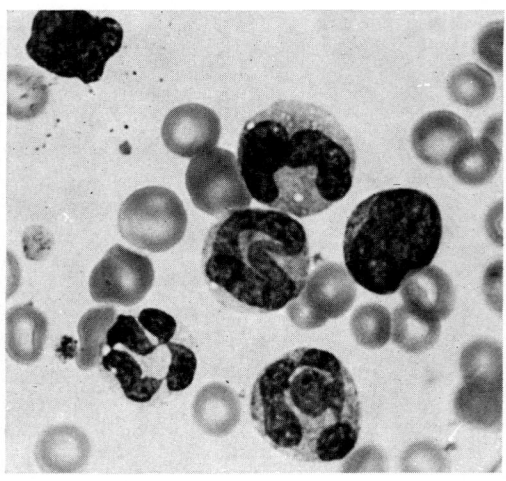

Fig. 32–26. Blood in canine granulocytic leukemia. Neutrophils vary in size and shape of the nucleus. Some cells have monocytoid characteristics. ×2,700.

dogs, while lymphoma is more common in older dogs.

Clinical Signs. Progressive weakness and weight loss over a period of several months are common complaints. In addition, anorexia, vomiting, polydipsia, polyuria, diarrhea, and anemia are present in various combinations. Physical examination commonly reveals a slight to moderate lymphadenopathy of peripheral nodes, and abdominal palpation reveals the existence of splenomegaly and sometimes hepatomegaly.

Unique and misleading clinical signs may develop as a result of neoplastic cell invasion of a great variety of tissues and organs. An example was encountered in a 4-year-old male Doberman pinscher dog (Theilen and Schalm, 1970; Table 32-13). This dog's illness began with the sudden onset of conjunctivitis, prominent membrana nictitans, icterus, recurrent vomiting, and depression. One week later, the dog was unable to close its mouth (Fig. 32-25). Other signs at this time were fever and abdominal tenderness.

Paralysis of the lower jaw distracted attention from the true nature of the disease until blood examination revealed the problem to be myelogenous leukemia. Most organs were found to be involved in the neoplastic process, but of special significance was tumorous involvement of the fifth, seventh, and ninth cranial nerve sheaths. Another interesting feature, noted at necropsy, was a greenish

coloration of the tumor tissue referred to as chloroma or chlorleukemia. The greenish pigmentation is due to myeloperoxidase. Chloroma was also seen in a 7-year-old female Irish Setter (Table 32-13).

Hematology of Granulocytic Leukemia. A truly leukemic blood has been a common finding in the dog with granulocytic leukemia. At some phase of the disease, the blood may not be diagnostic for leukemia. This was the case in a German shorthair pointer (Table 32-13) in which the leukocyte count was 10,800, with a left shift to metamyelocytes. Examination of bone marrow cytology revealed normal cellularity, but 17.0% of nucleated cells were myeloblasts, promyelocytes, and neutrophilic myelocytes. This marrow cytology indicated a disturbance in both maturation and release of neutrophilic granuocytes to the blood.

The typical blood picture of granulocytic leukemia is a neutrophilia with disorderly left shift to myeloblasts (Plate XXIII-1). The neutrophils exhibit considerable variation in shape and size (Fig. 32-26), and is some instance hypersegmentation of the mature neutrophils is a prominent feature (Fig. 32-27). Neoplastic neutrophils are susceptible to rapidly occurring degenerative changes with aging of the withdrawn blood sample (Schalm, 1980i). The degenerative changes consist of vacuolation of the cytoplasm and

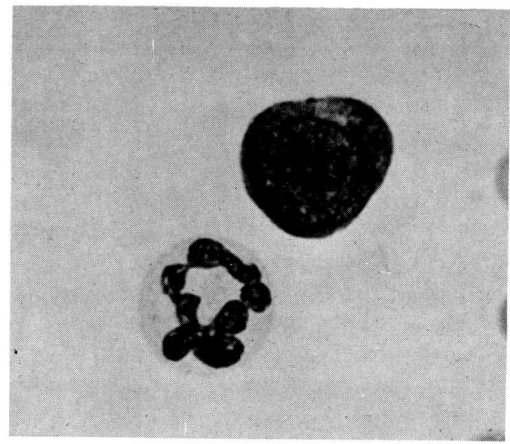

Fig. 32–27. Blood in canine granulocytic leukemia. A myeloblast and a hypersegmented neutrophil. ×2,700.

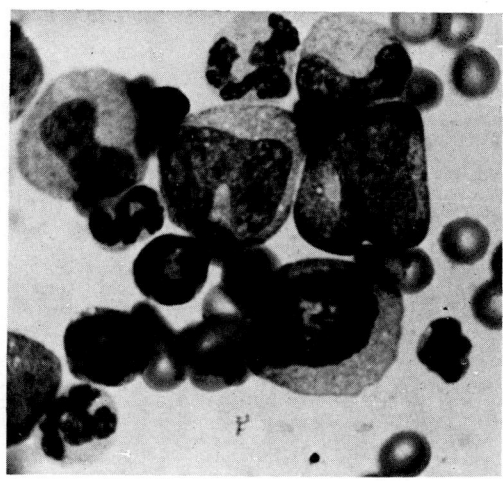

Fig. 32–29. Bone marrow in canine granulocytic leukemia, suggesting existence of two separate cell lines, normal and neoplastic. ×2,700.

possible shrinkage of the cell (Fig. 32-28). These changes in cell morphology make it difficult to differentiate degenerating neoplastic neutrophils from monocytes. Degenerative changes take place within 1 hour of withdrawal of blood from the animal.

Two cell lines of neutrophilic granulocytes in the blood may be suggested by the occurrence of neutrophils of normal morphology and the somewhat larger basophilic cells with bizarre nuclear patterns. The coexistence of a neoplastic cell line and a normal cell line may seem even more likely after examination of aspirated bone marrow, where large granulocytes in several stages of maturation are ad-

mixed with neutrophils undergoing a normal maturation (Fig. 32-29). In the event the neoplastic cells are too primitive or bizarre (Plate XXIII–2, XXIII–3) to be classified unequivocally as granulocytes, their granulocytic origin can be verified by application of cytochemical stains (Chapter 33). Granulocytes from the progranulocytic stage onward normally demonstrate a profusion of peroxidase-positive granules scattered over the nucleus and cytoplasm (Fig. 32-30). Cells of lymphocytic origin do not have peroxidase-positive granules, while monocytes may present a few such granules but usually far fewer than are

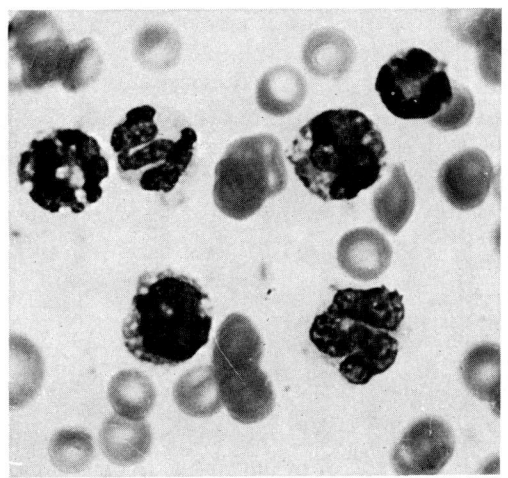

Fig. 32–28. Same blood as Fig. 32–26 after aging for 2 hours. Note shrinkage and vacuolation of neutrophils. ×2,700.

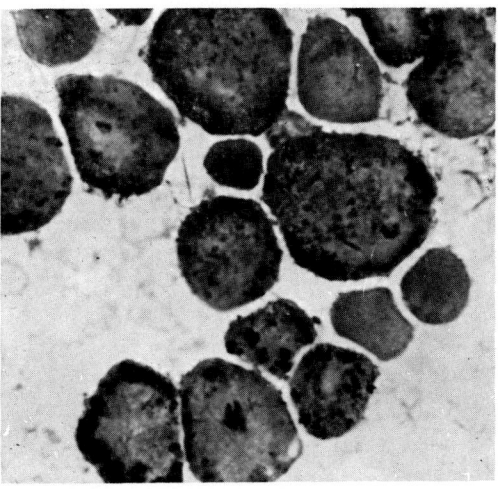

Fig. 32–30. Peroxidase-positive cells in the bone marrow in granulocytic leukemia of the dog. ×27,000.

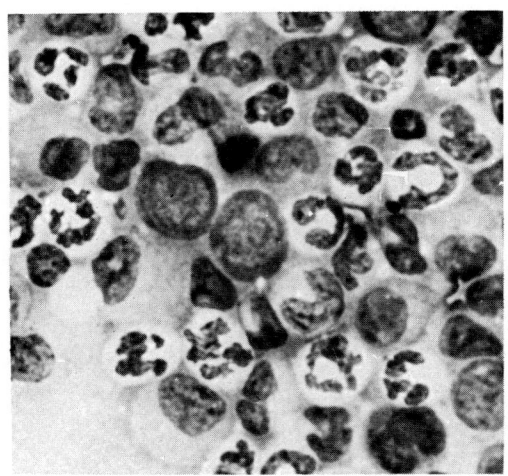

Fig. 32–31. Lymph node impression smear in canine granulocytic leukemia. All cells are of the granulocytic maturation series. ×1,400.

presented by neutrophils. On rare occasion, the neoplastic cells in blood and bone marrow do not resemble granulocytes (Plate XXIII-5), and they are peroxidase-negative. A positive reaction for alkaline phosphatase (Plate XXIII–6) is viewed as evidence that the cells are leukemic granulocytes (Chapter 33).

Massive displacement of the bone marrow by neoplastic granulocytes (Plates XXIII-4) leads to a marked reduction in erythrocyte production, so anemia is a common feature of the hemogram of myelogenous leukemia. In some instances, the anemia is so severe that the circulating erythrocytic mass is less than 10% of peripheral blood volume (Table 32-13). Similarly, megakaryocytopoiesis may be depressed, resulting in thrombocytopenia. Extramedullary hematopoiesis in the liver, spleen, and lymph nodes is a common histologic finding but is inadequate to correct the developing anemia. Stained films of material aspirated from enlarged lymph nodes may reveal large numbers of neutrophilic granulocytes in various stages of maturation (Fig. 32-31).

Monocytic and Myelomonocytic Leukemias

Monocytic and myelomonocytic leukemias have also been found to occur in the dog; several cases of spontaneously occurring (Barthel, 1974; Green and Barton, 1977; Grindem, 1985; Jain et al., 1981; Linnabary et al., 1978;

Latimer and Dykstra, 1984, Mackey et al., 1975; Ragan et al., 1976) and radiation-induced (Dungworth et al., 1969; Fritz et al., 1970; Shifrine et al., 1973; Tolle et al., 1979) disease have been reported. Myelomonocytic leukemia cells allografted prenatally in developing purebred beagle fetuses elicited tumor formation postnatally in some pups (Shifrine and Bryant, 1976).

Monocytic or myelomonocytic leukemia, like myelogenous leukemia, is a disease of young dogs. The diagnosis of monocytic leukemia is generally made when increased numbers of mature and immature monocytes are found in the circulation and bone marrow unassociated with inflammatory or other conditions known to induce monocytosis. The diagnosis of myelomonocytic leukemia is considered when the bone marrow abounds with an admixture of blast cells having features of myeloblasts and having monocytoid appearance, and the blood contains numbers of similar cells (Plates XXIV–1 through XXIV–4). In most cases, accurate identification of the cell type is difficult in Romanowsky-stained blood and bone marrow films. In such cases cytochemical staining for neutrophilic and monocytic markers (see Chapter 33) provides helpful information about lines of cellular differentiation (Plates XXIV–5, XXIV–6). For example, cytochemical characterization of blood and bone marrow cells for alkaline phosphatase and nonspecific esterase (α-naphthyl acetate esterase and α-naphthyl butyrate esterase) led to diagnosis of acute myelomonocytic leukemia in five dogs (Jain et al., 1981). Similar observations have been made in other studies (Latimer and Dykstra, 1984). Ultrastructure features of leukemic cells from dogs with myelomonocytic, monocytic, and lymphocytic leukemias have been compared (Grindem, 1985; Latimer and Dykstra, 1984).

Megakaryocytic Leukemia

This is an extremely rare form of MPD. Three cases of megakaryocytic leukemia (Holscher et al., 1978; Nielsen, 1970; Rudolph and Hübner, 1972) and a case of MPD with megakaryocytic predominance in association with occult dirofilariasis (Harvey et al., 1982) have been reported in the dog. The case described by Holscher and coworkers concerned a 2-year-old male Afghan dog that was anorexic and had progressive weakness in the rear legs. No abnormalities were detected in lateral spinal and pelvic radiographs. Blood urea nitrogen (BUN), and serum glutamic-pyruvic transaminase (SGPT) were within normal range. PCV was 18%, and WBC count was 5,723/μl. Many blast cells but no platelets were seen in blood film, and a diagnosis of myelomonocytic leukemia was made on the basis of a bone marrow biopsy. The dog was euthanized at the owner's request after supportive therapy for 10 days did not result in improvement.

Necropsy findings included marked hepatosplenomegaly and slightly enlarged superficial and visceral lymph nodes. Histopathologic examination of bone marrow specimens revealed numerous (>80%) megakaryocytes and their precursors and scarce myeloid and erythroid elements. Megakaryocytic cells were also found in other tissues such as the lymph nodes, spleen, liver, lungs, and kidneys. Cytochemical staining of bone marrow and lymph node smears revealed these cells to be strongly positive for PAS reaction, diffusely positive for an α-naphthyl acetate esterase, weakly sudanophilic, and negative for naphthol AS-D chloracetate esterase. These histologic and cytochemical findings supported the diagnosis of megakaryocytic leukemia and not of myelomonocytic leukemia.

Basophilic and Mast Cell Leukemias

True basophilic leukemia has been reported in two dogs (Alroy, 1972; MacEwen et al., 1975).

Mast cells are normally found in the tissues and must be distinguished from the basophil leukocyte when found in the blood. They differ from the basophil granulocyte (Plate VII-5) in that the mast cell nucleus is round and often covered by densely stained, blackish purple granules that also fill the cytoplasm. In some instances of neoplastic transformation of mast cells to form mastocytomas, the neoplastic mast cells may appear in the blood in considerable numbers, giving rise to a mast cell leukemia (Fig. 32-32). Two cases of mast cell leukemia are briefly described.

An intact female cocker spaniel, 13 years

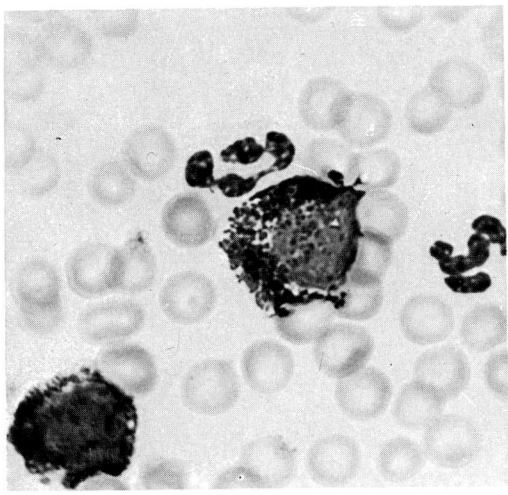

Fig. 32–32. Mast cells in blood of a dog with extensive mast cell neoplasia. ×2,700.

old, was admitted having been treated a month before for extensive subcutaneous edema of the left axillary region. The swelling reappeared 5 days before the present admission. Other signs were complete anorexia, polydipsia, polyuria, and severe vomiting. Rectal temperature was 103.8°F; the pulse was 160/minute and described as weak and thready; respiration was panting.

There was a 1-cm pigmented cutaneous tumor on the left side of the lower lip and a 2-cm tumor anterior to the sternum on the mid-line. A firm subcutaneous mass was present on the left side lateral to the mammary line with cords of tissue and extensive edema. Multiple tumors involved the first, second, and fourth left mammary glands and the second right gland. Lymph nodes were of normal size, with the exception of the left prescapular node. During 2 days of observation before the dog died, pyrexia and vomiting persisted. Two hemograms revealed total leukocyte counts of 18,600 and 35,400/μl of blood with 18.5% and 40.5% mast cells (Fig. 32-32), respectively. A bone marrow sample contained 60.4% mast cells (Fig. 32-33).

At necropsy, the mucosa of the pylorus contained many focal ulcerations, and a 3-mm perforating ulcer was present in the duodenum about 8 cm from the pylorus. It is possible that these lesions were the result of histamine release from the large concentration of mast cells in the body. Liver and spleen

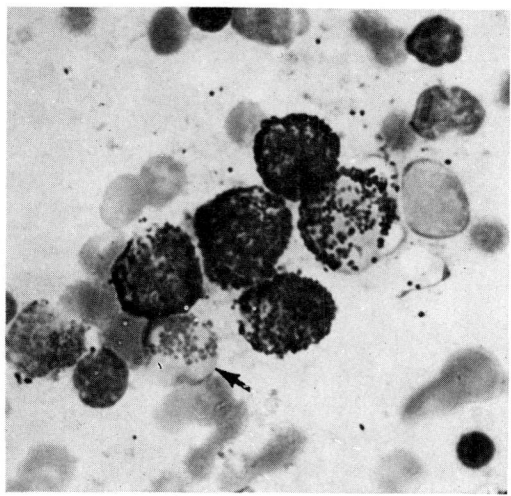

Fig. 32–33. Bone marrow invaded by mast cells in mast cell leukemia and neoplasia in the dog. Same dog as Fig. 32–32. Arrow points to an eosinophil. ×2,700.

were enlarged and invaded by neoplastic cells. Sections of mammary gland tumors contained no gland tissue but instead masses of neoplastic cells. The pathologic diagnosis was malignant mast cell tumor.

A male standard poodle, 5 years old, was presented with the history of lethargy and poor appetite. Examination disclosed a slight nasal discharge, slightly inflamed pharynx, a temperature of 102.4°F, and some reluctance to walk. There were no skin tumors, and peripheral lymph nodes were not enlarged. Two days later the dog was more depressed. A blood sample taken at that time showed a total leukocyte count of 34,700/μl and a PCV value of 37%. The differential leukocyte count revealed 40% mast cells. A bone marrow aspiration demonstrated a predominance of mast cells.

The dog was destroyed, and necropsy revealed somewhat enlarged liver, spleen, and kidneys and markedly enlarged mesenteric lymph nodes. Histologic examination of tissue sections demonstrated foci of mast cells in the liver (Fig. 32–34), spleen, and lymph nodes. A lymph node section was overrun by neoplastic cells and presented areas having a "starry sky" appearance and a mixture of eosinophils and mast cells. The diagnosis was malignant mast cell tumor with accompanying mast cell leukemia.

Mast cell tumors are common in dogs, but

an accompanying mast cell leukemia is rarely seen (Davies et al., 1981; Fowler et al., 1966; Leser et al., 1981). The poodle described here was unusual in that it did not have skin tumors or other peripheral tissue involvement. Others have described similar cases of mast cell neoplasia unaccompanied by skin involvement and with or without systemic mastocytosis (Davies et al., 1981). Mast cell leukemia with systemic mastocytosis is said to be more common in cats than in dogs (Davies et al., 1981)

Erythremic Myelosis and Erythroleukemia

Liu and Carb (1968) described "erythroblastic leukemia" in an 8-year-old male dachshund. The disease was characterized by severe refractory anemia, appearance of nucleated erythrocytes without reticulocytosis in peripheral blood, extensive proliferation of erythroblastic cells in the bone marrow with arrested maturation of erythroid cells, and marked splenomegaly with atrophy of follicles and diffuse infiltration by immature erythroid cells and megakaryocytes. The WBC counts varied between 5,000 and 15,250/μl in 12 blood examinations. PCV values varied between 6% and 12% except when increased by transfusion. Blood platelet counts on three occasions were 270,000, 126,000, and 262,000/μl.

A case of erythroleukemia in a 6-year-old boxer was described by Perk (1980). The dog had a WBC count of 19,917/μl, RBC count of 2.71 million/μl, and platelet count of 2,000/μl. Blood film contained many abnormal mature and immature nucleated erythrocytes and left shift to promyelocytes.

A case of myelofibrosis accompanied by erythremic myelosis has been reported (Thompson and Johnstone, 1983).

Radiation-Induced Hematopoietic Neoplasias

Andersen and Johnson (1962) described an erythroblastic malignancy in a female beagle that had received a total dose of 300 r of whole body x-radiation and that died 5 years later at the age of 5 years and 8 months. Necropsy findings included splenomegaly and multiple metastatic foci in the liver, lymph nodes, and lungs. The outstanding histologic finding was

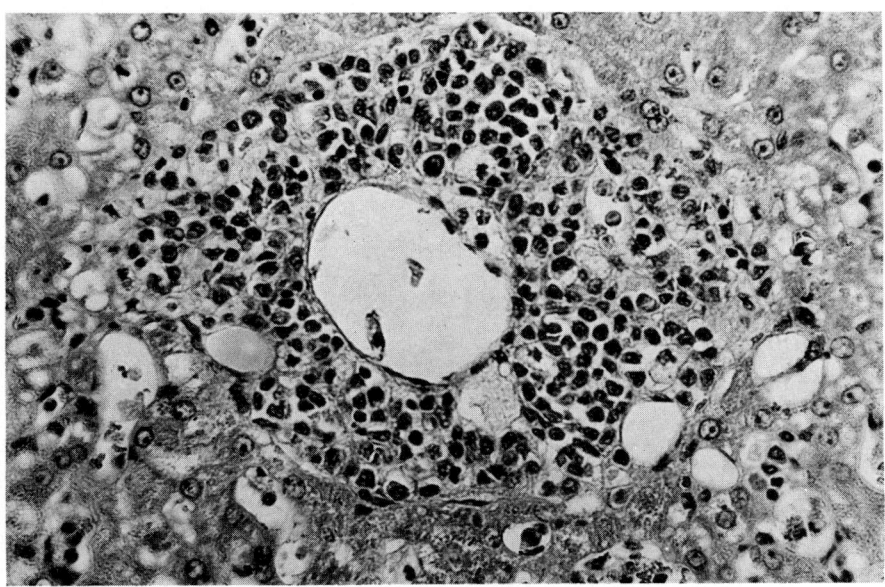

Fig. 32–34. Liver section from a poodle with mast cell leukemia. Accumulation of mast cells around a large vein is shown. H & E stain, ×250.

the presence of large numbers of neoplastic erythroid cells within both small and large blood vessels of all major organs. Anaplastic cells were especially conspicuous as small masses or clusters within organs having a rich sinusoidal bed.

Blood films prepared before necropsy revealed some erythroblasts containing bluish nucleoli, although more mature nucleated erythrocytes were the most frequent cell types. A unique cell type seen in tissue sections was a multinucleated giant cell in which each nucleus was surrounded by distinct cytoplasm, giving the appearance of a cluster or colony of cells. Multinucleated cells of this type were found only in bone marrow, while single and binucleated erythroid neoplastic cells occurred in tissues or other organs. These findings would be compatible with a diagnosis of acute erythremic myelosis as described in humans.

Eleven cases of MPD occurred in a group of 24 beagles exposed to ^{60}Co-gamma-irradiation (5r/22-hour day) for duration of life beginning from 13 months of age (Tolle et al., 1977). Five of the 11 dogs showed erythroleukemia characterized by marked myeloid and erythroid hyperplasia of the bone marrow, with maturation arrest of the erythroid elements. The terminal blood picture was that

of marked anemia and thrombocytopenia, with circulating erythroid precursors and abnormal red cell morphology. Hepatosplenomegaly was seen in four of five cases, although extensive leukemic infiltration was seen in all cases.

Dungworth et al. (1969) have described a granulocytic MPD in beagles exposed to ^{90}Sr from mid-gestation to 1.5 years of age. A dose-related increase in incidence was noted. The most acute cases were characteristic of granulocytic leukemia, while the more chronic disorders were not frank leukemias but bore some resemblance to myelofibrosis with myeloid metaplasia. The acute form has a clinical course of <100 days and was characterized by massive granulocytic proliferation in bone marrow and spleen with overwhelming preponderance of primitive cells at one or both sites. The most severely affected dogs also had extensive infiltration in the liver, lymph nodes, and lungs. The blood was not leukemic, but anemia was evident. The more chronic disorder lasted between 240 and 624 days in five beagles.

There was a slight elevation in WBC count with left shift, anemia with prominent anisocytosis and poikilocytosis, terminal thrombocytopenia, hyperplastic bone marrow with little or no shift toward greater numbers of immature granulocytes, and a mild myeloid metaplasia in the spleen and elsewhere with proportions of cell lines resembling normal patterns in bone marrow.

Additional observations on radiation-induced myelomonocytic leukemia and erythroleukemia have been described in the dog (Fritz et al., 1970; Shifrine et al., 1973; Seed et al., 1977; Tolle et al., 1979).

Micromegakaryocytes and megakaryocytes were found in the peripheral blood as a pre-leukemic phase to myelogenous leukemia in three dogs exposed to continuous whole body ^{60}Co gamma irradiation (Tolle et al., 1983). A case of acute megakaryoblastic leukemia in a young dog exposed continuously to whole body ^{60}Co gamma irradiation was described recently (Cain et al., 1985). The diagnosis was based on cytomorphologic, cytochemical, and tissue culture studies.

THE BOVINE LEUKEMIA COMPLEX

The lymphocyte is the cell most commonly involved in the leukemia complex of cattle. A C-type oncornavirus, designated bovine leukemia virus or BLV, is universally accepted as the agent causing abnormal proliferation of lymphocytes leading to a benign persistent lymphocytosis (PL) or a malignant, tumor-forming disease commonly referred to as enzootic bovine leukosis or "adult" form of lymphoma. Some recent reviews discuss various aspects of the BLV infection (Ferrer, 1980; J.M. Miller, 1980; Miller and van der Maaten, 1982; Straub, 1981) and the relationship between PL and lymphoma (Ferrer et al., 1979).

The Bovine Leukemia Virus

Persistent Lymphocytosis, Lymphoma, and BLV Infection

Bovine leukemia virus is regarded as an exogenous virus (Deschamps et al., 1981). It can infect lymphocytes of a variety of species in vitro, but in vivo infectivity or oncogenicity is relatively limited. Inoculation of virus-containing cultured lymphocytes into calves and sheep produced PL, lymphocytic leukemia, or lymphoma in some of the inoculated animals (Kenyon et al., 1981; Miller et al., 1972; Olson et al., 1972; Olson and Baumgartner,

1976), thereby demonstrating a causal relationship between BLV and the leukemia complex. Similar inoculations into goats (Hoss and Olson, 1974) and chimpanzees (van der Maaten and Miller, 1976) were infective but not oncogenic. It was recently reported, however, that a goat inoculated with BLV-infected sheep lymphocytes died 8 years later with lymphoma of BLV origin (Olson et al., 1981).

The bovine leukemia virus is highly prevalent in cattle with PL and lymphoma (Ferrer et al., 1974). It has been concluded that BLV is the cause of both PL and lymphoma and that genetic constitution plays an important role in the development of both conditions, but each is a separate and distinct response to the virus (Ferrer et al., 1979). Although PL precedes usually by several years the development of lymphoma in two out of three cases, most cattle with PL never develop lymphoma (Ferrer, 1979). PL can be distinguished from transient lymphocytosis of other causes by demonstration of an increase for at least 3 months in the absolute number of lymphocytes of greater than 3 standard deviations above the mean normal number for the breed and age of the animal.

In both PL and lymphoma, the abnormally proliferating cells are glucocorticoid sensitive B-lymphocytes, whereas most normal bovine lymphocytes are relatively steroid resistant T cells (Bloom et al., 1979). The prime producer of BLV appears to be the B-lymphocytes (Paul et al., 1977). Studies with immunologic markers of lymphocytes indicated that cows with PL had about 3–4 times more lymphocytes with surface Fc receptors and membrane IgG and cows with lymphoma had a lower percentage of similar cells than normal cows (Kumar et al., 1978).

Natural Incidence of BLV Infection

Natural infection by BLV can be demonstrated by direct laboratory manipulations or indirectly by serologic techniques. Direct procedures include demonstration of BLV in cultured lymphocytes by electron microscopy, immunofluorescence or immunoperoxidase staining, and a more sensitive syncytia infectivity assay (Ferrer, 1980). Cattle infected with BLV produce antibodies to several BLV antigens and also have virus-neutralizing antibodies.

Demonstration of virus particles by electron microscopy was accomplished in short-term phytohemagglutinin-stimulated lymphocyte cultures from cattle with lymphoma (Miller et al., 1969). This was confirmed in subsequent studies of virus isolations from short-term and long-term cultures and by transmission experiments. The virus apparently infects only lymphocytes and is not demonstrable by direct examination of uncultured lymphocytes or neoplastic tissue. Failure to demonstrate presence of the virus without cultivation may be due to a factor in infected cattle that inhibits virus replication (Baliga and Ferrer, 1977). BLV-associated antigens were detectable in cultured lymphocytes as early as 3 hours after incubation, with maximum presence of antigen at 10–20 hours (Driscoll and Olson, 1977).

Several serologic procedures for detection of BLV infection are available including immunodiffusion, immunofluorescence, radioimmunoassay, and others (Burny et al., 1978; Ferrer, 1980). Serologic tests are generally used to detect herd infections. For example, the agar gel immunodiffusion test (AGID) utilizing BLV glycoprotein gp51 is specific, sensitive, and simple for herd surveys and is commercially available (L.D. Miller, 1980). A positive serologic test in the adult animal generally indicates BLV infection, but several points are to be considered in interpretation of AGID test results (Thurmond and Burridge, 1982). BLV-infected cattle may not develop detectable antibodies for as long as 49 days after initial infection, and circulating BLV antibodies in infected cattle may decline at parturition. Calves born of BLV-infected dams may give a false positive reaction up to 6 months of age as a result of absorption of anti-BLV antibodies from colostrum consumed at birth. In such cases, direct demonstration of virus is necessary to establish BLV infection. Results of serologic testing and direct viral demonstration procedures may not correlate completely because of variations in sensitivity as well as limitations of the techniques.

Incidence of BLV infection among dairy cattle in leukemia-free herds ranged from 2–16% while in herds with histories of lymphoma the incidence of positive reactors was 24–42% (Olson et al., 1973). In a closed herd of 765 dairy cattle with a history of multiple cases of leukemia, BLV antibodies were detected in 59% of newborn calves, 43% of first lactation cows, and 72% of older cows (Ferdinand et al., 1979). In a herd comprised of both grade and purebred cattle, the incidence of BLV infection was greater among the purebred animals (Evermann et al., 1980). Purebred cattle tend to be kept longer than grade cows; thus age may have contributed to the higher infection rate among the purebreds. Bulls and cows appear to be equally susceptible to infection with BLV (Baumgartener et al., 1975; Evermann et al., 1980). Incidence of infection was found to be low in beef herds, 1.2% and 2.6% in two separate surveys (Baumgartener et al., 1975; van der Maaten and Miller, 1979).

Mode of Natural Transmission of BLV Infection

Vertical (prenatal or congenital) transmission of BLV from infected dam to the calf *in utero* occurs infrequently (Ferrer et al., 1976; van der Maaten et al., 1981), but may involve 15–20% of the calves (Piper et al., 1975). Venereal transmission through BLV-infected semen used for artificial insemination does not occur (Thurmond and Burridge, 1982). Calves from lymphoma-free herds foster-nursed for 10 weeks on BLV-infected cows did not become infected. However, when such calves were maintained in prolonged contact with BLV-infected animals, horizontal (postnatal or between animals) spread of the infection was demonstrated by the development of precipitating viral antibodies in well over half of the animals (Piper et al., 1975).

Close physical contact between infected animals and susceptible cattle appears to be the single most important prerequisite to transmission of BLV infection (Thurmond and Burridge, 1982). Infection with BLV through contact exposure increases progressively with age (Ferdinand et al., 1979; Ferrer et al., 1976). Horizontal spread of BLV infection increases with increase in cattle density as in winter months (Wilesmith et al., 1980).

Since BLV particles are seldom produced in vivo, it was conjectured that cattle become infected through exposure to blood or secretions or excretions containing infected lymphocytes rather than the virus as particles. The concept that BLV might be transmitted via blood-sucking insects was supported by the recovery of BLV-infected lymphocytes from the mid-guts of horseflies (tabanids) (Bech-Nielsen et al., 1978; Ferrer, 1980) and by experimental transmission of BLV infection to sheep by tabanids (Ohshima et al., 1981). It was also suggested that consideration should be given to mechanical transmission during surgical procedures such as dehorning and castrations (Ferrer, 1980).

Significance of BLV Infection

Infection with BLV does not mean that the animal will develop PL or lymphoma (Ferrer, 1979). Although BLV infection is widespread, particularly in multiple-case lymphoma herds, tumor development or leukemia is relatively rare (Ferrer, 1980). Most BLV-infected cattle remain asymptomatic and economically productive. Comparative studies have shown no significant differences in milk production, reproductive efficiency, longevity, or mastitis incidence between BLV-infected and noninfected animals within the same herds (Huber et al., 1981; Langston et al., 1978). Thus detection of BLV infection does not constitute a diagnosis of lymphoma. The latter is demonstrated by blood, bone marrow, and other cytologic examinations.

Lymphoproliferative Disorders

Lymphoma affects cattle of all breeds and ages but is more common in dairy cattle and after 5 years of age. Lymphoblastic lymphoma and leukemia have been described in fetuses stillborn in the eighth month of gestation (Hatziolos, 1960; Sheriff and Newlands, 1976). Lymphoma has also been observed on occasion in newborn and growing calves (Bendixen, 1959; Chander et al., 1977; Simon and Brewer, 1963).

Different Forms of Bovine Lymphoma

Two main forms of lymphoma have been recognized. *Enzootic bovine leukosis* (EBL) is by far the most prevalent in the United States, many European countries, and other parts of the world. It is often referred to as the "adult"

form of lymphoma and manifests as multiple incidences in a herd. The *sporadic form* is rare, occurs randomly, and is comprised of three clinicopathologic forms designated "calf," "adolescent-thymic," and "cutaneous" lymphomas. Recent studies support the view that PL and the adult form of lymphoma or EBL are caused by BLV, whereas none of the three sporadic forms appears to be associated with the BLV infection (Devare et al., 1977; Ferrer, 1980). Occasionally the adult form of lymphoma occurs sporadically; such cases are unassociated with BLV infection.

The calf form is characterized by generalized lymphadenopathy with gross changes in the bone marrow, liver, and spleen as common additional features. The abomasum, intestine, skeletal muscle, and spinal epidural space are not involved. It is seen in calves between 1 and 6 months of age. Lymphocytic leukemia is often present in these animals.

The adolescent-thymic form is observed in beef and dairy cattle 6 to 30 months of age. The main pathologic changes are a massive infiltration of the thymus and frequent involvement of bone marrow. Regional lymph nodes are also affected, but generalized lymphadenopathy is uncommon. The condition is encountered more often in beef than in dairy cattle. Dyspnea and bloating are common clinical signs.

The cutaneous form is rare and occurs in cattle 1–3 years of age. It is characterized by a nodular leukemic infiltration of the dermis. Metastases to lymph nodes and other organs occur in latter stages.

The adult form is seen in cattle 2 to 18 years of age, but usually in cattle over 3 years of age and most frequently between 5 and 8 years of age. About 65% of cases are encountered in herds having more than one occurrence of clinical lymphoma (Theilen et al., 1964). Such herds are called multiple-incidence herds.

The adult form of lymphoma is characterized by widespread lymphadenopathy with frequent involvement of the heart, abomasum, and intestine. The bone marrow, thymus, and liver are less frequently involved.

Clinical Signs in the Adult Form of Lymphoma

Bovine lymphoma is characteristically an afebrile disease, although elevations in body

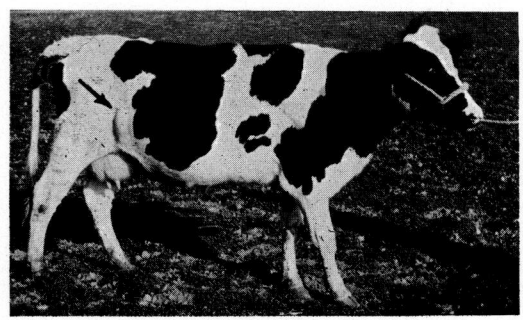

Fig. 32–35. Appearance on admission of the cow whose hemograms are presented in Table 32–14. The bilateral enlargement of prefemoral nodes *(arrow)* on admission subsided as the cow entered a period of temporary remission of clinical signs of lymphoma.

temperature may be encountered. The terminal tumor phase may appear suddenly, with rapid wasting and sudden death.

Because of the marked involvement of a variety of tissues and organs (Table 32-14), clinical signs may be quite variable. Bilateral enlargement of superficial nodes may be the first detectable abnormality, although in some instances only a single external node is involved, and in other cases no enlargement of external lymph nodes occurs. When lymphoma is suspected, rectal palpation of the pelvic and abdominal organs and tissues may reveal extensive neoplastic masses.

When the abomasum is infiltrated by neoplastic cells, the clinical signs may suggest a chronic indigestion. The myocardium is also a favored site for neoplastic cell infiltration, and when chronic indigestion and cardiac abnormality coexist, the resulting clinical signs may suggest traumatic pericarditis. The pressure of neoplastic masses on nerves of the spinal cord produces partial or complete paralysis, depending on the location of the tumorous masses. In rare cases, the subcutaneous tissues and skin may be involved, with a considerable number of nodules of varying sizes. Infiltration of neoplastic lymphocytes into the mammary gland has been reported (Boyd et al., 1947). A rare case of lymphoma with tumor tissue limited to the brain in a Shorthorn heifer has been reported (Smith and Anderson, 1977).

Anemia may develop when the tumor phase is protracted or when blood loss takes place from an ulcerated gastrointestinal tract.

Several factors tend to rule against the development of severe anemia: *(A)* the often rapid development of the terminal tumor phase, *(B)* the long life span of 160 days for the bovine erythrocyte, and *(C)* the rarity of bone marrow involvement in the adult form of lymphoma (Theilen et al., 1964; Weber, 1963).

Duration of illness among 45 lymphomatous adult cattle was reported to be 1 to 4 months (Olson et al., 1970). We observed an interesting case of clinical lymphoma in a 7-year-old grade Holstein-Friesian cow (Fig. 32-35) with bilateral enlargement of the prefemoral lymph nodes followed by remission of at least 7 months' duration (Table 32-14). At the end of that period, signs of lymphoma gradually reappeared, and during the last month of observation, there was an acute fulmination of clinical and hematologic signs. Details on this case have been described (Theilen et al., 1960).

Table 32–15 lists the percentage involvement of various organs in two studies examining 63 cases (Marshak et al., 1962) and 40 cases (Dungworth et al., 1968) of lymphoma. The main difference between the two reports was the much greater involvement of the abomasum among the 40 cases investigated in the latter study. Two of the cases of abomasal involvement were detected only on histologic examination, while in the remainder the abomasum was grossly involved. The right auricle of the heart is particularly vulnerable to neoplastic involvement. Marshak and coworkers (1962) concluded that cardiac failure is a major cause of death in the adult form of lymphoma.

Chromosomal abnormalities were detected in 75% of cattle with the adult form of lymphoma (Hare et al., 1967); the most conspicuous abnormality was hyperploidy. Karyotypic observations on different animals and cells from different sites suggested clonal origin of the disease. Leukotic cattle are immunosuppressed in that they usually exhibit absence of IgM (Trainen and Klopfer, 1971), impaired primary immune response (Trainen et al., 1976), and in vitro defects of the cellular immune system (Muscoplat et al., 1974; Weiland and Straub, 1976). This immunosuppressive activity was thought to be at least

Table 32–14. Hemograms of a Case of Lymphoma[a] in a 7-year-old Holstein-Friesian Cow Kept under Observation for 13 Months During Which a Period of Remission Occurred in the Clinical Picture

							Differential Leukocyte Count (%)						
Date	PCV (%)	WBC/μl	Band	Neutrophils	Blast	Prolymphocytes	Atypical Lymphocytes	Lymphocytes	Monocytes	Eosinophils	Basophils	Degenerated Cells
Nov. 18	26	9,850	0	55.0	0	14.0	0	14	15.0	2.0	0	0
Dec. 2	28	10,800	0	4.5	0	5.0	7.5	57.0	10.5	13.5	0	2.0
Jan. 7	31	22,000	0	18.5	0	5.0	0	62.0	4.0	10.5	0	0
Mar. 18	30.5	11,850	0	38.0	1.0	1.0	0	47.0	2.0	10.0	1.0	0
Apr. 29	32	9,400	0	27.0	0		4.0	63.5	0.5	5.0	0	0
June 12	30	12,400	0	27.0	0		3.0	64.0	1.5	4.0	0	0
July 15	36	8,600	0	31.0	0		2.0	59.0	5.0	2.5	0	0.5
Aug. 12	35	10,850	0	35.5	0		1.5	57.0	3.5	2.5	0.5	0
Oct. 6	36	12,200	0	30.5	0		2.0	54.0	8.0	5.5	0	0
Nov. 25	33	28,050	0.5	9.0	0		56.0	31.0	1.5	2.0	0	0
Dec. 10	21.5	95,000	0.5	2.0	0		85.5	11.5	0	0.5	0	0
Dec. 14	28	143,000	0	4.0	0		94.0	2.0	0	0	0	0
Dec. 18	23	142,000	0	3.0	0		88.0	9.0	0	0	0	0

[a]Necropsy revealed the following to be involved: all lymph nodes, tongue, abomasum, spleen, myocardium, uterus, ureters, lungs, and kidneys.

Table 32–15.   Percentage Involvement of Various Organs and Tissues in the Adult Form of Bovine Lymphoma Reported in Two Sources

Organs	Marshak et al., 1962[a]	Dungworth, 1968
Lymph nodes	95	95
Heart	89	87
Kidney and ureter	59	45
Abomasum	57	85
Uterus and cervix	51	50
Spinal cord	49	—
Intestine	46	48
Liver	37	—
Spleen	27	30
Urinary bladder	21	—
Epidural fat	—	52
Skeletal muscles	—	36
Rumen, reticulum, and omasum	21	—
Gall bladder	11	—
Lungs	8	—
Ovary	5	—
Adrenal medulla	3	—

[a]63 cases examined.
[b]40 cases examined.

partly related to inhibition of lymphocyte blastogenesis by substances present in sera of cows with lymphoma (Jacobs et al., 1980).

The Role of Hematology in Diagnosis of Bovine Leukemia

The use of total and differential leukocyte counts as an aid to diagnosis of bovine leukemia requires knowledge of the normal changes in circulating lymphocyte numbers with advancing age. Theilen et al. (1964) presented statistical data on lymphocyte numbers in Holstein-Friesian cattle as influenced by age (Table 32-16). Jersey and Guernsey cattle revealed similar patterns.

The demonstration of antibodies to BLV in cattle is evidence of presence of the virus in positively reacting animals. Such tests applied to entire herds are useful to demonstrate the incidence of infection and for use in selection of infected animals for further study.

However, as already stated, infection by BLV does not mean that persistent lymphocytosis or lymphoma is present or will necessarily develop at a later time (Ferrer, 1980). Hence various hematologic keys developed for detection of PL now appear to have limited value as indicators of BLV infection (Bendixen, 1957, 1959, 1963; Goetze et al., 1953, 1954).

Diagnosis of PL is to be based on repeated demonstration of a significant lymphocytosis, due principally to lymphocytes of normal morphology, occurring in a clinically normal animal. Lymphoma is mainly a tumor-forming disease and is not regularly associated with lymphocytosis or abnormal (primitive) lymphocytes in the blood (Figs. 32-36, 32-37). In cases of suspected lymphoma, such abnormal lymphocytes should be carefully looked for because they are diagnostic. Examples of total and differential leukocyte

Table 32–16.   Statistics of Normal Lymphocyte Count (in Thousands) by Age for California Holstein-Friesian Cattle[a]

Age	No. of Samples	$\overline{X}$	Sx	C.V.	95% Limits ($\overline{X}$ + 1.96 Sx)	99.74% Limits ($\overline{X}$ + 3.00 Sx)
0–6 mo	146	5.15	1.32	25.6	2.56–7.74	1.19–9.11
6–12 mo	98	6.41	1.55	24.1	3.37–9.45	1.76–11.06
1–2 yr	49	5.99	1.69	28.2	2.68–9.30	0.92–11.06
2–3 yr	64	4.29	1.16	27.0	2.01–6.57	0.81–7.77
3–4 yr	162	4.01	0.99	24.7	2.07–5.95	1.04–6.98
4–5 yr	176	3.42	1.04	30.4	1.39–5.45	0.30–6.54
Over 5 yr	488	3.08	0.96	31.2	1.19–4.97	0.20–5.96

[a]From Theilen et al., 1964; courtesy of *Health Laboratory Science*.

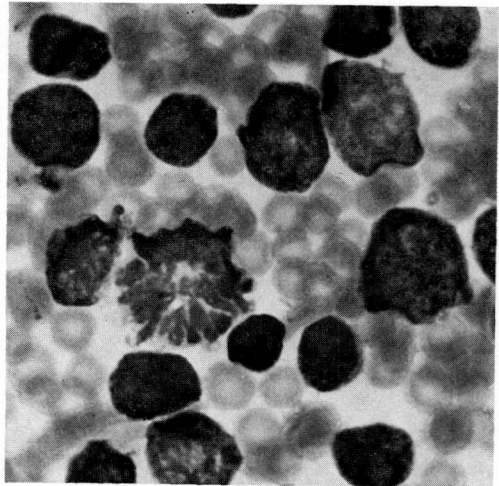

Fig. 32–36. Blood in lymphocytic leukemia in a cow with a total leukocyte count of 880,000/μl. Note mitotic figure and marked variation in size of lymphocytes. ×2,700.

counts in 10 cases of lymphoma are presented in Table 32-17. These hemograms were selected to demonstrate the great variation in cytology of blood in lymphoma.

Weber (1963) summarized the hematologic findings in bovine lymphoma as follows; Mitotic figures, lymphoblasts, and mononuclear cells with multiple asymmetrically lobed nuclei are frequently observed in the blood of cattle with the leukemic form of lymphoma. In approximately 55% of lymphoma cases, the

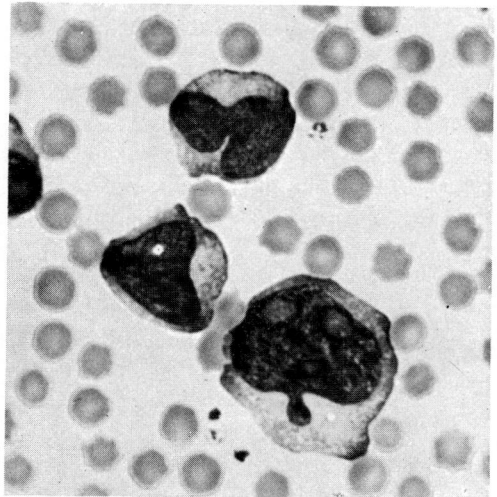

Fig. 32–37. Blood in lymphoma from the cow pictured in Fig. 32–35 and representative of hemograms in Table 32–14. Lymphoblast and atypical lymphocytes (Reider forms). ×2,700.

hemogram reveals a mild to moderate leukocytosis with an absolute increase in lymphocytes. A normal hemogram is present in 10–30% of cases. Leukemia is encountered in 5–10% of cases.

In conclusion, the examination of blood cytology has an important part to play in confirming a diagnosis of lymphoma, particularly in the individual animal presenting clinical signs suggestive of the disease. A negative finding in blood, however, does not necessarily exclude the possibility of lymphoma. Also, a few abnormal lymphocytes may sometimes be found in normal cattle and animals with PL.

THE LEUKEMIA COMPLEX IN THE HORSE

Neoplasia involving cells of the hematopoietic system of the horse is limited almost exclusively to lymphoid system. Lymphoma is the predominant neoplastic change, whereas lymphocytic leukemia is infrequent and myelogenous leukemia is extremely rare. Cause is unknown although virus-like particles were observed in lymph node sections in lymphoblastic lymphoma in a foal that died within 4 hours of its birth (Tomlinson et al., 1979).

Lymphoproliferative Disorders

Lymphoma has not been encountered as frequently in the horse as in the dog, cat, and cow. A survey of international veterinary literature up to 1973 showed that fewer than 100 cases of equine lymphoma had been reported (Neufeld, 1973). Since then several other case reports have been published (Greene and Donovan, 1977; Hoven and Franken, 1983; Kadota, 1981; Rebhun and Bertone, 1984; Roberts, 1977). The medical records at the Veterinary Medical Teaching Hospital (VMTH), University of California, Davis, covering the period 1957–1977 revealed 40 cases of equine lymphoma and 1 case of MPD classified as granulocytic leukemia (Theilen and Madewell, 1979). Various anatomic forms of lymphoma included the multicentric (most common), cutaneous, alimentary, mediastinal, and miscellaneous types. Eleven of the 40 cases (27.5%) were characterized by mul-

Table 32–17. Hemograms in 10 Cases of Bovine Lymphoma

Case No.	Age	Sex	PCV (%)	WBC/μl	Differential Leukocyte Count (%)							
					Band	Neut.	Pro-lymph.	Lymph.	Mono.	Eos.	Bas.	D.C.
53L40	5 wk	F	12	2,050	18.0	2.0	28.0	50.0	2.0	0	0	0
57L1672	8 mo	F	34.5	8,400	0	15.0	0	80.0	4.0	1.0	0	0
56L15	2½ yr	M	42	5,250	0	21.5	0	59.5	5.5	13.0	0.5	0
56L937	3 yr	F	28.5	6,800	0	47.5	0	33.0	14.0	5.5	0	0
961A	4 yr	F	28	175,000	0	6.0	83.0	6.0	0	0	0	5.0
53L114	5 yr	F	28	12,450	0	72.0	0	15.0	11.0	1.0	0	1.0
57L1400	Mature	F	34	20,700	0	51.5	0	42.0	6.5	0	0	0
RJO-68	Mature	F	34	19,100	0.5	3.0	16.0	79.5	0	1.0	0	0
RJO-329	Mature	F	35	145,000	0	2.0	57.0	39.0	0	0	0	2.0
UCV-65	Mature	F	25.5	198,750	0	14.0	2.5	38.5	45.0	0	0	0

tiple dermal and subcutaneous tumors, some of which exhibited a tendency to regress and reappear over a period of months. This special type of lymphoma is diagnosed by histologic examination of biopsied tumor tissue.

The clinical picture of equine lymphoma is varied, and differential diagnosis may be difficult. It seems probable that most cases of lymphoma in the horse could be diagnosed antemortem through a combination of cytologic examinations of blood, bone marrow, aspirated fluid from an enlarged lymph node or an effusion fluid (Schalm, 1981; Schalm and Carlson, 1982).

The following discussion is based on study of 14 horses with forms of lymphoma other than the cutaneous type and relevant literature reports.

Vital Statistics

Age. In rare instances, lymphoma has developed in fetal life and has been diagnosed at birth (Tomlinson et al., 1979) or has been found to be the cause of illness during the first year of life (Dewes and Blakeley, 1980). The VMTH medical records revealed the mean age of 39 horses with lymphoma to be 9.3 years with a range of 1 to 21 years. It was concluded that lymphoma usually occurs in horses 5 years of age and older, although the disease has been seen in foals. Among the 14 lymphomatous horses selected for our discussion, the range in age was 1 to 17 years with a median of 6 and a mean of 6.9 years. A mean age of 10 years was reported by others for 16 cases of lymphoma in the horse (Hoven and Franken, 1983).

Sex and Breed. A distorted pattern of distribution by sex existed among the small group of 14 horses; 11 horses were females and 3 were geldings. In the larger group of 40 horses (Theilen and Madewell, 1979), in which sex and age were recorded, there were 18 females, 5 intact males, and 16 geldings; sex was not recorded for one. Data gathered in the survey of international veterinary literature (Neufeld, 1973) on lymphoma in horses revealed, among 22 such horses, 7 females, 3 intact males, and 12 geldings. No sex predilection for lymphoma is demonstrated when the data from the three sources are combined. The findings then are 36 females and 39 males. In contrast, 13 out of 16 cases of lymphoma involved females in the study reported by Hoven and Franken (1983).

Among 40 horses with lymphoma (Theilen and Madewell, 1979) various breeds were recorded as follows: 14 quarter horses, 6 Thoroughbreds, 3 Arabians, 1 Standardbred, 1 Appaloosa, and 15 crossbreds.

Clinical Signs of Lymphoma

Peripheral lymphadenopathy was present in 10 of the 14 horses (71.4%), being generalized in 4 horses and limited to one or two nodes in 6 horses. Weight loss, sometimes rapid (within 3 weeks) or more protracted, was present in 8 horses (57.1%). Ventral edema, involving the cervical and pectoral regions, occurred in 6 horses (42.8%) and was associated in 4 horses with pleural effusions of 4–22 liters. Respiratory distress, ranging from coughing to frank dyspnea, was present in 6 horses (42.8%). An elevated rectal temperature of 103–107°F (39.4–41.7°C) was recorded in 5 horses (35.7%). Pale mucous membranes were seen in 5 horses (35.7%) in association with advanced anemia. Rectal palpation revealed pelvic and abdominal masses in 2 horses (14.3%). A tumor mass, rapidly growing over 6–8 weeks, occurred in the left neck region of one horse.

Hematologic Findings

Severe to modest suppression of erythropoiesis was present in half of the 14 horses with lymphoma. An increase in total plasma proteins (8.3–12.2 g/dl) was present in 8 (57.1%) of the horses. The highest value of 12.2 g/dl was characteristic of a monoclonal gammopathy, with 8.0 g/dl of β-globulin produced by protein-secreting neoplastic lymphoid cells. Plasma fibrinogen was elevated (0.6–0.9g/dl) in 6 (42.8%) of the horses with lymphoma.

Immature lymphocytes, indicative of lymphocytic leukemia, were present in the circulation of only 4 (28.6%) of the 14 lymphomatous horses. Only one of these 4 horses had leukemic blood, with a total leukocyte count of 41,600/µl, of which 31,000 cells were lymphocytes. In the 3 other horses with circulating immature lymphocytes, total leukocyte counts ranged from 1,800 (as a result of neutropenia) to 7,000/µl of blood. A moderate leukocytosis, due to neutrophilia, was seen in 5 horses. Neutrophilia was present also in other horses in which the total leukocyte count did not exceed the normal range. Thus a nonspecific neutrophilia was a common finding among the 14 horses, although 2 horses experienced both neutropenia and thrombocytopenia as a result of marrow displacement by neoplastic lymphocytes. Immune-mediated hemolytic anemia and immune-mediated thrombocytopenia have been observed in association with lymphoma in horses (Reef et al., 1984).

Lymphocytic leukemia in association with lymphoma has been observed in several case reports (Greene and Donovan, 1977; Madewell et al., 1982; Neufeld, 1973) and a case of primary lymphoid leukemia without discrete tumorous masses has been reported (Roberts, 1977). In such cases either the blood is overtly leukemic, or it contains immature or atypical lymphocytes. Hypercalcemia was observed in a horse with lymphoma (Esplin and Taylor, 1977).

Bone Marrow

Bone marrow of 6 horses was examined, 5 antemortem and 1 at necropsy, with the finding of massive displacement of normal marrow cytology by neoplastic lymphocytes in one-half of the marrow (Schalm, 1981; Schalm and Carlson, 1982). Findings in the remaining 3 marrows were: increased erythropoiesis in a horse with a PCV of 30%, decreased erythropoiesis in a horse with a PCV of 13% (nonresponsive anemia), and a normal cytologic pattern. These findings indicated that the bone marrow is not regularly infiltrated by neoplastic cells in equine lymphoma.

Lymph Node Cytology

Lymph nodes were sampled by needle aspiration in 4 horses. The small quantity of fluid available was filmed and stained as for blood. In each of four samples, a diagnosis of lymphoma was made on the basis of the presence of large, pleomorphic lymphoid cells (Schalm, 1981; Schalm and Carlson, 1982). The usual pattern was an admixture of lymphoblasts, prolymphocytes, some plasma cells, and a few normal mature lymphocytes. Mitotic figures were usually present in small numbers. In the presence of lymphadenopathy, examination of lymph node cytology can be a satisfactory procedure for verification of lymphoma.

Effusion Fluid

Pleural effusion fluid was aspirated from 4 horses. Total nucleated cell counts ranged from 5,700 to 103,600/µl. Differential cell counts revealed between 53 and 93% of cells to be lymphoid types (Schalm, 1981; Schalm and Carlson, 1982). These cells varied in size from normal lymphocytes to large, pleomorphic cells, with an occasional bizarre giant form. Mitotic figures were usually present in small numbers.

Necropsy Findings

Of the 14 horses, 1 died and 13 were destroyed for postmortem examination. An anterior mediastinal mass was present in 10 horses (71.4%), and 3 of the same horses also had tumor masses in the abdominal cavity. The spleen was either enlarged or nodular or

Table 32–18. Hemograms from a Case of Myelomatosis in the Horse

	Date		
	July 8	Oct. 13	Oct. 16
RBC ($\times 10^6/\mu$l)	2.70	1.13	1.06
PCV (%)	16	7.5	8
Hb (g/dl)	5.4	2.5	2.7
MCV (fl)	59	66	75
MCHC (%)	34	33	34
WBC/μl	3,200	6,000	6,400
WBC (%)			
Metamyelocytes	0.0	0.0	12.5
Band	3.0	2.0	22.0
Neutrophils	68.0	77.0	32.0
Lymphocytes	24.0	20.0	30.5
Monocytes	1.0	0.5	2.5
Eosinophils	3.0	0.0	0.0
Basophils	1.0	0.0	0.0
Unclassified	0.0	0.5	0.5

both in 8 horses (57.1%). The liver and lungs were sometimes involved with metastatic tumor foci. No organ or tissue appears to be protected against the infiltration of neoplastic lymphoid cells in equine lymphoma.

Multiple Myeloma

Multiple myeloma is very rare in the horse; only three cases have observed (Cornelius et al., 1959; Jacobs et al., 1983; Markel and Dorr, 1986).

The first report of multiple myeloma from our clinic was of a case in a 16-year-old Thoroughbred gelding (Cornelius et al., 1959). The patient was admitted with a history of lameness and weakness of 2 days' duration following heavy work. The right foreleg exhibited marked edema and tenderness. Examination of the blood (Table 32–18) revealed a severe macrocytic anemia. The clinical condition improved after symptomatic treatment for 2 weeks, although the severe anemia persisted. The horse was sent home with instructions recommending rest and improved nutrition. At first the horse gained weight, but 3 months later, a partial paralysis developed, and he was unable to rise. After 48 hours, the horse was able to stand again but showed irregular anorexia, loss of weight, and edema of all extremities and the intermandibular space. Other clinical signs were systolic murmur, jugular pulse, heart rate of 100/minute, moist rales over the ventral two-thirds of the lungs, a fetid breath, and pale mucous membranes.

Two examinations of peripheral blood were made prior to sacrificing the animal, and bone marrow was aspirated from the tuber coxae. The anemia was more severe now and continued to be macrocytic-normochromic. The leukocyte picture was one of leukopenia and a relative neutrophilia. The bone marrow findings provided the diagnosis of myeloma, as plasma cells accounted for 65% of the nucleated cells of the marrow (Fig. 32-38). There was a marked deficiency of precursors for both the granulocytic and erythrocytic series.

Electrophoretic separation of the serum proteins on filter paper revealed the presence of an abnormal myeloma β-globulin, which was estimated to be 8.4 g/dl. A marked deficiency of albumin and α-globulin was observed (Fig. 32–39). The Bence Jones protein commonly found in the urine in myeloma was not present in urine collected at necropsy.

Only the femur and humerus clearly showed gross lesions, but by microscopic examination, the ribs and vertebral column were found to be involved. All bone sections examined showed extensive replacement of normal marrow elements by plasma cells. Although the lymph nodes were not enlarged, all sections examined microscopically showed an almost complete replacement of lymphocytes by myeloma cells of the type seen in the bone marrow.

A more recent case from our clinic involved a 22-year-old Arabian mare with a history of chronic weight loss and progressive worsening of upper airway stridor (Markel and Dorr, 1986). Abnormal hematologic findings included mild anemia (PCV 30%), slight neutrophilia (12,834 cells/μl) and hyperproteinemia (13.8 g/dl). Bone marrow contained over 15% well-differentiated plasma cells with a myeloid:erythroid ratio of 1.5:1 and adequate numbers of megakaryocytes. A monoclonal gammopathy of IgG(T) (9.8 g/dl) was detected by single radial immunodiffusion assay; IgG, IgM, and IgA levels were markedly reduced. Bence Jones protein was not detected in the urine, and osteolytic lesions were not seen in any of the bones examined. Histopathologic examination revealed widespread plasma cell infiltration of bronchial, mesenteric, and renal lymph nodes, bone

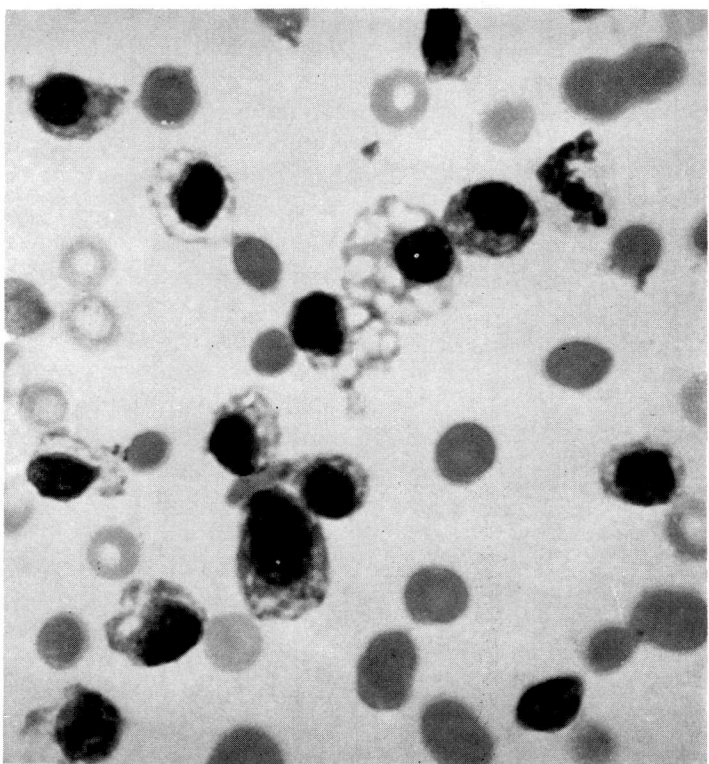

Fig. 32–38.   Myelomatous plasma cells with characteristic foamy cytoplasm in bone marrow aspirated from the tuber coxae of a horse with myelomatosis. ×2,700. (From Cornelius et al., 1959; courtesy of *Cornell Veterinarian*.)

marrow, spleen, liver, pituitary and adrenal glands, and the tongue.

Myeloproliferative Disorders

Two cases of myelogenous leukemia (Searcy and Orr, 1981; Theilen and Madewell, 1979), two cases of eosinophilic leukemia (Lewis and Leitch, 1975; Morris et al., 1984), and one case each of monocytic leukemia (Burkhardt et al., 1984) and myelomonocytic leukemia (Brumbaugh et al., 1982) have been reported. Brief remarks are made about some of these case reports.

The case report of myelomonocytic leukemia was from our clinic (Brumbaugh et al., 1982). It involved a 5-year-old quarter horse stallion with a history of depression and weight loss of at least 3 weeks' duration. Clinical and laboratory findings included splenomegaly, lymphadenopathy, coagulopathy, and bacteremia. Hematologic findings included severe normocytic-normochromic anemia, thrombocytopenia, monocytosis, and a left shift occasionally up to the pro-

myelocyte stage. The serum lysozyme concentration was increased, suggesting increased turnover of myelomonocytic cells. The bone marrow contained many immature cells of the myeloid series with a myeloid:erythroid ratio of 30.5:1. The horse died after a few days of hospitalization.

Necropsy findings included generalized lymphadenopathy and hemorrhages throughout the body. Histopathologic examination revealed primitive and myeloblastic cells in several tissues including the lymph nodes, spleen, liver, kidneys, lungs, and myocardium. The diagnosis of myelomonocytic leukemia was based on hematologic, enzymatic (lysozyme levels), and histopathologic findings.

Laboratory findings in a case of monocytic leukemia in a 6-year-old Hassian gray gelding included marked normocytic-normochromic anemia, leukocytosis with marked monocytosis, latex-particle phagocytosis by leukemic leukocytes, and positive staining of leukemic cells for α-naphthyl acetate esterase (a mon-

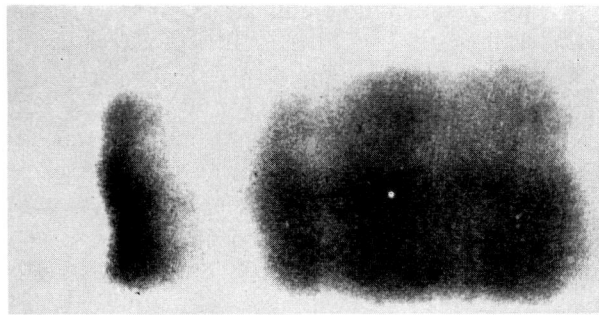
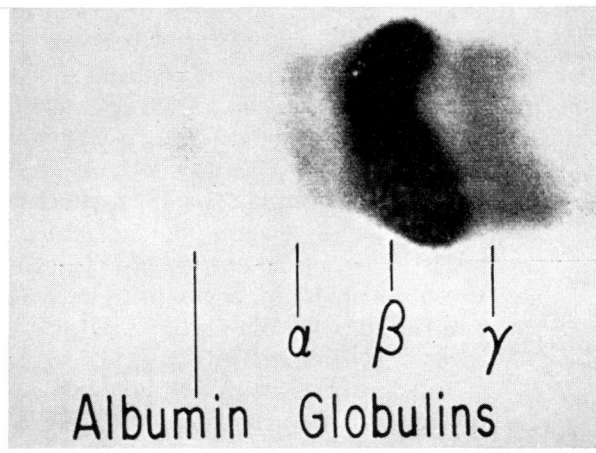

Fig. 32–39. Paper electrophoretic separation of equine serum proteins. *A*, normal control horse; *B*, horse with myelomatosis exhibiting an abnormal beta myeloma protein, hypoalbuminemia, and hypo-alpha-globulinemia. (From Cornelius et al., 1959; courtesy of *Cornell Veterinarian*.)

ocyte marker) and weak staining for chloroacetate esterase (a neutrophil marker). Leukemic cells showed surface features (prominent ruffles and ridge-like profiles) of monocytoid cells. Prominent pathologic findings were lymphadenopathy, splenomegaly, and massive infiltration with monocytoid cells of various parenchymatous organs and bone marrow (Burkhardt et al., 1984).

Eosinophilic leukemia was diagnosed in a 4-year-old Thoroughbred filly (Lewis and Leitch, 1975) and a 10-month-old Standardbred colt (Morris et al., 1984) based on blood and bone marrow findings of slight to marked eosinophilia with immature and atypical cells and excluding other possible causes of reactive eosinophilia. Other hematologic findings included marked anemia and thrombocytopenia. Bone marrow was markedly hyperplastic with highly aberrant eosinophils and showed secondary myelophthisis.

THE LEUKEMIA COMPLEX IN OTHER SPECIES

Leukemia is rare in other animal species. Sporadic cases have been reported in sheep,

pigs (Bostock and Owen, 1973), water buffaloes (Singh et al., 1979), and goats. Multiple incidences of lymphoma (enzootic leukemia) have been described in sheep (Boyt et al., 1976; Enke et al., 1961; Ulbrich et al., 1970), and an unusual occurrence of a hereditary form of lymphoma has been reported in the pig (Head et al., 1974).

Goat

Lymphoma is rare in the goat. Clinicopathologic findings of a case observed in our clinic are presented below:

A 3-year-old female Saanen-Nubian crossbred goat was the second case of lymphoma to develop among animals of a goat dairy. The course of the disease from first clinical signs was approximately 45 days. The patient had milked up to 10 days prior to death. One blood examination was made, and a moderate anemia was demonstrated by the following findings; RBC, 11 million/μl; PCV, 18.5%; and hemoglobin, 6.8g/dl. The WBC count was slightly above normal at 15,100/μl. The differential leukocyte count was band neutrophils, 2%; mature neutrophils, 31%;

lymphocytes, 61%, of which 13% consisted of large, atypical, and some binucleated forms; and monocytes, 6%.

The patient was afebrile and maintained an appetite up to the day before death. There was open-mouth breathing throughout, which became more pronounced 24 hours prior to death. At necropsy, all lymph nodes were enlarged.

A case of lymphoma in a Nubian goat with normal WBC count and absence of atypical lymphocytes was described recently (Baker and Sherman, 1982).

Myelofibrosis associated with pancytopenia has been observed in some newborn pygmy goats at our clinic (Dr. Nancy East, personal communication). Although a genetic association seems possible, its etiology and myeloproliferative nature remain to be investigated.

Sheep

The incidence of lymphoma in sheep slaughtered in abattoirs has generally been 5–20 per million, although incidences as high as 160 per million have been reported from certain parts of the world (Bostock and Owen, 1973). Monlux et al. (1956) reported 19 cases of lymphoma and 2 cases of myeloma among 1.1 million sheep slaughtered in the Denver, Colorado, area in 1953 and 1954.

Lymphoma in sheep occurs most commonly in adult animals without sex and breed predilection. Sporadic cases (Anderson and Jarrett, 1968) as well as multiple incidence herds (Boyt et al., 1976; Enke et al., 1961; Ulbrich et al., 1970) have been described. Horizontal transmission was suspected in a multiple incidence herd (Boyt et al., 1976). A pathologic study of 40 cases of ovine lymphoma revealed several anatomic forms, primarily the multicentric type, followed by the alimentary (mesenteric) form and rarely thymic and skin forms (Johnstone and Manktelow, 1978). Tissues most commonly involved, in decreasing order, were the lymph nodes, spleen, liver, kidney, small intestine, and heart.

Ovine lymphoma is caused by a C-type oncornavirus, and BLV is oncogenic for sheep. Inoculation of 40 ml heparinized blood from three leukotic cattle into newborn lambs was found to produce leukosis in 8 of 27 lambs within 10–24 months (Wittmann and Urbaneck, 1970). Subsequently, inoculation of BLV into neonatal lambs was found to induce leukemia or lymphoma (Olson and Baumgartener, 1976; Olson et al., 1972). Persistent leukocytosis, but not lymphoma, developed in sheep inoculated with cell-free extracts of spontaneously occurring lymphoma in sheep, and virus-like particles, unlike those of typical oncornaviruses, were observed in phytohemagglutinin (PHA)-stimulated lymph node cultures of some of these sheep (Johnstone and Manktelow, 1978, Johnstone et al., 1979). In other studies, however, C-type particles were observed in PHA-stimulated cultures of lymphocytes from affected sheep from a flock of enzootic leukemia (Paulsen et al., 1972; Weiss et al., 1971). Virus isolated from sheep lymphocyte cultures was found to produce lymphoma in experimentally inoculated sheep (Paulsen et al., 1972, 1975b) and appeared to have morphologic and biochemical characteristics of other oncornaviruses (Paulsen et al., 1975a). Reverse transcriptase activity and particles of retroviral density were demonstrated in short-term lymphoid tissue culture of a case of ovine lymphoblastic leukemia (Tomley et al., 1983b).

Pig

The incidence of lymphoma in pigs in abattoirs in the United States and certain countries of Western Europe ranged between 3 and 25 per million (Bostok and Owen, 1973). The disease appears to occur mainly in young animals (<6 months of age) before maturity, without sex or breed predilection.

Natural cases of lymphoma in pigs occur sporadically (Anderson and Jarrett, 1968; Fisher and Olander, 1978). Clinical signs in affected animals include ataxia or paralysis, enlarged superficial lymph nodes, particularly submandibular or prescapular lymph nodes, anorexia, loss of body weight, dyspnea, tachycardia, and sudden death. The diagnosis of lymphoma is difficult to make from blood examination because many animals have normal WBC counts and abnormal lymphocytes may not be present (Renier et al., 1966). A leukemic phase may occur terminally. Among various anatomic forms of lymphoma, the multicentric form is the most common, followed by the thymic form (Anderson and Jarrett, 1968). The liver, spleen, and kidneys are most often infiltrated when the disease is widespread. Histologically, characterization of cell types in 200 cases of porcine lymphomas revealed 42% to be lymphocytic, 34% lymphoblastic, 15% "histiocytic," and 9% mixed types (Migaki, 1969).

A hereditary form of lymphoma has been described in a breeding stock of Large White Pigs in Great Britain (Campbell, 1977; Head et al., 1974; McTaggart et al., 1971). The mode of inheritance was autosomal recessive, and all cases occurred in pigs under 6 months of age. Affected animals showed stunted growth, pot belly, and some enlargement of superficial lymph nodes. The WBC counts were moderately elevated, but lymphocyte numbers constituted up to 80% of the leukocyte counts along with a variable proportion of lymphoblasts and large undifferentiated cells. Multicentric lymphoid tumors were found in the lymph nodes, particularly those draining the gut and lungs (e.g., gastrosplenic, mesenteric, and bronchial lymph nodes). The disease was detected as early as 6-12 weeks of age by the presence of abnormal cells in the peripheral blood. In addition, anemia and thrombocytopenia developed in terminal stages. The bone marrow was virtually replaced by tumor cells, and spread of tumor cells to other organs was detected by histologic examination. The thymus was always involuted. Most of the affected animals died by 120 days, although some survived for 4-6 months; they rarely lived beyond 15 months of age and never attained sexual maturity. Affected animals at 10-24 weeks of age had increased serum γ-globulin levels and IgG heavy chain and light chain components in their serum and urine (Imlah et al., 1979) suggestive of the B-cell type of lymphoma.

Experimental transmission of swine lymphoma by inoculation of neonatal piglets was studied (Case and Simon, 1968). Lymphocytosis developed in inoculated pigs, but not in controls, at 1-6 months of age. Lymphocytic leukemia developed in 1 of 56 pigs exposed to gamma-radiation from ^{60}Co (Trum and Carll, 1957). Exposure of 665 swine to ^{90}Sr re-sulted in development of lymphoproliferative disorders in 18 animals and myeloproliferative disorders in 32 animals (Howard et al., 1968).

Myelogenous leukemia has also been reported in the pig. An early report consisted of a case of granulocytic leukemia with splenomegaly in a slaughtered 210-pound pig (Langham and Hallman, 1939). A case of poorly differentiated myeloid leukemia in a 3-day-old piglet (Allsup et al., 1981) and a case of eosinophilic leukemia (Kashima and Nomura, 1982) were described recently. Granulocytic sarcoma was detected in a pig after necropsy (Fisher and Olander, 1978).

A C-type virus was found in tissues or cell lines from swine with myeloproliferative disorders, thereby indicating that a virus might be associated with the observed lesions (Frazier et al., 1979). Serologic examination of random pig populations indicated that swine leukemia virus is not widespread and may be an endogenous virus that is serologically different from the BLV (Busse et al., 1978).

THERAPY OF LYMPHOPROLIFERATIVE AND MYELOPROLIFERATIVE DISORDERS

Lymphoma, lymphocytic leukemias, myelogenous leukemias, and other hematopoietic neoplastic diseases remain essentially uncurable by currently available means. The primary aim of cancer therapy in such patients, therefore, is to control the disease process as much as possible and prolong the life of the patient. Treatment of hematopoietic malignancies primarily involves chemotherapy, immunotherapy, radiation, and marrow transplantation. The purpose of various treatments is to destroy leukemic clones of cells and allow propagation of normal hematopoietic cells. In veterinary medicine, canine and feline patients with these diseases are being treated by a variety of means, while treatment of bovine and equine patients is generally not attempted, primarily for economic reasons. While chemotherapy in human leukemia may prolong life for several years in certain cases, in animals it may extend life by only 10-14 months (Madewell,

1985). Prolonged survival without therapy is rare (Harvey et al., 1981).

The drugs in use for the treatment of neoplasia, including hematopoietic malignancies, have been discussed (Cardeilhac, 1970; Henderson, 1983a, b; Theilen and Madewell, 1979; Wintrobe et al., 1981), and some are listed in Table 32-19. These drugs are broadly categorized as "cycle-dependent" drugs, which selectively kill cells in mitotic and DNA synthetic phases, and "non-cycle-dependent" agents, which kill cells in all phases of the cell cycle. This distinction is, however, not absolute. Based on the belief that the primary defect in leukemia is the lack of stem cell maturation, drugs inducing cellular differentiation and maturation in vitro may also be used for therapy of leukemias; these drugs have included cytosine arabinoside (ara-C) in low doses, *cis*-retinoic acid, and prednisone (Sachs, 1978).

Antineoplastic agents are more effective when used in combination, and substitution of other drugs should be made when the animal becomes refractory to the initial therapy or shows signs of drug toxicity. The reason for the relative success of combination therapy is that different drugs attack tumor cells at different stages of the cell cycle and by different mechanisms, thereby effecting possibly a synergistic action and a higher rate of tumoricidal effect with minimal toxicity (DeVita and Schein, 1973). Unless every neoplastic cell is destroyed, relapses may occur after discontinuation of therapy, or a refractoriness to chemotherapeutic drugs eventually develops, and the disease becomes progressive again.

Protocols for induction of remission, maintenance of remission, and reinduction of remission have been developed. Reinduction of remission is always difficult and sometimes unattainable. Remission rates and periods of complete remission have varied in different hematopoietic malignancies in humans and animals. Initial doses of drugs should be large enough to produce remissions rapidly; the dose should then be reduced to the level that will maintain remission as long as possible.

Chemotherapy of human leukemias has been summarized (Henderson, 1983a,b; Rundles, 1983; Wintrobe et al., 1981). Drugs commonly used in treatment of AML in humans include ara-C, 5-azacytidine, 6-thioguanine (TG), 6-mercaptopurine (MP), daunorubicin (DNR), and doxorubicin (DOX). Cytosine arabinoside in combination with DNR or DOX and with or without TG have been most successful in inducing initial remission (Henderson, 1983a). Remission rates of about 70% and median survival of about 10–12 months have been achieved, with over 20% of patients liv-

Table 32–19. Some Drugs Used for Chemotherapy of Canine and Feline Hematopoietic Malignancies

Drug	Indications[a]	Dose[b]
Busulphan (Myleran)	MPD	3–4 mg/m^2, orally, per day
Chlorambucil (Leukaran)	LPD	2 mg/m^2, orally, alternate days
Cyclophosphamide (Cytoxan)	LPD	50 mg/m^2, IV or orally, 3–4 days a week
Cytosine arabinoside (Cytosar)	LPD, MPD	100 mg/m^2, IV or SC, for 2–4 days
Doxorubicin (Adriamycin)	LPD	30 mg/m^2, IV, every 21 days
L-asparaginase	LPD	10,000–40,000 units, SC or IP, once or twice weekly, 15 min after giving antihistamine
Melphalan (Alkeran)	Myeloma	1.5 mg/m^2, orally, per day for 7–10 days every 2–3 weeks
6-Mercaptopurine	LPD, MPD	50 mg/m^2, orally, per day
Methotrexate	LPD, MPD	2.5 mg/m^2, orally, 2–3 times a week
Nitrogen mustard (Mustargen)	LPD	5 mg/m^2, orally or IV, per day or in divided dosage for 2–4 days
Prednisone	LPD	10–40 mg/m^2, orally, per day for 7 days then one-half the dose alternate days
Vinblastine (Velban)	LPD	2 mg/m^2, IV, once a week
Vincristine (Oncovin)	LPD	0.5 mg/m^2, IV, once a week

[a]LPD, lymphoproliferative disorder; MPD, myeloproliferative disorder.

[b]m^2, meter body surface area; IV, intravenous; SC, subcutaneous. For additional information on dosage of various drugs, see Madewell, 1985; Theilen and Madewell, 1979; and other references cited in the text.

ing for 5 years or longer after diagnosis. High dose ara-C and m-AMSA (an acridine derivative) have been used to treat relapsed patients with 70% success (Hines et al., 1981). Chemotherapy followed by compatible bone marrow transplantation in younger patients has been highly successful in achieving long-term remission.

More progress has been made in treatment of human ALL, particularly in children 2–10 years of age. Drugs commonly used in treatment of ALL in humans include prednisone, vincristine, L-asparaginase, DNR or DOX, methotrexate (MTX), MP, ara-C, and cyclophosphamide. Most successful remissions have been achieved with a combination of vincristine and prednisone plus DNR or asparaginase or both (Henderson, 1983b). Remission rates of 95% or more have been obtained in children compared to 72% in adults. Children on combination chemotherapy have a median survival of more than 5 years compared to a median survival of about 2 years for adults. Remission maintenance therapy has included DOX, MP, MTX, and cyclophosphamide in combination with drugs used for initial remission, radiation therapy, and immunotherapy.

Chronic lymphocytic leukemia in humans is treated using chlorambucil or cyclophosphamide singly or in combination with prednisone or vincristine or both (Rundles, 1983). Doxorubicin, procarbazine, and bleomycin have also been used in various combinations. Leukapheresis has been performed to decrease the circulating mass of leukocytes. Radiation therapy has been given to treat enlarged lymph nodes and splenomegaly in lymphoma patients. Cranial radiation and intrathecal administration of chemotherapeutic drugs may be necessary to control meningeal leukemia.

A variety of treatment programs involving single, sequential, and combination therapy have been developed for canine and feline patients (Bowlen et al., 1980; Cotter, 1983a; Crow, 1982; Crow et al., 1977b; Culvert and Leifer, 1981; MacEwen et al., 1977b, 1981a; Madewell, 1975; Theilen and Madewell, 1979; Theilen et al., 1977; Weller et al., 1980a). These programs are constantly being modified with experience to increase therapeutic

effectiveness with minimal side effects. In dogs and cats, remission rates have generally been higher and survival rates longer with lymphoproliferative disorders than with myeloproliferative disorders. Partial or complete response rates of 75–80% have been reported for lymphomatous dogs (Madewell, 1985) and of 50–60% for lymphomatous cats (Theilen and Madewell, 1979). Primary and secondary macroglobulinemias in dogs have been treated with melphalan, chlorambucil and prednisone, with survival times of over 1 year (MacEwen et al., 1977a; Matus and Leifer, 1985).

Immunotherapy has been used to induce a systemic antitumor immune response by the patient. Immunotherapy with an autogenous vaccine (injection of chemically modified tumor cell extracts in Freund's complete adjuvant) has been found beneficial when given following cytoreductive chemotherapy (Crow et al., 1977b; Theilen et al., 1977; Weller et al., 1980a). The prolonged survival was attributed to nonspecific immunostimulation by Freund's complete adjuvant rather than to tumor-specific vaccine (Weller et al., 1980a). However, the effectiveness of immunotherapy (i.e., maintenance of remission and prolongation of survival time) was found to depend partly on the number of tumor cells present at the onset of immunotherapy. Intralymphatic administration of a tumor cell vaccine as a maintenance therapy for lymphoma in dogs has been found to increase median survival (Jeglum, 1985). A temporary remission of 19 months' duration was obtained in a leukemic dog treated with fresh blood constituents (MacEwen et al., 1981b).

Newer means of immunotherapy using monoclonal antibodies, interferons, and interleukins are being developed in human medicine with great hopes of curing cancer. Their use in animals remains to be investigated.

Whole body radiation alone has been used to treat lymphoma in dogs, but prolonged periods of remission have been observed in lymphoma dogs treated with combination chemotherapy followed by total body radiation and transplantation of autologous bone marrow (Bowles et al., 1980; Weiden et al., 1979). Allogeneic bone marrow transplantation is also being performed to treat feline leukemia.

General experience has been that prospective clinical staging of lymphoma (Squire et al., 1973) has prognostic significance following various forms of therapy (Cotter, 1983a; Crow et al., 1977b; MacEwen et al., 1981a; Theilen et al., 1977; Weller et al., 1982b). Also, response to therapy varies among animals, probably because of heterogeneity of the disease process. Some other factors influencing prognosis include size and age of the animal, presence of paraneoplastic syndrome and other concurrent disease, and location and extent of the neoplastic process. The ideal canine patient is one in which the diagnosis has been made in the early stage of the disease and in which generalized spread of neoplastic cells to visceral organs has not taken place. With major organ involvement, the mass of neoplastic tissue is too large to be destroyed.

Normally functioning kidneys are important to therapeutic success, for with regression of large tumor masses, nitrogenous waste products are released and must be excreted. Blood urea nitrogen should be determined both before and during treatment to monitor kidney function. Treatment with allopurinol is not recommended in dogs because hyperuricemia seen in leukemic humans receiving chemotherapy is not a major problem in the dog (Leifer and Matus, 1985). Blood cytology should also be monitored routinely. A significant change in kidney function or evidence of developing thrombocytopenia, leukopenia, or anemia should call for immediate reduction in dose or discontinuance of the cytotoxic drugs. Whole blood transfusion or blood component therapy may be given to control anemia, neutropenia, thrombocytopenia, and coagulopathies. Prophylactic use of antibiotics reduces the risk of infections during cancer therapy.

The treatment of leukemia and lymphoma with cytotoxic drugs may produce signs of intoxication during the period of rapid regression of neoplastic tissue. The principal sign is depression. Other chronic signs of drug toxicity are sepsis, bone marrow suppression, gastrointestinal irritation, hemorrhagic cystitis, and alopecia. Hence proper supportive care is essential for successful management of the patient under treatment. Adequate supportive care is also necessary to control complications of the neoplastic disease per se, e.g., immune-mediated hemolytic anemia, immune-mediated thrombocytopenia, myelophthisis, hypercalcemia, monoclonal gammopathies, and central nervous system dysfunctions.

Myelotoxicity is a common problem in cancer chemotherapy. For example, reversible myelosuppression occurs with use of cyclophosphamide, ara-C, nitrogen mustard, busulphan, DNR, DOX, TG, and MP. Megaloblastic changes in erythroid cells are seen when folic acid antagonists such as MTX are given. Bleomycin and, in most cases, vincristine and L-asparaginase do not produce hematopoietic toxicity. Myelosuppression precedes changes in blood cell counts; hence it is generally detected when leukocyte counts drop progressively below 3,500/µl and platelet counts decrease below 50,000/µl.

Corticosteroids used in combination with cytotoxic drugs may prevent to a large extent the depression of hematopoiesis through their stimulatory effect on bone marrow. Severe anemia, leukopenia, or thrombocytopenia, in properly controlled drug administration, is not a common occurrence. In fact, platelet numbers have been observed to increase in the circulation in some dogs during therapy in which prednisolone was employed in combination with vincristine or cyclophosphamide or both. Appearance of Howell-Jolly bodies and/or nucleated erythrocytes in peripheral blood during therapy is conjectured to be an expression of suppression of the "pitting" function of the spleen primarily by action of administered corticosteroids (Fig. 13–21).

REFERENCES

Titles in parentheses are English translations of foreign language titles.

Ackerman, N., and Madewell, B.R.: Thoracic and Abdominal Radiographic Abnormalities in the Multicentric Form of Lymphosarcoma in Dogs. J. Amer. Vet. Med. Ass., *176*:36, 1980.

Allsup, T.N., et al.: Myeloid Leukosis in a Piglet. Vet. Rec., *108*:231, 1981.

Alroy, J.: Basophilic Leukemia in a Dog. Vet. Pathol., 9:90, 1972.

Andersen, A.C., and Johnson, R.M.: Erythroblastic Malignancy in a Beagle. J. Amer. Vet. Med. Ass., *141*:944, 1962.

Anderson, L.J., and Jarrett, W.H.: Lymphosarcoma (Leukemia) in Cattle, Sheep, and Pigs in Great Britain. Cancer, *22*:398, 1968.

Anderson, L.J., et al.: Feline Leukemia-Virus Infection of Kittens: Mortality Associated with Atrophy of the Thymus and Lymphoid Depletion. J. Natl. Cancer Inst., *47*:807, 1971.

Anonymous: National Cancer Institute Sponsored Study of Classification of Non-Hodgkin's Lymphomas: Summary and Description of a Working Formulation for Clinical Usage. Cancer, *49*:2112, 1982.

Baker, J.C., and Sherman, D.M.: Lymphosarcoma in a Nubian Goat. Vet. Med. Small Anim. Clin., *77*:557, 1982.

Baliga, V., and Ferrer, J.E.: Expression of the Bovine Leukemia Virus and Its Internal Antigen in Blood Lymphocytes. Proc. Soc. Exp. Biol. Med., *156*:388, 1977.

Barr, R.D., and Watt, J.: Preliminary Evidence for the Common Origin of a Lympho-Myeloid Complex in Man. Acta Haematol., *6029*, 1978.

Barthel, C.H.: Acute Myelomonocytic Leukemia in a Dog. Vet. Pathol.,*11*:79, 1974.

Baumgartener, L.E., et al.: Survey for Antibodies to Leukemia (C-type) Virus in Cattle. J. Amer. Vet. Med. Ass.,*166*:249, 1975.

Bech-Nielsen, S., et al.: Natural Mode of Transmission of the Bovine Leukemia Virus: Role of Blood Sucking Insects. Amer. J. Vet. Res., *39(7)*:1089, 1978.

Bendixen, H.J.: Studies on Leukosis in Cattle. 1. The Occurrence and Distribution of Cattle Leukosis. Nord. Vet. Med., *9*:1, 1957.

Bendixen, H.J.: Studies on Leukosis in Cattle. 3. Control of Leukosis Herds Using Hematological Examination. Nord. Vet. Med., *11*:733, 1959.

Bendixen, H.J.: Preventive Measures in Cattle Leukemia: Leukosis Enzootica Bovis. Ann. N.Y. Acad. Sci., *108*:1241, 1963.

Bennett, J.M., et at.: Proposals for the Classification of the Acute Leukaemias. Brit. J. Haematol., *33*:451, 1976.

Bennett, J.M., et al.: A Variant For of Hypergranular Promyelocytic Leukaemia (M3). Brit. J. Haematol., *44*:169, 1980.

Bennett, J.M., et al.: The Morphologic Classification of Acute Lymphoblastic Leukaemia: Concordance among Observers and Clinical Correlations. Brit. J. Haematol., *47*:553, 1981.

Bennett, J.M., et al.: Proposals for the Classification of the Myelodysplastic Syndromes. Brit. J. Haematol., *51*:189, 1982.

Bennett, J.M., et al.: Proposed Revised Criteria for the Classification of Acute Myeloid Leukemia. Annals Intern. Med., *103*:626, 1985.

Benveniste, R.E., et al.: Evolution of Type C Viral Genes: Origin of Feline Leukemia Virus. Science, *190*:886, 1975.

Berard, C.W., et al: Immunologic Aspects and Pathology of the Malignant Lymphomas. Cancer, *42*:911, 1978.

Bernard, J.: Preleukemic State. Blood Cells, 2:5, 1976.

Bernhard, W.: The Detection and Study of Tumor Viruses with the Electron Microscope. Cancer Res., *20*:712, 1960.

Bloom, J.C., et al.: Glucocorticoid Effects on Peripheral Blood Lymphocytes in Cows Infected with Bovine Leukemia Virus. Blood, *53*:899, 1979.

Bostock, D.E., and Owen, L.N.: Porcine and Ovine Lymphosarcoma: A Review. J. Natl. Cancer Inst., *50*:933, 1973.

Bowles, C.A., et al.: Autologous Bone Marrow Transplantation following Chemotherapy and Irradiation in Dogs with Spontaneous Lymphomas. J. Natl. Cancer Inst., *65*:615, 1980.

Boyd, W.L., et al.: Leucemic Lymphoblastoma in a Cow with Involvement of the Udder. Amer. J. Vet. Res., *8*:330, 1947.

Boyt, W.P., et al.: Enzootic Leucosis in a Flock of Sheep in Rhodesia. Vet. Rec., *98*:112, 1976.

Braund, K.G., et al.: Neurologic Manifestations of Monoclonal IgM Gammopathy Associated with Lymphocyte Leukemia in a Dog. J. Amer. Vet. Med. Ass., *172*:1407, 1978.

Brumbaugh, G.W., et al.: Myelomonocytic Myeloproliferative Disease in a Horse. J. Amer. Vet. Med. Ass., *180*:313, 1982.

Burkhardt, E., et al.: Monocytic Leukemia in a Horse. Vet. Pathol., *21*:394, 1984.

Burmester, B.R., et al.: The Oncogenic Spectrum of Two "Pure" Strains of Avian Leukosis. J. Natl. Cancer Inst., *23*:277, 1959.

Burny, A., et al.: Bovine Leukemia Virus Involvement in Enzootic Bovine Leukosis. Adv. Cancer Res., *28*:251, 1978.

Busse, C., et al.: Further Investigations on the Porcine Lymphoma C-type Particle (PLCP) and the Possible Biological Significance of the Virus in Pigs. Ann. Rech. Vet., *9*:651, 1978.

Cain, G.R., et al.: Radiation-Induced Megakaryoblastic Leukemia in a Dog. Vet. Path., *22*:641, 1985.

Campbell, J.G.: The Ultrastructure of a Porcine Hereditary Lymphoma with Some Observations on Cell Cultures and Enzyme Cytochemistry. J. Pathol., *122*:191, 1977.

Cardeilhac, P.T.: Recent Approaches to the Treatment of Neoplastic Disease of Animals. J. Amer. Vet. Med. Ass., *156*:355, 1970.

Case, M.T., and Simon, J.: Transmission Studies of Swine Lymphosarcoma: Hematologic and Pathologic Changes in Pigs Inoculated with Whole Cell Suspensions. Amer. J. Vet. Res., *29*:263, 1968.

Castro-Malaspina, H., and Moore, M.: Pathophysiological Mechanisms Operating in the Development of Myelofibrosis: Role of Megakaryocytes. Nouv. Rev. Fr. Hematol., *24*:221, 1982.

Catovsky, D.: Symposium: Classification of Leukemia. 1. The Classification of Acute Leukemia. Pathology, *14*:277, 1982.

Chander, S., et al.: Bovine Lymphosarcoma in Twin Calves. Can. J. Comp. Med., *41*:274, 1977.

Chapman, A.L., et al.: An Electron Microscopic Study of the Cell Types in Canine Lymphoma and Leukaemia. J. Comp. Pathol., *91*:331, 1981.

Chew, D.J., et al.: Pseudo Hyperparathyroidism in a Cat. J. Amer. Anim. Hosp. Ass., *11*:46, 1975.

Cohen, H., et al.: Pathogenesis of a Transplanted Canine Lymphocytic Leukemia. Cancer, *33*:1313, 1974.

Cooper, B.J., and Watson, A.D.J.: Myeloid Neoplasia in a Dog. Aust. Vet. J., *51*:150, 1975.

Cornelius, C.E., et al.: Plasma Cell Myelomatosis in a Horse. Cornell Vet., *40*: 478, 1959.

Cotter, S.M.: Update on Feline Leukemia. Proc. Amer. Anim. Hosp. Ass., 46th Annu. Meeting, New Orleans, p. 119, 1979a.

Cotter, S.M.: Anemia Associated with Feline Leukemia Virus Infection. J. Amer. Vet. Med. Ass., *175*:1191, 1979b.

Cotter, S.M.: Treatment of Lymphoma and Leukemia wiith Cyclophosphamide, Vincristine and Prednisone. I. Treatment of Dogs. J. Amer. Anim. Hosp. Ass., *19*:159, 1983a.

Cotter, S.M.: Treatment of Lymphoma and Leukemia with Cyclophosphamide, Vincristine, and Prednisone. II. Treatment of Cats. J. Amer. Anim. Hosp., *19*:166, 1983a.

Cotter, S.M., and Essex, M: Feline Acute Lymphoblastic Leukemia and Aplastic Anemia. Amer. J. Pathol., *87*:265, 1977.

Cotter, S.M., et al.: Association of Feline Leukemia Virus with Lymphosarcoma and other Disorders in the Cat. J. Amer. Vet. Med. Ass., *166*:449, 1975.

Croce, C.M., et al.: Molecular Basis of Human B Cell Neoplasia. Blood, *65*:1, 1985.

Crow, S.E.: Lymphosarcoma (Malignant Lymphoma) in the Dog: Diagnosis and Treatment. Comp. Cont. Educ. Pract. Vet., *4*:283, 1982.

Crow, S.E., et al.: Feline Reticuloendotheliosis: A Report of Four Cases. J. Amer. Vet. Med. Ass., *170*:1329, 1977a.

Crow, S.E., et al.: Chemoimmunotherapy for Canine Lymphosarcoma. Cancer, *40*:2102, 1977b.

Culvert, C.A., and Leifer, C.E.: Doxorubicin for Treatment of Canine Lymphosarcoma after Development of Resistance to Combination Chemotherapy. J. Amer. Vet. Med. Ass., *179*:1011, 1981.

Dameshek, W.: Some Speculation on the Myeloproliferative Syndromes. Blood, *6*:372, 1951.

Dameshek, W.: Sideroblastic Anaemia: Is This a Malignancy? Brit. J. Haematol., *11*:52, 1965.

Dameshek, W.: The Di Guglielmo Syndrome Revisited. Blood, *34*:567, 1969.

Dameshek, W., and Gunz, F.: Leukemia, 2nd ed., Grune & Stratton, New York, 1964.

Davies, A.P., et al.: Noncutaneous Systemic Mastocytosis and Mast Cell Leukemia in a Dog: Case Report and Literature Review. J. Amer. Anim. Hosp. Ass., *17*:361, 1981.

Deschamps, J. et al.: Experiments with Cloned Complete Tumor-Derived Bovine Leukemia Virus Information Prove that the Virus is Totally Exogenous to Its Target Animal Species. J. Virology, *40*:605, 1981.

Devare, S.G., et al.: Evaluation of Radioimmunoprecipitation for the Detection of Bovine Leukemia Virus Infection in Domestic Cattle. J. Immunol., *119*:277, 1977.

DeVita, V.T., and Schein, P.S.: The Use of Drugs in Combination for the Treatment of Cancer. New Eng. J. Med., *288*:998, 1973.

Dewes, H.F., and Blakeley, J.A.: Lymphosarcoma in a Thoroughbred Filly. N.Z. Vet. J., *28*:82, 1980.

Di Guglielmo, G.: Richerche di Hematologia. I. Un Caso dei Eritroluecemia. Folia Med., *13*:386, 1917.

Dorn, C.R., et at.: Epizootiologic Characteristics of Canine and Feline Leukemia and Lymphoma. Amer. J. Vet. Res., *28*:993, 1967.

Dorn, C.R., et al.: Survey of Animal Neoplasms in Alameda and Contra Costa counties, California. II. Cancer Morbidity in Dogs and Cats from Alameda County. J. Natl. Cancer Inst., *40*:307, 1968.

Dreyfus, B.: Preleukemic States. Blood Cells, *2*:33, 1976.

Driscoll, D.M., and Olson, C.: Bovine Leukemia Virus–Associated Antigens in Lymphocyte Cultures. Amer. J. Vet. Res., *38*:1897, 1977.

Dungworth, D.L., et al.: Early Detection of the Lesions of Bovine Lymphosarcoma. In Leukaemia in Animals and Man. Proc. 3rd Intl. Symp. on Comparative Leu-

kaemia Res., Paris, 1967. Bendixen, H.J., ed., Bibl. Haematol. *31*:206–211, Karger, Basel N.Y., 1968.

Dungworth, D.L., et al.: Development of a Myeloproliferative Disorder in Beagles Continuously Exposed to ⁹⁰Sr. Blood, *34*:610, 1969.

Ellermann, IV., and Bang, O.: Experimentelle Leukamie bei Huhnern. Zentralbl. Bakteriol. Abt. I. (Orig.) *46*:595, 1908.

Enke, K.H, et al.: Ein Kauistischer Beitrug zur lymphatischen Leukose des Schafes. Dtsch. Tierärztl. Wochenschr., *68*:359, 1961.

Esplin, D.G., and Taylor, J.L.: Hypercalcemia in a Horse with Lymphosarcoma. J. Amer. Vet. Med. Ass., *170*:180, 1977.

Essex, M.E.: Feline Leukemia: A Naturally Occurring Cancer of Infectious Origin. Epidemiol. Rev., *4*:189, 1982.

Essex, M., and Francis, D.: The Risk to Humans from Malignant Diseases of Their Pets: An Unsettled Issue. J. Amer. Anim. Hosp. Ass., *12*:386, 1976.

Essex, M., et al.: Naturally Occurring Persistent Feline Oncorna Virus Infections in the Absence of Disease. Infect. Immun., *11*:470, 1975a.

Essex, M., et al.: Feline Oncorna Virus–Associated Cell Membrane Antigen. IV. Antibody Titers in Cats with Naturally Occurring Leukemia, Lymphoma, and Other Diseases. J. Natl. Cancer Inst., *55*:463, 1975b.

Essex, M., et al.: Immune Response to Leukemia Virus and Tumor-Associated Antigens in Cats. Cancer Res., *36*:640, 1976.

Essex, M., et al.: Horizontal Transmission of Feline Leukemia Virus under Natural Conditions in a Feline Leukemia Cluster Household. Intl. J. Cancer, *19*:90, 1977.

Evermann, J.F., et al.: Prevalence of Bovine Leukemia Virus Antibody in Seven Herds of Holstein-Friesian Cattle. J. Amer. Vet. Med. Ass., *177*:549, 1980.

Eyestone, W.H.: Myelogenous Leukemia in the Cat. J. Natl. Cancer Inst., *12*:599, 1951.

Falconer, G.J., et al.: A Case of Erythremic Myelosis in a Cat. N.Z. Vet. J., *28*:83, 1980.

Ferdinand, G.A.A., et al.: Antibodies to Bovine Leukemia Virus in a Leukosis Dairy Herd and Suggestions for Control of the Infection. Can. J. Comp. Med., *43*:173, 1979.

Ferrer, J.F.: Bovine Leukosis: Natural Transmission and Principles of Control. J. Amer. Vet. Med. Ass., *175*:1281, 1979.

Ferrer, J.F.: Bovine Lymphosarcoma. Adv. Vet. Sci. Comp. Med., *24*:2, 1980.

Ferrer, J.F., et al.: Studies on the Relationship between Infection with Bovine C-type Virus, Leukemia, and Persistent Lymphocytosis in Cattle. Cancer Res., *34*:893, 1974.

Ferrer, J.F., et al.: Natural Mode of Transmission of the Bovine C-type Leukaemia Virus. Bibl. Haematol., *43*:235, 1976.

Ferrer, J.F., et al.: Relationship between Lymphosarcoma and Persistent Lymphocytosis in Cattle: A Review. J. Amer. Vet. Med. Ass., *175*:705, 1979.

Fisher, L.F., and Olander, H.J.: Spontaneous Neoplasms of Pigs: A Study of 31 Cases. J. Comp. Pathol., *88*:505, 1978.

Fisher, W.B., et al.: "Preleukemia" A Myelodysplastic Syndrome Often Terminating in Acute Leukemia. Arch. Intern. Med., *132*:226, 1973.

Flecknell, P.A., et al.: Myelosclerosis in a Cat. J. Comp. Pathol., *88*:627, 1978.

Fowler, E.H., et al.: Mast Cell Leukemia in Three Dogs. J. Amer. Vet. Med. Ass., *149*:281, 1966.

Francis, D.P., et al.: Excretion of Feline Leukaemia Virus by Naturally Infected Pet Cats. Nature, *269*:252, 1977.

Francis, D.P., et al.: Feline Leukemia Virus Infections: The Significance of Chronic Viremia. Leukemia Res., *3*:435, 1979.

Fraser, C.J., et al.: Acute Granulocyte Leukemia in Cats. Amer. Vet. Med. Ass., *165*:355, 1974.

Frazier, M.E., et al.: Comparative Studies on Cell Lines Established from Normal and Radiation-Exposed Miniature Swine. In Vitro, *15*:1001, 1979.

Fritz, T.E., et al.: Myeloproliferative Disease in Beagle Dogs Given Protracted Whole-Body Irradiation or Single Doses of ^{114}Ce. In Myeloproliferative Disorders of Animals and Man. Clarke, W.J., et al., eds. Natl. Tech. Service Conf. 680529, Springfield, Va., 1970.

Gallo, R.C., and Meyskens, F.L.: Advances in the Viral Etiology of Leukaemia and Lymphoma. Semin. Haematol., *15*:379, 1978.

Gallo, R.C., and Wong-Staal, F.: Retroviruses as Etiologic Agents of Some Animal and Human Leukemias and Lymphomas and as Tools for Elucidating the Molecular Mechanisms of Leukemogenesis. Blood, *60*:545, 1982.

Garner, R.M., and Lingeman, C.H.: Mast-Cell Neoplasms of the Domestic Cat. Path. Vet., *7*:517, 1970.

Gilmore, C.E., and Holzworth, J.: Naturally Occurring Feline Leukemia: Clinical, Pathologic, and Differential Diagnostic Features. J. Amer. Vet. Med. Ass., *158*:1013, 1971.

Gilmore, C.E., et al.: Reticuloendotheliosis: A Myeloproliferative Disorder of Cats: A Comparison with Lymphocytic Leukemia. Path. Vet., *1*:161, 1964.

Goetze, R., et al.: Zu, Diagnose der Leukose des Rindes. Mhefte. Tierhk., *5*:201, 1953.

Goetze, R., et al.: Die Leukose des Rindes, ihre Hamatologische und Klinische Diagnose. Mh. Veterinaermed., *9*:517, 1954.

Goh, K., et al.: Chromosomal Aberrations in Leukemic Cats. Cornell Vet., *71*:43, 1981.

Graf, T., and Stehelin, d.: Avian Leukemia viruses: Oncogenic and Genome Structure. Biochim. Biophys. Acta, *651*:245, 1982.

Green, R.A., and Barton, C.L.: Acute Myelomonocytic Leukemia in a Dog. J. Amer. Anim. Hosp. Ass., *13*:708, 1977.

Greenberg, P.L.: The Smoldering Myeloid Leukemic States: Clinical and Biologic Features. Blood, *61*:1035, 1983.

Greene, P.D., and Donovan, L.A.: Lymphosarcoma in a Horse. Can. Vet. J., *18*:257, 1977.

Grindem, C.B.: Ultrastructural Morphology of Leukemic Cells from 14 Dogs. Vet. Pathol., *22*:456, 1985.

Grindem, C.B., et al.: Morphologic Classification and Clinical and Pathological Characteristics of Spontaneous Leukemia in 17 Dogs. J. Amer. Anim. Hosp. Ass., *13*:708, 1977.

Grindem, C.B., et al.: Morphological Classification and Clinical and Pathological Characteristics of Spontaneous Leukemia in 10 Cats. J. Amer. Anim. Hosp. Ass., *21*:221, 1985a.

Grindem, C.B., et al.: Cytochemical Reactions in Cells from Leukemic Cats. Vet. Clin. Path., *14*(3):6, 1985b.

Gross, L.: "Spontaneous" Leukemia Developing in C3H Mice following Inoculation, in Infancy, with AK-Leukemic Extracts, or AK-Embryos. Proc. Soc. Exp. Biol. Med., *76*:27, 1951a.

Gross, L.: Pathogenic Properties, and "Vertical" Transmission of Mouse Leukemia Agent. Proc. Soc. Exp. Biol. Med., *78*:342, 1951b.

Gross, L.: How Many Different Viruses Causing Leukemia in Mice? Acta Haematol., *32*:44, 1964.

Grossman, B., et al.: Hypercalcemia Associated with T-Cell Lymphoma-Leukemia. Amer. J. Clin. Pathol., *75*:149, 1981.

Gruffydd-Jones, T.J., et al.: Clinical and Radiological Features of Anterior Mediastinal Lymphosarcoma in the Cat: A Review of 30 Cases. Vet. Rec.,*104*:304, 1979.

Hardy, W.D., Jr.: Epidemiology of Primary Neoplasms of Lymphoid Tissues in Animals. In Immunopathology of Lymphoreticular Neoplasms. Twomey, J. J., and Good, R.A., eds. Plenum, New York, pp. 129–180, 1978.

Hardy, W.D., Jr.: Facts about the FeLV FOCMA and FIP Tests: Feline Leukemia Update. Abstrs., from Calif. Vet., *33*:19, 1979, in J. Amer. Vet. Med. Ass., *176*:634, 1980.

Hardy, W.D., Jr.: Hematopoietic Tumors of Cats. J. Amer. Anim. Hosp. Ass., *17*:921, 1981a.

Hardy, W.D., Jr.: Feline Leukemia Virus Non-Neoplastic Diseases. J. Amer. Anim. Hosp. Ass., *17*:941, 1981b.

Hardy, W.D., Jr.: The Feline Leukemia Virus. J. Amer. Anim. Hosp. Ass., *17*:951, 1981c.

Hardy, W.D., Jr., et al.: Detection of the Feline Leukemia Virus and Other Mammalian Oncorna Viruses by Immunofluorescence. In Unifying Concepts of Leukemia, Bibl. Haematol., no. 39 Dutcher, R.M., and Chieco-Bianchi, R., eds. Karger, Basel, N.Y., pp. 778–799, 1973a.

Hardy, W.D., Jr., et al.: Horizontal Transmission of Feline Leukaemia Virus. Nature, *244*:266, 1973b.

Hardy, W.D., Jr., et al.: Prevention of the Contagious Spread of Feline Leukaemia Virus and Development of Leukaemia in Pet Cats. Nature, *263*:326, 1976.

Hardy, W.D., Jr., et al.: A Feline Leukaemia Virus– and Sarcoma Virus–Induced Tumour-Specific Antigen. Nature, *270*:249, 1977a.

Hardy, W.D., Jr., et al.: The Epidemiology of Feline Leukemia Virus. Cancer, *39*:1850, 1977b.

Hare, W.C.D., et al.: A Survey of Chromosomal Findings in 47 Cases of Bovine Lymphosarcoma (Leukemia). J. Natl. Cancer Inst., *38*:383, 1967.

Harmon, D.C.: The Leukemias. In Hematology. Beck, W.S., ed. The MIT Press, Cambridge, p. 323, 1985.

Harvey, J.W.: Myeloproliferative Disorders in Dogs and Cats. Vet. Clin. North Amer.: Small Anim. Pract., *11*:349, 1981.

Harvey, J.W., et al.: Feline Myeloproliferative Disease. Changing Manifestations in the Peripheral Blood. Vet. Pathol., *15*:437, 1978.

Harvey, J.W., et al.: Well-Differentiated Lymphocytic Leukemia in a Dog: Long-Term Survival without Therapy. Vet. Pathol., *18*:37, 1981.

Harvey, J.W., et al.: Myeloproliferative Disease with Megakaryocytic Predominance in a Dog with Occult Dirofilariasis. Vet. Clin. Pathol., *11*:5, 1982.

Hathway, J.E.: Feline Anemia. Vet. Clin. North Amer., *6*:495, 1976.

Hatziolos, B.C.: Lymphoblastic Lymphoma in a Bovine Fetus. J. Amer. Vet. Med. Ass., *136*:369, 1960.

Head, K.W., et al.: Hereditary Lymphosarcoma in a Herd of Pigs. Vet. Rec., *95*:523, 1974.

Heath, H., III, et al.: Canine Lymphosarcoma: A Model for Study of the Hypercalcemia of Cancer. Calcif. Tissue Int., *30*:127, 1980.

Henderson, E.S.: Acute Myelogenous Leukemia. In

Hematology 3rd ed. Williams, W.J., et al., eds. McGraw Hill, New York, ch. 28, 1983a.

Henderson, E.S.: Acute Lymphocytic Leukemia. *In* Hematology 3rd ed. Williams, W.J., et al., eds. McGraw Hill, New York, ch. 114, 1983b.

Henness, A.M., and Crow, S.E.: Treatment of Feline Myelogenous Leukemia: Four Case Reports. J. Amer. Vet. Med. Ass., 171:263, 1977.

Henness, A.M., et al.: Monocytic Leukemia in Three Cats. J. Amer. Vet. Med. Ass., 170:1325, 1977.

Herz, A., et al.: C-type Virus Particles Demonstrated in Bone Marrow Cells of a Cat With Myeloproliferative Disease, Calif. Vet., 23(4):16, 1969a.

Herz, A., et al.: Demonstration of C-type Virus Particles, Toxoplasma gondii and Hemobartonella felis in a Cat with a Myelo-Proliferative Disorder. Calif. Vet., 23(8):18, 1969b.

Herz, A., et al.: C-type Virus in Bone Marrow Cells of Cats with Myeloproliferative Disorders. J. Natl. Cancer Inst., 44:339, 1970.

Hines, J.D., et al.: High-Dose Cytosine Arabinoside (Ara-C) and m-AMSA in Refractory Acute Nonlymphocytic Leukemia (ANLL). Blood, 58:142a, 1981.

Hinshaw, V.S., and Blank, H.F.: Isolation of Feline Leukemia Virus from Clinical Specimens. Amer. J. Vet. Res., 38:55, 1977.

Hirsch, V.M., et al.: Comparison of ELISA and Immunofluorescence Assays for Detection of Feline Leukemia Virus Antigens in Blood of Cats. J. Amer. Anim. Hosp. Ass., 18:933, 1982.

Hodgkins, E.M., et al.: Chronic Lymphocytic Leukemia in the Dog. J. Amer. Vet. Med. Ass., 177:704, 1980.

Hoerni, B., et al.: Les Réticulopathies: Animales de Type Hodgkinien. Bull. Cancer, 57:37, 1970.

Holmberg, C.A., et al.: Feline Malignant Lymphomas: Comparison of Morphologic and Immunologic Characteristics. Amer. J. Vet. Res., 37:1455, 1976a.

Holmberg, C.A., et al.: Canine Malignant Lymphomas: Comparison of Morphologic and Immunologic Parameters. J. Natl. Cancer Inst., 56:125, 1976b.

Holscher, M.A., et al.: Megakaryocytic Leukemia in a Dog. Vet. Pathol., 15:562, 1978.

Holzworth, J.: Leukemia and Related Neoplasms in the Cat. II. Malignancies Other than Lymphoid. J. Amer. Vet. Med. Ass., 136:107, 1960.

Hoover, E.A., and Kociba, G.J.: Bone Lesions in Cats with Anemia Induced by Feline Leukemia Virus. J. Natl. Cancer Inst., 53:1277, 1974.

Hoover, E.A., et al.: Erythroid Hypoplasia in Cats Inoculated with Feline Leukemia Virus. J. Natl. Cancer Inst., 53:1271, 1974.

Hoss, H.E., and Olson, C.: Infectivity of Bovine C-Type (Leukemia) Virus for Sheep and Goats. Amer. J. Vet. Res., 35:633, 1974.

Hoven, R. Van Den, and Franken, P.: Clinical Aspects of Lymphosarcoma in the Horse: A Clinical Report of 16 Cases, Equine Vet. J., 15:49, 1983.

Howard, E.B., et al.: Experimental Myeloproliferative and Lymphoproliferative Diseases of Swine. *In* Leukemia in Animals and Man, Bendixen, W.J., ed. Karger, Basel, pp. 255–262, 1968.

Huber, N.L., et al.: Bovine Leukemia Virus Infection in a Large Holstein Herd: Prospective Comparison of Production and Reproductive Performance in Antibody-Negative and Antibody-Positive Cows. Amer. J. Vet. Res., 42:1477, 1981.

Hurvitz, A.L.: Fine Structure of Cells from a Cat with Myeloproliferative Disorder. Amer. J. Vet. Res., 31:747, 1970.

Idowu, L.: Observations on the Chromosomes of a Lymphosarcoma in a Dog. Vet. Rec., 99:103, 1976.

Ihle, J.N., et al.: The Immune Response to C-type Viruses and Its Potential Role In Leukemogenesis. Curr. Top. Microbiol. Immunol., 101:31, 1982.

Imlah, P., et al.: Serum Gamma Globulin Levels and the Detection of I.G. Heavy Chain and Light Chain in the Serum and Urine of Cases of Pig Hereditary Lymphosarcoma. Eur. J. Cancer, 15:1337, 1979.

Jacobs, R.M., et al.: Inhibition of Lymphocyte Blastogenesis by Sera from Cows with Lymphoma. Amer. J. Vet. Res., 41:372, 1980.

Jacobs, R.M., et al.: Monoclonal Gammopathy in a Horse with Defective Hemostasis. Vet. Pathol., 20:643, 1983.

Jain, N.C., et al.: Clinico-Pathological Findings and Cytochemical Characterization of Myelomonocytic Leukaemia in Five Dogs. J. Comp. Pathol., 91:17, 1981.

Jarrett, O.: Natural History of Feline Leukaemia Virus. J. Small Anim. Pract., 16:409, 1975.

Jarrett, O.: Recent Advances in the Epidemiology of Feline Leukaemia Virus. Vet. Ann., 23:287, 1983.

Jarrett, O., et al.: The Frequency of Occurrence of Feline Leukaemia Virus Subgroups in Cats. Int. J. Cancer, 21:334, 1978.

Jarrett, O., et al.: Detection of Transient and Persistent Feline Leukaemia Virus Infections. Vet. Rec., 110:225, 1982a.

Jarrett, O., et al.: A Comparison of Three Methods of Feline Leukaemia Virus Diagnosis. Vet. Rec. 110:325, 1982b.

Jarrett, W.F.H.: Viruses and Leukaemia. Brit. J. Haematol., 25:287, 1973.

Jarrett, W.F.H., et al.: Leukaemia in the Cat: Transmission Experiments with Leukaemia (Lymphosarcoma). Nature, 202:566, 1964a.

Jarrett, W.F.H., et al.: A Virus-Like Particle Associated with Leukaemia (Lymphosarcoma). Nature, 202:567, 1964b.

Jarrett, W.F.H., et al.: Leukaemia and Lymphosarcoma in Animals and Man. I. Lymphosarcoma or Leukaemia in Domestic Animals. Vet. Rec., 79:693, 1966.

Jarrett, W., et al.: Vaccination against Feline Leukaemia Virus Using a Cell Membrane Antigen System. Int. J. Cancer, 16:134, 1975.

Jeglum, K.A.: Immunomodulation of Hematopoietic Tumors. Vet. Clin. North Amer. (Small Anim. Pract.), 15:817, 1985.

Johnstone, A.C., and Manktelow, B.W.: The Pathology of Spontaneously Occurring Malignant Lymphoma in Sheep. Vet. Pathol., 15:301, 1978.

Johnstone, A.C., et al.: Persistent Lymphocytosis and Virus-like Particles in Lymphocytes of Sheep Inoculated with Cell-Free Extracts Derived from Ovine Malignant Lymphomas. J. Pathol., 128:183, 1979.

Joiner, G.N., et al.: A Case of Chronic Granulocytic Leukemia in a Dog. Can. J. Comp. Med., 40:153, 1976.

Kadota, K.: Patho-Morphological Observations of Equine Leukemia Complex. Jpn. Vet. Res., 29:22, 1981.

Kashima, T., and Nomura, T.: A Case of Myeloid Leukaemia (Eosinophilic) in Swine. Jpn. J. Vet. Sci., 44:529, 1982.

Kass, L.: Enzymatic Abnormalities in Erythroleukemia. Acta Haematol., 59:302, 1978.

Kass, L.: Leukemia: Cytology and Cytochemistry. J.B. Lippincott, Philadelphia, 1982.

Kenyon, S.J., et al.: Induction of Lymphosarcoma in Sheep by Bovine Leukemia Virus. J. Natl. Cancer Inst., 67:1157, 1981.

Knospe, W.H., and Gregory, S.A.: Smoldering Acute Leukemia. Arch. Intern. Med., *127*:910, 1971.

Kobilinsky, L., et al.: Hypocomplementemia Associated with Naturally Occurring Lymphosarcoma in Pet Cats. J. Immunol., *122*:2139, 1979.

Kumar, S.P., et al.: Frequency of Lymphocytes Bearing Fc Receptors and Surface Membrane Immunoglobulins in Normal, Persistent Lymphocytotic and Leukemic Cows. Amer. J. Vet. Res., *39*:1, 1978.

Langham, R.F., and Hallman, E.T.: Chronic Myeloid Leukemia of a Hog. J. Amer. Vet. Med. Ass., *94*:653, 1939.

Langston, A., et al.: Comparison of Production Variables of Bovine Leukemia Virus Antibody-Negative and Antibody-Positive Cows in Two California Dairy Herds. Amer. J. Vet. Res., *39*:1093, 1978.

Latimer, K.S., and Dykstra, M.J.: Acute Monocytic Leukemia in a Dog. J. Amer. Vet. Med. Ass., *184*:852, 1984.

Leifer, C.E., and Matus, R.E.: Lymphoid Leukemia in the Dog: Acute Lymphoblastic Leukemia and Chronic Lymphocytic Leukemia. Vet. Clin. North Amer. (Small Anim. Pract.), *15*:723, 1985.

Leifer, C.E.: Chronic Myelogenous Leukemia in the Dog. J. Amer. Vet. Med. Ass., *183*:686, 1983.

Leser, S.J., et al.: Disseminated Anaplastic Mastocytoma with Terminal Mastocythemia in a Dog. J. Amer. Anim. Hosp. Ass., *17*:355, 1981.

Lewis, H.B., and Leitch, M.: A Case of Granulocytic Leukemia in the Horse. *In* Proc. 1st Int. Symp. Equine Hematol. Kitchen, H., and Krehbiel, J.D., eds. Amer. Assoc. Equine Practitioners, Golden, Colo., pp. 141–143, 1975.

Lieberman, M., and Kaplan, H.S.: Leukemogenic Activity of Filtrates from Radiation-Induced Lymphoid Tumors of Mice. Science, *130*:387, 1959.

Lillie, R.D.: Mast Myelocyte Leukemia in a Cat. Amer. J. Pathol., *7*:713, 1931.

Linnabary, R.D., et al.: Acute Myelomonocytic Leukemia in a Dog. J. Amer. Anim. Hosp. Ass., *14*:71, 1978.

Liu, Si-Kwang, and Carb, A.V.: Erythroblastic Leukemia in a Dog. J. Amer. Vet. Med. Ass., *152*:1511, 1968.

Livingston, D.M., and Todaro, G.J.: Endogenous type C Virus from a Cat Cell Clone with Properties Distinct from Previously Described Feline Type C Virus. Virology, *53*:142, 1973.

Loeb, W.F., et al.: Myelomonocytic Leukemia in a Cat. Vet. Pathol., *12*:464, 1975.

Lucke, V.M.: Basophilic (Mast-Cell) Leukaemia in the Domestic Cat. J. Pathol. Bact., *88*:596, 1964.

Lukes, R.J.: The Immunologic Approach to the Pathology of Malignant Lymphomas. Amer. J. Clin. Pathol., *72*:657, 1979.

Lukes, R.J., et al.: Canine Lymphomas Histologically Indistinguishable from Burkitt's Lymphoma. Lancet, *2*:389, 1966.

Lutz, H., et al.: Humoral Immune Reactivity to Feline Leukemia Virus and Associated Antigens in Cats Naturally Infected with Feline Leukemia Virus. Cancer Res., *40*:3642, 1980a.

Lutz, H. et al.: Detection of Feline Leukemia Virus Infection. Feline Pract., *10(4)*:13, 1980b.

MacEwen, E.G.: Treatment of Basophilic Leukemia in a Dog. J. Amer. Vet. Med. Ass., *166*:376, 1975.

MacEwen, E.G., et al.: Hyperviscosity Syndrome Associated with Lymphocytic Leukemia in Three Dogs. J. Amer. Vet. Med. Ass., *170*:1309, 1977a.

MacEwen, E.G., et al.: Diagnosis and Treatment of Canine Hematopoietic Neoplasms. Vet. Clin. North Amer., *7*:105, 1977b.

MacEwen, E.G., et al.: Cyclic Combination Chemotherapy of Canine Lymphosarcoma. J. Amer. Vet. Med. Ass., *178*:1178, 1981a.

MacEwen, E.G., et al.: Temporary Plasma-Induced Remission of Lymphoblastic Leukemia in a Dog. Amer. J. Vet. Res., *42*:1450, 1981b.

Mackey, L.J. et al.: Monocytic Leukaemia in the Dog. Vet. Rec., *96*:27, 1975.

Mackey, L.J., and Jarrett, W.F.H.: Two Populations of Lymphocytes in a Cat. Vet. Rec., *96*:41, 1975.

Mackey, L.J., et al.: Anemia Associated with Feline Leukemia Virus Infection in Cats. J. Natl. Cancer Inst., *54*:209, 1975.

Madewell, B.R.: Chemotherapy for Canine Lymphosarcoma. Amer. J. Vet. Res., *36*:1525, 1975.

Madewell, B.R.: Canine Lymphoma. Vet. Clin. North Amer. (Small Anim. Pract.), *15*:709, 1985.

Madewell, B.R., and Feldman, B.F.: Characterization of Anemias Associated with Neoplasia in Small Animals. J. Amer. Vet. Med. Ass., *176*:419, 1980.

Madewell, B.R., and Jarrett, O.: Recovery of Feline Leukemia Virus from Non-Viremic Cats. Vet. Rec., *112*:339, 1983.

Madewell, B.R., et al.: Hematologic Abnormalities Preceding Myeloid Leukemia in Three Cats. Vet. Pathol., *16*:510, 1979.

Madewell, B.R., et al.: Serum Concentrations of Immunoglobulins G, A, and M in Dogs with Neoplastic Disease. Amer. J. Vet. Res., *41*:720, 1980.

Madewell, B.R., et al.: Lymphosarcoma with Leukemia in a Horse. Amer. J. Vet. Res., *43*:807, 1982.

Madewell, B.R., et al.: Mast Cell Phagocytosis of Red Cells in a Cat. Vet. Pathol., *20*:638, 1983.

Maede, Y., and Murata, H.: Erythroleukemia in a Cat with Special Reference to the Fine Structure of Primitive Cells in Its Peripheral Blood. Jpn. J. Vet. Sci., *42*:531, 1980.

Mandel, M.P., et al.: Endogenous RD-114 Virus of Cats: Absence of Antibodies to RD-114 Envelope Antigens in Cats Naturally Exposed to Feline Leukemia Virus. Infect. Immun., *24*:282, 1979.

Markel, M.D., and Dorr, T.E.: Multiple Myeloma in a Horse. J. Amer. Vet. Med. Ass., *188*:621, 1986.

Marshak, R.R., et al.: Studies on Bovine Lymphosarcoma. I. Clinical Aspects, Pathological Alterations and Herd Studies. Cancer Res., *22*:202, 1962.

Mathes, L.E., et al.: Immunosuppressive Properties of a Virion Polypeptide, a 15,000-Dalton Protein, from Feline Leukemia Virus. Cancer Res., *39*:950, 1979.

Matus, R.E., and Leifer, C.E.: Immunoglobulin-Producing Tumors. Vet. Clin. North Amer.: Small Anim. Pract., *15*:741, 1985.

Matus, R.E., et al.: Acute Lymphoblastic Leukemia in the Dog: A Review of 30 Cases. J. Amer. Vet. Med. Ass., *8*:859, 1983.

McTaggart, H.S., et al.: Evidence for a Genetic Factor in the Transmission of Spontaneous Lymphosarcoma (Leukaemia) of Young Pigs. Nature, *232*:557, 1971.

Medway, W., and Rapp, J.P.: A Case of Chronic Granulocytic Leukemia with Thrombocytopenic Purpura in a Dog. Cornell Vet., *52*:247, 1962.

Meier, H.: Neoplastic Diseases of the Hematopoietic System (So-Called Leukosis-Complex) in the Dog. Zentralbl. Veterinärmed., *4*:633, 1957.

Meier, H., and Gourley, G.: Basophilic (Myelocyte) or Mast Cell Leukemia in a Cat. J. Amer. Vet. Med. Ass., *130*:33, 1957.

Meier, H., and Patterson, D.F.: Myelogenous Leukemia in a Cat. J. Amer. Vet. Med. Ass., *128*:211, 1956.

Mertelsmann, R., et al.: Morphological Classification, Response to Therapy, and Survival in 263 Adult Patients with Acute Nonlymphoblastic Leukemia. Blood, *56*:773, 1980.

Michel, R.L., et al.: Megakaryocytic Myelosis in a Cat. J. Amer. Vet. Med. Ass., *168*:1021, 1976.

Migaki, G.: Hematopoietic Neoplasms of Slaughter Animals. *In* Comparative Morphology of Hematopoietic Neoplasms. Natl. Cancer Inst. Monogram., *32*:121, 1969.

Miller, J.M.: Bovine Lymphosarcoma. Modern Vet. Pract., *61*:588, 1980.

Miller, J.M., and van der Maaten, M.J.: Bovine Leukosis: Its Importance to the Dairy Industry in the United States. J. Dairy Sci., *65*:2194, 1982.

Miller, J.M., et al.: Virus-like Particles in Phytohemagglutinin-Stimulated Lymphocyte Cultures with Reference to Bovine Lymphosarcoma. J. Natl. Cancer Inst., *43*:1297, 1969.

Miller, L.D.: Export Testing for Enzootic Bovine Leukosis. J. Amer. Vet. Med. Ass., *177*:620, 1980.

Miller, L.D., et al.: Inoculation of Calves with Particles Resembling C-type Virus from Cultures of Bovine Lymphosarcoma. J. Natl. Cancer Inst., *48*:423, 1972.

Monlux, A.W., et al.: A Survey of Tumors Occurring in Cattle, Sheep, and Swine. Amer. J. Vet. Res., *17*:646, 1956.

Morris, D.D., et al.: Eosinophilic Myeloproliferative Disorder in a Horse. Amer. Vet. Med. Ass., *185*:993, 1984.

Moulton, J.E., and Bostick, W.L.: Canine Malignant Lymphoma, Simulating Hodgkin's Disease in Man. J. Amer. Vet. Med. Ass., *132*:204, 1958.

Muscoplat, C., et al.: Characteristics of Lymphocyte Response to Phytomitogens: Comparison of Responses of Lymphocytes from Normal and Lymphocytotic Cows. Amer. J. Vet. Res., *35*:1053, 1974.

Nalbandian, R.M., et al.: Myeloid Megakaryocytic Hepatosplenomegaly: Case Study with a Proposed System of Matrix Classification of the Myeloproliferative Disorders. Amer. J. Clin. Pathol., *49*:535, 1968.

Neil, J.C., and Onions, D.E.: Feline Leukemia Viruses: Molecular Biology and Pathogenesis. Anticancer Res., *5*:49, 1985.

Neufeld, J.L.: Lymphosarcoma in the Horse: A Review. Can. Vet. J., *14*:129, 1973.

Nielsen, S.W.: Myeloproliferative Disorders in Animals. *In* Myeloproliferative Disorders of Animals and Man, Clark et al., eds. National Technical Information Service, Springfield, Va. 297–313, 1970.

Nielsen, S.W.: Classification of Tumors in Dogs and Cats. J. Amer. Anim. Hosp. Ass., *19*:13, 1983.

Niman, H.L., et al.: RD-114 and Feline Leukaemia Virus Genome Expression in Natural Lymphomas of Domestic Cats. Nature, *266*:357, 1977.

O'Connor, G.T., et al.: Childhood Lymphoma Resembling "Burkitt Tumor" in the United States. Cancer, *18*:411, 1965.

Ohshima, K., and Miura, S.: Mast-Cell Leukosis in Cats: A Report of Two Cases. Jpn. J. Vet. Sci., *27*:233, 1965.

Ohshima, K., et al.: Evidence on Horizontal Transmission of Bovine Leukemia Virus Due to Blood-Sucking Tabanid Flies. Jpn. J. Vet. Sci., *43*:79, 1981.

Olsen, R.G., et al.: New Approach to Feline Leukemia Immunoprevention: Soluble Tumor Cell Vaccine. Calif. Vet., *34(3)*:11, 1980.

Olson, C., and Baumgartener, L.E.: Pathology of Lymphosarcoma in Sheep Induced with Bovine Leukemia Virus. Cancer Res., *36*:2365, 1976.

Olson, C., et al.: Progress on Transmission of Bovine Lymphosarcoma. *In* Comparative Leukemia Research 1969. Bibl. Haematol., no. 36, Dutcher, R.M., ed. Karger, Basel, N.Y., pp. 476–492, 1970.

Olson, C., et al.: Transmission of Lymphosarcoma from Cattle to Sheep. J. Natl. Cancer Inst., *49*:1463, 1972.

Olson, C., et al.: Evidence of Bovine C-type (Leukemia) Virus in Dairy Cattle. J. Amer. Vet. Med. Ass., *163(4)*:355, 1973.

Olson, C., et al.: Goat Lymphosarcoma from Bovine Leukemia Virus. J. Natl. Cancer Inst., *67*:671, 1981.

Onions, D.: B- and T-Cell Markers on Canine Lymphosarcoma Cells. J. Natl. Cancer Inst., *59*:1001, 1977.

Onions, D.: RNA-Dependent DNA Polymerase Activity in Canine Lymphosarcoma. Brit. J. Cancer, *16*:343, 1980.

O'Reilly-Felice, C., et al.: Viral Antigen-Antibody Complexes in Sera of Cats with Lymphosarcoma. Fed. Proc., *39*:682, 1980.

O'Rourke, L., and Jain, N.C.: Erythrophagocytosis by Feline Mast Cells. Unpublished observations, 1982.

Paul, F.S., et al.: Evidence for the Replication of Bovine Leukemia Virus in the B Lymphocytes. Amer. J. Vet. Res., *38*:873, 1977.

Paulsen, J., et al.: C-type Virus Particles in Phytohemagglutinin-Stimulated Lymphocyte Cultures with Reference to Enzootic Lymphatic Leukosis in Sheep. Med. Microbiol. Immunol., *158*:105, 1972.

Paulsen, J., et al.: Comparative Studies on Ovine and Bovine C-type Particles. *In* Comparative Leukemia Research 1975. Clemmesen, J., and Yohn, D.S., eds. Karger, Basel, N.Y., 1975a.

Paulsen, J., et al.: (Experimental Transmission of Lymphocytic Leucosis in Sheep.) Zentralbl. Veterinärmed. B., *22*:737, 1975b.

Payne, L.N.: Viral Lymphomagenesis in the Domestic Fowl: A Review. Proc. Roy. Soc. Med., *70*:559, 1977.

Pedersen, N.C., et al.: Studies of Naturally Transmitted Feline Leukemia Virus Infection. Amer. J. Vet. Res., *38*:1523, 1977.

Pedersen, N.C., et al.: Safety and Efficacy Studies of Live- and Killed-Feline Leukemia Virus Vaccines. Amer. J. Vet. Res., *40*:1120, 1979.

Perk, K.: Myeloproliferative Syndrome in a Dog. Refuah Vet., *37*:49, 1980.

Piper, C.E., et al.: Seroepidemiological Evidence for Horizontal Transmission of Bovine C-type Virus. Cancer Res., *35*:2714, 1975.

Pollet, L., et al.: Blast Crisis in Chronic Myelogenous Leukaemia in a Dog. J. Small Anim. Pract., *19*:469, 1978.

Ragan, H.A., et al.: Acute Myelomonocytic Leukemia Manifested as Myeloproliferative Anemia in a Dog. J. Amer. Vet. Med. Ass., *169*:421, 1976.

Rappaport, H.: Tumors of the Hematopoietic Systems. *In* Atlas of Tumor Pathology, Fascicle no. 8, Armed Forces Institute of Pathology, Washington D.C., 1966.

Raskin, R.E., and Krehbiel, J.D.: Myelodysplastic Changes in a Cat with Myelomonocytic Leukemia. J. Amer. Vet. Med. Ass., *187*:171, 1985.

Rebhun, W.C., and Bertone, A.: Equine Lymphosarcoma. J. Amer. Vet. Med. Ass., *184*:720, 1984.

Reef, V.B., et al.: Lymphosarcoma and Associated Immune-Mediated Hemolytic Anemia and Thrombocytopenia in the Horse. J. Amer. Vet. Med. Ass., *184*:313, 1984.

Renier, F., et al.: Quelques Considerations sur les Leucoses Porcines. Nouv. Rev. Fr. Hematol., 6:239, 1966.

Ricci, P., et al.: Clinical Contribution to the Knowledge of Hemopoietic Dysplasias: Long Term Follow-Up of 13 Patients with Refractory Anemia. Acta Haematol., 60:10, 1978.

Roberts, M.C.: A Case of Primary Lymphoid Leukaemia in a Horse. Equine Vet. J., 9:216, 1977.

Roggli, V.L., and Saleem, A.: Erythroleukemia: A Study of 15 Cases and Literature Review. Cancer, 49:101, 1982.

Rojko, J.L., et al.: Pathogenesis of Experimental Feline Leukemia Virus Infection. J. Natl. Cancer Inst., 63:759, 1979.

Roperto, F., et al.: Hodgkin's Disease in a Cat. Zentralbl. Veterinärmed., 30:182, 1983.

Roscher, A.A., et al.: Acute Myelogenous Leukemia with Histopathological Studies following Total Body Irradiation of a Dog. J. Amer. Vet. Med. Ass., 136:491, 1960.

Rosenthal, R.C.: Epidemiology of Canine Lymphosarcoma. Comp. Cont. Educ. Pract. Vet., 4:855, 1982.

Rosin, A.: Neurologic Disease Association with Lymphosarcoma in Ten Dogs. J. Amer. Vet. Med. Ass., 181:50, 1982.

Rous, P.: Transmission of a Malignant New Growth by Means of a Cell-Free Filtrate. JAMA, 56:198, 1911.

Rudolph, R., and Hübner, C.: Megakaryocyte Leukosis in a Dog. Kleintierpraxis, 17:9, 1972.

Rundles, R.W.: Chronic Lymphocytic Leukemia. In Hematology, 3rd ed. Williams, W.J., et al., eds. McGraw Hill, New York, ch. 115, 1983.

Sachs, L.: The Differentiation of Myeloid Leukaemic Cells: New Possibilities for Therapy. Brit. J. Haematol., 40:509, 1978.

Sanal, S.M., et al.: Pseudoleukemia: When "Leukemia" Is Not Leukemia. Postgrad. Med., 65:143, 1979.

Sarma, P.S., and Log, T.: Subgroup Classification of Feline Leukemia and Sarcoma Viruses by Viral Interference and Neutralization Tests. Virology, 54:160, 1973.

Sarma, P.S., et al.: Differential Host Range of Viruses of Feline Leukemia-Sarcoma Complex. Virology, 64:438, 1975.

Schalm, O.W.: Histiocytic Medullary Reticulosis, Canine Pract., 5(4):42, 1978.

Schalm, O.W.: Manual of Feline and Canine Hematology. Veterinary Practice Publishing, Santa Barbara, Calif., 1980. a, p. 123; b, pp. 65, 69; c, pp. 65, 71; d, pp. 65, 73; e,p. 95; f, pp. 91, 97; g, pp. 96–97; h, pp. 211–216; i, p. 209.

Schalm, O.W.: Lymphosarcoma in the Horse. Equine Pract., 3(2):23, 1981.

Schalm, O.W., and Carlson, G.P.: The Blood and Blood-Forming Organs. In Equine Medicine and Surgery. Mansmann, R.A., et al., eds. American Veterinary Publications, Santa Barbara, Calif., p. 377, 1982.

Schalm, O.W., and Switzer, J.W.: Bone Marrow Disease in the Cat. I. Atypical Granulocytic Leukemia. Calif. Vet., 22(4):24, 1968.

Schalm, O.W., and Theilen, G.H.: Myeloproliferative Disease in the Cat, Associated with C-type Leukovirus Particles in Bone Marrow. J. Amer. Vet. Med. Ass., 157:1686, 1970.

Schmidt, R.E., et al.: Megakaryocytic Myelosis in Cats: Review and Case Report. J. Small Anim. Pract., 24:759, 1984.

Schneider, R.: Comparison of Age- and Sex-Specific Incidence Rate Patterns of the Leukemia Complex in the Cat and the Dog. J. Natl. Cancer Inst., 70:971, 1983.

Searcy, G.P., and Oer, J.P.: Chronic Granulocytic Leukemia in a Horse. Can. Vet. J., 22:148, 1981.

Seawright, A.A., and Grono, L.R.: Malignant Mast Cell Tumour in a Cat with Perforating Duodenal Ulcer. J. Pathol. Bact., 87:107, 1964.

Seed, T.M., et al.: Irradiation-Induced Erythroleukemia and Myelogenous Leukemia in the Beagle Dog: Hematology and Ultrastructure. Blood, 50:1061, 1977.

Sheriff, D., and Newlands, R.W.: A Case of Focal Leukaemia in a Calf. Vet. Rec., 98:174, 1976.

Shifrine, M., and Bryant, B.J.: Leukemia Allotransplants in Canine Fetuses: Influence of Host Age and Immune Responsiveness. Proc. Soc. Exp. Biol. Med., 151:307, 1976.

Shifrine, M., et al.: Transplantation of Radiation-Induced Canine Myelomonocytic Leukemia. Haematologica, 39:158, 1973.

Simon, J., and Brewer, R.L.: Lymphosarcoma in a Calf. J. Amer. Vet. Med. Ass., 142:1388, 1963.

Simon, J., Small, E., and Jaeschke, W.: Hodgkin's Disease in a Dog. J. Amer. Vet. Med. Ass., 145:231, 1964.

Simon, N. and Holzworth, J.: Eosinophilic Leukemia in a Cat. Cornell Vet., 57:579, 1967.

Singh, B., et al.: Clinicopathological Studies on Lymphosarcoma in Indian Buffaloes (Bubalis bubalis). Zentralbl. Veterinärmed., 26:468, 1979.

Skelley, J.F.: Clinico-Pathologic Conference, School of Vet. Univ. of Pennsylvania. J. Amer. Vet. Med. Ass., 142:646, 1963.

Smith, B.P. and Anderson, M.: Lymphosarcoma of the Brain in a Heifer. J. Amer. Vet. Med. Ass., 170:333, 1977.

Squire, R.A., et al.: Clinical and Pathologic Study of Canine Lymphoma: Clinical Staging, Cell Classification and Therapy. J. Natl. Cancer Inst., 51:565, 1973.

Stann, S.E.: Myelomonocyte Leukemia in a Cat. J. Amer. Vet. Med. Ass., 174:722, 1979.

Strandstrom, H.V., and Rimaila-Parnanen, E.: Canine Atypical Malignant Lymphoma. Amer. J. Vet. Res., 40:1033, 1979.

Straub, O.C.: Enzootic Bovine Leukosis. In Virus Diseases of Food Animals. Vol. 20. Gibbs, E.P.S., Academic Press, New York, pp. 683–718, 1981.

Sutton, R.H., et al.: Myeloproliferative Disease in the Cat: A Granulocytic and Megakaryocytic Disorder. N.Z. Vet. J., 26:273, 1978.

Theilen, G.H., and Madewell, B.R.: Leukemia-Sarcoma Disease Complex, In Veterinary Cancer Medicine, Theilen and Madewell, eds. Lea & Febiger, Philadelphia, 1979.

Theilen, G.H., and Schalm, O.W.: Myeloproliferative Disease in the Dog: A Case Report of Granulocytic Leukemia. Calif. Vet., 24(10):10, 1970.

Theilen, G.H., et al.: Bovine Lymphosarcoma: Temporary Spontaneous Remission in a Cow. Cornell Vet., 50:429, 1960.

Theilen, G.H., et al.: Bovine Lymphosarcoma in California. I. Epizootiologic and Hematologic Aspects. Health Lab. Sci., 1:96, 1964.

Theilen, G.H., et al.: Chemoimmunotherapy for Canine Lymphosarcoma. J. Amer. Vet. Med. Ass., 170:607, 1977.

Thompson, J.C., and Johnstone, A.C.: Myelofibrosis in the Dog: Three Case Reports. J. Small Anim. Pract., 24:589, 1983.

Thurmond, M.C., and Burridge, M.J.: Application of Research to Control of Bovine Leukemia Virus Infection and to Exportation of Bovine Leukemia Virus-free Cattle and Semen. J. Amer. Vet. Med. Ass., *181*:1531, 1982.

Tolle, D.V., et al.: Radiation-Induced Erythroleukemia in the Beagle Dog. Amer. J. Pathol., *87*:499. 1977.

Tolle, D.V., et al.: Acute Monocytic Leukemia in an Irradiated Beagle. Vet. Pathol., *16*:243, 1979.

Tolle, D.V., et al.: Circulating Micromegakaryocytes Preceding Leukemia in Three Dogs Exposed to 2.5R/Day Gamma Radiation. Vet. Pathol., *20*:111, 1983.

Tomley, F.M., et al.: Retrovirus Particles Associated with Canine Lymphosarcoma and Leukaemia. Brit. J. Cancer, *45*:644, 1982.

Tomley, F.M., et al.: Reverse Transcriptase Activity and Particles of Retroviral Density in Cultured Canine Lymphosarcoma Supernatants. Brit. J. Cancer, *47*:277, 1983a.

Tomley, F.M., et al.: Reverse Transcriptase Activity in a Case of Ovine Lymphoblastic Leukaemia. Res. Vet. Sci., *34*:50, 1983b.

Tomlinson, M.J., et al.: Lymphosarcoma with Virus-like Particles in a Neonatal Foal. Vet. Pathol., *16*:629, 1979.

Torres, J., Jr., et al.: The Fine Structure of Canine Lymphoma and Lymphocytic Leukemia. Anat. Rec., *184*:548, 1976.

Trainen, A., and Klopfer, U.: Immunofluorescent Studies of Lymph Nodes and Spleen of Leukotic Cattle for Cells Producing IgM and IgG. Cancer Res., *31*:1968, 1971.

Trainen, A., et al.: IgG and IgM Antibodies in Normal and Leukemic Cattle. J. Comp. Pathol, *86*:571, 1976.

Trum, B.F., and Carll, W.T.: Lymphatic Leukemia in a Hog following Atomic Exposure to Gamma Radiation: A Case Report. J. Amer. Vet. Med. Ass., *131*:448, 1957.

Tsujimoto, H., et al.: Monocytic Leukemia in a Cat. Jpn. J. Vet. Sci., *43*:957, 1981.

Ulbrich, F., et al.: (Observations on a Flock of Sheep with Leucosis.) Tierärz. Umschau, *25*:277, 1970.

Valli, V.E., et al.: Histology of Lymphoid Tumors in the Dog, Cat, and Cow. Vet. Pathol.,*18*:494, 1981.

Van der Maaten, M.J., and Miller, J.M.: Serological Evidence of Transmission of Bovine Leukemia Virus to Chimpanzees. Vet. Microbiol., *1*:351, 1976.

Van der Maaten, M.J., and Miller, J.M.: Appraisal of Control Measure for Bovine Leukosis. J. Amer. Vet. Med. Ass., *175*:1287, 1979.

Van der Maaten, M.J., et al.: In Utero Transmission of Bovine Leukemia Virus. Amer. J. Vet. Res., *42*:1052, 1981.

Virchow, R.: Weisses Blut and Milztumoren. Med. Ztg., *15*:157, 1846. (Cited by Wintrobe et al., 8th ed., p. 1483, ref. 33.)

Ward, J.M., et al.: Myeloproliferative Disease and Abnormal Erythrogenesis in the Cat. J. Amer. Vet. Med. Ass., *155*:879, 1969.

Weber, W.T.: Hematologic Aspects of Bovine Lymphosarcoma. Ann. N.Y. Acad. Sci., *108*:1270, 1963.

Weiden, P.L., et al.: Prolonged Disease-Free Survival in Dogs with Lymphoma after Total Body Irradiation and Autologous Marrow Transplantation: Consolidation of Combination-Chemotherapy-Induced Remission. Blood, *54*:1039, 1979.

Weiden, P.O., et al.: Immune Reactivity in Dogs with Spontaneous Malignancy. J. Natl. Cancer Inst., *53*:1049, 1974.

Weiland, F., and Straub, O.C.: Differences in the in Vitro Response of Lymphocytes from Leukotic and Normal Cattle to Concanavalin A. Res. Vet. Sci., *20*:340, 1976.

Weiss, E., et al.: C-type Virus Particles in Blood Lymphocyte Culture from Two Sheep with Persistent Lymphocytosis. Zentralbl. Veterinärmed., *18*:244, 1971.

Weiss, M.A.: The First Real Human Type-C Retrovirus. Immunol. Today, *3*:61, 1982.

Weiss, R.: A Virus Associated With Human Adult T-Cell Leukaemia. Nature, *294*:212, 1981.

Weksler, M.E., et al.: Immune Complex Disease in Cancer. Clin. Bull., *5*:109, 1975.

Weller, R.E.: Paraneoplastic Disorders in Dogs with Hematopoietic Tumors. Vet. Clin. North Amer.: Small Anim. Pract., *15*:805, 1985.

Weller, R.E.: Chemoimmunotherapy for Canine Lymphosarcoma: A Prospective Evaluation of Specific and Nonspecific Immunomodulation. Amer. J. Vet. Res., *41*:516, 1980a.

Weller, R.E., et al.: Histologic Classification as a Prognostic Criterion for Canine Lymphosarcoma. Amer. J. Vet. Res., *41*:1310, 1980b.

Weller, R.E., et al.: Myeloblastic Leukemia and Leukemic Meningitis in a Dog. Mod. Vet. Pract., *61*:42, 1980c.

Weller, R.E., et al.: Canine Lymphosarcoma and Hypercalcaemia: Clinical Laboratory and Pathologic Evaluation of Twenty-four Cases. J. Small Anim. Pract., *23*:649, 1982a.

Weller, R.E., et al.: Chemotherapeutic Responses in Dogs with Lymphosarcoma and Hypercalcemia. Amer. J. Vet. Res., *181*:891, 1982b.

Wells, G.A.H.: Hodgkin's Disease-Like Lesions in the Dog. J. Pathol., *112*:5, 1974.

Wittmann, W., and Urbaneck, D.: (The Transmissibility of Bovine Leucosis to Sheep). Mh. Veterinaermed., *25*:218, 1970. Vet. Bull., 41, Abstr. No. 339.

Wilesmith, J.W., et al.: Some Observations on the Epidemiology of Bovine Leucosis Virus in a Large Dairy Herd. Res. Vet. Sci., *28*:10, 1980.

Wintrobe, M.M., et al.: Clinical Hematology, 8th ed., Lea & Febiger, Philadelphia, 1981.

Zawidzka, Z.Z., et al.: Erythremic Myelosis in a Cat: A Case Resembling Di Guglielmo's Syndrome in Man. Path. Vet., *1*:530, 1964.

33

Cytochemistry of Normal and Leukemic Leukocytes

CYTOCHEMICAL OBSERVATIONS ON
  LEUKOCYTES OF HUMANS AND
  ANIMALS 910
  Acid Phosphatase 910
  Alkaline Phosphatase 914
  Esterases 915
  Methyl Green–Pyronin Reaction 919
  Periodic Acid–Schiff Reaction 919
  Peroxidase 920
  Sudanophilia 921
  Terminal Deoxynucleotidyl Transferase 921
  Other Cytochemical Markers 922
  Summary of Cytochemical Markers in
    Classification of Leukemias 923

SOME COMMONLY USED CYTOCHEMICAL
  TECHNIQUES IN HEMATOLOGY 924
  General Comments 924
  Acid Phosphatase 926
  Alkaline Phosphatase 927
  α-Naphthyl Acetate Esterase 928
  α-Naphthyl Butyrate Esterase 929
  Chloroacetate Esterase 929
  Combined Technique for Nonspecific
    Esterase and Chloroacetate Esterase 930
  Methyl Green–Pyronin Staining 930
  Periodic Acid–Schiff Reaction 931
  Peroxidase 932
  Sudan Black B Staining 933

Investigations into the biochemical characteristics of leukocytes represent attempts to explore the metabolic pathways that can be expected to undergo alterations under the impact of disease. Several sensitive histochemical techniques have provided valuable information about the cytochemical makeup and metabolic activities of different leukocytes. The most important application of these techniques has been in characterization of undifferentiated and acute (blast cell) leukemias. Enzyme cytochemistry makes possible delineation of specific cellular features important in differentiating acute lymphocytic leukemia (ALL) and acute myelogenous leukemia (AML), and it is superior to morphologic subclassification of the myelogenous leukemias (Bennett and Reed, 1975).

Considerable information is available concerning cytochemical characteristics of human leukocytes in health and disease. By comparison, little is known about animal leukocytes, although some species differences have been noted (Table 33–1), and some observations have been made on leukemic patients. The following is a brief discussion of some commonly used cytochemical techniques in hematologic investigations and their application to blood of common domestic animals. The reader is referred to various general references on use of these techniques in human hematology (Bover, 1964; Cline, 1981; Hayhoe, 1960; Hayhoe and Quaglino, 1980; Hayhoe et al., 1960; Kass, 1982; Li and Yam, 1982; Shibata et al., 1985; Sun et al., 1985; Wulff, 1967) and on their application to veterinary hematology (Bauer-Sic, 1963; Facklam and Kociba, 1985; Grindem et al., 1985; Jain, 1968, 1969, 1970, 1971; Jain et al., 1981; Osbaldiston et al., 1978; Rudolph and Schnabl, 1979; Tschudi et al., 1977; Tsujimoto et al., 1983).

Clinical application of leukocyte cytochemistry, particularly in diagnosis and classification of human leukemias (Tables 33–2 and 33–3), has been made by both light and electron microscopic techniques. Some pertinent references are: Beckstead and Bainton, 1980; Bell et al., 1981; Bennett, 1982; Bover, 1964; Catovsky, 1980; Cawley and Burns, 1980; Cline, 1981; Crockard, 1984; Drexler et al., 1984; Hayhoe, 1984; Hayhoe and Quaglino,

Table 33–1. Comparative Cytochemical Properties of Leukocytes of Six Animal Species

Cytochemical Marker	Cell Type[a]	Dog	Cat	Horse	Cow	Sheep	Goat
Acid phosphatase	N	±[b]	±	±	±	±	±
	L	±	±	±	±	±	±
	M	±	±	±	±	±	±
	E	±	+	±	±	±	±
Alkaline phosphatase	N	−	−	+	+	+	+
	L	−	−	−	−	−	−
	M	−	−	−	−	−	−
	E	±	+	+	+	−	−
	B	. . .	±	−	±	. . .	. . .
Chloroacetate esterase	N	+	+	+	+	+	+
	L	−	−	±	±	−	−
	M	−	−	+	±	±	±
	E	−	−	−	−	−	−
	B	. . .	+	. . .	. . .	. . .	. . .
Glycogen	N	+	+	+	+	+	+
	L	±	−	±	±	±	−
	M	±	−	±	±	±	±
	E	±	±	±	±	±	±
Nonspecific esterase (NAE or NBE)	N	−	−	±	−	−	±
	L	±	±	±	±	±	±
	M	±	±	±	±	±	+
	E	−	−	+	±	−	±
	B	−	−	. . .	. . .	. . .	. . .
Peroxidase	N	+	+	+	+	+	+
	L	−	−	−	−	−	−
	M	±	−	±	−	−	−
	E	+	−	+	+	+	+
	B	. . .	−	−	. . .	. . .	. . .
Sudanophilia	N	+	+	+	+	+	+
	L	−	−	−	−	−	−
	M	±	±	±	±	−	±
	E	+	+	+	+	+	+

[a] N, neutrophil; L, lymphocyte; M, monocyte; E, eosinophil; B, basophil.
[b] −, negative staining; ±, positive or negative staining; +, positive staining; . . ., cell not seen.
NAE, α-naphthyl acetate esterase
NBE, α-naphthyl butyrate esterase

1980; Kass, 1982; Nelson, 1976; Nemoto et al., 1983; Schmalzl et al., 1978; Schwarze, 1980; Scott, 1978; Shaw, 1976; Srivastava et al., 1983; Stuart et al., 1975; Sun et al., 1985. Cytochemistry is being used increasingly in diagnosis of leukemias in animals (Boudreaux et al., 1984; Burkhardt et al., 1984; Facklam and Kociba, 1985; Grindem et al., 1985; Jain et al., 1981; Madewell et al., 1979; Rudolph and Schnabl, 1979; Weller et al., 1980). See Chapter 32 for additional comments on leukemic animals.

CYTOCHEMICAL OBSERVATIONS ON LEUKOCYTES OF HUMANS AND ANIMALS

Acid Phosphatase

Acid phosphatase (ACP) activity in leukocytes appears in granular form. The number of ACP-positive granules in animal leukocytes varies as follows: few in neutrophils and few to many in eosinophils, lymphocytes, and monocytes (Fig. 33–1G–K). Feline eosinophils exhibit numerous ACP-positive granules that often seem to fill the cytoplasm (Fig. 33–1I). Lymphocytes and monocytes in general seem to have more ACP activity than neutrophils. Human studies have shown that macrophages and osteoclasts reveal intense staining; monocytes, plasma cells, and megakaryocytes have moderate activity; mature and immature neutrophils have moderate to weak activity; and little activity is present in normal lymphocytes and nucleated erythroid cells (Cline, 1981). Macrophages may show granular as well as diffuse staining (Schwarze, 1980). Platelets are ACP-positive. ACP activity in immature megakaryocytes is

Table 33–2. Cytochemical Reactions of Leukocytes in Human Patients with Leukemias

Cytochemical Marker	Lymphocytic Leukemia	Myelogenous Leukemia	Monocytic Leukemia	Erythremic Myelosis or Erythroleukemia
Acid phosphatase	Negative/positive, granular, unipolar in T cells	Positive, diffuse or granular	Positive, diffuse or unipolar	Negative/positive, unipolar
Alkaline phosphatase	Negative	Decreased	Negative	Negative
β-glucuronidase	Negative/positive, chunk-like in T cells			
Chloroacetate esterase	Negative	Positive	Negative	Negative
α-Naphthyl acetate esterase	Negative/positive, unipolar, chunk-like, NaF-resistant	Negative	Positive, diffuse, NaF-sensitive	Negative/positive, diffuse
Acid α-naphthyl acetate esterase	Positive, focal, chunk-like in T cells	Negative	Negative/positive	Negative
α-Naphthyl butyrate esterase	Negative/positive, unipolar, chunk-like, NaF-resistant	Negative	Positive, diffuse, NaF-sensitive	
PAS	Negative/positive, coarse, block-like granules	Negative/positive, diffuse fine granules	Negative/positive, diffuse fine granules	Positive, large aggregates or diffuse
Peroxidase	Negative	Positive	Negative/weak positive	Negative
Pyroninophilia	Negative/positive	Negative	Negative	Positive
Sudanophilia	Negative	Positive	Negative/positive	Negative

usually resistant to fixation by methanol, while that in mature megakaryocytes and platelets is methanol-sensitive (Markovic and Schulman, 1977).

In ultrastructural studies, ACP activity in neutrophils was localized in primary and tertiary granules (Wetzel, 1970). Because of greater contribution of the primary granules to ACP activity, the enzyme activity is higher in younger granulocytes than in mature ones. Cytochemical studies of leukemic monoblasts and promonocytes have indicated that ACP and nonspecific esterase (NSE) activities manifest earlier than myeloperoxidase and lysozyme activities (Catovsky et al., 1978b; O'Brien et al., 1980).

Leukocytes are assessed not only for the presence of ACP activity, but also for its pattern of distribution and resistance to tartaric acid. ACP-positive lymphocytes may reveal one or more spot-like granules or multiple small to medium-sized granules localized in the Golgi zone or distributed in the cytoplasm in a circular or semicircular pattern (Schwarze, 1980). Normal human T- and B-

lymphocytes may or may not show significant differences in the degree and pattern of ACP activity (Catovsky, 1980: Liu et al., 1982).

The pattern of ACP activity within the lymphocytes has been correlated with various types of lymphoproliferative disorders. A strong focal, spot-like, paranuclear, ACP-positive reaction is considered highly characteristic of acute T-cell malignancies (Catovsky, 1975, 1980; Catovsky et al., 1974, 1978a; Savage et al., 1981; Schwarze, 1980), although a granular pattern has also been observed (Sondergaard-Petersen and Boesen, 1979; Telek et al., 1983). In comparison, a semicircular pattern of ACP-positive cytoplasmic granules is characteristic of B-cell malignancies (Schwarze, 1980), although a diffuse, weak, or undetectable enzyme activity may be seen in some cases of chronic lymphocytic leukemia (CLL) of B-cell type (Douglas et al., 1973; Li et al., 1970a).

Acid phosphatase activity in myeloid cells shows varying intensity of diffuse or diffuse and granular reaction in acute myelogenous leukemia (AML) and acute myelomonocytic

Table 33–3. Biochemical and Cytochemical Characteristics of Various Subclasses of Lymphoid Leukemias in Humans[a]

Cytochemical Marker	cALL	nALL	pre-T-ALL	T-ALL	T-CLL	pre-B-ALL	B-ALL	B-CLL	References
Adenosine deaminase[b]	I	II		III	II	II	Normal	D	van Laarhoven and De Bruyn, 1983; Vertongen et al., 1984
Adenylate kinase[b]		II		Normal		II	Normal	II	van Laarhoven and De Bruyn, 1983
Hexosaminidase[b]	+			-	Normal		-	D	Dunn and Maurer, 1982
5'-Nucleotidase[b]	I	I		DDD	Normal	II	DDD	DD/I	van Laarhoven and De Bruyn, 1983; Gutensohn et al., 1983; Vertongen et al., 1984
Purine nucleoside phosphorylase[b]	High	Normal		D	D	slight D	I/D	D	Reaman et al., 1981; van Laarhoven and De Bruyn, 1983; Vertongen et al., 1984
Terminal deoxynucleotidyl transferase[b]	+	+	?	+	-	+	-	-	Gaedicke and Drexler, 1982; Muehleck et al., 1983; Schumacher et al., 1983
Acid α-naphthyl acetate esterase[c]	-	-	++	++	-/±	-	-	-/D	Crockard et al., 1982; Gaedicke and Drexler, 1982; Girino et al., 1982
α-Naphthyl butyrate esterase[c]				+	+			-/D	Girino et al., 1982
Acid phosphatase[c]	-/±	±	±/+	++	+/++	-	±/+	-	Crockard et al., 1982; Gaedicke and Drexler, 1982; Girino et al., 1982
β-Glucuronidase[c]			++	++	++	-			Crockard et al., 1982
β-Glucosaminidase[c]			++	++	++	--		-/D	Crockard et al., 1982; Girino et al., 1982
Periodic acid–Schiff reaction[c]	-/++	-/++		-/+			+		Gaedicke and Drexler, 1982

[a] ALL, acute lymphoblastic leukemia; CLL, chronic lymphocytic leukemia; cALL, common cell ALL; nALL, null or non-T non-B cell ALL; T, T-lymphocyte; B, B-lymphocyte; pre-T, pre-T cell; pre-B, pre-B cell. Enzyme activity graded as -, absent; ±, weak; +, moderate; ++, strong; I, slight increase; II, moderate increase; III, marked increase; D, slight decrease; DD, moderate decrease; DDD, marked decrease.
[b] Biochemical determinations.
[c] Cytochemical determinations.

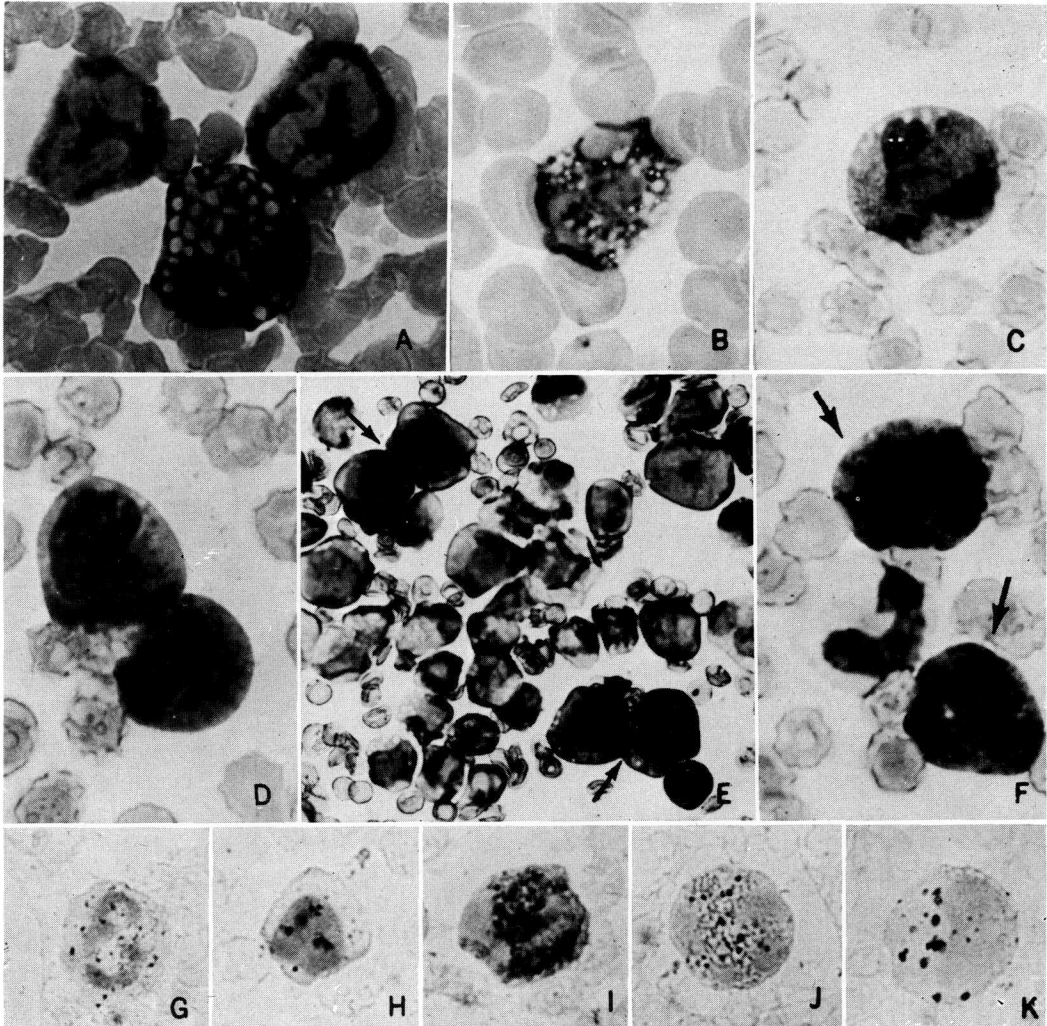

Fig. 33–1. Blood *(A–D, G–K)* and bone marrow *(E,F)* films stained for enzymes in leukocytes and their precursors. *A,* Two neutrophils and an eosinophil in equine blood with strong alkaline phosphatase activity. *B,* Canine eosinophil with moderate ALP activity, *C,* ALP-positive feline eosinophil. *D,* Two myelocytes exhibiting ALP activity in blood from a dog with granulocytic leukemia. *E* and *F,* ALP-positive *(arrows)* neutrophilic granulocytes in the bone marrow aspirate of a dog with granulocytic leukemia (same animal as in *D*); an ALP-negative band neutrophil is also present in *F.*

Acid-phosphatase-positive black granules are present in a canine neutrophil *(G),* in a feline lymphocyte *(H)* and eosinophil *(I),* in an ovine eosinophil *(J),* and in an ovine monocyte *(K).* (Figs. *A–C* and *G–K* from Jain, 1970; courtesy of *Folia Haematologica.*)

leukemia (AMMoL) and intense diffuse activity in acute monocytic leukemia (AMoL) compared to purely granular activity in acute lymphoblastic leukemia (ALL) (Stuart et al., 1975; Telek et al., 1983). Myelomatous plasma cells, in addition to granular ACP activity, may show intense, chunk-like aggregates with perinuclear or unipolar distribution (Kass, 1982). Intense focal ACP activity has been observed in erythroid precursors in erythroleukemia (Kass, 1982).

Acid phosphatase occurs in several iso-zyme forms, many of which appear to be rather cell-specific in that isozymes 2 and 4 occur in neutrophils, 4 in monocytes, 3 in lymphocytes and platelets, 3b in primitive blasts, and 5 in hairy cells, epitheliod cells, osteoclasts, and Gaucher cells (Li et al., 1970a, 1970b; Li and Yam, 1982; Radzun et al., 1980). Isozyme 5 is resistant to L(+)-tartaric acid. Thus different leukocytes can be distinguished on the basis of their ACP isozyme patterns and tartrate sensitivity.

Isozyme patterns of ACP have been studied

in human lymphocytic (Gaedicke and Drexler, 1982) and nonlymphocytic leukemias (Woessner et al., 1979). Tartrate-resistant, ACP-positive cells are highly characteristic of human patients with hairy cell leukemia (Cline, 1981; Yam et al., 1971b). ACP-positive cells of this type but with a less intense staining reaction were found in some cases of prolymphocytic leukemia of the B- or T-cell type and Sézary syndrome (Li and Yam, 1982; Schwarze, 1980).

Alkaline Phosphatase

Alkaline phosphatase (ALP) activity is present in neutrophils of humans, rabbits, rats, guinea pigs, horses, cows, sheep, goats, and monkeys, but not in those of dogs, cats, or mice (Fig. 33–1A; Plate X–1; Table 33–1) (Jain, 1968, 1970). Mature neutrophils of the dog and cat seem inherently deficient in ALP (Jain, 1971). Similarly, no ALP activity is found in mature or immature neutrophils in blood of dogs and cats with leukemoid reaction or leukocytosis with left shift from nonmalignant causes (Jain, 1967a) or in neutrophils of dogs given corticosteroids (Jain, 1971). This is in contrast to findings reported for humans and rabbits in which ALP activity of neutrophils is increased in many physiologic and pathologic conditions associated with leukocytosis and following administration of progesterone, estrogen, ACTH, glucocorticoids, epinephrine, and other steroids (Ebadi and McCoy, 1966; Okun and Tanaka, 1978; Valentine et al., 1957).

Alkaline phosphatase activity in eosinophils is strong in the horse, moderate in the cow, and trace to modest in the dog and cat (Figs. 33–1B, C; Plate X–2). The number of ALP-positive eosinophils in the dog is related neither to a particular clinical condition nor to an absolute increase in eosinophil numbers (Jain, 1967a). Careful differentiation of eosinophils is essential to avoid confusing them with ALP-positive neutrophils, particularly in the dog and cat in which neutrophils are normally ALP-negative. Examples of such misinterpretations can be found in the literature (Abul-Fadl and Scott, 1969). Basophils may reveal some ALP activity in the cytoplasm (Plate X–3), while monocytes and lymphocytes have been uniformly negative. ALP activity in eosinophils and basophils is located in the cytoplasm, not the granules.

In bone marrow smears of healthy dogs and cats, ALP activity can be found in less than 1% of immature cells of the neutrophil series as early as the myelocyte or perhaps promyelocyte stage. ALP-positive cells of the eosinophil series comprise up to 2 to 10% of the myeloid cells in an individual dog or cat. In addition, there are a few large rarely occurring, strongly ALP-positive immature cells that cannot be identified with certainty. ALP activity in cells of the neutrophilic, but not eosinophilic, series of these two species decreases with maturation so that it is absent in almost all metamyelocytes and in all bands and segmenters (Jain, 1971). On the contrary, immature cells of the neutrophil series, myelocytes to band cells, in the horse and cow are ALP-positive and often reveal increasingly greater activity with maturation. Progressive maturation of granulocytes in humans is associated with an increase in ALP activity (Bondue et al., 1980; Valentine, 1960). Observations on rats indicate that ALP activity of neutrophils is higher in the bone marrow than in the peripheral blood (Williams et al., 1978).

Controversy prevails regarding the precise location of ALP within the neutrophil. Ultrastructural cytochemical studies have demonstrated ALP in secondary (specific) granules of rabbit and human neutrophils (Bainton and Farquhar, 1968; Ullyot and Bainton, 1974). However, it was conjectured that the enzyme is present in secondary granules in latent (inactive) form which becomes demonstrable only after its activation in some unknown manner. In other studies, ALP was shown to be present in the plasma membrane of human (Borgers et al., 1978a) and rat (Williams et al., 1979) neutrophils. Recently, neutrophil ALP was shown to be associated with special membranous organelles termed "phosphasomes" (Rustin and Peters, 1979). Our efforts to localize ALP in specific granules or other cytoplasmic organelles of bovine neutrophils by electron microscopy have so far been unsuccessful for unknown reasons, although the enzyme can be demonstrated consistently in cytoplasmic granules of these cells with various light microscopic techniques.

Cytochemical studies of human leukocytes have shown that the determination of ALP activity of circulating neutrophils can be used as a diagnostic aid in many hematologic and nonhematologic disorders. For instance, it can facilitate differentiation of chronic myelogenous leukemia (CML) from leukemoid reaction or neutrophilic leukocytosis associated with nonmalignant causes (Kaplow, 1968; Koler et al., 1958; Mitus et al., 1958; Okun and Tanaka, 1978). ALP activity is generally markedly decreased or absent in the former, while it is normal or remarkably increased in the latter class of patients. However, ALP activity in patients with CML is often significantly increased during blast crisis, bacterial infection, pregnancy, and remission following drug therapy (Hayhoe et al., 1964; Hellmann and Goldman, 1980; Okun and Tanaka, 1978). ALP in neutrophils seems to be distinctly different from other tissue-specific isozymes of ALP (Miller et al., 1983). A unique ALP isoenzyme appears in leukocytes of CML patients with blast crisis (Miller et al., 1984) and in serums of some patients with AML (Leroux-Roels et al., 1982). Leukocytic ALP activity varies independently of serum ALP activity (Tanaka et al., 1960).

The cause of reduced leukocyte ALP in CML has been investigated. Ultrastructural studies have shown that the low ALP activity reflects an enzyme deficiency rather than absence of specific granules (Ullyot and Bainton, 1974). Evidence has been presented to indicate that reduced ALP activity may be due partly to increasing immaturity of circulating neutrophils (Bondue et al., 1980; Pedersen and Hayhoe, 1971) and partly to external influences (Chiyoda and Kinugasa, 1978; Hellmann and Goldman, 1980; Rustin et al., 1980; Sato et al., 1982; Schiffer et al., 1979).

Granulocytic leukemia occurs more commonly in the dog and cat than in other animal species. As mentioned above, neutrophils in these two species are devoid of ALP activity irrespective of the total leukocyte count or left shift from nonmalignant causes. In contrast, some ALP-positive mature and/or immature neutrophils (Fig. 33–1D) may be found in blood films of dogs and cats with granulocytic or myelomonocytic leukemia (Jain and Kono, unpublished observations; Jain et al., 1981;

Madewell et al., 1979; Weller et al., 1980). Bone marrow smears of such patients usually contain a significantly greater number of ALP-positive immature neutrophils than normal bone marrow (Figs. 33–1E, F; Plate XXIII-6). These findings indicate that determination of neutrophil ALP activity in blood and bone marrow of dogs and cats is of great value in differential diagnosis of doubtful cases of myeloid leukemias.

In recent years, some ALP activity has been demonstrated in the plasma membrane of lymphocytes from rats, mice, calf thymus, and normal and some leukemic people by cytochemical and more sensitive biochemical techniques (Catovsky, 1980; Foa et al., 1979; Kramers et al., 1978; Nanba et al., 1977; Poppema et al., 1978; Schwarze, 1980). Cytochemically, such ALP-positive cells display predominantly small granules on the cell membrane but not in the cytoplasm. Another unique enzyme recognized by its substrate specificity and called "N-alkaline phosphatase" has been demonstrated in neoplastic human B- and T-lymphocytes, but not in normal or stimulated lymphocytes and cells of AML or CML (Neumann et al., 1976, 1979). Similar observations have not been made in veterinary medicine.

Esterases

Esterases of different substrate specificities have been found in various leukocytes (Li et al., 1973). The enzyme demonstrated in neutrophils by using naphthol AS-D chloroacetate is presently referred to as chloroacetate esterase (CAE) or specific esterase (Kass, 1979, 1982). Nonspecific esterases present in the mononuclear phagocytes are usually referred to by their specific substrates, that is α-naphthyl acetate esterase (NAE) for the enzyme demonstrated by using α-naphthyl acetate as a substrate and α-naphthyl butyrate esterase (NBE) for the enzyme demonstrated by using α-naphthyl butyrate (Cline, 1981). NBE has also been referred to as lipase (Ansley and Ornstein, 1970). This classification of leukocyte esterases into specific and nonspecific categories should be regarded as arbitrary; specificity is relative to the substrate being used to demonstrate a particular esterase, and in that respect the enzymes demonstrated in both neutrophils and monocytes could be considered specific. It is best to describe each leukocyte esterase with respect to the substrate being used for its demonstration.

Leukocyte esterases differ with regard to their pH optima, sensitivity to inhibitors, and distribution or pattern of localization within the cell. The pattern of staining also differs with the dye used; e.g., fast garnet GBC gives a punctate reaction product, while hexazotized pararosanilin yields a diffuse reaction product (Kass, 1979). Species variations have been reported with regard to the incubation time and pH of the incubation mixture for staining NAE and CAE in animal leukocytes (Osbaldiston et al., 1978).

Nine isozymes of esterases have been described for human leukocytes (Li and Yam, 1982). Isozymes 1, 2, 7, 8, and 9 are found in neutrophils and mast cells and are demonstrated by CAE at pH 7.0 to 7.6. Isozymes 3, 4, 5 and 6 are found in monocytes, megakaryocytes, platelets, and plasma cells; they are demonstrated by NAE at pH 6.0 to 6.3 and are fluoride-sensitive. NBE is said to detect isozymes 2 and 4, while acid-NAE reaction in lymphocytes is believed to detect isozymes 2 and 6. In another study, a fluoride-sensitive NBE was found to be the major isozyme of human monocytes (Yurno and Mastropaolo, 1981).

Leukemic cells may synthesize newer isozymes in addition to producing large amounts of normally occurring isozymes. Based on isozyme patterns of leukemic human leukocytes, myelomonocytic leukemia was considered a monocytoid variant of myeloblastic leukemia, and, similarly, erythroleukemia was thought to be an erythroid variant of myeloblastic leukemia (Kass, 1978b, 1979; Kass and Peters, 1977, 1978). Furthermore, erythroleukemia was considered to constitute a transitory phase in the evolution of AML or AMMoL (Kass, 1977, 1978a, 1978b).

Chloroacetate Esterase

Chloroacetate esterase (CAE) in human neutrophils has a pH optimum of 7 to 7.6 and is fluoride-resistant (Li et al., 1973). In general, CAE follows patterns of sudanophilia and peroxidase (PO) reaction, and so it ap-

pears to be associated with primary granules. Thus CAE activity decreases with cell division and maturation from the promyelocyte stage to the mature neutrophil stage (Kass, 1982). In humans, monocytes, eosinophils, lymphocytes, plasma cells, and erythroid precursors are CAE-negative, while mast cells are CAE-positive. CAE activity is considered more specific for granulocytes than PO activity or sudanophilia (Kass, 1979). A weak CAE activity may be seen in leukemic myeloblasts and monoblasts, although normally these cells are CAE-negative (Kass, 1982). Localized perinuclear CAE activity is seen in erythroid precursors in erythremic myelosis and erythroleukemia (Kass, 1975, 1977, 1978a). Although some investigators have observed CAE activity in lymphocytes (Muller et al., 1981), this has not been the general experience.

Chloroacetate esterase activity among leukocytes of various animal species is moderate to strong in neutrophils, slight in lymphocytes and monocytes of some species, and absent in eosinophils (Table 33–1). Although neutrophils usually contain many lightly or moderately stained granules, occasionally they exhibit a strong reaction in the dog, horse, cow, and sheep.

The morphology of CAE-positive granules varies with the staining technique; neutrophils may show discrete, small to large, round or rod-shaped granules or fuzzy granularity (Figs. 33–2G, H). CAE activity of animal neutrophils, like human neutrophils, generally corresponds to their PO activity and sudanophilia. Some positively-stained lymphocytes and monocytes may be found in the cow. Equine monocytes invariably show a slight positive reaction, and a similar reaction may be seen in an occasional lymphocyte. Feline basophils show a marked CAE activity (Plate X–10); the basophil granules are large, round, and intensely stained (Fig. 33–2I) compared to small, moderately stained neutrophil granules.

Nonspecific Esterases

Nonspecific esterases in human monocytes and macrophages have a pH optimum of 6.0 to 6.3 and they are fluoride-sensitive. The NAE is strong in monocytes, macrophages, megakaryocytes, and platelets. Basophils and

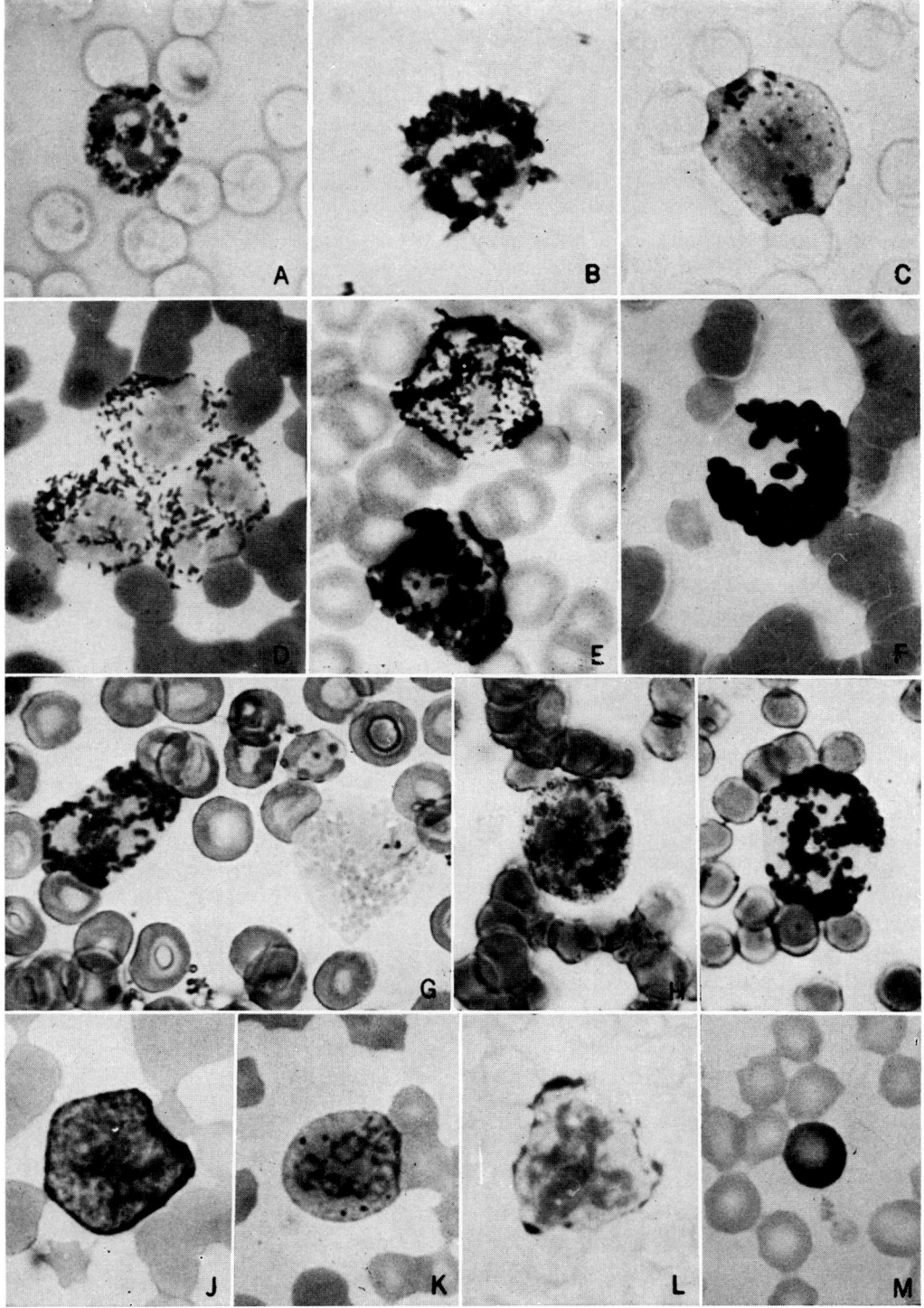

Fig. 33–2. Peroxidase-positive granules in a feline neutrophil *(A)*, in a canine eosinophil *(B)*, and in a canine monocyte *(C)*. Sudanophilic granules in three equine neutrophils *(D)*, in a canine neutrophil *(E,* upper cell) and eosinophil *(E,* lower cell), and in an equine eosinophil *(F)*. Naphthol AS-D chloroacetate esterase activity in a canine neutrophil *(G,* left cell), in an equine neutrophil *(H)*, and in a feline basophil *(I)*; the cell on the right in *G* is a negatively stained canine eosinophil. Periodic acid–Schiff reaction for glycogen in equine neutrophils *(J and K;* the cell in *K* also contains a few large glycogen droplets), in an ovine monocyte *(L)* with marginal staining and in an immature erythrocyte in blood from a week-old calf *(M)*. (Figs. *A, B,* and *D–K* from Jain, 1970; courtesy of *Folia Haematologica*.)

plasma cells may also stain positive, and lymphocytes may show a localized staining. Neutrophils are generally NAE-negative. An esterase activity demonstrable by using naphthol-AS (or AS-D) acetate follows a similar pattern. NBE activity, although weaker, is considered highly specific for the mononuclear phagocytes (Li et al., 1973).

Determination of the presence of these enzymes has been useful in differential diagnosis of AML, AMMoL, and AMoL. The presence of blasts or immature cells reactive for NSE, either NAE or NBE, is considered suggestive of monocytic involvement, whereas the presence of CAE-positive cells suggests granulocytic involvement, and a combination of both enzyme markers is indicative of myelomonocytic leukemia (Cline, 1981; Gordon and Hubbard, 1978, 1979; Tavassoli et al., 1979). However, about a third of human patients with acute promyelocytic leukemia may show moderate to strong NSE activity (Jain and Bennett, 1985; Tomonaga et al., 1985).

NAE activity in human lymphocytes generally appears as one or two focal coarse spots or small to medium-sized granules with focal, circular, or semicircular distribution, whereas monocytes and their precursors usually show a diffuse localized staining with or without some granular reaction (Schwarze, 1980). In ultrastructural studies, NAE activity in guinea pig and human leukocytes was found not in lysosomes but on the cell surface and on clusters of cytoplasmic vesicles of lymphocytes and mononuclear phagocytes (Monahan et al., 1981). The distribution of positively stained clusters of cytoplasmic vesicles in human lymphocytes and mononuclear phagocytes was consistent with staining patterns observed with the light microscope. A strong diffuse NAE activity, moderately resistant to sodium fluoride (NaF), was observed in erythroid precursors in erythroleukemia and megaloblastic anemia in humans (Rosenszajn et al., 1962). NAE-positive blast cells have been found in a few cases of human ALL (Shaw and Ishmael, 1975).

The pattern of distribution of the reaction product indicative of NAE activity has been used to characterize certain subpopulations of human lymphocytes, although observations vary with regard to typical patterns (Catovsky, 1980; Higgy et al., 1977; Pangalis et al., 1978; Pinkus et al., 1979; Schwarze, 1980). A strong spot-like or globular pattern is considered specific for T-lymphocytes, particularly T cells with Fc receptors for IgM (helper cells), while a granular pattern characterizes non-T, non-B cells (Higgy et al., 1977), some B cells (Grossi et al., 1978), and T cells with Fc receptors for IgG, i.e., Tg or suppressor cells (Manconi et al., 1979; Quesada and Murphy, 1982). Stimulated T cells have been found to lack NAE activity, while stimulated B cells show a positive reaction (Totterman et al., 1977). Unipolar distribution of NAE activity has been reported for leukemic cells in T-lymphocyte ALL (T-ALL), "histiocytic" lymphoma, multiple myeloma, and plasma cell leukemia (Bainton and Bozdech, 1979; Gaedicke and Drexler, 1982; Kass, 1982). A positive NBE staining was seen in hairy cells (Higgy et al., 1978).

An acid-NAE activity has been demonstrated at pH 5.8 in murine (Mueller et al., 1975) and human T-lymphocytes in blood (Knowles et al., 1978; Kulenkampff et al., 1977; Ranki et al., 1976) and tissues (Pinkus et al., 1979). A comparison with other markers of T cells revealed that acid-NAE is the most reliable cytochemical marker for human T-cell lymphomas and T helper cells (Schwarze, 1980). Normal B-lymphocytes usually give a negative reaction for acid-NAE, but a positive reaction may be seen in stimulated B-lymphocytes and in some cases of B-cell lymphomas. Monocytes give a diffuse weak reaction for acid-NAE activity.

Nonspecific esterase activity of leukocytes of various animal species has been determined (Table 33–1; Plate X-9). Neutrophils of the dog, cat, cow, and sheep lack both NAE and NBE activity, whereas those of the horse and goat may occasionally reveal a few positive granules. Lymphocytes of these species have been mostly negative, but an occasional cell may show a few positive granules. Monocytes of the dog, cat, and cow may give a modest positive reaction, whereas those of the horse stain faintly. Monocytes of the goat characteristically reveal a strong positive reaction. NSE-positive monocytes usually show a diffuse, smooth cytoplasmic reactivity, but sometimes granular or clumpy staining may be seen. It has been reported that in the dog focal, dot-like NAE-activity may be used to identify T cells in contrast to the diffuse positive reaction characteristically seen in monocytes (Wulff et al., 1981). Eosinophils of the dog and cat are negatively stained, while those of the cow and goat may occasionally show a few positive granules and those of the horse are invariably positive. Basophils of the dog and cat are negatively stained.

The possibility that NAE activity may be used as a marker for T-lymphocytes in various animal species has been investigated to a limited extent. It has been shown to be a specific marker for canine lymphocytes (Wulff et al., 1981), but not for feline (Dockrell et al., 1978) and ovine (Dixon and Moriarty, 1983) lymphocytes. Observations on bovine lymphocytes have been conflicting (Dhingra et al., 1982; Kajikawa et al., 1983; Yang et al., 1979).

Methyl Green–Pyronin Reaction

Methyl green specifically binds to DNA, while pyronin binds to RNA. Intense pyroninophilia is characteristic of plasma cells because of their abundant cytoplasmic RNA (Plate X-12). In addition, intense pyroninophilia is also seen in normal erythroid cells and megakaryocytes (Hayhoe and Quaglino, 1980; Kass, 1982). Similarly, most blasts cells stain with pyronin, but the staining reaction decreases with cell maturation. B-lymphocytes reveal a variable degree of pyroninophilia depending on their immunoglobulin synthetic activity. The pyroninophilic cells usually show diffuse cytoplasmic staining and occasionally a reticulated pattern. Pyronin may also react with cellular components other than RNA, e.g., eosinophil granules. Studies on human patients have revealed strong pyroninophilia of erythroid cells in erythroleukemia, of plasma cells in multiple myeloma and plasma cell leukemia, and of lymphoid cells during the leukemic phase of Burkitt's lymphoma (Kass, 1982).

Periodic Acid–Schiff Reaction

The periodic acid–Schiff (PAS) staining technique, a common method to demonstrate glycogen, demonstrates polysaccharides and glycoproteins. The presence of glycogen is recognized only when control preparations exposed to α-amylase or saliva before staining show negative or very little reaction.

Glycogen is present in the form of small distinct or indistinct PAS-positive granules in the cytoplasm of neutrophils of humans, horses, dogs, cats, cows, sheep, goats, guinea pigs, rats, and monkeys (Jain, 1969; Table 33–1; Plate X–11). In addition, an occasional neutrophil in common domestic animals contains a few large, deep red, coarse granules (Figs. 33–2*J*, *K*). Neutrophils of the dog, cat, and horse show a stronger PAS-positive reaction than those of other animal species. Staining intensity of cells of the granulocytic series increases with cell maturation, the myeloblast being PAS-negative, the promyelocyte and myelocyte being weakly positive, and the mature neutrophil being highly PAS-positive.

Lymphocytes, monocytes, and eosinophils have either no demonstrable glycogen or a very small amount (Table 33–1; Fig. 33–2*L*). PAS-positive reaction in lymphocytes and monocytes takes the form of a faint diffuse or fine to coarse granular staining. Platelets contain fine to small PAS-positive granules. Mature erythrocytes are PAS-negative; however, some immature erythrocytes in the newborn calf give a PAS-positive reaction (Fig. 33–2*M*; Jain, 1969). In normal bone marrow smears, megakaryocytes reveal a diffuse PAS-positive reaction, while erythroid cells are uniformly negative.

In human studies, it has been observed that erythroid precursors in patients with iron deficiency, β-thalassemia, and especially erythroleukemia are intensely PAS-positive; the early precursors exhibiting usually a granular reaction and the more mature precursors a diffuse reaction (Hayhoe and Cawley, 1972; Hayhoe and Quaglino, 1980; Kass, 1982; Quaglino and Hayhoe, 1960). It is also said that a chunk-like reaction is seen in erythroleukemia, while a diffuse pattern is seen in chronic erythremic myelosis. The megaloblasts of vitamin B_{12}–folate deficiency are PAS-negative. Glycogen content is decreased in CML, and it may be either decreased or increased in lymphoproliferative disorders (Efrati and Yaari, 1980; Gaedicke and Drexler, 1982).

The pattern of cytoplasmic PAS reactivity

has been used to characterize lymphocytic leukemias and their subtypes (Schwarze, 1980). Coarse, granular or block-like staining has been observed in a variable number of lymphocytes and lymphoblasts in ALL (Hayhoe and Cawley, 1972; Lilleyaman et al., 1979). Occasionally, the PAS-positive material may appear clumpy or globular. Globular or diffuse cytoplasmic staining may be seen in B-cell leukemias and plasma cells; diastase-resistant PAS-positive globules correspond to cytoplasmic immunoglobulin (Diebold et al., 1971; Dutcher and Fahey, 1960; Stein et al., 1972). Leukemic myeloblasts and monocytes give a fine, dust-like PAS-positive reaction (Kass, 1982).

We have not found PAS-positive erythroid precursors in feline patients diagnosed to have erythremic myelosis and erythroleukemia. Similarly, lymphocytes in several cases of canine and feline lymphocytic leukemia have not yielded PAS-positivity described above for leukemic human lymphocytes.

Peroxidase

Peroxidase (PO) activity is seen in neutrophils of all species and in eosinophils of all common domestic animals but the cat (Jain, 1967b; Table 33–1; Plates X–4, X–5, X–6). The eosinophil granules stain more intensely and are larger than the neutrophil granules (Figs. 33–2A, B). A few PO-positive small granules may be seen in monocytes of some species (Fig. 33–2C; Plate X–6). Human monocytes may show slightly granular or faint diffuse cytoplasmic staining (Cline, 1981). Basophils of the horse and cat are PO-negative, and this may be the case in other species. Lymphocytes in all species are PO-negative and so are erythroid cells in the bone marrow. Although platelets and megakaryocytes appear PO-negative by light microscopy, a PO-like activity has been demonstrated in these cells by electron microscopy (Breton-Gorius et al., 1978a, 1978b). The enzyme activity is localized in the endoplasmic reticulum and nuclear membrane of megakaryocytes and in the dense tubular system of platelets. Electron microscopic observations on rabbit and human leukocytes indicate that PO activity is present in primary granules of neutrophils (Bainton and Farquhar, 1968), in lysosomes of monocytes (Nichols et al., 1971), and in the matrix of crystalloid eosinophil granules (Bainton and Farquhar, 1970).

It has been shown that eosinophil PO is structurally, biochemically, antigenically, and genetically different from that in neutrophils and monocytes and that it resembles lactoperoxidase (Rytomaa and Teir, 1961; Wever et al., 1980). Eosinophil PO is resistant to inactivation by cyanide whereas neutrophil PO is not (Yam et al., 1971a). Neutrophil PO is highly bactericidal, and a similar but lesser functional activity has been demonstrated for eosinophil PO (Jong et al., 1980). Unstained granulocytes in mass have a greenish hue owing to their PO content. A form of granulocytic leukemia is referred to as chloroma because of the greenish color imparted by PO to the tissues (Chapter 32).

Peroxidase staining of mature and immature human neutrophils may vary in disease (Kitahara and Kushner, 1979), and hereditary deficiency may occur (Cline, 1981; Kass, 1982; also see p. 711). Negative staining of lymphoid cells is utilized for differentiation of ALL from AML. Myeloblasts are normally PO-negative, but in AML a proportion may reveal some PO activity. The PO activity is stronger in blasts of promyelocytic leukemia than in those of myeloblastic leukemia (Kass, 1982). In some cases of myelogenous leukemias, particularly during blast crisis of CML, and in some monoblastic leukemias, PO activity can be demonstrated only by electron microscopy (Catovsky, 1980). Peroxidase activity may be decreased in preleukemic syndromes (Cech et al., 1982), and it may even be absent in some neutrophils of patients with granulocytic leukemia (Bainton, 1975; Catovsky et al., 1972; Ullyot and Bainton, 1974) and in neutrophils with toxic granulation (Cline, 1981). Blast transformation of a well-differentiated monocytic leukemia in a human patient was accompanied by a deficiency of PO activity and loss of NBE reactivity (Rodgers et al., 1982). We have observed reduction or absence of PO activity in neutrophils of a few dogs with granulocytic leukemia and leukocytoses from other causes.

Ultrastructural cytochemical studies have shown that PO activity in myeloblasts is present in the nuclear membrane, rough endoplasmic reticulum (RER), and Golgi zone. Promyelocytes and promonocytes, in addition, show PO activity in primary granules and lysosomal granules, respectively (Ackerman and Clark, 1971; Bainton et al., 1971; Breton-Gorius, 1980; Breton-Gorius and Reyes, 1976; Nichols et al., 1971). Thus a decrease in the number of PO-positive granules with mitosis of neutrophil precursors is associated with lower PO activity in mature neutrophils than in the promyelocytes and myelocytes. As mentioned above, leukemic neutrophils may be deficient in primary granules or lack PO. Because of PO-negative staining on light microscopy, leukemic myeloblasts may resemble lymphoblasts, but such blast cells can be distinguished on electron microscopy by the presence of PO activity at locations mentioned above in the former but not the latter cells (Breton-Gorius, 1980; Reiffers et al., 1981; Wada, 1980a, 1980b). Remission rates and length of survival have been associated with cell maturity defined by PO activity of leukocytes of patients with myelogenous leukemia (Wada, 1980a, 1980b).

Sudanophilia

Sudan Black B stains various lipids including phospholipids, neutral fat, and sterols and probably some nonlipid cellular components (Hayhoe and Quaglino, 1980).

Sudanophilic granules are present in neutrophils of common domestic animals (Table 33–1). The granules are distinct, grayish-brown to black, and uniformly distributed (Figs. 33–2D, E; Plate X–7). They are usually rod-shaped and vary in number and size. The number of sudanophilic granules seems to decrease, while their staining intensity appears to increase, with mitosis and maturation of promyelocytes to mature neutrophils. Sudanophilia and PO positivity go hand in hand in neutrophils, eosinophils, and monocytes of most species. However, in early granulocytic precursors, a weak cytoplasmic sudanophilic staining may be apparent without PO activity, thereby indicating that during granulopoiesis sudanophilia manifests prior to PO positivity (Jain and Kono, unpublished observations).

The specific granules of eosinophils of all animals but the cat stain slightly brown to black (Figs. 33–2E, F). Monocytes may stain negative or have few small, round sudanophilic granules. Immature monocytes may show a positive staining (Cline, 1981). Lymphocytes and immature lymphoid cells, with rare exceptions (Ho et al., 1983; Stass et al., 1984; Tricot et al., 1982), are negative. This finding has been utilized in differentiation of ALL from AML or AMMoL. In AML, a variable proportion (5–90%) of blast cells may exhibit intense sudanophilia like that in mature neutrophils, and similarly some blast cells in AMMoL may show sudanophilia resembling that in normal monocytes (Cline, 1981).

Terminal Deoxynucleotidyl Transferase

Terminal deoxynucleotidyl transferase (TdT) is a unique DNA polymerase that catalyzes the synthesis of DNA sequence in the absence of DNA template. It can be detected in lymphoid cells by biochemical, immunofluorescent, electron microscopic, and histochemical methods (Bollum, 1979; Cousar et al., 1984). TdT is present in T-cell regions of lymph nodes and thymus and in a small number of bone marrow cells, but not in normal T- and B-lymphocytes in blood. TdT-positive cells are more numerous in the bone marrow of infants than of adults (Hoffbrand et al., 1982). In humans, TdT has been valuable in differentiating ALL from AML and for detection of lymphoblasts in extramedullary sites. Although TdT activity in blast cells at diagnosis varies widely (Hutton et al., 1982), about 94–96% of patients with ALL show high TdT activity (Beutler and Blume, 1979). TdT is considered a marker of ALL involving null cells, common lymphoid stem cells, pre-B cells, and T cells (Bollum, 1979; Folds et al., 1982; Gaedicke and Drexler, 1982; Muehleck et al., 1983; Schumacher et al., 1983). Lymphocytes from cases of B-CLL or T-CLL do not stain for TdT. About one-third of patients with lymphoid crisis of CML show TdT-positive cells. Significance of TdT in leukemic patients with regard to selection of therapy, prediction of prognosis, and detection of relapse is being investigated (Grever et al., 1983; Hutton et al., 1982). Similar studies on common domestic animals are lacking.

Other Cytochemical Markers

Enzymes of Purine Metabolism

Enzymes of purine metabolism have been measured in human studies mostly by biochemical methods. These measurements have been used primarily for differentiation of lymphocytic leukemias. Similar studies on animal patients are lacking.

5'-Nucleotidase. 5'-Nucleotidase (5'NT) causes dephosphorylation of 5'-nucleotides to corresponding nucleotides. It is an ectoenzyme present on the plasma membrane of lymphoid cells, and possibly a similar enzyme is present on many other tissue cells. 5'NT can be demonstrated by cytochemical, biochemical, and immunological methods. Normal thymic cells give a weak 5'NT activity, while higher activity is found in circulating T cells, and the highest activity is seen in B cells (Gaedicke and Drexler, 1982). About four times more 5'NT activity is present in peripheral blood B-lymphocytes than in T-lymphocytes (Hoffbrand et al., 1982). 5'NT activity is diminished in primary immune deficiency in humans. Human patients with leukemia may show normal or increased 5'NT activity in common ALL (cALL), normal or low activity in acute and chronic T-cell leukemias, increased activity in lymphoid crisis of CML, and decreased activity in some cases of acute and chronic B-cell leukemias, hairy cell leukemia, and Waldenström's macroglobulinemia (Dunn and Maurer, 1982; Gutensohn et al., 1983; Hoffbrand et al., 1982; Vertongen et al., 1984). 5'NT activity was found in blast cells from a case of megakaryoblastic leukemia (El-Mohandes and Hayhoe, 1983a) and in about 90% of myelomatous plasma cells, but not in nonmyelomatous plasma cells (El-Mohandes and Hayhoe, 1983b).

Adenosine Deaminase. Adenosine deaminase (ADA) catalyzes the conversion of adenosine to inosine. Its activity in serum, leukocytes, bone marrow, and lymphoid tissues has been measured by biochemical methods. ADA is present in blood and thymic lymphocytes (Gaedicke and Drexler, 1982), with highest activity in immature T cells and lowest in B cells (Dunn and Maurer, 1982). Deficiency of ADA has been associated with primary combined immune deficiency in humans;

ADA seems to be essential for differentiation and functional competence of lymphoid cells, particularly T cells. ADA activity is considerably high in T-ALL and increased in other types of T-cell leukemias, cALL, non-T non-B cell leukemia (nALL), and lymphoid crisis of CML (Grever et al., 1983; Ma et al., 1983; Sylwestrowicz et al., 1982). ADA activity is normal in B-ALL and subnormal in B-CLL (Vertongen et al., 1984). About 50% of patients with AML show moderate elevations in ADA activity (Hoffbrand et al., 1982). Elevated levels of ADA activity have been used as a guide in treatment of lymphoid leukemia with deoxycoformycin, an ADA inhibitor (Hoffbrand et al., 1982).

Purine Nucleoside Phosphorylase. Purine nucleoside phosphorylase (PNP) catalyzes conversion of purine nucleosides to their complementary bases, e.g., inosine to hypoxanthine. Its presence in lymphocytes can be demonstrated by cytochemical and biochemical methods and may be used as a marker to distinguish T and B cells. T-lymphocytes are PNP-positive and may show increasing activity with cell maturation, while most normal B cells are PNP-negative. Thus PNP positivity varies directly with the proportion of T cells and indirectly with the number of B cells (Borgers et al., 1978b). Absence of PNP in T-lymphocytes has been associated with primary immune deficiency of T-cell functions. Human patients with leukemia may show high PNP activity during lymphoblastic crisis of CML and a decrease in T-ALL (Sylwestrowicz et al., 1982). PNP activity is normal in nALL, increased or decreased in B-ALL and decreased in T-ALL, T-CLL, and B-CLL (Ma et al., 1983; Reaman et al., 1981; van Laarhoven and De Bruyn, 1983).

Other Enzymes

Several other enzyme markers of normal and leukemic cells have been determined in human studies, some with relatively less defined diagnostic significance (Hayhoe and Quaglino, 1980).

Enzymatic markers for histiocytes include lysozyme, α_1-antitrypsin and α_1-antichymotrypsin (Isaacson and Jones, 1983). Lysozyme is elevated in serums of patients with AMoL and to a lesser extent in AML (Stjernholm et al., 1972). Serum lysozyme concentration was significantly elevated in a horse diagnosed as having myelomonocytic leukemia (Brumbaugh et al., 1982). Increased serum lysozyme activity has been reported in dogs not only with myelogenous and myelomonocytic leukemia (Shifrine et al., 1973), but also with neoplastic diseases other than myeloproliferative disorders (Feldman et al., 1981).

Staining patterns of β-glucuronidase activity have been used to characterize myeloid and lymphoid leukemias (Stuart et al., 1975; Telek et al., 1983). Coarse granular positivity was seen in ALL, whereas a diffuse or diffuse and finely granular positivity was seen in AML, AMMoL and AMoL. β-glucuronidase, phosphorylase, and dehydrogenases were recently demonstrated in normal feline blood and bone marrow cells (Tsujimoto et al., 1983).

Dipeptidylaminopeptidase IV (DAP IV) is considered a reliable marker for T helper (Tμ) lymphocytes and their malignancies in humans (Feller et al., 1982). It can be demonstrated by both cytochemical and biochemical methods in about 90% of Tμ cells, but not in B cells or other bone marrow cells. DAP IV activity was found in lymphoid cells of about 83% cases of T-CLL and about 60% cases of T-ALL.

Levels of lysosomal enzymes β-hexosaminidase and α-mannosidase were significantly elevated in AMoL and AMMoL and somewhat higher in other myeloid leukemias compared to normal granulocytes (Besley et al., 1983).

An aminocaproate esterase has been demonstrated in human mast cells but not in leukocytes (Hayhoe and Quaglino, 1980; Li and Yam, 1982).

Acetylcholinesterase activity is demonstrated in megakaryocytes of rats, cats (Jackson, 1973), and dogs (Joshi and Jain, 1977).

Summary of Cytochemical Markers in Classification of Leukemias

Cytochemistry is being used increasingly in diagnosis of blastic forms of leukemias where distinction between lymphoid and myeloid lineage becomes extremely difficult from cell morphology in Romanowsky-stained blood and bone marrow smears. It should be realized, however, that although certain specific cytochemical properties have been discovered for various hematopoietic cells and their malignancies (Tables 33–2 and 33–3), because of developmental abnormalities such as asynchrony of maturation and enzyme expression in leukemic cells, cytochemical heterogeneity and irregularities may be encountered in leukemia making it difficult to predict the proper cell lineage with certainty. For example, PO-deficient neutrophils may be found in myelogenous leukemia (Bainton, 1975; Catovsky et al., 1972), and a subnormal number of NSE-positive and PO-positive monocytes may be seen in monocytic leukemias (van Furth and van Zwet, 1983). It is because of such singular observations that a cytochemical profile is developed using multiple cytochemical criteria and newer cell markers are constantly sought for differential diagnosis of hematopoietic malignancies. It is emphasized that a specific cytochemical finding is seldom suggestive of a neoplastic process per se; most often it discriminates only the cell lineage and to a certain extent cell maturity.

Myeloid leukemias can be distinguished from lymphocytic leukemias based on reactivity for ALP, PO, esterases, and Sudan black B. Neutrophils and their precursors stain for PO and CAE and exhibit sudanophilia forming the basis for recognition of myeloid leukemia. In humans, ALP activity is decreased during CML, while it is increased during blast crisis of CML. In the dog and cat, increased neutrophil ALP can be considered predictive of myeloid leukemia because it is usually increased during myelogenous and myelomonocytic leukemias. Monocytes and their morphologically recognizable precursors in normal or leukemic patients are identified by strong diffuse positivity for NAE or NBE, weak or no PO activity, and absence of ALP and CAE reactions. Diagnosis of myelomonocytic leukemia entails finding enzymatic markers of both cell lineages. Species differences should be given consideration in this respect, particularly with regard to CAE which is present, although at a low level, in equine and ruminant monocytes (Table 33–1). Lymphocytes are uniformly negative or exhibit little reaction for the aforementioned cytochemical markers except NSE. NSE activity in lymphocytes varies with their subclass, and the pattern of staining is often distinctive (focal or coarsely granular) compared to that in monocytes (diffuse cytoplasmic staining).

Lymphocytic leukemias and lymphomas are currently being classified using immunologic markers. Cytochemical and biochemical determinations are also being used to characterize various lymphoid malignancies. Enzymes of purine metabolism and several lysosomal enzymes have been measured to differentiate lymphoid and nonlymphoid leukemias and to subclassify lymphocytic leukemias. Results have been somewhat contradictory, but with multiple enzymatic determinations some distinction has been achieved, although specific criteria for more precise differentiation remain to be developed. Observations on commonly used biochemical and cytochemical markers in characterization of lymphoid leukemias are summarized in Table 33–3, and further information can be found in recent reports and reviews (Crockard, 1984; Crockard et al., 1982; Drexler et al., 1984; Gaedicke and Drexler, 1982; Girino et al., 1982; Matutes et al., 1983; van Laarhoven and De Bruyn, 1983; Vertongen et al., 1984).

In general, TdT is considered to be a marker for most lymphoblastic leukemias. Acid hydrolases such as ACP, β-glucuronidase, β-glucosaminidase, and NSE show stronger activity in T cells than in B cells. Positive reactions for these enzymes are seen in acute and chronic T-cell leukemias in contrast to weak or negative staining in B-cell leukemias. Patterns of cytoplasmic staining for ACP have been described to distinguish various subtypes of lymphoid leukemias. Hairy cell leukemia is particularly characterized by a strong tartrate-resistant ACP activity. Enzymes of purine metabolism such as 5'NT, ADA, and PNP have been utilized mostly as markers for lymphoid cells, and levels of these enzymes have been found to increase or decrease in various lymphocytic leukemias (Table 33–3). ADA activity is higher in T cells at various stages of maturation than in B cells, 5'NT activity is high in pre-B cells, and PNP activity is high in cALL. Deficiencies of each of these enzymes have been associated with primary immune deficiencies in humans.

Differentiation of B-CLL to plasma cell leukemia is accompanied by increases in ACP, acid-NAE, PNP, and thymidine phosphorylase activity (Srivastava and Han, 1984). Plasma cells also show strong β-glucuronidase activity. Myelomatous but not normal plasma cells exhibit 5'NT activity (El-Mohandes and Hayhoe, 1983b).

Azurophilic cytoplasmic granules in leukemic blast cells are generally considered indicative of a myeloid lineage. However, such granules may also be found in lymphoid cells. Lymphoid cells with azurophilic granules and indented nuclei have been referred to as large granular lymphocytes (LGLs) and immunologically characterized as natural killer (NK) cells (Timonen et al., 1981). Leukemia involving such LGLs has been recognized as a morphologic subgroup of lymphoid leukemia called granular acute lymphoblastic leukemia (G-ALL). Cytochemically granular lymphoblasts were found to exhibit PAS-positive reaction and ACP, NAE, and NBE activity; weak to negative reaction for β-glucuronidase; and negative reaction for PO and CAE. Sudan black B reaction was often negative, and TdT activity was present (Fuchs et al., 1984; Stein et al., 1983). Evidence has been presented to indicate that cytoplasmic granules of NK cells play a role in the cytolytic activity of these cells because absence of such granules is associated with impaired natural killing activity of NK cells (Kay and Zarling, 1984).

SOME COMMONLY USED CYTOCHEMICAL TECHNIQUES IN HEMATOLOGY

General Comments

Application of cytochemistry to hematology (Bover, 1964; Hayhoe and Quaglino, 1980; Hayhoe et al., 1964; Kass, 1982; Sun et al., 1985) is based on principles and techniques of histochemistry (Pearse, 1968, 1972). Following are brief comments of a general nature and a description of some commonly used cytochemical techniques adapted for use in veterinary hematology. Information presented is drawn from literature as well as from our experience with blood and bone marrow of various animal species (Jain, 1967a, 1967b,

1968, 1969, 1970, 1971, unpublished observations; Jain et al., 1981; Osbaldiston et al., 1978; Rudolph and Schnabl, 1979; Tschudi et al., 1977). A summary of these techniques is presented in Table 33–4.

It is highly recommended that cytochemical procedures on blood and bone marrow specimens be performed on coverslip smears rather than on slides. This not only conserves the use of expensive chemicals, but provides superior cellular distribution and morphology. Smears may be made from fresh, unanticoagulated blood or from blood anticoagulated with EDTA or heparin. Buffy coat smears may be prepared when total leukocyte count is low or when a search is to be made for rare cells. Thin, good quality smears are preferred. The smears should be fixed immediately and fixation carried no longer than the time specified for each technique because longer fixation may cause enzyme inactiva-

tion. The fixative should be checked periodically for adequacy of cell preservation. Fixed smears can be kept in a freezer for several weeks without loss of enzyme activity. This is advantageous, for a batch of smears may be accumulated to stain, particularly if cytochemical staining is performed infrequently.

The incubation medium, in most cases, needs to be prepared fresh and should always be filtered before use. It should be kept in screw-capped jars (Columbia dishes) and used as directed. Species variations may be encountered with regard to times of fixation and incubation necessary to delineate a particular enzyme activity. Shorter incubation time may give negative results, while longer incubation may introduce diffusion artifacts. Proper controls should be incorporated routinely, and specific enzyme inhibitors may be used to identify certain cell types.

Appearance of colored reaction product in

Table 33–4. Summary of Various Cytochemical Techniques

Cytochemical Marker	Fixative	Substrate or Principal Stain	Coupling Dye	Reaction Product	References
Acid phosphatase	None or citrated methanol	Naphthol AS-MX phosphate	Fast red violet LB	Red	Kaplow and Burstone, 1964
Alkaline phosphatase	Formalin-methanol	Naphthol AS-BI phosphate	Fast red violet LB	Red	Kaplow, 1955
Chloroacetate esterase	Formalin-methanol	Naphthol AS-D-chloroacetate	Fast garnet GBC	Reddish orange	Bauer-Sic, 1963
Nonspecific esterase:					
NAE	Formalin-acetone	α-naphthyl acetate	Hexazotized pararosanilin	Red	Yam et al., 1971a
NBE	Formalin-acetone	α-naphthyl butyrate	Hexazotized pararosanilin	Red	Ansley and Ornstein, 1970
Combined CAE and NSE	Formalin-acetone	α-naphthyl acetate or butyrate and	Hexazotized pararosanilin	Red	Yam et al., 1971a
		Naphthol AS-BI-chloroacetate	Fast blue BBN	Blue	
Glycogen	Absolute methanol	Schiff's reagent	. . .	Magenta	Hayhoe, 1960, and Bauer-Sic, 1963
Peroxidase	Formalin-ethanol	H_2O_2, benzidine dihydrochloride	. . .	Greenish blue	Kaplow, 1965
	Formalin-acetone	3-Amino-9-ethylcarbazole	. . .	Reddish brown	Graham et al., 1965
Pyroninophilia	Carnoy's solution	Pyronin Y	. . .	Red	Perry and Reynolds, 1956
Sudanophilia	Formalin vapor	Sudan black B	. . .	Brown to black	Sheehan and Storey, 1947

CAE, chloroacetate esterase; NAE, α-naphthyl acetate esterase; NBE, α-naphthyl butyrate esterase; NSE, nonspecific esterase.

a cell indicates that the particular enzyme or nonenzymatic component is present in the cell, but its specific site may not be obvious. Mounted smears should be examined as soon as possible because colors in some preparations fade upon storage. To alleviate this problem, smears should be mounted only when they are to be examined. Unmounted stained smears can be stored at room temperature for several years without deterioration of colors. Achieving satifactory counterstaining remains a constant hurdle to overcome in many cytochemical procedures.

The degree of positivity as well as the pattern of staining are important criteria of subjective evaluation. These may vary with species, techniques, batches of dyes, and laboratories. A positive staining may be qualitatively graded from trace to strong, and a variety of patterns such as granular or diffuse and focal or disseminated may be recognized.

A semi-quantitative score may be obtained by grading the degree of positive reaction for comparative evaluation. For example, alkaline phosphatase or peroxidase activity of neutrophils is often assessed by scoring 100 consecutive neutrophils including band cells from 0 to 4 + on the basis of staining intensity and then calculating a total score for comparison with the laboratory's normal range (Jain, 1968). Scoring is time-consuming and varies with staining techniques, different batches of dyes, and laboratories. In most cases determination of the overall degree of staining, the proportion and types of cells exhibiting positivity, and the stage of maturation of positive cells is sufficient to provide clues to diagnosis of leukemia or establish cell lineage.

Cytophotometric methods have been developed for more precise quantitative evaluation of certain cellular components, e.g., DNA, and in a number of cases biochemical measurements can be performed. Specific cytochemical reactions of various leukocytes form the basis of some recently developed automated instruments for differential leukocyte counts. Certain cytochemical techniques may also be performed in conjunction with electron microscopy to delineate the specific cytologic location of enzymatic activity or nonenzymatic constituent.

Acid Phosphatase (Kaplow and Burstone, 1964)

Principle

Acid phosphatase hydrolyzes naphthol AS-MX phosphate releasing insoluble naphthol and phosphate. The naphthol complexes at acid pH with diazonium salt forming a colored product at the site of enzyme activity.

Solutions

Incubation Mixture

Naphthol AS-MX phosphate	2 mg
N,N-dimethylformamide	0.1 ml
0.1 M Citrate buffer, pH 5.2	24 ml
Fast red violet LB salt	15 mg

Dissolve napthol AS-MX phosphate in N,N-dimethylformamide. Then add the buffer and fast red violet salt. Filter and use immediately. Tartaric acid (200 mg) may be added to the above medium to inhibit the enzyme activity; the same could also be accomplished by using the tartaric acid solution described below.

0.1 M Citrate Buffer, pH 5.2

A. 0.2 M Citric acid:

Citric acid	4.20 g
Distilled water (q.s.)	100 ml

B. 0.2 M Sodium citrate:

Sodium citrate ($Na_3C_6H_5O_7 \cdot 2H_2O$)	58.82 g
Distilled water (q.s.)	1 L

Mix 18 ml of solution A and 32 ml of solution B, adjust pH to 5.2 with solution A or solution B, then double the volume with distilled water.

0.2 M Tartaric Acid (Kass, 1982)

L(+)-Tartaric acid	3 g
Distilled water	50 ml
1 N NaOH	35 ml

Adjust pH to 4.9 with 1 N NaOH, then bring volume to 100 ml with distilled water. Add 1 ml per 9 ml of the incubation medium to use as an inhibitor of acid phosphatase activity.

Glycerin Jelly (Raphael, 1976)

Gelatin	5 g
Glycerol	35 ml
Distilled water	65 ml
Merthiolate	10 mg

Soak the gelatin in distilled water for 1 hour at room temperature, add the glycerol and merthiolate, and heat to 60°C. Stir constantly until solution is smooth. Filter if necessary, and store in 5-ml volumes in screw-capped tubes in refrigerator at 4°C. To use, melt the glycerin jelly by heating in a water bath or incubator at 60°C. To avoid the formation of air bubbles in the mounted specimen, do not shake or stir the melted jelly prior to use. Warming the slide on a hot plate before applying the melted jelly may facilitate proper mounting of specimen.

Mayer's Hematoxylin

Hematoxylin ....1 g
Distilled water.........................1 L
Sodium iodate........................ 0.2 g
Aluminium potassium sulfate ....50 g

Add hematoxylin to 500 ml distilled water, heat just to boiling, and add another 500 ml distilled water. Then add sodium iodate and aluminium potassium sulfate. Shake well and filter. Store in a dark brown bottle at room temperature. Filter before use.

Saturated Solution of Lithium Carbonate

Procedure

1. Prepare thin coverslip blood and bone marrow smears.
2. Incubate unfixed smears in freshly prepared and filtered incubation mixture for 4 to 5 hours at 37°C. Use smears less than 24 hours old to get the best results. Control smears are incubated in medium without the substrate, and sensitivity to tartaric acid is determined by incubating smears in medium containing L(+)-tartaric acid.
3. Wash in running tap water for 20 seconds and air-dry.
4. Counterstain with Mayer's hematoxylin for 4 to 8 minutes. Dip the smear in saturated solution of lithium carbonate to improve nuclear staining.
5. Rinse in tap water, air-dry, and mount in glycerin jelly.

Results

A positive reaction is indicated by red precipitate in the cytoplasm. The pattern and intensity of the reaction product are variable. A slight to modest positive reaction may be seen in neutrophils, eosinophils, lymphocytes, and monocytes of various animal species (Figs. 33–1G–K).

Alkaline Phosphatase (Kaplow, 1955)

Several techniques are available (Bover, 1964; Kaplow, 1955, 1968; Rutenberg et al., 1965), but that of Kaplow (1955) is preferred for better color contrast and is described below.

Principle

Alkaline phosphatase hydrolyzes naphthol AS-BI phosphate to aryl naphtholamide and phosphate. The former component couples with a diazonium salt such as fast red violet LB salt, forming an insoluble colored product at the site of enzyme activity (Cline, 1981).

Fixative

Formalin (37% formaldehyde).......... 1 part
Absolute methanol.................. 9 parts

Keep in freezer. Make fresh fixative every 3 weeks.

Buffered formalin acetone (p. 928) may also be used as a fixative for alkaline phosphatase.

Solutions

Incubation Mixture (Kaplow, 1955)

Naphthol AS-BI phosphate .... 1 mg
N,N-Dimethylformamide ....0.1 ml
0.05 M Propanediol buffer, pH 9.75 .....12 ml
Fast red violet LB salt .... 8 mg

Dissolve naphthol AS-BI phosphate in N,N-dimethylformamide. Then add the buffer and fast red violet salt. Shake vigorously for 30 seconds, filter, and use. Control medium is prepared by deleting the substrate, naphthol AS-BI phosphate.

0.05 M Propanediol Buffer

A. 0.2 M Propanediol stock solution:
   2-Amino-2-methyl-1,3 propanediol .. 10.5 g
   Distilled water .... 500 ml (q.s.)
B. Working solution:
   Stock solution A ....25 ml
   0.1 N HCl ....5 ml
   Distilled water ....70 ml

Procedure

1. Fix freshly prepared coverslip smears for 10 seconds in cold (−5 to −10°C) formalin-methanol. Longer fixation may inactivate the enzyme in some species.
2. Wash for 1 minute in running tap water and air-dry. Fixed smears may be stored in freezer up to 1 month.
3. Incubate at room temperature for 10 minutes (for most species) or longer (up to 1 hour for cats and dogs) in freshly prepared incubation medium. The time may be varied as desired for the species concerned. Place control smears in an incubation medium without the substrate.

4. Wash in running tap water for 10 to 15 seconds and air-dry.
5. Counterstain with Mayer's hematoxylin (p. 927) for 10 minutes. Dip the smear in saturated solution of lithium carbonate to improve nuclear staining.
6. Rinse in tap water, air-dry, and mount in glycerin jelly (p. 926).

Results

A positive reaction is indicated by red precipitate in the cytoplasm (Plate X–1). A moderate to strong reaction is characteristic of neutrophils of common domestic animals except the dog and cat whose neutrophils are ALP-negative. Eosinophils of some species may give a slight to modest reaction and basophils in a few species may stain slightly positive (Plates X–2, X–3). Lymphocytes and monocytes are uniformly negative. A horse or cow blood film may be stained simultaneously as a positive control while cat and dog blood films are being stained for neutrophil ALP.

α-Naphthyl Acetate Esterase (Yam et al., 1971a)

Principle

The nonspecific esterases hydrolyze synthetic esters, e.g., α-naphthyl acetate or butyrate, to liberate α-naphthol, which complexes with a diazonium salt to produce an insoluble colored product at or near the site of enzyme activity (Kass, 1979). NAE can be demonstrated at alkaline as well as acid pH; the latter is preferred for localizing NAE in lymphocytes.

Fixative

Buffered Formalin-Acetone, pH 6.6
Na_2HPO_4. . . . . 0.1 g
KH_2PO_4 . . . . 0.5 g
Deionized water . . . . .150 ml
Absolute acetone .225 ml
Formalin . . . . .125 ml

Adjust pH to 6.6 with 1 N NaOH or HCl. Store at 4°C.

Solutions

Pararosanilin Solution
Basic fuchsin (C.I. 42500) . . . . .1 g
Distilled water. . . . . .20 ml
HCl (concentrated). . . . . .5 ml

Dissolve basic fuchsin by gentle warming in water, add HCl, cool, and filter. Store at room temperature. Solution is good for 2 months.

Incubation Mixture

A. In beaker 1, phosphate buffer:
   $M/15$ Na_2HPO_4 (4.73 g/500 ml) . . . . . . 8.7 ml
   $M/15$ KH_2PO_4 (4.54 g/500 ml) . . . . 1.3 ml
B. In beaker 2:
   Pararosanilin solution. . . . . 0.3 ml
   4.0% $NaNO_2$ (freshly prepared) . . . . . 0.3 ml
   Mix and allow to react for 1 minute.
C. In beaker 3:
   α-Naphthyl acetate . . . . 10.0 mg
   Ethylene glycol monomethyl ether (2-methoxyethane) . . . . 0.5 ml

Add contents of beaker 1 to beaker 2, and add the mixture to beaker 3; mix and adjust pH to 6.1 (range 5.8–6.2) with 1.0 N NaOH. Filter and use. The solution is clear yellow.

Procedure

1. Fix freshly prepared smears in cold (-4 to $-10°C$) formalin-acetone for 30 seconds to 1 minute.
2. Wash 5 to 6 times with distilled water and air-dry.
3. Incubate in freshly prepared, filtered incubation mixture for 30 minutes to 1 hour at room temperature. Place control smears in the incubation medium to which NaF (15 mg/10 ml) has been added and mixed immediately prior to use.
4. Wash 5 to 6 times with distilled water.
5. Counterstain with methyl green (p. 930) for 10 minutes.
6. Rinse in water, air-dry, and mount with Pro-Texx mounting medium (Scientific Products).

Results

A positive reaction is indicated by reddish staining in the cytoplasm (Plate X–9). Lymphocytes and monocytes may reveal a slight to strong positive staining. Positively stained lymphocytes show a focal or coarse granular reactivity, while monocytes generally show a diffuse reaction. The enzyme activity in monocytes is fluoride-sensitive compared to that in lymphocytes. Neutrophils and eosinophils in most species stain negative, and basophils are nonreactive.

α-Naphthyl Butyrate Esterase (Ansley and Ornstein, 1970)

Principle

Same as that for NAE.

Fixative

Buffered formalin acetone, pH 6.6 (p. 928)

Solutions

Pararosanilin solution (p. 928)

1.0% α-Naphthyl Butyrate Solution
α-Naphthyl butyrate . . . . 1 g
Diethylene glycol . . . . 100 ml

Store solution at −4°C.

Incubation Mixture

A. In beaker 1, phosphate buffer:
   0.1 M Na$_2$HPO$_4$ . . . . 1.5 ml
   0.1 M KH$_2$PO$_4$ . . . . 8.5 ml

B. In beaker 2:
   1.0% α-Naphthyl butyrate . . . . 0.5 ml
   Diethylene glycol . . . . 0.5 ml

C. In beaker 3:
   Pararosanalin solution . . . . 0.2 ml
   4.0% NaNo$_2$ (freshly prepared) . . . . . 0.2 ml
   Mix and allow to react for 1 minute.

To beaker 3, first add contents of beaker 2 and then rinse beaker 2 with buffer from beaker 1 and add to beaker 3. Mix for 30 seconds. Add 10 ml of 0.1 M KH$_2$PO$_4$ (8.71 g/500 ml). Adjust pH to 6.1 (range 5.8–6.2) with 1.0 N HCl. Filter and use. Final incubation medium is straw color.

Procedure

1. Fix fresh smears in cold, buffered formalin-acetone fixative for 30 seconds to 1 minute.
2. Wash 5 to 6 times with distilled water and air-dry.
3. Incubate in freshly prepared, filtered incubation mixture for 1 to 2 hours at room temperature in covered Columbia jar. Mix solution by inversion several times during incubation period. Place control smears in the incubation medium to which NaF (15 mg/10 ml) has been added and mixed prior to use.
4. Wash 5 to 6 times with distilled water.
5. Counterstain with methyl green (p. 930) for 10 minutes.
6. Rinse, dry, and mount in mounting medium.

Results

A positive reaction is indicated by color at the site of enzyme activity in the cytoplasm (Plate X–8). Cellular distribution is similar to that for NAE.

Chloroacetate Esterase (CAE) (Bauer-Sic, 1963)

Principle

The esterase hydrolyzes naphthol AS-D chloroacetate to liberate naphthol, which complexes with a diazonium salt to produce an insoluble colored product at the site of enzyme activity (Kass, 1979).

Fixative

Cold formalin-methanol (p. 927)

Solutions

Incubation Mixture

A. Naphthol AS-D chloroacetate . . . . 20 mg
   Acetone . . . . 1 ml

Mix napthol AS-D chloroacetate in acetone.

B. Fast garnet GBC salt . . . . 20 mg
   Distilled water . . . . 10 ml
   0.1 M barbital buffer, pH 7.4 . . . . 10 ml

Mix Fast Garnet in distilled water, add the buffer, and mix for about 30 seconds. Then add solution B to solution A at once, mix, and filter.

0.1 M Barbital Buffer, pH 7.4

A. 0.2 M Sodium barbital:
   Sodium barbital . . . . 20.618 g
   Distilled water . . . . 500 ml

B. 0.2 N HCl

Mix 50 ml of solution A and 32 ml of solution B, adjust pH to 7.4, and then bring the volume to 100 ml with distilled water.

Procedure

1. Fix fresh smears for 20 seconds in cold (−4 to −10°C) formalin-methanol (p. 927).
2. Wash for 1 minute in running tap water and air-dry.
3. Incubate for 45 minutes in freshly prepared incubation mixture.
4. Wash in running tap water for 1 minute and air-dry.
5. Counterstain with Mayer's hematoxylin (p. 927) for 4 to 8 minutes.

6. Dip in saturated lithium carbonate 3 times to improve nuclear stain.
7. Rinse in water, air-dry, and mount in glycerin jelly (p. 926).

Results

A positive staining is indicated by reddish orange precipitate at the site of enzyme activity in the cellular organelles, primarily cytoplasmic granules. Neutrophils regularly give a moderate to strong reaction, while eosinophils are negative and basophils of the cat uniquely stain strongly positive (Plate X–10). Lymphocytes and monocytes in some species may give a slight reaction.

Combined Technique for Nonspecific Esterase and Chloroacetate Esterase (Yam et al., 1971a)

Princple

The smears are first stained for NSE, either NAE or NBE, and then for CAE using coupling dyes to yield reaction products of different colors.

Solution

Incubation Mixture for CAE
Naphthol AS-D chloroacetate . . . . 1.0 mg
N,N-Dimethyl formamide . . . . 0.5 ml
M/15 Phosphate buffer, pH 7.4 . . . . 9.5 ml
Fast blue BBN . . . . 5.0 mg

Mix, filter, and use immediately. The phosphate buffer is freshly prepared by mixing 8.1 ml of M/15 Na_2HPO_4 and 1.9 ml M/15 KH_2PO_4 (see p. 928)

Procedure

1. Stain for NAE following steps 1 through 4 given on p. 928 or for NBE following steps 1 through 4 given on p. 929.
2. Wash smears 3 times with distilled water.
3. Incubate for 10 minutes to 1 hour at room temperature in the incubation mixture described above.
4. Wash 5 to 6 times with distilled water.
5. Counterstain with methyl green (p. 930) for 10 minutes.
6. Rinse, air-dry, and mount with Pro-Texx mounting medium.

Results

A positive reaction for NSE is indicated by red color and for CAE by blue color in the cytoplasm (Plate X–9). Generally, neutrophils stain for CAE, whereas lymphocytes and monocytes reveal NSE activity.

Methyl Green–Pyronin Staining (Perry and Reynolds, 1956)

Principle

Methyl green binds specifically to highly polymerized DNA, whereas pyronin principally stains lower polymers of RNA and some other cellular components. Pyronin is less specific than methyl green, but in combination with ribonuclease treatment of smears, it specifically localizes RNA (Hayhoe and Quaglino, 1980).

Fixative

Carnoy's solution
Absolute ethanol . . . . 60 ml
Chloroform . . . . 30 ml
Glacial acetic acid . . . . 10 ml

Solutions

Methyl Green
Methyl green . . . . 2 g
Distilled water . . . . 100 ml

Dissolve methyl green in water and place in a Buckner funnel. Mark the level of solution. Add chloroform to extract methyl violet, an impurity in the dye. Shake several times for a few minutes each time. Allow chloroform to settle, then drain the chloroform layer. Add more chloroform to the stain and continue extraction procedure until the chloroform layer is clear; usually 3 extractions are sufficient. Store extracted methyl green in a glass, stoppered bottle at room temperature.

Pyronin Y
Pyronin Y . . . . 2 g
Distilled water . . . . 100 ml

Extract impurities in the same manner as for methyl green.

Methyl Green–Pyronin Stain
Methyl green solution . . . . 7.5 ml
Pyronin solution . . . . 12.5 ml
Distilled water . . . . 30.0 ml

Procedure

1. Fix smears in Carnoy's solution for 10 minutes.

2. Rinse in 95% ethanol for a few seconds.
3. Rinse in distilled water for a few seconds and air-dry. Place control smears for RNA in a ribonuclease solution (10 mg ribonuclease in 10 ml of distilled water) for 1 hour at 37°C (use water bath), wash in running water for 1 minute, and drain carefully.
4. Stain in methyl green–pyronin for 30 minutes.
5. Rinse fast (for 2 seconds) in distilled water.
6. Rinse for 5 seconds in a mixture of acetone and butyl alcohol (equal parts).
7. Rinse for 5 seconds in normal butyl alcohol.
8. Drain dry and mount in Pro-Texx mounting medium.

Results

A positive reaction for DNA is indicated by greenish color and a positive reaction for RNA by reddish color in the cell (Plate X–12). A slight to modest cytoplasmic pyroninophilia is typical of lymphocytes. Plasma cells stain strongly. Eosinophil granules also appear pyroninophilic, probably because of nonspecific reactivity with their major basic protein.

Periodic Acid–Schiff Reaction (Bauer-Sic, 1963; Hayhoe, 1960)

Principle

Periodic acid oxidizes glycols and related compounds to dialdehydes which react with leucofuchsin (the Schiff's reagent) to release fuchsin and stain cellular components (Hotchkiss, 1948). Glycogen is believed to be present when positive staining is evident in smears only when a control smear exposed to α-amylase or diastase shows very little or no reaction.

Fixative

Absolute methanol. Formalin-ethanol (p. 932) may also be used.

Solutions

Periodic Acid
Periodic acid . . . . .1 g
Distilled water (q.s.) . . . . .100 ml

Keep refrigerated in dark.

Schiff's Reagent (Kodousek, 1969)
Basic fuchsin . . . . .1 g
Absolute ethanol . . . . .10 ml
Distilled water. . . . . .186 ml
Sodium or potassium metabisulfite . . . . .5 g
HCl (concentrated, S.G. 1.19) . . . . .3.4 ml
Sodium dithionite . . . . 0.25 g
Activated pulverized charcoal. . . . . .2 g

Dissolve ground basic fuchsin in ethanol in a 250-ml flask. Shake gently for a few minutes. Then add cold (20°C) distilled water, followed in sequence by dry metabisulfite, HCl, and dithionite. Add charcoal, stir for 3 minutes, and filter through #2 filter paper. The reagent can be used immediately or stored for months in a dark bottle wrapped in foil in the refrigerator. The reagent is usually clear, but it may have a slight pinkish tinge or the latter may be acquired upon storage. The reagent is good if a few drops in 10 ml of 4% formalin turn purple and not blue.

Potassium Metabisulfite–Water
10% Potassium metabisulfite . . . . .5 ml
1 N HCl . . . . .5 ml
Distilled water 90 ml

Procedure

1. Keep smears at least for 48 or preferably 72 hours at room temperature before staining.
2. Fix smears in absolute methanol for 10 minutes.
3. Rinse 3 to 4 times in distilled water. Incubate control smears in filtered saliva (use #4 filter paper) for 30 minutes or 1.0% aqueous α-amylase (diastase) for 1 hour at 37°C and wash in water for 1 minute.
4. Treat with periodic acid for 10 minutes at room temperature. Use periodic acid solution only once.
5. Rinse 3 to 4 times in distilled water.
6. Incubate in Schiff's reagent for 30 minutes at room temperature. Films previously stained by a Romanowsky stain can also be stained with PAS reagent. In such instances, skip steps 1 through 3.
7. Rinse in 2 changes of potassium metabisulfite-water, about 15 seconds each. Discard after use.
8. Place in distilled water for 5 minutes.
9. Counterstain with methyl green (p. 930) for 8 minutes.
10. Rinse fast in tap water, air-dry, and mount in Pro-Texx mounting medium.

Results

A positive staining is indicated by magenta color in the cytoplasm (Plate X–11). Neutrophils contain usually fine and sometimes coarse positive granules. Eosinophils give a slight intergranular cytoplasmic staining. A few coarse granules or patchy staining may be found in occasional monocytes and lymphocytes.

Peroxidase

Several staining methods are available to demonstrate peroxidase activity in leukocytes. Those found satisfactory by us are described. Kaplow's technique gives better staining for myeloperoxidase than that of Sato and Sekiya (Frankel and Reitman, 1963), and the reagent is stable for reuse over a period of several months. Although these two techniques provide the best visual localization of myeloperoxidase activity, because of carcinogenic potential of the benzidine, other techniques have been developed (Elias, 1980; Hanker et al., 1977; Kaplow, 1975). Our experience with these techniques has been limited, but a technique using 3-amino-9-ethylcarbazole as an incubation medium has been found suitable (Graham et al., 1965).

TECHNIQUE 1: Benzidine Stain (Kaplow, 1965)

Principle

The peroxidase oxidizes benzidine or other substrates in the presence of H_2O_2 so that a greenish blue compound of the dye is localized at the site of enzyme activity (Kaplow, 1965).

Fixative

Formalin (37% formaldehyde) . . . . 1 part
Absolute ethanol . . . . 9 parts

Keep at room temperature.

Solutions

Incubation Mixture
Ethyl alcohol (30%) . . . . 100 ml
Benzidine dihydrochloride . . . . 0.3 g
$ZnSO_4 \cdot 7H_2O$ (0.132 M) 3.8% w/v . . . . 1.0 ml
Sodium acetate ($NaC_2H_3O_2 \cdot 3H_2O$) . . . . 1.0 g
Hydrogen peroxide (3%) . . . . 0.7 ml
NaOH (1.0 N) . . . . 1.5 ml
Safranin O . . . . 0.2 g

Add the reagents in the order listed, mixing well after each addition. The benzidine salt may contain a small amount of inert residue which will not go into solution. A precipitate forms upon addition of the zinc sulfate. This dissolves upon addition of the remaining reagents. Omit the safranin if a nuclear counterstain is not required. The final pH is 6.00 ± 0.05. Filter the solution and store it in a capped Columbia jar or bottle at room temperature. The same solution can be reused repeatedly for up to 6 months.

Procedure

1. Fix smears for 15 seconds at room temperature in formol-ethanol. Unfixed smears may be stored at room temperature in darkness for 4 to 6 days.
2. Wash for 15 to 30 seconds in running water. Shake off excess water.
3. Place wet smear in incubation medium in a Columbia jar for 30 seconds at room temperature. Bovine blood films and milk smears may require longer (90 seconds) incubation.
4. Wash for 5 to 10 seconds in running tap water, air-dry, and mount in glycerin jelly (p. 926).

For greater nuclear details, stained smears may be counterstained in 1% aqueous cresyl violet acetate for 1 minute, or in freshly diluted Giemsa stain for 10 minutes prior to mounting in glycerin jelly. Wright stain is less satisfactory as a counterstain.

Results

A positive reaction is indicated by greenish blue precipitate at the site of enzyme reaction in the cytoplasm (Plate X–6). Nuclei and erythrocytes stain red by the safranin. Neutrophils consistently give a moderate to strong reaction, and an intense staining is seen in eosinophils of most species. Cat eosinophils are distinctly negative. Monocytes may show a slight staining reaction, whereas lymphocytes and basophils are negative.

TECHNIQUE 2: 3-Amino-9-ethylcarbazole Stain (Graham et al., 1965).

Principle

Peroxidase catalyzes the oxidation of 3-amino-9-ethylcarbazole by H_2O_2, yielding an insoluble colored reaction product.

Fixative

Buffered formalin-acetone, pH 6.6 (p. 928)

Solutions

0.02 M Acetate Buffer, pH 5.0 to 5.2
Sodium acetate ($NaC_2H_3O_2 \cdot 3H_2O$) .... 0.2722 g
Distilled water........................75 ml

Adjust pH to 5.0 to 5.2 using acetic acid and bring total volume to 100 ml.

0.3% Hydrogen Peroxide
H_2O_2 (30%).........................0.1 ml
Distilled water.......................9.9 ml

Store in a brown bottle at 4°C.

Incubation Mixture
3-amino-9-ethylcarbazole .... 2.0 mg
Dimethyl sulfoxide....................1.2 ml
0.02 *M* Acetate buffer .... 10.0 ml
0.3% H_2O_2 .... 0.08 ml

Mix and filter before use. Carbazole must be pulverized and completely dissolved for consistent staining.

Procedure

1. Fix thin smears in cold buffered formalin acetone for 15 seconds.
2. Wash smears gently for 15 to 30 seconds in running tap water and air-dry.
3. Place smears in incubation medium in a Columbia jar for 2½ minutes at room temperature.
4. Wash gently for 10 to 15 seconds in running tap water.
5. Counterstain with Mayer's hematoxylin (p. 927) for 8 minutes, then dip three times in saturated lithium carbonate solution.
6. Wash well with tap water, air-dry, and mount in glycerin jelly (p. 926).

Results

A positive reaction is indicated by reddish-brown granulation (Plates X–4, X–5). The distribution of positive reaction is identical to that seen with benzidine methods.

Sudan Black B Staining (Sheehan and Storey, 1947)

Principle

Sudan black B has affinity principally for phospholipids, neutral fat, and sterols. The mechanism of staining is unknown.

Fixative

Formalin

Solutions

Incubation Mixture

A. Stock Sudan black B solution:
Sudan black B .... 0.3 g
Absolute ethanol ....30 ml

The dye must dissolve completely—leave the mixture at room temperature for a day or two, with frequent shaking or heating if necessary.

B. Stock buffer solution:
   (a) Crystalline phenol .... 16 g
           Absolute ethanol ....100 ml
   (b) Disodium phosphate ($Na_2HPO_4 \cdot 12H_2O$)
                               0.3 g
      Distilled water ....100 ml

Prepare both solutions, and add (a) to (b).

C. Working staining solution:
Sudan black B (Solution A)..........60 ml
Buffer (Solution B).................40 ml

Mix well and filter by suction (if necessary). The stain is ready to use. It can be stored at room temperature for weeks, but becomes weaker.

Procedure

1. Fix dry thin smears in formaldehyde vapor for 5 to 10 minutes. To do this, place a few drops of formalin in a Petri dish containing a single layer of glass beads. Place smears over the glass beads to avoid direct contact with the formalin, and close the lid.
2. Wash in running tap water for 1 minute.
3. Stain in buffered Sudan black B solution for 30 minutes. Longer time is needed if stain is old or not properly dissolved.
4. Place in 70% ethanol for 2 minutes to remove excess dye.
5. Wash in running water for 1 minute.
6. Counterstain with Wright stain allowing 10 to 12 minutes each in stain and in buffer. Mayer's hematoxylin (p. 927) may also be used.
7. Air-dry and mount in Pro-Texx mounting medium.

Results

A positive staining is indicated by brownish-black to black coloration of the organelles, principally cytoplasmic granules (Plate X–7). Distribution of sudanophilia corresponds to positivity for peroxidase. Thus neutrophils uniformly reveal a moderate to strong positive staining, and eosinophils of most species give a slight to moderate staining. Cat eosinophils are uniformly negative. Monocytes may occasionally show a slight reaction, whereas lymphocytes are negative.

REFERENCES

Abul-Fadl, Y., and Scott, R.B.: Effect of Estrogen and Progesterone on Leukocyte Glycogen and Alkaline Phosphatase in Dogs. Proc. Soc. Exp. Biol. Med., *132*:193, 1969.

Ackerman, G.A., and Clark, M.A.: Ultrastructural Localization of Peroxidase Activity in Normal Human Bone Marrow Cell. Z. Zellforsch., *117*:463, 1971.

Ansley, H., and Ornstein, L.: Enzyme Histochemistry and Differential White Cell Counts on the Technicon Hemalog D: Advances in Automate Analysis. Technicon International Congress, *1*:437, 1970.

Bainton, D.F.: Abnormal Neutrophils in Acute Myelogenous Leukemia: Identifcaiton of Subpopulations Based on Analysis of Azurophil and Specific Granules. Blood Cells, *1*:191, 1975.

Bainton, D.F., and Bozdech, M.J.: Fine Structure Localization of α-Naphthyl Esterase in Human Lymphocytes. Clin. Res., *27*:634, 1979.

Bainton, D.F., and Farquhar, M.G.: Differences in Enzyme Content of Azurophil and Specific Granules of Polymorphonuclear Leukocytes. II. Cytochemistry and Electron Microscopy of Bone Marrow Cells. J. Cell. Biol., *39*:299, 1968.

Bainton, D.F., and Farquhar, M.G.: Segregation and Packaging of Granule Enzymes in Eosinophilic Leukocytes. J. Cell Biol., *45*:54, 1970.

Bainton, D.F., et al.: The Development of Neutrophilic Polymorphonuclear Leukocytes in Human Bone Marrow. J. Exp. Med. *134*:907, 1971.

Bauer-Sič, P.: (Cytochemistry of Bovine Leucocytes in Health and Leucosis.) Zentralbl. Veterinärmed., *10*:365, 1963.

Beckstead, J.H., and Bainton, D.F.: Enzyme Histochemistry on Bone Marrow Biopsies: Reactions Useful in the Differential Diagnosis of Leukemia and Lymphoma Applied to 2-Micron Plastic Sections. Blood, *56*:386, 1980.

Bell, A., et al.: Use of Cytochemistry and FAB Classification in Leukemia and Other Pathological States. Amer. J. Med. Technol., *47*:431, 1981.

Bennett, J.M.: Leukemia Morphology and Cytochemistry. *In* Leukemia. 4th ed. Gunz, F.W., and Henderson, E.S., eds. Grune & Stratton, Orlando, Fla., 1982.

Bennett, J.M., and Reed, C.E.: Acute Leukemia Cytochemical Profile: Diagnostic and Clinical Implications. Blood Cells, *1*:101, 1975.

Besley, G., et al.: Correlation of Lysosomal Enzyme Abnormalities in Various Forms of Adult Leukaemia. J. Clin. Pathol., *36*:1000, 1983.

Beutler, E., and Blume, K.G.: Terminal Deoxynucleotidyl Transferase: Biochemical Properties, Cellular Distribution and Hematological Significance. Prog. Hematol., *11*:47, 1979.

Bollum, F.J.: Terminal Deoxyribonucleotidyl Transferase as a Hematopoietic Cell Marker. Blood, *54*:1203, 1979.

Bondue, H., et al.: Leucocyte Alkaline Phosphatase Activity in Mature Neutrophils of Different Ages. Scand. J. Haematol., *24*:51, 1980.

Borgers, M., et al.: Alkaline Phosphatase Activity in Human Polymorphonuclear Leukocytes. Histochem. J., *10*:31, 1978a.

Borgers, M., et al.: Purine Nucleoside Phosphorylase in Chronic Lymphocytic Leukemia (CLL). Blood, *52*:886, 1978b.

Boudreaux, M.K., et al.: Intravascular Leukostasis in a Horse with Myelomonocytic Leukemia. Vet. Pathol., *21*:544, 1984.

Bover, G.F.: Atlas of Blood Cytology: Cytomorphology, Cytochemistry, and Cytogenetics. Grune & Stratton, New York, 1964.

Breton-Gorius, J.: The Value of Cytochemical Peroxidase Reactions at the Ultrastructural Level in Haematology. Histochem. J., *12*:127, 1980.

Breton-Gorius, J., and Reyes, F.: Ultrastructure of Human Bone Marrow Cell Maturation. Int. Rev. Cytol., *46*:251, 1976.

Breton-Gorius, J., et al.: The Blast Crisis of Chronic Granulocytic Leukaemia: Megakaryoblastic Nature of Cells as Revealed by the Presence of Platelet-Peroxidase. A Cytochemical Ultrastructural Study. Brit. J. Haematol., *39*:295, 1978a.

Breton-Gorius, J., et al.: Megakaryoblastic Acute Leukemia. Identification by the Ultrastructural Demonstration of Platelet Peroxidase. Blood, *51*:45, 1978b.

Brumbaugh, G.W., et al.: Myelomonocytic Myeloproliferative Disease in a Horse. J. Amer. Vet. Med. Ass., *180*:313, 1982.

Burkhardt, E., et al.: Monocytic Leukemia in a Horse. Vet. Pathol., *21*:394, 1984.

Catovsky, D.: Antibody to Terminal Deoxynucleotidyl Transferase. Proc. Natl. Acad. Sci., *72*:4119, 1975.

Catovsky, D.O.: Leucocyte Enzymes in Leukaemia. Top. Rev. Haematol., *1*:157, 1980.

Catovsky, D., et al.: Myeloperoxidase-Deficient Neutrophils in Acute Myeloid Leukaemia. Scand. J. Haematol., *9*:142, 1972.

Catovsky, D., et al.: Cytochemical Profile of B and T Leukemia Lymphocytes with Special Reference to Acute Lymphoblastic Leukemia. J. Clin. Pathol., *27*:767, 1974.

Catovsky, D., et al.: The Acid Phosphatase Reaction in Acute Lymphoblastic Leukaemia. Lancet, *1*(8067):749, 1978a.

Catovsky, D., et al.: Cytochemistry: An Aid to the Diagnosis and Classification of the Acute Leukaemias. Recent Results Cancer Res., *64*:108, 1978b.

Cawley, J.C., and Burns, G.F.: The Cytochemistry of Human Lymphoreticular Subpopulations. Immunology Today, *1*:85, 1980.

Cech, P., et al.: Partial Myeloperoxidase Deficiency. Acta Haematol., *67*:180, 1982.

Chiyoda, S., and Kinugasa, K.: Alkaline Phosphatase Activity in Chronic Myelogenous Leukaemia Cells in Cultures. II. Suppressive Effect of Plasma. Acta Haematol. Jpn., *41*:564, 1978.

Cline, M.J.: Histochemical Reactions of Leukocytes. *In* Methods in Hematology. Vol. 3. Leukocyte Function. Cline, M.J., ed. Churchill Livingstone, New York, p. 130, 1981.

Cousar, J.B., et al.: Peripheral Blood and Bone Marrow Involvement by Non-Hodgkin's Lymphoma: Morphological, Immunological and Cytochemical Features. Prog. Clin. Pathol., *9*:173, 1984.

Crockard, A.D.: Cytochemistry of Lymphoid Cells: A

Review of Findings in the Normal and Leukaemic State. Histochem. J., *16*:1027, 1984.

Crockard, A., et al.: Cytochemistry of Acid Hydrolases in Chronic B- and T-Cell Leukemias. Amer. J. Clin. Pathol., *78*:437, 1982.

Dhingra, V.K., et al.: Demonstration of Acid α-Naphthyl Acetate Esterase Activity in Bovine Lymphocytes and Monocytes or Macrophages. Res. Vet. Sci., *33*:26, 1982.

Diebold, J., et al.: Syndrome Lymphoproliferatif avec Production de Macroglobuline IgM Purement Intracellulaire. Nouv. Rev. Fr. Hematol., *11*:429, 1971.

Dixon, R.J., and Moriarty, K.M.: α-Naphthyl Acetate Esterase Activity Is Not a Specific Marker for Ovine T Lymphocytes. Vet. Immunol. Immunopathol., *4*:505, 1983.

Dockrell, H.M., et al.: Cytochemical Identification of T and B Cells in Situ in Mouse Lymphoid Tissue and Lymph Nodes from the Rat, Gerbil, and Cat. Ann. Immunol., *129C*:617, 1978.

Douglas, S.D., et al.: Lymphocyte Lysosomes and Lysosomal Enzymes in Chronic Lymphocytic Leukemia. Blood, *41*:511, 1973.

Drexler, H.G., et al.: Enzymes Markers in Acute Leukemias: Advances during the Last Decade. J. Natl. Cancer Inst., *72*:1283, 1984.

Dunn, N.L., and Maurer, H.M.: Enzyme Alterations in Leukemic Cells. Amer. J. Hematol., *13*:343, 1982.

Dutcher, T.F., and Fahey, J.L.: Immunocytochemical Demonstration of Intranuclear Localization of 18S Gamma Macroglobulin in Macroglobulinemia of Waldenström. Proc. Soc. Exp. Biol. Med., *103*:452, 1960.

Ebadi, M., and McCoy, E.: Progesterone-Mediated Increases of Leucocyte Alkaline Phosphatase in Rabbits. Biochim. Biophys. Acta, *130*:502, 1966.

Efrati, P., and Yaari, A.: Evaluation of the Periodic-Acid-Schiff (PAS) Reaction in Mature Neutrophil Granulocytes from Peripheral Blood by a Scanning Microdensitometer (M-85, Vickers). Haematologica, *65*:168, 1980.

Elias, J.M.: A Rapid, Sensitive Myeloperoxidase Stain Using 4-Chloro-1-Napthol. Amer. J. Clin. Pathol., *73*:797, 1980.

El-Mohandes, E.A.-M., and Hayhoe, F.G.J.: 5'-Nucleotidase Activity of Megakaryoblasts in a Case of Acute Megakaryoblastic Leukaemia. Brit. J. Haematol., *53*:523, 1983a.

El-Mohandes, E.A.-M., and Hayhoe, F.G.J.: 5'-Nucleotidase Activity in Myeloma Cells. Clin. Lab. Haematol., *5*:265, 1983b.

Facklam, N.R., and Kociba, G.J.: Cytochemical Characterization of Leukemic Cells from 20 Dogs. Vet. Pathol., *22*:363, 1985.

Feldman, B.F., et al.: Serum Lysozyme (Muramidase) Activity in Dogs with Neoplastic Disease. Amer. J. Vet. Res., *42*:1319, 1981.

Feller, A.C., et al.: Enzymecytochemical Heterogeneity of Human Chronic T-Lymphocytic Leukemia as Demonstrated by Reactivity to Dipeptidylaminopeptidase IV (DAP IV; EC 3.4.14.4). Leukemia Res., *6*:801, 1982.

Foa, R., et al.: Alkaline Phosphatase in Human Lymphocyte Subpopulations. Experientia, *35*:269, 1979.

Folds, J.D., et al.: Simultaneous Evaluation of Terminal Deoxynucleotidyl Transferase and Myeloperoxidase in Leukemia. Amer. J. Haematol., *12*:391, 1982.

Frankel, S., and Reitman, S.: Gradwohl's Laboratory Method and Diagnosis. Vol. 2, 6th ed. Mosby, St. Louis, p. 1144, 1963.

Fuchs, C.A.R., et al.: Granular Acute Leukaemia Not Always of Myeloid Origin. Lancet 1(8377):636, 1984.

Gaedicke, G., and Drexler, H.G.: The Use of Enzyme Marker Analysis for Subclassification of Acute Lymphocytic Leukemia in Childhood. Leukemia Res., *6*:437, 1982.

Girino, M., et al.: Correlation between Cytochemical and Immunological Markers of CLL. Haematologica, *67*:946, 1982.

Gordon, D.S., and Hubbard, M.: Surface Membrane Characteristics and Cytochemistry of the Abnormal Cells in Adult Acute Leukemia. Blood, *51*:681, 1978.

Gordon, D.S., and Hubbard, M.R.: Neutrophilic Nonspecific Esterase: Reply. Blood, *53*:340, 1979.

Graham, R.C., Jr., et al.: Cytochemical Demonstration of Peroxidase Activity with 3-Amino-9-Ethylcarbazole. J. Histochem. Cytochem., *13*:150, 1965.

Grever, M.R., et al.: Adenosine Deaminase and Terminal Deoxynucleotidyl Transferase: Biochemical Markers in the Management of Chronic Myelogenous Leukemia. Cancer Res., *43*:1442, 1983.

Grindem, C.B., et al.: Cytochemical Reactions in Cells from Leukemic Cats. Vet. Clin. Path., *14*(3):6, 1985.

Grossi, C.E., et al.: Morphological and Histochemical Analyses of Two Human T-Cell Subpopulations Bearing Receptors for IgM and IgG. J. Exp. Med., *147*:1405, 1978.

Gutensohn, W., et al.: Evaluation of 5'-Nucleotidase as Biochemical Marker in Leukemias and Lymphomas. Klin. Wochenschr., *61*:57, 1983.

Hanker, J.S., et al.: A New Specific Noncarcinogenic Reagent for Demonstration of Horseradish Peroxidase. Histochem. J., *9*:789, 1977.

Hayhoe, F.G.J.: Leukaemia: Research and Clinical Practice. Chap. 5. J. & A. Churchill, London, 1960.

Hayhoe, F.G.J.: Cytochemistry of the Acute Leukemias. Histochem. J., *16*:1051, 1984.

Hayhoe, F.G.J., and Cawley, J.C.: Acute Leukemia: Cellular Morphology, Cytochemistry and Fine Structure. Clin. Haematol., *1*:49, 1972.

Hayhoe, F.G.J., and Quaglino, D.: Haematological Cytochemistry. Churchill Livingstone, Edinburgh, 1980.

Hayhoe, F.G.J., et al.: Consecutive Use of Romanowsky and Periodic-Acid-Schiff Technique in the Study of Blood and Bone Marrow Cells. Brit. J. Haematol., *6*:23, 1960.

Hayhoe, F.G.J., et al.: The Cytology and Cytochemistry of Acute Leukaemias. London, HMSO, 1964.

Hellmann, A., and Goldman, J.M.: Alkaline Phosphatase Activity of Chronic Granulocytic Leukaemia Neutrophils in Agar Culture. Scand. Haematol., *34*:237, 1980.

Higgy, K.E., et al.: Discrimination of B, T and Null Lymphocytes by Esterase Cytochemistry. Scand. J. Haematol., *18*:437, 1977.

Higgy, K.E., et al.: Identification of the Hairy Cells of Leukaemic Reticuloendotheliosis by an Esterase Method. Brit. J. Haematol., *38*:99, 1978.

Ho, F.C.S., et al.: Non-Specificity of Sudan Black B in the Diagnosis of Acute Myeloid Leukaemia. Brit. J. Haematol., *53*:171, 1983.

Hoffbrand, A.V., et al.: Enzyme Patterns in Normal Lymphocyte Subpopulations, Lymphoid Leukaemias and Immunodeficiency Syndromes. Clin. Haematol., *11*:719, 1982.

Hotchkiss, R.D.: A Microchemical Reaction Resulting in the Staining of Polysaccharide Structures in Fixed Tissue Preparations. Arch. Biochem., *16*:131, 1948.

Hutton, J.J., et al.: Prognostic Significance of Terminal Deoxynucleotidyl Transferase Activity in Childhood Acute Lymphoblastic Leukemia: A Prospective Analysis of 164 Patients. Blood, 60:1267, 1982.

Isaacson, P.G., and Jones, D.B.: Immunohistochemical Differentiation between Histiocytic and Lymphoid Neoplasms. Histochem. J., 15:621, 1983.

Jackson, C.W.: Cholinesterase as a Possible Marker for Early Cells of the Megakaryocytic Series. Blood, 42:413, 1973.

Jain, N.C.: Alkaline Phosphatase Activity in the Canine and Feline Granulocytes. Vet. Rec., 81:266, 1967a.

Jain, N.C.: Peroxidase Activity in Leukocytes of Some Animal Species. Folia Haematol., 88:297, 1967b.

Jain, N.C.: Alkaline Phosphatase Activity in Leukocytes of Some Animal Species. Acta Haematol., 39:51, 1968.

Jain, N.C.: Glycogen Content of Leukocytes of Some Animal Species. Acta Haematol., 41:249, 1969.

Jain, N.C.: A Comparative Cytochemical Study of Leukocytes of Some Animal Species. Folia Haematol., 94:49, 1970.

Jain, N.C.: Alkaline Phosphatase Activity in Leukocytes of Dogs and Cats. Blut, 22:133, 1971.

Jain, N.C., and Bennett, J.M.: Nonspecific Esterase in Acute Promyelocytic Leukemia. Unpublished observations, 1985.

Jain, N.C., et al.: Clinical-Pathological Findings and Cytochemical Characterization of Myelomonocytic Leukaemia in 5 Dogs. J. Comp. Pathol., 91:17, 1981.

Jong, E., et al.: Bactericidal Activity of Eosinophil Peroxidase. J. Immunol., 124:1378, 1980.

Joshi, B.C., and Jain, N.C.: Experimental Immunologic Thrombocytopenia in Dogs: A Study of Thrombocytopenia and Megakaryocytopoiesis. Res. Vet. Sci., 22:11, 1977.

Kajikawa, O., et al.: Use of Alpha-Naphthyl Acetate Esterase Staining to Identify T Lymphocytes in Cattle. Amer. J. Vet. Res., 44:1549, 1983.

Kaplow, L.S.: A Histochemical Procedure for Localizing and Evaluating Leukocyte Alkaline Phosphatase Activity in Smears of Blood and Marrow. Blood, 10:1023, 1955.

Kaplow, L.S.: Simplified Myeloperoxidase Stain Using Benzidine Dihydrochloride. Blood, 26:215, 1965.

Kaplow, L.S.: Leukocyte Alkaline Phosphatase Cytochemistry: Applications and Methods. Ann. N.Y. Acad. Sci., 155:911, 1968.

Kaplow, L.S.: Substitute for Benzidine in Myeloperoxidase Stains. Amer. J. Clin. Pathol., 63:451, 1975.

Kaplow, L.S., and Burstone, M.S.: Cytochemical Demonstration of Acid Phosphatase in Hematopoietic Cells in Health and in Various Hematological Disorders Using Azo Dye Techniques. J. Histochem. Cytochem., 12:805, 1964.

Kass, L.: Cytochemical Abnormalities of Atypical Erythroblasts in Acute Erythremic Myelosis. Acta Haematol., 54:321, 1975.

Kass, L.: Esterase Activity in Erythroleukemia. Amer. J. Clin. Pathol., 67:368, 1977.

Kass, L.: Enzymatic Abnormalities in Erythroleukemia. Acta Hematol., 59:302, 1978a.

Kass, L.: Preleukemic Disorders. Charles C Thomas, Springfield, Ill., 1978b.

Kass, L.: Cytochemistry of Esterases. CRC Crit. Rev. Clin. Lab. Sci., 10:205, 1979.

Kass, L.: Leukemia: Cytology and Cytochemistry. J.B. Lippincott, Philadelphia, 1982.

Kass, L., and Peters, C.L.: Nonspecific Esterase Activity in Pernicious Anemia and Chronic Erythremic Myelosis: A Cytochemical and Electrophoretic Study. Amer. J. Clin. Pathol., 68:273, 1977.

Kass, L., and Peters, C.L.: Esterases in Acute Leukemia: A Cytochemical and Electrophoretic Study. Amer. J. Clin. Pathol., 69:57, 1978.

Kay, N.E., and Zarling, J.M.: Impaired Natural Killing Activity in Patients with Chronic Lymphocytic Leukemia Is Associated with a Deficiency of Azurophilic Cytoplasmic Granules in Putative NK Cells. Blood, 63:305, 1984.

Kitahara, M., and Kushner, J.P.: Acquired Myeloperoxidase Deficiency and Recurrent Infections in a Patient with Acute Myelomonocyte Leukemia. Cancer, 44:2244, 1979.

Knowles, D.M., et al.: The Demonstration of α-Naphthyl Acetate Esterase Activity in Human Lymphocytes: Usefulness as a T-Cell Marker. Cell. Immunol., 35:112, 1978.

Kodousek, R.: A New, Rapid Method of Preparing Schiff's Reagent. Histochem. J., 1:277, 1969.

Koler, R.D., et al.: Myeloproliferative Diseases: Diagnostic Value of the Leukocyte Alkaline Phosphatase Test. Amer. J. Clin. Pathol., 30:295, 1958.

Kramers, M.T.C., et al.: Cell Membrane Enzymes. II. Alkaline Phosphatase and Alkaline Phosphodiesterase I in Normal and Leukaemic Lymphocytes. Brit. J. Haematol., 40:111, 1978.

Kulenkampff, J., et al.: Acid Esterase in Human Lymphoid Cells and Leukaemic Blasts: A Marker for T lymphocytes. Brit. J. Haematol., 36:231, 1977.

Leroux-Roels, G.G., et al.: A Novel Alkaline Phosphatase Isozyme in 4 Patients with Acute Non-Lymphocytic Leukemia: Its Nature, Origin and Clinical Significance. Oncodevel. Biol. Med., 3:31, 1982.

Li, C.Y., and Yam, L.T.: Histochemical and Immunologic Features of Leukemic Cells. Clinical Lab. Annual, 1:73, 1982.

Li, C.Y., et al.: Acid Phosphatase Isoenzyme in Human Leukocytes in Normal and Pathologic Conditions. J. Histochem. Cytochem., 18:473, 1970a.

Li, C.Y., et al.: Studies of Acid Phosphatase Isozymes in Human Leukocytes: Demonstration of Isozyme Cell Specificity. J. Histochem. Cytochem., 18:901, 1970b.

Li, C.Y., et al.: Esterases in Human Leukocytes. J. Histochem. Cytochem., 21:1, 1973.

Lilleyaman, J.S., et al.: PAS in Relapsing LbL. Scand. J. Haematol., 23:30, 1979.

Liu, P.I., et al.: Determination of Acid Phosphatase Activity in Normal Human Lymphocytes. Ann. Clin. Lab. Sci., 12:11, 1982.

Ma, D.D.F., et al.: Comparison of Purine Degradative Enzymes and Terminal Deoxynucleotidyl Transferase in T Cell Leukemias and in Normal Thymic and Post-Thymic T Cells. Brit. J. Haematol., 54:451, 1983.

Madewell, B.R., et al.: Hematologic Abnormalities Preceding Myeloid Leukemia in Three Cats. Vet. Pathol., 16:510, 1979.

Manconi, P.E., et al.: α-Naphthyl Acetate Esterase Activity in Human Lymphocytes: Distribution in Lymphocyte Subpopulations and in Mitogen-Activated Cells. Scand. J. Immunol., 9:99. 1979.

Markovic, O.S., and Schulman, N.R.: Megakaryocyte Maturation Indicated by Methanol Inhibition of an Acid Phosphatase Shared by Megakaryocytes and Platelets. Blood, 50:905, 1977.

Matutes, E., et al.: Ultrastructural Cytochemistry of Chronic T-Cell Leukemias: A Study with Four Acid Hydrolases. Histochem. J. 15:895, 1983.

Miller, D.M., et al.: Leukocyte Alkaline Phosphatase: Another Organ-Specific Alkaline Phosphatase. Amer. J. Hematol., 15:171, 1983.

Miller, D.M., et al.: Altered Isozyme Patterns of Leucocyte Alkaline Phosphatase in Disease States. Brit. J. Haematol., 57:145, 1984.

Mitus, W.J., et al.: Alkaline Phosphatase of Mature Neutrophils in Chronic Forms of the Myeloproliferative Syndrome. Amer. J. Clin. Pathol., 30:285, 1958.

Monahan, R.A., et al.: Ultrastructural Localization of Nonspecific Esterase Activity in Guinea Pig and Human Monocytes, Macrophages, and Lymphocytes. Blood, 58:1089, 1981.

Muehleck, S.D., et al.: Terminal Deoxynucleotidyl Transferase (TdT)-Positive Cells in Bone Marrow in the Absence of Hematopoietic Malignancy. Amer. J. Clin. Pathol., 79:277, 1983.

Mueller, J., et al.: Nonspecific Acid Esterase Activity: A Criterion for Differentiation of T and B Lymphocytes in Mouse Lymph Nodes. Eur. J. Immunol., 5:270, 1975.

Muller, J., et al.: Nonspecific Esterase in Human Lymphocytes. Int. Arch. Allergy Appl. Immunol., 64:410, 1981.

Nanba, K., et al.: Alkaline Phosphatase–Positive Malignant Lymphoma: A Subtype of B-Cell Lymphomas. Amer. J. Clin. Pathol., 68:535, 1977.

Nelson, D.A.: Cytomorphological Diagnosis of the Acute Leukemias. Semin. Oncol., 3:201, 1976.

Nemoto, K., et al.: Studies on Aminopeptidase Activity in Acute Non-Lymphocytic Leukemia: The Relation to Peroxidase Reaction. Acta Pathol. Jpn., 33:495, 1983.

Neumann, H., et al.: Comparative Study of Alkaline Phosphatase Activity in Lymphocytes, Mitogen-Induced Blasts, Lymphoblastoid Cell Lines, Acute Myeloid Leukemia, and Chronic Lymphatic Leukemia Cells. Proc. Natl. Acad. Sci., 73:1432, 1976.

Neumann, H., et al.: N-Alkaline Phosphatase: A Potential Disease Marker for Lymphoproliferative Disorders. Brit. J. Haematol., 41:519, 1979.

Nichols, B.A., et al.: Differentiation of Monocytes: Origin, Nature, and Fate of Their Azurophil Granules. J. Cell Biol., 50:498, 1971.

O'Brien, M., et al.: Ultrastructural Cytochemistry of Leukaemic Cells: Characterization of the Early Small Granules of Monoblasts. Brit. J. Haematol., 45:201, 1980.

Okun, D.B., and Tanaka, K.R.: Leukocyte Alkaline Phosphatase. Amer. J. Hematol., 4:293, 1978.

Osbaldiston, G.W., et al.: Cytochemical Demonstration of Esterases in Peripheral Blood Leukocytes. Amer. J. Vet. Res., 39:683, 1978.

Pangalis, G.A., et al.: Cytochemical Findings in Human Nonneoplastic Blood and Tonsillar B and T Lymphocytes. Amer. J. Clin. Pathol., 69:314, 1978.

Pearse, A.G.E.: Histochemistry, Theoretical and Applied. Vol. 1, 3rd ed., Little, Brown, Boston, 1968. Vol. 2, 3rd ed., Williams & Wilkins, Baltimore, 1972.

Pedersen, B., and Hayhoe, F.G.J.: Cellular Changes in Chronic Myeloid Leukaemia. Brit. J. Haematol., 21:251, 1971.

Perry, S., and Reynolds, J.: Methyl-Green-Pyronin as a Differential Nucleic Acid Stain for Peripheral Blood Smears. Blood, 11:1132, 1956.

Pinkus, G.S., et al.: α-Naphthyl Acetate Esterase Activity: A Cytochemical Marker for T Lymphocytes. Amer. J. Pathol., 91:17, 1979.

Poppema, S., et al.: Alkaline Phosphatase Positive Lymphoma: Functional and Morphological Aspects. Z. Immun. Forsch., 154:351, 1978.

Quaglino, D., and Hayhoe, F.G.J.: Periodic-Acid-Schiff Positivity in Erythroblasts with Special Reference to Di Guglielmo's Disease. Brit. J. Haematol., 6:26, 1960.

Quesada, J.R., and Murphy, S.G.: Histochemical Patterns of Human T Lymphocyte Subpopulations with Nonspecific Esterase Staining. Int. Arch. Allergy Appl. Immunol., 68:138, 1982.

Radzun, H.J., et al.: Lysosomal Acid Phosphatase: Activity and Isozymes in Separated Normal Human Blood Cells. Clin. Chim. Acta, 102:227, 1980.

Ranki, A., et al.: Identification of Resting Human T and B Lymphocytes by Acid α-Naphthyl Acetate Esterase Stain Combined with Rosette Formation with Staphylococcus aureus Strain Cowan 1. Scand. J. Immunol., 5:1129, 1976.

Raphael, S.S.: Lynch's Medical Laboratory Technology. W.B. Saunders, Philadelphia, p. 936, 1976.

Reaman, G.H., et al.: Lymphoblast Purine Pathway Enzymes in B-Cell Acute Lymphoblastic Leukemia. Blood, 58:331, 1981.

Reiffers, J., et al.: Ultrastructural Cytochemical Prospective Study of Adult Acute Lymphoblastic Leukemia: Detection of Peroxidase Activity in Patients Failing to Respond to Treatment. Cancer, 48:927, 1981.

Rodger, G.M., et al.: Blastic Transformation of a Well-Differentiated Monocytic Leukemia: Changes in Cytochemical and Cell Surface Markers. Leukemia Res., 4:613, 1982.

Rosenszajn, L., et al.: The Esterase Activity in Megaloblasts, Leukemic and Normal Hematopoietic Cells. Brit. J. Haematol., 14:605, 1962.

Rudolph, R., and Schnabl, W.: Histochemical, Enzyme Histochemical and Electron Microscopic Studies in Blood Leukocytes from Clinically Healthy and Leukaemic Sheep. Vet. Med. Rev., 2:140, 1979.

Rustin, G.J.S., and Peters, T.J.: Studies on the Subcellular Organelles on Neutrophils in Chronic Granulocytic Leukaemia with Special Reference to Alkaline Phosphatase. Brit. J. Haematol., 41:533, 1979.

Rustin, G.J.S., et al.: An Extrinsic Factor Controls Neutrophil Alkaline Phosphatase in Chronic Granulocytic Leukaemia. Brit. J. Haematol., 45:381, 1980.

Rutenberg, A.M., et al.: An Improved Histochemical Method for the Demonstration of Leukocyte Alkaline Phosphatase Activity: Clinical Application. J. Lab. Clin. Med., 65:698, 1965.

Rytomaa, T., and Teir, H.: Relationship between Tissue Eosinophils and Peroxidase Activity. Nature, 192(Oct.):271, 1961.

Sato, N., et al.: Factor(s) Responsible for the Increase in Alkaline Phosphatase Activity of Post-Mitotic Granulocytes from Normal Individuals and Patients with Chronic Myeloid Leukemia. Blood, 59:141, 1982.

Savage, R.A., et al.: Acid Phosphatase Staining Pattern as an Indicator of T-Cell Acute Leukemia. Amer. J. Clin. Pathol., 76:760, 1981.

Schiffer, C.A., et al.: Increased Leukocyte Alkaline Phosphatase Activity following Transfusion of Leukocytes from a Patient with Chronic Myelogenous Leukemia. Amer. J. Med., 66:519, 1979.

Schmalzl, F., et al.: Detection of Cytochemical and Morphological Anomalies in "Preleukemia." Acta Haematol., 59:1, 1978.

Schumacher, H.R., et al.: Terminal Deoxynucleotidyl Transferase (TdT): Serial Observations on Patients with Leukemia. Amer. J. Med. Sci., 286:18, 1983.

Schwarze, E.-W.: Cytochemical Methods. *In* Malignant Lymphoproliferative Diseases. van den Tweel, J.G., et al., eds. Martinus Nijhoff, Boston, pp. 137–148, 1980.

Scott, C.S.: Cytochemical Applications in Haematology, with Particular Reference to Acute Leukaemias: A Review. Med. Lab. Sci., 35:111, 1978.

Shaw, M.T.: The Cytochemistry of Acute Leukemia: A Diagnostic and Prognostic Evaluation. Semin. Oncol., 3:219, 1976.

Shaw, M.T., and Ishmael, D.R.: Acute Lymphocytic Leukemia with Atypical Cytochemical Features. Amer. J. Clin. Pathol., 63:415, 1975.

Sheehan, H.L., and Storey, G.W.: An Improved Method of Staining Leucocyte Granules with Sudan Black B.: J. Pathol., Bact., 59:336, 1947.

Shibata, A., et al.: Recommended Methods for Cytological Procedures in Haematology. Clin. Lab. Haematol., 7:55, 1985.

Shifrine, M., et al.: Lysozyme (Muramidase) Activity in Canine Myelogenous Leukemia. Amer. J. Vet. Res., 34:695, 1973.

Sondergaard-Petersen, H., and Boesen, A.M.: Three Different Acid Phosphatase Patterns in Leukaemic Lymphoid T-Cells. Scand. J. Haematol., 23:51, 1979.

Srivastava, B.I.S., and Han, T.: Alterations in Enzyme Expression on 12-O-Tetradecanoylphorbol-13-Acetate-Induced Differentiation of Chronic Lymphocytic Leukemia Cells. FEBS Lett., 170:152, 1984.

Srivastava, B.I.S., et al.: Cytochemical Comparison of Immunologically Characterized Human Leukaemia/Lymphoma Cell Lines Representing Different Levels of Maturation. Brit. J. Cancer, 47:771, 1983.

Stass, S.A., et al.: Sudan Black B Positive Acute Lymphoblastic Leukemia. Brit. J. Haematol., 57:413, 1984.

Stein, H., et al.: Malignant Lymphoma of B-Cell Type. Lancet, 2(7782):855, 1972.

Stein, P., et al.: Granular Acute Lymphoblastic Leukemia. Amer. J. Clin. Pathol., 79:426, 1983.

Stjernholm, R.L., et al.: Carbohydrate Metabolism by Leukocytes. Enzyme, 13:7, 1972.

Stuart, J., et al.: Enzyme Cytochemistry of Blood and Marrow Cells. Histochem. J., 7:471, 1975.

Sun, T., et al.: Atlas of Cytochemistry and Immunochemistry of Hematologic Neoplasms. American Society of Clinical Pathologists Press, Chicago, 1985.

Sylwestrowicz, T., et al.: 5'-Nucleotidase, Adenosine Deaminase and Purine Nucleoside Phosphorylase Activities in Acute Leukaemia. Leukemia Res., 6:475, 1982.

Tanaka, K.R., et al.: Diseases or Clinical Conditions Associated with Low Leukocyte Alkaline Phosphatase. New Engl J. Med., 262:912, 1960.

Tavassoli, M., et al.: Cytochemical Diagnosis of Acute Myelomonocytic Leukemia. Amer. J. Clin. Pathol., 72:59, 1979.

Telek, B., et al.: Differential Diagnostic Value of Acid Phosphatase and β-Glucuronidase in Acute Leukaemia. Blut, 46:67, 1983.

Timonen, T., et al.: Characteristics of Human Large Granular Lymphocytes and Relationship to Natural Killer and K Cells. J. Exp. Med., 153:569, 1981.

Tomonaga, M., et al.: Cytochemistry of Acute Promyelocytic Leukemia (M3): Leukemic Promyelocytes Exhibit Heterogeneous Patterns in Cellular Differentiation. Blood, 66:350, 1985.

Totterman, T.H., et al.: Expression of Acid α-Naphthyl Acetate Esterase Marker by Activated and Secondary T Lymphocytes in Man. Scand. J. Immunol., 6:305, 1977.

Tricot, G., et al.: Sudan Black B Positivity in Acute Lymphoblastic Leukaemia. Brit. J. Haematol., 51:615, 1982.

Tschudi, P., et al.: Cytochemical Staining of Equine Blood and Bone Marrow. Equine Vet. J., 9(4):205, 1977.

Tsujimoto H., et al.: A Cytochemical Study on Feline Blood Cells. Jpn. J. Vet. Sci., 45:373, 1983.

Ullyot, J.L., and Bainton, D.F.: Azurophil and Specific Granules of Blood Neutrophils in Chronic Myelogenous Leukemia: An Ultrastructural and Cytochemical Analysis. Blood, 44:469, 1974.

Valentine, W.N.: The Metabolism of the Leukemic Leukocyte. Amer. J. Med., 28:699, 1960.

Valentine, W.N., et al.: The Relationship of Leukocyte Alkaline Phosphatase to "Stress," to ACTH, and to Adrenal 17-OH-Corticosteroids. J. Lab. Clin. Med., 49:723, 1957.

van Furth, R., and Zwet, T.: Cytochemical, Functional, and Proliferative Characteristics of Promonocytes and Monocytes from Patients with Monocytic Leukemia. Blood, 62:298, 1983.

van Laarhoven, J.P.R.M., and De Bruyn, C.H.M.M.: Purine Metabolism in Relation to Leukemia and Lymphoid Cell Proliferation. Leukemia Res., 7:451, 1983.

Vertongen, F., et al.: Enzymes of Purine Metabolism in B-Chronic Lymphocytic Leukemia. Amer. J. Hematol., 17:61, 1984.

Wada, J.: Ultrastructural Peroxidase Cytochemistry of Leukemic Cell. I. Classification of Acute Myelogenous Leukemia. Keio J. Med., 29:163, 1980a.

Wada, J.: Ultrastructural Peroxidase Cytochemistry of Leukemic Cells. II. Blast Crisis of Chronic Myelogenous Leukemia. Keio J. Med., 29:175, 1980b.

Weller, R.E., et al.: Myeloblastic Leukemia and Leukemic Meningitis in a Dog. Mod. Vet. Pract., 61:42, 1980.

Wetzel, B.K.: The Fine Structure and Cytochemistry of Developing Granulocytes with Special Reference to the Rabbit. Chap. 33. *In* Regulation of Hematopoiesis. Vol. 2. Gordon, A.S., ed. Appleton-Century-Crofts, New York, p. 769, 1970.

Wever, R., et al.: Characterization of the Peroxidase in Human Eosinophils. Eur. J. Biochem., 108:491, 1980.

Williams, D.M., et al.: A Comparison Using Quantitative Enzyme Cytochemistry between Leukocyte Alkaline Phosphatase Levels in Bone Marrow and Blood of the Rat. Brit. J. Haematol., 40:119, 1978.

Williams, D.M., et al.: Light Microscope and Electron Microscope Alkaline Phosphatase Cytochemistry of Rat Bone Marrow Leucocytes. J. Histochem. Cytochem., 27:665, 1979.

Woessner, S., et al.: Isozymes of Acid Phosphatase in Nonlymphoid Acute Leukemia. Acta Haematol., 61:85, 1979.

Wulff, H.R.: Morphological and Histochemical Features of Leucocytes in Experimental Inflammation and in Disease. Munksgaard, Copenhagen, 1967.

Wulff, J.C., et al.: Nonspecific Acid Esterase Activity as a Marker for Canine T Lymphocytes. Exp. Hematol., 9:865, 1981.

Yam, L.T., et al.: Cytochemical Identification of Monocytes and Granulocytes. Amer. J. Clin. Pathol., 55:283, 1971a.

Yam, L.T., et al.: Tartrate-Resistant Acid Phosphatase Isoenzyme in the Reticulum Cells of Leukemic Reticuloendotheliosis. New Engl. J. Med., *284*:357, 1971b.

Yang, T.J., et al.: Acid α-Naphthyl Acetate Esterase: Presence of Activity in Bovine and Human T and B Lymphocytes. Immunol., *38*:85, 1979.

Yurno, J., and Mastropaolo, W.: Nonspecific Esterases of the Formed Elements: Zymograms Produced by pH 9.5 Polyacrylamide Gel Electrophoresis. Blood, *58*:939, 1981.

34

The Plasma Proteins, Dysproteinemias, and Immune Deficiency Disorders

FACTORS GOVERNING PLASMA PROTEIN CONCENTRATIONS 942
  Hormonal Control 943
  Dietary Factors 943
  Stress Factors 943
  Hemoconcentration 944
  Pregnancy and Lactation 944
  Age 945

PLASMA PROTEINS 945
  Prealbumin 945
  Albumin 947
  Fibrinogen 947
  Glycoproteins 948
  Transferrin 948
  Haptoglobin and Hemopexin 948
  Ceruloplasmin 949
  C-Reactive Protein 950
  α-Fetoprotein 950
  Lipoproteins 950

IMMUNOGLOBULINS 951
  Basic Structure 951

Classes of Immunoglobulins 952
Species Differences 954

METHODOLOGY 955
  Total Protein Concentrations 955
  The Electrophoretic Techniques 956

DYSPROTEINEMIAS 957
  Changes in Albumin Concentrations 960
  Changes in Fibrinogen Levels 960
  Changes in α- and β-Globulins 962
  Changes in γ-Globulins 964
  The Gammopathies 964
  Plasma Proteins in Selected Conditions 971

IMMUNE DEFICIENCY DISORDERS 976
  Clinical Signs and Diagnostic Approach 977
  Primary Immune Deficiency Disorders 978
  Secondary Immune Deficiency Disorders 979
  Immune Deficiencies of Undefined Origin 981

Proteins are polymers of some 22 amino acids linked linearly by peptide bonds in various combinations. Their functional specificity is determined by the sequence of amino acids and their architectural conformation. They are present in the plasma and all living cells. Each tissue synthesizes its own characteristic proteins, some of which remain within the synthesizing cell. The liver occupies a central role in protein anabolism and catabolism. It synthesizes serum albumin, many coagulation factors, and most of the α- and β-globulins.

Functionally, plasma proteins are involved in nutrition, maintenance of osmotic pressure, buffering, transport of smaller ions and molecules, hemostasis, and resistance to infection.

Nearly 80% of the body's protein stores are found in striated muscle, skeleton, and skin. The structural proteins are among the last components to be "consumed" by the starving animal. Thus, in general, the body tends strongly to conserve its proteins. There is no storage of protein in times of dietary excess, however. Any excess of amino acids over the level necessary to maintain the circulating pool and for new protein synthesis is quickly converted to carbohydrate or fat and utilized for energy.

In disease, other signs will generally become evident before changes in plasma protein concentrations take place. Alterations in plasma protein concentrations must be examined in light of the entire complex of clinical and laboratory findings before any diagnosis or prognosis can be given.

Table 34–1.   The Principal Plasma Proteins and a Brief Statement of Their Functions

Plasma Protein	Function
Albumin	Osmostic function; amino acid pool; transporter of other anions and cations; most abundant protein in plasma
In α-Globulin Zone	
α_1-Lipoprotein	Transports fats, lipids, fat-soluble vitamins, and hormones
α_1-Acid glycoprotein	Function unknown; increased in inflammatory, degenerative, and neoplastic disease
α_1-Glycoprotein	Function unknown
Transcortin	Binds and transports cortisol
Thyroxin-binding globulin	Binds thyroxin
Gc-globulins	Group-specific, genetically determined proteins; function unknown
Haptoglobin	Binds free hemoglobin
Ceruloplasmin	Glycoprotein that binds copper
Cholinesterase	Enzyme that degrades acetylcholine
α_2 Macroglobulin	Binds insulin
α_2-Lipoprotein	Transports lipids
Erythropoietin	Erythropoietic function
In β-Globulin Zone	
β-Lipoprotein	Transports glycerides and other lipids
Transferrin	Binds iron
Hemopexin	Binds heme
Fibrinogen	Essential to blood clotting
Plasminogen	Proenzyme form of plasmin
Partly in β-Globulin Zone, Mostly in γ-Globulin Zone	
IgG, IgA, IgM, IgD, IgE	Antibody activity

The plasma proteins are a group of heterogeneous molecules with known as well as poorly defined characteristics and functions. A list of some of the principal plasma proteins and their functions is given in Table 34–1. Their complexity is well demonstrated by the technique of immunoelectrophoresis, through which as many as 35 distinct proteins can be recognized in the blood serum (Fig. 34–1).

Through the technique of starch-gel electrophoresis, multiple molecular forms of individual proteins can be demonstrated. The synthesis of some polymorphic proteins is genetically controlled, and their determination has been a valuable aid in breed studies and the establishment of parentage. Proteins involved include prealbumin, postalbumin, albumin, transferrin, haptoglobin, group-specific α_2-globulin, β-lipoproteins, blood group substances, and certain enzymes.

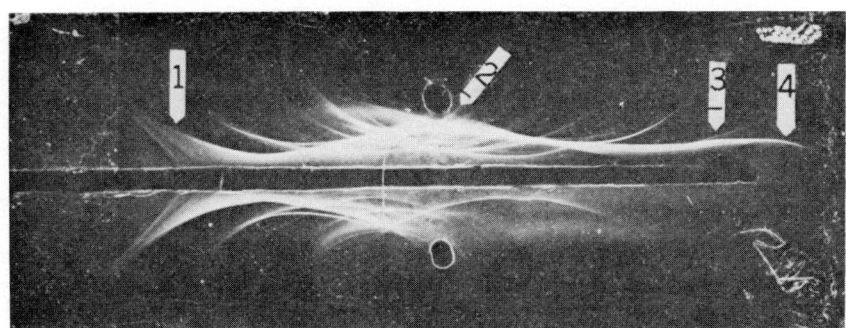

Fig. 34–1.   Immunoelectrophoresis of cow and precolostral calf serum. The glass slide was coated with a thin film of agar, and two holes separated by a trench were punched out. Cow serum was added to the top well, and precolostral calf serum was added to the bottom well. An electric current was applied across the ends of the slide for electrophoresis. After electrophoretic migration, rabbit antibovine serum was applied to the middle trench. The slide was incubated in a moist chamber to allow the immune precipitating arcs to develop. The slide was dried and stained for protein. Migration is from right to left. Identified are (1) serum albumin, (2) IgM, (3) IgG–1, and (4) IgG–2. Only a part of the 35 lines discussed in the text are resolved here from adult serum, illustrating the fact that antisera vary in their content of antibodies to individual serum protein antigens. Note the absence of immune globulins in the precolostral calf serum.

FACTORS GOVERNING PLASMA PROTEIN CONCENTRATIONS

The total protein in the body represents a balance between anabolism and catabolism. Plasma protein concentrations reflect a balance between filtration into the capillaries and return from the tissues via the lymph. This balance depends on the colloidal osmotic pressure and the circulatory dynamics—i.e., the tendency for blood to attract fluids from the tissues due to colloidal osmotic pressure and the opposing hydrostatic pressure of blood tending to force fluids into the tissue spaces.

The concentration of protein in the plasma at any given time is a function of hormonal balance, nutritional status, water balance, and other factors affecting the state of health. The rate of turnover of the various proteins varies from species to species (Table 34–2). There is a direct correlation between half-life of a protein and body size (Allison, 1960), the turnover being much faster in smaller animals.

Compartmentalization studies indicate that extravascular protein concentrations are much greater than vascular. For example, the extravascular:vascular ratio for albumin was found to be 2.90 in horses (Mattheeuws et al., 1966), 2.58 in cattle (Cornelius et al., 1962), and 1.71 in young pigs (Dich and Nielson, 1963).

In addition to normal catabolism by the liver, kidney, and other tissues, there is a constant loss of plasma proteins into the gut. It is not known whether plasma proteins move into the intestines by passive transudation or by active secretion.

It is generally believed that plasma protein concentrations regulate metabolic rate—i.e., as the concentration of albumin or γ-globulin increases, the absolute and fractional degradative rate also increases. Conversely, there is a prolongation of the half-life in hypoproteinemia (Rothschild et al., 1966a). In turn-

Table 34–2. Half-Life of Serum Proteins of Various Animals (Data Abstracted from the Literature)

Species	Protein	T½ (days)	Method	Reference
Sheep	Albumin	14–28	[131]I	Campbell et al. (1961)
Young swine	Albumin	8.2	[131]I	Dich and Neilson (1963)
Cattle	Albumin	16.5	[131]I	Cornelius et al. (1962)
	γ-Globulin	21.2		Dixon et al. (1952)
Dairy cows	Albumin	15	[14]C	Cornelius et al. (1959a)
Cow	Albumin	20.7	[131]I	Dixon et al. (1953)
Human	Albumin	15.0	[131]I	Dixon et al. (1953)
	γ-Globulin	20.0	[131]I	Dixon et al. (1952)
Dog	Albumin	8.2	[131]I	Dixon et al. (1953)
	γ-Globulin	8.0	[131]I	Dixon et al. (1952)
Rabbit	Albumin	5.7	[131]I	Dixon et al. (1953)
	γ-Globulin	5.7	[131]I	Dixon et al. (1952)
Guinea pig	Albumin	2.8	[131]I	Allison (1960)[a]
	γ-Globulin	5.4	[131]I	Dixon et al. (1952)
Rat	Albumin	2.5	[131]I	Allison (1960)
	γ-Globulin	5.5		
Mouse	Albumin	1.9	[131]I	Allison (1960)[a]
	γ-Globulin	1.9	[131]I	Dixon et al. (1952)
Baboon	Albumin	16	[131]I	Cohen (1956)
	γ-Globulin	12		
Dog	Albumin	23.3 ± 4	[35]S	Bruenger et al. (1967)
	α_1-Globulin	12.8 ± 1.4	[35]S	
	β_1-Globulin	13.5 ± 1.5	[35]S	
	β_2-Globulin	15.6 ± 0.9	[35]S	
	γ-Globulin	19.5 ± 2.2	[35]S	
Horse				
Normal	Albumin	19.4	[131]I	Mattheeuws et al. (1966)
Splenectomized	Albumin	17.3	[131]I	
Hypoalbuminemic	Albumin	14.5	[131]I	

[a]A part of Allison's data came from the work of others and was abstracted from the literature.

over studies in humans (Margen and Tarver, 1956), calculations revealed that if albumin synthesis were suddenly reduced by 50% and the normal rate of catabolism and loss were to continue, it would take 16 days for a 20% decrease of serum albumin to occur.

Hormonal Control

Protein concentrations are influenced or regulated by hormones. Hormones are either anabolic or catabolic. Growth hormone acts to increase deposition of protein in the tissues and diminish nitrogen excretion. Insulin is required for normal action of growth hormone. The androgens and estrogens are also anabolic, resulting in protein deposition in the liver, muscle, and accessory sex glands. Thyroid hormone at normal physiologic doses is anabolic, but higher doses are catabolic. The glucocorticoids result in protein consumption for gluconeogenesis; hence they are catabolic. Effects of glucocorticoids on the bovine immune system have been reviewed (Roth and Kaeberle, 1982).

Dietary Factors

The protein requirements for animals vary from species to species. For example, ruminants can be maintained on protein-free rations. The rumen flora can synthesize the animal's amino acid needs from nonprotein nitrogenous sources such as ammonium salts or urea.

Dietary requirements vary with age. The young need dietary protein for growth, whereas adults need it to maintain existing tissues. Additional demands are imposed during pregnancy and lactation. The concept has also been developed that an amino acid balance is needed in dietary protein; proteins vary greatly in their amino acid composition and nutritional adequacy (reviewed elegantly by Allison, 1957).

In humans, the disease kwashiorkor is characterized by a marked reduction in total plasma protein levels, albumin, and many enzymes. It is caused by a dietary deficiency of protein and some degree of caloric imbalance. There is no animal equivalent to this disease. It is perhaps redundant to mention that protein levels fall in animals on low protein diets. Dietary restriction of protein in the dog leads

to marked hypoalbuminemia (Weech et al., 1935; Zeldis et al., 1945) and reduction in total circulating hemoglobin (Weech et al., 1937). Dietary protein levels ranging from 8.3% to 16.0% crude protein led to no detectable changes in serum proteins in horses (Fonnesbeck and Symons, 1969). Restricted protein intake in chickens leads to depressed levels of total serum protein due to decreased albumin. The globulin is not significantly affected (Leveille et al., 1961).

Certain disease states can markedly influence the utilization of dietary protein. For example, the intestinal breakdown of dietary protein is a prerequisite for absorption. This is a function of pancreatic enzymes and enzymes of the mucosal cells of the gut wall. Therefore, any degenerative changes of the gut or severe pancreatic disease (lack of trypsin) can lead to malabsorption syndromes.

Stress Factors

Stress in several forms alters the total plasma protein concentration. *Febrile illness* causes a loss of nitrogen associated with a rise in energy output and an increase in adrenocortical activity, resulting in gluconeogenesis and diversion of amino acids to antibody formation. *Cold* causes increased urinary nitrogen output and induces an increase in heat output, leading to a temporary alteration in plasma protein concentration. Local vascular changes responsible for the signs of inflammation lead to loss of proteins, particularly albumin, into tissue fluids in *tissue injury*. In this situation, tissue cathepsins break down the infiltrating plasma proteins into smaller fragments, leading to an increase in effective extravascular osmotic pressure. Movement of fluid from vascular to extravascular spaces in order to equilibrate the osmotic pressure changes between the two compartments results in edema. *Hemorrhage* leads to protein loss and reduced blood volume. Replacement of volume by rapid movement of fluid into the vascular system leads to a temporary reduction of plasma protein concentration. The hallmark of blood loss is an accompanying hypoproteinemia (Appendix Cases 20 and 23). The existence of anemia with normal or elevated total plasma protein concentration indicates that the anemia is not likely due to hemorrhage (Appendix Case 5).

It has been shown in dogs that after hemorrhage at least 50% of the albumin appears to be replaced within 24 hours (Wasserman et al., 1956). This replacement comes from extravascular sources, principally the lymph (Cope and Litwin, 1962). Others have shown that during a 74-minute period of bleeding of dogs in which 48% of the circulating plasma and 47% of total protein were removed, 29% of the plasma and 14% of the protein were replaced (Deavers et al., 1963). To aid in further conservation, liver anabolism of albumin is stepped up and catabolism is slowed down during hemorrhage. A part of the control has been ascribed to the albumin concentration within the hepatic interstitial space (Rothschild et al., 1966b).

The ability of the animal to maintain normal protein levels in the face of significant loss has been further demonstrated by plasmapheresis experiments in humans (Simson et al., 1966) and dogs (Orentreich et al., 1968), in which normal protein levels were found in the face of weekly removal of as much as a liter of plasma in humans and $\frac{1}{2}$ to 1 liter of blood in dogs.

Hemoconcentration

Loss of water due to dehydration leads to elevation of total plasma proteins through concentration in a reduced blood volume. In this instance, there will be an elevation of both albumin and globulin, i.e., the albumin:globulin (A/G) ratio will be normal. Thus the clinician should be aware that an absolute hypoproteinemia may exist, even though the plasma proteins are in the normal range, due to lowered plasma volume. In the horse, splenic contraction forces a large mass of erythrocytes into the circulation, suddenly increasing circulating blood volume. This is accompanied by a small rise in plasma proteins, possibly due to movement of water out of the blood to compensate partially for the sudden blood-volume increase (Carroll et al., 1965).

Pregnancy and Lactation

In studies on cows in which the movement of protein from blood into colostrum was quantitated (Larson and Kendall, 1957), it was found that at about 2 months before parturition, the protein level in the blood started increasing as a consequence of increasing levels of β_2- and γ_1-globulins. About 4 weeks before parturition, the proteins reached a maximum, and then started decreasing to a minimum at parturition. This drop coincided with the movement of blood proteins into colostrum. The level of serum albumin and β_1- and γ_2-globulins did not change appreciably. Serum albumin levels were found to decrease from 5 weeks before calving to 10 weeks after calving (Rowland and Manston, 1983).

There are three major immunoglobulins (Igs) in colostrum: IgG, IgM, and IgA, with IgG comprising about 65–90% of the total Ig level (Tizard, 1982). Some breed differences have been found in serum and colostrum Ig levels in cows (Logan et al., 1981; Muller and Ellinger, 1981). The Ig level of mammary secretion decreases gradually as production changes from colostrum to milk. Thus milk contains comparatively lower levels of Igs. IgG_1 predominates in milk of ruminants and IgA in nonruminant domestic animals. Most of the IgG_1 is transported selectively into the mammary gland of ruminants, while some of it may be synthesized locally as is IgA (Chang et al., 1981). This selective transport may be a property of the Fc region of the IgG_1 (Micusan and Borduas, 1976). Bovine colostrum contains IgM associated with secretory component, and certain colostrum may be deficient in IgA (Seto et al., 1977). The Ig content of equine colostrum is predominantly IgG and IgG(T), although smaller amounts of IgM, IgA, and aggregating Ig have been found (Rumbaugh et al., 1979). The IgG level of equine colostrum decreases within 24 hours of foaling to <25% of that present at foaling (Pearson et al., 1984). The Ig levels in colostrum of sows is influenced by a variety of factors; IgA is particularly influenced by breed and number of parturitions (Inoue, 1981a) and IgM by the season, breed, and vaccination history (Inoue, 1981b).

Specific serum Ig levels in relation to parturition and lactation have been studied by many workers. Serum IgG_1 levels decline before parturition, particularly during colostrum formation. As a result, the half-life of serum IgG_1 in prepartum cows is much shorter (5–6) than that of cows in normal lactation (about 10 days) (Sasaki et al., 1976). This shorter half-life is associated with selective transfer of the IgG_1 into the mammary secretion. In one study (Williams and Millar, 1979), serum IgG_1 and IgM levels were decreased and IgG_2 levels were increased from about 4 weeks before calving through 8 (for IgG_1 and IgM) to 12 weeks (for IgM) after calving. In another study (Guidry et al., 1980), serum IgA and to a lesser extent IgM levels were elevated at parturition and showed a significant decline postpartum. Serum IgA continued to decrease for 30 days and then increased from days 60 to 180 of lactation. Although serum IgG_1 increased gradually during the postpartum period and early lactation, all Igs generally remained constant during most of the lactation (240 days) and increased during late lactation. IgG_1 levels are higher in colostrum and milk of third and fourth lactation cows compared to cows in first lactation (Caffin et al., 1983; Devery-Pocius and Larson, 1983).

In sheep, a fall in the globulin concentration in the latter stage of pregnancy, probably associated with colostrum formation, was also noted (Dalgarno et al., 1950; Fell et al., 1968). Selective transfer of IgG_1 into the colostrum is reflected in reduced serum half-life—3.7 days during late pregnancy versus 8 days in nonpregnant adult ewes (Cripps and Lascelles, 1974). The decrease in serum IgG and IgM of ewes at lambing is followed by a slow recovery, most within 2–3 months and complete within 5–6 months in lactation (Ciupercescu, 1977). A similar decrease in serum γ-globulins during pregnancy and lactation was seen in goats (Vihan and Sahni, 1981).

Age

Serum protein concentration increases with age in most species; it is lowest during fetal life and remarkably low at birth. An increase is apparent soon after colostrum consumption, and subsequently it rises as the newborn begins to synthesize Igs. Adult levels are reached by about 6 months to 1 year of age depending on the animal species. Total plasma protein concentrations are higher in older animals.

Colostrum ingestion and absorption by the neonate lead to increased blood levels of γ-globulins and temporary proteinuria (Pierce, 1961). Electrophoresis of neonatal serum affords an effective way to determine whether the animal has absorbed colostrum, since elevated γ-globulin is markedly evident in various species when colostral Igs have been absorbed (Figs. 34–2 and 34–3). Absorption of colostral Igs by newborn calves has been reviewed (Bush and Staley, 1980), and the role of membrane receptors in selective absorption of Igs has been discussed (Staley and Bush, 1985).

Immunoglobulin levels in precolostral and postcolostral calf serums have been measured (LaMotte, 1977; Naylor et al., 1977). The three major Igs—IgM, IgG_1, and IgG_2—may be detected in precolostral calf serum (LaMotte, 1977). Serum Igs peak in colostrum-fed calves 18–30 hours after birth, the IgM and IgA peaking earlier than the IgG_1 and IgG_2 (Ishikawa and Konishi, 1982). There is a gradual decrease at 1–5 weeks, depending on the half-life of Igs, and this is followed by a gradual increase. The half-life of IgG_1 in calves is 11.5 ± 0.6 days (Sasaki et al., 1977). Calves vary widely in their concentration of serum Igs. This variation may be related to a variety of factors including the amount of colostrum ingested per unit body weight, the concentration of Ig in the colostrum fed, the time when suckling commenced after birth, environmental temperature, and dietary factors (Bush and Staley, 1980; Fellah and Stott, 1981; Stott, 1980; Stott et al., 1979a, b, c). The newborn calf begins to synthesize IgM as early as 1 week of age, IgG_1 and IgG_2 within 2 weeks, and IgA not until 7–9 weeks. Age-related increases were reported in IgG_2 levels for cattle (Williams and Millar, 1978) and in β- and γ-globulins for dogs (Barsanti et al., 1977).

PLASMA PROTEINS

Plasma proteins other than immunoglobulins are described under this section, while immunoglobulins are described in the next section. Discussion is limited to certain major and minor plasma proteins.

Prealbumin

Prealbumin is synthesized by the liver. It has a molecular weight (MW) of

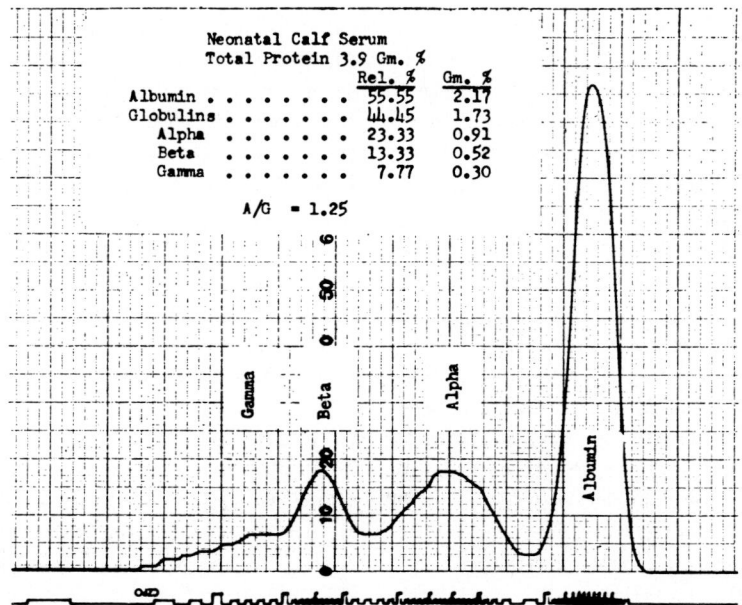

Fig. 34–2. Electrophoretic pattern of neonatal calf serum before colostrum ingestion. Note the virtual absence of γ-globulin. The calf was bled 5 minutes after parturition.

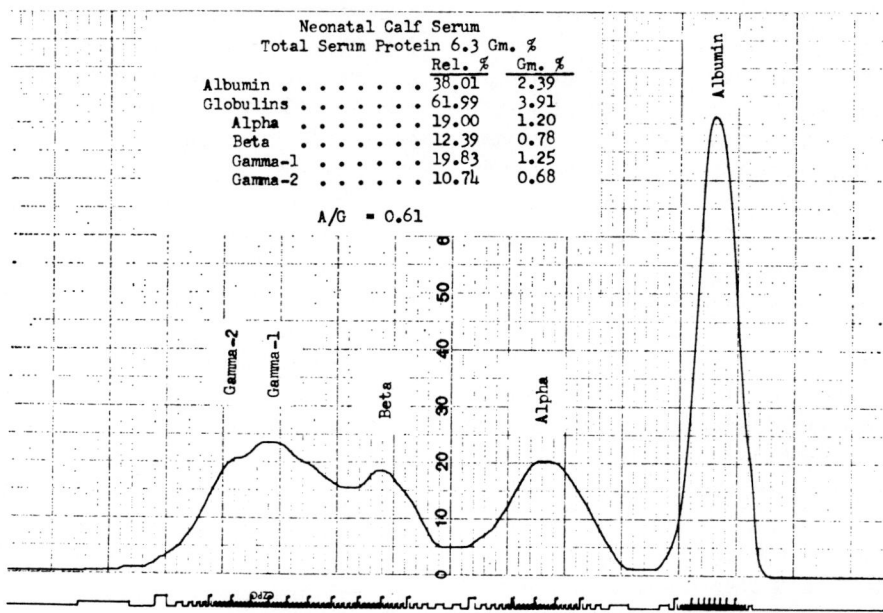

Fig. 34–3. Electrophoretic pattern of serum from the same calf shown in Fig. 34–2 after colostrum ingestion and absorption. The calf was 24 hours old at the time of bleeding.

50,000–60,000 and is found in human and some animal plasma. Prealbumin binds thyroxin (both T_4 and T_3) to serve as a transport protein. Thyroxin in plasma is also transported bound to albumin and thyroxin-binding globulins (MW 54,000–65,000). A prealbumin-like protein that migrates in the α_2 region to transport thyroxin has been described in the dog (Fex et al., 1977). Prealbumin also binds retinol-binding protein (MW 21,000), the protein that binds vitamin A (retinol) and is responsible for the transport of vitamin A from the liver (Blombäck and Hanson, 1979). A decrease in prealbumin level may suggest impaired liver function, although it may also be decreased in nephrotic syndrome (Helen et al., 1975). Prealbumin is found at a significantly higher concentration in healthy foals than in mares and is elevated in horses with acute infections, laminitis, and malignant tumors (Ek, 1980).

Albumin

Albumin is the most abundant of the plasma proteins. Thus it is a readily available pool of amino acids suitable to meet tissue needs. It is composed of 585 amino acid residues and has a molecular weight of 66,300. It is one of the most soluble plasma proteins, but being a larger molecule it normally is retained by the capillaries. Albumin is the first protein to be lost from the blood during tissue injury. Albumin is important in the regulation and maintenance of colloidal osmotic pressure of the blood. The large number of reactive groups on the albumin molecule cause it to bind reversibly with a large number of anions and cations. Thus albumin has an important transport function. Albumin transports free fatty acids; the bile acids; bilirubin; the porphyrins; ketosteroids; many drugs, such as penicillin, aspirin, and the barbiturates; histamine; and cations and trace elements such as calcium, copper, and zinc.

Albumin is synthesized by the liver and catabolized by a variety of tissues. The mechanism for the control of synthesis is not known, although it is frequently mentioned that control may lie in colloidal osmotic pressure changes. Because there is constant exchange between intravascular and extravascular spaces, it has been suggested that albumin synthesis may be sensitive to albumin concentrations within the interstitial space of the liver (Rothschild et al., 1966b). Similarly, albumin synthesis is inversely related to its extravascular concentration (Blombäck and Hanson, 1979). Albumin synthesis is also influenced by the state of nutrition, the hormonal balance, and the general condition of the liver. For example, its synthesis is diminished during fasting or malnutrition, hypothyroidism, and cirrhosis. The half-life of albumin varies with the species; e.g., it is 1.2 days for the mouse, 8.2 days for the dog, 15 days for humans, 19.4 days for the horse, and 20.7 days for the cow. However, the absolute amount of albumin synthesized daily is relatively constant in all species including humans (150–200 mg/kg body wt/day).

Correct interpretation of serum total calcium values requires adjustment of serum total calcium levels for serum albumin or total protein concentration (Meuten et al., 1982). A positive linear relationship was found between serum albumin and total calcium and between total protein and total calcium. A correction formula for calcium was derived on the basis of the concentration of albumin: adjusted calcium (mg/dl) = calcium (mg/dl) − albumin (g/dl) + 3.5. Similar correction on the basis of serum protein concentration was: adjusted calcium (mg/dl) = calcium (mg/dl) − 0.4 [total serum protein (g/dl)] + 3.3. Hypercalcemia was not associated with hyperalbuminemia or hyperproteinemia.

Fibrinogen

Fibrinogen is primarily concerned with hemostasis; it serves as the substrate for thrombin in the formation of fibrin. It has also been thought to play some role in wound healing and defense against infections by providing a fibrin meshwork to serve as a scaffolding for tissue growth and as a barrier for spread of bacteria.

Fibrinogen is a glycoprotein with about 4–5% carbohydrate and a molecular weight of 340,000. It is a very heterogeneous protein consisting of different molecules that may separate into distinct fractions. The fibrinogen molecule is a dimer, each half consisting of three polypeptide chains interconnected by disulfide bonds; its molecular formula is (α, β, and γ)₂. The fibrinogen–fibrin transformation occurs after removal of two acidic peptides (fibrinopeptides A and B) from the NH_2-terminal portions of the α- and β-chains.

Fibrinogen is produced by microsomes of the hepatic parenchymal cells, where it is stored until required. Fibrinogen has a much shorter half-life than other plasma proteins (2.5–4.5 days in the dog), and its rate of formation is governed by the plasma concentration. Fibrinogen is also found in the lymph, connective tissues, and interstitial spaces. Broad ranges of normal fibrinogen levels stated in grams per deciliter of plasma have been established by us as follows: cat, 0.05–0.30; dog and horse, 0.10–0.50; and cow, 0.30–0.70. Plasma fibrinogen concentrations may reach or exceed the maximum normal for the cow for several days after parturition.

Glycoproteins

Glycoproteins are proteins conjugated with carbohydrate. These include γ-globulins, ceruloplasmin, haptoglobin, α₂-macroglobulin, and α₁-acid mucoprotein or seromucoid. All the electrophoretic fractions of serum except albumin contain carbohydrate. There is no generally accepted terminology or standardized method for determination of serum glycoproteins. The most commonly used method in clinical medicine is electrophoresis on cellulose acetate or other support medium; instead of being stained for protein, the strips are stained for carbohydrate with periodic acid–Schiff reagent. There is a large body of literature in clinical medicine on glycoproteins wherein different components have been measured with specific chemical reagents. These include the orcinol-H_2SO_4 method for protein-bound hexose, Ehrlich's reagent for hexosamine, cysteine for fucose, and diphenylamine for "sialic acid." Functions of this heterogeneous group of substances are not known in all instances.

Marked variations in serum glycoprotein content may occur in both physiologic and pathologic states. Levels have been reported for normal and diseased animals (Cornelius et al., 1960; Cornelius and Kaneko, 1963). Plasma levels of glycoproteins appear to parallel the degree of inflammation and degenerative changes. Electrophoretically, glyco-protein in the α₂-globulin zone is in greatest concentration and seems to show the greatest change in disease. (See Winzler, 1955, for discussion and methods.) Some of the glycoproteins are recognized as "acute phase reactants or proteins" and are described separately below. Some recent reviews provide details of a variety of plasma proteins of defined and undefined functions (Schwick and Haupt, 1981; Swain et al., 1980).

Transferrin

Transferrin is the only protein in the plasma that transports iron. It is a glycoprotein composed of one polypeptide chain. Species variations occur in the molecular weight (77,000–90,000) and the number of iron-binding sites (one or two). Generally, each molecule of transferrin binds two atoms of ferric (Fe^{3+}) iron through tyrosine residues. Normally, about one-third of the plasma transferrin is saturated with iron and provides about two-thirds of the iron needed for erythropoiesis. Transferrin under normal conditions is not catabolized when it delivers iron. The plasma half-life is 8–9 days. Several genetic variants of transferrin can be separated on starch gel electrophoresis. Antibacterial and antiviral activities have been ascribed to transferrin.

Transferrin is synthesized in the liver and possibly in the spleen, lymph nodes, bone marrow, and intestinal mucosa. Transferrin levels increase in iron-deficiency states and pregnancy and decrease in diseases such as pernicious anemia, liver disease, and acute and chronic active infections. Transferrin levels may also be altered during leukemia (Swain et al., 1980). Transferrin levels in foals are high at birth and increase during the first three weeks of the neonatal period after a transient fall during the first 48 hours of life (Csontos et al., 1984).

Haptoglobin and Hemopexin

Both haptoglobin and hemopexin are carbohydrate-rich (about 19–20%) glycoproteins synthesized in the liver. Haptoglobin consists of four polypeptide chains, has a molecular weight of 99,000, and plasma half-life of 2–4 days. It occurs in one monomeric and two polymeric forms and exhibits genetic polymorphism. Hemopexin consists of one polypeptide chain and has a molecular weight of 57,000.

Haptoglobin specifically binds free hemoglobin in stoichiometric proportion, but the hemoglobin tetramer must dissociate into dimeric form before binding. The hemoglobin–haptoglobin complex is rapidly removed (T½, 20–30 mins) from the circulation by the Kupffer cells (Hershko et al., 1972). Free hemoglobin in excess of that needed to saturate all the plasma haptoglobin is excreted by the kidneys, resulting in hemoglobinuria. Some of the excess hemoglobin breaks down in the circulation, liberating heme which is then oxidized to hematin. This hematin binds with hemopexin (found in the β-globulin zone), and the hematin–hemopexin complex is removed slowly (T½, 7–8 hr) from the plasma by the hepatocytes. Excess hematin not bound by hemopexin is bound to serum albumin, forming a complex called ferrihemalbumin (methemalbumin). The hemalbumin complex is removed from the circulation at a considerably slower rate (T½, 22 hrs) than the hematin-hemopexin complex (T½, <7–8 hrs). For additional comments on catabolism of free hemoglobin see Chapter 19.

Plasma haptoglobin and hemopexin levels are markedly reduced in hemolytic anemias and during ineffective erythropoiesis. Human studies have shown that haptoglobin levels may be age-related, being low in the young and high in people in their sixties, and that levels may decrease during pregnancy, severe malnutrition, hyperparathyroidism, and corticosteroid therapy (see Swain et al., 1980). Haptoglobin is an important acute phase protein; hence its levels are invariably elevated from increased synthesis during acute and chronic active inflammatory conditions (Pinters, 1971). Haptoglobin migrates in the α_2-globulin region, and so an increase of α_2-globulin in the serum electrophoretogram in many inflammatory diseases reflects changes primarily due to haptoglobin (Busby and Travis, 1978). It may also increase from trauma, after surgery, and during hematopoietic malignancies.

Serum haptoglobin levels have been measured in several animal species (Furukawa and Sugiyama, 1984; Harvey and Gaskin, 1978; Makimura and Suzuki, 1982; Richter and Wagner, 1974; Sheldrick et al., 1982; Travis, 1977). Normal cattle have no or small amounts of serum haptoglobin, whereas cattle suffering from severe inflammatory diseases such as mastitis, pyometra, and traumatic reticulitis have greatly elevated levels (Makimura and Suzuki, 1982). The serum haptoglobin level is increased in horses with infection (Sheldrick et al., 1982). Serum levels of a hemoglobin reactive protein, presumably haptoglobin, were increased in all of 17 cattle with a clinical picture and leukograms typical of bacterial infection and in nearly 50% of cattle that had aborted recently (Blackshaw, 1979). Gamma-irradiation and turpentine-induced inflammation caused increases in serum haptoglobin levels in sheep, goats, and cattle (Travis, 1977). In cats, recurrent intravascular hemolysis (as in autoimmune hemolytic anemia and haemobartonellosis) was associated with a reduction in serum haptoglobin level, which became normal within 2 days, whereas an increase occurred from splenectomy, abscess formation, feline infectious peritonitis, and upper respiratory infections (Harvey and Gaskin, 1978).

Ceruloplasmin

Ceruloplasmin is a glycoprotein synthesized by the liver. It has a molecular weight of 124,000–134,000 and plasma half-life of 5–7 days. It carries over 90% of plasma copper and donates it to the liver and other tissues. It plays an important role in copper homeostasis and in mobilizing iron (see p. 664). As an acute phase protein, its synthesis is increased in acute inflammatory conditions and bacterial, viral, and parasitic infections. Elevated levels have also been found in some other conditions including leukemia, solid tumors, and biliary cirrhosis (Swain et al., 1980). Decreased ceruloplasmin levels may be found during malnutrition, malabsorption, nephrosis, and Wilson's disease (liver disease associated with copper toxicosis).

C-Reactive Protein

C-reactive protein is one of the well-characterized human serum proteins found to increase during inflammatory conditions. The name signifies its pure polypeptide nature and the property of nonimmunologic precipitation with the somatic C-polysaccharide of pneumococci in the presence of Ca^{++}. The C-reactive protein (molecular weight, about 21,000) consists of five identical subunits, each consisting of 187 amino acids and held together by noncovalent bonds. The serum concentration of C-reactive protein increases quickly and up to several-hundred-fold during bacterial infections, inflammatory conditions, and other pathologic conditions. Thus determination of serum levels of C-reactive protein has some diagnostic importance. Normal dogs contain 5 mg/L of C-reactive protein in serum, and the level increases as early as 4 hours after a major surgery (Caspi et al., 1984).

In recent years, it has been shown that C-reactive protein may have some functional significance in the regulation of inflammatory process and microbial defense through a variety of its properties such as activation of complement by the classical pathway, promoting phagocytosis, inhibition of platelet aggregation and release of mediators, interaction with certain subpopulations of T-lymphocytes, and some other physiochemical interactions (Schwick and Haupt, 1981).

α-Fetoprotein

Human α-fetoprotein (AFP) is a single-chain glycoprotein with a molecular weight of about 60,000–70,000. It is one of the most prominent plasma proteins found in the early fetal life of humans, reaching peak levels about the middle trimester. Then its concentration declines considerably by birth so that it is present only in trace amounts during neonatal life. It is synthesized by various tissues including the yolk sac, liver, gastrointestinal tract, and placenta (Schwick and Haupt, 1981). Based on its structural, immunologic, and certain functional similarities to albumin, it has been suggested that α-fetoprotein during fetal life may serve functions similar to those of serum albumin in adult life. In adult life, its concentration has been found to increase remarkably in primary carcinoma of the liver. A slight but transient increase may also occur during metastatic malignancies of the liver and inflammatory liver and gastrointestinal diseases. AFP of fetal origin is also found in the serum of healthy pregnant women, the highest level being detected during the middle trimester, and increased levels are found in certain pathologic pregnancies (Lai et al., 1978a).

α-Fetoprotein is present in fetal plasmas of various animal species including the cow (Abe et al., 1976; Baetz et al., 1981; Lai et al., 1978b; Smith et al., 1979), horse (Lock et al., 1978), sheep (Lai, et al., 1978a), and pig (Carlsson et al., 1976; Fujimoto et al., 1984; Stone and Christenson, 1982). Two molecular variants of AFP are found in cattle. One of these, the α_1-fetoprotein, has a molecular weight of 68,000 and amino acid composition similar to other mammalian α_1-fetoprotein and is immunochemically related to human α_1-fetoprotein. The equine AFP has a molecular weight of 70,000–75,000 and migrates in the α_2-region. It cross-reacts with bovine and porcine AFP. AFP concentration in equine fetal plasma was highest at mid-gestation, declined markedly by birth, and was undetectable after 24 days of life. The porcine AFP has a molecular weight of 75,000–80,000. In the sheep, cow, and pig, fetal AFP is highest during early gestation and then declines rapidly before birth irrespective of fetal weight or maturity. Determination of AFP levels in bovine fetal plasma was not found diagnostic for fetal disease or death. Serum AFP levels in pregnant ewes were lower than in pregnant women.

Lipoproteins

The plasma lipids—glycerides, cholesterol and its esters, and phospholipids—are insoluble in water. In blood they are transported combined with specific proteins (apolipoproteins) as micellar or macromolecular lipoproteins (LPs). It is generally accepted that LPs are spherical particles having a lipoprotein membrane consisting of phospholipids, "free" cholesterol, and protein (apolipoprotein) and a "nucleus" made of triglycerides and esterified cholesterol. The LPs can be separated into several classes based on their density, which is mainly due to lipid content, or electrophoretic mobility, which is a function of their structural protein. Four major classes of LPs are recognized: high-density LPs, low-density LPs, very low density LPs, and chylomicra. Electrophoretically, the first three migrate, respectively, as α-LP, β-LP, and pre-β-LP, whereas chylomicra do not migrate and remain at the origin. The electrophoretic mobilities of α-, β-, and pre-β-LPs are determined by the three predominant apoproteins, apoA, apoB, and apoC, respectively. The high-density LPs are composed primarily of cholesterol, the low-density LPs mainly of cholesterol and some triglycerides, the very low density LPs mostly of triglycerides and some cholesterol, and chylomicra principally of triglycerides.

Lipoproteins are synthesized in the liver and/or intestine. Quantitation of various classes of LPs in human medicine has claimed the attention of several workers, who have shown an association between disease states and changes in the lipoprotein profile. Acquired and genetic abnormalities of LPs have been described (Blombäck and Hanson, 1979). In normal animals (horses, sheep, pigs, dogs), the α-LPs are in higher concentration than the β-LPs (Campbell, 1963). Species and individual variations in LP profiles have been observed (Bartley, 1980). Changes in lipoprotein and lipid profiles have been reported for developing pigs (Johansson and Karlsson, 1982).

IMMUNOGLOBULINS

Basic Structure

Immunoglobulins are glycoproteins comprised of 82–96% protein and 4–18% carbohydrate. The biologic properties of the Ig molecules are ascribed primarily to their polypeptide structure. An Ig molecule is basically bilaterally symmetrical and appears to be a Y-shaped structure on electron microscopy. It is comprised of four polypeptide chains held together by covalent and disulfide bonds. Two of the chains are long, each having a molecular weight of 50,000 and being comprised of 446 amino acid residues in identical sequence (Edelman, 1973); these are called "heavy" chains. In comparison, the other two chains are small, each having a molecular weight of 25,000 and an identical sequence of 214 amino acid residues (Edelman, 1973); these are called "light" chains. The entire Ig monomer is a 7S molecule with a molecular weight of 180,000.

Based on relative variability of heterogeneity of amino acid sequences, each light chain has a "variable region," comprised of about half a chain length toward the amino terminal end, and a "constant region" of equal length toward the carboxyl end. Similarly, each heavy chain is comprised of one constant region and three variable regions of approximately equal lengths. Within the variable regions, certain portions have exceedingly variable amino acid sequences; these are called "hypervariable regions." These various regions contribute to the structural and functional heterogeneity of the Ig molecules. The hypervariable regions of the light and heavy chains, at the amino terminal ends, together carry the antigen-binding sites. Thus antigenic specificity of an Ig molecule is determined by innumerable amino acid sequences in the hypervariable region. Secondary functions of the Ig molecule, such as complement fixation, are the property of the terminal constant region of the heavy chains. The hinge region has high protein content and facilitates extension of the antigen-binding portions of the Ig molecule.

Papain, a proteolytic enzyme, splits the Ig molecule in such a manner that two Fab (antigen-binding) fragments and one Fc (crystallizable) fragment are obtained. In contrast, pepsin treatment splits the molecule at a slightly higher location resulting in two Fab fragments held together, the F(ab)'$_2$ fragment, and breaks down the Fc region into small peptides.

Five major classes of Igs have been identified in human serum. A similar existence is generally anticipated for various animal species (Tables 34–3 and 34–4). These Igs have been defined by antigenic differences in the constant region of the heavy chains. The specific heavy chains are designated as gamma (γ), mu (μ), alpha (α), delta (δ), and epsilon (ε), respectively, for IgG, IgM, IgA, IgD, and IgE molecules. The light chains are divided into two classes, namely, kappa (κ) and lambda (λ). An Ig molecule contains only a single type of light chain, never both. Both types are found in the same individual, but their ratio may vary from species to species, e.g., 2:1 in humans. Antigenic determinants (differences) of the heavy and light chains are

Table 34–3. Classes and Subclasses of Immunoglobulins in Domestic Animals and Humans

Species	IgG	IgA	IgM	IgE	IgD
Horses[a]	Ga, Gb, Gc, G(B), G(T)a, G(T)b	A	M	E[b]	?
Cattle	G1, G2, G3[c]	A	M	E	?
Buffaloes	G1, G2, G3[d]	A1, A2	M	?	?
Sheep	G1, G1a, G2, G3[c]	A1, A2	M	E	?
Goats	G1, G2, G3[c]				
Pigs[e]	G1, G2, G3, G4	A1, A2	M	E	?
Dogs	G1, G2a, G2b, G2c	A	M	E	?
Cats	G1, G2	A	M	E	?
Chickens	G1, (G2, G3)?	A	M	?	D
Humans	G1, G2, G3, G4	A1, A2	M	E	D

Modified from Tizard, 1982.
[a]A gamma 10S molecule and two immunoglobulins of fast mobility have been reported.
[b]Suter and Fey, 1981, 1983.
[c]Babel and Lang, 1976.
[d]Kulkarni et al., 1973.
[e]A gamma 18S molecule and a 4S "half" Ig molecule have also been reported.

responsible for the *isotypes* of Igs found in all animals of the same species. Similarly, antigenic determinants of the constant region of the polypeptide chains form the basis of *allotypes* of Igs found in some individuals of the same species, while antigenic determinants of the variable regions (antigen-combining sites) form the basis of Ig *idiotypes* found in an individual animal.

Classes of Immunoglobulins

The various classes of Igs are characterized according to physiochemical, electrophoretic, immunochemical, and functional properties.

IgG

IgG is the major Ig of blood serum in the adult of various species and is the component responsible for most of the humoral immunity of the organism. The IgG is a 7S molecule with a molecular weight of 180,000, electrophoretic mobility in the γ region, and biologic half-life of approximately 20 days. Being a smaller molecule, IgG readily permeates blood vessels and can be found in various body fluids in minute quantities in health and in larger amounts during inflammatory conditions. It is the only Ig that can cross placenta and is found in fetal serum of certain animal species (dogs, cats, and rodents) and humans. It is the primary Ig in the colostrum and is responsible for natural passive immunity in the neonatal calf, foal, lamb, kid, and piglet.

The IgG molecules have several biologic activities including opsonization, agglutination, precipitation, and complement fixation. They contain the majority of antibacterial, antiviral, and antitoxic antibodies. Neutrophils and macrophages have receptors to bind the Fc region of the IgG molecule. Effective complement fixation requires the binding of IgG molecules to specific antigens in close proximity

Table 34–4. Serum Immunoglobulin Levels (mg/dl) in Domestic Animals and Humans[a]

Species	IgG	IgM	IgA	IgG(T)	IgG(B)	IgE
Horse	1,000–1,500	100–200	60–350	100–1,500	10–1,000	—
Bovine[b]	1,700–2,700	250–400	10–50	—	—	<50[c]
Buffaloes[d]	2,331	253	—	—	—	—
Sheep	1,700–2,000	150–250	10–50	—	—	—
Pigs	1,700–2,900	100–500	50–500	—	—	—
Dogs	1,000–2,000	70–270	20–150	—	—	2.3–42
Chickens	300–700	120–250	30–60	—	—	—
Humans	800–1,600	50–200	150–400	—	—	0.002–0.05

[a]All data, except bovine IgE, and buffalo Igs, from Tizard, 1982.
[b]Cattle show very significant seasonal differences in serum Ig levels.
[c]6-months old, parasite-free calves, <50 U/ml; adult dairy cattle, <40 U/ml (Gershwin and Dygert, 1983).
[d]Mean values from Mulbagal, 1983.

so as to form dimers, and it has become apparent that certain subclasses of IgG either do not fix complement or are less efficient in this regard. Various subclasses of IgG have been recognized on the basis of serologic and physiochemical differences in the constant region of the light chain, and they also differ in biologic activities.

IgM

IgM is a 19S molecule with a molecular weight of 900,000, electrophoretic mobility in the β to fast-γ regions, and biologic half-life of about 5 days. It typically exists as a pentamer composed of five 7S subunits similar to IgG. The heavy chain ends of the subunits are interconnected by disulfide bonds, and a glycopeptide J chain unites two of the subunits to complete a circular structure. The J chains are synthesized by the plasma cells, have a molecular weight of 15,000, and are unusually rich in aspartic acid and glutamic acid. An intact IgM molecule is elaborated by the plasma cells. It is found in fetal and precolostral foal serum.

IgM is the second major Ig of the serum, and remains confined primarily to the vascular system because of its molecular size. It is typically the first Ig to increase in concentration in serum during the primary immune response. It also increases during the secondary immune response, but is usually exceeded by the IgG synthesized during this phase of the immune response.

Various biologic activities of the IgM are similar to those of the IgG. As a pentamer, though, it has 10 binding sites and is functionally much more efficient, e.g., one molecule of IgM can fix complement. It should be mentioned, however, that in humans some non-complement-fixing IgM has been found under certain conditions. An IgM molecule is reduced by 2-mercaptoethanol so that it no longer reacts in agglutination and complement fixation tests, but is still able to bind antigen.

IgM molecules contain "natural" antibodies for Gram-negative bacteria, blood-group isoantibodies, rheumatoid factors, and antinuclear and other antibodies. They are of minor importance in toxin neutralization. IgM monomers (7S) have been found on antigen-responsive B- and T-lymphocytes, where they are thought to regulate the immune response. Secretory IgM with bound secretory component has been found in body secretions (Thompson and Reynolds, 1977). It may play a compensatory role in disorders associated with IgA deficiency because increased synthesis of secretory IgM was found to occur in such conditions.

IgA

IgA is a carbohydrate-rich Ig forming a minor component of the blood serum, but a major component of various external secretions (tears, saliva, and respiratory and gastrointestinal secretions) in most species. It exhibits electrophoretic mobility in the β to fast-γ regions and has a biologic half-life of 6 days. The IgA monomer is a 7S molecule with a molecular weight of 160,000, but it tends to polymerize forming 11S dimers, 13S trimers, and higher polymers. The dimeric form, interconnected by a J chain, predominates in serums of most animal species in contrast to the monomeric form, which constitutes about 90% of the human serum IgA.

The secretory IgA is an 11S molecule composed of two monomers, a J chain, and a secretory component and has a molecular weight of 400,000. The secretory component (MW 70,000) is synthesized by intestinal epithelial cells near the mucous membrane and also by the hepatocytes. It enables the IgA molecules elaborated locally in the intestinal lymphoid tissue to be transported across the mucosa into the gut. It also makes the IgA molecule resistant to proteolysis by digestive enzymes. The hepatic secretory component allows secretion of serum IgA into the bile. The secretory component is not essential for transport of IgA into the circulation. The secretory component may be found free and also bound to IgM, but not to IgG and IgE, in body secretions.

IgA plays an important role in local defense by protecting various body surfaces, e.g., the intestinal, respiratory and urogenital tracts, the mammary gland, and the eye, from bacterial and viral invasion. It prevents bacterial adherence by binding to glycoproteins essential for colonization. The IgA has virus neutralization and agglutinating activities, can fix complement, but only by the alternate pathway, has no or limited opsonic activity, and is not bactericidal (Knop and Rowley, 1974; Tizard, 1982). Specific IgA antibodies present in colostrum provide passive immunity to the newborn against neonatal bacterial and viral infections (Inoue, 1981a).

IgD

IgD is a 7–8S molecule with a molecular weight of 180,000, electrophoretic mobility in the fast γ region, and biologic half-life of 2–8 days. It is found in trace amounts in human serum and on about 15% of human B-lymphocytes. It has been found in chickens but not so far in other species. Its function is unknown, although it has been shown to have some antibody activity and is thought to be involved in differentiation of B-lymphocytes.

IgE

IgE is an 8S molecule with a molecular weight of 190,000, an electrophoretic mobility into the fast γ region, and biologic half-life of 1–5 days. IgE occurs in extremely low concentration in serum, and so it has been difficult to demonstrate. However, its concentration in nasopharyngeal secretions is higher than in the serum. Increasing amounts of IgE are produced in response to many parasitic infestations and allergens (antigens stimulating the production of IgE). Most cattle infested with gastrointestinal nematodes and cestodes have total serum IgE levels higher than those of normal controls (Gershwin and Dygert, 1983). An interesting observation has been that helminth parasites induce a substantial increase in IgE production, but only a portion of it is specific to parasitic antigens, while the rest is directed to non-parasitic antigens (Urban, 1982).

IgE mediates the type I hypersensitivity reaction (allergies and anaphylaxis) and is referred to as a reagin or reaginic antibody. It is a non-complement-fixing antibody, but its Fc region uniquely binds to the mast cells and basophils (i.e., it is homocytotropic) and triggers an immediate degranulation of these cells after combining with specific antigens. The IgE is also unique in that it is destroyed when serum is heated at 56°C for 30 minutes.

β₂-Microglobulin

β₂-Microglobulin is a polypeptide (MW 118,000) found free in serum and body fluids such as milk, colostrum, and urine and bound to the surface membrane of many cells of several species (see review by Groves and Greenberg, 1982). Thus β₂-microglobulin is related to both immune and histocompatibility antigen systems. In part, it structurally resembles IgG. Thus it can fix complement and bind to Fc receptors on cells of the mononuclear phagocyte system. The amount of β₂-microglobulin in body fluids is several times greater than in normal serum, and its level may increase in disease.

Species Differences

All animal species contain species-specific IgG, IgM, and IgA, whereas IgE has so far been identified in some animal species and IgD in the chicken only. Species differences (Table 34–3) have been found in the number and types of subclasses of various Igs (Barlough et al., 1981; Butler, 1983; Roberts, 1975; Wells et al., 1981). In general, immunoglobulin levels in serum (Table 34–4) and body fluids vary with the species and age (Barta, 1981). Newborn animals differ from adults in that they are hypogammaglobulinemic.

Species differences have also been noted with regard to biologic activities and body distribution of some of the Igs. For example, equine IgG(T) has a higher carbohydrate content, does not fix complement, and is found in body secretions in high concentration. Its half-life in the body is about 20 days in the newborn foal, which is very similar to that of IgG (Macdougall and Dunlop, 1974). Bovine IgG₁ constitutes about half of the serum IgG and is the major secretory Ig in the milk. It migrates faster than IgG₂ toward the anode in agar gel electrophoresis. Biologic activities of bovine IgG₁ and IgG₂ are essentially similar, but the former does not promote phagocytosis by monocytes and neutrophils (McGuire and Musoke, 1981) and the latter does not fix complement. Cattle have been found to have hereditarily high or low serum levels of IgG₂. Breed differences have been reported in Ig levels of newborn lambs (Halliday, 1976) and horses (McGuire and Poppie, 1973).

Various immunoglobulins are found in body secretions and in the intestine in different concentrations. They may originate locally or are serum-derived. In pigs from birth to 10 weeks of age IgG was the major Ig in nasal secretions, although a transient increase in IgA occurred during the first week of life (Morgan and Bourne, 1981). Species differences occur in the ratio of IgG and IgA in bronchioalveolar secretions compared to secretions of the upper respiratory tract, which contain relatively more IgA (Wilkie and Markham, 1981).

Because of selective transfer of Igs from the circulation into the mammary glands, colostrum of all the major domestic animals is rich in IgG, which comprises 60–90% of the total Ig level. Colostrum also contains higher amounts of other Igs. In comparison, milk predominantly contains IgG (specifically IgG_1) in ruminants and IgA in humans, primates, and some nonruminant domestic animals. In cats, IgG predominates in the serum, colostrum, and milk, and IgA forms a major component in other body secretions (Yamada et al., 1984).

For additional information on Igs of domestic animals see the immunology texts by Outteridge (1985) and Tizard (1982) and specific reports and reviews (Allen and Dalton, 1975; Babel and Lang, 1976; Barlough et al., 1981; Bonk et al., 1982; Butler, 1983; Changiago et al., 1978; Crips et al., 1985; Gershwin and Dygert, 1983; McGuire and Musoke, 1981; Mulbagal, 1983; Mulbagal and Keshavmurthy, 1983; Roberts, 1975; Schultz, 1978; Setcavage and Kim, 1976; Suter and Fey, 1981, 1983; Wells et al., 1981).

METHODOLOGY

Plasma or serum protein concentrations can be determined by a variety of methods. Total protein concentration can be determined by the Kjeldahl, biuret, Lowery, or refractometric methods. The Kjeldahl method is a reference method for analytical protein chemistry, but is not practical in a clinical diagnostic laboratory. Levels of individual proteins can be determined by electrophoretic and immunochemical methods. Specific techniques are also available to determine concentrations of certain individual plasma or serum proteins, e.g., albumin, various immunoglobulins, transferrin, ceruloplasmin, and haptoglobin.

Total Protein Concentrations

Several adequate methods are available to the veterinarian for determining total serum or plasma protein concentrations. If a spectrophotometer is available, the biuret or the Lowery method (Lowery et al., 1951) is quite satisfactory. The reagents needed for the biuret method are inexpensive and readily available. This method requires a larger volume of serum or plasma (1 ml minimum) than the Lowery method (0.2 ml) and is relatively less sensitive (minimum detectable protein concentration is about 25 mg/dl). The principal reagent for the Lowery method (Folin and Ciocalteu phenol reagent) is commercially available. This method is specially suited for extremely low concentration (0.1 mg/dl) of protein, as in the cerebrospinal fluid. The refractometric method is perhaps the most practical, since only a drop of sample is required, and a determination can be made in seconds (see Chapter 2). Although it is the least sensitive method, measuring 100 mg/dl of proteins or over, it provides satisfactory values for routine diagnostic work.

Several colorimetric systems are now available at a reasonable cost for doing simple blood chemistries (Green et al., 1982; Kaneko, 1980). With these systems, albumin is generally determined by a dye-binding method, and total protein by the biuret test or a modification of it. Globulin content is determined by subtracting albumin concentration from serum protein value, and the A/G ratio is calculated. A rough estimate of the globulin content of serum can be obtained by salt precipitation. Depending on the animal species, a certain amount of sodium-, ammonium-, or zinc-sulfate is added to serum. This precipitates globulins, but not albumin. The amount of globulins then can be estimated colorimetrically from a suitable standard. This procedure has been refined to detect immunoglobulins in serums of newborn calves, foals, and lambs. A glutaraldehyde coagulation test has been used to detect hypoproteinemia in neonates (Larsson, 1985; O'Rourke and Satterfield, 1981; Tennant et al., 1979).

The Electrophoretic Techniques

At an alkaline pH (usually pH 8.6), the serum proteins have a net negative charge; hence they migrate from cathode to anode in an electrical field. Because the charge density of individual proteins varies, they can be separated from each other by the technique of electrophoresis.

The most common method in use in clinical medicine is zone electrophoresis, wherein the serum is placed on a supporting medium such as filter paper or, more commonly, cellulose acetate, and less commonly agarose, starch, or polyacrylamide gels. Results obtained by various electrophoretic techniques may differ significantly with regard to proportions of various protein fractions resolved, making it difficult to compare data obtained by different techniques.

Cellulose acetate electrophoresis, being simple and accurate, is currently in vogue, but agarose electrophoresis is claimed to provide better resolution and yield more fractions (Keay, 1982; Kristensen and Barsanti, 1977). After electrophoretic separation, the proteins on cellulose acetate membranes are stained by any number of specific protein stains. One can also stain selectively for glycoproteins and lipoproteins. After rinsing and destaining, the proteins appear as bands (zones) representative of albumin and the various globulins (Fig. 34–4). It must be kept in mind that with the exception of albumin, the bands are made up of a group of individual proteins (see Table 34–1). The proteins are quantitated by a recording and integrating spectrophotometer. Albumin, being strongly electronegative, migrates farthest toward the anode, whereas globulins, being variably weakly negative, move in succession as α-, β-, and γ-globulins. The value for each component is calculated as a percentage of the total and is converted to an absolute amount after determination of the total serum protein concentration by a standard method.

Although there is a certain degree of arbitrariness in assigning zones to the various globulin classes, a common practice at the Veterinary Medical Teaching Hospital, University of California, Davis, is to determine the mid-point of the electrophoretogram from

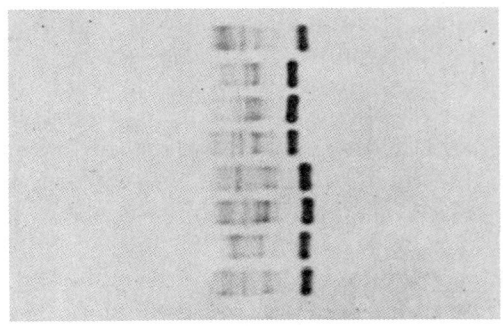

Fig. 34–4. Cellulose acetate strip on which eight serums have been applied, separated by electrophoresis, and stained for protein. These particular serums are from animals from the Los Angeles zoo. Migration is from left to right. Top to bottom: African lion, white-handed gibbon, another white-handed gibbon, gorilla, cheetah, jaguar, leopard, and domestic cat. Note the faster migration of the albumin band (dark band on the extreme right) of the Felidae. Note also the heterogeneity with regard to concentration and relative mobility of the various globulins. (From Carroll et al., 1967; courtesy of the *American Journal of Veterinary Clinical Pathology.*)

the anodal base of the albumin to the cathodal base of the slow γ-globulin; the mid-point lies between the α$_2$ and β$_1$ regions or in that vicinity (Kaneko, 1980).

There are many variables inherent in the method. It is almost mandatory that for comparative evaluation each worker or laboratory establish their own set of normals for each species, using the same technique. Accurate quantitation of the protein patterns is perhaps not an absolute necessity. After a certain degree of expertise has been acquired, major changes in the patterns will be readily recognized. Commercial laboratories are usually equipped to do electrophoresis. However, the veterinarian should do his or her own interpretations in view of the variability among species (Fig. 34–5, *A–D*).

The mobility of the various globulins and of albumin varies from species to species. This variation can be seen rather dramatically in zoo animals (Fig. 34–4). Depending on the animal species and technical considerations, various globulin fractions on cellulose acetate electrophoresis resolve into one or two distinct zones. Among common domestic animals, canine serums usually show two α-, one or two β-, and two γ-globulins (Fig. 34–5C). Equine serums characteristically are resolved into two α-, two β-, and one γ-globulin (Fig. 34–5D). Bovine serums generally resolve into single α-, β-, and γ-globulin zones (Fig. 34–5A), although resolution of the γ-zone into γ-₁ and γ₂ is not uncommon. Feline (Fig. 34–5B), ovine, and caprine serums may resolve into one or two α and β regions and one γ zone. Electrophoresis of plasma or hemolyzed serum may yield somewhat different distribution. For example, plasma shows a prominent γ₁ peak due to migration of fibrinogen in that region, and hemolyzed serum or plasma exhibits slurring or prominence of the β-globulin peaks due to the presence of free hemoglobin and increases in α₂ region due to formation of haptoglobin-hemoglobin complexes (Amog et al., 1977).

Immunochemical methods are highly specific and sensitive, but require highly monospecific reagents (antibodies) to each of the proteins to be detected for the species concerned (see review by Barta, 1981). Immunoelectrophoresis, which involves gel electrophoresis followed by immunodiffusion, is a simple procedure to demonstrate the presence of various plasma proteins, particularly immunoglobulins, but it is not quantitative. The single radial immunodiffusion technique (Mancini's method) is simple and sensitive for quantitation of various proteins, particularly immunoglobulins, and results are available within 24–72 hours. Rocket immunoelectrophoresis (electroimmunodiffusion) is another simple and rapid quantitative procedure. It is as accurate or better than the radial immunodiffusion method. Radioimmunoassay and enzyme-linked immunosorbent assay (ELISA) are very sensitive procedures for detection of minute quantities of various proteins.

DYSPROTEINEMIAS

The term *dysproteinemia* literally means a derangement of the protein content of the blood. It includes an abnormality of the total protein content as well as that of individual proteins. An appreciation of the derangement requires determination of total plasma or serum protein concentration, plasma fibrinogen level, serum protein electrophoresis, and A/G ratio.

Hypoproteinemia is a reduction in serum or plasma protein concentration below the min-

imum normal level for the species. The converse is *hyperproteinemia.* Hypoproteinemia may entail diminution of serum levels of albumin or globulins or both. Hyperproteinemia, by comparison, usually involves increases in globulin levels. The relative concentration of individual proteins may change without an alteration in the total amount (normoproteinemia). This condition can have its origin in several mechanisms, including metabolic, physiologic, and pathologic. The most obvious is noted from a study of A/G ratios. It can be taken as a rule of thumb that when globulins rise, there will be a concomitant drop in albumin concentration. An absolute rise in albumin is rarely, if ever, seen. The exact mechanism whereby this change in relative concentrations of proteins occurs has not been satisfactorily explained, although the seat of control may be in the liver. In vitro studies with liver homogenates and ¹⁴C-labeled amino acids and albumin have shown that albumin can serve as a substrate for globulin production (Roberts and Kelley, 1956) but probably only at the amino acid level (Campbell and Stone, 1957). Because there is an absolute need for the maintenance of colloidal osmotic pressure, the regulating mechanism may be related to this need.

Before it can be determined whether a given animal is hyperproteinemic or hypoproteinemic, several factors must be considered. Of particular importance is the *age* of the animal. Total protein concentrations are low in the newborn of most species, commonly being less than 5 g/dl of plasma. Colostrum consumption causes a temporary elevation (Figs. 34–2 and 34–3). Thereafter, the total plasma proteins increase gradually with age to a normal range of 6.0–7.5 g/dl. In lactating cows, levels of 8.0–8.5 g/dl are not uncommon, especially in the summer.

A dog 8 to 10 years old would normally be expected to have total proteins between 7.0–8.0 g/dl, whereas dogs under 6 months of age would be expected to have levels of 6.0–6.5 g/dl. On this basis, a dog 8–10 years of age with total plasma proteins of 6.5 g/dl or less should be classed as hypoproteinemic.

The *state of hydration* of an animal is also an important consideration. It is imperative that

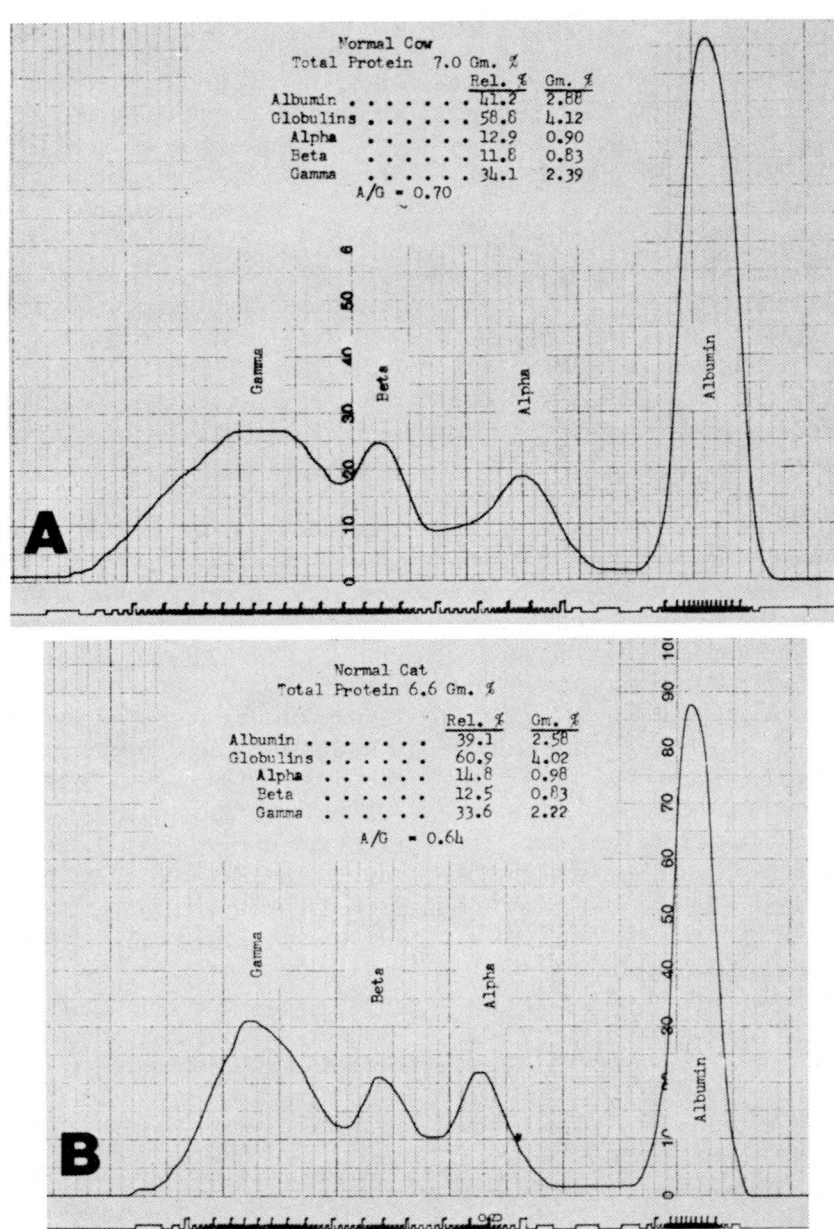

Fig. 34–5. Representative electrophoretograms of serums from normal animals: A, cow; B, cat; C, dog; D, horse.

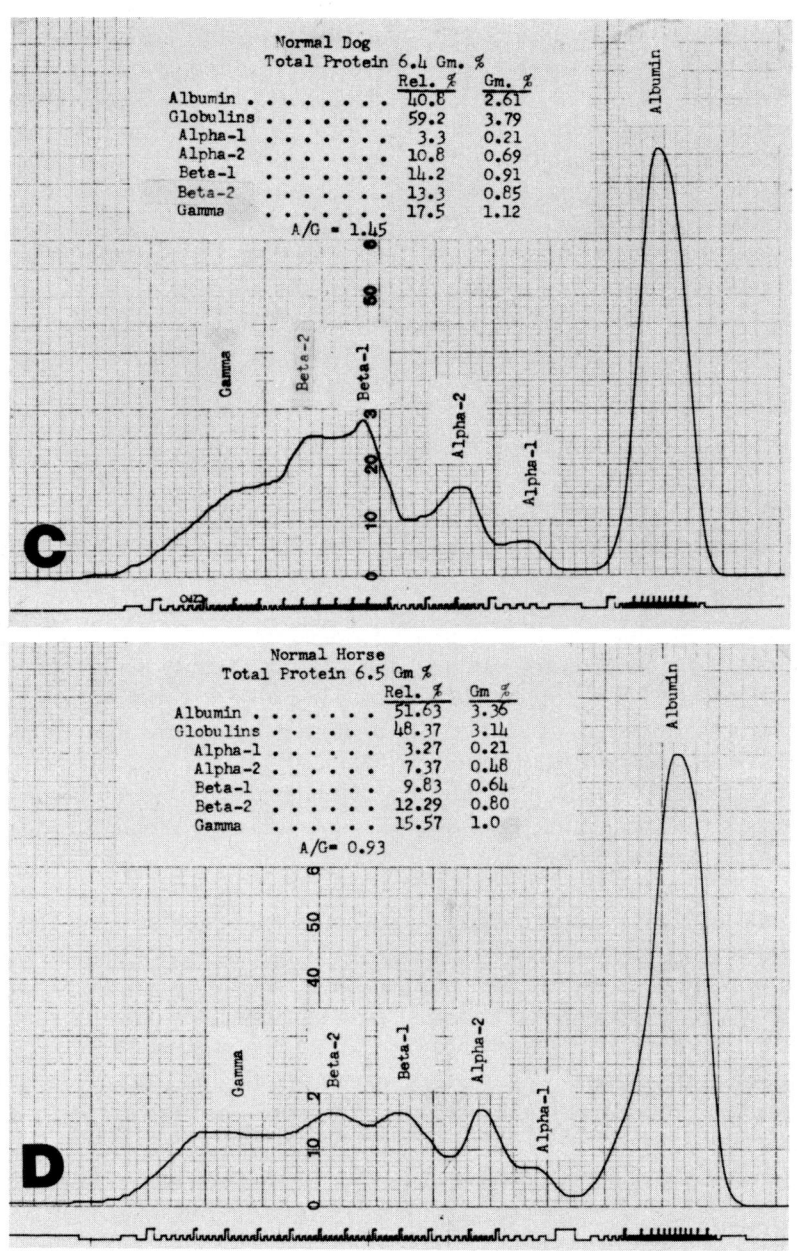

Fig. 34–5.   *Continued.*

the plasma protein concentration be considered along with the hematocrit. If there is a hyperproteinemia with a normal A/G ratio and a significantly elevated PCV, the high protein concentration is most likely a consequence of dehydration. When the PCV is significantly elevated and plasma proteins remain within the normal range, splenic contraction is strongly indicated (Schalm, 1970a). In contrast, hypoproteinemia with normal A/G ratio and a significantly diminished PCV is a consequence of either blood loss or fluid therapy. Hypoproteinemia from fluid loss only could have normal to elevated PCV values depending on the degree of fluid loss.

Changes in Albumin Concentrations

Albumin constitutes about 35–50% of total serum proteins in various animals in contrast to 60–67% in humans and nonhuman primates (Kaneko, 1980). *Hypoalbuminemia* is more common than hyperalbuminemia. Hypoalbuminemia may be a result of decreased synthesis, increased loss, increased catabolism, or pathologic body distribution. Albumin synthesis is diminished in cirrhosis, malnutrition, and reduced intestinal absorption. Increased body loss of albumin is common through the gut and kidneys, and a significant amount can be lost through the skin, as in burn patients. Increased catabolism may be a result of hormonal disturbances such as Cushing's disease and hyperthyroidism, trauma, and infection. Abnormal body distribution of albumin may occur because of changes in capillary permeability or colloidal osmotic pressure as in patients with extensive burns, cardiac disease, or ascites.

Hyperalbuminemia is usually a result of hemoconcentration because a true increase in serum albumin concentration does not occur.

Changes in Fibrinogen Levels

Plasma fibrinogen levels are not affected by age, sex, exercise, repeated bleeding, or hemorrhage, but they can be altered by only moderate inflammatory states. Plasma fibrinogen commonly increases in inflammatory, suppurative, traumatic, and neoplastic diseases. Increased synthesis is probably involved in such cases. Fibrinogen is elevated in moderate liver damage, whereas severe liver damage causes a decrease. In disseminated intravascular coagulation (DIC) and fibrinolysis, fibrinogen levels decline due to increased consumption and catabolism (see Chapter 14; Appendix Case 26). Congenital afibrinogenemia and hypofibrinogenemia are rare conditions described in humans. Functionally defective fibrinogen (dysfibrinogenemia) as a hereditary defect has also been described in humans, but not in animals.

The plasma protein:fibrinogen ratio (PP:F) is useful in interpretation of disease in the presence of dehydration. This concept is based on the fact that hemoconcentration also produces a relative elevation of fibrinogen. The ratio is obtained by subtracting the fibrinogen from the total plasma protein concentration and then dividing the remainder by the amount of fibrinogen. Some normal values for fibrinogen and the PP:F ratios are given in Table 34–5. A PP:F ratio of less than 15:1 indicates a relative increase in fibrinogen over plasma protein. A ratio below 10:1 indicates a marked increase in fibrinogen. The ratio rises steadily with age because of increasing levels of plasma proteins, while fibrinogen concentrations remain relatively constant.

Results in representative diseases in dogs are presented in Table 34–6. Massive liver involvement (Dogs 1 and 2) brought about reduced fibrinogen levels. In addition to these selected examples in Table 34–6, in 16 dogs with lymphoma, the plasma proteins varied from 5.5–7.7 g/dl (ave. 6.7), and fibrinogen ranged from 0.05–0.6 g/dl (ave. 0.30); in 15 dogs with distemper, the plasma proteins ranged from 4.5–8.3 g/dl (ave. 6.5), and fibrinogen concentrations varied from 0.20–0.80 g/dl (ave. 0.45). Nine of the latter values were within the normal range. Eighteen dogs with kidney problems and elevated blood urea nitrogen had plasma protein concentrations of 6.5–10.9 g/dl (ave. 8.2), and fibrinogen ranged from 0.20–1.30 g/dl (ave. 0.75). The PP:F ratio ranged from 4.7–31.0 among the eighteen dogs, with an average of 11.4:1. In inflammatory and suppurative diseases, fibrinogen is elevated but not always in direct relationship to the severity of the disease. Malignancies in some instances have

Table 34–5. Total Protein and Fibrinogen Concentration in Blood Plasma of Normal Dogs, Calves, Cows, Foals, and Horses

Animal	Number	Age	Plasma Proteins (g/dl) Range	Mean	Fibrinogen (g/dl) Range	Mean	Protein:Fibrinogen Ratio Range	Mean
Dog	11	8 wk	5.0–6.5	5.7	0.1–0.3	0.2	19–50:1	27.5:1
	11	10–12 wk	5.5–6.5	6.2	0.2–0.4	0.23	15–31:1	29.8:1
	9	4–6 mo	6.3–7.0	6.7	0.1–0.3	0.22	20–68:1	30.5:1
	9	1–1½ yr	6.5–7.7	7.1	0.1–0.4	0.23	17–66:1	34.5:1
	9	2–3½ yr	6.9–7.8	7.5	0.1–0.3	0.2	25–74:1	36.4:1
Calf	16[a]	Newborn	4.0–5.3	4.7	0–0.4	0.19	10–52:1	19.0:1
	5	2–7 days	4.7–5.3	4.9	0.2–0.4	0.3	12–30:1	15.3:1
Cow	6[b]	Mature	6.8–8.0	7.3	0.2–0.6	0.4	10–37:1	18.2:1
Thoroughbred Foal	12	1 day	5.1–6.8	5.7	0.2–0.4	0.27	17–30:1	22.9:1
	12	1 wk	5.4–6.9	6.2	0.3–0.5	0.37	12–22:1	17.5:1
	10[c]	1 mo	5.5–7.0	6.9	0.3–0.5	0.43	10–20:1	13.9:1
	4[c]	2 mo	6.2–6.8	6.5	0.5	0.5	11–13:1	12.1:1
Horse								
Thoroughbred	7	1½–7 yr	6.8–7.8	7.2	0.2–0.4	0.27	18–34:1	26.7:1
Quarter horse	5	2–7 yr	6.6–7.1	6.8	0.2–0.3	0.22	21–34:1	31.8:1
Appaloosa	1	3 yr	7.2	—	0.2	—	35:1	—

Modified slightly from Schalm et al., 1970; courtesy of *The California Veterinarian*.
[a]Newborn calves were colostrum-deprived and mostly taken by caesarean section at term.
[b]37 separate determinations on the six cows.
[c]A number of the original 12 foals developed a mild respiratory disease with increases of fibrinogen to between 0.60 and 0.80 g/dl.

Table 34–6. Examples of Plasma Protein:Fibrinogen Ratios in Various Clinical Entities of the Dog

Dog No.	Age (yr)	Sex	Clinical Entity	PCV (%)	Icterus Index Units	WBC/μl	Plasma Proteins (g/dl)	Fibrinogen (g/dl)	PP:F Ratio
1	12	XF	Carcinoma of the pancreas and liver	36	15	22,400	6.0	0.05	119
2	7	F	Hepatic lipidosis and myocardial necrosis	34	10	29,500	5.3	0.1	52
3	3	M	Granulocytic leukemia and anemia	19	2	78,700	6.7	0.2	32
4	4	M	Lymphosarcoma	30	5	44,600	6.5	0.3	20
5	<1	M	Distemper	41	2	4,600	6.9	0.4	16
6	5	F	Pyometra	40	2	40,300	8.6	0.5	16
7	13	M	Mastocytoma and anemia	22	5	55,200	7.9	0.7	10
8	8	XF	Distemper and peritonitis	43	7.5	34,300	6.4	0.8	7
9	4	M	Chronic interstitial nephritis and uremia	36	2	11,800	9.5	0.9	10
10	12	M	Neoplastic abdominal mass	47	5	37,500	9.4	1.0	8
11	4	M	Gastric and pancreatic necrosis	50	5	55,200	9.9	1.1	8
12	7	M	Invasive squamous cell carcinoma of pharynx and facial bones	35	2	16,100	9.5	1.2	7

Modified slightly from Schalm, 1970b; courtesy of *The California Veterinarian*.

been associated with high fibrinogen levels in dogs. The reason for the commonly observed elevated plasma fibrinogen in chronic nephritis in the dog is not understood (Appendix Case 4).

Plasma fibrinogen levels observed in representative diseases of horses are given in Table 34–7. In a few cases of liver disease and in many cases of colic, fibrinogen levels were normal. Fractures and bacterial infections were associated with distinctly elevated fibrinogen levels.

Fibrinogen levels in representative diseases of cats are shown in Table 34–8. Of 729 fibrinogen determinations in cats, 16.6% were 0.50 g/dl or greater. (Table 34–9).

Because blood samples from cattle were usually submitted only in cases of severe disease, a rather selective list of conditions with elevated fibrinogen levels is given in Table 34–10 (see also Table 34–9).

Changes in α- and β-Globulins

A decrease in albumin and increase in α-globulin is noted in many instances. Being an acute phase protein, α-globulin is increased in acute inflammatory conditions such as acute hepatitis and acute glomerulonephritis and in nephrotic syndrome. In humans, this change is noted in pneumonia, scarlet fever, rheumatic fever, streptococcal infections, diabetes, tonsillitis, Hodgkin's disease, hyperthyroidism, thyroiditis, malaria, and certain carcinomas.

Experimentally, α-globulin was shown to increase in dogs deliberately injured with turpentine treatment, heat, cold, or fractures (Chanutin and Gjessing, 1946). The increase in α_2-globulin was attributed to an increase in the lipoprotein components (Gjessing et al., 1947). A selective, twofold elevation of α_2-globulin was observed in dogs given cortisone or cortisone and cholesterol (Bossak et al., 1955), and again it was suggested that this elevation may have been due to lipoprotein.

Altered α-globulin concentrations in cattle were observed when albumin and globulin levels were measured in cows producing different amounts of milk (Herz and Hod, 1969). It was found that increasing albumin levels usually resulted in a decrease in α-globulin values and an increase in the ratio between the two.

Elevated levels of α_2-globulins with normoproteinemia have been reported in cases of canine mastocytoma (Howard and Kenyon, 1965). The increased protein was shown to be a glycoprotein, and there was a direct correlation between the concentration of the glycoprotein and the extent of tumor development. Increases in serum α_2- and β-globulins have been reported in dogs with a va-

Table 34–7. Examples of Plasma Protein:Fibrinogen Ratios in Various Clinical Entities of the Horse

Horse No.	Age (yr)	Sex	Clinical Entity	PCV (%)	WBC/μl	N:L Ratio[a]	Plasma Proteins (g/dl)	Fibrinogen (g/dl)	PP:F Ratio
1	5	M	Massive liver necrosis	48	10,400	2.2	7.8	0.3	25
2	10	F	Colic	43	10,300	6.3	8.0	0.4	19
3	6	M	Pleuritis and anemia	19	6,400	3.5	8.7	0.5	16
4	23	F	Inguinal abscess	36	17,800	14.1	8.7	0.6	13
5	5	F	Abdominal abscess	32	27,700	11.0	9.8	0.7	13
6	3	M	Strangles.	32	24,200	4.7	6.3	0.8	7
7	1½	F	Abdominal abscesses and peritonitis	28	6,900	1.2	8.0	0.9	8
8	12	XM	Abdominal abscess	26	17,000	5.8	9.0	1.0	8
9	2	M	Fracture of metacarpus	37	17,900	10.4	6.7	1.0	6
10	3	M	Bacterial pleuritis	48	8,100[b]	3.1	9.9	1.1	8
11	3	F	Pseudomonas infection of guttural pouch	34	10,700	4.8	10.2	1.2	7
12	½	M	Salmonellosis	45	12,200[b]	2.2	8.4	1.9	4

Slightly modified from Schalm, 1970b; courtesy of *The California Veterinarian.*
[a]N:L ratio greater than 2 indicates increased numbers of neutrophils in relation to lymphocytes or a decreased number of lymphocytes without a similar change in neutrophil numbers.
[b]Toxic degenerative left shift.

Table 34–8.   Examples of Plasma Protein:Fibrinogen Ratios in Various Clinical Entities of the Cat

No.	Age (yr)	Sex	Clinical Entity	PCV (%)	WBC/μl	Plasma Proteins (g/dl)	Fibrinogen (g/dl)	PP:F Ratio
1	7	XM	Adenocarcinoma of jejunum	50	7,700	7.2	0.1	71.0
2	2	M	Infectious peritonitis	28	6,350	7.8	0.2	38.0
3	1	M	Infectious anemia	12	6,100	7.6	0.3	24.3
4	Mature	F	Panleukopenia	30	700	7.6	0.3	24.3
5	2½	M	Myeloproliferative disease	13	14,800	6.6	0.3	21.0
6	8	XF	Lymphosarcoma	27	21.900	8.8	0.4	21.0
7	10	M	Pyelonephritis	42	8,250	9.5	0.5	18.0
8	1	M	Infectious peritonitis	20	8,500	8.0	0.6	11.7
9	2	XF	Steatitis	33	68,600	5.3	0.7	6.6
10	2	M	Otitis interna	39	350	9.0	0.8	10.2
11	4	XM	Urethral obstruction	41	45,000	9.9	0.9	10.0
12	16	XF	Systemic infection, undetermined cause	30	46,000	8.0	1.1	6.3

Slightly modified from Schalm, 1970c; courtesy of *The California Veterinarian*.

Table 34–9.   Species Differences in Percentage Distribution of Plasma Fibrinogen Concentrations in Routine Blood Samples from Clinical Material

Species	Number of Plasma Samples	Fibrinogen (g/dl)						
		0–0.05	0.1	0.2–0.4	0.5	0.6–0.7	0.8–0.9	1.0–2.0
Cat	729	3.4	21.7	58.2	10.3	4.9	1.1	0.3
Dog	1,585	0.4	8.3	64.5	12.1	10.3	3.8	0.5
Horse	982	0.0	2.2	63.3	13.9	11.4	6.1	3.0
Cow	1,034	0.0	0.7	13.2	14.4	25.6	20.0	26.1

Slightly modified from Schalm 1970, courtesy of *California Veterinarian*.

Table 34–10.   Examples of Plasma Protein:Fibrinogen Ratios in Various Clinical Entities of the Cow

No.	Age (yr)	Sex	Clinical Entity	Verification	WBC/μl	Plasma Proteins (g/dl)	Fibrinogen (g/dl)	PP:F Ratio
1	2	M	Necrotic laryngitis	Clinical	9,300	8.9	1.0	7.9
2	4	F	Acute mastitis, 3rd day	Clinical	12,100	6.8	1.1	5.2
3	4	F	Pharyngeal abscess	Clinical	8,800	8.6	1.2	6.2
4	5	F	Traumatic reticulitis	Rumenotomy	19,900	8.9	1.2	6.4
5	Mature	F	Chronic gastroenteritis	Necropsy	7,800	6.9	1.3	4.3
6	2½	F	Pyelonephritis	Necropsy	7,400	8.5	1.3	5.5
7	3	F	Endocarditis	Necropsy	12,900	11.2	1.4	7.0
8	10	F	Fibrinous pneumonia	Clinical	4,100	9.0	1.5	5.0
9	5	F	Traumatic reticuloperitonitis	Rumenotomy	13,800	9.5	1.5	5.3
10	1	F	Necrotic glossitis	Clinical	29,900	11.3	1.6	6.1
11	1	XM	Necrotic rumenitis	Necropsy	4,600	8.8	1.8	3.9
12	2	F	Peritonitis	Rumenotomy	16,900	12.6	2.0	5.3

Slightly modified from Schalm, 1970c; courtesy of *The California Veterinarian*.

riety of neoplasms (Phillips et al., 1978). Dogs with lymphoma were reported to have increased levels of IgM (Madewell et al., 1980).

In leukemic cattle, there may be a moderate increase in α_2-globulin, and IgM production is often significantly impaired (Jacobs et al., 1980; Tranin et al., 1976), although an increase may be seen in some cases, particularly in cows with high numbers of lymphocytes (Pierce et al., 1977). Cows with lymphoma were found to have lower serum albumin and variable globulin levels without a particular pattern (see Liberg, 1977, for reference).

Because one of the α_2-globulins is haptoglobin, haptoglobulin is regularly absent in hemolytic disease, presumably because it is removed from the circulation at a rate exceeding its production.

Increases in β-globulins have been observed in active liver disease, suppurative dermatologic conditions, and occasionally in nephrotic syndrome. Polyclonal gammopathy may involve increases of IgM.

An increase in both β_2- and γ_1-globulins, leading to what has been termed "beta-gamma bridging," is considered almost pathognomonic for chronic active hepatitis and is occasionally seen in lymphoma (Kaneko, 1980). It results from an increase in IgA, IgM, or both.

Changes in γ-Globulins

Hypogammaglobulinemia is natural during fetal life and in newborns. Low levels of immunoglobulins are found in postcolostral serums and during the first few months of life. Animals with immune deficiency disorders are particularly hypogammaglobulinemic. Calves with total plasma protein concentration of <6.0 g/dl before weaning were found to have higher frequency of disease (Naylor et al., 1977). It was also reported that calves with low serum IgG (c. 1,267 mg/dl) had higher morbidity, requiring early and frequent treatments, than calves with high (c. 2,698 mg/dl) IgG levels (Davidson et al., 1981). Decreased γ-globulin levels in the adult animal may occur as a result of physiologic conditions (e.g., before parturition in the cow) or pathologic conditions (e.g., immunodeficiencies of various types; see p. 976).

Hypergammaglobulinemia is described

Table 34–11.   Various Plasma Cell Dyscrasias[a]

Primary monoclonal gammopathies
   Myeloma
   Waldenström's macroglobulinemia
   Solitary plasma cell tumor or plasmacytoma
   Heavy chain disease
   Light chain disease
   Lymphoma
   Chronic lymphocytic leukemia
Secondary monoclonal gammopathies
   Nonlymphoid malignancies
   Monocytic leukemias
   Hepatobiliary diseases
   Rheumatoid diseases
   Chronic inflammation
Benign monoclonal gammopathy
   Transient
   Persistent

[a]Modified from Stites et al., 1984.

under the heading Gammopathies, below. A simple test for hypergammaglobulinemia in cattle has been proposed (Sandholm, 1974). Mix 2.5 ml of a 1.2% glutaraldehyde solution with 1 mg/ml of Na_2EDTA and an equal quantity of fresh blood, directly from the vein. After 15 minutes at room temperature, the blood with hypergammaglobulinemia will coagulate, while normal blood will flow upon tilting of the tube. Formaldehyde may be substituted for glutaraldehyde, but use of the latter is preferred (Liberg et al., 1975).

The Gammopathies

Gammopathies are a heterogeneous group of diseases characterized by the presence of highly elevated levels of immunoglobulins in blood. The gammopathies are classified as monoclonal or polyclonal on the basis of the relative spreading of the γ-globulin zone on serum electrophoresis. An abnormally elevated, heterogeneous, broad-based sawtooth pattern indicates a polyclonal gammopathy, whereas a sharp, narrow-based, church-spire pattern indicates a monoclonal gammopathy. Polyclonal gammopathies are generally characteristic of benign plasma cell proliferation in response to a persistent antigenic stimulation. Polyclonal gammopathies are seen in chronic infections, chronic inflammatory diseases, immune-mediated diseases, and occasionally in lymphoma. In contrast, monoclonal gammopathies are found in association with a variety of plasma cell and lymphocytic dyscrasias, usually of obscure etiology (Table

34–11). Monoclonal gammopathies are seen in about 5% of dogs with lymphoproliferative disorders (MacEwen et al., 1977). Clinicopathologic manifestations of monoclonal gammopathy vary with the degree of plasma cell proliferation, tissue infiltration, and paraproteinemia.

A monoclonal gammopathy results from a malignant or "benign" proliferation of a single clone of lymphoid cells characteristically secreting massive amounts of a single protein species (Appendix Case 38). Gammopathies involving malignant proliferation of more than one clone of cells have been reported in humans, but they are extremely rare. A case of polyclonal gammopathy in a dog with plasma cell dyscrasia has been reported (DiBartola and Reynolds, 1982).

The terms "paraprotein" and "paraproteinemia" were coined to indicate the presence of "foreign" proteins in patients with various plasma cell dyscrasias (Apitz, 1940). The protein has also been called myeloma protein, M-protein, or M-component. Chemical analysis of the abnormally increased protein revealed that the molecules were structurally homogeneous and similar to normal γ-globulin. Indeed, it was through the study of these molecules that immunochemists were able to deduce the structural features of the immunoglobulins. Although the conditions are called gammopathies, it must be emphasized that the increased globulin may migrate in the β zone or even in the slow α zone on electrophoresis (Figs. 34–6 through 34–8). Electrophoretically, IgG migrates in the γ region, IgA in the β region, IgM in β to fast γ regions, and IgD and IgE in the fast γ region. It should also be mentioned that serum protein abnormalities in gammopathies not only may consist of excessive amounts of a complete immunoglobulin, but also may include free kappa or lambda chains or fragments of heavy chains which may not be recognized on electrophoresis (Wintrobe et al., 1981).

Gammopathies have been described in the dog (Braund et al., 1979; Cordy, 1957; Finnie and Wilks, 1982; Groulade, 1965b; Holmes et al., 1964; Hurvitz et al., 1970; MacEwen et al., 1977; Mejia et al., 1979; Miller et al., 1982; Orr et al., 1981; Osborne et al., 1968; Shepard et al., 1972; Shull et al., 1978; Takahashi et al., 1980; Virella et al., 1977; Williard et al., 1981), cat (Farrow and Penny, 1971; Hribernik et al., 1982; Holzworth and Meier, 1957; Mills et al., 1982; Williams and Goldschmidt, 1982), horse (Cornelius et al., 1959b; Perryman and McGuire, 1980; Schalm et al., 1974), and ox (Pedini and Romanelli, 1955). Clinicopathologic manifestations of monoclonal gammop-

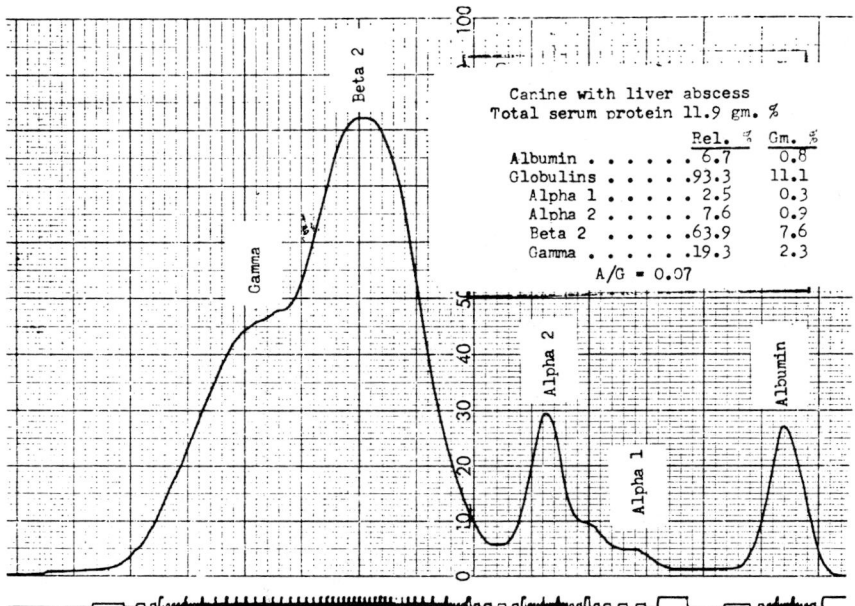

Fig. 34–6. Electrophoretic tracing of the serum of a dog with a liver abscess showing a polyclonal gammopathy.

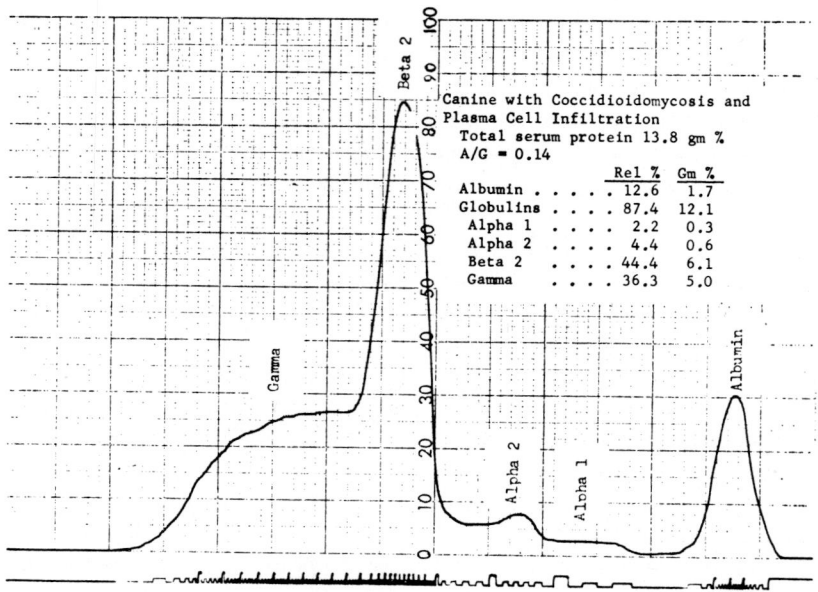

Fig. 34–7. Electrophoretic tracing of serum of a dog diagnosed as having coccidioidomycosis and plasma cell infiltration of internal organs, leading to a diagnosis of myelomatosis.

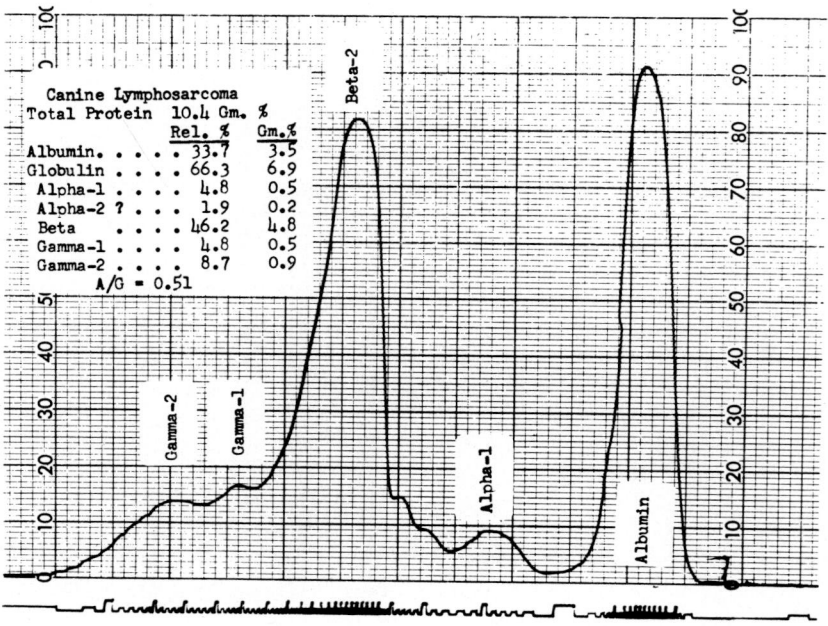

Fig. 34–8. Protein concentrations and electrophoretic tracing of serum from a dog with lymphosarcoma.

athy vary with the degree of plasma cell proliferation, tissue infiltration, and paraproteinemia.

Laboratory investigation of a patient suspected to have a monoclonal gammopathy should include complete blood analysis, bone marrow biopsy, serum chemistries, hemostatic profile, serum viscosity, radiographic examination, urinalysis, and immunologic tests. Serum protein electrophoresis should be followed by immunoelectrophoresis to identify the abnormal immunoglobulin and then single radial immunodiffusion to quantitate various immunoglobulins. Serum should be separated at 37°C to avoid cryoprecipitation of certain immunoglobulins. In rare cases of "nonsecretory" myeloma, serum protein analyses may be nondiagnostic (MacEwen et al., 1984a). In such cases bone marrow smears should be examined by immunofluorescence to define the intracellular location of monoclonal immunoglobulin. Plasma cell infiltration of the bone marrow is focal in various plasma cell dyscrasias; hence a random marrow aspirate may appear nondiagnostic.

Bence Jones proteins may be found in the urine in plasma cell myeloma but not in Waldenström's macroglobulinemia, and so testing for Bence Jones proteins is one way to differentiate between the two conditions. The Bence Jones proteins consist of monoclonal kappa or lambda light chains. Although the Bence Jones proteins in urine can be demonstrated by heat precipitation (precipitating when heated to 50–60°C at pH 4.5–5.0 and redissolving at 90–100°C), they are best demonstrated by electrophoretic techniques. The urine sample often needs to be concentrated before analysis. The Bence Jones proteins are present in the urine of 55–80% of human patients (Wintrobe et al., 1981) and in less than 10% of canine patients with myeloma. Bence Jones protein was detected in the urine of some myeloma cats (Barlough et al., 1981).

Multiple Myeloma

In humans, multiple myeloma or simply myeloma is characterized by the finding of increased levels of a monoclonal protein in serum (or urine) associated with increased numbers (>15–20%) of plasma cells in the bone marrow and typical lytic bone lesions. Myeloma has been described in the dog (Bloom, 1946; Braund et al., 1979; Cordy, 1957; Finnie and Wilks, 1982; Holmes et al., 1964; Miller et al., 1982; Orr et al., 1981; Osborne et al., 1968; Shepard et al., 1972; Shull et al., 1978; Takahashi et al., 1980; Virella et al., 1977), cat (Barlough et al., 1981; Farrow and Penny, 1971; Holzworth and Meier, 1957; Mills et al., 1982), horse (Cornelius et al., 1959b; Jacobs et al., 1983; Markel and Dorr, 1986), and rabbit (Pascal, 1961). In each instance, plasma cell tumors usually infiltrated the bone marrow. Serum protein analyses in early studies have been minimal except that in most instances, markedly elevated γ-globulin levels were found. Bence Jones proteinuria was found in only some patients (Dewhirst et al., 1977; Hurvitz et al., 1971). In rare instances, the tumor may arise at extramedullary sites as solitary plasmacytoma and may metastasize later (Lester and Mesfin, 1980; MacEwen et al., 1984b).

Other laboratory and clinical findings in human and various animal patients are as follows: The concentration of immunoglobulins other than the paraprotein is generally decreased because of diminished immune response. Anemia (nonresponsive), azotemia, and hypercalcemia are common, and thrombocytopenia and other hemostatic defects may be found. Leukopenia due to neutropenia may be encountered. Erythrocyte sedimentation rate is generally elevated. Splenomegaly and hepatomegaly may be present. Abnormalities of plasma cell morphology are also evident in patients with myeloma. "Flame cells," i.e., plasma cells with reddish cytoplasmic staining at the periphery (Plates XIII–7, XIII–8, XIII–9) and "thesaurocytes" (storage cells) have been described in cases of IgA myeloma. Plasma cells with distinct nucleoli, excessive cytoplasm, or multiple nuclei may be evident. Plasma cell leukemia in myeloma is extremely rare (Takahashi et al., 1980) and probably indicates a terminal event.

Frequent complications are recurrent infections from diminished immune response and impaired phagocytic activity; acute or chronic renal failure primarily from excretion of myeloma proteins; lameness, bone pain, and pathologic fractures from bone marrow infiltration by malignant plasma cells and osteolysis; hypercalcemia from release of an osteoblast activating factor by tumor cells; spinal cord compression and peripheral neuropathy from plasma cell infiltration; hyperviscosity syndrome from the presence of excessive paraprotein; bleeding tendency as a result of thrombocytopenia and hemostatic defects; and myelogenous or myelomonocytic leukemia as a progression of the disease. Renal insufficiency and neurologic manifestations are more common in humans than in dogs (Osborne et al., 1968). Neurologic signs were observed in a dog with monoclonal IgM gammopathy associated with lymphocytic leukemia (Braund et al., 1978) and in a dog with IgA myeloma associated with cryoglobulinemia (Braund et al., 1979).

The serum paraprotein in more than 50% of human cases of myeloma is IgG, in about 20% of cases IgA, and in about 1% of cases IgD (Wintrobe et al., 1981). About 20% of cases exhibit only light chains; in such cases a prominent monoclonal spike is not seen. In the IgD myeloma, total serum proteins and monoclonal protein levels are usually not very high. The patients with only light chain disease present with renal failure and absence of serum paraprotein and often have Bence Jones proteinuria and lytic bone lesions. Heavy chain disease is rare and is characterized by incomplete heavy chains in serum and possibly in the urine. About 1% of the myeloma patients show no paraprotein in the serum (nonsecretors). The immunologic distribution of animal patients with myeloma is not known because case reports are limited, but the trend suggests that the IgG type predominates, whereas the IgA type is infrequent (Dewhirst et al., 1977; Takahasi et al., 1980). Elevations in IgM are discussed under Waldenström's Macroglobulinemia and Hyperviscosity Syndrome (next two sections).

Although plasma cell myeloma cannot be completely treated, about 70% of human patients respond with a mean life span of 30 months to irradiation and chemotherapy with melphalan, cyclophosphamide, and prednisone (Wintrobe et al., 1981). Supportive treatment is crucial for patient survival.

Waldenström's Macroglobulinemia

Monoclonal increase in IgM is referred to as macroglobulinemia. Waldenström's macroglobulinemia is a primary disorder of this nature. It may also occur secondary to lymphoma, infections, and inflammation and sometimes as a benign monoclonal gammopathy.

Waldenström's macroglobulinemia has been described in the dog (Groulade, 1965b; Hurvitz et al., 1970). The disease is characterized by lassitude, bleeding, retinal hemorrhage, distension of retinal veins, and enlarged lymph nodes and spleen. The bleeding tendency is thought to be due to the effects of anoxia, clotting abnormalities, and thrombocytopenia. Laboratory findings include marked hyperproteinemia with a sharply defined β or γ peak on electrophoresis. The plasma is quite viscous, which contributes to the eye problem.

Bone marrow aspirates of human patients with this disease may yield "dry tap" or contain lymphocytoid rather than plasmacytic cells. The disease differs from myeloma in that there are no bone lesions. Bence Jones proteinuria is less common. Human patients are given frequent plasmapheresis and treated with low doses of chlorambucil. A combination chemotherapy including cyclophosphamide, melphalan, and prednisolone is instituted in nonresponsive cases. Death is commonly due to infection resulting from depression of normal antibody production.

We have had several cases in dogs of marked hyperproteinemia in which the increased protein was a β-globulin. The *first case* was that of a 2-year-old male pointer. The dog had a history of weight loss, anorexia, lethargy, and hair loss. A radiograph revealed a mass in the area of the liver. Liver function tests were normal. On the day of admission, the urine had a specific gravity of 1.019, protein was $4+$, and bile $2+$. Six days later, a hemogram revealed a slight leukocytosis, due principally to neutrophilia and monocytosis. The dog was also anemic. The most striking feature of the case was a β_2-proteinemia of 7.6 g/dl (Fig. 34–6). Serum proteins were 11.9 g/dl, and albumin was 0.8 g/dl, giving an A/G ratio of 0.07. The dog died 1 week after ad-

Table 34–12. Hematologic Findings in a Dog with a Plasma Cell Dyscrasia

RBC × 10⁶/μl	3.59
WBC/μl	23,500
Band neutrophils	470
Neutrophils	19,035
Monocytes	1,175
Eosinophils	705
Lymphocytes	1,197
Plasma cells	Rare
Total plasma protein	12.2 g/dl
Fibrinogen	0.2 g/dl
Reticulocytes	1.6%

mission. At necropsy, the principal lesions were abscesses of the liver of bacterial origin.

The *second case* was that of a 6½-year-old spayed female cocker-poodle cross. The dog was presented to the clinic with a history of pustular skin lesions and anemia of 4½ months' duration. Examination revealed enlarged lymph nodes, anemia, and the presence of circulating plasma cells. The latter finding led the clinician to suspect myelomatosis. Material from a skin lesion was cultured, and *Coccidioides immitis* was isolated. The serum was also positive for coccidioidal antibodies in the complement-fixation test. Hematologic findings the day after admission are given in Table 34–12. The urine had a specific gravity of 1.021 and was negative for Bence Jones protein, but had 2 + albumin.

The electrophoretic pattern for serum is shown in Fig. 34–7. At 1 week, impression smears of enlarged lymph nodes after biopsy revealed many plasma cells. Bone marrow aspiration revealed scattered clusters of plasma cells. Necropsy was performed at the third week. In addition to the skin lesions, scattered foci of plasma cells were found in the kidney, pancreas and its adjacent lymph node, the myocardium, adrenals, mammary gland, inguinal lymph node, spleen, and bone marrow. Evidence of membranous glomerulonephritis was also present. A diagnosis of *myelomatosis* was given, although Bence Jones proteinuria was not found.

The *third case* was a 4-year-old Belgian sheepdog with a history of weight loss for 6 weeks, dysuria, progressive uremia, respiratory distress, conjunctivitis, and vomiting. Laboratory findings on admission were: blood urea nitrogen, 182 mg/dl; creatinine, 7.5 mg/dl; WBC, 17,000/μl; urinalysis, 4 + protein

and many RBC and WBC. The dog was destroyed, and necropsy revealed *lymphoma*. The serum protein values and electrophoretogram are shown in Fig. 34–8. (This case is discussed in greater detail in Chapter 32.)

The *fourth case* involved a 4-year-old male collie. The dog was presented to the clinic with a history of diarrhea and weakness. Two years before, the dog had a tonsil removed, and a diagnosis of lymphoma was made by an MD pathologist. On admission to our clinic, the dog appeared weak. Palpation revealed an enlarged liver and spleen. Splenomegaly and hepatomegaly were verified by radiography. Hemograms made during the hospital stay were normal, except that the blood film appeared to be coated with a substance suspected of being protein and a clear halo was observed around the neutrophils. Plasma alkaline phosphatase and glutamic-pyruvic transaminase (SGPT) were elevated (314 and 185 UI/L, respectively). Total serum protein concentration on the third day was 10.9 g/dl. Fractionation by electrophoresis revealed a markedly elevated β-globulin peak in a concentration of 8.06 g/dl (Fig. 34–9). Plasma fibrinogen level was less than 50 mg/dl. The deteriorating condition of the dog and obvious liver involvement prompted euthanasia. At necropsy, the mesenteric lymph nodes, liver, and spleen were all found to be involved with *lymphocytic neoplasia*.

The serum protein profile of this last case was typical of that observed in Waldenström's macroglobulinemia. This case in the dog is interesting in that depressed fibrinogen and elevated alkaline phosphatase and SGPT all indicate liver involvement, although serum albumin was in the normal range. The dog was hypogammaglobulinemic, a common finding in human lymphoma (Green et al., 1966), but the markedly elevated β-globulin may well represent IgM often associated with liver necrosis. A part of this elevated globulin may also be due to β-lipoprotein.

Hyperviscosity Syndrome

Hyperviscosity syndrome (HVS) has been observed in the dog and cat. In the dog, as in humans, it is primarily associated with IgM, less commonly with IgA, and rarely with IgG paraproteins. Thus HVS is not only a

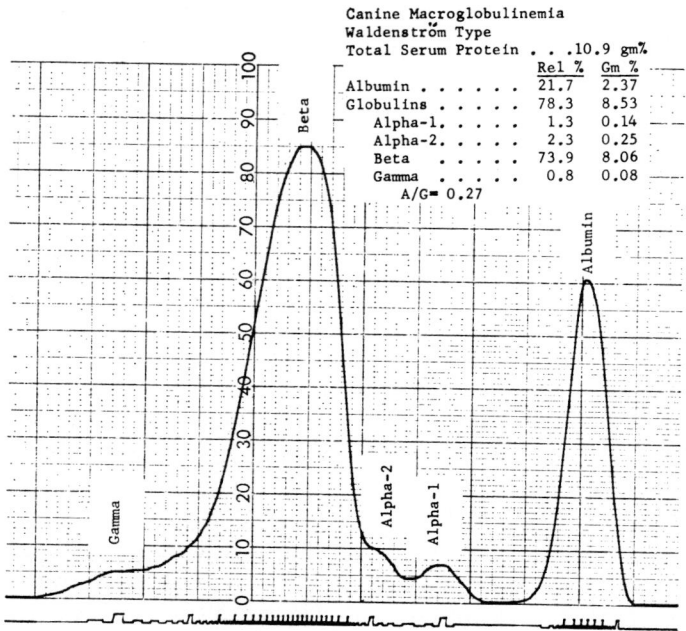

Canine Macroglobulinemia
Waldenström Type
Total Serum Protein . . .10.9 gm%

	Rel %	Gm %
Albumin	21.7	2.37
Globulins	78.3	8.53
Alpha-1.	1.3	0.14
Alpha-2.	2.3	0.25
Beta	73.9	8.06
Gamma	0.8	0.08
A/G= 0.27		

Fig. 34–9. Serum protein profile from a dog with lymphosarcoma.

manifestation of Waldenström's macroglobulinemia (Hurvitz et al., 1970; Mejia et al., 1979), but it may also be seen in certain cases of myeloma, particularly those having polymeric IgA (Matus et al., 1983; Miller et al., 1982; Shepard et al., 1972; Shull et al., 1978; Virella et al., 1977) and in lymphoma and lymphocytic leukemia with macroglobulinemia (Braund et al., 1978; MacEwen et al., 1977; Williams and Goldschmidt, 1982; Williard et al., 1981). HVS may also accompany benign monoclonal gammopathy, and cryoglobulinemia may be an additional cause (Hurvitz et al., 1977; Wintrobe et al., 1981). HVS associated with IgG myeloma was reported in a cat (Hribernik et al., 1982). Weekly or biweekly plasmapheresis, chemotherapy, and treatment with penicillamine or other chelating agents to reduce aggregation of paraproteins are various means of palliative therapy in HVS. The long-term prognosis is still poor.

The hematocrit is the most important single factor influencing whole blood viscosity (Preston, 1979). Plasma fibrinogen and certain Igs influence plasma and in turn whole blood viscosity. Thus flow characteristics of blood are affected by the red cell count as well as plasma viscosity. In paraproteinemia, altered plasma viscosity and aggregation of erythrocytes may significantly alter blood flow. Plasma viscosity in macroglobulinemias and myelomatosis is elevated because of extremely high concentrations of serum paraproteins and physical properties of the Igs involved (Preston, 1979). The IgM not only is a macromolecule, but also has a high intrinsic viscosity. The IgA and to some extent IgG_3 tend to form high-molecular-weight complexes (polymers) and raise plasma viscosity at relatively lower concentrations than IgM.

Increased plasma viscosity and aggregation of erythrocytes decrease blood flow and tissue perfusion. This is associated with a spectrum of clinical signs that include abnormalities of cardiovascular, neurologic, and renal functions as well as of hemostasis and immune mechanisms. For example, cardiomegaly, distended tortuous appearance of retinal veins, and neurologic manifestations may be present to a varying degree at admission. The paraproteins may interact with various coagulation factors. They may also interfere with platelet functions, thus adding to bleeding tendency from thrombocytopenia and clotting defects. Retinal hemorrhages and bleeding from mucous membranes are common.

Some advances have been made in treatment of patients with HVS. In a recent report

(Matus et al., 1983) of HVS associated with IgA monoclonal gammopathy in three dogs, continuous plasmapheresis and alkylation therapy with melphalan and cyclophosphamide induced sustained remission in each patient. Clinical signs associated with HVS resolved, and normal serum protein levels were attained.

Aleutian Disease in Mink

A plasma cell dyscrasia was first observed on a mink ranch in Oregon in a mutation that led to a lack of vigor. The syndrome, now called Aleutian disease, is characterized by plasma cell infiltration of the liver, kidney, and other organs, widespread periarteritis, glomerulonephritis, and hyperproteinemia. Aleutian disease of mink has been compared to disseminated lupus erythematosus of humans (Leader et al., 1963; Obel, 1959; Thompson and Aliferis, 1964; Wagner, 1963). The electrophoretic patterns in this disease are striking in that they appear as tracings of normal serum, only in the reverse order: The γ-globulin concentration is like that of albumin of normal serum, as seen in monoclonal gammopathy (Henson et al., 1961). Marked hypoalbuminemia accompanies the increased serum γ-globulin. Neither Bence Jones proteinuria nor lytic bone lesions are seen. The disease is transmissible with crude organ suspensions and cell-free tissue filtrates (Trautwein and Helmboldt, 1962) and may be transmitted to humans (Chapman and Jimenez, 1963). The responsible agent is a parvovirus called Aleutian disease virus, which replicates in macrophages in vivo (Porter et al., 1980). A similar disease has also been described in ferrets (Porter et al., 1982). A case of plasma cell myeloma in a ferret was recently reported (Methiyapun et al., 1985).

Benign Monoclonal Gammopathy

In humans, benign monoclonal gammopathy is characterized by the presence of a monoclonal protein in the serum or urine unassociated with other manifestations of a plasma cell dyscrasia (Wintrobe et al., 1981). Plasma cells in the bone marrow are normal to <10% of all nucleated marrow cells and show normal morphology. Such patients are prone to develop myeloma, which may take more than two decades, but this does not happen in all cases. The patients with high or increasing serum paraprotein levels, low serum levels of normal immunoglobulins, and significant Bence Jones proteinuria are more likely candidates. In more than 95% of cases, the amount of M-protein does not change significantly over the years. Most cases of benign monoclonal gammopathy are secondary to a variety of conditions including chronic suppurative process, autoimmune diseases, immunodeficiency states, hematologic malignancies, and other tumors. Some age relationship has been noted, and genetic factors may play a part as well.

Plasma Proteins in Selected Conditions

Early studies (reviewed by Liberg, 1977) on patterns of serum protein fractionations indicated that an acute inflammation, especially in the dog and pig, was reflected by an increase in α-globulin, a subacute inflammation by an increase in α- and γ-globulins, and a chronic inflammation by an increase in γ-globulin. A decrease in albumin fraction was noted with simultaneous increase chiefly in γ-globulins. Recently, agarose electrophoresis of serums from adult cattle revealed an increase primarily of the α-globulins in acute inflammatory conditions, e.g., acute traumatic peritonitis, and an elevation of globulins in general and of γ-globulins in particular in chronic inflammatory diseases and infections, e.g., chronic peritonitis, mastitis, pneumonia, laminitis, urinary tract infections, and abscesses (Liberg, 1977). Such a general trend in deviations of plasma protein concentrations may manifest in a variety of diseases in different animal species (Appendix Case 61). A brief description of selected examples of abnormalities of plasma proteins follows.

Gastrointestinal Disorders

Excessive loss of protein into the gut is one of the major pathophysiologic disorders in several conditions in which the intestinal tract is involved. In humans, the term "protein-losing gastroenteropathy (or enteropathy)" has been coined (Anonymous, 1959) to describe a syndrome associated with a group of diseases with no common etiology or pathogenesis. The clinical appearance may be one of idiopathic hypoproteinemia with lethargy, weight loss, and perhaps subcutaneous edema, ascites, and hydrothorax. Protein loss into the gut can be detected by measuring fecal excretion of ^{51}Cr-labeled albumin (Barton et al., 1978) and by other methods (Waldmann, 1966). Protein-losing enteropathies have been described in the dog (Barton et al., 1978; Tams and Twedt, 1981) and horse (Meuten et al., 1978).

That the gastrointestinal (GI) tract is involved in significant protein metabolism has been difficult to prove because protein is recycled. Once excreted into the gut, proteins are degraded and resorbed as amino acids by the mucosal cells lining the tract (Waldmann, 1966). The magnitude of the contribution of the GI tract to catabolism of proteins in humans, although a subject of controversy, may amount to between 10% and 60% of total albumin catabolism (Waldmann, 1966). In dogs, it was found that some 10% of total metabolic albumin degradation took place in the stomach, 40% in the small intestine, and 4% in the colon (Glenert et al., 1962). As much as three-fourths of albumin catabolism in the dog occurs in the GI tract (Wetterfors, 1964).

Loss of plasma proteins into the GI tract may increase markedly secondary to conditions leading to obstruction of the GI lymphatics, which produces loss of lymph into the intestinal lumen, or in disorders of the mucosal cells such as inflammation or ulceration. In humans, such conditions as hypotrophic or ulcerative gastritis, stomach polyps or cancer, idiopathic steatorrhea or sprue, intestinal lymphangiectasia, ulcerative colitis, and congestive heart failure are among some 40 disorders in which excessive protein loss occurs in the intestine (Jeffries et al., 1962; Peeters, 1963; Waldmann, 1976).

Total serum protein concentration in several cases of gastrointestinal diseases in dogs are shown in Fig. 34–10. The marked hypoproteinemia is evident. With only one exception, the A/G ratios were much lower than normal, suggesting several possibilities, one of which is the selective movement of albumin into the gut. Kaneko and coworkers (1965) have described three cases of sprue with malabsorption syndrome in the dog.

In intestinal lymphangiectasia, dilated lym-

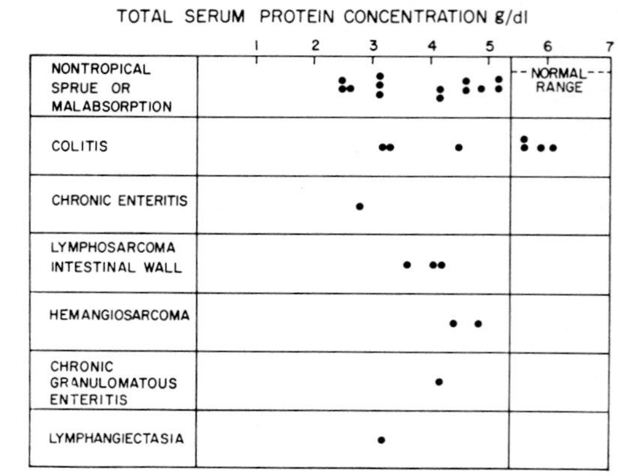

TOTAL SERUM PROTEIN CONCENTRATION g/dl

	1	2	3	4	5	6	7
NONTROPICAL SPRUE OR MALABSORPTION						NORMAL RANGE	
COLITIS							
CHRONIC ENTERITIS							
LYMPHOSARCOMA INTESTINAL WALL							
HEMANGIOSARCOMA							
CHRONIC GRANULOMATOUS ENTERITIS							
LYMPHANGIECTASIA							

Fig. 34–10. Some gastrointestinal disease of dogs causing hypoproteineima.

phatic channels of the bowel wall are characteristic. In this instance, protein and lymphocyte-rich lymph are lost into the intestinal tract and serous cavity, and lymphocytopenia is common. Although rare in animals, such cases have been reported (Campbell et al., 1968; McDonald, 1982; Nielsen and Andersen, 1967), and a case is recorded in Appendix Case 39.

Congestive heart failure and other cardiac problems in humans lead to GI protein loss due to dilated intestinal lymphatic channels as a result of abnormal blood pressure changes. Furthermore, there may be an accompanying significant alteration of liver function.

Loss of protein during inflammation or ulceration of the GI tract could well lead to impaired absorption as well as increased protein loss due to injured mucosal cells. This mechanism may be potentiated by intestinal parasites (Barton et al., 1978). Preferential loss of globulins may also occur from the GI tract. For example, diminished total serum protein concentration in diarrheic calves was associated with decreases in both β- and γ-globulins up to 2 weeks of age and with loss of only β-globulins at 3–6 weeks of age (Borg, 1983).

Johne's disease of cattle leads to intestinal protein loss, a part of which has been ascribed to lymphangiectasia (Neilsen and Andersen, 1967), since dilation and occlusion of submucosal and subserosal lymph vessels were present in this condition. A case considered typical of Johne's disease is documented (Appendix Case 70). The need for an effective method of diagnosing Johne's disease has prompted workers to do extensive studies on serum glycoproteins and plasma enzymes (Patterson and Sweasey, 1968; Patterson et al., 1969).

Parasitism

Parasitic infestations of ruminants have a profound effect on plasma proteins. Apart from frank blood loss by the sucking parasites, such as *Haemonchus* and *Ostertagia*, diseases caused by parasites common to lambs, calves, sheep, and cattle produce nutritional hypoproteinemia due to the animal's decreased food and water consumption. Excessive water loss in the feces reduces the amount of protein resorbed from the gut because the animal is unable to resorb either water or protein. Haemonchosis causes a mild gastritis, whereas *Trichostrongylus axei* larvae can cause acute catarrhal gastritis; thus all degrees of protein loss can occur from the abomasum. Oesophagostomiasis causes loss of plasma into the cecum and colon (Bremner, 1969). Massive losses of albumin in sheep have been reported in experimentally induced oesophagostomiasis (Dobson, 1965). Total plasma protein slowly declined, owing to loss of albumin and α- and β-globulins. Loss of albumin as great as 1 g/dl was reported. Decreased A/G ratios due to relative increase in globulins have been reported in heavily parasitized lambs (Turner and Wilson, 1960; Wilson and Turner, 1965).

Experimental infestations of calves with *Trichostrongylus axei* produced an absolute reduction in all serum protein components, although there was an increase in relative concentration of α_2-globulin (Leland et al., 1959). Total protein levels of 6–7 g/dl fell to as low as 3 g/dl in the calves. *Haemonchus placei, Oesophagostomum radiatum*, and *Bunostomum phlebotomum* (Bremner, 1960) and ostertagiasis in cattle (Halliday et al., 1968) also induced hypoproteinemia and hypoalbuminemia. Our own data on plasma protein levels in trichostrongylosis of cattle show a range of 2.8–5.4 g/dl of plasma, with an average of 4.4 g/dl (see also Appendix Case 71).

Metabolic studies have shown that there was an increased fractional catabolic rate for albumin in ostertagiasis of cattle. Although albumin levels were low in trichostrongylosis, the turnover rates were similar to those of control cattle (Cornelius et al., 1962).

Total serum protein concentration is increased in horses with helminthiasis, probably as a result of an increase in β-globulins, although albumin is diminished (Patton et al., 1978). IgG(T) is increased fourfold in ponies chronically infected with *Strongylus vulgaris* (Patton et al., 1978) and significantly increased in horses and ponies grazing on pastures contaminated with intestinal parasite eggs and larvae (Kent and Blackmore, 1985).

Groulade (1965a) reported on leishmaniasis in dogs in which broad fluctuations in serum protein concentrations were observed during the course of the disease. In this condition, albumin would drop by as much as 30% of normal, whereas γ-globulin would increase by as much as 31% of normal, even though the total protein remained within normal limits. We have observed two cases of leishmaniasis in the dog in which moderate to marked hyperproteinemia was a consistent feature for a period of several months.

Dogs naturally infected with *Dirofilaria immitis* were reported to have significantly higher serum β-globulins levels than uninfected dogs (Barsanti et al., 1977).

Serum Ig and complement levels may also be altered during parasitism. Although catabolism of Igs and complement components (C1 and C3) is enhanced in trypanosomiasis (Neilsen et al., 1978), serum levels of IgG and IgM are elevated while levels of IgA, IgE, C1, and C3 are depressed. Sheep experimentally infected with *Trypanosoma congolense* developed increased levels of IgM and IgG within few weeks of infection (Mackenzie et al., 1979).

Liver Disease

Because the liver plays a central role in both anabolism and catabolism of plasma proteins, it is not unreasonable to expect that plasma protein analysis would be useful in detecting liver injury. Unfortunately, protein fractionation is of little value in detecting the degree of lost function, making a differential diagnosis of jaundice, or establishing presence of parenchymal damage. Liver damage does produce characteristic changes in plasma proteins. However, these changes appear late in the process and may be more prognostic than diagnostic. Other function tests are indicated for detecting liver disease.

In hepatitis, cirrhosis, or carcinoma, the characteristic though not universal finding is depressed albumin and elevated γ-globulins. We have observed animals with acute toxic hepatopathy in which albumin was markedly depressed and γ-globulins were markedly elevated. The fall in albumin is due to failure of synthesis by the hepatic parenchyma. However, the remarkable regenerative power of the liver is such that significantly depressed albumin synthesis is generally found only in a chronic process such as diffuse fibrosis or chronic hepatitis.

In humans, significantly depressed albumin levels and elevated γ-globulin levels are taken as a rather grave prognostic sign (Post and Patek, 1942). The reason for the elevated γ-globulin levels has not been determined, although consideration has been given to the possibility of an immune response to tissue breakdown products.

In puppies experimentally infected with hepatitis virus, abnormal increases in α- and β-globulins were noted (Larin, 1959). Albumin decrease was not observed during the febrile stage but albumin levels were considerably lower in the convalescent period or after complete recovery. Elevated α-globulin in a majority of cases was seen only in the later stages of the disease. Another report (Beckett et al., 1964) described an increase of α-globulins but not of β-globulins and a significant decrease in albumin during the early stages, to some 75% of normal at 1 week after infection. Elevated transaminases (SGPT and SGOT) were found only during the acute phase.

In humans, a progressive alteration of plasma proteins is found in viral hepatitis, occlusion icterus, compensated cirrhosis, decompensated cirrhosis, and hepatic coma (Muting and Reckowski, 1965). The alteration takes the form of decreased serum albumin and prothrombin and increased levels of γ-globulins.

Kidney Disease

The potential for loss of protein in kidney disease is quite substantial. The rate of urinary protein excretion is dependent upon the glomerular filtration rate, the permeability of the glomerular membrane, the rate of absorption in the glomerular membrane, the rate of absorption in the tubules, and the rate at which the tubules dispose of absorbed protein. The first proteins to leak through the glomerular membranes are albumin and α-globulin. The β- and γ-globulins leak through when the damage is greater. Collectively, the proteins of urine are called albumin by custom.

In dogs, chronic interstitial nephritis (end stage kidney disease) is a common finding. However, significant changes in plasma proteins are not found, except that an unexplained hyperfibrinogenemia is a common finding. Hyperproteinemia, however, may occur because of dehydration. Glomerular nephritis, on the other hand, results in significant loss of protein, particularly albumin, and hypoproteinemia is the usual finding (see Appendix Case 4).

The etiology of glomerular nephritis is well described by Dixon (1967): Immunoglobulins arising as a result of an infection combine with antigen in vivo, and the antigen-antibody complexes lodge on the glomerular basement membrane. These complexes activate complement and thereby generate factors chemotactic for leukocytes. Injury is instituted when the proteolytic enzymes of disintegrated leukocytes, particularly neutrophils, act on the basement membrane.

Renal lesions in dogs with pyometra were attributed to this mechanism (Obel et al., 1964). It was felt that the antigen either was bacterial or derived from damaged tissue originating in the uterus. However, in this instance, the dogs had hyperproteinemia due mostly to elevated γ-globulins.

Nephrosis

The designation *nephrosis* was introduced in human medicine to describe patients with edema, proteinuria, hypoproteinemia, and lipemia. The term *nephrotic syndrome* is now used to describe a variety of renal disorders in which proteinuria is severe enough to lead to hypoproteinemia. Indeed, the loss of as much as 40 g of protein per day is not uncommon. The cause may be metabolic disease such as diabetes, or it may be mechanical, as from a renal thrombus. A frequent cause is an infection or a drug idiosyncrasy, and more attention is being given to the possibility of an immunologic reaction.

The electrophoretic pattern is one of marked reduction in serum albumin and elevation of the α_2-globulin peak. The former results from proteinuria despite enhanced production of serum albumin by the liver (Blahd et al., 1955). The latter is due to an increase in α-lipoprotein.

Fifteen cases diagnosed as nephrosis have been described in dogs (Moegle et al., 1956); the common findings were edema (mostly ascites), chronic catarrhal gastritis, and proteinuria. Plasma protein concentrations generally were quite low, most due to depressed albumin and γ-globulin. In most instances, α_2-globulin and β-globulins were elevated. In addition, 22 instances of uremia in dogs were documented in which the plasma protein concentrations were not unusual. In six dogs in which both the kidney and liver were damaged, increased γ-globulin was observed. The authors concluded that electrophoresis of serum was a valuable tool in distinguishing the nephrotic syndrome from other forms of kidney disease.

Effect of Infection on Serum Proteins

The clinician is constantly confronted with the need to differentiate between an infectious process and other causes of disease. Unfortunately, an examination of serum protein profiles will furnish little help in this regard. Although antibodies are globulins, some of which can become elevated following an infection, more often than not there is no relationship between antibody titers and serum protein changes. Extensive increase in globulins have not always been associated with the development of immunity, and hyperimmunization can cause an increase in nonspecific globulins as well as specific antibodies (Gourvitch, 1956). The effects of an infection or bacterial toxins on a target organ such as liver or kidney, however, may alter the serum protein concentrations significantly.

In acute febrile infections, the principal changes are a decrease in albumin and most frequently an increase in α-globulin. This is especially evident if one determines glycoprotein levels by electrophoresis. However, these changes are observed after injury, surgery, or neoplastic disease and are probably related to adrenal stimulation and protein catabolism following the stress. In chronic infections and especially if abscess formation occurs and provides a constant and potent source of antigen, a marked rise in γ-globulin can result. In this event, there is invariably a concomitant decrease in albumin.

Hyperproteinemia, principally due to increase in γ-globulins, occurred in goats chronically infected with *Corynebacterium pseudotuberculosis* (Desiderio et al., 1979).

The heterogeneous nature of antibody molecules has already been alluded to. The type of antibody present in the serum at any given time depends on several factors. In general, the first antibodies to appear in the plasma after most antigenic exposures are globulins with β mobility (IgM). These decline to low levels or disappear in a few weeks, but in the meantime, antibodies with γ mobility (IgG) make their appearance. These persist. The animal responds to a second exposure to antigen by making IgG. In either case, the IgG may be γ_1- or γ_2-molecules. Some antigens evoke only IgM response.

Viral and Rickettsial Diseases

As a rule, viral and rickettsial infections do not produce significant changes in either relative or absolute amount of plasma proteins, even though antibody titers may be elevated. (See Dimopoullos, 1961, for an early review.) These include infections with western and Venezuelan equine encephalomyelitis virus, Japanese B encephalitis, influenza, foot-and-mouth disease, vascular stomatitis, and Newcastle disease. In fact, studies with infectious bronchitis of chickens indicated a reverse correlation between virus neutralization titers and γ-globulin concentrations (Dimopoullos and Cunningham, 1956).

Early studies on equine infectious anemia (EIA) indicated that there was a progressive increase in globulin and decrease in albumin following experimental inoculation of horses. A significant increase in total protein was not observed. Later work (McGuire et al., 1970) indicated that persistent viremia in EIA is associated with hypergammaglobulinemia due to elevated IgG and IgG(T). Early increases in globulin were associated with IgM, which decreased to normal during the infection.

Feline Infectious Peritonitis (FIP). In this viral disease (Zook et al., 1968), total serum proteins can attain very high levels (Appendix Case 45). A record-breaking 14 g/dl was observed in one case in which γ-globulin comprised 60% of the total (Fig. 34–11). Electrophoresis of the peritoneal fluid offers a diagnostic aid (Fig. 34–12). In 35 cats with FIP in our clinic, plasma proteins averaged 8.3 ± 1.1 g/dl and ranged from 6.4–11.0 (Schalm, 1971). The case illustrated in Fig. 34–11 was not included in the study.

Tropical Canine Pancytopenia. This disease, observed in military dogs in the tropics, is characterized by marked serum protein changes (Burghen et al., 1971). In the terminal stages of the naturally acquired disease, marked elevation in γ-globulin level is observed, with a concomitant depression in albumin. In experimentally infected pups, elevated α_2-glycoproteins were observed during the febrile stage, followed by a gradual rise in γ-globulin.

Germfree Animals

The intestinal flora contribute significantly to the serum protein concentrations, as evidenced by comparison of germfree with conventional animals. The globulin concentrations are much lower in the germfree animals (Gustafsson and Laurell, 1958; Travnicek and Mandel, 1982; Wagner and Wostmann, 1961). Exposing them to conventional animals for 1 week brought about an elevation in α_2-globulin, followed in the second week by an increase in the β fraction. Only after more than 2 weeks did the serum γ-globulin increase; there was a concomitant decrease in serum albumin (Wostmann and Gordon, 1960). In germfree and conventionally raised ruminants (goats and sheep), no significant differences were found in albumin and α- and β-globulin concentrations, whereas a significant increase in γ-globulin occurred with age in conventional animals but not in germfree animals (Wostmann, 1961). Thus total protein concentration is lower in germfree animals for the first few weeks of life.

IMMUNE DEFICIENCY DISORDERS

The importance of humoral and cellular defense mechanisms for the well-being of an individual has been amply demonstrated. Thus it is obvious that any disturbance of these vital body components would be incompatible with survival. Indeed, it has been

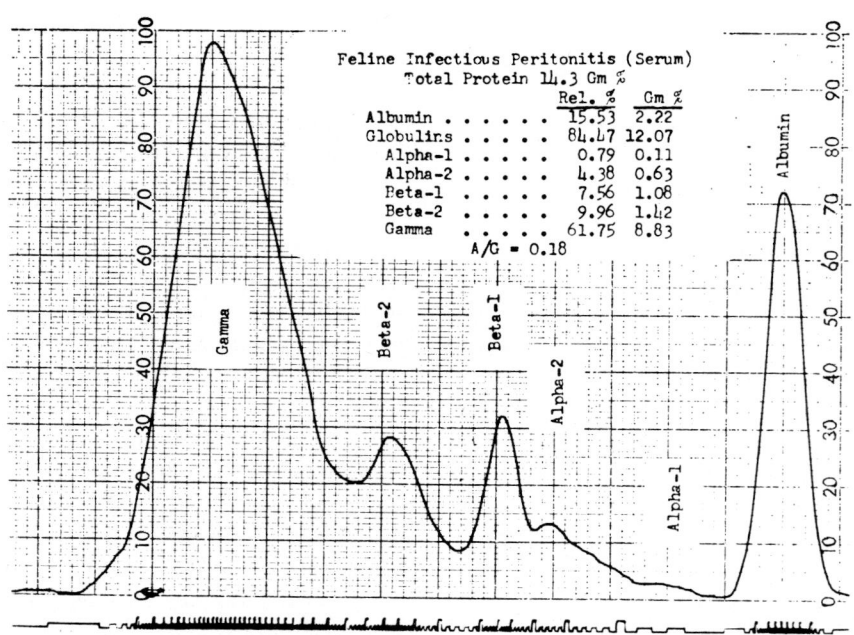

Feline Infectious Peritonitis (Serum)
Total Protein 14.3 Gm %

	Rel. %	Gm %
Albumin	15.53	2.22
Globulins	84.47	12.07
Alpha-1	0.79	0.11
Alpha-2	4.38	0.63
Beta-1	7.56	1.08
Beta-2	9.96	1.42
Gamma	61.75	8.83

A/G = 0.18

Fig. 34–11. Electrophoretic pattern of serum of a cat with feline infectious peritonitis.

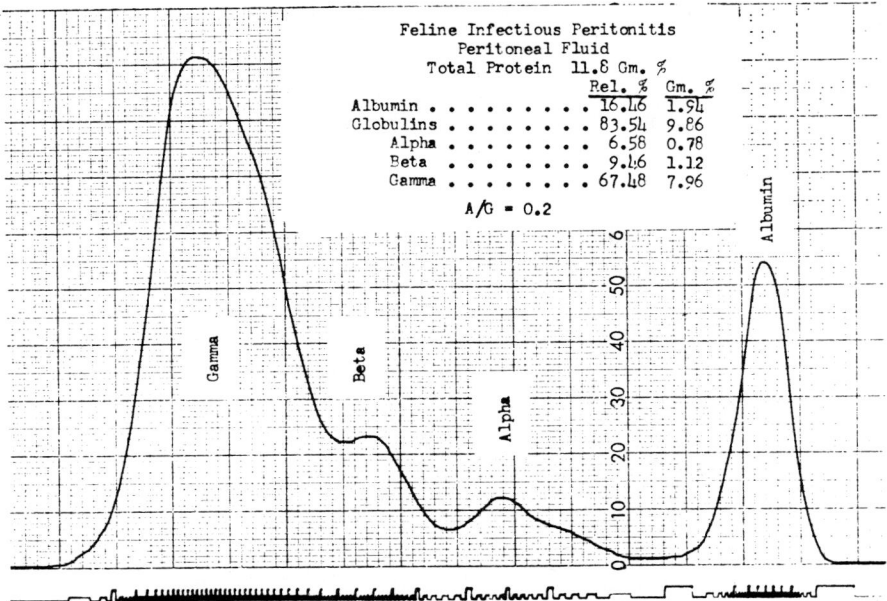

Fig. 34–12. Electrophoretic pattern of peritoneal fluid from a cat with feline infectious peritonitis (same cat as in Fig. 34–11).

shown in humans and several animal species that inadequacies of the phagocytic cells, lymphocytes, and complement components are associated with increased susceptibility to infections and sometimes death. Immune deficiency disorders in the broadest sense include disorders of these cellular and humoral defense systems, but it would seem more appropriate and congruous with the prefix to be somewhat restrictive and consider only disorders associated with the immune system, i.e., the lymphocytes, immunoglobulins, and complement components, although they may all present a similar clinical picture. This more restrictive approach has been taken for the discussion to follow.

Information presented is derived largely from reviews of immune deficiency disorders in humans (Horowitz and Hong, 1977; Rosen, 1980) and various animal species (Hammer et al., 1981; Letvin et al., 1983; McGuire and Perryman, 1981; Perryman 1979, 1982; Perryman and McGuire, 1980). The reader is referred to Chapters 26 and 29, respectively, for disorders associated with abnormalities of the neutrophils and the mononuclear phagocyte system.

Clinical Signs and Diagnostic Approach

Primary immune deficiencies arise as a result of hereditary defects in the immune system, while immune deficiencies associated with or developing as a result of a known disease condition are considered secondary. The former usually manifest at birth or during early postnatal life, while the latter may occur at any age. Primary immune deficiencies have been reported in horses and cattle, and secondary immune deficiencies from a variety of causes including drug therapy are being recognized increasingly in various animal species.

Clinical signs most commonly associated with a disturbance of the immune system include: infections during neonatal life, particularly during the first 6 weeks; recurrent infections or poor response to appropriate antibiotic therapy; increased susceptibility to minor pathogens or unusual organisms such as *Pneumocystis carinii*; and systemic illness following vaccination with a live virus vaccine.

Diagnostic evaluation of the suspected immune-deficient patient should be directed at defining the possible cellular or humoral defect. A systematic approach is therefore necessary after an initial laboratory data base has been established. As a minimum, initial laboratory evaluation should include hematologic examination, estimation of total serum proteins, and protein electrophoresis. Both Band T-lymphocyte functions should be evaluated to determine humoral and cell-mediated defects of the lymphoid system (see Chapter 30). B-lymphocyte function can be evaluated by serum electrophoresis, immunoelectrophoresis, and quantitation of serum immunoglobulin levels by single radial immunodiffusion; by quantitation of B-lymphocytes in blood and lymph nodes by defining various surface markers; and by determining immune response following injection of certain antigens such as heterologous red cells and keyhole limpet hemocyanin. Cell-mediated immunity can be evaluated by quantitation of T-lymphocytes in blood by the E-rosette method; by determining in vitro blastogenic response to certain mitogens, e.g., phytohemagglutinin and Con A; and by performing certain in vivo determinations such as skin sensitization and rejection of allogenic skin grafts. Whenever possible, histologic examination of lymphoid tissues, particularly the thymus, spleen, lymph nodes, and gut-associated lymphoid tissue, should be made in all cases of immune deficiency disorders. Total hemolytic complement may be assayed and, when appropriate antiserums are available, single radial immunodiffusion may be performed to determine deficiency of complement components. Evaluation of the phagocytic system would require quantitation of neutrophils in blood and bone marrow and an assessment of their functional attributes such as chemotaxis, phagocytosis, and bactericidal activity. The nitro blue tetrazolium reduction test and electron microscopy may be performed to assess metabolic and structural defects, respectively.

Primary Immune Deficiency Disorders

Combined Immune Deficiency in Arabian Foals

Combined immune deficiency (CID) is a hereditary functional disorder of T- and B-lymphocytes recognized for the first time in Arabian foals in 1973. It is inherited as an autosomal recessive trait and occurs in pure or part Arabian foals. The natural incidence is estimated at 2.3–2.7% without any sex predilection. The newborn foal appears normal at birth and remains healthy up to 2 months

of age. The foal becomes susceptible to infection as circulating immunoglobulins that had been acquired through colostrum consumption diminish. Death usually occurs within 5 months, frequently from bacterial infections, equine adenovirus, and the protozoan, *P. carinii*. Necropsy findings characteristically reveal a poorly developed lymphoid system. Grossly the thymus appears poorly developed, and the spleen may be normal to subnormal. Histologically the thymus, spleen, and lymph nodes show absence of lymphoid cells including plasma cells. A similar condition has been recognized in children. CID was also diagnosed in an Appaloosa foal (Perryman et al., 1984a).

The diagnosis of CID can be made at birth by finding at least two of the following three criteria: (1) lymphopenia (<1,000/µl), (2) absence of circulating IgM, and (3) hypoplastic lymphoid tissues, e.g., thymus (Perryman, 1979; Appendix Case 59). Hematologic examination reveals marked lymphopenia, with counts usually <500/µl of blood. The normal number of lymphocytes at birth to 21 days of age is much higher (4,119 ± 1,649/µl). The peripheral blood lymphocytes lack various in vitro and in vivo functional criteria of B and T cells. Neutrophils and monocytes are present in normal numbers and are functionally competent. Serum complement level is normal, and plasma corticosteroid levels are not elevated (Magnuson et al., 1980).

The normal equine fetus begins to synthesize IgM at 190 days of gestation so that a small amount (0.08–0.2 mg/ml) is present in serum at birth and slightly higher levels (0.1–0.5 mg/ml) are detected at 1–21 days of life. The absence of IgM in precolostral foal serum is diagnostic of primary immune deficiency. In suckled CID foal serum, IgM and IgA concentrations decline rapidly because of shorter half-life; hence an absence or low levels of IgM and IgA at a later date are also diagnostic. Secretory IgA was absent in CID foals over 2 months in age (Buening et al., 1978).

Pathogenesis of CID remains to be elucidated. Studies on children with CID indicate an association with abnormalities of purine metabolism due to absence of adenosine deaminase and purine nucleosidase phosphorylase. Although an abnormality of purine metabolism has been detected in Arabian foals with CID (Splitter et al., 1980), further investigations are needed to establish its association with the disease. No treatment is available at present. Attempts to transplant fetal liver or thymus, bone marrow, and cultured thymic cells have been unsuccessful or only partially successful (Campbell and Studdert, 1983).

Lethal Trait A-46 in Black Pied Danish Cattle

A lethal primary immune deficiency of T cells has been described in Black Pied Danish cattle of Friesian ancestry (Andersen et al., 1970). It is an autosomal recessive trait. The calves are normal at birth, but develop characteristic skin lesions at 4–8 weeks of age and die by the age of 4 months. The skin lesions are characterized by exanthema, alopecia, and parakeratosis. The animals are highly susceptible to infection. Generalized hypoplasia of lymphoid tissue, particularly of the T regions, is seen in the thymus, spleen, lymph nodes, and gut-associated lymphoid tissue. Cellular immunity is markedly reduced, whereas humoral immune response is undisturbed. A unique characteristic of the disorder is that affected calves respond to zinc therapy with complete recovery (Brummerstedt et al., 1971).

Complement Deficiency

Deficiency of several complement components has been detected in inbred strains of certain laboratory animals including mice, guinea pigs, rabbits, rats, and hamsters (Hammer et al., 1981). These animals are valuable for research on pathogenesis of disease processes because complement is important in host defense. An inherited deficiency of C3 was recently reported in some Brittany spaniel dogs bred to develop a colony to study canine spinal muscular dystrophy (Blum et al., 1985; Winkelstein et al., 1981, 1982). This deficiency was inherited as an autosomal recessive trait unrelated to the primary disease and susceptibility to renal disease was increased. Recurrent bacterial infections were common in these dogs. An interesting finding was that although levels of immunoreactive

C3 were extremely low, some (about 10% of normal) functional hemolytic "C3-like" activity was still present in the serum. Hematologic parameters were normal, and humoral antibody response was unaltered.

Other Conditions

A report implicating a sex-linked primary immune deficiency of lymphocyte function was reported in 6 male miniature dachshunds (Farrow et al., 1972). The dogs were found to develop fatal pneumonia due to *P. carinii* infection at 9–12 weeks of age.

Thymic hypoplasia, as a result of growth hormone insufficiency, was described in weimaraner dogs (Roth et al., 1980). Postnatal growth was slow, and thymus glands were small. Serum protein concentration, lymphocyte numbers in blood, and immune response were normal, but T-cell function was subnormal. Increased susceptibility to infection was common. Injection of thymosin caused clinical improvement, whereas stimulation of growth hormone production by clonidine hydrochloride was absent.

Secondary Immune Deficiency Disorders

Several conditions have been recognized in various species, but only a few will be described below.

Failure of Passive Transfer of Maternal Immunoglobulin

Failure of passive transfer of maternal immunoglobulin is the most common form of immune deficiency in foals (LeBlanc and Asbury, 1985; McClure et al., 1985; McGuire et al., 1975) and is also reported to occur in calves (McGuire et al., 1976), lambs (McGuire et al., 1983; Sawyer et al., 1977), piglets (Yaguchi et al., 1980), and goat kids. It may be complete or partial. It is the most common cause of neonatal infection and early deaths of the young in most species, particularly the horse and cow. Affected foals may develop omphalophlebitis, septic arthritis, and respiratory infections. Neonatal septicemia and diarrhea are common in calves.

Maternal antibodies provide immediate protection to the neonate from environmental pathogens until its own immune system begins to function adequately. Studies with calves have shown that such antibodies are not only bactericidal, but they are also essential for expression of normal phagocytic activity of neutrophils in the newborn. High serum Ig, particularly IgM, protects calves against death from neonatal salmonellosis by a nonspecific means (Fisher et al., 1976).

Some knowledge of the normal immune status of the newborn is essential to understanding problems associated with this type of immune deficiency. Maternal antibodies are acquired by the newborn foal, calf, lamb, piglet, and kid through consumption of colostrum within the first 24 hours of birth. In utero transfer of maternal antibodies does not occur in these animals because of their unique placental patterns and probably for reasons unknown. For example, the newborn foal is generally agammaglobulinemic at birth in that it usually has no IgG, although a small amount of IgM is present and occasionally trace levels of IgG may be found. Similarly, the fetal lamb normally synthesizes IgM and sometimes IgG_1 at late term, but not IgG_2 or IgA (Fahey and Brandon, 1978). Therefore colostrum consumption and absorption of immunoglobulins are essential to passive transfer of maternal immunity.

The intestinal epithelium of the newborn absorbs all immunoglobulins from colostrum, predominantly during the first 6 hours and at gradually diminishing levels only up to 24–48 hours of age (Cabello and Levieux, 1980; Logan et al., 1978; Sawyer et al., 1977). Some selectivity of absorption between individual classes of Igs has been observed in different species, and discontinuance of absorption occurs at different times depending on the Ig type. Subsequent inability of immunoglobulin absorption has been associated with rapid replacement of the intestinal epithelial cells during this period. Evidence has been presented to support the concept that the transfer process is mediated by membrane receptors for IgG and its Fc fragment on absorptive cells of the fetal membranes and neonatal gut (Schlamowitz, 1976; Staley and Bush, 1985).

In the newborn pig, preferential transport of IgG by a micropinocytotic process in the intestinal tract, particularly the proximal small intestine, was demonstrated (Leary and Lecce, 1979). Such selective absorption of Igs does not occur in lambs and calves; in foals, it has been reported to occur in some studies (Cabello and Levieux, 1980) but not in others (Medeiros et al., 1975). The level of passive immunity in the newborn is influenced by a variety of factors (Cabello and Levieux, 1980; Edwards et al., 1982; Halliday and Williams, 1979). Additional information can be found elsewhere (Jeffcott, 1975; Micusan et al., 1976; Perryman et al., 1980; Prokesova et al., 1981; Sawyer et al., 1977, 1978).

Normally, serum immunoglobulin levels of the foal of 24 hours of age are comparable to the adult levels. The foal begins to synthesize its own immunoglobulins by 2 weeks of life and gradually replaces the diminishing maternal antibodies which catabolize at varying rates. Thus the serum immunoglobulin levels of the foal initially decline to reach a nadir by 2 months of age and then increase again to adult levels by the sixth month. Similar observations have been reported for the calf and lamb.

Mare's colostrum is rich in IgG and IgG(T) and contains some IgM and IgA. Immunodeficient foals have very low serum levels of both IgG and IgG(T). It has been shown that serum Ig levels of 400 mg/dl or more indicate adequate absorption of colostral immunoglobulins in the foal, whereas 0–200 mg/dl constitute failure of transport and values between 200 and 400 are suggestive of partial failure. Inadequate transfer of maternal immunoglobulins to the newborn can result from a variety of causes. The most common cause in foals is colostrum that is deficient or low in IgG (<1,000 mg/dl) as from dripping mares. Inability to ingest sufficient colostrum within the first 24 hours or delayed ingestion is another cause. Malabsorption may also account for some failure of transport of sufficient immunoglobulins. In one study this was found to occur in 14% of lambs (Sawyer et al., 1977).

Prompt diagnosis and management of immune-deficient animals is important to protect from possible infections. Immunoglobulin deficiency from passive transfer in the newborn can be detected by quantitation of postcolostral serum immunoglobulin levels. This can be achieved by single radial immunodiffusion, serum electrophoresis and immunoelectrophoresis, refractometry, and Ig precipitation tests such as the zinc sulfate turbidity test.

The zinc sulfate turbidity test is the most practical means of field screening for Ig deficiency in newborn foals (Rumbaugh and Ardans, 1979; Rumbaugh et al., 1979). To perform this test, prepare zinc sulfate solution by dissolving 250 mg zinc sulfate in 1 liter of boiled water. Allow it to cool and store in a tightly capped, dark glass bottle. Add 0.1 ml of serum to 1.0 ml of distilled water in a test tube, mix, and then add 5 ml of zinc sulfate solution and mix again. After 1 hour, read optical density in a spectrophotometer at 485 nm and compare with the standard curve to obtain Ig concentration. The appearance of cloudiness or opacity is sufficient evidence that the foal suckled and absorbed colostrum.

The zinc sulfate turbidity test has also been used to test Ig levels in neonatal lambs (Logan and Irwin, 1977; Reid and Martinez, 1975) and calves (Reid and Martinez, 1975). In calves, the sodium sulfate precipitation test was found most useful for identifying complete failure of passive transfer (Igs, <800 mg/dl), although partial failure could be detected by the glutaraldehyde coagulation test (Igs, 800–1,600 mg/dl) (Hopkins et al., 1984). An ammonium sulfate precipitation test was similarly used to estimate serum immunoglobulins in neonatal pigs (Yaguchi et al., 1980). The A:G ratio was found useful in assessing adequate absorption of colostrum antibody in the newborn foal (Bauer et al., 1985).

Once a failure of transport problem is diagnosed, forced colostrum (200–300 ml) feeding can be attempted, or plasma or serum (20 ml/kg body weight) rich in immunoglobulins (maternal or frozen pool) can be given intravenously. The colostrum, plasma, and serum given should be checked for antierythrocyte antibodies to avoid fatal incompatible transfusion reaction.

Other Conditions

Several infectious diseases have been found to induce secondary immune deficiencies of either T or B cell functions or both. For example, equine herpesvirus I infection of Thoroughbred foals during the later part of ges-

tation may destroy lymphoid tissues resulting in secondary immune deficiency at birth (Bryans et al., 1977). Bovine viral diarrhea in calves suppresses both T and B cell functions, whereas cattle with Johne's disease and calves with lymphoma show primarily reduced T-cell activity. Acquired humoral deficiency was reported in a cow with *Eperythrozoon wenyoni* and *Trypanosoma theileri* infections (Baket et al., 1982). Canine distemper is associated with suppression of both T and B cell functions (Stevens and Osburn, 1976), while *Demodex canis* inhibits T-cell function. A serum factor was found responsible for immune deficiencies associated with Johne's disease in cattle and demodicosis in dogs. Immunosuppression has been observed in cats infected with feline leukemia virus and panleukopenia virus.

Immune Deficiencies of Undefined Origin

Agammaglobulinemia

Agammaglobulinemia was found in two Thoroughbreds and a Standardbred horse (Perryman, 1979; Perryman and McGuire, 1980). A sex-linked origin was suggested by the fact that all three cases were males. A deficiency of B-lymphocytes was indicated by extremely low or no serum immunoglobulin levels, functional evaluation, and histologic finding of absence of plasma cells and germinal centers. Normal T-lymphocyte functions were indicated by adequate responses to phytohemagglutinin and skin sensitization. Repeated infections and poor response to therapy were common. Death occurred by 17–18 months of age.

Selective Immunoglobulin Deficiencies

Several cases of selective IgM deficiency were described in Arabian and quarter horses (Perryman et al., 1977; Perryman and McGuire, 1980). Very low or no serum IgM was found, but levels of IgG and complement components, numbers of B- and T-lymphocytes, and response to phytohemagglutinin were normal. Clinical manifestations included poor growth and recurrent respiratory infections, beginning within the first month of life, with death occurring usually at 4–8 months of age and occasionally by 2 years.

Klebsiella sp. was isolated from joint fluids, bronchial lymph nodes, or tracheal washings from three foals (Perryman et al., 1977). Acquired IgM deficiency has been observed in horses with lymphoma (Perryman and McGuire, 1980); in such cases, it may be associated with neoplasia of suppressor T cells (Perryman et al., 1984b).

Selective IgM deficiency was found in two Doberman pinschers, but an association with clinical disease was not seen as long as IgG and IgA levels were within normal range (Plechner, 1979). A deficiency of IgA was detected in the German shepherd dogs as a breed characteristic (Whitbred et al., 1984) and in Beagle dogs from a large breeding colony (Felsburg et al., 1985).

A selective deficiency of IgG_2 was described in Red Danish Milk cattle (Mansa, 1965). Affected cattle showed increased susceptibility to gangrenous mastitis and pyogenic bacterial infections such as bronchopneumonia, peritonitis, and abomasoenteritis.

Transient Hypogammaglobulinemia

Delayed onset of postnatal immunoglobulin synthesis leading to hypogammaglobulinemia was observed in Arabian foals (Perryman and McGuire, 1980). Serum IgG and IgG(T) levels were very low at two months of age, and significant synthesis did not occur until 3 months of age, with normal response occurring by 3.5 months. Systemic bacterial and adenovirus infections were common during this undefined hypogammaglobulinemic state.

Acquired Immune Deficiency Syndrome

A naturally occurring immunodeficiency syndrome having certain clinicopathologic and immunologic features in common with the recently recognized acquired immune deficiency syndrome (AIDS) in humans has been reported in macaque (Letvin et al., 1983) and rhesus (Henrickson et al., 1983; Osborn et al., 1983) monkeys. Affected animals develop chronic diarrhea and wasting and exhibit hematologic abnormalities such as anemia, neutropenia, and bizarre immature monocytes in peripheral blood, abnormal liver function tests, and diminished T-cell responses. Death occurs from unusual disease,

neoplasia, or opportunistic infections. The etiologic agent has been defined as a type D retrovirus (Marx et al., 1984) and its nucleotide sequence has been determined (Power et al., 1986). The mechanism of T-cell deficiency remains unknown.

REFERENCES

(Titles in parentheses are English translations of foreign language titles.)

Abe, T., et al.: The α-Fetoprotein Level in the Sera of Bovine Fetuses and Calves. Jpn. J. Vet. Sci., *38*:339, 1976.

Allen, P.Z., and Dalton, E.J.: Studies on Equine Immunoglobulins. IV. Immunoglobulins of the Donkey. Immunology, *28*:187, 1975.

Allison, A.C.: Turnovers of Erythrocytes and Plasma Proteins in Mammals. Nature, *188*:37, 1960.

Allison, J.B.: Nitrogen Balance and the Nutritive Value of Proteins. J. Amer. Med. Ass., *164*:283, 1957.

Amog, V.M., et al.: Comparison of Electrophoretograms of Normal Canine Serums and Plasma and of Serum and Plasma of Hemolyzed Specimens. Amer. J. Vet. Res., *38*:387, 1977.

Anderson, I., et al.: Evidence of a Lethal Trait, A 46, in Black Pied Danish Cattle of Friesian Descent. Nord. Vet. Med., *22*:473, 1970.

Anonymous: Protein-Losing Gastroenteropathy. Lancet. *1*:351, 1959.

Apitz, K.: Die Paraproteinasen (uber die Storung des Eiweisstoffwechsels bei Plasmocytosis.) Virchows Arch. (Pathol. Anat), *306*:631, 1940.

Babel, C.L., and Lang, R.W.: Identification of a New Immunoglobulin Subclass in Three Ruminant Species. Fed. Proc., *35*:272, 1976.

Baetz, A., et al.: Plasma α-Fetoprotein Concentration in Pregnant Cows before Abortion or Parturition. Clin. Biochem., *27*:1039, 1981.

Baket, D.C., et al.: Hemoparasitism, Humoral Immunodeficiency, and an IgG1 Fragment in a Cow. J. Amer. Vet. Med. Ass., *181*:480, 1982.

Barlough, J.E., et al.: The Immunoglobulins of the Cat. Cornell Vet., *71*:397, 1981.

Barsanti, J.A., et al.: Analysis of Serum Proteins, Using Agarose Electrophoresis in Normal Dogs and in Dogs Naturally Infected with Dirofilaria immitis. Amer. J. Vet. Res., *38*:1055, 1977.

Barta, O.: Laboratory Techniques of Veterinary Clinical Immunology: A Review. Comp. Immunol. Microbiol. Infect. Dis., *4*:131, 1981.

Bartley, J.C.: Lipid Metabolism and Its Disorders. *In* Clinical Biochemistry of Domestic Animals. 3rd ed. Kaneko, J.J., ed. Academic Press, New York, 1980.

Barton, C.L., et al.: The Diagnosis and Clinicopathological Features of Canine Protein-Losing Enteropathy. J. Amer. Anim. Hosp. Ass., *14*:85, 1978.

Bauer, J.E., et al.: Serum Protein Reference Values in Foals during the First Year of Life: Comparison of Chemical and Electrophoretic Methods. Vet. Clin. Pathol., *14*(1):14, 1985.

Beckett, S.K., et al.: Blood Glucose, Serum Transaminase and Electrophoretic Patterns of Dogs with Infectious Canine Hepatitis. Amer. J. Vet. Res., *25*:1186, 1964.

Blackshaw, C.: The Measurement of Serum Haemoglobin

Reactive Protein in Selected Groups of Cattle and Its Use in Clinical Practice. N.Z. Vet. J., 27:103, 1979.

Blahd, W.H., et al.: The Turnover Rate of Serum Albumin in the Nephrotic Syndrome as Determined by I[131]-Labelled Albumin. J. Lab. Clin. Med., 46:747, 1955.

Blombäck, B., and Hanson, L.A.: Plasma Proteins. John Wiley & Sons, New York, 1979.

Bloom, F.: Intramedullary Plasma Cell Myeloma Occurring Spontaneously in a Dog. Cancer Res., 6:718, 1946.

Blum, J.R., et al.: The Clinical Manifestations of a Genetically Determined Deficiency of the Third Component of Complement in the Dog. Clinical Immunol. Immunopathol., 34:304, 1985.

Bonk, R.J., et al.: Radial Immunodiffusia for the Evaluation of Immunoglobulin Levels in Beagle Dogs. Clin. Chem., 28:1640, 1982.

Borg, L.: (Measurement of Total Protein and Immunoglobulin Content of the Blood Serum of Diseased Calves up to 12 Weeks Old by Means of Refractometry, Biuret Method, Electrophoresis and Nephelometry). Inaug. Diss. Hanover, 143 pp., 1981. Vet. Bull. 53, Abstr. No. 4769, 1983.

Bossak, E.T., et al.: Effect of Cortisone on Plasma Globulins in the Dog: Studies by Paper Electrophoresis. Proc. Soc. Exp. Biol. Med., 88:634, 1955.

Braund, K.G., et al.: Neurologic Manifestations of Monoclonal IgM Gammopathy Associated with Lymphocytic Leukemia in a Dog. J. Amer. Vet. Med. Ass., 172:1407, 1978.

Braund, K.G., et al.: Neurologic Complications of IgA Multiple Myeloma Associated with Cryoglobulinemia in a Dog. J. Amer. Vet. Med. Ass., 174:1321, 1979.

Bremner, K.C.: Relative Influence of Three Gastrointestinal Nematodes in Cattle on the Concentrations of Haemoglobin and Serum Protein in the Host. Nature, 212:429, 1960.

Bremner, K.C.: Hypoproteinemia in Oesophagostomiasis. Exp. Parasitol., 25:382, 1969.

Bruenger, F.W., et al.: Half-Periods of Serum Proteins in the Dog. Amer. J. Vet. Res., 28:1699, 1967.

Brummerstedt, E., et al.: The Effect of Zinc on Calves with Hereditary Thymus Hypoplasia (Lethal Trait A 46). Acta Pathol. Microbiol. Scand., 791:686, 1971.

Bryans, J.T., et al.: Neonatal Foal Disease Associated with Prenatal Infection by Equine Herpesvirus I. J. Equine Med. Surg., 1:20, 1977.

Buening, G.M., et al.: Immunoglobulins and Secretory Component in the External Secretions of Foals with Combined Immunodeficiency. Infect. Immun., 19:695, 1978.

Burghen, G.A., et al.: Development of Hypergammaglobulinemia in Tropical Canine Pancytopenia. Amer. J. Vet. Res., 32:749, 1971.

Busby, W.H., Jr., and Travis, J.C.: Structure and Evolution of Artiodactyla Haptoglobins. Comp. Biochem. Physiol., 60B:389, 1978.

Bush, L.J., and Staley, T.E.: Absorption of Colostral Immunoglobulins in Newborn Calves. J. Dairy Sci., 63:672, 1980.

Butler, J.E.: Bovine Immunoglobulins: An Augmented Review. Vet. Immunol. Immunopathol., 4:43, 1983.

Cabello, G., and Levieux, D.: Comparative Absorption of Colostral IgG1 and IgM in the Newborn Calf. Effects of Thyroxine, Cortisol and Environmental Factors. Ann. Rech. Vet., 11:1, 1980.

Caffin, J.P., et al.: Physiological and Pathological Factors Influencing Bovine Immunoglobulin G$_1$ Concentration in Milk. J. Dairy Sci., 66:2161, 1983.

Campbell, E.A.: The Serum Lipoproteins of the Domestic Animals. Res. Vet. Sci., 4:56, 1963.

Campbell, P.N., and Stone, N.E.: The Role of Serum Albumin as a Precursor of the Soluble Tissue Proteins and the Serum Globulins of the Rat Bearing Liver Tumors. Biochem. J., 66:669, 1957.

Campbell, R.M., et al.: Passage of Plasma Albumin into the Intestine of Sheep. J. Physiol., 158:113, 1961.

Campbell, R.S.F., et al.: Intestinal Lymphangiectasia in a Dog. J. Amer. Vet. Med. Ass., 153:1050, 1968.

Campbell, T.M., and Studdert, M.J.: Reconstitution of Primary, Severe, Combined Immunodeficiency in Man and Horse. Comp. Immunol. Microbiol. Infect. Dis., 6:101, 1983.

Carlsson, R.N.K., et al.: Isolation and Characterization of α-Fetoprotein from Foetal Pigs. Int. J. Biochem., 7:13, 1976.

Carroll, E.J., et al.: Endotoxemia in a Horse. J. Amer. Vet. Med. Ass., 146:1300, 1965.

Caspi, D., et al.: Isolation and Characterization of C-Reactive Protein from the Dog. Immunology, 53:307, 1984.

Chang, C.C., et al.: Immune Response in the Bovine Mammary Gland after Intestinal, Local, and System Immunization. Infect. Immun., 31:650, 1981.

Chaniago, T.D., et al.: Immunoglobulins in Blood Serum of Foetal Pigs. Aust. Vet. J., 54:30, 1978.

Chanutin, A., and Gjessing, E.C.: Electrophoretic Analysis of Sera of Injured Dogs. J. Biol. Chem., 165:421, 1946.

Chapman, I., and Jimenez, F.A.: Aleutian-Mink Disease in Man. New Eng. J. Med., 269:1171, 1963.

Ciupercescu, D.D.: Dymanics of Serum Immunoglobulin Concentrations in Sheep during Pregnancy and Lactation. Res. Vet. Sci., 22:23, 1977.

Cohen, S.: Plasma Protein Distribution and Turnover in the Female Baboon. Biochem. J., 64:286, 1956.

Cope, O., and Litwin, S.B.: Contribution of the Lymphatic System to the Replenishment of the Plasma Volume following a Hemorrhage. Ann. Surg., 156:655, 1962.

Cordy, D.R.: Plasma Cell Myeloma in a Dog. Cornell Vet., 47:498, 1957.

Cornelius, C.E., and Kaneko, J.J.: Clinical Biochemistry of Domestic Animals. Academic Press, New York, p. 276, 1963.

Cornelius, C.E., et al.: The Use of Glycine-1-C14 in the Measurement of Serum Protein Turnover Rates in Dairy Cows. Amer. J. Vet. Res., 20:44, 1959a.

Cornelius, C.E., et al.: Plasma Cell Myelomatosis in a Horse. Cornell Vet., 49:478, 1959b.

Cornelius, C.E., et al.: Seromucoid Levels in Normal and Hospitalized Domestic and Exotic Animal Species. Amer. J. Vet. Res., 21:1095, 1960.

Cornelius, C.E., et al.: Distribution and Turnover of Iodine-131-Tagged Bovine Albumin in Normal and Parasitized Cattle. Amer. J. Vet. Res., 23:837, 1962.

Cripps, A.W., and Lascelles, A.K.: The Biological "Half-lives" of IgG1 and IgG2 in Young Milk-Fed Lambs and in Non-Pregnant Colostrum-Forming Sheep. Aust. J. Exp. Biol. Med. Sci., 52:717, 1974.

Cripps, A.W., et al.: Quantitation of Sheep IgG$_1$, IgG$_2$, IgA, IgM, and Albumin by Radioimmunoassay. Vet. Immunol. Immunopathol., 8:137, 1985.

Csontos, G., et al.: Serum Transferrin Concentration in Foals. Acta Physiol. Hung., 63:223, 1984.

Dalgarno, A., et al.: The Effect of High- and Low-Plane Feeding on the Serum Protein Levels of Pregnant

Ewes, Foetuses, and Young Lambs. Biochem. J., 46:162, 1950.

Davidson, J.N., et al.: Relationship between Serum Immunoglobulin Values and Incidence of Respiratory Disease in Calves. J. Amer. Vet. Med. Ass., 179:708, 1981.

Deavers, S., et al.: Movement of Fluid, Albumin, and Globulins with Overtransfusion and Hemorrhage. Amer. J. Physiol., 205:995, 1963.

Desiderio, J.V., et al.: Serum Proteins of Normal Goats and Goats with Caseous Lymphadenitis. Amer. J. Vet. Res., 40:400, 1979.

Devery-Pocius, J.E., and Larson, B.L.: Age and Previous Lactations as Factors in the Amount of Bovine Colostral Immunoglobulins. J. Dairy Sci., 66:221, 1983.

Dewhirst, M.W., et al.: Idiopathic Monoclonal (IgA) Gammopathy in a Dog. J. Amer. Vet. Med. Ass., 170:1313, 1977.

DiBartola, S.P., and Reynolds, H.A.: Hypoglycemia and Polyclonal Gammopathy in a Dog with Plasma Cell Dyscrasia. J. Amer. Vet. Med. Ass., 180:1345, 1982.

Dich, J., and Nielson, K.: Metabolism and Distribution of ^{131}I-Labelled Albumin in the Pig. Can. J. Comp. Med. Vet. Sci., 27:269, 1963.

Dimopoullos, G.T.: Serum Protein and Antibody Studies in Viral Diseases: A Review. Ann. N.Y. Acad. Sci., 94:149, 1961.

Dimopouollos, G.T., and Cunningham, C.H.: Electrophoretic and Serum Neutralization Studies of Infectious Bronchitis of Chickens. Amer. J. Vet. Res., 17:755, 1956.

Dixon, F.J.: Glomerulonephritis and Immunopathology. Hosp. Pract., 2(11):35, 1967.

Dixon, F.J., et al.: The Half-Life of Homologous γ Globulin (Antibody) in Several Species. J. Exp. Med., 96:313, 1952.

Dixon, F.J., et al.: Half Lives of Homologous Serum Albumins in Several Species. Pro. Soc. Exp. Biol. Med., 83:287, 1953.

Dobson, C.: Serum Protein Changes Associated with Oesophagostomum columbianum Infections in Sheep. Nature, 207:1304, 1965.

Edelman, G.M.: Antibody Structure and Molecular Immunology. Science, 180:830, 1973.

Edwards, S.A., et al.: Factors Affecting Levels of Passive Immunity in Dairy Cows. Brit. Vet. J., 138:233, 1982.

Ek, N.: Concentration of Serum Prealbumin (PR) Protein in Sick Horses and Its Correlation to Blood Leucocyte Count and Albumin Content in Serum. Acta Vet. Scand., 21:482, 1980.

Fahey, K.J., and Brandon, M.R.: Synthesis of Immunoglobulin by Normal and Antigenically Stimulated Fetal Sheep. Res. Vet. Sci., 25:218, 1978.

Farrow, B.R.H., and Penny, R.: Multiple Myeloma in a Cat. J. Amer. Vet. Med. Ass., 158:606, 1971.

Farrow, B.R.H., et al.: Pneumocystis Pneumonia in the Dog. J. Comp. Path., 82:447, 1972.

Fell, B.F., et al.: Quantitative Changes Occurring in the Serum Proteins During Lactation in the Ewe. Res. Vet. Sci., 9:563, 1968.

Fellah, A., and Stott, G.H.: Immunoglobulin Absorption in Calves Related to the Colostral Immunoglobulin Concentration. J. Dairy Sci., 64:172, 1981.

Felsburg, P.J., et al.: Selective IgA Deficiency in the Dog. Clin. Immunol. Immunopathol., 36:297, 1985.

Fex, G., et al.: Purification of Prealbumin from Human and Canine Serum Using a Two-Step Affinity Chromatographic Procedure. Eur. J. Biochem., 75:181, 1977.

Finnie, J.W., and Wilks, C.R.: Two Cases of Multiple Myeloma in the Dog. J. Small Anim. Pract., 23:19, 1982.

Fisher, E.W., et al.: Studies on Neonatal Calf Diarrhoea. IV. Serum and Faecal Immune Globulins in Neonatal Salmonellosis. Brit. Vet. J., 132:39, 1976.

Fonnesbeck, P.V., and Symons, L.D.: Effect of Diet on Concentration of Protein, Urea Nitrogen, Sugar and Cholesterol of Blood Plasma of Horses. J. Anim. Sci., 28:216, 1969.

Fujimoto, T., et al.: Serum Concentration and Properties of Fetoprotein and Serum Level of Albumin in Suckling Piglets. Res. Vet. Sci., 36:212, 1984.

Furukawa, T., and Sugiyama, F.: Isolation of Feline Plasma Hemopexin. Jpn. J. Vet. Sci., 46:877, 1984.

Gershwin, L.J., and Dygert, B.S.: Development of a Semiautomated Microassay for Bovine Immunoglobulin E: Definition and Standardization.. Amer. J. Vet. Res., 44:891, 1983.

Gjessing, E.C., et al.: Fractionation, Electrophoresis, and Chemical Studies of Proteins in Sera of Control and Injured Dogs. J. Biol. Chem., 170:551, 1947.

Glenert, J., et al.: The Albumin Transfer from Blood to Gastrointestinal Tract in Dogs. Acta Chir. Scand., 124:63, 1962.

Gourvitch, A.E.: Relation between the Formation of Specific and Nonspecific Serum α-Globulins. Clin. Chim. Acta, 1:101, 1956.

Green, I., et al.: Hypergammaglobulinemia with Late Development of Lymphosarcoma. Arch. Intern. Med., 118:592, 1966.

Green, S.A., et al.: A Comparison of Chemical and Electrophoretic Methods of Serum Protein Determinations in Clinically Normal Domestic Animals of Various Ages. Cornell Vet., 72:416, 1982.

Groulade, P.: Clinique Canine. Vol. 1. Librairie Maloine, Paris, p. 9, 1965a.

Groulade, P.: Clinique Canine. Vol. 1. Librairie Maloine, Paris, p. 84, 1965b.

Groves, M.L., and Greenberg, R.: β$_2$-Microglobulin and Its Relationship to the Immune System. J. Dairy Sci., 65:317, 1982.

Guidry, A.J., et al.: IgA, IgG1, IgG2, IgM, and BSA in Serum and Mammary Secretion throughout Lactation. Vet. Immunol. Immunopathol., 1:329, 1980.

Gustafsson, B.E., and Laurell, C.B.: γ-Globulins in Germ-Free Rats. J. Exp. Med., 108:251, 1958.

Halliday, G.J., et al.: Parasitic Hypoalbuminaemia: Studies on Type II Ostertagiasis of Cattle. Res. Vet. Sci., 9:224, 1968.

Halliday, R.: Variations in Immunoglobulin Concentrations in Finnish X Dorset Horn Lambs. Res. Vet. Sci., 21:331, 1976.

Hammer, C.H., et al.: Complement Deficiencies of Laboratory Animals. In Immunologic Defects in Laboratory Animals. 2. Gershwin, M.E., Merchant, B., eds. Plenum Press, New York, pp. 207–240, 1981.

Harvey, J.W., and Gaskin, J.M.: Feline Haptoglobin. Amer. J. Vet. Res., 39:549, 1978.

Helen, P.L., et al.: A Study of Prealbumin in Health and Disease by Polyacrylamide Gel Electrophoresis. Indian J. Med. Res., 63:273, 1975.

Henrickson, R.V., et al.: Epidemic of Acquired Immunodeficiency in Rhesus Monkeys. Lancet, 1(8321):388, 1983.

Henson, J.B., et al.: Hypergammaglobulinemia in Mink. Proc. Soc. Exp. Biol. Med., 107:919, 1961.

Hershko, C., et al.: Storage Iron Kinetics. II. The Uptake

of Hemoglobin Iron by Hepatic Parenchymal Cells. J. Lab. Clin. Med., *80*:624, 1972.

Herz, A., and Hod, I.: The Albumin/α-Globulin Ratio in Various Physiological States in Cattle. Brit. Vet. J., *125*:326, 1969.

Holmes, D.D., et al.: Myelosarcoma (Plasma-Cell Type) in a Dog. J. Amer. Vet. Med. Ass., *145*:234, 1964.

Holzworth, J., and Meier, H.: Reticulum Cell Myeloma in a Cat. Cornell Vet., *47*:302, 1957.

Hopkins, F.M., et al.: Failure of Passive Transfer in Calves: Comparison of Field Diagnosis Methods. Mod. Vet. Pract., *65*:625, 1984.

Horowitz, S.D., and Hong, R.: The Pathogenesis and Treatment of Immunodeficiency. Monogr. Allergy, *10*:1–198, 1977.

Howard, E.B., and Kenyon, A.J.: Canine Mastocytoma: Altered α-Globulin Distribution. Amer. J. Vet. Res., *26*:1132, 1965.

Hribernik, T.N., et al.: Serum Hyperviscosity Syndrome Associated with IgG Myeloma in a Cat. J. Amer. Vet. Med. Ass., *181*:169, 1982.

Hurvitz, A.I., et al.: Macroglobulinemia with Hyperviscosity Syndrome in a Dog. J. Amer. Vet. Med. Ass., *157*:455, 1970.

Hurvitz, A.I., et al.: Bence-Jones Proteineima and Proteinuria in Dog. J. Amer. Vet. Med. Ass., *159*:1112, 1971.

Hurvitz, A.I., et al.: Monoclonal Cryoglobulinemia with Macroglobulinemia in a Dog. J. Amer. Vet. Med. Ass., *170*:511, 1977.

Inoue, T.: Possible Factors Influencing Immunoglobulin. A Concentration in Swine Colostrum. Amer. J. Vet. Res., *42*:533, 1981a.

Inoue, T.: Possible Factors Influencing the Immunoglobulin M Concentration in Swine Colostrum. Amer. J. Vet. Res., *42*:1429, 1981b.

Ishikawa, H., and Konishi, T.: Changes in Serum Immunoglobulin Concentrations of Young Calves. Jpn. J. Vet. Sci., *44*:555, 1982.

Jacobs, R.M., et al.: Serum Electrophoresis and Immunoglobulin Concentrations in Cows with Lymphoma. Amer. J. Vet. Res., *41*:1942, 1980.

Jacobs, R.M., et al.: Monoclonal Gammopathy in a Horse with Defective Hemostasis. Vet. Pathol., *20*:643, 1983.

Jeffcott, L.B.: The Transfer of Passive Immunity to the Foal and Its Relation to Immune Status after Birth. J. Reprod. Fertil. Suppl., *23*:727, 1975.

Jeffries, G.H., et al.: Plasma Proteins and the Gastrointestinal Tract. New Eng. J. Med., *266*:652, 1962.

Johansson, M.B.N., and Karlsson, B.W.: Lipoprotein and Lipid Profiles in the Blood Serum of the Fetal, Neonatal and Adult Pig. Biol. Neonate, *42*:127, 1982.

Kaneko, J.J.: Clinical Biochemistry of Domestic Animals. 3rd ed. Ch. 3. Academic Press, New York, p. 97, 1980.

Kaneko, J.J., et al.: Malabsorption Syndrome Resembling Nontropical Sprue in Dogs. J. Amer. Vet. Med. Ass., *46*:463, 1965.

Keay, G.: Serum Protein Values from Clinically Normal Cats and Dogs Determined by Agarose Gel Electrophoresis. Res. Vet. Sci., *33*:343, 1982.

Kent, J.E., and Blackmore, D.J.: Turbidimetric Measurement of IgG(T) in the Serum of Healthy Thoroughbreds and Ponies. Equine Vet. J., *17*:119, 1985.

Knop, J.G., and Rowley, D.: The Antibacterial Efficiencies of Ovine IgA, IgM, and IgG. J. Infect. Dis., *130*:368, 1974.

Kristensen, F., and Barsanti, J.A.: Analysis of Serum Pro-

teins in Clinically Normal Pet and Colony Cats, Using Agarose Electrophoresis. Amer. J. Vet. Res., *38*:399, 1977.

Kulkarni, B.A., et al.: Immunoglobulins of the Indian Buffalo. Indian J. Biochem. Biophys., *10*:216, 1973.

Lai, P.C.W., et al.: Fetal-Maternal Distribution of Ovine α-Fetoprotein. Amer. J. Physiol., *235*:E27, 1978a.

Lai, P.C.W., et al.: Bovine-Fetus-Specific Serum Proteins: Purification and Characterization of α₁-Fetoprotein and Immunochemical Identification of α₂- and β-Fetoproteins. Biochim. Biophys. Acta, *535*:138, 1978b.

LaMotte, G.M.: Total Serum Protein, Serum Protein Fractions and Serum Immunoglobulins in Colostrum-Fed and Colostrum-Deprived Calves. Amer. J. Vet. Res., *38*:263, 1977.

Larin, N.M.: The Mechanism of Immunity in Canine Virus Hepatitis. Brit. Vet. J., *115*:35, 1959.

Larson, B.L., and Kendall, K.A.: Changes in Specific Blood Serum Protein Levels Associated with Parturition in the Bovine. J. Dairy Sci., *40*:659, 1957.

Larsson, B.: The Relationship between Total Protein in Serum, Glutaraldehyde Coagulation Test and Disease in Feedlot Calves. Nord. Vet. Med., *37*:90, 1985.

Leader, R.W., et al.: Structural and Histochemical Observations of Liver and Kidney in Aleutian Disease in Mink. Amer. J. Pathol., *43*:33, 1963.

Leary, H.L., Jr., and Lecce, J.G.: The Preferential Transport of Immunoglobulin G by the Small Intestine of the Neonatal Pig. J. Nutr., *109*:458, 1979.

LeBlanc, M.M., and Asbury, A.C.: Treatment of Foals with Failure of Passive Antibody Transfer Using Plasma Obtained by Plasmapheresis. J. Equine Vet. Sci., *5*:78, 1985.

Leland, S.E., Jr., et al.: Studies on Trichostrongylus axei (Cobbold, 1879). III. Blood and Plasma Volume, Total Serum Protein, and Electrophoretic Serum Fractionation in Infected and Uninfected Calves. Exp. Parasitol., *8*:383, 1959.

Lester, S.J., and Mesfin, G.M.: A Solitary Plasmacytoma in a Dog with Progression to a Disseminated Myeloma. Can. Vet. J., *21*:284, 1980.

Letvin, N.L., et al.: Acquired Immunodeficiency Syndrome in a Colony of Macaque Monkeys. Proc. Nat. Acad. Sci., *80*:2718, 1983.

Leveille, G.A., et al.: Dietary Protein and Its Effects on the Serum Proteins of the Chicken. Ann. N.Y. Acad. Sci., *94*:265, 1961.

Liberg, P.: Agarose Gel Electrophoresis Fractionation of Serum Proteins in Adult Cattle. Acta Vet. Scand., *18*:335, 1977.

Liberg, P., et al.: The Value of the Glutaraldehyde and Formaldehyde Tests in Evaluation of the Globulin Level in Bovine Blood. Acta Vet. Scand., *16*:236, 1975.

Lock, T.F., et al.: Equine α-Fetoprotein: Isolation and Characterization. Ch. 21. *In* Equine Infectious Diseases. IV. Proc. 4th Int. Conf. Equine Infect. Dis., p. 201, 1978.

Logan, E.F., and Irwin, D.: Serum Immunoglobulin Levels in Neonatal Lambs. Res. Vet. Sci., *23*:389, 1977.

Logan, E.F., et al.: Absorption of Colostral Immunoglobulins by the Neonatal Calf. Brit. Vet. J., *134*:258, 1978.

Logan, E.F., et al.: Colostrum and Serum Immunoglobulin Levels in Jersey Cattle. Brit. Vet. J., *137*:279, 1981.

Lowery, O.A., et al.: Protein Measurement with the Folin Phenol Reagent. J. Biol. Chem., *193*:265, 1951.

Macdougall, D.F., and Dunlop, E.M.: The Metabolism

of IgG(T) in the Newborn Foal. Res. Vet. Sci., *17*:260, 1974.

MacEwen, E.G., et al.: Hyperviscosity Syndrome Associated with Lymphocytic Leukemia in Three Dogs. J. Amer. Vet. Med. Ass., *170*:1309, 1977.

MacEwen, E.G., et al.: Nonsecretory Multiple Myeloma in Two Dogs. J. Amer. Vet. Med. Ass., *184*:1283, 1984a.

MacEwen, E.G., et al.: Extramedullary Plasmacytoma of the Gastrointestinal Tract in Two Dogs. J. Amer. Vet. Med. Ass., *184*:1396, 1984b.

MacKenzie, P.K.I., et al.: Serum Immunoglobulin Levels in Sheep during the Course of Naturally Acquired and Experimentally Induced Trypanosomiasis. Brit. Vet. J., *135*:178, 1979.

Madewell, B.R., et al.: Serum Concentrations of Immunoglobulins G, A, and M in Dogs with Neoplastic Disease. Amer. J. Vet. Res., *41*:720, 1980.

Magnuson, N.S., et al.: Total Plasma Corticoid Concentrations in Horses with Combined Immunodeficiency. Amer. J. Vet. Res., *41*:826, 1980.

Makimura, S., and Suzuki, N.: Quantitative Determinations of Bovine Serum Haptoglobin and Its Elevation in Some Inflammatory Disease. Jpn. J. Vet. Sci., *44*:15, 1982.

Mansa, B.: Hypo-7s-α-Globulinaemia in Mature Cattle. Acta Pathol. Microbiol. Scand., *63*:153, 1965.

Margen, S., and Tarver, H.: Competitive Studies on the Turnover of Serum Albumin in Normal Human Subjects. J. Clin. Invest., *35*:1161, 1956.

Markel, M.D., and Dorr, T.E.: Multiple Myeloma in a Horse. J. Amer. Vet. Med. Ass., *188*:621, 1986.

Marx, P.A., et al.: Simian AIDS: Isolation of a Type D Retrovirus and Transmission of the Disease. Science, *223*:1083, 1984.

Mattheeuws, D.R.G., et al.: Compartmentalization and Turnover of 131I-Labeled Albumin and γ-Globulin in Horses. Amer. J. Vet. Res., *27*:699, 1966.

Matus, R.E., et al.: Plasmapheresis and Chemotherapy of Hyperviscosity Syndrome Associated with Monoclonal Gammopathy in the Dog. J. Amer. Vet. Med. Ass., *183*:215, 1983.

McClure, J.J., et al.: Immunodeficiency Manifested by Oral Candidiasis and Bacterial Septicemia in Foals. J. Amer. Vet. Med. Ass., *186*:1195, 1985.

McDonald, J.: Protein-Losing Enteropathy Due to Lymphangiectasia. Canine Pract., *9*(5):22, 1982.

McGuire, T.C., and Musoke, A.J.: Biologic Activities of Bovine IgG Subclasses. *In* The Ruminant Immune System. Butler, J.E., et al., eds. Plenum Press, New York, p. 359, 1981.

McGuire, T.C., and Perryman, L.E.: Combined Immunodeficiency of Arabian Foals. *In* Immunologic Defects in Laboratory Animals. Vol. 2. Gershwin, M.E., and Merchant, B., eds. Plenum Press, New York, pp. 185–203, 1981.

McGuire, T.C., and Poppie, M.J.: Hypogammaglobulinemia and Thymic Hypoplasia in Horses: A Preliminary Combined Immunodeficiency Disorder. Infect. Immun., *8*:272, 1973.

McGuire, T.C., et al.: Immunoglobulin Composition of the Hypergammaglobulinemia of Equine Infectious Anemia. Fed. Proc., *29*:435, 1970.

McGuire, T.C., et al.: Hypogammaglobulinemia Predisposing to Infection in Foals. J. Amer. Vet. Med. Ass., *166*:71, 1975.

McGuire, T.C., et al.: Failure of Colostral Immunoglobulin Transfer in Calves Dying from Infectious Disease. J. Amer. Vet. Med. Ass., *169*:713, 1976.

McGuire, T.C., et al.: Failure in Passive Transfer of Immunoglobulin G1 to Lambs: Measurement of Immunoglobulin G1 in Ewe Colostrums. Amer. J. Vet. Res., *44*:1065, 1983.

Medeiros, L.F., et al.: Colostrum Ingestion and Age connected with Physiological Variations upon the Electrophoretogram of Newborn Thoroughbred Horses. Comp. Biochem. Physiol., *50A*:595, 1975.

Mejia, E.B., et al.: Macroglobulinemia in a Dog. Can. Vet. J., *20*:28, 1979.

Methiyapun, S., et al.: Spontaneous Plasma Cell Myeloma in a Ferret (Mustela putorius furo). Vet. Pathol., *22*:517, 1985.

Meuten, D.J., et al.: Chronic Enteritis Associated with Malabsorption and Protein-Losing Enteropathy in the Horse. J. Amer. Vet. Med. Ass., *172*:326, 1978.

Meuten, D.J., et al.: Relationship of Serum Total Calcium to Albumin and Total Protein in Dogs. J. Amer. Vet. Med. Ass., *180*:63, 1982.

Micusan, V.V., and Borduas, A.G.: Preferential Transport into Colostrum of Fc Fragment Derived from Serum IgG₁ Immunoglobulin in the Goat. Res. Vet. Sci., *21*:150, 1976.

Micusan, V.V., et al.: The Role of Colostrum on the Occurrence of Immunoglobulin G Subclasses and Antibody Production in Neonatal Calves. Can. J. Comp. Med., *40*:184, 1976.

Miller, C., et al.: IgA Multiple Myeloma with Multi-System Manifestations in the Dog.: A Case Report. J. Amer. Anim. Hosp. Ass., *18*:53, 1982.

Mills, J.N., et al.: A Case of Multiple Myeloma in a Cat. J. Amer. Anim. Hosp. Ass., *18*:79, 1982.

Moegle, H., et al.: (Studies on Serum Proteins in Dogs with Renal Disease, with Special Reference to the Nephrotic Syndrome.) Zentralbl. Veterinärmed., *3*:662, 1956.

Morgan, K.L., and Bourne, F.J.: Immunoglobulin Content of the Respiratory Tract Secretions of Piglets from Birth to 10 Weeks Old. Res. Vet. Sci., *31*:40, 1981.

Mulbagal, A.N.: Studies on Serum Immunoglobulins of Buffalo (Bos bubalus bubalis): Quantitation of IgG₁, IgG₂, and IgM. Trop. Vet. J., *1*(2):23, 1983.

Mulbagal, A.N., and Keshavmurthy, B.S.: Physiochemical Studies on Serum Immunoglobulins IgG₁ and IgG₂ of Buffalo (Bos bubalus bubalis). Trop. Vet. J., *1*(2):26, 1983.

Muller, L.D., and Ellinger, D.K.: Colostral Immunoglobulin Concentrations among Breeds of Dairy Cattle. J. Dairy Sci., *64*:1727, 1981.

Muting, D., and Reckowski, H.: Protein Metabolism in Liver Disease. *In* Progress in Liver Diseases. Vol. 2. Popper, H., and Schaffner, F., eds. Grune & Stratton, New York, p. 84, 1965.

Naylor, J.M., and Kronfeld, D.S.: Refractometry as a Measure of the Immunoglobulin Status of the Newborn Dairy Calf: Comparison with the Zinc Sulfate Turbidity Test and Single Radial Immunodiffusion. Amer. J. Vet. Res., *38*:1331, 1977.

Naylor, J.M., et al.: Plasma Total Protein Measurement for Prediction of Disease and Mortality in Calves. J. Amer. Vet. Med. Ass., *171*:635, 1977.

Nielsen, K., and Anderson, S.: Intestinal Lymphangiectasia in Cattle. Nord. Vet. Med., *19*:31, 1967.

Nielsen, K., et al.: Changes in the Catabolism of Serum Immunoglobulins and Complement Components in Infected Cattle. Immunology, *35*:811, 1978.

Obel, A.L.: Studies on a Disease in Mink with Systemic

Proliferation of the Plasma Cells. Amer. J. Vet. Res., 20:384, 1959.

Obel, A.L., et al.: Light and Electron Microscopical Studies of the Renal Lesion in Dogs with Pyometra. Acta Vet. Scand., 5:146, 1964.

Orentreich, N., et al.: Intensive Chronic Plasmapheresis in Dogs. Amer. J. Vet. Res., 29:1929, 1968.

O'Rourke, K.I., and Satterfield, W.C.: Glutaraldehyde Coagulation Test for Detection of Hypogammaglobulinemia in Neonatal Nondomestic Ruminants. J. Amer. Vet. Med. Ass., 179:1144, 1981.

Orr, C.M., et al.: Plasma Cell Myeloma with IgG Paraproteinaemia in a Bitch. J. Small Anim. Pract., 22:31, 1981.

Osborn, K.G., et al.: Simian Acquired Immunodeficiency Syndrome (SAIDS) in Rhesus Monkeys. Proc. 34th Annu. Meeting Amer. Coll. Vet. Pathol. and Meeting Amer. Soc. Vet. Clin. Pathol., San Antonio, p. 117, Nov. 29–Dec. 2, 1983.

Osborne, C.A., et al.: Multiple Myeloma in the Dog. J. Amer. Vet. Med. Ass., 153:1300, 1968.

Outteridge, P.M.: Veterinary Immunology. Academic Press, Orlando, Florida, 1985.

Pascal, R.R.: Plasma Cell Myeloma in the Brain of a Rabbit. Cornell Vet., 51:528, 1961.

Patterson, D.S.P., and Sweasey, D.: An Electrophoretic Study of Serum Glycoproteins in Clinical Johne's Disease of Cattle. Res. Vet. Sci., 9:319, 1968.

Patterson, D.S.P., et al.: Plasma Enzyme and Glycoprotein Changes in Experimental Mycobacterium johnei Infection in Calves. J. Comp. Pathol., 79:79, 1969.

Patton, S., et al.: Increase of Immunoglobulin T Concentration in Ponies as a Response to Experimental Infection with the Nematode Strongylus vulgaris. Amer. J. Vet. Res., 39:19, 1978.

Pearson, R.C., et al.: Times of Appearance and Disappearance of Colostral IgG in the Mare. Amer. J. Vet. Res., 45:186, 1984.

Pedini, B., and Romanelli, V.: I. Plusmocitoma negli Animali domestici. Osservazioni e Considerazioni su di un Caso Riscontrato nel Vitello. Arch Vet. Ital., 6:193, 1955.

Peeters, H., ed.: Protein Losing Diseases. In Protides of the Biological Fluids. Elsevier, New York, Section B., p. 168, 1963.

Perryman, L.E.: Primary and Secondary Immune Deficiencies of Domestic Animals. Adv. Vet. Sci. and Comp. Med., 23:23, 1979.

Perryman, L.E.: Mechanisms of Immune Deficiency Diseases of Animals. J. Amer. Vet. Med. Ass., 181:1097, 1982.

Perryman, L., and McGuire, T.C.: Evaluation for Immune System Failures in Horses and Ponies. J. Amer. Vet. Med. Ass., 126:1374, 1980.

Perryman, L.E., et al.: Selective Immunoglobulin M Deficiency in Foals. J. Amer. Vet. Med. Ass., 170:212, 1977.

Perryman, L.E., et al.: Ontogeny of Lymphocyte Function in the Equine Fetus. Amer. J. Vet. Res., 41:1197, 1980.

Perryman, L.E., et al.: Combined Immunodeficiency in an Appaloosa Foal. Vet. Pathol., 21:547, 1984a.

Perryman, L.E., et al.: Biochemical and Functional Characterization of Lymphocytes from a Horse with Lymphosarcoma and IgM Deficiency. Comp. Immunol. Microbiol. Infect. Dis., 7:53, 1984b.

Phillips, R.K., et al.: Electrophoretic Evaluation of Sera from Dogs with Cancer. Amer. J. Vet. Res., 39:1482, 1978.

Pierce, A.E.: Further Studies on Proteinuria in the Newborn Calf. J. Physiol., 156:136, 1961.

Pierce, K.R., et al.: Serum Immunoglobulin Concentrations of Cattle in a Herd with Bovine Leukosis. Amer. J. Vet. Res., 38:771, 1977.

Pinters, J.: The Biological Genetic and Clinicopathological Aspects of Haptoglobin. Ser. Haematol., 4:12, 1971.

Plechner, A.J.: IgM Deficiency in Two Doberman Pinschers. Mod. Vet. Pract., 60:150, 1979.

Porter, D.D., et al.: Aleutian Disease of Mink. Adv. Immunol., 29:261, 1980.

Porter, H.G., et al.: Aleutian Disease in Ferrets. Infect. Immun., 36:379, 1982.

Post, J., and Patek, A.J.: Serum Proteins in Cirrhosis of the Liver. I. Relation to Prognosis and to Formation of Ascites. Arch. Intern. Med., 69:67, 1942.

Power, M.D., et al.: Nucleotide Sequence of a Type D Rebovirus SRV-1 Etiologically Linked with the Simian Acquired Immunodeficiency Syndrome. Science, 231:1567, 1986.

Preston, F.E.: Hyperviscosity and Other Complications of Paraproteinemia. J. Clin. Pathol., 32, Suppl. No. 13, p. 85, 1979.

Prokesova, L., et al.: Ontogeny of Immunoglobulin Synthesis. Production of IgM, IgG and IgA in Pig Foetuses. Dev. Comp. Immunol., 5:491, 1981.

Reid, J.F.S., and Martinez, A.A.: A Modified Refractometer Method as a Practical Aid to the Epidemiological Investigation of Disease in the Neonatal Ruminant. Vet. Rec., 96:177, 1975.

Richter, H., and Wagner, H.: (Haptoglobin in Domestic Animals. II. Qualitative Determination in Blood Plasma and Serum, Using Various Techniques.) Arch. Exp., 28:491, 1974.

Roberts, M.C.: Equine Immunoglobulins and the Equine Immune System. Vet. Annual, 15:192, 1975.

Robert, S., and Kelley, M.B.: Metabolism of Plasma Proteins in Vitro. J. Biol. Chem., 222:555, 1956.

Rosen, F.S.: Immune Deficiencies: An Overview. In Biological Basis of Immunodeficiency. Gelfand, E.W., and Dosch, H.M., eds. Raven Press, New York, pp. 1–14, 1980.

Roth, J.A., and Kaeberle, M.L.: Effect of Glucocorticoids on the Bovine Immune System. J. Amer. Vet. Med. Ass., 180:894, 1982.

Roth, J.A., et al.: Thymic Abnormalities and Growth Hormone Deficiency in Dogs. Amer. J. Vet. Res., 41:1256, 1980.

Rothschild, M.A., et al.: Factors Regulating Serum Protein Metabolism. In Protides of the Biological Fluids. Peeters, H., ed. Elsevier, New York, p. 267, 1966a.

Rothschild, M.A., et al.: Role of Hepatic Interstitial Albumin in Regulating Albumin Synthesis. Amer. J. Physiol., 210:57, 1966b.

Rowlands, G.J., and Manston, R.: Decline of Serum Albumin Concentration at Calving in Dairy Cows: Its Relationship with Age and Association with Subsequent Fertility. Res. Vet. Sci., 34:90, 1983.

Rumbaugh, G.E., and Ardans, A.A.: Field Determination of the Immune Status of the Newborn Foal. Equine Pract., 1(4):37, 1979.

Rumbaugh, G.E., et al.: Identification and Treatment of Colostrum-Deficient Foals. J. Amer. Vet. Med. Ass., 174:273, 1979.

Sandholm, M.: (Detection of Hypergammaglobulinemia in Cattle under Conditions of Practice.) Tierarztl. Prax., 2:237, 1974. Vet. Bull 45, Abstr. No. 480, 1975.

Sasaki, M., et al.: Production and Turnover of IgG1 and IgG2 Immunoglobulins in the Bovine around Parturition. J. Dairy Sci., 59:2046, 1976.

Sasaki, M., et al.: Immunoglobulin IgG1 Metabolism in Newborn Calves. J. Dairy Sci., *60*:623, 1977.

Sawyer, M., et al.: Passive Transfer of Colostral Immunoglobulins from Ewe to Lamb and Its Influence on Neonatal Lamb Mortality. J. Amer. Vet. Med. Ass., *171*:1255, 1977.

Sawyer, M., et al.: Ontogeny of Immunity and Leukocytes in the Ovine Fetus and Elevation of Immunoglobulins Related to Congenital Infection. Amer. J. Vet. Res., *39*:643, 1978.

Schalm, O.W.: Clinical Significance of Plasma Protein Concentration. J. Amer. Vet. Med. Ass., *157*:1627, 1970a.

Schalm, O.W.: Plasma Proteins:Fibrinogen Ratios in Disease in the Dog and Horse. Part II. Calif. Vet., *24*:19, April, 1970b.

Schalm, O.W.: Plasma Proteins:Fibrinogen Ratios in Routine Clinical Material from Cats, Dogs, Horses, and Cattle. Part III. Calif. Vet., *24*:6, June, 1970c.

Schalm, O.W.: Feline Infectious Peritonitis: Vital Statistics and Laboratory Findings. Calif. Vet., *25*:6, Oct., 1971.

Schalm, O.W., et al.: Plasma Protein:Fibrinogen Ratios in Dogs, Cattle, and Horses. Part I. Calif. Vet., *24*:9, Feb., 1970.

Schalm, O.W., et al.: Idiopathic Gammopathy and Plasmacytosis in a Horse. Calif. Vet., *28*:13, 1974.

Schlamowitz, M.: Membrane Receptors in the Specific Transfer of Immunoglobulins from Mother to Young. Immunol. Commun., *5*(6):481, 1976.

Schultz, R.D.: Laboratory Diagnosis of Immunological Disorders in the Dog and Cat. Cornell Vet., *68*(suppl. no. 7):235, 1978.

Schwick, H.G., and Haupt, H.: Purified Human Plasma Proteins of Unknown Function. Jpn. J. Med. Sci., *34*:299, 1981.

Setcavage, T.M., and Kim, Y.B.: Characterization of Porcine Serum Immunoglobulins IgG, IgM and IgA and the Preparation of Monospecific Anti-Chain Sera. Immunochemistry, *13*:643, 1976.

Seto, A., et al.: Immunoglobulin M Associated with Secretory Component and Immunoglobulin A Deficiency in Bovine Colostrum. Amer. J. Vet. Res., *38*:1895, 1977.

Sheldrick, R., et al.: Haemoglobin Binding Capacity of Serum as an Indicator in Infection in the Horse. Vet. Rec., *111*:128, 1982.

Shepard, V.J., et al.: Gamma A Myeloma in a Dog with Defective Hemostasis. J. Amer. Vet. Med. Ass., *160*:1121, 1972.

Shull, R.M., et al.: Serum Hyperviscosity Syndrome Associated with IgA Multiple Myeloma in Two Dogs. J. Amer. Anim. Hosp. Ass., *14*:58, 1978.

Simson. L.R., et al.: The Long-Term Effects of Repeated Plasmapheresis. Amer. J. Clin. Pathol., *45*:367, 1966.

Smith, K.M., et al.: Distribution of α-Fetoprotein in Fetal Plasma, Allantoic Fluid, Amniotic Fluid, and Maternal Plasma of Cows. J. Reprod. Fertil., *57*:235, 1979.

Splitter, G.A., et al.: Combined Immunodeficiency of Horses: A Review. Dev. Comp. Immunol., *4*:21, 1980.

Staley, T.E., and Bush, L.J.: Receptor Mechanisms of the Neonatal Intestine and Their Relationship to Immunoglobulin Absorption and Disease. J. Dairy Sci., *68*:184, 1985.

Stevens, D.R., and Osburn, B.I.: Immune Deficiency in a Dog with Distemper. J. Amer. Vet. Med. Ass., *168*:493, 1976.

Stites, D.P., et al.: Basic and Clinical Immunology. 5th ed. Lang Medical Publications, Los Altos, Calif. p. 454, 1984.

Stone, R.T., and Christenson, R.K.: The Relationship of Fetal Weight to Serum Albumin and α-Fetoprotein in Swine. J. Anim. Sci., *55*:818, 1982.

Stott, G.H.: Immunoglobulin Absorption of Calf Neonates with Special Consideration of Stress. J. Dairy Sci., *63*:681, 1980.

Stott, G.H., et al.: Colostral Immunoglobulin Transfer in Calves. I. Period of Absorption. J. Dairy Sci., *62*:1632, 1979a.

Stott, G.H., et al.: Colostral Immunoglobulin Transfer in Calves. II. The Rate of Absorption. J. Dairy Sci., *62*:1766, 1979b.

Stott, G.H., et al.: Colostral Immunoglobulin Transfer in Calves. III. Amount of Absorption. J. Dairy Sci., *62*:1902, 1979c.

Suter, M., and Fey, H.: Isolation and Characterization of Equine IgE. Zentralbl. Veterinärmed., *28B*:414, 1981.

Suter, M., and Fey, M.: Further Purification and Characterization of Horse IgE. Vet. Immunol. Immunopathol., *4*:545, 1983.

Swain, B.K., et al.: Genetic Variation in Serum Proteins in Relation to Diseases. Med. Biol., *58*:246, 1980.

Takahashi, K., et al.: IgG Type Myeloma in a Dog. Jpn. J. Vet. Sci., *42*:271, 1980.

Tams, T.R., and Twedt, D.C.: Canine Protein-Losing Gastroenteropathy Syndrome. Comp. Cont. Educ. Pract. Vet., *3*:105, 1981.

Tennant, B., et al.: Use of the Glutaraldehyde Coagulation Test for Detection of Hypogammaglobulinemia in Neonatal Calves. J. Amer. Vet. Med. Ass., *174*:848, 1979.

Thompson, G.R., and Aliferis, P.: A Clinical-Pathological Study of Aleutian Mink Disease. Arthritis Rheum., *7*:521, 1964.

Thompson, R.E., and Reynolds, H.Y.: Isolation and Characterization of Canine Secretory Immunoglobulin M. J. Immunol., *118*:323, 1977.

Tizard, I.: An Introduction to Veterinary Immunology. 2nd. ed. W.B. Saunders, Philadelphia, 1982.

Tranin, Z., et al.: IgG and IgM Antibodies in Normal and Leukemic Cattle. J. Comp. Pathol., *86*:571, 1976.

Trautwein, G.W., and Helmboldt, C.F.: Aleutian Disease of Mink. I. Experimental Transmission of the Disease. Amer. J. Vet. Res., *23*:1280, 1962.

Travis, J.C.: Immunochemical Comparison of Human and Goat Haptoglobin and α₂-Macroglobulin. Comp. Biochem. Physiol., *56B*:347, 1977.

Travnicek, J., and Mandel, L.: Haematology of Conventional and Germfree Minnesota Piglets. II. Serum Proteins and Immunoglobulins. A. Versuchstierkd., *24*:308, 1982.

Turner, J.H., and Wilson, G.I.: The Effect of Three Different Exposures to Parasitism on the Serum Proteins of Shropshire Lambs. J. Parasitol., *46*:29, No. 5, Sect. 2, 1960.

Urban, J.F., Jr.: Cellular Basis of the Nonspecific Potentiation of the Immunoglobulin E Response after Helminth Parasite Infection. Vet. Parasitol., *10*:131, 1982.

Vihan, V.S., and Sahni, K.L.: Note on the Quantitative Changes Occurring in the α-Globulin Level during Pregnancy and Lactation. Indian J. Anim. Sci., *51*(10):992, 1981.

Virella, G., et al.: Multiple Myeloma IgA Cryoglobulinemia and Serum Hyperviscosity in a Dog. Int. Arch. Allergy Appl. Immunol., *55*:537, 1977.

Wagner, B.M.: Aleutian Disease of Mink. Arthritis Rheum, *6*:369, 1963.

Wagner, M., and Wostmann, B.S.: Serum Protein Fractions and Antibody Studies in Gnotobiotic Animals

Reared Germfree or Monocontaminated. Ann. N.Y. Acad. Sci., *94*:210, Art. 1, 1961.

Waldmann, T.A.: Protein-Losing Enteropathy. Gastroenterology, *50*:422, 1966.

Waldmann, T.A.: Protein Losing Gastroenteropathies. *In* Gastroenterology. Bochus, H.L., ed. W.B. Saunders, Philadelphia, pp. 361–384, 1976.

Wasserman, K., et al.: Kinetics of Vascular and Extravascular Protein Exchange in Unbled and Bled Dogs. Amer. J. Physiol., *184*:175, 1956.

Weech, A.A., et al.: Nutritional Edema in the Dog. I. Development of Hypoproteinemia in a Diet Deficient in Protein. J. Exp. Med., *61*:299, 1935.

Weech, A.A., et al.: Nutritional Edema in the Dog. V. Development of Deficits in Erythrocytes and Hemoglobin on a Diet Deficient in Protein. J. Clin. Invest., *16*:719, 1937.

Wells, P.W., et al.: Equine Immunology: An Introductory Review. Equine Vet. J., *13*:218, 1981.

Wetterfors, J.: The Normal Passage of Serum-Albumin into the Gastrointestinal Tract and Its Role in the Catabolism of Albumin. Acta Med. Scand., *176*:787, 1964.

Whitbred, T.J., et al.: Relative Deficiency of Serum IgA in the German Shepherd Dog: A Breed Abnormality. Res. Vet. Sci., *37*:350, 1984.

Wilkie, B.N., and Markham, R.J.F.: Bronchoalveolar Washing Cells and Immunoglobulins of Clinically Normal Calves. Amer. J. Vet. Res., *42*:241, 1981.

Williams, D.A., and Goldschmidt, M.H.: Hyperviscosity Syndrome with IgM Monoclonal Gammopathy and Hepatic Plasmacytoid Lymphosarcoma in a Cat. J. Small Anim. Pract., *23*:311, 1982.

Williams, M.R., and Millar, P.: Changes in IgG2 Levels with Age in British Cattle. Res. Vet. Sci., *25*:82, 1978.

Williams, M.R., and Millar, P.: Changes in Serum Immunoglobulin Levels in Jerseys and Friesians Near Calving. Res. Vet. Sci., *26*:81, 1979.

Williard, M.D., et al.: Serum and Urine Protein Abnormalities Associated with Lymphocytic Leukemia and Glomerulonephritis in a Dog. J. Amer. Anim. Hosp. Ass., *17*:381, 1981.

Wilson, G.I., and Turner, J.H.: Serum Protein Studies on Sheep and Goats: Studies on Targhee Lambs Raised under Varied Exposure to Parasitism. Amer. J. Vet. Res., *26*:645, 1965.

Winkelstein, J.A., et al.: Genetically Determined Deficiency of the Third Component of Complement in the Dog. Science, *212*:1169, 1981.

Winkelstein, J.A., et al.: Genetically Determined Deficiency of the Third Component of Complement in the Dog: In Vitro Studies of the Complement System and Complement-Mediated Serum Activities. J. Immunol., *129*:2598, 1982.

Wintrobe, M.M., et al.: Clinical Hematology. 8th ed. Lea & Febiger, Philadelphia, 1981.

Winzler, R.J.: Determination of Serum Glycoproteins. *In* Methods of Biochemical Analysis. Vol. 2. Glick, D., ed. Interscience, New York, p. 279, 1955.

Wostmann, B.S., and Gordon, H.A.: Electrophoretic Studies on the Serum Protein Pattern of the Germfree Rat and its Changes upon Exposure to a Conventional Bacterial Flora. J. Immunol., *84*:27, 1960.

Yaguchi, H., et al.: Studies on the Relationship between the Serum γ-Globulin Levels of Neonatal Piglets and Their Mortality during the First Two Months of Life: An Evaluation for the Ammonium Sulfate Reaction. Brit. Vet. J., *136*:63, 1980.

Yamada, T., et al.: Immunoglobulin Compositions of the Feline Body Fluids. Jpn. J. Vet. Sci., *46*:791, 1984.

Zeldis, L.J., et al.: Plasma Protein Metabolism-Electrophoretic Studies: Chronic Depletion of Circulating Proteins during Low Protein Feeding. J. Exp. Med., *82*:157, 1945.

Zook, B.C., et al.: Ultrastructural Evidence for the Viral Etiology of Feline Infectious Peritonitis. Path. Vet., *5*:91, 1968.

35

Immunohematology

RED CELL ANTIGENS AND BLOOD GROUPS
IN VARIOUS ANIMAL SPECIES   991

BLOOD TRANSFUSION   993

HEMOLYTIC DISEASE OF THE
NEWBORN   996

LEUKOCYTE ANTIGENS AND ANTIBODIES
AND HISTOCOMPATIBILITY
ANTIGENS   998
Leukocyte Antigens in Humans   998
Leukocyte Antibodies in Humans   1000
Techniques to Detect Leukocyte Antigens
and Antibodies and Histocompatibility
Antigens   1000
Leukocyte and Histocompatibility Antigens
in Various Animal Species   1000
Histocompatibility or Transplantation
Antigens and Their Significance 1003

THE ANTILYMPHOCYTE SERUM   1004

PLATELET ANTIGENS AND
ANTIBODIES   1005
Neonatal Thrombocytopenic Purpura in
Pigs   1006

BONE MARROW TRANSPLANTATION   1006

AUTOIMMUNE HEMATOLOGIC
DISORDERS   1007
Autoimmune Hemolytic Anemia   1007
Autoimmune Thrombocytopenia   1018
Autoimmune Neutropenia   1025

THE LE CELL PHENOMENON AND
ANTINUCLEAR ANTIBODIES   1026
Canine Systemic Lupus
Erythematosus   1027

Immunohematology is a branch of medicine dealing with diseases of the blood whose cause, pathogenesis, or clinical manifestations have been shown to be determined by an antigen-antibody reaction. It has emerged as a distinct discipline during the last three decades and is gaining prominence in human medicine largely because of extensive investigations of blood group systems and transplantation antigens and because of important advances in recognition of the immunologic basis of disease. A similar expansion of veterinary immunohematology is under way. Knowledge of red cell antigens belonging to the different blood group systems of common domestic animals is constantly expanding. Extensive blood group studies in cattle and horses have essentially provided genetic markers that could potentially type each individual animal of the species. Moreover, the development of more potent reagents and a variety of highly sensitive testing systems clearly indicate that there are additional red cell antigens yet to be discovered.

Originally, the field of immunohematology was concerned primarily with blood grouping and related phenomena such as blood transfusion and hemolytic disease of the newborn. Now it has a wider horizon, encompassing tissue transplantation and various immune-mediated hematologic disorders. With the increase of interest in organ transplantation, the need has arisen to type tissues so that donors and recipients can be matched. Numerous transplantation antigens have been found in humans and various animal species, particularly the dog and pig, which have been used as models for transplantation studies. Most of these antigens are also present on lymphocytes and platelets. The importance of blood groups and leukocyte and platelet antigens is being extensively studied in humans and animals as the fields of organ transplantation and immunogenetics continue to expand.

Development of extremely sensitive serologic techniques, together with advances in understanding the role of complement and antibody in the pathogenesis of disease, have established the immunologic origin of certain hematologic disorders. Autoimmune hemolytic anemia is the classic example.

Several topics of interest in immunohematology are discussed in this chapter to provide a general understanding of this discipline in veterinary medicine and to stimulate further interest.

RED CELL ANTIGENS AND BLOOD GROUPS IN VARIOUS ANIMAL SPECIES

The present knowledge of blood group antigens dates back to the year 1900, when Landsteiner discovered the ABO antigens in humans and Ehrlich and Morgenroth reported finding antigenic dissimilarities of red cells of goats. Numerous red cell antigens have since been discovered in humans and animals. However, the real impetus to animal blood grouping was provided by the investigations of Irwin, Ferguson, and Stormont at the University of Wisconsin in the late 1930s and 1940s (Ferguson, 1955). Earlier studies on animal blood groups have been reviewed (Cohen, 1962; Ferguson, 1955; Wiener, 1943). A general description of blood groups of animals and related topics can be found in many recent publications (Andresen, 1984; Auer and Bell, 1980, 1981; Colling and Saison, 1980a; Ejima et al., 1980b; Khanna et al., 1979; Moore, 1976b; Moor-Jankowski and Wiener, 1972; Osterhoff, 1980; Rasmusen, 1969; Scott, 1975; Stormont, 1973, 1979, 1982; Stormont and Suzuki, 1980; Storset, 1977; Tizard, 1982; Zaleski et al., 1983). Observations on apes and monkeys (Socha, 1980), turkeys (Law, 1974), and chickens (Abplanalp et al., 1976) have been described. Information on human blood groups can be found in texts on immunohematology (Bryant, 1982; Zmijewski, 1978).

Erythrocytes of common domestic animals possess several species-specific antigens belonging to many blood group systems (Table 35–1). These antigens in different species are arbitrarily designated using the same letter system, which does not imply that the antigens are related; e.g., antigen A of dogs is not the same as the A antigen of humans. The

lack of uniformity in nomenclature and availability of specific antisera are real deterrents to advancement of blood group research, although new blood group factors are being discovered.

Blood group antigens are inherited as simple Mendelian dominant characters, with a few exceptions; e.g., the O determinant of sheep is inherited as a recessive to R (Stormont, 1951). All blood group genes but one are located on autosomes; the exception is the gene for a sex-linked antigen (Xg^a) of humans, which is located on the X chromosome. They may be inherited independently or as an inclusion group (e.g., in antigens BKG of cattle, K makes its appearance only in the presence of B and G), and they are phenotypic expressions of a di-, tri-, or multi-allelic system (Stormont, 1973). Antigens believed to be products of allelic or closely linked genes are classified together in a blood group system. Many blood group systems in various animal species are comprised of several blood group antigens. The B system of cattle, with over a thousand different alleles, is the most complex blood group system known in any species.

Antigens of all blood group systems in an individual are present on every one of its erythrocytes, with each blood group system occupying innumerable separate locations on the erythrocyte surface. The antigens are thought to be arranged in a more or less regularly patterned mosaic structure on the cell surface (Wiener and Wexler, 1963). Some of the erythrocyte antigens are also present, although in weaker concentrations, on platelets and leukocytes and in other body tissues.

Certain blood group substances can be found in soluble form in blood plasma, saliva, milk, gastric juice, meconium, seminal fluid, and ovarian-cyst fluid. Notable examples are the J antigen of cattle (Stormont, 1949), the R and O antigens of sheep (Rendel, 1957), the A and O antigens of pigs (Goodwin and Coombs, 1956; Saison and Ingram, 1962), Tr (Bowdler et al., 1971) and O (Colling and Saison, 1980b) antigens of dogs, and the Lewis antigen in humans. The Tr antigen in dogs is serologically related to human A antigen and is similar to bovine J, sheep R, and pig A antigens (Bowdler et al., 1971). Serum and red

Table 35–1.   Blood Group Systems and Related Phenomena in Humans and Animals

Species	Blood Group Systems	Blood Group Factors	Techniques Generally Used for Blood Typing	Soluble Blood Group Factors in Body Fluids	Natural Alloantibodies in Serum	Transfer of Antibodies to the Young	Causes of Isoimmune Hemolytic Anemia
Humans	14	100+	Agglutination	A, B, H, Lewis	Anti-A Anti-B	In utero	Pregnancy Transfusion
Cattle	12	80+	Hemolytic	J	Anti-J	Colostrum	Vaccination
Sheep	8	30+	Hemolytic Agglutination	R, O	Anti-R Anti-O	Colostrum	. . .
Horses	8	30+	Hemolytic Agglutination	. . .[a]	Anti-A	Colostrum	Vaccination Pregnancy Transfusion
Pigs	15	65+	Agglutination Hemolytic Antiglobulin	A, O	Anti-A Anti-E	Colostrum	Vaccination Breeding Transfusion
Bison	7	15+	Hemolytic	?	?	?	. . .
Dogs	11	15+	Agglutination Hemolytic Antiglobulin	Tr, O	Anti-B Anti-D Anti-Tr	Colostrum	Experimental only
Cats	2	2	Hemolytic Agglutination	?	Anti-A Anti-B	Colostrum	Pregnancy Experimental
Chickens	12	30+	Agglutination	?	?	?	. . .
Turkeys	7	12+	Agglutination	?	?	?	. . .

[a] . . . , not described.

cells of water buffaloes were found to have a J substance serologically related to that of cattle (Khanna et al., 1979). Suppressive genes in the homozygous state can inhibit production of soluble blood group substances; e.g., the i gene in sheep and s gene in pigs inhibit production of R and AO antigens, respectively.

Soluble blood group substances are produced in the tissues, secreted into the blood plasma, and then acquired by red cells in the circulation. Similarly, red cells of an animal lacking such an antigen can be coated with the respective antigen in vitro by incubation of red cells in plasma containing the soluble blood group substance. Erythrocytes of different ages may vary in their activity of acquired blood group factors as indicated by the increasing concentration of J antigen on bovine red cells of increasing senescence (Krötlinger et al., 1980).

Isolation of blood group factors from body fluids in pure form has made possible the characterization of their chemical nature and structure. The chemical structures of A, B, H, and Lewis substances from red cells of humans have been determined and compared (Watkins, 1966). The antigens A and B from red cells appear to be glycolipids, whereas those from secretions are glycoproteins.

However, the serologic specificity in either case is determined by the carbohydrate structure. Similar studies on animal blood groups are being initiated. The J blood group substance of bovine red cells is a lipid, while that in serum is found in lipid as well as nonlipid fractions; the lipid J substance is a glycosphingolipid, while the nonlipid J substance is probably a glycoprotein (Thiele et al., 1979). Cattle F, V, and epsilon 1 antigens were found in a sialic acid–rich fraction of the red cell membrane protein (Spooner and Maddy, 1971). The Forssman antigen present on erythrocytes of many species is a glycolipid; erythrocytes of horses, dogs, cats, and mice are Forssman-positive, whereas those of humans, cows, pigs, rabbits, and rats are Forssman-negative (Tizard, 1982).

Blood group antigens vary in antigenicity. Naturally occurring antibodies to some red cell antigens can be found, though irregularly, in normal animals that lack the respective antigens. Examples are anti-J in cattle, anti-R in sheep, anti-C in horses, anti-A in cats, and anti-A in pigs (Table 35–1). These antibodies are produced from natural exposure of the animal to similar or identical antigenic determinants (heterophil antigens) in nature. Seasonal variations may occur in levels of natural alloantibodies.

Specific antiserums or reagents for blood typing purposes can be prepared from such a natural source, but natural antibodies in animals are found against only a few antigens and are generally present in low concentrations. Hence almost all reagents for blood grouping in animals are obtained by planned alloimmunization; a few are obtained by heteroimmunization. Monospecific typing reagents are prepared by proper absorption to eliminate undesirable antibodies. Although most of the reagents are species-specific, some can be used to type certain blood groups in other species because of their cross-reactivity; e.g., anti-J of cattle can be used to type A-positive pigs (Andersen, 1962), and sheep antibodies can be used to type goat red cells (Eyquem et al., 1962; Nguyen, 1977). Some lectins have also been found to agglutinate canine red cells (Ikemoto et al., 1981; Stieler, 1979).

Techniques used for animal blood typing have been concisely outlined (Rasmusen, 1969) and vary with the species in question (Table 35–1). Saline agglutination, a satisfactory method for typing human blood, is of limited use in animal blood typing. The hemolytic test system is the method of choice for typing cattle, sheep, and goat blood because red cells of these species are not prone to agglutinate, even when sensitized with multiple doses of blood-typing antibodies (Stormont, 1962, 1973) or after removal of sialic acid residues by prolonged treatment with neuraminidase (Green and Spooner, 1977). This may be due to deep-seated antigens on the erythrocyte surface of these animals, as shown by Coombs et al. (1951) for bovine erythrocytes. Saline agglutination, however, can be used for grouping dog and pig red cells. Agglutination can be enhanced by incorporating dextran and serum albumin in the test system (Rubinstein et al., 1968) or by using papainized (Jorgensen et al., 1979) or trypsinized red cells (Edebo et al., 1980). Hemolytic and saline agglutination tests are used simultaneously in some species, such as the horse. The antiglobulin test may also be used for blood typing in some animals, e.g., the pig and dog (Colling and Saison, 1980a: Rubinstein et al., 1968; Suzuki et al., 1975).

It is very important to have an appropriate source of complement in carrying out the hemolytic test. Fresh rabbit serum is generally used, but certain reagents react better in the presence of guinea pig serum (Stormont, 1962). The serum has to be absorbed at 4° C with red cells of the species concerned to remove Forssman antibodies before it is used as a complement source. Hemolytic tests must be conducted and interpreted carefully. Erythrocytes of certain horses are intrinsically susceptible to lysis by autologous or homologous serum in the absence of complement (Suzuki and Stormont, 1972). Similarly, canine red cells are vulnerable to hemolysis when washed and suspended in virtually any neutral medium (Stormont, 1973).

The importance of blood groups in genetics and breeding is well known. Monozygotic twins can be differentiated from dizygotic twins by demonstration of blood group chimerism in the latter and not the former (Owen, 1945). Blood groups may also serve as markers for inheritance of certain biochemical and physiologic characteristics. For example, sheep with the gene for red cell antigen M also have the gene for high K^+ content in the erythrocyte (Rasmusen and Hall, 1966; Tucker, 1976). Intracellular transport of certain amino acids in sheep red cells is closely associated with the blood group C locus (Tucker et al., 1980). The potassium level of bovine red cells may be controlled by certain S system antigens (Rasmusen et al., 1974). Stress susceptibility and hemorrhagic diathesis in pigs were associated with H blood types (Rasmusen, 1977). Significance of human ABO antigens in transplantation has become established in recent years. The importance of blood groups in animals in this regard remains to be investigated further. The significance of blood groups in blood transfusion and in hemolytic disease of the newborn is discussed below.

BLOOD TRANSFUSION

Transfusion therapy is basically an attempt to replace blood or its components when life is threatened without such a restoration. Undoubtedly, it is often a life-saving measure, but it has the potential of doing as much harm as the condition it is designed to alleviate.

While this should not deter the use of transfusion in clinical practice when indicated, transfusion should be instituted with extreme caution and care. An effective and safe transfusion requires an accurate knowledge of the condition to be treated, determination of specific transfusion requirements, and cognizance of hazards and benefits associated with such a therapy (Masouredis, 1983). The book of Mollison (1983) on blood transfusion in humans is recommended for a thorough understanding of this subject.

Platelet and leukocyte transfusions in humans have been reviewed (Kelton and Blajchman, 1979; Luban, 1983; Miller and Harmon, 1983). General reviews on blood transfusions in animals may be seen for specific information (Archer and Franks, 1961; Byars and Divers, 1981; Killingsworth, 1984; Norsworthy, 1977; Owen and Glen, 1972; Pichler and Turnwald, 1985a, b; Schmotzer et al., 1985; Wright, 1962a, b). A method for exchange transfusion in foals has been described (Roberts and Archer, 1966). Successful results of exchange transfusions in dogs with a dextran-hemoglobin complex have been reported (Tam et al., 1978). The possibility of interspecies transfusion was investigated by Clark and Kiesel (1963). Some observations on granulocyte transfusions in animals have been reported (Harvath et al., 1976).

Blood for transfusion may be collected in acid-citrate-dextrose (ACD) or citrate-phosphate-dextrose (CPD) solution and used fresh or stored in cold (<10° C) up to 3 weeks for use as needed. Canine blood stored in CPD solution is more efficient in delivering oxygen than that stored in ACD solution (Ou et al., 1975). A new storage medium for canine blood was described to provide adequate preservation up to 6 weeks (Smith et al., 1978). Feline blood can be stored in ACD solution at 4° C for at least 30 days (Marion and Smith, 1983b). Survival of erythrocytes decreases with increase in storage temperature and time (Shields, 1972). Donor animals may be maintained as a ready source of fresh blood. Donor dogs and cats should be splenectomized to detect otherwise inapparent blood parasites and they should be blood typed to avoid incompatibility at least of the A blood type. They should be kept in excellent health and current on necessary vaccinations. A nutritious diet and hematinics should be provided for optimum erythropoiesis. These animals should not be bled too frequently to avoid development of iron-deficiency anemia. Dogs can tolerate repeated withdrawal of 13–17 ml blood/kg body weight every 3–4 weeks (Grunbaum and Gotter, 1973).

Transfusion of fresh compatible whole blood or erythrocytes provides full benefit of the therapy, in that infused red cells circulate in the recipient for almost their normal life span. On the other hand, incompatible erythrocytes are destroyed quickly by antibodies reactive against them that are present in the recipient at the time of transfusion or that develop shortly thereafter. Intravascular hemolysis occurs when highly incompatible red cells are infused. This process is complement-mediated and takes place within minutes of initiation of the transfusion. It is recognized by the immediate appearance of mild to severe signs of anaphylactic shock, followed by hemoglobinemia and hemoglobinuria. A massive hemolysis may be accompanied by abnormal bleeding due to consumption coagulopathy. In minor incompatibilities, the erythrocytes are destroyed slowly as antibodies against them are produced by the recipient over a period of 4–14 days. This is accompanied by a progressive anemia, icterus, and a positive direct antiglobulin test. Clinical signs and laboratory findings in either event vary with the degree of incompatibility, amount of blood transfused, and the animal species involved. Blood should be warmed to body temperature prior to transfusion and should be given slowly, particularly when stored blood is used. Patients should be watched carefully for early signs of anaphylaxis, in which case transfusion should be stopped immediately and adequate therapy should be instituted.

Red cell survival has been measured in some transfusion studies (Kallfelz and Whitlock, 1973; Kallfelz et al., 1978; Koichev, 1975, Marion and Smith, 1983a). Transfusion reactions have been investigated in dogs (Dudok de Wit et al., 1967; Killingsworth, 1984; Swisher et al., 1962; van Bree et al., 1977; Yamamoto, 1980; Young et al., 1949b, 1952), cattle (van der Walt and Osterhoff, 1969a, b), cats (Auer et al., 1982; Auer and Bell, 1983), pigs (Goodwin and Coombs, 1956; Talbot and Andresen, 1964), horses (Hata, 1973), goats (Fitzsimmons et al., 1967), and water buffaloes (Koichev, 1975).

Sensitivity to plasma proteins is generally responsible for allergic reactions seen following a transfusion. Sensitivity to leukocytes and platelets is the most common cause of a febrile reaction in humans. The sensitivity usually develops after several transfusions; however, pregnant or multiparous women may react to the first or second transfusion. The sensitivity also causes a significant reduction in graft survival (Storb et al., 1972), because leukocytes and platelets carry histocompatibility antigens.

Transmission of infection, e.g., infectious hepatitis in humans, is a serious complication of blood transfusion. Examples in veterinary medicine include parasitic diseases such as haemobartonellosis, toxoplasmosis, anaplasmosis, babesiosis, trypanosomiasis, theileriasis, and sarcocystosis, and viral diseases such as infectious hepatitis and feline leukemia virus (FeLV) infection.

Blood typing and cross-matching to select a proper donor–recipient pair is a step to safeguard against a severe transfusion reaction. Blood typing may not be feasible in general veterinary practice because of a lack of suitable reagents. Cross-matching is the most practical approach. A common procedure is saline agglutination (see Chapter 2), but it may be inadequate for certain species or under certain circumstances. For instance, hemolytic tests should be used for horses and cattle to select suitable donors, and it may be necessary to use the direct antiglobulin test to demonstrate the presence of nonagglutinating anti–red cell IgG antibodies in animals given multiple transfusions.

It is a generally accepted principle in veterinary medicine that the first transfusion can be given safely without regard to blood typing and cross-matching, while subsequent transfusions require a proper match. It is best to give properly matched blood to females even the first time to avoid primary sensitization, which carries a risk of birth of offspring that may develop hemolytic disease (see below).

Some reports on the danger of transfusion reactions following the first transfusion or after compatibility testing have appeared in recent years. In studies from Australia, it was reported that about 50–60% of group B cats may experience a severe transfusion reaction even the first time when given as little as 1 ml of a 50% suspension of group A red cells (Auer et al., 1982; Auer and Bell, 1983). No transfusion reaction was seen in group A cats given group B cells. The chance of incompatible transfusion reaction was calculated at 3 in 8 cats from the frequency of blood groups A (75%) and B (25%) and the chance (50%) of cross-transfusion ($\frac{3}{4} \times \frac{1}{4} \times \frac{2}{1}$). Blood transfusion experiments in horses indicated that despite compatibility testing, one horse died of anaphylactic shock and another was severely affected after a second transfusion 1 month later (Kallfelz et al., 1978).

Autotransfusion has been attempted in some species (Crowe, 1980; Northway, 1977; Pontois, et al., 1977). Autotransfusion avoids risks of alloimmunization to blood components, transmission of disease, and incompatible transfusion reactions. In addition, the patient itself serves as a ready source of compatible blood. In vivo survival of autologous red cells was found to be considerably longer than that of the allogeneic red cells (Gimlette, 1978; Gulliani et al., 1975). Blood for autotransfusion may be collected during surgery for immediate retransfusion or obtained prior to surgery and stored for later use. Autologous canine red cells may be stored in ACD solution for up to 6 weeks without significant reduction in viability (Owen and Holmes, 1972). Complications of autotransfusion include intravascular hemolysis, disseminated intravascular coagulation (DIC), microembolism, sepsis, and tumor metastasis (Zenoble and Stone, 1978).

Some general points and precautions to be considered while instituting transfusion therapy in animals are given below (Andresen, 1984):

1. Avoid transfusion of A-positive blood in cats (Auer et al., 1982), A-positive pig blood, J-positive cattle blood, R-positive sheep blood, and A- or C-positive horse blood in order to prevent shock or early

destruction of erythrocytes by naturally occurring alloantibodies (Table 35–1).

2. Potent antigens present on donor cells but absent in the recipient would evoke antibody formation at the first transfusion and reduce survival of donor cells in the recipient. Examples are certain E and K antigens in pigs, A antigens in dogs and horses, and certain B antigens in cattle and sheep.

3. Another transfusion given 4 days or more after the first carries a risk of a transfusion reaction.

4. If the donor erythrocytes lack antigens or have weak antigens (e.g., antigens B, D, and E in dogs), normal or significant survival of the transfused cells may be anticipated.

5. Plasma transfusion, for the first time, is considered safe, because (a) natural alloantibodies to red cell antigens rarely occur, (b) such antibodies, when present, are generally in low titers, and (c) in pigs, sheep, and cattle, soluble antigens present in the plasma of the recipient and corresponding to natural antibodies occurring in the donor plasma (Table 35–1) would cause neutralization of the donor antibodies.

6. Plasma and colostrum from suitable dams can be stored frozen to give to foals deficient in immunoglobulins (Rumbaugh et al., 1979).

HEMOLYTIC DISEASE OF THE NEWBORN

Hemolytic disease of the newborn or neonatal isoerythrolysis (NI) is a consequence of maternal alloimmune blood group antibodies gaining access to the circulation of the fetus or newborn and destroying its erythrocytes. The principle involved is that the dam becomes sensitized to "foreign" red cell antigens in one or more of the following ways: from the leakage of fetal red cells through placenta during pregnancy and at parturition; after immunization with homologous tissue vaccines or vaccines containing blood components; or after injection of incompatible blood or blood products. The dam consequently synthesizes antibodies against such antigens and remains sensitized indefinitely. Mares have been found to produce antibodies to fetal red cells as early as 56 days postconception (Tizard, 1982). Cows vaccinated with red cell alloantigens may continue to produce alloantibodies for years (in one case, 7 years) after the last inoculation (Stormont, 1977). Such antibodies enter the circulation of the fetus via transplacental passage, depending on the type of placentation, or are acquired by the newborn after colostrum consumption (Table 35–1) (Simpson-Morgan and Smeaton, 1972). Once in the blood of the fetus or the newborn, these antibodies react with specific antigens on the erythrocytes, producing an accelerated red cell destruction. Generally, the first offspring is born unaffected, but subsequent ones are affected, the severity becoming greater with the number of pregnancies involving the same sire or another sire of identical blood group. If the dam becomes sensitized through vaccination or blood transfusions, the chances are that the first offspring will be affected.

The disease has been recognized in humans and horses for the last two centuries, yet the exact etiology was not established until 1941, when Levine and coworkers demonstrated that alloimmunization with the Rh antigen is the cause of erythroblastosis fetalis in the human newborn. Subsequently, alloimmunization was found to be the cause of hemolytic disease in the newborn mule (Caroli and Bessis, 1947), horse (Bruner et al., 1948), and pig (Doll and Brown, 1954).

The incidence of NI is estimated at 8–10% in mules, 0.05–1.0% in Thoroughbred foals (Tizard, 1982), and sporadic in ponies (Clarke, et al., 1978). NI has been recognized as a problem in calves from cows vaccinated for anaplasmosis or babesiosis (Dennis et al., 1970; Dimmock and Bell, 1970; Osterhoff and Vos, 1977; Searl, 1971, 1980). Natural NI is extremely rare in the dog (Young, et al., 1951) and cat (Cain and Suzuki, 1985). An important feature of feline NI was that the affected kittens were from primiparous queens. The disease has been produced experimentally in the pig (Bruner et al., 1949), dog (Young, et al., 1949a, 1951), cow (Dimmock et al., 1976; Dowsett et al., 1978; Langford et al., 1971; Stormont, 1972), cat (Tizard, 1982), horse

(Becht et al., 1983), and chicken (Tizard, 1982).

The reader is referred to the excellent monograph of Roberts (1957) on comparative aspects of hemolytic disease in humans and animals, and additional information may be found in general (Rasmusen, 1969; Stormont, 1975) and specific reports on hemolytic disease in the calf (Searl, 1971; Stormont, 1977), piglet (Cop, 1969), and foal (Bailey, 1982; Clarke et al., 1978; Cox, 1984; A.M. Scott, 1978; Scott and Jeffcott, 1978).

The antigens commonly associated with alloimmunization of the dam and causing hemolytic disease of the newborn have been identified in certain species. In the horse, antigens most often involved in NI include Aa, Ca, Qa, and Ac, while antigens Da, Dc, Ka, Qb, Qc, and Ua are of minor importance (Bailey, 1982; Cox, 1984; Scott and Jeffcott, 1978; Stormont, 1977). In the pig, antigens involved have been of the blood group systems B, E, F, K, and L (Abe et al., 1970; Andresen and Baker, 1963; Cop, 1969; Meyer et al., 1969; Saison and Ingram, 1962). In the cow, these have been antigens of the A and F-V systems (Tizard, 1982), and in the dog, it is antigen A (Christian et al., 1949; Young et al., 1949a, 1951).

Natural antibodies to certain blood groups are found in the serum of some animal species (Table 35–1) and may appear in the colostrum, e.g., anti-A in pigs, anti-J in cattle, and anti-R in sheep. However, offspring of such dams are not affected. This is thought to be due to the absence of the corresponding antigen on erythrocytes at the time of birth and the presence of the soluble blood group factor in the gastric juice and plasma of the newborn. The former makes the red cells refractory to the antibody, and the latter may neutralize the ingested antibody, first in the stomach and then in the circulation. Absorption of maternal anti-E_a antibodies from the colostrum did not cause hemolytic anemia in E_a-positive piglets, although the red cells were found to be Coombs-positive for 1 week (Linklater, 1972). Bailey (1982) performed a thorough study of anti–red cell antibodies in the serum and colostrum of mares and its relationship to NI. Serum contained antibodies to many red cell antigens, but most commonly to the antigen Ca. Although anti-Ca antibodies were also most frequent in colostrum and were found in high titers, they were not associated with NI. NI developed in a foal consuming colostrum containing anti-Aa. Anti-Qa was not found. In comparison, in a study of 67 cases of NI in horses, Cox (1984) found a high association of the disease with anti-Aa (27 cases), anti-Ca (18 cases), anti-Qa (10 cases) and anti-Ac (5 cases). Observations on breed differences in natural occurrence of anti–red cell antibodies in horses and ponies and their relevance to NI have been made (Bailey, 1982; Clarke et al., 1978; Cox, 1984; Scott and Jeffcott, 1978).

Antibodies in the serum, colostrum, and early milk of the dam and in the serum of the newborn can be detected by appropriate serologic tests. The colostrum usually contains higher concentrations of the antibody than the serum. Sensitization of erythrocytes of the newborn can be demonstrated by the complement-mediated hemolytic test or the direct antiglobulin test (see Chapter 2). For example, to diagnose NI in a calf, prepare a 2.5–3% suspension of saline-washed red cells of the affected calf. To 0.1 ml of the cell suspension, add an equal amount of fresh rabbit serum (complement). Check for hemolysis after incubation at 23–30° C for 1 hour (Stormont, 1977). The antibody can be eluted from the erythrocytes by heat (50–56° C) and is generally of the IgG class.

Animals are generally born healthy but develop the hemolytic syndrome within a few hours to days after ingestion of colostrum. Affected animals show mild to severe signs typical of hemolytic anemia—weakness, hemoglobinemia, hemoglobinuria, pale mucous membranes, and icterus (Appendix Case 58). Neutrophils and monocytes with phagocytosed erythrocytes and sideroleukocytes may be found in anemic and icteric foals (Sonoda et al., 1972). Piglets with NI may also show thrombocytopenic purpura and neutropenia (Linklater et al., 1973). Piglets may also develop neonatal isoimmune (alloimmune) thrombocytopenia from absorption of colostral antiplatelet antibodies (Linklater, 1971).

Severity of NI depends on (a) concentration of the antibody in the serum and colostrum of the dam; (b) the amount of antibody entering the serum of the newborn (this would depend on the amount of colostrum ingested and the absorptive capacity of the digestive tract of the young); and *(c)* the nature of the antigen–antibody reaction. Severely affected animals may die within 24 hours from acute respiratory distress, but death in the majority of untreated cases occurs within 2–6 days. Death is attributed to DIC resulting from activation of the coagulation system by the lysed red cells (Dimmock et al., 1976; Tizard, 1982). At necropsy, hepatomegaly and splenomegaly may be found, and histopathologic examination reveals degenerative changes in the liver and kidneys. Some animals may recover within a few weeks. The natural incidence of the disease varies with the species and may be influenced by the geographic distribution of different blood group factors in a random animal population. The occurrence and incidence of NI in calves was shown to be directly related to the number of doses of anaplasma vaccine injected and their proximity to calving (Searl, 1980).

Treatment of the affected animal consists of blood transfusion, given intravenously or intraperitoneally. An exchange transfusion may be given when the red cell parameters fall below a critical level for the species. Roberts and Archer (1966) stated that an exchange transfusion should be performed in the foal as soon as the red cell parameters fall to or below the following: PCV, 10%; RBC count, 2 million/μl; and hemoglobin, 4 g/dl. They also advise exchange transfusion when bilirubin is above 18–20 mg/dl. A healthy, compatible horse is an ideal donor, but difficult to find. Alternatively, thoroughly washed (at least three times with isotonic saline) red cells of the dam may be transfused with favorable results (Scott and Jeffcott, 1978). Corticosteroids may be given to reduce immune elimination of red cells.

The possibility of an offspring experiencing hemolytic disease can be determined by testing the sire's red cells against the dam's serum during pregnancy. In case of a positive finding, foster-feeding the young for the first 2 days before allowing it to suckle the dam would preclude development of the hemolytic disease. Such animals should be given antibiotics as a prophylactic measure against bacterial infections. A practical approach to prevention of sensitization of women and development of hemolytic disease of the newborn has been to inject anti-Rh antibodies to mothers at risk soon after delivery.

LEUKOCYTE ANTIGENS AND ANTIBODIES AND HISTOCOMPATIBILITY ANTIGENS

The knowledge of leukocyte antigens and antibodies has evolved for the most part from studies in humans. Numerous leukocyte antigens have been recognized in humans over the last two decades, and similar studies on various animal species have been initiated or expanded. Various leukocyte antigens include histocompatibility or transplantation antigens, blood group or red cell antigens, leukocyte-specific antigens, and some unidentified antigens. Transplantation antigens may be defined as those antigens on the cells and tissues that, after grafting, induce an immune response in the host resulting in a rejection phenomenon (Kissmeyer-Nielsen and Thorsby, 1970). Such antigens have been found on leukocytes of humans and many animal species. A few lymphocyte-specific and neutrophil-specific antigens have also been recognized in humans, but these are not considered transplantation antigens. Human leukocytes have been found to contain several blood group factors in minute quantities, but the evidence is equivocal except for antigens A and B (Dausset and Tangün, 1965; Walford, 1969). In animal studies, porcine red cell antigens of systems A, E, G, and N (Newman and Antczak, 1983; Simon and Hojny, 1972), bovine B system and J antigens (Schmid et al., 1978), and ovine B system and R antigens (Schmid et al., 1978) have been found on lymphocytes of the respective species.

Leukocyte Antigens in Humans

Current universal interest in leukocyte antigens began following demonstration of the human leukocyte antigen "Mac" by Dausset, the antigens 4[a] and 4[b] by van Rood, and the antigens LA1 and LA2 by Payne (van Rood and Eernisse, 1968) and their recognition as potential transplantation antigens. The World Health Organization and International Histocompatibility Workshops have contributed immensely to development and standardization in this field. Well-defined human leukocyte (lymphocyte) antigens (HLA) are considered gene products of four separate loci designated HLA-A, HLA-B, HLA-C, and HLA-D (Terasaki et al., 1981). Antigens of the first three loci are recognized by serologic tests (e.g., lymphocyte cytotoxicity test), while HLA-D antigens are defined by mixed lymphocyte reaction (culture), or MLR. Hence they are, respectively, also known as serologically defined (SD) and lymphocyte-defined (LD) antigens. Some HLA-D antigens present on B-lymphocytes are also detected by serologic tests; these are called HLA-DR (for D-related) antigens, and some such antigens have also been found in dogs, pigs, and cattle (Newman and Antczak, 1983). Each HLA locus controls inheritance of many antigens. At an International Histocompatibility Workshop, well-defined antigens are given their proper locus designations, while newly recognized antigens are assigned a "w" (for "workshop") prefix until further confirmation.

Several excellent monographs and reviews summarize early (Killman, 1960; Kissmeyer-Nielsen and Thorsby, 1970; van Rood and Eernisse, 1968; Walford, 1960, 1969) and more recent (Ferrone and Soldheim, 1982; Gotze, 1977; Kissmeyer-Nielsen, 1981; Parham and Strominger, 1982; Perkins, 1979; Rodey, 1981; Terasaki et al., 1981; van Rood et al., 1984) literature on this subject. Proceedings of recent histocompatibility workshops should be consulted for current updates of this ever growing field of immunohematology.

The knowledge of inheritance of HLA antigens has greatly expanded in recent years. The HLA loci are situated in close proximity on a small segment of the short arm of chromosome 6. This genetic region is termed the major histocompatibility complex (MHC), and its gene products constitute the major histocompatibility system (MHS). Several minor histocompatibility systems have also been recognized. Observations in humans and animals indicate that the MHC region also contains immune-response genes and genes for some complement components and select red cell enzymes. These findings form the basis of recognition of different regions within the MHC in various species: The Class I region controls antigens demonstrated serologically (HLA-A, HLA-B, and HLA-C antigens) and playing a predominant role in transplantation; the Class II region controls antigens demonstrated by MLR (HLA-D antigens), immune responsiveness to particulate antigens, and graft versus host reaction; and the Class III region controls expression of certain complement components (Svejgaard et al., 1983; van Dam, 1981).

The antigens at each HLA locus are controlled by mutually exclusive multiple allelomorphic genes. This means that in a given instance only one allele is present at each locus on each chromosome of the pair. Therefore, phenotypically, only two antigens from each locus (A, B, C, or D) can be present in an individual, and a parent can thus pass on to a child only one antigen from each locus. Thus if there are four siblings, each will have a 1 in 4 or 25% probability of being identical to another sibling. This chromosomal combination of genetic determinants from each locus (from one parent) is called a *haplotype* and is significant in organ transplantation. Because of linkage disequilibrium, certain combinations of HLA loci antigens (haplotypes) occur much more frequently than expected by chance (Terasaki et al., 1981).

Various human leukocyte antigens form a component of the cell surface membrane with some subcellular location. Highly purified, soluble HLA-A and HLA-B antigens seem to be composed of two asymmetric polypetide chains, one larger (molecular weight 43,000) and the other smaller (MW 12,000) bound by noncovalent bonds. The larger chain has some carbohydrate residues and carries the HLA specificity, whereas the smaller chain is a β_2-microglobulin. This structural configuration indicates some homology between antigens of these loci and the IgG molecule. HLA-DR antigens similarly have two chains (MW 35,000 and 28,000), but lack the β_2-microglobulin. Biochemical characterization of some MHS antigens in the dog, pig, and cow has yielded generally similar information (Newman and Antczak, 1983).

Leukocyte Antibodies in Humans

Leukocyte antibodies are, in almost all instances, acquired by alloimmunization. *Acquired isoantibodies* to leukocytes develop after multiple transfusions, during pregnancy (usually in multiparous females), after immunization with skin grafts or leukocytes, and after organ transplantation. The frequency of encountering leukocyte antibodies increases with the number of transfusions or pregnancies. Serums from such individuals have been generally used for leukocyte typing, but they are usually multispecific, i.e., they carry antibodies to several leukocyte antigens. However, serums from multiparous women are less multispecific. Serums having a narrower or limited specificity can best be obtained by planned immunization of subjects lacking the antigens against which antiserum is to be developed. A "monospecific" serum for leukocyte typing is prepared by repeated absorptions with leukocytes from many (at least 30) individuals. Similar procedures have been used to obtain antibodies for leukocyte typing in animals.

The occurrence of *natural isoantibodies* to leukocytes has not been conclusively demonstrated. *Autoantibodies* to leukocytes have been found in human patients with connective-tissue diseases, cirrhosis, viral infections, leukemia, and drug allergy (Killman, 1960; Logue and Shimm, 1980). Neutropenia or agranulocytosis has been observed in association with such autoantibodies in some cases (Finch, 1983; Logue and Shimm, 1980).

Leukocyte antibodies in vitro inhibit mobility and phagocytic activity and induce cytopathic changes leading to leukocytolysis and in vivo produce leukopenia. A febrile reaction and anaphylaxis may develop following an intravenous injection of a potent antileukocyte serum. These effects of antileukocyte antibodies are not species-specific, for a certain degree of cross-reactivity has been found.

Techniques to Detect Leukocyte Antigens and Antibodies and Histocompatibility Antigens

Several techniques have been used to detect leukocyte antigens and antibodies (Ferrone and Soldheim, 1982; Zmijewski, 1978). Those commonly used are leukoagglutination, lymphocyte-cytotoxicity, and complement-fixation tests (see Kissmeyer-Nielsen and Thorsby, 1970 for details). These techniques vary in sensitivity, and it is said that no single technique is completely suitable. However, the lymphocyte-cytotoxicity test is at present the method of choice. Reliable and simple microprocedures have been developed to conserve "monospecific" antiserums (0.001 ml). This has been a major achievement in the field of tissue typing, and consequently the micro-lymphocytotoxicity test is used as an international standard method. As mentioned previously, this test detects antigens of the HLA-A, -B, and -C systems or corresponding antibodies. It also detects HLA-DR antigens present on B-lymphocytes and monocytes, but not on T-lymphocytes, granulocytes, platelets, or erythrocytes (Kissmeyer-Nielsen, 1981).

The degree of compatibility between two individuals (histocompatibility matching) without regard to knowledge of their HLA identity can be assessed by the MLR test.

Leukocyte and Histocompatibility Antigens in Various Animal Species

Some human leukocyte antigens are partially or wholly represented on leukocytes of several animal species (Walford, 1960). Many human leukocyte and platelet alloantigens are shared by nonhuman primates (Hiller and Shulman, 1969). This has given impetus to immunization of nonhuman primates, for instance, the chimpanzee, to obtain monospecific antileukocyte serums for HLA typing of humans. Normal sera from parous cows have been found to cross-react with antigens of the HLA system and other human leukocyte antigens (Iha et al., 1973; Newman and Antczak, 1983). Cross-reactivity between some HLA antigens and streptococcal M proteins has been demonstrated (Hirata and Terasaki, 1970).

Research on leukocyte antigens in various animal species over the last decade has unveiled several antigenic systems in common domestic animals (Newman and Antczak, 1983; van Dam, 1981; Vriesendorp, 1979; Vriesendorp et al., 1972). These antigens seem to constitute an MHS, which is referred to by an acronym specific for each species. Although the basis for formulation of such an acronym has been inconsistent, it has followed a pattern similar to the HLA system in humans (Table 35–2). Evidence for existence of these systems evolved from demonstration of various antigens by serologic, graft-survival, MLR, and immunogenetic studies.

International conferences and workshops are being held to standardize methodology and develop a unifying system of nomenclature of lymphocyte antigens of various animal species. This has entailed comparison of established methods used in HLA typing, testing a panel of selected lymphocyte samples against well-defined lymphocytic alloantisera from different laboratories, and performing computer analyses to detect patterns defining distinct specificities. Evidence from genetic studies, when available, is also included to substantiate these findings. Brief comments about the MHS in various domestic animals are given below; for details see recent reviews (Dixon, 1982; Newman and Antczak, 1983; van Dam, 1981; Vriesendorp, 1979; Zaleski et al., 1983).

Typing reagents have been obtained from a variety of sources such as planned immunization (skin grafts and lymphocyte preparations), pregnant females, and colostrum

(Amorena and Stone, 1982; Cohen and Kozaki, 1969; Cullen et al., 1982; Ejima et al., 1980a; Epstein et al., 1968; Lazary et al., 1980a, b; Newman and Antczak, 1983). Lymphocyte cytotoxic antibodies, presumably resulting from transplacental immunization of the fetus, have been found in sera of parous females of different animal species with a frequency of about 85–100% in horses (Newman and Antczak, 1983; Zachary, 1983), 57% in ewes (Cullen et al., 1982), 45% in cows (Amorena and Stone, 1982), and 20% in goats (Newman and Antczak, 1983). Antilymphocyte antibodies may be found in 30–40% first-calf heifers (Newman and Antczak, 1983); these antibodies are of the IgG and IgM types (Newman and Hines, 1980). A newborn calf may acquire cytotoxic antibodies from colostrum consumption (Amorena and Stone, 1982). Bovine red cell typing reagents have been found to contain antibodies against lymphocyte antigens, but the two groups of antibodies seem to be directed against distinct cellular antigens rather than antigens in common (Ostrand-Rosenberg and Stormont, 1974).

The Committee on Nomenclature of DLA [dog lymphocyte antigen] Determinants (Anonymous, 1977) recognized three Class I loci (DLA-A, B, C) and one Class II locus (DLA-D). Subsequently, one more Class II

Table 35–2. Major Histocompatibility System (MHS) in Different Animal Species[a]

Species	Term for MHS	Loci or antigens defined[b]
Cattle	BoLA	17 specificities recognized; 1 to 2 SD loci and 2 LD loci suggested
Chicken	B	15 SD antigens
Chimpanzee	ChLA	14 SD antigens on 2 loci; 5 antigens on 1 LD locus
Dog	DLA	19 antigens on 3 SD loci; 10 antigens on 2 LD loci
Goat	GLA	9 SD antigens on 2 loci; 1 LD locus antigen recognized
Guinea pig	GPLA	6 SD antigens on 2 loci; 3 LD antigens on 3 loci; 1 DR antigen
Horse	ELA	11 specificities—10 on 1 locus and 1 on another
Human	HLA	3 SD loci and 1 LD locus on chromosome 6
Mouse	H-2	Many antigens; 3 SD loci (K, D, L) and 2 LD loci (A, E) on chromosome 17
Rabbit	RLA	About 10 SD antigens on 2 loci; 5 antigens on 1 LD locus
Rat	RT1	13 SD antigens on 2 loci; 12 LD antigens on 2 loci
Rhesus monkey	RhLA	24 SD antigens on 2 SD loci; 1 more SD locus postulated; 1 major LD locus and 1 minor LD locus
Sheep	OLA	12 antigens on 2 loci; 1 other antigen recognized
Swine	SLA	20 SD antigens on 3 loci; 6 LD antigens on 1 LD locus

[a]Modified from van Dam, 1981, with additional information from Anonymous, 1982; Bull, 1983; Newman and Antczak, 1983; Stear and Spooner, 1981; van Dam et al., 1979; Vriesendorp, 1979; Zaleski et al., 1983.
[b]SD, serologically defined or Class I; LD, lymphocyte-defined or Class II; DR, D-related antigens demonstrated serologically or Class III antigens.

locus (DLA-E) was described (Vriesendorp, 1979). The number of antigens demonstrated for these loci so far have been: DLA-A, 8 antigens; DLA-B, 7 antigens; DLA-C, 4 antigens; DLA-D, 9 antigens; and DLA-E, 1 antigen (Newman and Antczak, 1983). Phenotypic expression of Class I DLA antigens varies greatly among dogs of various breeds, particularly between mongrels and purebred beagles (Newman and Antczak, 1983). The importance of DLA antigens in organ transplantation has been demonstrated in several studies (see next section).

In the first bovine lymphocyte antigen (BoLA) workshop, 11 specificities were recognized (Spooner et al., 1979). In the second BoLA workshop, 10 of the 11 specificities were confirmed and an additional 6 specificities were designated (Anonymous, 1982). Two of the additional specificities formed subgroups of a previously defined specificity (W6), and 4 were new. The data from this workshop were consistent with the hypothesis that BoLA antigens are controlled by a series of codominant alleles at a single autosomal locus. However, some workers have suggested the possibility of three to four loci (Stear et al., 1982; van Dam, 1981). Significant breed differences have been found in the frequency of various BoLA antigens (Newman and Antczak, 1983; Stear et al., 1982). Bovine lymphocytes were also found to have the J substance, and some cross-reactions have been detected between HLA and BoLA systems.

As many as 26 distinct swine lymphocyte antigens (SLA) have been defined (Renard et al., 1982), and some soluble SLA antigens have been found in plasma or serum of pigs (Chardon et al., 1977). All of these antigens are also present on platelets. There is some evidence that some erythrocyte antigens (of A, E, G, and N systems) are also shared by lymphocytes (Newman and Antczak, 1983; Simon and Hojny, 1972). In addition to the clinical application of SLA antigens in pigs, i.e., in choosing pigs as experimental models for organ transplantation, it is becoming increasingly apparent that SLA antigens are also important in breeding and selection of pigs.

Six lymphocyte specificities, W1 through W6, were defined during the first international workshop on lymphocyte alloantigens of the horse (Bull, 1983). It was concluded that the specific antisera defined alleles of a single genetic region, the ELA region, and that this genetic region probably constitutes the MHC in the horse. Five additional antigens were defined at the second international workshop (Newman and Antczak, 1983). Thus a total of 11 antigens were defined; of these, 10 antigens, W1 through W10, are believed to be present on one locus (Ely-1) and 1 antigen on a locus (Ely-2) not linked to the ELA region. Sixteen antigens possibly belonging to three separate loci were described in a recent study (Zachary, 1983). The ELA antigens are also present on platelets but not on erythrocytes. ELA antibodies have been found in sera of 85–100% of multiparous and primiparous mares sampled within two weeks of foaling, and in colostrum of about 43% of mares (Newman and Antczak, 1983; Zachary, 1983). Foals nursing on such mares did not show any pathologic changes.

Numerous lymphocyte antigens have been detected in the sheep (Cullen et al., 1982; Forschner, 1975; Schmid et al., 1975; Stear and Spooner, 1981). Family studies indicate that many of these antigens fall under a single genetic system controlled by the autosomal codominant genes of at least two linked loci (Cullen et al., 1982; Stear and Spooner, 1981). Sheep lymphocyte antigens constitute the OLA (ovine lymphocyte antigens) system. Over 50% of pregnant ewes may contain cytotoxic antibodies in their sera (Newman and Antczak, 1983).

Studies on goats have been limited. The MHS of goats seems to consist of at least two SD and one LD loci with several different specificities (van Dam et al., 1979, 1980). Cytotoxic antibodies were found in postpartum serums of about 20% of does (Newman and Antczak, 1983).

A preliminary study of the feline histocompatibility system (Pollack et al., 1982) indicated that unlike most species, cats do not appear to develop lymphocyte cytotoxic antibodies in response to pregnancy or transfusion, although some cats have natural allolymphocytotoxic antibodies. Cats also show only relatively weak MLR between unrelated cats of different breeds.

Histocompatibility or Transplantation Antigens and Their Significance

The ABO and HLA antigens are strong transplantation antigens in humans because they are present, although in differing concentrations, in many tissues including the skin, kidneys, heart, liver, lungs, leukocytes, and platelets. Neutrophils contain far fewer antigens than lymphocytes. Soluble HLA antigens are found in plasma and urine. The HLA antigens are not found on erythrocytes, although some may be present on reticulocytes. In mice, H-2 antigens are found on red cells.

The significance of histocompatibility antigens varies (Parham and Strominger, 1982). It is becoming increasingly apparent that they play a central role in immune responses through regulation of T-lymphocyte responses (see Chapter 30). The HLA system is the most polymorphic system known in humans (Terasaki et al., 1981). Hence lymphocyte antigens, like red cell antigens, appear to be suitable markers for anthropologic studies and paternity testing. Similarly, ancestral relationships of different breeds of an animal may be investigated. In animal species, correlations of these antigens with certain physiologic traits such as body weight and productivity and breeding are also being made. Information summarized below emphasizes the importance of histocompatibility antigens in various clinical situations in human medicine.

It is now accepted that ABO compatibility is a prerequisite for transplantation. The importance of HLA antigens as the histocompatibility antigens has been demonstrated in numerous in vitro and in vivo experiments. Survival of skin grafts and kidney transplants is longer in HLA-identical siblings. The correlation between the HLA typing and the survival of skin grafts is better in HLA-compatible siblings than in HLA-compatible unrelated individuals. This is explained by the assumption that the latter may have differences with regard to transplantation antigens that cannot be detected by present methods. It has become evident in recent years that HLA-B antigens are more important in graft survival than are antigens of A and C loci, and that HLA-D and HLA-DR are important for survival of renal grafts.

Transplantation experiments in dogs have shown that DLA typing is of some value in graft survival. Allografts of skin, small bowel, kidney, heart, liver, pancreas, and bone marrow from DLA-identical littermates survived significantly longer than grafts from DLA-nonidentical littermates (Dausset et al., 1971; Rapaport et al., 1972; Vriesendorp et al., 1972). Epstein and coworkers (1971) reported a significantly improved survival of irradiated dogs receiving a marrow graft when donor and recipient typed identical in the cytotoxicity test with four serums the authors had produced. This was true for both littermate and unrelated donor–recipient combinations. A few dogs were alive well beyond 1 year. When an intensive course of immunosuppression with methotrexate was given after grafting, it was possible to prolong the life of dogs receiving grafts from mismatched, unrelated dogs.

It is obvious, therefore, that histocompatibility testing is of great importance in selecting suitable donors for allografting. Although it may not always be possible to have a perfect match, selection of compatible donors can reduce the need for immunosuppressive therapy.

As mentioned earlier, transfusions can induce formation of leukocyte antibodies as a result of an immunologic response directed against "foreign" alloantigens on the leukocytes and platelets. Histocompatibility testing is valuable in selecting compatible donors, particularly if the patient is to be given repeated transfusions. Such testing would probably also minimize rejection phenomena if the patient were to receive an organ transplant. Survival of marrow grafts is considerably reduced in dogs receiving a single or multiple blood transfusions (Storb et al., 1972). The presence of preformed lymphocytotoxic antibodies in some recipients has been associated with hyperacute rejection of kidney transplants in humans. Similarly, leukocyte antibodies are implicated in causation of most instances of febrile transfusion reactions.

Leukocyte antibodies found in serums of pregnant and multiparous women are formed during pregnancy in response to "foreign" HLA antigens on the fetal cells. The majority of these antibodies are of the IgG type and can, therefore, cross the placental barrier. It may be anticipated that these antibodies would cause a serious problem in the developing fetus. However, the reaction is both mild and rare. HLA antibodies have not been found to produce neonatal leukopenia, although they may induce *neonatal thrombocytopenia* or *isoimmune neonatal purpura.* Non-HLA antibodies have been shown to be involved in the development of *isiommune neonatal neutropenia.* Similar studies on animal species have revealed leukocyte antibodies and associated leukopenia in newborns in some instances, e.g., in pigs (Linklater, 1973), calves (Dimmock et al., 1976), and foals (Leidl et al., 1980; Schmid et al., 1980).

Observations are being made on the relationship of certain HLA antigens to susceptibility to disease in humans (Perkins, 1979; Svejgaard et al., 1983). In general, more correlations have been found with HLA-D/DR antigens than with HLA-A and HLA-B antigens. Two examples are given: the HLA-B8, DR3 haplotype is associated with many autoimmune diseases; and about 90% of patients with ankylosing spondylitis have HLA-B27 antigen, whereas controls show an incidence of only 9.4%. Studies in mice have shown that a relationship exists between the MHS (the H-2 system) and malignancy (Walford, 1969). Similar disease associations are being investigated in other animal species; some observations have been made in dogs, pigs, and cattle (Newman and Antczak, 1983).

THE ANTILYMPHOCYTE SERUM

Interest in the antilymphocyte serum (ALS) as a potent immunosuppressive agent in transplantation immunity has gained prominence since the demonstration of its usefulness in suppressing a delayed hypersensitivity reaction (Inderbitzin, 1956; Waksman et al., 1961) and homograft rejection (Woodruff and Anderson, 1963). A monograph and several reviews have been written about the ALS (James, 1968; Shanfield and MacLean, 1969;

Sheil and Rogers, 1969; Taub, 1970; Vegh and Petri, 1978; Wolstenholme and O'Connor, 1967; Woodruff, 1971).

ALS has been prepared using lymphoid cells and their subcellular fractions. Sources of lymphoid cells have been the lymph nodes, spleen, thymus, thoracic duct, blood, and cultured lymphocytes. Immunization with splenic cells regularly results in the production of hemagglutinins and platelet antibodies, which are difficult to absorb without a reduction in immunosuppressive activity. A variety of routes of immunization, injection schedules, and animal species have been used. The use of adjuvants yields more effective but toxic antiserums. Antiserums harvested earlier during the course of the immunization period have fewer side effects than serums obtained after a prolonged immunization. Heterologous antiserums seem to be more effective immunosuppressants than alloimmune antiserums. ALS is species-specific, but some cross-reactivity may exist. Purified IgG, obtained from ALS after proper fractionations and after absorption with extracts of the liver, lungs, kidneys, or bone marrow, appears to have increased specificity and reduced toxicity.

In vitro effects of ALS are as follows: (1) agglutination of lymphocytes without involvement of C', but cytotoxic in the presence of C'; (2) inhibition of antibody production by lymphoid cells; (3) rendering lymphocytes more liable to phagocytosis by macrophages and reducing their functional activity in in vitro tests; (4) inhibition of contact action by sensitized lymphocytes on target cells; and (5) stimulation of lymphoid cells to synthesize RNA and DNA and to undergo mitosis.

A single parenteral injection of ALS produces a rapid but transient lymphopenia due to a decrease in the number of small lymphocytes. Such an effect may persist for 24 hours. Repeated ALS administration may cause a sustained lymphopenia associated with a depletion of the paracortical (thymus-dependent) regions of the lymph nodes, but continual ALS administration may result in lymphoid hyperplasia. Prolonged ALS therapy results in replacement of long-lived, thymus-dependent lymphocytes in the blood by short-lived lymphocytes.

Clinical applications of ALS include its use to delay homograft rejection, to induce specific immunologic tolerance, to suppress or abolish preexisting delayed hypersensitivity, and to treat some autoimmune disorders. These applications are based on observations of in vivo effects of the ALS, such as prolonged survival of skin, renal, cardiac, and corneal grafts; abolition of skin manifestations of delayed hypersensitivity to tuberculin; inhibition of the primary humoral antibody response with little or no effect on the secondary response; reversal of established rejection phenomenon; abolition of immunologic memory; induction of tolerance to transplantation antigens across strain and even species barriers; loss of capacity of lymphoid cells from ALS-treated animals to cause graft versus host reaction; and some beneficial effects in treatment of autoimmune disease involving cellular immunity. ALS is of little value in immune reactions where humoral antibodies play a major role. Thymectomy or treatment with other immunosuppressive agents such as radiation, corticosteroids, and drugs such as methotrexate potentiate the immunosuppressive effect of ALS if given before the antiserum. Administration of ALS for several days before establishing a graft, followed by a prolonged postoperative treatment, is said to give best results. ALS has been found to be effective when given subcutaneously, intramuscularly, intraperitoneally, or intravenously. Toxic reactions are seen when ALS is given by any of these routes, but crude serum is especially dangerous if given intravenously or intraperitoneally. A purified IgG fraction is reasonably well tolerated.

Side effects of the ALS treatment are development of sensitization to the heterologous protein, which may result in an anaphylactic reaction, serum sickness, and nephritis; severe depression of the bone marrow, resulting in anemia and thrombocytopenia; enhanced tumor growth; increased susceptibility to bacterial and viral infections; development of a wasting syndrome; acute localized pain and swelling caused by intramuscular injections; and fever and hypotension caused by intravenous injections.

PLATELET ANTIGENS AND ANTIBODIES

The literature on platelet antigens and antibodies has been reviewed (Klein and Blajchman, 1982; Majsky, 1969; Miller and Harmon, 1983). Human platelets, like leukocytes, contain (a) blood group antigens A and B and possibly others; (b) all currently known HLA-A antigens, most HLA-B antigens, and some HLA-C antigens; and (c) some platelet-specific antigens. Well-identified platelet-specific antigens and their alleles (in parentheses) are: DUZO; Zw (Zw[a], Zw[b]) or Pl[A] (Pl[A1], Pl[A2]); Ko (Ko[a], Ko[b]); and Pl[E] (Pl[E1], Pl[E2]). A new platelet-specific antigen called Bak[a] was recently reported (von dem Borne et al., 1980). Some of the antigens of human platelets are also shared by platelets of animal species such as the pig, sheep, cattle, and dog. Antigens Pl[A1] and Pl[E1] are found on platelets of monkeys, dogs, and rabbits. Many platelet antigens were found in early studies on pigs (Lie, 1966) and cattle (Millot, 1966); whether these are all histocompatibility antigens or represent also some platelet-specific antigens remains to be determined.

Isoantibodies reacting with platelets may develop after blood transfusions, pregnancy, leukocyte or platelet injections, and skin or organ grafting. Although the thromboagglutination test can detect some antibodies, the complement-fixation test is the method of choice to detect platelet antigens and antibodies. Transplacental alloimmunization of the mother to fetal platelet antigens or HLA-A antigens has been reported to cause *neonatal isoimmune purpura* in human newborns. The platelet-specific antigens DUZO and Pl[A1] and the transplantation antigen HLA-A2 are frequently associated with such alloimmunization of the mother. Infants become thrombocytopenic shortly after birth. Neonatal thrombocytopenia has also been found in association with the antigen Bak[a]. Neonatal thrombocytopenia may also develop in a child born of a mother with autoimmune thrombocytopenia (Kernoff et al., 1979) which is discussed later in this chapter.

Platelet alloantibodies in humans reduce survival of grafts and intravascular life span of platelets carrying the corresponding antigens. Rare cases of what is called *posttransfusion purpura* (PTP) have been encountered in humans; in this condition, sensitization to the transfused platelets develops, resulting in destruction of platelets (of both the donor and the recipient) and purpura in the sensitized individual. Such a reaction has been seen in Zw^a-negative recipients 1 week after transfusion of Zw^a-positive blood. The mechanism involved is not definitely known. Similar observations have been made on dogs and pigs. Baldini (1965) noted development of thrombocytopenia upon injection of homologous platelets in some dogs alloimmunized with platelets from the same donor. Posttransfusion purpura was reported to develop in a pig immunized with platelets from another pig (Linklater, 1977).

Neonatal Thrombocytopenic Purpura in Pigs

Thrombocytopenic purpura in piglets has been reported to occur as a result of maternal alloimmunization (Saunder et al., 1966; Stormorken et al., 1963) and sensitization induced by blood transfusions (Cop, 1969). Details of clinical findings have been given (Dimmock et al., 1982; Lie, 1968; Saunders and Kinch, 1968). Agglutinating antibodies against thrombocytes of the piglet and sire can be demonstrated in the serum of the dam. Antibodies in the colostrum have not been detected because of technical difficulties, although other serologic tests in addition to thromboagglutination have been found to detect anti-porcine-platelet antibodies in serum (Linklater and Imlah, 1974). Sensitization of the sow persists indefinitely and may affect subsequent litters even if the sire is changed (Saunders and Kinch, 1968). Although a relationship between red cell and platelet antigens has not been established, alloantibodies to certain red cell antigens (mainly of the E, but also of K and L systems) were found in about 50% of sows having litters affected with thrombocytopenia (Linklater, 1971).

The piglets are generally born healthy, although an occasional piglet may be thrombocytopenic and purpuric at birth. The platelets decrease in number abruptly after 5–9 days, reaching the lowest level at 10–13 days and completely disappearing in some piglets at 1–2 days before death. The thrombocytopenia results from both platelet destruction and impaired marrow production. Abnormalities in coagulation tests corresponding to a low platelet count may be found (Stormorken et al., 1963). The thrombocytopenia is accompanied by subcutaneous hemorrhage along the ventral abdominal wall and medial aspects of the legs and behind the ears. A concurrent anemia, sometimes accompanied by leukopenia, may develop in some piglets. Death may occur within a few days in severely involved cases or by 2–3 weeks of age. Lesions at necropsy are typical of hemorrhagic diathesis (Nordstoga, 1965). The most outstanding finding upon histopathologic examination is a complete or almost complete absence of megakaryocytes in the bone marrow. Surviving pigs appear clinically and hematologically normal by 16 weeks of age (Dimmock et al., 1982).

BONE MARROW TRANSPLANTATION

Bone marrow transplantation has emerged during the last decade as the treatment of choice for human patients with lethal primary immunodeficiencies, severe aplastic anemia, and congenital aregenerative anemias. It is also being performed with success in human patients with acute leukemias and in patients with other congential and acquired disorders of hematopoiesis. Thus bone marrow transplantation has rather vast potential for treatment of a variety of lethal hematologic and immunologic diseases associated with abnormalities of hematopoietic stem cells or their milieu. Progress in marrow transplantation has been achieved through a better understanding of histocompatibility antigens, development of methods to achieve adequate immunosuppression and control infection, and supportive care.

The reader is referred to recent reviews on various aspects of bone marrow transplantation (Atkinson, 1984; Dinsmore and O'Reilly, 1982; Dupont et al., 1981; Gale and Fox, 1980; James and Odom, 1983; Santos and Kaizer, 1982; Storb, 1983; Storb and Thomas, 1983; Thomas et al., 1975; van Rood et al., 1984). Observations on bone marrow transplantation after radiation injury have been compiled

(Balner, 1977). Successful marrow transplantation for a hematopoietic stem cell disorder in the dog (see Chapter 4) and for certain genetic disorders in the cat (Haskins et al., 1983; Thrall, 1983) have been performed in recent years.

Bone marrow transplantation has been performed using autologous, syngeneic, or allogeneic marrow grafts. Autotransplantation and transplantations between HLA-identical siblings or identical twins are invariably successful. Major problems with bone marrow transplantation arise from the graft versus host disease (GVHD) that leads to rejection of the graft when donor and recipient are genetically different. This has been shown in human studies as well as in canine and murine models of bone marrow transplantation. The lymphoid cells of an immune-competent host recognize the graft as "nonself" and develop an immunologically destructive reaction against the graft. Destruction of all host lymphocytic tissue by total body x-radiation or other immunosuppressive conditioning regimens leads to acceptance of an allogeneic graft, but unless donor and recipient are histocompatible, the repopulated donor-type lymphoid cells mount an immune response against the host and cause a GVHD, producing destruction of the host's tissues. Loss of weight, diarrhea, organ dysfunction, interstitial pneumonia, and infection lead to death in the acute and chronic GVHD. Infections usually involve opportunistic organisms, e.g., *Pneumocystis carinii* and cytomegalovirus.

The severity of the GVHD increases with disparity in histocompatibility. Animal experiments have shown that the GVHD is reduced and survival of the recipient is increased if a donor is matched with the recipient at the MHC (Thomas et al., 1975). Human patients are matched for antigens of the HLA-A, B, and D loci, but complete identity is rarely found. Furthermore, GVHD also occurs in over 50% of cases of HLA identity (Dinsmore and O'Reilly, 1982); perhaps this indicates nonidentity in many more yet to be identified HLA antigens, a role for some minor histocompatibility antigens, or importance of some other unknown factors. New approaches are being sought to prevent GVHD and prolong graft survival. The recent use of cyclosporin A for prevention of GVHD through improved immunosuppression and the encouraging results with transplantation of histocompatible marrow selectively depleted of immunocompetent cells could expand the use of marrow transplantation and bring greater success. It has also become evident that infusion of immunocompetent T cells in recipients of marrow transplants reduces the risk of GVHD; bacterial flora, particularly enterobacteriaceae, augment the disease because it is minimal in germfree animals; and success of bone marrow transplantation decreases with increase in age of the patient (Dinsmore and O'Reilly, 1982).

AUTOIMMUNE HEMATOLOGIC DISORDERS

Immune-mediated hematologic disorders can be broadly categorized in two groups. One group comprises conditions induced by alloantibodies (isoantibodies), which may occur naturally or develop after exposure to alloantigens (isoantigens). Examples include neonatal isoerythrolysis or hemolytic disease of the newborn, neonatal thrombocytopenia, neonatal leukopenia, and hemolytic transfusion reactions. These have been discussed in previous sections of this chapter. The other group is composed of conditions caused by autoantibodies produced against self-antigens at some time during the postnatal immunologic mature life of an individual (Petz, 1980). Examples of this category are autoimmune hemolytic anemia (AIHA), autoimmune thrombocytopenia (AITP), autoimmune neutropenia, and certain drug-induced hemolytic anemias, thrombocytopenias, and leukopenias. Each of these conditions have been reported in humans (Frank et al., 1977; Petz, 1980; Swisher and Burka, 1977b), and some have been found in animals (Dodds, 1983; Halliwell, 1982; Jain and Switzer, 1981; Leidl et al., 1980; Linklater, 1973; Switzer and Jain, 1981).

Autoimmune Hemolytic Anemia

Autoimmune hemolytic anemia has been reported in the dog (Avolt et al., 1973; Bennet, 1981; Bull et al., 1971; Bundza et al., 1976;

Feldman, 1982; Ford, 1980; Halliwell, 1978, 1982; Harvey, 1980; Lapras and Oudar, 1971; Lewis et al., 1963; Maggio, 1979b; Marks, 1981; Mori, 1972; Rebar and Lewis, 1979; Schalm, 1975; Slappendel, 1979; Slappendel et al., 1975; Stockham et al., 1980; Utroska, 1976; Werner, 1980), cat (Faircloth and Montgomery, 1981; Heise et al., 1973; Maggio, 1979a; Perman, 1977; Scott et al., 1973; Schrader and Hurvitz, 1983; Sodikoff and Custer, 1966; Utroska, 1980; Werner, 1980), horse (Anderson, 1974; Collins, 1975; Farrelly et al., 1966; Lokhorst and Breukink, 1975; Moriarty et al., 1976; Sutton et al., 1978; Weiser et al., 1983) and ox (Dixon et al., 1978; Valli and Erb, 1977). Several reviews are available on this disease in humans (Dacie, 1970; Dacie and Worlledge, 1969; Horwitz, 1979a, b; Leddy and Swisher, 1971; Petz, 1980; Swisher, 1977b) and animals (Dodds, 1983; Ford, 1980; Halliwell, 1982; Jain, 1975; Lapras and Oudar, 1971; Perman and Schall, 1983; Schalm, 1975; Switzer and Jain, 1981).

AIHA is a consequence of red cell destruction mediated by autologous antierythrocyte antibodies (Frank et al., 1977; Petz, 1980). Hence, AIHA is characterized by an increased destruction of erythrocytes in vivo and the presence of autoantibody against the patient's own erythrocytes. The anemia is usually responsive in that it is accompanied by increased polychromasia, reticulocytosis, normoblastemia, and bone marrow erythroid hyperplasia. Associated findings may also include jaundice, hemoglobinemia, hemoglobinuria, elevated indirect bilirubin, and increased fecal stercobilin, depending on the extent and mode of red cell destruction. The presence of spherocytosis and increased osmotic fragility are further indications of immune-mediated hemolytic process.

Essential to the definitive diagnosis of AIHA is the demonstration of autoantibodies to erythrocytes. The classical procedure used for this purpose is the Coombs antiglobulin test (see Chapter 2). One should be aware, however, that due to limitations in the sensitivity of the Coombs test, extremely low levels of antibody may escape detection (Avolt et al., 1973; Cooper, 1977; Feldman, 1982; Gilliland et al., 1971), constituting the so-called "Coombs-negative AIHA." Such Coombs-

negative cases of AIHA should be investigated with more sensitive methods to detect antierythrocyte antibodies (Campbell et al., 1984a; Feldman, 1982; Kaplan and Quimby, 1983).

Classification

AIHA is generally classified on the basis of etiology and thermal reactivity of the autoantibody involved. The former entails defining the occurrence of AIHA by itself or in association with other diseases. AIHA resulting from antibody formation unassociated with a known cause is considered primary or idiopathic, while that having a well-defined disease association is considered secondary or symptomatic. The latter category includes AIHA seen in association with lymphoproliferative disorders; connective tissue diseases, e.g., systemic lupus erythematosus (SLE); viral, bacterial, and parasitic infections; and certain chronic inflammatory conditions (Lewis et al., 1963, 1965a; Lewis and Schwartz, 1971; Slappendel, 1979; Swisher and Burka, 1977b; Switzer and Jain, 1981).

What provokes an individual to develop antibodies to its own tissue remains unknown. It may involve an interplay of various factors such as immunologic, genetic, viral, hormonal, and other factors (Dodds, 1983; Theofilopoulos and Dixon, 1982). In the broadest sense it is hypothesized that this process may involve a change in the antigenicity of red cells or a change in the immune status (humoral as well as cellular) of the individual. Sometimes it may involve destruction of red cells as innocent bystanders or by cross-reactive antibodies. The continuing investigations on the etiopathogenesis of autoantibody formation may reveal that most cases of AIHA are secondary in one form or the other.

Antibodies involved in AIHA are primarily of IgG and IgM types (Greene et al., 1977; Halliwell, 1978; Horwitz, 1979a, b; Jain, 1975; Perman, 1977; Petz, 1980; Rebar and Lewis, 1979; Slappendel, 1979; Swisher and Burka, 1977a, b; Werner, 1980). These are often referred to as warm- and cold-reactive antibodies, respectively. The warm antibody is optimally active at 37° C, whereas the cold antibody is most active at 2–10° C but has a thermal reactivity up to 30–32° C. Most cases of AIHA involve IgG antibody and in some cases both IgG and IgM; IgM alone is rarely found (Petz, 1980; Slappendel et al., 1975; Switzer and Jain, 1981). The IgG in humans is often non-complement-fixing (Dacie, 1970) and infrequently complement-fixing (Leddy and Swisher, 1971). Low levels of cold antibody (cold agglutinins) may occur naturally in some people (Leddy and Swisher, 1971), dogs, and horses (Switzer and Jain, 1981) and are usually of no clinical concern. Cold agglutinins as a cause of AIHA have been described in the dog (Slappendel et al., 1975), cat (Schrader and Hurvitz, 1983), and horse (Moriarty et al., 1976). The development of a cold hemagglutinin has been reported during leptospirosis in sheep and is incriminated as a cause of hemolytic anemia associated with this disease (Bhasin et al., 1971). Rare cases of AIHA may be associated with IgA (Englefriet et al., 1968; Halliwell, 1982; Slappendel, 1979).

It is advantageous while diagnosing AIHA to determine whether the disease is primary or secondary and what type(s) of antibodies are involved, for this information may dictate the mode and course of therapy. Resolution of secondary AIHA depends on the nature of primary disease. General experience has been that cold agglutinin disease is less responsive to corticosteroid therapy and splenectomy than the warm antibody type of AIHA. A classification of AIHA in dogs based on autoantibody type with some prognostic relevance has been described (Halliwell and Werner, 1979; Werner, 1980).

Clinical Observations

Reports of AIHA in dogs indicate that either sex may be affected and that there is a broad age and breed involvement (Bull et al., 1971; Halliwell, 1978; Lewis et al., 1963; Rebar and Lewis, 1979; Werner, 1980). A higher occurrence in females and a familial tendency in poodles, cocker spaniels, and Irish setters has been reported (Dodds, 1977; Jacobs et al., 1984; Quimby et al., 1978). Our observations on 77 dogs diagnosed as having AIHA revealed no breed predilection or obvious gender pattern, but a significant correlation between age and gender was noted (Switzer and Jain, 1981). In dogs less than 1 year old, only males were affected, while more females were affected with increase in age; e.g., in the 4- to 7-year-old group, females predominated over males by a ratio of 2:1.

Clinical signs have been presented in Chapter 24 and also summarized in literature reports (Perman, 1977; Perman and Schall, 1983; Schalm, 1975; Switzer and Jain, 1981; Werner, 1980, 1983). Generally they vary with the rapidity and severity of the onset of AIHA. In most cases, the sudden appearance of a progressive anemia is noted. Anorexia and lethargy are the most common clinical complaints. Increased water intake and emesis are often reported by the owner, followed in several days by weakness, staggering, and collapse. The most prominent physical finding is pale mucous membranes. Jaundice, hepatomegaly, and splenomegaly are frequently present. Frank intravascular hemolysis, although infrequent, will be indicated by hemoglobinemia and hemoglobinuria. Increased heart rate with weak rapid pulse and a low-grade systolic heart murmur may be heard and may be associated with abnormal electrocardiographic findings in degenerative carditis associated with prolonged severe anemia. Increased respiratory rate, especially with excitement or exertion, will be observed. If thrombocytopenia is present, petechiae, epistaxis, and retinal hemorrhages may be evident. Melena, frank bleeding from the bowel, and hematuria are often noted in cases of severe AITP. The body temperature may be elevated, especially if infection is present. Weakness may be moderate to profound. Syncopal episodes may be reported and are not to be confused with epileptic seizures.

The animal should undergo thorough physical examination for abdominal tumors, pyometra, and other conditions. In most instances, there is no previous clinical association with the current clinical complaint. The history should be taken carefully to determine if any toxic substance or medication has been given. The ambient temperature should be taken into consideration when patients are suspected of having cold agglutinin disease. Skin lesions (necrosis and gangrene), especially on the nose, pinnae, tail, and toes, may be seen with cold agglutinin disease (Slappendel, 1979). These result from obstruction of microcirculation from agglutinated red cells due to high titered antibody reactive at temperatures below 30–32° C.

The differential diagnosis of AIHA must include and distinguish between other causes of hemolytic disease in the animal species under investigation (see Chapters 23 and 24 for various causes).

Laboratory Findings

Severe hemolysis is indicated by hemoglobinemia, hemoglobinuria, bilirubinemia (due mostly to indirect-reacting bilirubin), increased levels of serum lactic dehydrogenase, and decreased levels of serum haptoglobin (Petz, 1980; Schalm, 1975). Hemoglobinemia and a high icteric index are seen in early stages when antibody-coated red cells and spherocytes undergo massive destruction in the circulation and in the mononuclear phagocyte system (MPS), respectively. The findings disappear as the number of spherocytes is reduced. The presence of spherocytes in blood films is strongly suggestive of immune-mediated red cell destruction.

Blood from patients with cold agglutinins undergoes intense autoagglutination upon storage at 4° C and usually at room temperature (Fig. 20–8), but not above 30–32° C; the agglutination is reversible at 37° C (Pruzanski and Shumak, 1977; Rebar and Lewis, 1979). Placing a large drop of blood on a microscope slide aids in the detection of microagglutination. Cold agglutination can be distinguished from the rouleaux by diluting the sample 1:1 with normal saline or by placing the blood sample in the refrigerator (4° C) and then examining the vial; the former disaggregates rouleaux and the latter accentuates cold agglutination.

In the stained blood film, there is usually evidence of a bone marrow response to anemia manifested by reticulocytosis, polychromasia, and the presence of nucleated red blood cells. The number of nucleated cells may be extremely high, which, when accompanied by a left shift, may suggest a leukoerythroblastic reaction. Spherocytes are invariably present (Plate XVII–4), and clumps of agglutinated red cells (Plate XVII–5) are usually seen when cold agglutinins are involved. The reticulocyte count will vary, depending

on the duration of illness, degree of response, and severity of the anemia (Schalm, 1975; Werner, 1980). If erythropoiesis is not impaired, the patient will show an elevated reticulocyte count within 3–5 days of an acute hemolytic episode. The bone marrow aspirate will reflect increased erythropoiesis and a decreased myeloid:erythroid ratio. The mean corpuscular volume may be elevated, depending on the degree of reticulocytosis. Failure of an adequate reticulocyte response may be indicative of inhibition of erythropoietic activity due to specific antibody-mediated bone marrow suppression (Rebar and Lewis, 1979; Schalm, 1975; Stockham et al., 1980; Switzer and Jain, 1981; Switzer et al., 1966; Werner, 1980), or it may be due to lack of specific nutrients (such as folic acid) needed for rapid erythropoiesis required for compensated bone marrow response to anemia. The reticulocyte response is temporarily reduced following blood transfusion (Schalm, 1975; Fig. 35–1).

The leukocyte count is frequently elevated with a slight to marked neutrophilia and left shift. There may be moderate monocytosis and thrombocytopenia. Plasma protein concentration is generally within the normal range, and fibrinogen concentration may be slightly elevated (Schalm, 1975). Erythrocyte sedimentation rate (ESR) may be elevated or reduced in response to the disease process or degree of reticulocytosis, respectively. Erythrocyte osmotic fragility is increased and often parallels the degree of spherocytosis (Schalm, 1975; Switzer and Jain, 1981). This may be helpful in the management of the patient because osmotic fragility tends to become normal as recovery takes place (see Chapter 24); conversely, during crisis, it becomes markedly increased.

The presence of autoagglutination of red cells and spherocytosis on the blood film should enable the practitioner to arrive at a tentative diagnosis of AIHA with reasonable confidence. Serologic diagnosis is based on the demonstration of immune antibodies on the red cells or in patient's serum by the Coombs antiglobulin test. Typical cases give a positive direct Coombs test. The direct Coombs test was positive for about two-thirds and negative for about one-third of the 65

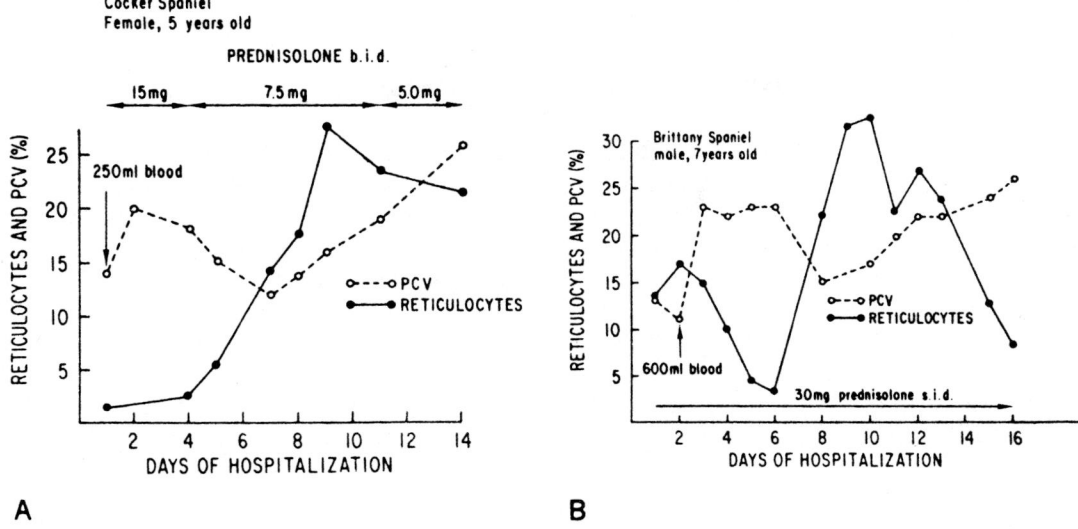

Fig. 35–1. Influence of whole blood transfusion on PCV and reticulocyte numbers of dogs with AIHA. *A,* A 250-ml transfusion increased the initial PCV of this dog from 14% to 20%, which gradually fell to 12% over the next 4 days. Initial reticulocyte count was 1.6%, but its rapid increase was delayed until after the fifth day. A significant reticulocytosis probably would have occurred early if the transfusion had been withheld. *B,* A 600-ml transfusion in this patient increased the PCV from 11% to 23%, at which level it remained for 4 days. This transfusion dramatically reduced the reticulocyte count from a 17% level to less than 2%, thereby indicating inhibition of reticulocytosis and probably diminished erythropoiesis. Subsequent drop in PCV from 23% to 15% between the sixth and eighth days was associated with a heightened reticulocytosis into the circulation to attain a peak of 31.4% on the tenth day. (From Schalm, 1975; courtesy of *Canine Practice.*)

canine patients examined at the Veterinary Medical Teaching Hospital at the University of California, Davis (VMTH-UCD) (Switzer and Jain, 1981). In the latter instances, other clinical and laboratory tests were used to arrive at a diagnosis of "Coombs-negative AIHA." These tests showed the presence of hemoglobinemia, autoagglutination of red cells, spherocytes, and a persistently high number of reticulocytes. In several instances, diagnosis was based on exclusion of other causes of hemolytic anemia and on responsiveness to corticosteroid therapy. Such cases also occur in humans, as mentioned above.

Other laboratory tests that may be helpful in management of AIHA patients include the lupus erythematosus (LE) cell test and antinuclear antibody (ANA) test if SLE is suspected; bone marrow examination, particularly in unresponsive or leukopenic patients (Cline and Golde, 1978; Stockham et al., 1980; Switzer and Jain, 1981; Switzer et al., 1966); serum biochemical survey to assess liver and kidney disease; urinalysis for the detection of cystitis or renal disease; stool examination for occult blood and parasites; and blood examination for dirofilariasis. Cardiopulmonary examination for carditis and pulmonary disease are indicated as part of a thorough medical examination.

Coombs Antiglobulin Test

Confirmatory diagnosis of AIHA is based on demonstration of a positive antiglobulin (Coombs) test (see Chapter 2 for the method). The direct Coombs test (DCT) demonstrates the presence of antierythrocyte antibody or activated complement components on the surface of the patient's cells. The indirect Coombs test (ICT) reveals the presence of antierythrocyte antibody in serum or in eluates prepared from the patient's red cells. IgG antibody, but not the C' components, can be eluted from erythrocytes by heat, mild acid, or certain organic solvents and can be stored frozen for years (Leddy and Swisher, 1971). A suspension of washed red cells of the patient (in DCT) or of normal homologous washed red cells exposed to the patient's serum (in ICT) is allowed to react with species-specific antiglobulin to induce visible agglutination of red cells. IgG or complement

(C'3)-coated red cells do not ordinarily undergo saline agglutination.

Red cell suspensions for the Coombs test must be obtained from blood anticoagulated with EDTA because EDTA is anticomplementary and prevents in vitro binding of C' to erythrocytes. Clotted blood kept in the refrigerator will have red cells coated with C'3, and such cells will give a false positive reaction with anti-C' reagent. Enzyme-treated red cells are more susceptible to C'-lysis and yield a higher degree of positivity in the ICT (Feldman, 1982). Enzyme-treated red cells may also be used to detect cold agglutinins (Roelcke et al., 1979).

Titers or scores of a Coombs test may be helpful in following progress of an individual patient. In humans, remission is frequently associated with a decrease in antibody titer. However, with cold antibody, thermal reactivity of the antibody is more important than the titer in this regard (Petz, 1980). In certain instances of cold agglutinin disease, it may be necessary to conduct the Coombs test at 4° C as well as at 37° C (Bundza et al., 1976).

Three patterns of positive Coombs reactions are obtained when the test is performed with specific antiserums such as anti-IgG and anti-C'. These patterns indicate that erythrocytes may be coated with IgG alone, C' alone, or both IgG and C'. In most cases of AIHA in humans the erythrocytes are coated with both IgG and C', but in as many as 25% of the cases, they are coated with IgG or C' alone (Swisher, 1977b). Hence use of a polyspecific antiserum containing both anti-IgG and anti-C' is recommended. Because IgM is capable of activating C', its role in AIHA can be assessed easily by using anti-C' to detect C'3 components on the patient's red cells. The identical situation prevails for animals, but it must be remembered that species-specific antiglobulin and anti-C'3 reagents are needed.

In our study involving 32 canine patients from VMTH-UCD, 60% gave a positive DCT with anticanine globulin (Switzer and Jain, 1981). A polyspecific antiserum containing both anti-IgG and anti-C'3 is now available for canine use. Direct Coombs tests were performed on all 32 dogs using this polyspecific reagent, simultaneously with monospecific anti-IgG and anti-C'3 reagents (Table 35–3). It was found that red cells of 81.2% of the dogs had IgG and 68.8% had C'; IgG alone was detected on red cells of 31.2% of the dogs and C' alone on 18.8%. Comparable findings were reported by Slappendel (1979).

IgG and C'3b, alone or in combination, generally participate in a positive direct Coombs test. If C'3 sensitization has occurred as a result of IgG activation, reactivity tends to persist even in the absence of IgG (low titer IgG). Persistent chronic AIHA with negative antiglobulin tests may continue to occur in the presence of less than 500 molecules of IgG per cell required for a positive antiglobulin test (Cooper, 1977; Gilliland et al., 1971). The numbers of molecules of IgG and IgM found necessary to give a positive direct Coombs test in the guinea pig were 12,000 and 50, respectively (Schreiber and Frank, 1972a, b).

Gilliland and coworkers (1970) have described an extremely sensitive method to detect minute quantities of red cell–bound IgG not detectable by other methods. A papain agglutination test to detect minute amounts of antierythrocyte antibodies is described in Chapter 2.

Coombs tests are presently performed in cats and horses using species-specific anti-IgG only, and positive cases have been found. Anti-C' should also be used if available. As more specific reagents become available commercially for general use in veterinary practice, more information will become available for other species of animals.

Interpretation of the Coombs test results requires an understanding of the mechanisms of antibody and complement associations with the red cells, circumstances leading to and the types of immune responses, and therapeutic consequences (Jain, 1975; Perman, 1977). A host of conditions have been found to give a positive Coombs test, either with anti-IgG or anti-C'3, in dogs and cats (Cotter, 1979; Halliwell, 1982; Medleaw and Miller, 1983; Slappendel, 1979; Werner, 1980). These include a variety of neoplastic, infectious, parasitic, inflammatory, and other immune-mediated diseases. A positive DCT is also obtained in patients with hemolytic transfusion reaction and in neonatal isoerythrolysis.

False negative and false positive results

Table 35–3. Patterns of Results of Direct Coombs Tests[a] for 32 Canine Patients with Autoimmune Hemolytic Anemia

Anti-IgG and Anti-C'3 Reagents	Anti-IgG Reagent	Anti-C'3 Reagent	Number of Cases	% of Total
+	+	+	16	50
+	+	−	10	31.2
+	−	+	6	18.8
100%	81.2%	68.8%		

From Switzer and Jain, 1981; courtesy of *Veterinary Clinics of North America, Small Animal Practice.*

[a]All reagents from Miles Laboratories, Inc. Direct Coombs tests were performed at 37°C.

may be obtained because of modified patient status, sample handling, and laboratory manipulations (Jain, 1975; Werner, 1980). In cases of drug-induced AIHA, the offending drug must be incorporated in the test system; otherwise the test may yield negative results. Some patients exhibiting signs of AIHA repeatedly yield negative Coombs test results, whereas some normal individuals with no signs of anemia may give a weakly positive reaction. A negative Coombs test does not necessarily rule out AIHA (Appendix Case 31), particulary when antierythrocyte antibodies are below the threshold of sensitivity of antiglobulin reagents (Avolt et al., 1973; Cooper, 1977; Gilliland et al., 1971; Halliwell, 1982; Medleau and Miller, 1983; Rosse, 1977). Prozone reactions may also contribute to negative results unless antiserum is diluted 1:4, 1:8, and 1:16 in performing the Coombs test (Halliwell, 1982; Medleau and Miller, 1983). Dissociation of IgG from the red cell surface in vitro may give a negative DCT with anti-IgG.

A patient's pattern of antiglobulin reaction may change during the course of disease and may become negative after prolonged therapy with corticosteroids or immunosuppressive drugs. In other cases, the DCT may remain positive even after complete remission from anemia. The DCT is sometimes positive during the clinical course, whereas the ICT may or may not be positive. However, both tests are almost always positive at the onset of acute hemolysis in humans (Dacie and Worlledge, 1969; Worlledge, 1967). Detection of antibody in the serum (indirect test) depends on the total amount present and its binding affinity for homologous red cells. DCT with anti-C' is often positive at a time when there is no clinical or other evidence of hemolysis (Dacie and Worlledge, 1969).

Cold agglutinating antibody is capable of fixing C' at temperatures below 30–32° C and lysing red cells at pH 6.5–7 in vitro. Because the antibody usually fixes C'3 and C'4, a positive direct Coombs test with anti-C' reagent is obtained in most instances. The antibody is not detected with anti-IgM serum because the IgM is eluted from the erythrocytes at 37° C in vivo and during washing of red cells in vitro. In contrast, the C' components are irreversibly bound to the red cells.

Pathogenesis of AIHA

Production of Autoantibody. The pathogenesis of AIHA involves circumstances leading to the formation of the autoantibody and the associated red cell destruction. The underlying mechanisms for the formation of autoantibody remain unknown, while some insight has been gained about red cell destruction.

In general, two major hypotheses or views prevail concerning the development of autoantibodies (Carpenter and Rabin, 1983), in this instance to erythrocytes. According to one view, a fundamental change occurs in the erythrocyte membrane, resulting in the formation of a new or "altered" antigen or unmasking a hidden antigen that subsequently stimulates the normal immune apparatus to synthesize antierythrocyte antibodies. Modification of the red cell antigen may be evoked by such factors as drugs, chemicals, viruses, and bacteria. Vos et al. (1971) have presented evidence indicating that a defect of the structural composition of the rhesus genome may be involved in the initial development of autoantibody in certain cases of AIHA in humans. It has been conjectured that these antibodies react with some fundamental ("core") structural units or precursor substances in the red cell related to the Rh system (Wiener et al., 1953). The majority of cold agglutinins in humans are directed against I-antigen, and some are directed against i-antigen.

The second view holds that somehow a spontaneous change occurs in the normal immune apparatus, which then recognizes normal erythrocyte antigens as foreign and produces antibodies. In other words, natural tolerance to certain self-erythrocyte antigens is terminated. This represents the development of "forbidden" clones of cells as proposed by Burnet (1957). This may occur when there is a generalized hyperactivity of the immune system, such as in malignant lymphoproliferative disorders, and probably in some other disorders (Dacie, 1970). It is also suspected that patients developing AIHA may be genetically prone to form autoantibodies (Dacie, 1970). Occurrence of AIHA in the NZB/BL hybrid of mice is well known, and certain breeds of dogs have been found to have a higher incidence of immune-mediated hematologic disorders (Dodds, 1983). Other factors predisposing to autoantibody production include sex of the individual, virus infection, vaccination, hormonal status, drug reactions, stress, and disease state (Dodds, 1983).

Current investigations on factors regulating immune responses have indicated that imbalances of immunoregulatory mechanisms involving lymphocytes concerned with antibody production and cellular immunity may be associated with expression of autoimmunity (Carpenter and Rabin, 1983; Kurlander and Rosse, 1979; Theofilopoulos and Dixon, 1982).

Mechanism of Red Cell Destruction. Red cell destruction in vivo is a consequence of direct lysis or erythrophagocytosis, or both (Cooper, 1977; Corbeil, 1978; Frank et al., 1977; Petz, 1980; Rosse, 1977; Rosse and Adams, 1980). Intravascular hemolysis is associated with C'-fixing antibodies, whether IgG or IgM, that cause activation of all complement components from C'1 to C'9 and the presence of antibody in very high titers. Two adjacent red cell–bound IgG molecules are re-

quired to initiate complement activation, while a single IgM molecule can efficiently initiate such an activation. As many as 90,000 C'3 molecules per red cell are believed necessary to result in a single complete lesion necessary for cell lysis (Rosse, 1977).

IgG is an inefficient activator of complement and, therefore, phagocytosis is the usual mode of red cell destruction when this antibody is involved. In comparison, IgM is a more efficient activator of complement, but even with this antibody, intravascular hemolysis is highly variable, from none or little to severe (Rosse and Adams, 1980). Frank hemolysis is rare, but when observed, is generally proportional to the amount of antibody in circulation, its thermal amplitude and binding to the red cell surface, and the degree of C' activation (Petz, 1980; Rosse and Adams, 1980). A role for lymphocytes in cell-mediated lysis of antibody-coated human erythrocytes has also been suggested (Kurlander and Rosse, 1979).

Erythrophagocytosis is associated with a relatively low concentration of IgG antibodies alone or in combination with partial activation of C' to C'3b on the red cell surface. Complement fixation up to the C'3b stage is ineffective in causing frank hemolysis but sufficient to promote phagocytosis. Macrophages have receptors for IgG and C'3b. Hence adherence of IgG- and C'3b-coated red cells occurs while these cells are passing through organs rich in the MPS, particularly the spleen. This interaction of red cells and MPS leads to partial or complete erythrophagocytosis. The former results in formation of spherocytes (Plate XVII–4; Figs. 20–8F and 35–2), and the latter contributes to bilirubinemia. Spherocytes are relatively rigid (less deformable), and their osmotic fragility is greatly increased (Figs. 20–10 through 20–13). Hence their intravascular life span is shortened because they cannot withstand trauma of the microcirculation, particularly in the spleen.

Removal of red cells in the absence of C' activation requires extensive coating by IgG. Removal of IgM-sensitized red cells is entirely C'-dependent. Attachment of IgM alone is inconsequential because macrophages lack appropriate IgM receptors. Complement acti-

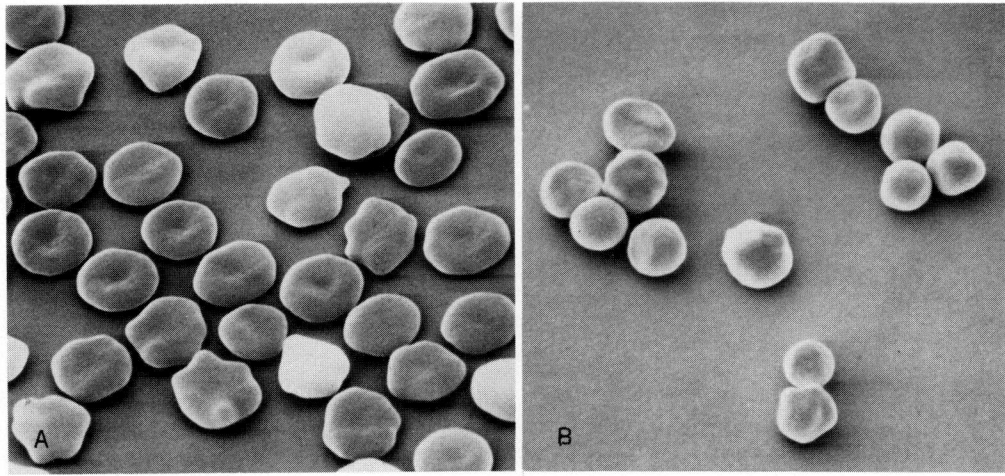

Fig. 35–2. Feline normal biconcave discocytic erythrocytes *(A)* compared with spherocytes *(B)* from a cat with autoimmune hemolytic anemia. A few slightly crenated cells are also present in *A*. Scanning electron photomicrographs. Both × 3,600.

vation in AIHA is usually through the classic pathway, although other mechanisms may also be involved (Corbeil, 1978). Degradation of the C′3b molecule abolishes its opsonic activity. Although neutrophils also have receptors for IgG and C′3 and can be shown to phagocytize opsonized red cells and platelets in vitro, they uniquely do not exhibit these properties in vivo.

Erythrophagocytosis occurs predominantly in the spleen, liver, and bone marrow, occasionally in the lymph node, and rarely in the peripheral blood. The major site of red cell removal varies with the type and degree of red cell coating. It has been shown that erythrocytes sensitized with IgG alone or with IgG and C′3b are removed primarily by the spleen, whereas those coated with C′3b resulting from activation of IgM are removed primarily by the liver (Frank et al., 1977). However, red cells having both IgG and C′3b are also likely to be removed by macrophages throughout the body and at a rate greater than when each is present singly (Petz, 1980). The rate of removal of red cells is also influenced by the antibody titer and the rate of blood flow through the liver and spleen (Frank et al., 1977; Schreiber and Frank, 1972a, b). Normal erythrocytes transfused into AIHA patients become coated with the autoantibody and are readily removed (Leddy and Swisher, 1971). Therefore, blood transfusion in AIHA

should be avoided as much as possible. It has also been shown that macrophages from human patients with AIHA may exhibit greater phagocytic activity for red cells than macrophages from normal persons (MacKenzie, 1975). Enhancement of macrophage activity in experimental studies was shown to increase removal of red cells coated with IgG and C′ or with C′ alone by the spleen and liver, respectively (Frank et al., 1977). In contrast, therapy with corticosteroid reduced in vivo clearance of such cells.

Donath-Landsteiner Antibody-Mediated AIHA

A rare autoimmune hemolytic syndrome seen in humans and characterized by an acute, intermittent, massive hemolysis that appears after exposure to cold temperatures is due to the Donath-Landsteiner (D-L) antibody. The D-L antibody is also referred to as a biphasic antibody because chilling at 0° C followed by warming to 30–37° C is often the best method to demonstrate hemolysis in vitro. The antibody and early components of C′ are fixed to the red cell surface at low temperatures (<20° C), whereas at 37° C, the antibody readily dissociates from the red cells, but fixation of further C′ components proceeds, resulting in lysis. The D-L antibody is of the IgG class and is rarely present in high titers. It is usually directed against P antigen

(Worlledge, 1967). Erythrocytes from a patient during and shortly after recovery from an acute attack of hemolysis frequently give a positive DCT with anti-C' reagents. A positive reaction with anti-IgG is obtained only if all the test procedures are carried out at 10° C or below. This type of AIHA has not been reported in animals.

Drug-Induced AIHA

Several drugs have been found to cause AIHA or to result in a positive antiglobulin test in humans (Leddy and Swisher, 1971; Swisher, 1977b). The mechanisms involved in the autoimmune response are varied (Petz and Fudenberg, 1975) and appear to follow along the lines of drug-induced AITP (discussed later in this chapter). Two cases of acute hemolytic anemia possibly induced by levamisole therapy for adult heartworms in the dog have been reported (Atwell et al., 1979).

Therapy

Details of therapy of AIHA in animal patients have been published (Halliwell, 1982; Switzer and Jain, 1981; Werner, 1980). The primary goals in therapy are to manage the anemic crisis, inhibit red cell destruction, and reduce production of autoantibodies. Intensive care consisting of warmth, oxygen, intravenously administered fluids, and blood transfusion may be required in the most severe cases. Avoidance of cold is essential in dogs with cold agglutinin disease.

Corticosteroids are the drugs of choice for treatment in immune-mediated diseases, including AIHA and AITP. They appear to reduce immune-mediated destruction of red cells (or of platelets in the case of AITP) in several ways: by suppression of phagocytic activity of macrophages of the MPS, particularly in the spleen and liver; reduction of antibody production; increased catabolism of immunoglobulins; and decrease in antibody avidity to red cells (or platelets). Experimental studies have shown that corticosteroids are most effective in reducing clearance of IgG-sensitized red cells and moderately effective when sensitization is with IgG and C'3 (Frank et al., 1977). Thus in clinical practice, corticosteroid therapy may be expected to be more effective in warm-antibody-type AIHA without significant C' involvement. In comparison, when cold agglutinins are involved, very high levels of corticosteroids are given but with less success.

Initially, dexamethasone is given intravenously at 1–2 mg/kg body weight as needed. Then prednisone is given at 2–4 mg/kg body weight, orally, once or twice daily as indicated. Corticosteroids are continued at a high level until signs of remission are indicated by an increasing PCV. Normlly, a positive response to therapy should be seen within the first seven days. The dosage of corticosteroids is tapered down at weekly intervals until a maintenance dosage is reached for the next 30 days. With continued remission, the dosage is further reduced to an alternate-day therapy for the next 60 days, at which time therapy may be discontinued. Response is monitored by determining PCV in case of AIHA and platelet counts in case of AITP. Our experience has been that at least 90–120 days of therapy are not uncommon in the great majority of cases of AIHA. Since relapses are common, a definite schedule of laboratory testing is important and must be stressed with the client.

Cyclophosphamide (Cytoxan) is a potent antimetabolite that has been used successfully in the treatment of AIHA (Halliwell and Werner, 1979). Its beneficial effect is mediated through reduction in antibody production. In response to corticosteroid therapy, the PCV should stabilize, usually within 3–5 days, and a clinical remission of anemia can be expected in 1–4 weeks. Failure to obtain a satisfactory remission in these patients makes them suitable candidates for cyclophosphamide therapy. It may be preferable to begin cyclophosphamide therapy at the onset in the more severe cases of AIHA. In some instances, it may be necessary to continue cyclophosphamide for several months, particularly where relapse is frequent. The recommended dosage of cyclophosphamide is 50 mg/m² body surface area, given orally, daily for 4 consecutive days per week, and repeated in weekly cycles until remission is evident. Although cyclophosphamide is a potentially toxic drug, its use in AIHA has been generally excellent. Antibiotics are suggested when infections are present or suspected (as in fever of unknown origin) and when vigorous immunosuppressive therapy is instituted. Hematuria and cystitis are frequent complications.

Additional immunosuppressive drugs such as azathioprine (Immuran) and 6-mercaptopurine may prove beneficial in the treatment of immune-mediated diseases and associated red cell aplasia (Erslev, 1983; Pedersen, 1978).

Heparin therapy may be used to reduce massive red cell destruction and prevent DIC (Bardana et al., 1970; Heine et al., 1964; Ten Pas and Monto, 1966). Although there is disagreement on the value of heparin as an anticomplementary agent to treat patients in anemic crisis, some very impressive results have been documented. In our experience (Switzer and Jain, 1981), heparin has been valuable in certain critical cases with plunging PCV values. The use of heparin is not to be taken lightly in view of some of the hazards reported. Heparin can be safely used if clotting time is monitored. Suggested starting dose is 10,000 IU (100 mg)/kg body weight, subcutaneously or intravenously b.i.d. or t.i.d., every 4–6 hours. Clotting time should be checked before each subsequent dosage is administered, and the dosage should be adjusted to obtain a Lee-White clotting time of 20–30 minutes. A major disadvantage that has been reported is the occurrence of rebound hemolysis upon cessation of heparin therapy (Bardana et al., 1970; Heine et al., 1964; Ten Pas and Monto, 1966), but this has not been our experience. It is believed that heparin therapy may be preferable to the risks of transfusion in dogs and cats with AIHA. If bleeding is encountered with heparin therapy, injectable protamine sulfate may be administered.

Blood transfusion is recommended only in life-threatening, severe anemic states. The benefit of transfusion therapy must be weighed against the risks involved in the patient with AIHA. Transfused cells may be rapidly destroyed by the patient's antibodies and result in serious transfusion reaction, DIC, and renal failure. Blood used for transfusion must be cross-matched with the recipient's serum and red cells. The intravenous administration of dexamethasone prior to transfusion is suggested to minimize risk of reactions. Warming the blood to body temperature prior to transfusion will also minimize reactions, especially in patients with cold agglutinin disease. The amount of blood to be administered depends on the size of the patient and the degree of anemia. As a general rule, 2 ml of blood given per kg body weight will increase the PCV by 1%. It is generally considered that patients with a PCV of 20% or more are not in critical need of blood transfusion and should not be subjected to the risks associated with transfusion.

Splenectomy may be indicated in situations of persistent relapse or inadequate response to prolonged corticosteroid and immunosuppressive therapy. Patients exhibiting extravascular hemolysis (primarily due to warm antierythrocytic antibodies) and hypersplenism are the most likely candidates. Before splenectomy, the patient must be stabilized. The clinical results of splenectomy have not been as beneficial in animals as they have been in humans (Halliwell, 1982; Petz, 1980). Splenectomy removes a major site of accelerated destruction of antibody-sensitized red cells as well as a major site of antibody production. In time these functions are taken over by other similar sites in the body and relapses continue to occur despite splenectomy. Secondary hemolytic disease due to haemobartonellosis or babesiosis is a frequent sequela of splenectomy (Rebar and Lewis, 1979).

Other supportive therapy such as a nutritious, high protein diet, folic acid and B-complex vitamins, and other drugs may be given to meet the demands of increased erythropoiesis. Myelostimulatory therapy may prove beneficial in AIHA associated with poorly responsive bone marrow and red cell aplasia (Erslev, 1983; Stockham et al., 1980; Switzer and Jain, 1981). Anabolic steroids may stimulate erythropoiesis through several mechanisms including stimulation of erythropoietin production or its effect. In addition, it has been shown that androgenic or anti-estrogenic substances play a role in delaying the onset of autoimmunity in NZB/NZW hybrid mice (Duvic et al., 1978; Melez et al., 1978).

Early detection and prompt institution of treatment is important if terminal anemic crisis is to be prevented. Corticosteroids and cyclophosphamide remain the therapeutic drugs of choice in the management of immune-mediated disorders. A therapeutic regimen of sufficient length and intensity is required to secure remission and to prevent relapse. Long-term or lifelong therapy is often necessary in these patients. Despite intensive care, death loss may be as high as 38%, particularly within the first few days of illness and often in association with other complicating diseases such as nephritis, hepatitis, carditis, and other immune-mediated disorders (Switzer and Jain, 1981).

In cats, the prognosis may be more guarded or poor, particularly in view of the association with feline oncornavirus infection or other bone marrow disorders. However, the therapy is similar to that instituted in dogs, and prolonged corticosteroid therapy may produce long-term remission of clinical anemia. Remissions in excess of 5 years have been obtained by us in cats with FeLV-associated AIHA, even though the FeLV test remained positive (Switzer and Jain, 1981).

Autoimmune Thrombocytopenia

Autoimmune thrombocytopenia has been recognized as a distinct entity in the dog. It also occurs in the cat and horse. AITP in these species is characterized by: (1) clinical signs of thrombocytopenia, such as hemorrhages into the skin and tissues and from body orifices; (2) coagulation defects related to thrombocytopenia, such as prolonged bleeding time and poor clot retraction; (3) hematologic abnormalities such as severe to moderate thrombocytopenia, often blood loss anemia, and signs of increased erythropoiesis; and (4) an absence or decreased number of megakaryocytes in the bone marrow during the early phase and an increased number during the compensatory phase. Megakaryocytes may also show morphologic abnormalities. Serologic diagnosis of AITP currently involves demonstration of antiplatelet antibody in serum by a platelet factor-3 (PF–3) test or enzyme-linked immunosorbent assay (ELISA) and on bone marrow megakaryocytes by a technique of direct immunofluorescence (see Chapter 2).

AITP in Humans

The occurrence of autoimmune thrombocytopenia as a distinct clinical entity in humans was long suspected but not clearly established until 1951, when Harrington and coworkers presented convincing evidence for the involvement of an autoantibody in causation of idiopathic thrombocytopenia in some patients. Since then, several workers have substantiated this claim and have made extensive studies of the antibody involved, its detection, and clinical and therapeutic aspects of AITP (Dixon et al., 1975; Karpatkin, 1971, 1978, 1980; Karpatkin et al., 1972, 1977; Kelton and Gibbons, 1982; Leporrier et al., 1979; Shulman et al., 1965; van Boxtel et al., 1975).

The diagnosis of AITP or idiopathic thrombocytopenia (ITP) in humans has been generally by exclusion of other causes of thrombocytopenia, although several positive criteria have also been suggested (Dixon and Rosse, 1975; Karpatkin, 1980; McMillan, 1978; Mueller-Eckhardt, 1977; Wintrobe et al., 1981). Other causes of thrombocytopenia include disorders of production (such as drug therapy or hypoplastic or aplastic marrow); preferential distribution of platelets in the spleen (as in hypersplenism); and increased platelet utilization or destruction (as in disseminated intravascular coagulation) (Aster, 1977; McMillan, 1978; Wintrobe et al., 1981). Characteristic hematologic findings in AITP include thrombocytopenia, reduced platelet survival, and normal or usually increased megakaryocytes in bone marrow. Platelet volume is increased from increased numbers of circulating young platelets (megathrombocytes).

Clinically AITP in humans may manifest as an acute, chronic, or intermittent disorder (Karpatkin, 1980; Mueller-Eckhardt, 1977; Wintrobe et al., 1981). Acute AITP is seen primarily in children. It is usually self-limiting, with spontaneous remissions occurring in most cases within a few weeks to months. Chronic AITP has a prolonged course and is most often seen with a preferential sex distribution in females, with a female:male ratio of 2–4:1 (Karpatkin, 1980). Intermittent thrombocytopenia may occur at any age and is characterized by cycles of thrombocytopenia at intervals of 3–6 months or more. A positive diagnosis of AITP is made upon demonstration of either antiplatelet antibody in serum or increased levels of platelet-associated IgG in the absence of sepsis or hypergammaglobulinemia (Karpatkin, 1980). The term ITP is reserved for those 10–15% of cases in which antiplatelet antibody is not demonstrated. ITP has also been reported as a hereditary disorder in humans (Stuart et al., 1978).

AITP in Domestic Animals

AITP in dogs was suspected in early studies of patients with concurrent thrombocytopenia and AIHA or SLE and in those having a corticosteroid-responsive thrombocytopenia (Lewis, 1965; Lewis et al., 1965b; Schalm and Ling, 1970; Schalm, 1971). Adaptation of a PF–3 test by Wilkins and coworkers (1973) and Joshi and Jain (1976a) led to demonstration of an antiplatelet antibody in serums of about 60% of thrombocytopenic canine patients. Joshi and Jain also reported on the use of an immunofluorescence test to detect antiplatelet antibody associated with bone marrow megakaryocytes (Plate XII–12). Thus AITP was established as a distinct disease entity in the dog. In recent years, AITP has also been found to occur in the cat (Jain and Switzer, 1981; Joshi et al., 1979) and horse (Dodds and Wilkins, 1977; Jain and Switzer, 1981) but less frequently than in the dog. The following clinical description of the disease as it occurs in the dog is derived mainly from our observations (Jain and Switzer, 1981). Clinical signs and therapy for one canine patient are described in Chapter 17. General reviews and reports on AITP and ITP in animals are available (Byars and Greene, 1982; Clark et al., 1980; Dodds, 1983; Halliwell, 1982; Jain and Switzer, 1981; Williams and Maggio-Price, 1984).

Classification of AITP

Acquired AITP may be primary or idiopathic, or it may be secondary or symptomatic to other diseases (Aster, 1977). Our observations on canine patients indicate that secondary AITP is about three times more prevalent than primary AITP and spontaneous remission of thrombocytopenia may occur in some cases of primary AITP (Jain and Switzer, 1981). Secondary AITP in dogs has been seen in association with AIHA, SLE, ehrlichiosis, DIC, multiple myeloma, myelogenous leukemia, lymphoma, solid tumors, severe generalized exfoliative dermatitis, nephropathy, portocaval shunt, possible Cushing's disease, and von Willebrand's disease. Such an association, however, is not seen in every case of the conditions listed, and other conditions may be found with such an association. Some such associations have also been observed in other studies (Wilkins et al., 1973). AITP in association with SLE was seen in a cat (Jain and Switzer, 1981). Antiplatelet antibody in serum or increased levels of platelet-associated IgG have been found in humans with thrombocytopenia associated with a variety of conditions including lymphoproliferative and myeloproliferative disorders, SLE, thrombotic thrombocytopenic purpura, bacterial, protozoal, and viral infections, and tumors and following therapy with certain drugs (Dixon and Rosse, 1975; Hedge et al., 1977; Kaden et al., 1979; Karpatkin, 1978; Karpatkin et al., 1977; Kelton and Gibbons, 1982; Kelton et al., 1979; Morrison et al., 1978).

These observations on human and animal patients indicate possible immune pathogenesis (at least in part) of thrombocytopenias associated with other diseases. In view of these observations, all patients with ITP or thrombocytopenia associated with other diseases should be examined, if possible, for evidence of immune-mediated platelet destruction.

Clinical Observations

Clinical signs of AITP are identical to those of thrombocytopenia in general. Signs of purpura are present in severely thrombocytopenic patients (platelet counts of <20,000/µl of blood). Petechiae may be seen in oral, gingival, nasal, and vaginal mucous membranes. With ecchymoses, they also may be seen on the skin over the abdominal areas, inner aspects of thighs and forelimbs, and in the ear canal. Bleeding may occur following the slightest trauma, such as during grooming. Epistaxis, melena, hematuria, scleral hemorrhage, and hyphema may be found. Bleeding from body orifices is more prevalent than tissue hemorrhages, and in some cases there may be no signs of bleeding (Jain and Switzer, 1981).

Signs of anemia may be apparent in patients with significant blood loss. The type of bleeding often provides an important clue as to the cause of bleeding. Large subcutaneous hemorrhages and acute pulmonary bleeding are often associated with acute poisoning with warfarin. In hemophilia, blood-filled, swollen, painful joints may be noted in addition to large subcutaneous or deep muscle hemorrhages. A thorough physical and laboratory examination is therefore necessary to determine the exact cause of a bleeding tendency. It should be remembered that stress on blood vessels plays a significant role in enhancing bleeding in the thrombocytopenic state, and bleeding episodes are much more common in the thrombocytopenic dog than in the thrombocytopenic cat (see Chapter 17). A variety of nonspecific clinical signs such as fever, increased thirst, anorexia, and lethargy may be found in these patients.

A thorough history and physical examination should be conducted to determine secondary causes of thrombocytopenia and duration and extent of bleeding when present. Differential diagnosis of AITP should include other causes of thrombocytopenia such as infectious agents, estrogen toxicity, DIC, drug sensitivity, myeloproliferative disorders, and lymphoproliferative disorders, particularly those with bone marrow involvement (see Chapter 18). A systemic approach to laboratory diagnosis of AITP should then be followed.

Sex, age, and breed distribution was determined for 28 dogs found to be positive for antiplatelet antibody (Jain and Switzer, 1981). In this group, females exceeded males by nearly two to one. Ages ranged from 1–12 years, with 21 of the 28 dogs being over 4 years of age. Sixteen different breeds were involved, with Standard poodles (five cases) and German shepherd dogs (four cases) being the most frequently affected.

Hematologic Findings

The characteristic finding is, of course, thrombocytopenia, with platelet counts most often below 50,000/µl of blood. A mild to severe blood loss anemia may be indicated by reduction in both red cell parameters (PCV, hemoglobin, and red blood cell count) and total plasma protein concentration. Some anemic dogs may present evidence of increased erythropoietic response such as polychromasia, reticulocytosis, and macrocytic hypochromic erythrocytes. Nucleated red cells may be found in some cases, particularly in those with erythrogenic response to anemia. The ESR is variable, and icteric index is generally normal. Total and differential leukocyte counts are variable. Leukocytosis, neutrophilia with slight to moderate left shift, and monocytosis may occur in some dogs, particularly in those briskly responding to anemia. A few dogs may have leukopenia, lymphopenia, or eosinopenia.

The number of mature and immature megakaryocytes in the bone marrow is generally reduced in severely thrombocytopenic dogs (Joshi and Jain, 1976a). In smears of marrow aspirates from ribs, normally there are about 70–84% mature and 16–30% immature megakaryocytes, with a ratio of 2.35–5.25:1. In AITP, the ratio of mature to immature cells is usually below unity (0.17–0.85:1). Morphologic abnormalities are also evident in mature and immature megakaryocytes. The cytoplasm shows excessive foaminess, vacuolation, and reduction in or absence of granularity. The nucleus may exhibit karyolysis. In rare instances, the marrow may be devoid of megakaryocytes at initial examination. Examination of blood films taken during the uncompensated or compensated thrombocytopenic state reveals microthrombocytes as well as megathrombocytes. The former type of platelet morphology results from fragmentation of circulating platelets (Khan et al., 1975), while the latter represents young forms of platelets (Karpatkin, 1978).

Megakaryocytes of dogs with AITP give a moderate to strong cytoplasmic immunofluorescence for IgG (Plate XII–12) in contrast to the negative fluorescence of megakaryocytes from normal dogs or dogs with non-immune-mediated thrombocytopenia (Joshi and Jain, 1976a). The positive immunofluorescence is reduced or disappears following therapy with corticosteroids and/or other immunosuppressive drugs. Positive megakaryocyte immunofluorescence has also been observed in human patients with AITP (McMillan et al., 1978).

Cats with AITP may show similar blood and bone marrow abnormalities.

Detection of Antiplatelet Antibody

A variety of tests have been introduced to detect circulating or platelet-bound antiplatelet antibody (Harmon and Miller, 1981; Kelton and Gibbons, 1982; Schiffer and Young, 1983). Primarily these include methods to detect (a) complement fixation by or complement-mediated lysis of platelets, (b) platelet alteration or injury, and (c) immunoglobulin binding to platelets or megakaryocytes. Detection of platelet-bound IgG or antiplatelet antibody in serum by an immunofluorescence or ELISA technique is gaining prominence in human medicine. Such developments in veterinary diagnostics are being introduced (Bloom et al., 1985; Campbell, et al., 1984b). See Chapter 2 for a description of a PF-3 test to detect antiplatelet antibody in serum (Jain and Kono, 1980) and for a direct immunofluorescence technique to demonstrate antiplatelet antibody associated with megakaryocytes (Joshi and Jain, 1976a, b). Our observations on canine patients indicate that the latter technique is much more sensitive than the former for detection of antiplatelet antibody in that more positive test results are obtained with it than with the former (Jain and Switzer, 1981).

Specimens for demonstration of antiplatelet antibody should ideally be collected prior to institution of corticosteroid and/or immunosuppressive therapy, for negative results may be obtained due to reduction in antibody levels. However, collection of specimens from a patient recently placed on such a therapy may still be fruitful in that antiplatelet antibody was detected in some dogs given corticosteroid therapy, with or without cyclophosphamide, for as long as 3 weeks (Jain and Switzer, 1981). It was also found that an antiplatelet antibody test may remain positive even when platelet counts have increased to within the normal range (Jain and Switzer, 1981). Such patients are probably in a "compensated thrombocytolytic state," i.e., they have a subclinical compensated AITP wherein increased bone marrow production keeps up with increased peripheral destruction of platelets (Karpatkin, 1980). It is believed that such patients are probably prone to easy bruising and extremely vulnerable to thrombocytopenia from secondary causes.

Pathogenesis of AITP

Circumstances leading to the formation of autologous antiplatelet antibody have not been fully delineated except in certain cases of drug-induced thrombocytopenias (Mueller-Eckhardt, 1977; Wintrobe et al., 1981). In general, the mechanisms of formation of autoantibodies to platelets may be similar to those described above for AIHA. Briefly these include (a) modification of platelet antigens or unmasking of cryptic platelet antigens so that they are recognized as "foreign" by the immune system, (b) selective modification of the immune system or formation of abnormal "clones" of lymphoid cells which recognize normal platelet antigens as "nonself," and (c) abnormalities of immunoregulatory cells. Defects in cellular immunity have recently been found in some humans with AITP (Karpatkin, 1978; Morimoto et al., 1980). Formation of cross-reactive antibodies or hapten mechanisms involving platelets in an antibody response may also be involved in immune destruction of platelets. The spleen and bone marrow are important sites for production of antiplatelet antibodies (McMillan, 1977).

The antiplatelet antibody has specificity for antigens associated with platelets and megakaryocytes (Karpatkin and Siskind, 1974; McMillan et al., 1978), although it may vary in its ability to bind to platelets from different individuals (Donnell et al., 1976; Karpatkin et al., 1977). The autoantibody directed against platelet antigens may be IgG or IgM, one or the other predominating, and rarely IgA (Dixon and Rosse, 1975; Dodds and Wilkins, 1977; Hauch and Rosse, 1977; Karpatkin, 1978; Nel et al., 1983; Veenhoven et al., 1980). The antiplatelet IgG may be either complement-fixing or non-complement-fixing (Dixon and Rosse, 1975; Hauch and Rosse, 1977; Veenhoven et al., 1980).

Thrombocytopenia is due primarily to the sequestration and destruction of platelets in the MPS. Macrophages phagocytize antibody- and C'-coated platelets analogous to erythrophagocytosis in AIHA (McMillan, 1977). Fragmented platelets (microthrombocytes) and fragmented red cells have been found, respectively, in blood of such patients (Karpatkin, 1978; Khan et al., 1975). Platelets that are heavily coated with antibody are removed by the liver, whereas lightly coated ones are destroyed in the spleen (Dixon and Rosse, 1975; Kernoff et al., 1980; McMillan, 1977). Because of its unique functional and anatomic structure, the spleen is the major site of platelet destruction. Normal preferential pooling of platelets, local high concentration of antiplatelet antibody from synthesis by lymphoid cells, an environment rich in highly phagocytic macrophages, almost stagnant blood flow, and tortuous pathway of blood circulation all contribute to intrasplenic platelet sensitization and phagocytosis (McMillan, 1977). Recently it was shown that platelets are trapped by pseudopods of splenic macrophages and are phagocytized as whole elements (Luk et al., 1980). Their degradation in phagolysosomes of macrophages is incomplete and results in formation of myelin-like figures that accumulate in large numbers in these cells. Such cells appear as large, foamy, "sea-blue histiocytes." It was suggested that this phenomenon has immunologic significance in providing a constant source of antigen for macrophage-lymphocyte interaction in the formation of antiplatelet antibodies. Phagocytosis of antibody-coated platelets by neutrophils can be demonstrated in vitro (Shebani and Jain, 1983).

Reduction in effective megakaryocytopoiesis from destruction of productive (mature) megakaryocytes in the bone marrow also contributes to thrombocytopenia in dogs (Joshi and Jain, 1976a, b). Platelets and megakaryocytes have been shown to share common antigens, and antiplatelet antibody has been found to bind to megakaryocytes (Joshi and Jain, 1976b; McMillan et al., 1978). Dogs injected with rabbit anti-canine-platelet antibody or its IgG fraction, but not IgM fraction, developed thrombocytopenia within hours (Joshi and Jain, 1976b). In addition, the number of megakaryocytes in the bone marrow was reduced, and morphologic abnormalities appeared in both mature and immature meg-

akaryocytes. Attachment of the IgG antibody to platelets in blood and to megakaryocytes in bone marrow was demonstrated by immunofluorescence (Plate XII–12). Disappearance of antiplatelet antibody from the circulation was followed by recovery within 5–7 days. Altered thrombopoiesis as a cause of thrombocytopenia was suggested in a report on humans with AITP (McMillan et al., 1978). Production of antiplatelet antibody has been shown in marrow culture. Hence it was suggested that local production of antiplatelet antibody, and presumably antimegakaryocytic antibody, could be expected to cause megakaryocyte damage and intramedullary platelet destruction (McMillan et al., 1978).

Antiplatelet antibody in serum and that bound to platelets has been quantitated (Dixon and Rosse, 1975; Dixon et al., 1975; Hedge et al., 1977; Leporrier et al., 1979; Luiken et al., 1977; Veenhoven et al., 1980). Serum levels of antiplatelet antibody vary widely and show little or no relationship to platelet counts or clinical response to therapy (Dixon and Rosse, 1975). In comparison, the amount of platelet-associated IgG generally correlates inversely with platelet counts and seems to have some clinical usefulness. It has been estimated that each normal human platelet has <0.4 pg of surface-bound IgG. Various degrees of platelet IgG coating were found in patients with ITP. Patients with more than 1.1 pg of IgG per platelet were found to be generally unresponsive to prednisone therapy and splenectomy, those with between 0.4 and 1.0 pg IgG per platelet were invariably responsive, and those with no demonstrable increase in platelet surface IgG had thrombocytopenia of very long duration (5–20 years), showed absence of increased megakaryocytopoiesis, and were unresponsive to all modes of therapy (administration of prednisone and immunosuppressive agents, and splenectomy). Poor prognosis was indicated in patients with persistently high platelet-associated IgG, despite continued corticosteroid therapy (Goudemand et al., 1979). Higher values of platelet-associated IgG were found in acute ITP than in chronic ITP (Goudemand et al., 1979). In some patients, platelets were found to be coated with antiplatelet antibody, but thrombocytopenia was absent. Functional defects of platelets may be found in such patients. Some recent studies have questioned the significance of increased levels of platelet-associated IgG because it is not confined to AITP (Nel et al., 1983; Pfueller et al., 1981). Similar observations for canine patients with AITP may become available with the use of a recently described method to measure platelet-associated immunoglobulin in this species (Bloom et al., 1985).

Most patients with ITP were found to have circulating immune complexes (Clancy et al., 1980). Immune complexes capable of interaction with platelets and C'-fixation have been found in patients with SLE with or without thrombocytopenia (Dixon and Rosse, 1975). The role of cellular immunity and immune complexes in platelet destruction, however, remains to be further investigated.

It has been suggested that the purpura associated with thrombocytopenia may be a consequence of damage to the vessel wall by antibodies directed against the capillary endothelium (Morrison and Baldini, 1969). Dogs sensitized to allogeneic aorta endothelium were found to exhibit a significantly reduced survival of injected allogeneic platelets.

Drug-Induced AITP

Many drugs are implicated in immunologic destruction of platelets in humans (Aster, 1977; Hackett et al., 1982; Karpatkin et al., 1977; Petz and Fudenberg, 1975). Drug-induced thrombocytopenia has been seen in dogs (see Chapter 17 and Appendix Case 23). Long-term administration of gold compounds in dogs was associated with a dose-dependent immune-mediated thrombocytopenia (Bloom et al., 1985).

Sensitivity to a drug usually develops after continued therapy and persists indefinitely after termination of the therapy. The onset of thrombocytopenia is usually rapid and may be accompanied by a generalized purpura or bleeding. Discontinuation of the drug results in an increase in the platelet count, usually within 7–10 days. Plasma from a sensitized individual induces thrombocytopenia in a normal individual, provided the drug in question is given to the recipient before or shortly after the plasma injection.

The antibodies involved in the drug-induced AITP are largely of the IgG class, although IgM antibodies may sometimes occur simultaneously (Eisner and Shahidi, 1972; Zeigler et al., 1979). In contrast to classical AITP, the antibody in the drug-induced AITP is demonstrable only in the presence of the drug or its metabolite. For example, if a PF-3 test is to be conducted, it must be performed in the presence of the drug; otherwise the test may be negative. The antibody is remarkably drug-specific; e.g., antiquinidine antibodies do not react with quinine, a levorotatory isomer of quinidine.

Mechanisms of antibody formation and platelet destruction have been studied in detail for quinine, quinidine, and sedormid. Ackroyd (1962) thoroughly investigated sedormid sensitivity and established the antibody nature of the factor involved. The antibody was found to react with platelets only in the presence of the drug. It caused platelet agglutination and lysis, C'-fixation by platelets, and inhibition of clot retraction. Ackroyd postulated that the drug, acting as a hapten, conjugated with the circulating platelets and that the drug–platelet complex acted as an antigen to produce specific antibodies. The antibodies reacted with the drug–platelet complex and not with the platelets alone.

Miescher and Straessle (1956) proposed an alternative mechanism, suggesting that the drug may initially bind to a plasma antigen or a "carrier," forming a primary antigen. Antibodies formed against such an antigen may react with the drug even in the absence of the "carrier" molecule. Formation of the drug-antibody complexes in the circulation may involve platelets secondarily by having a specific affinity for the platelet membrane (innocent bystander). This may result in thrombocytopenia due to lysis through C'-fixation. This hypothesis was supported by Shulman (1964), who further showed that (a) the drug alone has a weak affinity for the platelets, (b) an excess of the drug does not interfere with the absorption of drug-antibody complexes onto the platelets, and (c) the drug-antibody complexes have a great affinity for the platelets. Eisner and Shahidi (1972) reported that, in certain instances, a drug metabolite, rather than the drug itself, may be the antigenic substance producing antibodies involved in the drug-induced AITP.

Therapy

Therapeutic management is generally similar to that of patients with AIHA. Prognosis is favorable with early diagnosis, particularly in cases of primary AITP, and prompt initiation of adequate therapeutic measures. Long-term therapy is indicated in many cases, because relapses may occur upon termination of therapy (such a case is described in Chapter 17). Transfusion of fresh platelets (suspended in donor's plasma) is becoming practical with advances in techniques of platelet isolation and preservation. Fresh whole blood, no more than 12 hours old, must be used to insure platelet viability. Spontaneous remissions have been noted in a few humans with AITP (Dixon and Rosse, 1975), and acute AITP of children is generally self-limiting (Mueller-Eckhardt, 1977; Wintrobe et al., 1981). Spontaneous remissions may also occur in thrombocytopenic canine patients with primary AITP (Jain and Switzer, 1981). Therapy of AITP and ITP in humans has been discussed (Ahn et al., 1984; Harrington et al., 1983; Karpatkin, 1980; Kelton and Gibbons, 1982; Martin et al., 1984).

Canine patients with antiplatelet antibody may be categorized as "responders" or "nonresponders" to various forms of corticosteroid and immunosuppressive therapy (Jain and Switzer, 1981). Corticosteroids are the drug of choice for initial therapy of AITP or ITP. The mode of action is similar to that outlined earlier in this chapter for AIHA. In addition, they promote reduction of capillary fragility with the restoration of normal bleeding time. The dosage of corticosteroids is as for AIHA, but it is reduced or increased according to the patient's response. Because of the high frequency of relapses, platelet counts must be monitored frequently (weekly to monthly), especially after any reduction in corticosteroid therapy. A decrease in the platelet count may be detected from 1–4 weeks after cessation of corticosteroid therapy and is often evident before the onset of clinical bleeding.

Prednisone therapy may be expected to increase platelet counts significantly by the third day of therapy and, in responding dogs,

platelet counts may attain normal or higher levels in 5–7 days. Remissions may occur, but antiplatelet antibody may still persist in some cases (Dixon and Rosse, 1975; Jain and Switzer, 1981). In an occasional dog, the platelet counts may remain in the 100,000–200,000 range, but physical improvement is attained. In nonresponders, platelet counts remain below 100,000, or no real increase in platelet number occurs even after as long as 2 weeks of therapy. Among the dogs with positive PF-3 tests, the number of nonresponders may equal or exceed that of the responder dogs. It has been reported that only 36–44% of human patients with AITP respond to corticosteroid therapy (Karpatkin, 1980). Also, it has been reported that continued high doses of corticosteroids may cause an impaired thrombocyte production from excessive protein catabolism (Cohen and Gardner, 1961).

Cyclophosphamide (Cytoxan) may be given in conjunction with corticosteroid therapy, particularly when the response to corticosteroids is not seen within the first 3–5 days. Cyclophosphamide is given at the rate of 50 mg/m² body surface area daily, for 4 consecutive days per week, and repeated weekly until response is noted. Platelet counts may be expected to rise within the normal range in responder dogs within 5–6 days, whereas nonresponders may show low platelet counts for as long as 12 days. Cyclophosphamide should be withdrawn from the treatment program as soon as possible, owing to its cytotoxic and immunosuppressive actions, which can lead to undesirable side effects. The patient is maintained on corticosteroid therapy after the withdrawal of cyclophosphamide.

Vincristine (Oncovin) has proved to be a valuable drug in the management of ITP (Ahn et al., 1974). Dosage in the dog has been 0.2–0.6 mg/m² given intravenously at 7 to 10-day intervals (Jain and Switzer, 1981; Greene et al., 1982); the lower dose is preferred. Its use is generally indicated in cases resistant to corticosteroid administration or combined corticosteroid and cyclophosphamide therapy. The mode of action is believed to be direct stimulation of platelet production by megakaryocytes in the bone marrow. Vincristine is secondarily effective in suppressing antibody production; a decrease in platelet-associated IgG has been noted after vincristine therapy (Luiken et al., 1977).

Thrombocytopenic canine patients treated with vincristine may be expected to respond by increasing platelet counts usually within 3–5 days, sometimes dramatically to levels exceeding 1 million/μl of blood within 7–10 days (Greene et al., 1982; Jain and Switzer, 1981). An occasional patient may take longer to respond or require more than one treatment. No response may be evident in some cases even after repeated vincristine or other immunosuppressive therapy. Such observations have also been made in human studies.

A novel approach to therapy of thrombocytopenic human patients resistant to such conventional modes of therapy has been administration of allogenous platelets loaded with vinblastine or vincristine (Ahn et al., 1978; Nenci et al., 1981). Allogeneic platelets are first incubated in vitro with the vinka alkaloid and then infused into the patient. We have successfully treated one canine patient with vincristine-loaded platelets (Helfand et al., 1984).

Secondary infections are frequently associated with potent immunosuppressive therapy; hence careful attention to any signs of infection and periodic urine checks are required. Antibiotic therapy is to be guided according to organisms involved and their antibiotic sensitivity.

Splenectomy should be considered in selected cases in which recurrent thrombocytopenia is present. In any event, surgery should not be performed until bleeding is under control. About 60–75% of humans with AITP have been found to respond to splenectomy (Dixon and Rosse, 1975; Karpatkin, 1980). Splenectomy is indicated in patients with thrombocytopenia of more than 6 months' duration (Karpatkin, 1980). Platelet counts then return to normal levels, although antiplatelet antibody may persist in some cases; subsequently, 20–30% of splenectomized patients undergo relapse. Beneficial effects of splenectomy are attributed to removal of an important site of platelet pooling and destruction (Freedman and Karpatkin, 1975) as well as that of antiplatelet antibody synthesis (McMillan, 1977). Relapse is due to formation of antibodies at other sites, such as the bone marrow and lymph nodes, and destruction of sensitized platelets by the MPS at sites other than the spleen. Splenectomized individuals are at high risk of infection. The usefulness of splenectomy in therapy of AIHA and AITP in dogs and cats needs to be evaluated in a well-designed study on a large number of patients because the available information is insufficient to draw valid conclusions (Feldman et al., 1985; Williams and Maggio-Price, 1984). It is believed that splenectomy may be adjunctive to immunosuppressive therapy rather than curative.

Autoimmune Neutropenia

Antibodies to neutrophils can be detected by several methods, and human cases of autoimmune neutropenia (AIN) have been reviewed (Clay and Kline, 1981; Finch, 1983; Killmann, 1960; Logue and Shimn, 1980; Madyastha et al., 1982; McCullough, 1983; Verheught et al., 1978). AIN results from the action of an antibody directed against antigens located on the neutrophils. The antibody is specific for neutrophils as opposed to HLA antileukocyte antibody. The latter has been implicated in rare cases of allogeneic neonatal neutropenia in children, although such cases may also occur from in utero transfer of autoantibody to neutrophils. AIN may occur at any age. Typical manifestations of AIN include fever and recurrent infections associated with neutropenia. Transfusion of plasma containing antineutrophil antibody into a normal recipient is often associated with a temporary neutropenia and a febrile reaction, but sometimes a more severe transfusion reaction may occur. Transfusion of granulocyte-poor blood does not produce these reactions.

AIN has not been investigated in animals as much as in humans, although occasional case reports on immune-mediated leukopenias and granulocyte transfusion have appeared in the veterinary literature (Bull, 1980; Dimmock et al., 1976; Leidl et al., 1980; Linklater, et al., 1973; Schmid et al., 1980). Leukoagglutination and indirect immunofluorescence techniques have been adapted to detect the presence of antineutrophil antibody in feline serum (Chickering et al., 1985).

THE LE CELL PHENOMENON AND ANTINUCLEAR ANTIBODIES

The designation *LE cell* refers to a leukocyte, mainly neutrophil, containing a large, homogeneous or amorphous, light blue or pink cytoplasmic inclusion body of nuclear origin. The LE cell phenomenon was first observed by Hargraves in 1943 (but reported in 1948) as occurring in bone marrow preparations of persons suffering from lupus erythematosus (LE); hence the name of the cell (Hargraves, 1969). This disease of humans was originally considered a dermatologic problem, but after recognition of its systemic nature, the condition was called disseminated or systemic lupus erythematosus (SLE). It is an immune-mediated, multisystem inflammatory disease of the connective tissues (collagen disease) involving a variety of tissues and organs. Arthritis, arthralgia, photosensitivity, hepatitis, pleurisy, pericarditis, valvular lesions, AIHA, thrombocytopenia, and leukopenia may be associated in various combinations with SLE. In addition, the plasma of about 10–20% of SLE patients contains "lupus anticoagulants" whose nature is incompletely known (Shapiro and Thiagarajan, 1982). These anticoagulants appear to be immunoglobulins and cause prolongation of all phospholipid-dependent coagulation tests, namely, prothrombin time (PT), partial thromboplastin time (PTT), and Russell's viper venom time (RVVT), with the greatest prolongation occurring in the PTT. Diagnosis of SLE is challenging and requires demonstration of several laboratory and clinical abnormalities. It has been stated that no single test or combination of tests would permit a diagnosis of SLE in the absence of clinical signs (Willkens et al., 1968).

The LE cell may be found in diseases other than SLE, yet it continues to serve as an important indicator of SLE and closely allied disorders. Although the LE cells were originally seen in bone marrow films, it is now known that the formation of LE cells is mainly an in vitro phenomenon (Holman, 1960). Several laboratory techniques have been developed for the demonstration of LE cells; the one used in our laboratory is described in Chapter 2.

The formation of LE cells depends on an IgG antibody to deoxyribonucleoprotein (DNP) that can be absorbed by bare nuclei (Blondin and McDuffie, 1970; Holman and Kunkel, 1957). The phenomenon can be induced in vitro using serums of patients with SLE and normal marrow or buffy coat cells. The antibody is not species-specific and does not show any cellular or organ specificity. The development of the LE cell involves two steps. First, the anti-DNP antibody combines with nuclei of injured or nonviable leukocytes, resulting in nuclear swelling and altered stainability. In the second step, viable neutrophils are attracted to the altered nuclear material, and engulfment ensues. The result is the appearance within the leukocyte cytoplasm of a round, homogeneous mass, about the size of a lymphocyte nucleus, that takes the nuclear stain but lacks the normal chromatin pattern of a viable nucleus (Plate XI–3). LE cell formation must be distinguished from simple nucleophagocytosis (tart cells, named after the patient in whom these cells were first found), in which case the phagocytosed nuclear mass retains its normal morphologic features and usually has a darker staining rim. Although LE cell formation typically involves neutrophils, the nuclear mass may be phagocytosed by other cells, including eosinophils, basophils, monocytes, lymphocytes, and even plasma cells (Ogryzlo, 1956).

Phagocytosis of the altered nuclear mass leading to LE cell formation occurs only when sufficient IgG anti-DNP antibody is present along with complement. The IgG anti-DNP antibody in low concentrations produces only the nuclear alteration known as "extracellular material" (ECM) or "hematoxylin bodies" (Golden and McDuffie, 1967; Blondin and McDuffie, 1970). IgM anti-DNP antibody does not produce LE cells even at a very high concentration, although formation of ECM is seen. Inability of the IgM anti-DNP antibody to produce LE cells is probably due to its incapacity to fix complement (Blondin and McDuffie, 1970), although IgM is normally an excellent C'-fixing antibody. Thus IgG anti-DNP antibody produces both LE cells and ECM, depending on the amount of the antibody present, while IgM anti-DNP antibody induces only ECM formation. An amorphous ECM may be surrounded by many leukocytes, which form a collar or "rosette" (Plate XIV–12). The rosette is not acceptable per se as evidence of a positive LE test, but it is highly suggestive of the presence of the anti-DNP antibodies in the test serum. It has been reported that platelet factors may contribute to LE cell formation, for the intensity of LE cell formation is proportionate to the number of platelets present (Miale, 1982). A negative result in the LE cell test is not necessarily meaningful, because the concentration of anti-DNP antibodies varies and decreases as the disease enters a quiescent phase or during therapy with corticosteroids. When LE cells have been found in canine blood, it has required a tedious search in all but a few instances (Schalm and Ling, 1970). LE cells were found in synovial fluid of a dog with polyarthritis associated with SLE (Slappendel et al., 1972).

In addition to anti-DNP antibodies, the serum of patients with SLE may contain antinuclear antibodies (ANAs) against various cellular components including DNA, histone, nucleolus, and RNA. These antibodies can be demonstrated by an indirect immunofluorescence test (see Chapter 2). The anti-DNA antibody reacts with free DNA, as well as with DNA-protein complex, but it does not induce the formation of LE cells. It is more specific for SLE, has a higher association with an acute disease, and occurs in almost all patients with SLE (Niejadlik, 1971). However, a positive test may occur in diseases other than SLE. A relationship between the titer of the ANA and the disease activity has been shown (Ritchie, 1967), and a high or rising titer is considered diagnostic of SLE (Niejadlik, 1971). Granulocyte-specific IgG and IgM ANA antibodies have been found in human patients with rheumatoid arthritis (Wink, 1980).

Miale (1982) has recently summarized observations on LE cell and ANA tests in humans as follows: The pattern of immunofluorescence of a positive ANA (and its clinical correlation, given in parenthesis) may be diffuse (common in SLE, particularly the mild form), peripheral (usually in the acute phase of SLE), speckled (in scleroderma), or nucleolar (in collagen diseases other than SLE). Neither the titer nor the pattern of ANA alone is diagnostic. Mixed patterns may occur, and a pattern may change with serum dilution. The LE cell test is positive at best in 80% of SLE cases. It does not correlate with clinical severity of the disease. In comparison, the ANA test is positive in almost all cases; thus a negative ANA test, with rare exceptions (Fessel, 1978), rules out SLE. The LE cell test becomes negative following spontaneous or steroid-induced remissions, whereas the ANA test is not influenced by steroid treatment, although titers decrease in remission. The ANA test is always positive in drug-induced SLE, while the LE cell test may be positive or negative. Some recent reviews may be seen for additional information on ANA (Lorincz et al., 1981; Tan, 1982; Weiss et al., 1983).

Observations on a large population of dogs with a variety of diseases indicated that the ANA test was useful in supporting the diagnosis of SLE only when both antibody titer and staining pattern were taken into consideration (Quimby et al., 1980). The LE cell test was specific, but not sensitive when used to confirm a diagnosis of SLE. Our observations in canine patients similarly indicate that the ANA test has greater positivity than the LE cell test and that the pattern of fluorescence may change with serum dilution (Jain, unpublished observations). The pattern of fluorescence is usually of the ring type or diffusely speckled, and high titers may sometimes be found in normal dogs (Halliwell, 1981). Both ANA and LE cell tests are negative in human (Miale, 1982) and canine (Halliwell, 1981; Walton et al., 1981) cases of discoid lupus erythematosus. Antinuclear antibodies of several specificities may be found in dogs with SLE (Costa et al., 1984).

Canine Systemic Lupus Erythematosus

Lewis and coworkers (Lewis, 1965; Lewis and Borel, 1971; Lewis and Schwartz, 1971; Lewis et al., 1963; 1965a, b, 1973) were the first to describe naturally occurring SLE in dogs and to develop a breeding colony of such dogs. The following brief description of SLE is from their reported findings. The disease in dogs, as in humans, involves several body systems, usually affecting young adult females and often terminating in renal failure. A typical patient with SLE sequentially or simultaneously develops AIHA, thrombocytopenic purpura, and glomerulonephritis. Symmetrical polyarthritis, dermatitis, or thyroiditis may also occur in some cases. A variety of skin lesions have been reported in other spontaneous cases of SLE in dogs (D.W. Scott, 1978; Werner, 1983).

The diagnosis of SLE is substantiated by positive results of tests for LE cells, ANA, complement-fixing antibodies to DNA-histone complexes, and rheumatoid factor. Multiple serologic abnormalities may be found in the progeny of dogs with SLE. The development of ANA appears to be unrelated to the incidence of a positive LE cell test. About 10% of the dogs may be positive for rheumatoid factor.

Breeding trials suggested transmission of the disease by a factor from dog to dog by extragenetic mechanisms. Subsequent transmission experiments showed that a transmissible agent (probably a virus) induces serologic abnormalities of SLE in normal dogs and mice and that it spreads by both horizontal and vertical routes (Lewis et al., 1973). A female predisposition has been reported (Moraillon, 1978; Quimby et al., 1980). Ovariectomy seemed to prevent the development of SLE (Quimby et al., 1980). Studies in mice suggest that a deficiency of suppressor T cell function may be involved in development of SLE (Krakauer et al., 1976).

Schalm and Ling (1970) and Schalm (1978) have reported clinical and hematologic findings in dogs with positive LE cell tests (Table 35–4). Hemolytic anemia and thrombocytopenia, prominent features of canine SLE as reported by Lewis and coworkers (Lewis, 1965; Lewis et al., 1965b), were not significant findings in these dogs. Similarly, glomerulonephritis was suspected in only one dog (dog 6, Table 35–4) on the basis of 4+ proteinuria. Other hematologic findings included a consistently high corrected ESR, high total plasma protein concentration, and

Table 35–4. Principal Clinical and Hematologic Signs in Dogs with Positive LE Cell Test[a]

Dog Number	1	2	3	4	5	6	7	8
Clinical Number	113999	105399	112378	112835	114182	106219	115063	112308
Breed[b]	GSX	Basenji	GS	Cocker	GS	GS	Doberman	GS
Sex	F	F	F	M	M	M	M	M
Age	14 mo	16 mo	2 yr	5½ yr	8 yr	10 yr	9 yr	7 yr
Muscle wasting	+	—	+	+	+	—	—	—
Lameness	+	+	+	+	+	+	+	+
Joint swellings	+	+	+	—	—	—	—	—
Edema of limbs	+	±	—	—	+	+	. . .	+
Pyrexia	+	+	+	+	—	—	—	+
Heart murmur	—	+	—	+	—	—	—	—
Proteinuria	+	—	. . .	±	—	4+	+	+
Lymphadenopathy	—	—	—	+	+	+	—	+
Hyperkeratosis	—	—	—	nose	inguinal	—	—	—
PCV (mean %)	34	37	36	27	51	47	50	40
RBC sed. rate (mean corrected)	23+	33+	1−	30+	. . .	26+	3+	12+
Neutrophilia	+	+	+	+	—	+	—	—
Lymphopenia	+	—	—	—	—	—	—	—
Plasma protein (g/dl)	7.7	7.3	7.0	7.2	9.0	8.3[c]	7.8	6.6
Fibrinogen (g/dl)	0.45	0.45	0.30	0.40	0.30	0.42	0.30	0.30
Coombs test	—	2+	—	3+	—	—	—	—
LE cell test	+	+	+	+	+	+	+	+
Antinuclear antibody test	. . .	+	—	+	. . .	. . .	. . .	. . .
Diagnosis	SLE	polyarthritis	polyarthritis	arthritis (SLE)	SLE	glomerulonephritis	myopathy	SLE

[a]From Schalm and Ling, 1970; courtesy of *The California Veterinarian*.
[b]GS, German shepherd; GSX, Crossbred, shepherd-type.
[c]Globulin 5.6 g/dl.

normal fibrinogen level. Neutropenia was seen in five dogs, but lymphopenia was not found to be a part of the syndrome. Hematologic changes have been varied in other cases of SLE, with primary findings being neutrophilic leukocytosis, hyperfibrinogenemia, and hyperproteinemia primarily due to hypergammaglobulinemia of polyclonal pattern (Werner, 1983). Comments on occurrence of ANA and LE cells in dogs with SLE have been made in the preceding section. A case of SLE in a female Besenji dog is described in Appendix Case 30 and Appendix Case 29 describes some other features of the disease. For additional information on canine SLE see other reports (Halliwell, 1981; Moore, 1976a; Scott et al., 1979, 1983; Werner, 1983).

Several cases of SLE have been reported in the cat (Faircloth and Montgomery, 1981; Gabbert, 1983; Heise et al., 1973; Scott et al., 1979; Slauson et al., 1971), and Appendix Case 51 describes SLE with AIHA in a domestic shorthair cat (Heise et al., 1973). Cats in these reports have shown either a positive or negative LE cell test and ANA titers from negative to 1:40. Immune-complex glomerulonephritis was prominent in one case with a positive LE cell test, and thrombocytopenia was seen in an another case.

Guidelines for therapy of SLE are similar to those for AIHA and AITP, discussed earlier in this chapter. Canine patients with SLE respond to corticoid therapy (Halliwell, 1981; Lewis et al., 1963, 1965b; Schalm and Ling, 1970; Slappendel et al., 1972). The rate of corticoid administration is important. Initial doses of 2–4 mg/kg body weight daily, in divided doses, and maintenance levels of 0.5 mg/kg daily have given good results. The latter is important to avoid relapse. It is also important to give antibiotics in conjunction with initial steroid therapy. Other immunosuppressive drugs such as cyclophosphamide and azathioprine have been used in steroid refractory cases or when AIHA was also present. Vincristine is given when thrombocytopenia is also evident. Plasmapheresis may be performed to aid treatment of dogs with immune-mediated diseases like SLE (Matus et al., 1985). Details of clinical management of human SLE patients have been provided (Schur, 1983).

REFERENCES

Abe, T., et al.: A Subclinical Case of Hemolytic Disease of Newborn Pigs Caused by Anti-Ea. Jpn. J. Vet. Sci., *32*:139, 1970.

Abplanalp, H., et al.: Distribution of Blood Group Alleles in Inbred Lines of Chickens Derived from a Common Base Population. Poultry Sci., *55*:2005, 1976.

Ackroyd, J.F.: The Immunologic Basis of Purpura Due to Drug Hypersensitivity. Proc. Roy. Soc. Med., *55*:30, 1962.

Ahn, Y.S., et al.: Vincristine Therapy of Idiopathic and Secondary Thrombocytopenia. New Eng. J. Med., *291*:376, 1974.

Ahn, Y.S., et al.: The Treatment of Idiopathic Thrombocytopenia with Vinblastine-Loaded Platelets. New Eng. J. Med., *298*:1101, 1978.

Ahn, Y.S., et al.: Immunosuppressant Therapy of Idiopathic Thrombocytopenic Purpura. Springer Semin. Immunopathol., *7*:35, 1984.

Ahn, Y.S., et al.: The Treatment of Idiopathic Thrombocytopenia with Vinblastine-Loaded Platelets. New Eng. J. Med., *298*:1101, 1978.

Amorena, B., and Stone, W.H.: Sources of Bovine Lymphocyte Antigen (BOLA) Typing Reagents. Anim. Blood Groups Biochem. Genet., *13*:81, 1982.

Anderson, L.: Idiopathic Autoimmune Haemolytic Anaemia in a Horse. N.Z. Vet. J., *22*:102, 1974.

Andresen, E.: Blood Groups in Pigs. Ann. N.Y. Acad. Sci., *97*:205, 1962.

Andresen, E.: Blood Groups, Immunogenetics, and Biochemical Genetics. *In* Dukes' Physiology of Domestic Animals. 10th ed. Swenson, M.J., ed. Cornell Univ. Press, Ithaca, N.Y., pp. 51–67, 1984.

Andresen, E., and Baker, L.N.: Hemolytic Disease in Pigs Caused by Anti-Ba. J. Amin. Sci., *22*:720, 1963.

Aner, L., and Bell, K.: Transfusion Reactions in Cats Due to AB Blood Group Incompatibility. Res. Vet. Sci., *35*:145, 1983.

Anonymous: Report of the IUIS Committee on Nomenclature of DLA Determinants. Transplant. Proc., *9*:1909, 1977.

Anonymous: Proceedings of the Second International Bovine Lymphocyte Antigen (BOLA) Workshop. Anim. Blood Groups Biochem. Genet., *13*:33, 1982.

Archer, R.K., and Franks, D.: Blood Transfusion in Veterinary Practice. Vet. Rec., *73*:657, 1961.

Aster, R.H.: Disorders of Hemostasis: Quantitative Platelet Disorders. *In* Hematology. 2nd ed. Williams, W.J., et al., eds. McGraw-Hill, New York, pp. 1317–1360, 1977.

Atkinson, K.: Clinical Bone Marrow Transplantation: Current Status. Transplant. Proc., *16*:1009, 1984.

Atwell, R.B., et al.: Haemolytic Anaemia in Two Dogs Suspected to Have Been Induced by Levamisole. Aust. Vet. J., *55*:292, 1979.

Auer, L., and Bell, K.: The AB Blood Group System in the Domestic Cat. Anim. Blood Groups Biochem. Genet., *11*(suppl. 1):63, 1980.

Auer, L., and Bell, K.: The AB Blood Group System of Cats. Anim. Blood Groups Biochem. Genet., *12*:287, 1981.

Auer, L., and Bell, K.: Transfusion Reactions in Cats Due to AB Blood Group Incompatibility. Res. Vet. Sci., *35*:145, 1983.

Auer, L., et al.: Blood Transfusion Reactions in the Cat. J. Amer. Vet. Med. Ass., *180*:729, 1982.

Avolt, M.D., et al.: Autoimmune Hemolytic Anemia in a Dog. J. Amer. Vet. Med. Ass., *162*:45, 1973.

Bailey, E.: Prevalence of Anti–red Blood Cell Antibodies in the Serum and Colostrum of Mares and Its Relationship to Neonatal Isoerythrolysis. Amer. J. Vet. Res., 43:1917, 1982.

Baldini, M.: Acute "ITP" in Isoimmunized Dogs. Ann. N.Y. Acad. Sci., 124:543, 1965.

Balner, H.: Bone Marrow Transplantation and Other Treatment after Radiation Injury. Nijhoff Medical Division, The Hague, 1977.

Bardana, E.J., Jr., et al.: The Use of Heparin in Autoimmune Hemolytic Disease. Blood, 35:377, 1970.

Becht, J.L., et al.: I. Experimental Production of Neonatal Isoerythrolysis in the Foal. II. Evaluation of a Series of Testing Procedures to Predict Neonatal Isoerythrolysis in the Foal. Cornell Vet., 73:380–402, 1983.

Bennet, D.: Primary Autoimmune Haemolytic Anaemia in the Dog. Vet. Rec., 109:150, 1981.

Bhasin, J.L., et al.: Properties of a Cold Hemagglutinin Associated with Leptospiral Hemolytic Anemia of Sheep. Infect. Immun., 3:398, 1971.

Blondin, C., and McDuffie, F.C.: Role of IgG and IgM Antinuclear Antibodies in Formation of Lupus Erythematosus Cells and Extracellular Material. Arthritis Rheum., 13:786, 1970.

Bloom, J.C., et al.: Gold-Induced Immune Thrombocytopenia in the Dog. Vet. Pathol., 22:492, 1985.

Bowdler, A.J., et al.: Tr: A Canine Red Cell Antigen Related to A Antigen of Human Red Cells. Vox Sang., 20:542, 1971.

Bowdler, A.J., et al.: Representation of the ABH Blood Group System in the Dog. Vox Sang., 24:228, 1973.

Bruner, D.W., et al.: Icteric Foals. J. Amer. Vet. Med. Ass., 112:440, 1948.

Bruner, D.W., et al.: Blood Factors and Baby Pig Anemia. J. Amer. Vet. Med. Ass., 115:94, 1949.

Bryant, N.J.: An Introduction to Immunohematology. 2nd ed. Saunders, Philadelphia, 1982.

Bull, R.W.: Granulocyte Transfusions in the Septic Puppy. Vet. Clin. Path., 9:48, 1980.

Bull, R.W., ed.: Joint Report of the First International Workshop on Lymphocyte Alloantigens of the Horse, Held 24–29 October 1981. Anim. Blood Groups Biochem. Genet., 14:119, 1983.

Bull, R.W., et al.: Autoimmune Hemolytic Disease in the Dog. J. Amer. Vet. Med. Ass., 159:880, 1971.

Bundza, A., et al.: Haemobartonellosis in a Dog in Association with Coombs' Positive Anemia. Can. Vet. J., 17:267, 1976.

Burnet, F.M.: A Modification of Jerne's Theory of Antibody Production Using the Concept of Clonal Selection. Aust. J. Sci., 20:67, 1957.

Byars, T.D., and Divers, T.J.: Clinical Use of Blood Transfusions. Calif. Vet., 35:14, 1981.

Byars, T.D., and Greene, C.E.: Idiopathic Thrombocytopenic Purpura in the Horse. J. Amer. Vet. Med. Ass., 180:1422, 1982.

Cain, G.R., and Suzuki, Y.: Presumptive Neonatal Isoerythrolysis in Cats. J. Amer. Vet. Med. Ass., 187:46, 1985.

Campbell, K.L., et al.: Application of the Enzyme-Linked Immunosorbent Assay to Detect Canine Erythrocyte Antibodies. Amer. J. Vet. Res., 45:747, 1984a.

Campbell, K.L., et al.: Application of the Enzyme-Linked Immunosorbent Assay to Detect Platelet Antibodies. Amer. J. Vet. Res., 45:2561, 1984b.

Caroli, J., and Bessis, M.: Sur la cause et le traitement de l'ictère grave des muletons nouveau-nés. C.R. Acad. Sci., 224:969, 1947.

Carpenter, A.B., and Rabin, B.S.: Autoimmunity in Immunopathology. Clin. Lab. Med., 3:745, 1983.

Chardon, P., et al.: Presence of Soluble SLA Histocompatibility Antigen in Pig Plasma. Anim. Blood Groups Biochem. Genet., 8:139, 1977.

Chickering, W.R., and Prasse, K.W.: Immune Mediated Neutropenia in Man and Animals: A Review. Vet. Clin. Path., 10:6, 1981.

Chickering, W.R.: Development and Clinical Application of Methods for Detection of Antineutrophil Antibody in Serum of the Cat. Amer. J. Vet. Res., 46:1809, 1985.

Christian, R.M., et al.: Hemolytic Anemia in Newborn Dogs Due to Absorption of Isoantibody from Breast Milk during the First Day of Life. Science, 110:443, 1949.

Clancy, R., et al.: Autosensitization and Immune Complexes in Chronic Idiopathic Thrombocytopenic Purpura. Clin. Exp. Immunol., 39:17, 1980.

Clark, C.H., and Kiesel, G.K.: Longevity of Red Blood Cells in Interspecies Transfusion. J. Amer. Vet. Med. Ass., 143:400, 1963.

Clark, H.C., et al.: Idiopathic Thrombocytopenic Purpura: A Review and Case Report. Vet. Med. Small Anim. Clin., 75:427, 1980.

Clarke, C.A., et al.: Symposium: Haemolytic Disease of the Newborn Foal. J. Roy. Soc. Med., 71:574, 1978.

Clay, M.E., and Kline, W.E.: Neutrophil Antibodies: Detection and Clinical Application. Amer. J. Med. Tech., 47:805, 1981.

Cline, M.J., and Golde, D.W.: Immune Suppression of Hematopoiesis. Amer. J. Med.: 64:301, 1978.

Cohen, C., ed.: Blood Groups in Infrahuman Species. Ann. N.Y. Acad. Sci., 97:1–328, 1962.

Cohen, I., and Kozaki, M.: The Production of Isoantibodies in Littermate Dogs after Allogeneic Skin Grafting. Transplantation, 7:468, 1969.

Cohen, P., and Gardner, F.H.: The Thrombocytopenic Effect of Sustained High-Dosage Prednisone Therapy in Thrombocytopenic Purpura. New Eng. J. Med., 265:611, 1961.

Colling, D.T., and Saison, R.: Canine Blood Groups. 1. Description of New Erythrocyte Specificities. Anim. Blood Groups Biochem. Genet., 11:1, 1980a.

Colling, D.T., and Saison, R.: Canine Blood Groups. 2. Description of a New Allele in the Tr Blood Group System. Anim. Blood Groups Biochem. Genet., 11:13, 1980b.

Collins, J.: Autoimmune Hemolytic Anemia in the Horse. Proc. First Intl. Symp. Equine Hematology, East Lansing, Mich., p. 342, May 28–30, 1975.

Coombs, R.R.A., et al.: Factors Influencing the Agglutinability of Red Cells. II. The Agglutination of Bovine Red Cells Previously Classified as "Inagglutinable" by the Building up of an "Antiglobulin:Globulin Lattice" on the Sensitized Cells. Brit. J. Exp. Pathol., 32:195, 1951.

Cooper, R.A.: Destruction of Erythrocytes. In Hematology. 2nd ed. Williams, W.J., et al., eds. McGraw-Hill, New York, pp. 216–230, 1977.

Cop, W.A.G.: Blood Group Antagonism in Newborn Piglets. Neth. J. Vet. Sci., 2:66, 1969.

Corbeil, L.B.: Role of the Complement System in Immunity and Immunopathology. Vet. Clin. North Amer., 8:585, 1978.

Costa, O., et al.: Specifications of Antinuclear Antibodies Detected in Dogs with Systemic Lupus Erythematosus. Vet. Immunol. Immunopathol., 7:369, 1984.

Cotter, S.M.: Anemia Associated with Feline Leukemia

Virus Infection. J. Amer. Vet. Med. Ass., *175*:1191, 1979.

Cox, L.A.: A Survey of Equine Red Blood Cell Antibody Frequencies and Their Relevance to Neonatal Isoerythrolysis. M.S. thesis, Univ. of California, Davis, 1984.

Crowe, D.T., Jr.: Autotransfusion in the Trauma Patient. Vet. Clin. North Amer. (Small Anim. Pract.), 10:581, 1980.

Cullen, P.R., et al.: Sheep Lymphocyte Antigens: A Preliminary Study. Anim. Blood Groups Biochem. Genet., *13*:149, 1982.

Dacie, J.V.: Autoimmune Haemolytic Anemias. Brit. Med. J., 2:381, 1970.

Dacie, J.V., and Worlledge, S.M.: Auto-Immune Hemolytic Anemias. In Progress in Hematology. Vol. 6. Brown, E.B., and Moore, C.V., eds. Grune and Stratton, New York, p. 82, 1969.

Dausset, J., and Tangün, Y.: Leucocyte and Platelet Groups and Their Practical Significance. Vox Sang., 10:641, 1965.

Dausset, J., et al.: Histocompatibility Studies in a Closely Bred Colony of Dogs. III. Genetic Definition of the DL-A System of Canine Histocompatibility, with Particular Reference to the Comparative Immunogenicity of the Major Transplantable Organs. J. Exp. Med., *134*:1222, 1971.

Dennis, R.A., et al.: Neonatal Immunohemolytic Anemia and Icterus of Calves. J. Amer. Vet. Med. Ass., *156*:1861, 1970.

Dimmock, C.K., and Bell, K.: Haemolytic Disease of the Newborn in Calves. Aust. Vet. J., *46*:44, 1970.

Dimmock, C.K., et al.: The Experimental Production of Haemolytic Disease of the Newborn in Calves. Res. Vet. Sci., *20*:244, 1976.

Dimmock, C.K., et al.: Isoimmune Thrombocytopenic Purpura in Piglets. Aust. Vet. J., *59*:157, 1982.

Dinsmore, R., and O'Reilly, R.J.: Bone Marrow Transplantation: Current Status. Pathobiology Annual, *12*:213, 1982.

Dixon, J.B.: Transplantation Immunology: A Review of Some Biological and Veterinary Implications. 1. Detection and Inheritance of Some Antigens Affecting Graft Survival. Vet. Res. Commun., 5:205, 1982.

Dixon, P.M., et al.: Bovine Autoimmune Haemolytic Anaemia. Vet. Rec., *103*:155, 1978.

Dixon, R.H., and Rosse, W.F.: Platelet Antibody in Autoimmune Thrombocytopenia. Brit. J. Haematol., *31*:129, 1975.

Dixon, R., et al.: Quantitative Determination of Antibody in Idiopathic Thrombocytopenic Purpura. Correlation of Serum and Platelet-Bound Antibody with Clinical Response. New Eng. J. Med., *292*:230, 1975.

Dodds, W.J.: Autoimmune-Mediated Disease and Other Causes of Immune-Mediated Anemia: An Overview. J. Amer. Anim. Hosp. Ass., *13*:437, 1977.

Dodds, W.J.: Immune-Mediated Diseases of the Blood. Adv. Vet. Sci. Comp. Med., *27*:163, 1983.

Dodds, W.J., and Wilkins, R.J.: Animal Model: Canine and Equine Immune-Mediated Thrombocytopenia and Idiopathic Thrombocytopenic Purpura. Amer. J. Pathol., 2:489, 1977.

Doll, E.R., and Brown, R.G.: Isohemolytic Disease of Newborn Pigs. Cornell Vet., *44*:86, 1954.

Donnell, R.L., et al.: Different Antiplatelet Antibody Specificities in Immune Thrombocytopenic Purpura. Brit. J. Haematol., *66*:147, 1976.

Dowsett, K.F., et al.: Haemolytic Disease in Newborn Calves. Aust. Vet. J., *54*:65, 1978.

Dudok de Wit, C., et al.: The Practical Importance of Blood Groups in Dogs. J. Small Anim. Pract., 8:285, 1967.

Dupont, B., et al.: Bone Marrow Transplantation for Correction of Severe Aplastic Anemia and Primary Immunodeficiency. Ann. Clin. Res., *13*:358, 1981.

Duvic, M., et al.: Effect of the Anti-Estrogen, Nafoxidine, on NZB/W Autoimmune Disease. Arthritis Rheum., *21*:414, 1978.

Edebo, L., et al.: Serological and Physiochemical Reactivity of Bovine Erythrocytes before and after Trypsin Treatment. Scand. J. Immunol., *12*:193, 1980.

Ehrlich, P., and Morgenroth, J.: Ueber Haemolysine. Ber. Klin. Wschr., *37*:453, 1900.

Eisner, E.V., and Korbitz, B.C.: Quinine-Induced Thrombocytopenic Purpura Due to an IgM and an IgG Antibody. Transfusion, *12*:317, 1972.

Eisner, E.V., and Shahidi, N.T.: Immune Thrombocytopenia Due to a Drug Metabolite. New Eng. J. Med., *287*:376, 1972.

Ejima, H., et al.: Studies on Dog Lymphocyte Antigen (DLA) System: Cytotoxic Antibodies of Serum Produced by Allo-Skin Transplantation and Pregnancy in Bitches. Jpn. J. Vet. Sci. 42:83, 1980a.

Ejima, H., et al.: Comparison Test of Antibodies for Dog Blood Grouping. Jpn. J. Vet. Sci., *42*:435, 1980b.

Engelfriet, C.P., et al.: Autoimmune Haemolytic Anaemias: I. Serological Studies with Pure Antiimmunoglobulin Reagents. Clin. Exp. Immunol., 3:605, 1968.

Epstein, R.B., et al.: Cytotoxic Typing Antisera for Marrow Grafting in Littermate Dogs. Transplantation, 6:45, 1968.

Epstein, R.B., et al.: Relation of Canine Histocompatibility Testing to Marrow Grafting. Transplant. Proc., 3:161, 1971.

Erslev, A.: Aplastic Anemia. In Hematology. 3rd ed. Williams, W.J., et al., eds. McGraw-Hill, New York, p. 151, 1983.

Eyquem, A., et al.: Blood Groups in Chimpanzees, Horses, Sheep, Pigs, and Other Mammals. Ann. N.Y. Acad. Sci., *97*:320, 1962.

Faircloth, J.C., and Montgomery, J.K.: Systemic Lupus Erythematosus in a Cat Presenting with Autoimmune Hemolytic Anemia. Feline Pract., *11*(2):22, 1981.

Farrelly, B.T., et al.: Autoimmune Haemolytic Anaemia (AHA) in the Horse. Irish Vet. J., *20*:42, 1966.

Feldman, B.F.: Use of Low Ionic Strength Solution in Combination with Papain Treated Red Cells for the Detection of Canine Erythrocytic Autoantibodies. J. Amer. Anim. Hosp. Ass., *18*:653, 1982.

Feldman, B.F., et al.: Splenectomy as Adjunctive Therapy for Immune-Mediated Thrombocytopenia and Hemolytic Anemia in the Dog. J. Amer. Vet. Med. Ass., *187*:617, 1985.

Ferguson, L.C.: The Blood Groups of Animals. Adv. Vet. Sci., 2:106, 1955.

Ferrone, S., and Soldheim, B.G., eds.: HLA typing: Methodology and Clinical Aspects. CRC Press, Boca Raton, Fla., 1982.

Fessel, W.J.: ANA-Negative Systemic Lupus Erythematosus. Amer. J. Med., *64*:80, 1978.

Finch, S.C.: Neutropenia. In Hematology. 3rd ed. Williams, W.J., et al., eds. McGraw-Hill, New York, p. 773, 1983.

Fitzsimmons, W.M., et al.: Blood Transfusion and Red Cell Survival in the Goat. Brit. Vet. J., *123*:192, 1967.

Ford, R.B.: Immune-Mediated Hemolytic Anemia: A Clinical Review. Calif. Vet., *34*:13, 1980.

Forschner, J.: Lymphocyte Antigens in Sheep. Inaug. Diss., 1975.

Frank, M.M., et al.: Pathophysiology of Immune Hemolytic Anemia. Ann. Int. Med., 87:210, 1977.

Freedman, M.L., and Karpatkin, S.: Heterogeneity of Rabbit Platelets. V. Preferential Splenic Sequestration of Megathrombocytes. Brit. J. Haematol., 31:255, 1975.

Gabbert, N.H.: Systemic Lupus Erythematosus in a Cat with Thrombocytopenia. Vet. Med. Small Anim. Clin., 78:77, 1983.

Gale, R.P., and Fox, C.F.: Biology of Bone Marrow Transplantation. Academic Press, New York, 1980.

Gilliland, B.C., et al.: The Detection of Cell-Bound Antibody on Complement-Coated Human Red Cells. J. Clin. Invest., 49:898, 1970.

Gilliland, B.C., et al.: Red-Cell Antibodies in Acquired Hemolytic Anemia with Negative Antiglobulin Serum Tests. New Eng. J. Med., 285:252, 1971.

Gimlette, T.M.D.: Transfusion of Autologous and Allogeneic Chromium-51 Labelled Red Cells in Ponies. J. Roy. Soc. Med., 71:576, 1978.

Golden, H.E., and McDuffie, F.C.: Role of Lupus Erythematosus Factor and Accessory Serum Factors in Production of Extracellular Nuclear Material. Ann. Intern. Med., 67:780, 1967.

Goodwin, R.F.W., and Coombs, R.R.A.: The Blood Groups of the Pig. IV. The A Antigen–Antibody System and Haemolytic Disease in Newborn Piglets. J. Comp. Pathol., 66:317, 1956.

Gotze, D.: The Major Histocompatibility System in Man and Animals. Springer-Verlag, New York, 1977.

Goudemand, J., et al.: La detection des anticorps anti-plaquettaries dans le purpura thrombopenique. Nouv. Rev. Fr. Hematol., 21:47, 1979.

Green, J.R., and Spooner, R.L.: Ox Erythrocyte Agglutinability. 4. The Effect of Neuraminidase Treatment on the Agglutinability of Cells and Ghosts. Anim. Blood Groups Biochem. Genet., 8:25, 1977.

Greene, C.E., et al.: Cold Hemagglutinin Disease in a Dog. J. Amer. Vet. Med. Ass., 170:505, 1977.

Greene, C.E., et al.: Vincristine in the Treatment of Thrombocytopenia in Five Dogs. J. Amer. Vet. Med. Ass., 180:140, 1982.

Grunbaum, E.-G., and Gotter, J.: Blood Transfusion in the Dog. I. Obtaining Blood from Permanent Donors. Arch. Exp. Vet., 27:825, 1973.

Gulliani, G.L., et al.: Survival of Chromium-51-Labeled Autologous and Homologous Erythrocytes in Goats. Amer. J. Vet. Res., 36:1469, 1975.

Hackett, T., et al.: Drug-Induced Platelet Destruction. Semin. Thromb. Hemost., 8:116, 1982.

Halliwell, R.E.W.: Autoimmune Disease in the Dog. Adv. Vet. Sci. Comp. Med., 22:222, 1978.

Halliwell, R.E.W.: Skin Diseases Associated with Autoimmunity. Part II. The Nonbullous Autoimmune Skin Diseases. Comp. Cont. Educ. Pract. Vet., 3:156, 1981.

Halliwell, R.E.W.: Autoimmune Diseases in Domestic Animals. J. Amer. Vet. Med. Ass., 181:1088, 1982.

Halliwell, R.E.W., and Werner, L.L.: Autoimmune Disease. In Canine Medicine and Therapeutics. Chandler, E.A., et al., eds. Blackwell Scientific Publications, Oxford, pp. 216–218, 1979.

Hargraves, M.M.: Discovery of the LE Cell and Its Morphology. Mayo Clin. Proc., 44:579, 1969.

Harmon, J.A., and Miller, W.V.: Platelet Antibodies: Their Detection and Significance. Amer. J. Med. Tech., 47:797, 1981.

Harrington, W.J., et al.: Demonstration of Thrombocytopenic Factor in the Blood of Patients with Thrombocytopenic Purpura. J. Lab. Clin. Med., 38:1, 1951.

Harvath, L., et al.: Combined Pre-Immunization and Granulocyte Transfusion Therapy for Treatment of Pseudomonas Septicemia in Neutropenic Dogs. J. Lab. Clin. Med., 87:840, 1976.

Harvey, J.W.: Canine Hemolytic Anemias. J. Amer. Vet. Med. Ass., 176:970, 1980.

Haskins, M.E., et al.: Bone Marrow Transplantation in the Cat. Proc. 34th Amer. Coll. Vet. Pathol. and Annu. Meeting Amer. Soc. Vet. Clin. Pathol. p. 19, San Antonio, Texas, Nov. 29–Dec. 2, 1983.

Hata, R.: Clinical and Hematological Observations on Experimental Repeated Blood Transfusions in Horses. Jpn. J. Vet. Res., 21:97, 1973.

Hauch, T.W., and Rosse, W.F.: Platelet-Bound Complement (C3) in Immune Thrombocytopenia. Blood, 50:1129, 1977.

Hedge, V.M., et al.: Platelet Antibodies in Thrombocytopenic Patients. Brit. J. Haematol., 35:113, 1977.

Heine, von, K.M., et al.: Die Heparin-behandlung bei erworbener Hemolytischer Anamie. Acta Haematol., 32:27, 1964.

Heise, S.C., et al.: Lupus Erythematosus with Hemolytic Anemia in the Cat. Feline Pract., 3:314, 1973.

Helfand, S., et al.: Vincristine-Loaded Platelet Therapy for Idiopathic Thrombocytopenia in a Dog. J. Amer. Vet. Med. Ass., 185:224, 1984.

Hiller, M.C., and Shulman, N.R.: Characteristics of Leukocyte and Platelet Antigens Shared by Nonhuman Primates and Man. Ann. N.Y. Acad. Sci., 162:429, 1969.

Hirata, A.A., and Terasaki, P.I.: Cross-Reactions between Streptococcal M Proteins and Human Transplantation Antigens. Science, 168:1095, 1970.

Holman, H.R.: The LE Cell Phenomenon. Ann. Rev. Med., 11:231, 1960.

Holman, H.R., and Kunkel, H.G.: Affinity between the Lupus Erythematosus Serum Factor and Cell Nuclei and Nucleoprotein. Science, 126:162, 1957.

Horwitz, C.A.: Autoimmune Hemolytic Anemia. 1. Warm Antibody Type. Postgrad. Med., 66:167, 1979a.

Horwitz, C.A.: Autoimmune Hemolytic Anemia. 3. Cold Antibody Type. Postgrad. Med., 66:189, 1979b.

Iha, T.H., et al.: Cross-Reactions of Cattle Lymphocytotoxic Sera with HL-A and Other Human Antigens. Tissue Antigens, 3:291, 1973.

Ikemoto, S., et al.: Genetic Studies of New Blood Group C System on Red Cells of Beagles. Jpn. J. Vet. Sci., 43:429, 1981.

Inderbitzin, T.: The Relationship of Lymphocytes: Delayed Cutaneous Allergic Reaction and Histamine. Int. Arch. Allergy, Appl. Immunol., 8:150, 1956.

Jacobs, R.M., et al.: Use of a Microtiter Coombs' Test for Study of Age, Gender, and Breed Distributions in Immunohemolytic Anemia of the Dog. J. Amer. Vet. Med. Ass., 185:66, 1984.

Jain, N.C.: Autoimmune Hemolytic Anemia. Canine Pract., 2:30, 1975

Jain, N.C., and Kono, C.S.: The Platelet Factor 3 Test for Determination of Canine Antiplatelet Antibody. Vet. Clin. Path., 9:10, 1980.

Jain, N.C., and Switzer, J.W.: Autoimmune Thrombocytopenia in Dogs and Cats. Vet. Clin. North Amer. (Small Anim. Pract.), 11:421, 1981.

James, K.: Anti-Lymphocyte Serum. Clin. Chim. Acta, 22:101, 1968.

James, W.D., and Odom, R.B.: Graft-v-Host Disease. Arch. Dermatol., *119*:683, 1983.

Jorgenesen, J., et al.: The Influence of Ionic Strength and Incubation Time on the Sensitivity of Methods Using Papainized Red Cells. Vox Sang., *37*:111, 1979.

Joshi, B.C., and Jain, N.C.: Detection of Antiplatelet Antibody in Serum and on Megakaryocytes of Dogs with Autoimmune Thrombocytopenia. Amer. J. Vet. Res., *37*:681, 1976a.

Joshi, B.C., and Jain, N.C.: Experimental Immunologic Thrombocytopenia in Dogs: A Study of Thrombocytopenia and Megakaryocytopoiesis. Res. Vet. Sci., *22*:11, 1976b.

Joshi, B.C., et al.: Autoimmune Thrombocytopenia in a Cat. J. Amer. Anim. Hosp. Ass., *15*:585, 1979.

Kaden, B.R., et al.: Immune Thrombocytopenia in Lymphoproliferative Disease. Blood, *53*:545, 1979.

Kallfelz, F.A., and Whitlock, R.H.: Survival of ^{59}Fe-Labeled Erythrocytes in Cross-Transfused Bovine Blood. Amer. J. Vet. Res., *34*:1041, 1973.

Kallfelz, F.A., et al.: Survival of ^{59}Fe-Labeled Erythrocytes in Cross-Transfused Equine Blood. Amer. J. Vet. Res., *39*:617, 1978.

Kaplan, A.V., and Quimby, F.W.: A Radiolabeled Staphylococcal Protein Assay for Detection of Antierythrocyte IgG in Warm Agglutinin Autoimmune Hemolytic Anemia in Dogs and Man. Vet. Immunol. Immunopathol., *4*:307, 1983.

Karpatkin, S.: Autoimmune Thrombocytopenic Purpura. Amer. J. Med. Sci., *261*:127, 1971.

Karpatkin, S.: Platelet Antibodies in Autoimmune Thrombocytopenia and Drug-Dependent Thrombocytopenia. Cell-Mediated Immunity. HLA Phenotypes. Evan's Syndrome. Prog. Clin. Biol. Res., *28*:193, 1978.

Karpatkin, S.: Autoimmune Thrombocytopenic Purpura. Blood, *56*:329, 1980.

Karpatkin, S., and Siskind, G.W.: Studies on the Specificity of Antiplatelet Autoantibodies. Proc. Soc. Exp. Biol. Med., *147*:715, 1974.

Karpatkin, S., et al.: Cumulative Experience in the Detection of Antiplatelet Antibody in 234 Patients with Idiopathic Thrombocytopenic Purpura, Systemic Lupus Erythematosus and Other Clinical Disorders. Amer. J. Med., *52*:776, 1972.

Karpatkin, M., et al.: The Platelet Factor 3 Immunoinjury Technique Re-evaluated. Development of a Rapid Test for Antiplatelet Antibody. Detection in Various Clinical Disorders, Including Immunologic Drug-Induced and Neonatal Thrombocytopenias. Lab. Clin. Med., *89*:400, 1977.

Kelton, J.G., and Blajchman, M.A.: Platelet Transfusions. Can. Med. Ass. J., *121*:1353, 1979.

Kelton, J.G., and Gibbons, S.: Autoimmune Platelet Destruction: Idiopathic Thrombocytopenic Purpura. Semin. Thromb. Hemost., *8*:83, 1982.

Kelton, J.G., et al.: Elevated Platelet-Associated IgG in the Thrombocytopenia of Septicemia. New Eng. J. Med., *300*:760, 1979.

Kernoff, L.M., et al.: Neonatal Thrombocytopenia Complicating Autoimmune Thrombocytopenia in Pregnancy: Evidence for Transplacental Passage of Antiplatelet Antibody. Ann. Intern. Med., *90*:55, 1979.

Kernoff, L.M., et al.: Influence of the Amount of Platelet-Bound IgG on Platelet Survival and Site of Sequestration in Autoimmune Thrombocytopenia. Blood, *55*:730, 1980.

Khan, I., et al.: Microthrombocytosis and Platelet Fragmentation Associated with Idiopathic/Autoimmune Thrombocytopenic Purpura. Brit. J. Haematol., *31*:449, 1975.

Khanna, N.D., et al.: Blood Group Studies in Indian Buffaloes. I. Blood Factors: Their Detection and Frequencies. Indian Vet. J., *56*:916, 1979.

Killingsworth, C.R.: Use of Blood and Blood Components for Feline and Canine Patients. J. Amer. Vet. Med. Ass., *185*:1452, 1984.

Killmann, S.: Leukocyte Agglutinins. Blackwell Scientific Publications, Oxford, 1960.

Kissmeyer-Nielsen, F.: The HLA System: An Overview. Triangle, *20*(3):59, 1981.

Kissmeyer-Nielsen, F., and Thorsby, E.: Human Transplantation Antigens. Transplant. Rev., *4*:1, 1970.

Klein, C.A., and Blajchman, M.A.: Alloantibodies and Platelet Destruction. Semin. Thromb. Hemost., *8*:105, 1982.

Koichev, K.: Capability of Cattle and Buffaloes for Post-transfusion Isoerythroimmunization and the Significance of the Immune Antibodies for Blood Transfusion. J. Anim. Health Prod., *3*:1, 1975.

Koichev, K.: Survival of the Transfused Homologous Erythrocytes in Cattle. J. Anim. Health Prod., *4*:1, 1976.

Krakauer, R.S., et al.: Loss of Suppressor T Cells in Adult NZB/NZW Mice. J. Exp. Med., *144*:662, 1976.

Krötlinger, F., et al.: Bovine J Blood-Group Activity in the Lipids of Erythrocytes of Different Age. Blut, *40*:417, 1980.

Kurlander, R.J., and Rosse, W.F.: Lymphocyte-Mediated Lysis of Antibody Coated Human Red Cells in the Presence of Human Serum. Blood, *53*:1197, 1979.

Landsteiner, K.: Zur Kenntnis der antiformertastiven, lytischen und agglutinierenden Wirkungen des Blutserums und der Lymphe. Zentralbl. Bakteriol. Parasitol. Abt. I. Orig., *27*:357, 1900.

Langford, G., et al.: Haemolytic Disease of Newborn Calves in a Dairy Herd in Queensland. Aust. Vet. J., *47*:1, 1971.

Lapras, M., and Oudar, J.: Autoimmune Diseases of Animals: The Present State of Knowledge. Vet. Med. Rev., *2*:248, 1971.

Law, G.R.J.: Blood Typing of Turkeys Revisited. Anim. Blood Groups Biochem. Genet., *5*(suppl. 1):17, 1974.

Lazary, S., et al.: Equine Leukocyte Antigen System. I. Serological Studies. Transplantation, *30*:203, 1980a.

Lazary, S., et al.: Equine Leukocyte Antigen System. II. Serological and Mixed Lymphocyte Reactivity Studies in Families. Transplantation, *30*:210, 1980b.

Leddy, J.P., and Swisher, S.N.: Acquired Immune Hemolytic Disorders. *In* Immunological Diseases. Vol. 2. 2nd ed. Samter, M., ed. Little Brown, Boston, p. 1083, 1971.

Leidl, W., et al.: Neonatal Isoimmune Leukopenia in Foals. Berl. Münch. Tierärztl. Wochenschr., *93*:141, 1980.

Leporrier, M., et al.: Detection and Quantification of Platelet Bound Antibodies with Immunoperoxidase. Brit. J. Haematol., *42*:605, 1979.

Levine, P., et al.: The Role of Isoimmunization in the Pathogenesis of Erythroblastosis fetalis. Amer. J. Obstet. Gynecol., *42*:925, 1941.

Lewis, R.M.: Clinical Evaluation of the Lupus Erythematosus Cell Phenomenon in Dogs. J. Amer. Vet. Med. Ass., *147*:939, 1965.

Lewis, R.M., and Borel, Y.: Canine Rheumatoid Arthritis: A Case Report. Arthritis Rheum., *14*:67, 1971.

Lewis, R.M., and Schwartz, R.S.: Canine Systemic Lupus

Erythematosus: Genetic Analysis of an Established Breeding Colony. J. Exp. Med., *134*:417, 1971.

Lewis, R.M., et al.: A Syndrome of Autoimmune Hemolytic Anemia and Thrombocytopenia in Dogs. Proc. Annu. Meeting Amer. Vet. Med. Ass., *100*:140, 1963.

Lewis, R.M., et al.: Autoimmune Disease in Domestic Animals. Ann. N.Y. Acad. Sci., *124*:178, 1965a.

Lewis, R.M., et al.: Canine Systemic Lupus Erythematosus. Blood, *25*:143, 1965b.

Lewis, R.M., et al.: Canine Systemic Lupus Erythematosus: Transmission of Serologic Abnormalities by Cell-Free Filtrates. J. Clin. Invest., *5*:1893, 1973.

Lie, H.: The Complexity of Platelet Antigens in Pig. *In* Xth European Conference on Animal Blood Groups and Biochemical Polymorphism. Institut National De La Recherche Agronomique, Paris, 1966.

Lie, H.: Thrombocytopenic Purpura in Baby Pigs: Clinical Studies. Acta Vet. Scand., *9*:285, 1968.

Linklater, K.A.: Iso-antibodies to Red Cell Antigens in Pigs' Sera. 1. Iso-immunisation of Pregnancy in Sows. 2. The Incidence of Iso-antibodies to Red Cell Antigens in the Sera of Adult Pigs. Anim. Blood Groups Biochem. Genet., *2*:201, 1971.

Linklater, K.A.: Iso-antibodies to Red Cell Antigens in Pigs' Sera. 3. The Effect of Maternal Red Cell Iso-antibodies on the Red Cells of Piglets. Anim. Blood Groups Biochem. Genet., *3*:77, 1972.

Linklater, K.A.: Post-Transfusion Purpura in a Pig. Res. Vet. Sci., *22*:257, 1977.

Linklater, K.A., and Imlah, P.: Serologic Techniques for the Detection of Antibodies to Porcine Thrombocytes. 1. The Agglutination, Fluorescent Antibody and Immunodiffusion Techniques. 2. The Complement Fixation and Antiglobulin Consumption Techniques. Anim. Blood Groups Biochem. Genet., *5*:29, 41, 1974.

Linklater, K.A., et al.: Haemolytic Disease of the Newborn, Thrombocytopenic Purpura and Neutropenia Occuring Concurrently in a Litter of Piglets. Brit. Vet. J., *129*:36, 1973.

Logue, G.L., and Shimm, D.S.: Autoimmune Granulocytopenia. Ann. Rev. Med., *31*:191, 1980.

Lokhorst, H.M., and Breukink, H.J.: Auto-Immune Hemolytic Anemia in Two Horses. Tijdschr. Diergeneeskd., *100*:752, 1975.

Lorincz, L.L., et al.: Antinuclear Antibodies. Int. J. Dermatol., *20*:401, 1981.

Luban, N.L.C.: Transfusion Therapy with Platelets and Leukocytes. Pediatr. Ann. *12*:437, 1983.

Luiken, G.A., et al.: Platelet-Associated IgG in Immune Thrombocytopenic Purpura. Blood, *50*:317, 1977.

Luk, S.C., et al.: Platelet Phagocytosis in the Spleen of Patients with Idiopathic Thrombocytopenic Purpura (ITP). Histopathology, *4*:127, 1980.

MacKenzie, M.R.: Monocyte Sensitization in Autoimmune Hemolytic Anemia. Clin. Res., *23*:132A, 1975 (abstr.).

Madyastha, P.R., et al.: Autoimmune Neutropenia in Early Infancy: A Review. Ann. Clin. Lab. Sci., *12*:356, 1982.

Maggio, L.: Anemia in the Cat. Comp. Cont. Educ. Small Anim. Pract., *1*:114, 1979a.

Maggio, L.: Anemia in the Dog. Comp. Cont. Educ. Small Anim. Pract., *1*:474, 1979b.

Majsky, A.: Antigenicity of Blood Platelets. Curr. Top. Microbiol. Immunol., *50*:138, 1969.

Marion, R.S., and Smith, J.E.: Survival of Erythrocytes After Autologous and Allogeneic Transfusion in Cats. J. Amer. Vet. Med. Ass., *183*:1437, 1983a.

Marion, R.S., and Smith, J.E.: Posttransfusion Viability of Feline Erythrocytes Stored in Acid-Citrate-Dextrose Solution. J. Amer. Vet. Med. Ass., *183*:1459, 1983b.

Marks, D.L.: Autoimmune Hemolytic Anemia in a Dog. Vet. Med. Small Anim. Clin., *76*:1607, 1981.

Martin, J.N., Jr., et al.: Autoimmune Thrombocytopenic Purpura: Current Concepts and Recommended Practices. Amer. J. Obstet. Gynecol., *150*:86, 1984.

Masouredis, S.P.: Preservation and Clinical Use of Whole Blood. *In* Hematology. 3rd ed. Williams, W.J., et al., eds. McGraw-Hill, New York, p. 1529, 1983.

Matus, R.E., et al.: Plasmapheresis in Five Dogs with Systemic Immune-Mediated Disease. J. Amer. Vet. Med. Ass., *187*:595, 1985.

McCullough, J.: Granulocyte Antigen Systems and Antibodies and Their Clinical Significance. Human Pathol., *14*:228, 1983.

McMillan, R.: The Pathogenesis of Immune Thrombocytopenic Purpura. CRC Crit. Rev. Clin. Lab. Sci., *8*:303, 1977.

McMillan, R.: Diagnostic Approach to Immune Thrombocytopenia. Prog. Clin. Biol. Res., *28*:215, 1978.

McMillan, R., et al.: Antibody against Megakaryocytes in Idiopathic Thrombocytopenic Purpura. J. Amer. Med. Ass., *239*:2640, 1978.

Medleau, L., and Miller, W.H.: Immunodiagnostic Tests for Small-Animal Practice. Comp. Cont. Educ. Pract. Vet., *5*:705, 1983.

Melez, K.A., et al.: Modification of Murine Lupus by Sex Hormones. Ann. Immunol., *129*:707, 1978.

Meyer, R.C., et al.: A Hemolytic Neonatal Disease in Swine Associated with Blood Group Incompatibility. J. Amer. Vet. Med. Ass., *154*:531, 1969.

Miale, J.B.: Laboratory Medicine. *In* Hematology. 6th ed. C.V. Mosby, St. Louis, 1982.

Miescher, P., and Straessle, R.: Experimentelle Studien uber den Mechanismus der Thrombocyten Schadigung durch antigen-antikorper Reacktionen. Vox Sang., *1*:83, 1956.

Miller, W.V., and Harmon, J.A.: Platelet Serology and Transfusion. Human Pathol., *14*:221, 1983.

Millot, P.: Groups Thrombocytaires chez les Bovins. *In* Xth European Conference on Animal Blood Groups and Biochemical Polymorphism. Institut National de la Recherche Agronomique, Paris, p. 129, 1966.

Mollison, P.L.: Blood Transfusions in Clinical Medicine. Blackwell Scientific Publications, Oxford, 1983.

Moor-Jankowski, J., and Wiener, A.S.: Red Cell Antigens of Primates. *In* Pathology of Simian Primates. Part 1. General Pathology., Fiennes, R., ed. S. Karger, Basel, 1972.

Moore, D.J.: Canine Systemic Lupus Erythematosus: The Disease, Clinical Manifestations and Treatment. J. South Afr. Vet. Ass., *47*:267, 1976a.

Moore, D.J.: The Blood Grouping Systems of Dogs. J. South Afr. Vet. Ass., *47*:282, 1976b.

Moraillon, R.: Disseminated Lupus Erythematosus in the Dog. Recueil de Médecine Vétérinaire, *154*:587, 1978.

Mori, K.: Hematological Observation of Experimental Immuno-Hemolyic Anemia in a Dog. Jpn. J. Vet. Res., *20*:85, 1972.

Moriarty, K., et al.: An Anaemic State in a Horse Associated with a Cold-Reacting Antibody. N.Z. Vet. J., *24*:85, 1976.

Morimoto, C., et al.: Cell-Mediated Immunity to Platelets in SLE Patients with Thrombocytopenia: Two Different Types of Lymphocyte Stimulation. Clin. Immunol. Immunopathol., *15*:1, 1980.

Morrison, F.S., and Baldini, M.G.: Antigenic Relationship between Blood Platelets and Vascular Endothelium. Blood, *33*:46, 1969.

Morrison, J., et al.: Elevated Platelet-Associated IgG in Thrombotic Thrombocytopenic Purpura. J. Amer. Med. Ass., *239*:2242, 1978.

Mueller-Eckhardt, C.: Idiopathic Thrombocytopenic Purpura (ITP): Clinical and Immunologic Considerations. Semin. Thromb. Hemost., *3*:125, 1977.

Nel, J.D., et al.: Platelet-Bound IgM in Autoimmume Thrombocytopenia. Blood, *61*:119, 1983.

Nenci, G.G., et al.: Infusion of Vincristine-Loaded Platelets in Acute ITP Refractory to Steroids: An Alternate to Splenectomy. Acta Haematol., *66*:117, 1981.

Newman, M.J., and Antczak, D.F.: Histocompatibility Polymorphisms of Domestic Animals. Adv. Vet. Sci. Comp. Med., *27*:1, 1983.

Newman, M.J., and Hines, H.C.: Stimulation of Maternal Anti-Lymphocyte Antibodies by First Gestation Bovine Fetuses. J. Reprod. Fertil., *60*:237, 1980.

Nguyen, T.C.: Further Investigations on the Relationship between Groups of Sheep and Goats. Anim. Blood Groups Biochem. Genet., *8*(suppl. 1):11, 1977.

Niejadlik, D.C.: Antinuclear Antibodies: Role in Diagnosing Systemic Lupus Erythematosus. Postgrad. Med., *50*:273, 1971.

Noda, H., and Watanabe, Y.: Relationships between Blood Groups and Hemolytic Disease of Newborn Foal. Jpn. J. Zootech. Sci., *46*:180, 1975.

Nordstoga, K.: Thrombocytopenic Purpura in Baby Pigs Caused by Maternal Isoimmunization. Path. Vet., *2*:601, 1965.

Norsworthy, G.D.: Blood Transfusions in the Cat. Feline Pract., *7*:29, 1977.

Northway, R.B.: Autologous Blood Transfusion in Dogs and Cats. Vet. Med. Small Anim. Clin., *72*:1006, 1977.

Ogryzlo, M.A.: Morphology of the L.E. Cell Phenomenon. Seminar Rep. (Fall 1956), pp. 13–16.

Osterhoff, D.R.: Two Decades of Immunogenetical Research in the Republic of South Africa. Zietschrift fur Tierzuchtung und Züchtungsbiologie, *97*:196, 1980.

Osterhoff, D., and Vos, A.J.D.: Isoimmune Group Antibodies in Cattle after the Use of a Blood Vaccine. J. South Afri. Vet. Med. Ass., *48*:137, 1977.

Ostrand-Rosenberg, S., and Stormont, C.: Bovine Leukocyte Antigens. Anim. Blood Groups Biochem. Genet., *5*:231, 1974.

Ou, D., et al.: Effect of Storage on Oxygen Dissociation of Canine Blood. J. Amer. Vet. Med. Ass., *167*:56, 1975.

Owen, R. ap. R., and Glen, J.B.: Factors to Be Considered When Making Canine Blood Products Available for Transfusion. Vet. Rec., *91*:406, 1972.

Owen, R. ap. R., and Holmes, P.H.: An Assessment of the Viability of Canine Blood, Stored under Normal Veterinary Hospital Conditions. Vet. Rec., *90*:231, 1972.

Owen, R.D.: Immunogenetic Consequences of Vascular Anastomoses between Bovine Twins. Science, *102*:400, 1945.

Parham, P. and Strominger, J., eds.: Histocompatibility Antigens: Structure and Function. Chapman and Hall, London, 1982.

Pedersen, N.C.: Immunosuppressive Drugs and Their Role in the Treatment of Immunologic Diseases in the Dog. Gaines Symposium, Tuskegee, Ala., 1978.

Perkins, H.A.: Concise Review: Current Status of the HLA System. Amer. J. Hematol., *6*:285, 1979.

Perman, V.: The Anemic Cat. In Scientific Proc. 44th Annu. Mtg. Amer. Anim. Hosp. Ass., pp. 51–59, 1977.

Perman, V., and Schall, W.D.: Diseases of the Red Blood Cells. In Textbook of Veterinary Internal Medicine. 2nd ed. Ettinger, S.J., ed. W.B. Saunders, Philadelphia, pp. 1938–2000, 1983.

Petz, L.D.: Acquired Immune Hemolytic Anemia. New York, Churchill Livingstone, 1980.

Petz, L.D., and Fudenberg, H.H.: Immunologic Mechanisms in Drug-Induced Cytopenias. Prog. Hematol., *9*:185, 1975.

Pfueller, S.L., et al.: Relationship of Raised Platelet IgG in Thrombocytopenia to Total Platelet Protein Content. Brit. J. Haematol., *49*:293, 1981.

Pichler, M., and Turnwald, G.H.: Blood Transfusion in the Dog and Cat. I. Physiology, Collection, Storage, and Indications for Whole Blood Therapy. Comp. Cont. Educ. Pract. Vet., *7*:64, 1985a.

Pichler, M., and Turnwald, G.H.: Blood Transfusion in the Dog and Cat. II. Administration, Adverse Effects and Component Therapy. Comp. Cont. Educ. Pract. Vet., *7*:115, 1985b.

Pollack, M.S., et al.: Preliminary Studies of the Feline Histocompatibility System. Immunogenetics, *16*:339, 1982.

Pontois, M., et al.: Autotransfusion. Rev. Med. Vet., *128*:905, 1977.

Pruzanski, W., and Shumak, K.H.: Biological Activity of Cold-Reacting Auto-Antibodies. New Eng. J. Med., *297*:538 (pt. 1), 297: 583: (pt. 2), 1977.

Quimby, F.W., et al.: Selected Autoimmune Disease in the Dog. Vet. Clin. North Amer., *8*:665, 1978.

Quimby, F.W., et al.: Efficacy of Immunoserodiagnostic Procedures in the Recognition of Canine Immunologic Diseases. Amer. J. Vet. Res., *41*:1662, 1980.

Rapaport, F.T., et al.: Induction of Unresponsiveness by Total Body Irradiation in Bone Marrow Transplantation in Dogs. Nature, *235*:190, 1972.

Rasmusen, B.A.: Blood Groups and Incompatibility Testing. In A Textbook of Veterinary Clinical Pathology. Medway, W., et al., eds. Williams & Wilkins, Baltimore, p. 282, 1969.

Rasmusen, B.A.: H Blood Types, Stress Susceptibility and Hemorrhagic Diathesis in Pigs. Anim. Blood Groups Genet., *8*(suppl. 1):44, 1977.

Rasmusen, B.A., and Hall, J.G.: Association between Potassium Concentration and Serological Type of Sheep Red Blood Cells. Science, *151*:1551, 1966.

Rasmusen, B.A., et al.: The Relationship between the S System of Blood Groups and Potassium Levels in Red Blood Cells of Cattle. Anim. Blood Groups Biochem. Genet., *5*:95, 1974.

Rebar, A.H., and Lewis, H.: Blood Cells in Disease. In Canine Medicine. 4th ed. Catcott, E.J., ed. American Veterinary Publications, Santa Barbara, Calif., pp. 969–1034, 1979.

Renard, C., et al.: The Pig Histocompatibility System SLA: Serological Study on a Group of Antigenic Specificities. Anim. Blood Groups Biochem. Genet., *13*:161, 1982.

Rendel, J.: Further Studies on Some Antigenic Characters of Sheep Blood Determined by Epistatic Action of Genes. Acta Agr. Scand., *7*:224, 1957.

Ritchie, R.F.: The Clinical Significance of Titered Antinuclear Antibodies. Arthritis Rheum., *10*:544, 1967.

Roberts, E.J., and Archer, R.K.: Current Methods for the

Diagnosis and Treatment of Haemolytic Disease in the Foal. Vet. Rec., *79*:61, 1966.

Roberts, G.F.: Comparative Aspects of Haemolytic Disease of the Newborn. William Heinemann Medical Books, London, 1957.

Rodey, G.E.: Current Understanding of the Complexity of the HLA Antigen System. Prog. Clin. Biol. Res., *58*:135, 1981.

Roelcke, D., et al.: Human Cold Agglutinins against "Cryptic" Erythrocyte Antigens. Blut, *39*:217, 1979.

Rosse, W.F.: Complement. *In* Hematology. 2nd ed. Williams, W.J., et al., eds. McGraw-Hill, New York, pp. 87–99, 1977.

Rosse, W.F., and Adams, J.P.: The Variability of Hemolysis in the Cold Agglutinin Syndrome. Blood, *56*:409, 1980.

Rubinstein, M., et al.: Isohemagglutinins and Histocompatibility in the Dog. Transplantation, *6*:961, 1968.

Rumbaugh, G.E., et al.: Identification and Treatment of Colostrum-Deficient Foals. J. Amer. Vet. Med. Ass., *174*:273, 1979.

Saison, R., and Ingram, D.G.: A Report on Blood Groups in Pigs. Ann. N.Y. Acad. Sci., *97*:226, 1962.

Santos, G.W., and Kaizer, H.: Bone Marrow Transplantation in Acute Leukemia. Semin. Hematol., *19*:227, 1982.

Saunders, C.N., and Kinch, D.A.: Thrombocytopenic Purpura of Pigs. J. Comp. Pathol., *78*:513, 1968.

Saunders, C.N., et al.: Thrombocytopenia Purpura in Pigs. Vet. Rec., *79*:549, 1966.

Schalm, O.W.: The Blood Platelets (Thrombocytes): II. The Thrombocytopathies. Calif. Vet., *25*(6):6, 1971.

Schalm, O.W.: Autoimmune Hemolytic Anemia in the Dog. Canine Pract., *2*:37, 1975.

Schalm, O.W.: Lupus Erythematosus (LE) Cells in the Dog. Canine Pract., *5*:20, 1978.

Schalm, O.W., and Ling, G.V.: The L.E. Cell Phenomenon in the Dog. Calif. Vet., *24*(12):20, 1970.

Schiffer, C.A., and Young, V.: Detection of Platelet Antibodies Using a Micro-Enzyme-Linked Immunosorbent Assay (ELISA). Blood, *61*:3111, 1983.

Schmid, D.O., et al.: Lymphocyte Antigens in Sheep. Zentralbl. Veterinärmed., *22B*:386, 1975.

Schmid, D.O., et al.: Red Cell Associated Antigens of the B Blood Group System on Bovine and Sheep Lymphocytes. Anim. Blood Groups Biochem. Genet., *9*:47, 1978.

Schmid, D.O., et al.: Neonatal Isoimmune Leucopenia in the Foal. Anim. Blood Groups Biochem. Genet., *11*(suppl. 1):19, 1980.

Schmotzer, W.B., et al.: Time-Saving Techniques for the Collection, Storage, and Administration of Equine Blood and Plasma. Vet. Med., *80*:89, 1985.

Schrader, L.A., and Hurvitz, A.I.: Cold Agglutinin Disease in a Cat. J. Amer. Vet. Med. Ass., *183*:121, 1983.

Schreiber, A.D., and Frank, M.M.: Role of Antibody and Complement in the Immune Clearance and Destruction of Erythrocytes. I. In Vivo Effects of IgG and IgM Complement-Fixing Sites. J. Clin. Invest., *51*:575, 1972a.

Schreiber, A.D., and Frank, M.M.: Role of Antibody and Complement in the Immune Clearance and Destruction of Erythrocytes. II. Molecular Nature of IgG and IgM Complement-Fixing Sites and Effect of Their Interaction with Serum. J. Clin. Invest., *51*:583, 1972b.

Schur, P.H.: The Clinical Management of Systemic Lupus Erythematosus. Grune & Stratton, New York, 1983.

Scott, A.M.: Blood Typing in Horses. Vet. Annual., *15*:181, 1975.

Scott, A.M.: Principal Red-Cell Antigens Responsible for Haemolytic Disease of the Newborn Foal: Naturally-Occurring Antibodies in Thoroughbreds. J. Roy. Soc. Med., *71*:581, 1978.

Scott, A.M., and Jeffcott, L.B.: Haemolytic Disease of the Newborn Foal. Vet. Rec., *103*:71, 1978.

Scott, D.W.: Immunologic Skin Disorders in the Dog and Cat: Symposium on Practical Immunology. Vet. Clin. North Amer. (Small Anim. Pract.), *8*:641, 1978.

Scott, D., et al.: Autoimmune Hemolytic Anemia in the Cat. J. Amer. Anim. Hosp. Ass., *9*:530, 1973.

Scott, D.W., et al.: A Glucocorticoid-Responsive Dermatitis in Cats, Resembling Systemic Lupus Erythematosus in Man. J. Amer. Anim. Hosp. Ass., *15*:157, 1979.

Scott, D.W., et al.: Canine Lupus Erythematosus. I. Systemic Lupus Erythematosus. J. Amer. Anim. Hosp. Ass., *19*:461, 1983.

Searl, R.C.: Neonatal Isoerythrolysis in the Bovine. Biochem. Rev., *34*(2):3, 1971.

Searl, R.C.: Use of an Anaplasma Vaccine as Related to Neonatal Isoerythrolysis. Vet. Med. Small Anim. Clin., *75*:101, 1980.

Shanfield, I., and MacLean, L.D.: Antilymphocyte Serum: Present Status. Can. Med. Ass. J., *100*:925, 1969.

Shapiro, S.S., and Thiagarajan, P.: Lupus Anticoagulants. *In* Progress in Hemostasis and Thrombosis. Vol. 6. Spaet, T.H., ed. Grune & Stratton, New York, pp. 263–285, 1982.

Shebani, O., and Jain, N.C.: In Vitro Phagocytosis of Antibody-Coated Canine Platelets by Autologous Neutrophils. Vet. Clin. Path., *12*:23, 1983.

Sheil, A.G.R., and Rogers, J.H.: Antilymphocyte Serum: A Review with Report of the Current Clinical Situation in Australia. Med. J. Aust., *56*:1370, 1969.

Shields, C.E.: Application of Isotopic Methods for Measuring Post-Transfusion Survival of Stored Blood in Dogs. Lab. Anim. Sci., *22*:196, 1972.

Shulman, N.R.: A Mechanism of Cell Destruction in Individuals Sensitized to Foreign Antigens and Its Implications in Autoimmunity. Ann. Intern. Med., *60*:506, 1964.

Shulman, N.R., et al.: Similarities between Known Antiplatelet Antibodies and the Factors Responsible for Thrombocytopenia in Idiopathic Purpura: Physiologic, Serologic, and Isotopic Studies. Ann. N.Y. Acad. Sci., *124*:499, 1965.

Simon, M., and Hojný, J.: A Study of Lymphocyte Antigens in Pigs by Means of Anti-Erythrocyte Reagents. *In* XII European Conference on Animal Blood Groups and Biochemical Polymorphism. Kovács. G., and Papp, M., eds. W. Junk N.V., The Hague, and Académiai Kiadó, Budapest, p. 369, 1972.

Simpson-Morgan M.W., and Smeaton, T.C.: The Transfer of Antibodies by Neonates and Adults. Adv. Vet. Sci., *16*:355, 1972.

Slappendel, R.J.: The Diagnostic Significance of the Direct Antiglobulin Test (DAT) in Anemic Dogs. Vet. Immunol. Immunopathol., *1*:49, 1979.

Slappendel, R.J., et al.: Canine Systemic Lupus Erythematosus Treated with Prednisone. Zentrabl. Veterinärmed., *19A*(1):23, 1972.

Slappendel, R.J., et al.: Cold Hemagglutinin Disease in a Toy Pinscher Dog. Tijdschr. Diergeneeskd., *100*:445, 1975.

Slauson, D.O., et al.: Naturally Occurring Immune Complex Glomerulonephritis in the Cat. J. Pathol., *103*:131, 1971.

Smith, J.E., et al.: A New Storage Medium for Canine Blood. J. Amer. Vet. Med. Ass., *172*:701, 1978.

Socha, W.W.: Blood Groups of Apes and Monkeys: Current Status and Practical Applications. Lab. Anim. Sci., *30*:698, 1980.

Sodikoff, L.H., and Custer, M.A.: Secondary Autoimmune Hemolytic Anemia in Cats. J. Amer. Anim. Hosp. Ass., *2*:20, 1966.

Sonoda, M., et al.: Clinical and Hematological Studies on Hemolytic Icterus of Foals. Exp. Reports Equine Health Lab., *9*:103, 1972.

Spooner, R.L., and Maddy, A.H.: The Isolation of Ox Red Cell Membrane Antigens: Antigens Associated with Sialoprotein. Immunology, *21*:809, 1971.

Spooner, R.L., et al.: Analysis of Alloantisera against Bovine Lymphocytes: Joint Report of the 1st International Bovine Lymphocyte Antigen (BOLA) Workshop. Anim. Blood. Groups Biochem. Genet., *15*:63, 1979.

Stear, M.J., and Spooner, R.L.: Lymphocyte Antigens in Sheep. Anim. Blood Groups Biochem. Genet., *12*:265, 1981.

Stear, M.J., et al.: Two Closely Linked Loci and One Apparently Independent Locus Code for Bovine Lymphocyte Antigens. Tissue Antigens, *20*:289, 1982.

Stieler, C.M.: Identification of Erythrocytic Types in Dogs by Antisera and Lectins. Diss. Abstr., *39B*:3687, 1979.

Stockham, S.L., et al.: Canine Autoimmune Hemolytic Disease with a Delayed Erythroid Regeneration. J. Amer. Anim. Hosp. Ass., *16*:927, 1980.

Storb, R.: Human Bone Marrow Transplantation. Transplant. Proc., *15*:1379, 1983.

Storb, R., and Thomas, E.D.: Allogeneic Bone-Marrow Transplantation. Immunol. Rev., *71*:77, 1983.

Storb, R., et al.: The Effect of Prior Blood Transfusions on Hemopoietic Grafts from Histoincompatible Canine Littermates. Transplantation, *14*:248, 1972.

Stormont, C.: Acquisition of the J Substance by the Bovine Erythrocyte. Proc. Natl. Acad. Sci. USA, *35*:232, 1949.

Stormont, C.: An Example of a Recessive Blood Group in Sheep. Genetics, *36*:577, 1951.

Stormont, C.: Current Status of Blood Groups in Cattle. Ann. N.Y. Acad. Sci., *97*:251, 1962.

Stormont, C.J.: Hemolytic Diseases of Newborn Calves. Fed. Proc., *31*(2):761, 1972.

Stormont, C.J.: A Survey of Blood Groups in Several Species of Animals Used in Medical Research. In National Conference on Research Animals in Medicine. Jan. 28–30, 1972. Dept. Health Educ. and Welfare pub. no. (NIH) 72–181, 1973.

Stormont, C.J.: Neonatal Isoerythrolysis in Domestic Animals: A Comparative Review. Adv. Vet. Sci. Comp. Med., *19*:23, 1975.

Stormont, C.J.: The Etiology of Bovine Neonatal Isoerythrolysis. Bovine Practitioner, *12*:22(Nov.), 1977.

Stormont, C.J.: Positive Horse Blood Typing. Part 2. Blood Typing. Equine Pract., *1*(5):48, 1979.

Stormont, C.J.: Blood Groups in Animals. J. Amer. Vet. Med. Ass., *181*:1120, 1982.

Stormont, C.J., and Suzuki, Y.: Canine Blood Groups. In The Canine as a Biomedical Research Model: Immunological, Hematological, and Oncological Aspects. Shifrine, M., and Wilson, F.D., eds. Tech. Info. Center/U.S. Dept. Energy, pp. 127–133, 1980.

Stormorken, H., et al.: Thrombocytopenic Bleedings in Young Pigs Due to Maternal Isoimmunization. Nature, *198*:1116, 1963.

Storset, A.: Blood Groups in Horses. Norsk, Veterinaertidsskrift, *89*(1):6, 1977.

Stuart, M.J., et al.: Chronic Idiopathic Thrombocytopenic Purpura: A Familial Immunodeficiency Syndrome. J. Amer. Med. Ass., *239*:939, 1978.

Sutton, R.H., et al.: Autoimmune Haemolytic Anaemia in a Horse. N.Z. Vet. J., *26*:311, 1978.

Suzuki, Y., and Stormont, C.: Genetic control of an in Vitro Autolytic Factor in Horse Red Cells. In XII European Conference on Animal Blood Groups and Biochemical Polymorphism. Kovács, G., and Papp, M., eds. W. Junk N.V., The Hague, and Académiai Kiadó, Budapest, p. 525, 1972.

Suzuki, Y., et al.: New Antibodies in Dog Blood Groups. Transplant. Proc., *7*:365, 1975.

Svejgaard, A., et al.: HLA and Disease 1982: A Survey. Immunol. Rev., *70*:193, 1983.

Swisher, S.N., and Burka, E.R.: Cryopathic Hemolytic Syndromes. In Hematology. 2nd ed. Williams, W.J., et al., eds. McGraw-Hill, New York, pp. 596–600, 1977a.

Swisher, S.N., and Burka, E.R.: Acquired Hemolytic Anemia Due to Warm Reacting Autoantibodies. In Hematology. 2nd ed. Williams, W.J., et al., eds. McGraw-Hill, New York, pp. 585–596, 1977b.

Swisher, S.N., et al.: In Vitro and in Vivo Studies of the Behavior of Canine Erythrocyte-Isoantibody Systems. Ann. N.Y. Acad. Sci., *97*:15, 1962.

Switzer, J.W., and Jain, N.C.: Autoimmune Hemolytic Anemia in Dogs and Cats. Vet. Clin. North Amer. (Small Anim. Pract.), *11*:405, 1981.

Switzer, J.W., et al.: Clinicopathologic Conference. J. Amer. Vet. Med. Ass., *149*:774, 1966.

Talbot, R.B., and Andresen, E.: Influence of Blood Group Antibodies on Survival of Transfused Erythrocytes in Pigs. Amer. J. Vet. Res., *25*:1556, 1964.

Tam, S.-C., et al.: Blood Replacement in Dogs by Dextran-Hemoglobin. Can. J. Biochem., *56*:981, 1978.

Tan, E.M.: Autoantibodies to Nuclear Antigens (ANA): Their Immunobiology and Medicine. Adv. Immunol., *33*:167, 1982.

Taub, R.N.: Biologic Effects of Heterologous Antilymphocyte Serum. Prog. Allergy, *14*:208, 1970.

Ten Pas, A., and Monto, R.W.: The Treatment of Autoimmune Hemolytic Anemia with Heparin. Amer. J. Med. Sci., *251*:63, 1966.

Terasaki, P.I., et al.: Serology of HLA. Transplant. Proc., *13*:900, 1981.

Theofilopoulos, A.N., and Dixon, F.J.: Autoimmune Disease Immunopathology and Etiopathogenesis. Amer. J. Pathol., *108*:319, 1982.

Thiele, O.W., et al.: Studies on the Chemical Nature of the Lipidic J Blood-Group Substance of Cattle. Anim. Blood Groups Biochem. Genet., *10*:1, 1979.

Thomas, E.D., et al.: Bone-Marrow Transplantation. New Eng. J. Med., *292*:832, 895, 1975.

Thrall, M.A.: Unpublished observations, 1983.

Tizard, I.R.: An Introduction to Veterinary Immunology. 2nd ed. W.B. Saunders, Philadelphia, p. 285, 1982.

Tucker, E.M.: Some Physiological Aspects of Genetic Variation in the Blood of Sheep. Anim. Blood Groups Biochem. Genet., *7*:207, 1976.

Tucker, E.M., et al.: Close Linkage between the C Blood Group Locus and the Locus Controlling Amino Acid Transport in Sheep Erythrocytes. Anim. Blood Groups Biochem. Genet., *11*:119, 1980.

Utroska, B.: Autoimmune Hemolytic Anemia Associated with Lupus Erythematosus (in a Dog). Vet. Med. Small Anim. Clin., *71*:1247, 1976.

Utroska, B.: Autoimmune Hemolytic Anemia in Sibling Cats. Vet. Med. Small Anim. Clin., 75:1699, 1980.

Valli, V.E.O., and Erb, H.N.: Idiopathic Immune Hemolytic Anemia with Deficient Remodeling of Medullary Bone in a Holstein Calf. Can. Vet. J., 18:222, 1977.

van Boxtel, C.J., et al.: Immunofluorescence Microphotometry for the Detection of Platelet Antibodies. III. Demonstration of Autoantibodies against Platelets. Scand. J. Immunol., 4:657, 1975.

van Bree, H., et al.: Blood Transfusion in Dogs. I. Blood Groups, Incompatibility and Clinical Indications. Vlaams Diergeneeskindig Tijschrift, 46:26, 1977.

van Dam, R.H.: Definition and Biological Significance of the Major Histocompatibility System (MHS) in Man and Animals. Vet. Immunol. Immunopathol., 5:517, 1981.

van Dam, R.H., et al.: The Histocompatibility Complex GLA in the Goat. Anim. Blood Groups Biochem. Genet., 10:121, 1979.

van Dam, R.H., et al.: The Major Histocompatibility Complex in the Goat (GLA). Anim. Blood Groups Biochem. Genet., 11(suppl.):55, 1980.

van der Walt, K., and Osterhoff, D.R.: Blood Transfusion in Cattle with Special Reference to the Influence of Blood Group. I. Single Transfusions into Young Animals and Pregnant Cows. J.S. Afr. Vet. Med. Ass., 40:107, 1969a.

van der Walt, K., and Osterhoff, D.R.: Blood Transfusion in Cattle with Special Reference to the Influence of Blood Groups. II. Repeated Blood Transfusions. J.S. Afr. Vet. Med. Ass., 40:265, 1969b.

van Rood, J.J., and Eernisse, J.G.: The Detection of Transplantation Antigens in Leukocytes. Semin. Hematol., 5:187, 1968.

van Rood, J.J., et al.: New Facts on HLA Genetics: Are They Relevant in Bone Marrow Transplantation? Semin. Hematol., 21:65, 1984.

Veenhoven, W.A., et al.: Platelet Antibodies in Idiopathic Thrombocytopenic Purpura. Clin. Exp. Immunol., 39:645, 1980.

Vegh, P., and Petri, G.: The Use of Antilymphocyte Serum. Panminerva Med., 20(1):39, 1978.

Verheugt, F.W.A., et al.: Autoimmune Granulocytopenia: The Detection of Granulocyte Autoantibodies with the Immunofluorescence Test. Brit. J. Haematol., 39:339, 1978.

von dam Borne, A.E.G.K., et al.: Baka: A New Platelet Specific Antigen Involved in Neonatal Allo-immune Thrombocytopenia. Vox Sang., 39:113, 1980.

Vos, G.H., et al.: Specificity and Immunoglobulin Characteristics of Autoantibodies in Acquired Hemolytic Anemia. J. Immunol., 106:1172, 1971.

Vriesendorp, H.M.: Application of Transplantation Immunology in the Dog. Adv. Vet. Sci. Comp. Med., 23:229, 1979.

Vriesendorp, H.M., et al.: Polymorphism of the DL-A System. Transplantation, 14:299, 1972.

Waksman, B.H., et al.: The Use of Specific "Lymphocyte" Antisera to Inhibit Hypersensitive Reactions of the "Delayed" Type. J. Exp. Med., 114:997, 1961.

Walford, R.L.: Leukocyte Antigens and Antibodies. Grune & Stratton, New York, 1960.

Walford, R.L.: The Isoantigenic Systems of Human Leukocytes: Medical and Biological Significance. Ser. Haematol., 2(2):1, 1969.

Walton, D.K., et al.: Canine Discoid Lupus Erythematosus. J. Amer. Anim. Hosp. Ass., 17:851, 1981.

Watkins, W.M.: Blood-Group Substances. Science, 152:172, 1966.

Weiser, G., et al.: Erythrocyte Volume Distribution Analysis and Hematologic Changes in Two Horses with Immune-Mediated Hemolytic Anemia. Vet. Pathol., 20:424, 1983.

Weiss, R.A., et al.: Diagnostic Tests and Clinical Subsets in Systemic Lupus Erythematosus: Update 1983. Ann. Allergy, 51:135, 1983.

Werner, L.L.: Coombs Positive Anemia in the Dog and Cat. Comp. Cont. Educ. Small Anim., 2:96, 1980.

Werner, L.L.: Immunologic Diseases Affecting Internal Organ Systems. In Textbooks of Veterinary Internal Medicine. Vol. 2. Diseases of the Dog and Cat. Ettinger, S.J., ed. W.B. Saunders, Philadelphia, ch. 83. p. 2158, 1983.

Wiener, A.S.: Blood Groups and Transfusion. 3rd ed. Hafner Publishing Co., New York, 1943.

Wiener, A.S., and Wexler, I.B.: An Rh-Hr Syllabus. Grune & Stratton, New York, 1963.

Wiener, A.S., et al.: Studies on Autoantibodies in Human Sera. J. Immunol., 71:58, 1953.

Wilkins, R.J., et al.: Immunologically Mediated Thrombocytopenia in the Dog. J. Amer. Vet. Med. Ass., 163:277, 1973.

Williams, D.A., and Maggio-Price, L.: Canine Idiopathic Thrombocytopenia: Clinical Observations and Long-Term Follow-Up in 54 Cases. J. Amer. Vet. Med. Ass., 185:660, 1984.

Willkens, R.F., et al.: Comparative Evaluation of Antinuclear Factor Tests in Rheumatic Disorders. Med. Clin. North Amer., 52:559, 1968.

Wink, A.: Granulocyte-Specific Antinuclear Antibodies. Allergy, 35:263, 1980.

Wintrobe, M.M., et al.: Clinical Hematology. 8th ed. Lea & Febiger, Philadelphia, 1981.

Wolstenholme, G.E.W., and O' Connor, M., eds.: Antilymphocyte Serum. Little, Brown & Co., Boston, 1967.

Woodruff, M.F.A.: Antilymphocyte Serum and Its Mode of Action. Transplant. Proc., 3:34, 1971.

Woodruff, M.F.A., and Anderson, N.A.: Effect of Lymphocyte Depletion by Thoracic Duct Fistula and Administration of Antilymphocytic Serum on the Survival of Skin Homografts in Rats. Nature, 200:702, 1963.

Worlledge, S.: Auto-Immunity and Blood Diseases. Practitioner, 199:171, 1967.

Wright, J.N.: Some Incompatibilities in the Blood of Cattle. Cornell Vet., 52:327, 1962a.

Wright, J.N.: Blood Incompatibilities in the Dog. Cornell Vet., 52:523, 1962b.

Yamamoto, K.: Experimental Studies on Blood Transfusion into Dogs: Blood Groups and Clinical and Hematological Findings on Transfusion Using Erythrocytes. Jpn. J. Vet. Res., 28:52, 1980.

Young, L.E., et al.: Hemolytic Disease in Newborn Dogs following Isoimmunization of the Dam by Transfusion. Science, 109:630, 1949a.

Young, L.E., et al.: Hemolytic Reactions Produced in Dogs by Transfusion of Incompatible Dog Blood and Plasma. Blood, 4:1218, 1949b.

Young, L.E., et al.: Hemolytic Disease in Newborn Dogs. Blood, 6:291, 1951.

Young, L.E., et al.: Blood Groups in Dogs: Their Significance to the Veterinarian. Amer. J. Vet. Res., 13:207, 1952.

Zachary, A.A.: An Immunogenetic Study of the Equine

Leukocyte Antigen (ELA) System. Diss. Abstr. B, 43:3481, 1983.

Zaleski, M.B., et al.: Immunogenetics. Pitman, Boston, 1983.

Zeigler, Z., et al.: Immune Hemolytic Anemia and Thrombocytopenia Secondary to Quinidine: In Vitro Studies of the Quinidine-Dependent Red Cell and Platelet Antibodies. Blood, 53:396, 1979.

Zenoble, R.D., and Stone, E.A.: Autotransfusion in the Dog. J. Amer. Vet. Med. Ass., 172:1411, 1978.

Zmijewski, C.M.: Immunohematology. 2nd ed. Appleton-Century-Crofts, New York, 1978.

36

Blood Pictures in Some Common Diseases of Domestic Animals

CHRONIC RENAL FAILURE IN THE DOG   1040

CANINE LEPTOSPIROSIS   1043

CANINE DISTEMPER   1046

INFECTIOUS CANINE HEPATITIS   1049

PYOMETRA IN THE DOG   1051

CANINE CUSHING'S SYNDROME (HYPERADRENOCORTICISM)   1054

HYPOADRENOCORTICISM (ADDISON'S DISEASE) IN THE DOG   1059

HYPOTHYROIDISM IN THE DOG   1063

CANINE AND EQUINE EHRLICHIOSIS   1066

CANINE LEISHMANIASIS   1068

FELINE INFECTIOUS PERITONITIS   1068

FELINE PANLEUKOPENIA   1071

HEMOGRAMS IN ACUTE AND CHRONIC INFLAMMATORY DISEASES IN CATTLE   1074

ACUTE BOVINE MASTITIS   1076

EXPERIMENTAL COLIFORM MASTITIS   1078

The purpose of this chapter is to outline briefly the characteristic clinical and laboratory findings in some common diseases. It should be recalled that laboratory data are of greatest value when combined with a complete history and a thorough physical examination. A blood study represents the situation at the moment the blood is drawn; the laboratory data become increasingly meaningful as tests are repeated so that the progress of the disease can be followed. The Appendix cases that follow this chapter generally include multiple hemograms to show progress in representative diseases of individual patients.

CHRONIC RENAL FAILURE IN THE DOG

A distinction has been made in recent years between renal disease and renal failure. Renal disease (injury) may vary in extent and therefore may be reversible or irreversible and may or may not manifest renal dysfunction. Renal failure, on the other hand, is evident when about two-thirds of the functional renal mass has been compromised. The classic hemato-logic abnormality of a progressive nonresponsive anemia of renal disease is associated with chronic renal failure ("end stage" kidney disease or renal failure); the present discussion is limited to this form of advanced renal insufficiency. Chronic renal failure in dogs and cats may be caused by a variety of primary glomerular, tubular, interstitial, or vascular disorders, which may be congenital or acquired (Osborne et al., 1983). The etiology of such disorders is also varied and commonly includes immune, infectious, and toxic mechanisms. Diseases of the kidney (Cowgill, 1983) and pathophysiology of renal disease, renal failure, and uremia have been thoroughly discussed (Osborne et al., 1983). Table 36–1 lists selected hemograms on dogs with chronic renal failure, and details of a dog with acute renal failure are given in Appendix Case 2.

Chronic renal failure may occur at any age, but is more common after 5 years of age. The renal cortical hypoplasia may occur as a congenital condition, and therefore the signs of chronic renal failure may be seen at an early age (Finco et al., 1970; Persson et al., 1961). The most common forms of chronic renal dis-

Table 36-1. Biochemistry and Hematology of Chronic Renal Failure in the Dog

Age (yr)	Sex	Clinical Type[a]	Urine Specific Gravity	Urine Protein	BUN	Creatinine	Ca	P	Fibrinogen (g/dl)	Protein (g/dl)	ESR (cor)	PCV (%)	WBC/μl	Band	Neutrophils	Lymphocytes	Monocytes	Eosinophils	Basophils
1	F	P	1.009	1+	120	—	12.1	10.2	0.8	8.4	27+	25	30,300	0	21,059	2,575	6,060	606	0
1	M	I	1.004	2+	157	—	11.6	11.4	1.0	8.0	33+	38	10,800	0	8,748	810	810	378	54
2	F	PG	1.008	2+	141	6.4	13.3	14.0	0.7	6.8	27+	23	12,100	0	8,470	2,057	726	847	0
3	F	PO	1.012	1+	360	13.0	8.2	21.0	0.7	9.4	27+	21	7,700	38	6,699	423	539	0	0
4	M	IO	1.009	1+	103	—	10.8	5.9	0.7	7.2	33+	24	16,300	81	11,247	1,304	3,260	245	163
5	M	G	1.008	1+	144	6.0	4.6	18.8	0.7	6.1	9+	10	18,400	0	17,204	184	920	92	0
5	M	I	1.013	—	156	28.0	6.9	28.0	0.5	8.7	42+	36	9,000	0	8,190	495	315	0	0
6	F	G	1.017	4+	177	3.8	7.9	17.6	0.7	5.2	1+	37	10,900	109	9,374	545	763	109	0
7	M	P	1.011	2+	204	—	13.0	14.2	0.7	10.9	24+	44	31,100	0	27,213	311	3,577	0	0
7	M	IO	1.013	4+	282	4.4	6.2	20.8	0.6	7.3	—	22	8,300	83	7,262	83	830	41	0
8	M	IO	1.013	2+	136	—	10.9	11.2	0.8	8.5	25+	28	16,500	0	13,860	165	2,475	0	0
8	F	I	1.010	2+	277	15.6	4.5	30.0	0.7	8.1	35+	29	21,800	0	19,838	872	981	109	0
9	F	G	1.013	3+	205	—	—	—	0.9	8.4	27+	43	15,800	395	13,746	395	1,264	0	0
10	F	PG	1.011	2+	150	7.7	—	15.3	0.4	7.9	16+	26	9,500	142	7,362	522	1,377	95	0
11	F	G	1.013	4+	265	—	6.6	17.8	1.3	7.5	34+	39	18,700	0	16,082	281	1,963	374	0
15	M	G	1.010	2+	169	—	—	—	0.3	9.0	8+	50	14,300	429	11,011	858	1,215	787	0

[a]P = pyelonephritis; I = interstitial nephritis; G = glomerulonephritis; O = osteodystrophy fibrosa.

ease, based on histopathologic diagnosis, have been nearly equally distributed among interstitial nephritis, glomerulonephritis, and pyelonephritis. Examples of these three common forms are presented in Table 36–1. Findings on urine analysis, biochemical tests, and hematologic studies have been similar, regardless of pathologic diagnosis. Similar findings were reported by Osborne et al. (1969a).

The functional reserve capacity of the kidney is of such magnitude that clinical signs of renal disease may not become apparent until 60–75% of the renal parenchyma has become incapacitated (Osborne, 1970; Osborne et al., 1983). Blood urea nitrogen (BUN) and creatinine concentrations increase when the glomerular filtration rate falls below the level necessary for maintenance of homeostasis (Appendix Case 5). The resulting uremia is accompanied by a reduced capacity of the kidney tubules to dilute or concentrate the urine to meet the water needs of the body. Failure on the part of the tubules to excrete inorganic phosphate and potassium or to retain sodium are features common to failing kidney function.

Clinical signs resulting from failure of kidney function are polydipsia, polyuria, vomiting, uremic breath, ulceration of oral mucous membranes, pale mucous membranes reflecting anemia, weight loss, weakness, and, in some instances, central nervous system disturbances.

Urine specific gravity becomes fixed in the range of the glomerular filtrate (1.010 ± 0.002). Proteinuria is variable, depending on the degree of glomerular involvement. In glomerulonephritis, the daily loss of albumin in the urine may be of such magnitude as to result in hypoproteinemia from hypoalbuminemia (Appendix Case 4). Renal amyloidosis is another form of chronic renal disease characterized by marked proteinuria and hypoproteinemia (Osborne et al., 1969b). Failure to excrete inorganic phosphate leads to hyperphosphatemia and a distortion of the normal calcium:phosphorus ratio of 3:1. This leads to a chain of events whereby blood calcium concentration is reduced, which in turn stimulates the parathyroid glands to secrete parathormone. Calcium is then mobilized from the bones, particularly from the man-

dible. The jawbones may become soft and rubbery, producing the condition referred to as "rubber jaw" or "renal rickets." The bone structure is replaced by fibrous tissue, giving rise to the designation *osteodystrophy fibrosa*. The calcium removed from the skeleton may succeed in overcoming the hypocalcemia, but the Ca:P ratio remains distorted (Table 36–1). Calcium is deposited in the soft tissue and is grossly visible at necropsy, particularly in intercostal musculature.

The hemogram (Table 36–1) is commonly characterized by a normocytic-normochromic anemia, a high corrected erythrocyte sedimentation rate (ESR), hyperfibrinogenemia, and marked lymphopenia. The anemia, when it exists, is due to depressed erythropoiesis, with the PCV generally being in the range of 20–30%. In dogs that survive for many months, the anemia may be progressive, and PCV may fall as low as 10% (Appendix Case 5). Anemia may sometimes be masked by dehydration associated with renal failure. Highly echinocytic red cells referred to as "burr cells" may be seen in advanced cases of uremia (Chapter 20). Bone marrow cytology reveals hypoplasia of the erythrocytic maturation series leading to an elevated M:E ratio (Table 4–9). Granulopoiesis is not affected, although some abnormal cells may be seen.

Pathophysiologic mechanisms of anemia include reduced erythropoietin production by diseased kidneys, hypoproliferation of erythroid progenitors in bone marrow from toxic uremic substances, and reduced red cell life span. Other contributing factors include iron deficiency from chronic blood loss or impaired absorption, myelofibrosis secondary to renal osteodystrophy, and chronic infection and malnutrition. Blood loss through gastrointestinal hemorrhage, seen in humans, is not usually a part of the clinical syndrome of chronic renal failure in the dog. See Chapter 25 for additional comments on mechanisms of anemia in chronic renal disease.

Total plasma protein concentration is commonly in excess of 7.5 g/dl, except in those instances of glomerulonephritis in which significant daily loss of albumin in the urine has taken place. This latter situation seemed to have existed in the 6-year-old and one of the

5-year-old dogs in Table 36–1. The hyperproteinemia may be a reflection of a modest dehydration, but to some extent it is also due to the increase in plasma fibrinogen. Most dogs with chronic renal failure have elevated plasma fibrinogen levels, possibly in response to development of vascular lesions (Kelly, 1967) or other inflammatory lesions. The significantly elevated ESR characteristic of chronic renal failure in the dog may be related in part to the hyperfibrinogenemia. Glomerular fibrin deposition occurs in chronic glomerulonephritis as well as chronic interstitial nephritis by unknown mechanisms but may involve activation of coagulation cascade by immune complexes lodged in the glomeruli (Wright et al., 1976).

The total leukocyte count is variable, commonly in the high normal range, with an occasional dog exhibiting leukocytosis. Leukopenia is rarely seen. On differential leukocyte count, a neutrophilia and monocytosis may be seen associated with eosinopenia or persistence of eosinophils within the mid-normal range. Infrequently, a temporary eosinophilia occurs. Neutrophilia with left shift is common in acute pyelonephritis and kidney abscesses. The most consistent and characteristic feature of the differential leukocyte count in chronic renal failure is a marked lymphopenia. In very young dogs, the existing lymphopenia may not appear as impressive as in older dogs because absolute lymphocyte numbers in health are higher in young dogs (see Chapter 4). When neutrophilia, monocytosis, and eosinopenia accompany the lymphopenia, the action of corticosteroids of stress may be suspected. However, marked lymphopenia exists irrespective of other signs of the stress pattern due to depression of lymphopoiesis by the uremic toxins.

The observations of Holman (1944) support this concept. He produced renal insufficiency in dogs with uranium nitrate, mercury bichloride, or bilateral nephrectomy and observed the effect of the developing uremia on the lymphocytic tissues. Gross and histologic changes interpreted as "exhaustion atrophy" were consistent findings in lymph nodes, spleen, thymus, Peyer's patches, and solitary lymphoid follicles in a group of 78 adult dogs. The lymphocyte number in blood fell to an average of 32% below the normal control level. Lymphopenia is also seen in uremic cats. Lymphopenia in uremic humans involves decreases of both T- and B-lymphocytes (Anagnostou et al., 1981).

Some acquired coagulopathies have also been defined in recent studies on human and canine patients with uremia (Anagnostou et al., 1981; Remuzzi et al., 1979). Platelets acquire reversible qualitative defects of reduced availability of platelet factor 3 (PF-3) and decreased adhesiveness and aggregation. These changes are attributed to circulating uremic toxins, namely, guanidinosuccinic acid and hydroxyphenolacetic acid in dogs (Anagnostou et al., 1981) and prostacyclin in humans (Remuzzi et al., 1979). Platelet dysfunction may manifest as prolonged bleeding time and elevated clot retraction time and is reversed when uremia is controlled by dialysis or diet. Activation of clotting factors leading to thromboembolism has also been observed in human and canine patients with certain types of glomerulonephropathy. Although exact mechanisms remain unknown, a contributing factor may be diminished levels of antithrombin III from excessive renal loss.

CANINE LEPTOSPIROSIS

Leptospirosis in the dog is due primarily to *Leptospira canicola* and *Leptospira icterohemorrhagiae*. Clinically inapparent, but serologically detectable infections may occur with some other serotypes (Chapter 23). The disease is more severe in infections with *L. icterohemorrhagiae* than in those with *L. canicola*.

Clinical Signs

Leptospirosis in the dog may vary from a mild form that goes undetected to an acute septicemic form characterized by sudden onset leading to kidney failure and death. The most common clinical signs are listlessness or depression, varying from mild to marked, partial to complete anorexia, increased thirst, vomiting of bile-stained mucus, conjunctival congestion, and a variety of signs indicative of muscle stiffness and pain. Palpation may elicit pain over the lumbar region and may also reveal a tense, painful abdomen. Jaundice may occur in about 15% of cases due to

L. canicola infection, while it may be seen in up to 70% of cases from infection with *L. icterohemorrhagiae* (Farrow and Love, 1983). The body temperature may have passed its peak by the time of presentation of the dog to the veterinarian. In experimentally produced leptospirosis, the rectal temperature may be 105.0°F, occasionally as high as 107.0°F, with rapid decline usually within 24 hours. Data on 18 dogs, 12 males and 6 females, aged 2 months to 7 years, are summarized in Table 36–2.

Diagnosis

An attempt should be made to demonstrate leptospirae in blood, urine, or tissue material by dark-field examination, culture, or animal transmission (Chapter 23). Urine examination is performed using uncentrifuged specimen or the supernatant of a centrifuged sample; it is rarely necessary to employ urinary sediment for this purpose. The various leptospirae are indistinguishable on morphologic basis. In experimentally produced leptospirosis, leptospiruria was first detected on the seventh day postinoculation, and the urine was positive for leptospirae in 72–78% of examinations made over 80–100 days (Taylor et al., 1970).

A confirming diagnosis is based on the demonstration of a rise in serum antibody titer between two samples taken 10 days to 2 weeks apart. On occasion, there may be no evidence of antibody titer in the first serum sample, but the diagnosis is confirmed when the second serum sample demonstrates the presence of antibodies against the leptospiral antigen. The serologic data presented in Table 36–2 are based on the microscopic agglutination test; the highest titers obtained to *L. canicola* and *L. icterohemorrhagiae* are recorded. In some instances, a second blood sample was not submitted either because the dog was not returned for a progress check or because it had died. In those instances, the demonstration of leptospirae in the urine was recorded as evidence of infection.

Antibody cross-reaction occurs between *L. canicola* and *L. icterohemorrhagiae*, but titers for the former are greater than for the latter organism (Table 36–2). In experimental infection of dogs, agglutinins were demonstrated

between the fourth and seventh days after inoculation with *L. icterohemorrhagiae* and between the sixth and eleventh days after inoculation with *L. canicola*. The titers tended to reach their peak during the third week and began to decline after the sixth or seventh week (Monlux, 1948). Dogs inoculated with *L. canicola* had leptospiremia on day 4 and irregularly thereafter (12–13% positive tests) during an observation period extending over 80–100 days (Taylor et al., 1970).

Clinical Pathology

Clinico-pathologic findings were variable and were influenced to some extent by the stage of the disease on initial examination. Since the kidneys are the major target organ of the leptospirae, many of the clinical signs were referable to failing kidney function. The proximal portion of convoluted tubules is particularly involved, showing changes characteristic of degeneration and atrophy (Monlux, 1953). BUN and creatinine become elevated as tubular function fails and the glomerular filtration rate decreases. Two dogs, admitted early in the course of the disease, had a BUN value falling within the normal range of 10-28 mg/dl. In 4 dogs, the range was 32-93 mg, while in 12 dogs, the BUN was 100–300 mg. Despite the low BUN value in some dogs, evidence of tubular injury is seen in a low urine specific gravity (<1.015) and, in some instances, is suggested by the presence of reducing substances (positive reaction for sugar) in the urine. Proteinuria is also a prominent finding.

Icterus has not been a common finding among dogs admitted to the Veterinary Medical Teaching Hospital, University of California, Davis (VMTH-UCD) with *L. canicola* infection. One dog with marked icterus is described in Appendix Case 3. When leptospirosis was first detected and described in California, icterus characterized the disease in 48.6% of the dogs (Meyer et al., 1939).

Some dehydration was usually reflected in a total plasma protein concentration in excess of 7.5 g/dl; in one instance a PCV in excess of 50% was noted. The acute inflammatory nature of leptospirosis resulted in plasma fibrinogen levels in excess of 0.4 g/dl (range, 0.5–0.9 g) in the majority of dogs, and in many dogs

Table 36–2. The Clinical Pathology of Canine Leptospirosis

						Plasma			Urine			Serology (titer)			Differential Leukocyte Count in Absolute Numbers/μl						
Age	Sex	Temp. (°F)	PCV (%)	ESR (cor)	Icterus Index	Protein (g/dl)	Fibrinogen (g/dl)	BUN (mg/dl)	Specific Gravity	Sugar	Dark Field[a]	L. canicola	L. icterohaemorrhagiae	WBC/μl	Band	Neutrophils	Lymphocytes	Monocytes	Eosinophils	Basophils
2 mo	M	101.2	36	4–	10	6.1	0.5	300	1.017	1+	–	1:1,280	1:640	24,800	124	21,328	868	2,480	0	0
3 mo	F	100.5	44	5–	20	9.4	0.4	260	1.012	2+	–	1:3,000	1:300	13,400	0	9,916	2,211	1,206	67	0
4 mo	F	104.6	36	–	2	7.6	0.8	13	1.014	trace	+	1:300	1:100	25,200	756	16,884	2,142	5,418	0	0
7 mo	F	105.3	36	–	2	7.6	0.9	14	1.008	–	+	1:5,120	1:640	25,100	251	15,939	4,141	4,769	0	0
8 mo	M	101.4	39	40+	2	9.5	0.4	116	1.014	–	+	1:10,240	1:5,120	11,000	0	6,490	2,145	110	2,200	55
9 mo	M	101.4	40	9–	2	8.0	0.3	200	1.016	2+	+	1:40	–	13,100	0	10,349	1,310	1,244	196	0
10 mo	F	102.1	39	39+	2	7.8	0.4	33	1.007	–	+	1:3,000	1:1,000	23,500	702	14,040	4,329	3,861	468	0
10 mo	M	–	46	–	5	8.9	0.6	184	1.021	–	+	–	–	22,400	448	15,344	1,904	4,704	0	0
12 mo	M	101.6	31	42+	2	8.1	0.5	176	1.013	trace	c	1:10,240	1:5,120	16,300	0	9,210	1,630	570	4,564	326
14 mo[b]	M	101.0	43	–	2	8.6	0.7	225	1.014	trace	+	1:2,560	1:1,280	52,700	1,054	41,370	790	9,486	0	0
14 mo	M	101.7	40	25+	2	8.3	0.4	32	1.007	trace	–	1:1,000	–	25,600	2,432	19,200	2,304	1,664	0	0
16 mo[b]	M	103.0	49	–	2	8.4	0.6	145	1.021	trace	+	1:320	1:40	40,000	1,000	35,400	600	3,000	0	0
18 mo	M	102.7	45	28+	2	8.9	0.5	78	1.010	3+	+	1:10,240	1:1,280	64,500	11,610	44,505	967	7,417	0	0
3 yr[b]	M	103.0	46	11+	10	11.5	0.8	300	1.019	1+	+	–	–	15,400	462	13,167	693	1,078	0	0
3 yr	F	102.5	54	6+	2	11.4	0.7	133	1.019	1+	–	1:20,480	1:2,560	19,100	382	17,095	477	1,146	0	0
3 yr	M	101.6	46	20+	2	9.6	0.9	100	1.009	–	–	1:640	1:320	30,100	0	23,628	2,408	4,063	0	0
5 yr	F	100.2	45	3–	5	7.7	0.5	148	1.007	2+	+	1:1,280	1:640	13,400	134	11,189	536	536	1,005	0
7 yr	M	102.0	40	28+	7.5	9.3	0.8	93	1.010	2+	–	1:320	1:320	32,300	161	28,585	3,068	484	0	0

a +, *Leptospirae* seen.
b Died.
c Dark field examination negative, but urine culture positive for *Leptospirae*.

a significantly elevated corrected ESR was seen, although in some dogs the corrected ESR had a negative value.

The total leukocyte count was variable but generally ranged from high normal to a modest leukocytosis of 20,000–40,000/μl. Two dogs had leukocyte counts in excess of 50,000. Neutrophilia with a variable left shift limited to band forms was a fairly consistent finding. A tendency for an absolute lymphopenia, absolute monocytosis, and eosinopenia was characteristic of the differential leukocyte count of old dogs. In dogs less than 1 year old, the lymphopenia was less obvious, because the normal absolute lymphocyte number is generally high in young dogs (see Chapter 4).

CANINE DISTEMPER

Canine distemper was diagnosed in 64 dogs by clinical signs, and the diagnosis was verified by demonstration of typical inclusion bodies in conjunctival scrapings (Goss et al., 1948), in blood neutrophils (Cello et al., 1959), or, on histopathologic examination, in tissues (Watson and Plummer, 1942) of dogs that died or were euthanized. Generally the dogs had been ill for 2–4 weeks or longer before being admitted to the hospital. Clinical signs in order of frequency of occurrence were (a) ocular and nasal discharge; (b) coughing and/or abnormal lung sounds, dyspnea, and pneumonia; (c) central nervous system signs such as convulsions, chorea, and champing or frothing from the mouth; (d) hardening of the foot pads; and (e) anorexia, vomiting, and diarrhea. In addition, all dogs exhibited a variable degree of depression or lethargy. Fever was the most consistent sign, with temperature elevations generally falling between 103.0°F and 105.0°F. Age ranged from 6 weeks to 8 years, with two-thirds of the dogs between 2 and 12 months of age. However, 10 of the 64 dogs were over 2 years of age. No sex predilection was evident. Experimental studies have shown that transplacental infection may occur (Krakowka et al., 1977).

Hemograms of the 64 dogs have been grouped on the basis of total leukocyte count in Table 36–3 as follows: leukopenia, 8 dogs; low normal count, 20 dogs; high normal count, 21 dogs; and leukocytosis, 15 dogs. In all groups, the extremes of the ranges for erythrocyte parameters indicated anemia in some dogs and dehydration in others. In general, the means for erythrocyte count, hemoglobin concentration, and PCV were on the low side of their normal ranges; this was attributable mainly to the immaturity of many dogs. The mean values for total plasma proteins were normal in view of the youth of most of the dogs. Hypoproteinemia was present in a few dogs, and hyperproteinemia (dehydration) in others. Plasma fibrinogen concentration revealed a trend toward a modest elevation, with means at the high normal values of 0.4–0.5 g/dl. ESR varied from 39− to 37+. Some of the larger negative corrected values for ESR were associated with plasma protein concentrations of <6.0 g/dl.

Leukopenia (WBC <6,000/μl) was present in only 12.5%, and leukocytosis (WBC >17,500/μl) occurred in 23.4% of the dogs. Among the 15 dogs with leukocytosis, the mean total leukocyte count ws 30,620 ± 10,663/μl of blood. Many dogs had been sick for several weeks and may have had complications from bacterial infections. Forty-one dogs had total leukocyte counts within the broad normal range of 6,000–17,000/μl. Leukopenia is believed to occur during the early stage of the disease and is followed by leukocytosis from secondary bacterial infection.

The most consistent feature of the differential leukocyte count was a marked *lymphopenia*, while the patterns presented by all other leukocytes were variable. The marked lymphopenia is an expression of widespread atrophy and necrosis in lymphocytic tissue produced by the virus.

Lauder and coworkers (1954) reported on the clinical and pathologic findings in 50 dogs with naturally acquired distemper. During the acute phase, there was depletion of lymphocytes and degenerative changes in lymph nodes, spleen, and tonsils, accompanied by hypertrophy of reticulum cells. After about 5 weeks, regeneration was observed in the form of new lymphoid follicles in which lymphoblasts and lymphocytes were prominent. Gibson and coworkers (1965) reported gross atrophy of the thymus, lymphoid depletion, and reticular cell hyperplasia in all lymphocytic

Table 36-3. Hemograms in Canine Distemper Grouped on the Basis of Total Leukocyte Count as Leukopenia, Low Normal, High Normal, and Leukocytosis

No. Dogs	Hemogram Class	RBC (×10⁶/μl)	Hb (g/dl)	PCV (%)	Plasma[a] Proteins (g/dl)	Fibrinogen (g/dl)	WBC/μl	Differential Leukocyte Count in Absolute Numbers/μl Band Neutrophils	Neutrophils	Lymphocytes	Monocytes	Eosinophils	Basophils
8	**Leukopenia**												
	Range	4.12–7.50	8.6–18.0	26–50	6.0–8.3	0.4–0.6	1,300–5,500	0–690	720–4,977	27–360	120–1,240	0–55	0–27
	Mean ±1 SD	5.61±1.31	12.0±2.8	36±8	(6) 6.9±0.8	(5) 0.5±0.1	3,863±1,586	237±249	2,858±1,533	227±118	513±334	9±18	3±9
20	**Low normal**												
	Range	3.08–8.25	6.7–18.1	23–54	5.3–7.6	0.1–0.8	6,000–9,500	0–1,974	998–8,052	44–1,653	484–7,315	0–585	0–88
	Mean ±1 SD	5.48±1.33	12.1±3.0	37±8	(10) 6.6±0.9	(9) 0.4±0.2	8,185±1,206	349±504	5,737±1,705	582±423	1,384±1,464	99±171	7±21
21	**High normal**												
	Range	3.74–9.30	7.1–19.6	23–58	4.5–9.4	0.2–0.6	9,900–15,300	0–2,632	6,720–12,852	54–994	288–2,550	0–610	0
	Mean ±1 SD	5.87±1.5	13.1±3.5	40±10	(15) 6.6±1.2	(11) 0.4±0.1	11,980±1,512	400±600	9,880±1,463	441±249	1,145±552	98±161	0
15	**Leukocytosis**												
	Range	3.50–6.70	7.5–16.9	25–49	4.9–8.8	0.2–0.8	18,000–53,000	0–10,822	8,640–42,480	0–2,976	481–9,824	0–1,800	0–343
	Mean ±1 SD	5.61±0.9	13.1±2.2	40±6	(11) 6.8±1.0	(10) 0.6±0.2	30,620±10,663	1,922±3,032	24,593±9,270	577±734	2,845±2,310	221±496	35±94
64	**All classes**												
	Range	3.08–9.3	6.7–19.6	23–58	4.5–9.4	0.1–0.8	1,300–53,000	0–10,822	720–42,480	0–2,976	120–9,824	0–1,800	0–343
	Mean ±1 SD	5.67±1.3	12.7±3.1	38±8	(42) 6.7±1.0	(35) 0.5±0.2	14,148±10,846	720±1,676	11,153±9,086	490±467	1,539±1,620	116±282	11±50

[a]Number of parentheses represents number of samples when less than the total for the group.

tissues examined in gnotobiotic dogs with experimentally produced distemper. Tajima and coworkers (1971) found necrosis, reticular cell hyperplasia, giant cells, and intranuclear inclusions in the lymph nodes of minks exposed to the canine distemper virus. In similar recent experimental studies in dogs, massive lymphoid necrosis was associated with depletion of both T- and B-lymphocytes in conventionally raised animals but not in gnotobiotic dogs; repopulation of lymphoid tissues occurred in subacutely infected or convalescent dogs; and cellular as well as humoral immunity was suppressed in surviving animals (Krakowka et al., 1980). These reports indicate that the virus multiplies in lymphocytic tissues and causes depletion of lymphocytes, which is responsible in turn for the characteristic lymphopenia of canine distemper. Because of the serious depression of lymphopoiesis, lymphocyte numbers in peripheral blood remain at low levels for considerable periods of time in dogs convalescing from canine distemper.

Cerebrospinal fluid from dogs with distemper encephalitis may have elevated protein and mononuclear cells, and in some cases only protein is elevated (Farrow and Love, 1983). Dogs infected with distemper virus have significantly reduced serum calcium concentrations associated with parathyroid dysfunction, and this may contribute to neurologic disturbances of canine distemper infection (Weisbrode and Krakowka, 1979).

Distemper Inclusions in Erythrocytes and Leukocytes

It is well known that distemper inclusions can be found in stained smears of scrapings from the conjunctiva and tonsils. Viral antigen can be demonstrated in such cellular materials by immunofluorescence. On rare occasions, an inclusion body has been detected in immature erythrocytes and leukocytes in blood of dogs with distemper. Usually, there has been the accompanying description of hardening of the foot pads. The inclusions, when evident in peripheral blood, can also be observed in erythroid cells of the bone marrow. The reason for the occurrence of distemper inclusions in various blood elements is unknown.

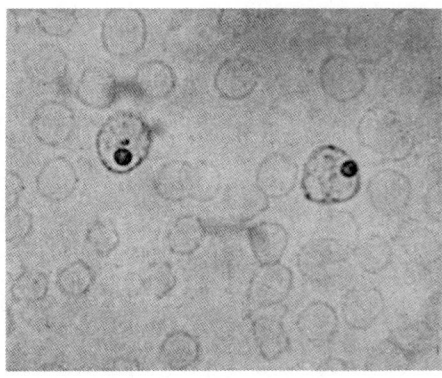

Fig. 36–1.   Inclusion bodies in young red blood cells in canine distemper. New methylene blue stain applied to dry unfixed blood film. (See also Appendix Case 37.)

In the routinely stained blood film, the inclusions in young erythrocytes stain variously from pale blue to reddish purple (Plate XVIII-9) and vary in size and location. They can be readily distinguished from Howell-Jolly bodies because they are larger and stain less intensely. With new methylene blue stain, their association with reticulocytes is obvious (Fig. 36–1). In target cells, the inclusion may be seen in the central bull's-eye, and in other forms of leptocytes, it may be present in the displaced portion of hemoglobin such as the bar extending across the middle of the cell.

Distemper inclusions may also be seen in an occasional neutrophil and lymphocyte in blood and bone marrow as circumscribed or diffuse reddish objects in the cytoplasm (Plate XIV–7; Figs. A-1 through A-5, Appendix). Electron microscopy has revealed the inclusions in erythrocytes and leukocytes to be aggregates of filamentous viral structures (nucleocapsid tubules) compatible with canine distemper virus (see Appendix Case 37; Figs. A-5 and A-6). Watson and Wright (1974a, b) have provided excellent light and electron photomicrographs and descriptions of distemper inclusions in leukocytes of three dogs. In each case inclusion bodies were seen not throughout the course of the disease but only during certain periods. The inclusions were more frequent in lymphocytes than in neutrophils, and more leukocytes were found to contain inclusions on electron microscopy than by light microscopy.

INFECTIOUS CANINE HEPATITIS

Infectious canine hepatitis (ICH or *Rubarth's disease)* is an acute infectious disease caused by an adenovirus. It may affect dogs of all ages but, like canine distemper, is generally seen in young dogs (Table 36–4). In the early stages, the clinical signs may be confused with those of distemper and leptospirosis. Some very suggestive signs are acute onset, swollen red tonsils, pain on placing pressure over the liver, and high temperature in the early stages, reaching 105–106°F. Other signs are pronounced apathy or lethargy, anorexia, abnormal thirst, vomiting that may become blood-stained terminally, and melena. Petechial hemorrhages may be seen in mucocutaneous areas, and prolonged bleeding may be observed from sites of venipuncture. Icterus may develop but is rare. During the recovery period, a keratoconjunctivitis and corneal edema in one or both eyes develops in about 30% of the dogs; this results in what is commonly referred to as "blue eye." Death may occur suddenly in 4 or 5 days, or recovery may be rapid. Specific diagnosis can be made at necropsy on demonstration of intranuclear inclusions in liver cells (Coffin, 1952; Flint, 1953; Pay, 1950; Smith, 1951). New methylene blue in physiologic saline can be used to stain the inclusion bodies (Klopfer, 1969).

A marked prolongation of bleeding time may occur on about the third day of illness and persist throughout the febrile period. Liver damage may interfere with prothrombin and fibrinogen production, while heparin may be liberated from damaged liver tissue (Poppensiek, 1952). Decreased platelet numbers were associated with a prolonged clotting time and poor clot retraction (Coffin and Cabasso, 1953). Lindblad and Bäckgren (1964) infected dogs experimentally and observed degenerative changes in megakaryocytes of rib sections between the fourth and seventh days postinoculation. A marked decrease in platelet counts occurred at the same time, falling in some dogs to less than 20,000/μl. There was a gradual increase of platelet counts among surviving dogs, with normal values being attained by the twelfth day. Experimental studies (Wigton, 1978; Wigton et al., 1976) showed that the hemostatic defect in

ICH is a manifestation of virus-induced disseminated intravascular coagulation (DIC) characterized by thrombocytopenia, abnormal platelet function, appearance of schistocytes, prolonged one-stage prothrombin time and activated partial thromboplastin time, normal thrombin time, decreased factor VIII activity, and increased fibrinogen degradation products. Platelet survival was reduced and ultrastructural features of young and altered platelet morphology were evident. The DIC was most probably initiated by virus-induced endothelial disruption, for ICH has particular tropism for endothelial cells.

Eleven cases of ICH are described in Table 36–4. Acute illness, fever, tonsillitis, liver pain, or development of keratoconjunctivitis during convalescence were clinical signs used as a basis for diagnosis. None of the dogs died; therefore, the diagnosis by demonstration of liver inclusion bodies was lacking. The data relative to plasma proteins and fibrinogen are also lacking because these tests were introduced into our routine laboratory procedures after admission of the 11 dogs to the hospital. Perhaps because of widespread vaccination against ICH, the disease is currently rarely seen at the VMTH-UCD.

Icterus index was within the normal range for all dogs. Although some dehydration may have existed, it was not clearly reflected in an elevated PCV, except for Dog 9. Only Dogs 2 and 3 had an elevated ESR. Because plasma proteins, particularly fibrinogen and globulins, are involved in elevating ESR, while albumin decreases the settling rate, it is not unusual to have negative corrected ESR in dogs 1–2 months of age (see Chapter 4).

The leukogram is typically one of leukopenia to low normal total leukocyte counts; the range for the total leukocyte count in the 11 dogs was 1,800–9,500 with a mean value of 5,900/μl. Lindblad and Bäckgren (1964), in experimentally produced ICH, observed total leukocyte counts to range from 2,400–10,400/μl (mean 4,300) in 17 dogs. Smith (1951) infected 17 mongrel pups, 2–4 months of age, and observed a decrease in total leukocytes to between 5,000 and 6,000/μl by the fifth to sixth day. In our observations (Table 36–4), neutrophils and lymphocytes were decreased, lymphocytes more markedly than

Table 36–4. Infectious Canine Hepatitis—Natural Infections

Dog No.	Sex	Age (mo)	Temp. (°F)	PCV (%)	Icterus Index Units	ESR (corrected)	WBC/µl	Differential Leukocyte Count										
								Neutrophils				Lymphocytes		Monocytes		Eosinophils		Unclassified Cells	
								Band		Mature									
								No.	%	No.	%	No.	%	No.	%	No.	%	No.	%
1	F	8	103.4	45	5	5 –	1,800	0	0	972	54.0	702	39.0	108	6.0	18	1.0	0	0
2	M	30	104.5	48	5	18 +	3,800	38	1.0	3,116	82.0	494	13.0	114	3.0	38	1.0	0	0
3	F	8	106.0	43	5	12 +	4,900	147	3.0	0	0	441	9.0	3,773	77.0	0	0	539	11.0
4	M	1½	104.0	37	5	6 –	4,900	0	0	2,891	59.0	956	19.5	857	17.5	123	2.5	73	1.5
5	M	15	103.5	44	2	1 +	5,200	676	13.0	2,808	54.0	1.092	21.0	624	12.0	0	0	0	0
6	F	2½	103.6	36	5	0	6,000	0	0	4,080	68.0	840	14.0	1,020	17.0	60	1.0	0	0
7	M	2	102.5	37	5	13 –	6,800	34	0.5	5,508	81.0	714	10.5	544	8.0	0	0	0	0
8	M	22	104.0	46	5	2 +	7,000	210	3.0	4,095	58.5	1,260	18.0	875	12.5	140	2.0	420	6.0
9	F	21	105.4	60	5	0	7,200	540	7.5	4,716	65.5	1,188	16.5	684	9.5	72	1.0	0	0
10	M	2	103.0	40	5	7 –	7,700	0	0	2,194	28.5	3,427	44.5	539	7.0	616	8.0	924	12.0
11	F	2	103.4	35	5	13 –	9,500	0	0	6,697	70.5	1,568	16.5	1,188	12.5	47	0.5	0	0

neutrophils. Monocytes generally remained within the normal range, but some confusion existed with respect to classification of leukocytes in Dog 3. We are of the opinion that in ICH both lymphocytes and monocytes tend to stain dark blue, making it difficult at times to classify them properly. Some of the cells were left unclassified in Dogs 3, 4, 8, and 10. Further observations indicated that the dark-staining lymphoid/monocytoid cells occur early in the course of the disease and are replaced by normal lymphocytes and monocytes as convalescence begins (Schalm, 1979a). Wigton and coworkers (1976) described similar changes in lymphocyte morphology, characterized by increased size, deep basophilic cytoplasm, and azurophilic granules, by 60 hours of experimental infection. Such cells predominated until death in fatally infected dogs. Hodgman and Larin (1953) stated that leukocytosis accompanied by lymphocytosis associated with a marked increase in young lymphocytes develops after the sixth day. McSherry and Smith (1953) observed in two experimentally infected dogs the occurrence of marked neutrophilia and lymphocytosis during the recovery period. Total leukocyte count increased to between 20,000 and 40,000/μl before returning to normal levels.

Other clinicopathologic features of ICH are albuminuria and sometimes bilirubinuria. The disease spreads primarily through the urine, and the virus has been isolated from urine for as long as 160 days after inoculation of susceptible animals (Poppensiek and Baker, 1951). The appearance of nucleated red cells unaccompanied by reticulocytes in peripheral blood and mild to severe nonresponsive anemia with normoproteinemia have been observed in experimentally infected dogs (Wigton et al., 1976). Serum biochemical determinations revealed elevated levels of serum glutamic-pyruvate transaminase (SGPT), lactate dehydrogenase (LDH), and alkaline phosphatase within 3–4 days of infection.

PYOMETRA IN THE DOG

Pyometra is a disease encountered most commonly in the aging female dog. Among 50 dogs with pyometra, 39 (78%) were in the age range of 5–14 years.

Clinical Signs

Occasionally the owner reports having observed signs suggestive of estrus occurring several weeks to a month previously (Appendix Case 12). This is generally followed by persistent vaginal discharge varying from slight to copious. In some dogs, the lips of the vulva are swollen, and several mammary glands may be enlarged. In those instances where the cervix remains closed, the retention of the purulent exudate within the uterine horns causes enlargement of the abdomen. When systemic toxemia develops, the clinical signs may suggest chronic renal disease, e.g., polydipsia, polyuria, vomiting, depression, and dehydration.

Pyometra is considered to be a consequence of a hormone imbalance in which hyperplastic changes occur in the endometrium (Talanti, 1959; Whitney, 1956). When compounds of progesterone, such as medroxyprogesterone acetate or hydroxyprogesterone acetate, were used to suppress estrus, a few bitches so treated displayed a vaginal discharge associated with filling of the uterus with exudate as a result of development of cystic endometrial hyperplasia (Anderson et al., 1965; Brodey and Fidler, 1966). We have observed development of the typical pyometra syndrome in several dogs treated with synthetic progesterone to prevent estrus; surgical removal of the uterus and ovaries was necessary.

The purulent exudate that forms in the uterus in pyometra is rarely sterile. A considerable mixture of bacteria may be cultured, e.g., staphylococci, streptococci, coliforms, and *Proteus vulgaris*. *Escherichia coli* is perhaps the most frequent secondary bacterial invader, and it was found to be present in almost all cases of pyometra, whether the cervix was open or sealed (Renton et al., 1971).

Clinical Pathology

Hemograms of 16 dogs with pyometra are arranged in sequence of the total leukocyte count in Table 36–5. Leukopenia (Dog 1) is an infrequent finding and occurs in association with the most extreme systemic toxemia. A degenerative left shift (Dogs 2 and 6) is en-

Table 36–5.   The Hemogram in Pyometra in the Dog

Dog No.	Age (yr)	Temp. (°F)	Clinical Comments	Plasma					Differential Leukocyte Count in Absolute Number/μl						
				PCV (%)	ESR (cor.)	Protein (g/dl)	Fibrinogen (g/dl)	WBC/μl	Myelocytes	Metamyelocytes	Bands	Neutrophils	Lymphocytes	Monocytes	Eosinophils
1	12	105.4	Mucoid discharge	40	—	7.9	0.7	4,200[a]	42	420	2,772	rare	840	126	0
2	4	103.0	Dead pup removed	32	37+	7.3	0.7	8,500	340	680	3,910	1,700	1,615	170	85
3	6	101.0	Open pyometra	41	5−	7.7	0.2	12,300	0	0	0	7,995	1,907	431	1,968
4	9	101.0	Open pyometra	36	4−	8.5	0.2	13,500	0	0	135	9,315	2,295	1,283	472
5	7	103.0	Copious discharge	40	34+	7.0	0.6	18,500	0	185	1,572	12,580	1,202	2,682	277
6	2	104.0	Ruptured uterus	57	—	9.5	0.7	18,800[a]	376	1,692	9,024	5,452	2,256	0	0
7	12½	101.4	Yellow, bloody discharge	26	32+	8.0	0.6	28,300	0	283	6,368	16,131	2,122	2,972	424
8	12½	102.2	Copious discharge	33	24+	7.8	0.4	29,000	0	145	2,320	20,155	1,595	3,915	870
9	14	102.0	Purulent, bloody discharge	37	—	8.0	0.5	37,300	187	0	7,273	24,059	1,492	4,289	0
10	5	102.0	Received promone uterus distended	40	37+	8.6	0.5	40,300[a]	0	3,425	11,485	13,501	3,425	6,649	1,813
11	7	102.8	Copious discharge	33	—	7.8	0.3	43,000[a]	1,505	4,730	13,545	19,350	3,225	645	0
12	11	102.4	Mucopurulent discharge	39	42+	7.8	0.5	44,100	0	661	7,938	28,003	1,543	5,733	220
13	12	102.3	Heavy discharge	27	33+	8.4	0.5	49,100	982	7,365	16,694	21,850	736	1,473	0
14	2	101.0	Both horns extremely enlarged	40	—	8.5	0.5	53,000	rare	4,505	10,865	27,825	3,180	5,565	1,060
15	12	102.5	Closed pyometra	31	35+	9.3	0.5	76,200	0	1,905	2,667	64,770	1,143	5,715	0
16	7	99.4	Closed pyometra	42	38+	8.0	0.6	98,200	0	7,365	24,059	57,938	982	7,856	0

[a]Neutrophils appear toxic.

countered somewhat more frequently than frank leukopenia. In other instances, a leukocytosis occurs, but immature neutrophils may equal or exceed the number of mature cells (Dogs 10 and 11). This type of leukocytic response is interpreted as a pseudo-degenerative left shift, rather than a true degenerative left shift which characteristically has total leukocyte count below or within the normal range (see Chapter 31). It is speculated that in such cases granulopoiesis has been stimulated from the chronic course of the disease, but because of absorption of increased amounts of chemotactic and neutrophil releasing factor(s) produced in the diseased uterus, an unusual demand is placed on the bone marrow, thereby forcing an imbalanced, heightened release of immature granulocytes into the circulation (Appendix Case 13). Therefore, a marked leukocytosis with "degenerative left shift pattern" is seen in the peripheral blood despite an enhanced marrow myeloid activity. This could either resolve with improvement or terminate in myeloid hypoplasia. Similar findings may also be recorded in pyometra in the cat (Appendix Case 47).

The retention of a purulent exudate in the uterus exerts a chemotactic effect on neutrophil leukocytes. The magnitude of the total leukocyte count in pyometra may be in part a reflection of the degree of closure of the cervix. Drainage of the exudate through an open cervix reduces the chemotactic effect on neutrophils, and thus the total leukocyte count in peripheral blood may remain within the normal range (Dogs 3 and 4). Total leukocyte counts in pyometra as reported by others are similar to the range of counts in Table 36–5 (Åsheim, 1964; Renton et al., 1971).

Total leukocyte counts of 25,000/μl or greater, with mature neutrophils outnumbering immature forms (Dogs 7, 8, and 9), are typical of a regenerative left shift (Appendix Case 12). In some instances, leukocyte counts of 40,000/μl of blood or more with left shift to include myelocytes are suggestive of a leukemoid reaction (Dogs 11 and 13). In pyometra associated with a closed cervix, the total leukocyte count may approach 100,000 (Dogs 15 and 16). After surgical removal of the uterus, the total leukocyte count may exceed the preoperative level for several days—e.g., postoperative counts were 55,900 on day 1 (Dog 4); 74,600 on day 3 (Dog 13); and 130,000 on day 1 and 26,500 on day 4 (Dog 16).

Lymphocyte, monocyte, and eosinophil numbers vary depending on the degree of stress or toxemia. In most instances, as in other chronic suppurative diseases, lymphocyte numbers remain within their normal range, except when depressed by severe stress (Dogs 1, 13, and 16), and monocyte numbers are generally significantly elevated, as in most chronic diseases involving suppuration. In a group of 24 other dogs with pyometra, the mean absolute monocyte count was 5,250 ± 3,700 SD. Eosinophilia may be present, possibly in response to the decomposition of tissue.

Pyometra in other species may not elicit a leukocytosis that is common in canine pyometra. For example, mares with pyometra had leukocyte counts usually within but occasionally below the normal range as a result of a neutropenia that was associated, in some instances, with lymphopenia (Hughes et al., 1979). Monocytes and eosinophils, within the normal range initially, increased gradually to attain high normal or greater values. A mild normocytic-normochromic amenia also developed in some mares.

A slight to modest normocytic-normochromic anemia (PCV <36%) may accompany canine pyometra, possibly as a combined effect of loss of erythrocytes by diapedesis into the exudate and toxic depression of erythropoiesis (anemia of chronic disease). PCV values of 36–40% may in reality reflect the existence of a borderline anemia that is masked by some dehydration. The corrected ESR is commonly significantly elevated (Table 36–5).

Total plasma protein concentration suggests a slight to moderate hyperproteinemia. Total plasma protein in excess of 8.0 g/dl may be the result of hemoconcentration, but, considering the advanced age of most dogs with pyometra, the increase may be due to hyperglobulinemia. Plasma fibrinogen concentration is usually at the maximum normal of 0.5 g/dl or is increased to between 0.6 and 0.7 g/dl. The hyperfibrinogenemia may influence to some extent the markedly elevated ESR. Hypoalbuminemia seen in some cases of pyometra has been attributed to decreased production by the liver rather than to renal loss (Børresen and Skrede, 1980).

The kidneys exhibit evidence of nephrotoxic injury described as membranous glomerulonephritis or mixed proliferative and membranous (immune complex–induced) glomerulonephritis with associated tubular atrophy presumably the result of obliteration of glomeruli. Plasma cells may be found surrounding glomeruli. Obel and coworkers (1964), in describing these lesions in 23 dogs with pyometra, suggested that an immunobiologic process was involved in production of these histopathologic changes in the kidneys. In a subsequent study, liver and kidney lesions found in canine pyometra were attributed to deposition of immune complexes (*E. coli* antigen and antibody) in these organs (Sandholm et al., 1975). Whitney (1969) was of the opinion that the polydipsia and polyuria common to pyometra can be explained by the lowered ability of the kidneys to concentrate urine.

Although histopathologic changes occur in the kidneys, the BUN level is not regularly elevated. In 16 dogs listed in Table 36–5, the BUN was above the maximum normal of 28 mg/dl of plasma in only 4 (25%), and in these dogs, the values were 35, 47, 69, and 83 mg/dl. The BUN at these levels could reflect hemoconcentration or decomposition of the purulent exudate. Renton and coworkers (1971), however, reported BUN values to be >60 mg in 8 of 28 dogs with pyometra, with values as high as 240 and 310 mg in 2 of the dogs. Considering the advanced age of many dogs with pyometra, one might expect the existence of renal lesions due to causes other than pyometra.

CANINE CUSHING'S SYNDROME (HYPERADRENOCORTICISM)

A syndrome of polydipsia, polyuria, and polyphagia accompanied by bilaterally symmetrical hair loss over areas of the body receiving the greatest wear and muscle wasting leading to development of a pendulous abdomen characterizes a disorder caused by hyperadrenocorticism and commonly referred to as Cushing's syndrome. Observations on 117 cases of canine Cushing's syndrome (Ling et al., 1979) indicated that poodles, dachshunds, and boxers of all ages are at increased risk, as are dogs of all breeds 6 years of age or older. No sex preference is noted. Most frequent abnormalities in laboratory data include lymphopenia; eosinopenia; elevations in serum alkaline phosphatase, γ-glutamyl transferase (GGT), SGPT, and cholesterol; increased bromsulphalein (BSP, sulfobromophthalein) dye retention; and decreased urine specific gravity. About 50% of dogs may exhibit urinary tract infections.

The disease is the result of hypercorticosteroidism from either bilateral hyperplasia of the adrenal cortex secondary to excessive secretion of ACTH by pituitary or ectopic endocrine tumors, or an "autonomous" (functional) neoplasm of the adrenal cortex (Feldman, 1983). Adrenal hyperplasia is seen in about 80% of cases, while adrenocortical neoplasia accounts for 10–15% of cases of canine hyperadrenocorticism (DiBartola, 1979).

Cushing's syndrome has been observed in cats, with signs similar to those seen in dogs but with less remarkable clinicopathologic changes except for blood glucose, which is invariably elevated (Feldmanm 1983). A case of pituitary adrenocorticotropin–dependent Cushing's syndrome was reported in a horse, with clinical, biochemical, and hematologic features similar to canine Cushing's syndrome (Moore et al., 1979).

Several recent excellent reviews and case reports are available on canine Cushing's syndrome (DiBartola, 1979; Feldman, 1983; Ling et al., 1979; Peterson, 1984; Willeberg and Priester, 1982).

Correlation of Laboratory Data and Clinical Signs

Results of tests on urine and blood serum or plasma of nine dogs with Cushing's syndrome are summarized in Table 36–6.

A low specific gravity of the urine is a generally observed characteristic, and most dogs have some degree of proteinuria. The urine specific gravity for six of the nine dogs was in the range of 1.003–1.012, while the specific gravity of three urines fell within the normal range. Polydipsia and polyuria may be of such magnitude as to be compatible with a

Table 36-6.   Biochemical Evaluation of Blood and Urine in Canine Hyperadrenocorticism (Cushing's Syndrome)

Entity Tested		Dog Number									Normal Range
	1	2	3	4	5	6	7	8	9		
Urine specific gravity	1.003	1.039	1.018	1.032	1.007	1.010	1.008	1.012	1.008		1.015–1.045
Proteinuria	0	1+	2+	3+	1+	1+	0	2+	0		none
Blood urea nitrogen (mg/dl)	7.0	10.0	8.2	8.0	13.0	9.5	15.0	22.4	9.0		10–28
SGPT (IU/L)	48.0	77.0	—	36.0	185.0	3.6	30.0	27.0	4.0		4.8–24
Alkaline phosphatase (IU/L)	304.0	442.0	10.2	367.0	54.7	2.8	94.0	134.0	11.6		20–156
Bromsulphalein (% at 30 min)	3	5	—	5	10	5	0	6	2		5% at 30 min
Glucose (mg/dl)	104.0	116.0	—	126.0	122.0	119.0	122.0	149.0	163.0		65.0–118.0
Cholesterol (mg/dl)	348.0	379.0	334.0	554.0	270.0	293.0	236.0	403.0	515.0		135.0–270.0
Serum sodium (mEq/L)	—	—	151	—	155	160	—	150	—		141–152
Serum potassium (mEq/L)	—	—	4.9	—	3.0	4.5	—	5.0	—		4.4–5.7
Serum chloride (mEq/L)	—	—	112	—	113	—	—	104	—		105–115
Plasma corticoids (µg/dl)											
Pre-ACTH	3.2	9.8	—	6.5	6.2	8.4	12.3	4.2	11.2		1.0–7.0
Post-ACTH (2 hr)	41.0	40.0	—	>50.0	>30.0	54.0	98.0	21.0	31.2		7.5–18.0[a]
Post-dexamethasone	0.5	3.3	—	—	—	1.8	—	1.2	—		0.2–0.8[a]
Post-o,p'DDD therapy	0.2	0.5	—	3.7	—	1.4	0.95	0.8	—		decreased
Urinary 17-KGS (mg/24 hr)											
Pre-ACTH	—	—	8.0	—	—	—	—	—	—		2.13–6.98[b]
Post-ACTH	—	—	24.0	—	—	—	—	—	—		2.85–11.15[b]

[a]Martin et al., 1971.
[b]Siegel, 1968a.

diagnosis of diabetes insipidus (Coffin and Munson, 1953).

BUN was below the stated normal range in six of the nine dogs, and it was slightly above the maximum in one dog. Some evidence of hepatopathy was reflected in five of eight dogs tested, although the BSP excretion test results were normal in seven of the eight dogs tested. Dog 5 had the highest SGPT value (185 IU/L), and the BSP retention was 10% at 30 minutes.

The liver shows what has been termed "steroid hepatopathy," which is characterized by hepatomegaly and centrilobular vacuolation of hepatocytes probably from accumulation of water as a result of ionic imbalances, perivacuolar glycogen accumulation within hepatocytes, and focal centrilobular necrosis (Rijnberk et al., 1968; Rogers and Ruebner, 1977; Strombeck, 1979; Thompson et al., 1971). The hepatopathy is reversible.

Blood cholesterol levels exceeded the normal maximum of 270 mg/dl in six dogs, with a range of 293–554 mg. Hypercholesterolemia has been reported to be a common finding (Martin et al., 1971; Rijnberk et al., 1968; Siegel et al., 1970). Alkaline phosphatase was elevated in three dogs, with levels ranging from 304–442 IU/L. Elevations in serum alkaline phosphatase concentration are due to an increase in steroid-induced isoenzyme of alkaline phosphatase of hepatic origin (Dorner et al., 1974). There is a lack of evidence of primary bone disease (Martin et al., 1971), but osteoporosis and metastatic calcification are frequently seen (Rijnberk et al., 1968).

Muscle wasting, weakness, and relaxation lead to development of a "potbellied" appearance that is characteristic of the canine Cushing's syndrome. Catabolism of muscle protein leads to gluconeogenesis and an increase in plasma glucose levels above the maximum normal of 118 mg/dl in most dogs. Blood glucose levels ranging from 119–163 mg/dl were recorded for Dogs 4 through 9 (Table 36–6). Serum electrolytes have generally been found to fall within their normal ranges (Capen et al., 1967; Martin et al., 1971; Rijnberk et al., 1968; Siegel et al., 1970). However, increased serum sodium and decreased serum potassium may be found in some dogs (Dogs 5 and 6).

Hematology of Canine Cushing's Syndrome (Table 36–7)

The administration of ACTH or corticosteroids to normal dogs produces a leukocytosis characterized by neutrophilia, monocytosis, lymphopenia, and eosinopenia (Fig. 4–2). A similar leukocyte pattern might be expected a priori in hyperadrenocorticism. Perhaps this typical steroid pattern exists during the initial stages of the disease. However, among the nine dogs with verified Cushing's syndrome, only Dogs 2 and 5 exhibited a typical steroid leukocyte pattern. Dog 8 had the anticipated differential leukocyte pattern but without accompanying leukocytosis, whereas all dogs exhibited lymphopenia and eosinopenia. A small number of basophils were present in Dog 4. A few basophils have been seen even in the absence of eosinophils in some dogs with Cushing's syndrome (Appendix Cases 8 and 9).

In summary, lymphopenia and eosinopenia are the only consistent changes characteristic of the leukogram in hyperadrenocorticism. In a study of 117 canine cases of Cushing's syndrome, 80% of the patients exhibited eosinopenia and lymphopenia, while leukocytosis was seen in 24% of the cases (Ling et al., 1979).

Considering the advanced age of most of the dogs, total plasma protein concentration of less than 7.0 g/dl would indicate that a borderline hypoproteinemia existed in Dogs 5, 6, and 7. Perhaps this was an expression of the catabolic action of glucocorticoids on protein. Only Dog 9 had hyperproteinemia. Plasma fibrinogen remained within the broad normal range of 0.2–0.5 g/dl, with the exception of Dog 5, in which plasma fibrinogen was 0.7 g/dl.

Dogs 2 and 5 had PCV values of 37% and 36%, respectively, indicating a borderline anemia. Otherwise, PCV values ranged between 44% and 58%. Rijnberk and coworkers (1968) noted elevated PCV values in 33% of their dogs with hyperadrenocorticism. ESRs were significantly elevated in Dogs 2, 5, and 9. Although the ESR was limited to 5+ in Dog 9, this was highly significant at a PCV of 57%. The 1+ and 2+ ESR values of Dogs 6 and 3 were also significant, in view of PCV

Table 36–7. Hemograms in Canine Hyperadrenocorticism (Cushing's Syndrome)

Entity	Dog Number								
	1	2	3	4	5	6	7	8	9
Breed	Corgi	Beagle	Boxer	Chihuahua	Poodle	Terrier	Dachshund	Dachshund	Dachshund
Sex	F	M	F	M	XF	XF	M	F	F
Age (yrs)	1	6	7	8	10	10	12	6	11
RBC ($\times 10^6$/µl)	7.24	4.82	7.39	7.32	4.67	8.00	6.18	8.07	8.19
Hb (g/dl)	17.7	12.7	16.3	18.5	12.1	18.8	15.2	15.3	18.5
PCV (%)	50	37	51	58	36	53	44	44	57
MCV (fl)	69.0	76.7	69.0	79.2	77.0	66.2	71.1	54.5	69.5
MCHC (%)	35.0	34.3	35.9	31.8	33.6	35.4	34.5	34.7	32.4
Plasma proteins (g/dl)	6.8	7.2	7.5	7.8	6.9	6.8	6.5	7.3	9.1
Fibrinogen (g/dl)	0.2	0.5	0.4	0.3	0.7	0.5	0.3	0.4	0.4
Icterus index units	2	2	2	2	2	2	2	2	2
ESR (corrected)	1+	39+	2+	1	42+	1+	6+	6+	5+
Nucleated RBC/100 WBC	0	0	0	1	2	0	0	0	0
WBC/µl	11,000	32,300	13,400	12,100	20,500	12,100	7,000	16,400	12,650
Band neutrophil	0	807	201	181	1,332	544	805	1,394	0
Mature neutrophil	9,625	28,585	11,189	10,588	17,015	11,011	4,550	13,038	10,626
Lymphocyte	715	1,292	1,072	666	512	242	490	492	1,075
Monocyte	660	1,615	871	484	1,435	302	1,120	1,394	948
Eosinophil	0	0	67	121	205	0	35	82	0
Basophil	0	0	0	60	0	0	0	0	0
Leukocytes (%)									
Band neutrophil	0	2.5	1.5	1.5	6.5	4.5	11.5	8.5	0
Mature neutrophil	87.5	88.5	83.5	87.5	83.0	91.0	65.0	79.5	84.0
Lymphocyte	6.5	4.0	8.0	5.5	2.5	2.0	7.0	3.0	8.5
Monocyte	6.0	5.0	6.5	4.0	7.0	2.5	16.0	8.5	7.5
Eosinophil	0.0	0.0	0.5	1.0	1.0	0.0	0.5	0.5	0.0
Basophil	0.0	0.0	0.0	0.5	0.0	0.0	0.0	0.0	0.0

values of 53% and 51%, respectively. A mild polycythemia observed in some dogs has been attributed to respiratory problems associated with obesity or excessive production of androgens by hyperplastic or neoplastic cortical tissue (Feldman, 1983).

Corticosteroid Levels in Plasma and Urine

Although canine Cushing's syndrome can be diagnosed provisionally from history and clinical signs supported by results of laboratory tests, a more certain diagnosis can be made through measurement of corticosteroids in plasma or urine before and after injection of ACTH (Martin et al., 1971; Rijnberk et al., 1968; Siegel, 1965, 1968a). The intramuscular injection of ACTH gel is followed by a modest rise in plasma 17-hydroxycorticosteroids in normal dogs and by a considerably greater increase in dogs with hyperadrenocorticism (Table 36–6). The same is true of the excretion of 17-ketogenic steroids (17-KGS) in the urine (Dog 3, Table 36–6). These determinations of 17-KGS in plasma and urine have now been supplanted by measurements of plasma cortisol described below.

Several excellent reports are available regarding measurement and significance of plasma cortisol levels in diagnosis of canine Cushing's syndrome. The following summation is largely from reports by Feldman (1983, 1985a), which are recommended for further information and appropriate references. Total blood cortisol levels can be measured by three methods: fluorescence, competitive protein binding, and radioimmunoassay. The last two are more precise and generally yield lower values than those obtained by a fluorescence assay. Hence data from different reports or laboratories should be compared in view of the method used for cortisol assay. Blood sample collection and processing are important factors influencing plasma levels of cortisol; heparin should be used as anticoagulant, and plasma should be separated as soon as possible because the red cells may absorb some cortisol (Lester et al., 1981). Cortisol levels are reduced in refrigerated samples, but not in frozen samples.

Basal cortisol concentration in dogs with Cushing's syndrome varies from within the normal range to significantly elevated. Therefore other diagnostic strategies have been devised. Cushing's syndrome in dogs is diagnosed by performing an ACTH stimulation test and/or a low-dose dexamethasone suppression test. Then a high-dose dexamethasone test is performed and/or endogenous plasma ACTH concentrations are measured to differentiate pituitary-dependent hyperadrenocorticism from that due to adrenal tumor (Feldman, 1985a, b; Peterson, 1984).

The ACTH stimulation test assesses additional secretory ability of the adrenal in response to pharmacologic doses of ACTH. Plasma cortisol levels are determined before and 1 or more hours after an injection of exogenous ACTH intramuscularly. In one protocol, 0.25 mg of a synthetic ACTH, cosyntropin (Cortrosyn, Organon Diagnostics), is given and a postinjection sample is obtained 1 hour later. Normal dogs have a basal cortisol concentration of 1–7 µg/dl and post-ACTH stimulation cortisol concentration of 7–15 µg/dl. Similar values for dogs with hyperadrenalism are, respectively, 1–10 µg/dl and >20 µg/dl. About 15–20% of Cushing's dogs may show normal ACTH stimulation. Thus neither basal cortisol levels nor the rise in cortisol levels after ACTH injection completely distinguishes normal dogs from those with adrenal disease. Dogs with hypoadrenalism do not respond to ACTH stimulation; pre- and post-ACTH cortisol values are <3–4 µg/dl. The ACTH stimulation test has also been performed in the cat to assess adrenal function (Peterson et al., 1984).

The dexamethasone suppression test utilizes the principle of diminished production of cortisol as a result of feedback inhibition of ACTH secretion. Preinjection and 8-hour-postinjection samples are collected. The low-dose dexamethasone suppression test (0.01 mg/kg body weight given intravenously) is associated with a reduction in plasma levels of cortisol in normal animals, but usually (in about 95% cases) not in those with Cushing's syndrome, irrespective of the cause. The 8-hour-postinoculation plasma cortisol level is <1.4 µg/dl in the former and >1.4 µg/dl in the latter.

The high-dose dexamethasone suppression

test (0.1 mg/kg body weight given intravenously) is performed to distinguish patients with pituitary-dependent hyperadrenocorticism (diminished cortisol output) from those with functional adrenal tumor (no effect). Suppression is defined as a cortisol concentration of <50% of basal value at 8 hours postinjection. However, it has been observed that about 25% of dogs with pituitary-dependent Cushing's syndrome do not show suppression with high dose dexamethasone.

Measurement of endogenous ACTH levels (Feldman, 1983, 1985a, b) is considered most reliable to distinguish canine patients with pituitary-dependent hyperadrenocorticism (elevated ACTH levels, >40 pg/ml) from those with functional adrenal tumor (diminished ACTH levels, <20 pg/ml; normal ACTH values, 20–100 pg/ml).

A combined dexamethasone and ACTH stimulation test has been described to assess pituitary gland and adrenal gland responses in a single trial within a few hours (Eiler and Oliver, 1980; Feldman, 1985a).

The dexamethasone suppression test measuring diminished secretion of urinary 17-hydroxycorticosteroids has been used in diagnosis of Cushing's syndrome in humans (Liddle, 1960). All patients with bilateral adrenal hyperplasia experienced a decrease in secretion of 17-hydroxycorticosteroids, while patients with adrenocortical tumors did not. The effects of the dexamethasone suppression test on four dogs are recorded in Table 36–6. The results suggest that these dogs had ACTH-dependent bilateral adrenal hyperplasia.

Administration of *o,p'*-DDD in dogs causes atrophy of the adrenal cortex and consequently a marked decrease in the secretion of 17-hydroxycorticosteroids and cortisol. Six dogs with hyperadrenocorticism were treated with *o,p'*DDD (Table 36–6); the dose was 50 mg/kg, given s.i.d. orally for 5–10 days. A rapid fall in plasma 17-hydroxycorticosteroids was demonstrated, with lowest levels attained by the time of the last dose. Lymphocyte and eosinophil numbers usually increased in the blood during treatment. See recent reports for a detailed discussion of the treatment of canine Cushing's syndrome with

*o,p'*DDD (David, 1983; Feldman; 1983; Peterson, 1984).

HYPOADRENOCORTICISM (ADDISON'S DISEASE) IN THE DOG

Atrophy of the adrenal cortices is the principal cause of hypoadrenocorticism in the dog, although it may occur less frequently from diminished secretion of ACTH. The lack of adrenocortical secretion leads to the insidious development of a chain of events characterized by *(a)* muscle weakness; *(b)* gastrointestinal disturbances such as anorexia, emesis, and bloody diarrhea; *(c)* loss of body water through failure of the kidneys to retain sodium and chloride; *(d)* tachycardia and bradycardia due to failure of the kidneys to excrete potassium; and *(e)* severe dehydration leading to hypotension and elevation of BUN. Depression, weak pulse, and eventual collapse are common accompanying clinical signs. Differential diagnosis includes kidney disease and gastrointestinal disease.

Adrenal insufficiency is most commonly seen in the female, intact or spayed, particularly in dogs less than 5 years old; it occurs as early as 1 year of age (Siegel, 1968b). Marshak and coworkers (1960) presented the first complete clinical and laboratory investigation of adrenal insufficiency in the dog. Morales and Nielsen (1970) briefly summarized nine literature reports involving 32 dogs and added a description of two cases of their own. Mulnix (1971) described eight dogs with hypoadrenocorticism and discussed therapy with deoxycorticosterone acetate (DOCA) and the long-acting deoxycorticosterone pivalate. The latter slow-release corticoid is used in conjunction with a liberal daily intake of salt in the diet (Siegel, 1968b, 1971). The disease has been reviewed recently (Feldman, 1983; Feldman and Peterson, 1984; Feldman and Tyrrell, 1977; Hill, 1979; Rakich and Lorenz, 1984; Schaer and Chen, 1983; Willard et al., 1982).

Laboratory data on five dogs with adrenal insufficiency are summarized in Tables 36–8 (hematology) and 36–9 (clinical chemistry). All five dogs were referrals with a history of illness of 8 days' to 3 months' duration. Two hemograms are presented for each dog to

Table 36–8. Hemograms of Dogs with Adrenocortical Insufficiency upon Admission and after Hydration[a]

Dog number	1		2		3		4		5		
Sex	Male		X Female		Female		Female		Female		
Age	1 yr		8 yr		4 yr		2 yr		1 yr		Normal Range
Hospital day number	1	9[b]	1	7	1	4	1	4[c]	1[d]	6	
RBC ($\times 10^6$/µl)	7.34	5.26	9.40	5.60	5.01	4.10	4.53	2.82	6.79	4.72	5.5–8.5
Hemoglobin (g/dl)	17.2	11.7	21.6	12.5	10.9	9.2	9.9	6.7	15.4	11.1	12.0–18.0
PCV (%)	51.0	35.0	67.0	39.0	35.0	27.0	29.0	20.0	48.0	32.0	37.0–55.0
MCV (fl)	69.4	66.5	71.1	69.6	69.9	65.9	64.0	70.9	70.6	67.7	60.0–77.0
MCHC (%)	33.7	33.4	32.2	32.1	31.1	34.1	34.1	33.5	32.0	34.6	32.0–36.0
Reticulocytes (%)	—	rare	0.0	0.0	0.6	3.0	rare	0.0	—	0.0	0.0–1.5
Plasma proteins (g/dl)	7.1	6.0	6.2	5.4	9.4	6.9	8.3	4.9	7.9	5.8	6.0–8.0
WBC/µl	50,900	30,800	9,700	14,600	14,800	19,600	11,200	8,400	16,600	7,300	6,000–17,000
Bands	255	6,930	0	0	74	196	392	336	415	219	0–300
Neutrophils	38,175	16,324	5,577	12,337	7,770	9,898	9,072	7,518	14,442	5,621	3,000–11,500
Lymphocytes	5,090	2,926	3,104	1,606	5,698	7,546	1,120	336	747	438	1,000–4,800
Monocytes	3,818	4,158	242	657	888	1,274	616	168	996	985	150–1,350
Eosinophils	3,563	462	776	0	370	588	0	42	0	37	100–1,250
Basophils	0	0	0	0	0	98	0	0	0	0	rare

[a] From Keeton, et al., 1972; courtesy of The California Veterinarian.
[b] Dog on steroid therapy.
[c] Dog had received blood transfusion one day before and was on steroids.
[d] Steroids had been administered one day before admission by referring veterinarian.

Table 36–9. Initial Serum Electrolyte and Blood Urea Nitrogen Determinations and Other Test Results Obtained from Dogs with Adrenocortical Insufficiency[a]

	Dog Number					Normal Range[b]
	1	2	3	4	5	
Serum sodium (mEq/L)	127.5	110.0	124.0	107.0	128.0	141.0–152.0
Serum potassium (mEq/L)	8.5	5.9	4.8	7.7	6.7	4.4–5.7
Serum chloride (mEq/L)	98.0	88.0	89.0	70.0	96.0	105.0–115.0
Na:K ratio	15.0:1	18.6:1	25.8:1	13.9:1	19.1:1	27.0:1–32.3:1
BUN (mg/dl)	102.0	24.3	72.0	145.0	19.0	10.0–28.0
Plasma cortisol (µg/dl)	0.40	—	—	—	0.35	1.0–7.0[c]
Urinary 17-ketogenic steroids (mg/24 hr)	—	—	<1	—	—	1.13–3.67
Thorn test (response of blood eosinophils to ACTH)	—	—	Negative	Negative	—	70% decrease @ 7 hr

[a]From Keeton, et al., 1972; courtesy of *The California Veterinarian.*
[b]Normal ranges from Kaneko, 1980b.
[c]From Feldman, 1985b.

demonstrate the disease pattern on admission and after hydration and therapy. Upon initial clinical examination, all five dogs were dehydrated. Following hydration, the erythrocyte parameters fell, revealing slight to marked anemia in all but Dog 2. The anemia was normocytic normochromic, and the absence of a significant reticulocyte response indicated depression of erythrogenesis. Hemoconcentration resulting from dehydration also masked the significant hypoproteinemia in Dogs 2, 4, 5. Loss of protein into the gut due to gastrointestinal disturbances may account for the hypoproteinemia.

In the absence of glucocorticoid action, the total and differential leukocyte pattern characteristic of the "stress phenomenon" would not be expected. Thus persistence of lymphocytes and eosinophils and absence of neutrophilia in an obviously clinically stressed dog could be expected in adrenocortical insufficiency. This clear-cut pattern was seen on admission only in Dogs 2 and 3. Only Dog 1 presented eosinophilia on admission, although an absolute eosinophilia was noted in Dogs 3 and 5 during their period of hospitalization (values not shown). Furthermore, a progress check 6 weeks after the initial hemogram on Dog 4 revealed an absolute eosinophilia. Thus eosinophilia was an inconstant finding in this series of cases. Lymphocyte numbers in the initial hemogram were within their normal range in two dogs, below normal in one dog (Dog 5), which had received steroid therapy on the day before admission to our hospital, and above normal in two dogs (Dogs 1 and 3). Owing to the poor clinical condition of all dogs upon entry, a typical stress-related lymphopenia would have been anticipated in the presence of a normally functioning adrenal gland. Similar hemogram findings have also been reported by Feldman and Tyrrell (1977). Thus normal eosinophil counts and normal or elevated lymphocyte numbers in sick dogs should alert one to include hypoadrenocorticism in the differential diagnosis.

In the presence of a functioning adrenal cortex, an intramuscular injection of ACTH should cause a reduction in lymphocytes and eosinophils as well as an increase in neutrophils and monocytes (Thorn et al., 1948). The Thorn test was conducted on Dogs 3 and 4, and no decrease in eosinophils could be demonstrated, thereby indicating an unresponsive adrenal cortex. (See also Appendix Case 10). The neutrophil:lymphocyte ratio in normal dogs may increase significantly (30% over basal value) prior to development of eosinopenia and by 2–4 hours after an injection of 10 units of aqueous ACTH intramuscularly (Osbaldiston and Greve, 1978).

Initial serum electrolyte levels (Table 36–9) were compatible with hypoadrenocorticism. The presence of hyponatremia, hypochloremia, and hyperkalemia was clearly demonstrated. Mulnix (1971) found the serum sodium and potassium concentrations and the Na:K ratio (Wilkinson, 1969) to be the most useful laboratory findings in the diagnosis of hypoadrenocorticism in the dog. The Na:K ratios fell significantly below the normal minimum of 27.0:1.0 in all dogs, a result of mineralocorticoid (aldosterone) deficiency. Significant elevations of BUN reflected a developing renal failure, the result of decreased stores of body water, leading to hemoconcentration, hypotension, and circulatory collapse. Some atypical cases of canine hypoadrenocorticism have been reported in which abnormal electrolyte concentrations were not seen (Rogers et al., 1981). Diagnosis in such cases was based on lack of response to ACTH stimulation, rather than on serum electrolyte concentrations.

Plasma cortisol and urinary 17-hydroxycorticosteroids have been measured to evaluate adrenal function. Plasma corticoid levels were measured in Dogs 1 and 5 and found to be less than 50% of the minimum normal value of 1.0 µg/dl. Urinary 17-ketogenic steroids were ascertained in Dog 3 and were found to be decreased, as expected in adrenal cortical insufficiency.

Dogs with hypoadrenocorticism show below normal levels of plasma cortisol in response to exogenous injection of ACTH in contrast to significantly elevated levels observed in normal dogs and dogs with Cushing's syndrome (Feldman, 1983; Feldman, 1985a; Lester et al., 1981). It has been stressed that three criteria should be established for interpretation of plasma cortisol levels in diagnosis of normal and hypoadrenalism: baseline values, post-exogenous ACTH levels, and increment of change between the two values (Feldman, 1983). An abnormality in any one of the three criteria would suggest hypoadrenocorticism. In addition, plasma ACTH levels are significantly elevated in dogs with hypoadrenocorticism from primary adrenal insufficiency, while decreased levels are seen in patients with secondary adrenal insufficiency, i.e., pituitary failure (Feldman, 1983).

Primary hypoadrenocorticism was diagnosed in a cat based on laboratory findings of hyponatremia, hypochloremia, hyperkalemia, azotemia, hypophosphatemia, subnormal ACTH stimulation response, and markedly elevated endogenous ACTH concentration (Johnessee et al., 1983). Hematologic findings were unremarkable.

HYPOTHYROIDISM IN THE DOG

The clinical syndrome of frank hypothyroidism in the dog generally includes weight gain to the point of excessive obesity associated with lethargy, listlessness, or sleepiness. The most common additional complaint is a progressive thickening, wrinkling, and scaliness of the skin associated with seborrhea, which imparts a greasy feel and an undesirable odor; sometimes there is pigmentation. These changes in texture of the skin are accompanied by bilateral thinning of the hair coat leading to alopecia. The patient may scratch itself constantly, but this is not a common complaint. In some cases, exuding lesions form and crust over, and when they are removed, the hair pulls away. Hypothyroidism in dogs is mainly due to acquired primary destructive processes from undefined causes or immune mechanisms. Clinical and laboratory features of thyroid disease in the dog and cat have been discussed (Belshaw, 1983; Chastain, 1982; Kaneko, 1980a; Stogdale, 1980).

A number of laboratory tests are available to evaluate thyroid function (Belshaw, 1983; Ferguson, 1984; Kaneko, 1980a; Lothrop et al., 1984). These tests measure the plasma concentration of the thyroid gland hormones, thyroxine (T_4) and triiodothyronine (T_3), bound to plasma proteins or determine the

uptake of ^{131}I by the thyroid gland 72 hours after injection of the isotope. Thyroid hormone bound to plasma proteins is biologically inactive and constitutes over 99% of the circulating hormone. Biopsy of the thyroid gland or histopathologic examination of tissue removed at necropsy represents an additional procedure for verification of the functional state of the gland. Thyroid scintigraphy is a recently introduced, extremely useful method for diagnosing thyroid disorders in dogs and cats (Belshaw, 1983).

Various methods of measuring T_4 such as serum protein-bound iodine (PBI) and competitive protein binding assays have now been supplanted by a highly sensitive, specific, and accurate radioimmunoassay (Kaneko, 1980a). The test is available in a kit form, and there is no interference with iodine or iodine-containing compounds which occurs with the PBI assay. Plasma T_3 can similarly be measured by radioimmunoassay, but its determination is considered of little additional value when T_4 assay can be performed. Normal canine T_4 and T_3 values are, respectively, 0.6–3.6 µg/dl and 82–138 ng/dl (Kaneko, 1980b) and similar values are reported for the cat (Belshaw, 1983). A variety of factors can cause spurious changes in circulating thyroid hormone concentrations (Evinger and Nelson, 1984; Ferguson, 1984).

The response of the thyroid gland to stimulation by exogenous thyroid-stimulating hormone (TSH) can be determined by T_4, PBI, or ^{131}I assay or scintigraphic imaging. One protocol for its use in the dog recommends injecting 10 IU of TSH intramuscularly and determining pre- and 4-hour-postinjection T_4 values. The test enables the clinician to differentiate between primary and secondary (pituitary-induced) hypothyroidisms and to distinguish primary hypothyroidism from drug-induced (phenylbutazone and glucocorticoids) diminution of plasma T_4. TSH stimulation in normal dogs causes an increase in T_4 values to about 3.0–6.5 µg/dl (about double the high normal value), whereas in primary hypothyroidism, the increase is rarely more than 0.2 µg/dl above the basal value (Belshaw, 1983). Dogs with drug-induced lowering of T_4 give a response generally similar to that of normal dogs. An unequivocally low T_4 at zero hour together with a significant TSH response suggests pituitary hypofunction. Dogs with secondary hypothyroidism show a variable response (Evinger and Nelson, 1984). The TSH-stimulation test has also been used to assess thyroid function in cats (Hoenig and Ferguson, 1983) and horses (Held and Oliver, 1984). A thyrotropin releasing hormone (TRH) response test is being developed to assess thyroid function in the dog and cat (Lothrop et al., 1984).

Hemograms and blood cholesterol concentrations of 11 dogs with hypothyroidism are presented in Table 36–10. In this group of dogs, females predominated, and ages ranged from 2–10 years. The diagnosis of hypothyroidism was verified by the demonstration of atrophy of the thyroid gland in 7 dogs, by decreased uptake of ^{131}I in 3 dogs, and by T_4 column chromatography in 1 dog. A slight to modest anemia (PCV <36%) was demonstrated in 7 dogs, and an eighth dog had a PCV of 37% and was considered to have a borderline anemia. The anemia was normocytic-normochromic in 9 dogs and slightly macrocytic-normochromic in dogs 5 and 9. The MCHC of dogs 10 and 11 was slightly high from hemolysis of the samples. Anemia was more obvious (PCV 25–30%) in hypothyroid dogs described in a recent report (Chastain, 1982). The anemia of hypothyroidism may be due to the reduced metabolic rate or possibly to a decrease in direct action of thyroxine on erythropoiesis (Hollander et al., 1967). Cline and Berlin (1963) investigated erythropoiesis and erythrocyte survival in 7 dogs with hypothyroidism due to exposure to radioiodine. Anemia developed slowly and resulted in a decrease in PCV of 18–35% and red cell mass of 22–52% of control values. Plasma volume decreased by only 19%. The anemia resulted from diminished erythrocyte production; erythrocyte life span was unaffected.

Erythrocyte morphology in hypothyroidism is characteristic of a depression anemia. Reticulocyte numbers remain low, and there is a lack of polychromasia. Leptocytes may be prominent, and their presence in large numbers may cause a diphasic ESR, as occurred in Dog 6. A significantly high positive corrected ESR value was observed in 7 of the 11 dogs. Alterations in the skin from any cause have been associated with an elevated ESR in many instances in the dog. In addition, pathologic changes that could influence ESR have been described in blood vessel walls in the hypothyroid dog (Clark and Meier, 1958).

Total leukocyte number varied from low normal (8,300/μl) to moderate leukocytosis (36,500/μl) in the 11 dogs. Only Dog 10 exhibited the stress pattern typical of increased secretion of adrenal glucocorticoid. One might expect a leukocyte pattern opposite to the stress reaction as a result of the decreased metabolic rate; such was the case in Dogs 2 through 7. A leukocytosis due to neutrophilia with slight left shift, increased monocytes, normal or high lymphocyte numbers and normal or increased eosinophils, as seen in Dogs 8, 9, and 11, would suggest a response to changes in the devitalized skin due to infection. Plasma proteins may be elevated by an increase in γ-globulin in response to the microbial activity that leads to pustular dermatitis (Appendix Case 6).

An increase in blood cholesterol concentration above the normal range of 135–270 mg/dl of plasma was observed in most of the dogs tested (Table 36–10). The cholesterol levels ranged from 260–1,454 mg/dl. Thyroid hormone exerts an anabolic as well as catabolic effect on cholesterol metabolism. Hypercholesterolemia of hypothyroidism is attributed to a greater decrease in the rate of destruction and intestinal excretion of cholesterol than decrease in the hepatic synthesis (Rosenman et al., 1952). It should be noted that hypercholesterolemia can occur in a variety of other situations such as nephrotic syndrome, hepatopathy, diabetes mellitus, Cushing's syndrome, and corticoid therapy, and from diets rich in animal fat. Although cholesterol concentration is useful in diagnosing hypothyroidism in only about 60% of cases (Kaneko, 1980a), it has been found to be a very useful indicator to monitor therapy of hypothyroid dogs (Baker, 1971). A fasting hypercholesterolemia of >500 mg/dl in the absence of diabetes mellitus and in the presence of clinical signs of hypothyroidism is highly suggestive of hypothyroidism.

Chronic fluoride toxicity (fluorosis) in cattle has been associated with hypothyroidism, anemia, and eosinophilia (Hillman et al.,

Table 36–10. The Hemogram in Hypothyroidism in the Dog

Dog No.	Sex	Age (yr)	Thyroid Function Tests[a]	Cholesterol (mg/dl)	RBC (×10⁶/µl)	Hb (g/dl)	PCV (%)	MCV (fl)	MCHC (%)	ESR (cor.)	WBC/µl	Neutrophils Band	Neutrophils Mature	Lymphocyte	Monocyte	Eosinophil
1	F	2	$T_4 = 0$	—	4.08	8.5	27	66.1	31.5	28+	13,300	133	10,308	864	1,724	266
2	F	4	$^{131}I = 0\%$	300	6.0	12.5	37	61.7	33.8	5−	8,900	0	6,185	2,047	489	178
3	XF	5	atrophy	470	5.7	10.2	31	54.4	32.9	21+	8,650	0	6,055	1,816	788	0
4	M	5	atrophy	1454	4.6	9.8	30	65.2	32.7	37+	8,300	0	5,810	1,909	498	83
5	F	5	atrophy	446	5.0	13.3	40	80.0	33.2	—	9,000	45	5,850	2,160	765	180
6	F	5	atrophy	740	4.2	10.0	30	71.4	33.3	diphasic 20+	14,250	0	7,339	4,346	1,211	1,354
7	XM	6	atrophy	400	4.6	10.2	32	69.6	31.0	26+	6,900	0	5,072	1,587	138	103
8	F	7	atrophy	322	5.2	11.8	35	67.3	33.7	2+	21,050	105	14,630	4,210	1,579	526
9	F	8	$^{131}I = 1.0\%$	508	5.2	13.5	41	79.8	32.0	0	22,200	222	15,762	2,664	1,110	2,442
10	F	9	$^{131}I = 1.0\%$	260	6.1	15.0	41	67.2	36.6	27+	28,100	422	25,009	842	1,545	281
11	XM	10	atrophy	262	3.2	8.8	24	75.0	36.7	29+	36,500	1,643	29,747	2,190	2,555	365

Differential Leukocytes, Absolute Numbers/µl (columns Band, Mature, Lymphocyte, Monocyte, Eosinophil)

[a] T_4 normal 0.6–3.6 µg/dl (Kaneko, 1980b); ^{131}I normal uptake 10% to 40% (Kaneko, 1980a).

1979). Clinical complaints in cattle ingesting excessive fluoride included inanition, anorexia, reduced milk production, infertility, lameness, and high mortality. Urine, teeth, and bone levels of fluoride were highly elevated. Classical dental and bone lesions of fluoride toxicity were observed; dental lesions varied from bilateral pitting, mottling, and hypoplasia of enamel to brown to black severe wear, and bone lesions comprised of severe exostosis.

Hyperthyroidism has been recognized in the dog and more recently in the cat (Holzworth et al., 1980; McMillan and Sherding, 1981), but hematologic findings are generally unremarkable. Experimental hypothyroidism in dogs was associated with a decrease in PCV from 39 ± 2% to 29 ± 3%, while no significant change occurred in hyperthyroid dogs (Chaiyabutr, 1981).

CANINE AND EQUINE EHRLICHIOSIS

Rickettsia canis was the name used in the older literature for the causative agent of a tick-borne anemia of dogs characterized by fever and weight loss (Malherbe, 1948; Neitz and Thomas, 1938). Later, this agent was designated *Ehrlichia canis* (Coles, 1953; Philip, 1953). Ehrlichiosis may occur in acute, subacute, or chronic form, and is common in tropical and subtropical countries having the appropriate tick vector, *Rhipicephalus sanguineus*. Domestic dogs and wild canines serve as the vertebrate hosts. *E. canis* was first detected in the United States as a mixed infection with *Babesia canis* (Ewing, 1963; Ewing and Buckner, 1965). In general, pure canine ehrlichiosis has been described as a relatively mild disease, while in dogs presenting a concomitant infection with *B. canis*, a grave and often fatal illness results.

Diagnosis is based on demonstration of the organism in blood, bone marrow, or biopsy specimens of other tissues and/or of antibodies in serum by an indirect immunofluorescence test (Ristic et al., 1972). Antibodies to *E. canis* may develop by 7–28 days of infection (Pyle, 1980), and it is important to recognize that seropositive dogs may not show clinical signs of the disease (Keefe et al., 1982). Tetracycline is the drug of choice for treatment

of ehrlichiosis. Several reports describe observations on natural and experimental infections in dogs (Buhles et al., 1974, 1975; Burghen et al., 1971; Ewing, 1969; Huxsoll, 1976; Huxsoll et al., 1970, 1972; Kuehn and Gaunt, 1985; Pyle, 1980; Reardon and Pierce, 1981a, b; Van Heerden, 1982; Walker et al., 1970; Wilkins et al., 1967).

E. canis occurs in the blood, bone marrow, and other tissues, particularly the lungs. In the blood, it is found as cytoplasmic inclusions primarily in monocytes and lymphocytes (Ewing et al., 1971). The organisms appear in Wright-stained blood or bone marrow films as single or multiple aggregates of fine bluish to slightly azurophilic coccoid or rod-shaped structures (elementary bodies) forming inclusions (morulae) in the cytoplasm of afflicted leukocytes (Plates XIII–5, XIII–6, XIV–4). Care should be exercised to avoid confusion with distemper inclusions, which may on rare occasions be seen in leukocytes of a dog infected with distemper virus (Figs. A1–A4, Appendix). Electron microscopy revealed the *Ehrlichia* inclusions in monocytes to be membrane-bound structures containing many elementary bodies, each of which presented a double membrane, and comprised of fine fibrils and granules (Simpson, 1972).

Wilkins and coworkers (1967) described a new and highly fatal disease that appeared in Singapore in late 1963 among military dogs. In the initial stages, high fever (106°F) was seen, and as the disease progressed, there were signs of hemorrhagic episodes characterized by epistaxis and ecchymotic and petechial hemorrhages in the skin and mucous membranes, sometimes accompanied by edema of the limbs and scrotum. In some instances, there was sudden death with but few clinical signs, although necropsy revealed widespread hemorrhages. The hemogram revealed anemia, neutropenia, and thrombocytopenia. Blood clotting was delayed, and prolonged bleeding occurred at injection sites. Although some dogs appeared to recover, relapses were common. The authors thought that the disease was probably caused by a previously unidentified virus. Huxsoll and coworkers (1970, 1972) called the new disease "tropical canine pancytopenia" and assigned *E. canis* as the etiologic agent. They found German shepherd dogs to be more severely affected in experimental transmission trials than beagles and mongrel dogs. Intracytoplasmic inclusions of *E. canis* were demonstrated in monocytes in capillary blood smears prepared during the early stages of the disease. The inclusions were more readily found in impression smears prepared from lung tissue and in some instances from the liver, spleen, and kidneys.

The characteristic pancytopenia of ehrlichiosis is attributed to marrow hypoplasia (Buhles et al., 1975), but its pathogenesis is not definitely known. In experimental infections marked thrombocytopenia (10,000-35,000/μl) and slight to moderate leukopenia (3,100-7,000/μl) are evident 10–14 days after infection, while a mild to moderate anemia (PCV 25–35%) develops 20–28 days after infection (Pyle, 1980). Severe leukopenia and anemia in certain cases may develop after several weeks. Thrombocytopenia can be attributed to megakaryocytic hypoplasia (Buhles et al., 1975) and reduced platelet survival (Pierce et al., 1977). The latter may, at least in part, be immune-mediated because a positive platelet factor-3 test for antiplatelet antibodies has been obtained in some natural cases of canine ehrlichiosis (Codner et al., 1985; Jain unpublished observations; Jain and Switzer, 1981). The anemia may be due to several mechanisms including blood loss from thrombocytopenia, bone marrow suppression, and immune-mediated red cell destruction (Buhles et al., 1975; Werner, 1980). Depletion of granulocytic precursors contribute to leukopenia (Buhles et al., 1975), but some other factors may also be involved. The total leukocyte count was found to be of significant prognostic value in that mortality was high in dogs with counts of <2,000/μl (Van Heerden, 1982).

Additional findings on some infected dogs have included hypergammaglobulinemia and hyperviscosity syndrome (Burghen et al., 1971; Hoskins et al., 1983; Reardon and Pierce, 1981a), hypoalbuminemia and elevated SGPT (Reardon and Pierce, 1981a), antinuclear antibodies (Codner et al., 1985), reduced platelet survival (Pierce et al., 1977), impaired platelet function and consumption of complement (Kuehn and Gaunt, 1985; Lov-ering et al., 1980), increased number of plasma cells and megakaryocytes in bone marrow (Kuehn and Gaunt, 1985), and Coombs-positive anemia (Heald, 1984; Kuehn and Gaunt, 1985; Werner, 1980).

Harvey and coworkers (1978) observed thrombocytopenia in dogs in association with cyclic infection from a rickettsial agent other than *E. canis*. The causative organism was recently named *E. platys*, and an indirect immunofluorescence test was described for its serologic diagnosis (French and Harvey, 1983; Fig. 17–6).

Ehrlichia equi (Lewis et al., 1975) causes a peracute disease of horses, characterized by high fever, anorexia, depression, limb edema, ataxia, leukopenia, and thrombocytopenia (Gribble, 1969; Stannard et al., 1969). The disease was described first from California, where it is endemic in certain areas, but sporadic cases in other parts of the United States have been observed in recent years (Brewer et al., 1984; Madewell and Gribble, 1982). The organism presents elementary bodies and morula-like structures in the cytoplasm of neutrophils (Plates XIV–1, XIV–2, XIV–3) and occasionally in eosinophils during the period of pyrexia. The host specificity of *E. equi* is broad in that several animal species—dogs, cats, sheep, goats, and nonhuman primates—can acquire infection, while the canine organism infects only domestic and wild canines (Gribble, 1969; Harvey et al., 1979; Lewis et al., 1975; Madewell and Gribble, 1982). Natural infection of two dogs from *E. equi* has been observed at the VMTH-UCD (Madewell and Gribble, 1982). Thus *Ehrlichia* morulae found primarily in canine neutrophils and eosinophils and causing a mild disease (Ewing et al., 1971) are considered to represent infection by *E. equi*.

Potomac horse fever is caused by an *Ehrlichia* serologically related to *E. sennetsu* (Holland et al., 1985). Affected horses are leukopenic. The organism has not been found in circulating leukocytes in stained blood films, but it can be observed in cultured blood monocytes.

Ehrlichia organisms have been described as the cause of tick-borne fever of sheep and cattle. Foggie (1951) presented an excellent color plate showing various morphologic features of the intracytoplasmic inclusions in neutrophils and monocytes of sheep. The disease in sheep is characterized by a marked transient thrombocytopenia and neutropenia (Foster and Cameron, 1968).

CANINE LEISHMANIASIS

Leishmaniasis has been reported in dogs imported into the United States from Greece (Gleiser et al., 1957; Schalm, 1979b; Theran and Ling, 1967; Thorson et al., 1955). Infection rates as high as 40% have been reported in Greece (Levine, 1961). The dog may be considered as a reservoir host, and *Phlebotomus* sand flies are suspected as vectors for transmission of the parasite to both dogs and humans (Kudo, 1966). *Leishmania* are intracellular parasites in macrophages and may occasionally appear in circulating monocytes and neutrophils. *Leishmania donovani* may cause either visceral or cutaneous leishmaniasis in the dog, and the disease is usually chronic (Levine, 1961). Visceral leishmaniasis is the most common form in dogs.

Presenting clinical signs in infected dogs have been variable and have included weight loss, lameness, intermittent pyrexia, central nervous system disturbances, skin ulceration, epistaxis, lymphadenopathy, and hepatomegaly. Anemia may be present; it may be regenerative or nonregenerative. Total and differential leukocyte counts may be normal, or a left shift may be present with normal leukocyte count. Leukopenia, lymphopenia, and thrombocytopenia may be seen in more severe cases. Serum globulins are elevated and albumin is decreased. Serum tryptophan concentration is decreased because of increased consumption by *Leishmania* (Longstaffe and Guy, 1985).

Diagnosis is based on finding macrophages filled with the amastigote form of the parasite, Leishman-Donovan bodies, in Wright or Giemsa stained smears or biopsies from lymph nodes, spleen, or bone marrow. Immunofluorescence and ELISA tests can be performed to detect specific antibody in cytologically negative cases of leishmaniasis (Longstaffe and Guy, 1985; Reiter et al., 1985).

In experimental dogs, the infection was completely controlled by stibogluconate so-

dium (Pentostam), 10 or 50 mg/Kg body weight daily, given intravenously for two periods of 10 days at 10-day intervals (Reiter et al., 1985).

A significant finding in two dogs observed at the VMTH-UCD was hyperproteinemia, 11.0 and 13.0 g/dl of plasma, respectively, of which 7.4 g and 10.8 g was γ-globulin. *Leishmania* were demonstrated either by culture methods or by observation in tissue sections, particularly of the liver but also of many other organs such as the spleen, lymph nodes, intestine, skin, synovial membranes, and bone marrow. The rounded leishmanial stage of the organism is observed within fixed and free macrophages. Following is a brief description of another dog with leishmaniasis observed at our clinic (Schalm, 1979b).

A long-haired male dachshund, 3 years and 9 months old, was born in Greece and resided in Athens for 16 months before being brought to the United States, first to Alabama and then to California. About 29 months after leaving Greece, the dog was admitted to the VMTH-UCD. It had been on prednisone therapy for 1 year for the treatment of polyarthritis. The dog was exhibiting depression, muscle atrophy, fever (103.2°F), fresh blood in feces, generalized lymphadenopathy, a swollen right carpal joint, and generalized seborrhea with hair loss over the chest, abdomen, and hips.

Blood examination demonstrated a normocytic-normochromic anemia (PCV 32%) with reticulocyte count of 0.5%. The total leukocyte count was 9,000/μl with a left shift to metamyelocytes and a lymphopenia. Platelet count was not done, but seemed to be adequate from examination of the blood film. There was hypoproteinemia at 5.6 g/dl. Scanning the stained blood film revealed a single neutrophil with an inclusion later identified as *L. donovani*. *Leishmania* were subsequently demonstrated in biopsy materials from the colon, skin, joint fluid and synovial membrane, bone marrow, and additionally in the spleen at necropsy. The dog died 16 days after admission to the hospital.

FELINE INFECTIOUS PERITONITIS

Feline infectious peritonitis (FIP) was described as a distinct entity by Wolfe and Griesemer (1966); they subsequently described the gross and histopathologic lesions (Wolfe and Griesemer, 1971). Zook and coworkers (1968) and Ward and coworkers (1968) presented ultrastructural evidence of a viral etiology. The virus is classified as a coronavirus. Based on a wide spectrum of abnormalities, in addition to peritonitis, associated with infection from this virus, "feline coronaviral disease" has been suggested as a more suitable name (Farrow and Love, 1983).

FIP has been reported more frequently in males than in females (70–80% of cases) (Robison et al., 1971; Schalm, 1971; Wolfe and Griesemer, 1966) and mostly in young (<3 years of age) cats (Wilkinson, 1979). Spontaneous recovery is rare. Temporary improvement may occur during continuous therapy with corticosteroids and other immunosuppressive drugs such as cyclophosphamide. Most commonly, clinical signs persist or recur and lead eventually to death or to a request for euthanasia of an emaciated, dehydrated cat.

Two clinicopathologic forms of FIP are recognized. The outstanding clinical feature in a majority of cats is an accumulation of a viscous, usually clear but sometimes flaky fluid in the abdominal cavity and less frequently in the thoracic cavity. This represents the so called "wet" or effusive form of FIP (Appendix Case 45). Despite the presence of peritonitis, abdominal palpation is not painful. Persistent fever, anorexia, and weight loss are accompanying clinical signs. In addition, icterus, vomiting, diarrhea, and periorchitis are exhibited by some cats. The "dry" or granulomatous form of FIP is most difficult to diagnose. It is characterized by little or no exudate in body cavities and granulomatous lesions primarily in parenchymatous organs, uveal tract, brain, and spinal cord.

The disease has been found in domestic as well as wild cats. It was transmitted experimentally by a variety of routes with an incubation period ranging from 1–33 days (mean 14 days) (Wilkinson, 1979). The incubation period of the spontaneously occurring disease is unknown but may be longer. A high proportion of inapparent infection is detected by serologic examination of random healthy cats (9–60% positive) and cats from catteries

with a history of FIP (about 80–90% positive) (Farrow and Love, 1983). Interpretation of the serum FIP antibody test has been controversial. It has been suggested that this test is not diagnostic for FIP, but is indicative of a past viral infection (Weiss and Scott, 1980). Cats with enteric coronavirus infection may give positive antibody titers against FIP virus. However, in conjunction with clinicopathologic abnormalities, a positive antibody test (indirect fluorescent antibody titers of >1:100) supports a diagnosis of FIP. Concurrent infection with *Haemobartonella felis* or feline leukemia virus (FeLV) may occur in cats with FIP.

An immune-complex pathogenesis of FIP has been suggested; it has found support in findings such as circulating immune complexes, deposition of immune complexes in the kidneys and livers of infected cats, diminution of blood complement levels, and shorter survival of kittens seropositive to FIP virus than of those seronegative to FIP virus (Jacobse-Geels, 1982; Pedersen and Boyle, 1980; Weiss et al., 1980). Recent reviews give additional information on FIP (August, 1984; Farrow and Love, 1983; Horzinek and Osterhaus, 1979; Pedersen, 1983, 1984; Weiss and Scott, 1980; Wilkinson, 1979).

Hematologic data (Table 36–11) on FIP were developed from jugular blood of 26 cats and capillary blood from an ear vein of 9 cats. The PCV values of the 35 cats ranged from 12–50%, with a mean of 26.2%. Anemia was present in 43% of the cats as a result of depressed erythrogenesis as evidenced by normocytic normochromic erythrocytic indexes (MCV 46.2 ± 4.4 fl and MCHC 31.4 ± 1.9%). The icterus index was above normal (10–50 units) in 15 of 29 cats. Increased icterus index is of hepatic origin and is due to extension of the inflammatory process to involve the liver. Focal hepatic necrosis was reported in 20% of cats with FIP (Wolfe and Griesemer, 1971), and jaundice was seen in 20% of another group of cats (Robison et al., 1971). Experimental infection in kittens produces a progressive normocytic normochromic anemia with red cell morphology characterized by poikilocytosis and anisocytosis (Weiss and Scott, 1981).

Hypergammaglobulinemia from increases

Table 36–11. The Hemogram in Feline Infectious Peritonitis (35 Cats)[a]

Item	Minimum	Maximum	Median	Mean	Standard Deviation	No. of Cats
Erythrocytes ($\times 10^6$/μl)	3.21	9.88	5.50	5.71	1.64	34
Hemoglobin (g/dl)	4.6	15.1	8.5	8.2	2.3	34
PCV (%)	12.0	50.0	26.5	26.2	7.5	35
MCV (fl)	37.3	58.5	45.6	46.2	4.4	34
MCH (pg)	11.2	17.4	14.3	14.5	1.4	34
MCHC (%)	28.3	38.3	31.0	31.4	1.9	34
Icterus index units	2.0	50.0	5.0	7.5	10.0	29
Plasma proteins (g/dl)	6.4	11.0	8.0	8.3	1.1	26
Fibrinogen (g/dl)	0.10	0.70	0.40	0.40	0.18	26
Leukocytes/μl	1,700	52,000	12,800	18,000	11,500	34
Band neutrophils	0	13,450	1,000	1,750	2,600	33
Mature neutrophils	1,088	40,300	11,500	15,400	9,300	33
Lymphocytes	0	3,750	450	769	770	33
Monocytes	0	1,470	250	384	382	33
Eosinophils	0	294	0	34	79	33
Basophils	0	220	0	13	42	33
Leukocytes (%)						
Band neutrophils	0	38.0	6.0	8.9	9.2	33
Mature neutrophils	50.0	96.0	82.5	83.3	11.3	33
Lymphocytes	0	20.5	3.5	4.8	4.7	33
Monocytes	0	8.0	1.5	2.5	2.3	33
Eosinophils	0	2.0	0	0.2	0.5	33
Basophils	0	0.5	0	0.06	0.16	33

[a]From Schalm, 1971; courtesy of *The California Veterinarian.*

in both β- and γ-globulins is characteristic of FIP (Disque et al., 1968; Hardy and Hurvitz, 1971; Robison et al., 1971; Ward and Pederson, 1969; Wilkinson, 1979). Total plasma proteins in 26 of our cats ranged from 6.4–11.0 g/dl, mean 8.3 g/dl. An extreme of 14.0 g/dl was recorded in an additional cat subsequently admitted to the hospital. Fractionation of the serum of this last cat (Fig. 34–11) revealed the γ-globulin fraction to be 9.0 g. Hardy and Hurvitz (1971) reported a range of total protein of 6.0–12.0 g/dl, mean 9.0 g/dl, in nine cats with FIP. In FIP, fibrinogen is involved in formation of the characteristic fibrinous exudate in the abdominal and pleural cavities. Among 26 cats (Table 36–11) plasma fibrinogen was within the normal range of 0.05–0.3 g/dl in 11 cats (42.3%). In the remaining 15 cats, plasma fibrinogen ranged between 0.4 and 0.7 g/dl. The mean value for all 26 cats was 0.40 ± 0.18 g/dl.

Total leukocyte counts in 34 cats with FIP ranged from leukopenia (1,700) to marked leukocytosis (52,000); the mean count was 18,000 ± 11,500/μl. These findings compared favorably with results from 48 cats in the Boston area (Robison et al., 1971). Generally there is a neutrophilia with modest left shift consisting of band neutrophils. The most char-

acteristic feature of the leukogram in FIP is a marked lymphopenia. There is also an eosinopenia, while monocytes commonly remain within their normal range. A leukopenia may occur in terminal or fulminating cases (Horzinek and Osterhaus, 1979). These changes in peripheral blood may be associated with development of necrosis in bone marrow and lymphoid depletion in lymph nodes, spleen, and thymus (Ward et al, 1974). Infection with feline enteric coronavirus, which is antigenically similar to FIP virus and induces enteritis but not FIP in young cats, is associated with leukopenia primarily due to neutropenia during the febrile and diarrheic phases (Pedersen et al., 1981).

Recent experimental studies on FIP have demonstrated significant clotting abnormalities suggestive of DIC, e.g., prolonged prothrombin and partial thromboplastin times, reduced coagulation factors VII, VIII, IX, X, XI, and XII, elevated fibrin and/or fibrinogen degradation products, and thrombocytopenia (Weiss and Scott, 1980; Weiss et al., 1980). Some of these abnormalities were also found in natural cases of FIP. Serum biochemistry and urinalysis may reflect changes associated with liver disease (e.g., elevated bilirubin, SGPT, serum glutamic oxaloacetate transaminase, sorbitol dehydrogenase, lactic dehydrogenase, and alkaline phosphatase) and kidney disease (e.g., high BUN and creatinine and proteinuria), depending on the extent of specific organ involvement.

Composition of the Exudate

Exudates from the abdominal cavity of 22 cats and from the thoracic cavity of 1 cat were analyzed for specific gravity, protein concentration, and total and differential cell counts (Table 36–12). Abdominal fluid volume has been reported to vary from 15–1,000 ml (Wolfe and Griesemer, 1966; Robison et al., 1971). The exudate differs from that of a suppurative process in that cellular content is low (6,300 ± 5,400/μl) and clotting may occur on exposure to air. The neutrophil is the major cell type (73 ± 20%), except that in long-standing cases mononuclear cells may predominate. High protein content (5.9 ± 0.7 g/dl) characterizes the fluid as a true exudate, and globulin is the main protein fraction (Hardy and O'Reilly, 1969). Immune-mediated vasculitis is responsible for the protein-rich exudate. One of our cats with a total plasma protein concentration of 14 g/dl had 11.8 g of protein in the abdominal exudate, and fractionation of this protein revealed 1.9 g of albumin and 9.9 g of globulin, of which 8.1 g was γ-globulin.

FELINE PANLEUKOPENIA

Feline panleukopenia (infectious enteritis) is a highly contagious viral disease of young cats; it is characterized by extreme leukopenia and a high mortality rate. Feline panleukopenia virus is a parvovirus; hence the disease is also called feline parvovirus infection. Bentinck-Smith (1949) reported the following clinical signs among 574 cases of feline panleukopenia: anorexia, 80.1%; emesis, 67.9%; prostration, 50.7%; and diarrhea, 24.0%. Ad-

ditional signs reported by Carpenter (1971) were high fever, dehydration, and excessive gas and liquid in the gastrointestinal tract, with death sometimes occurring within 24 hours of admission to the hospital. Bloody diarrhea, persistent vomiting, necrotic and ulcerative oral lesions, and anemia may develop in more protracted cases. Intensive fluid therapy to combat dehydration and electrolyte loss and antibiotics to control bacterial infection are indicated. Cats recovering from a recent infection become carriers and shed the virus in feces and urine for months. In addition, the virus may also persist in the cat's environ for months. Transmission of the virus usually occurs by direct contact, but fleas and other biting insects may also be involved (Kahn, 1978).

Infection usually occurs by ingestion or inhalation, although other routes can also produce infection. The virus multiplies first in the lymphoid tissue and then invades the intestinal mucosa by hematogenous route (Carlson et al., 1977). Striking absence of enteric involvement in germfree cats in early experiments indicated an association of enteric lesions with resident microbial flora in naturally infected cats. The disease in germfree cats otherwise paralleled the naturally occurring disease, except that there was no death (Rohovsky and Fowler, 1971). Recent observations indicate that the severity of the enteric lesions is dependent upon the mitotic activity of the intestinal crypt epithelium which, in turn, is related to a mitotic stimulatory action of resident enteric bacteria (Kahn, 1978). The virus has an affinity for rapidly dividing cells. Thus the germfree animals, lacking enteric bacteria, show very little mitotic activity in intestinal crypt epithelium and hence absence of enteric lesions. Recent reviews give additional information on feline panleukopenia (Farrow and Love, 1983; Kahn, 1978; Timoney, 1976).

Table 36–12. Cell and Protein Composition of the Exudate in FIP (23 Cats)[a]

	Specific Gravity	Protein (g/dl)	RBC (×10³/μl)	Nucleated Cells (/μl)	Neutrophils (%)	Small Mononuclears (%)	Large Mononuclears (%)
Range	1.0203–1.0275	4.5–7.7	2–350	700–22,900	13.0–99.0	0–39.0	0–65.0
Mean	1.0232	5.9	42	6,300	73.0	11.5	15.3
1 SD	0.0017	0.7	80	5,400	20.4	10.8	13.3

[a]From Schalm, 1971; courtesy *The California Veterinarian.*

Newberne et al. (1957) reported an incubation period of 4–8 days in the experimentally produced disease in conventional cats. They reported the average daily total leukocyte count to decrease from 12,512 to 2,897/μl on the day of sacrifice. Bone marrow changes were characterized by diminution of cellular elements, vacuolation, and apparent replacement with fat. In germfree cats and specific pathogen–free cats leukopenia developed within 2–4 days of experimental infection (Carlson et al., 1977). Similar observations on two experimentally infected cats are summarized in Appendix Case 54. Langheinrich and Nielsen (1971) described their bone marrow findings as follows: depression of myelopoiesis, depopulation of the reticular meshwork, sinusoidal congestion and edema, and serous atrophy of fat cells. There is good evidence from peripheral blood studies to indicate that erythropoiesis and megakaryocytopoiesis are also markedly depressed, leading to development of anemia and thrombocytopenia in the more protracted cases. The most immediate and marked effect observed in peripheral blood is the depletion of leukocytes, neutrophils being depressed to the greatest degree. Extensive blood and bone marrow findings, supportive of these observations, on natural and experimental cases of feline panleukopenia have been reported by others (Ichijo et al., 1976).

Lawrence and coworkers (1940) described the disease under the name infectious feline agranulocytosis. They found the average total leukocyte count of 113 cats at the height of the disease to be 1,350/μl, but 22 of the cats had counts of from 0–200 leukocytes. Because of the very marked reduction in neutrophil numbers, the other leukocytes appear completely out of proportion to their true distribution when the differential count is expressed in percentage (Table 36–13). A marked lymphopenia also exists, but the few lymphocytes remaining in the circulation may represent 70–80% of lymphocytes in the differential leukocyte count (Cats 2, 5, 7, 8, and 9). Dogs with parvovirus infection similarly develop marked leukopenia due to neutropenia and lymphopenia. The eosinophil granulocyte appears to be somewhat more resistant to the effects of the virus than the

neutrophil. Cats with *E. coli* enteritis and salmonellosis, presenting features clinically similar to those of feline panleukopenia, can be distinguished by the presence of leukopenia and neutropenia in the latter.

During convalescence, granulopoiesis becomes reestablished, and the bone marrow initially contains only the precursors of the granulocytes. A few of these enter the circulation, and a marked left shift, suggestive of a degenerative left shift, is seen in the blood (Cats 10 and 12, Table 36–13). Table 5–2 presents the differential leukocyte distribution in blood of a cat in convalescence. Initially, the immature neutrophils released to blood are giant forms with bizarre nuclear patterns (Figs. 5–4, 5–5, 5–6, and Plates XV–8, XV–9, XV–10). With each successive day, however, neutrophil morphology improves so that by the fourth or fifth day, the neutrophils in blood are of normal size and appearance.

The leukopenia with marked left shift characteristic of early convalescence from panleukopenia must be distinguished from a similar pattern that may develop in other diseases that seriously depress granulopoiesis, e.g., subleukemic granulocytic leukemia and some instances of massive displacement of the bone marrow in lymphoma. This can be done by sequential blood film examination or bone marrow aspiration. Blood cytology associated with a convalescent marrow progresses rapidly toward normal, while such progress is not evident when granulopoiesis is more permanently suppressed, either by neoplasia or by a toxemic maturation arrest. Cats in the convalescent stage of panleukopenia may be presented to the veterinarian for diagnosis; it is therefore important to recognize the bizarre cells as belonging to the neutrophilic series and to demonstrate the return to normal on subsequent days. Riser (1947) showed that in surviving cats the leukocyte count rapidly increased and could exceed the maximum normal value in 3 or 4 days. Some examples from our observations are given in Table 36–14.

Total plasma protein concentration has commonly been between 7.0 and 8.0 g/dl, with an occasional cat having a protein level of 9.0 g/dl. Considering that most cats developing panleukopenia are 6 months of age or younger (Table 36–13), these levels reflect the

Table 36–13. Hemograms in Feline Panleukopenia

Cat No.	Age (mo)	Temp. (°F)	PCV (%)	WBC/ μl	Differential Leukocyte Count																
					Neutrophils						Lymphocyte		Monocyte		Eosinophil		Unclassified		Degenerated	
					Metamyelocyte		Band		Mature											
					No.	%	No.	%	No.	%	No.	%	No.	%	No.	%	No.	%	No.	%
1	3	—	—	150	0	0.0	0	0.0	3	2.0	27	18.0	117	78.0	3	2.0	0	0.0	0	0.0
2	6	—	39	600	0	0.0	0	0.0	12	2.0	432	72.0	108	18.0	48	8.0	0	0.0	0	0.0
3	6	104.0	36	600	0	0.0	0	0.0	0	0.0	324	54.0	24	4.0	252	42.0	0	0.0	0	0.0
4	8	105.8	30	700	0	0.0	14	2.0	196	28.0	315	45.0	70	10.0	0	0.0	28	4.0	77	11.0
5	6	105.0	35	1,000	0	0.0	10	1.0	50	5.0	860	86.0	70	7.0	10	1.0	0	0.0	0	0.0
6	6	—	27	900	0	0.0	0	0.0	18	2.0	486	54.0	126	14.0	270	30.0	0	0.0	0	0.0
7	17	105.0	41	1,500	0	0.0	0	0.0	150	10.0	1,200	80.0	90	6.0	60	4.0	0	0.0	0	0.0
8	3	—	37	1,500	0	0.0	0	0.0	240	16.0	1,200	80.0	60	4.0	0	0.0	0	0.0	0	0.0
9	5	106.5	30	1,500	0	0.0	15	1.0	0	0.0	1,110	74.0	120	8.0	255	17.0	0	0.0	0	0.0
10	5	103.8	—	1,800	252	14.0	324	18.0	684	38.0	504	28.0	36	2.0	0	0.0	0	0.0	0	0.0
11	36	106.0	39	2,200	0	0.0	0	0.0	1,166	53.0	374	17.0	198	9.0	132	6.0	154	7.0	176	8.0
12	6	107.2	43	2,100	420	20.0	189	9.0	126	6.0	63	3.0	819	39.0	483	23.0	0	0.0	0	0.0

Table 36–14.   Examples of Changes in Leukocyte Counts (/μl of blood) during Convalescence from Feline Panleukopenia

Initial Count	Subsequent Count	Days Later
300	1,500	1
100	6,250	2
100	6,000	4
400	22,800	5
750	36,000	5
1,100	36,100	5

developing dehydration. Plasma fibrinogen is also commonly in excess of the normal range; values of 0.4–1.0 g/dl have been observed in many cats with clinically diagnosed panleukopenia. The icterus index may be normal, but 7.5, 10, and 20 units have been recorded among our feline patients.

HEMOGRAMS IN ACUTE AND CHRONIC INFLAMMATORY DISEASES IN CATTLE

Total plasma proteins in mature cattle range from 7.0–8.5 g/dl and plasma fibrinogen ranges from 0.3–0.7 g/dl. Total plasma proteins (including fibrinogen) increase rapidly (relative increase) in dehydration and more slowly (absolute increase) when globulins increase in response to some forms of hepatopathy and infections. Fibrinogen increases in response to almost any systemic disorder in cattle, and a major elevation is anticipated in both acute and chronic inflammatory diseases. Fibrinogen levels in excess of 1.0 g/dl commonly have been associated with inflammatory lesions, and the values have at times exceeded 2.0 g/dl. Because of the influence of dehydration on plasma protein and fibrinogen levels, it was found convenient to express the relationship as a ratio of plasma proteins to fibrinogen (PP:F). A ratio of 10:1 or less has been interpreted as demonstrating a significant increase in fibrinogen above any elevation due to dehydration. For details, see Chapter 34.

Table 36–15 presents hemograms of 20 cattle with a variety of acute and chronic inflammatory diseases. The diagnosis was verified in each instance either by surgery (traumatic reticulitis, ruptured urinary bladder) or at necropsy of those animals in an advanced stage of disease. The hemograms are listed in order of increasing plasma fibrinogen level. The ma-

jority of cattle with fibrinogen levels of 1.4 g/dl or more also had significantly elevated total plasma proteins (see also Table 34–8).

Response of the bovine neutrophilic leukocyte to inflammatory disease is discussed in Chapter 7. In evaluating the total and differential leukocyte counts in bovine blood, the following guidelines are recommended:

leukocytosis	= WBC >12,000/μl of blood
leukopenia	= WBC <4,000
neutrophilia	= neutrophils >4,000
left shift	= immature neutrophils >200
lymphopenia	= lymphocytes <2,500
monocytosis	= monocytes >850

Table 36–15 shows that 13 cattle (65%) with serious inflammatory problems had total leukocyte counts of less than 10,000/μl. The differential leukocyte counts in 9 of these 13 cattle revealed neutrophilia and/or a left shift. In two of the cattle (numbers 13 and 16) the neutrophils were described as toxic. These examples indicate that in cattle the differential leukocyte count is considerably more indicative of the possible presence of an inflammatory lesion than the total leukocyte count. Fibrinogen concentration was elevated in all cases, and the low PP:F ratios verified the marked increase in fibrinogen in relation to total plasma protein. The data relative to plasma fibrinogen levels are a valuable addition to the bovine hemogram and could stand alone as indicative of the possibility of a serious internal inflammatory lesion. See Chapter 7 for a discussion of the influence of acute indigestion on plasma fibrinogen levels and total and differential leukocyte counts.

Frank lymphopenia was encountered in 6 (30%) of the 20 cattle (Table 36–15). If lymphopenia is defined as <3,000 lymphocytes, rather than <2,500, then 50% of the cattle would be classified as lymphopenic. The number of monocytes was of little value to interpretation, while 75% of the cattle could be regarded as having had an eosinophilia.

Table 36–15. Hemograms in a Variety of Acute and Chronic Diseases of Cattle; Diagnosis Verified by Surgery or Necropsy

| Animal Number | Sex | Age (yr) | Clinical Condition | Plasma | | | WBC/μl | Differential Leukocyte Count in Absolute Numbers/μl | | | | | | | |
				Proteins (g/dl)	Fibrinogen (g/dl)	PP:F Ratio		Myelocytes	Meta-myelocytes	Bands	Neutrophils	Lymphocytes	Monocytes	Eosinophils	Basophils
1	F	5	Peritonitis	6.3	1.0	5.3:1	26,700	934	1,203	7,209	11,614	2,803	2,937	0	0
2	F	6	Intussusception	9.8	1.1	7.9:1	6,700	201	402	2,345	1,809	1,809	134	0	0
3	F	3	Ruptured bladder	8.7	1.2	6.2:1	8,500	0	0	808	3,782	2,880	935	85	0
4	F	2	Traumatic pericarditis	7.2	1.2	5.0:1	21,300	0	0	532	17,466	2,237	746	213	106
5	F	5	Traumatic reticulitis	8.9	1.2	6.4:1	19,900	0	0	0	4,776	14,825	0	299	0
6	M	4	Pharyngeal abscess	8.6	1.2	6.1:1	8,800	0	0	0	5,236	3,080	264	220	0
7	F	2½	Pyelonephritis	8.5	1.3	6.3:1	7,400	0	0	94	3,182	3,367	444	222	111
8	F	1	Necrotizing nephrosis	8.8	1.3	5.7:1	5,300	0	0	0	1,299	3,683	318	0	0
9	F	4	Pyelonephritis	9.7	1.4	5.9:1	5,700	0	0	0	2,023	3,249	371	57	0
10	F	3	Endocarditis	11.2	1.4	7.0:1	12,900	0	0	0	6,257	5,676	774	193	0
11	F	1½	Traumatic reticulitis	11.8	1.5	6.9:1	19,500	0	0	390	14,430	4,388	292	0	0
12	F	8	Intussusception	9.2	1.5	5.1:1	9,600	0	0	576	6,096	2,688	240	0	0
13	F	2	Pyelonephritis	12.5	1.5	7.3:1	6,200	0	0	217[a]	3,875[a]	1,860	248	0	0
14	F	5	Traumatic reticulitis	10.0	1.6	5.3:1	8,300	0	0	1,411	4,150	2,366	290	83	0
15	M	½	Pyelonephritis	10.4	1.7	5.1:1	6,000	0	0	0	2,520	3,420	60	0	0
16	M	¾	Mycotic rumenitis and peritonitis	8.2	1.7	3.8:1	5,000	100[a]	400[a]	300[a]	0	4,200	0	0	0
17	F	5	Traumatic peritonitis	13.2	1.8	6.3:1	7,400	0	0	518	4,366	2,146	370	0	0
18	M	2	Brain abscess	9.6	1.9	4.0:1	11,300	0	0	0	7,684	2,825	791	0	0
19	M	2½	Urolithiasis and ruptured bladder	11.1	1.9	4.8:1	7,600	0	38	3,040	2,584	1,444	456	38	0
20	F	2	Peritonitis and dead fetus	12.6	2.0	5.3:1	16,900	0	0	85	10,900	5,577	253	85	0

[a] Neutrophils toxic.

An early diagnosis in traumatic lesions of the bovine reticulum is important so that the foreign body may be surgically removed before extensive peritonitis with abscess formation or pericarditis complicates the condition. Clinical signs common to traumatic gastritis are anorexia, marked reduction in milk secretion, sluggish rumen activity, normal or elevated body temperature, and evidence of pain (grunt) upon application of pressure over the xiphoid region. Many of these same signs are common to simple indigestion, and therefore laboratory reports should help in making a diagnosis. Table 36–16 lists percentage distributions of leukogram abnormalities, using the guidelines outlined above for evaluation of the leukogram, in 50 cattle with traumatic reticulitis and 8 with traumatic pericarditis. It can be seen that the leukogram is more reliable as an indicator of the existence of an inflammatory lesion in cows displaying an elevation of body temperature above 102.5°F. Furthermore, in the more serious lesion of traumatic pericarditis, there was less occurrence of leukocytosis, but left shift was more significant as an indicator of a serious problem. A case of traumatic reticulitis with splenitis is presented in Appendix Case 67.

ACUTE BOVINE MASTITIS

Acute mastitis in the cow may be caused by a variety of bacterial organisms, but the most common are *Staphylococcus aureus*, *E. coli*, *Enterobacter aerogenes* (previously designated *Aerobacter aerogenes)*, and *Pseudomonas aeruginosa*. *S. aureus* is generally responsible for the gangrenous types of mastitis, although it is also commonly associated with a mild chronic mastitis.

Pattison and coworkers (1950), who studied experimental mastitis due to *Streptococcus agalactiae* in goats, remarked that after inoculation there was a severe leukopenia and concomitant shift to the left. Holman (1955), in discussing the blood picture of the cow, made the statement that a marked leukopenia is seen over a short period in experimental mastitis, the leukocyte count falling to about 2,000 with a return to normal in a few hours. Cole and Easterbrooks (1958) have reported on the leukopenia of acute mastitis. Theilen et al. (1959) made observations on the hematology of acute mastitis in 62 cows, of which 8 cases were gangrenous. Data on representative cases of acute bovine mastitis are summarized in Table 36–17.

Cows with acute mastitis are generally toxemic and depressed, and the blood picture taken early in the disease, that is, during the first 24–48 hours, often is one of marked leukopenia (Fig. 7–3). The general pattern of leukocyte response in acute mastitis appears to be as follows: Within hours of the onset, a decrease of both neutrophils and lymphocytes takes place. If this decrease is great enough, the total leukocyte count may fall below the normal minimum of 4,000/μl of blood. Total leukocyte counts of less than 1,000 have been recorded (Appendix Case 6). In other cases, the total leukocyte count remains within the normal range, but in all probability, it is considerably lower than the normal for the particular animal in question, and thus a relative leukopenia exists.

The leukopenic state persists from a few hours to a few days, depending on the severity of the mastitis and the success of treatment. The neutrophils reappear, with a variable number of immature forms. The extent of this shift to the left is influenced by severity

Table 36–16. Frequency of Certain Hemogram Abnormalities in Traumatic Reticulitis and Pericarditis in Cattle

	Traumatic Reticulitis Temperature °F		Traumatic Pericarditis
	<102.5° (26 Cattle)	>102.5° (24 Cattle)	(8 Cattle)
Leukocytosis	35%	62%	37%
Neutrophilia	80%	80%	63%
Left Shift	11%	40%	88%
Leukopenia	0	8%	0
Lymphopenia	11%	33%	37%
Monocytosis	77%	96%	87%

Table 36–17. Hemograms in Representative Cases of Acute Bovine Mastitis

Case No. and Breed	Age (yr)	Type of Infection	Date	WBC/μl	Percentage Distribution of Leukocyte Types								Comments on Clinical Examination			
					Myelocytes	Metamyelocytes	Bands	Neutrophils	Lymphocytes	Monocytes	Eosinophils	Basophils	Temp. (°F)	Pulse	Respiration	Other
GTS-6 Jersey	8	E. aerogenes	3/ 8/57	1,300	0	0	1.0	19.0	77.0	3.0	0	0	108.8	108	58	Severe, responded to two treatments.
		S. aureus	3/ 9/57	2,850	0	0	0	6.0	63.5	24.5	6.0	0	102.2	80	28	
SD-520 Guernsey	5	Sterile sample	10/22/56	2,800	0	0.5	10.0	5.5	62.0	9.0	13.0	0	101.5	86	25	Moderately severe; responded to two treatments.
			10/24/56	8,000	0	2.0	14.0	44.0	27.0	9.0	3.0	1.0	101.0	75	25	
UCD-127 Holstein-Friesian	14	E. coli	10/ 2/56	2,950	0	2.0	5.0	2.0	66.0	17.0	8.0	0	104.8	100	100	Severe, responded slowly, treated for 2 weeks continuously. Liver biopsy showed micro-abscesses.
			10/ 3/56	3,950	0	3.0	9.5	4.0	63.5	18.0	2.0	0	104.4	100	80	
			10/ 8/56	4,450	0	0	12.0	39.0	36.0	11.0	2.0	0	104.1	90	60	
			10/15/56	9,500	0	0	0.5	51.5	24.5	23.5	0	0	105.5	96	80	
			10/23/56	8,350	0	0	1.5	50.5	23.0	13.5	11.0	0	103.0	86	24	
			11/23/56	7,050	0	0	0	35.0	50.0	5.0	10.0	0	101.4	80	24	
			3/12/57	1,800	0	0	1.0	2.0	83.0	12.0	2.0	0	105.0	100	—	Severe; did not respond to treatment. Liver biopsy showed severe lipidosis. Animal died.
			3/13/57	1,350	0	0	0	1.0	85.0	6.0	8.0	0	104.2	—	—	
UCD-65 Jersey	10	E. coli	3/14/57	2,850	0	0	0	1.0	82.0	8.0	9.0	0	104.8	—	—	
			3/15/57	3,250	14.0	20.0	5.0	0	51.0	7.0	3.0	0	100.0	—	—	
			3/16/57	6,300	0	7.0	0	0	84.0	9.0	0	0	100.0	—	—	
			3/18/57	7,800	4.0	23.0	8.0	7.0	51.0	7.0	0	0	101.4	—	—	
FJH-451 Holstein-Friesian	3	S. aureus (gangrene)	5/20/58	5,600	0	1.0	7.0	33.0	50.0	0	9.0	0	103.0	80	32	Two quarters gangrenous; responded to antibiotics and mammectomy.
			5/21/58 a.m.	8,250	10.0	17.5	4.5	13.0	40.0	7.0	8.0	0	101.5	100	28	
			5/21/58 p.m.	10,700	5.5	31.5	8.5	14.0	34.0	6.0	0.5	0	—	—	—	
			5/22/58	9,000	3.5	5.5	23.0	24.5	36.0	3.5	4.0	0	100.2	70	28	
			6/ 6/58	5,100	0	0	0	20.0	67.0	10.0	3.0	0	101.3	70	28	
UCVA	6	S. aureus (gangrene)	10/ 2/57	4,000	22.5	22.0	15.0	2.0	28.5	10.0	0	0	100.0	180	80	Severe gangrenous mastitis. Cow died in 24 hours.

of the mastitis and degree of initial neutropenia. Thus the shift is generally more extreme in gangrenous mastitis than in nongangrenous acute mastitis. In peracute coliform mastitis, though, the initial neutropenia and subsequent left shift are both of marked degree (see UCD-65, Table 36–17). With the appearance of the shift to the left, the total leukocyte count increases, although it seldom exceeds the maximum normal.

This blood picture gives the impression of a degenerative left shift, but such a leukocytic pattern in acute bovine mastitis does not necessarily indicate a grave prognosis. The differential leukocyte count returns to normal in a few days or a week as the generalized clinical signs subside. In animals that recover more slowly, the shift to the left persists for a longer period.

Initial plasma fibrinogen levels in acute mastitis are commonly in the range of 0.5–0.8 g/dl. In subsequent days, if the inflammatory process does not subside, plasma fibrinogen may increase to levels of 1.0–1.2 g/dl. Part of the increase may be relative, due to advancing dehydration, but the greater portion is representative of an absolute increase in fibrinogen.

A hemolytic anemia due to direct action of staphylococcal toxins on erythrocytes has been observed infrequently in gangrenous mastitis.

EXPERIMENTAL COLIFORM MASTITIS

The normal lactating mammary gland is an ideal organ in which to investigate the complex events of the developing inflammatory reaction and to correlate changes occurring in the total and differential distribution of leukocytes in peripheral blood (Schalm et al., 1964, 1971).

Acute coliform mastitis is in reality an endotoxemia. Upon death of coliform bacteria within the mammary gland, endotoxin is released and, if enough is released, signs of toxemia make their appearance—fever, increased heart rate, leukopenia, muscular tremors, depression, anorexia, and local tissue swelling due to edema.

The elapsed time between introduction of viable *E. aerogenes* or *E. coli* into the cistern of

the gland, via the teat orifice, and the appearance of signs of mastitis are conditioned by the number of organisms introduced. A single injection of approximately 100 organisms into normal lactating quarters caused an acute mastitis in 12 hours, while a dose of 1 million organisms produced a peracute mastitis within 4–6 hours. A preexisting infiltration of neutrophils into the milk at levels as low as 300,000–500,000 cells/ml of foremilk led to immediate destruction of *E. aerogenes* when introduced in small numbers and significantly modified the reaction to exposures of 1 million or more viable organisms. Thus a preexisting leukocytosis in the milk, even of low order, was found to be highly protective against multiplication of coliform organisms within such glands.

The interaction between *E. aerogenes* introduced into a normal lactating mammary quarter and the infiltrating leukocytes is graphically portrayed in Fig. 36–2. After a morning milking, 500,000 *E. aerogenes* were introduced into the gland cistern of one mammary quarter via the teat orifice. After brief massage of the gland to distribute the inoculum throughout the residual milk, a few ml of milk was removed to establish the initial bacterial population and cell count (Fig. 36–2 at the 0 hour). At hourly intervals, 10 ml of milk was withdrawn for additional bacteria and cell counts, and rectal temperatures were recorded. During the first 5 hours, *E. aerogenes* increased from 4,300 to 94,500/ml of milk. Infiltration of neutrophils first became apparent at the fifth hour, when the cell count was recorded at 1 million/ml. However, centrifugation of the milk and preparation of stained films of the sediment revealed neutrophils in small number by the third hour, along with evidence of phagocytosis of *E. aerogenes* (Fig. 36–3). The neutrophil count in milk increased rapidly after the fifth hour, and at the same time further multiplication of *E. aerogenes* was brought under control, as shown by the precipitous decline in numbers of viable bacteria. Clinical signs of acute mastitis made their appearance at the time of massive destruction of the bacterial population. At the sixth hour, body temperature started its rapid ascent; other signs of systemic effect were increased heart rate (84/minute), marked depression,

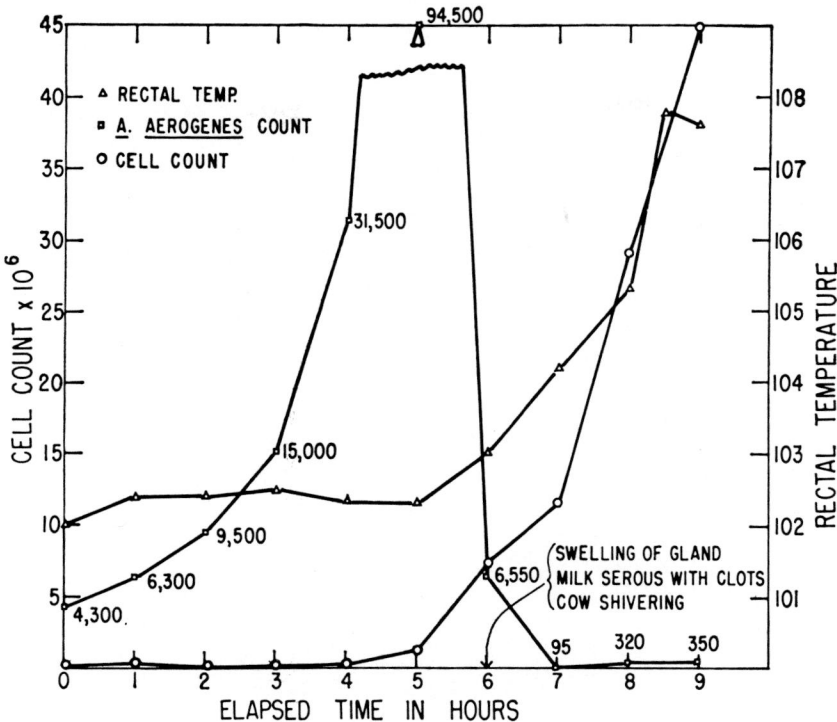

Fig. 36–2. Demonstration of sequential events in the interaction between *Enterobacter aerogenes,* introduced at a level of 500,000 organisms into a normal lactating mammary quarter, and infiltrating neutrophils attracted into the gland by the developing bacterial population. (From Schalm et al., 1964; courtesy of the *American Journal of Veterinary Research.*)

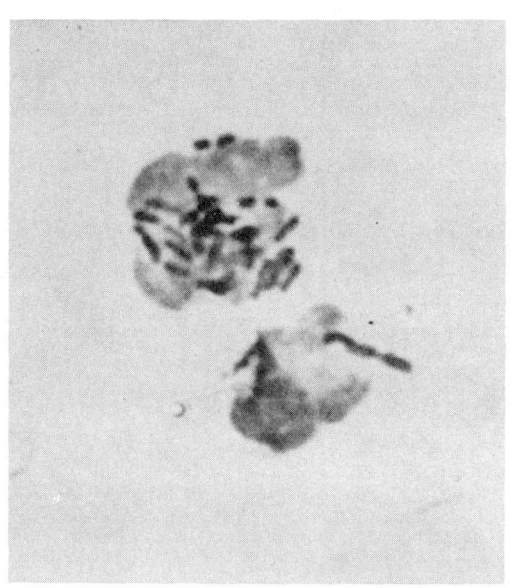

Fig. 36–3. Phagocytosis of *E. aerogenes* by infiltrating neutrophils at the third hour after the introduction of 500,000 organisms into a normal lactating mammary gland.

and violent muscular tremors. Local signs at the sixth hour were beginning of swelling of the gland and a change in gross appearance of the secretion from milk-like to a watery fluid containing visible particles. The crisis was reached at about the eighth hour, when body temperature was 107.8°F and heart rate, 116/minute; there were continuing muscular tremors and drooling, and the gland was firm and warm. By the ninth hour, considerable improvement was noted. The cow was more alert, and the quarter had started to soften. At this time the cow was milked, and the volume obtained was 85% of the normal production. At the next milking, 12 hours later, the volume of milk obtained was 50% of normal, and all signs of systemic reaction had disappeared. The rapid disappearance of systemic signs of toxemia indicated effective control on further unlimited multiplication of *E. aerogenes* within the udder.

The cell count in foremilk reached a peak of over 100 million/ml at the second milking after inoculation and then declined rapidly.

Table 36–18. Sequential Leukograms before and after Introduction of 2.3 Million *Enterobacter aerogenes* into Three Lactating Quarters of Third Lactation Cow 2414

| Elapsed Time | Temp. (°F) | WBC/μl of Blood | Neutrophils | | | | Lympho-cytes | Mono-cytes | Eosino-phils | Baso-phils | Unclassi-fied | Direct Eosinophil count |
			Myelo-cyte	Meta-myelocyte	Band	Mature						
−18 hr	—	9,600	0	0	0	4,320	3,360	816	1,008	96	0	—
0 hr	101.5	6,600	0	0	0	2,673	2,904	561	363	99	0	311
+ 3 hr	101.8	6,100	0	0	0	2,257	2,562	854	427	0	0	422
+ 6 hr	106.4	2,900	0	0	58	580	2,059	0	203	0	0	244
+10 hr	105.2	1,850	0	0	55	777	999	0	18	0	0	83
+24 hr	106.0	2,650	0	26	291	424	1,802	79	26	0	0	11
+31 hr	106.2	2,200	22	66	110	198	1,584	154	22	0	44	6
+48 hr	101.4	4,300	215	387	774	387	2,064	129	301	0	43	189
+72 hr	100.8	8,100	81	202	688	3,280	2,065	1,134	567	81	0	266
+96 hr	101.4	8,200	0	82	492	3,280	2,706	1,312	328	0	0	178
+ 6 days	101.6	7,650	0	114	229	3,480	2,830	765	153	76	0	189
+ 9 days	—	8,750	0	0	0	4,812	2,975	612	262	87	0	188

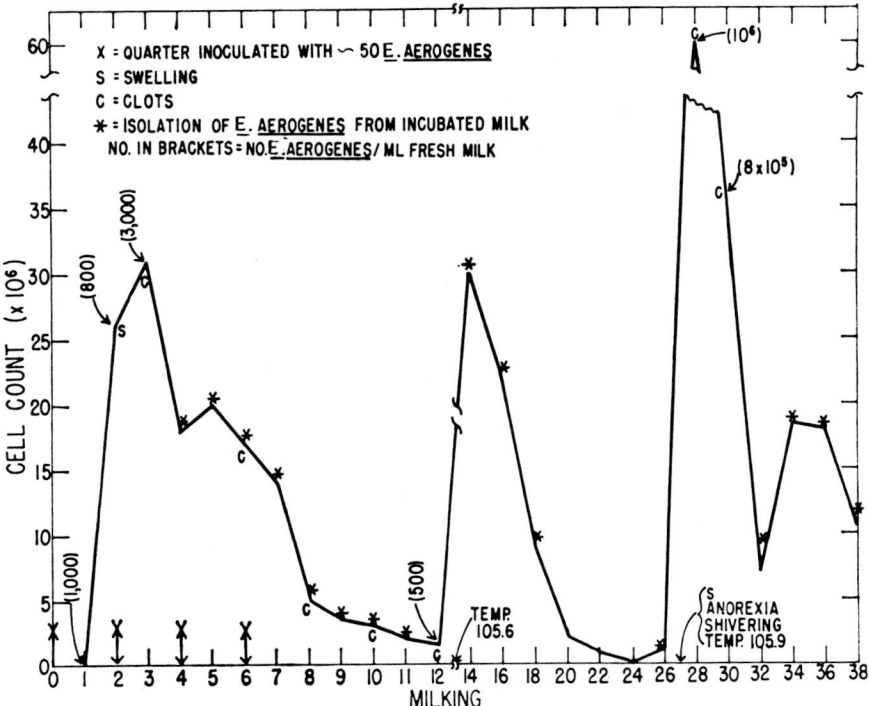

Fig. 36–4.   A demonstration of the interrelationship between *Enterobacter aerogenes* numbers, cell numbers, and the development of repeated acute episodes of inflammation in a lactating mammary quarter exposed to four daily injections of approximately 50 viable organisms per dose. (From Schalm et al., 1964; courtesy of the *American Journal of Veterinary Research.*)

At 1 week after inoculation, the cell count in foremilk was less than 100,000/ml. The continuing presence of *E. aerogenes* in small numbers could be demonstrated only by incubation of the milk prior to culturing on blood agar. The rapid decline in leukocyte numbers in milk before complete destruction of all *E. aerogenes* permitted a recidivation of acute coliform mastitis on the ninth day after inoculation, with temperature increase to 103°F and exudation of neutrophils into the milk to levels of 89 million/ml. Five days after the recidivation, the cell count in milk had declined to less than 100,000/ml and *E. aerogenes* had disappeared from the gland. Repeated episodes of acute inflammatory responses may occur when coliform organisms persist in a lactating gland in the presence of a too rapid decline in numbers of infiltrating leukocytes (Fig. 36–4).

The massive infiltration of neutrophils into the mammary gland in acute mastitis places significant drain on the neutrophils in peripheral blood and bone marrow. In coliform mastitis, endotoxin per se may have a leu-

kopenic effect by causing agglutination and sequestration of leukocytes within capillary beds. Furthermore, the corticosteroids of stress intensify the initial leukopenia by producing both lymphopenia and eosinopenia. The changes in total and differential leukocyte counts during development of and recovery from experimental coliform mastitis are shown in Table 36–18. It is of special interest that the entire leukocytic response in peripheral blood did not exceed the maximum normal range for total leukocyte numbers in the cow. However, with depletion of mature neutrophils, a significant left shift developed that reached its peak at the 48th hour. With return of body temperature to normal, the total and differential leukocyte counts also rapidly returned to normal levels.

For additional information on granulokinetics in coliform mastitis and endotoxemia see comments in Chapters 7, 26, and 31.

REFERENCES

Anagnostou, A., et al.: Hematologic Consequences of Renal Failure. *In* The Kidney. Vol. 2, 2nd ed. Brenner,

B.M., and Rector, F.C., eds. W.B. Saunders, Philadelphia, 1981.

Anderson, R.K., et al.: Utero-Ovarian Disorders Associated with Use of Medroxyprogesterone in Dogs. J. Amer. Vet. Med. Ass., *146*:1311, 1965.

Åsheim, Å.: Comparative Pathophysiological Aspects of the Glomerulonephritis Associated with Pyometra in Dogs. Acta Vet. Scand., *5*:188, 1964.

August, J.R.: Feline Infectious Peritonitis: An Immune-Mediated Coronavirus Vasculitis. Vet. Clin. North Amer. (Small Anim. Pract.), *14*:971, 1984.

Baker, H.J.: Laboratory Evaluation of Thyroid Function. *In* Current Veterinary Therapy. Vol. 4. Small Animal Practice. Kirk, R.W., ed. W.B. Saunders, Philadelphia, p. 595, 1971.

Belshaw, B.E.: Thyroid Diseases. *In* Textbook of Veterinary Internal Medicine. Vol.2. 2nd ed. Ettinger, S.J., ed. W.B. Saunders, Philadelphia, ch. 67, p. 1592, 1983.

Bentinck-Smith, J.: Feline Panleukopenia (Feline Infectious Enteritis): A Review of 574 Cases. N. Amer. Vet., *30*:379, 1949.

Børresen, B., and Skrede, S.: Pyometra in the Dog: A Pathophysiological Investigation. V. The Presence of Intrahepatic Cholestasis and an "Acute Phase Reaction." Nord. Vet. Med., *32*:378, 1980.

Brewer, B.D., et al.: Ehrlichiosis in a Florida Horse. J. Amer. Vet. Med. Ass., *185*:446, 1984.

Brodey, R.S., and Fidler, I.J.: Clinical and Pathologic Findings in Bitches Treated with Progestational Compounds. J. Amer. Vet. Med. Ass., *149*:1406, 1966.

Buhles, W.C., Jr., et al.: Tropical Canine Pancytopenia: Clinical, Hematologic, and Serologic Response of Dogs to Ehrlichia canis Infection, Tetracycline Therapy, and Challenge Inoculation. J. Infect. Dis., *130*:357, 1974.

Buhles, W.C., Jr., et al.: Tropical Canine Pancytopenia: Role of Aplastic Anemia in the Pathogenesis of Severe Disease. J. Comp. Pathol., *85*:511, 1975.

Burghen, G.A., et al.: Development of Hypergammaglobulinemia in Tropical Canine Pancytopenia. Amer. J. Vet. Res., *32*:749, 1971.

Capen, C.C., et al.: Neoplasm in the Adenohypophysis of Dogs. Path. Vet., *4*:301, 1967.

Carlson, J.H., et al.: Feline Panleukopenia. I. Pathogenesis in Germfree and Specific Pathogen–Free Cats. Vet. Pathol., *14*:79, 1977.

Carpenter, J.L.: Feline Panleukopenia: Clinical Signs and Differential Diagnosis. J. Amer. Vet. Med. Ass., *158*:857, 1971.

Cello, R.M., et al.: The Occurrence of Inclusion Bodies in the Circulating Neutrophils of Dogs with Canine Distemper. Cornell Vet., *49*:127, 1959.

Chaiyabutr, N.: Changes of Renal Functions in Experimental Hyperthyroid and Hypothyroid Dogs. Acta Vet. (Beograd), *31*:251, 1981.

Chastain, C.B.: Canine Hypothyroidism. J. Amer. Vet. Med. Ass., *181*:349, 1982.

Clark, S.T., and Meier, H.: A Clinico-Pathological Study of Thyroid Disease in the Dog and Cat. I. Thyroid Pathology. Zentralbl. Veterinärmed., *5*:17, 1958.

Cline, M.J., and Berlin, N.I.: Erythropoiesis and Red Cell Survival in the Hypothyroid Dog. Amer. J. Physiol., *204*:415, 1963.

Codner, E.C., et al.: Atypical Findings in 16 Cases of Canine Ehrlichiosis. J. Amer. Vet. Med. Ass., *186*:166, 1985.

Coffin, D.L.: The Rapid Diagnosis of Contagious Canine Hepatitis from Autopsy Material. J. Amer. Vet. Med. Ass., *120*:287, 1952.

Coffin, D.L., and Cabasso, V.J.: The Blood and Urine Findings in Infectious Canine Hepatitis. Amer. J. Vet. Res., *14*:245, 1953.

Cole, E.J., and Easterbrooks, H.L.: Leukopenia Associated with Acute Bovine Mastitis. J. Amer. Vet. Med. Ass., *133*:163, 1958.

Coles, J.D.W.A.: Classification of Rickettsiae Pathogenic to Vertebrates. Ann. N.Y. Acad. Sci., *56*(art. 3):457, 1953.

Cowgill, L.D.: Diseases of the Kidney. *In* Textbook of Veterinary Internal Medicine. Vol. 2., 2nd ed. Ettinger, S.J., ed. W.B. Saunders, Philadelphia, ch. 74, p. 1793, 1983.

Davis, L.E.: *o,p'*-DDD (Mitotane) Treatment of Canine Pituitary-Dependent Hyperadrenocorticism. J. Amer. Vet. Med. Ass., *182*:527, 1983.

DiBartola, S.P.: Canine Hyperadrenocorticism: A Brief Review. Calif. Vet., *33*:13, 1979.

Disque, D.F., et al.: Feline Infectious Peritonitis. J. Amer. Vet. Med. Ass., *152*:372, 1968.

Dorner, J.L., et al.: Corticosteroid Induction of an Isozyme of Alkaline Phosphatase in the Dog. Amer. J. Vet. Res., *35*:1457, 1974.

Eiler, H., and Oliver, J.: Combined Dexamethasone Suppression and Cosyntropin (Synthetic ACTH) Stimulation Test in the Dog: New Approach to Testing of Adrenal Gland Function. Amer. J. Vet. Res., *41*:1243, 1980.

Evinger, J.V., and Nelson, R.W.: The Clinical Pharmacology of Thyroid Hormones in the Dog. J. Amer. Vet. Med. Ass., *185*:314, 1984.

Ewing, S.A.: Observations on Leukocytic Inclusion Bodies from Dogs Infected with Babesia canis. J. Amer. Vet. Med. Ass., *143*:503, 1963.

Ewing, S.A.: Canine Ehrlichiosis. Adv. Vet. Sci. Comp. Med., *13*:331, 1969.

Ewing, S.A., and Buckner, R.G.: Manifestations of Babesiosis, Ehrlichiosis, and Combined Infections in the Dog. Amer. J. Vet. Res., *26*:815, 1965.

Ewing, S.A., et al.: A New Strain of Ehrlichia canis. J. Amer. Vet. Med. Ass., *159*:1771, 1971.

Farrow, B.R.H., and Love, D.N.: Bacterial, Viral, and Other Infectious Problems. *In* Textbook of Veterinary Internal Medicine. Vol. 1. 2nd ed. Ettinger, S.J., ed. W.B. Saunders, Philadelphia, ch. 27, p. 269, 1983.

Feldman, E.C.: The Adrenal Cortex. *In* Textbook of Veterinary Internal Medicine. Vol. 2. 2nd ed. Ettinger, S.J., ed. W.B. Saunders, Philadelphia, ch. 69, p. 1650, 1983.

Feldman, E.C.: Evaluation of a Combined Dexamethasone Suppression/ACTH Stimulation Test in Dogs with Hyperadrenocorticism. J. Amer. Vet. Med. Ass., *187*:49, 1985a.

Feldman, E.C.: Personal communication, 1985b.

Feldman, E.C., and Peterson, M.E.: Hypoadrenocorticism. Vet. Clin. North Amer. (Small Anim. Pract.), *14*:751, 1984.

Feldman, E.C., and Tyrrell, J.B.: Hypoadrenocorticism. Vet. Clin. North Amer. (Small Anim. Pract.), *1*:555, 1977.

Ferguson, D.C.: Thyroid Function Tests in the Dog: Recent Concepts. Vet. Clin. North Amer. (Small Anim. Pract.), *14*:783, 1984.

Finco, D.R., et al.: Familial Renal Disease in Norwegian Elkhound Dogs. J. Amer. Vet. Med. Ass., *156*:747, 1970.

Flint, J.C.: Canine Distemper-Hepatitis Complex. J. Amer. Vet. Med. Ass., *122*:110, 1953.

Foggie, A.: Studies on the Infectious Agent of Tick-Borne Fever in Sheep. J. Pathol. Bacteriol., *63*:1, 1951.

Foster, W.N.M., and Cameron, A.E.: Thrombocytopenia in Sheep Associated with Experimental Tick-Borne Fever Infection. J. Comp. Pathol., *78*:251, 1968.

French, T.W., and Harvey, J.W.: Serologic Diagnosis of Infectious Cyclic Thrombocytopenia in Dogs Using an Indirect Fluorescent Antibody Test. Amer. J. Vet. Res., *44*:2407, 1983.

Gibson, J.P., et al.: Experimental Distemper in the Gnotobiotic Dog. Path. Vet., *2*:1, 1965.

Gleiser, C.A., et al.: Visceral Leishmaniasis in a Dog Imported into the United States. Amer. J. Trop. Med. Hyg., *6*:227, 1957.

Goss, L.W., et al.: Inclusion Bodies, with Special Application to Clinical Diagnosis of Canine Distemper. J. Amer. Vet. Med. Ass., *112*:236, 1948.

Gribble, D.H.: Equine Ehrlichiosis. J. Amer. Vet. Med. Ass., *155*:462, 1969.

Hardy, W.D., Jr., and Hurvitz, A.I.: Feline Infectious Peritonitis: Experimental Studies. J. Amer. Vet. Med. Ass., *158*:994, 1971.

Hardy, W.D., Jr., and O'Reilly, W.J.: Clinicopathologic Conference: Feline Infectious Peritonitis and Pleuritis. J. Amer. Vet. Med. Ass., *155*:1728, 1969.

Harvey, J.W., et al.: Cyclic Thrombocytopenia Induced by a Rickettsia-like Agent in Dogs. J. Infect. Dis., *137*:182, 1978.

Harvey, J.W., et al.: Ehrlichiosis in Wolves, Dogs, and Wolf-Dog Crosses. J. Amer. Vet. Med. Ass., *175*:901, 1979.

Heald, R.D.: Ehrlichia-Associated Coombs-Positive Anemia in a Dog. Canine Pract., *11*(2):34, 1984.

Held, J.P., and Oliver, J.W.: A Sampling Protocol for the Thyrotropin Stimulation Test in the Horse. J. Amer. Vet. Med. Ass., *184*:326, 1984.

Hill, F.W.G.: Adrenocortical Insufficiency in the Dog. Vet. Annual, *19*:223, 1979.

Hillman, D., et al.: Hypothyroidism and Anemia Related to Fluoride in Dairy Cattle. J. Dairy Sci., *62*:416, 1979.

Hodgman, S.F.J., and Larin, N.M.: Diagnosis of Canine Virus Hepatitis (Rubarth's Disease). Vet. Rec., *65*:447, 1953.

Hoenig, M., and Ferguson, D.C.: Assessment of Thyroid Functional Reserve in the Cat by the Thyrotropin-Stimulation Test. Amer. J. Vet. Res., *44*:1229, 1983.

Holland, C.J., et al.: Isolation, Experimental Transmission, and Characterization of Causative Agent of Potomac Horse Fever. Science, *227*:522, 1985.

Hollander, C.S., et al.: Repair of the Anemia and Hyperlipidemia of the Hypothyroid Dog. Endocrinology, *81*:1007, 1967.

Holman, H.H.: The Blood Picture of the Cow. Brit. Vet. J., *111*:440, 1955.

Holman, R.L.: Renal Injury and Lymphatic Atrophy: Lymphopenia and Atrophy of Lymphatic Tissue Associated with Acute Renal Insufficiency in Dogs. Arch. Pathol., *37*:124, 1944.

Holzworth, J., et al.: Hyperthyroidism in the Cat: Ten Cases. J. Amer. Vet. Med. Ass., *176*:345, 1980.

Horzinek, M.C., and Osterhaus, A.D.M.E.: The Virology and Pathogenesis of Feline Infectious Peritonitis. Arch. Virol., *59*:1, 1979.

Hoskins, J.D., et al.: Serum Hyperviscosity Syndrome Associated with *Ehrlichia canis* Infection in a Dog. J. Amer. Vet. Med. Ass., *183*:1011, 1983.

Hughes, J.P., et al.: Pyometra in the Mare. J. Reprod. Fertil. (Suppl.), *27*:321, 1979.

Huxsoll, D.L.: Canine Ehrlichiosis (Tropical Canine Pancytopenia): A Review. Vet. Parasitol., *2*:49, 1976.

Huxsoll, D.L., et al.: Tropical Canine Pancytopenia.. J. Amer. Vet. Med. Ass., *157*:1627, 1970.

Huxsoll, D.L., et al.: Laboratory Studies of Tropical Canine Pancytopenia. Exp. Parasitol., *31*:53, 1972.

Ichijo, S., et al.: Clinical and Hematological Findings and Myelograms in Feline Panleukopenia. Jpn. J. Vet. Sci., *38*:197, 1976.

Jacobse-Geels, H., et al.: Antibody, Immune Complexes, and Complement Activity Fluctuations in Kittens with Experimentally Induced Feline Infectious Peritonitis. Amer. J. Vet. Res., *43*:666, 1982.

Jain, N.C., and Switzer, J.W.: Autoimmune Thrombocytopenia in Dogs and Cats. Vet. Clin. North Amer. (Small Anim. Pract.), *11*:421, 1981.

Johnessee, J.S., et al.: Primary Hypoadrenocorticism in a Cat. J. Amer. Vet. Med. Ass., *183*:881, 1983.

Kahn, D.E.: Pathogenesis of Feline Panleukopenia. J. Amer. Vet. Med. Ass., *173*:628, 1978.

Kaneko, J.J.: Thyroid Function. *In* Clinical Biochemistry of Domestic Animals. 3rd ed. Kaneko, J.J., ed. Academic Press, New York, ch. 12, p. 491, 1980a.

Kaneko, J.J.: Clinical Biochemistry of Domestic Animals. Academic Press, New York, pp. 792–797, 1980b.

Keefe, T.J., et al.: Distribution of Ehrlichia canis among Military Working Dogs in the World and Selected Civilian Dogs in the United States. J. Amer. Vet. Med. Ass., *181*:236, 1982.

Keeton, K.S., et al.: Adrenocortical Insufficiency in the Dog. Calif. Vet., *26*(6):12, 1972.

Kelly, D.F.: Aspects of Canine Renal Pathology. J. Small Anim. Pract. *8*:329, 1967.

Klopfer, U.: A Quick Method for Demonstrating Inclusion Bodies of Infectious Canine Hepatitis in Liver Smears. Vet. Med. Small Anim. Clin., *64*:158, 1969.

Krakowka, S., et al.: Experimental and Naturally Occurring Transplacental Transmission of Canine Distemper Virus. Amer. J. Vet. Res., *38*:919, 1977.

Krakowka, S., et al.: Canine Distemper Virus: Review of Structural and Functional Modulations in Lymphoid Tissues. Amer. J. Vet. Res., *41*:284, 1980.

Kudo, R.R.: Protozoology. 5th ed. Charles C Thomas, Springfield, 1966.

Kuehn, N.F., and Gaunt, S.D.: Clinical and Hematologic Findings in Canine Ehrlichiosis. J. Amer. Vet. Med. Ass., *186*:355, 1985.

Langheinrich, K.A., and Nielsen, S.W.: Histopathology of Feline Panleukopenia: A Report of 65 Cases. J. Amer. Vet. Med. Ass., *158*:863, 1971.

Lauder, I.M., et al.: A Survey of Canine Distemper. Vet. Rec., *66*:623, 1954.

Lawrence, J.S., et al.: Infectious Feline Agranulocytosis. Amer. J. Pathol., *16*:333, 1940.

Lester, S.J., et al.: A Rapid Radioimmunoassay Method for the Evaluation of Plasma Cortisol Levels and Adrenal Function in the Dog. J. Amer. Anim. Hosp. Ass., *17*:121, 1981.

Levine, N.D.: Protozoan Parasites of Domestic Animals and Man. Burgess Publ. Co., Minneapolis, 1961.

Lewis, G.E., Jr., et al.: Experimentally Induced Infection of Dogs, Cats, and Nonhuman Primates with Ehrlichia equi, Etiologic Agent of Equine Ehrlichiosis. Amer. J. Vet. Res., *36*:85, 1975.

Liddle, G.W.: Tests of Pituitary-Adrenal Suppressibility in the Diagnosis of Cushing's Syndrome. J. Clin. Endocrinol., *20*:1539, 1960.

Lindblad, G., and Bäckgren, A.W.: Megakaryocytes, Thrombocytes, and Blood-Clotting Time in Dogs with Experimental Contagiosa Canis. Acta Vet. Scand., *5*:370, 1964.

Ling, G.V., et al.: Canine Hyperadrenocorticism: Pretreatment Clinical and Laboratory Evaluation of 117 Cases. J. Amer. Vet. Med. Ass., *174*:1211, 1979.

Longstaffe, J.A., and Guy, M.W.: Leishmaniasis in Dogs. Vet. Annual., *25*:358, 1985.

Lothrop, C.D., Jr., et al.: Canine and Feline Thyroid Function Assessment with Thyrotropin Releasing Hormone Response Test. Amer. J. Vet. Res., *45*:2310, 1984.

Lovering, S.L., et al.: Serum Complement and Blood Platelet Adhesiveness in Acute Canine Ehrlichiosis. Amer. J. Vet. Res., *41*:1266, 1980.

Madewell, B.R., and Gribble, D.H.: Infection in Two Dogs with an Agent Resembling Ehrlichia equi. J. Amer. Vet. Med. Ass., *180*:512, 1982.

Malherbe, W.D.: The Diagnosis and Treatment of Rickettsiosis in Dogs. J.S. Afr. Vet. Med. Ass., *19*:135, 1948.

Marshak, R.R., et al.: Observations on a Case of Primary Adrenocortical Insufficiency in a Dog. J. Amer. Vet. Med. Ass., *136*:274, 1960.

Martin, S.L., et al.: Laboratory Evaluation of Adrenocortical Function in Dogs. *In* Current Veterinary Therapy. Vol. 4. Small Animal Practice. Kirk, R.W., ed. W.B. Saunders, Philadelphia, p. 589, 1971.

McMillan, F.D., and Sherding, R.G.: Feline Hyperthyroidism. Feline Pract., *11*(5): 25, 1981.

McSherry, B.J., and Smith, D.L.T.: Hematological Changes Noted in Three Dogs Experimentally Infected with the Virus of Infectious Canine Hapatitis. Cornell Vet., *43*:104, 1953.

Meyer, K.F., et al.: Canine Leptospirosis in the United States. J. Amer. Vet. Med. Ass., *95*:710, 1939.

Monlux, A.W.: The Histopathology of Nephritis of the Dog. I. Introduction. II. Inflammatory Interstitial Diseases. Amer. J. Vet. Res., *14*:425, 1953.

Monlux, W.S.: Leptospirosis. III. The Clinical Pathology of Canine Leptospirosis. Cornell Vet., *38*:109, 1948.

Moore, J.N., et al.: A Case of Pituitary Adrenocorticotropin-Dependent Cushing's Syndrome in the Horse. Endocrinology, *104*:576, 1979.

Morales, G.A., and Nielsen, S.W.: Canine Adrenocortical Atrophy: Review of Literature and a Report of Two Cases. J. Small Anim. Pract., *11*:257, 1970.

Mulnix, J.A.: Hypoadrenocorticism in the Dog. Amer. Anim. Hosp. Ass. J., *7*:220, 1971.

Neitz, W.O., and Thomas, A.D.: Rickettsiosis in the Dog. J.S. Afr. Vet. Med. Ass., *9*:166, 1938.

Newberne, J.W., et al.: Studies on Clinical and Histopathological Aspects of Feline Panleukopenia (Infectious Enteritis). Southwestern Vet., *10*:111, 1957.

Obel, A.L., et al.: Light and Electron Microscopical Studies of the Renal Lesion in Dogs with Pyometra. Acta Vet. Scand., *5*:146, 1964.

Osbaldiston, G.W., and Greve, T.: Estimating Adrenal Cortical Functions in Dogs with ACTH. Cornell Vet., *68*:308, 1978.

Osborne, C.A.: Urologic Logic-Diagnosis of Renal Disease. J. Amer. Vet. Med. Ass., *157*:1656, 1970.

Osborne, C.A., et al.: Reversible versus Irreversible Renal Disease in the Dog. J. Amer. Vet. Med. Ass., *155*:2062, 1969a.

Osborne, C.A., et al.: Amyloid Nephrotic Syndrome in the Dog. J. Amer. Vet. Med. Ass., *154*:1545, 1969b.

Osborne, C.A., et al.: Pathophysiology of Renal Disease,

Renal Failure, and Uremia. *In* Textbook of Veterinary Internal Medicine. Vol. 2. 2nd ed. Ettinger, S.J., ed. W.B. Saunders, Philadelphia, ch. 73, p. 1733, 1983.

Pattison, I.H., et al.: Studies on Experimental Streptococcal Mastitis. I. Inoculation of Large Numbers of Streptococcus agalactiae into the Teat Canal of Goats. J. Comp. Pathol., *60*:71, 1950.

Pay, T.W.F.: Infectious Canine Hepatitis (Hepatitis Contagiosa Canis, Rubarth). Vet. Rec., *62*:551, 1950.

Pedersen, N.C.: Feline Infectious Peritonitis and Feline Enteric Coronavirus Infections. Part 2. Feline Infectious Peritonitis. Feline Pract., *13*(5):5, 1983.

Pedersen, N.C.: Pathogenic Difference between Various Feline Coronavirus Isolates. Adv. Exp. Med. Biol., *173*:365, 1984.

Pedersen, N.C., and Boyle, J.F.: Immunologic Phenomena in the Effusive Form of Feline Infectious Peritonitis. Amer. J. Vet. Res., *41*:868, 1980.

Pedersen, N.C., et al.: An Enteric Coronavirus Infection of Cats and Its Relationship to Feline Infectious Peritonitis. Amer. J. Vet. Res., *42*:368, 1981.

Persson, F., et al.: Renal Cortical Hypoplasia in Dogs: A Clinical Study of Uraemia and Secondary Hyperthyroidism. Acta Vet. Scand., *2*:68, 1961.

Peterson, M.E.: Hyperadrenocorticism. Vet. Clin. North Amer. (Small Anim. Pract.), *14*:731, 1984.

Peterson, M.E., et al.: Adrenal Function in the Cat: Comparison of the Effects of Cosyntropin (Synthetic ACTH) and Corticotropin Gel Stimulation. Res. Vet. Sci., *37*:331, 1984.

Philip, C.B.: Nomenclature of Rickettsiaceae Pathogenic to Vertebrates. Ann. N.Y. Acad. Sci., *56*(art. 3):484, 1953.

Pierce, K.R., et al.: Acute Canine Ehrlichiosis: Platelet Survival and Factor 3 Assay. Amer. J. Vet. Res., *38*:1821, 1977.

Poppensiek, G.C.: Virus Diseases of Dogs: With Special Reference to Infectious Hepatitis. Vet. Med., *47*:282, 1952.

Poppensiek, G.C., and Baker, J.A.: Persistence of Virus in Urine as a Factor in Spread of Infectious Hepatitis in Dogs. Proc. Soc. Exp. Biol. Med., *77*:279, 1951.

Pyle, R.L.: Canine Ehrlichiosis. J. Amer. Vet. Med. Ass., *177*:1197, 1980.

Rakich, P.M., and Lorenz, M.D.: Clinical Signs and Laboratory Abnormalities in 23 Dogs with Spontaneous Hypoadrenocorticism. J. Amer. Anim. Hosp. Ass., *20*:647, 1984.

Reardon, M.J., and Pierce, K.R.: Acute Experimental Canine Ehrlichiosis. I. Sequential Reaction of the Hemic and Lymphoreticular System. Vet. Pathol., *18*:48, 1981a.

Reardon, M.J., and Pierce, K.R.: Acute Experimental Canine Ehrlichiosis. II. Sequential Reaction of the Hemic and Lymphoproliferative System of Selectively Immunosuppressed Dogs. Vet. Pathol., *18*:384, 1981b.

Reiter, I., et al.: (Leishmania Infection in the Dog: Course of Infection, Diagnosis and Experimental Treatment of Beagles Experimentally Infected with L. donovani [Calcutta Strain].) Berl. Munch. Tierärztl. Wochenschr., *98*:40, 1985.

Remuzzi, G., et al.: Bleeding in Renal Failure: A Possible Role of Vascular Protacycline (PG12). Clin. Nephrol., *12*:127, 1979.

Renton, J.P., et al.: Pyometra in the Bitch. J. Small Anim. Pract., *12*:249, 1971.

Rijnberk, A., et al.: Spontaneous Hyperadrenocorticism in the Dog. J. Endocrinol., *41*:397, 1968.

Riser, W.H.: The Behavior of the Peripheral Blood Elements in Panleukopenia (Agranulocytosis) of the Domestic Cat. Amer. J. Vet. Res., 8:82, 1947.

Ristic, M., et al.: Serological Diagnosis of Tropical Canine Pancytopenia by Indirect Immunofluorescence. Infect. Immun., 6:226, 1972.

Robison, R.L., et al.: Naturally Occurring Feline Infectious Peritonitis: Signs and Clinical Diagnosis. J. Amer. Vet. Med. Ass., 158:981, 1971.

Rogers, W.A., and Ruebner, B.H.: A Retrospective Study of Probable Glucocorticoid-Induced Hepatopathy in Dogs. J. Amer. Vet. Med. Ass., 170:603, 1977.

Rogers, W., et al.: Atypical Hypoadrenocorticism in Three Dogs. J. Amer. Vet. Med. Ass., 179:155, 1981.

Rohovsky, M.W., and Fowler, E.H.: Lesions of Experimental Feline Panleukopenia. J. Amer. Vet. Med. Ass., 158:872, 1971.

Rosenman, R.H., et al.: The Mechanism Responsible for the Altered Blood Cholesterol Content in Deranged Thyroid States. J. Clin. Endocrinol., 12:1287, 1952.

Sandholm, M., et al.: Pathogenesis of Canine Pyometra. J. Amer. Vet. Med. Ass., 167:1006, 1975.

Schaer, M., and Chen, C.L.: A Clinical Survey of 48 Dogs with Adrenocortical Hypofunction. J. Amer. Anim. Hosp. Ass., 19:443, 1983.

Schalm, O.W.: Feline Infectious Peritonitis. Calif. Vet., 25:6, Oct., 1971.

Schalm, O.W.: Special Characteristics of Lymphocytes and Monocytes in Infectious Canine Hepatitis. Canine Pract. 6(1):51, 1979a.

Schalm, O.W.: Uncommon Hematologic Disorders: Spirochetosis, Trypanosomiasis, Leishmaniasis, Pelger-Huët Anomaly. Canine Pract., 6(6):46, 1979b.

Schalm, O.W., et al.: Pathogenesis of Experimental Coliform (Aerobacter aerogenes) Mastitis in Cattle. Amer. J. Vet. Res., 25:75, 1964.

Schalm, O.W., et al.: Experimentation in Mastitis. *In* Bovine Mastitis. Lea & Febiger, Philadelphia, ch. 12, 1971.

Siegel, E.T.: Determination of 17-Hydroxycorticosteroids in Canine Urine. Amer. J. Vet. Res., 26:1152, 1965.

Siegel, E.T.: Assessment of Pituitary-Adrenal Gland Function in the Dog. Amer. J. Vet. Res., 29:173, 1968a.

Siegel, E.T.: Hypoadrenocorticalism. *In* Current Veterinary Therapy. Vol. 3. Small Animal Practice. Kirk, W.R., ed. W.B. Saunders, Philadelphia, p. 553, 1968b.

Siegel, E.T.: Adrenal Insufficiency, p. 593. In Current Veterinary Therapy. IV. Small Animal Practice. R.W. Kirk (ed.) W.B. Saunders Co., Philadelphia, 1971.

Siegel, E.T., et al.: Cushing's Syndrome in the Dog. J. Amer. Vet. Med. Ass., 157:2081, 1970.

Simpson, C.F.: Structure of Ehrlichia canis in Blood Monocytes of a Dog. Amer. J. Vet. Res., 33:2451, 1972.

Smith, D.L.T.: Observations on Infectious Canine Hepatitis. Amer. J. Vet. Res., 12:38, 1951.

Stannard, A.A., et al.: Equine Ehrlichiosis: A Disease with Similarities to Tick-Borne Fever and Bovine Petechial Fever. Vet. Rec., 84:149, 1969.

Stogdale, L.: The Diagnosis and Treatment of Canine Hypothyroidism. J. S. Afr. Vet. Ass., 51:46, 1980.

Strombeck, D.R.: Small Animal Gastroenterology. Stonegate Publishing, Davis, Calif., 1979.

Tajima, M., et al.: Light and Electron Microscopic Studies of Lymph Node of Mink Exposed to Canine Distemper Virus. Amer. J. Vet. Res., 32:913, 1971.

Talanti, S.: Observation on Pyometra in Dogs, with Reference to the Hypothalamic-Hypophysial Neurosecretory System. Amer. J. Vet. Res., 20:41, 1959.

Taylor, P.L., et al.: Serologic, Pathologic, and Immunologic Features of Experimentally Induced Leptospiral Nephritis in Dogs. Amer. J. Vet. Res., 31:1033, 1970.

Theilen, G.H., et al.: Bovine Hematology. I. Leukocyte Response to Acute Bovine Mastitis. J. Amer. Vet. Med. Ass., 135:481, 1959.

Theran, P., and Ling, G.V.: Canine Visceral Leishmaniasis. J. Amer. Vet. Med. Ass., 150:82, 1967.

Thompson, S.W., et al.: Vacuoles in the Hepatocytes of Cortisone-Treated Dogs. Amer. J. Pathol., 63:135, 1971.

Thorn, G.W., et al.: A Test for Adrenal Cortical Insufficiency: The Response to Pituitary Adrenocorticotropic Hormone. J. Amer. Med. Ass., 137:1005, 1948.

Thorson, R.E., et al.: A Report of a Case of Imported Visceral Leishmaniasis of a Dog in the United States. Amer. J. Trop. Med. Hyg., 4:18, 1955.

Timoney, J.F., Jr.: Panleukopenia. Vet. Clin. North Amer. (Small Anim. Pract.), 6:385, 1976.

Van Heerden, J.V.: A Retrospective Study on 120 Natural Cases of Canine Ehrlichiosis. J. S. Afr. Vet. Ass., 53:17, 1982.

Walker, J.S., et al.: Clinical and Clinicopathologic Findings in Tropical Canine Pancytopenia. J. Amer. Vet. Med. Ass., 157:43, 1970.

Ward, B.C., and Pederson, N.: Infectious Peritonitis in Cats. J. Amer. Vet. Med. Ass., 154:26, 1969.

Ward, J.M., et al.: An Observation of Feline Infectious Peritonitis. Vet. Rec., 83:416, 1968.

Ward, J.M., et al.: Feline Infectious Peritonitis: Experimental Evidence for Its Multiphasic Nature. Amer. J. Vet. Res., 35:1271, 1974.

Watson, A.D.J., and Wright, R.G.: The Ultrastructure of Cytoplasmic Inclusions in Circulating Lymphocytes in Canine Distemper. Res. Vet. Sci., 17:188, 1974a.

Watson, A.D.J., and Wright, R.G.: The Ultrastructure of Inclusions in Blood Cells of Dogs with Distemper. J. Comp. Pathol., 84:417, 1974b.

Watson, E.A., and Plummer, P.J.G.: Distemper Inclusion Bodies. Amer. J. Vet. Res., 3:350, 1942.

Weisbrode, S.E., and Krakowka, S.: Canine Distemper Virus–Associated Hypocalcemia. Amer. J. Vet. Res., 40:147, 1979.

Weiss, R.C., and Scott, F.W.: Laboratory Diagnosis of Feline Infectious Peritonitis. Feline Pract., 10(2):16, 1980.

Weiss, R.C., and Scott, F.W.: Pathogenesis of Feline Infectious Peritonitis: Nature and Development of Viremia. Amer. J. Vet. Res., 42:383, 1981.

Weiss, R.C., et al.: Disseminated Intravascular Coagulation in Experimentally Induced Feline Infectious Peritonitis. Amer. J. Vet. Res., 41:663, 1980.

Werner, L.L.: Coombs-Positive Anemias in the Dog and Cat. Comp. Cont. Educ., 2:96, 1980.

Whitney, J.C.: "Pyometra" in the Bitch (with Special Reference to the Pathology of the Condition). Brit. Vet. J., 112:25, 1956.

Whitney, J.C.: Polydipsia and Its Relationship to Pyometra. J. Small Anim. Pract., 10:486, 1969.

Wigton, D.H.: Platelet Turnover, Function and Ultrastructure in Infectious Canine Hepatitis. Vet. Clin. Pathol., 7(2):16, 1978.

Wigton, D.H., et al.: Infectious Canine Hepatitis: Animal Model for Viral-Induced Disseminated Intravascular Coagulation. Blood, 47:287, 1976.

Wilkins, J.H., et al.: A New Canine Disease Syndrome. Vet. Rec., 81:57, 1967.

Wilkinson, G.T.: Feline Infectious Peritonitis. Vet. Annual, *19:*269, 1979.

Wilkinson, J.S.: Endocrine Disease. *In* Veterinary Clinical Pathology. Medway, W., et al., eds. Williams & Wilkins, Baltimore, p. 181, 1969.

Willard, M.D., et al.: Canine Hypoadrenocorticism: Report of 37 Cases and Review of 39 Previously Reported Cases. J. Amer. Vet. Med. Ass., *180:*59, 1982.

Willeberg, P., and Priester, W.A.: Epidemiological Aspects of Clinical Hyperadrenocorticism in Dogs (Canine Cushing's Syndrome). J. Amer. Anim. Hosp. Ass., *18:*717, 1982.

Wolfe, L.G., and Griesemer, R.A.: Feline Infectious Peritonitis. Path. Vet., *3:*255, 1966.

Wolfe, L.G., and Griesemer, R.A.: Feline Infectious Peritonitis: Review of Gross and Histopathologic Lesions. J. Amer. Vet. Med. Ass., *158:*987, 1971.

Wright, N.G., et al.: Chronic Renal Failure in Dogs: A Comparative Clinical and Morphologic Study of Chronic Glomerulonephritis and Chronic Interstitial Nephritis. Vet. Rec., *98:*288, 1976.

Zook, B.C., et al.: Ultrastructural Evidence for the Viral Etiology of Feline Infectious Peritonitis. Path. Vet., *5:*91, 1968.

Appendix

INTRODUCTION

The purpose of the Appendix is to demonstrate basic principles in the responses of the different domestic animals to disease as revealed in blood and bone marrow. The brief histories and summaries of clinical findings, complete hemograms, and suggestions for interpretation provide a means whereby typical situations can be discussed in greater depth than was possible in the general text. Throughout the various chapters, the reader is repeatedly referred to the Appendix for demonstration of the point under consideration.

For the most part, the title for each Appendix case suggests the principal feature to be demonstrated. As an example, Case 1 concerns a dog with a mastocytoma in which the initial hemogram was markedly lipemic. The case was selected not because the hemogram in mastocytoma is unique, but rather to explain the basis for the lipemia and accompanying hemolysis. The basic principle involved is applicable to all bloods regardless of primary nature of the disease. Specific names of diseases have been used as titles when changes in the blood are uniquely characteristic of the disease. Thus chronic interstitial nephritis, hypothyroidism, and Cushing's syndrome in the dog; infectious anemia and panleukopenia in the cat; and anaplasmosis and congenital porphyria in the cow are named specifically.

Emphasis is given to the anemic state in all animals. It is of prime importance to differentiate, for purposes of therapy and prognosis, the blood loss and hemolytic anemias from the secondary anemias resulting from depression of erythrogenesis in chronic diseases. The former commonly have a favorable prognosis, since treatment is often possible, while prognosis in the face of a progressive secondary anemia is generally unfavorable.

Attention is directed to a unique feature in equine hematology (Case 55): peripheral blood rarely displays the usual signs of anemia in remission (polychromasia and reticulocytosis) seen in the other domestic animals.

Responses in the leukogram characteristic of the species are demonstrated specifically. The changes in the differential leukocyte count in all animals in response to the corticoids of stress are neutrophilia, lymphopenia, and eosinopenia. In the dog, this triad is accompanied by monocytosis, often of marked degree. In the cow, the initial neutrophilia is often masked by a rapid draining of neutrophils from blood into the developing lesion (Case 66). A systemic toxemia commonly occurs in diseases affecting cats of all ages. A response typical of the species is depression of granulopoiesis with significant morphologic changes in cells of the neutrophil series. These changes lead to "toxic" signs in the cytoplasm, often accompanied by giant cells presenting bizarre nuclear patterns (Cases 40, 41). The lymphopenia of stress is most prominently displayed by the dog. In protracted disease, lymphopenia may be profound in the dog (Cases 1 and 4), and thus this leukocyte is useful to prognosis. Failure of lymphocytes to return to normal levels despite therapy is to be viewed as an unfavorable sign in all animals.

The means and ranges for normal values of

the hemogram in the dog, cat, cow, sheep, goat, horse, and pig are presented in Tables 1–3 and 1–4. Frequent reference to these data, when studying the Appendix cases, will in time lead to ready recall of the limits of the normal without need of reference. Once the normal values become fixed in the mind, interpretation of the hemogram becomes more sophisticated and profitable.

A LISTING OF CASES BY ANIMAL SPECIES

DOG   Page

1. Postprandial Lipemia in a Case of Mastocytoma 1089
2. Dehydration in Acute Nephritis with Uremia 1090
3. Icterus and Uremia in Acute Leptospirosis 1092
4. Hypoproteinemia and Hyperfibrinogenemia in Glomerulonephritis 1093
5. Chronic Interstitial Nephritis or End-Stage Kidney Disease 1094
6. Hypothyroidism 1094
7. Diabetes Mellitus with Lipemia 1096
8. Canine Cushing's Syndrome 1097
9. Cushing's Syndrome with Unique Erythrocyte Response 1098
10. Addison's disease (Hypoadrenocorticism) 1099
11. Thrombocytopenia and Intensified Granulopoiesis due to Hyperestrogenism 1100
12. Regenerative Left Shift in Pyometra 1102
13. Degenerative Left Shift in Pyometra 1102
14. Leukocytosis and Left Shift in Hepatic Cell Carcinoma 1104
15. Leukemoid Reaction in Chronic Peritonitis 1105
16. Granulocytic Leukemia 1106
17. Polycythemia Vera 1107
18. Secondary Polycythemia due to Tetralogy of Fallot 1108
19. Acute Internal Blood Loss in Hemangiosarcoma 1109
20. Blood Loss from Gastrointestinal Hemorrhage 1111
21. Dicumarol (Warfarin) Poisoning 1111
22. Rodenticide and Aspirin Intoxication 1113
23. Thrombocytopenic Purpura, Possibly Due to Sensitivity to Administered Drugs 1113
24. Idiopathic Thrombocytopenic Purpura (Hypersplenism) 1114
25. Disseminated Intravascular Coagulation 1116
26. Epistaxis Associated with Nasal Carcinoma and Terminal Fibrinolysis 1117
27. Hemophilia B 1118
28. Circulating Inhibitor of Coagulation 1119
29. Amyloidosis Associated with Leukopenia, Anemia, Thrombocytopenia, and a Positive Test for Antinuclear Antibodies 1119
30. Systemic Lupus Erythematosus 1121
31. Early Autoimmune Hemolytic Anemia 1123
32. Autoimmune Hemolytic Anemia 1124
33. Microcytic Hypochromic Anemia in Chronic Blood Loss 1125
34. Microcytic Hypochromic Anemia Due to Subacute Blood Loss 1126
35. Chronic Lead Poisoning 1127
36. Salmon Poisoning 1129
37. Canine Distemper: Viral Inclusions in Erythrocytes and Leukocytes 1130
38. Plasma Cell Myeloma and Glomerulonephritis 1130
39. Lymphangiectasia 1132

CAT

40. Abnormal Granulopoiesis in Acute Toxemic Disease 1133
41. Marked Leukopenia with Rapid Remission 1134
42. Severe Dehydration and Response to Corticosteroids 1135
43. Leukopenia and Anemia in Toxoplasmosis 1137
44. Lymphopenia and Anemia in Chronic Peritonitis................................. 1138
45. Feline Infectious Peritonitis 1138
46. Progressive Anemia in Adenocarcinoma of the Small Intestine 1140
47. Pyometra with Systemic Toxemia 1140
48. Anemia and Leukopenia in Lymphosarcoma...................................... 1142
49. Lymphadenopathy and Neutropenia Associated with *Chlamydia*-like Organisms and Terminal Neoplasia.. 1143
50. Myeloproliferative Disorder with a Period of Remission and Relapse Two Years Later.. 1144
51. Lupus Erythematosus with Autoimmune Hemolytic Anemia 1146
52. Feline Infectious Anemia (Haemobartonellosis)................................. 1148
53. Experimentally Induced Feline Infectious Anemia (FIA)......................... 1148
54. Experimentally Induced Panleukopenia 1150

HORSE

55. Response to Massive Hemorrhage 1150
56. Hemolytic Anemia Associated with Heinz Body Formation in Phenothiazine Toxicosis 1152
57. Equine Infectious Anemia.. 1153
58. Neonatal Isoerythrolysis in a Foal... 1154
59. Combined Immune Deficiency in an Arabian Foal 1155
60. Severe Lymphopenia Associated with Fibrinous Pericarditis and Bronchitis 1156
61. Hyperglobulinemia in Chronic Dermatitis 1157
62. Extreme Leukocytosis Associated with Pyelonephritis 1158
63. Degenerative Left Shift with "Toxic" Neutrophils in Perforation of the Rectum 1158
64. Icterus and Lipemia Associated with Hepatic Lipidosis 1160
65. Acute Salmonellosis 1160

COW

66. Leukopenia and Left Shift in Acute Mastitis 1162
67. Neutrophilia and Lymphocytosis in Traumatic Reticulitis and Splenitis 1163
68. Dehydration in Traumatic Reticulitis 1164
69. The Hematology of Anaplasmosis 1165
70. Johne's Disease 1165
71. Trichostrongyloidosis 1165
72. Congenital Porphyria (Pink Tooth) 1167

SHEEP

73. Haemonchosis 1168

Case 1 (Dog). Postprandial Lipemia in a Case of Mastocytoma

A male Bedlington terrier, 11 years old, was referred for biopsy of a recurrent neoplasm. Large masses were present in the left inguinal region and in the right dorsal pelvis. The neoplasm was a mastocytoma.

Interpretation

1. This case of lipemia resulted from the dog having had a meal of standard dog food

Case 1 (Dog). Mastocytoma

	March 7 (2 p.m.)		March 8 (8:30 a.m.)	
Erythrocytes				
RBC ($\times 10^6/\mu$l)	6.05		6.00	
Hemoglobin (g/dl)	16.0		15.4	
PCV (%)	41.0 (low due to hemolysis)		45.0	
MCV (fl)	67.7		75	
MCHC (%)	39.0 (high due to hemolysis)		34.2	
Erythrocyte sed. rate/1 hr	32/9 = 23+		26/5 = 21+	
Anisocytosis	slight		slight	
Polychromasia	slight		slight	
Leukocytes		%		%
WBC/μl	14,800		18,400	
Neutrophils	11,618	78.5	14.904	81.0
Lymphocytes	962	6.5	828	4.5
Monocytes	2,072	14.0	2,300	12.5
Eosinophils	148	1.0	276	1.5
Basophils	0	0.0	92	0.5
Plasma				
Total protein	8.1 (not valid due to lipemia)		7.2	
Icterus index units	Markedly lipemic and hemolyzed		2 (no lipemia or hemolysis)	
Cholesterol	200 mg/dl		—	

about 2 to 3 hours before arrival at the clinic and the drawing of the blood sample for the first hemogram. The second blood sample was taken the following morning, at least 15 hours after the last food intake. The lipemia had disappeared by that time.

2. Erythrocytes in lipemic blood are readily hemolyzed unless the blood is drawn and handled with great care. The lipids in the plasma render the RBC more susceptible to hemolysis. With free hemoglobin in the plasma, the MCHC is erroneously high because the formula for MCHC places the free hemoglobin into the remaining erythrocytes of the lowered PCV.

3. The lipids increase the refractive index, and this gives an erroneously high value for plasma proteins.

4. Features of the hemogram common to malignancies are a significantly elevated corrected erythrocyte sedimentation rate, neutrophilia, lymphopenia, monocytosis, and variable eosinophil numbers.

5. In some instances of mastocytoma, an increase in basophils has been recorded, but basophilia is not a common finding in this type of neoplastic disease.

Case 2 (Dog).   Dehydration in Acute Nephritis with Uremia

A male toy terrier, 3 years old, had been vomiting for 3 days. He was reluctant to walk because of muscle stiffness. The dog was treated with antibiotics and sent home. However, the condition worsened overnight, and he was returned the following day. The body temperature was within normal range throughout his stay in the hospital.

Therapy consisted of antibiotics and fluids. Recovery was slow.

Interpretation

1. The hemograms are representative of an acute disease accompanied by progressive dehydration.

2. The initial hemogram revealed maximum normal levels for erythrocytes, hemoglobin, and PCV, but when viewed in light of the acute nature of the disease and the above-normal plasma proteins, it became apparent that considerable hemoconcentration existed. Despite fluid therapy, evidence of hemoconcentration persisted through Feb. 6, when the last hemogram was obtained. The dog was not released until Feb. 15.

3. The high corrected value for erythrocyte sedimentation rate in the face of a PCV of 52% pointed to the extreme severity of the disease at the first hemogram. The corrected value of 1+ the following day was as significant as the previously recorded 21+. With increasing PCV, there is marked interference with settling of the erythrocytes. Any settling when the PCV exceeds 50% is clinically significant.

4. The leukocytosis and changing patterns in differential leukocyte distribution revealed marked systemic stress (extreme lymphopenia), with monocytosis increasing to a peak 24 hours later. The increase in lymphocyte numbers in the leukogram of Feb. 6 gave limited encouragement to an interpretation that systemic stress was decreasing. However, the reduction of BUN from 172.5 mg/dl to 19.1 mg/dl was an encouraging sign.

Case 2 (Dog).   Acute Nephritis

	Jan. 29		Jan. 30		Feb. 6	
Erythrocytes						
RBC ($\times 10^6/\mu$l)	8.65		9.55		8.75	
Hemoglobin (g/dl)	18.1		19.7		20.6	
PCV (%)	52.0		57.0		57.0	
MCV (fl)	60.1		59.7		65.1	
MCHC (%)	34.8		34.6		36.1	
Erythrocyte sed. rate/1 hr	21/0 = 21+		1/0 = 1+		0/0 = 0	
Anisocytosis	slight		slight		slight	
Polychromasia	rare		rare		slight	
Leukocytes		%		%		%
WBC/μl	26,200		28,500		37,700	
Neutrophils	24,297	93.5	22,658	79.5	33,930	90.0
Lymphocytes	393	1.5	1,282	4.5	1,696	4.5
Monocytes	1,310	5.0	4,560	16.0	1,696	4.5
Eosinophils	0	0.0	0	0.0	377	1.0
Plasma						
Proteins (g/dl)	8.2		10.6		8.0	
Icterus index units	5		10		7.5	
Blood urea nitrogen (mg/dl)	—		172.5		19.1	

Case 3 (Dog).   Acute Leptospirosis

	Sept. 22	Sept. 23	Sept. 24	Sept. 27	Sept. 28	Oct. 4	Oct. 20
Erythrocytes ($\times 10^6/\mu$l)	5.18	5.03	4.75	4.29	4.18	4.49	3.84
Hemoglobin (g/dl)	11.6	11.4	10.8	9.7	9.2	10.0	8.3
PCV (%)	36.0	36.0	32.0	30.0	29.0	31.0	26.0
MCV (fl)	69.4	71.5	67.3	69.9	69.3	69.0	67.7
MCH (pg)	32.2	31.6	33.7	32.3	31.7	32.2	31.9
MCHC (%)	22.3	22.6	22.7	22.6	22.0	22.2	16.1
Erythrocyte sed. rate/1 hr	4–	11–	—	8+	—	18–	—
Icterus index units	10	25	20	50	>100	7.5	2
Plasma proteins (g/dl)	6.1	6.7	6.8	8.2	6.9	7.1	5.3
Plasma fibrinogen (g/dl)	0.5	0.4	—	0.6	0.3	0.5	0.2
Nucleated RBC/100 WBC	1.5	0	0	0	0	0	0
Anisocytosis	slight	slight	slight	slight	slight	slight	moderate
Polychromasia	slight	slight	slight	slight	slight	slight	slight
Howell-Jolly bodies	few	0	few	0	few	0	few
Reticulocytes (%)	—	—	5.7	7.5	3.4	7.4	3.6
Platelets/μl	low	29,000	few	—	55,000	—	—
WBC/μl (corrected)	24,800	31,000	24,000	22,700	20,800	16,200	11,900
Band neutrophils	124	155	600	454	416	81	297
Segmenter neutrophils	21,328	24,180	18,240	18,500	15,808	12,879	6,723
Lymphocytes	868	2,945[a]	3,120	1,248	2,184	2,511	3,272
Monocytes	2,480	3,720	1,920	2,497	1,976	729	1,071
Eosinophils	0	0	0	0	416	0	535
Basophils	0	0	120	0	0	0	0
Unclassified cells	rare	0	0	0	0	0	0
Blood urea nitrogen (mg/dl)	—	210	136	68.5	32.0	45.5	17.0
Urine specific gravity	—	1.017	—	—	—	—	—
Urine bilirubin glucuronide	—	4+	—	—	—	—	—
Urine urobilinogen	—	0	—	—	—	—	—
SGPT (IU/L)	—	107.5	—	16	—	—	—
SGOT (IU/L)	—	—	—	7	—	—	—

[a]Many lymphocytes dark-staining.

Case 3 (Dog). Icterus and Uremia in Acute Leptospirosis

An 8-week-old male boxer dog was presented with a history of sneezing, listlessness, and anorexia. Body temperature was 101.2°F, heart rate was 160/min, and respiratory rate was 25/min. There was a mucoid discharge from the eyes. Lung sounds were normal. A tentative diagnosis of early distemper was made. Conjunctival scrapings for distemper inclusion bodies were negative. A hemogram (Sept. 22) revealed leukocytosis with stress pattern and an icterus index of 10 units. The following were noted the next day: body temperature of 100°F, clinical icterus, bilateral nasal discharge, and diarrhea. The mucoid ocular discharge was less pronounced, and anorexia persisted. The provisional diagnosis was changed to possible leptospirosis, and therapy was administered. Leptospirae were not demonstrated on dark-field examinations of urine sediment made on Sept. 23 and again on Sept. 28. Serum titers (Sept. 29) of 1:320 for *L. canicola* and 1:160 for *L. icterohemorrhagiae* increased to 1:1,280 and 1:640, respectively, by Oct. 20, thereby establishing the diagnosis of acute leptospirosis. Body temperature did not exceed 102.2°F throughout hospitalization from Sept. 22 through Oct. 5. The dog was in good health and had gained 15 pounds when presented on Oct. 20 for the withdrawal of blood for the serum test for *Leptospira* antibodies. The illness was monitored by laboratory studies throughout hospitalization.

Interpretation

1. The pup was 8 weeks old on admission. Hemoconcentration from dehydration elevated the values for RBC, PCV, Hb, and plasma proteins above the normal mean values for a young pup (see Table 4–2).
2. Erythrocyte parameters diminished gradually while icterus index increased gradually over a period of 6 days. Although the increasing icterus index might appear to have been due to erythrocyte destruction resulting in lowering of RBC, Hb, and PCV values, this is not the most likely explanation for these changes. Fluid therapy was administered daily between Sept. 24 and Oct. 1 to combat dehydration, and in amounts that would dilute the blood and reduce the erythrocyte number per µl. One would expect, however, that plasma proteins would also be diluted, but the total plasma protein concentration increased. Despite this inconsistency, it is not likely that an icterus index of greater than 100 units would result from the limited decrease in RBC numbers seen here. Reticulocyte numbers were slightly above average for the age of the dog, indicating a mild response to a borderline anemia that was masked by dehydration on admission.
3. The dog became more anemic between Oct. 4 and Oct. 20 when at home. Icterus index was normal during this period. The dog gained 15 pounds after recovery from acute leptospirosis. The demands of growth on expansion of the vascular system may have exceeded the ability of hematopoietic activity to supply the required number of erythrocytes to maintain a normal circulating RBC mass. Plasma proteins also became reduced to their lowest levels, suggesting that the dog was properly hydrated on Oct. 20.
4. An icterus index of 10 units on admission was clinically significant and preceded the appearance of clinically detectable icterus by 24 hours. It is felt that most of the rise in icterus index to >100 units over a 6-day period was a reflection of residual liver damage from initial acute necrosis. The SGPT value of 107.5 IU/liter on Sept. 23 established the fact that acute liver necrosis had taken place. One wonders if the change in erythrocyte sedimentation rate from a negative corrected value to a positive (8+) corrected value on Sept. 27 might have been a reflection of a temporary decrease in plasma albumin as a result of liver damage. Albumin is one plasma protein that retards RBC sedimentation. If albumin concentration was reduced while fibrinogen increased (0.6 g/dl), this could explain the temporary change in ESR. The inconsistency here is the increased concentration of total plasma proteins to 8.2 g/dl on that day. This would not appear to support a concept of possible reduction of plasma albumin. Another possibility, and perhaps the more likely one, is that the 8.2 g predicted as protein by a refractive index measurement was not all protein but was due to something else in the plasma (lipids) resulting from the hepatitis. We have some evidence to the effect that in hepatitis the refractometric method of estimating plasma proteins may yield erroneously high readings.
5. The markedly elevated blood urea nitrogen (Sept. 23) was conjectured to be due to a combination of kidney damage in acute leptospirosis and dehydration resulting in reduced blood flow through the kidneys. With hydration and other therapy, the BUN gradually fell to normal levels by Oct. 20.
6. The total and differential leukocyte counts on admission (Sept. 22) were typical of neutrophilia, monocytosis, lymphopenia, and eosinopenia of stress of acute disease. The rapid return of lymphocytes to normal absolute values was an encouraging sign that appeared before other elements of the hemogram reflected beginning subsidence of the acute phase of the disease. The dark staining of lymphocytes on Sept. 23, with the first upsurge of lymphocytes, may have been

more a reflection of immaturity than of toxic effects.

7. Blood platelet counts were below normal for all of the period of hospitalization. The counts remained above the level of 20,000/μl, below which bleeding is most commonly seen. Also, the fact that the dog was caged and depressed limited stress on blood vessels, which would tend to decrease episodes of bleeding in a thrombocytopenic dog.

Case 4 (Dog). Hypoproteinemia and Hyperfibrinogenemia in Glomerulonephritis

A 6-year-old Shetland sheepdog had been vomiting for 3 weeks and had lost weight over a period of 6 months. Physical examination revealed a thin, apprehensive dog in a fair state of hydration. Body temperature was 100.8°F, pulse rate was 160/min, and respiration was 16/min. The owner stated that polydipsia had been noted over a period of a few weeks.

Initial laboratory data indicated a diagnosis of chronic nephritis, possibly glomerulonephritis. Therapy was directed toward increasing urine flow and reducing the level of blood urea nitrogen. Fluid therapy was administered daily, mannitol diuresis was conducted twice, and peritoneal dialysis was carried out daily from May 8 through May 12. Prednisolone, approximately 0.5 mg/pound of body weight b.i.d., was initiated on May 9. Antibiotics and other therapeutics were also given daily. The effects of fluid therapy, dialysis,

and prednisolone administration are reflected in the sequential hemograms and the BUN determinations. Therapy did not bring sufficient improvement to recommend its continuation. The owner requested that the dog be destroyed.

Necropsy. The kidneys were swollen and pale. The capsule peeled easily. On cut surface, the cortex bulged, and glomeruli were prominent. There was intercostal mineralization. Microscopic examination revealed relatively avascular and diffusely hyalinized glomeruli. Bowman's capsules were thickened, and diffusely hyalinized and presented numerous adhesions. Cortical tubules were moderately dilated and lined with somewhat atrophic epithelium. There were perivascular accumulations of neutrophil leukocytes and mononuclear cells in the interstitial tissues, particularly in the lower cortical area. The pelvis of the kidney appeared essentially normal.

Interpretation

1. In chronic nephritis with uremia, the following findings are common in the hemogram: anemia, a significantly elevated corrected erythrocyte sedimentation rate, elevated plasma fibrinogen, and an absolute lymphopenia.
2. RBC, Hb, and PCV were at their minimum normal levels in the first hemogram. The existence of a moderate anemia became apparent as hemoconcentration was reduced by fluid therapy. The anemia was normo-

Case 4 (Dog). Glomerulonephritis

	May 3		May 10		May 11		May 12	
RBC ($\times 10^6$/μl)	5.18		4.35		4.30		4.24	
Hemoglobin (g/dl)	12.4		10.8		9.9		10.0	
PCV (%)	37.0		31.0		29.0		29.0	
MCV (fl)	71.4		71.2		67.4		68.3	
MCH (pg)	23.9		24.8		23.0		23.5	
MCHC (%)	33.5		34.8		34.1		34.4	
Erythrocyte sed. rate/1 hr	14/13 = 1+		61/24 = 37+		61/28 = 33+		—	
Icterus index	2		2		2		2	
Plasma proteins (g/dl)	5.2		5.0		5.1		4.6	
Fibrinogen (g/dl)	0.7		0.9		1.0		1.0	
Reticulocytes (%)	—		0		0.2		0	
Anisocytosis	slight		slight		slight		slight	
Polychromasia	none		none		none		none	
WBC/μl	10,900		6,100		8,100		21,400	
		%		%		%		%
Band neutrophils	109	1.0	671	11.0	648	8.0	749	3.5
Segmenters	9,374	86.0	4,331	71.0	5,751	71.0	18,932	88.0
Lymphocytes	545	5.0	854	14.0	729	9.0	107	0.5
Monocytes	763	7.0	244	4.0	972	12.0	1,712	8.0
Eosinophils	109	1.0	0	0.0	0	0.0	0	0.0
Blood urea nitrogen (mg/dl)	181.5		135		122		104	
Creatinine (mg/dl)	3.8		3.8		—		3.0	
Urine specific gravity	1.017		—		—		1.017	
Urine protein	4+[a]		—		—		2+	
Blood calcium (mg/dl)	7.9		—		—		—	
Blood phosphorus (mg/dl)	17.6		—		—		—	

[a]Urine protein on May 7 = 1.2 g/24 hr. An immune panel of Coombs' test, antinuclear antibody test, and LE cell test, also conducted on May 7, was negative.

cytic-normochromic, indicating that it was the result of depression of erythrogenesis. This was further substantiated by the absence or very low level of reticulocytes in peripheral blood.

3. The ESR was prevented from expressing its true level in the initial hemogram. During hydration, the markedly elevated ESR in the face of hypoproteinemia can best be explained on the basis of hyperfibrinogenemia, a common finding in chronic nephritis, and the hypoalbuminemia resulting from loss of albumin into the urine. The loss of albumin into the urine was significant, as demonstrated by 1.2 g/24-hour urine sample on May 7. Fibrinogen increases sedimentation rate, while albumin decreases it.

4. Dysfunction of the kidneys was demonstrated by a BUN of 181.5 mg/dl of serum, creatinine of 3.8 mg/dl, a marked retention of phosphorus, and a compensatory decrease in serum calcium, leading to the intercostal mineralization noted at necropsy.

5. The hypoproteinemia and 4+ proteinuria pointed to glomerulonephritis rather than chronic interstitial nephritis. In the latter form of nephritis, total plasma protein is commonly normal or somewhat elevated.

Case 5 (Dog). Chronic Interstitial Nephritis (CIN) or End Stage Kidney Disease

A male cocker spaniel, 8 to 9 years old, had an illness diagnosed as chronic interstitial nephritis characterized by a slowly progressive uremic condition and an advancing normocytic-normochromic anemia. A number of hemograms were made over a period of a year to follow the progress of the disease. The parts of the hemogram most influenced by CIN, as well as blood urea nitrogen levels, are presented.

Interpretation

1. A chronic anemia, which became progressively more severe, was present through the entire year of observations. For a brief period in June and July, erythropoiesis became more active, and this resulted in a temporary increase in PCV and stabilized the hemoglobin concentration at 5.9 g/dl for approximately 4 months. The more active erythropoiesis during this period is shown by the increase in reticulocytes in peripheral blood to about 5.0%. The larger size of the immature erythrocytes brought the mean erythrocyte size (MCV) to the maximum normal of 75 to 78 fl.

2. By December 12, kidney function had become less effective, for the blood urea nitrogen had doubled, and by May 26, 1964, the patient was entering the terminal stage of uremia. Vomiting, polydipsia, polyuria, nocturia, and a uremic breath were present. Up to this time, despite the progressive anemia and prolonged elevation of the blood urea nitrogen, the dog had appeared sufficiently normal that the owner was convinced the ailment was only minor.

3. The erythrocyte sedimentation rate was significantly elevated throughout. This is a typical finding in CIN.

4. The total leukocyte count was variable, with a distinct leukocytosis and neutrophilia on July 5. The medical record did not make note of any change in the physical signs at that time. In general, an increase of total leukocyte numbers into the high normal (15,000 to 18,000) range can be anticipated in CIN, with the increase attributable to neutrophilia and monocytosis.

5. A lymphopenia is characteristic of CIN, especially when a significant uremia is present. Absolute lymphocyte numbers were at the bottom of the normal range (1,000/μl) or significantly below the minimum normal number throughout the entire year.

6. Plasma protein concentrations were determined by the refractometer method. Protein concentrations remained in the middle to high normal range except terminally. The terminal values are not entirely valid because of interference by lipids.

Case 6 (Dog). Hypothyroidism

A spayed female cocker spaniel was presented with a complaint of a skin disorder. There was a pustular dermatitis, several spots of alopecia over the back, and a seborrheic odor. In addition, the dog was obese and listless. Both thyroid glands were enlarged but movable. Hypothyroidism was suspected. A very low level of thyroid gland activity was demonstrated by the limited uptake (2.5%) of ^{131}I. By the method used, an uptake of 10–40% is expected in the presence of normally functioning thyroid glands in the dog. Cholesterol levels in hypothyroidism are usually above the normal range of 135–270 mg/dl for the dog. A serum cholesterol level of 338 mg/dl was found in this patient. A skin biopsy was described as "thin atrophic epidermis with degenerative changes in the hair follicles compatible with hypothyroidism." The patient was placed on thyroxin therapy. Considerable clinical improvement was noted within 3 weeks. Two hemograms during the period of application of diagnostic tests were consistent with the diagnosis of hypothyroidism. (See Chapter 36.)

Interpretation

1. Hypothyroidism is often associated with a borderline normocytic, normochromic anemia. Thyroxin is one of the hormones involved in the control of erythrogenesis, hence anemia results from diminished red cell production.

Case 5 (Dog). Chronic Interstitial Nephritis (CIN)

| Date | PCV (%) | Hb (g/dl) | MCV (fl) | Reticulocytes (%) | ESR (cor.) | Plasma Protein (g/dl) | WBC/µl | Differential leukocyte count/µl | | | | Blood Urea Nitrogen (mg/dl) |
								Neutrophils	Lymphocytes	Monocytes	Eosinophils	
5/10/63	27	9.1	69.2	0.8	32+	7.5	7,550	5,014	1,320	1,026	190	58.8
6/10/63	18	6.2	78.0	1.6	19+	6.8	7,600	5,244	1,026	912	418	57.0
6/20/63	17	5.9	74.8	5.2	17+	6.7	8,700	7,000	610	830	260	56.5
7/ 5/63	20	5.9	75.0	4.8	26+	6.8	5,700	23,772	385	1,413	130	46.2
9/17/63	19	5.9	66.0	0.6	22+	7.7	5,600	3,836	1,008	504	252	59.6
12/12/63	14	4.7	68.0	rare	17+	7.7	16,700	12,525	1,085	2,756	334	101.3
5/26/64	13	4.2	80.7	2.2	lipemic	8.9	11,400	8,210	740	1,710	740	149.2
6/16/64	10	3.1	68.0	0.8	10+	8.4	12,700	9,842	318	2,286	254	199.5

Case 6 (Dog).   Hypothyroidism

	February 25		March 10	
Erythrocytes				
RBC ($\times 10^6/\mu l$)	5.50		5.85	
Hemoglobin (g/dl)	10.5		11.9	
PCV (%)	34.0		34.5	
MCV (fl)	62.0		59.0	
MCHC (%)	31.0		34.5	
Erythrocyte sed. rate/1 hr	55/18 = 37+		52/18 = 34+	
Reticulocytes (%)	1.0		—	
Nucleated RBC/100 WBC	none seen		0.5	
Anisocytosis	slight		slight	
Polychromasia	slight		slight	
Leptocytes	prominent		prominent	
RBC "punched-out" centers	prominent		prominent	
RBC agglutination	present		present	
Leukocytes		%		%
WBC/μl	15,700		17,100	
Band neutrophils	2,041	13.0	770	4.5
Neutrophils	9,498	60.5	12,825	75.0
Lymphocytes	3,532	22.5	2,736	16.0
Monocytes	628	4.0	770	4.5
Eosinophils	0	0.0	0	0.0
Plasma				
Protein (g/dl)	8.6		9.1	
Icterus index units	2		5	

2. A high positive corrected erythrocyte sedimentation rate is commonly found. Occasionally, when leptocytes are very prominent, a diphasic reaction is seen. The elevated ESR may be referable to the changes occurring in the skin, and hyperproteinemia.

3. Total leukocyte count is variable in hypothyroidism. A neutrophilia with modest left shift, as seen in this case, is one of the patterns to be anticipated. Lymphocyte numbers are generally well within the normal range, as in this case, and eosinophils are usually present.

4. The elevated plasma protein level may have been due to an increase in globulins in response to the microbial activity in the skin that resulted in pustular dermatitis.

Case 7 (Dog). Diabetes Mellitus with Lipemia

A spayed female mongrel dog, 6 years old, had become obese over a 6-month period with spontaneous occurrence of cataracts within the last month. Polydipsia, polyuria, and occasional vomiting were additional clinical signs. The first hemogram was lipemic with hemolysis resulting from an increased susceptibility to hemolysis in the presence of a lipemic plasma. The urine had a high specific gravity and gave 4+ reactions for both sugar and acetone. Blood sugar was 265 mg/dl and serum cholesterol was 398 mg/dl. The dog was treated with 6 units of insulin at 5 p.m. on Feb. 20. The insulin dose was increased as follows: 9 units, Feb. 21 through 23; 12 units, Feb. 24 through

26; 14 units, Feb. 27 through March 2. Then the insulin dose was reduced as follows: 12 units, March 3 through 5; 9 units, March 6 through 9; and 8 units on March 10 and thereafter. The patient was discharged on March 13.

Interpretation

1. The hemogram of Feb. 20 is affected by both hemoconcentration and lipemia. The latter is a direct result of faulty fat metabolism in the face of inability to metabolize sugar. Hemolysis is generally present in significantly lipemic blood. This is due to an increased susceptibility of erythrocytes to hemolysis when chylomicra are present in the plasma in large numbers. The hemolysis occurs after the blood is drawn and its occurrence is enhanced by physical force applied to the sample, e.g., shaking as in mixing or forcing the blood through the needle into the vial. This renders the MCHC abnormally high. Prediction of plasma proteins is also in error since the visible lipids increase the refractive index.

2. Lymphopenia and eosinopenia on Feb. 20 indicate a severe systemic stress. Return of these cells in normal numbers as seen on Feb. 24 can be correlated with a significant improvement in the general well-being of the dog even though blood glucose remained significantly elevated at that time. However, the parenteral use of insulin brought about an improvement in water balance, disap-

Case 7 (Dog).   Diabetes Mellitus

	Feb. 20		*Feb. 21*		*Feb. 24*	
Erythrocytes						
RBC ($\times 10^6/\mu$l)	8.55		7.60		6.55	
Hemoglobin (g/dl)	20.6		14.9		16.0	
PCV (%)	55.0		47.0		46.0	
MCV (fl)	64.3		61.8		70.2	
MCHC (%)	37.4		31.7		34.8	
Erythrocyte sed. rate/1 hr	1/0 = 1+		1/3 = 2–		1/4 = 4–	
RBC morphology	Marked rouleaux, slight polychromasia		"punched-out" centers are a prominent feature		Moderate aniso-cytosis	
Leukocytes		%		%		%
WBC/μl	10,050		13,550		16,800	
Band neutrophils	100	1.0	203	1.5	84	0.5
Neutrophils	7,487	74.5	10,433	77.0	10,668	63.5
Lymphocytes	704	7.0	1,084	8.0	2,268	13.5
Monocytes	1,708	17.0	1,219	9.0	2,772	16.5
Eosinophils	50	0.5	610	4.5	924	5.5
Unclassified cells	0	0.0	0	0.0	84	0.5
Plasma						
Plasma proteins (g/dl)	11.0 (spurious)		7.0		7.7	
Icterus index units	Lipemic, hemolysis		5		2	
Urine						
Specific gravity	1.032		—		>1.050	
Acetone	4+		—		Trace	
Sugar	4+		—		3+	
Blood Serum						
Cholesterol (mg/dl)	398		230		342	
Serum protein (g/dl)	—		5.65		—	
Blood urea nitrogen (mg/dl)	—		—		3.6	

Case 7 (Dog).   Blood Glucose

	(mg/dl)
Feb. 20	265
Feb. 21	147
Feb. 24	232
Feb. 25	235
Feb. 26	262
Feb. 28	71
Mar. 2	59
Mar. 5	73
Mar. 9	138
Mar. 13	134

pearance of the lipemia, and a fall in blood glucose levels.

Case 8 (Dog).   Canine Cushing's Syndrome

A male Boston terrier had developed alopecia over the past 1½years. Recently, polydipsia and polyuria became prominent clinical signs, and the abdomen developed a "potbellied" appearance. The alopecia was bilaterally symmetrical over the shoulders, back, tail, and thighs. The skin was atrophic with a doughy texture, and there were whitish nodules in the skin about the ears and also in the left thoracic region. The testicles were small and firm. The tonsils were of normal size, but the superficial lymph nodes appeared to be somewhat enlarged.

Interpretation

1. The hemogram in canine Cushing's syndrome is typical of hyperactivity of the adrenal cortex. The main features of such hemograms are neutrophilia, monocytosis, frank lymphopenia, and eosinopenia.
2. Evidence of greater than normal erythropoiesis is to be expected in the form of variable polychromasia and reticulocytosis, although the PCV may reflect anemia, normal levels of circulating RBC, or very rarely, polycythemia.
3. An elevated erythrocyte sedimentation rate is commonly encountered and may be due to the changes in the skin. However, in this dog, ESR was not significantly elevated, except in the initial hemogram. A diphasic erythrocyte sedimentation was seen when evidence of erythropoiesis was most marked (July 22).
4. Moderate to marked leptocytosis in view of MCV and MCHC within normal ranges and prominence of "punched out" red cells seem to reflect the chronic nature of the disease.

Case 8 (Dog). **Canine Cushing's Syndrome**

	May 15, 1963	July 22, 1963	Aug. 2, 1963	Feb. 11, 1964
Erythrocytes				
RBC ($\times 10^6/\mu l$)	6.91	5.20	4.60	6.80
Hemoglobin (g/dl)	17.0	12.8	9.6	15.4
PCV (%)	49.0	36.0	30.0	42.0
MCV (fl)	70.9	69.2	65.2	61.8
MCHC (%)	34.7	35.5	32.0	36.7
Erythrocyte sed. rate/1 hr.	5/1 = 4+	9/14 = 5− (diphasic)	30/26 = 4+	10/8 = 2+
Reticulocytes (%)	—	—	4.0	
Anisocytosis	slight	moderate	moderate	slight
Polychromasia	slight	moderate	moderate	slight
Leptocytes	moderate	moderate	many	many
RBC "punched-out" centers	prominent	prominent	prominent	prominent
Leukocytes	%	%	%	%
WBC/μl	8,550	11,900	19,800	21,800
Band neutrophils	0 0.0	119 1.0	198 1.0	0 0.0
Neutrophils	7,310 85.0	9,877 83.0	17,622 89.0	18,748 86.0
Lymphocytes	427 5.0	476 4.0	594 3.0	545 2.5
Monocytes	812 9.5	1,428 12.0	1,386 7.0	2,398 11.0
Eosinophils	0 0.0	0 0.0	0 0.0	0 0.0
Eosinophils (direct count)	0 —	— —	6 —	— —
Basophils	0 0.0	0 0.0	0 0.0	109 0.5
Plasma				
Protein (g/dl)	7.6	6.6	6.6	6.7
Icterus index units	10	2 (cloudy)	2	2

Other Tests

Iodine-[131] uptake for thyroid gland function was 8.7% on May 15 and 9.13% on Sept. 26, indicating thyroid gland activity.

Blood cholesterol levels were above normal at 366 mg/dl on May 15 and 290 mg/dl on Sept. 26.

Case 9 (Dog). Cushing's Syndrome with Unique Erythrocyte Response

A female dachshund, 6 years old, had developed an abnormal skin texture over a period of 5 months. Other clinical signs were polydipsia, enlarged abdomen, and bilateral alopecia. The latter had existed for over 2 years. The dog had been treated with thyroxin, cortisone, and digitalis without benefit. The dog was hospitalized for diagnostic tests. The urine specific gravity was 1.010 to 1.016 but was normal in other respects. A blood urea nitrogen of 14.0 mg/dl indicated normal kidney function. Normal thyroid gland activity was indicated by a ^{131}I uptake of 12.5%. A blood serum alkaline phosphatase test resulted in the exceedingly high value of 500 Bodansky units, pointing to the possible existence of abnormal metabolism in the bones. A radiograph demonstrated slight decalcification of the thoracic and lumbar vertebrae, with calcification taking place in a majority of the intervertebral discs. The radiologist's comment was, "This appears to be a case of Cushing's syndrome." The several hemograms developed during the period of hospitalization were consistent with a diagnosis of Cushing's syndrome with the unique added feature of large numbers of nucleated erythrocytes in peripheral blood.

Interpretation

1. Features in the hemograms consistent with a hyperactive adrenal cortex are neutrophilia, monocytosis, low normal lymphocytes, eosinopenia, and signs of increased erythrogenesis despite the generally high normal circulating erythrocyte volume.

2. The positive erythrocyte sedimentation rate in the face of the high normal PCV values of 47% to 49% is significant. With the fall of PCV to 34% in the last hemogram, the high positive corrected ESR value became strikingly apparent. An elevated ESR is a common finding in Cushing's syndrome.

3. Basophil leukocytes may be present in peripheral blood in small numbers in some canine patients with this disease; the cause remains unknown.

4. Hyperactivity of the adrenal cortex stimulates erythropoiesis. Thus reticulocytosis and polychromasia are to be anticipated. However, the large number of nucleated erythrocytes observed in this case was unique. The life span of the erythrocyte is probably less than normal in Cushing's syndrome, for the PCV is seen to undulate between borderline anemia and values approaching polycythemia.

Case 9 (Dog). **Cushing's Syndrome with Unique Erythrocyte Response**

	July 12		July 18		July 24		August 2	
Erythrocytes								
RBC ($\times 10^6/\mu$l)	7.08		6.75		6.80		4.56	
Hemoglobin (g/dl)	16.4		15.9		16.0		10.1	
PCV (%)	48.0		47.0		49.0		34.0	
MCV (fl)	67.8		69.6		72.0		74.5	
MCHC (%)	34.2		33.8		32.6		29.7	
Erythrocyte sed. rate/1 hr	—		10/3 = 7+		7/1 = 6+		58/17 = 41+	
Reticulocytes (%)	—		4.8		4.0		5.6	
Nucleated RBC/100 WBC	56.5		20		16.5		5	
Anisocytosis	moderate		slight		moderate		marked	
Polychromasia	moderate		moderate		moderate		moderate	
RBC "punched-out" centers	2+		3+		3+		2+	
Leukocytes		%		%		%		%
WBC/μl	11,718		31,700		33,100		47,000	
Band neutrophils	58	0.5	317	1.0	331	1.0	8,460	18.0
Neutrophils	9,843	84.0	28,312	89.0	27,473	83.0	33,840	72.0
Lymphocytes	1,464	12.5	1,109	3.5	1,324	4.0	1,410	3.0
Monocytes	351	3.0	1,426	4.5	2,648	8.0	3,055	6.5
Eosinophils	0	0.0	0	0.0	0	0.0	0	0.0
Basophils	0	0.0	317	1.0	1,324	4.0	235	0.5
Degenerated cells	0	0.0	317	1.0	0	0.0	0	0.0
Plasma								
Protein (g/dl)	8.5		7.8		7.8		7.4	
Icterus index units	2		5		5		2	

Case 10 (Dog).
Addison's Disease (Hypoadrenocorticism)

A 4-year-old spayed female miniature poodle was presented with a history of listlessness, poor stamina, some vomiting, shaking, and desire to hide under the bed. The dog had a history of allergic dermatitis every summer that was treated with corticosteroids. There were no abnormal findings on physical examination except for depression and dehydration. Body temperature was normal. The dog was retained for observation.

Interpretation

1. A rapidly advancing dehydration, associated with prerenal uremia due to hypovolemic shock and renal failure, was apparent from the physical condition of the dog as well as from blood urea nitrogen—72 mg/dl on admission, which advanced to 123.7 mg/dl within 24 hours.
2. The PCV on admission did not indicate the degree of anemia that existed because it was elevated by the hemoconcentration resulting from dehydration. The plasma proteins, at 9.4 g/dl, gave support to the concept of advanced dehydration.
3. The differential leukocyte count was not typical of a state of stress. In fact, the mean normal absolute number of neutrophils, the marginal lymphocytosis, and persistence of eosinophils were the first indication of the possibility of a hypofunctioning adrenal cortex.
4. Serum electrolyte analysis added support to

the possibility of Addison's disease. The low sodium value was characteristic of hypofunction of the adrenal cortex. As a result of loss of sodium in the urine, the dog was unable to maintain its normal body water and thus entered a hypovolemic state, leading to renal failure and uremia. Potassium level was in the high normal range. It was watched closely throughout the study of the patient since the adverse effect of hyperkalemia on the heart is a common cause of death in Addisonian crisis.

5. To relieve the advancing uremia, peritoneal dialysis was conducted on June 6 and 7, and, in addition, 200 ml of half-strength physiologic saline solution and 2.5% dextrose was given subcutaneously each day; an additional 400 ml was administered on June 8. During this time, the dog's condition was monitored daily by laboratory tests. Results on June 11 indicated that the uremia had been relieved and that normal water balance had been achieved (plasma proteins 6.9 g/dl). The neutrophilia and slight left shift noted at this time may have been caused by the peritoneal dialysis.
6. On June 10, salt administration was started in the form of 0.5 g t.i.d. with adequate availability of fresh drinking water. On June 13, the dog was permitted to go home to await laboratory results on testing the urine for 17-ketogenic steroids.
7. The dog was readmitted June 19 for further study and treatment. Salt intake was in-

Case 10 (Dog). Addison's Disease

	June 5		June 11		June 19–20		August 26	
Erythrocytes								
RBC ($\times 10^6/\mu l$)	5.01		3.84		3.77		7.07	
Hemoglobin (g/dl)	10.9		8.9		9.4 (lipemic)		14.1	
PCV (%)	35.0		27.0		25.0		45.0	
MCV (fl)	69.9		70.3		66.3		63.6	
MCHC (%)	31.1		33.0		37.6 (lipemic)		31.3	
Erythrocyte sed. rate/1 hr	26/6 = 10+		18/32 = 14−		25/36 = 11−		15/5 = 10+	
Anisocytosis	slight		slight		slight		slight	
Polychromasia	slight		slight		no comment		—	
Reticulocytes (%)	0.6		1.4		1.2		—	
Leukocytes		%		%		%		%
WBC/μl	14,800		19,700		22,800		15,200	
Band neutrophils	74	0.5	2,265	11.5	798	3.5	76	0.5
Neutrophils	7,770	52.5	13,593	69.0	12,654	55.5	9,804	64.5
Lymphocytes	5,698	38.5	2,069	10.5	7,182	31.5	4,560	30.0
Monocytes	888	6.0	493	2.5	1,254	5.5	608	4.0
Eosinophils	370	2.5	1,281	6.5	912	4.0	152	1.0
Basophils	0	0.0						
Plasma								
Proteins (g/dl)	9.4		6.9		6.5		6.8	
Fibrinogen (g/dl)	0.4		0.4		0.3		0.4	
Icterus index	2		5		—		2	
Blood urea nitrogen (mg/dl)	72.0		14.5		13.3		13.0	
Sodium (mEq/L)	124.0		127.0		135.0		142.0	
Potassium (mEq/L)	4.0		4.5		5.6		5.0	
Chloride (mEq/L)	89.0		93.0		97.0		111.0	
Blood urea nitrogen (mg/dl)	123.7		—		—		—	
17-ketogenic steroids in 24 hours	—		<1 mg		<1 mg		—	
24-hr urine volume	—		100 ml		84 ml		—	

Case 10. Thorn Test for Adrenal Cortex Function

	Standard Test—20 units of ACTH given intramuscularly at 8:00 a.m. 8:00 a.m.	7 hr post-ACTH	Prolonged Test—results following 20 units of ACTH gel given intramuscularly daily for 3 days
Total WBC/μl	16,600	14,600	16,800
Neutrophils	9,379	8,468	8,064
Lymphocytes	5,395	4,455	6,216
Monocytes	1,079	803	1,764
Eosinophils	747	876	588

creased to 0.5 g q.i.d. on June 21. A Thorn test for evaluation of adrenal cortex function was conducted on June 24; results indicated no response to the standard test of 20 units of ACTH administered intramuscularly. However, since in chronic hypofunction of the adrenal cortex, a single injection of ACTH may not be adequate to stimulate the cortex, continuous stimulation over a 3-day period was conducted; this also failed to bring a response. The response of a normal adrenal cortex to ACTH injection would be neutrophilia, monocytosis, lymphopenia, and eosinopenia. These changes did not occur, and thus the existence of hypoadrenocorticism was verified. Furthermore, the test for 17-ketogenic steroids in urine revealed excretion of less than 1.0 mg in 24 hours. Normal excretion is approximately 1.0 to 4.0 mg in 24 hours.

8. Specific hormone therapy was started on June 24 with continuation of oral salt intake at 0.5 g daily. The dog was permitted to go home with periodic return for evaluation. The last evaluation on August 26 revealed that relative normalcy had been attained. (Deoxycorticosterone pivalate in the form of a 30-day repositol was given by deep intramuscular injection; this treatment was to be continued at monthly intervals by the referring veterinarian. Low-level doses of prednisolone were advised as needed to treat the original complaint of dermatitis.)

Case 11 (Dog). Thrombocytopenia and Intensified Granulopoiesis Due to Hyperestrogenism

A 4-year-old female Saint Bernard dog was admitted to the hospital with a history of infertility

Case 11 (Dog). Hyperestrogenism

	Nov. 9	Nov. 10	Nov. 11	Nov. 12	Nov. 15	Nov. 17	Nov. 20	Nov. 24	Dec. 6	Jan. 28 (estrus)
RBC ($\times 10^6/\mu l$)	5.90	5.58	5.58	5.31	5.54	5.90	5.70	6.12	6.30	6.89
Hemoglobin (g/dl)	14.5	13.7	13.6	12.7	13.6	14.1	15.1	14.9	15.6	16.9
PCV (%)	41.0	39.0	37.0	36.0	39.0	40.0	42.0	43.0	45.0	45.0
MCV (fl)	69.4	69.8	66.3	67.7	70.3	67.7	73.6	70.2	71.4	65.3
MCHC (%)	35.3	35.1	36.7	35.2	34.8	35.2	35.9	34.6	34.6	37.5
MCH (pg)	24.5	24.5	24.3	23.9	24.5	23.8	26.4	24.3	24.7	24.5
ESR/1 hour	16/9=7+	36/11=25+	0/13=13−	2/14=12−	5/11=6−	4/10=6−	2/8=6−	0/7=7−	8/5=3+	—
Icterus index	hem.	2	2	2	2	2	2	2	hem.	hem.
Plasma proteins (g/dl)	7.9	7.5	7.4	7.3	7.2	7.1	7.0	7.1	7.0	8.0
Plasma fibrinogen (g/dl)	0.3	0.4	0.4	0.4	0.3	0.3	0.3	0.2	0.2	—
WBC/μl	63,500	75,200	48,000	37,500	10,800	11,800	7,900	4,100	9,500	8,700
Metamyelocytes	635	0	0	0	0	0	0	0	0	0
Bands	11,450	3,384	2,880	1,125	0	59	0	82	0	0
Neutrophils	46,037	69,184	40,560	33,938	7,074	7,375	4,740	1,968	5,510	6,047
Lymphocytes	3,492	752	1,440	1,125	1,674	1,829	1,659	1,722	2,992	1,827
Monocytes	1,587	1,504	1,920	937	270	118	0	41	285	348
Eosinophils	317	376	1,200	375	1,782	2,419	1,501	287	712	478
Basophils	0	0	0	0	0	0	0	0	0	0
Thrombocytes/μl	decreased	same	35,000	30,000	30,000	65,000	109,000	78,000	80,000	normal distribution
Anisocytosis	slight	slight	slight	slight	slight	slight	slight	slight	slight	slight
Blood urea nitrogen (mg/dl)	12.0	—	—	—	—	—	—	—	—	—
Fecal occult blood	—	—	—	4+	—	—	—	—	—	—
Urine specific gravity	—	1.036	—	—	—	—	—	—	—	—

and a vaginal discharge. Physical examination revealed a healthy bitch with no abnormalities other than a swollen vulva and a noncopious brownish vaginal discharge. The first hemogram was typical of pyometra, but this diagnosis was not supported by radiography. One finding in the first hemogram that was not typical of pyometra was a possible thrombocytopenia based on scarcity of platelets in the stained blood film. Upon further questioning of the owner, it was learned that the dog was under treatment for infertility. A veterinarian had given intramuscular injections of 5 mg of estradiol on Oct. 18 and Oct. 25, followed on Nov. 1 with 50 mg of diethylstilbestrol repositol and 5-mg tablets of stilbestrol to be given orally s.i.d. The dog had received eight tablets up to the time of present admission. Further treatment with estrogens was stopped and antibiotic therapy was initiated for treatment of vaginitis.

Interpretation

1. Estrogen has a marked effect on bone marrow cytology. The first hemogram was typical of cytologic changes seen in hyperestrogenism leading to neutrophilia with left shift and thrombocytopenia. Estrogen administration also produces lymphocytosis and monocytosis (see Chapter 17).
2. Withdrawal of estrogen therapy resulted in a temporary marked lymphopenia and a gradual reduction of neutrophil and monocyte numbers to normal levels by the end of the first week. An eosinophilia developed during the second week and then subsided. Neutropenia was noted at the end of the second week, after which recovery took place although neutrophils remained on the low side of the mean normal value of 7,000/μl.
3. Thrombocytopenia persisted through the first month. Circulating platelet levels were not reduced to the point where spontaneous bleeding occurred. However, the finding of 4+ occult blood in the stool pointed to the possibility of some bleeding into the gut.
4. The fall in PCV from 41% to 36% and a gradual increase to 45% suggests that some blood loss and replacement had occurred. MCV, MCH, and MCHC, however, were consistently within the normal ranges, as were total plasma proteins and plasma fibrinogen.
5. The dog was seen again on Feb. 22. The PCV had increased to 52%, thrombocyte distribution was normal, and leukocyte total and differential counts were similar to those of Jan. 28. The dog was found to be pregnant. Permanent bone marrow damage from estrogen administration appeared to have been averted.
6. Without knowledge that this dog had been receiving estrogen therapy, the presenting signs and initial hemogram would have presented a difficult problem of interpretation.

Case 12 (Dog). Regenerative Left Shift in Pyometra

A female weimaraner, 9 years old, was presented with a complaint of urinary incontinence associated with polydipsia. She had given birth to her last litter some 5 years earlier. According to the owner, the dog had shown signs suggestive of estrus about 1 month before. There had been no history of vomiting.

Physical Examination. The dog was obese and presented a distended, painful abdomen. The rectal temperature was 103°F, pulse 172/min, and respiration was rated as fast. The conjunctivae were congested, and there was evidence of dehydration.

Radiographic Examination. Both uterine horns were very much enlarged.

Interpretation

1. A borderline anemia that commonly accompanies pyometra was probably masked by some hemoconcentration. The above-normal plasma protein concentration was possibly both relative (from hemoconcentration) and absolute (from increase in production of globulins in response to the suppurative inflammatory process).
2. The very high positive value for corrected erythrocyte sedimentation rate is to be anticipated in pyometra.
3. The marked leukocytosis with left shift indicates that the bone marrow has adjusted to accelerated granulopoiesis in response to continual heavy demands for neutrophils. The signs of "toxicity" in neutrophils suggest exposure to metabolic and bacterial toxins produced in conjunction with pyometra. The initial hemogram can be distinguished from the leukocytosis and left shift of an acute disease process, such as leptospirosis, by the persistence of lymphocytes and eosinophils. These latter cell types have become diminished in the second hemogram as a result of the stress of surgery. The monocytosis of the level seen here is common to pyometra.
4. The elevated blood urea nitrogen is referable to the decomposition of body protein associated with the suppurative process within the uterus and also to the dehydration.
5. An increase in WBC, due to an increase in the neutrophil leukocytes, is a common finding during the first days after surgery for pyometra.

Case 13 (Dog). Degenerative Left Shift in Pyometra

A female miniature poodle, 3 years old, was presented with a complaint of anorexia, depression, and polydipsia. The owner stated that the dog had exhibited signs of estrus 3 weeks previously. Rectal temperature was 104°F, pulse 118, hydration appeared to be good, and a mass about the size of a

Case 12 (Dog).   Regenerative Left Shift in Pyometra

	October 28 (Admission date)		November 1 (2nd day postsurgery)	
Erythrocytes				
RBC ($\times 10^6/\mu$l)	6.10		6.00	
Hemoglobin (g/dl)	13.2		13.6	
PCV (%)	41.0		43.0	
MCV (fl)	67.0		71.6	
MCHC (%)	32.2		31.6	
Erythrocyte sed. rate/1 hr	42/9 = 33+		—	
Anisocytosis	slight		slight	
Polychromasia	slight		slight	
Leukocytes		%		%
WBC/μl	59,500		66,000	
Myelocytes	298	0.5	330	0.5
Metamyelocytes	7,438	12.5	1,320	2.0
Band neutrophils	17,850	30.0	7,260	11.0
Neutrophils	23,800	40.0	46,860	71.0
Lymphocytes	3,272	5.5	1,320	2.0
Monocytes	5,950	10.0	6,270	9.5
Eosinophils	892	1.5	330	0.5
Degenerated cells	0	0.0	2,310	3.5
Toxic signs	Neutrophils are large with basophilic, foamy cytoplasm			
Plasma				
Protein (g/dl)	8.3		8.0	
Icterus index units	10 (slight hemolysis)		—	
Blood urea nitrogen (mg/dl)	29.8		46.2	

Case 13 (Dog).   Degenerative Left Shift in Pyometra

	October 24		October 28		November 5	
Erythrocytes						
RBC ($\times 10^6/\mu$l)	6.95		5.90		6.70	
Hemoglobin (g/dl)	6.0		12.5		13.9	
PCV (%)	46.0		42.0		44.0	
MCV (fl)	66.2		71.2		65.7	
MCHC (%)	34.8		29.7		31.6	
Erythrocyte sed. rate/1 hr	40/4 = 36+		42/8 = 34+		31/6 = 25+	
Nucleated RBC/100 WBC	0		0		0.5	
Anisocytosis	slight		slight		slight	
Leukocytes		%		%		%
WBC/μl	14,800		17,000		33,200	
Metamyelocytes	814	5.5	0	0.0	1,826	5.5
Band neutrophils	3,700	25.0	935	5.5	11,122	33.5
Neutrophils	8,066	54.5	12,155	71.5	12,118	36.5
Lymphocytes	1,628	11.0	2,380	14.0	2,324	7.0
Monocytes	444	3.0	1,360	8.0	4,482	13.5
Eosinophils	74	0.5	85	0.5	0	0.0
Unclassified cells	74	0.5	0	0.0	332	1.0
Degenerated cells	0	0.0	85	0.5	996	3.0
Toxic signs in neutrophils	basophilic cytoplasm		none		slight basophilia of the cytoplasm	
Plasma						
Protein (g/dl)	8.0		7.9		7.5	
Icterus index units	2		7.5		5.0	
Blood urea nitrogen (mg/dl)	6.3		—		6.8	

golf ball could be palpated in the abdomen. No diarrhea or vomiting had been observed.

Radiographic Examination. Enlarged uterine horns were demonstrated.

Therapy. The record indicates that treatment was limited to antibiotics administered twice daily between October 25 and 31, after which the dog was permitted to go home, with antibiotic therapy to be continued by the owner. The patient was returned November 5 for removal of the uterus. Three hemograms were obtained covering the period from first entry to return for surgery.

Interpretation

1. The plasma proteins were at the maximum and above maximum normal concentrations. Since pyogenic bacteria are often associated with pyometra, an absolute increase in plasma proteins may develop as a result of hyperglobulinemia. Serum protein fractionation would be required to demonstrate this occurrence. Plasma proteins also increase relatively in hemoconcentration. However, the low blood urea nitrogen and lack of signs of dehydration on physical examination suggested that the dog was in water balance.

2. The high positive corrected erythrocyte sedimentation rate points to a significant tissue derangement somewhere in the body. In this instance, it was inflammation of the uterus.

3. The left shift without significant elevation in total neutrophils reflected a state of toxemia with some depression of granulopoiesis. This depression of maturation of neutrophils is further demonstrated by the persistence of basophilia (bluish staining) of the cytoplasm.

4. Administration of antibiotics appeared to lessen the toxemia, for the left shift was receding and the signs of toxicity in neutrophils had disappeared in the second hemogram. However, the improvement in general well-being did not persist for long. On Nov. 5 a leukocytosis was demonstrated in which immature neutrophils outnumbered the mature neutrophils (degenerative left shift) pointing to a demand for neutrophils that could not be met by the bone marrow. This is generally interpreted as a poor prognostic sign.

5. Lymphocytes remaining within the normal range despite signs of systemic stress is a common finding in chronic suppurative diseases.

6. A monocytosis is a characteristic feature of pyometra. However, this feature did not express itself until the third hemogram. Perhaps the initial toxemia depressed production of monocytes as well as of granulocytes.

Case 14 (Dog).   Leukocytosis and Left Shift in Hepatic Cell Carcinoma

A spayed female Labrador retriever, 10 years old, had been sick for approximately 18 days when referred on Feb. 16. On arrival, clinical signs were fever (104°F), labored breathing, and a painful, distended abdomen. Respiratory distress was evident in all positions, with some relief when lying down. There was a generalized increase in bronchovesicular sounds, especially on the left side. The condition became progressively worse until death 16 days later.

Necropsy Report: Liver enlarged, especially right portion, weight 3 pounds; many adhesions to intestines and omentum. Right kidney was half normal size, while left kidney was twice normal size. The microscopic examination revealed necrosis of kidney tubules and infiltration by mononuclear cells. The liver presented degeneration and necrosis of parenchymal cells with clusters and sheets of well-defined neoplastic cells. In some areas, the neoplastic tissue appeared to be forming ducts.

Interpretation

1. Icterus index above 7.5 units is abnormal for the dog. The icterus index score of 15 units, taken together with the low plasma proteins on first hemogram, would point to liver involvement. The elevated SGPT verified that liver necrosis was present. The subsequent increase in plasma proteins may have been due to an absolute increase in globulins. The increasing plasma protein concentration does not appear to have been due to hemoconcentration, since the PCV was not significantly increased simultaneously.

2. The greater part of the plasma bilirubin gave an indirect reaction to the van den Bergh test. This would indicate decreased liver uptake of free bilirubin due to hepatic cell insufficiency. The negative urobilinogen in the urine on three separate occasions pointed to the possibility of bile duct closure. The presence of bile pigments (conjugated bilirubin) in large amounts in the urine also indicated bile duct occlusion.

3. The marked leukocytosis with left shift, marked monocytosis and significantly elevated erythrocyte sedimentation rate further reflect response to tissue destruction and the seriousness of the problem. The increasing numbers of lymphocytes would tend to support the conclusion that systemic stress was lessening, but other elements of the leukogram could not support such interpretation.

4. The presence of microcytic hypochromic red cells with slightly below normal hemoglobin concentration suggested the possibility of a borderline anemia. An anemia of this kind may develop from interference with iron utilization in a variety of chronic diseases in-

Case 14 (Dog). Hepatic Cell Carcinoma

	February 16		February 21		February 26	
Erythrocytes						
RBC ($\times 10^6/\mu l$)	6.5		6.65		6.3	
Hemoglobin (g/dl)	11.5		11.7		13.4	
PCV (%)	38.0		38.0		39.0	
MCV (fl)	58.5		57.0		61.9	
MCHC (%)	30.3		30.8		34.4	
Erythrocyte sed. rate/1 hr	52/12 = 40+		38/12 = 26+		50/11 = 39+	
Nucleated RBC/100 WBC	1		0		0	
Anisocytosis	slight		slight		slight	
Polychromasia	slight		slight		slight	
Leukocytes		%		%		%
WBC/μl	42,700		40,900		60,500	
Metamyelocytes	1,495	3.5	818	2.0	907	1.5
Band neutrophils	9,607	22.5	3,681	9.0	6,353	10.5
Neutrophils	19,001	44.5	26,176	64.0	40,232	66.5
Lymphocytes	1,708	4.0	2,250	5.5	3,025	5.0
Monocytes	10,675	25.0	7,362	18.0	9,377	15.5
Eosinophils	0	0.0	0	0.0	302	0.5
Unclassified cells	213	0.5	409	1.0	302	0.5
Degenerated cells	0	0.0	204	0.5	0	0.0
Plasma						
Proteins (g/dl)	4.8		7.9		8.1	
Icterus index units	15		10		10	
Other Tests						
Blood urea nitrogen (mg/dl)	32		30		33	
SGPT (IU/L)	63		—		150	
van den Bergh:						
Total bilirubin (mg/dl)	0.7		—		—	
Direct reacting	0.2		—		—	
Indirect reacting	0.5		—		—	
Urine						
Specific gravity	1.030		1.021		1.024	
Protein	3+		2+		negative	
Bile	3+		3+		3+	
Urobilinogen	negative		negative		negative	
WBC/high dry field	10–15		0–4		10	
Casts/low-power field	occasional		occasional		5 coarse granular	

cluding neoplasias of the type present in this patient.

Case 15 (Dog).   Leukemoid Reaction in Chronic Peritonitis

A spayed female mixed-breed terrier, 5½ years old, had exhibited polydipsia, polyuria, and severe incontinence for 2 months. On arrival, the temperature was 101.9°F, pulse 160/minute, and respiration approximately 60/minute. The palpable lymph nodes were of normal size, the mucous membranes were somewhat pale, and the abdomen was distended. An attempt at fluid aspiration from the peritoneal cavity was unsuccessful. The hemograms revealed increasing leukocytosis with left shift, pointing to the possibility of suppuration. An exploratory laparotomy revealed an extensive granulomatous peritonitis involving all serous surfaces in the abdominal cavity. Nocardiosis was suspected but not definitely verified. The patient died on the seventh day after surgery. Necropsy findings failed to elucidate the cause of the peritonitis.

Interpretation

1. The first hemogram directed attention to the possibility of a chronic infection with associated normocytic-normochromic anemia from toxic depression of erythropoiesis. The marked left shift without significant elevation of total leukocyte numbers indicated toxic depression of granulopoiesis.

2. The very marked increase in total leukocyte count in the second hemogram, with immature neutrophils outnumbering the mature neutrophils, without an apparent significant change in the physical condition of the dog, caused some thought to be given to the possibility of a granulocytic leukemia.

Case 15 (Dog).   Chronic Peritonitis

	November 5		November 15		November 19	
Erythrocytes						
RBC ($\times 10^6/\mu$l)	4.10		3.9		3.75	
Hemoglobin (g/dl)	10.6		8.6		8.4	
PCV (%)	29.0		25.0		25.0	
MCV (fl)	70.7		64.1		66.6	
MCHC (%)	36.6		34.4		33.6	
Erythrocyte sed. rate/1 hr	62/28 = 34+		69/36 = 33+		69/36 = 33+	
Nucleated RBC/100 WBC	0		0		0	
Reticulocytes (%)	0.2		1.0		—	
Anisocytosis	slight		slight		slight	
Polychromasia	rare		slight		slight	
Leptocytosis	moderate		moderate		moderate	
Leukocytes		%		%		%
WBC/μl	26,800		104,000		61,400	
Myeloblasts	rare		rare		rare	
Progranulocytes	268	1.0	rare		rare	
Myelocytes	402	1.5	1,040	1.0	307	0.5
Metamyelocytes	2,814	10.5	23,400	22.5	6,140	10.0
Band neutrophils	4,556	17.0	36,920	35.5	20,569	33.5
Neutrophils	8,978	33.5	38,480	37.0	26,402	43.0
Lymphocytes	2,412	9.0	1,560	1.5	4,298	7.0
Monocytes	7,236	27.0	2,600	2.5	2,456	4.0
Eosinophils	0	0.0	0	0.0	0	0.0
Unclassified cells	134	0.5	0	0.0	1,228	2.0

Leukocyte morphology: The cytoplasm is blue to gray and somewhat granular in metamyelocytes and most band neutrophils. These are signs of toxic interference with maturation. An occasional neutrophil presents a double nucleus. This reflects failure of the cell to divide after division of the nucleus. It is an additional indication of toxemic disease.

	November 5	November 15	November 19
Plasma			
Protein (g/dl)	7.5	6.9	6.9
Icterus index units	2	2	2
Urine			
Specific gravity	1.007	—	1.002

However, the evidence of toxemic disease as revealed by basophilia and double nuclei in neutrophils continued to support the original conclusion that the disease was of inflammatory nature.

3. The progressive anemia, marked leukocytosis, "toxic" neutrophils, and immature neutrophils in excess of mature forms called for an unfavorable prognosis.

Case 16 (Dog).   Granulocytic Leukemia

A spayed female German shepherd, 2½ years old, had exhibited anorexia, depression, and signs of anemia about 6 months previously. It was given a blood transfusion and appeared to improve to near normal. The illness made its appearance again with extreme weakness, anemia, and temperature elevations of 103° to 105°F. A stained blood film was sent to us for examination and consultation. It was apparent from the film that the condition possibly was an infrequently occurring form of leukemia involving the neutrophilic granulocytes. The dog was hospitalized; it died within 2 weeks. Temperature during this period was undulating between 101.7° and 104.4°F. Three blood transfu-

sions of 250 ml each were administered during this period, and antibiotics were given twice daily.

Necropsy. The integument was icteric. The liver was mottled, yellow, and softened and histologically presented central necrosis and many portal and sinusoidal accumulations of immature to mature cells of the granulocytic series. The spleen was 30 cm long by 13 cm at the widest part and weighed 400 g. There was intense infiltration of the pulp by the neoplastic cells. Tonsils and lymph nodes were also heavily infiltrated, as was the cortical region of the kidneys. The central portion of the thyroid gland was invaded with the type cells. Diagnosis: Granulocytic leukemia.

Interpretation

1. Granulocytic leukemia is an infrequently encountered form of the leukemia complex. Note that the hemograms in this case show some similarity to those in Case 15.
2. The marked fall in total blood leukocyte count in a period of 5 days is interesting. However, all stages in the maturation series of the granulocytes persisted. Such extreme variations in leukocyte numbers may occur

Case 16 (Dog).   Granulocytic Leukemia

	May 23		May 28		Bone Marrow Aspiration May 23	No.	%
Erythrocytes							
RBC (($\times 10^6/\mu$l)	1.21		2.52		Rubriblast	0	0.0
Hemoglobin (g/dl)	2.7		5.5		Prorubricyte	0	0.0
PCV (%)	9		17		Basophilic rubricyte	7	1.4
MCV (fl)	74.4		67.5		Polychromatophilic rub.	1	0.2
MCHC (%)	30.0		32.4		Metarubricyte	5	1.0
Erythrocyte sed. rate/1 hr	88/73 = 15+		73/58 = 15+		Total erythrocytic =	13	2.6
Anisocytosis	marked		moderate				
Reticulocytes	0		0		Myeloblast	0	0.0
Nucleated RBC	rare		none		Progranulocyte	18	3.6
					Myelocyte, neut.	55	11.0
Leukocytes		%		%	Myelocyte, eos.	6	1.2
WBC/μl	116,000		18,750		Metamyelocyte, neut.	40	8.0
Blast cells	3,712	3.2	562	3.0	Metamyelocyte, eos.	12	2.4
Progranulocytes	2,784	2.4	656	3.5	Band, neutrophils	39	7.8
Myelocytes	2,784	2.4	1,218	6.5	Band, eosinophils	4	0.8
Metamyelocytes	1,160	1.0	843	4.5	Neutrophils	284	56.8
Band neutrophils	812	0.7	562	3.0	Eosinophils	0	0.0
Neutrophils	53,940	46.5	6,375	34.0	Mitotic neutrophils	2	0.4
Lymphocytes	22,852	19.7	7,781	41.5	Degenerated neut.	8	1.6
Monocytes	26,216	22.6	375	2.0	Total granulocytic	468	93.6
Eosinophils	464	0.4	0	0.0			
Degenerated cells	0	0.0	281	1.5	M:E ratio = 468/13 = 36:1.0		
Unclassified cells	1,276	1.1	93	0.5	Hematogones	7	1.4
Thrombocytes	abnormal morphology				Lymphocytes	3	0.6
					Monocytes	2	0.4
Icterus index units	2		not recorded		Degenerated cells	7	1.4
						19	3.8

as a result of cyclic fluctuations in production and release of granulocytes from the bone marrow as reported in humans with myelogenous leukemia. A second bone marrow examination on May 28 would have been interesting to evaluate for this purpose.

3. The extreme anemia and marked depression of erythrogenesis as observed in the bone marrow should be noted.

4. Although a platelet count was not done, thrombocytopenia is to be anticipated in granulocytic leukemia, and in some such cases platelet morphology may be abnormal.

5. The differential cell count of bone marrow demonstrated marked proliferation of granulocytic series cells and marked suppression of erythrocytic maturation series (Plate XXIII–4).

Case 17 (Dog).   Polycythemia Vera

An intact female Old English sheepdog, 14 months old, was referred with a tentative diagnosis of polycythemia vera. Laboratory data accompanying the dog indicated a PCV of 80.3% and a WBC of 19,500/μl of blood.

On admission, the body temperature was 101.2°F, and the pulse rate was 100/min. The conjunctival and oral mucous membranes were intensely red, the result of engorgement of the blood vessels. The dog weighed 21.8 kg.

Hemograms. The admission hemogram agreed with the accompanying laboratory data in that the PCV was 83%, Hb was 29.6 g/dl; RBC count was 13.78 $\times$ 10^6/μl; WBC was 9,900/μl; and a modest thrombocytopenia of 94,000/μl was present. Numerous hemograms were made on this dog to follow results of phlebotomy. Five representative hemograms are presented.

Radiography revealed hypervascularity of lung fields, hepatomegaly, and possibly a minor degree of right heart enlargement. Cardiac evaluation results were within normal limits.

Blood gas values were Po_2 90.0 mmHg; Pco_2, 24.5 mmHg; pH, 7.60; CO_2CT, 19.3 mM/L; and HCO_3, 18.7 mEq/L.

Blood volume studies with Evans blue and ^{51}Cr gave plasma volume of 54.0 ml/kg, RBC volume of 106.0 ml/kg, and total blood volume of 160.0 ml/kg. Normal blood volume is usually 80 to 90 ml/kg.

Erythrocyte fragility test was normal, with beginning hemolysis at 0.55% and complete hemolysis at 0.30% buffered NaCl solution.

Erythrocyte kinetics. Erythrocyte ^{51}Cr T$\frac{1}{2}$ = 56 days. ^{59}Fe transfer rate was 8.88 mg/100 ml/day.

Treatment. Reduction of erythrocyte volume was accomplished by periodic phlebotomy. Beginning on April 10 and continuing through April 16, 300 ml of blood was withdrawn on six separate occasions. On April 13 and 16, blood was removed both

Case 17 (Dog).   **Polycythemia Vera**

	March 23		March 30		April 9		April 17		April 24	
Erythrocytes										
RBC ($\times 10^6/\mu$l)	13.78		12.94		13.92		7.30		7.07	
Hemoglobin (g/dl)	29.6		28.0		27.6		14.5		14.8	
PCV (%)	83.0		80.0		80.0		43.0		45.0	
MCV (fl)	60.2		61.8		57.5		58.9		63.6	
MCHC (%)	35.6		35.0		34.5		33.7		32.9	
MCH (pg)	21.4		21.6		19.9		19.9		20.9	
Erythrocyte sed. rate/1 hr	0		0		0		0/7 = 7−		not recorded	
Nucleated RBC/100 WBC	0		2		0		0		0	
Reticulocytes (%)	—		0.8		—		0.8		—	
Anisocytosis	slight		slight		slight		slight		slight	
Polychromasia	slight		slight		slight		slight		slight	
Leukocytes		%		%		%		%		%
WBC/μl	9,900		8,600		10,300		9,300		10,300	
Band neutrophils	0	0.0	172	2.0	0	0.0	0	0.0	0	0.0
Neutrophils	5,940	60.0	5,504	64.0	5,099	49.5	5,766	62.0	5,459	53.0
Lymphocytes	2,673	27.0	2,150	25.0	4,120	40.0	2,371	25.5	3,039	29.5
Monocytes	693	7.0	688	8.0	618	6.0	558	6.0	463	4.5
Eosinophils	594	6.0	86	1.0	463	4.5	605	6.5	1,287	12.5
Basophils	0	0.0	0	0.0	0	0.0	0	0.0	51	0.5
Plasma										
Total plasma proteins (g/dl)	7.0		6.8		6.7		4.6		6.7	
Fibrinogen (g/dl)	0.2		0.2		0.2		0.1		0.3	
Icterus index units	2 (slight hemolysis)		2 (slight hemolysis)		5 (slight hemolysis)		5		5	
Thrombocytes/μl	94,000		90,000		—		—		352,000	

in the morning and again in the afternoon. The PCV was reduced from 83.0% to 45.0%. The dog was discharged on April 29. The referring veterinarian reported an increase in PCV to 57% on May 13 and to 72% by June 29. By the periodic removal of 500 ml of blood, the PCV was maintained at 40% to 52%. A lapse of 6 to 8 weeks between phlebotomies resulted in the elevation of the PCV to 70%.

Interpretation

1. A marked polycythemia was evident in the initial hemogram. Leukocytosis and thrombocytosis, however, were not present as is commonly the case in polycythemia vera of humans (see Chapter 21).
2. The arterial O_2 tension was normal (Po_2 = 90 mmHg) indicating that the polycythemia was primary and not due to a lowered O_2 tension secondary to lung or cardiac disease. The normal radiographic and cardiovascular findings confirmed the absence of lung or cardiac disease.
3. The erythrocyte and plasma volume studies indicated an absolute increase in RBC and total blood volume characteristic of polycythemia vera.
4. The erythrocyte fragility was normal, although the erythrocyte half-life of 56 days was somewhat longer than normal. The ^{59}Fe transfer rate indicated a marked acceleration of erythropoiesis, which further characterizes polycythemia vera.

5. The accelerated rate of erythrocyte production in the presence of a normal arterial O_2 tension and an increased red cell mass support the diagnosis of polycythemia vera.
6. In addition, blood erythropoietin levels can be measured to determine the erythropoietin-independent nature of primary polycythemia vera.
7. The hypoproteinemia on April 17 was the result of circulatory loss as well as hemodilution in response to repeated phlebotomy between April 13 and 16.

Case 18 (Dog).   Secondary Polycythemia Due to Tetralogy of Fallot

A 4-year-old intact English bulldog, weighing 20 kg, was presented with the complaint of dyspnea, cyanosis, polyphagia, polydipsia, and polyuria. Body temperature was normal.

Physical Examination. Dyspnea was not noticeable at rest, but cyanosis due to engorgement of blood vessels was marked. The pulse rate was 150/min, and respiratory rate was 29/min and of the abdominal type. There was a grade-2 systolic heart murmur heard over the left chest at the fourth interspace. The dog would walk only a few steps and then rest. An initial hemogram revealed a PCV of 83%, RBC of 13.06 × $10^6/\mu$l and Hb of 28.2 g/dl.

Cardiac Angiography. Multiple films were taken at 0.5-sec intervals after injection of a contrast medium through a catheter placed into the right ventricle. The findings were consistent with the pres-

Case 18 (Dog). **Polycythemia Due to Tetralogy of Fallot**

	Dec. 16, 1968		Jan. 24, 1969		Feb. 27, 1969[a]		April 16, 1969		July 9, 1969	
Erythrocytes										
RBC ($\times 10^6/\mu$l)	13.06		13.26		7.49		12.81		14.52	
Hemoglobin (g/dl)	28.2		26.6		14.8		21.6		20.3	
PCV (%)	83		83		49		69[b]		68	
MCV (fl)	63.5		62.6		65.4		53.9		46.8	
MCH (pg)	21.6		20.0		19.7		16.1		13.9	
MCHC (%)	34.0		32.0		30.2		31.3		29.9	
RBC sed. rate/1 hr	0/0 = 0		—		0/1 = 1−		0/0 = 0		0/0 = 0	
Nucleated RBC /100 WBC	2		1		0		0		0	
Anisocytosis	slight		slight		slight		slight		slight	
Polychromasia	slight		slight		slight		slight		slight	
Leukocytes		%		%		%		%		%
WBC/μl (corrected)	11,862		8,700		22,000		7,400		7,200	
Band neutrophils	0	0.0	261	3.0	330	1.0	74	1.0	72	1.0
Neutrophils	10,319	87.0	6,699	77.0	17,820	81.0	3,848	52.0	4,896	68.0
Lymphocytes	1,186	10.0	783	9.0	990	4.5	1,332	18.0	864	12.0
Monocytes	0	0.0	783	9.0	2,640	12.0	592	8.0	576	8.0
Eosinophils	355	3.0	174	2.0	220	1.0	1,554	21.0	792	11.0
Plasma										
Plasma proteins (g/dl)	9.5		7.2		6.9		7.8		8.2	
Fibrinogen (g/dl)	0.5		0.3		0.5		0.3		0.4	
Icterus index units	hemolyzed		5		5		5		5	
Blood urea nitrogen (mg/dl)	31.8		30.0		—		39.0		—	
Urine										
Specific gravity	1.008		1.010		—		1.028		—	
Protein	1+		1+		—		2+		—	

[a]After withdrawal of 1,100 ml of blood and corrective surgery (blood withdrawn over 10-day period).
[b]After withdrawal of 1,100 ml of blood between April 18 and 25, PCV was 44% on April 29.

ence of a right-to-left shunt through a septal defect with marked holdup of the contrast medium within the pulmonary artery. The changes were compatible with tetralogy of Fallot.

Blood Volume. Plasma volume based on Evans blue was 62.5 ml/kg. The RBC volume was determined with ^{51}Cr to be 100.5 ml/kg. Total blood volume was 163.0 ml/kg. Normal blood volume is usually reported to be 80 to 90 ml/kg. Arterial blood oxygen saturation was 65% and 69% in two blood gas studies.

Other Findings. The dog developed a persistent ulcer of the right cornea, and urine analysis indicated continuous mild proteinuria associated with blood urea nitrogen levels of 23.2 to 48.6 mg/dl. Erythrocyte osmotic fragility test was normal, and ^{51}Cr T½ was 28 days.

Treatment. Phlebotomies were performed as follows: Feb. 10, 200 ml; Feb. 11, 250 ml; Feb. 13, 400 ml; and Feb. 19, 250 ml. The dog was hydrated on Feb. 14 with 500 ml of lactated Ringer's solution b.i.d. and 500 ml on Feb. 15, s.i.d. On Feb. 25, corrective surgery was attempted; the left pulmonary artery was anastomosed to the descending aorta. Temporary improvement followed, but polycythemia developed again, with PCV attaining a value of 69% by April 16. Periodic phlebotomy was employed to maintain the PCV between 50% and 60%. The dog collapsed and died on the following Jan. 28, 1 hour after a routine phlebotomy.

Interpretation

1. Compensatory polycythemia developed as a result of the right-to-left shunt of blood, which allowed a portion of venous blood to bypass the lungs, resulting in hypoxemia. The low arterial oxygen saturation of 65% and 69% reflected the failure of all blood to circulate through the lungs.
2. The increase in erythrocyte number and total volume to compensate for the induced hypoxemia was reflected in the congested and cyanotic mucous membranes.
3. Erythrocyte size (MCV) was minimum normal and microcytic at times. This possibly reflected a compensating effect due to the markedly increased numbers of erythrocytes. MCHC and MCH decrease in parallel with repeated blood withdrawal, suggesting some depletion of body iron stores.
4. Total leukocyte count was mostly in the low normal range, with persistent lymphopenia. The stress pattern of neutrophilia, monocytosis, and lymphopenia was manifested in the hemogram of Feb. 27, taken 2 days after the attempt at corrective surgery.

Case 19 (Dog). **Acute Internal Blood Loss in Hemangiosarcoma**

A male cocker spaniel, 7 years old, was presented because of abdominal enlargement of 1

Case 19 (Dog).   Hemangiosarcoma

	Jan. 22		Jan. 28		Jan. 30	
Erythrocytes						
RBC ($\times 10^6/\mu$l)	1.83		2.30		1.08	
Hemoglobin (g/dl)	4.5		5.9		2.5	
PCV (%)	18.0		20.0		11.0	
MCV (fl)	98.3		87.0		102.0	
MCHC (%)	25.0		29.5		22.7	
Erythrocyte sed. rate/1 hr	markedly diphasic		2/49 = 47 −		1/76 = 75 −	
Reticulocytes (%)	24.8		20.2		33.2	
Nucleated RBC/100 WBC	8.5		24.5		15.5	
Anisocytosis	marked		marked		marked	
Polychromasia	marked		marked		marked	
Howell-Jolly bodies	few		few		few	
Leptocytes (macrocytic)	many		moderate		moderate	
Leukocytes		%		%		%
WBC/μl (corrected)	28,700		14,100		28,500	
Band neutrophils	1,004	3.5	141	1.0	2,280	8.0
Neutrophils	22,099	77.0	10,716	76.0	22,800	80.0
Lymphocytes	1,722	6.0	2,044	14.5	570	2.0
Monocytes	3,875	13.5	1,199	8.5	2,280	8.0
Eosinophils	0	0.0	0	0.0	0	0.0
Degenerated cells	0	0.0	0	0.0	570	2.0
Plasma						
Protein (g/dl)	8.1		7.7		6.7	
Icterus index units	10		10		7.5	

Rib marrow at necropsy

Rubriblasts	4	0.8%
Prorubricytes	11	2.2
Basophilic rubricytes	53	10.6
Mitotic rubricytes	2	0.4
Polychromatic rubricytes	219	43.8
Mitotic polychromatic rubricytes	4	0.8
Metarubricytes	10	2.0
Total erythrocytic cells	303	60.6
Myeloblasts	1	0.2
Progranulocytes	4	0.8
Myelocytes, neutrophilic	23	4.6
Myelocytes, eosinophilic	1	0.2
Metamyelocytes, neutrophilic	31	6.2
Band neutrophils	30	6.0
Band eosinophils	2	0.4
Neutrophils	24	4.8
Total granulocytic cells	116	23.2
Hematogones	9	1.8
Lymphocytes	0	0.0
Plasma cells	1	0.2
Monocytes	1	0.2
RE nuclei	9	1.8
Degenerated cells	61	12.2
Total other cells	81	16.2

Myeloid:erythroid ratio = 0.38:1.0

week's duration. Appetite was normal. The dog was less active than usual but not listless. The mucous membranes were pale; there was an inspiratory dyspnea, the temperature was 102.4° F, pulse 126/min. The distended abdomen was not painful on palpation and did not appear on first examination to contain an excess of fluid. The first hemogram, however, demonstrated a well-advanced macrocytic hypochromic anemia with intense erythrogenesis. This directed attention to the likelihood of blood loss into the abdominal cavity. An attempt at paracentesis produced 5 ml of blood fluid (Jan. 23) that compared favorably with peripheral blood with respect to erythrocyte content. The dog's condition deteriorated during the following week. Finally, on Jan. 30 an exploratory laparotomy was performed. Numerous blood-filled, pea- to grape-size tumor implants were found throughout the peritoneal cavity. Euthanasia was performed.

Necropsy. In addition to the extensive distribution of tumor implants in the peritoneal cavity, tumor implants were scattered throughout the lungs and were associated with bleeding into the thoracic cavity. Neoplastic foci were present also in the hepatic and sternal lymph nodes. The spleen and liver were not involved. The primary site was not definitely established.

Interpretation

1. The very intense bone marrow response to compensate for the continuing escape of erythrocytes into the body cavities and tissues was reflected in the massive movement of large, immature erythrocytes (reticulocytes) into the circulation. This movement was reflected in the stained blood film by the macrocytic leptocytes, many of which stained blue or gray as a result of incomplete hemoglobin synthesis. Bone marrow taken from a rib at necropsy further exhibited the intense erythrogenesis in the M:E ratio of 0.38:1.0. It is of interest that most of the cells were in the polychromatic rubricyte stage, and a few were in the final nucleated metarubricyte stage. This indicates that under the intense demand for erythrocytes in peripheral blood, the cells were released primarily as polychromatophilic erythrocytes and bypassed the metarubricyte stage.
2. The diphasic erythrocyte sedimentation rate in the first hemogram and the large negative value for the corrected rates in the second and third hemograms are an expression of the nonclumping characteristic of immature RBCs (Plate I-2).
3. A neutrophilia with left shift of magnitudes far greater than that seen here may be anticipated in association with intensification of erythrogenesis of the degree displayed.
4. The progressive loss of blood is also reflected in the falling plasma proteins.

5. The final hemogram reflects the crisis of Jan. 30 in the extremely low RBC, PCV, and hemoglobin concentration. The severe systemic stress was also expressed in the frank lymphopenia.
6. Despite the very large loss of erythrocytes into the body cavities and tissues, the icterus index remained low. The urine gave a very strong reaction for bile pigment. Thus, much of the conjugated bilirubin from hemoglobin degradation was escaping into the urine.

Case 20 (Dog). Blood Loss From Gastrointestinal Hemorrhage

An intact male beagle, 11 years old, was referred with the accompanying history: The dog was treated with antibiotics for a cough considered to be due to bronchitis. The coughing disappeared in 1 week, but later the owner noticed that the dog was very weak. The consulting veterinarian found the dog to be anemic and noticed some blood in its stool. Over a period of 3 weeks, iron, vitamin B_{12}, and three whole-blood transfusions were administered. There was no vomiting or diarrhea, and the dog seemed to improve. For 3 days before admission, however, the dog had been anorectic and unable to walk.

Interpretation

1. The hemogram was representative of blood loss due to a bleeding intestinal tumor. The significant findings were an advanced anemia in remission, as indicated by macrocytic hypochromic erythrocytes (MCV and MCHC), accompanied by active reticulocytosis (32.0%) and the occurrence of nucleated erythrocytes in peripheral blood. In addition, the stained film revealed moderate anisocytosis and polychromasia.
2. Total plasma proteins of 6.4 g/dl further substantiated blood loss. The normal value for an 11-year-old dog would be 7.5 g/dl or greater.
3. The presence of a significant lesion was indicated by the elevated fibrinogen and a positive corrected erythrocyte sedimentation rate. A negative corrected value would be the rule in the face of 32% reticulocytes in the absence of a serious lesion.
4. The nature of the feces further indicated bleeding. Existence of a neoplasm was verified by the barium series. The dog made an uneventful recovery after removal of the tumor.

Case 21 (Dog). Dicumarol (Warfarin) Poisoning

A male Labrador retriever, 3 months old, was presented with a history of having been seen eating warfarin. The dog was severely depressed, had been vomiting, and was constipated; the mucous

Case 20 (Dog). Gastrointestinal Hemorrhage

	Admission Hemogram	Other Data
Erythrocytes		
RBC ($\times 10^6/\mu$l)	2.04	
Hemoglobin (g/dl)	4.6	
PCV	17.0	
MCV (fl)	83.3	
MCHC (%)	27.1	
RBC sed. rate/1 hr	65/58 = 7+	
Reticulocytes (%)	32.0	Many thrombocytes seen on blood film
Nucleated RBC/100 WBC	10.5	Coombs test: negative
Anisocytosis	moderate	LE cells: none seen
Polychromasia	moderate	Fecal examination: Blackish-green (tarry) color; no
Hypochromasia	moderate	parasitic ova seen; occult blood test = 4+
Leptocytosis	marked	
Howell-Jolly bodies	few	
Leukocytes		%	
WBC/μl (corrected)	17,800	
Band neutrophils	356	2.0	
Neutrophils	12,282	69.0	
Lymphocytes	1,513	8.5	GI tract barium series: detected a mass occluding the
Monocytes	3,204	18.0	ascending duodenum
Eosinophils	445	2.5	
			Histopathology: a leiomyoma with ulcerated bleeding
			surface
Plasma		
Icterus index units	2	
Plasma proteins (g/dl)	6.4	
Fibrinogen (g/dl)	0.7	
Blood urea nitrogen (mg/dl)	23.2	

membranes were pale, but there was no external evidence of hemorrhage. The pulse was 180/minute, respiration 56/minute, and temperature was 102.4° F. A blood transfusion of 120 ml ws administered immediately, as was vitamin K. The only hemogram was taken the following day (Nov. 3), and considerable difficulty was experienced in controlling bleeding from the venipuncture. A hematoma formed extending from the olecranon to distal to the carpus. Three days later, another hematoma was observed on the right flank. The dog exhibited signs of pain when moving that may have been referable to the escape of blood into the joints. On Nov. 7, the mucous membranes again appeared pale, pulse was 220/minute, and rectal temperature was 102.6° F. A second transfusion of

100 ml of whole blood was given, but the clinician in charge did not submit a sample to the laboratory for a hemogram. Recovery thereafter was rapid and uneventful.

Interpretation

1. The toxic effect of dicumarol is an interference with the enzyme system needed to recycle vitamin K required as a cofactor for activation of precursor forms of coagulation factors produced by the liver—factors II, VII, IX, and X. See Chapter 14 for diagnostic tests and therapy of vitamin K antagonism.

2. The hemogram is typical of a blood-loss disease with escape of blood from the body or into the tissues. This is reflected in the well-

Case 21 (Dog). Dicumarol Poisoning

	Nov. 3			
Erythrocytes		*Leukocytes*		%
RBC ($\times 10^6/\mu$l)	1.69	WBC/μl (corrected)	14,200	
Hemoglobin (g/dl)	4.2	Band neutrophils	355	2.5
PCV (%)	15.0	Neutrophils	7,881	55.5
MCV (fl)	88.7	Lymphocytes	4,686	33.0
MCHC (%)	28.0	Monocytes	1,136	8.0
Icterus index units	7.5	Eosinophils	0	0.0
Nucleated RBC/100 WBC	2.5	Degenerated cells	142	1.0
Reticulocytes (%)	9.2			
Anisocytosis	moderate	Thrombocytes/μl	74,000	
Polychromasia	moderate	Plasma proteins (g/dl)	5.2	

advanced anemia and low total plasma protein concentration.

3. Bone marrow response to the blood loss into the tissues was indicated by the presence in peripheral blood of macrocytic erythrocytes (MCV 88.7 fl), polychromasia, and reticulocytosis of 9–10%.

4. The leukogram did not suggest a severe systemic stress, as neutrophils were not elevated and both lymphocytes and monocytes were in their high normal range. Eosinophils are not normally present in large numbers in young dogs. Thus the absence of this cell from the differential leukocyte count does not necessarily mean depression by natural corticoids.

5. The thrombocytopenia can be explained on the basis of blood loss and consumption to prevent blood loss.

Case 22 (Dog). Rodenticide and Aspirin Intoxication

A 4-year-old poodle was referred for evaluation of purpura. The owners remarked that previously she appeared to bruise easily, but they had noticed more bruising during the past 5 days. She had been spayed 2 years before and had had dental extractions 1 year before, both without difficulties. History included involvement in a bicycle accident 10 months before and subsequent occasional pain during ambulation.

Laboratory findings included: platelet count, 280,000/μl; bleeding time, 65 min (control up to 8 min); prothrombin time (PT), 65 sec (control 12 sec); partial thromboplastin time (PTT), 60 sec (control 28 sec); thrombin time (TT), 12 sec (control 11.5 sec); and Stypven (Russell's viper venom) time, 38 sec (control 15 sec). Liver function and enzyme tests were all normal. Coagulation factor assays revealed values of: normal, >70%; Factor II, 10%; Factor V, 76%; Factor VII, 15%; Factor VIII, 86%; Factor IX, 25%; and Factor X, 15%.

Interpretation

1. Coumarin (warfarin) intoxication was diagnosed from the abnormal test results of PT, PTT, and Stypven time and diminished concentrations of vitamin K-dependent coagulation factors II, VII, IX, and X. Since fibrinogen is not affected, TT was normal.

2. A deficiency of vitamin K-dependent coagulation factors does not affect the platelet or vascular phases of hemostasis, and because the platelet count was normal, the prolonged bleeding time thus was surprising. During the office visit, the owners were asked if the dog had received any "drugs" recently. They said no. After the test results were examined, the owners were again asked the same question, and again a negative reply was elicited. When asked if aspirin had been administered, the reply was "Of course, we gave her an aspirin whenever she had difficulty walking and have been doing so since the bicycle accident." Owners sometimes fail to concede that aspirin is a drug. Aspirin, salicylates in general, and phenylbutazone affect platelet function by inhibiting prostaglandin synthesis, and thus adenosine diphosphate (ADP) release, for the life of the circulating platelet. Consequently bleeding time is prolonged.

3. Therapy in dogs for coumarin toxicosis is directed at replacing vitamin K. Vitamin K_1 is administered orally or subcutaneously (never intravenously or intramuscularly because of dangers of anaphylaxis and intramuscular hemorrhage) at a dosage of 2 mg/kg divided twice daily for 5 days. There is no therapy except for "tincture of time" for excessive aspirin ingestion. Fresh plasma is given intravenously when a coumarin toxicosis patient is hemorrhaging. (See Chapter 14 for details of vitamin K therapy.)

Case 23 (Dog). Thrombocytopenic Purpura, Possibly Due to Sensitivity to Administered Drugs

A male Samoyed, 1½ years old, had been hit by an automobile 7 months earlier. The dog had lost its left ear, and a hole remained over the left frontal sinus. The tissue wounds had healed rapidly, but the bone injury with opening into the sinus persisted. The dog was in excellent condition, and no presurgical hemogram was requested. On March 4, periosteal strips and rib bone were removed from three ribs on the left side and laid down in a lattice held in place over the head wound by connective tissue. Bleeding from the left nostril was noticed for 24 hours, but it was not extensive. Penicillin, streptomycin, and chlorpromazine were administered twice daily. The dose of chlorpromazine was 100 mg the first day, increased to 150 mg total daily dose on the second and third day, after which it was discontinued. The antibiotics were discontinued on the sixth day. On the seventh day, a hematoma formed (200 cc) in the region of the head wound; the following day, the dog was coughing, and many hemorrhages occurred in the skin over the body. At this time, the temperature was 103.3° F, pulse 160/min and respiration 80/min. The first hemogram obtained at this time demonstrated complete absence of thrombocytes and a marked bone marrow response to blood loss. Further treatment was directed at controlling hemorrhage and giving blood transfusions as needed.

Interpretation

1. Cause of the spontaneous development of thrombocytopenia was not apparent but was thought possibly to have been the result of response to drugs and/or antibiotics in a particularly sensitive dog.

2. All responses in the hemogram were those to be anticipated following massive hemor-

Case 23 (Dog). **Thrombocytopenic Purpura**

	March 13 (2nd hemogram)		March 15 (4th hemogram)		March 16 (5th hemogram)		March 21 (9th hemogram)		April 8 (19th hemogram)	
Erythrocytes										
RBC ($\times 10^6/\mu$l)	2.03		2.45		4.00		4.25		4.93	
Hemoglobin (g/dl)	4.4		5.5		8.6		10.5		11.3	
PCV (%)	17.0		20.0		29.0		35.0		38.0	
MCV (fl)	83.7		81.6		72.5		82.3		77.0	
MCHC (%)	25.9		27.5		29.7		30.0		29.7	
Erythrocyte sed. rate/1 hr	not done		9/49 = 40−		22/28 = 6−		16/16 = 0 diphasic		8/12 = 4−	
Reticulocytes (%)	19.0		27.0		15.0		5.6		not done	
Nucleated RBC/100 WBC	7.5		18.0		6.0		0.5		none seen	
Anisocytosis	prominent		prominent		prominent		moderate		slight	
Polychromasia	prominent		prominent		moderate		slight		slight	
Howell-Jolly bodies	few		few		few		none seen		none seen	
Thrombocytes	none seen		none seen		few present		numerous		numerous	
Leukocytes		%		%		%		%		%
WBC/μl (corrected)	67,400		73,900		53,100		44,000		16,800	
Metamyelocytes	2,022	3.0	739	1.0	0	0.0	0	0.0	0	0.0
Band neutrophils	6,066	9.0	7,760	10.5	1,328	2.5	440	1.0	0	0.0
Neutrophils	46,169	68.5	50,621	68.5	43,011	81.0	33,660	76.5	12,180	72.5
Lymphocytes	6,403	9.5	4,065	5.5	1,858	3.5	1,980	4.5	2,772	16.5
Monocytes	6,740	10.0	9,977	13.5	6,638	12.5	7,920	18.0	588	3.5
Eosinophils	0	0.0	369	0.5	265	0.5	0	0.0	1,260	7.5
Unclassified cells	0	0.0	369	0.5	0	0.0	0	0.0	0	0.0

Blood administered = 250 ml, Mar. 12; 450 ml, Mar. 13; 400 ml, Mar. 15.

Plasma										
Protein (g/dl)	5.0		5.6		6.9		5.8		6.0	
Icterus index units	hemolyzed		hemolyzed		hemolyzed		2		2	

Coagulation Studies

Lee and White	12½ minutes	— — — —
Clot retraction	None (repeated March 19 with good retraction in 90 minutes; control 60 minutes: test conducted at 37° C).	

rhage, e.g., macrocytic hypochromic erythrocytes, prominent anisocytosis and polychromasia, reticulocytosis, occurrence of rubricytes in peripheral blood, leukocytosis with left shift, and low plasma proteins. The initial lymphocytosis was unexplained in view of the clinical state of the dog, which would normally be associated with stress.

3. Two weeks after chlorpromazine administration was stopped and 11 days after antibiotics were stopped, numerous platelets were present in the circulation. Thus platelet numbers increased rapidly after their first appearance in the blood on March 16.

4. Recovery was uneventful after the return of platelets in normal numbers to the circulation.

Case 24 (Dog). Idiopathic Thrombocytopenic Purpura (Hypersplenism)

A white miniature poodle, female, 2 years old, was referred on July 22 with the history of bleeding from the upper gums since May 10 following an injury to the tissues while chewing on a bone. The dog had been under treatment for 3 months for an

anemia associated with thrombocytopenia and leukocytosis characterized by a regenerative left shift. The body temperature was normal on all examinations. Treatment had consisted of vitamins (including vitamin C), hematinics, and corticoids, with no improvement. Fecal examination had been negative for parasite ova but strongly positive for occult blood. However, with bleeding in the mouth, the latter reaction would be anticipated from the continuous swallowing of blood. The dog had been kept in the house with no opportunity to consume chemical poisons, and there was no history of therapeutic use of drugs prior to first detection of the anemia. A radiograph on July 7 had revealed an enlarged spleen.

On arrival, the rectal temperature was 103.2° F, pulse 200/min, and respiration rapid. The elevated temperature was perhaps referable to excitement from a 100-mile car ride and the high ambient temperature. Under hospitalization, the temperature fluctuated between 98.3° and 102.4° F. The mucous membranes were white, there was bleeding from the margins of the gums around the upper incisors, large ecchymotic hemorrhages were present over the body, especially in the inguinal and axillary

Case 24 (Dog). **Bone Marrow Nucleated Cell Count (July 24)**

Erythrocytic Series			Granulocytic Series			Other Cells		
Rubriblast	3	0.6%	Myeloblast	3	0.6%	Hematogone	5	1.0%
Prorubricyte	1	0.2	Progranulocyte	11	2.2	Lymphocytes	7	1.4
Basophilic rubricyte	23	4.6	Myelocyte (neut.)	14	2.8	Plasma cell	1	0.2
Polychrom. rubricyte	88	17.6	Myelocyte (eos.)	7	1.4	Monocyte	3	0.6
Metarubricyte[a]	112	22.4	Metamyelocyte (neut.)	48	9.6	RE nuclei	5	1.0
Mitotic rubricyte	3	0.6	Metamyelocyte (eos.)	3	0.6	Mitotic cell	1	0.2
Total erythroid =	230	46.0	Band neutrophil	80	16.0	Degenerated	4	0.8
			Segmenter neutrophil	74	14.8	Megakaryocytes	0	0.0
			Eosinophil	4	0.8	Total other =	26	5.2
M:E ratio = 1.05:1.0			Total granulocytic =	244	48.8			

Peripheral blood total leukocyte count = 52,500 with 74.5% neutrophils.

[a]Polychromatophilic

areas, and the spleen appeared to be moderately enlarged.

Preliminary blood studies (July 22) indicated the blood type to be A positive, Coombs test negative, advanced anemia in active remission, an absence of thrombocytes in the stained blood film and no megakaryocytes on scanning of the entire stained film of bone marrow aspirated from the iliac crest. Blood clotting and coagulation tests (July 24) indicated normal coagulation—Lee and White method, 6 minutes; prothrombin time, 8.5 seconds

(control, 8.0 seconds)—but the clot remained soft with no retraction in 24 hours. The latter finding correlated with an absence of thrombocytes in the blood. On the basis of history and blood studies, it was concluded that the spleen was possibly actively involved in causing the thrombocytopenia. Splenectomy was performed on July 24 and was accompanied by transfusion of blood during surgery. The following day, the routine administration of antibiotics was initiated, and 7.5 mg of prednisolone was given orally b.i.d. Bleeding from the

Case 24 (Dog). **Idiopathic Thrombocytopenic Purpura in Hypersplenism**

	July 22		July 27		Aug. 3		Aug. 18		Sept. 23	
Erythrocytes										
RBC ($\times 10^6/\mu l$)	1.75		1.25		1.81		3.70		6.70	
Hemoglobin (g/dl)	4.9		2.3		4.0		8.8		13.9	
PCV (%)	18.0		11.0		18.0		27.0		42.0	
MCV (fl)	102.8		88.0		99.4		72.8		62.7	
MCHC (%)	27.2		20.9		22.2		32.6		33.1	
MCH (pg)	28.0		18.4		22.1		21.0		20.7	
ESR/1 hr	1/54 = 53−		2/76 = 74−		2/55 = 53− (diphasic)		5/32 = 27− (diphasic)		0/8 = 8−	
Reticulocytes (%)	56.8		18.0		8.8		7.6		2–3/oil field	
Nucleated RBC	27.5		8.0		0.5		0.0		0.0	
Anisocytosis	moderate		marked		moderate		moderate		slight	
Polychromasia	marked		marked		moderate		moderate		slight	
H-J bodies	few		few		few		rare		moderate	
Thrombocytes	none		none		63,000/μl		numerous		normal numbers	
Leukocytes		%		%		%		%		%
WBC/μl	52,500 (corrected)		119,500 (corrected)		78,000 (corrected)		21,350		11,900	
Metamyelocyte	0	0.0	2,390	2.0	0	0.0	0	0.0	0	0.0
Band neutrophils	2,362	4.5	19,718	16.5	390	0.5	214	1.0	60	0.5
Neutrophils	36,750	70.0	75,882	63.5	56,550	72.5	17,400	81.5	6,962	58.5
Lymphocytes	788	1.5	1,792	1.5	rare	0.0	1,815	8.5	2,082	17.5
Monocytes	8,138	15.5	18,552	15.5	21,060	27.0	1,922	9.0	1,309	11.0
Eosinophils	525	1.0	0	0.0	0	0.0	0	0.0	1,488	12.5
Degenerated cells	3,938	7.5	0	0.0	0	0.0	0	0.0	0	0.0
Blast cells	rare	0.0	598	0.5	0	0.0	0	0.0	0	0.0
Unclassified cells	0	0.0	0	0.0	0	0.0	0	0.0	0	0.0
Plasma										
Protein (g/dl)	5.4 (spurious)[a]		4.0		7.0		6.5		7.5	
Icterus index units	lipemic		10		5		5		2	

[a]Not valid because of lipemic plasma.

mouth stopped on July 29, and the general condition continued to improve until Aug. 4, when depression became apparent. The depression persisted; a radiograph of the abdomen (Aug. 10) indicated the possibility of adhesions between loops of the intestine. An exploratory laparotomy revealed a mass of necrotic fat, 6 × 3 inches, at the site of the previous surgery. Rapid recovery followed removal of the necrotic fat mass. A progress check on Sept. 23 revealed that the dog had been active and was gaining weight but that the white hair had started to fall out and was being replaced by red hair; there was some spotty skin pigmentation.

Simultaneous intensification of granulopoiesis and erythropoiesis renders the M:E ratio invalid as an indicator of the degree of erythropoietic activity in the bone marrow. Neutrophils in peripheral blood were 3.5 times the maximum normal. The M:E divided by 3.5 = 0.30; a M:E of 0.30 would approximate the anticipated bone marrow activity based upon degree of erythrocyte immaturity in peripheral blood.

Histopathology of Spleen. There was depletion of mature lymphoid elements; the red pulp was hyperactive and contained large numbers of hematopoietic cells, including primitive RE cells. Megakaryocytes were scarce to absent.

Interpretation

1. Thrombocytes play a significant role in the sealing of ruptured capillary walls. In the absence of thrombocytes, hemorrhages occur in regions of the body that are easily traumatized, e.g., the mouth and ventral abdominal wall.

2. Absence of thrombocytes in stained films of blood, failure of clot retraction, and absence of megakaryocytes in bone marrow films demonstrated that bleeding in this dog was the result of thrombocytopenia. The history suggested that the primary cause was hypersplenism.

3. Blood morphology indicated extreme activity of the bone marrow to meet the demand for erythrocytes. Maturation time was shortened with release of macrocytic erythrocytes containing an above-normal quantity of hemoglobin by weight (MCH) but below-normal on a volume basis (MCHC). The marked changes in both the erythrocytic (decrease in the reticulocyte count) and leukocytic (marked leukocytosis) values, as noted on July 27, were referable to the blood transfusion and splenectomy, respectively, on July 24. After July 28, bleeding stopped, and a return of the erythrocytic series to normal followed.

4. The corrected erythrocyte sedimentation rate resulted in a large negative value. This is to be anticipated on the basis of immaturity of the RBC and low plasma proteins.

5. Plasma protein concentration of 5.4 g/dl (July 22) was rendered invalid by the lipemic plasma. The plasma protein concentration of 4.0 g/dl on July 27 was valid. Low plasma proteins are to be anticipated in chronic blood loss.

6. A leukocytosis with left shift is ordinarily anticipated when the bone marrow response to anemia is extreme, as in this case. The great increase in total leukocyte count, with doubling of neutrophils and monocytes on July 27, is referable both to the surgical removal of the spleen and in greater measure to the twice-daily administration of prednisolone. In the dog, corticoids produce neutrophilia and monocytosis and a fall in lymphocytes and eosinophils. The lymphocytes revealed a temporary increase after surgery despite prednisolone therapy. This might be explained by some slight improvement in general well-being following removal of the spleen, despite the fact that the anemic state appeared to have worsened. The nearly complete absence of lymphocytes on Aug. 3 correlates well with the developing fat necrosis and marked depression. On Aug. 1, prednisolone therapy was reduced to 5.0 mg twice daily; this therapy was stopped after Aug. 10. The hemogram of Aug. 18 was interpreted as reflecting favorable convalescence, and the dog was released.

7. The progress check on Sept. 23 revealed a favorable hemogram. Howell-Jolly bodies were present in every microscopic field of the stained blood film. Removal of the spleen or suppression of splenic function by steroid therapy may be followed by occurrence of Howell-Jolly bodies in circulating erythrocytes. The spleen normally removes these nuclear remnants through its pitting function. (See Chapter 13 for additional details.) Small Heinz bodies were demonstrated with new methylene blue stain to be present in a majority of the erythrocytes. This was conjectured to be another sign of absence of splenic function.

Case 25 (Dog). Disseminated Intravascular Coagulation

An urgent consultation was requested for a patient in the intensive care unit. A 7-year-old, mixed breed, spayed female had returned from surgery following an extensive bowel resection for carcinoma. Over a 24-hour period she had received 3 units of blood as treatment for mild preoperative anemia and extensive blood loss during surgery. She had received 2 of these 3 units during the 30 minutes immediately following surgery. Oozing was noted from the abdominal drain tube following surgery and following venipuncture. There was no previous history of bleeding, and a coagulogram performed 24 hours before surgery was normal. Petechiae and purpura were noted on the lower limbs.

Laboratory values included: hemoglobin, 11 g/dl; WBC, 15,500/μl with 80% neutrophils, 15% lymphocytes, and 3% monocytes; platelet count, 25,000/μl; bleeding time, not performed; prothrombin time (PT), 23 sec (control 12 sec); partial thromboplastin time (PTT), 48 sec (control 21 sec); thrombin time (TT) 19 sec (control 12 sec); and fibrin and fibrinogen degradation products (FDPs), 15 μg/ml (control, <10 μg/ml). Chest radiographs suggested no abnormalities, and blood culture was negative.

Interpretation

1. Based on the patient's history, clinical signs, and laboratory test results, disseminated intravascular coagulation (DIC; consumption coagulopathy) was diagnosed.
2. Common laboratory abnormalities in DIC include a profound thrombocytopenia, mild anemia, prolonged coagulation screening tests (PT, PTT, and TT), elevated FDPs, and fractured red cells known as schistocytes.
3. A bleeding time was not performed in this patient because of the thrombocytopenia. Thrombocytopenia always prolongs the bleeding time. It should be noted that the petechiae and purpura present on the lower hind limbs resulted from the severe thrombocytopenia.
4. DIC is never a primary event; it is always secondary to a primary or inciting event. In this case, several inciting events are suggested. These include tumor, surgical trauma, and perhaps transfusion hemolysis.
5. Treatment of DIC is complex and is discussed in Chapter 14. The basic therapeutic principles include removal or mitigation of the primary or inciting cause, establishing microvascular blood flow through fluid administration, inhibiting hemostasis through the use of aspirin (platelet prostaglandin inhibition) and heparin (activation of the circulatory inhibitor antithrombin III), and blood transfusion.

Case 26 (Dog). Epistaxis Associated with Nasal Carcinoma and Terminal Fibrinolysis

A spayed female beagle, 10 years old, was observed to snort after ingestion of food and water. One month later, the snorting was accompanied by sneezing of blood. Several weeks later, intermittent epistaxis was found to be associated with neoplasia of the turbinate bones. The dog was referred for diagnostic consultation and possible surgery. Several hemograms and clotting tests were conducted over a period of 4 days, during which time intermittent and severe bleeding from the nose continued. A biopsy of the tumor mass revealed it to be an undifferentiated carcinoma. The dog was destroyed, and necropsy revealed neoplastic cells to be present in local lymph nodes, the lungs, and the marrow of several bones examined. Infarcts and amyloidosis were observed in the spleen, heart, and kidneys. In addition, there was an acute necrotizing pancreatitis.

Interpretation

1. Continuous blood loss was reflected in the reduction of RBC count, Hb concentration, and PCV.
2. Failure of erythrogenesis to keep pace with the blood loss was evident from the modest reticulocytosis, insignificant increase in MCV, and the M:E ratio of 1.9:1.0. The inadequate response of erythrogenesis may have reflected reduced erythopoietin production by the kidneys, which were affected by amyloidosis, or neoplastic cell metastasis to the bone marrow. However, no neoplastic cells were seen in aspirated marrow from the iliac crest, although they were found on histopathologic examination. The elevated blood urea nitrogen lends support to the probable existence of reduced kidney function.
3. Plasma protein concentration was low on admissin at 6.3 g/dl, and the further reduction to 5.8 g/dl resulted from both continuing blood loss and hemodilution from movement of fluid from the tissues into the blood to maintain blood volume. The disappearance of plasma fibrinogen was of special significance in understanding the intermittent epistaxis and fibrinolysis.
4. The prolonged blood-clotting tests and dissolution of the blood clot in the clot retraction test were directly related to the hypofibrinogenemia. Breakdown products of tumor tissue may release tissue-activator substances into the blood, leading to DIC and fibrinolysis, both of which would cause fibrinogenemia.
5. In hemorrhage due to primary fibrinolysis, it is common in humans for the blood platelet count to be within the normal range. The modest thrombocytopenia of 115,000/μl in this dog may have been due to a combination of factors, namely, continuous loss through epistaxis, utilization of platelets in intravascular coagulation, leading to formation of infarcts noted at necropsy, and reduced megakaryopoiesis. Megakaryocytes were seen on scanning of the film of aspirated marrow.
6. The diphasic ESR and large negative corrected ESR value can be explained by the presence of a modest number of reticulocytes and the hypofibrinogenemia.
7. The leukocytosis in the admission hemogram, with neutrophilia, monocytosis, eosinopenia, and low lymphocyte numbers, represents in part the effect of corticoids of stress and also a reaction to inflammatory

Case 26 (Dog).   Nasal Carcinoma and Terminal Fibrinolysis

	July 28		July 29		July 31	
Erythrocytes						
RBC ($\times 10^6/\mu$l)	3.02		2.57		2.08	
Hemoglobin (g/dl)	6.1		4.8		4.0	
PCV (%)	20.0		17.0		15.0	
MCV (fl)	66.2		66.1		72.1	
MCH (pg)	22.0		18.6		19.2	
MCHC (%)	30.5		28.2		26.6	
Nucleated RBC/100 WBC	1.0		rare		4.5	
Reticulocytes (%)	9.2		14.6		11.4	
RBC sed. rate/1 hr	8/49 = 41 − (diphasic)		5/58 = 53 − (diphasic)		—	
Anisocytosis	slight		slight		moderate	
Polychromasia	moderate		moderate		moderate	
Hypochromasia	—		slight		moderate	
Leptocytes	few		moderate		few	
Leukocytes		%		%		%
WBC/μl (corrected)	45,900		37,500		61,700	
Band neutrophils	918	2.0	188	0.5	2,160	3.5
Mature neutrophils	39,704	86.5	32,063	85.5	49,360	80.0
Lymphocytes	1,607	3.5	750	2.0	2,160	3.5
Monocytes	3,672	8.0	2,813	7.5	7,404	12.0
Eosinophils	0	0.0	1,688	4.5	617	1.0
Plasma						
Total protein (g/dl)	6.3		6.9		5.8	
Fibrinogen (g/dl)	0		0		0	
Icterus index units	2		2		2	
Other Tests						
Thrombocytes/μl	—		115,000		—	
M:E ratio	—		—		1.9:1.0	
Blood urea nitrogen (mg/dl)	200		79.5		—	

	Patient	Control	Patient	Control
Lee and White coagulation time	15 min	7 min 36 sec	—	—
Prothrombin time	2 min	6.5 sec	—	—
Partial thromboplastin time	3 min	35.0 sec	—	—
Clot retraction test	—		abnormal, clot almost completely dissolved (fibrinolysis)	normal, firm

response and tissue destruction associated with neoplasia. The increase in eosinophils in subsequent hemograms indicates the probable release of histamine from either the tumor tissue or the necrotizing pancreatitis or both. The increase in lymphocytes on July 31 is unexplained, unless it represents increasing numbers of lymphocytes added to blood as thoracic duct lymph flow increased to maintain the rapidly falling blood volume.

Case 27 (Dog).   Hemophilia B

A 9-month-old male golden retriever was presented because of a swollen, painful left knee joint of 1 day's duration. The dog's owners related previous problems with joints and occasional hematuria. There was no history of epistaxis, gastrointestinal bleeding, purpura, polydipsia, or polyuria. Physical examination was normal other than abnormalities noted in association with the left knee. Aspiration of the joint revealed frank blood (hemarthrosis).

Laboratory findings included: hemoglobin, 10.5 g/dl with normocytic-normochromic red cell indices; platelet count, 175,000/μl; bleeding time, 5 min (normal to 9 min); prothrombin time (PT), 13 sec (control 12 sec); partial prothrombin time (PTT), 60 sec (control 32 sec); and thrombin time (TT), 12 sec (control 12 sec).

Interpretation

1. A mild normocytic-normochromic anemia may be seen in disorders of hemostasis when bleeding is infrequent and of a lesser magnitude. The bleeding in this case was associated with defective hemostasis from a coagulation protein (factor) disorder, as was evident from the normal platelet count and

bleeding time. Platelet functional disorders will also prolong the bleeding time.

2. A prolonged PTT with normal PT and TT indicates an intrinsic pathway defect. Results of all screening coagulation factor tests must be compared to values established within individual laboratories or to control values derived from similar animals, i.e., matched by age, weight, and sex. When a patient's value exceeds a control value by a ratio of more than 1:1.3, the prolongation is considered significant. In this case, the ratio was 1:1.88.

3. A defect of intrinsic pathway includes factors XII, XI, IX, and VIII. Factor XII (Hageman factor) deficiency, while causing prolonged PTTs, does not cause bleeding problems as activation of factor XI occurs through a contact activation similar to that of factor XII. Hence factor XII deficiency may be eliminated. Although factor XI deficiency has been reported in the dog, it is rare. Factor VIII (factor VIII:C) deficiency (hemophilia A) is the most common, and factor IX deficiency (hemophilia B) is the second most common sex-linked coagulation protein deficiency. However, in order to establish which factor is the cause of prolonged PTT, factor XI, IX, and VIII:C analyses must be performed.

4. A factor analysis revealed the patient had less than 15% of the normal factor IX concentration, indicating a diagnosis of hemophilia B. (See Chapter 14 for inheritance and therapy of hemophilias A and B.)

Case 28 (Dog). Circulating Inhibitor of Coagulation

A 2-year-old Doberman, known to have factor VIII deficiency (hemophilia A) was presented because of right hind leg pain of sudden onset. He had been treated with cryoprecipitate by the owners. Recently, however, this therapy had no obvious beneficial effect. During the past few hours the intensity of pain had increased and the leg was carried in a flexed position. A tender mass was palpated in the right iliac fossa.

Laboratory findings included: hemoglobin, 11.5 g/dl; platelet count, 300,000/μl; bleeding time, <5 min; partial prothrombin time (PTT), 66 sec (control 22 sec); factor VIII assay, 1% (normal 70–120%).

A dose of cryoprecipitate calculated to produce a factor VIII:C concentration of 50% was infused. Twenty minutes later, the PTT was 60 sec (control 22 sec), and PTT performed with equal parts of normal and patient plasma was 61 sec.

Interpretation

1. Hemophilia A was evident from the factor VIII concentration of 1%.
2. The history of bleeding despite infusion of cryoprecipitate and failure of cryoprecipitate infusion to normalize PTT suggested the possibility of a plasma inhibitor (antibody) active against factor VIII:C. This was further substantiated by the persistence of prolonged PTT in a mixing study in which normal plasma added to the patient plasma did not correct PTT as expected. The PTT exhibits normal time when factor concentrations are >20%; in the present case assuming the normal plasma had 100% of the normal factor VIII:C concentration and the patient had a 1% concentration, the resultant mixture should have approximated 50% of normal concentration and resulted in normal PTT.

3. Some inhibitors may be time-dependent; hence mixing studies are often conducted over several hours. Equal parts of patient and control plasma are mixed and a PTT is performed. A normal result suggests a true factor deficiency or the presence of a time-dependent inhibitor. The mixture is then incubated at 37° C for several hours. During this period PTT is performed at 30-minute intervals. Any prolongation of the PTT by more than a few seconds suggests a time-dependent coagulation protein inhibitor.

4. Although immunosuppressive therapy has been attempted to suppress the inhibitor concentration, this form of therapy offers only transient relief, and most patients succumb at an early age.

5. The normal bleeding time suggests normal platelet function, thus von Willebrand's disease could be tentatively eliminated as a second or concurrent disease.

Case 29 (Dog). Amyloidosis Associated with Leukopenia, Anemia, Thrombocytopenia, and a Positive Test for Antinuclear Antibodies

A 6-year-old Border collie female was referred with a history of periodic episodes of bloody diarrhea. Physical examination revealed the dog to be in poor flesh with thinning of the hair coat in some body areas and a 2-cm pale pink area of alopecia on the face caudal to the nose (collie nose). The teeth were loose, and there was a foul breath. Body temperature was normal. The dog was killed on April 28.

Treatment from April 9 through April 15 was limited to 400,000 units of penicillin orally t.i.d. From April 15 onward, after two positive tests for antinuclear antibodies, 10 mg of prednisolone b.i.d. was added to the therapy. Because of a temperature increase to 102.6° on April 12 and 13 and further increase to 104.0° F on the 14th, tetracycline was substituted for penicillin. The temperature returned to normal thereafter.

Necropsy. The most significant lesions were those of amyloidosis of the kidneys. All glomeruli were involved in diffuse amyloid deposits. The spleen also contained deposits of amyloid, and foci of extramedullary hematopoiesis were present, as

Case 29 (Dog).   Amyloidosis

	April 6		April 10		April 13		April 27	
Erythrocytes								
RBC ($\times 10^6/\mu$l)	4.13		4.41		4.26		3.07	
Hemoglobin (g/dl)	9.2		11.2		9.9		7.6	
PCV (%)	30.0		32		30.0		23.0	
MCV (fl)	72.6		72.6		70.4		74.9	
MCHC (%)	30.7		35.0		33.0		33.0	
Nucleated RBC/100 WBC	3		2.0		rare		none	
Reticulocytes (%)	3.4		6.0		3.6		1.8	
RBC sed. rate/1 hr	60/26 = 34+		45/22 = 23+		42/26 = 16+		24/40 = 16+	
Anisocytosis	slight		moderate		slight		slight	
Polychromasia	slight		slight		slight		rare	
Leukocytes		%		%		%		%
WBC/μl (corrected)	3,300		4,200		2,800		11,500	
Myelocytes	759	23.0	0	0.0	0	0.0	0	0.0
Metamyelocytes	759	23.0	42	1.0	0	0.0	0	0.0
Band neutrophils	561	17.0	378	9.0	140	5.0	287	2.5
Neutrophils	99	3.0	588	14.0	140	5.0	8,625	75.0
Lymphocytes	693	21.0	630	15.0	476	17.0	403	3.5
Monocytes	429	13.0	2,562	61.0	1,988	71.0	2,185	19.0
Eosinophils	0	0.0	0	0.0	56	2.0	0	0.0
Basophils	0	0.0	0	0.0	0	0.0	0	0.0
Plasma								
Protein (g/dl)	7.4		7.2		7.1		5.8	
Fibrinogen (g/dl)	0.8		0.6		0.6		0.6	
Icterus index units	2		2		2		2	
Other								
Thrombocytes/μl	42,000		—		—		33,000	
Blood urea nitrogen (mg/dl)	22.5		22.5		59.0		85.0	
Urine protein	4+		4+		4+		4+	
Serum albumin (g/dl)	1.0		—		—		1.4	
Serum globulin (g/dl)	5.0		—		—		3.0	
Coombs test	—		negative		negative		—	
LE cell test	—		negative		negative		negative	
Antinuclear antibodies	—		4+		4+		—	

April 7, Bone Marrow Aspiration

	%		%
Rubriblast	0.0	Myeloblast	1.4
Prorubricyte	0.6	Progranulocyte	7.8
Basophilic rubricyte	5.0	Myelocyte, neutrophilic	7.8
Polychromatophilic rubricyte	10.8	Myelocyte, eosinophilic	0.8
Metarubricyte	6.0	Metamyelocyte, neutrophilic	28.2
Mitotic rubricyte	0.4	Metamyelocyte, eosinophilic	0.8
Total erythrocytic	22.8	Band, neutrophilic	16.2
		Band, eosinophilic	1.4
Lymphocyte	7.8	Neutrophil	1.0
Plasma cell	0.2	Eosinophil	0.4
Monocyte	0.8	Total granulocytic	65.8
Macrophage	1.0		
Mitotic cell	1.2	M:E = 2.88:1.0	
RE nuclei	0.4		
Megakaryocytes, present			

well as hyperplasia of the reticuloendothelial cells. The liver exhibited lipidosis.

Interpretation

1. The anemia, leukopenia, thrombocytopenia, markedly elevated erythrocyte sedimentation rate, proteinuria, and hyperglobulinemia recorded on admission (April 8), taken together with the 4 + reaction for antinuclear antibodies, supported a diagnosis of systemic lupus erythematosus (SLE). The skin lesion on the caudal portion of the nose (collie nose) appeared *a priori* to be part of the syndrome of SLE.

2. The episodes of bloody diarrhea in the history of the dog may have been due to periods of thrombocytopenia considerably lower than platelet counts of 33,000 and 42,000/μl recorded during hospitalization.

3. Renal amyloidosis was responsible for the gradually increasing concentrations of blood urea nitrogen and for the loss of protein in the urine that led to hypoalbuminemia. Amyloidosis is not characteristic of systemic lupus erythematosus, although glomerular lesions occur in SLE. It is possible that the amyloidosis was secondary and was superimposed on the SLE kidney lesions, thus increasing loss of protein in the urine.

4. An above-normal plasma fibrinogen level is a common finding in kidney disease.

5. Significant changes were seen in the final hemogram. These were influenced in part by the steroid therapy and in part by the advancing kidney damage. Beginning on April 22, it was noted that the dog was consuming large quantities of water. It appears that this large volume of water intake may have caused hemodilution, for PCV became reduced to 23%, and total plasma proteins became reduced to 5.8 g/dl. The changes in the total and differential leukocyte counts from leukopenia with degenerative left shift to a normal number of neutrophils, monocytosis, and continuing lymphopenia can be attributed to the response to steroid therapy. Although steroid therapy generally can be expected to reverse a thrombocytopenia in autoimmune disease, no increase in thrombocytes was noted in the last and final hemogram.

6. Examination of bone marrow aspirated from the iliac crest, on the day after admission of the dog to the hospital, gave interesting findings in view of the neutropenia and degenerative left shift in peripheral blood. The granulocytic elements presented a picture of hypercellularity with a greater number of progranulocytes and neutrophilic metamyelocytes than commonly present in normal bone marrow aspirates. Furthermore, maturation ceased at the band neutrophil stage, suggesting that the granulocytes were being destroyed in the bone marrow before attaining the mature neutrophil stage. The ineffective granulopoiesis in turn may have stimulated the hypercellularity and left shift within the granulocytic cell series. The eosinophils were unusual, in that some of them presented a few but very large granules. An occasional eosinophil presented a single large granule. Maturation in the erythrocytic series was normal, but cell numbers were reduced in comparison to the granulocytic series. Numerous megakaryocytes were seen on scanning of the film, but an ineffective thrombopoiesis or accelerated platelet destruction may have been in effect since thrombocytopenia was evident in the peripheral blood on April 27.

7. The LE cell test is commonly but not always positive in SLE. Perhaps failure to observe LE cells in this dog was due to the markedly reduced numbers of neutrophils available for formation of LE cells. (See Chapter 35.)

Case 30 (Dog). Systemic Lupus Erythematosus

An intact female basenji, weight 16 pounds, was admitted with a complaint of swollen joints and lameness. One month earlier, a marble-sized swelling had appeared on the right hock. Pain was evident, since the dog avoided placing weight on the leg. Later swellings involved the carpal joints also, and at times the dog was unable to rise and would cry when moved. Body temperature had been recorded at 104° F for the previous few days. The referring veterinarian had the dog on antibiotic therapy. There was generalized radiolucency of the metaphyseal regions of the long bones. Tentative diagnoses were (a) generalized joint infection, (b) osteomyelitis, and (c) bacterial endocarditis. The patient was seen on nine occasions between July 31, 1968, and May 13, 1970. Initially, antibiotic therapy, mainly chloromycetin, but changed later to penicillin and streptomycin, was the principal therapeutic measure. The swellings receded, and the radiographs of the bones became normal. The patient appeared improved until Jan. 1, 1970 when lameness reappeared. At this time, the dog's temperament was described as "grouchy," the carpal joints were swollen and painful, the right stifle joint was definitely larger than the left, rectal temperature was 104.4° F, and the submandibular lymph node was somewhat enlarged. There had been difficulty with swallowing, and an ulcer was found in the oral mucous membrane. Joint fluid was negative for bacteria but contained 70,000 somatic cells/μl, of which 97% were neutrophils. Chloromycetin therapy was changed to penicillin and streptomycin. There was no improvement when the dog was seen again on Feb. 18, 1970. At this time, all joints were distended, a systolic mitral murmur was noted, and the temperature was 103.8° F. Systemic lupus erythematosus was sus-

Case 30 (Dog).   Systemic Lupus Erythematosus

	July 31, 1968		Aug. 19, 1968		Jan. 30, 1970		Mar. 3, 1970		May 13, 1970	
Erythrocytes										
RBC ($\times 10^6/\mu$l)	5.17		5.07		5.41		5.68		6.09	
Hemoglobin (g/dl)	11.8		11.4		13.5		13.8		—ᵃ	
PCV (%)	37		36		41		42		45	
MCV (fl)	71.6		71.0		75.8		73.9		73.9	
MCHC (%)	31.9		31.7		32.9		32.9		—ᵃ	
Erythrocyte sed. rate/1 hr	43/13 = 30+		43/4 = 39+		46/9 = 37+		3/8 = 5−		10/5 = 5+	
Leukocytes		%		%		%		%		%
WBC/μl	28,600		17,800		36,100		33,300		20,700	
Band neutrophils	429	1.5	178	1.0	0	0.0	499	1.5	103	0.5
Neutrophils	22,880	80.0	12,371	69.5	31,768	88.0	30,969	93.0	18,216	88.0
Lymphocytes	3,432	12.0	2,937	16.5	1,625	4.5	333	1.0	1,242	6.0
Monocytes	1,573	5.5	801	4.5	2,166	6.0	1,499	4.5	1,139	5.5
Eosinophils	286	1.0	1,513	8.5	541	1.5	0	0.0	0	0.0
Plasma										
Plasma proteins (g/dl)	7.1		7.4		7.3		7.2		—ᵃ	
Fibrinogen (g/dl)	0.4		0.3		0.7		0.2		—ᵃ	
Icterus index units	5		2		2		2		very lipemic	
Other Tests										
Urine protein	negative		negative		negative		negative		—	
Reticulocytes (%)	rare		—		—		6.6		—	
Joint fluid WBC/μl	147,000		—		70,000		—		—	
Joint fluid, bacteria	none		—		none		—		—	
Coombs test	—		—		—		2+		—	
LE cells	—		—		—		positive		—	
Antinuclear antibody testᵇ	—		—		—		negative		—	

Serum protein, Feb. 18, 1970: albumin = 2.0 g, globulin = 4.3 g.

ᵃNot valid because of marked lipemia.
ᵇBy latex agglutination test available commercially.

pected. Therapy was changed to 250 mg of chloromycetin and 5 mg of prednisolone t.i.d. On this therapy, marked improvement resulted. The body temperature became normal, and joint swellings receded. Chloromycetin was stopped and prednisolone reduced to 5 mg b.i.d. On April 13, prednisolone was further reduced to 5 mg s.i.d., and on May 13 to 2.5 mg s.i.d. On May 16, the dog was vomiting and depressed; it died the following day. An autopsy was not permitted.

Interpretation

1. The episodic nature of systemic lupus erythematosus was demonstrated in this patient with the apparent return to normal health for a period of over a year, followed by a reappearance of severe, noninfectious inflammation of the joints and pyrexia.
2. Although clinical signs of bone and joint involvement had disappeared when the dog was seen on Aug. 19, the PCV remained at the minimum of the normal range, and the high corrected erythrocyte sedimentation rate indicated that an underlying disease process persisted. At this time, an eosinophila was noted, but neutrophils had become reduced to the maximum of the normal range.

3. The disease flareup in Jan. 1970 was accompanied by an increase in plasma fibrinogen. This was the only time in the blood studies that an above-normal plasma fibrinogen level was found. The leukocyte total and differential counts indicated a severe stress response with persistence of eosinophils. The persistence of eosinophils suggested that histamine release was in excess of the capacity of the natural corticoids to neutralize it.
4. Treatment with prednisolone was followed by disappearance of the strongly positive erythrocyte sedimentation rate, and eosinophils disappeared from the blood. The total and differential leukocyte counts on Mar. 3, 1970, were typical of the anticipated response to steroid therapy in the dog, namely, neutrophilia, monocytosis, lymphopenia, and eosinopenia. On this date, Coombs test and a search for LE cells were conducted for the first time. Both tests were found to be positive. Normally, steroid therapy reduces the positive reaction to these antibody tests. Low sensitivity of the ANA latex agglutination may have been the cause of negative results for antinuclear antibodies.
5. Clinical improvement was apparent on May

13, but the dog died suddenly from an acute illness on May 17. The hemogram of May 13 revealed a change in erythrocyte sedimentation rate to 5+, and the blood was very lipemic. It is suspected that these may have been signs of the impending acute disease, which may have been acute pancreatitis.

Case 31 (Dog). Early Autoimmune Hemolytic Anemia

A female Pomeranian, 4 years old, was seen early, perhaps within 24 hours of the beginning of an autoimmune hemolytic crisis. The dog had no history of a previous illness. It was a closely watched house pet. The dog was seldom permitted outside. The owners noticed that the dog seemed to be weak on Jan 24. It was taken to a veterinarian, who found the PCV to be 12%. He suggested that the dog be taken to the university clinic. On arrival on Jan. 25, the dog was calm and in generally good condition with the following findings: pale and icteric mucous membranes, PCV 12%, rectal temperature 104.5° F, rapid respiration, and enlarged spleen. After the first hemogram, 130 ml of whole blood was administered. No additional blood was given throughout the course of hospitalization.

Prednisolone therapy IM was begun at 1 mg/lb total daily dose (7.5 mg given b.i.d.). On Jan. 29, the dose was increased to 10 mg b.i.d.

Interpretation

1. This patient was seen in the beginning state of autoimmune hemolytic anemia (AIHA). The diagnosis was in doubt at the time of the first hemogram because of a negative direct Coombs test. It was necessary to make the diagnosis on the basis of uniform dark staining of the erythrocytes (spherocytes). Gross agglutination of erythrocytes was not present (see Chapter 35).
2. The neutrophilia with left shift and monocytosis were characteristic of AIHA, but the high normal absolute lymphocyte number was not consistent with an acute stress response. The significantly increased neutrophil and monocyte numbers in response to the steroid therapy was as anticipated (Jan. 27 through Feb. 3), but the absolute lymphocyte number did not fall to lymphopenic levels until after the fourth day on steroid therapy.
3. A reticulocytosis failed to develop during the

Case 31 (Dog). Early Autoimmune Hemolytic Anemia

	Jan. 25		Jan. 27		Jan. 28		Jan. 31[a]		Feb. 3[b]	
Erythrocytes										
RBC ($\times 10^6/\mu l$)	1.86		2.05		1.75		1.69		2.82	
Hemoglobin (g/dl)	4.0		4.8		3.6		3.9		7.0	
PCV (%)	12		13		12		12		25	
MCV (fl)	64.5		63.4		68.5		71.0		88.6	
MCHC (%)	33.3		36.9		30.0		32.5		28.0	
MCH (pg)	21.5		23.4		20.6		23.1		24.8	
ESR/1 hr	—		79/70 = 9+		80/73 = 7+		—		35/36 = 1−	
Reticulocytes (%)	none		none		0.4		22.4		24.6	
Nucleated RBC/100 WBC	none		none		0.5		17		7.5	
Anisocytosis	slight		slight		moderate		marked		marked	
Polychromasia	rare		none		rare		marked		marked	
Other	no agglu- tination		moderate leptocytes		some macrocytes		few H-J		—	
Spherocytes	moderate		moderate		some		few		rare	
Leukocytes		%		%		%		%		%
WBC/μl	24,500		43,500		48,600		32,300		34,800	
Metamyelocytes	735	3.0	435	1.0	486	1.0	0	0.0	0	0.0
Bands	2,695	11.0	5,438	12.5	5,103	10.5	2,099	6.5	2,784	8.0
Neutrophils	15,680	64.0	30,667	70.5	34,263	70.5	25,194	78.0	24,708	78.0
Lymphocytes	3,553	14.5	2,610	6.0	1,458	3.0	646	2.0	1,218	3.5
Monocytes	1,837	7.5	4,350	10.0	6,804	14.0	4,361	13.5	5,916	17.0
Eosinophils	0	0.0	0	0.0	486	1.0	0	0.0	0	0.0
Basophils	0	0.0	0	0.0	0	0.0	0	0.0	174	0.5
Platelets/μl	—		—		331,000		—		271,000	
Plasma										
Icterus index units	hemolyzed		50		15		—		2	
Plasma protein (g/dl)	7.8		7.3		6.3		—		6.3	
Fibrinogen (g/dl)	0.8		0.7		0.6		—		0.5	
Coombs test	negative		—		—		—		—	

[a]Excessive EDTA.
[b]Feb. 1: PCV 17%; reticulocytes, 19%.

first 4 days of therapy. The clinician in charge decided to increase the dose of steroid on the fifth day. At that time (Jan. 29), however, a blood film stained with new methylene blue revealed beginning reticulocytosis, and by Jan. 31, reticulocytosis was a prominent feature of the stained blood film.

4. The 5-day-delay in appearance of reticulocytes in peripheral blood indicated that the first hemogram was representative of the earliest stage of hemolytic crisis in AIHA. It requires 4 to 5 days for a significant reticulocytosis to develop after an initial massive blood loss or erythrocyte destruction from any cause.

5. The dog was released to the owners on Feb. 3 with directions for gradual reduction of the steroid dose to a maintenance level to be administered every 48 hours.

Case 32 (Dog).   Autoimmune Hemolytic Anemia

A spayed beagle terrier female, 5 years old, was referred with the following brief medical history: On May 22, she was listless, exhibiting pharyngitis and a temperature of 104° F. Treatment consisted of antibiotics and B-complex vitamins. The dog had displayed anorexia, and on May 27 it was noted that she was eating a little. At that time, the temperature was 102.5° F. On June 18, the condition worsened; anorexia, vomiting, listlessness, evidence of severe anemia, and red urine were all noted. The hematocrit test revealed a PCV of 11.0% and a buffy coat of 2.0 mm. Antibiotics, liver extract, and iron were administered intramuscularly. The next day, the dog was referred for diagnosis and treatment.

On arrival, the dog was depressed and pale and exhibited a fast, thready pulse and a temperature of 102° F. The initial hemogram (June 19) revealed advanced anemia in remission, with evidence of spherocytes. A urine analysis revealed a reddish-brown color, 4+ albumin, and 4+ occult blood. Coombs test was positive. Blood from six donor dogs was submitted for compatibility tests, and only one was found suitable for transfusion.

Treatment.   Oral prednisolone was given twice daily beginning with 20 mg/dose on June 20 through June 24; the dose was continued twice daily but was reduced to 10 mg through June 28; thereafter, 5 mg of prednisolone was administered twice daily. This dose was to be continued by the

Case 32 (Dog).   Autoimmune Hemolytic Anemia

	June 19		June 23 preoperative (Blood transfusion given)		June 23 postoperative		June 25		June 29	
Erythrocytes										
RBC ($\times 10^6/\mu$l)	1.22		1.10		3.48		4.05		3.10	
Hemoglobin (g/dl)	3.1		3.6		8.8		9.9		8.5	
PCV (%)	13		15		30		33		29	
MCV (fl)	106.5		136.4		86.2		81.5		93.5	
MCHC (%)	23.8		24.0		29.3		30.0		29.3	
MCH (pg)	25.4		32.7		25.3		24.4		27.4	
ESR/1 hr	—		—		3/26 = 23− diphasic		1/20 = 19−		0/28 = 28−	
Reticulocytes (%)	25.2		54.4		11.2		23.5		2.18	
Nucleated RBC/100 WBC	24.0		14.5		25.5		11.5		20.5	
Anisocytosis	marked		marked		marked		marked		marked	
Polychromasia	marked		marked		moderate		marked		moderate	
Spherocytes	present		present		present		prominent		present	
H-J bodies	few		few		few		few		few	
Leukocytes		%		%		%		%		%
WBC/μl (corrected)	71,500		63,500		27,000		46,200		23,600	
Metamyelocytes	357	0.5	1,588	2.5	405	1.5	0	0.0	0	0.0
Band neutrophils	2,145	3.0	8,255	13.0	2,160	8.0	924	2.0	118	0.5
Neutrophils	60,060	84.0	42,228	66.5	19,980	74.0	33,264	72.0	16,756	71.0
Lymphocytes	0	0.0	952	1.5	945	3.5	1,155	2.5	1,062	4.5
Monocytes	8,937	12.5	10,478	16.5	3,510	13.0	10,857	23.5	5,664	24.0
Eosinophils	0	0.0	0	0.0	0	0.0	0	0.0	0	0.0
Plasma										
Proteins (g/dl)	7.6		7.4		7.0		7.0		6.7	
Icterus index units	hemolyzed		10 (hemolyzed)		10 (hemolyzed)		10		5 (hemolyzed)	
Other										
Coombs test	+		—		—		+		+	
LE cell test	—		negative		—		—		—	
Thrombocytes	normal		normal		normal		normal		normal	

owner after release of the patient. The spleen was removed on June 23. The dog was bright and active when released to the owner on July 3.

Pathologist's description of the spleen: not enlarged, sinuses clearly distended, follicles not hyperplastic and often show plasma cell increase, the latter cell type also being frequent as clumps in the red pulp. Hemosiderin is fairly abundant in fixed phagocytes. No megakaryocytes observed.

Interpretation

1. In AIHA, the erythrocytes become coated with specific IgG antibody and/or C3b and are consequently destroyed intravascularly or through phagocytosis in the mononuclear phagocyte system or by both processes. Partial erythrophagocytosis results in formation of spherocytes. The spherocyte appears smaller and more darkly stained than normal erythrocytes (Plate XVII–4). Spherocytes are inflexible cells that become trapped in the microcirculation of the spleen, where they are destroyed.

2. The centers of erythrogenesis are responsive to the hemolytic anemia. Within a few days of initial massive destruction of erythrocytes, the blood picture is typical of anemia in remission, as seen in the admission hemogram of this patient (MCV 106.5 fl, reticulocytes 25.2%, and marked anisocytosis and polychromasia).

3. The marked neutrophilia with left shift, monocytosis, lymphopenia, and eosinopenia were in response to the natural corticoids of stress. The extreme neutrophilia was also a reflection, in part, of granulopoiesis acting in concert with erythropoiesis in response to the intense stimulation of hematopoiesis by the rapidly developing hemolytic anemia. Intense monocytosis, in part, may also be a reflection of enhanced activity of the mononuclear phagocyte system to destroy antibody-coated red cells.

4. Corticosteroid therapy is given at 1–2 mg/lb body weight initially at a higher dose level until hemolysis stops and the PCV has increased to minimum normal levels. This is followed by gradual reduction of dose to a maintenance level of 5 to 10 mg (depending on weight of the dog) once daily and then to once every 2 days. By giving the maintenance dose at 48-hour intervals, the side effects of polydipsia and polyuria are less in evidence. A relapse of AIHA may occur within 3 weeks after maintenance therapy is discontinued.

5. Splenectomy should be reserved for those cases in which steroid or immunosuppressive therapy is ineffective. Also, transfusion of whole blood should be withheld, except for the most advanced cases of anemia. It was noted that only one blood among six

donor dogs was compatible with the patient. Dogs given multiple blood transfusion may become sensitized to a degree that no compatible donor blood can be found should a transfusion be needed later to preserve life.

6. See Chapter 35 for a discussion on various aspects of AIHA.

Case 33 (Dog). Microcytic Hypochromic Anemia in Chronic Blood Loss

A male English pointer, 4 years old, was presented with a complaint of loss of blood in the stools for the past 3½ years. The initial hemogram verified the existence of an advanced anemia in which erythrocyte morphology and bone marrow differential cell counts were typical of iron-deficiency anemia. Fresh blood was observed to be present in the stools. The condition was diagnosed as a case of ulcerative colitis. Treatment consisted of daily administration of a hematinic and salicylazosulfapyridine* from Jan. 4 through Feb. 6. The bleeding was controlled and the anemia corrected itself.

Interpretation

1. In chronic blood loss leading to iron deficiency, hemoglobin synthesis is delayed, leading to buildup of metarubricytes in the bone marrow and production of microcytic hypochromic erythrocytes. In the dog, MCV is less than 60 fl, MCHC is less than 30%, and MCH is less than 15 pg (Plate XVII–1, 2).

2. The number of erythrocytes is not reduced to the same degree as the hemoglobin concentration. This is because, in an iron-deficient state, the body tends to produce more smaller red cells (microcytosis), probably to carry oxygen more efficiently, than normal size cells deficient in hemoglobin (hypochromasia). Therefore, the erythrocyte count does not reflect the true state of the anemia. With erythrocytes of normal size, the 4.1 × 10^6/μl counted in the first hemogram would yield a PCV of 24%. However, because of the small size of the erythrocytes, the PCV was 18%.

3. Peripheral blood contained about 7% reticulocytes, thereby indicating active erythrogenesis. However, these erythrocytes were defective and could not withstand the wear and tear of circulation. Early fragmentation of erythrocytes was reflected in the presence of poikilocytes in the initial hemograms.

4. The less-than-normal plasma protein concentration was as expected in continuous blood loss.

5. The effect of therapy was dramatic. Blood loss was gradually reduced and, within 2 weeks the hemoglobin concentration had

---

*Annals of Internal Medicine, 51:879, 1959.

Case 33 (Dog). Microcytic Hypochromic Anemia

	Jan. 3		Jan. 17		Jan. 28		Jan. 30	
Erythrocytes								
RBC ($\times 10^6/\mu l$)	4.10		5.35		6.25		7.25	
Hemoglobin (g/dl)	4.6		10.3		11.8		13.2	
PCV (%)	18		35		38		41	
Erythrocyte sed. rate/1 hr	7/55 = 48−		1/16 = 15−		0/12 = 12−		0/9 = 9−	
MCV (fl)	43.9 (microcytic		65.4 (normocytic		60.8 (normocytic		56.5 (microcytic	
MCHC (%)	25.5	hypo-chromic)	29.4	hypo-chromic)	31.1	normo-chromic)	32.2	normo-chromic)
MCH (pg)	11.2		19.2		18.8		18.2	
Reticulocytes	7.3		0.2		2.0		—	
Nucleated RBC/100 WBC	1		0		0		0	
Anisocytosis	moderate		slight		slight		moderate	
Polychromasia	moderate		slight		slight		slight	
Poikilocytosis	moderate		slight		slight		none	
Leptocytosis	marked		marked		marked		moderate	
Howell-Jolly bodies	none		few		rare		none	
Hypochromasia	prominent		moderate		slight		none	
Leukocytes		%		%		%		%
WBC/μl	17,500		5,000		5,200		5,600	
Neutrophils	13,038	74.5	2,125	42.5	2,418	46.5	2,632	47.0
Lymphocytes	2,100	12.0	1,875	37.5	1,300	25.0	1,568	28.0
Monocytes	1,487	8.5	700	14.0	546	10.5	644	11.5
Eosinophils	787	4.5	300	6.0	936	18.0	728	13.0
Basophils	0	0.0	0	0.0	0	0.0	28	0.5
Degenerated cells	0	0.0	0	0.0	0	0.0		
Unclassified cells	88	0.5	0	0.0	0	0.0		
Plasma								
Total protein (g/dl)	5.6		6.6		6.4		6.7	
Icterus index units	2		2		2		5	
Blood urea nitrogen (mg/dl)	—		11.0		—		—	
Fecal Examination					(Jan. 23)		(Feb. 1)	
Parasite ova	few *Trichuris* and coccidia		few *Trichuris*		*Trichuris* rare		No ova seen	
Occult blood test	4+		3+		fresh blood		4+	

Bone marrow evaluation, aspiration from iliac crest on Jan. 3 (500 cells differentiated)

Rubriblast	1.0%	Myeloblast	0.8%	Lymphocytes	8.4%
Prorubricyte	2.6	Progranulocyte	0.6	Monocytes	2.2
Basophilic rubricyte	16.6	Neutrophilic myelocyte	1.6	Plasma cells	0.6
Polychromatic rubricyte	8.8	Eosinophilic myelocyte	0.6	RE nuclei	2.0
Metarubricyte	16.0	Neutrophilic metamyelocyte	5.0	Degenerated	2.8
Mitotic figure	0.6	Neutrophilic band cells	6.4	Total other cells	16.0
Total erythrocytic	45.6	Neutrophils mature	22.6		
		Eosinophils	0.8		
M:E ratio = 0.84:1.0		Total granulocytic	38.4		

more than doubled. By the end of the fourth week, all values of the hemogram were within the normal range, with the exception of the leukocyte count. A leukopenia was evident from January 17 onward and was due essentially to a neutropenia. It was speculated that this was a direct result of the daily administration of salicylazosulfapyridine.

Case 34 (Dog). Microcytic Hypochromic Anemia Due to Subacute Blood Loss

A male springer spaniel, 2 years old, was presented on Sept. 18 exhibiting extreme weakness, very pale mucous membranes, temperature 99.2° F, and a pulse rate of 168/min. The severe anemia was due to subacute blood loss from a heavy infestation with the bloodsucking flea, *Echidnophaga gallinacea.*

A blood transfusion of 250 ml was administered immediately, the fleas were removed, and a hematinic of high iron content was given orally. The dog was maintained under observation to follow the remission of the anemia in both blood and bone marrow. The latter was aspirated from the iliac crest.

Interpretation

1. The PCV of 9.0% and the microcytic hypochromic erythrocytes indicated that the

Case 34 (Dog). **Microcytic Hypochromic Anemia**

	Sept. 18		Sept. 25		Oct. 1		Oct. 5		Oct. 12	
Erythrocytes										
RBC ($\times 10^6$/μl)	1.94		3.20		5.03		6.58		8.09	
Hemoglobin (g/dl)	2.25		5.30		7.63		8.63		10.80	
PCV (%)	9.0		20.0		29.0		37.0		38.0	
MCV (fl)	46.4		62.5		57.7		56.2		46.9	
MCHC (%)	25.0		26.5		26.3		23.3		28.4	
Erythrocyte sed. rate/1 hr	diphasic		diphasic		8/28 = 20−		0/13 = 13−		0/12 = 12−	
Reticulocytes (%)	2.3		6.7		2.3		—		—	
Nucleated RBC/100 WBC	4.0		5.0		1.0		0		0	
Anisocytosis	prominent		prominent		moderate		moderate		slight	
Polychromasia	moderate		moderate		slight		slight		slight	
Hypochromasia	prominent		prominent		prominent		prominent		moderate	
Leukocytes		%		%		%		%		%
WBC/μl (corrected)	25,650		12,050		9,100		12,550		11,350	
Band neutrophils	1,539	6.0	241	2.0	637	7.0	251	2.0	113	1.0
Neutrophils	20,520	80.0	6,748	56.0	5,187	57.0	7,530	60.0	4,880	43.0
Lymphocytes	1,795	7.0	4,579	38.0	2,821	31.0	3,263	26.0	4,880	43.0
Monocytes	1,795	7.0	361	3.0	273	3.0	627	5.0	794	7.0
Eosinophils	0	0.0	120	1.0	182	2.0	878	7.0	340	3.0
Unclassified cells	0	0.0	0	0.0	0	0.0	0	0.0	340	3.0

Bone Marrow	September 18 %	October 1 %	*Bone Marrow*	September 18 %	October 1 %
Rubriblasts	0.9	1.3	Myeloblasts	0.3	0.4
Prorubricytes	2.5	2.7	Progranulocytes	0.6	0.5
Rubricytes	11.8	19.0	Neutrophilic myelocytes	0.7	1.1
Metarubricytes	36.1	43.0	Neutrophilic metamyelocytes	2.4	2.4
Total erythroid cells	51.3	66.0	Band neutrophils	8.0	9.3
			Neutrophils	18.4	8.8
Lymphocytes	4.0	4.1	Eosinophilic metamyelocytes	0.0	0.3
Monocytes	0.7	0.2	Band eosinophils	0.0	0.3
Unclassified	2.0	0.5	Eosinophils	0.0	0.1
Degenerated	11.6	6.0	Total granulocytic	30.4	23.2
Myeloid:erythroid ratio	0.59:1.0	0.35:1.0			

anemia was due to blood loss leading to iron deficiency and inadequate hemoglobin synthesis. It is important to note that with a slowly developing anemia, the PCV may become reduced to a very low level before the dog is presented to the veterinarian. In another dog, with a similar history of heavy flea infestation, the PCV was 5.0% on admission to the clinic. In slowly developing anemia, the vascular system makes adjustments to use the reduced number of erythrocytes more efficiently, e.g., hypertrophy of the heart, increased heart rate, constriction of the vascular beds in all but the vital organs, and increased depth of respiration.

2. The myeloid:erythroid ratio was typical of iron deficiency in that a majority of the nucleated erythrocytes were in the metarubricyte stage. Because of lack of iron the synthesis of hemoglobin occurs at a slow pace; hence the nucleus is retained longer than in the normal maturation sequence.

3. A marked depletion of body iron was indicated by the persistence of microcytic hypochromic erythrocytes, even though the anemia had essentially corrected itself by the final hemogram on Oct. 12. It may take months to replenish body stores of iron and reestablish normal erythrogenesis.

4. The initial leukogram was typical of a stress reaction. The relief felt systemically from administration of the blood transfusions and removal of the fleas was reflected in the fall in total leukocyte count, neutrophils, and monocytes and the increase in lymphocytes and eosinophils in the subsequent hemograms.

Case 35 (Dog). **Chronic Lead Poisoning**

A male wire-haired terrier, 10½ months of age and weighing about 16 pounds, was first seen by the referring veterinarian on Oct. 21. The owner complained that the dog was not eating and was displaying signs of nervous irritation. Despite symptomatic treatment and hospitalization on two occasions, the illness continued, and vomiting was observed on Dec. 15. The body temperature was within the normal range throughout this period. On Dec. 31, the patient developed running and champing fits (it had been vaccinated for canine distemper the previous June). The following day,

Case 35 (Dog).   Chronic Lead Poisoning

	Jan. 3	Jan. 5	Jan. 6	Jan. 14	Jan. 26
RBC ($\times 10^6/\mu l$)	7.45	—	6.75	6.37	6.72
Hemoglobin (g/dl)	14.3	—	13.4	13.5	12.5
PCV (%)	45.0	—	39.0	39.0	39.0
MCV (fl)	60.4	—	57.7	61.2	58.0
MCHC (%)	31.7	—	34.3	34.6	32.0
Erythrocyte sed. rate/1 hr	—	—	10−	18+	10−
Icterus index units	1.0	—	<5.0	<5.0	<5.0
Reticulocytes (%)	—	1.7	3.2	—	—
Nucleated erythrocytes	53/100 WBC	48/100	89/100	1/100	2/100
Target cells	+ + +		no record made of erythrocyte morphology		+ + +
Poikilocytes	+ +		Jan. 5, 6, 14		+ +
Polychromasia	+				+
WBC/μl (corrected)	10,000	17,300	18,000	28,400	20,300
Metamyelocytes	1.0%	—	1.0%	0.0%	0.0%
Bands	3.0	—	10.0	2.0	3.0
Neutrophils	64.0	—	66.0	81.0	74.0
Lymphocytes	18.0	—	16.0	5.0	13.0
Monocytes	10.0	—	3.0	8.0	7.0
Eosinophils	3.0	—	4.0	2.0	3.0
Unclassified cells	1.0	—	0.0	2.0	0.0

January 7: Bone Marrow Aspiration

	(%)
Myeloblasts	0.2
Progranulocytes	1.5
Myelocytes (neutrophilic)	3.4
Myelocytes (eosinophilic)	0.3
Metamyelocytes (neutrophilic)	3.8
Bands (neutrophilic)	13.8
Bands (eosinophilic)	0.3
Neutrophils	12.8
Total myeloid cells =	36.1
Prorubricytes	1.7
Rubricytes	11.2
Metarubricytes	47.0
Total erythroid cells	59.9
Other cells	4.0

M:E = 0.60:1.0

the patient was admitted to the clinic of the School of Veterinary Medicine.

Physical examination revealed an alert, thin, and somewhat dehydrated animal. A routine blood examination revealed a blood picture that was unusual in that there were 53 nucleated erythrocytes per 100 leukocytes but no other evidence of red cell regeneration. In searching for a probable explanation for the high level of nucleated red cells, attention was turned to the spleen. Physical examination had not detected any abnormality of the spleen, so a radiograph was requested. The diagnosis became apparent from the radiograph, for a dense object was revealed to be present in the stomach. A piece of lead, 1 inch square, was removed surgically. The diagnosis was chronic plumbism.

Treatment was directed at withdrawal of the lead by administration of the calcium salt of ethylenediaminetetraacetate (CaEDTA). The details of this treatment and results have been reported (J. Amer. Vet. Med. Ass., 128:295, 1956). The patient was

discharged on Jan. 30, but was readmitted Mar. 26. Polydipsia, anorexia, and vomiting had persisted during most of this period. On re-entry, the patient was moribund, the pulse rate was 200/min, and the body temperature was 105° F. The patient died, and on necropsy the kidneys revealed tissue changes suggestive of leptospirosis. Chemical analysis indicated high levels of lead in the urine, kidneys, liver, and bones.

Interpretation

1. Note the very high level of nucleated erythrocytes in the blood in the absence of frank anemia and out of proportion to the reticulocyte count. This is characteristic of lead poisoning in the dog.
2. Also note that basophilic stippling of erythrocytes, another characteristic finding in lead poisoning, was not observed at any time.
3. Although a frank anemia is not apparent, the M:E ratio of 0.60:1 indicates active erythrogenesis, but the presence of poikilocytes in

peripheral blood suggests a shorter life span of erythrocyte. Lead poisoning produces a defect in erythrocyte maturation, and microcytosis (MCV 57.7–61.2 fl) seen in this case may be a reflection of such an interference. For details on lead poisoning, see Chapter 24.

Case 36 (Dog). Salmon Poisoning—A Rickettsial Disease Caused by *Neorickettsia helminthoeca*

A male Gordon setter, 3 months of age, was presented for its final distemper vaccination. At that occasion there was a complaint of weight loss, anorexia, diarrhea, and conjunctivitis. Physical examination revealed enlarged cervical and popliteal lymph nodes and a rectal temperature of 102.8° F. The feces were bloody, and an occasional egg of the fluke *Nanophyetus salmincola* was found. The dog had eaten steelhead trout 2 weeks previously. Treatment to combat dehydration, diarrhea, and infection over a 5-day period brought about recovery.

Interpretation

Salmon poisoning of dogs is a disease indigenous to the Pacific Coast from northwestern California to southwestern Washington (Farrel et al., J. Amer. Vet. Med. Ass., *127*:241, 1955).

1. Presenting clinical signs were typical of salmon poisoning, i.e., anorexia, depression, dehydration, severe bloody diarrhea, fever, and lymphadenopathy.

2. Aspiration of a lymph node failed to demonstrate *Neorickettsia helminthoeca*; however, the finding of eggs of the fluke *Nanophyetus salmincola* (which is thought to constitute the reservoir of infections) on fecal examination was incriminating evidence of salmon poisoning, particularly in view of the typical clinical signs.

3. The progressive fall in PCV was a response to the daily administration of fluids to combat dehydration and to stimulate urine flow. The unmasked anemia was normocytic-normochromic without signs of remission.

4. The negative corrected value for erythrocyte sedimentation rate was consistent with the existence of hypoproteinemia and a normal plasma fibrinogen concentration.

5. The icterus index was clinically significant and increased from 10 to 25 units. A test for evidence of liver necrosis (SGPT) on the third day gave results within the normal range. The bilirubinemia may have resulted from swelling of liver cords with compression of bile canaliculi as a result of hypoxemia from anemia.

6. The differential leukocyte count on admission (Dec. 1) was of particular interest in view of the lymphocytosis with many large abnormal forms of lymphocytes and the monocytosis with many large, vacuolated cells (Plate XI–6). It is of interest that Farrell et al. (J. Amer. Vet. Med. Ass., *152*:370, 1968) also commented that lymphocytes were

Case 36 (Dog). Salmon Poisoning

	Dec. 1		Dec. 2		Dec. 3	
Erythrocytes						
RBC ($\times 10^6/\mu$l)	5.16		4.15		3.89	
Hemoglobin (g/dl)	10.7		8.1		7.9	
PCV (%)	34		27		25	
MCV (fl)	65.9		65.1		64.3	
MCHC (%)	31.4		30.0		31.6	
ESR/1 hr	0/18 = 18−		10/32 = 22−		4/36 = 32−	
Reticulocytes (%)	0.1		0.0		0.0	
Anisocytosis	slight		slight		slight	
Leukocytes		%		%		%
WBC/μl	31,200		43,000		26,100	
Band neutrophils	1,248	4.0	3,293	7.5	131	0.5
Mature neutrophils	16,380	52.5	30,511	69.5	17,878	68.5
Lymphocytes	11,232	36.0[a]	9,439	21.5[a]	4,306	16.5
Monocytes	2,340	7.5[a]	659	1.5	3,784	14.5
Mast cells	—		rare			
Plasma						
Total protein (g/dl)	4.4		4.3		4.9	
Fibrinogen (g/dl)	0.3		0.3		0.2	
Icterus index units	10		20		25	
Other Tests						
Blood urea nitrogen (mg/dl)	—		36.0		28.5	
SGPT (IU/L)	—		—		13.0	

[a]Many large abnormal forms of lymphocytes and monocytes (Plate XI–6).

large and some had indented nuclei and a faint basophilic staining of the cytoplasm.

7. The pathology of this disease in dogs has been described by D.R. Cordy and J.R. Gorham (Amer. J. Pathol., 26:617, 1950). The in vitro cultivation of *Neorickettsia helminthoeca* has been discussed by Brown et al. (Amer. J. Vet. Res., 33:1695, 1972).

Case 37 (Dog). Canine Distemper: Viral Inclusions in Erythrocytes and Leukocytes

A female Australian shepherd dog, 2 years old, was referred with a history of coughing and sneezing for 2 weeks. It had been on antibiotic therapy during the 2-week period without improvement. The dog had not received any vaccinations. On admission, the rectal temperature was 103° F, emaciation and depression were evident, there was a nasal exudate, and the footpads were dry and hard. The rectal temperature remained between 102.8° and 103.2° F during the following 3 days. On the fourth day of hospitalization, the temperature dropped to 99.9° F; the dog was exhibiting opisthotonos and nystagmus. The dog was euthanized. The pathologic diagnosis was canine distemper with demyelinating encephalitis. Numerous intranuclear inclusion bodies typical of canine distemper were seen.

Interpretation

1. Inclusions in immature erythrocytes occasionally have been encountered in association with canine distemper. The erythrocytic inclusion has been demonstrated in reticulocytes (Fig. 36–1) with new methylene blue stain. The inclusions also are demonstrable with Wright-Leishman stain (Plate XVIII–9). A typical erythrocytic inclusion as seen in this case is shown in Fig. A–1.

2. Cytoplasmic viral inclusions in leukocytes generally require a special staining procedure (Schorr stain) for their demonstration. On rare occasions, however, leukocyte inclusions in canine distemper may be seen in the routinely stained blood film. The cytoplasmic inclusion in neutrophils has appeared as a discrete round or oval structure (Figs. A–1 and A–2). In lymphocytes and monocytes, the inclusions have tended to be larger and more diffuse (Figs. A–3 and A–4) and appear light red (Plate XIV–7).

3. Electron microscopy revealed the inclusions in erythrocytes and leukocytes of the patient under consideration to be viral structures compatible with canine distemper (Figs. A–5 and A–6).

4. The marked absolute lymphopenia observed in the two hemograms was characteristic of canine distemper (Chapter 36).

Case 38 (Dog). Plasma Cell Myeloma and Glomerulonephritis

A 6-year-old male Scottish terrier was presented on Jan. 19 with the complaint of vomiting and difficulty in walking. The dog was unable to hold its head in a central position and appeared to be weak and unbalanced. Palpation detected a mass in the middle left abdomen. An exploratory laparotomy revealed an enlarged spleen with infarction, hematoma, and massive intra-abdominal hemorrhage. Splenectomy was performed. Histopathologic examination of the splenic tissue revealed large areas of hemorrhage and accumulations of round cells, with vesicular nuclei and prominent nucleoli, resulting in separation and compression of splenic follicles. Numerous megakaryocytes and extramedullary hemopoiesis were evident.

After removal of the spleen, the dog's condition improved and there was gain in weight, but a slight head tilt to the left persisted. On April 12, the dog

Case 37 (Dog). Canine Distemper

	Oct. 16		Oct. 19	
RBC ($\times 10^6/\mu$l)	4.46		4.91	
Hemoglobin (g/dl)	10.1		11.4	
PCV (%)	30.0		34.0	
MCV (fl)	67.2		69.2	
MCH (pg)	22.6		23.2	
MCHC (%)	33.6		33.5	
Erythrocyte sed. rate/1 hr.	—		44/18 = 26+	
Icterus index units	2		hemolysis	
Plasma proteins (g/dl)	6.3		7.3	
Fibrinogen (g/dl)	0.4		0.5	
Reticulocytes (%)	0.8		1.7	
WBC/μl	13,200	%	16,300	%
Neutrophils	11,550	87.5	12,062	74.0
Lymphocytes	528	4.0	489	3.0
Monocytes	1,122	8.5	3,749	23.0

Inclusion bodies present in a few erythrocytes and in the cytoplasm of some neutrophils, lymphocytes, and monocytes.

Only one neutrophil seen with a cytoplasmic inclusion, and rare erythrocyte with an inclusion.

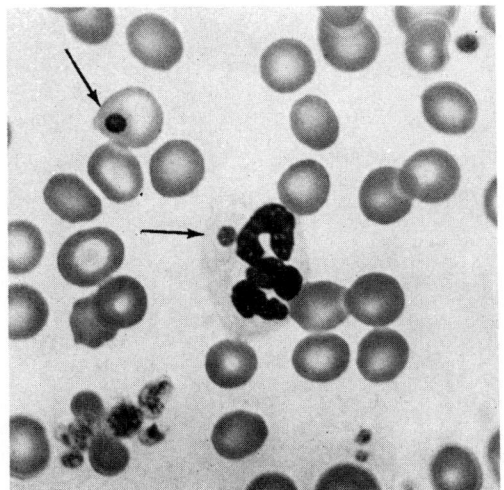

Fig. A–1. Viral inclusions in an erythrocyte and neutrophil. ×2,320.

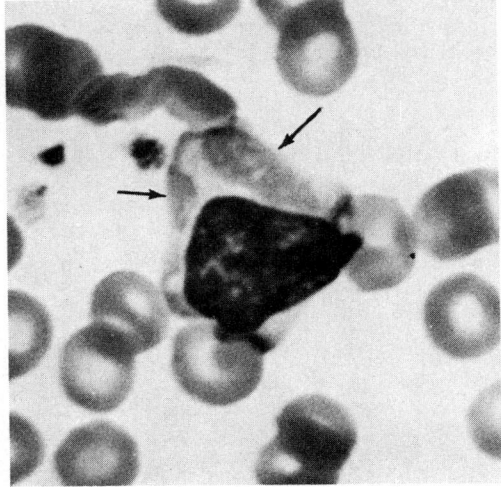

Fig. A–3. Viral inclusions in a lymphocyte. ×3,870.

was readmitted to the hospital with a history of poor appetite, polydipsia, and polyuria for the preceding 2 weeks and vomiting for the preceding 2 days. Laboratory findings were similar to those of the first admission. On the basis of all available data, multiple myeloma was suspected, and a skeletal survey was made. Decreased bone density was noted in the proximal right tibia, distal right femur, and dorsal spine of the second lumbar vertebra. Euthanasia was recommended.

Necropsy. The liver was somewhat enlarged, the kidneys were small and pale with atrophic cortices, and the mesenteric and colonic lymph nodes were slightly enlarged. On histopathologic examination of selected tissues, myeloma plasma cells were observed in the myocardium, liver, and bone marrow. There were several myeloma cell foci in the cortex of the kidney, and, in addition, many

glomeruli were small with thickened tufts and some clumps of amyloid. A diagnosis of plasma cell myeloma and glomerulonephritis was made.

Interpretation

1. On first admission (Jan. 19), an anemia in remission was in evidence. The low plasma fibrinogen concentration and thrombocytopenia gave rise to speculation of internal bleeding due to disseminated intravascular coagulation. This concept was supported by the observation of infarction and massive hematoma of the spleen.
2. The most significant feature of the initial laboratory study was the demonstration of a dysproteinemia due to marked elevation of γ-globulin. The finding of a proliferation of abnormal and immature cells in the spleen pointed to the existence of a neoplastic, glob-

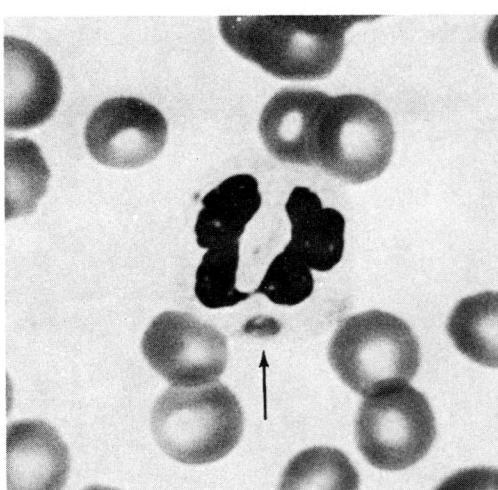

Fig. A–2. Viral inclusion in a neutrophil. ×3,870.

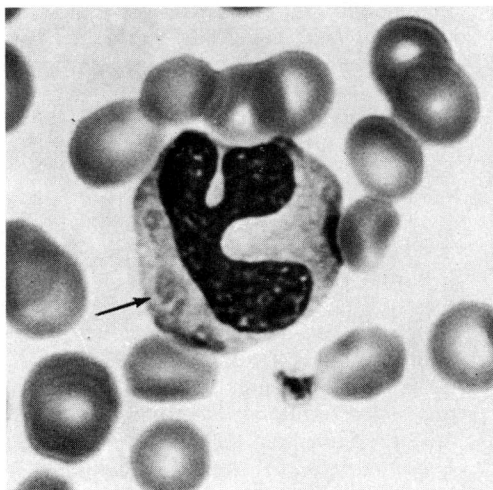

Fig. A–4. Viral inclusions in a monocyte. ×3,870.

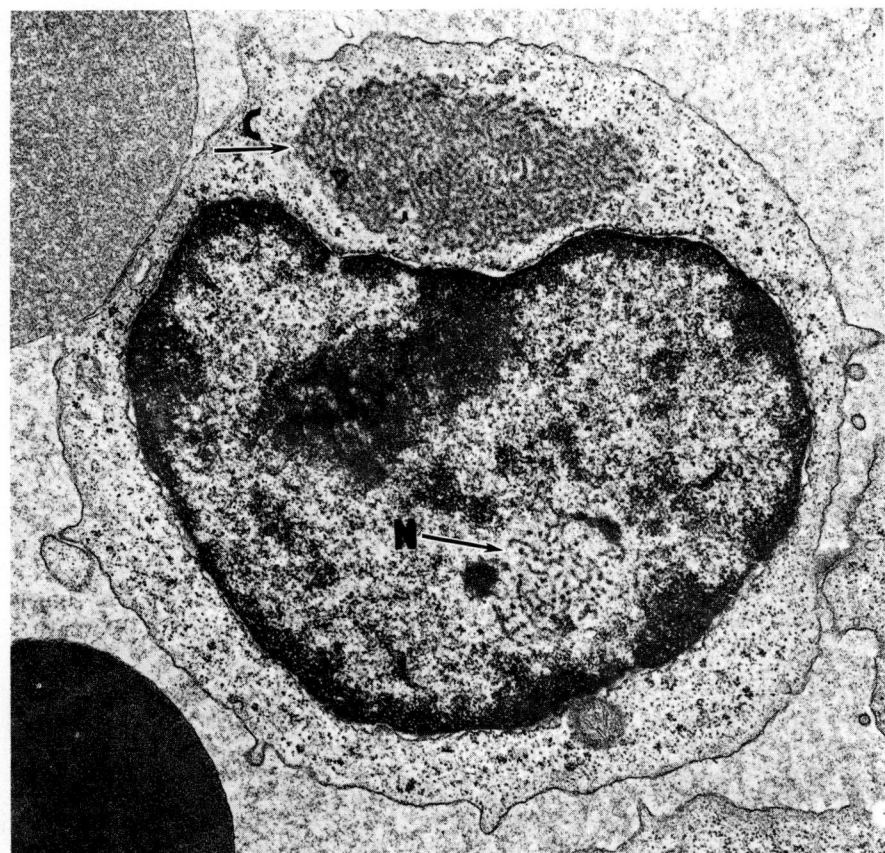

Fig. A–5.   Filamentous viral structures, compatible with canine distemper virus, are present in the nucleus *(N)* and cytoplasm *(C)* of a lymphocyte (×16,500). Compare with Fig. A–3.

ulin-secreting plasma cell population, as supported by subsequent findings.

3. Removal of the spleen and the transfusion of whole blood during surgery led to an increase in erythrocyte number, PCV, and hemoglobin and a decrease in total plasma proteins, as demonstrated in the hemogram of Jan. 26 and the protein fractionation pattern on Jan. 29.

4. The improvement in health was temporary; in 2 months, the dog was exhibiting signs of general poor health. Laboratory studies on April 12 revealed advanced nonresponsive anemia and marked dysproteinemia characterized by a monoclonal gammopathy (Chapter 34). A test for Bence Jones protein was negative, but a bone scan by radiography indicated decreased density of several bones, thereby lending support to a diagnosis of multiple myeloma. Bence Jones proteinuria is found only in some cases of canine multiple myeloma. (See Chapter 34.)

5. The anemia and thrombocytopenia of April 12 may be attributed to replacement of normal marrow cells by malignant cells. The el-

evated SGPT and low plasma fibrinogen may be explained by the extensive infiltration of the liver by malignant plasma cells. Protein fractionation revealed a monoclonal gammopathy (Fig. A–7).

6. The blood urea nitrogen and creatinine values did not reflect the considerable glomerular changes observed on histopathologic examination of the kidneys, but 1+ proteinuria at urine specific gravity of 1.016 is consistent with kidney lesions.

Case 39 (Dog).   Lymphangiectasia

A 10-year-old male German shepherd dog had a 6-year history of gastrointestinal problems dating from surgical correction of a gastrosplenic torsion. In August 1968, the dog developed diarrhea and anemia. It was given antibiotics, an anticholinergic, and pancreatic enzymes per os. A dietary change was recommended. There was no response, so it was admitted to the university clinic in October. On admission, the dog had diarrhea, anorexia, and malaise. An intensive study was made, and it was concluded that the dog had a gluten-induced enteropathy resulting in malab-

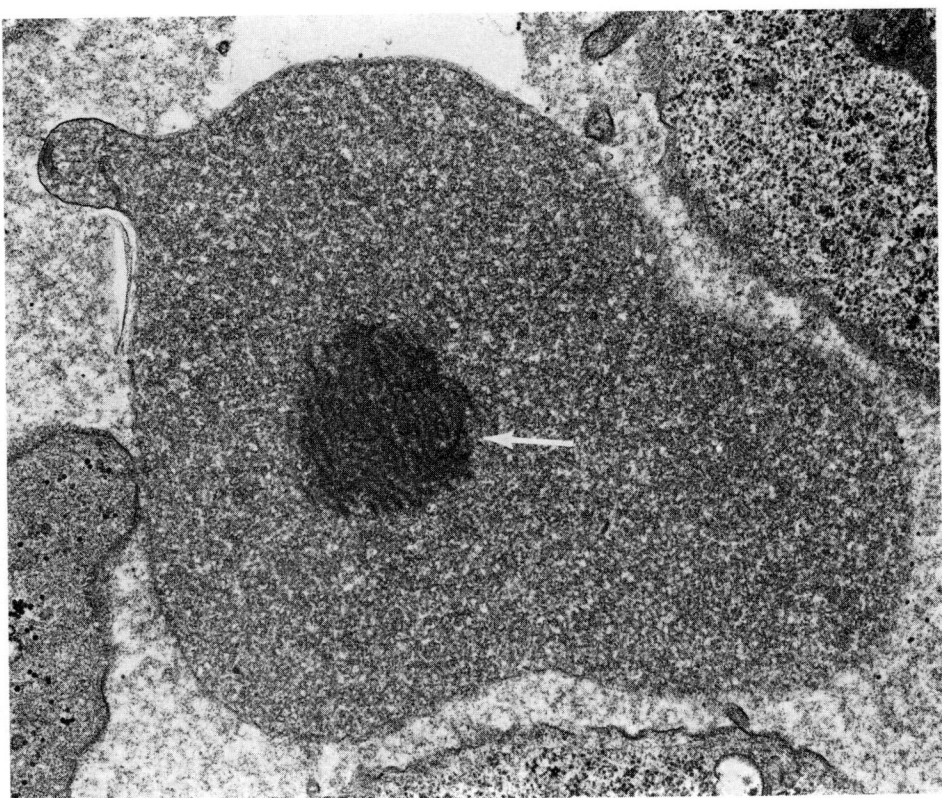

Fig. A–6. A filamentous viral structure in an erythrocyte (×23,000). Compare with Fig. A–1. (Figs. A–5 and A–6 courtesy of Dr. David H. Gribble.

sorption. After the dog was placed on a gluten-free diet, an immediate improvement was noted, and the dog was sent home. It was readmitted in February 1969, when the owners noted that the dog was losing weight. In March 1969, an intestinal biopsy demonstrated excessive swelling of the intestinal lymphatics. A diagnosis of lymphangiectasia was made.

The serum protein profiles are given in the table.

The dog was treated with methischol (Armour) and was kept on the gluten-free diet, but it died in April 1969 from a gastric torsion.

Although only two serum protein fractionations were done, there is a strong possibility that the dog had been hypoproteinemic for a long time. The severe lymphopenia suggests the possibility of loss of lymph into the gut. A similar case has been reported by Campbell et al. (J. Amer. Vet. Med. Ass., *153*:1050, 1968).

Case 40 (Cat).   Abnormal Granulopoiesis in Acute Toxemic Disease

A male seal-point Siamese, 5 years old, was presented exhibiting signs of dyspnea, increased vesicular sounds, depression, dehydration, and a temperature of 103.6° F. Antibiotics and multivitamins were administered daily. Recovery was rapid and uneventful. The hemograms are of in-terest in view of the marked change in the leukogram within a 4-day period.

Interpretation

1. The cat characteristically expresses the severity of a disease process in changes in the morphology of the neutrophil granulocyte. In toxemic diseases, there may be complete depression of granulopoiesis, initially, leading to leukopenia, followed by remission with a marked left shift and "toxic" neutrophils. The toxic state is shown in increased size of neutrophils, bizarre nuclear patterns, sometimes giant forms, and basophilia of the cytoplasm. The cytoplasm is very granular and diffusely bluish. As the toxemia decreases, the succeeding generations of neutrophils are more normal in size, and the cytoplasm presents its normal pinkish granularity with residual deposits of angular to round bluish structures called Döhle bodies (Plate IX–2).

2. Changes in neutrophil morphology occur rapidly as the toxemia is brought under control. Examination of the stained blood film taken daily from capillary blood of the ear is a rapid and practical means for evaluation of the progress in toxemic diseases of the cat.

Case 38 (Dog). Plasma Cell Myeloma and Glomerulonephritis

	Jan. 19		Jan. 26		April 12	
Erythrocytes						
			(postsplenectomy)			
RBC ($\times 10^6/\mu$l)	2.86		5.05		2.65	
Hb (g/dl)	7.3		11.3		5.1	
PCV (%)	20		35		17	
MCV (fl)	69.9		69.3		64.1	
MCH (pg)	25.5		22.3		19.2	
MCHC (%)	36.5		32.2		30.0	
ESR/1 hr	67/49 = 18+		21/16 = 5+			
Reticulocytes (%)	10.8		5.2		2.5	
Nucleated RBC/100 WBC	4		0		5	
Anisocytosis	moderate		slight		moderate	
Polychromasia	moderate		slight		slight	
Leukocytes		%		%		%
WBC/μl (corrected)	10,800		23,600		7,100	
Band neutrophils	324	3.0	1,062	4.5	284	4.0
Mature neutrophils	7,938	73.5	17,818	75.5	4,118	58.0
Lymphocytes	1,134	10.5	1,298	5.5	2,201	31.0
Monocytes	1,296	12.0	3,422	14.5	426	6.0
Eosinophils	0	0.0	0	0.0	71	1.0
Plasma cells	108	1.0	0	0.0	0	0.0
Plasma						
Protein (g/dl)	14.1		7.8		14.9	
Fibrinogen (g/dl)	0.1		0.2		<0.1	
Icterus index units	7.5		2		slight hemolysis and lipemia	
Other Tests						
Platelets	56,000		—		24,000	
Urine specific gravity	1.016		—		1.013	
Creatinine (mg/dl)	—		—		0.8	
Blood urea nitrogen (mg/dl)	—		—		30.0	
Proteinuria	1+		—		1+	
Bence Jones protein	—		—		negative	
SGPT (IU/L)	—		—		45.5	

Serum Protein Fractionation (g/dl)			
	Jan. 19	Jan. 29	April 12 (see Fig. A–7)
Total protein	13.9	6.8	14.7
Albumin	1.9	3.6	1.93
Globulin	12.0	3.2	12.77
alpha-1	0.2	0.7	0.13
alpha-2	0.3	—	0.09
beta-1	0.9	0.1	} 0.44
beta-2	0.6	0.7	
gamma-1	5.3	0.6	} 12.11
gamma-2	4.7	1.1	
A:G ratio	0.16:1.0	1.12:1.0	0.15:1.0

Immune panel

Antinuclear antibody test = negative
Coombs test = negative
LE cells = negative

Case 41 (Cat). Marked Leukopenia with Rapid Remission

A castrated male seal-point Siamese, 3½ years old, was presented exhibiting signs of anorexia, nausea characterized by bile-stained vomitus, and bloody diarrhea. One popliteal lymph node was enlarged. There was evidence of dehydration, and the temperature was 102.6° F. The cat had been vaccinated against panleukopenia virus at 2 months of age. Therapy consisted of antibiotics, multivitamins, and fluids. A total of 150 ml of 5% dextrose was given between Oct. 24 and Oct. 27. The cat was considerably improved by October 28, and it was able to go home on the seventh day from admission.

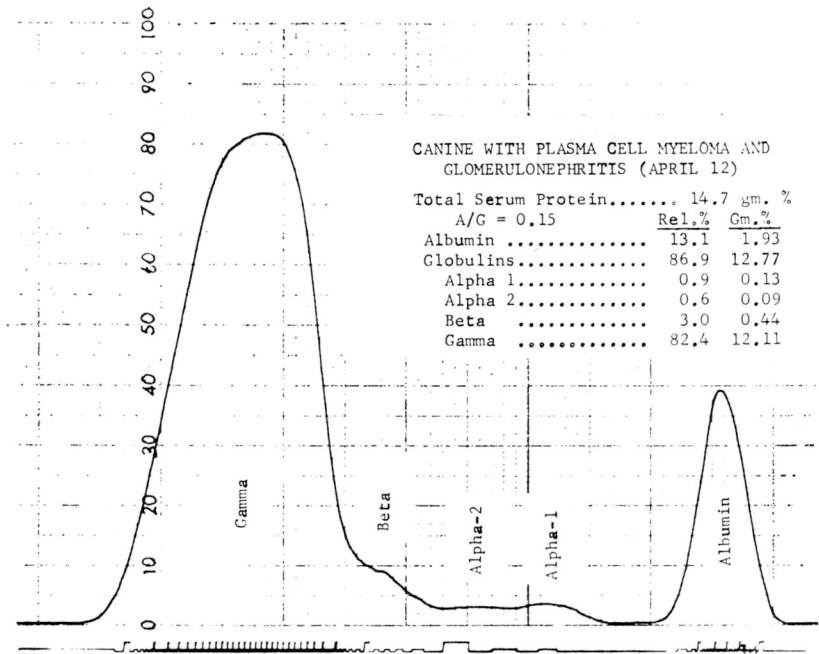

CANINE WITH PLASMA CELL MYELOMA AND
GLOMERULONEPHRITIS (APRIL 12)

	Rel.%	Gm.%
Total Serum Protein....... 14.7 gm. %		
A/G = 0.15		
Albumin	13.1	1.93
Globulins.............	86.9	12.77
Alpha 1.............	0.9	0.13
Alpha 2.............	0.6	0.09
Beta	3.0	0.44
Gamma	82.4	12.11

Fig. A–7. Protein fractionation demonstrating a monoclonal gammopathy in a dog with plasma cell myeloma.

Bone marrow aspiration on Oct. 26 revealed a nearly complete absence of mature neutrophils. The cells of the granulocytic series were large, with many metamyelocytes appearing as large as the progranulocytes. The impression gained was that maturation of the nucleus proceeded directly from the progranulocyte stage without division of the cell. Thus the cells were large and the cytoplasm remained basophilic. There was a distinct lack of cells within the erythrocytic maturation series.

Interpretation

1. The disease produced a depression of all leukocyte types as well as cells of the erythrocytic maturation series. The bone marrow and blood findings on Oct. 26 were typical of the cellular patterns to be seen during the early recovery stage from panleukopenia virus infection.
2. Marrow suppression of erythropoiesis was not reflected as frank anemia because of the considerably long life span of red cells com-

pared to that of the neutrophils, which can be depleted within a few days of inhibition of granulopoiesis. The rebound of the erythrocytic series followed a few days later. There was evidence of red blood cell production and release to peripheral blood on Oct. 30.
3. This sequence of hemograms clearly reveals the speed with which neutrophilic granulocytes of the cat enter a remission phase after a marked neutropenia in an acute disease process.

Case 42 (Cat). Severe Dehydration and Response to Corticosteroids

A female Siamese cat, 2 years old, was presented with a complaint of anorexia, vomiting, and constipation. It had been vaccinated against panleukopenia virus. Clinical signs on entry were a temperature of 103° F, depression, dull appearance to the eyes, and a dry nose. Therapy consisted of the daily administration of antibiotics, corticosteroids,

Case 39 (Dog). Lymphangiectasia

	10/68	2/69	Lymphocyte counts		
				Rel. %	Total
Total protein	2.9 g/dl	3.2 g/dl	10/11/68	3.0	549
Albumin	1.0	1.1	10/16/68	1.5	253
Globulin	1.9	2.1	2/20/69	1.0	196
alpha-1	0.1	0.1			
alpha-2	0.5	0.3			
beta-1	0.7	0.8			
gamma	0.6	0.9			

Case 40 (Cat).   Abnormal Granulopoiesis

	April 27		May 1	
Erythrocytes				
RBC ($\times 10^6/\mu l$)	8.30		6.95	
Hemoglobin (g/dl)	10.1		10.8	
PCV (%)	36.0		32.0	
MCV (fl)	43.4		46.0	
MCHC (%)	28.0		33.7	
Anisocytosis	slight		slight	
Howell-Jolly bodies	occasional		rare	
Heinz bodies	rare		rare	
Leukocytes		%		%
WBC/μl	41,200		27,300	
Progranulocytes	206	0.5	0	0.0
Myelocytes	618	1.5	0	0.0
Metamyelocytes	1,442	3.5	0	0.0
Band neutrophils	8,034	19.5	0	0.0
Neutrophils	28,016	68.0	22,796	83.5
Lymphocytes	2,678	6.5	3,549	13.0
Monocytes	206	0.5	273	1.0
Eosinophils	0	0.0	410	1.5
Basophils	0	0.0	136	0.5
Unclassified cells	0	0.0	136	0.5
Neutrophil morphology	Large cells, many with bizarre coiled nuclei and basophilic, granular cytoplasm. (Plate IX–3)		Essentially normal in size and appearance. Cytoplasm has the normal dust-like, pinkish granulation with only an occasional tiny bluish granule	

Case 41 (Cat).   Marked Leukopenia

	October 24		October 26		October 30	
Erythrocytes						
RBC ($\times 10^6/\mu l$)	9.25		7.4		5.75	
Hemoglobin (g/dl)	12.7		12.4		10.0	
PCV (%)	34		34		28	
MCV (fl)	36.7		45.9		48.7	
MCHC (%)	37.3		36.5		35.7	
Icterus index units	—		2		—	
Nucleated RBC/100 WBC	0		0		2.5	
Anisocytosis	slight		slight		moderate	
Howell-Jolly bodies	none		few		few	
Heinz bodies	few		rare		none	
Polychromasia	none		none		moderate	
Leukocytes		%		%		%
WBC/μl (corrected)	1,300		5,200		22,900	
Progranulocytes	0	0.0	52	1.0	0	0.0
Myelocytes	0	0.0	26	0.5	0	0.0
Metamyelocytes	0	0.0	26	0.5	0	0.0
Band neutrophils	0	0.0	260	5.0	229	1.0
Neutrophils	312	24.0	1,716	33.0	16,259	71.0
Lymphocytes	806	62.0	1,430	27.5	5,611	24.5
Monocytes	169	13.0	1,066	20.5	458	2.0
Eosinophils	13	1.0	312	6.0	229	1.0
Basophils	0	0.0	0	0.0	0	0.0
Unclassified cells	0	0.0	208	4.0	0	0.0
Degenerated cells	0	0.0	104	2.0	114	0.5
Neutrophil morphology	Larger than normal; blue, granular cytoplasm		Larger than normal with basophilic cytoplasm		Essentially normal	

Case 42 (Cat). Dehydration and Response to Corticosteroids

	March 20		*March 25*		*April 3*	
Erythrocytes						
RBC ($\times 10^6/\mu$l)	11.65		8.30		6.66	
Hemoglobin (g/dl)	17.6		12.1		11.5	
PCV (%)	59.6		39.0		35.0	
MCV (fl)	50.6		46.9		52.5	
MCHC (%)	29.8		31.0		32.8	
Erythrocyte morphology	extreme rouleaux		normal		normal	
Heinz bodies	few		few		few	
Leukocytes		%		%		%
WBC/μl	14,700		48,200		28,700	
Band neutrophils	441	3.0	241	0.5	287	1.0
Neutrophils	12,495	85.0	45,308	94.0	26,547	92.5
Lymphocytes	1,544	10.5	723	1.5	1,004	3.5
Monocytes	73	0.5	0	0.0	430	1.5
Eosinophils	147	1.0	1,928	4.0	430	1.5
Leukocyte morphology	All neutrophils are very large; some giant forms, with coiled bizarre nuclei; some Döhle bodies (Plate XV–10).		Neutrophils are large; many with hypersegmentation of the nucleus. Cytoplasm has normal staining characteristics.		Essentially normal, but some large cells remain.	
Other Tests						
Fecal examination	no parasite ova seen					
Urine: Specific gravity	1.045		1.012			
Protein	2+		negative			
Indican	3+		negative			
Blood urea nitrogen	March 22 = 58 mg/dl					

and fluids. The specific cause of the disease was not determined.

Interpretation

1. The extreme degree of dehydration was clearly reflected in the first hemogram by a PCV of 59.6%; erythrocyte number and hemoglobin concentration were elevated proportionately.

2. In the second hemogram, made 5 days later, the PCV had been reduced to 39% by the administration of 1,000 ml of fluids. This suggests that the loss of water from the circulation in this cat had reached the near-fatal level of 35%.

3. The first hemogram revealed an absolute lymphocyte count bordering on lymphopenia. The effect of steroid therapy on total and differential leukocyte numbers is clearly demonstrated in the second hemogram, namely, marked leukocytosis, neutrophilia, lymphopenia, and monocytopenia. Instead of the anticipated eosinopenia, the cat presented an unexplained eosinophilia. From these results it can be seen that steroid therapy complicates interpretation of the leukogram (Fig. 5–3).

Case 43 (Cat). Leukopenia and Anemia in Toxoplasmosis

A male, domestic shorthair cat was first seen when 1 year of age. At this time, there was re-spiratory distress and a corneal ulcer of the left eye. At the age of 2 years, there was a complaint of coughing with increasing frequency over the past year. The first hemogram was made at this time (July 15). Three months later, Oct. 25, the cat was presented with a complaint of vomiting for the past 3 days. The temperature was 102.0° F, respiration 20/min, and pulse 128/min. Antibiotics were administered and were continued throughout this terminal period. The temperature increased to 103° and then to 104° F with death occurring on Dec. 9.

Necropsy. Gross examination revealed pulmonary congestion and edema, and microscopically there was evidence of interstitial pneumonia with areas of acute necrosis. Numerous macrophages were present containing structures characteristic of *Toxoplasma gondii*. Toxoplasma organisms were also observed in lymph node sections. The liver was pale and presented numerous red pinpoint foci of acute focal coagulative necrosis, probably from terminal bacterial invasion.

Interpretation

1. A slight to borderline anemia was in evidence throughout, although on Oct. 25, the red cell values were within the lower normal range. The increasing MCV and moderate to marked anisocytosis may suggest a regenerative response to anemia, but in the absence of a significant polychromasia or reticulo-

Case 43 (Cat).   Toxoplasmosis

	July 15		October 25		November 9		December 3	
Erythrocytes								
RBC ($\times 10^6/\mu$l)	4.45		5.55		3.20		3.85	
Hemoglobin (g/dl)	8.1		9.1		6.0		8.1	
PCV (%)	24.0		30.0		18.0		25.0	
MCV (fl)	53.0		54.0		56.0		64.0	
MCHC (%)	33.0		30.0		33.0		32.0	
Icterus index units	2		—		—		—	
Nucleated RBC/100 WBC	0.5		0		2.5		0	
Anisocytosis	marked		slight		moderate		moderate	
Polychromasia	none		none		slight		none	
Howell-Jolly bodies	few		few		moderate		few	
Heinz bodies	none		few		rare		rare	
Other RBC features	crenation		none		poikilocytes		poikilocytes	
Leukocytes		%		%		%		%
WBC/μl (corrected)	4,400		4,600		9,700		2,200	
Band neutrophils	88	2.0	138	3.0	0	0.0	44	2.0
Neutrophils	3,740	85.0	3,588	78.0	7,954	82.0	1,782	81.0
Lymphocytes	308	7.0	598	13.0	1,310	13.5	176	8.0
Monocytes	154	3.5	276	6.0	388	4.0	198	9.0
Eosinophils	22	0.5	0	0.0	48	0.5	0	0.0
Basophils	0	0.0	0	0.0	0	0.0	0	0.0
Degenerated cells	88	2.0	0	0.0	0	0.0	0	0.0
Neutrophil morphology	Occasional Döhle body		Döhle bodies prominent		Less toxic appearing		Döhle bodies moderately prominent	

cytosis these findings are to be viewed as interference with erythropoiesis leading to some maturation arrest and production of macrocytic red cells. The presence of poikilocytes terminally indicated a shortened life span of the erythrocytes.

2. Leukopenia due essentially to marked lymphopenia and later to neutropenia was characteristic of the disease. For a brief period after antibiotic therapy was started, the neutrophils and lymphocytes increased, but this was followed shortly by a more marked depression of these cells. Signs of toxic changes in neutrophils were limited to the presence of Döhle bodies. (Retrak, M., and Carpenter, J.: Feline Toxoplasmosis. J. Amer. Vet. Med. Ass., 146:728, 1965.)

Case 44 (Cat).   Lymphopenia and Anemia in Chronic Peritonitis

A male domestic shorthair cat, 1 year old, was presented with a history of anorexia and listlessness of 2 to 3 weeks' duration. The temperature was 105° F, pulse rapid and weak; hyperpnea and painful abdomen were also noted. A radiograph revealed fluid in the abdominal cavity. The fluid was found to be a purulent exudate with 60,500 white cells/μl of which half were neutrophils. No bacteria were observed in the stained film, and no bacteria grew on aerobic culturing of the exudate. Therapy was limited to daily administration of antibiotics. The hemograms reveal steady improve-

ment, but despite this progress the owner requested that the cat be destroyed.

Necropsy. Organizing fibrinopurulent peritonitis of unknown cause.

Interpretation

1. A borderline anemia was present that was masked initially by some dehydration. On improvement in the clinical well-being, the PCV fell to 23%.
2. The most significant value in the hemogram was the change in absolute lymphocyte numbers from a state of lymphopenia to the high normal range in a 4-day period. This was a reflection of the improved clinical condition following antibiotic therapy. Prognosis was excellent for an uneventful recovery. The return of lymphocytes to peripheral blood on administration of therapy indicated that this most likely was not feline infectious peritonitis of viral origin. Furthermore, the purulent nature of the peritoneal exudate was not typical of FIP.
3. The neutrophilia with slight left shift to band cells and few Döhle bodies were in response to suppurative inflammation.

Case 45 (Cat).   Feline Infectious Peritonitis

An intact female domestic shorthair, 10 months old, was presented with a complaint of anorexia, temperature 105°F, congested mucous membranes, purulent exudate from the eyes, and central nervous system signs characterized by turning

Case 44 (Cat). **Chronic Peritonitis**

	April 16		April 18		April 19		April 20	
Erythrocytes								
RBC ($\times 10^6/\mu l$)	6.80		7.1		8.0		4.55	
Hemoglobin (g/dl)	8.7		10.0		9.7		7.6	
PCV (%)	27.0		30.0		28.0		23.0	
MCV (fl)	39.7		42.2		35.0		50.5	
MCHC (%)	32.2		33.3		34.6		33.0	
Nucleated RBC/100 WBC	2		0		1		4.5	
Crenation	prominent		none		none		moderate	
Anisocytosis	slight		slight		slight		moderate	
Polychromasia	slight		none		rare		slight	
Howell-Jolly bodies	few		few		rare		rare	
Bowl-shaped RBC	none		many		slight		none	
Leukocytes		%		%		%		%
WBC/μl (corrected)	22,550		36,900		39,600		18,525	
Band neutrophils	1,465	6.5	533	1.5	1,188	3.0	93	0.5
Neutrophils	18,378	81.5	31,918	86.5	30,888	78.0	10,929	59.0
Lymphocytes	1,465	6.5	3,690	10.0	6,534	16.5	6,298	34.0
Monocytes	902	4.0	184	0.5	594	1.5	1,204	6.5
Eosinophils	0	0.0	553	1.5	198	0.5	0	0.0
Basophils	0	0.0	0	0.0	198	0.5	0	0.0
Degenerated cells	338	1.5	0	0.0	0	0.0	0	0.0
Neutrophil morphology	Few Döhle bodies		Few Döhle bodies		Few Döhle bodies		Essentially normal pinkish granular cytoplasm	

the head to one side. No treatment was administered. Temperature remained between 103.0° and 104.8°F for 16 days and then fell to 101.4–102.5°F. The patient was observed over a period of 55 days and then was euthanized.

Bone Marrow Aspirated from Dorsal Femur, April 22. Early stages of the erythrocytic series were lacking and only limited numbers of late stages were present. Progranulocytes and myelocytes pre-

sented abnormal cytoplasmic vacuolation. Mature neutrophils appeared normal in number and morphology. M:E ratio was estimated to be 5.0:1.0.

Necropsy Findings. Multiple whitish foci and plaques were distributed over the entire peritoneal surface. The pleura also was covered with whitish foci. The mesenteric nodes were enlarged and reddish gray.

Histopathology. Numerous pyogranulomas

Case 45 (Cat). **Feline Infectious Peritonitis**

	March 18		April 22		May 12	
Erythrocytes						
RBC ($\times 10^6/\mu l$)	4.95		3.25		4.25	
Hemoglobin (g/dl)	6.3		5.6		7.0	
PCV (%)	20.0		19.0		22.0	
MCV (fl)	40.4		58.5		51.8	
MCHC (%)	31.5		29.5		31.8	
Nucleated RBC/100 WBC	1.0		none seen		none seen	
Reticulocytes (%)	rare		rare		rare	
Anisocytosis	slight		slight		slight	
Polychromasia	none		none		none	
Heinz bodies	rare		few		rare	
Leukocytes		%		%		%
WBC/μl (corrected)	9,850		10,850		5,900	
Band neutrophils	2,659	27.0	217	2.0	118	2.0
Neutrophils	6,403	65.0	10,036	92.5	5,428	92.0
Lymphocytes	788	8.0	217	2.0	236	4.0
Monocytes	0	0.0	217	2.0	59	1.0
Eosinophils	0	0.0	163	1.5	59	1.0
Plasma						
Proteins (g/dl)	—		9.8		9.8	
Fibrinogen (g/dl)	—		0.3		0.3	
Icterus index units	—		2		2	

were scattered throughout the omentum but were largely centered on blood vessels. Giant cells were present, and the tissue was edematous. Pyogranulomatous cuffs were present in the meninges, medulla, and cerebrum. Similar pyogranulomatous vessel lesions occurred in the kidneys and mesenteric lymph nodes.

Interpretation

1. The virus of feline infectious peritonitis depresses both erythropoiesis and lymphopoiesis; hence there is a normocytic-normochromic anemia and lymphopenia.
2. Granulopoiesis was not stimulated as in bacterial infections, and at the terminal stage of the disease, absolute neutrophil numbers in the circulation were less than the mean normal value. This was probably a reflection of suppression of marrow granulocytopoiesis from marrow necrosis as a terminal event.
3. Icterus index was normal, but in some cases of FIP it is elevated from liver involvement.
4. Total plasma protein was increased at 9.8 g/dl, possibly due to a combination of dehydration and hypergammaglobulinemia characteristic of the disease (Fig. 34–11). Plasma fibrinogen remained within the normal range.
5. The exudate that forms in the abdominal cavity and on occasion in the thoracic cavity is typical of the disease. The exudate is commonly voluminous, clear to slightly cloudy, and viscous, and it may clot on exposure to air. There is a high protein content consisting mainly of γ-globulin. The exudate is nonsuppurative; the total leukocyte count is low (6,300 ± 5,400/µl in 22 cats with FIP; see also Chapter 36).

Case 46 (Cat).   Progressive Anemia in Adenocarcinoma of the Small Intestine

A female seal-point Siamese cat, 11½ years old, was first presented on August 7 with a complaint of vomiting sporadically over a period of 2 weeks. An essentially normal hemogram (Aug. 8) was observed. The cat was treated as an outpatient, but vomiting started again about 3 weeks later, and by September 19 hardly any food could be retained. The cat entered the clinic again on Oct. 14. The 2-hour film after barium administration exhibited a dilatation of the small intestine anterior to a narrow band of intestinal constriction. The cat died on Oct. 20.

Necropsy Report.   Adenocarcinoma of the intestine causing incomplete obstruction was present. There was a mild nephrosis, and the liver and spleen contained extensive deposits of hemosiderin.

Interpretation

1. The hemogram of September 19 revealed Heinz bodies in profusion and of such large

size to be readily visible in the Wright-Leishman-stained blood film. Thereafter, a progressive anemia developed with no evidence of remission. The pathologist's report indicated extensive deposits of hemosiderin in the liver and spleen from erythrocyte destruction in macrophages. It would appear that destruction of the erythrocytes containing large Heinz bodies enhanced the development of anemia of chronic disease. Heinz body anemia is typically hemolytic and regenerative. Reticulocytopenia and absence of polychromasia indicate inability of the bone marrow to respond. In the presence of depressed erythropoiesis, the anemia persists and becomes progressively more severe.
2. The progressive fall in eosinophils with terminal neutrophilia and lymphopenia were an expression of a marked systemic stress.

Case 47 (Cat).   Pyometra with Systemic Toxemia

A domestic shorthair female cat, 18 months old, was presented with a history of suspected abortion. Three days before admission to the hospital, a purulent exudate was detected coming from the vulva. This was associated with complete anorexia and limited intake of water. Physical examination revealed marked depression, temperature of 100.4°F, pulse rate of 168/min, icteric mucous membranes, and evidence of dehydration. Abdominal palpation revealed an enlarged uterus associated with the purulent vulvar discharge. A diagnosis of pyometra was made. Surgery was delayed until the cat's condition could be improved by administration of fluids and antibiotics. Blood studies were conducted to evaluate the cat's progress.

Interpretation

1. Pyometra is rarer in the cat than in the dog. Although clinical history and physical findings indicated pyometra, the marked leukopenia on admission caused speculation concerning the possibility of a complication of panleukopenia.
2. The icterus was an unusual and persistent finding. No tests were conducted to determine the nature of the icterus. The extreme systemic toxemia may have produced a severe liver involvement.
3. Dehydration was indicated by clinical findings and the blood urea nitrogen of 79 mg/dl of plasma.
4. Fluids were administered to correct dehydration. The cat was overhydrated, as indicated by the fall in plasma proteins from 7.4 to 4.8 g/dl in the first 24 hours of therapy. A comparable reduction was seen in RBC number, hemoglobin concentration, and PCV.
5. Hydration and antibiotic therapy relieved the toxemia and permitted re-establishment

Case 46 (Cat).   Adenocarcinoma

	August 8	September 19	October 15	October 17
Erythrocytes				
RBC ($\times 10^6/\mu l$)	8.10	9.00	5.05	3.65
Hemoglobin (g/dl)	13.8	15.1	7.3	6.0
PCV (%)	41.0	41.0	22.0	18.0
MCV (fl)	50.6	45.5	43.6	49.3
MCHC (%)	33.6	36.8	33.2	33.3
Nucleated RBC/100 WBC	0	0	4.5	0
Icterus index units	—	—	—	15
Reticulocytes (%)	—	—	—	none seen
Anisocytosis	slight	slight	Slight to moderate variation in cell size, with many erythrocytes presenting "punched-out" centers. No polychromasia.	
Polychromasia	none	none		
Howell-Jolly bodies	few	few		
Other	—	Heinz bodies distinctly observable in Wright-Leishman-stained film.		
Heinz bodies	few	numerous, very large	numerous	numerous, large

Leukocytes		%		%		%		%
WBC/μl	20,300		18,100		16,900		22,300	
Band neutrophils	0	0.0	452	2.5	85	0.5	112	0.5
Neutrophils	15,225	75.0	14,752	81.5	12,590	74.5	20,404	91.5
Lymphocytes	2,741	13.5	1,900	10.5	3,251	19.0	1,561	7.0
Monocytes	812	4.0	91	0.5	507	3.0	0	0.0
Eosinophils	1,320	6.5	724	4.0	507	3.0	223	1.0
Basophils	102	0.5	0	0.0	0	0.0	0	0.0
Degenerated cells	102	0.5	181	1.0	0	0.0	0	0.0
Neutrophil morphology	normal		normal		normal		normal	

Case 47 (Cat).   Pyometra

	May 24	May 25	May 30	June 5[a]
Erythrocytes				
RBC ($\times 10^6/\mu l$)	6.39	4.88	5.24	6.18
Hemoglobin (g/dl)	9.2	7.4	7.8	9.8
PCV (%)	31.0	23.0	26.0	29.0
MCV (fl)	48.5	47.1	49.6	46.9
MCH (pg)	14.3	15.2	14.9	15.8
MCHC (%)	29.7	32.2	30.0	33.8
Anisocytosis	slight	slight	slight	moderate
Howell-Jolly bodies	occasional	few	few	few
Heinz bodies	few	few	moderate	moderate

Leukocytes					%		%
WBC/μl	400	400	35,600		28,500	
Myelocytes			356	1.0	0	0.0
Metamyelocytes			3,026	8.5	0	0.0
Bands	Too few cells for differential leukocyte counts.		15,486	43.5	855	3.0
Mature neutrophils			12,282	34.5	22,800	80.0
Lymphocytes			1,602	4.5	2,565	9.0
Monocytes			1,602	4.5	1,283	4.5
Eosinophils			1,068	3.0	997	3.5
Basophils			178	0.5	0	0.0

Plasma				
Total proteins (g/dl)	7.4	4.8	5.0	—
Fibrinogen (g/dl)	0.5	0.4	0.2	—
Icterus index units	20	20	50	—

Other Tests				
Platelets/μl	—	very few	45,000	below normal
Blood urea nitrogen (mg/dl)	79	19	—	—

[a]Capillary blood from ear vein taken on 3rd day after removal of the uterus.

of granulopoiesis. On the sixth day (May 30), a leukocytosis with marked left shift was seen. At this time, immature neutrophils outnumbered the mature neutrophils, and the cytoplasm of neutrophils remained basophilic. This differential leukocyte pattern is anticipated during the early phase of recovery of granulopoiesis following severe depression.

6. The small number of blood platelets in stained blood films and a count of 45,000/μl on May 30 indicated depression of megakaryopoiesis as well as granulopoiesis.

7. On June 5, the third day after removal of the uterus, a leukocytosis persisted. The neutrophils were mostly mature, and lymphocytes and eosinophils were at normal levels. These were signs of convalescence.

Case 48 (Cat). Anemia and Leukopenia in Lymphosarcoma

A male domestic shorthair cat, 9 months old, was presented with a complaint of lethargy and some loss of appetite of 1 week's duration.

Physical Examination. Temperature of 103.5°F, enlarged lymph nodes, tenderness of abdominal area, some palpable nodules in the abdomen, and a dry, nonproductive cough were noted. An initial hemogram at this time revealed a low total leukocyte count mainly due to a well-advanced lymphopenia. Antibiotics were administered, and there appeared to be an immediate improvement. However, 5 weeks later, the cat returned to the clinic exhibiting coughing, weakness, anorexia, and a body temperature of 104°F. The patient was hospitalized for observation and treatment. Body temperature dropped to 102.6°F for a few days and then increased to between 104° and 106°F. Death came on the tenth day of hospitalization (April 18).

Necropsy. Lymphosarcomatous process involved all layers of the intestine in the region of the jejunum, producing a constriction and dilatation. The contents were dark and tarry from hemorrhage originating in the area of dilatation. Neoplastic nodules were present in the spleen and liver, and the lymph nodes were mildly enlarged throughout the cadaver. In the spleen, macrophages were filled with hemosiderin.

Interpretation

1. Progressive anemia was associated with the formation of Heinz bodies in the erythrocytes. These bodies were of sufficient size to cause destruction of the erythrocytes. The pathologist's comment concerning the presence of macrophages filled with hemosiderin supports the opinion that the spleen or mononuclear phagocyte system in general was destroying erythrocytes. There was no evidence of remission of the anemia.

2. Progressive nonregenerative anemia and marked lymphopenia are common findings in feline lymphosarcoma.

3. Proliferation of neoplastic lymphocytes in the bone marrow may cause development of progressive anemia and neutropenia.

Case 48 (Cat). Lymphosarcoma

	February 28		April 8		April 12		April 15	
Erythrocytes								
RBC ($\times 10^6/\mu$l)	6.25		4.01		3.95		3.45	
Hemoglobin (g/dl)	10.5		7.4		5.9		5.0	
PCV (%)	32		22		18		15	
MCV (fl)	51.2		54.8		45.5		43.5	
MCHC (%)	32.8		33.6		32.8		33.3	
Nucleated RBC/100 WBC	1		1		2		1	
Reticulocytes (NMB stain)[a]	none seen		none seen		none seen		none seen	
Heinz bodies (NMB stain)[a]	moderate number		moderate number		moderate number		moderate number	
Anisocytosis	slight		slight		slight		slight	
Polychromasia	none		slight		none		none	
Poikilocytosis	few		few		few		few	
Howell-Jolly bodies	few		few		few		few	
Leukocytes		%		%		%		%
WBC/μl	6,900		1,600		3,300		1,800	
Band neutrophils	0	0.0	16	1.0	33	1.0	72	4.0
Neutrophils	5,279	76.5	960	60.0	2,046	62.0	1,260	70.0
Lymphocytes	1,000	14.5	528	33.0	858	26.0	252	14.0
Monocytes	517	7.5	48	3.0	132	4.0	162	9.0
Eosinophils	35	0.5	32	2.0	0	0.0	0	0.0
Unclassified cells	0	0.0	16	1.0	165	5.0	36	2.0
Degenerated cells	69	1.0	0	0.0	66	2.0	18	1.0
Neutrophil morphology	normal		normal		normal		Few Döhle bodies	

[a]Fig. 2–25:3.

4. This case illustrates the difficulty often encountered in diagnosis of lymphosarcoma from blood examination only. Lymphopenia may be seen in as many as 50% of the cats and 25% of the dogs with lymphosarcoma. (See Chapter 32.)

Case 49 (Cat). Lymphadenopathy and Neutropenia Associated with *Chlamydia*-like Organisms and Terminal Neoplasia

A 3-year-old domestic shorthair cat was presented exhibiting marked enlargement of all peripheral lymph nodes. The cat was somewhat thin; rectal temperature was 102.5°F, pulse 180/min, and respiratory rate 18/min. An impression smear from a lymph node biopsy presented many small, mature lymphocytes and a moderate number of histiocytic cells, some of which contained a cytoplasmic vacuole with elementary bodies suggestive of *Chlamydia* or *Rickettsia* (Plate XIV–6). Similar inclusions have been seen in neutrophil leukocytes of other cats (Plate XIV–5).* Histologic examination of the lymph node revealed prominent lymphoid follicles consisting of normal-appearing lymphocytes and some larger reticular-type cells, indicating a reactive lymph node with no evidence of neoplasia.

A bone marrow aspiration was found to be cel-

---

*Ward, J.M., Smith, R., and Schalm, O.W.: Inclusions in Neutrophils of Cats with Feline Infectious Peritonitis. J. Amer. Vet. Med. Ass., *158*:348, 1970.

lular with abnormal granulopoiesis and erythroid hypoplasia. The M:E ratio was 27.5:1.0. There were few mature neutrophils, while large precursor forms through myelocytes were numerous and were accompanied by some giant metamyelocytes and band forms (Plate XV–8, 9) with bizarre nuclear patterns (maturation arrest). Small mature lymphocytes made up 44% of the bone marrow cytology. Megakaryocytes, plasma cells, mitotic cells, and macrophages were seen on scanning of the film. Some phagocytosis of erythrocytes was also seen. The iron stain was negative.

Interpretation

The cat exhibited a progressive fall in PCV from 33 to 22% over a period of 18 days. On admission (April 29), the peripheral blood neutrophil count was approaching neutropenia, and it became neutropenic 11 days later, at which time there was an increase in monocytes with a rare monocyte containing cytoplasmic elementary bodies suggestive of *Chlamydia* or possibly *Rickettsia*. Between April 29 and May 7, no treatment was given. Between May 8 and May 17, an antibiotic was administered subcutaneously b.i.d. The rectal temperature remained at the level of 102.0–102.2°F until May 12, when it fell to between 101.4° and 101.6°F. Generalized lymphadenopathy, depression, and anorexia persisted throughout the 18 days of observation, although the hemogram of May 17 demonstrated a rise in circulating neutrophils. The cat was released to its owner but was returned 4 months later for euthanasia. The necropsy report

Case 49 (Cat). Chlamydia-Like Organisms and Neoplasia

	April 29 (Jugular blood)		May 10 (Capillary blood)		May 17 (Capillary blood)	
Erythrocytes						
RBC ($\times 10^6/\mu l$)	7.14		6.05		5.40	
Hemoglobin (g/dl)	11.0		8.0		7.6	
PCV (%)	33.0		24.0		22.0	
MCV (fl)	46.2		39.6		40.7	
MCH (pg)	15.4		13.2		14.0	
MCHC (%)	33.3		33.3		34.5	
Nucleated RBC/100 WBC	rare		0		1	
Reticulocytes (%)	0.8		—		—	
Plasma						
Icterus index units	2		—		—	
Total proteins (g/dl)	8.0		—		—	
Fibrinogen (g/dl)	0.1		—		—	
Leukocytes		%		%		%
WBC/μl	7,500		6,100		8.500	
Band neutrophils	37	0.5	183	3.0	213	2.5
Neutrophils	2,587	34.5	1,098	18.0[a]	4,745	55.5
Lymphocytes	4,312	57.5	3,233	53.0	3,035	35.5
Monocytes	375	5.0	1,342	22.0[b]	470	5.5
Eosinophils	187	2.5	152	2.5	42	0.5
Basophils	0	0.0	91	1.5	42	0.5

[a]Occasional large toxic neutrophil.
[b]Rare monocyte with large cluster of *Chlamydia*-like organisms (Plate XIV–6).

classified the condition as a myeloproliferative syndrome, associated with lymphadenopathy. The bone marrow was hypercellular with many large primitive cells with large nucleoli. In addition, some megakaryocytes appeared larger than normal. Similar abnormal cells (possibly tumor cells) were found in sheets in the lymph nodes, spleen, liver, and kidneys.

Case 50 (Cat). Myeloproliferative Disorder with a Period of Remission Followed by a Relapse Two Years Later

A 5-year-old castrated male Persian cat was first seen by the referring veterinarian on Jan. 30, 1968. Clinical signs were listlessness, anorexia, fever (104.5°F), anemia (PCV 14%) and leukopenia (WBC 3,000/μl). Treatment consisted of vitamins, antibiotics, and glucocorticoids without significant improvement. On Mar. 1, 1968, the cat was referred to the Veterinary Medical Teaching Hospital (VMTH). Blood examination on admission revealed a PCV of 14% and a leukocyte count of 4,300/μl with a marked left shift. A bone marrow aspiration on Mar. 6 contained megaloblastoid (giant) rubricytes (Figs. A–8 and A–9), indicating the probable existence of a myeloproliferative disorder involving the erythrocytic maturation series and leading to ineffective erythropoiesis.

Two blood transfusions of 40 ml each were administered on Mar. 11 and 13. A blood examination on Mar. 18 revealed no change in PCV and a leukocyte count of 3,600/μl with a differential count of 94% mature lymphocytes and 6% mature neutrophils. The attending clinician administered vitamin B_{12} by intramuscular injection and folic acid by mouth on the assumption that the macrocytic rubricytes and erythrocytes (Fig. A–9) observed in

the bone marrow may have been an expression of a deficiency of these vitamins. The cat improved and was released to the owner with a recommendation for continuing home treatment with a complete hematinic. The cat made an apparent recovery, for it was not seen again by the original referring veterinarian until Feb. 19, 1970. Clinical signs at that time were anorexia, fever (105°F), and anemia (PCV 15%). Antibiotics, vitamins, steroids, and a whole-blood transfusion were administered, but the cat's condition continued to decline. It was referred to the VMTH on Apr. 7, 1970. On admission, the PCV was found to be 6.0%; because of the extreme weakness and cachexia of the patient, euthanasia was recommended. A bone marrow sample was taken for comparison with the cytology seen 2 years before. This bone marrow sample was also examined by electron microscopy, and C-type viral particles were demonstrated.

Bone Marrow Cytology on March 6, 1968. The marrow sample was not very cellular. There was an almost complete absence of granulocytic-series cells. This correlated with the marked leukopenia on Mar. 1 and 18. The erythrocytic maturation series exhibited reduced numbers of nucleated cells with many abnormal forms. Some prorubricytes had small, chromatin-deficient nuclei and considerably more cytoplasm than normal for the stage of maturation. There were normal polychromatophilic rubricytes and metarubricytes and nearly as many giant rubricytes (Figs. A–8 and A–9) associated with a scattering of macrocytic erythrocytes. The giant rubricytes and erythrocytes were either normochromic or polychromatophilic. In some instances, the cytoplasm of a giant rubricyte had a muddy appearance suggesting abnormal hemoglobinization. Rare instances of phagocytosed rub-

Case 50 (Cat). Myeloproliferative Disorder

	March 1, 1968		March 18, 1968		April 7, 1970	
RBC ($\times 10^6$/μl)	3.25		2.47		1.11	
Hemoglobin (g/dl)	4.1		4.8		1.8	
PCV (%)	14.0		14.0		6.0	
MCV (fl)	43.1		56.7		54.1	
MCHC (%)	29.3		34.3		30.0	
Reticulocytes (%)	0		few		few	
Nucleated RBC/100 WBC	0		16		3	
Anisocytosis	slight		moderate		marked	
Polychromasia	none		rare		moderate	
		%		%		%
Leukocytes/μl	4,300		3,600		23,900	
Blasts	rare	—	0	0.0	0	0.0
Progranulocytes	rare	—	0	0.0	0	0.0
Myelocytes	43	1.0	0	0.0	0	0.0
Metamyelocytes	215	5.0	0	0.0	0	0.0
Band neutrophils	430	10.0	0	0.0	359	1.5
Mature neutrophils	946	22.0	216	6.0	21,151	88.5
Lymphocytes	1,720	40.0	3,384	94.0	1,553	6.5
Monocytes	215	5.0	0	0.0	478	2.0
Eosinophils	43	1.0	0	0.0	359	1.5
Unclassified cells	430	10.0	0	0.0	0	0.0
Degenerated cells	258	6.0	0	0.0	0	0.0

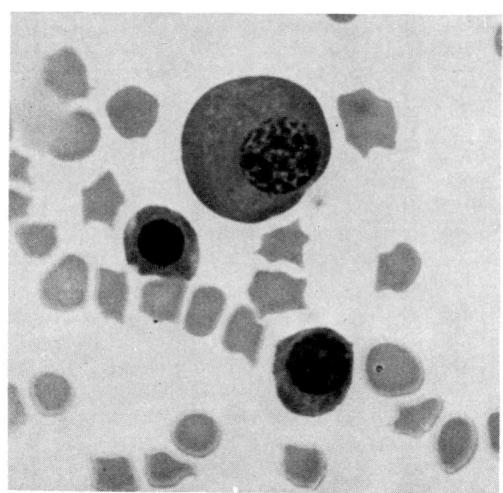

Fig. A–8. Bone marrow (Mar. 6, 1968) showing a megaloblastoid polychromatophilic rubricyte and two rubricytes of normal size and morphology. ×3,000.

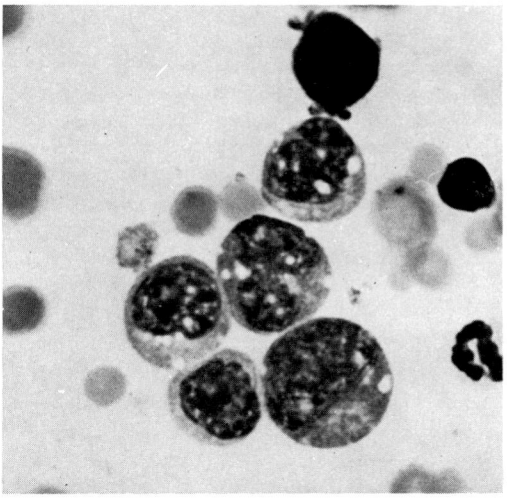

Fig. A–10. Bone marrow (Apr. 7, 1970) showing vacuolation and coarse chromatinization of granulocytic precursor cells. ×3,000.

ricytes and erythrocytes were seen. One small cluster of agglutinated polychromatophilic erythrocytes was encountered. There were considerable numbers of free, degenerating nuclei, each containing a nucleolus, thereby indicating their origin from blast cells.

Bone Marrow Cytology on April 7, 1970. The marrow sample was very cellular with numerous granulocytic series cells, many of which were vacuolated and presented coarse nuclear chromatin (Fig. A–10). All features described in the first marrow sample for the erythrocytic maturation series were prominent in this marrow. A significant additional finding was the existence of clusters of agglutin-

ated polychromatophilic erythrocytes with rubricytes included in some clusters (Fig. A–11).

Necropsy. The carcass exhibited a moderately severe weight loss. The liver was of normal size, and it was not infiltrated by hematopoietic cells. The spleen was slightly enlarged, and there was prominent congestion of the red pulp. A significant finding was extensive erythrophagocytosis in the spleen and lymph nodes (Plate XVII–6). Bone marrow cytology was characterized by densely packed blast cells with prominent nuclei and nucleoli. Mitotic figures were plentiful. Small numbers of erythrocytic, granulocytic, and megakaryocytic maturation forms were present in the marrow.

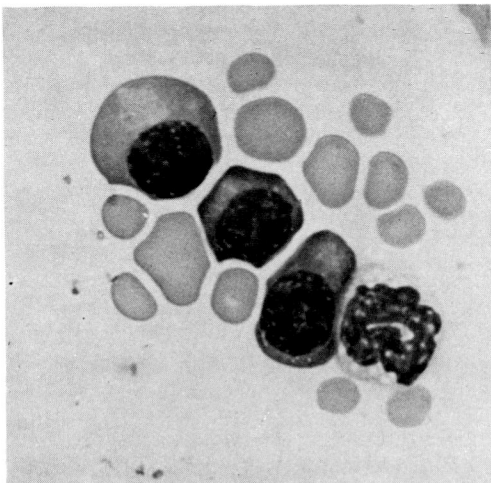

Fig. A–9. Bone marrow (Mar. 6, 1968) demonstrating size variations of polychromatophilic rubricytes and of erythrocytes. A vacuolated neutrophil is also seen. ×3,000.

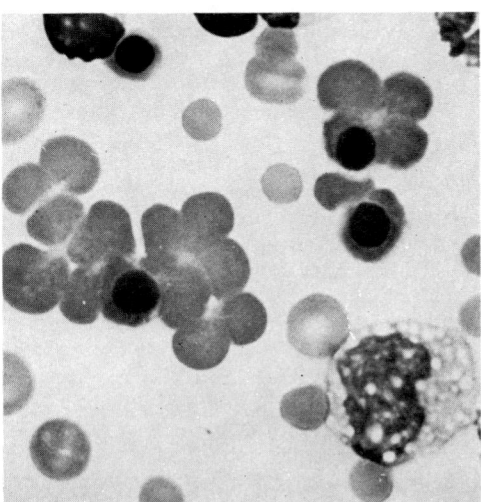

Fig. A–11. Bone marrow (Apr. 7, 1970) demonstrating agglutination of polychromatophilic erythrocytes, several normal metarubricytes, and a vacuolated myelocyte. ×3,000.

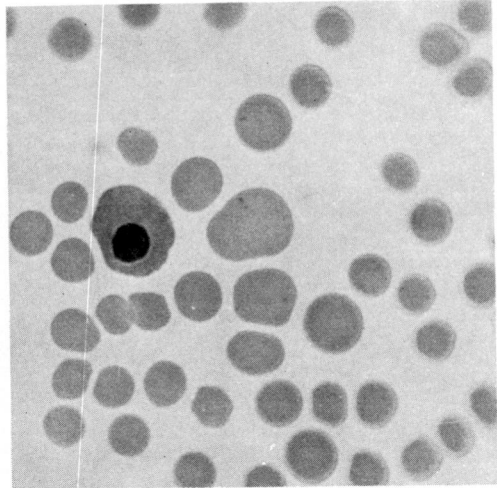

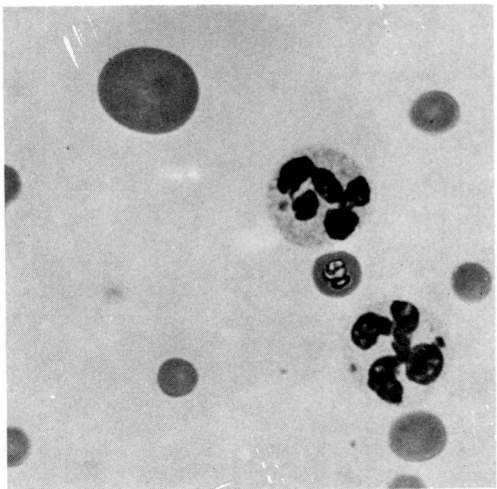

Fig. A–12. Blood (Apr. 7, 1970) showing a macrocytic metarubricyte and marked anisocytosis of normochromic erythrocytes. ×3,000.

Fig. A–13. Blood (Apr. 7, 1970) presenting a giant polychromatophilic erythrocyte and 2 neutrophils with cytoplasmic Döhle bodies. ×3,000.

Interpretation

1. Megaloblastoid rubricytes have been a feature of feline marrow cytology in instances of erythremic myelosis and erythroleukemia (Chapter 32), and thus their presence in the bone marrow on first admission (Figs. A–8 and A–9) led to the opinion that there was evidence of a myeloproliferative disease.
2. Deficiencies of vitamin B_{12} and folic acid lead to defective synthesis of nucleoprotein, resulting in ineffective erythropoiesis. Prorubricytes and basophilic rubricytes may be present in the marrow in numbers out of proportion to normal numbers as mitosis is delayed (Plate XIX–1). Synthesis of hemoglobin without cell division may lead to megaloblastoid polychromatophilic and normochromic rubricytes. In addition, however, macrometamyelocytes and hypersegmented neutrophils are to be anticipated. In the cat under consideration, there was on first admission a paucity of granulocytes in the marrow, with considerable vacuolation of the few neutrophils that were present (Fig. A–9).
3. The fact that the cat responded to injectable vitamin B_{12}, folic acid by mouth, and home therapy with a hematinic would seem to indicate that a beginning myeloproliferative disorder on first admission may have been complicated by a vitamin deficiency.
4. On second admission, 2 years later, the blood revealed marked anisocytosis (Fig. A–12), and neutrophils contained Döhle bodies (Fig. A–13). In the bone marrow, granulopoiesis was active, but many cells presented clumped nuclear chromatin and vacuolation (Fig. A–10). Megaloblastoid rubricytes were present in even greater numbers

than on first admission, but in addition there were clusters of agglutinated polychromatophilic erythrocytes and metarubricytes (Fig. A–11). This was a significant feature, for immature erythrocytes normally do not participate in formation of agglutinated masses. It was interpreted as indicative of an immune response to the erythrocytes. The marked erythrophagocytosis observed in the spleen and lymph nodes (Plate XVII–6) lends support to this concept. A direct Coombs test, if performed, probably would have confirmed such an occurrence.
5. If a deficiency of either vitamin B_{12} or folic acid existed on first admission, the resulting defect in marrow cytology may have provided an opportunity for the C-type feline leukemia virus to become established within marrow cells and to produce after 2 years the rapidly developing terminal anemia from a combination of ineffective erythropoiesis and marked erythrophagocytosis.

Case 51 (Cat). Lupus Erythematosus with Autoimmune Hemolytic Anemia

A spayed domestic shorthair cat, 2 years old, with no history of prior illness, developed anorexia, depression, and weakness on Jan. 14. Physical examination on Jan. 22 revealed a thin, alert cat with pale mucous membranes, a rectal temperature of 103°F, a heart rate of 200/min, and enlarged submaxillary lymph nodes. Autoagglutination of erythrocytes was noted on the side wall of the blood vial and agglutinated clumps of four to five cells, including polychromatophilic erythrocytes, were observed in the stained blood film. An autoimmune disease was suspected. Extensive studies were conducted between Jan. 22 and May 16 with the cat under close supervision both in the

Case 51 (Cat). Lupus Erythematosus

	Jan. 22	Feb. 23	Mar. 22	Apr. 4	May 16[a]
Erythrocytes					
RBC ($\times 10^6/\mu$l)	2.65	7.65	2.60	3.62	1.50
Hb (g/dl)	4.5	10.1	3.7	7.0	2.8
PCV (%)	15.0	33.0	13.0	21.0	9.0
MCV (fl)	56.6	43.1	50.3	58.0	60.0
MCH (pg)	16.9	13.2	14.2	19.3	18.7
MCHC (%)	30.0	30.6	28.5	33.3	31.1
ESR/1 hr	7/64 = 57−	3/20 = 17−	—	—	—
Nucleated RBC/100 WBC	64	0	17	23	12
Reticulocytes (%)	many	—	11.0	30.2	3.0
Spherocytes	+	0	+	0	0
Anisocytosis	marked	slight	moderate	moderate	moderate
Polychromasia	marked	slight	moderate	marked	slight
Leukocytes					
Leukocytes/μl	9,300	11,400	5,200	16,800	12,100
Band neutrophils	0	57	0	420	121
Mature neutrophils	1,581	8,037	312	6,972	3,025
Lymphocytes	6,417[b]	2,736	4,056	7,476	6,655[b]
Monocytes	1,209	342	832	1,260	1,936[c]
Eosinophils	0	114	0	672	363
Basophils	93	114	0	0	0
Other Tests					
Plasma proteins (g/dl)	10.6	8.9	10.3	10.0	—
Fibrinogen (g/dl)	0.2	0.1	0.1	0.1	—
Icterus index units	15	2	10	5	—
Platelets	377,000	many	many	many	many
BUN (mg/dl)	18.0	28.0	23.0	—	—
Urine protein	3+	1+	1+	—	—

[a]Capillary blood from ear vein. Other hemograms made on jugular blood.
[b]Some immature lymphocytes present.
[c]Occasional monocyte with phagocytosed erythrocyte.

hospital and at home. Five hemograms, representing significant changes in the medical progress, are presented from among 22 blood studies conducted during the course of the disease.

Interpretation

The icterus index of 15 units, autoagglutination of erythrocytes, and evidence of intensified erythropoiesis (Jan. 22) pointed to lysis of erythrocytes as an explanation for the anemia. An erythrocyte

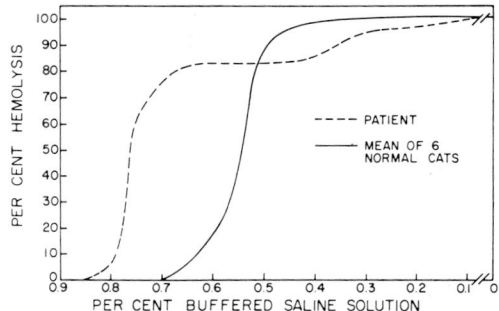

Fig. A–14. Demonstration of markedly reduced erythrocyte osmotic resistance to hypotonic saline solution in a cat with autoimmune hemolytic anemia.

fragility test demonstrated 62% lysis at 0.75% buffered NaCl solution (Fig. A–14). Examination for lupus erythematosus cells (Chapter 2) revealed many clusters of typical LE cells (Fig. A–15). The total plasma protein concentration of 10.6 g/dl and fractionation of the serum proteins demonstrated 81.1% (9 g) to be globulin, of which 3.2 g consisted of a mixture of β- and γ_1-globulin and 5.2 g was γ_2-globulin (Fig. A–16). This supported a diagnosis of autoimmune hemolytic anemia associated with systemic lupus erythematosus. Additional support for an autoimmune process existed in the relatively high absolute lymphocyte number (6,417/μl), some of which were immature. A lymph node biopsy revealed greatly increased populations of lymphocytes and some plasma cells characteristic of lymphocytic tissue reacting to antigenic stimulation.

Therapy. In addition to multivitamins and antibiotics, prednisolone (4.5 mg) was given by intramuscular injection b.i.d. for the first 2 days; this was followed by 5.0 mg b.i.d. orally through Jan. 30. Thereafter, the dose of steroid was gradually reduced, and finally all medication was stopped on Feb. 23. Blood morphology had returned to normal by Feb. 23, with the exception of a persisting, although somewhat reduced, hyperproteinemia. Medication was stopped to determine if

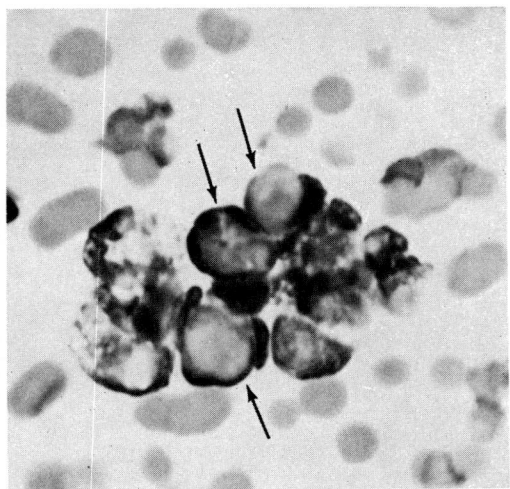

Fig. A–15. A cluster of neutrophils, three of which are LE cells *(arrows)* from a cat with autoimmune hemolytic anemia. Also shown are two clumps of agglutinated erythrocytes with polychromatophilic erythrocytes included within the clumps. × 2,250.

a relapse would occur in the absence of steroid administration. On March 22, which was 28 days after stopping steroid therapy, the cat was readmitted in acute hemolytic crisis. The PCV was 13% but fell to 9% over the next 5 days. Bilirubinemia and marked hyperproteinemia were present again. Steroid therapy was reinstituted, but the cat failed to make a full recovery. The cat's condition began to deteriorate rapidly in early May, and on May 16 the PCV was 9%. The cat died the next day.

Necropsy. The principal gross findings were enlargement of the liver, spleen, and lymph nodes. The peritoneum was moist and yellow. Lymph node cytology was characterized by immature lymphocytes, some plasma cells, and prominent reticulum cells. Tissue changes in the spleen, liver, and lymph nodes were suggestive of a severe reaction to antigenic stimulation. It was conjectured that antibodies reacting with erythrocytes led to a rapidly developing terminal anemia from extensive erythrophagocytosis (Fig. A–17). There was evidence of glomerulonephritis with hyalinization of glomeruli and thickening of Bowman's capsule. The bone marrow was hypercellular because of marked intensification of erythropoiesis. (See also Heise, S.C., et al.: Lupus Erythematosus with Hemolytic Anemia in a Cat. Feline Pract., 3(3):6, 1973.)

Case 52 (Cat). Feline Infectious Anemia (Haemobartonellosis)

A male domestic shorthair cat, 7 months old, was referred for diagnosis and treatment of a chronic anemia. The referring veterinarian had administered a blood transfusion 2 weeks previously, and vitamin B_{12} and iron had been given at weekly intervals.

Physical Examination. The cat appeared normal except for pale mucous membranes. The temperature was 101.4°F on admission, and during the 6 days of hospitalization it was 101.7–102.4°F. A few coccidia were found on fecal examination. Three hemograms were obtained over a 6-day period. The first two verified the existence of an anemia in which the erythrocytes were bordering on being macrocytic. The third hemogram was diagnostic for *Haemobartonella felis*. The diagnosis was verified additionally by transmission of the disease by introduction of 0.5 ml of blood into the peritoneal cavity of a normal 7-month-old male cat (see Case 53).

Interpretation and Remarks

1. This series of hemograms clearly demonstrates the difficulty of diagnosis of feline infectious anemia in the chronic state on the basis of demonstration of *Haemobartonella felis* in the stained blood film. Often several sequential hemograms are necessary before the parasite is observed in peripheral blood.
2. Moderate anisocytosis and polychromasia on Nov. 19 indicated beginning remission of the anemia. The marked increase in absolute lymphocyte count at this time reflected the decrease in systemic stress.

Case 53 (Cat). Experimentally Induced Feline Infectious Anemia (FIA)

A normal male cat, 7 months old, had been raised from birth in the experimental animal house. In preparation for receiving 0.5 ml of blood intraperitoneally from a natural infection with *Haemobartonella felis* (Case 52), the cat was placed in a cardboard box and brought to the laboratory. The box was placed on the floor where the cat remained for about 30 minutes before the inoculation was made. These details are important to an understanding of the hemogram on day zero. The new experience and new noises apparently frightened the recipient cat, bringing on a "physiologic" leukocytosis. The recipient cat was brought to the laboratory every day so that the progress of the developing infection could be followed. The cat soon became accustomed to this routine. It is probable that the hemogram taken on the fifth day postinoculation was more representative of the normal.

Interpretation

1. Physiologic leukocytosis in the cat, as observed on day zero, is characterized by an increase of neutrophils and lymphocytes in large-vessel blood, a consequence of the flushing out of leukocytes from small capillaries and, perhaps, of increased flow of lymph into the circulation. The increased force and rate of the heart in fright brings about these changes. (See Chapter 5.)
2. *Haemobartonella felis* appeared in peripheral

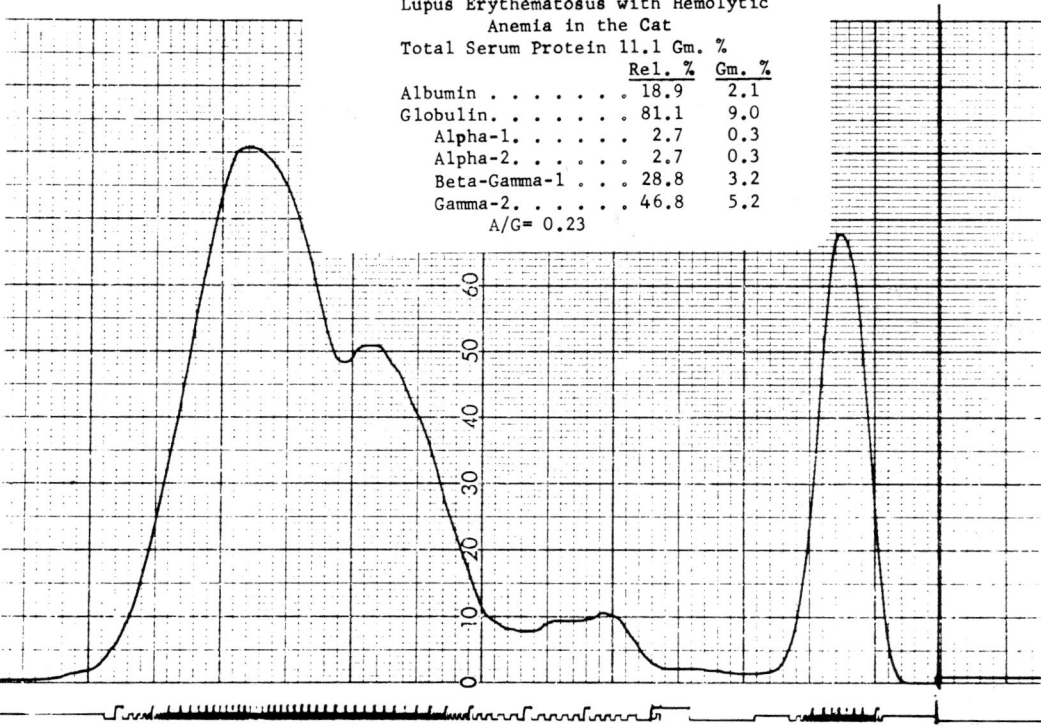

Lupus Erythematosus with Hemolytic
Anemia in the Cat
Total Serum Protein 11.1 Gm. %

	Rel. %	Gm. %
Albumin	18.9	2.1
Globulin	81.1	9.0
Alpha-1	2.7	0.3
Alpha-2	2.7	0.3
Beta-Gamma-1	28.8	3.2
Gamma-2	46.8	5.2

A/G= 0.23

Fig. A–16. Demonstration of a polyclonal gammopathy in a cat with autoimmune hemolytic anemia.

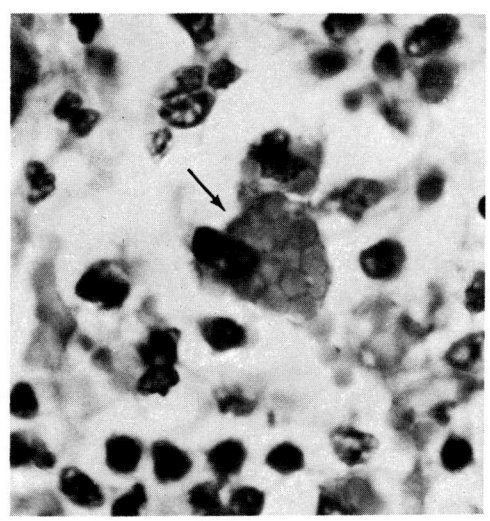

Fig. A–17. Spleen section of a cat with autoimmune hemolytic anemia showing a macrophage engorged with erythrocytes. ×2,700.

blood in very small numbers on the third day postinoculation. Thereafter, it was readily found in the blood through the eighteenth day, when the numbers began to diminish. Three weeks later, the PCV had returned to 41%, and *H. felis* had disappeared.

3. The first real evidence of a developing anemia was seen on the eighth day, when a reduction in PCV was noted. The PCV continued to fall during the next 7 days to the lowest level observed, 16%. Despite the rapid decline in PCV and hemoglobin, clinical icterus was not observable. This is also true in most natural cases of FIA.

4. Four days after the first significant drop in PCV and hemoglobin, the release of immature red cells to the blood in response to the anemia was indicated by an increase of MCV to 45 fl. The mean erythrocyte size increased steadily, thereafter, reaching a peak of 86 fl on the twenty-second day. Macrocytosis and polychromasia were accompanied by a fall in MCHC to a low of 23% on the twenty-fifth day. Immature erythrocytes contain less Hb than mature RBC on a volume basis (MCHC) but more Hb than mature cells on a weight basis (MCH).

5. The leukograms were not unusual, except for modest stimulation of granulopoiesis. Absolute lymphocyte numbers remained well within the normal range and then exceeded

Case 52 (Cat). Feline Infectious Anemia

	November 14		November 15		November 19	
Erythrocytes						
RBC ($\times 10^6/\mu l$)	4.20		3.40		3.20	
Hemoglobin (g/dl)	7.20		6.60		5.60	
PCV (%)	23.0		20.0		18.0	
MCV (fl)	54.8		58.8		56.3	
MCHC (%)	31.3		33.0		31.1	
Nucleated RBC/100 WBC	2.5		4.0		2.0	
Anisocytosis	slight		slight		moderate	
Polychromasia	slight		slight		moderate	
Howell-Jolly bodies	none seen		few		few	
Haemobartonella felis	none seen		none seen		few ring forms	
Leukocytes		%		%		%
WBC/μl (corrected)	4,680		4,368		13,328	
Band neutrophils	0	0.0	0	0.0	133	1.0
Neutrophils	2,761	59.0	1,791	41.0	6,397	48.0
Lymphocytes	1,778	38.0	2,446	56.0	5,864	44.0
Monocytes	94	2.0	131	3.0	600	4.5
Eosinophils	23	0.5	0	0.0	133	1.0
Unclassified cells	23	0.5	0	0.0	200	1.5
Neutrophil morphology	Döhle bodies		Döhle bodies		Essentially normal	

the normal maximum levels on the sixteenth through the eighteenth day.

6. Feline infectious anemia became complicated by severe pneumonitis with secondary bacterial infection which may account for the marked leukocytosis with left shift beginning on the 21st day.

Case 54 (Cat). Experimentally Induced Panleukopenia

A half dozen cats, about 6 months of age, were exposed to panleukopenia virus under controlled experimental conditions. The influence of the developing disease on the leukogram is shown with data developed from daily blood studies on two of the cats. Both cats were sacrificed for histopathologic examination. (For a discussion of panleukopenia, see Chapter 36 and Table 5–2.)

Interpretation

1. Both cats exhibited a larger number of circulating lymphocytes than neutrophils at the zero hour. This suggests that both cats were apprehensive relative to their new environment, with "physiologic" leukocytosis resulting. This experience points to the importance of allowing time for newly acquired cats to become adjusted to the new environment before initiating experiments in which the hemogram is used as one measure of effects produced.
2. In both cats, the lymphocytes were reduced initially to a greater extent than the neutrophils. However, due to the "physiologic" leukocytosis, the base level of absolute lymphocytes was distorted.
3. Once leukocyte numbers began to fall, the

developing leukopenia advanced rapidly, reaching its lowest level in 6 to 8 days. At the most advanced stage of leukopenia, the differential leukocyte count stated in percentage gives a false impression of relative proportion of various leukocytes when viewed without reference to the total leukocyte numbers/μl.

Case 55 (Horse). Response to Massive Hemorrhage

A quarter horse crossbred, male, 7 years old, was operated upon for removal of the penis. On Feb. 6, 4 days before surgery, a blood sample was submitted for a presurgical hemogram. The penis was removed on Feb. 10. The sheath and surrounding tissues became markedly edematous. On Feb. 19, the suture line ruptured and the wound began to bleed profusely. Considerable blood was lost before bleeding was brought under control. The blood was examined eight times during the next 20 days to follow the replacement of erythrocytes and to demonstrate the unique difference between the horse and other domestic mammals in blood morphology during remission of anemia.

Interpretation

1. It is characteristic of the horse to retain erythrocytes in the bone marrow until hemoglobin synthesis is complete. The only sign of anemia in remission is the presence of erythrocytes that are somewhat larger than normal. The difference in size of the young red blood cells and the mature cell is usually not great. For this reason, it is difficult to determine with certainty from a single hemogram the intensity of the erythrogenic response to

Case 53 (Cat).   Experimentally Induced Feline Infectious Anemia

Elapsed time in days	PCV (%)	Hb (g/dl)	MCV (fl)	MCHC (%)	Nucleated RBC/100 WBC	H. felis	WBC/μl	Differential Leukocyte Count in Absolute Numbers/μl					
								Band	Neut.	Lymph.	Mono.	Eos.	Bas.
0	40	14.3	40	35.8	0	0	22,600	0	10,396	11,300	226	452	226
1	38	—	—	—	0	none	kitten frightened, physiologic						
2	38	—	—	—	0	none	leukocytosis at 0 time						
3	—	—	—	—	0	rare							
4	42	—	—	—	0	moderate							
5	37	12.0	39	32.4	0	many	15,000	0	8,550	4,800	825	825	0
7	37	12.8	39	34.6	0	moderate	16,400	0	9,430	5,740	246	902	82
8	33	11.4	41	34.5	0	many	14,500	435	10,150	3,190	435	290	0
9	31	10.7	41	34.5	0	many	13,700	68	8,288	4,178	685	411	68
10	27	8.8	39	32.6	0	many	11,100	55	5,717	3,830	1,110	388	0
11	21	6.6	41	31.4	0	many	12,200	224	6,954	4,819	122	61	0
12	22	6.2	45	28.2	0	many	10,600	106	6,042	3,922	159	371	0
14	18	5.5	52	30.6	1.5	many	8,400	126	2,604	4,704	84	546	336
15	16	4.9	51	30.6	3	many	14,200	355	4,970	7,455	497	213	710
16	16	4.9	52	30.6	2[a]	many	19,700	296	8,175	9,554	591	689	394
17	16	4.7	53	29.4	3[a]	many	17,200	516	6,192	9,288	344	602	258
18	19	5.7	55	30.0	1.5[a]	many	18,800	2,068	6,956	8,366	658	752	0
21	18	4.2	75	23.3	8.5[b]	few	37,900	marked left shift, pneumonitis					
22	17	4.2	86	24.7	12[b]	few	29,300	2,344	18,166	6,886	1,025	732	147
23	16	3.9	82	24.4	6[b]	moderate	48,280	left shift includes metamyelocytes					
25	16	3.7	80	23.0	11[b]	moderate	41,300	left shift includes metamyelocytes					

[a]Moderate anisocytosis and polychromasia.
[b]Marked anisocytosis and polychromasia.

Case 54 (Cat). Experimentally Induced Panleukopenia

Elapsed time (hr)	WBC/μl	Band Neutrophils		Neutrophils		Lymphocytes		Monocytes		Eosinophils		Basophils	Other
		No.	%	No.	%	No.	%	No.	%	No.	%		
Cat 1													
0	11,550	0	0.0	4,158	36.0	6,294	54.5	173	1.5	924	8.0	0	0
24	12,800	128	1.0	4,416	34.5	6,912	54.0	192	1.5	1,024	8.0	0	128
48	15,700	79	0.5	4,867	31.0	9,027	57.5	314	2.0	1,177	7.5	0	235
72	4,700	47	1.0	3,995	85.0	329	7.0	47	1.0	235	5.0	0	47
96	3,500	0	0.0	1,855	53.0	1,557	44.5	35	1.0	52	1.5	0	0
120	2,700	0	0.0	1,606	59.5	931	34.5	0	0.0	148	5.5	0	13
144	2,200	11	0.5	1,001	45.5	1,089	49.5	0	0.0	99	4.5	0	0
168	350	0	0.0	14	4.0	245	70.0	7	2.0	84	24.0	0	0
192	200	too few cells, 15 lymphocytes and 1 eosinophil found on entire blood film.											
Cat 2													
0	29,000	292	1.0	11,020	38.0	13,630	47.0	725	2.5	3,045	10.5	0	292
24	20,000	400	2.0	8,400	42.0	8,400	42.0	700	3.5	2,100	10.5	0	0
48	11,000	0	0.0	6,600	60.0	2,420	22.0	55	0.5	1,815	16.5	0	110
72	5,500	55	1.0	3,575	65.0	935	17.0	0	0.0	935	17.0	0	0
96	3,400	17	0.5	2,261	66.5	935	27.5	34	1.0	85	2.5	0	68
120	5,300	159	3.0	3,948	74.5	980	18.5	0	0.0	212	4.0	0	0
144	900	0	0.0	9	1.0	648	72.0	0	0.0	243	27.0	0	0

an anemia. Reticulocyte counts cannot be employed as an index since only an occasional reticulocyte can be found even in association with the most intense response to blood loss.

2. The MCV may be of some help when the mean red blood cell size approaches 60 fl.
3. The total leukocyte count did not deviate significantly from the normal. The differential leukocyte counts were essentially also normal.
4. Bone marrow examination may be performed to evaluate erythropoiesis in the horse. A regenerative anemia is indicated by a reticulocyte count in bone marrow of >5%, while a low M:E ratio may not necessarily reflect increased erythrogenesis in this species. (See Chapter 6.)

Case 56 (Horse). Hemolytic Anemia Associated with Heinz Body Formation in Phenothiazine Toxicosis

A male Morgan horse, 2½ years old, was admitted on Oct. 4 exhibiting clinical signs of hemolytic anemia. The horse had been losing weight for about 1½ months when the owner decided to treat it for parasites using phenothiazine. It was stated that after the first dose of phenothiazine, which was mixed with the grain feed, the horse refused to eat the grain on subsequent days. The history was incomplete relative to the exact quantity of phenothiazine consumed or the elapsed time between administration of the anthelmintic and appearance of the hemolytic anemia.

Physical examination on admission revealed icteric mucous membranes, a temperature of

Case 55 (Horse). Massive Hemorrhage

	Feb. 6	Days Posthemorrhage							
		1	3	4	6	8	10	14	20
Erythrocytes (×10⁶/μl)	7.75	2.25	2.06	2.64	3.0	3.15	3.71	4.20	4.90
Hemoglobin (g/dl)	13.7	3.7	3.7	4.9	5.8	7.4	6.9	9.6	9.0
PCV (%)	38.0	11.5	11.5	15.0	18.0	21.0	20.0	25.0	28.0
MCV (fl)	49.0	51.1	55.8	56.8	60.0	66.6	53.9	59.5	57.1
MCHC (%)	36.0	32.2	32.2	32.7	32.2	35.2	34.5	38.4	32.1
MCH (pg)	17.8	16.4	17.9	18.5	19.3	23.5	18.6	22.8	18.3

Erythrocyte morphology: On the first day following hemorrhage, the erythrocytes were few in number in the stained blood film. Many red blood cells presented "punched-out" centers, meaning that the cell had retained the bowl shape assumed during circulation through the smallest capillaries. Beginning with the third day and increasing in prominence thereafter, macrocytic normochromic erythrocytes were present in peripheral blood. This was the only evidence of increased erythropoiesis and release of new erythrocytes to the circulation in response to the blood loss. By the 20th day, the majority of erythrocytes appeared macrocytic. No polychromasia, nucleated erythrocytes, or reticulocytes were seen. Howell-Jolly bodies were few in number.

WBC/μl		7,400	13,700	8,300	8,500	10,500	7,500	6,600	7,100	10,600

Case 56 (Horse). Hemolytic Anemia Associated with Heinz-Body Formation in Phenothiazine Toxicosis

Date	RBC ($\times 10^6/\mu l$)	Hb (g/dl)	PCV (%)	MCV (fl)	MCHC (%)	Icterus Index Units	Reticulo-cytes (%)	Nucleated RBC/100 WBC	Heinz Bodies	Macro-cytic RBC	WBC/μl
10/4	2.76	5.5	14.0	50.7	39.3	75	0.0	0	4+	2+	19,000
10/6	2.08	4.3	11.0	52.9	39.1	100	0.0	0	4+	2+	22,300
10/9	2.37	4.5	14.0	59.1	32.2	75	0.0	0	few	2+	17,200
10/11	2.05	4.3	13.0	63.4	33.1	25	0.0	0	few	3+	16,300
10/14	2.01	4.3	14.0	69.7	30.7	30	0.2	0.5	rare	4+	16,800
10/18	2.55	5.1	16.5	64.7	30.9	10	0.0	0	none	4+	7.400
10/20	3.00	6.3	18.0	60.0	35.0	7.5	0.0	0	none	2+	8,700
10/23	4.15	8.0	23.0	55.4	34.8	20	0.0	0	none	2+	11,500
10/25	4.64	9.0	25.0	53.9	36.0	15	0.0	0	none	2+	16,800

100.3°F, heart rate of l60/min, and respiration of 50/min. Blood examinations were conducted 19 times between Oct. 4 and Oct. 27 because of the unusual morphology of the erythrocytes. New methylene blue stain demonstrated more clearly than Wright-Leishman stain the large number of erythrocytes involved with Heinz-body formation (Fig. 2–25:5).

Interpretation

1. The initial blood film of Oct. 4, stained by Wright-Leishman method, revealed moderate anisocytosis and many erythrocytes with "punched-out" centers; many erythrocytes presented at one edge a small round structure (Heinz body) that stained the same as the erythrocyte and appeared to be in the process of being extruded. Careful inspection gave the impression that the Heinz body was attached to the parent cell by one or two delicate fibrils (Fig. 24–2). Occasionally, Heinz bodies were found free in the plasma.

2. The characteristic erythrocyte morphology, with formation of Heinz bodies, was produced experimentally in a horse by administering a greater than therapeutic dose of phenothiazine and repeating it on four occasions over a 3-week period.

3. In both the natural case of hemolytic anemia and the experimentally produced case, the cyanmethemoglobin method gave a higher hemoglobin value than actually existed. When the diluted blood specimen was centrifuged before determination of light transmission, the hemoglobin value was reduced as much as 0.5 g. The Heinz bodies affected the optical density of the sample, for they remained in suspension after lysis of the erythrocytes by the cyanide reagent. The high hemoglobin value of uncentrifuged hemolyzed sample resulted in a high MCHC (note the Oct. 4 and 6 hemograms). When Heinz bodies were no longer present in numbers in the blood, the MCHC became reduced. The lowest levels of MCHC recorded between Oct. 14 and 18 were a reflection of release of young erythrocytes to blood as the anemia entered the phase of remission.

4. This natural case of hemolytic anemia followed by remission demonstrates clearly the singular phenomenon of failure of the horse to develop reticulocytosis or polychromasia in peripheral blood during remission of anemia due to severe blood loss or destruction (see also Case 55).

5. A leukocytosis was observed initially. This was due entirely to a neutrophilia. All other leukocyte types remained within the normal range.

6. High icterus index in the face of markedly low PCV on Oct. 4, 6, and 9 is probably related to hemolytic destruction of red cells, but these values must be interpreted with caution because the horse uniquely develops marked elevations in icterus index during anorexia or systemic illness. (See Chapter 6.)

Case 57 (Horse). Equine Infectious Anemia

An 8-year-old male quarter horse was presented with the history of having a temperature of 105–106°F for 5 days in the fourth week of November. The patient had received 18,000,000 units of penicillin and a total of 2,500 grains of triple-sulfa. The clinical signs exhibited at that time were slight icterus, weakness, and poor appetite. Improvement occurred within 5 days. The animal became sick again in February and it was presented to the clinic on February 19. At that time, the clinical findings were as follows: body temperature 106.8°F, mucous membranes congested and icteric, abdomen tucked-up and sensitive to palpation, gait wobbly and shuffling behind; the general condition, however, was good.

Interpretation

1. A progressive normocytic-normochromic anemia was produced by repeated episodes of hemolytic disease. The icterus index was above normal for the PCV at all times (see normal values in Chapter 6, p. 160) and increased in degree with periodic intensification of red blood cell destruction.

2. The periodic episodes of fever were related to intensification of erythrocyte destruction.

3. The viral nature of the disease was reflected

Case 57 (Horse).   Equine Infectious Anemia

	Feb. 24	March 1	April 13	April 16	April 21
Erythrocytes ($\times 10^6/\mu l$)	9.10	8.54	5.90	5.64	3.8
Hemoglobin (g/dl)	12.25	10.9	7.13	8.3	6.09
PCV (%)	36.0	36.0	23.0	24.0	17.0
MCV (fl)	39.5	42.1	38.9	42.5	44.7
MCHC (%)	34.0	30.3	31.0	34.6	35.8
Icterus index units	20	100	100	20	50

Erythrocyte morphology essentially normal, no young forms

		%		%		%		%		%
WBC/μl	6,100		5,800		1,950		4,950		4,550	
Band neutrophils	0	0.0	0	0.0	58	3.0	0	0.0	0	0.0
Neutrophils	2,440	40.0	3,364	58.0	1,014	52.0	1,831	37.0	1,592	35.0
Lymphocytes	2,379	39.0	2,204	38.0	760	39.0	1,930	39.0	2,366	52.0
Monocytes	976	16.0	232	4.0	117	6.0	990	20.0	591	13.0
Eosinophils	305	5.0	0	0.0	0	0.0	99	2.0	0	0.0
Degenerated cells	0	0.0	0	0.0	0	0.0	50	1.0	0	0.0
Unclassified cells	0	0.0	0	0.0	0	0.0	50	1.0	0	0.0

Temperature readings in °F were:

February		*March*		*March*		*April*	
20th (a.m.)	107.0	1st (a.m.)	101.8	10th–16th	99.4–100.0	1st–3rd	99.0–100.0
(p.m.)	105.2	(p.m.)	99.6	17th–25th	no record	4th	103.3
21st (a.m.)	102.5	2nd (a.m.)	101.6	26th	104.0	5th	106.7
(p.m.)	104.4	(p.m.)	101.2	27th	106.3	6th–11th	99.2– 99.6
23rd–27th		3rd–6th	99.0– 99.4	28th	104.3	12th	103.5
	99.6–101.2	8th	103.6	29th	100.0	13th	107.0
28th (a.m.)	106.8	9th (a.m.)	103.0	30th	99.2	14th–19th	99.6–100.8
(p.m.)	107.3	(p.m.)	101.6	31st	99.0	20th	106.8
						21st	101.2
						22nd	104.4

Record of April 12:   There has been a gradual decline in condition; horse now is quite thin. Swelling of the scrotum was noticed today. This swelling was firm in nature.

   April 20:   Patient very weak, scrotum greatly enlarged and edematous; also, there is edema around the muzzle, and the mucous membranes are icteric.

   April 22:   Euthanasia and necropsy.

in the nearly constant neutropenia and marked lymphopenia on April 13.

4. Ventral edema is to be anticipated in equine infectious anemia. In this horse, edema of the scrotum and muzzle were observed. Both serum proteins and the albumin:globulin ratio were noted to be low:
   March 10: 6.2 g/dl;   A:G = 0.44:1.0
   April 21:   5.6 g/dl;   A:G = 0.32:1.0
5. See Chapter 23 for a discussion of equine infectious anemia.

Case 58 (Horse).   Neonatal Isoerythrolysis in a Foal

A 3-day-old male foal was presented with the chief complaints of weakness and slight icterus the previous night and marked icterus, dark urine, and loose yellow feces on the day of presentation. The foal was listless and too weak to stand. Its temperature was 103°F, pulse 130/min, and respiration 40/min. Initial CBC showed PCV 16%, total plasma protein 5.7, and icterus index >100 units. A diagnosis of neonatal isoerythrolysis (NI) was made. Serum chemistries included: SGOT, 235 U/L; SGPT 13 U/L; LDH, 717 U/L; alkaline phosphatase, 637 U/L; total bilirubin, 28.8 mg/dl; BUN, 23 mg/dl; glucose, 440 mg/dl; cholesterol, 199 mg/dl; inor-

ganic phosphorus, 4.2 mg/dl; Ca^{++}, 9.8 mg/dl; albumin, 2.6 g/dl; and total protein 4.9 g/dl. Significant changes on Aug. 8 were an increase in SGOT to 541 U/L and a decrease in glucose to 155 mg/dl.

Therapy consisted of administering 4 L of dextrose-saline, washed red cells from 2 L of mare's blood, phenylbutazone, antibiotics, and dexamethasone. One liter of mare's milk was fed by stomach tube on the first day of hospitalization. The foal's condition improved by the next day, and it began to nurse. However, it developed diarrhea and became febrile again on Aug. 4, with body temperature ranging between 103 and 104.6°F until Aug. 6. Clinical dehydration was not observed. With continued antibiotic therapy, gradual improvement occurred after Aug. 7, although mucous membranes were still orangish on Aug. 11. A transfusion of 900 ml of plasma was given on Aug. 11, and the foal was sent home on Aug. 12. The foal was normal on Aug. 25.

Interpretation

1. Marked anemia and icterus during the first few days of life are suggestive of neonatal isoerythrolysis (NI). An icterus index of 50 to 100 units with red cell values within the normal range is to be anticipated in newborn

Case 58 (Horse).   Neonatal Isoerythrolysis in a Foal

	Aug. 1, 1977 (3 days old)		Aug. 3		Aug. 8		Aug. 10	
Erythrocytes								
RBC ($\times 10^6/\mu$l)	3.86		5.55		5.32		4.7	
Hemoglobin (g/dl)	5.7		9.2		8.9		7.7	
PCV (%)	16		26		27		24	
MCV (fl)	41.5		46.8		50.8		51.1	
MCHC (%)	35.6		35.4		32.9		32.1	
MCH (pg)	14.8		16.6		16.7		16.4	
Anisocytosis	Slight		Slight		Slight		Slight	
Crenation							Marked	
Leukocytes								
WBC/μl	12,500	%	15,500	%	3,100	%	6,800	%
Band neutrophils	688	5.5	310	2.0	0	0.0	0	0.0
Neutrophils	7,500	60.0	13,098	84.5	589	19.0	3,298	48.5
Lymphocytes	1,687	13.5	1,627	10.5	2,325	75.0	2,992	44.0
Monocytes	2,625[a]	21.0	465	3.0	186	6.0	510	7.5
Platelets/μl	Present		Present		Present		Present	
Plasma								
Icterus index (units)	>100		50		50		75	
Total protein (g/dl)	5.7		5.8		4.0		3.5	
Fibrinogen (g/dl)	0.4		0.4		0.3		0.3	
Total bilirubin (mg/dl)	28.8		18.8					

[a]Rare cell with phagocytosed RBC.

foals as a result of their inability to conjugate and excrete bilirubin because of immaturity of the liver (see Chapters 6 and 19).

2. The increase in PCV on Aug. 3 is an effect of blood transfusion. Adequate survival of mare's red cells, as expected, is reflected in stabilization of PCV in subsequent hemograms.

3. A gradual increase in MCV indicates accelerated effective erythropoiesis in response to anemia. In the absence of reticulocyte response in the horse, such changes in MCV can be a valuable aid in assessing response to anemia.

4. Although increases in icterus index values usually parallel elevations in serum bilirubin concentrations, the degree of bilirubinemia cannot be assessed accurately from a subjective reading of the icterus index, particularly when it has reached its maximum (100 units) or when interference in light transmittance (lipemia or hemolysis) is encountered. Total bilirubin content, and if possible direct and indirect bilirubin, should be determined for proper evaluation. Kernicterus (bilirubin encephalopathy) may develop from persistent accumulation of exceedingly high amounts of bilirubin in the circulation.

5. The finding of a rare monocyte with a phagocytosed red cell in the circulation signifies immune-mediated destruction of red cells by the mononuclear phagocyte system. Spherocyte formation follows partial erythrophagocytosis and may be encountered occasion-

ally in NI. Similarly, indications for intravascular hemolysis are hemoglobinemia and hemoglobinuria, which may be observed in cases of NI. Corticosteroids are the mainstay of therapy to control immune-mediated red cell destruction in isoimmune or autoimmune hemolytic anemia.

6. Hypoproteinemia is anticipated in a newborn even after colostrum consumption. Marked decreases in total plasma protein concentrations on Aug. 8 and 10 seem to be related primarily to protein loss associated with diarrhea and to some extent inanition.

7. Leukopenia, primarily from neutropenia, on Aug. 8 probably indicates endotoxemia developing in association with diarrhea from intestinal infection. Monocytopenia in the horse is considered an expression of stress effect from an acute disease such as endotoxemia (Chapter 6). The increase in neutrophils on Aug. 10 was a favorable sign.

Case 59 (Horse).   Combined Immune Deficiency in an Arabian Foal

A male Arabian foal, about 2 weeks old, was presented with a 1 week history of respiratory distress and nasal discharge. The foal did not suckle colostrum until about 8 hours after birth. Physical examination revealed cyanotic mucous membranes, abnormal inspiratory and expiratory sounds, with both rales and rhonchi present. Temperature was 102°F, pulse 150/min, and respiration 50/min. Increased pulmonary densities, compatible with bronchopneumonia, were seen on radiologic examination of the chest.

Case 59 (Horse).   Combined Immune Deficiency in an Arabian Foal

	Aug. 6, 1981
Erythrocytes	
RBC (× 10⁶/μl)	8.66
Hemoglobin (g/dl)	11.7
PCV (%)	36
MCV (fl)	41.6
MCHC (%)	32.5
MCH (pg)	13.5
Anisocytosis	Slight
Leukocytes	
WBC/μl	12,300 %
Neutrophils	11,316 92
Lymphocytes	rare, seen on scanning
Monocytes	984 8
Eosinophils	0 0
Platelets/μl	Present in adequate numbers
Plasma	
Icterus index (units)	5
Total protein (g/dl)	6.6
Fibrinogen (g/dl)	0.8
Serum IgG (mg/dl)	355
Serum IgM (mg/dl)	0

Cytologic examination of the tracheal wash revealed many neutrophils, rarely with intracellular bacilli and cocci, and occasional macrophages. *E. coli* and *Actinobacillus* were cultured from the tracheal wash. Serologic examination demonstrated absence of IgM and 355 mg/dl of IgG. Results of the hematologic examination are shown in the table. A diagnosis of combined immune deficiency (CID), with a partial failure of passive transfer based on the low IgG levels, was made. Virus isolations and indirect immunofluorescence tests were negative for equine herpesvirus 1 and adenovirus.

Because of its acute condition, the foal was placed under intensive care and given oxygen, fluids, hyperalimentation, antibiotics (potassium penicillin and gentamicin) and aminophylline. However, because of its progressively deteriorating condition, the foal was euthanized the next day.

Necropsy. All lymph nodes appeared smaller than normal, were difficult to locate, and showed absence of differentiation between cortex and medulla on cut surface. The thymus weighed 15 g, was almost gelatinous, and showed marked interlobular edema. The spleen was very meaty and lacked obvious follicles on cut surface. Histopathologic examination of various lymphoid organs such as the thymus, lymph nodes, and spleen revealed mainly reticular stroma and total absence of lymphocytic elements. The respiratory system showed lesions of severe, acute, patchy bronchopneumonia and severe, necrotizing diffuse bronchitis and bronchiolitis. Histologic changes were compatible for an adenovirus infection, although virologic ex-

amination for it was negative. The liver showed moderate, multifocal necrosis and diffuse hepatocellular lipidosis. Diffuse nonsuppurative enteritis was also present. Cryptosporidiosis and *Pneumocystis carinii,* common to CID in humans and animals, were not observed in this foal.

Interpretation

1. Foals with CID generally develop complications from secondary bacterial, viral, and/or protozoan infections within a few weeks to a few months of birth.
2. The clinical history and signs and the breed and age of the animal indicated a tentative diagnosis of CID.
3. Severe absolute lymphopenia and absence of IgM were consistent with a diagnosis of CID, and this was further substantiated by necropsy findings of marked lymphoid hypoplasia. (See Chapter 34.)
4. A history of delayed colostrum consumption coupled with <400 mg/dl of serum IgG levels suggest the possibility of a partial failure of passive transfer of immunoglobulins. However, some consideration should be given to catabolic disappearance of maternal IgG over the 2 weeks of life of the foal, which would tend to reduce its serum IgG level from that attained after colostral consumption. The diagnosis of partial or complete failure of transfer of immunoglobulins generally entails measuring IgG concentrations in serums collected within the first 24–48 hours of birth. (See Chapter 34.)
5. The elevated fibrinogen concentration and neutrophilia were indicative of response to acute inflammation from secondary infection. Absence of left shift indicated that the foal was able to meet the increased functional demand for neutrophils without depletion of body reserves of mature neutrophils.
6. Red cell parameters were within the normal range for a foal less than 1 month old.

Case 60 (Horse).   Severe Lymphopenia Associated with Fibrinous Pericarditis and Bronchitis

A female Standardbred horse, 15 years old, had been sick for 2 weeks with signs of coughing, diarrhea, and weight loss. Upon examination, the rectal temperature was 100°F, pulse 61/min, and respiration 24/min. There was ventral edema to the thickness of about 3 inches and fluid in the thoracic cavity. The latter was tapped and 2 gallons of reddish fluid removed. A jugular pulse was evident that diminished upon removal of the 2 gallons of fluid. The horse was hospitalized and treated daily with antibiotics. Since no improvement resulted, permission was obtained to destroy the horse.

Necropsy. The epicardium was completely covered with a fibrinous exudate. The pericardium was thickened and coarsely granular. The lung tis-

Case 60 (Horse).   Fibrinous Pericarditis and Bronchitis

	September 30		October 2		October 7	
Erythrocytes						
RBC ($\times 10^6/\mu l$)	7.05		6.05		6.50	
Hemoglobin (g/dl)	11.5		9.5		10.1	
PCV (%)	35.0		29.0		30.0	
MCV (fl)	49.6		47.9		46.1	
MCHC (%)	32.8		32.7		33.7	
Leukocytes		%		%		%
WBC/μl	23,900		18,400		17,900	
Band neutrophils	359	1.5	92	0.5	0	0.0
Neutrophils	22,705	95.0	16,744	91.0	16,916	94.5
Lymphocytes	597	2.5	644	3.5	447	2.5
Monocytes	239	1.0	644	3.5	268	1.5
Eosinophils	0	0.0	92	0.5	0	0.0
Basophils	0	0.0	184	1.0	268	1.5
Neutrophil morphology	Hypersegmented		Hypersegmented		Cytoplasm slightly blue, indicating beginning of "toxic" signs	
Plasma						
Proteins (g/dl)	7.5		7.7		8.3	
Icterus index units	20		25		30	

sues revealed patchy consolidation oriented about bronchioles.

Interpretation

1. A normocytic-normochromic anemia was evident by Oct. 2. The anemia was due in part to the loss of red blood cells into the thoracic cavity as indicated by the reddish color of the removed fluid. Inflammatory diseases of this type commonly depress erythrogenesis, which in turn enhances the development of anemia. Furthermore, the anemia was possibly more advanced than demonstrated since there was clinical evidence of a disturbance in water balance.

2. The icterus index increased progressively, and in the terminal stages, it exceeded normal values for the PCV. An above-normal icterus index is difficult to evaluate in the horse, since retention of bilirubin occurs readily in this species when food and water intake is significantly reduced. In the present case, the above-normal icterus index values may have resulted from destruction of red blood cells escaping into the fluid accumulating in the thoracic cavity.

3. A marked neutrophilia and marked lymphopenia that persisted despite antibiotic therapy were grave signs. Hypersegmentation of neutrophil nuclei indicated a retention of the neutrophil leukocyte in peripheral blood for a longer period than normal. It is conjectured that this is one of the effects of corticosteroids of stress whereby diapedesis of neutrophil leukocytes is partially prevented and the cells continue to age within the circulation.

4. It was surprising that plasma protein con-

centration was not found to be higher than 7.5–8.3 g/dl. The loss of protein into the thoracic cavity may have masked an anticipated absolute increase in protein in response to the extensive inflammatory process.

Case 61 (Horse).   Hyperglobulinemia in Chronic Dermatitis

A female quarter horse was under treatment for dermatitis characterized by alopecia, eczema, and pruritus. Examination of skin scrapings for bacteria, fungi, and parasites failed to reveal specific agents. No cause could be established from histologic study of skin biopsy material. Several hemograms were developed during the period of treatment. They were of interest from the point of view of increase in plasma proteins due to production of γ-globulin.

Interpretation

1. The circulating erythrocyte volume as reflected in RBC and PCV values remained at the minimum normal level. Hemoglobin concentration was below the minimum normal. A borderline normocytic hypochromic anemia existed initially as an anemia of chronic disease.

2. In the first hemogram, the plasma protein concentration was 11.6 g/dl. In chronic suppurative diseases in the horse, globulins often increase markedly, as in this case. The albumin fraction becomes reduced as a protective mechanism to maintain osmotic pressure of blood plasma within limits. The albumin:globulin ratio approximates 1.0:1.0 in health but becomes significantly less than unity (below 0.5:1.0) when hyperglobuline-

Case 61 (Horse). Hyperglobulinemia in Chronic Dermatitis

	February 13		February 20		February 27		March 11	
Erythrocytes								
RBC ($\times 10^6/\mu l$)	6.85		7.00		7.35		7.70	
Hemoglobin (g/dl)	9.8		10.5		10.0		11.1	
PCV (%)	33.0		32.0		32.0		33.0	
MCV (fl)	48.2		45.7		43.5		42.9	
MCHC (%)	29.7		32.8		31.3		33.6	
Leukocytes		%		%		%		%
WBC/μl	21,200		12,500		13,600		13,200	
Band neutrophils	424	2.0	0	0.0	0	0.0	0	0.0
Neutrophils	14,946	70.5	8,375	67.0	8,500	62.5	6,468	49.0
Lymphocytes	4,452	21.0	3,688	29.5	4,353	32.0	5,808	44.0
Monocytes	848	4.0	250	2.0	272	2.0	66	0.5
Eosinophils	318	1.5	125	2.0	272	2.0	528	4.0
Basophils	212	1.0	0	0.0	68	0.5	132	1.0
Degenerated cells	0	0.0	63	0.5	136	1.0	198	1.5
Plasma								
Protein (g/dl)	11.6		9.7		9.5		8.3 (March 4)	
Serum proteins (g/dl) (biuret)	10.0		—		—		8.1	
Albumin	1.2		—		—		1.7	
Globulin	8.8		—		—		6.4	
γ globulin	5.7		—		—		3.9	
A:G ratio	0.14:1.0		—		—		0.27:1.0	

mia develops. Plasma protein concentrations increase in dehydration, but under conditions of hemoconcentration, the A:G ratio is not significantly altered.

3. Serum protein concentration determined by the biuret method on Feb. 13 was found to be 10.0 g/dl, and protein fractionation demonstrated the A:G ratio to be 0.14:1.0. This finding demonstrated that the hyperproteinemia was absolute and not the result of hemoconcentration.

4. A total leukocyte count of 20,000+ is a significant leukocytosis in the horse. The first hemogram demonstrated a significant neutrophilia, with other leukocyte types remaining in the normal range, which probably reflected a response to an established inflammatory lesion.

Case 62 (Horse). Extreme Leukocytosis Associated with Pyelonephritis

A pregnant Arabian mare, 15 years old, had had a problem with abscesses over the chest and abdomen. Currently, her urine contained fresh blood. Rectal examination revealed a pregnancy of about 50 days' duration. The bladder felt normal to palpation, but a large mass in the area of the left kidney was detected. These findings were reported on Sept. 26, 1962. Treatment consisted of 3 million units of penicillin and 5 g of streptomycin repeated several times at daily intervals. The mare gained weight, and the urine was grossly normal by Oct. 4. She was discharged Oct. 10 as clinically improved. Blood and urine were rechecked on Dec. 7 and again the following year in Aug. 1963.

Interpretation

1. Leukocytosis of 51,500 in the horse is an extremely high count and is typical of a localizing suppurative inflammatory process. The lymphopenia and eosinopenia were referable to systemic stress, and the monocytosis suggests chronicity.

2. Total proteins in plasma and serum were elevated, principally by hyperglobulinemia in response to the suppurative inflammatory process. With convalescence, the albumin:globulin ratio returned to the low normal range.

3. Marked improvement was reflected in near normal urine on Oct. 9 and the return of lymphocytes in large numbers to peripheral blood. The reduction in monocytes and reappearance of eosinophils and basophils also verified the relief from systemic stress. A significant neutrophilia persisted on Oct. 9.

4. A borderline anemia of chronic inflammatory disease was evident in slightly below normal values for RBC, PCV, and hemoglobin in the Sept. 26 and Oct. 9 hemograms.

5. The final hemogram, developed 1 year after the onset of the disease, revealed a fall in circulating erythrocyte volume that perhaps was due to the recent termination of gestation with a normal foal. The mare, however, had been losing weight during the month before the last hemogram.

Case 63 (Horse). Degenerative Left Shift with "Toxic" Neutrophils in Perforation of the Rectum

A 14-year-old female horse of mixed breeding was presented with a history of perforation of the

Case 62 (Horse). **Leukocytosis with Pyelonephritis**

	Sept. 26, 1962		Oct. 9		Dec. 7		Aug. 1963	
Erythrocytes								
RBC ($\times 10^6/\mu$l)	6.3		6.4		7.75		6.60	
Hemoglobin (g/dl)	11.3		10.2		13.8		10.6	
PCV (%)	30		29		39		30	
MCV (fl)	47.6		45.3		50.3		45.5	
MCHC (%)	37.6		35.2		35.4		35.3	
Leukocytes		%		%		%		%
WBC/μl	51,500		21,400		13,100		12,400	
Band neutrophils	1,030	2.0	0	0.0	0	0.0	0	0.0
Neutrophils	46,608	90.5	16,050	75.0	8,253	63.0	8,370	67.5
Lymphocytes	1,802	3.5	4,280	20.0	4,061	31.0	3,348	27.0
Monocytes	2,060	4.0	642	3.0	458	3.5	558	4.5
Eosinophils	0	0.0	321	1.5	262	2.0	124	1.0
Basophils	0	0.0	107	0.5	66	0.5	0	0.0

Neutrophil morphology: No evidence of toxic changes, but the neutrophils appeared to be somewhat larger than normal on Sept. 26 and to be hypersegmented.

Plasma								
Plasma proteins (g/dl)	10.4		8.3		7.8		7.1	
Blood urea nitrogen (mg/dl)	24.1		22 (Oct. 2)		—		—	
Serum proteins (g/dl)	8.8		—		7.0		6.3	
Icterus index units	5		2		5		10	
Albumin:globulin ratio	0.17:1.0		—		0.89:1.0		0.75:1.0	
Urine								
Specific gravity	1.020		1.010		1.024		1.018	
Proteinuria	3+		1+		negative		negative	
Occult blood	3+		trace		negative		negative	
WBC/high-power field	50–100		none		none		none	
RBC/high-power field	numerous		5		none		none	

Case 63 (Horse). **Perforation of the Rectum**

	April 25		April 29		May 2		May 3	
Erythrocytes								
RBC ($\times 10^6/\mu$l)	10.25		10.00		10.30		10.50	
Hemoglobin (g/dl)	21.2		18.3		18.9		18.9	
PCV (%)	57.0		56.0		53.0		53.0	
MCV (fl)	55.6		56.0		51.5		50.5	
MCHC (%)	37.2		32.7		35.6		35.6	
Leukocytes		%		%		%		%
WBC/μl	3,400		6,700		13,000		9,300	
Progranulocytes	0	0.0	0	0.0	0	0.0	47	0.5
Myelocytes	68	2.0	0	0.0	0	0.0	0	0.0
Metamyelocytes	102	3.0	167	2.5	65	0.5	325	3.5
Band neutrophils	714	21.0	1,440	21.5	2,405	18.5	2,186	23.5
Neutrophils	1,938	57.0	3,116	46.5	7,410	57.0	4,510	48.5
Lymphocytes	408	12.0	1,374	20.5	3,120	24.0	2,139	23.0
Monocytes	136	4.0	502	7.5	0	0.0	93	1.0
Eosinophils	34	1.0	0	0.0	0	0.0	0	0.0
Basophils	0	0.0	33	0.5	0	0.0	0	0.0
Degenerated cells	0	0.0	67	1.0	0	0.0	0	0.0

Neutrophil morphology: Cytoplasm of the immature neutrophils was blue and granular; the cytoplasm of the mature cell presented a bluish background in which a variable number of pink granules were interspersed.

Plasma								
Protein (g/dl)	—		8.3		8.3		7.7	
Icterus index units	50		50		25		10	

rectum. The condition under which the perforation occurred was not stated. The horse was received on April 23 and died on May 4. The first hemogram was not obtained until 48 hours after the perforation had occurred.

Necropsy. A tear about 4 inches long was found in the wall of the rectum. A large organized pocket occurred at the site of the rent, and there were massive adhesions between the peritoneum and intestines. The liver was enlarged and of normal color, and thrombi were present in the portal veins. A large thrombus containing strongyle larvae was present at the origin of the iliac artery.

Interpretation

1. The initial PCV of 57% and hemoglobin concentration of 21.2 g/dl were an expression of hemoconcentration from dehydration and, perhaps, splenic contraction as a result of extreme stress. Some improvement in water balance appeared to be evident in subsequent hemograms.
2. The elevated icterus index of the first two hemograms is a common finding in the horse in diseases leading to anorexia and reduced water intake (Table 6–16).
3. The leukopenia, marked left shift, and "toxic" neutrophils of the first hemogram indicated the extremely serious nature of the disease. Although leukocyte numbers increased, including both neutrophils and lymphocytes, perhaps as a response to antibiotic therapy, the persistence of "toxic" cells called for a continuing grave prognosis.

Case 64 (Horse). Icterus and Lipemia Associated with Hepatic Lipidosis

A female pony, 6 years old, had suddenly stopped eating 7 days previously. It had lost nearly 100 pounds of weight. On admission, the clinical signs were depression, temperature of 102.3°F, pulse rate of 65/min, and respiratory rate of 102/min. A foal, 2 months of age, was at its side. The pony died on July 16.

Necropsy. The liver was about twice normal size, yellowish white in color, and very greasy. Histologically the hepatic cells were filled with large fat droplets and resembled adipose tissue. The collecting tubules of the medulla and cortex of the kidneys presented hydropic degeneration. The convoluted tubules exhibited similar changes, and many were prominently dilated. Hyalin casts, granular casts, cellular casts, and crystals suggestive of oxalate crystal were contained within the convoluted tubules. Pathologic diagnosis was hepatic lipidosis and nephrosis.

Interpretation

1. A markedly lipemic plasma in the horse generally has been found to be associated with severe hepatopathy. A white, opaque plasma in the horse is to be viewed as a grave sign.

2. The high icterus index in the absence of hemolytic disease was referable to the hepatopathy. However, hyperbilirubinemia is common in the horse in a variety of acute diseases involving the gastrointestinal tract or in diseases characterized by complete anorexia (Table 6–17).
3. The presence of lipids in visible form in the blood plasma increases the refractive index and renders the prediction of plasma protein concentration invalid.
4. Neutrophilia was accompanied by evidence of toxic granulation of the cytoplasm resulting from suppressed maturation in the bone marrow due to systemic toxemia.

Case 65 (Horse). Acute Salmonellosis

A thoroughbred female, 3 years old, was a nervous filly that had to be tranquilized for training. She was exhibiting signs of colic at 5 a.m. April 28. Upon admission to the teaching hospital, her rectal temperature was 100°F, and her pulse was 50/min, steady and strong. There were reduced gut sounds. Passage of a stomach tube released foul-smelling gas. Mucous-covered feces were in the rectum. Clinical dehydration was not apparent. Initial therapy consisted of a combination of dihydrostreptomycin and procaine penicillin G. On April 29, the filly appeared normal until 6:30 p.m., when profuse diarrhea was noted. However, the feces were formed again the next morning. At this time, there appeared to be a loss of appetite. By noon on April 30, she was kicking at her abdomen. An indwelling catheter was placed in the left jugular, and 9 liters of lactated Ringer's solution was administered over a 2-hour period. Profuse diarrhea was present on May 1 and persisted throughout a 5-day period. Diarrhea began to recede on May 6, with the first really formed feces on May 9. Therapy from May 1 through May 5 consisted of IV fluids, 8 to 12 liters b.i.d., basically lactated Ringer's fortified with potassium and sodium as needed to maintain electrolyte levels. In addition, fluids were given by stomach tube and fortified with NaCl, dextrose, and furazolidone. Group B *Salmonella* organisms in moderate numbers were isolated from the feces on May 1. Considerable improvement was noted on May 10, although some weight loss was evident and weakness was apparent.

Interpretation

1. The colicky signs noted on April 29 were probably due to the beginning enteritis from *Salmonella* infection.
2. Although the combination of dihydrostreptomycin and procaine penicillin G was the only treatment administered initially, the horse appeared to be clinically normal the following day. This improved clinical state was also reflected in the near normal blood picture. Lymphopenia and bilirubinemia

Case 64 (Horse). **Hepatic Lipidosis**

	July 10		July 11		July 12	
Erythrocytes						
RBC ($\times 10^6/\mu l$)	9.20		8.40		9.13	
Hemoglobin (g/dl)	15.4		15.4		14.4	
PCV (%)	40		40		40	
MCV (fl)	43.5		47.6		43.8	
MCHC (%)	38.5		38.5		36	
Nucleated RBC/100 WBC	0.5		0		0	
Leukocytes		%		%		%
WBC/μl	14,300		12,400		16,700	
Band neutrophils	0	0.0	124	1.0	0	0.0
Neutrophils	11,225	78.5	10,044	81.0	14,028	84.0
Lymphocytes	2,860	20.0	1,984	16.0	2,171	13.0
Monocytes	143	1.0	186	1.5	501	3.0
Eosinophils	71	0.5	62	0.5	0	0.0
Basophils	0	0.0	0	0.0	0	0.0
Neutrophil morphology:	Hypersegmentation of the nucleus is a prominent feature. The cytoplasm stains a faint pink and presents many large reddish-colored granules (toxic granulation) (see Plate XI–12).					
Plasma						
Protein (g/dl)	10.5		11.7		11.5	
Icterus index units	100 (lipemic)		50 (lipemic)		50 (lipemic)	

Case 65 (Horse). **Acute Salmonellosis**

	April 28	April 29	May 1	May 2	May 3	May 4	May 5	May 8
RBC ($\times 10^6/\mu l$)	11.0	8.89	10.20	9.74	13.14	14.80	13.06	8.92
Hb (g/dl)	16.9	13.7	14.4	16.3	19.5	21.1	19.2	14.4
PCV (%)	45	38	44	45	56	62	51	39
MCV (fl)	40.9	42.7	43.1	46.2	42.6	41.9	39.1	43.7
MCHC (%)	37.5	36.0	32.7	36.2	34.8	34.0	37.6	36.9
MCH (pg)	15.4	15.4	14.1	16.7	14.8	14.3	14.7	16.1
Icterus index units	100	50	50	75	75	50	75	10 slightly lipemic
Protein (g/dl)	6.9	6.2	7.1	7.1	8.0	8.7	7.7	5.8
Fibrinogen (g/dl)	0.4	0.2	0.6	0.8	1.2	1.4	1.3	0.8
WBC/μl	12,900	8,900	2,500	1,800	4,200	3,600	5,900	11,100
Myelocytes	0	0	25[a]	90[a]	126[a]	36[a]	0	0
Metamyelocytes	0	0	125[a]	270[a]	840[a]	396[a]	472[a]	0
Bands	387	0	1,450[a]	486[a]	756[a]	936[a]	1,298[a]	610
Neutrophils	10,385	6,898	150[a]	0	252[a]	0	1,180[a]	6,105
Lymphocytes	1,935	1,735	550	918	2,142	2,196	2,950	2,886
Monocytes	193	178	200	36	42	36	0	1,332
Eosinophils	0	89	0	0	0	0	0	167
Unclassified	0	0	0	0	42	0	0	0
Na (mEq/L)	141	—	135	125	120	131	133	134
K (mEq/L)	2.8	—	2.9	3.8	4.5	3.8	3.6	3.3
Cl (mEq/L)	105	—	100	95	90	94	101	101
pH	—	—	7.40	7.42	7.34	7.35	7.35	7.38
P_{CO_2}	—	—	37.5	33.0	32.5	35.0	37.5	42.0
HCO_3^- (mEq/L)	—	—	22.7	21.1	21.0	18.7	20.3	24.0
CO_2Ct (mmole/L)	—	—	23.6	21.9	21.8	19.6	21.3	25.0
Base excess (mEq/L)	—	—	−1	−2	−1	−5	−4	0

[a]Toxic cells (Plate XI–11).

were the only abnormalities noted, but the icterus index was reduced somewhat from the high level of the previous day.

3. Profuse diarrhea leading to dehydration was apparent on May 1 through May 5. The dehydrating effect of the diarrhea was partially controlled by massive fluid therapy given orally and by intravenous infusion. The peak of dehydration was on May 4, when the PCV was 62% and the plasma protein concentration was 8.7 g/dl. A comparison of these data with those of May 8, when convalescence was in evidence, reveals the severity of water loss despite the daily administration of more than 30 liters of fluids consisting of lactated Ringer's solution fortified with electrolytes for intravenous infusion and water fortified with NaCl and dextrose given by stomach tube.

4. Loss of the electrolytes, sodium and chlorine, was greatest on May 3, and blood pH dropped to its lowest level of 7.34 at that time. The massive fluid therapy contributed significantly to success in maintaining blood pH within reasonable limits.

5. Blood gas evaluation indicated a mild metabolic acidosis that was greatest on May 4 when dehydration was at its peak. Loss of the base HCO_3 into the gut was compensated for by reduction of carbonic acid through removal of CO_2 by increased respiration. This was reflected in the below-normal concentration of Pco_2 and CO_2Ct (CO_2 content) in the blood.

6. Plasma fibrinogen increased from 0.2 to 1.4 g/dl between April 29 and May 4, indicating a marked response of the liver to the acute enteritis.

7. Leukopenia due to decrease of all leukocyte types has been a constant feature of acute salmonellosis in the horse. Most spectacular was the marked suppression of granulopoiesis with exhaustion of the bone marrow pool of mature neutrophils. On May 2, no mature neutrophils were seen in the peripheral blood, and the total leukocyte count was at its lowest level of 1,800/μl.

8. Circulating leukocyte numbers started to increase on May 3, due mainly to a significant rise in lymphocytes. Since the increase in lymphocytes to more than 2,000/μl persisted through the following days, it is conjectured that this may have been the first sign of beginning improvement despite the apparent worsening of the state of hydration and the marked hyponatremia and hypochloremia on May 3 and the acidosis on May 4.

Case 66 (Cow). Leukopenia and Left Shift in Acute Mastitis

A Holstein cow was near the end of her first lactation when once-daily milking was practiced for a 2-week period followed by abruptly stopping further milk removal. All mammary quarters were normal at that time. Since the cow was part of a small herd established for research purposes, the plan was to follow blood morphology on a daily basis to note if the abrupt cessation of milk removal would be reflected in a stress pattern in peripheral blood. The last milking was on the morning of July 16. Blood and milk samples were drawn by the milker. *Escherichia coli* was present in the milk of the right front gland at this time, but little attention was given to this finding for it was assumed to be an extraneous contaminant. However, the hemogram of the following day, July 17, indicated the cow to be sick, although the milker had not noticed any significant change in her attitude. Body temperature was 107°F on the morning of July 18, but the mammary glands were not swollen. *E. coli* was isolated from the secretions of three of the mammary quarters. By July 20, the cow was recumbent and refused to rise. The two rear mammary quarters were swollen at this time. However, by July 23, the cow was well on the way to recovery. No therapy had been administered; therefore, the sequential hemograms reveal the typical leukocytic patterns to be anticipated in acute coliform mastitis followed by recovery.

Interpretation

1. Coliform organisms multiply rapidly in cell-free milk within the mammary gland. Eventually, the presence of the multiplying bacterial population brings on an exudation of neutrophils into the milk. The neutrophils participate in the destruction of the coliform bacteria by the process of phagocytosis. Death of the Gram-negative bacteria leads to release of endotoxin, which in turn precipitates the local and systemic signs of acute mastitis.

2. The movement of neutrophils in large numbers from blood to milk results in neutropenia. The bone marrow pool of mature neutrophils is also soon exhausted, and, therefore, a marked left shift is commonly seen in the cow in response to a developing inflammatory process. Endotoxin absorbed into the circulation may temporarily depress granulopoiesis, and then a severe neutropenia may persist for several days. Other leukocyte types also become reduced in numbers in blood in response to corticosteroids of stress. Thus the cow has no other way to respond to a developing acute inflammatory process but by almost complete disappearance of all leukocyte types from peripheral blood. New generations of neutrophils become available to peripheral blood by the fourth or fifth day from original stimulus. A delay in granulopoietic response may take place, as in this case, if the bone marrow cells have been injured by circulating toxin.

Case 66 (Cow). Acute Mastitis

Date	July 16[a]	July 17[a]	July 18	July 19	July 20	July 23
Body temp. (°F)	—	—	107	102.7	104.1	102.6
WBC/μl	9,400	2,850	800	1,500	1,700	8,500
Myelocytes	0	0		0	187	127
Metamyelocytes	0	0		0	391	2,082
Band neutrophils	0	0	too few cells	30	102	1,700
Neutrophils	2,538	342	for valid	90	85	1,062
Lymphocytes	5,358	1,995	differential	1,170	799	2,762
Monocytes	1,128	399	count	195	0	467
Eosinophils	188	144		15	51	85
Basophils	188	0		0	0	56
Degenerated cells	0	0		0	85	159
"Toxic" neutrophils	—	—	—	—	4+	4+
						(Plate XI–9)

[a]Cow was normal on this day.

For further discussion on leukocytic response in mastitis see Chapter 36.

Case 67 (Cow). Neutrophilia and Lymphocytosis in Traumatic Reticulitis and Splenitis

A Jersey cow, 6 years old, had calved 6 weeks previously. A sudden noticeable decline in milk production was followed in 3 days by moderate depression, a temperature of 105°F, pulse rate of 120/min, respiratory rate of 60/min, and evidence of pain on pressure over the xyphoid region. Rumen activity was depressed, but no abnormalities could be detected on rectal palpation. The cow had been under observation as a potential lymphosarcoma case because of a somewhat above-normal number of circulating lymphocytes. On the basis of the initial hemogram and previous history, a tentative diagnosis of lymphosarcoma with su-perimposed traumatic reticulitis was proposed. An exploratory laparotomy on Jan. 31 revealed the presence of adhesions between the liver and peritoneum, and palpable portions of the liver presented numerous small, hard nodules up to one-fourth inch in diameter. The cow continued to lose weight, and she was destroyed on Feb. 14.

Necropsy. There were three wires, one about 8 inches long, penetrating the wall of the reticulum. The liver was enlarged and presented numerous small nodules containing a thick, creamy exudate. The spleen was markedly enlarged and contained a fistulous tract 1½ cm in diameter throughout its length. The abdominal cavity contained up to 5 gallons of clear yellow fluid that coagulated upon exposure to air. Multiple abscesses were found in all lobes of the lungs. Histopathologic examination of numerous tissue sections did not reveal evidence of lymphosarcoma.

Case 67 (Cow). Traumatic Reticulitis and Splenitis

	January 26		January 28	
Erythrocytes				
RBC (×10⁶/μl)	—		4.40	
Hemoglobin (g/dl)	—		7.8	
PCV (%)	28.0		25.0	
MCV (fl)	—		56.8	
MCHC (%)	—		31.2	
Leukocytes		%		%
WBC/μl	63,000		33,200	
Band neutrophils	4,725	7.5	3,984	12.0
Neutrophils	21,735	34.5	5,644	17.0
Lymphocytes	35,595	56.5	23,240	70.0
Monocytes	630	1.0	0	0.0
Eosinophils	315	0.5	0	0.0
Degenerated cells	0	0.0	332	1.0
Leukocyte morphology	Band neutrophils tend toward a pale blue granular cytoplasm with an occasional small, darkly stained "toxic" granule. Lymphocytes present more cytoplasm and basophilia than normal, suggesting some immaturity of the cells.			
Plasma				
Protein (g/dl)	9.0		8.6	
Icterus index units	12		5	

Interpretation

1. A total leukocyte count of 63,000 is an unusually high count for the cow. In this instance, the hemogram was especially unusual in that there was a marked lymphocytosis. This was perhaps in response to the extensive involvement of the spleen in the traumatic lesion.
2. The chronic nature of the disease was evident on first hemogram in the distinct neutrophilia. The bone marrow had had time to respond with increased production and release of mature neutrophils with left shift limited to band neutrophils.
3. The elevated plasma protein concentration was probably absolute, although a minor increase may be relative to slight dehydration. Hyperproteinemia due to hyperglobulinemia is anticipated in response to the chronic inflammatory process. Plasma fibrinogen also increases significantly in inflammatory diseases.
4. Depression of erythropoiesis is common to chronic inflammatory diseases. The anemia was probably masked from dehydration as indicated by slightly elevated plasma protein on Jan. 26 and subsequent reduction in both PCV and plasma protein concentration on Jan. 28.

Case 68 (Cow). Dehydration in Traumatic Reticulitis

A Holstein cow, 3 to 4 years old, was due to calve in 2 weeks when she became depressed and bloated. The body temperature was 100.8°F, pulse rate was 88/min, and respiratory rate was 25/min. Dull sounds were heard on percussion of the abdomen and thorax on the right side. Gas and fluid were expelled on passage of a stomach tube. A tentative diagnosis of traumatic reticulitis was made, and a poor prognosis given. The cow was observed several times during the following week and treated symptomatically. On Dec. 11, three gallons of water were administered by stomach tube. At this time the cow was recumbent and her temperature was 98.8°F, pulse rate was 80/min, and her respiration was 40/min. The cow died on December 13.

Necropsy. Rumen and reticulum were fairly solidly filled. The intestines were almost entirely empty. A pocket 13 × 17 cm of fibrinonecrotic tissue containing a 7-cm-long wire was present between the reticulum and abomasum.

Interpretation

1. The progressive dehydration between Dec. 6 and 10 was revealed by significant increases in RBC, Hb, PCV, and plasma proteins.
2. While total leukocyte number was not impressive, a neutrophilia was evident. By the day of death, a degenerative left shift was precipitated. The progressive decrease in lymphocytes to levels of lymphopenia expresses the severe and continuing systemic stress.
3. Low eosinophil numbers were in response to the corticosteroids of stress, and the drop

Case 68 (Cow).   Dehydration in Traumatic Reticulitis

	Dec. 6		Dec. 10		Dec. 11		Dec. 13	
Erythrocytes								
RBC ($\times 10^6/\mu l$)	5.50		9.30		—		8.95	
Hemoglobin (g/dl)	9.3		14.6		14.8		14.8	
PCV (%)	28.0		42.0		43.0		44.0	
MCV (fl)	51.0		45.2		—		49.2	
MCHC (%)	33.2		34.8		34.4		33.6	
Erythrocyte morphology	normal		Moderate rouleau formation; also, many cells have become distorted to bowl-shape, as viewed on edge, producing an appearance of "punched-out" centers in full surface view.					
Leukocytes		%		%		%		%
WBC/μl	13,100		13,700		11,400		4,600	
Metamyelocytes	0	0.0	0	0.0	0	0.0	322	7.0
Band neutrophils	66	0.5	137	1.0	171	1.5	276	6.0
Neutrophils	8,450	64.5	10,070	73.5	8,949	78.5	1,886	41.0
Lymphocytes	4,192	32.0	2,946	21.5	1,710	15.0	2,024	44.0
Monocytes	328	2.5	548	4.0	570	5.0	46	1.0
Eosinophils	66	0.5	0	0.0	0	0.0	46	1.0
Neutrophil morphology	normal		normal		normal		immature forms are large with basophilic cytoplasm.	
Plasma								
Plasma proteins (g/dl)	8.6		11.7		11.5		10.0	
Icterus index units	10		10		15		7.5	

in monocytes to almost zero on the last day was a further expression of the rapid deterioration that was taking place in the defenses of the cow.

4. Moderate rouleau formation could have resulted from increased fibrinogen concentration (although not determined in this case) associated with the inflammatory lesion of this type.

Case 69 (Cow). The Hematology of Anaplasmosis

A Guernsey heifer was given 10 ml of blood by subcutaneous route from a cow that was a carrier of *Anaplasma marginale*. Blood drawn on the tenth and twelfth days postinoculation had a PCV of 31% and 32%, respectively, and it was also normal in all other respects as reflected in blood values up to the twenty-fifth day (see tabulated data). Compare the PCV, RBC, and MCV on the thirtieth and thirty-seventh days postinoculation. Note that the PCV is 13% on each day but the erythrocyte number became reduced by two-thirds in that 7-day period. The size of the red cell had almost tripled. While there had been continuing destruction of the infected red cells, the bone marrow had been releasing immature erythrocytes of large size (Plate XVIII–7). Thus a good bone marrow response was shown, and prognosis was favorable. The leukocytosis was consistent with an anticipated increase in granulopoiesis in hemolytic crisis or acute blood loss. Anaplasmosis in the recovery phase is a transitory macrocytic hypochromic anemia. The body temperature of 104.9°F on the thirtieth day was probably the result of rapid release of products of hemoglobin breakdown. A temperature rise is to be expected when large quantities of free hemoglobin or breakdown products of hemoglobin develop suddenly. This is an excellent example of how the bone marrow responds to massive blood loss or erythrocyte destruction. The greatest drop in PCV probably occurred on the 29th day, and it was 4 days later that the first real evidence of a significant release of young erythrocytes to peripheral blood was seen. This is indicated by the rise in MCV and the presence of polychromatophilic macrocytes in large numbers. Although the red cell number continued to fall, the mass of circulating red cells (PCV) became stabilized by the larger size of the erythrocytes. The crisis was met 10–11 days after erythrocyte destruction started (thirty-seventh day), after which red cell numbers increased and red cell size decreased. The polychromatophilic macrocytes disappeared from the circulation within a few days after the initial crisis had passed. (Note rapid drop of MCV and MCH on the forty-fifth and sixty-sixth days.) (See also Table 23–3.)

Case 70 (Cow). Johne's Disease

In a herd of dairy cattle, there was a history of illness characterized by anorexia, scouring, weight loss, and eventual death. Cows ranging in age from heifers to older cows were affected, and 25 cattle had been lost. An 8-year-old pregnant Guernsey cow in poor condition and in the fourth month of lactation was admitted to the clinic for diagnostic tests. Physical examination revealed a rough hair coat, pale mucous membranes, and grossly normal rectal mucosa from which acid-fast bacilli were cultured. A johnin skin test was positive. A urine sample was cloudy with a specific gravity of 1.018 and a 1+ test for protein.

The cow was euthanized, and necropsy revealed a disseminated interstitial nephritis and an infarct in the kidney. The intestinal wall was thickened, and the mucosa had a corrugated appearance throughout. There was obstruction of the lymphatics of the small intestine with an accumulation of giant cells in the submucosal lymphatics.

Interpretation

The hemogram reflected a chronic disease problem, as indicated by a PCV at the low normal level, a hemoglobin concentration below normal, and a differential leukocyte count indicating a neutrophilia and a monocytosis. There was a marked hypoalbuminemia from loss of protein into the intestine, but a fairly good level of total protein was maintained by a modest hyperglobulinemia, which was possibly a reflection of an immunologic response.

Case 71 (Cow). Trichostrongyloidosis

A Hereford steer, 1½ years old, representing one of a pair on dry pasture, was showing an edematous swelling under the jaw that was first noticed 3 weeks previously. The other steer was not involved, but both animals had been treated with phenothiazine by the owner when he first noticed the edematous swelling. The general condition of the patient was poor, and its body temperature was 102.4°F.

Interpretation

1. Trichostrongyloidosis in cattle often manifests as a depression anemia (normocytic normochromic) of advanced degree. The presence of normocytic hypochromic anemia in this patient may suggest progressively impaired iron utilization as in anemia of chronic disease. (See Chapter 22.)
2. In this disease, the leukocyte count is generally within the normal range, and there are no significant changes in the differential count. When the leukocyte picture is altered, it is in the direction shown by this case: leukocytosis with moderate neutrophilia.
3. The edema of the throat is associated with a fall in plasma proteins, as shown here. (See also Chapter 34.)

Case 69 (Cow). The Hematology of Anaplasmosis

Day Postinoculation	17th	21st	25th	26th	27th	30th	31st	32nd	33rd	35th	37th	39th	45th	66th
Erythrocytes (×10^6/µl)	—	—	7.25	6.55	6.15	3.16	2.58	2.12	1.67	1.24	1.11	1.41	2.42	4.88
Hemoglobin (g/dl)	12.0	11.4	13.0	10.7	9.7	4.4	3.8	3.4	3.4	3.4	3.4	3.8	5.0	7.9
PCV (%)	34.0	32.5	36.5	30.5	28.0	13.0	12.0	11.0	12.0	12.0	13.0	14.0	18.5	24.0
MCV (fl)	—	—	50.3	46.6	45.5	41.1	46.5	51.8	71.8	96.7	117.1	99.3	76.4	49.2
MCH (pg)	—	—	17.9	16.3	15.8	13.9	14.7	16.0	20.4	27.4	30.6	26.9	20.6	16.2
MCHC (%)	35.3	35.1	35.6	35.1	34.6	33.8	31.7	30.9	28.3	28.3	26.1	27.1	27.0	32.9
RBC with AB[a]	—	—	—	—	30% AB	—	50% AB	—	Many polychromatophilic macrocytes	—	—	Basophilic stippling		
Leukocytes	—	—	8,000	6,900	7,500	9,600	11,000	16,550	31,829	—	—	—	11,000	10,300
Physical condition	Normal	N	N	N	N	Marked depression, anorexia, constipation, and icterus			Down, emaciated, labored breathing			Up, eating a little		
Temperature (°F)	101.8	101.8	101.8	101.2	101.0	104.9	101.8	100.4	92.0	100.0	—	101.6	106.2	101.8
Pulse/min	80	84	80	76	84	132	144	152	120	100	—	96	88	80
Respiration/min	Normal	N	N	N	N	56	N	16	20	20	—	20	20	44

[a]AB = *Anaplasma marginale* bodies (Plate XVIII–7).

Case 70 (Cow).   Johne's Disease

Hemogram		Serum Protein Fractionation	
RBC ($\times 10^6/\mu l$)	4.80	Total protein (g/dl)	5.9
Hb (g/dl)	7.5	Albumin	1.0
PCV (%)	24	Globulin	4.9
Icterus index units	2	alpha	1.1
WBC/μl	12,700	beta	0.7
Band neutrophils	131	gamma	3.1
Neutrophils	7,112	A:G ratio	0.2 (normal =
Lymphocytes	3,933		0.86–1.18)
Monocytes	1,524		

Case 71 (Cow).   Trichostrongyloidosis

			Plasma Protein Analysis	
Erythrocytes ($\times 10^6/\mu l$)	2.5			
Hemoglobin (g/dl)	3.7		Total protein (g/dl)	2.8
PCV (%)	14.0		Albumin	1.8
MCV (fl)	56.2		Globulin	1.0
MCHC (%)	26.4		Alpha	0.3
Anisocytosis	moderate		Beta	0.6
Hypochromasia	moderate		Gamma	0.1
Leukocytes/μl	15,500	%	A:G ratio	1.8:1.0
Bands	155	1.0		
Neutrophils	7,750	50.0		
Lymphocytes	6,200	40.0	Fecal examination	
Monocytes	1,240	8.0	Flotation: Trichostrongyles 5/low power field	
Eosinophils	155	1.0	Stoll count: Trichostrongyles 500/g	

Case 72 (Cow).   Congenital Porphyria (Pink Tooth)

Calf 1: A Holstein female calf, 3 months of age, was presented with a complaint of skin lesions of 2 months' duration, dark urine, and poor growth. The white areas of the body over the back were scaly, crusty, and hairless (a result of photosensitization from porphyrins). The mucous membranes were pale, and the teeth were reddish brown and fluoresced in ultraviolet light (a result of uroporphyrin deposition in teeth and bones). All bones were found to be reddish brown at necropsy.

Calf 2: A grade, red and white Holstein female calf, 5½ months old, from another herd was referred with a history of paralysis of 2 weeks' duration. There were crusty, scaly areas around the nose and rectum and alopecia with skin necrosis

Case 72 (Cow).   Congenital Porphyria

	Calf 1			Calf 2	
	Feb. 4		Feb. 7	March 2	
Erythrocytes ($\times 10^6/\mu l$)	2.42		2.55	3.42	
Hemoglobin (g/dl)	5.0		4.8	6.7	
PCV (%)	15.0		14.0	21.0	
MCV (fl)	61.9		54.9	61.4	
MCHC (%)	33.3		34.2	31.9	
Reticulocytes (%)	2.8		—	3.6	
Nucleated erythrocytes	78/100 WBC		30/100 WBC	32/100 WBC	

Erythrocyte morphology in both calves was similar. There was marked polychromatophilia, basophilic stippling, poikilocytosis, and anisocytosis.

WBC/μl (corrected)	14,000		14,820	10,000	
		%		%		%
Band neutrophils	0	0.0	148	1.0	0	0.0
Neutrophils	2,380	17.0	1,334	9.0	2,500	25.0
Lymphocytes	8,120	58.0	6,817	46.0	5,700	57.0
Monocytes	3,360	24.0	4,743	32.0	1,800	18.0
Eosinophils	140	1.0	593	4.0	0	0.0
Unclassified cells	0	0.0	296	2.0	0	0.0
Degenerated cells	0	0.0	889	6.0	0	0.0
Icterus index units	<5		—	<5	

Case 73 (Sheep). Haemonchosis

Erythrocytes ($\times 10^6/\mu l$)	3.3	
Hemoglobin (g/dl)	2.9	
PCV (%)	11.5	
MCV (fl)	34.7	
MCHC (%)	25.2	
Icterus index units	<5	
Reticulocyte count (%)	5.7	
Nucleated erythrocytes	1/100 WBC	

Anisocytosis	moderate to marked	Basophilic stippling	marked
Poikilocytosis	moderate to marked	Polychromasia	moderate to marked
Hypochromasia	moderate to marked	H-J bodies	occasional

Leukocytes/μl	7,100	%
Bands	71	1.0
Neutrophils	2,698	38.0
Lymphocytes	3,905	55.0
Monocytes	177	2.5
Eosinophils	213	3.0
Degenerated cells	35	0.5

Fecal examination: McMaster count—84,000 eggs per gram, most of which were *Haemonchus contortus*.

and scaling over an area of white in the hip region. The teeth and bones were reddish brown. The urine contained a brownish pigment. The paralysis was due to a fracture of a lumbar vertebra; there were rib fractures as well.

Porphyrins. The urine of both calves contained large quantities of the abnormal isomeric uroporphyrin I and a high level of coproporphyrin. These large quantities of porphyrins arise in the bone marrow because of a deficiency of uroporphyrinogen III–cosynthetase. (See Chapter 24.)

Interpretation

1. The RBC, Hb, and PCV values indicate a well-advanced anemia in Calf 1 and a moderate anemia in Calf 2. The MCV indicates a macrocytic anemia; the mean red cell size is more than double the normal. The large numbers of polychromatophilic erythrocytes and nucleated red cells and basophilic stippling of erythrocytes indicate intense erythrogenesis, while the poikilocytosis points to shortened life span of the erythrocytes. Basophilic stippling of a bovine erythrocyte is shown in Plate XVIII–10.
2. Bone marrow from the iliac crest revealed a megaloblastic type of marrow. The nucleated red cells were typically large, with basophilic cytoplasm. The myeloid:erythroid ratio was estimated to be 0.1:1. An accurate determination was not possible because of the presence of large numbers of disintegrating blast-like cells and free nuclei.
3. Monocytosis is probably a reflection of chronic skin lesions.

Case 73 (Sheep). Haemonchosis

A 1-year-old male Suffolk sheep had been showing edema of head and throat for 2 days. On physical examination, the following were observed:

temperature 102.5°F, pulse 136/min, respiration 28/min, mucous membranes pale, pupils dilated, moderate degree of nasal exudate, and marked depression.

Interpretation

1. *Haemonchus contortus* is a bloodsucking parasite of the abomasum.
2. A macrocytic hypochromic anemia with active erythrogenesis is anticipated in acute blood loss from heavy infection with *H. contortus*, whereas a normocytic normochromic or hypochromic anemia develops in chronic infections. In the present case, the normocytic hypochromic anemia indicates a chronic rather than acute blood loss, while reticulocytosis, moderate to marked polychromasia, and basophilic stippling indicate active but inadequate red cell production. Together, these findings probably suggest a transitional phase of anemia from acute to chronic stage in which iron deficiency is setting in with diminution of erythropoiesis from progressive heavy parasitism. (See Chapter 22.)
3. The occurrence of many poikilocytes seems to be an expression of the inability of the newly formed erythrocytes to withstand the stress of circulation. This is common to anemia associated with iron deficiency from chronic blood loss. Thus anemia in this sheep may have resulted from both blood loss and shortened life span of newly formed erythrocytes.
4. Although plasma protein concentration was not determined in this case, the presence of edema of head and throat are most likely a manifestation of hypoproteinemia (hypoalbuminemia) associated with haemonchosis. (See Chapter 22.)

Index

Page numbers in *italics* refer to illustrations, roman numerals refer to plates, and those followed by the letter "t" indicate tables.

A antigen(s), 991, 992, 995-996
Abdominal exudate(s), cat, 1071
Abdominal lymphoma(s), 848
Abscess(es)
  liver, in dog, *965*
  neutrophil migration and, 690
  serum protein and, 975
Absolute leukocyte count(s), 824
Acanthocyte(s), *530, 534, 536, 538,* 540
  anemia and, 570
  cholesterol and, 544, 545
  echinocyte and, 541
  etymology of, 534t
Acaprin, 598
ACD. *See* Acid-citrate-dextrose
Acer rubrum, 642
Acetyl phenylhydrazine, 158
Acetylpromazine maleate, 142
Achlorhydria, 382
Achromatic lens(es), 21
Acid hydrolase, 684
α_1-Acid mucoprotein(s), 948
Acid α-naphthyl acetate esterase, 776, 911t, 912t, 915-919, 928
Acid phosphatase, 910-914, 910t, 912t
  neutrophils and, 685
  technique for, 926-927
Acid-citrate-dextrose, 994
Acidosis
  canine babesiosis and, 599
  horse, 166
  plasma volume and, 95
Acinonyx, 335t, 340-341
Acomys cahirinus, 310-311
ACP. *See* Acid phosphatase
Acquired coagulopathy(ies), 407-410
Acquired immune deficiency syndrome, 982
Acquired isoantibodies to leukocyte(s), 1000
Acridine, 598
ACTH. *See* Adrenocorticotropic hormone
Actin
  erythrocytes and, 532
  platelets and, 455
Activated clotting time, 421, 421t
Activated macrophage(s), 774
Activated partial thromboplastin time
  coagulopathy and, 419-420
  hemostasis and, 421-422
Activator, plasminogen, 399, 761t, 785
Acuminocyte(s), *530, 538,* 540

etymology of, 534t
Acute hemolytic anemia. *See* Hemolytic anemia(s)
Acute lymphoblastic leukemia, feline, 852
Acute lymphocytic leukemia
  canine, 874-876
  chemotherapy and, 899
  nonspecific esterase and, 918
  peroxidase and, 920
  sudanophilia and, 921
  terminal deoxynucleotidyl transferase and, 921
Acute monocytic leukemia
  acid phosphatase and, 911-913
  nonspecific esterase and, 918
Acute myelogenous leukemia
  acid phosphatase and, 911-913
  neutrophil abnormalities and, 716
  nonspecific esterase and, 918
  peroxidase and, 920
  sudanophilia and, 921
  terminal deoxynucleotidyl transferase and, 921
Acute myelomonocytic leukemia
  acid phosphatase and, 911-913
  dog, XXIV
  nonspecific esterase and, 918
  sudanophilia and, 921
Acute promyelocytic leukemia, 918
ADA. *See* Adenosine deaminase
ADCC. *See* Antibody-dependent cellular cytotoxicity
Addison's disease
  blood urea nitrogen and, 1061t
  dog, 1059-1063, 1099-1100
  hemogram and, 1060t
Adenocarcinoma(s), cat, 1140, 1141
Adenosine deaminase, 912t, 922
Adenosine diphosphate
  canine platelet and, 121
  hemostasis and, 389
  platelet aggregation and, 457, 461
Adenosine monophosphate, cyclic, 389
Adenosine triphosphate, 545, 551
Adenylate kinase, 912t
ADP. *See* Adenosine diphosphate
Adrenal gland(s)
  canine, 1054-1063
  pig leukocyte and, 249
Adrenalin. *See* Epinephrine
β-Adrenergic agent(s), degranulation and, 703
Adrenocortical insufficiency(ies)
  blood urea nitrogen and, 1061t
  dog, 1059-1063, 1099-1100

Adrenocortical insufficiency(ies) *(Continued)*
  hemogram and, 1060t
  screening for, 64
Adrenocorticosteroid(s). *See* Corticosteroid(s)
Adrenocorticotropic hormone
  blood corticosteroid and, 692, 765t
  canine Cushing's syndrome and, 1054-1056, 1058-1059
  cattle and, 198, 199, 200, 201
  dog and, 111, 112t, 1054-1056, 1058-1059
  eosinophils and, 64
  horse and, 163-166
  monocytes and, 119, 777-778
  pig and, 249
Adriamycin. *See* Doxorubicin
Adult hemoglobin, 518t. *See also* Hemoglobin(s)
Aedes, 268-269
Aepyceros melampus, 329, 333t
Aerobacter aerogenes
  bovine mastitis and, 1076
  cat endotoxemia and, 834t
Afibrinogenemia(s), 403t, 407
AFP. *See* α-Fetoprotein
African lion(s), 334t
A/G ratio. *See* Albumin:globulin ratio
Agammaglobulinemia, 981
Agar gel immunodiffusion test(s)
  bovine leukemia virus and, 885
  equine infectious anemia and, 618
Agarose electrophoresis, 956
Age, blood values and, 7
  cattle, 178-188, 181t, 182t, 187t, *187*
  dog, 109-111
  erythrocytes and, 104-107
  feline infectious anemia in, 604
  goat, 225
  horse, 148t, 151
  laboratory animal, 276
  monkey, 315
  mouse, 306
  pig, 244-245
  plasma proteins in, 945
  platelets in, 442
  sheep, 208-215, 210t, 211t, 213t
  total proteins in, 957-960
  water buffalo, 328
  Wintrobe index in, 104-107
Agglutination
  autoimmune hemolytic anemia and, 648, 1010
  cell counting error and, 52
  cold, 648, 1010
  leptospirosis and, 617
  papain-treated erythrocyte, 75
Agglutinin(s), 71-72. *See also* Agglutination
Aggregate reticulocyte(s), 62-63
Aggregation, platelet, 6, 457-458, 460-461
Aggregometer(s), 461
AGID. *See* Agar gel immunodiffusion test(s)
Agranulocyte(s), 7
Agranulocytosis, infectious feline, 1072
AID. *See* Anemia(s), inflammatory disease and
AIDS. *See* Acquired immune deficiency syndrome
AIHA. *See* Autoimmune hemolytic anemia
AIN. *See* Autoimmune neutropenia
AITP. *See* Autoimmune thrombocytopenia
Akita, 107
δ-ALA. *See* δ-Aminolevulinic acid
ALA dehydrase. *See* δ-Aminolevulinic acid dehydrase
ALAD. *See* δ-Aminolevulinic acid dehydratase
Albumin, 947. *See also* Albumin:globulin ratio
  changes in, 960
  equine multiple myeloma and, 893, *896*
  extravascular:vascular ratio for, 942
  fascioliasis and, 586
  half-life of, 947

horse, 160, 172t, 893, *896*
  mink, 317
  radioiodine labeled, 87, 93
  rat, 298
  replacement of, 944
  transport function of, 947
Albumin:globulin ratio, 955. *See also* Albumin
  dehydration and, 944
  dysproteinemia and, 957
  horse, 172t
  immunoglobulin deficiency and, 981
  mule, 340
Alder-Reilly anomaly, 716
Aleukemic leukemia, 838, 839
Aleutian disease of mink, 317-318, 971
Alimentary tract. *See* Gastrointestinal disease(s)
Alkaline phosphatase, 910t, 914-915
  eosinophils and, 737
  neutrophils and, 685
  technique for, 927-928
Alkeran. *See* Melphalan
ALL. *See* Acute lymphocytic leukemia
Allergy(ies). *See also* Hypersensitivity(ies);
      Sensitivity(ies)
  eosinophil and, 746
  immunoglobulin E and, 954
  transfusions and, 995
Allogenous platelet(s) loaded with vinblastine or
      vincristine, 1025
Alloimmunization with Rh antigen(s), 996
Allotype of immunoglobulin(s), 952
ALP. *See* Alkaline phosphatase
Alpaca(s), 336-337
  erythrocyte and, 528
Alpha₁-acid mucoprotein, 948
Alpha₁-antichymotrypsin, 714, 922
Alpha₁-antitrypsin, 714, 922
  clotting regulation and, 398
Alphadolone/alphaxalone acetate, 127
Alpha-fetoprotein, 950
Alpha-globulin(s), 941t
  changes in, 962-964
  equine multiple myeloma and, 893, *896*
  erythrocyte sedimentation rate and, 55
  horse and, 160, 893, *896*
Alpha-granule(s), megakaryocyte and, 436
Alpha-L-iduronidase, 716
Alpha₂-macroglobulin, 398, 714, 948
Alpha-mannosidase, 923
Alpha-naphthyl acetate esterase, 776, 911t, 912t, 915-919
  technique for, 928
Alpha-naphthyl butyrate esterase, 911t, 912t, 915-919
  technique for, 929
Alphaxalone/alphadolone acetate, 127
ALS. *See* Antilymphocyte serum
Altitude(s)
  cattle hemogram and, 193-194
  sheep hemoglobin and, 212, 215
Alveolar macrophage(s), 773
Amblyomma variegatum, 483
American black bear(s), 335t
Amicarbalide, 598
Amino acid(s), 940
  albumin and, 947
  hemoglobinopathy and, 520
  immunoglobulins and, 951
3-Amino-9-ethylcarbazole stain, 932-933
δ-Aminolevulinic acid, 514
δ-Aminolevulinic acid dehydrase, 515, 629
δ-Aminolevulinic acid dehydratase, 271
Ammonium sulfate precipitation test(s), 981
Ammotragus lervia, 329, 333t

Amphibian erythrocyte(s), 275
Amphophil, 281
Amphotericin B, 719
Amporolium poisoning, 483
Amyloidosis in dog(s), 1119-1121
ANA. *See* Antinuclear antibody(ies)
Anabolic steroid(s), 1017
Anabolism, 942
Anaerobic glycolysis
    lymphocytes and, 795
    macrophages and, 775
    neutrophils and, 684-685
    phagocytosis and chemotaxis and, 706
    platelets and, 454
Anaphylaxis, 835t, 836
    basophil degranulation and, 760, 761t, *764*
    blood transfusions and, 994
    eosinophilic chemotactic factor of, 760, 761t
    immunoglobulin E and, 954
    leukopenias and, 835t, 836
    slow reacting substance of, 746, 760, 761t
Anaplasma centrale, 590
Anaplasma marginale, 321, 590
    erythrocytes and, 501
Anaplasma ovis, 590
Anaplasmosis, 590-596, 591t, 592t, *593*, *594*
    blood film and, 60, *61*
    cow, 1165, 1166
    Eperythrozoa and, 609
    erythrocytes and, 501
    morphology in, 592-595
    sheep and goats and, 596
Anas platyrhynchos, 271
Ancylostoma caninum, 584-585
Androgen(s)
    autoimmune hemolytic anemia and, 1017
    erythropoiesis and, 370, 507-508
    plasma proteins and, 943
Anemia(s)
    amyloidosis with, 1119-1121
    aplastic, 665-668
    assessing response to, 3, 12
    autoimmune hemolytic. *See* Autoimmune hemolytic
        anemia
    bird, 267, 269, 270-271
    blood loss. *See* Blood loss anemia(s)
    bone marrow transplantation and, 118
    calf and, 181
    cat. *See* Anemia(s), cat
    cattle, 191, 194, 585, 586, 671
    classification of, 564-566, 565t
    clinical signs of, 563-564
    depression. *See* Depression anemia
    dog. *See* Anemia(s), dog
    elephant, 338
    equine infectious. *See* Equine infectious anemia
    erythrocyte osmotic fragility and, 554
    erythrocyte sedimentation rate and, 55
    erythrocytes in, 55, 554, 565t, 566-569, 571-572, XVII
    erythropoietin and, 504, 506-507
    Fanconi's, 666
    feline infectious, 602, 1148-1150, 1151
    goat, 226, 229, 230t, 235, 237
    Heinz bodies and. *See* Heinz body(ies)
    hypochromic macrocytic, 565, 566, 585, 656. *See also*
        Microcytic hypochromic anemia(s)
    hypoproliferative. *See* Hypoproliferative anemia(s)
    immune-mediated hemolytic. *See* Immune-mediated
        hemolytic anemia
    infectious. *See* Anemia(s), feline infectious; Equine
        infectious anemia
    inflammatory disease and, 668-669
    iron deficiency. *See* Iron deficiency anemia
    laboratory evaluation of, 566-571, 567t, 568t, *569*

lead poisoning and, 515, 628-632
    leukocyte response and, 827
    leukoerythroblastic, 825
    marrow examination in, 12
    macrocytic, 565, 566, 585, 656
    microcytic hypochromic. *See* Microcytic hypochromic
        anemia(s)
    neonatal. *See* Neonatal anemia(s)
    noninfectious hemolytic. *See* Noninfectious hemolytic
        anemia
    normochromic, 565-566. *See also* Normocytic
        normochromic anemia(s)
    packed cell volume and, 37
    pernicious, 381, 657
    pig, *See* Anemia(s), pig
    protein and, 508
    sheep, 209, 215, 585, 586, 626-628, 671
    sickle cell, 519-520. *See also* Sickle cell(s)
    spur-cell, 544-545
    Theileria parva and, 611
    treatment of, 571-572
    trypanosomiasis and, 614
Anemia(s), cat
    adenocarcinoma of small intestine and, 1140, 1141
    autoimmune hemolytic, 1146-1148
    feline infectious, 602, 1148-1150, 1151
    lupus erythematosus and, 1146-1148
    lymphosarcoma and, 1142-1143
    peritonitis and, 1138
    toxoplasmosis and, 1137-1138
Anemia(s), dog
    amyloidosis and, 1119-1121
    autoimmune hemolytic, 474t, 476, 648, 649t, 1007-
        1009, 1123-1125
    blood loss, 1125-1126
    erythrocytes and, 108
    idiopathic, 470t
    immune-mediated, 75
    inflammatory disease and, 668-669
    microcytic hypochromic, 583, *583*
    reticulocyte count and, 567t
    protein and, 508
Anemia(s), pig, 247, 248, 250, 252
    blood volume and, 245
    neonatal, 243-244
Anesthesia, 283
    blood loss and, 97
    horse and, 142, 143t
Angora goat(s), *233*, *234*
Anhydremia, 96
Anisocytosis, 6, 131
    cat, 131, 856
    cow, 194
    dog, 104
    goat, 234
Ankylosing spondylitis, 1004
Antagonism, vitamin K, 407-408, 417
Anteater(s), 338
Anterior vena cava, 25t, 26, 27
Antibiotic(s), phagocytosis and, 707, 719
Antibody(ies)
    anti-DNA, 78, 1026-1027
    anti-erythrocyte. *See* Antierythrocyte antibody(ies)
    antinuclear, 77-79
    antiplatelet. *See* Antiplatelet antibody(ies)
    to blood group antigens, 992-993, 992t
    to deoxyribonucleoprotein, 78, 1026-1027
    Factor VIII complex, 405-406
    feline oncornavirus cell membrane, 846-847
    IgG, 73, 74, 74t, 78
    leptospirosis and, 617
    leukocyte, 827, 1000-1003
    lymphocytes and production of, 807-808
    maternal, 479, 979-981
    warm-reactive, 1008, 1009

Antibody-dependent cellular cytotoxicity, 809
Anti-C, 73, 74, 74t
Anticanine globulin(s), 77
Antichalone(s), 696-697
Antichymotrypsin, 714, 922
Anticoagulant(s)
  avian blood samples and, 260
  blood collection and, 1, 2, 23-24
  Coombs test and, 73
  cross-matching blood and, 71, 72
  disseminated intravascular coagulopathy and, 413-415
  lupus, 1026
  marrow aspiration and, 66
  method for dispensing, 23-24, 25
  thrombus and, 417, 418t
Anti-DNA antibody(ies), 78, 1026-1027
Antierythrocyte antibody(ies), 73-75, 555, 592, 1008
  Anaplasma and, 592
  autoimmune hemolytic anemia and, 648
Anti-estrogenic substance(s), 1017
Antigen(s)
  factor VIII-related, 394, 406
  feline oncornavirus cell membrane, 846-847
  hemolytic disease of newborn and, 997
  immunoglobulins and, 951-952
  leukocyte, 827, 999, 1000-1003
  lymphocyte, 1002
  lymphocyte recirculation and, 803, 806
  lymphopoiesis and, 802
  macrophages and, 782
  monocytes and, 777
  neonatal isoerythrolysis and, 650, 996
  platelet, 1005-1006, 1021. *See also* Antiplatelet
    antibody(ies)
  red cell, 991-993
  Rh, 650, 996
  surface, 796, 797
  transplantation, 998, 1003-1004
Antigen-reactive T cell(s), 807
Antihemophilic factor(s), 394-395, 404-405, 406, 468
Anti-IgG, 73, 74, 74t, 1026
  antinuclear antibody and, 78
Anti-inflammatory steroid(s). *See* Corticosteroid(s);
    Steroid(s)
Antilope cervicapra, 329, 333t
Antilymphocyte serum, 1004-1005
Antimalarial drug(s), 269
Antimetabolite(s), 716. *See also* Antineoplastic agent(s);
    specific agent
Antineoplastic agent(s)
  leukemia complex and, 898
  neutrophils and, 716, 719
Antinuclear antibody(ies), 1026-1029, 1028t
  amyloidosis and, 1119-1121
  autoimmune hemolytic anemia and, 1011
  detection of, 77-79
Antinucleoprotein(s), 78
Antiplasmin, 398, 401
Antiplatelet antibody(ies), 75-77
  detection of, 1021
  formation of, 1021-1023
  immunofluorescence test and, 1019
  thrombocytopenia and, 479
Antiplatelet drug(s), thrombosis and, 417-418, 418t
Antiseptic(s), urinary, 131, 638
Antithrombin III
  clotting regulation and, 398
  disseminated intravascular coagulation and, 423
Antithymocyte antibody(ies), 796
Antitrypsin, 714, 922
  clotting regulation and, 398
Antiviral activity(ies) of neutrophil, 714
Aoudad, 329, 333t

Aperture(s), numerical, 22
Aplasia(s)
  of bone marrow, 666
  red cell, 665-668
Aplastic anemia(s), 665-668
Apochromatic lens(es), 21
Apolipoprotein(s), 950
Apoprotein(s), 951
Appaloosa horse(s), 149-163. *See also* Horse(s)
  normal values for, 149, 150t
APTT. *See* Activated partial thromboplastin time
Arabian horse(s), 149-163. *See also* Horse(s)
  combined immune deficiency in, 978
  hematology of, 152t
  normal values for, 149, 150t
Ara-C, 898, 899, 900
Arachidonic acid
  chemotaxis and, 700
  inflammatory response and, 713
  mast cells and basophils and, 761t
  platelets and, 452t, 455-456, 461
Argas persicus, 270
Arginase, 784
Arteritis, viral, 830
Arthritis, rheumatoid, 77, 507
Arthropod(s), theileriasis and, 610
Artifact(s), red cell morphology and, 6
Arylsulfatase, 716, 761t
Ascaris suum, 714
L-Asparaginase, 898, 899, 900
Aspirin
  albumin and, 947
  arachidonic acid metabolism and, 456
  bone marrow cytology of cat and, 137
  intoxication and, 1113
  neutrophil migration and, 692
  platelets and, 441, 462
  thrombosis and, 417-418, 418t
Ateless sp., 334t
Atherosclerosis, platelet and, 459-460
Auer body(ies), 715-716
Australian swamp buffalo, 329
Autoagglutination, 592, 598
Autoantibody(ies). *See* Autoimmune hematologic
    disorder(s)
  Anaplasma and, 592
  autoimmune hemolytic anemia and, 1013-1014
  equine infectious anemia and, 619
  leukocytes and, 1000
  platelet antigen and, 1021
Autoimmune hematologic disorder(s), 1007-1025
  antilymphocyte serum and, 1005
  hemolytic anemia in. *See* Autoimmune hemolytic
    anemia
  neutropenia in, 1025
  T cells and, 808
  thrombocytopenia in, 1018-1025. *See also*
    Autoimmune thrombocytopenia
Autoimmune hemolytic anemia, 1007-1018
  antinuclear antibody and, 77
  cat, 649t, 650, 1146-1148
  cell counting error and, 51
  classification of, 1008-1009
  clinical observations of, 1009-1010
  Coombs antiglobulin test in, 73, 74, 74t, 1011-1013,
    1013
  corticosteroids and, 649t, 650, 1016, 1017
  dog, 474t, 476, 648, 649t, 1007-1009, 1123-1125
  Donath-Landsteiner antibody-mediated, 1015-1016
  drug-induced, 1016
  laboratory findings of, 1010-1011. *See also*
    Autoimmune hemolytic anemia, Coombs
    antiglobulin test in

pathogenesis of, 1013-1015
platelet disorders and, 474t, 476
spherocyte and, 543
therapy of, 1016-1018
Autoimmune neutropenia, 1025
Autoimmune thrombocytopenia, 478-479, 1018-1025
antiplatelet antibody detection in, 75-77, 1021
classification of, 1019
clinical observations of, 1019-1020
corticosteroids and, 1024
in domestic animals, 1019
drug-induced, 1023-1024
hematologic findings in, 1020-1021
in humans, 1018-1019
megakaryocyte and, *434*
pathogenesis of, 1021-1023
therapy for, 1024-1025
Autologous red cell(s), sodium radiochromate labeling and, 93
Autotransfusion(s), 952
Avian hematology, 256-273
blood and, 256-258
blood elements and, 258-259, XXV
blood sampling and, 259-260
bone marrow and, 263-264, 364-365
erythrocytes and, 256, 257, 259, 261, 268, 269, 548
Heinz body anemia and, 270-271
hematopoiesis in marrow and, 263-264
hematopoietic neoplasias and, 264-268
lead poisoning and, 271
leukocyte count of, 261-263
leukocytes and, 257-258, 261
normal blood values and, 257t
parasites of, 268-270, XXV
spirochetosis and, 270
techniques and, 259-263
Avian malaria, 268-269
Aythya valisneria, 271
5-Azacytidine, 898
Azathioprine
autoimmune hemolytic anemia and, 1017
systemic lupus erythematosus and, 1029
Azure dye, 31
Azurophilic granule(s), 7, 15, 16, 683
blast cells with, 856, *856*
eosinophils and, 734
lymphocytes and, 119, 134, 159, 196, 220, 238, 252, 281, 287, 297, 318, 319, 328
monocytes and, 119, 159, 196, 238, 252, 297, 318, 319, 328
neutrophils and, 826
platelets and, 120, 136, 238, 252, 282, 288, 318, 328
scattered or uniformly distributed, 16

B antigen(s), 991, 996
B cell(s), 264, 790-791
antibody production and, 807-808
bird, 259, 264
blastogenesis and, 799-800
bovine leukemia virus and, 884
canine lymphocytic leukemia and, 874
characterization of, 795-798
immune deficiencies and, 978
immunoglobulin D and, 954
lymphokines and, 809
lymphopoiesis and, 801
migration of, 804
nonspecific esterase and, 918
plasma cells and, 808, 812-814
regulation of, 372
transformation of, 808
viral immunity and, 714
Babesiosis, 596-601, *597*

canine, 599
equine, 598, 601
feline, 601
Baboon(s)
blood collection and, 28
hematologic values of, 333t
Bacillary hemoglobinuria in sheep and cattle, 617-618, 618t
Bacillary spore(s), 17
Bacterial endotoxin, 831-836
Bacterial permeability increasing protein, 712
Bacterial pyrogen(s), 688
Bacterial septicemia or toxemia, 836
Bactericidal property
eosinophil and, 743
platelet as, 459
Bacteriostatic system in milk, 710
Bacterium(a)
endotoxins of, 831-836
hemolytic anemia and, 616-618
leukocytes and, 196, 826-827, 831-836
monocytes and, 780
neutrophils and, 719
oxygen metabolites and, 780
phagocytosis and, 707, 709
septicemia or toxemia and, 836
spleen and, 378
susceptibility to, 701
thrombocytopenia and, 473, 475
vascular response to, 712-714
Bacterium monocytogenes, 281
Bak^a antigen, 1005
Balance, water, 87-102. *See also* Blood volume(s)
Band 3 protein, 532
Band neutrophil(s), 13, 677
cat, 133, 135, *135*
cattle, 195
dog, 113
goat, 231
horse, 158
pig, *251*, 252
sheep, 218
Barbary sheep, 329, 333t. *See also* Sheep
Barbiturate(s)
albumin and, 947
horse and, 142
Barking deer, 321
Barr body(ies), 676
chromatin and, 115, *116*
Basenji
blood values and, 103, 105t, 109
pyruvate kinase deficiency in, 645
Basichromatin, 16
Basket cell(s), 7, 15
Basopenia, 765
Basophil(s), 7, 13, 756-767, 758t, *759*, 761t, *764*
avian, 263
biochemical composition of, 760
biologic properties of, 760-762
cat, 133-134
cattle, 195
dog, 119
functions of, 762-764
goat, 231, 238
guinea pig, 287
horse, 159
mink, 316t, 317
monkey, 314
morphology of, 757-760
mouse, 307
muskrat, 316t, 319
numbers of, 764-765
pig, 249, *251*, 252
production and distribution of, 756-757

Basophil(s) *(Continued)*
  rabbit, 281-282
  raccoon, 316t, 318
  rat, 296, 297
  sheep, 218, *219*, 220
  toxemic diseases and, 826
  water buffalo, 328
Basophilia, 765, 826, 829
  neutrophils and, 715
Basophilic leukemia, 839
  canine, 880-882, *881*, *883*
  feline, 865-867, *865*, *866*
Basophilic rubricyte(s), 12, 490, 658, V, VI
Basophilic stippling, 63, 578
  cat, 131
  cattle, 194
  dog, 629
  gerbil, 308
Basset hound(s)
  hereditary thrombopathia in, 468
  hospitalization and, 113
B-complex vitamin(s), 1017
Beagle(s), 103, 106t, 107, 109
Bear(s), 335t, 342
Bedlington terrier(s), 628
Bence Jones protein(s), 967
Bengal tiger(s), 334t
Benign monoclonal gammopathy, 971
  hyperviscosity syndrome and, 970
Bernard-Soulier syndrome, 453
Beta-adrenergic agent(s), degranulation and, 703
Beta-globulin(s), 941t, 962-964
  equine infectious anemia and, 618
  equine multiple myeloma and, 893, *896*
  foal serum protein and, 149
Beta-glucosaminidase, 912t
Beta-glucuronidase, 911t, 912t, 923
Beta-hexosaminidase, 912t, 923
Beta-lysin, 459
Beta₂-microglobulin, 954
BFU-E. *See* Burst forming unit erythroid
Biconcavity(ies), 528, *529*, 550
Bicytopenia(s), 665
Bilayer couple hypothesis, 544
Bilayer couple transformation(s), 544
Bile
  hemolytic anemia and, 571
  liver and, 380-381
Bile duct obstruction(s), 40
Bile pigment(s), 380, 522. *See also* Bilirubin
Bilirubin, 380
  anemia and, 571
  cattle serum, 188
  donkey serum, 339
  formation and excretion of, 522-525
  hemolytic disease of newborn and, 971
  horse, 159, 160
  liver and, 380
  metabolism of, 520-525
Bilirubinuria, 380
Biopsy(ies), bone marrow, 18-19
  needle for, 67
Bird(s). *See* Avian hematology
Bison, 329
Biuret method
  plasma protein concentration and, 57t
  for total proteins, 955
Black bear(s), 335t, 342
Black fly(ies), 269
Black Pied Danish cattle, lethal trait A-46 in, 979
Blackbuck(s), 329, 333t
Black-tailed deer, 321-322, 323t, 324-325t
Black-tongue syndrome, 659
Blast cell(s), 799-800, 810
  canine, 880

cat, *856*
  crisis and, 842, 915
  smoldering or aleukemic leukemia and, 867
Blast crisis, 842
  alkaline phosphatase and, 915
Blastogenesis. *See* Blast cell(s)
Blastogenic factor, 810
Bleeding, 96-99. *See also* Bleeding disorder(s)
  anemia and. *See* Blood loss anemia(s)
  autoimmune thrombocytopenic purpura and, 1019-1020
  blood volume and, 87
  chronic, 581-586
  dog, 1109-1112, 1125-1127
  fibrinolysis and, 402
  goat, 229, 230t, 235, *237*
  hemophilia A and, 404
  horse, 142-144, 145t
  liver disease and, 409
  thrombocytopenia and, 475-476
  thrombocytosis and, 469-470
Bleeding disorder(s)
  diagnosis of, 394t, 419-425
  disseminated intravascular coagulation and. *See* Disseminated intravascular coagulation
  Glanzmann's thrombasthenia as, 453, 468
  hereditary, 402-410
  megakaryocytes and, 433
  platelets and, 467
  poodle macrocytosis and, 662
  thrombocythemia as, 471-472
  thrombosis and, 415-419
  von Willebrand's disease as, 402-403, 403t, 405-406, 406t, 468-469
Bleeding time test(s), 420
Bleomycin, 899, 900
Blood. *See also* Blood cell(s); Blood picture(s) in diseases of domestic animals
  cat. *See* Feline blood
  cattle. *See* Bovine blood
  collection of, 1-2, 23-29. *See also* Blood sample(s); Collection of blood
  cross-matching of, 71-72, 951
  cytochemical reactions of. *See* Cytochemistry
  differential characteristics in domestic animals of, 5-7, 8t
  dog. *See* Canine blood
  examination of, 1-19. *See also* Blood sample(s)
  films stained for enzymes in, 913. *See also* Blood film(s)
  flow of, through microcirculation, 550
  handling of, 2, 28-29
  hematopoiesis and. *See* Hematopoietic system
  hemogram development and, 2-5
  leukocyte morphology of old, 5
  loss of. *See* Bleeding; Bleeding disorder(s); Hemorrhage
  microfilariae and, 79-82, 80t
  myeloproliferative disorders of cat and, 855t
  normal values and, 7-11, 8t, 9t, 10t. *See also* Blood value(s); specific species
  physiological considerations in interpretation of, 7
  separation of cells and plasma of, 28
  species variation and, 5-7
  spleen and circulation of, 375
  transfusion of. *See* Transfusion(s)
  wet-film method and, 59, *60*. *See also* Blood film(s)
Blood cell(s), XI, XII, XIII. *See also* Blood cell count(s); Blood picture(s) in diseases of domestic animals; specific species
  bird, 258-259, XXV
  canine, I, II, XII, XIII.
  cattle, 194-197.
  equine, XII.

feline, XII, XV.
goat, 232-238
in marrow aspirates, 12-15
mechanical trauma and, 6
pig, 250-252. *See also* Pig(s)
red. *See* Erythrocyte(s)
separation of plasma and, 28
sheep, 218-222
wet-film method and, 59, *60. See also* Blood film(s)
white. *See* Leukocyte(s)
Blood cell count(s), 2, 3, 45-48
DNA viscosity test and, 67-69, *68,* 69t
eosinophil leukocyte, 64-65
error in, 48, 51-52
hemocytometer method in, 45-48
nucleated erythrocytes in, 47
platelets and, 65-66
prenatal and early postnatal hematopoiesis and, 352
reticulocyte, 3, 62-63, 501, 567-568, 567t
sequence of, 28-29
units of measurement of, 2-3
Unopette method of, 48-49, *49*
Blood coagulation. *See* Coagulation
Blood component therapy, 414-415. *See also*
    Transfusion(s)
Blood dyscrasia(s). *See* Bleeding disorder(s)
Blood film(s), 2, 29-31. *See also* Stain(s)
cytochemistry and, 925, 926
examination of, 4t
methods of preparation of, 29-31
microfilariae and, 80
microscopy of, 35-36
new methylene blue stain and, 59-62, *61, 62,* 79, 80,
    81
Romanowsky stain and, 31-35
Wright-stained, 4t, 5
Blood granulocyte pool, total, 689
Blood group(s), 991-993, 992t
as markers for inheritance, 993
Blood loss. *See* Bleeding; Bleeding disorder(s);
    Hemorrhage
Blood loss anemia(s), 564, 577-581, 577t, 579t, 584-586
cat, 129
erythrocyte survival time and, 548
horse, 158, 1150-1152
water buffalo, 328-329
Blood morphology, species variation and, 5-7, 8t. *See
    also* Blood cell(s); Blood picture(s) in diseases of
    domestic animals; specific cell type
Blood parasite(s), 584-586, XIV, XVIII
anaplasmosis in, 590-596, 591t, 592t, *593, 594,*
avian, 268-270, XXV
babesiosis in, 596-501, *597*
blood film and, 60
blood loss anemia and, 584-586
cytauxzoonosis in, 615-616
depression anemia and, 671
eosinophil and, 743-746, *745,* 748-749
eperythrozoonosis in, 608-610, *608*
haemobartonellosis in, 602-608, *603,* 604t, *607*
immunoglobulin E and, 954
iron deficiency anemia and, 581
leukocyte response and, 827
neutrophils and, 714
plasma proteins and, 973
sarcocystosis in, 616
sheep hemoglobin and, 212, 671
spleen and, 378
theileriasis in, 610-612
thrombocytopenia and, 481
trypanosomiasis in, 612-615, *613*
Blood picture(s) in diseases of domestic animals, 1040-
    1086
acute bovine mastitis in, 1076-1078
Addison's disease in dog and, 1059-1063
canine Cushing's syndrome in, 1054-1059
canine distemper in, 1046-1048
canine ehrlichiosis in, 1066-1068
canine infectious hepatitis in, 1049-1051
canine leptospirosis in, 1043-1046
chronic renal failure in dog and, 1040-1043
equine ehrlichiosis in, 1066-1068
experimental coliform mastitis in, 1078-1081
feline infectious peritonitis in, 1068-1071, 1071t
feline panleukopenia in, 1071-1074
hyperadrenocorticism in, 1054-1059
hypoadrenocorticism in, 1059-1063
hypothyroidism in dog and, 1063-1066
inflammatory diseases in cattle in, 1074-1076
pyometra in dog and, 1051-1054
Blood restoration. *See* Transfusion(s)
Blood sample(s), 24-28
avian, 259-260
cat, 126
chinchilla, 319
elephant, 338
ferret, 315-317
guinea pig, 282
hamster, 308
handling of, 2
mink, 315-317
monkey, 311
mouse, 298
rabbit, 276
raccoon, 318
rat, 288-289
Blood smear(s). *See* Blood film(s)
Blood transfusion(s). *See* Transfusion(s)
Blood typing, 993
Blood value(s), 7-11, 8t, 9t, 10t. *See also* specific species
bird, 257, 257t, 261-263
cat, 10t, 127
dog, 10t, 104t
fetal. *See* Fetal blood value(s)
foal, 146-147, 147t
goat, 226
horse, 9t, 10t, 11, 146-147, 147t, 148t, 149, 150t
laboratory animal, 275
Long-Evans rat, 290t, 291t, 292t
pig, 240
seasonal. *See* Seasonal variation(s) in blood values
sex differences in. *See* Sex difference(s) in blood
    values
sheep, 10t, 208-218, 210t, 211t, 213t
Sprague-Dawley rat, 293t, 294t, 295t
Blood volume(s), 87-102
determination of, 87-93, 88t-91t, 94
foal, 146-147
goat, 89t, 94
neonate, 94-95
pathology and, 95-96
pig, 244-245
pregnancy and, 95
shock and, 97
Blue azo dye(s), 92
Blue stippling, cat reticulocyte and, 129, 131
Bluetongue virus, 830
Bobcat(s), 335t
Body mass, lean, 87
Body surface area(s), 87
Body fluid(s). *See also* Blood volume(s)
relative polycythemia and, 575
stain for, 62
Body weight, blood volume and, 87
BoLA. *See* Bovine lymphocyte antigen
Bolivian field mouse(mice), 310-311
Bone(s)
congenital porphyria and, 647
long, venous vasculature of, *361*

Bone marrow, 11-19, XI
  acute blood loss and, 580-581
  alkaline phosphatase and, 914
  anemia and, 566, 570-571
  antiplatelet antibody and, 77
  aspiration of, 18-19, 66-67
  basophils and, 764
  biopsy of, 18-19
  bird, 263
  cat. *See* Bone marrow, cat
  cattle, 197, 198t, 199t
  cell transit and, 362-364
  characteristics of, 12-15
  chinchilla, 319
  classification of cells in, 12-15
  cytology of, 15-17, X
  dog. *See* Bone marrow, dog
  dry tap and, 19
  eosinophils and, 240, 739, 742
  examination of, 11-18
  films stained for enzymes in, 913
  general comments about cytology of, 15-17
  goat, 238
  guinea pig, 288
  hamster, 310, 311t
  hematopoiesis and, 118, 350, 352, *353*, 359, 361-362
  horse, 161-163, 162t, 164t, 571, 892, V, VI, XII
  iron and, 12, 582, 583
  lymphocytes and, 16, 800-801, 806
  megakaryocytes and, 437
  monkey, 314-315
  monocytes and, 769-770
  mouse, 307
  myeloid:erythroid ratio and. *See* Myeloid:erythroid
      ratio
  neutrophil release and, 695-696
  neutrophil reserve of, 687-689, 692
  new methylene blue stain and, 62
  pig, 244, 250
  rabbit, 282, 283t
  rat, 298, 299t
  sheep, 222
  tally sheet for, 17, *18*
  transplantation of, 118, 1003, 1006-1007
  trypanosomiasis and, 614
  venous vasculature of, *361*
Bone marrow, cat, 137-138, 137t, XV
  erythremic myelosis and, 857
  erythroleukemia and, 859, *859*
  erythroleukemia changing to granulocytic leukemia
      and, 858t
  erythropoiesis in, IV, V
  granulocytopoiesis in, V
  hematopoiesis and, 352
  lymphoid malignancies and, 851-852, *851*
  myelomonocytic leukemia and, 861-863
  myeloproliferative disorders and, 855t
Bone marrow, dog, 121t, 122t, 123, XI, XII, XIII
  aspiration of, 66-67
  differential cell count and, 121t, 122t
  erythropoiesis in, IV, V
  granulocytic leukemia and, 879-880, *879*
  granulocytopoiesis in, V
  hematopoiesis and, *353*
  mast cell leukemia and, 881, *882*
  megakaryocytopoiesis in, III
  myeloid:erythroid ratio of, 18t
  poodle macrocytosis and, 661-662, *661*, 663t
Bone marrow pool, 692
Bone marrow reserve of neutrophils, 687-689
Bone marrow transplantation(s), 1006-1007
  cyclic hematopoiesis and, 118
  histocompatibility antigens and, 1003
Boophilus, 595, 596

Bordetella pertussis, 811
Borrelia anserina, 270
Bos indicus, 329, 333t
Bovidae, 329-336
Bovine blood. *See* Cattle
Bovine congenital porphyria, 548. *See also* Cattle
Bovine leukemia complex, 884-890
Bovine leukemia virus, 884-886
Bovine lymphocyte antigen, 1002
Bovine mastitis. *See* Mastitis, bovine
Bovine plumbism, 631
Bovine viral diarrhea, 830
  hematopoiesis and, 355-356, 356t, 357t
  immune deficiency and, 981
  impaired bactericidal activity and, 719
Boxer(s), 107
Boyden chamber, 698
BPA. *See* Burst promoting activity
Bracken fern poisoning
  aplastic anemia and, 666
  thrombocytopenia and, 481, 482
Bradykinin, 712
  eosinophil and, 746
Brassica, 640
Braunvieh cattle, 193
Breed difference(s)
  blood values and, 7. *See also* specific animal
  cattle hemogram and, 191-193
  dog and, 107
  horse and, 11, 154-155
  pig and, 247
Brilliant cresyl blue, 62
Bronchial mucus inhibitor, 714
Bronchitis in horse, 1156-1157
Brown bear(s), 342
Brown lemming, 311
Brown Swiss cattle, 193
Brownian movement, 59
Brucella, 780
  phagocytosis and, 703, 709
Bubalis bubalis, 322-329, 326t, 327t
Budding, platelet and, 453
Buffalo, water, 322-329, 326t, 327t
  blood volume and, 89t, 94, 95
  postparturient hemoglobinuria and, 643
Buffer(s), phosphate, 32
Buffy coat, 3
  trypanosomiasis and, 613-614
  Wintrobe hematocrit and, 37-39
Bunostomum phlebotomum, 973
Burkitt's lymphoma, canine, 876
Burr cell(s), 570
Burro, blood volume and, 90t, 94
Bursa of Fabricius, 264, 798
  chicken and, 373
  hematopoiesis and, 372
Burst forming unit erythroid, 368
Burst promoting activity, 368
  source of, 372
Bush baby(ies), 27-28
Busulphan, 898, 900

¹⁴C. *See* Carbon 14
C₁ inactivator(s), 398
C3, 73, 74
  inherited deficiency of, 979
  macrophages or monocytes and, 776, 780
C5a, degranulation and, 703, 706
Cabot's ring(s), 6
Cadmium, 664
CAE. *See* Chloroacetate esterase
Calcium

degranulation and, 703
  lymphoma and, 852, 871
  serum albumin and, 947
Calcium EDTA, 630. *See also*
      Ethylenediaminetetraacetate
Calf(ves). *See also* Cattle
  acute blood loss and, 578, 579t, 580
  anemia and, 181
  babesiosis and, 597
  leptospirosis in, 616
  maternal postparturient hemoglobinuria and, 642-643
  neutrophil reserve and, 688-689
  thrombocytopenia and, 483
California mastitis test(s), 68-69
Calomys callosus, 310-311
Calomys ducilla, 310-311
Camel(s), 331t, 333t, 336-337
  erythrocytes and, 275, 528
cAMP. *See* Cyclic adenosine monophosphate
Cancer(s). *See also* Carcinoma(s); Malignancy(ies);
      Neoplasia(s)
  lymphocyte recirculation and, 806, 807
  viral etiology of, 264
Candida albicans
  myeloperoxidase deficiency and, 711
  phagocytosis and, 718
Canidae, 337
Canine anemia. *See* Anemia(s), dog
Canine babesiosis, 599-601
Canine blood. *See* Dog(s)
Canine bone marrow. *See* Bone marrow, dog
Canine coronavirus, 830
Canine Cushing's syndrome, 1054-1059
  biochemical evaluation and, 1055t
  case report of, 1097, 1098, 1099
  hemograms and, 1057t
Canine cyclic hematopoiesis, 117-118
Canine distemper, 830, 1046-1048
  case report of, 1130
  hemograms in, 1047t
  immune deficiency and, 981
  inclusion body and, 1048
Canine ehrlichiosis, 1066-1068, XIV
Canine granulocytopathy syndrome, 719
Canine hyperadrenocorticism. *See* Canine Cushing's
      syndrome
Canine infectious hepatitis, 830, 1049-1051
  natural infections and, 1050t
Canine leishmaniasis, 1068
Canine leptospirosis, 616, 1043-1046
  clinical pathology of, 1045t
Canine leukemia complex, 869-884
  acute lymphocytic leukemia in, 874-876
  age and, 870
  basophilic leukemia in, 881-882, *881, 883*
  blood profile in lymphoma in, 870-871, 871t, 872t,
      873t
  breed predilection and, 870
  Burkitt's lymphoma in, 876
  clinical findings of, 869-870
  erythremic myelosis in, 882
  erythroleukemia in, 882
  granulocytic leukemia in, 690, 876-880, 877t, XXIII
  histopathology of, 873-874
  Hodgkin's disease in, 876
  immunology of, 873-874
  lymphocytic leukemia in, 874-876, 899, XXI
  lymphoproliferative disorders in, 869-876
  lymphosarcoma in, 480, *966, 969, 970*
  mast cell leukemia in, 880-882, *881, 883*
  megakaryocytic leukemia in, 880-881
  monocytic leukemia in, 880
  myelogenous leukemia in, 876-880, 877t, 915
  myelomonocytic leukemia in, 880

  myeloproliferative disorders in, 876-884
  pathogenesis of, 869
  plasma cell dyscrasia in, *966*, 968-969
  radiation-induced hematopoietic neoplasias in, 882-
      884
  sex and, 870
  viral etiology of, 869
Canine lymphosarcoma, 869-876, *966, 969, 970*
  thrombocytopenia and, 480
Canine mucopolysaccharidosis, XIII
Canine pancytopenia, tropical
  plasma proteins and, 976
  thrombocytopenia and, 480-481
Canine parvovirus, 830
Canine systemic lupus erythematosus, 1027-1029
Canis latrans, 337
Canis lupus, 335t, 337
Canvasback duck(s), lead poisoning and, 271
Capillary blood, 550
  babesiosis and, 598
  birds and, 260
Capillary endothelium, platelets and, 458
Capillary tube(s), plasma fibrinogen and, 58-59, *59*
Capsulated bacterium(a), phagocytosis and, 707
Capuchin, 334t
Caracal, 335t
Carbohydrate(s), erythrocyte membrane and, 531
Carbon 14 (^{14}C), 547-548
  camel erythrocyte and, 337
  horse, 155
  mouse erythrocyte and, 306
  pig, 247
Carcinoma(s). *See also* Cancer(s); Malignancy(ies);
      Neoplasia(s)
  dog, 1104-1105, 1117-1118
  of liver, 974
Caribou, 330t, 337
Carrier(s)
  anaplasmosis and, 595
  theileriasis and, 611
Castor bean(s), 640
Cat(s), 126-139
  acute blood loss and, 578
  autoimmune hemolytic anemia and, 649t, 650, 1146-
      1148
  babesiosis and, 601
  bacterial toxemia and septicemia and, 836
  basophilia and, 748t
  blood of, 8t, 127, XII, XV
  blood volume of, 88t, 94
  bone marrow of. *See* Bone marrow, cat
  collection of blood of, 25t, 26
  cytauxzoonosis and, 615-616
  defective microtubule assembly and, 717
  dehydration and, 1135-1137
  differential leukocyte number and, 9t
  elliptocyte and, 541
  endotoxemia and, 832, 832t
  eosinophilic granule and, 731, *734, 737*
  eosinophils and, 133, *340*, 748t
  erythremic myelosis and, 856-857, *857*
  erythrocytes and, 127-132, 528
  granulocytic leukemia in, XXII
  haemobartonellosis in, 554-555, 602-606, *603*, 604t
  Heinz bodies and, 130-131, 634-640, *635, 636, 639*,
      XVI
  hemoglobin and, 127, 128, 130-131, 518t
  infectious anemia of, 602, 1148-1150, 1151
  infectious peritonitis of. *See* Feline infectious
      peritonitis
  lead poisoning and, 632
  leukemia complex in, 844-869. *See also* Feline
      leukemia complex

Cat(s) *(Continued)*
 leukocyte count and, 9t, 10t, 11, 130t, 132-136, 823,
  VII, IX, XIV
 leukocytes of, 130t, 132-136, 823, VII, IX, XIV
 liver impression film and, *354*
 lymphocyte antigens of, 1002-1003
 marrow aspiration and, 67, *67*
 mucopolysaccharidosis in, 716
 myeloid:erythroid ratio of, 18t
 normal blood values of, 10t, 127
 oncornavirus cell membrane antigen and, 846
 panleukopenia and, 1071-1074, 1073t, 1074t
 platelets and, 136, 447, *449*, 469t
 plumbism and, 632
 postnatal blood changes in, 128t
 prenatal hematopoiesis and, 351-352
 reticulocytes and, 128-130, 500, 567, IV
 systemic lupus erythematosus and, 1029
 thrombocytopenia and, 473t, 476, 481
 thrombocytosis and, 470t
 Wintrobe hematocrit tube and abnormalities in blood
  of, I
Catabolism, 942
 hemoglobin and, 520-521, *521*
 mononuclear phagocyte system and, 522-523
Catalase
 macrophages and, 780
 microperoxisomes and, 683, 776
 monocytes and, 775
 phagocytes and, 710, 711
Catecholamine(s), 750
Cathepsin(s), 712, 713
Cationic protein(s)
 eosinophils and, 738
 inflammatory response and, 713
 microbicidal mechanisms of, 711
Cattle, 178-207
 acute blood loss and, 578, 579t, 580
 age and, 177-188, 181t, 182t, *187*, 187t
 altitude and, 193-194
 anaphylaxis and, 835t, 836
 anaplasmosis of, 590-596, 591t, 592t, *593*, *594*
 anemia and, 191, 194, 585, 586, 671
 babesiosis and, 596, 599
 bacillary hemoglobinuria in, 617-618, 618t
 Black Pied Danish, lethal trait A-46 in, 979
 blood of, 179, 180t
 blood collection in, 25t
 blood loss anemia and, 586
 blood volume in, 88t-89t, 94, 95
 bone marrow and, 197, 198t, 199t
 breed of, 191-193
 chemotaxis impairment and, 718
 coliform enteritis in, 202
 copper deficiency and, 662, 664-665
 corticosteroids and, 198-201
 dehydration and, 189, 1164-1165
 2,3-diphosphoglycerate and, 547
 double-muscling trait and, 185
 endotoxemia and, 201-204, 831-832, 832t
 environmental temperature and, 189-190
 eosinophils and, 186, 195, *744*
 eperythrozoonosis in, 608-610, *608*
 erythrocytes and, 179-181, 191-194, 528, 545, 546, 552
 erythropoiesis disorder and, 502
 haemobartonellosis in, 606-608
 Heinz bodies and, 634, 641
 hematocrit and, 188
 hemoglobin and, 190, 190t, 518t
 hemoglobinuria and, 185, 189, 617-618, 618t
 hypoproteinemia and, 585
 icterus index and, 188-189
 immunoglobulin G and, 955
 inflammatory disease and. *See* Cattle inflammatory
  disease(s)

 kale and, 634
 lactation and, 191
 lead poisoning and, 631
 leukemia complex in, 884-890
 leukocyte count in, 9t, 10t, 11, 823
 leukocytes and. *See* Leukocyte(s), cattle
 lymphocyte antigen and, 1002
 lymphocytes of, 186-187, 191, 192t, *193*, 196, 791-792,
  889t
 marrow aspiration and, 67
 mastitis of. *See* Mastitis, bovine
 molybdenosis and, 665, 665t
 mononuclear phagocyte system of, 770
 morphology of blood in, 8t, 194-197
 muscular activity and, 189
 myeloid:erythroid ratio and, 18t, 197
 neutrophils and. *See* Neutrophil(s), cattle
 nitrate poisoning and, 642
 normal blood values and, 10t
 parasitism and, 671
 parturition and, 191, 192t, *193*
 phagocytosis and, 707
 platelets of, 194, 447, *449*, 469t
 plumbism and, 631
 polycythemia and, 573-574
 porphyria and, 548, 646
 pregnancy and, 191
 prenatal hematopoiesis and, 352, 354-355
 psychologic factors and, 189
 reticulocytes and, 499-500
 sarcocytosis in, 616
 seasonal variation and, 189-190
 sex and, 191-193
 theileriasis and, 610, 611
 thrombocytopenia and disease in, 481, 483
 trichostrongyloidosis and, 585
 trypanosomiasis and, 612, 614
 virus diarrhea of. *See* Bovine viral diarrhea
 vitamin B_{12} deficiency and, 659
 water balance and, 189
Cattle inflammatory disease(s), 201, 1074-1076, 1075t
 bone marrow and, 197, 199t
 immature neutrophils and, 195
 mastitis and, 713, *713*
CBC. *See* Blood cell count(s); Complete blood count(s)
Cell(s). *See* specific cell type
Cell calculation(s). *See* Blood cell count(s)
Cell count(s). *See* Blood cell count(s)
Cell counter(s), electronic, 48-52, *49*. *See also* Coulter
  Counter(s)
Cell cycle time(s), 739
Cell differentiation, 369t
Cell line(s), 842, 853, *853*
Cell membrane(s). *See* Erythrocyte membrane(s)
Cell size(s), counting error and, 52
Cell transit
 bone marrow and, 362-364
 granulopoiesis and, 686-687, 687t
 neutrophil and, 433, *435*
Cell-mediated immunity, 790, 808-811
Cellulose acetate electrophoresis, 956
Central lymphoid organ(s), 798
Centrifugation
 goat blood and, 225-226, 229t
 trapped plasma and, 92-93
Cephalic vein(s), 25t, 26
Cercocebus sp., 334t
Ceruloplasmin, 714, 948, 949
 copper and, 664
 pig and, 244
Cervidae, 321-322, 323t, 324t-325t, 337
Cervus elaphus, 337
CFU-Eos. *See* Colony forming unit eosinophil(s)

CFU-GM. *See* Colony forming unit granulocyte-monocyte(s)
CFU-M. *See* Colony forming unit megakaryocyte(s)
CFU-S. *See* Colony forming unit in spleen
cGMP. *See* Cyclic guanosine monophosphate
CH. *See* Chédiak-Higashi syndrome
Chalone(s), 696-697
Charlais cattle, 193
Chédiak-Higashi syndrome
    Aleutian disease of mink and, 317, 318
    cattle, 197
    neutrophils and, 717, 719
    platelets and, 453, 454
Cheetah(s), 335t, 340
Chelation
    hyperviscosity syndrome and, 970
    lead poisoning and, 630
Chemical(s)
    aplastic anemia and, 666
    hemolytic anemia and, 627-632
    leukocyte response and, 827
Chemiluminescence, 705-706
Chemoattractant(s), phagocytosis and, 698, 699t
Chemokinesis, 698
Chemotactic deactivation, 718, 719
Chemotactic factor(s), 810. *See also* Chemotaxis
    inactivator(s) of, 718, 719
    neutrophil adherence and, 694-695
Chemotaxis, 741-742, 810
    defects of, 717-719
    energy source and, 684
    factors in, 699, 810
    monocytes and macrophages and, 776-777
    neutrophils and, 694-695, 698-701, 699t, 717-719, 761t
Chemotherapy. *See also* Cytotoxic drug(s); specific agent
    hyperviscosity syndrome and, 970
    leukemia complex and, 897-900
    toxicity of, 900
Chest fluid, lymphoproliferative disease and, 848, *849*
Chevrotain, 275
Chicken(s)
    bursa of Fabricius and, 373
    Leukocytozoon species and, 270
    normal blood values in, 257-258
    spirochetosis and, 270
    thymus and, 373
Chihuahua(s), 107
Chimpanzee(s), 334t
Chinchilla(s), 316t, 319
Chlamydia-like organism(s) in cat, 1143-1144
Chlorambucil, 898, 968
Chloramphenicol
    aplastic anemia and, 666
    bone marrow of cat and, 137-138
    phagocytosis and, 707, 719
Chloroacetate esterase, 910t, 911t, 915-919
    technique for, 929-930
Chlorpropmazine
    cattle hemogram and, 189
    thrombocytopenia in dog and, 478
Cholchicine, 700
Cholera, hog, 250, 829-830
    experimental, 249
Cholestasis, 160
Cholesterol
    acanthocytes and, 540, 544
    canine hypothyroidism and, 1064
    codocyte and, 540
    erythrocyte membrane and, 544
    erythrocyte osmotic fragility and, 552
    α-globulin and, 962
    membrane fluidity and, 545

phospholipid and. *See* Cholesterol-to-phospholipid ratio
Cholesterol-to-phospholipid ratio, 544
    acanthocyte and, 540
    anemia of liver disease and, 670
    erythrocyte and, 531-532
Chondroitin sulfate, 761t
Christmas disease, 402-403, 403t, 406
Chromatin
    nuclear. *See* Nuclear chromatin
    sex. *See* Sex chromatin
Chromium 51 (^{51}Cr). *See* Radiochromate
Chromosome, Philadelphia, 367
Chronic blood loss, 581-586. *See also* Blood loss anemia(s)
Chronic granulocytic leukemia, 690, 915
Chronic granulomatous disease, 710
Chronic interstitial nephritis, 669-670
    case report of, 1094, 1095
Chronic lead poisoning, 1127-1129
Chronic lymphocytic leukemia
    canine, 874-876
    chemotherapy and, 899
Chronic myelogenous leukemia, 690, 915
Chronic peritonitis, 1105-1106
CHS. *See* Chédiak-Higashi syndrome
Chylomicron(a), 950-951
    lipemic blood and, 60, *61*
    plasma compartment and, 40
    spectrophotometry and, 45
Chylothorax in dog, 640
Chymase, 761t
Chymotrypsin-like protease, 713
CID. *See* Combined immune deficiency
CIF. *See* Colony inhibitory factor(s)
CIN. *See* Chronic interstitial nephritis
Circulating erythrocyte volume, 140-144
Circulating inhibitor of coagulation, 1119
Circulating pool, neutrophil, 689
Circulating red cell mass, 94
Cirrhosis
    anemia of, 96
    plasma proteins and, 974
Citrate-phosphate-dextrose, 994
Classic hemophilia, 402-405, 403t, 406t
    case report of, 1118-1119
Cleaning of glassware, 22-23
CLL. *See* Chronic lymphocytic leukemia
Clostridium novyi, 617
Clot(s). *See also* Coagulation
    lysis of, 399-402
    platelet and retraction of, 456, 458
Clotting cascade(s), 419
Clotting factor(s). *See* Coagulation factor(s)
Clotting time(s), 420-421
Clumping, platelet, 120. *See also* Agglutination
Clydesdale horse(s), 156, 159
CMT. *See* California mastitis test(s)
Coagulation, 388-430
    biosynthesis and, 397-398
    bird, 257, 259
    cascade and, 419
    circulating inhibitor of, 1119
    diagnosis of disorder of, 394t, 419-425
    disorders of, 402-410. *See also* Bleeding disorder(s)
    disseminated intravascular. *See* Disseminated intravascular coagulation
    eosinophil and, 747
    factors of. *See* Factor(s), coagulation
    fibrinolysis and, 399-402, *339*, 401t
    platelets and, 391-392, 396-397, 456, 458
    primary hemostasis and, 389-391
    regulation of, 398-399
    schistocytes and, 542

Coagulation *(Continued)*
  systems interactions and, 395
  thrombosis and, 415-419
Coagulation factor(s)393-397, 396t
  III, 396
  V, 395, 397
  VII, deficiency of, 403t, 406-407
  VIII, 394-395
  VIII:C, 404
  VIII:RAg, 394, 404, 406, 468
  VIII:vWF, 404-405, 406
  X, 395, 403t, 407
  Xa, 395, 397
  XI, 403t, 407
  XII, 393-394, 407
  XIII, 425
  XIIIa, 396
  birds and, 259
  nomenclature for, 393
Coagulation factor VIII-coagulant, 394-395
Coagulation factor VIII-related antigen, 394, 404, 406, 468
Coagulation thrombus(i), 416
Coagulopathy(ies). *See also* Bleeding disorder(s)
  acquired, 407-410
  consumption. *See* Disseminated intravascular coagulation
  hereditary, 402-410, 403t
Cobalamin, 381. *See also* Vitamin B_{12}
Cobalt
  anemia and deficiency of, 665
  canine radiation-induced hematopoietic disorder and, 883, 884
  erythropoiesis and, 505-506, 509
  swine lymphoma and, 897
  vitamin B_{12} deficiency and, 659
Coccidioidomycosis, 586, *966*, 969
Codocyte(s), *535*, *537*, 540
  etymology of, 534t
Colchicine, 703
Cold, nitrogen loss and, 943
Cold agglutination, 648, 1010
Cold-blooded horse(s), 153t, 155. *See also* Horse(s)
Cold-reactive antibody(ies), 1008, 1009
Coliform enteritis in cattle, 202
Coliform mastitis in cattle, 202, 831. *See also* Mastitis, bovine
  experimental, 1078-1081
  leukogram and, 1080t
Colitis, ulcerative
  erythrogenesis and, 123
  excessive protein loss and, 972
Colitis X, 832
Collagen
  canine platelet and, 121
  coagulation and, 397
  hemostasis and, 389
Collagenase, 714
Collection of blood, 1-2, 23-29
  handling of specimen and, 2, 28-29
  microfilariae and, 79-82, 80t
  needle size for, 24-26, 25t
  site for, 24-26, 25t
  vacutainers for, 1, 2, 23, 26
Collie dog(s), 117-118
Colony forming unit in spleen, 366
Colony forming unit eosinophil(s), 739
Colony forming unit erythrocyte(s), 506
Colony forming unit granulocyte-monocyte(s), 368, 685, 769
Colony forming unit megakaryocyte(s), 368
  analogue and, 371-372
  megakaryocytopoiesis and, 431
Colony inhibitory factor(s), 696-697
Colony stimulating factor(s), 696-697, 770

  eosinophil, 740
  myeloid cell and, 370-371
  source of, 372
Colostrum
  antibodies and, 997
  cattle and, 187
  horse and, 146, 149, 980
  immunoglobulins and, 955, 980
  opsonic activity and, 707
  pig and, 241, 244
  protein and, 944
Columbiformes, 267
Combined immune deficiency, 978-979
  case report of, 1155-1156
Committed erythrocytic progenitor cell(s), 501-502. *See also* Colony forming unit erythrocyte(s)
Committed hematopoietic progenitor cell(s), 367-368
Committed lymphoid stem cell(s), 798
Committed progenitor cell(s), 367-368, 370-373, 501-502
Committee for Clarification of Nomenclature of Cells and Diseases of the Blood and Blood-Forming Organs, 12, 487
Committee on Nomenclature of DLA Determinants, 1001-1002
Compartment(s), distribution of fluid among, 97-98
Compartment transit time, 686-687, 687t
Compatibility, blood, 71-72, 951
Compensated hemolytic disorder(s), 589
Complement. *See also* C3
  chemotaxis and, 699
  Coombs antiglobin test and, 1011-1013
  deficiency of, 979
  degranulation and, 703, 706
  endotoxin and, 694
  eosinophils and, 741, 742, 751
  equine infectious anemia and, 619
  feline lymphoma and, 852
  phagocytosis and, 708
  platelet antigens and antibodies and, 1005
  receptors for, 776, 780
  systems interactions and, *395*
Complete blood count(s), 2. *See also* Blood cell count(s)
  sequence of, 28-29
  units of measurement of, 2-3
Compound 48/80, 712, 752
Con A. *See* Concanavalin
Concanavalin
  degranulation and, 703, 706
  T cells and, 798
Concavity, erythrocytes and, 528, *529*, 550
Condenser lens(es), 22
Congenital coagulation disorder(s), 402-410
Congenital erythroid hypoplasia of Diamond-Blackfan, 666
Congenital erythropoietic porphyria(s), 646-647
  case report of, 1165, 1167
Congenital iron deficiency anemia, 181, 581
Congenital porphyria(s), 646-647
  case report of, 1165, 1167
Congestive heart failure, 972
Conjugated bilirubin, 380, 523-524
Consumption coagulopathy. *See* Disseminated intravascular coagulation
Contact product, 76
Contact reaction, 394
Contractile protein(s), 455
Contraction(s) of spleen. *See* Splenic contraction(s)
Coombs test(s), 1008
  direct, 73-75, 74t, 1011-1013, *1013*
  false negative reactions in, 74
  indirect, 73-75, 1011
Coombs-negative autoimmune hemolytic anemia, 1008
Cooperia, 585
Copper

deficiency of, 244, 662, 664-665, 719
ceruloplasmin and, 949
erythropoiesis and, 509
hemolytic anemia and, 627-628
Copper:molybdenum ratio, 628
Coproporphyrin
heme synthesis and, 516
lead poisoning and, 629
Coronavirus, canine, 830
Corrected erythrocyte sedimentation rate, 54
Correction factor(s), blood volume and, 92, 93
Corticoid(s), ACTH administration and, 765t
Corticosteroid(s) or steroid(s)
antilymphocyte serum and, 1005
arachidonic acid metabolism and, 456
autoimmune hemolytic anemia and, 649t, 650, 1016, 1017
autoimmune thrombocytopenic purpura and, 1024
blood film and, *378*
canine Cushing's syndrome and, 1058-1059
canine erythrocyte and, 104
canine leukocyte and, 111, *111*, 112t
canine platelet and, 121
cat dehydration and, 1135-1137
cat leukocyte and, 134
cattle response to, 198-201
chemotaxis inhibition and, 719
with cytotoxic drugs, 900
direct Coombs test and, 1013
eosinophils and, 64, 750-751
erythropoiesis and, 370
α-globulin and, 962
hemolytic disease of newborn and, 998
horse and, 163-166, 165t
immune response and, 808
leukocytes and, 111, *111*, 112t, 825-826, 827
lymphocytes and, 119, 811-812
marrow reserve assessment and, 688
monocytes and, 119, 776, 777-778, 781
neutrophils and, 692-693, 716, 719
phagocytosis and, 708
pig and, 249
systemic lupus erythematosus and, 1029
water buffalo and, 329
Corticosterone, cattle response to, 198. *See also* Corticosteroid(s)
Cortisol. *See also* Corticosteroid(s)
cattle and, 186, 198
neutrophilia and, 692
Cortisone. *See also* Corticosteroid(s)
eosinophil count and, 64
α-globulin and, 962
Corynebacterium parvum, 697
Corynebacterium pseudotuberculosis
goat and, 232, 975
pony and, *173*
Coulter Channelyzer, 51
Coulter Counter(s), 48-52, *49*
cell count errors and, 51-52
diluent and, 51
lysing solution and, 51
platelets and, 65
model F, 50, 51
model F$_N$, 50, 51
model ZBI, *49*, 50, 51
threshold settings and, 50
Coumarin-type drug(s), thrombosis and, 418t
Counting chamber(s), 46-47
Coverslip(s)
care of, 22
method for smear making on, 29-30, *30*, *31*
Cow(s). *See* Cattle
Coyote(s), 337
CP. *See* Contact product

C-particle(s), 679
CPD. *See* Citrate-phosphate-dextrose
^{51}Cr or ^{59}Cr. *See* Radiochromate
C-reactive protein, 949-950
Crenation, 6, 59, *60*, 570
echinocyte and, 541
erythrocyte, 29
Critical hemolytic volume, 552
Crocuta crocuta, 335t, 341
Cross-matching, 71-72, 951
Crude oil, avian anemia and, 270-271
Cryohydrocyte, 534t
Cryoprecipitate infusion(s)
hemophilia A and, 404-405
von Willebrand's disease and, 406
Crystalloid granule(s), 737
CSF. *See* Colony stimulating factor(s)
CSF-Eos. *See* Eosinophil-colony stimulating factor
C-type oncornavirus
leukemia complex of cattle and, 884
ovine lymphoma and, 895-896
Culex, 268-269
Culicoides sp., 269
Cushing's syndrome, canine, 1054-1059
biochemical evaluation and, 1055t
case report of, 1097, 1098, 1099
hemograms and, 1057t
Cyanmethemoglobin, 3, 644
avian blood and, 261
spectrophotometry and, 44
Cyclic adenosine monophosphate
hemostasis and, 389
metabolism and, 706
neutrophils and, 692, 695
Cyclic guanosine monophosphate, 695
Cyclic hematopoiesis, 117-118
Cyclic parasitemia, 481. *See also* Blood parasite(s)
Cyclo-oxygenase activity, 456
17-β-Cyclopentylpropionate ester of α-estradiol, 477-478, 478t
Cyclophosphamide, 898, 899, 900
autoimmune hemolytic anemia and, 1016-1017, 1018
autoimmune thrombocytopenic purpura and, 1024
feline eosinophilic leukemia and, 865
hyperviscocity syndrome and, 971
plasma cell myeloma and, 968
systemic lupus erythematosus and, 1029
Waldenström's macroglobulinemia and, 968
Cyclosporin, 1007
Cytauxzoonosis, 615-616
Cytochalasin B, 700
Cytochemistry, 841t, 909-939, X
acid phosphatase in, 910-914, 910t, 912t, 926-927
alkaline phosphatase in, 914-915, 910t, 927-928
chloroacetate esterase in, 910t, 911t, 915-919, 929-930
classification of leukemia and, 923-924
comparative properties of species and, 910t
enzymes of purine metabolism in, 922
esterases in, 910t, 911t, 912t, 915-919, 928-930
leukemia classification by markers in, 923-924
methyl green-pyronin reaction in, 911t, 919, 930-931
α-naphthyl acetate esterase in, 910t, 911t, 912t, 915-919, 928
α-naphthyl butyrate esterase in, 910t, 911t, 912t, 915-919, 929
periodic acid-Schiff reaction in, 911t, 912t, 919-920, 931-932
peroxidase in, 910t, 911t, 920-921, 932-933
sudanophilia in, 910t, 911t, 921, 933-934
techniques in, 924-934, 925t
terminal deoxynucleotidyl transferase in, 912t, 921
Cytofibrinolysokinases, 399
Cytology, bone marrow, 11-19, 841t. *See also* Cytochemistry

Cytophotometric method(s), 926
Cytoplasm, 7
  asynchronous maturation of nucleus and, 16
  basophilia of, 16, 826
  foamy, 16, 715, 826
  lymphocytes and, 791, 792, *793*, *794*
  neutrophils and, 676, 715, 826
  plasma cell, 812
  prorubricyte, 492
  RNA in, pyronin and, 919
Cytoplasmic inclusion(s), blood film and, 62
Cytoplasmic organelle(s) in basophils, 760
Cytosar. *See* Cytosine arabinoside
Cytosine arabinoside, 898, 899, 900
  neutrophil abnormalities and, 716
Cytoskeletal protein(s), 532
Cytotaxigen, 698
Cytotaxin, 698
Cytotoxic drug(s), 900. *See also* Chemotherapy
  blood film and, *378*
Cytotoxicity
  lymphocyte and, 808
  macrophages and, 783-784
  neutrophil and, 714
Cytoxan. *See* Cyclophosphamide

Dachshund(s)
  hospitalization and, 113
  normal blood value range and, 107
Dacrocyte(s), *536*, *539*, 540
Dalmatian(s), 107
Dama dama, 337
Dama virginiana, 611
Danish cattle, lethal trait A-46 in, 979
DAP IV. *See* Dipeptidylaminopeptidase IV
Daunorubicin, 898, 899, 900
DCT. *See* Direct Coombs test
Deer, 321-322, 323t, 324-325t
  anaplasmosis and, 595
  erythrocytes and, 275, 321, *321*, *332*, 528
  fallow, 337
  hemoglobin and, 518t
  red, 337
  Theileria mutans and, 611
Deer mouse (mice), 310-311
Deformability
  erythrocytes and, 550-551
  intrinsic membrane, 551
Degenerated cell(s), 15
Degenerative left shift, 824, 828
  in perforation of rectum, 1158-1160
  in pyometra, 1102-1104
Degradation product(s)
  fibrin, 400, 424
  phagocytosis and, 702
Degranulation
  basophil, 763, *764*
  eosinophil, 738
  mast cell, 763
  phagocytosis and, 702-706
Dehydration, 7, 96
  cat, 1135-1137
  cattle, 189, 1164-1165
  dog, 1090, 1091
  plasma proteins and, 944
  relative polycythemia and, 575
  total proteins and, 957-960
Delayed hypersensitivity, 1005
Delta-aminolevulinic acid, 514
Delta-aminolevulinic acid dehydrase, 629
Delta-aminolevulinic acid dehydratase, 271
Demodectic mange, 800
Demodex canis, 981

Denaturation of hemoglobin, oxidative, 644
Dendritic platelet, 447, *447*
Deoxycorticosterone acetate, 1059
Deoxynucleotidyl transferase, terminal, 912t, 921
Deoxyribonucleic acid
  depressed synthesis of, 16
  granulopoiesis and, 686
  megakaryocytopoiesis and, 433
  prorubricytes and, 492, 495
  viscosity test and, 67-69, *68*, 69t
Deoxyribonucleic acid virus, 844
Deoxyribonucleoprotein, antibody to, 1026-1027
Depression anemia, 655-675
  aplastic anemia and, 665-668
  erythroid hypoplasia and, 668-671
  nutritional deficiency and, 655-665
Deprivation, water, 96
Derivative curve, osmotic fragility test and, 70
Dermacentor andersoni, 595
Dermacentor nitens, 601
Dermacentor occidentalis, 595
Dermatan sulfate, 761t
Dermatitis, horse, 1157-1158
Descicyte(s), 534t
Desiccytosis, 544
Deuterium oxide, 703
Dexamethasone
  autoimmune hemolytic anemia and, 1016
  cattle and, 199, 200, 200t, 201
  horse and, 163, 165t, 166
  neutrophilia and, 692
  pig and, 249
  water buffalo and, 329
Dextran
  exchange transfusions and, 994
  lymphocyte migration and, 806
DFP, chemotaxis and, 700
DF³²P. *See* Radioactive diisopropyl fluorophosphate
DHF. *See* Dihydrofolate
Diabetes mellitus in dog, 1096-1097
Diamidine, 598
Diamond-Blackfan congenital erythroid hypoplasia, 666
Diapedesis, 700
Diarrhea, bovine viral, 830
  hematopoiesis and, 355-356, 356t, 357t
  immune deficiency and, 981
  impaired bactericidal activity and, 719
Diathesis, hemorrhagic, 616
Dichromate cleaning solution(s), 22, 23
Dictyocaulus viviparus, 745
Dicumarol poisoning, 1111-1113
Diet(s). *See also* Nutritional deficiency(ies)
  autoimmune hemolytic anemia and, 1017
  iron and, 581, 582
  plasma proteins and, 943
Differential cell count(s), 5, 9t, 10t, 11, 35-36, 824. *See also* Blood cell count(s)
  avian, 262-263
  beagle and, 110t
  cattle and, 185-187, *187*, 187t
  dog and, 121t, 122t
  horse and, 147, 147t, 161-163, 162t, 164t
Diffuse intravascular thrombosis, 410. *See also* Disseminated intravascular coagulation
Dihydrofolate, 657-658, *658*
Diminazene aceturate, 598
Dipeptidylaminopeptidase IV, 923
Dipetalonema reconditum, 79-82, 80t
Diphasic erythrocyte sedimentation rate(s), 55
2,3-Diphosphoglycerate, 546-547
Diphosphopyridine nucleotide, 545-546
Dipyridamole, 418, 418t
  dog and, 121
  platelet release reaction and, 462

Direct blood film(s), microfilariae and, 80
Direct Coombs test, 73-75, 74t, 1011-1013, *1013*
Direct immunofluorescence, megakaryocyte and, 77
Direct matching, 43
Dirofilaria immitis, 79-80, 80t
  nitroblue tetrazolium reduction and, 115
  occult disease and, 82
  plasma proteins and, 973
Discocyte(s), 534t, 540, 544
Discocytic-echinocytic transformation(s), 544
Discocytic-stomatocytic transformation(s), 544
Disease(s)
  Addison's, 1059-1063, 1060t, 1061t, 1099-1100
  Aleutian, of mink, 317-318, 971
  Christmas, 402-403, 403t, 406
  Hodgkin's, 852, 876
  Hurler's, 716, 782
  Johne's. *See* Johne's disease
  Marek's, 264-266, 265t
  Newcastle, 215
  runt, 374
  von Willebrand, 402-403, 403t, 405-406, 406t, 468-469
Disseminated intravascular coagulation, 410-415, 411t, 412t
  case report of, 1116-1117
  hemolytic disease of newborn and, 998
  hemostatic tests for, 423-425
  schistocyte and, 542
  thrombocytopenia and, 480
  Trypanosoma congolense and, 483
Distemper, canine, 830, 1046-1048
  case report of, 1130
  hemograms in, 1047t
  immune deficiency and, 981
Distilled water, neutralization of, 32
D-L antibody. *See* Donath-Landsteiner antibody
DLA. *See* Dog lymphocyte antigen
DNA. *See* Deoxyribonucleic acid
DNR. *See* Daunorubicin
DOCA. *See* Deoxycorticosterone acetate
Dog(s), 103-125
  ACTH administration and, 765t
  acute blood loss and, 578
  Addison's disease in, 1059-1063, 1060t, 1061t, 1099-1100
  anemia and. *See* Anemia(s), dog
  autoimmune thrombocytopenia in, 1018-1025
  babesiosis and, 599-601
  bactericidal activity impairment and, 719
  basophilia and, 748t
  blood loss and, 97-99, 578
  blood volume of, 88t, 94, 95
  bone marrow of. *See* Bone marrow, dog
  carcinoma of, 1104-1105, 1117-1118
  chemotaxis impairment and, 718
  chylothorax in, 640
  collection of blood of, 25t, 26
  colony stimulating factor and, 697
  copper toxicosis and, 2628
  coronavirus and, 830
  Cushing's syndrome and, 1054-1059, 1055t, 1057t, 1097, 1098
  cyclic hematopoiesis in, 117-118
  cyclic neutropenia in, 701
  dehydration and, 1090, 1091
  dietary restriction of protein in, 943
  2,3-diphosphoglycerate and, 547
  disseminated intravascular coagulopathy and, 410-414, 411t
  distemper in. *See* Canine distemper
  Ehrlichia in, 599, 830, 1066-1068, XIII, XIV
  electrophoretic tracing of, 956, *965*, *966*
  elliptocytes and, 541
  eosinophilic granule and, 731-734, *732*, *733*, 737
  eosinophils and, 118-119, 748t
  erythremic myelosis and, 882
  erythrocyte membrane permeability and, 552
  erythrocyte osmotic fragility and, *109*, 553-554
  erythrocytes and, 103-109, 552, 553-554, 583, *583*, 1048
  erythropoietin production and, 505, 505t
  factor VII deficiency and, 403t, 406-407
  fibrinogen in, 122-123, 961t, 1093-1094
  folate deficiency in, 657
  granulocytic leukemia in, 690, 876-880, 877t, XXIII
  granulocytopathy syndrome of, 719
  haemobartonellosis in, 606, *607*, 607t
  Heinz bodies and, 640
  hemoglobin and, 104-108, 518t
  hemolytic disease of newborn and, 650
  hereditary thrombopathia in, 468
  hypoadrenocorticism in, 1059-1063, 1060t, 1061t, 1099-1100
  hypothyroidism and, 1063-1066, 1065t, 1094-1096
  idiopathic anemia in, 470t
  immunoglobulin A myeloma in, XIII
  infectious hepatitis and, 830, 1049-1051, 1050t
  kidney and, 669-670, 1040-1043, 1041t, 1094, 1095
  leishmaniasis and, 1068
  leptospirosis in, 616, 1043-1046, 1045t
  leukemia complex in. *See* Canine leukemia complex
  leukocyte count and, 9t, 10t, 11, 110t, 823
  leukocytes and, 109-119, 110t, 823, 1048, VII, XIV
  lupus erythematosus and, 1027-1029
  macrophages in, VIII
  marrow aspiration and, 66-67
  microfilariae in, 79-82, 80t
  monocytes and, 119, 771, *773*, VIII
  mucopolysaccharidosis and, XIII
  myeloid:erythroid ratio of, 18t
  neutrophils and. *See* Neutrophil(s), dog
  nicotinic acid-deficient diet in, 659
  normal blood values and, 10t, 104t
  pancytopenia and, 480-481, 976
  parvovirus and, 830
  physiologic and emotional leukocytosis in, 111-113, 113t, 114t
  plasma of, 11, 122-123
  platelets of, 119-122, *120*, 447, *449*, 469t
  polycythemia and, 573
  prenatal hematopoiesis and, 350-351
  pyometra and. *See* Pyometra, canine
  pyruvate kinase deficiency and, 645-646, 646t
  renal failure and, 1040-1043, 1041t
  reticulocytes and, 108, 500, 567t, 568
  reticulocytosis and, 568
  riboflavin deficiency in, 660
  spheroechinocytes and, 104
  stomatocytic erythrocyte and, 104
  thrombocytopenia and, 473t, 474t, *475*, 476-478, 480-481
  thrombocytosis and, 470-471, 470t, *471*
  toxic neutrophils in, 115, VIII
  venous hematocrit and, 93-94
  vitamin K antagonism and, 408
  von Willebrand's disease and, 402
  Waldenström's macroglobulinemia and, 968-969
  Wintrobe hematocrit and, I, II
Dog lymphocyte antigen, 1001-1002
Döhle body, 16, 826
  cat leukocyte and, 135
  neutrophils and, 715, *716*
Domestic animal(s). *See also* specific animal
  blood morphology of, 8t, 1040-1086. *See also* Blood picture(s) in disease of domestic animals
  erythrocytes and, 11
  leukocytes and, 9t, 10t, 11
  normal blood values of, 10t

Donath-Landsteiner antibody, 1015-1016
Donkey(s), 339-340
   babesiosis and, 601
   hematologic values of, 332t
Donor and recipient blood compatibility, 71-72, 951
Donor animal(s), 994
Double nucleus, 115
Double-muscling trait in cattle, 185
Doughnut-shaped nucleus, 115
Dourine, 612
Dove(s), 267, 270
DOX. *See* Doxorubicin
Doxorubicin, 898, 899, 900
DPG. *See* 2,3-Diphosphoglycerate
DPNH. *See* Diphosphopyridine nucleotide
Drabkin's solution, 44
Draught horse, 159. *See also* Horse(s)
Drepanocyte(s), *538, 540*
   etymology of, 534t
Drug(s), 900. *See also* specific agent
   aplastic anemia and, 666
   antimalarial, 269
   hemolytic anemia and, 627-632, 1016
   leukocytes and, 827
   thrombocytopenia and, 478-479, 1023-1024, 1113-1114
Drummond microcapillary hematocrit, 37
   microfilariae and, 80-81, *81*
Drumstick
   cat neutrophil and, 133
   chromatin and, 115, *116*
Duckling(s), 269
Duodenal iron absorption, 582
Duroc-Jersey pig, 242, 246t
DUZO antigens, 1005, 1006
Dye(s), azure, 31
Dysfibrinogenemia, 403t, 407
Dysproteinemia(s), 957-976
   albumin changes in, 960
   coagulopathy and, 410
   fibrinogen changes in, 960-962, 961t, 962t, 963t
   gammapathies in, 964-971
   gastrointestinal disorders and, 971-973
   germfree animals and, 976
   α- and β-globulin changes in, 962-964
   γ-globulin changes in, 964
   infection and, 975
   kidney disease and, 974
   liver disease and, 973-974
   nephrosis and, 974-975
   parasitism and, 973
   platelet disorder and, 467-468
   rickettsial disease and, 975-976
   viral disease and, 975-976

EACA. *See* Epsilon aminocaproic acid
East Coast fever, 483, 610
EBL. *See* Enzootic bovine leukosis
Eccentrocyte(s), 540-541
   entymology of, 534t
Eccymosis(es), thrombocytopenic purpura and, 1019.
      See also Thrombocytopenia; Thrombocytopenic
      purpura
ECF-A. *See* Eosinophil chemotactic factor of
      anaphylaxis
Echidnophaga gallinacea, 584
Echinocyte(s), *536, 538,* 541
   entymology of, 534t
ECM. *See* Extracellular material(s)
Ecotaxis lymphocyte, 806
ECP. *See* 17-β-Cyclopentylpropionate ester of α-
      estradiol; Eosinophilic cationic protein
EDTA. *See* Ethylenediaminetetraacetate
Efflux, neutrophil, 690

Effusion fluid(s), equine, 892
Eggshell(s), oxygen transport and, 258
Ehrlichia canis, 830, 1066-1068, XIII, XIV
   babesiosis and, 599
Ehrlichia equi, 1067, XIV. *See also* Ehrlichiosis
Ehrlichiosis
   canine, 480-481, 830, 976, 1066-1068, XIII, XIV
   equine, 481, *482,* 830, 1066-1068, XIV
EIA. *See* Equine infectious anemia
ELA. *See* Equine lymphocyte antigen
Elastase, 714
Electroimmunodiffusion, 957
Electron microscope
   anaplasmosis and, 593, *594*
   canine haemobartonellosis and, 606
   erythrocyte and, 491-495, *491, 492, 493, 494*
   haemobartonellosis and, 602, 606
   platelets and, 446-450, *447, 449*
Electronic cell counter(s), 48-52, *49. See also* Coulter
      Counter(s)
   platelets and, 65
Electrophoresis, 956-957, *958*
   agarose, 956
   cellulose acetate, 956
   of dog, 956, *965, 966*
   feline infectious peritonitis and, *976, 977*
   kidney disease and, 975
   serum protein, 967
   starch-gel, plasma proteins and, 941
   zone, 956
Electrophoretogram(s), *958. See also* Electrophoresis
Elephant(s), 338-339
   erythrocytes and, 275, 338
   hematologic values of, 333t
   leukocytes and, 338-339, VII
Elicited macrophage, 774
ELISA. *See* Enzyme-linked immunosorbent assay
Elk, 337
Elliptical red cell(s), 6, 528
Elliptocyte(s), 528, *530,* 541
   etymology of, 534t
EM pathway. *See* Embden-Meyerhof pathway
Embden-Meyerhof pathway, 545-546
Embryonic hemoglobin, 517, 518t
Emotion(s), blood value and, 7
   cat, 126, 132, 133t
   sheep, 214
Emperipolesis, 433, *435*
End stage kidney disease
   case report of, 1094, 1095
   plasma proteins and, 974
Endocytosis, 701, 702
Endomitosis, 15
Endoplasmic reticulum, lymphocytes and, 792, 794
Endoreduplication, megakaryocytopoiesis and, 433
Endothelium
   arachidonic acid metabolism and, 455
   disseminated intravascular coagulopathy and, 411-
      412
   hemostasis and, 389
   lymphocytes and, 804-805
   platelets and, 457, 458, 460-461
   vascular. *See* Vascular endothelium
   venous sinus and, 362-364
Endotoxin(s), 831-836
   cattle and, 201-204, 831-832, 832t
   chemotaxis inhibition and, 719
   cyclic hematopoiesis and, 118
   Escherichia coli. See Escherichia coli
   leukocyte response and, 827, 831-836
   leukopenias and, 831-836
   marrow reserve assessment and, 688
   neutrophils and, 693-695
   Salmonella typhosa, 688

thrombocytopenia and, 483
Entamoeba histolytica, 714
Enteritis
    granulomatous, *972*
    infectious, 1071-1074
    protein loss and, *972*
Enterobacter aerogenes
    bovine mastitis and, 1076, 1078-1081, *1081*
    horse endotoxemia and, 833t
Enterohepatic circulation, 524
Environmental temperature, cattle hemogram and, 189-190
Enzootic bovine leukosis, 886
Enzyme(s)
    epoxide reductase, 408
    erythrocyte autoantibody and, 75
    lymphocytes and, 794-795
    lysosomal, degranulation of, 702
    proteolytic, 784
    purine metabolism and, 922
    T cells and, 798
Enzyme-linked immunosorbent assay, 957
    feline leukemia virus and, 844, 845-846
    microfilariae and, 80, 81
Eo-GSF. *See* Eosinophil growth stimulating factor
Eosin, 31
Eosinopenia, 750-752
Eosinophil(s), 6-7, 13, 731-755
    age and, 111
    avian, 257, 261-263
    biochemical composition of, 737-739
    cat, 133, *340*, 748t
    cattle, 186, 195, *744*
    chemotaxis and, 741-742
    chicken, 262
    count of, 64-65
    disease and, 731
    dog, 118-119, 748t
    elephant, 339
    function of, 743-747
    goat, 231, 236-238
    guinea pig, 287
    histamine release and, 763
    horse, 158, 173
    Hyaena hyaena, 341, *341*
    large cat, *340*
    leukemoid blood picture and, 825
    metabolism and, 739
    mink, 316t, 317
    monkey, 314
    morphology of, 731-737, *732, 733, 734, 735, 736*
    mouse, 307
    muskrat, 316t, 319
    owl monkey, 276
    Pelger-Huët anomaly and, 117
    pig, 248, *251*, *252*, 737
    production of, 739-741
    rabbit, 281, *281*
    raccoon, 316t, 318
    rat, 296, 297
    regulation of, 371
    release of, 739-741
    sheep, 216, 218, *219*, *220*
    surface receptors and, 741
    tissue distribution and, 742-743
    toxemic diseases and, 826
    ultrastructure of, 735
    water buffalo, 328
Eosinophil chemotactic factor of anaphylaxis, 741, 760, 761t
Eosinophil degranulation, 738
Eosinophil growth stimulating factor, 740
Eosinophil releasing factor, 741
Eosinophil stimulation promotor, 742
Eosinophil colony stimulating factor, 740
Eosinophilia, 747-750, 748t
    interpretation of, 828
Eosinophilic cationic protein, 738
Eosinophilic granule(s), 118-119, 731-737, *732, 733, 734, 735, 736*
Eosinophilic leukemia, 839
    equine, 894
    feline, 863-865, 864t
    in pig, 897
Eosinophilopoietin, 371, 740
Eperythrozoon felis, 602
Eperythrozoon ovis, 609
Eperythrozoon parvum, 609
Eperythrozoon suis, 609
Eperythrozoon wenyoni, 608, 981
Eperythrozoonosis, 554-555, 608-610
Epinephrine
    cat reticulocyte and, 129
    dog platelet and, 121
    eosinopenia and, 750
    horse and, 142, 159
    neutrophils and, 691, 692
    platelets and, 441
Epistaxis with nasal carcinoma, 1117-1118
Epithelioid cell(s), 774-775
Epoxide reductase enzyme, 408
EPP. *See* Eosinophilopoietin
Epsilon 1 antigen, 992
Epsilon aminocaproic acid, 402
Epstein-Barr virus, 876
Equidae, 339-340
Equine babesiosis, 598, 601
Equine blood. *See* Horse(s)
Equine ehrlichiosis, 481, *482*, 830, 1066-1068
Equine infectious anemia, 63, 618-619
    case report of, 1153-1154
    plasma proteins and, 975
    thrombocytopenia and, 481
Equine influenza, 830
Equine leukemia complex, 890-894
Equine lymphocyte antigen, 1002
Equine plumbism, 630-631
ERF. *See* Eosinophil releasing factor
E-rosetting, 796, 797
Erysipelothrix rhusiopathiae, 249
Erythematosus, systemic lupus. *See* Lupus erythematosus, systemic; Lupus erythematosus cell
Erythremic myelosis, 853
    canine, 882
    chloroacetate esterase and, 916
    feline, 856-857, *857*
    term of, 853
Erythroblast(s), 12
Erythroblastic island, 488, *490*
Erythrocyte(s), 3, 12, 13, 104-107, *529, 530*
    abnormalities of, 532-545, 534t, *535-539*, XVIII
    acute blood loss and, 577-578
    agglutinated, 1010
    amphibian, 275
    anemia and, 55, 554, 565t, 566-569, 571-572, XVII. *See also* Anemia(s)
    antibody to, 73-75, 555, 592, 648, 1008
    antigen and, 991-993
    aplasia of, 665-666
    bird, 256, 257, 259, 261, 268, 269, 548
    blood volume and, 87
    bone marrow evaluation and, 15
    bovine viral diarrhea and, 356t, 357t
    buffy coat and, 38-39
    camel, 275, 336, *336*
    caribou, 337
    cat, 127-132, 340, 528

Erythrocyte(s) *(Continued)*
 cattle, 179-181, 191-194, 528, 545, 546, 552
 chevrotain, 275
 colony forming unit, erythropoietin and, 506
 counting of, 3, 45-52
 deer, 275, 321, *321*, 322, 528
 destruction of, 377, 550-556, 1014
 2,3-diphosphoglycerate and, 546-547
 disseminated intravascular coagulopathy and, 411
 distemper and, 1048
 dog, 103-109, 552, 553-554, 583, *583*, 1048
 donkey, 339
 elephant, 275, 338
 elliptical, 6, 528
 equine infectious anemia and, 619
 Felidae, 275
 fetal, antibodies to, 996
 fish, 275
 foal, 146
 fox, 320
 giraffe, 341
 goat, 11, 225-231, 227t, 229t, 528, 532
 guinea pig, 282-283, 284t
 Haemoproteus and *Parahaemoproteus* and, 269
 hamster, 308-310, 309t
 Heinz body and, 632-640
 heme synthesis and, 515
 hemocytometer and, 45-48
 horse and. *See* Erythrocyte(s), horse
 inclusion in, 6
 iron-deficient, 583
 koala, 275
 large cat, 340
 lead poisoning and, 630
 life span of, 155, 547-550, 549t, 583, 585
 macrocytic polychromatic, 578, 661
 maturation of, 12-13, 363-364. *See also* Erythropoiesis
 membrane of. *See* Erythrocyte membrane(s)
 metabolism of, 545-547
 mink, 316t, 317
 monkey, 311-313, 312t
 morphology of. *See* Erythrocyte morphology
 mouse, 299-306, 300t, 303t
 mule, 340
 muskrat, 316t, 319
 myeloproliferative disorder and, *859*
 nucleated. *See* Nucleated erythrocyte(s)
 osmotic fragility and. *See* Erythrocyte osmotic fragility
 papain-treated, agglutination of, 75
 parasites in. *See* Blood parasite(s)
 pig. *See* Pig erythrocyte(s)
 polychromatic, 6
 polycythemia and, 572-574, 572t
 prenatal, morphology and, 352, *353*, 354-359, *355*, 356t, *358*, *359*
 production of. *See* Erythropoiesis
 rabbit, 276-280, 277t
 raccoon, 316t, 318
 radiochromate labeled. *See* Radiochromate, erythrocytes labeled with
 rat, 289-296, 290t, 293t
 reptile, 275
 reticulocytes and, 499-501
 rouleau. *See* Rouleau formation
 sedimentation rate. *See* Erythrocyte sedimentation rate
 shapes of, 532-534, 534t, *535*, *536*, *537*, *538*, *539*, 552
 sheep. *See* Sheep erythrocyte(s)
 sodium radiochromate labeling and volume of. *See* Radiochromate, erythrocytes labeled with
 spleen and, 7, 142, 376-377, 575
 survival of, 545
 theileriasis and, 610
 transfusions and, 994

 trypanosomiasis and, 614
 variations in, 7, 8t
 volume of, 87-93, 94, 140-144, 552
 water buffalo, 322-326, *327*
 white rhino, 275
 zeta potential of surface of, 555
Erythrocyte(s), horse, 140-144, 141t, 150t, 151, 528
 age and, 151
 Arabian, 152t
 breed and, 11, 154-155
 cold-blooded, 153t
 foal, 146
 hemolytic anemia in viral disease and, 619
 morphology of, 155-158
 pregnancy and lactation and, 151
 seasonal differences in, 151-154
 sex differences and, 151
 thoroughbred and, 152t
 training and, 154
Erythrocyte index(ices), 4-5
 error in, 53
 Wintrobe, 52-53
Erythrocyte mass, 3
 neonate and, 94-95
 strenuous exercise and, 141-142, 141t
Erythrocyte membrane(s), 528, 531-532, *531*, 544
 destruction of, 551-554, *553*, *554*
 macrophages and, 781
 parasites and, 602
Erythrocyte morphology, 527-545
 anemia and, 569-570, *569*
 artifact and, 6
 cell membrane and, 528, 531-532, *531*, *532*
 dog, 103-104
Erythrocyte osmotic fragility, 69-71, 551-554, *553*, *554*
 cat, 132, *132*
 cattle, 181-185
 derivative curve of, 70
 dog, 108-109, *109*
 goat, 229-230
 Haemobartonella felis and, 605-606
 horse, 156
 lead poisoning and, 630
 pig, 248
 sheep, 214-215
 sigmoid curve of, 70
 sodium chloride solution and, 70, 70t
Erythrocyte pyrimidine-specific 5'nucleotidase, 629
Erythrocyte refractile. *See* Heinz body(ies)
Erythrocyte sedimentation rate, 5, 11, 53-56
 cat, 132
 corrected table for dog, 54-56
 diphasic, 55
 dog, 54-56, 108
 donkey, 339
 factors influencing, 54
 goat, 229
 horse, 155-156, 157t
 method for, 53-54
 monkey, 313
 pig, 248
 sheep, 214
Erythrocytosis, polycythemia and, 572
Erythroid burst forming unit, 368
Erythroid cell(s), 582
Erythroid ferritin, 582
Erythroid hypoplasia(s), 668-671
 of Diamond-Blackfan, 666
Erythroid progenitor cell(s), 488-490, *488*, 488t
 stimulation of, 370
Erythrokinetics, 501-503
Erythroleukemia
 canine, 882
 chloroacetate esterase and, 916

feline, 853, 857-859
isozyme and, 916
periodic acid-Schiff reaction and, 919
term of, 853
Erythrolysis, neonatal, 650, 1154-1155
Erythromycin, 707, 719
Erythrophagocytosis, 554-556, 1014-1015
autoimmune hemolytic anemia and, 648
feline mast cell leukemia and, 866
immunoglobulin G antibodies and, 1014-1015
myeloproliferative disease and, *859*
Erythropoiesis, 12-13, 17-18, 363-364, 487-513
anemia and, 570-571, 586, 655
bird, 263, 364
canine bone marrow and, IV, V
cat, 352, IV, V
equine bone marrow and, V, VI
erythrokinetics in, 501-503
factors influencing, 369t
fascioliasis and, 586
feline bone marrow and, IV, V
haemonchosis and, 585-586
iron deficiency and, 583
intraembryonic, dog and, 350
light microscopy and, 488-491, *490*
materials essential for, 508-509
myeloid:erythroid ratio and, 17-18
nomenclature and, 487-488, 489t
parasitism and, 585
regulation of, 503-508
reticulocyte and, 495-501, *497, 498*
secondary polycythemia and, 575
ultrastructure and, 491-495, *491-494*
yolk sac and, 352
Erythropoietic porphyria, congenital, 646-647, 1165,
    1167
Erythropoietin, 440, 503-507, *504,* 505t
acute blood loss and, 580
cat, 129
hematopoiesis and, 368
kidney and, 383
polycythemia and, 573
secondary polycythemia and, 575
sheep hemoglobin and, 215
source of, 372
Escherichia coli, 831, 832t
granulopoiesis and, 697
marrow reserve assessment and, 688
mastitis and, 1078-1081
microbicidal activity and, 712
neutrophil migration and, 694
peripheral leukocyte in cattle and, 202t
phagocytosis and, 708
superoxide anion and, 710
water buffalo and, 329
ESP. *See* Eosinophil stimulation promotor
ESR. *See* Erythrocyte sedimentation rate
Esterase(s), 776, 910t, 911t, 912t, 915-919, 928-930
Estrogen(s)
erythropoiesis and, 370, 508
excess, in dog, 1100-1102
plasma proteins and, 943
thrombocytopenia and, 475-478, 478t
Estrus, eosinophilia and, 750
Ether, 142
Ethyl alcohol, stain and, 32, 33
Ethylenediaminetetraacetate, 1, 23-24, 25t
avian blood and, 260
cat blood and, 126
Coombs test and, 73
cross-matching blood and, 71, 72
DNA viscosity test and, 68
erythrocyte shrinkage and, 53
lead poisoning and, 630

marrow aspiration and, 66, 67
method for dispensing, 23-24, *25*
platelet counting and, 65
Etiocholanolone, 688
Euarctos americanus, 335t
Euglobulin lysis, 401-402
Evans blue, 92, 93
Evoked macrophage(s), 774
Exchange transfusion, 994, 998
Excitement, blood values and
horse, 142
sheep, 214
Exercise, 7
horse, 141-142, 141t
neutrophilia and, 692
sheep erythrocytes and, 214
thrombocytosis and, 469
Exocytosis, 702, 763
Exogenous estrogen, 476-478, 478t
Extracellular material(s), 1026-1027
Extrahepatic cholestasis, 160
Extravascular fluid(s), blood loss and, 577
Extravascular hemolysis, 522
Extravascular:vascular ratio for albumin, 942
Exudate(s)
abdominal cavity and, 1071
macrophages in, 773

F_{cells}, 94
F antigen, 992
FAB. *See* French American British classification of
    leukemias
Fab fragment, 951
Factor(s), coagulation. *See* Coagulation factor(s)
Factor increasing monocytopoiesis, 770
Factor VIII-coagulant, 394-395
Factor VIII-related antigen, 394, 404, 406, 468
Fallot's tetralogy, 95, 1108-1109
Fallow deer, 337
Familial polycythemia, cow and, 574
Fanconi's anemia, 666
Fasciola gigantica, 549
Fasciola hepatica, 744, 745
Fascioliasis, 549, 586, 744, 745
Fasting hyperbilirubinemia, 160
Fc portion of immunoglobulin, 762, 797, 951
E, 762
G, 776
monocytes and macrophages and, 776
receptors for, 707, 780, 797, 918
Fc receptor, 707, 780, 797
nonspecific esterase and, 918
FDP. *See* Fibrin degradation product
Fear, cat blood values and, 126, 132, 133t
Febrile illness. *See* Fever(s)
Feces
blood test and, 571
parasitism and, 585
Felidae, 340-341
erythrocytes of, 275
Feline babesiosis, 601. *See also* Cat(s)
Feline blood. *See* Cat(s)
Feline bone marrow. *See* Bone marrow, cat
Feline haemobartonellosis, 554-555, 602-606, 604t, *606*
Feline infectious anemia, 602
case report of, 1148-1150, 1151
Feline infectious peritonitis, 830, XIV
case reports of, 1138-1140, 1068-1071, 1071t
exudate in, 1071t
hemogram and, 1070t
plasma proteins and, 976
Feline infectious peritonitis virus, 830

Feline leukemia complex, 844-869
  acute lymphoblastic leukemia in, 852
  basophilic leukemia in, 865-867, *865, 866*
  eosinophilic leukemia in, 863-865, 864t
  erythremic myelosis in, 856-857, *857*
  erythroleukemia in, 857-859
  feline leukemia virus and. *See* Feline leukemia virus
  feline oncornavirus cell membrane antigen and, 846
  granulocytic leukemia in, 860-863
  Hodgkin's disease and, 852
  incidence of infection in, 847
  iron particles in, 860
  lupus erythematosus cells and, 859-860
  lymphoma in, 847-849
  lymphocytic leukemia in, XXI
  lymphoproliferative disorders in, 847-852
  mast cell leukemia in, 865-867, *865, 866,* XXII
  megakaryocytic leukemia in, 867
  monocytic leukemia in, 863
  myelogenous leukemia in, 860-863
  myelomonocytic leukemia in, 863
  myeloproliferative disorders in, 852-869, XIX, XX
  phagocytosis of erythrocytes and, 859-860
  preleukemia in, 867-869, *868*
  smoldering leukemia in, 867-869, *868*
  thrombocytopenia and, 481
Feline leukemia virus, 844-847
  diagnosis of, 844-846
  diseases of, 846
  feline infectious peritonitis and, 1069
  immune deficiency and, 981
  incidence of, 847
  monocytes and macrophages and, 779
  spread of, 847
  subgroups of, 846
  thrombocytopenia and, 481
Feline oncornavirus cell membrane antigen, 846
Feline plumbism, 632
Felis sp, 334t, 335t, 340-341
FeLV. *See* Feline leukemia virus
Femur, marrow aspiration and, 66, *66, 67*
Ferrihemalbumin, 949
Ferritin, 382-383
  erythroid, 582
  erythroid precursor and, 495
  iron deficiency anemia and, 583-584
Fetal blood value(s), 350-359, 517, 518t
  cattle, 179
  elephant, 339
  foal, 146
  sheep, 208, 212t
Fetal erythropoiesis, 506
Fetal hemoglobin, 518t
  antibodies to, 996
  cat, 127
  elephant, 339
Fetal membrane(s), retained, 191, 192t, *193*
α-Fetoprotein, 950
Fetus. *See also* Fetal blood value(s)
  blood loss and, 97
  pig, 240-241
  trypanosomes and, 613
Fever(s)
  nitrogen loss and, 943
  serum protein and, 975
FIA. *See* Feline infectious anemia
Fibrin
  coagulation and, 396
  fibrinogen and, 947
  hemostasis and, 391
  stabilization test and, 425
Fibrin degradation product, 400, 424
Fibrin split product, 400
Fibrinogen, 2, 5, 58, 59, 947-948
  cat, 127t, 133-137

cattle, 179t, 188, 961t
  changes in, 960-962, 961t, 962t, 963t
  coagulation and, 396
  disseminated intravascular coagulation and, 424
  dog, 104t, 122-123, 961t, 1093-1094
  elevation of, 829, 1093-1094
  erythrocyte sedimentation rate and, 55
  goat, 226t, 232
  horse, 141t, 149, 161, 173t, 174, 961t
  pig, 140t, 250
  rat, 297
  refractometer and, 58-59
  sheep, 209t, 218
Fibrinolysis, 399-402, *400*
  disseminated intravascular coagulation and, 410, 424-425
  eosinophils and, 747
  hemostatic tests for, 423-425
  nasal carcinoma and, 1117-1118
  systems interactions and, *395*
Fibrinolytic factor(s), 779
Fibrinous pericarditis, 1156-1157
Fibrometer, antiplatelet antibody and, 76
Fibronectin, 780
Field mouse, Bolivian, 310-311
Filariasis
  bird, 270
  dog, 79-82, 80t
  eosinophilia and, 749
Film(s), blood. *See* Blood film(s)
FIM. *See* Factor increasing monocytopoiesis
FIP. *See* Feline infectious peritonitis
Fish erythrocytes, 275
Fitzgerald factor, 394
Flagellated protozoon(a), 612
Flame cell(s), 812, 967
Flaujeac factor, 394
Fletcher factor, 394
Fluid distribution, 97-98
Fluid mosaic model, erythrocyte and, 531
Fluid shift, 97-98
Fluke(s), liver, 586
Fluorescein isothiocyanate, 803
Fluorescence. *See also* Immunofluorescence
  antinuclear antibody and, 77, 78
  antiplatelet antibody and, 77, 1019
  lymphocytes and, 796
Fluoride toxicity, 1064
9α-Fluoro-16α-methylprednisoline
  horse and, 165t
  cattle and, 198, 200t
FMLP, 703
Foa-Kurloff body, 287
Foal(s)
  combined immune deficiency in, 978
  failure of passive transfer of maternal
    immunoglobulin in, 979
  normal blood values of, 146-147, 147t
FOCMA. *See* Feline oncornavirus cell membrane
    antigen
Folate. *See* Folic acid
Folic acid, 656-659
  autoimmune hemolytic anemia and, 1017
  deficiency of, 16-17
  erythropoiesis and, 509
  neutrophils and, 716, 719
  stomach and, 381
Follicles, hematopoiesis and, 379-380
Formaldehyde, 964
Formalin, 24
Forssman antigen, 992
Fox(es), 316t, 320, 320t, 335t
Fragiligraph, 71

Fragility, erythrocyte osmotic. *See* Erythrocyte osmotic fragility
Fragmentation, erythrocyte, 556
Fratercula arctica, 270
Free bilirubin, 380
French American British classification of leukemias, 840
Fresh plasma transfusion(s), 408. *See also* Transfusion(s)
Frustrated phagocytosis, 703
Furaxolidone, 483
Fur-bearing animal(s), 315-320, 316t
Furosemide, 95
Fusiform erythrocyte, 528
Fusocyte(s), *530, 538,* 540
  etymology of, 534t
FVIII:C. *See* Coagulation factor VIII-coagulant
FVIII:Rag. *See* Coagulation factor VIII-related antigen

G-6-PD. *See* Glucose-6-phosphate dehydrogenase
Galago crassicaudatus, 27-28
Gall body, 793
Galliform, 267
Gallus gallus domesticus, 257
GALT. *See* Gut-associated lymphoid tissue
Gamma globulin(s), 218, 948
  changes in, 964
  equine infectious anemia and, 618
  feline infectious peritonitis and, 1069
  foal serum protein and, 149
  goat, 232
  mink, 317
  mule, 340
  pig, 241, 250
  rat, 298
  transient decrease in, 982
Gamma radiation
  canine radiation-induced hematopoietic disorder and, 883, 884
  swine lymphoma and, 897
  thrombocytopenia and, 483
Gammopathy(ies) 964-971
  benign monoclonal, 970, 971
  polyclonal, 965
Gastroenteropathy(ies), protein-losing, 971-972
Gastrointestinal disease(s)
  bleeding tumor in, 581
  blood loss and, 97, 581, 1111, 1112
  horse, 169, 171t
  lead poisoning in dog and, 629
  plasma proteins in, 971-973
Gaucher's disease, 781-782
Gazelle(s), 333t
G-CSF. *See* Granulocyte-CSF
G:E ratio. *See* Granulocyte:erythrocyte ratio
Gelatinase, 714
Genetics
  blood group antigens and, 991, 993
  coagulopathy and, 402-410
  monocytes and macrophages and, 781
  platelets and, 453, 468-469
  spherocytosis and, 543
  stomatocytosis and, 543
  thrombopathia and, 468
Gentamicin, 707, 719
Gentian violet, 46
Gerbil(s), 308
German shepherd(s)
  babesiosis and, 600
  normal blood values and, 107
German trotter horse(s), 159
Germfree animal(s), 976
Gestation, 350-359. *See also* Fetal blood value(s)
Ghost(s), erythrocyte, 60, 63
Giant cell(s), 775

Giant neutrophil(s), bizarre, 826
Giemsa stain(s), 31-32, 33
Gigantocyte(s), 541
Giraffe(s), 330t, 333t, 341
Glanzmann's thrombasthenia, 453, 468
Glassware cleaning, 22-23
Globin synthesis, 516
Globulin(s), 948
  antiplatelet antibody and, 77
  cattle, 187
  equine infectious anemia and, 618
  erythrocyte sedimentation rate and, 55
  foal serum protein and, 149
  horse, 160, 1157-1158
  pig, 241, 250
  rabbit anticanine, 77
  rat, 298
α-Globulin(s), 941t
  changes in, 962-964
  equine multiple myeloma and, 893, *896*
  erythrocyte sedimentation rate and, 55
  horse, 160, 893, *896*
β-Globulin(s), 941t
  changes in, 962-964
  equine infectious anemia and, 618
  equine multiple myeloma and, 893, *896*
  foal serum protein and, 149
γ-Globulin(s), 218, 948
  changes in, 964
  equine infectious anemia and, 618
  feline infectious peritonitis and, 1069
  foal serum protein and, 149
  goat, 232
  mink, 317
  mule, 340
  pig and, 241, 250
  rat, 298
  transient decrease in, 982
Globulin permeability factor, 712
Glomerulonephritis
  dog, 1093-1094
  plasma proteins and, 974
Glucocerebroside, 781-782
Glucocorticoid(s)
  arachidonic acid metabolism and, 456
  plasma proteins and, 943
Glucosaminidase, 912t
Glucose-6-phosphate dehydrogenase
  erythrocyte metabolism and, 546
  pluripotential stem cell(s) and, 367
Glucuronidase, 911t, 912t, 923
Glucuronide, bilirubin, 524
Glutaraldehyde, 964, 981
Glutathione deficiency, 546, 640
Glutathione peroxidase, 546
  macrophages and, 780-781
  water buffalo and, 329
Glutathione reductase, 546
Glycine-2-^{14}C labeling of erythrocyte(s), 155, 247
Glycogen
  leukocytes and, 910t, 919-920
  platelets and, 454
Glycol methacrylate, 19
Glycolysis, anaerobic
  chemotaxis and phagocytosis and, 706
  lymphocytes and, 795
  macrophages and, 775
  neutrophils and, 684-685
  platelets and, 454
Glycophorin A, 532
Glycoprotein(s), 948
  platelet and, 451, 454-455
GM-CSF. *See* Granulocyte-macrophage-CSF

Goat(s), 225-239
    anaplasmosis and, 590-596, 591t, 592t, *593, 594*
    blood cell morphology and, 232-238
    blood collection from, 25t
    blood volume measurement and, 89t, 94
    bone marrow and, 238
    2,3-diphosphoglycerate and, 547
    eperythrozoonosis, 609
    erythrocyte membrane permeability and, 552
    erythrocytes and, 11, 225-231, 227t, 229t, 528, 532
    hemoglobin and. *See* Goat hemoglobin
    hemolysis and, 26, 229-230
    kale and, 634
    leukemia complex in, 894-895
    leukocyte count(s) and, 9t, 10t, 11
    leukocytes and, 228t, 231
    lymphocyte antigens of, 1002
    myeloid:erythroid ratio of, 18t, 238
    normal blood values and, 10t
    plasma and, 225, 229t, 232
    platelets of, 231, 238, 447, *449*, 469t
    sarcocytosis in, 616
    theileriasis and, 610
Goat hemoglobin, 226t, 227t
    blood loss anemia and, 230t
    centrifugation and, 229t
    packed cell volume and, 225-226
    polymerized, 234, *234, 235, 236*
    types of, 230-231, 518t
Gold compound(s), 1023
Goldberg refractometer(s), 56, *56*
Golden hamster(s), 308-310, 309t
Golgi complex
    eosinophil and, 736, 737
    plasma cells and, 812, *813*, 814
Gorilla(s), 334t
Gosling(s), 269
Gower's solution, 46
GP. *See* Glutathione peroxidase
GPF. *See* Granulocyte production factor
GR. *See* Glutathione reductase
Graft rejection, 1005, 1007
Gram-negative bacterium(a), 707, 709, 831-832. *See also*
        Bacterium(a)
Granulation. *See* Granule(s)
Granule(s), 7
    acid phosphatase-positive, 910-914
    alkaline phosphatase and, 914
    avian leukocyte and, 257, 258, 262-263
    azurophilic. *See* Azurophilic granule(s)
    basophil(s) and, 119, 159, 757-758
    cat leukocyte and, 133-134
    cat reticulocyte and, 129
    cattle eosinophil and, 195
    chinchilla leukocyte and, 319
    crystalloid, 737
    electron microscopy and, 679, *680*
    elephant leukocyte and, 339
    eosinophil(s) and, 118-119, 731-737, *732, 733, 734,
        735, 736*
    exocytosis of, 763
    giraffe neutrophil and, 341
    goat leukocytes and, 238
    guinea pig leukocyte and, 287, 288
    hamster leukocyte and, 310
    horse eosinophil and, 158
    lymphocytes and, 793
    lysosomal, 683-684
    mast cells and, 759-760
    α-, megakaryocyte and, 436
    mink leukocyte and, 317, 318
    monkey leukocyte and, 314
    mouse leukocyte and, 306, 307
    muskrat leukocyte and, 319
    peroxidase-positive, 917

pig leukocyte and, 252
    platelets and, 120
    pleomorphic, 679, *682*
    primary, 679, 683
    rabbit neutrophil and, 281
    raccoon leukocyte and, 318
    rat leukocyte and, 297
    secondary, 679
    sheep leukocyte and, 218, 220
    sudanophilic, 921
    tertiary, 679
    toxic. *See* Toxic granule(s)
    water buffalo leukocyte and, 328
Granulocyte(s), 7
    bone marrow and, 15
    cell transit and, 364
    leukemic, vacuolation of, 861, *862, 879*
    life span of, 686, 689
    maturation of, 13t, 16, 17-18, 118. *See also*
        Granulocytopoiesis
Granulocyte pool, total blood, 689
Granulocyte production factor, 696
Granulocyte-CSF, 371
Granulocyte:erythrocyte ratio, 17. *See also*
        Myeloid:erythroid ratio
Granulocyte-macrophage-CSF, 371
Granulocytic leukemia, 839, 876-880, 877t. *See also*
        Myelogenous leukemia
    alkaline phosphatase and, 915
    cat, 860-863, 862t, XXII
    chronic, 690, 915
    dog, 876-880, 877t, 1106-1107, XXIII
    pig, 897
    subleukemic, 862, 862t
Granulocytic progenitor cell migration, 367
Granulocytopoiesis. *See* Granulo(cyto)poiesis
Granulokinetics, neutrophils and, 685-695, 687t
Granulomatous disease
    chronic, 710
    monocytes and macrophages and, 778, 781
    protein loss and, *972*
Granulomatous enteritis, *972*
Granulo(cyto)poiesis, 13t, 118
    aberrant or abnormal, 16
    acute blood loss and, 580
    acute toxemic disease and, 1133, 1136
    bird, 263-264, 364
    canine bone marrow and, V
    degenerative left shift and, 824
    eosinophil and, 747
    equine bone marrow and, V, VI
    factors influencing, 369t
    feline bone marrow and, V
    hyperestrogenism and, 1100-1102
    myeloid:erythroid ratio and, 17-18
    neutrophils and, 685-695, 687t
    rat, 298
    regulation of, 370-371
    stimulators and inhibitors of, 696-698
Gray collie syndrome, 719
Gray fox, 320
Gray platelet syndrome, 453
Greyhound(s), 107
Grisson, 335t
Ground substance, 113-115, 119
Grouse, 270
Growth, hematopoiesis and, 359, 361, 362
Growth factor
    hematopoiesis and, 368
    monocyte/macrophage-derived, 785
Growth hormone
    erythropoiesis and, 370
    plasma proteins and, 943
Guanacos, 336-337

Guernsey cattle, 193
Guinea pig(s), 282-288
  anaphylactic degranulation and, *764*
  basophil culture and, 757
  blood volume measurement and, 91t, 94
  hemoglobin and, 518t
Gull(s), herring, 270
Gut-associated lymphoid tissue, 798

H antigen, 992
H₂O₂. *See* Hydrogen peroxide
Haematopinus eurysternus, 584
Haemobartonella canis
  babesiosis and, 599
  ultrastructure of, 606
Haemobartonella felis, 130, 554-555, 602-606, 604t, *606*,
    1069
  feline infectious peritonitis and, 1069
  Howell-Jolly body and, 130
Haemobartonellosis, 602-608, *603*, 604t, *607*, 607t
  babesiosis and, 599
  canine, 599, 606
  feline, 130, 554-555, 602-606, 604t, *606*, 1069
  feline infectious peritonitis and, 1069
  Howell-Jolly body and, 130
Haemonchosis, 585
  case report of, 1168
  plasma proteins and, 973
Haemoproteus, 269
Hageman factor, 393-394
  deficiency of, 407
  mast cells and basophils and, 761t
Half-time of disappearance
  eosinophil, 740
  neutrophil, 689, 690t, 693
Halothane, 142
Hamster(s), golden, 308-310, 309t
Handling of blood for laboratory study, 2, 23-29
Haplotype, 999
Haptoglobin, 520, 521-522, 948-949
Harris tissue culture system, 698
Hassall's corpuscle, 373
Hayem's solution, 46
Hb. *See* Hemoglobin(s)
HbF. *See* Fetal hemoglobin
HbS. *See* Sickle cell anemia
³H-DFP, 155
Heart failure, protein loss and, 972
Heartworm(s), 79-82, 80t
Heavy chain(s), 951
Heavy chain disease, 968
Heavy metal(s), monocytes and macrophages and, 781
Heinz body(ies), 6
  anemia and, 270-271, 570, 632-640, 1152-1153
  bird, 270-271
  blood film and, 60, *61*, 63
  cat, 130-131, 340, 634-640, *635*, *636*, *639*, XVI
  cow, 634, 641
  erythrocyte destruction and, 555
  hemoglobin concentration error and, 53
  horse, 1152-1153
  large cat and, 340
  permanent stain for, 63
  phenothiazine toxicosis and, 1152-1153
  spectrophotometry and, 45
  spleen and, 377-378
Helminthiasis, 585
  eosinophil and, 744, 748-749
Helper T cell(s), 807
Hemangiosarcoma(s)
  blood loss in, 1109-1111
  protein loss and, *972*
Hematin

hemoglobin study and, 43-44
hemolysis and, 521
hemopexin and, 949
Hematocrit, 36-41. *See also* Packed cell volume(s)
  Buffy coat, 37
  cattle, 188
  Drummond microcapillary, 37
  icterus index and, 39-40
  lipemia and, 40
  microhematocrit and, 41
  microfilariae and, 80-81
  plasma color, 40
  plasma fibrinogen and, 59
  venous, 93-96
  Wintrobe, 37
Hematocrit tube(s), 37
  care of, 22-23, *24*
  plasma fibrinogen and, 59
Hematofluorometer(s), modified, 271
Hematogone, 14
Hematologic technique(s), 20-86. *See also* Blood
    picture(s) in diseases of domestic animals;
    specific technique
  anticoagulants in, 23-24
  anti-erythrocyte antibody in, 73-75
  antinuclear antibody in, 77-79
  antiplatelet antibody in, 75-77
  avian, 259-263
  basophilic stippling in, 63
  blood cross-matching and, 71-72
  blood examination by wet-film method in, 59, *60*
  blood film preparation in, 29-31. *See also* Blood
    film(s)
  bone marrow aspiration and, 66-67
  canine blood for microfilariae and, 79-82, 80t
  cleaning of glassware in, 22-23
  collecting of blood in, 23-29
  Coombs test and, 73
  counting of cells in, 45-52. *See also* Blood cell count(s)
  cross-matching of blood and, 71-72
  cytochemistry in, 924-934, 925t. *See also*
    Cytochemistry
  DNA viscosity test in, 67-69, *68*, 69t
  electronic cell counters in, 48-52, *49*
  eosinophil leukocyte counting and, 64-65
  erythrocyte count in. *See* Erythrocyte(s)
  erythrocyte indexes in, 52-53
  erythrocyte osmotic fragility test in, 69-71
  erythrocyte sedimentation rate in, 53-56
  fibrinogen by refractometer in, 58-59
  handling of blood in, 23, 28-29
  Heinz body stain and, 63
  hematocrit in, 36-41. *See also* Hematocrit
  hemocytometer and, 45-48
  hemoglobin in, 3-4, 41-45
  immunofluorescence of megakaryotypes in, 77
  iron stain and, 64
  LE cell test in, 78
  leukocyte count. *See* Leukocyte count(s)
  methylene blue stain in, 59-62, *61*, *62*
  microfilariae and, 79-82, 80t
  microscope in, 21-22
  microscopic examination in, 35-36
  new methylene blue stain and, 59-62, *61*, *62*
  obtaining sample and, 24-28
  osmotic fragility test and, 69-71
  packed cell volume in, 36-41. *See also* Packed cell
    volume(s)
  papain agglutination in, 75
  plasma fibrinogen in, 58-59
  plasma protein in, 56-58
  platelet count and, 65-66
  platelet factor-3 test in, 75
  reticulocyte stain and count in, 62-63

Hematologic technique(s) *(Continued)*
  Romanowsky stain in, 31-35
  sideroleukocyte stain and, 63-64
  special stain procedures in, 62-64
  staining blood films in, 31-34. *See also* Stain(s)
  total leukocyte count in, 67-69, *68,* 69t
  total plasma protein in, 56-58
  transfusion cross-matching and, 71-72
  Unopette method in, 48
  wet-film method in, 59, *60*
  Wintrobe erythrocyte indexes in, 52-53
Hematology pipette(s), 22
Hematopoiesis, 15, 369-370. *See also* Hematopoietic
    system
  in avian marrow, 263-264
  cyclic, collie dog and, 117-118
  regulation of, 368-372
  spleen and, 307-308, 378-379
  mouse, 307-308
Hematopoietic humoral factor, 372
Hematopoietic inductive microenvironment, 369-370
Hematopoietic malignancy. *See* Malignancy(ies)
Hematopoietic progenitor cell, committed, 367-368
Hematopoietic stem cell, 366
Hematopoietic system, 350-387. *See also* Hematopoiesis
  bird and, 364-365
  bone marrow and, 359, 361-362
  cell transit from marrow and, 362-364
  growing and adult animal and, 359, 361-372
  intestinal mucosa and iron and, 382-383
  kidney and, 383
  liver and, 380-381
  lymphoid tissue and, 372-380
  mononuclear phagocyte system and, 380
  prenatal and early postnatal life and, 350-359
  regulation in, 368-372
  stem cell and, 365-368
  stomach and, 381-382
  thymus and, 373-375
Hematoxylin body(ies), 1026
Heme synthesis, 514-516
  iron and, 582
Hemoconcentration, 7, 37
  dehydration and, 96
  leptospirosis and, 616
  packed cell volume and, 37
  plasma proteins and, 944
Hemocytometer(s), 45-48
  avian leukocytes and, 261-262
  blood cell count error with, 48
  care of, 23
  erythrocyte count and, 45-48
  leukocyte count and, 45-48, 261-262
Hemodilution, 98
  acute blood loss and, 577
Hemoglobin(s), 2, 3, 7-11, 514-526
  adult, 516-519, 518t
  avian, 261
  bilirubin metabolism and, 520-525
  caribou, 337
  cat, 127, 128, 130-131, 518t
  cattle, 190, 190t, 518t
  codocyte and, 540
  deer, 321-322
  degradation and, 520-525
  determination of, 41-45
  dog, 104-108, 518t
  donkey, 340
  elephant, 338
  fetal. *See* Fetal hemoglobin
  fox, 320
  goat. *See* Goat hemoglobin
  guinea pig, 282
  hamster, 308
  horse, 140, 141t, 146, 151, 154, 518t

  iron deficiency and, 583
  methods for study of, 43t
  monkey, 313
  mouse, 299
  mule, 340
  osmotic fragility and, 552
  oxidative denaturation of, 644
  pig, 243-244, 518t
  protein and, 508-509
  rabbit, 280
  rat, 289, 296
  sheep, 212, 215, 518t
  synthesis of, 514-516, *515*
  types of, 516-519, 518t
Hemoglobin A
  cattle, 185
  goat, 230-231
  sheep, 215
Hemoglobin AB
  goat, 230-231
  sheep, 215
Hemoglobin ABC
  goat, 231
Hemoglobin B
  goat, 230-231
  sheep, 215
Hemoglobin BC
  goat, 231
Hemoglobin C
  goat, 230-231, 235
  sheep, 215
Hemoglobin F, 185
Hemoglobin N, 215
Hemoglobinemia
  autoimmune hemolytic anemia and, 1010
  plasma and, 521
Hemoglobin-O₂ dissociation curve, 258
Hemoglobinometer(s), 45
Hemoglobinopathy(ies), 519-520
Hemoglobinuria, 521
  cattle, 185, 189, 617-618, 618t
  Heinz bodies and, 634
  postparturient, 642-643
Hemogram(s), 2-5. *See also* specific test
  ACTH administration and, 765t
  sequential, 1
Hemolysin, cross-matching and, 71-72
Hemolysis. *See also* Hemolytic anemia(s)
  camel erythrocyte and, 336
  cat blood and, 132
  cattle, 185
  copper toxicity and, 628
  dog erythrocyte and, 108-109
  erythrocyte osmotic fragility test and, 69-71
  extravascular, 522
  goat, 26, 229-230
  guinea pig, 283
  intravascular, 520-522. *See also* Disseminated
    intravascular coagulation
  liver disease and, 670
  monkey, 313
  pig, 248
  rat, 296
  sheep, 214-215
Hemolytic anemia(s), 544
  acute, 564
  autoimmune. *See* Autoimmune hemolytic anemia
  bile excretion in, 571
  causes of, 590t
  crude oil ingestion and, 270
  erythrocyte survival time and, 548
  horse, 158, 642, 1152-1153
  immune-mediated. *See* Immune-mediated hemolytic
    anemia

infectious agents and. *See* Infectious agents in
    hemolytic anemia(s)
  leukocyte response and, 827
  noninfectious, 627-654. *See also* Noninfectious
    hemolytic anemia
  in phenothiazine toxicosis, 1152-1153
Hemolytic crisis, trypanosomes and, 612
Hemolytic disease(s)
  icterus index and, 40
  of newborn, 73, 650, 996-998, 1154-1155
Hemolytic test system for blood typing, 993
Hemolytic transfusion reaction(s), 74
Hemolytic volume, critical, 552
Hemoparasite(s), XVIII. *See also* Blood parasite(s)
Hemopexin, 521, 948-949
Hemophilia A, 402-405
Hemophilia B, 402-405, 403t, 406t
  case report of, 1118-1119
Hemorrhage. *See also* Bleeding
  anemia and, 564
  blood restoration and, 96-99
  compensatory mechanism and, 97
  gastrointestinal, 1111, 1112
  horse, 98-99, 1150-1152
  leptospirosis and, 616
  nitrogen loss and, 943
  thrombocytopenia and, 475-476
Hemorrhagic anemia(s). *See* Blood loss anemia(s)
Hemorrhagic diathesis, 616
Hemorrhagic disorder(s). *See* Bleeding disorder(s)
Hemosiderin, 382-383
  erythroid precursor and, 495
  in urine, 521
Hemostasis
  disseminated intravascular coagulation and, 423-425
  fibrin stabilization and, 425
  fibrinogen and, 947
  mammal and, 476
  platelet and, 457-458, 457
  primary, 389-391. *See also* Coagulation
  screening tests for, 421-423
  vessel wall injury and, 390, 391
HEp-2 tissue cell culture(s). *See* Human epithelioid
    tissue cell culture(s)
Heparin, 24, 25t
  autoimmune hemolytic anemia and, 1017
  avian blood and, 260
  basophils and mast cells and, 763-764
  blood collection and, 1, 2
  chemotaxis inhibition and, 719
  disseminated intravascular coagulopathy and, 414
  dog platelet and, 121
  epsilon aminocaproic acid and, 402
  lymphocyte migration and, 807
  lymphocytosis and, 811
  mast cells and basophils and, 761t
  thrombocytopenia and, 479
  thrombosis and, 418t
Hepatic cell carcinoma, 1104-1105. *See also* Liver
Hepatic lipidosis, 1160, 1161
Hepatitis
  canine infectious, 830, 1049-1051, 1050t
  lipemia in, 161
  plasma proteins and, 974
HEPTE, 455-456
Hereditary disease(s). *See* Genetics
Hereditary spherocytosis, 543
Hereditary stomatocytosis, 543
Hereditary thrombopathia, 468
Hereford cattle
  anaphylaxis and, 835t, 836
  hemogram and, 193
Hermansky-Pudlak syndrome, 453
Herpesvirus

bird, 264, 265t
  equine, 981
Herring gull, 270
HES. *See* Hypereosinophilic syndrome
HETE, 455-456
Heterophil(s), 7, 677
  bird, 257, 259, 262-263
  guinea pig, 287
  laboratory animal, 275-276
  mouse, 306
  rabbit, 281
  rat, 296, 297
HEV. *See* High endothelial venule
Hexosaminidase, 912t, 923
Hexose monophosphate pathway
  eosinophils and, 739
  neutrophils and, 684-685
Hibernating animal(s), 548
High endothelial venule, 804
High-density lipoproteins, 950-951
HIM. *See* Hematopoietic inductive microenvironment
Hippoboscidae, 269
Hippotigris sp, 333t
Histamine, 712
  albumin and, 947
  eosinophils and, 742, 746, 751-752
  inflammatory response and, 713
  mast cells and, 760
  monocytes and macrophages and, 784
  release of, 762-763
Histiocyte(s)
  enzymatic marker and, 922
  mononuclear phagocyte system and, 768
  sea-blue, 1022
Histiocytic medullary reticulosis, XIII
Histiocytosis in dog, XIII
Histocompatibility antigen, 998-1004
Histoplasma, 62
HLA. *See* Human leukocyte antigen(s)
HMP. *See* Hexose monophosphate pathway
HMW-kininogen, 394
Hodgkin's disease
  cat, 852
  dog, 876
Hog cholera, 250, 829-830
  experimental, 249
Holstein cattle, 184t, 189, 193
Homeostasis, regulation of, 695-698
Homograft rejection, 1005
Hookworm(s), 584-585
Hormone(s)
  erythropoiesis and, 370, 507-508
  plasma proteins and, 943
Horse(s), 140-177
  acute blood loss and, 578
  babesiosis and, 598, 601
  bacterial toxemia and septicemia and, 836
  bilirubin and, 524
  blood of, 169-174, 170t-172t, XII
  blood collection from, 25t
  blood morphology and, 8t
  blood volume of, 90t, 94, 95
  bone marrow and, 161-163, 162t, 164t, 571, 892, V,
    VI, XII
  breed of, erythrocytes and, 11
  circulating erythrocyte volume and, 140-144
  cold-blooded, 140, 153t
  corticosteroids and, 163-166, 165t
  2,3-diphosphoglycerate and, 547
  ehrlichiosis of, 481, 482, 830, 1066-1068, XIV
  electrophoresis of, 956, 958
  endotoxemia and, 832, 833t
  erythrocytes and. *See* Erythrocyte(s), horse
  fibrinogen and, 149, 161, 173t, 174, 961t

Horse(s) *(Continued)*
　foals, 144-149
　hematology of, 152t
　hemoglobin and, 140, 141t, 146, 151, 154, 518t
　hemogram of, 361t
　hemolytic anemia of, 158, 642, 1152-1153
　hemorrhage and, 98-99, 1150-1152
　herpesvirus and, 981
　hot-blooded. *See* Horse(s), hot-blooded
　immunoglobulin G and, 954
　impaired chemotaxis and, 718
　infectious anemia of. *See* Equine infectious anemia
　influenza of, 830
　lead poisoning and, 630-631
　leukemia complex in, 890-894
　leukocyte count and, 9t, 10t, 11, 141-142, 141t, 823
　leukocytes and, 158-159, 163-166, 165t, 173, 823, VII, XIV
　lymphocyte antigen of, 1002
　marrow aspiration and, 67
　myeloid:erythroid ratio of, 18t, 163, 164t
　myelomatosis and, 893t
　neonatal isoerythrolysis and, 650
　neutrophils and, 688, 701, 716
　normal blood values for, 10t, 141t, 149, 150t, 152t
　plasma protein and, 142, 144, 145t, 160-161, 172t, 961t
　platelets and, 6, 159, 447, *449*, 461, 469t
　plumbism and, 630-631
　quarter horse foals and, 144-149
　reticulocytes and, 156-158, 163, 499
　serum bilirubin and, 159
　strenuous exercise in, 141-142, 141t
　stress and, 163, 166-169
　thoroughbred foals and, 144-149
　thrombocytopenia and, 473t, 481
　thrombocytosis and, 470t
　transfusions and, 71-72
　trypanosomiasis and, 612
　vitamin B$_{12}$ and, 657
Horse(s), hot-blooded, 140, 149-163
　age and, 148t, 151
　bone marrow and, 161-163, 162t, 164t
　breed differences and, 154-155
　cold-blooded horse versus, 155
　corticosteroids and, 163-166, 165t
　erythrocytes and, 11, 140, 141t, 146, 151, 154, 155-158, 528, 619
　Heinz bodies and, 1152-1153
　lactation and, 151
　leukocytes and, 158-159
　normal values for, 9t, 10t, 11, 148t, 149, 150t
　plasma and, 159-161
　platelets and, 159
　pregnancy and, 151
　seasonal differences and, 151-154
　sex differences and, 151
　training and, 154
Horsefly(ies), 619
House fly(ies), 269
House sparrow(s), 270
Howell-Jolly body, 6, 661, *661*
　blood film and, 60
　cat, 130
　dog, 104
　horse, 155
^{3}HTdR. *See* Tritiated thymidine
Human epithelioid tissue cell culture(s), 78
Human leukocyte antigen(s), 999
Human serum albumin labeled with radioiodine, 87, 93
Humoral antibody(ies), 790
　macrophages and, 78
Humoral factor(s), 264
　hematopoietic, 372
　neutrophils and, 694, 696

Hurler's syndrome, 716, 782
HVS. *See* Hyperviscosity syndrome
Hyaenidae, 335t, 341
Hyalomma rufipes, 483
Hydration of animal. *See* Dehydration
Hydrochloric acid
　erythrocyte count and, 46
　iron and, 581-582
　leukocyte count and, 46
　stomach and, 382
Hydrocortisone, 690
　phagocytosis and, 708
Hydrocyte(s), 534t
Hydrocytosis, 534t, 543-544
Hydrogen peroxide
　macrophages and, 780-781
　methemoglobinemia and, 644
　phagocytosis and, 710
Hydrolase, acid, 684
Hyena(s), 335t, 341
Hyperadrenocorticism, 1054-1059
　biochemical evaluation and, 1055t
　hemograms and, 1057t
Hyperalbuminemia, 960
Hyperbilirubinemia, fasting, 160
Hypercalcemia, lymphoma and, 852, 871
Hypereosinophilia, 747-750
Hypereosinophilic syndrome, 749-750
Hyperestrogenism, 1100-1102
Hyperfibrinogenemia, 1093-1094
Hypergammaglobulinemia, 964
　feline infectious peritonitis and, 1069
Hyperglobulinemia in horse, 1157-1158
Hyperplasia, lymphoid, 600
Hyperproteinemia, 957
Hypersegmentation
　leukocyte, 115, *116*
　neutrophil, 659, 662, 826, 878, *879*
Hypersensitivity(ies). *See also* Allergy(ies); Sensitivity(ies)
　antilymphocyte serum and delayed, 1005
　basophils and, 762
　drug, in dog, 1113-1114
　immunoglobulin E and, 954
　mast cells and, 762
Hypersplenism
　case report of, 1114-1116
　platelets and, 441-442
　thrombocytopenia and, 475, 479-480
Hyperviscosity syndrome, 969-971
Hypervolemia, 87
Hypoadrenocorticism
　blood urea nitrogen and, 1061t
　dog, 1059-1063, 1060t, 1061t, 1099-1100
　hemogram and, 1060t
　screening for, 64
Hypoalbuminemia, 960
Hypobilirubinemia, 524
Hypochromasia, 583
Hypochromic anemia(s)
　macrocytic, 565, 566, 585, 656
　microcytic. *See* Microcytic hypochromic anemia(s)
Hypogammaglobulinemia, 964
　transient, 982
Hypophosphatemia, 643
Hypoplasia(s)
　of bone marrow, 666
　erythroid, 666, 668-671
Hypoproliferative anemia(s), 665-675
　aplastic anemia and, 665-668
　erythroid hypoplasia and, 668-671
　mineral deficiencies and, 662, 664-667
　nutritional deficiency and, 655-665. *See also* Nutritional deficiency(ies)

poodle macrocytosis and, 661-662
vitamin deficiency and, 660-661
Hypoproteinemia, 957
  acute blood loss and, 578
  dehydration and, 944
  dog, 1093-1094
  fascioliasis and, 586
  helminthiasis and, 585
  iron deficiency and, 583
  sheep, 218
Hyposegmentation of neutrophil, 826
Hypothyroidism
  anemia and, 671
  dog, 1063-1066, 1065t, 1094-1096
  hemogram and, 1065t
Hypovolemia, 87, 96-97
Hypovolemic shock, 96-97
Hypoxia
  erythropoietin and, 503, 505
  sheep hemoglobin and, 215

131I. *See* Radioiodine
Ia antigen
  lymphocytes and, 797
  macrophage and, 782
ICT. *See* Indirect Coombs test
Icterus. *See also* Icterus index
  bilirubin and, 524
  babesiosis and, 599, 601
  haemobartonellosis and, 605
  hepatic lipidosis in horse and, 1160, 1161
  leptospirosis in dog and, 1091, 1092-1093
  neutrophils and, 719
Icterus index, 3. *See also* Icterus
  cat, 136
  cattle, 188-189
  dog, 122
  fascioliasis and, 586
  foal, 147-149
  goat, 232
  hot-blooded horse, 159-160
  mouse, 307
  pig, 250
  rabbit, 282
  rat, 297
  sheep, 216
  Wintrobe hematocrit and, 39-41
Idiopathic anemia in dog, 470t
Idiopathic thrombocypenic purpura, 442, 472
  case report of, 1114-1116
α-L-Iduronidase, 716
Ig. *See* Immunoglobulin(s)
IgG antibody, 73, 1026
Iliac crest marrow aspiration, 66, *66*
Imidocarb
  anaplasmosis and, 595
  babesiosis and, 598, 599
Immune complex(es)
  autoimmune thrombocytopenic purpura and, 1023
  degranulation and, 703
  monocytes and macrophages and, 776
Immune deficiency disorder(s), 976-982
  clinical signs and diagnostic approach in, 977-978
  horse, case report of, 1155-1156
  primary, 978-979
  secondary, 979-981
  of undefined origin, 981-982
Immune response(s)
  cell-mediated, 808-811
  monocytes and macrophages and, 782
Immune surveillance, lymphocyte recirculation and, 803
Immune-mediated hemolytic anemia, 647-650, 649t

canine erythrocyte autoantibody and, 75
equine infectious anemia and, 619
newborn and, 73
Immune-mediated thrombocytopenia, 473, 478-479
Immunity
  cell-mediated, 790, 808-811
  newborn and, 979-981
  renal disease and, 670
  thymus and, 374
Immunoblasts, 814
Immunocompetent cells, 803
Immunocytes, 814
Immunoelectrophoresis, 957
  plasma proteins and, 941
Immunofluorescence
  antinuclear antibody and, 78
  antiplatelet antibody and, 77, 1019
  direct, 77
  equine infectious anemia and, 618
  immunoglobulin G and, 1020-1021
  indirect, 78
Immunoglobulin(s), 951-955. *See also* specific
    immunoglobulin
  antigenic specificity of molecule, 951
  basic structure of, 951-952
  classes and subclasses of, 951-954, 952t
  colostrum and, 944-945
  eosinophil and, 741
  Fc receptor for, 707, 797
  foal serum protein and, 149
  interstitial absorption of, 980
  lymphocytes and, 796
  maternal, failure of passive transfer of, 979-981
  plasma cells and, 814
  production of, 814
  selective deficiency of, 981-982
  serum levels of, 952t
  species differences and, 954-955
  surface, 796, 797
Immunoglobulin A, 953-954
  colostrum and, 944-945
  deficiency of, 982
  monocytes and macrophages and, 776
  and myeloma in dog, XIII
  neonatal serum and, 945
Immunoglobulin D, 954
Immunoglobulin E, 954
  monocytes and macrophages and, 776
Immunoglobulin G, 952-953
  autoimmune hemolytic anemia and, 1008, 1009
  autoimmune thrombocytopenia and, 1022
  cattle and, 955
  colostrum and, 944-945
  Coombs antiglobulin test and, 1011-1013
  foal serum protein and, 149
  immunofluorescence and, 1020-1021
  monocytes and macrophages and, 776
  neonatal serum and, 945
  opsonins and, 707
  phagocytosis and, 1014
  transient deficiency of, 982
Immunoglobulin G₁, 954
Immunoglobulin G₂, selective deficiency of, 982
Immunoglobulin G antibody, 73, 74, 74t, 78, 1026
Immunoglobulin M, 953
  autoimmune hemolytic anemia and, 1008, 1009
  colostrum and, 944-945
  erythrocytes coated with, 6
  foal serum protein and, 149
  hyperviscosity syndrome and, 969
  monocytes and macrophages and, 776
  neonatal serum and, 945
  nonspecific esterase and, 918
  opsonins and, 707

Immunoglobulin M *(Continued)*
  selective deficiency of, 981-982
  Waldenström's macroglobulinemia and, 968
Immunohematology, 990-1039
  antilymphocyte serum in, 1004-1005
  antinuclear antibodies in, 1026-1029
  autoimmune hematologic disorders in, 1007-1025. *See also* Autoimmune hematologic disorder(s)
  blood groups in, 991-993
  blood transfusions in, 993-996
  bone marrow transplantation in, 1006-1007
  hemolytic disease of newborn in, 996-998
  histocompatibility antigens in, 998-1004
  LE cell phenomenon and, 1026-1029, 1028t
  leukocyte antibodies and antigens in, 998-1004
  platelet antigens and antibodies in, 1005-1006
  red cell antigens in, 991-993
Immunologic tolerance, 1005
Immunoregulatory role of lymphocyte, 808
Immunosuppression
  antilymphocyte serum and, 1004
  autoimmune thrombocytopenic purpura and, 1024
  direct Coombs test and, 1013
  feline leukemia virus and, 846
  graft survival and, 1003
  leukemia complex and, 899
Immuran. *See* Azathioprine
Impala(s), 329, 333t
¹¹¹In. *See* Indium 111
Inclusion body(ies), 632. *See also* Heinz body(ies)
  canine distemper and, 1048
  new methylene blue stain and, 62
Incompatible erythrocyte, 994
Index(es), erythrocyte, 52-53
Indian water buffalo. *See* Water buffalo
Indigestion in cattle, 203t, 204
Indirect Coombs test, 73-75
  autoimmune hemolytic anemia and, 1011
Indirect immunofluorescence test, 78
¹¹¹Indium
  granulokinetics and, 686-687
  lymphokinetic studies and, 802, 803, 804
  neutrophil migration and, 690
  plasma volume and, 93
  platelet kinetics and, 441
Indomethacin, 694
Inducer T cell, 807
Ineffective erythropoiesis, 502
Infection(s)
  bacterial. *See* Bacterium(a)
  cat, 602. *See also* Feline infectious peritonitis
  eosinopenia and, 751-752
  equine infectious anemia and. *See* Equine infectious anemia
  erythrocyte sedimentation rate and. *See* Erythrocyte sedimentation rate
  hemolytic anemia and. *See* Infectious agents in hemolytic anemia(s)
  leukocytes and, 824, 826-827
  monocytosis and, 778
  neutrophil kinetics and, 693
  serum proteins and, 975
  sheep, 218
  spleen and, 378
  susceptibility to, 701
  thrombocytopenia and, 473, 475
  transfusions and, 995
  viral. *See* Virus(es)
Infectious agents in hemolytic anemia(s), 589-626
  bacterial infection and, 616-618
  blood parasites and, 596-616. *See also* Blood parasite(s)
Infectious enteritis, 1071-1074
Infectious hepatitis, canine, 830, 1049-1051
  natural infections and, 1050t

Infectious peritonitis, cat. *See* Feline infectious peritonitis
Inflammation(s)
  anemia and, 668-669
  cattle. *See* Cattle inflammatory disease(s)
  disseminated intravascular coagulopathy and, 411
  eosinophils and, 746, 751-752
  erythrocyte sedimentation rate and, 156
  leukocyte response and, 827
  lymphocyte recirculation and, 806
  monocytosis and, 778
  mononuclear phagocytes and, 771
  neutrophils and, 195, 690, 693, 712-714
  platelet and, 458-459
Influenza, equine, 830
Infusion(s). *See also* Transfusion(s)
  cryoprecipitate, 404-405, 406
  plasma, 415
Inheritance. *See* Genetics
Inhibitor(s)
  coagulation and, 398, 410, 414, 420
  lupus, 410
  plasma, 400-401
  thrombopoiesis and, 440
Injury(ies). *See* Trauma
¹¹¹In-oxine
  granulokinetics and, 686-687
  neutrophil migration and, 690
  platelet kinetics and, 441
Insect(s), equine infectious anemia and, 619
Insulin
  eosinopenia and, 750
  plasma proteins and, 943
Interferon, 810
  leukemia complex and, 899
  phagocytosis and, 708
  viral immunity and, 714
Interleukin(s), 810-811
  hematopoiesis and, 368
  leukemia complex and, 899
International Committee for the Nomenclature of Blood Clotting Factors, 393
International Committee on Standardization in Haematology, 87
Interstitial nephritis
  anemia and, 669-670
  case report of, 1094, 1095
  plasma proteins and, 974
Interstitial volume, 98
Intestinal obstruction, 95
Intestinal tract
  eosinophil and, 742-743
  Heinz bodies and, 638
  hematopoiesis and, 382-383
  plasma volume and obstruction of, 95
Intoxication. *See also* Toxicity
  rodenticide and aspirin, 1113
  water, 650-651
Intracellular fluid, 98
Intracellular hemolysis, 522
Intraerythrocytic defects, 643-647
Intrahepatic cholestasis, 160
Intramedullary phase, neutrophils and, 686-689
Intrauterine transfer of trypanosome, 613
Intravascular coagulation, disseminated. *See* Disseminated intravascular coagulation
Intravascular hemolysis, 520-522
  liver disease and, 670
Intravascular phase
  erythrocytes and, 548-550
  neutrophils and, 689-690
Intravascular thrombosis, diffuse, 410. *See also* Disseminated intravascular coagulation
Intrinsic factor, 657

Intrinsic membrane deformability, 551
Ionic transport, 543-544
Iron. *See also* Iron deficiency; Iron deficiency anemia
  absorption and transport of, 581-582
  cat with myeloproliferative disorder and, 860
  ceruloplasmin and, 949
  copper and, 664
  erythropoiesis and, 495, 509
  intestinal mucosa and, 382-383
  methemoglobin and, 643-644
  storage of, 382-383
  suckling pigs and, 243-244
  thrombocytosis and, 470
  transferrin and, 948
  vitamin B_6 deficiency and, 660
Iron deficiency, 17. *See also* Iron; Iron deficiency anemia
  anemia of inflammatory disease and, 669
  erythrogenesis and, 123
  goat, 226
  neutrophils and, 716, 719
  pig, 243-244
  thrombocyte production and, 440-441
Iron deficiency anemia, 581-584, 584t. *See also* Iron; Iron deficiency
  clinical and laboratory findings in, 582-584
  congenital, 181
  thrombocytosis and, 440, 470
Iron dextran
  cat and, 127
  goat and, 226
  pig and, 244
  sheep and, 209
Iron pyrophosphate, 244
Iron stain, 64
Iron sulfate, saturated solution of, 244
Irradiation. *See* Radiation
Isoantibody(ies) to leukocytes, 1000
Isoerythrolysis, neonatal, 73, 650, 996-998, 1154-1155
Isoimmune neonatal neutropenia, 1004
Isoimmune neonatal purpura, 479, 1004, 1005
Isoproterenol, 750
Isoton, 45, 50
Isotonic sodium chloride, 46, 48
Isotope(s). *See* specific isotope
Isotype of immunoglobulin(s), 952
Isozyme of esterase, 916
ITP. *See* Idiopathic thrombocytopenic purpura
Ivy bleeding time test, 420
Ixodid tick, 596
Ixodidae
  babesiosis and, 596
  theileriasis and, 610

J antigen, 991, 992, 995-996
J chain, 953
Jackrabbit(s)
  wild, 276, 280t
Jaguar(s), 334t
Jamshidi bone needle, 67
Jaundice, neutrophil activity and, 719. *See also* Icterus
Jaw paralysis, *878*
Jersey cattle, 182t, 183t, 193
Johne's disease
  case report of, 1165, 1167
  goat, 232
  immune deficiency and, 981
  protein loss and, 972
Jordon's anomaly, 717
Jugular vein, 25t, 26

K antigen, 991, 996
K cell(s). *See* Killer cell(s)
Kale, 640-641

Heinz bodies and, 634
Kallikrein, 712
  coagulation and, 394
Keratocyte(s), *536, 538*, 541
  etymology of, 534t
Ketamine, 4, 127
Kidney(ies)
  dog, 669-670, 1040-1043, 1041t, 1094, 1095
  erythrogenesis and, 123
  erythropoietin and, 504-505
  hematopoiesis and, 383
  leukemia therapy and, 900
  plasma proteins and, 974
Killer cell(s), 809
Kinetics
  eosinophil production, 739
  lymphocyte, 802
  monocytopoiesis, 769
  neutrophil, 685-695, 687t
  platelet, 441-442
Kinin, *395*, 761t
Kinkajou(s), 335t
Kitten(s)
  erythrocytes and, 127
  haemobartonellosis and, 605
Kjeldahl method for total proteins, 955
Knizocyte(s), *535, 537*, 541
  etymology of, 534t
Knott technique, modified, 80, 81-82
Ko antigens, 1005
Koala, 275
Koeppe's criterion for complete packing, 37
Krebs cycle, 545
Kupffer cell, 768
Kurloff's body, 793
  guinea pig and, 287-288, *288*
Kwashiorkor, 943

Labeling index, 686
Laboratory and miscellaneous animal(s), 274-349
  bovidae, 329-336
  camellidae, 336-337. *See also* Camel(s)
  canidae, 337
  cervidae, 321-322, 323t, 324t-325t, 337
  deer. *See* Deer
  elephantidae, 275, 333t, 338-339, VII
  equidae, 339-340
  felidae, 275, 340-341
  fur-bearing, 315-320, 316t
  gerbil, 308
  giraffidae, 330t, 333t, 341
  golden hamster, 308-310, 309t
  guinea pig. *See* Guinea pig(s)
  hyaenidae, 335t, 341
  monkey. *See* Monkey(s)
  mouse. *See* Mouse (mice)
  normal blood values of, 275
  rabbit. *See* Rabbit(s)
  rat. *See* Rat(s)
  tayassuidae, 333t, 341-342
  ursidae, 342
  water buffalo. *See* Water buffalo
  wild rodent species, 310-311
Lactation
  cattle hemogram and, 191
  goat erythrocyte and, 229
  mature hot-blooded horse and, 151
  pig, 245-247, 246t, 247t
  plasma proteins and, 944-945
Lactescence, plasma, 11
Lactic acid, phagocytosis and, 711
Lactoferrin, 684
  granulopoiesis and, 697-698

Lactoferrin *(Continued)*
  microbicidal mechanisms of, 711-712
Lama spp., 331t, 333t, 336-337
Lamb(s). *See also* Sheep
  hemograms and, 213t
  leptospirosis in, 616
Lamellipodium, 700
Larus argentatus, 270
Larva(ae), circulating, 82
Lazy leukocyte syndrome, 718
LD antigen(s). *See* Lymphocyte-defined antigen(s)
LE cell(s). *See* Lupus erythematosus cell
Lead poisoning
  anemia and, 515, 628-632
  bird, 271
  clinical signs of, 630
  dog, case report of, 1127-1129
  impaired bactericidal activity and, 719
Lean body mass, 87
Lecithin, 544-545
Lectin, 780
  lymphocyte migration and, 806
  macrophages and, 780
Lee-White clotting time test, 420-421
Left shift(s)
  acute blood loss and, 578
  cattle, 195
  definition of, 823
  degenerative, 823, 824, 1102-1104, 1158-1160
  degree of, 826
  dog, 115
  hepatic cell carcinoma and, 1104-1105
  mastitis and, 1162-1163
  pseudo, neutrophil and, 117
  pyometra and, 1102-1104
  rectal perforation and, 1158-1160
  regenerative, 823, 824, 1102, 1103
  sheep, 216
Leiomyoma(s), 581
Leishmaniasis
  canine, 1068
  phagocytosis and, 709, 780
  plasma proteins and, 973
Lemming, brown, 311
Lemmus trimucronatus alascensis, 311
Lemur(s), 276, 334t
Lens(es), microscope, 21-22
Leontocebus, 27-28
Leopard(s), 340
  hematologic values of, 334t, 335t
Leptocyte(s), 535, 537, 538, 539, 541-542
  anemia and, 570
  etymology of, 534t
Leptospirosis, 616-617
  case reports of, 1043-1046, 1045t, 1091, 1092-1093
Lethal trait A-46 in Black Pied Danish cattle, 979
Leukapheresis, 688-689
Leukeran. *See* Chlorambucil
Leukemia(s), 838-908
  acute lymphoblastic, 852
  acute lymphocytic, 874-876, 899, 918, 920, 921
  acute monocytic, 911-913, 918
  acute myelogenous, 716, 911-913, 918, 920, 921
  acute myelomonocytic, 911-913, 918, 921, XXIV
  acute promyelocytic, 918
  basophilic. *See* Basophilic leukemia
  bird, 267
  bovine, 884-890
  canine. *See* Canine leukemia complex
  cell properties and, 842
  chronic granulocytic, 690
  chronic lymphocytic, 874-876, 899, XXI
  chronic myelogenous, 915
  classification of, 840-841
  clonal origin of, 842-843

cytochemistry in diagnosis and classification of, 841t, 909- 910, 911t, 912t, 923-924
  eosinophilic, 839, 863-865, 864t, 894, 897
  equine, 890-894
  etiology of, 843-844
  feline. *See* Feline leukemia complex
  goat, 894-895
  granulocyte vacuolation and, 861, *862*, *879*
  granulocytic. *See* Granulocytic leukemia
  guinea pigs, 287
  incidence of, 843-844
  laboratory characterization of, 838-840
  leukemoid reaction and, 824-825
  leukocyte count and, 829
  lymphoblastic, 852, 924
  lymphocytic. *See* Lymphocytic leukemia(s)
  mast cell, 865-867, *865*, *866*, 880-882, *881*, *883*, XXII
  megakaryocytic, 867, 880-881
  monocytic, 839, 863, 880, 894, 911-913, 918, 923
  myelogenous. *See* Myelogenous leukemia
  myeloid. 698, 839, 897, 923, 924
  myelomonocytic. *See* Myelomonocytic leukemia
  pig, 896-897
  plasma cell, 924
  pluripotential stem cell and, 366-367
  sheep, 895-896
  subclassification of, 840-842
  subleukemic granulocytic, 862, 862t
  therapy of, 840-842
  transformations of cell lines and, 842
Leukemia virus, bovine, 884-886
Leukemia virus, feline. *See* Feline leukemia virus
Leukemia-associated inhibitory activity, 698
Leukemic cell(s)
  properties of, 842
  vacuolation of, 861, *862*, *879*
Leukemic leukemia, 838
Leukemogenic virus(es), 843-844
Leukemoid blood picture(s), 824-825
Leukemoid reaction in chronic peritonitis, 1105-1106
Leukergy, 52
Leukin, microbicidal mechanisms of, 711
Leukocyte(s), 6-7, 821-837. *See also* Leukocytosis;
      Leukopenia; specific leukocyte type
  acute blood loss and, 578
  anaphylaxis and, 836
  antibodies and. *See* Leukocyte antibody(ies)
  autoimmune hemolytic anemia and, 649, 649t
  bacteria and, 196, 826-827, 831-836
  basophil. *See* Basophil(s)
  birds, 257-258, 261-262
  blood film and, 60-62, *61*
  buffy coat and, 38
  cat, 130t, 132-136, 823, VII, IX, XIV
  cattle. *See* Leukocyte(s), cattle
  cell transit and, 364
  classification of, in response to disease, 823-826
  comparative properties of species and, 910t
  corticosteroids and, 111, *111*, 112t, 825-826, 827
  count of. *See* Leukocyte count(s)
  cytochemistry of, 909-939. *See also* Cytochemistry
  decrease in. *See* Leukopenia
  degenerative left shift of. *See* Left shift(s)
  disease process and response of, 826-827
  distemper and, 1048
  DNA viscosity test and, 67-69, *68*, 69t
  dog, 109-119, 110t, 823, 1048, VII, XIV
  elephant, 338-339, VII
  endotoxins and, 827, 831-836
  eosinophil. *See* Eosinophil(s)
  fox, 320
  goat, 228t, 231
  guinea pig, 283-288, 285t, 286t
  hamster, 309t, 310

hematopoiesis in prenatal and early postnatal life and, 352, 356-359
hemocytometer and count of, 45-48
heterophil. *See* Heterophil(s)
horse. *See* Leukocyte(s), horse
hypersegmentation and, 115, *116*
increase in. *See* Leukocytosis
interpretation of picture of, 827-829
isoantibodies in, 1000
laboratory animals and, 275
left shift of. *See* Left shift(s)
leukemoid blood picture and, 824-825
leukoerythroblastic reaction and, 825
leukopenias and, 829-836
locomotion of, 700
lymphocyte. *See* Lymphocyte(s)
mobilization of, 701
monkey, 313-314, 312t
mononuclear, 7
mouse, 301t, 302t, 304t, 305t, 306-307
neutrophil. *See* Neutrophil(s)
old blood and, 5
physiologic leukocytosis and. *See* Physiologic leukocytosis
pig, 241, 243, 245-249, 246t
polymorphonuclear, 7. *See also* Neutrophil(s)
pulmonary circulation and, 691
rabbit, 278t, 279t, 280-282
rat, 291t, 292t, 294t, 295t, 296-297
reserve of, 687-689
rickettsial infection and, 830-831
seasonal variation in, 109
septicemia and, 201, 836
sheep, 209, 210t, 215-216, 217t
species variation in, 821-823
stress and, 11
surface features of, 555, 679-682, *683*
transfusion of, 994
viral diseases and, 829-830
water buffalo, 327-329
zeta potential of surface of, 555
Leukocyte(s), cattle, 185-187, *187*, 187t, 823, VII
disease and, *196*, 201-204
morphology of, 195-197
parturition and, 191, 192t, *193*
Leukocyte(s), horse, 141t, 158-159, VII, XIV
corticosteroids and, 163-166, 165t
disease and, 169-174, *173*
foal and, 147, 147t
mature hot-blooded, 151, 154, 155
strenuous exercise and, 141-142, 141t
Leukocyte antibody(ies), 827, 998-1004
human, 998-999
techniques to detect, 1000
Leukocyte antigen(s), 998-1004
human, 1000
techniques to detect, 1000
Leukocyte count(s), 2, 3, 9t, 10t, 11. *See also* Blood cell count(s)
absolute, 824
avian, 261-263
cat, 9t, 10t, 11, 130t, 132-136, 823, VII, IX, XIV
cattle, 9t, 10t, 11, 823
differential. *See* Differential cell count(s)
DNA viscosity test, by, 67-69, *68*, 69t
dog, 9t, 10t, 11, 110t, 823
eosinophil, 64-65
hemocytometer and, 45-48
horse, 9t, 10t, 11, 141-142, 141t, 823
physiologic variations in. *See* Physiologic leukocytosis
relative, 824
species differences in, 7, 9t, 10t
stress effect on, 11

trends in, 828-829
Leukocytosis, 696, 823
diminishing, 828
dog, 113, 114t, 870, 873t, 1104-1105
hepatic cell carcinoma and, 1104-1105
horse, 169, 1158, 1159
physiologic. *See* Physiologic leukocytosis
pyelonephritis and, 1158, 1159
sheep, 215-216
Leukocytosis inducing factor, 696
Leukocytosis promoting factor, 696
Leukocytozoon species, 269-270
Leukoerythroblastic reaction, 570, 825
Leukokinin, 708
Leukopenia, 823, 829-836
age and, 109-111
amyloidosis and, 1119-1121
cat, 1134-1135, 1136, 1137-1138, 1142-1143
cattle, 201, 1162-1163
dog, 870, 873t, 1119-1121
foal, 147
inflammatory response in cattle and, 201
interpretation of, 828
leptospirosis and, 616
lymphoma and, 870, 873t
lymphosarcoma and, 1142-1143
mastitis and, 1162-1163
pig, 248
sheep, 216
toxoplasmosis and, 1137-1138
Leukopoietin G, 696
Leukosis
bird, 265t, 266-268
cattle, 187
Leukosis/sarcoma complex, avian, 265t, 266-268
Leukotaxine, 712
Levamisole
autoimmune hemolytic anemia and, 1016
chemotaxis and, 718
Lewis antigen, 991, 992, 995-996
Lidocaine, marrow aspiration and, 66, 67
LIF. *See* Leukocytosis inducing factor
Life span of erythrocyte(s), 155, 547-550, 549t, 583, 585
Light chain(s), 951-952
Light chain disease, 968
Light microscopy
erythropoiesis and, 488-491, *490*
neutrophils and, 676-677
Lion(s), 334t, 340-341, *340*
Lipemia(s). *See also* Lipid(s)
blood film and, 60, *61*
diabetes mellitus and, 1096-1097
hemoglobin concentration error and, 53
with hepatic lipidosis, 1160, 1161
hot-blooded horse and, 161
plasma compartment and, 40
postprandial, 11, 1089-1090
Lipid(s). *See also* Lipemia(s)
erythrocyte membrane and, 531-532
lipid A and, 694
mast cells and basophils and, 761t
monocytes and, 777
refractive index and, 56
Lipid A, 694
Lipid chemotactic factor, 761t
Lipidosis, hepatic, 1160, 1161
Lipoprotein(s), 950-951
LISS. *See* Low ionic strength solution(s)
Listeria
monocytes and, 281
phagocytosis and, 707, 709
Lithium
cyclic hematopoiesis and, 118
degranulation and, 703
granulopoiesis and, 697

Liver
    abscess of, in dog, *965*
    anemia and, 670-671
    carcinoma of, 1104-1105
    cat, 351-352, *354*
    coagulation and, 397, 399, 409-410, 409t
    equine infectious anemia and, 619
    flukes and, 586
    hematopoiesis and, 350, 351-352, *354*, 380-381
    impression smear of, *354*
    inflammation of. *See* Hepatitis
    lipidosis and, 1160, 1161
    plasma proteins and, 973-974
    platelet disorder and, 467
    thrombocytopenia and, 475
Liver fluke(s), 586
Llama(s), 331t, 333t, 336-337
Locomotion defect(s), 717-719
Loeffler's syndrome, 750
Long-Evans rat(s), 290t, 291t, 292t
Low ionic strength solution(s), 75
Low-density lipoprotein(s), 950-951
Lowry method for total proteins, 955
Loxodonta africana, 339
LPF. *See* Leukocytosis promoting factor
Lung(s)
    eosinophils and, 742
    leukocyte migration and, 691
Lungworm(s), swine, 287
Lupus anticoagulant, 1026
Lupus erythematosus, systemic, 77-79, 1026
    dog, 1121-1123
Lupus erythematosus cell, 77, 78-79, *79*, XIV
    autoimmune hemolytic anemia and, 1011, 1146-1148
    cat, 859, 1146-1148
    dog, 1121-1123
Lupus inhibitor, 410
Lymph node(s). *See also* Lymphadenopathy(ies)
    canine lymphoma and, 871
    cross section of, *379*
    equine, cytology of, 892
    granulocytic leukemia and, 880, *880*
    hematopoiesis and, 379-380
    lymphocytes and, 380, 805
    lymphoma and, 871, 892
    lymphopoiesis and, 801
    new methylene blue stain and, 62
    prenatal development of, 351
    Theileria parva and, 611
Lymphadenopathy(ies). *See also* Lymph node(s)
    cat, 1143-1144
    dog, 869
    horse, 891
Lymphangiectasia
    dog, 1132-1133
    protein loss and, 972
Lymphatic tissue(s), hematopoiesis and, 372-380
Lymphoblast(s), lymphoma and, 850-851, *850*
Lymphoblastic leukemia
    diagnosis of, 924
    feline, 852
Lymphocyte(s), 7, 14, 35, 36, 790-812. *See also*
        Lymphocytosis; Lymphopenia
    age and, 109-111
    antibodies and, 807-808
    avian, 257-258, 262-264
    B. *See* B cell(s)
    bone marrow and, 15, 16
    cat, 132, 134
    cattle, 186-187, 191, 192t, *193*, 196, 791-792, 889t
    chinchilla, 319
    classification of, 790
    corticosteroids and, 119, 811-812
    count of, 35, 36

criteria for characterization of, 791t
cytochemistry, 794, 795
dog, 119
ecotaxis, 806
elephant, 338, *338*
entry of, into lymph nodes, 805
foal, 147
functional differentiation of, *799*
functions of, 807-811
gerbil, 308
goat, 231, 238
guinea pig, 287
hot-blooded horse and, 158, 159
leukemoid blood picture and, 825
life span of, 803
lymph node and, 380, 805
lymphokinetics in, 802-803
lymphopoiesis and, 798-802
macrophage and, 782
mink, 316t, 317
monkey, 314, 315
morphology of, 790-794
mouse, 306-307
muscular activity and, 113, 113t
muskrat, 316t, 319
neutrophil ratio and. *See* Neutrophil:lymphocyte
        ratio
old blood sample and, 5
peripheral blood and, 792t, 811-812
pig, 248-249, *251*, 252, 805-806
pool of, 811
qualitative and quantitative differences of, 803
rabbit, 280, 281
raccoon, 316t, 318
rat, 297, *297*, 298
recirculation of, 803-807
regulation of, 372
sequential development of, *799*
sheep, 216, *219*, 220-222, *221*, 804
stimulation of, 800
subpopulation, 790-791, 791t, 792t, 795-798
supplementary, 805
T. *See* T cell(s)
theileriasis and, 610
transit time of, 804
ultrastructure of, 791, *793*, *794*
viral immunity and, 714
water buffalo and, 328
Lymphocyte antigen(s), 1001-1002
Lymphocyte cytotoxicity test, 999, 1000
Lymphocyte mitogenic factor, 810
Lymphocyte-defined antigen(s), 999
Lymphocyte:neutrophil ratio. *See*
        Neutrophil:lymphocyte ratio
Lymphocytic leukemia(s), 839
    acute, 874-876, 899, 918, 920, 921
    cat, XXI
    cattle, 196, 200
    chemotherapy and, 899
    chronic, 874-876, 899
    diagnosis of, 924
    dog, 874-876, XXI
    erythrogenesis and, 123
    horse, 892
    hyperviscosity syndrome and, 970
    nonspecific esterase and, 918
    peroxidase and, 920
    sudanophilia and, 921
    terminal deoxynucleotidyl transferase and, 921
Lymphocytosis, 811
    babesiosis and, 600
    canine lymphoma and, 870, 873t
    cattle, 186, 615, 1163-1164

hospitalization and, 113
persistent, 829
traumatic reticulitis and splenitis and, 1163-1164
trypanosomes and, 615
Lymphoid cell(s)
  babesiosis and, 600
  hematopoietic differentiation and, *366*
  tumors of, birds and, 264-268
Lymphoid hyperplasia, 600
Lymphoid leukemia, 698
Lymphoid leukosis, 265t, 266-268
Lymphoid malignancy(ies), feline, 849-852, 850t, *850,*
  851
Lymphoid organ(s)
  central, 798
  migration of lymphocytes through, 804-806
  peripheral, 798, 801-802
  primary, 798
  secondary, 798
Lymphoid tissue(s)
  hematopoiesis and, 372-380
  T- and B-lymphocytes in, 790-791, 796-797. *See also* B
    cell(s); T cell(s)
Lymphokine(s), 809-811
Lymphokinetics, 802-803
Lymphoma(s) or lymphosarcoma(s)
  alimentary or abdominal form of, 848
  bovine, 198, 200, 884, 886-890, 888t, 889t, *890*, 891t
  Burkitt's, 876
  canine, 480, 869-876, 871t, 872t, 873t, *966, 969, 970*
  classification of, 841-842
  clinical staging of, 900
  diagnosis of, 924
  equine, 890-893
  feline, 847-852, 1142-1143
  goat, 894
  hereditary form of, 897
  histopathologic and immunologic characterization of,
    873-874
  hyperviscosity syndrome and, 970
  leukocyte count and, 829
  lymphocyte production and, 802
  multicentric form of, 848
  ovine, 895-896
  pig, 896-897
  protein loss and, 972
  thymic form of, 848
Lymphopenia, 811
  age and, 111
  cat, 1138
  dog, 119, 870, 873t
  horse, 1156-1157
  lymphoma and, 870, 873t
  pericarditis and bronchitis and, 1156-1157
  peritonitis and, 1138
  persistent, 119
  radiation and, 667-668
Lymphopoiesis, 798-802
  blastogenesis and, 799-800
  bone marrow and, 800-801
  factors influencing, 369t
  hematopoietic inductive microenvironment and, 370
  long and short production pathways in, 799
  marrow, 801
  ontogeny and, 798-799
  peripheral lymphoid organs and, 801-802
  regulation of, 802
  thymus and, 801
Lymphoproliferative disorder(s), 267
  acid phosphatase and, 911
  bovine, 886-890
  canine, 869-876
  classification of, 841-842
  clonal, 807

equine, 890-893
feline, 847-852
therapy of, 897-900
Lymphosarcoma(s). *See* Lymphoma(s) or
  lymphosarcoma(s)
Lymphotoxin(s), 810
Lysis
  clot, 399-402
  erythrocyte destruction and, 551
Lysis time, euglobulin, 401-402
Lysosomal enzyme(s), 776, 779
  degranulation of, 702
  monocytes and macrophages and, 784
Lysosomal hydrolase, 784
Lysosome(s), neutrophil, 683-684, 712-714
Lysozyme(s), 683-684, 922-923
  microbicidal mechanisms of, 711

Macaca mulatta, 311-315, 312t
Macaque, 311-315, 312t
  immunodeficiency syndrome and, 982
Macrocyte(s), 502-503, *537, 539*, 542, 578. *See also*
  Reticulocyte(s)
  etymology of, 534t
  poodle macrocytosis and, 661-662, 663t
Macrocytic anemia(s), 565
  folic acid deficiency and, 656
  hypochromic, 566, 585
  normochromic, 565-566
Macrocytosis, poodle, 661-662, 663t
α_2-Macroglobulin, 714, 948
  clotting regulation and, 398
Macroglobulinemia, Waldenström's, 968-969, 970
Macrophage(s), 14, 829. *See also* Monocyte(s)
  activated, 783
  antibody production and, 807-808
  armed, 783
  canine, VIII
  definitions of, 774
  erythrocyte phagocytosis and, 555
  functions of, 778-785, 778t, 779t
  inflammation and, 458-459
  iron and, 582
  Kurloff cells and, 288
  lymphocytes and, 782
  membranes and, 781
  morphology of, 772-775, *773, 774*
  origin, development, and kinetics of, 770-771
  mouse peritoneal, 784
  resident, 774
Macrophage activating factor, 810
Macrophage-CSF, 371
Macrophage-lymphocyte interaction, 782
Macropolycyte(s), 716
MAF. *See* Macrophage activating factor
Major basic protein, 738, 746
Major histocompatibility complex, 999
Major histocompatibility system, 999, 1001, 1001t
Malabsorption syndrome(s), 943, 972
Malaria, avian, 268-269
Malay chevrotain, 275
Malaysian swamp buffalo, 329
Malignancy(ies). *See also* Leukemia(s); Neoplasia(s)
  anemia and, 671
  categorization of, 838, 839t
  erythropoietin and, 507
  leukocyte response and, 827, 1004
  radiation-induced, 882-884
  subclassification of, 840-842
Malignant histiocytosis, XIII
Mallard duck, 271
Mammary gland, macrophages and, 777
m-AMSA, 899

Mancini's method of radial immunodiffusion, 957
Mange, 800
Mannosidase, 923
Mare(s), colostrum of, 980. *See also* Horse(s)
Marek's disease, 264-266, 265t
Marginal pool of granulocyte(s), 689
Maroteaux-Lamy syndrome, 716
Marrow, bone. *See* Bone marrow
Marrow transit time, eosinophil and, 739-740
Mast cell(s), 756-767, 758t, 761t
  biochemical composition of, 760
  biologic properties of, 760-762
  blood basophil and, 756
  bone marrow and, 15
  eosinophils and, 744, 746
  functions of, 762-764
  granules and, 759-760
  morphology of, 757-760
  production and distribution of, 756-757
Mast cell leukemia
  canine, 880-882, *881, 883*
  feline, 865-867, *865, 866,* XXII
Mast cell mediator, 744, 746
Mastitic milk, neutrophils from, 707, 719
Mastitis, bovine, 1076-1081, 1162-1163
  bacterial phagocytosis and, 707, 719
  bone marrow response and, 197, 199t
  coliform, 831, 1078-1081
  experimental, 1078-1081
  hemogram and, 1077t
  left shift in, 1162-1163
  leukogram and, 1080t
  leukopenia and, 1162-1163
Mastocytemia, 829
Mastocytoma, postprandial lipemia and, 1089-1090
Match-stick form erythrocyte(s), 528
Maternal antibody(ies), 979-981
  thrombocytopenia in neonate and, 479
Maternal immunoglobulin transfer, 979-981
Maturation
  erythrocyte, 12-13, 363-364. *See also* Erythropoiesis
  granulocyte, 13t, 16, 17-18, 118. *See* Granulocytopoiesis
  megakaryocyte, 14t-15t, 435, *435, 436. See also* Megakaryocytopoiesis
May-Hegglin anomaly, 717
MBP. *See* Major basic protein
MCH. *See* Mean corpuscular hemoglobin
MCHC. *See* Mean corpuscular hemoglobin concentration
M-component, 965
M-CSF. *See* Macrophage-CSF
MCV. *See* Mean corpuscular volume
M:E ratio. *See* Myeloid:erythroid ratio
Mean corpuscular hemoglobin, 52
  anaplasmosis and, 592
  bird, 261
  cat, 127, 128, 129
  cattle, 179
  dog, 104, 107
  elephant, 338
  error in, 53
  fox, 320
  goat, 226
  horse, 151, 154
  mouse, 299
  pig, 245
  rat, 296
  sheep, 209
Mean corpuscular hemoglobin concentration, 52-53
  anaplasmosis and, 592
  anemia and, 565, 649, 649t
  bird, 256, 257-258, 259, 261
  Camellidae, 336

cat, 128
cattle, 179
dog, 104, 107
error in, 53
fox, 320
goat, 225-226, 229t
horse, 146, 151, 154
monkey, 313
mouse, 299
pig, 245
rabbit, 280
rat, 296
sheep, 209
Mean corpuscular volume, 52
  anaplasmosis and, 592
  anemia and, 565, 568-569, 604, 649, 649t
  bear, 342
  cat, 127, 128, 552
  cattle, 179
  clinical condition and, 58t
  dog, 104, 107
  elephant, 338
  error in, 53
  erythrocyte osmotic fragility and, 552
  fox, 320
  goat, 225-226, 229t
  guinea pig, 283
  hamster, 308
  horse, 146, 151, 154
  monkey, 311
  mouse, 299
  pig, 244, 245
  rat, 296
  sheep, 209
  water buffalo, 322
Mechanical fragility, 71
  canine erythrocyte and, 109
Mediator release, 762-763
Medullary reticulosis, histiocytic, XIII
Megakaryoblast(s), 14, 432
  ultrastructure and cytochemistry of, 434
Megakaryocyte(s), 14, *434*
  autoimmune thrombocytopenia and, 1018, 1019, 1020
  bone marrow and, 15
  colony forming unit, 368, 371-372, 431
  colony stimulating factor and, 372
  development and maturation of, 432
  direct immunofluorescence of, 77
  maturation of, 14t-15t, 435, *435, 436. See also* Megakaryocytopoiesis
  platelet product and, 437-439
  prenatal and early postnatal hematopoiesis and, 354, *354*
  reduction in effective, 1022
  thrombocythemia and, 471
Megakaryocytic leukemia
  canine, 880-881
  feline, 867
Megakaryocytopoiesis, 431-441
  in canine bone marrow, III
  cytomorphology of, 432-433
  regulation of, 369t, 371-372, 438-441
  ultrastructure and cytochemistry of, 433-436, *435*
Megaloblast(s), 17
  vitamin deficiency anemia and, 658
Megaloblastoid rubriblast(s), 858, *859*
Megalocyte(s), *537, 539,* 542
  etymology of, 534t
Megathrombocyte(s), 197, 454
Melphalan, 898
  hyperviscosity syndrome and, 971
  plasma cell myeloma and, 968
  Waldenström's macroglobulinemia and, 968
Melursus ursinus, 335t

Membrane(s)
 cholesterol, 544
 erythrocyte. *See* Erythrocyte membrane(s)
 lipids and, 531-532, 544
 macrophages and, 781
 phospholipid, 544
 platelets and, 453
 proteins and, 532, 628
Memory cell(s), 801
Menadione, 408
Menaquinone, 408
Mendelian inheritance of blood groups, 991
6-Mercaptopurine, 898, 899, 900
 autoimmune hemolytic anemia and, 1017
 neutrophil abnormalities and, 716
Mesenchymal cell(s), 756-757
Messenger RNA, 492, 495, 516
Metabolic acidosis
 canine babesiosis and, 599
 plasma volume and, 95
Metabolic burst, 706
Metabolic intoxication, leukocyte response and, 827
Metabolism, 739
 eosinophil, 739
 erythrocyte, 545-547
 hemolytic anemia and, 642-643
 lymphocyte, 795
 monocyte, 775
 neutrophil, 684
 plasma protein and, 942-943
Metachromasia, 757
Metagranuloblast(s), 263
Metamyelocyte(s), 13, 677
 basophilic, 13
 cat, 133
 cattle, 195
 dog, 115
 eosinophilic, 13
 monkey, 315
 pig, 252
Metarubricyte(s), 12, 490, *494*, 495-496, *496*
 bone marrow and, 15
 generation time of, 502
 iron deficiency anemia and, 583, XVII
 normochromatic, XIX
Metastasis, platelet and, 460
Methacrylate, 19
Methemalbumin, 949
Methemoglobinemia, 4, 546, 643-645
Methotrexate, 898, 899, 900
 antilymphocyte serum and, 1005
 graft survival and, 1003
 neutrophils and, 716, 719
Methyl alcohol in staining, 32, 33
Methyl green-pyronin reaction, 911t, 919
 avian leukosis and, 266
 technique for, 930-931
Methylene blue, 31-32
 cat hemolytic anemia and, 131
 Heinz bodies and, 638, *639*, 640
Methyl-tetrahydrofolate trap, 658
MHC. *See* Major histocompatibility complex
MHS. *See* Major histocompatibility system
Mice. *See* Mouse (mice)
Microbicidal activity(ies)
 monocytes and macrophages and, 779-781
 neutrophils and, 708-712, 708t, 719
Microbody(ies), 683, 684t
Microcapillary hematocrit, 37
 microfilariae and, 80-81, *81*
Microcirculation, 550
Microcyte(s), *535*, *537*, 542
 entymology of, 534t
Microcytic hypochromic anemia(s)

chronic blood loss and, 1125-1126
 copper deficiency and, 662
 dog, 583, *583*, 660, 1125-1127
 erythrocytes and, 583, *583*
 erythroid hypoplasia and, 668
 subacute blood loss and, 1126-1127
Microcytosis, 583
 cat, 127
 pig, 247
Microenvironment, hematopoietic inductive, 369-370
Microfilament(s)
 leukocyte movement and, 700
 platelets and, 451-452
Microfilaria(iae)
 bird, 270
 canine blood and, 79-82, 80t
 circulating larvae and, 82
Microglial cell(s), 768
β₂-Microglobulin, 954
Microhematocrit, 3, 41
Micro-lymphocytotoxic test, 1000
Microperoxisome, 683, 684t
Microscope(s), 21-22
Microscopy
 electron. *See* Electron microscope
 light, 488-491, *490*, 676-677
 platelets and, 446-450, *447*, *448*, *449*, *450*
 stained blood film, 35-36
Microthrombocyte(s), 453
Microtubule(s)
 erythrocyte and, 528
 leukocyte movement and, 700
Midge, 269
MIF. *See* Migration inhibition factor
Migration, neutrophil, 698-701, 699t
Migration inhibition factor, 719, 810
Migration pore(s), 695
Milk
 bacteriostatic system in, 710
 mastitic, neutrophils from, 707, 719
Mineral(s)
 deficiencies of, 662, 664-665
 erythrocyte production and, 509
Miniature swine, 245
Mink, 315-318, 971
Mirror(s), substage, 22
Mitosis(es), 14, 810
 granulopoiesis and, 686-687
Mitosis stimulating factor, 810
Mitotic figure(s), 14
Mixed lymphocyte reaction(s), 999
Mixed platelet thrombus(i), 416
MLR. *See* Mixed lymphocyte reaction(s)
MLR test. *See* Micro-lymphocytotoxic test
Molybdenosis, 548, 665, 665t
Molybdenum, 548, 664, 665
Monkey(s), 311-315, 312t
 blood collection and, 27-28
 blood volume measurement and, 91t, 94
Monoblast(s), 772
Monoclonal antibody(ies), leukemia complex and, 899
Monoclonal gammopathy(ies), 964-967
 benign, 970, 971
Monocyte(s), 7, 14. *See also* Macrophage(s);
   Monocytosis
 bird, 258, 262
 cat, 134
 cattle, 191, 192t, *193*, 196-197, 201
 chemotaxis of, 776-777
 corticosteroids and, 119, 776, 777-778, 781
 cytochemistry of, 775-776
 dog, 119, 771, *773*, VIII
 elephant, 338, *338*, 339, *339*
 function of, 778-788

Monocyte(s) *(Continued)*
  goat, 231, 238
  guinea pig, 287
  hamster, 310
  horse, 159, 169
  kinetics of, 769-770
  metabolism of, 775-776
  mink, 316t, 317
  monkey, 314
  morphology of, 771-772
  mouse, 307, *307*
  numbers of, in blood, 777-778
  nucleus of, 119
  old blood sample and, 5
  origin of, 769-770
  pig, *251*, 252
  rabbit, 281
  raccoon, 316t, 318
  rat, 296, 297
  sheep, 219, *220*, 222
  surface receptors, 776
  water buffalo, 328
Monocytic leukemia, 839
  acid phosphatase activity and, 911-913
  acute, 911-913, 918
  canine, 880
  diagnosis of, 923
  equine, 894
  feline, 863
  nonspecific esterase and, 918
Monocytoid cell(s)
  dog, 880
  cat, 861, *861*
Monocytopenia, 777-778
Monocytopoiesis, 769
  factors influencing, 369t
  inhibition of, 371, 770
Monocytosis, 777-778
  canine, 880
  corticosteroid-induced, 111, 198, 201
  interpretation of, 828-829
Monokine, 784
Mononuclear cell(s), 7. *See also* Mononuclear phagocyte
        system
  inflammation and, 771
  spleen and, 377
Mononuclear phagocyte system, 380, 768
  disseminated intravascular coagulopathy and, 415
  hematopoiesis and, 380
  hemoglobin catabolism and, 522-523
  inflammation and, 771
  platelets and, 442
  secretory product of, 779, 779t
Mordant for blood and tissue cell(s), 32
Morphology, 5-7, 8t. *See also* Blood cell(s); Blood
        picture(s) in disease of domestic animals; specific
        cell type
  artifact of, 6
Mosquito(es), avian malaria and, 268-269
Mott cell(s), 812
Mountain lion(s), 334t, 340-341, *340*
Mouse (mice), 298-308
  blood collection from, 25t, 26
  blood volume and, 91t, 94
  Bolivian field, 310-311
  colony stimulating factor and, 697
  deer, 310-311
  hemoglobin and, 518t
  monocytosis and, 778
  peritoneal macrophages and, 784
  spiny, 310-311
  thymectomized, 374
  vesper, 310-311
MP. *See* 6-Mercaptopurine
MPD. *See* Myeloproliferative disorder(s)

MPI. *See* Monocytopoiesis, inhibition of
MPO. *See* Myeloperoxidase
MPO-H_2O_2-halide system, 710
M-protein, 965
MPS. *See* Mononuclear phagocyte system
mRNA. *See* Messenger RNA
Mucopolysaccharide(s), basophil granules and, 757-758.
        See also Mucopolysaccharidosis(es)
Mucopolysaccharidosis(es), 716-717
  canine, XIII
  macrophages and, 782
Mucoprotein(s), 948
Mucosa, intestinal
  hematopoiesis and, 382-383
  iron absorption and, 582
Mucosal transferrin, 582
Mule(s), 339-340
  babesiosis and, 601
  hematologic values of, 332t
  neonatal isoerythrolysis and, 650
Mule deer, 321, 548
Multiple myeloma. *See* Myeloma(s)
Multipotential stem cell(s). *See* Pluripotent stem cell(s)
Muntiacus muntjak, 321
Muscular activity(ies)
  cattle hemogram and, 189
  horse lymphocytosis and, 166, 167-169, 168t
Muskrat(s), 316t, 318-319
Mustargen, 695, 898, 900
Mycobacterium, 780
  phagocytosis and, 703, 707, 709
Myeloblast(s), 13, 677
  electron microscopy and, 677-679, *678*
Myeloblastosis, 266-267
Myelocyte(s), 677
  basophilic, 13
  electron microscopy and, 679, *681*
  eosinophilic, 13
  neutrophilic, 13
Myelocyte sink, 687
Myelocytomatosis, 266-267
Myelodysplastic syndrome, feline, 867
Myelofibrosis
  feline, 854
  goat, 895
Myelogenous leukemia, 839, 876-880, 877t. *See also*
        Granulocytic leukemia
  acid phosphatase and, 911-913, 915
  acute, 716, 911-913, 918, 920, 921
  canine, 876-880, 877t
  chronic, 690, 915
  diagnosis of, 923
  equine, 894
  feline, 860-863
  neutrophil abnormalities and, 716
  nonspecific esterase and, 918
  peroxidase and, 920
  pig, 897
  sudanophilia and, 921
  terminal deoxynucleotidyl transferase and, 921
Myeloid cell(s)
  hematopoietic differentiation and, *366*
  stimulation of, 370
Myeloid leukemia, 839. *See also* Granulocytic leukemia;
        Myelogenous leukemia
  diagnosis of, 923, 924
  granulopoiesis and, 698
  pig, 897
Myeloid:erythroid ratio, 17-18, 18t
  cat, 137-138, 137t
  cattle, 18t, 197
  chinchilla, 319
  dog, 121t, 122t, 123
  gerbil, 308

goat, 18t, 238
guinea pig, 288
hamster, 310, 311t
hot-blooded horse, 163, 164t
monkey, 314-315
mouse, 307
pig, 18t, 250
rabbit, 282
rat, 298, 299t
sheep, 18t, 222
Myelokathexis, 695
Myeloma(s). *See also* Myelomatosis
    multiple, 893-894, 893t, *895*, *896*, 967-968
    plasma cell, 16, 812, 971, 1130-1132, 1134, 1135
Myeloma protein, 965
Myelomatosis, *966*, *969*. *See also* Myeloma(s)
Myelomonocytic leukemia, 839
    acid phosphatase and, 911-913
    acute, 911-913, 918, 921, XXIV
    diagnosis of, 923
    dog, 880, XXIV
    equine, 894
    feline, 863
    isozyme and, 916
    nonspecific esterase and, 918
    sudanophilia and, 921
Myeloperoxidase, 683
    deficiency of, 711
Myelopoiesis, 687
Myeloproliferative disorder(s)
    canine, 876-884
    cat. *See* Myeloproliferative disorder(s), cat
    equine, 894
    leukocyte count and, 829
    platelets and, 468
    polycythemia as, 573
    thrombocythemia as, 472-472
    thrombocytopenia and, 481
Myeloproliferative disorder(s), cat, 852-869, XIX, XX
    additional cytologic features of, 859-860
    case report of, 1144-1146
    gross features of, 860
    histology of, 860
    significant findings in, 855t
    therapy of, 897-900
    undifferentiated or poorly differentiated, 854-856
Myelosis, erythremic. *See* Erythremic myelosis
Myelotoxicity, 900
Myleran. *See* Busulfan
Myo-inositol pentaphosphate, 258
Myosin, platelet and, 455
Myrmecophaga tridactyla, 338

Na₂EDTA, 964. *See also* Ethylenediaminetetraacetate
NADH. *See* Nicotinamide-adenine dinucleotide, reduced
NADPH. *See* Nicotinamide-adenine dinucleotide phosphate
Nagana, 612
N-alkaline phosphatase, 915
Naphthol AS-D chloroacetate esterase, 915
    basophils and, 760
    monocytes and, 776
    neutrophils and, 685
α-Naphthyl acetate esterase, 776, 910t, 911t, 912t, 915-919
    technique for, 928
α-Naphthyl butyrate esterase, 910t, 911t, 912t, 915-919
    technique for, 929
Nasal carcinoma(s), 1117-1118
Nasal discharge, bacillary hemoglobinuria and, 617
Natt-Herricks's solution, 262
Natural killer cell(s), 809

NBT. *See* Nitro blue tetrazolium
Necropsy finding(s), equine, 892-893
Necrosis, intravascular coagulopathy and, 411
Necrotaxis, 777
Needle biopsy(ies), 18-19
Needle size(s), 24-26, 25t
Neonatal anemia(s)
    iron deficiency, 581, 584
    isoerythrolysis and, 650, 996-998, 1154-1155
    pig, 243-244
Neonatal isoerythrolysis, 650, 996-998
    case report of, 1154-1155
Neonatal isoimmune purpura, 1004, 1005
Neonatal neutropenia, 1004
Neonatal pig(s), 241-244
    erythrocyte metabolism in, 545
Neonatal purpura, 1004, 1005
Neonatal thrombocytopenia, 479
    leukocyte antibodies and, 1004, 1005
    pigs, 1006
Neonate(s)
    anemia of. *See* Neonatal anemia(s)
    bilirubin and, 524
    blood loss and, 97
    blood volume and, 94-95
    erythrocyte lipids and, 532
    hemolytic disease of, 73, 650, 996-998, 1154-1155
    immune status of, 979-981
    iron deficiency and, 584
    iron deficiency anemia and, 581
    isoerythrolysis of, 73, 650, 996-998, 1154-1155
    isoimmune purpura of, 1004, 1005
    neutrophils and, 718
    serum proteins of, 945, *946*
    thrombocytopenia of, 479, 1004, 1005, 1006
Neoplasia(s). *See also* Malignancy(ies)
    anemia and, 671
    Chlamydia-like organisms and, 1143-1144
    hematopoietic, categorization of, 838, 839t
    lymphocyte recirculation and, 806, 807
    radiation-induced hematopoietic, 882-884
    stem cell and, 367
    viral etiology of, 264
Neorickettsia helminthoeca, 1129-1130
Nephrectomy, erythropoietin production and, 505
Nephritis in dog(s)
    chronic interstitial, 669-670, 994, 1094, 1095
    plasma proteins and, 974
    uremia and dehydration of, 1090, 1091
Nephrosis, 974-975
Nephrotic syndrome, 974-975
Neuraminidase, 806, 807
Neurohormonal mechanism of neutrophil release, 696
Neutral protease, 713
Neutral stain(s), 32
Neutralization, distilled water, 32
Neutropenia
    autoimmune, 1025
    cyclic, 118
    isoimmune neonatal, 1004
    mechanisms of, 695
    terminal neoplasia and, 1143-1144
Neutrophil(s), 6-7, 35, 36, 676-730. *See also* Neutropenia; Neutrophilia
    abnormalities of, 714-719
    adherent properties of, 694-695
    age and, 109-111
    alkaline phosphatase in, 914
    antiviral activity and, 714
    band. *See* Band neutrophil(s)
    bizarre giant, 826
    cat, 132, 133, 135-136, *135*
    cattle. *See* Neutrophil(s), cattle
    cellular deformability and motility of, 696

Neutrophil(s) *(Continued)*
  chemotaxis and, 694-695, 698-701, 699t, 717-719, 761t
  chinchilla, 319
  corticosteroids and, 692-693, 716, 719
  count of, 35, 36
  cytochemistry and, 684-685
  cytotoxic effect and, 714
  dog. *See* Neutrophil(s), dog
  efflux and, 690
  embryonic hematopoiesis and, 352
  enzymatic and nonenzymatic constituents of, 683-684, 684t
  extravasation of, 700
  foamy blue cytoplasm of, 826
  functional abnormalities and, 717-719
  functions of, 701-714
  goat, 231, 236
  granulokinetics and, 685-695, 687t
  guinea pig, 287
  hamster, 310
  homeostasis regulation and, 695-698
  horse, 154, 158
  human, disorders of, 717t
  hyena, 341, *342*
  hypersegmentation of, 659, 662, 826, 878, *879*
  hyposegmentation of, 826
  inflammation and, 458-459, 712-714
  llama, 337
  locomotion defects and, 717-719
  loss of, 690
  lymphocyte ratio to. *See* Neutrophil:lymphocyte ratio
  lysosomal constituents and, 683-684, 712-714
  from mastitic milk, 707, 719
  metabolism and, 684-685
  metamyelocyte, 115
  microbicidal activity and, 708-712, 708t, 719
  migration into tissues and, 698-701, 699t
  mink, 316t, 317
  monkey, 313-314
  monocytes and, 771
  morphologic abnormalities, 714-717, 715t
  morphology of, 676-682
  mouse, 306
  muscular activity and, 113, 113t
  muskrat, 316t, 319
  of neonates, 718
  old blood sample and, 5
  oxygen consumption by, 710
  parasite destruction and, 714
  Pelger-Huët anomaly and, 117
  peroxidase-positive granule in, 917
  phagocytosis and, 701-708, 719
  pig, 248, 251, 252
  platelet satellitism and, 446
  production and release of, 695-698
  pseudo left shift and, 117
  rabbit, 280, 281
  raccoon, 316t, 318
  rat, 296,•297
  renal disease and, 670
  rodent, 276
  rosette of, 79
  segmented, 13, 676, VII. *See also* Neutrophil(s), hypersegmentation of
  sequential development of, 677
  sheep, 216, 218, *219, 220*
  shift of, 115, 690-695
  tissue injury and, 712-714
  toxemic diseases and, 826
  toxic. *See* Toxic neutrophil(s)
  transmigration of, 433, *435*
  ultrastructures, 677
  water buffalo, 328
Neutrophil(s), cattle, 195
  age and, 185
    endotoxemia and, 202
    mastitis and, 701, 707, 719, *1079*
    migration of, 693-694
    parturition and, 191, 192t, *193*
  Neutrophil(s), dog, 113-118
    bone marrow reserve of, 688-689
    function of, 701
    granulocytic leukemia and, 878, *879*
    maturation of, 687, 687t
    monocytes and, 771
    poodle macrocytosis and, 662
Neutrophil adherence factor, 692
Neutrophil chemoattractant, 698, 699t
Neutrophil chemotactic factor, 761t
Neutrophil count(s), 35, 36
Neutrophil efflux, 690
Neutrophil immobilizing factor, 719
Neutrophil protease, 713
Neutrophil releasing activity, 696
Neutrophil releasing factor, 696
Neutrophilia
  autoimmune hemolytic anemia and, 649, 649t
  chronic, half-time of disappearance and, 693
  granulocytic leukemia and, 878, *878*
  interpretation of, 828
  lymphoma and, 870, 873t
  mechanisms of, 690-695, 691t
  pseudo, 825
  regenerative left shift and, 824
  traumatic reticulitis and splenitis and, 1163-1164
Neutrophil:lymphocyte ratio, 216, 821, 822t
  cat, 822t
  cattle, 185-186
  dog, 822t
  donkey and mule, 340
  foal, 147
  hamster, 310
  horse, 169
  mink, 317
  monkey, 313, 315
  pig, 248
  rabbit, 280
  rat, 296-297
  reversal of, 829
New methylene blue, 59-62, *61, 62*
  Anaplasma, 60, *61, 593*
  body fluids, 62
  Chlamydia, 62
  chylomicra, 60, *61*
  cytoplasmic inclusions, 62
  Cryptococcus neoformans, 62
  Döhle bodies, 62
  Ehrlichia, 62
  Haemobartonella felis, 60
  Heinz body, 60, *61*, XVIII
  heterophil granules, 62
  Histoplasma, 62
  Howell-Jolly bodies, 60
  LE cells, 79
  leukocytes, 60, *61*, 62
  lymph node aspirate, 62
  microfilariae and, 80, *81*
  Piroplasma, 60
  reticulocytes, 60, *61*
  rickettsial bodies, 62
  thrombocytes, *61*, 62
  Toxoplasma, 62
  vaginal smears, 62
New Zealand White rabbit(s), 276, 277t, 278t, 279t
Newborn. *See also* Neonate(s)
  hemolytic disease of, 73, 650, 996-998, 1154-1155
  immune status of, 979-981
Newcastle disease virus, 215
NI. *See* Neonatal isoerythrolysis

Niacin, 509
Nicotinamide-adenine dinucleotide, reduced, 545
  methemoglobin and, 644
Nicotinamide-adenine dinucleotide phosphate, 546
  methemoglobin and, 644
Nicotinamide-adenine dinucleotide phosphate oxidase,
  710
Nicotinic acid
  erythropoiesis and, 509
  diet deficient in, 659
Niemann-Pick disease, 782
Nitrate or nitrite poisoning, 642
Nitro blue tetrazolium reduction
  infection and, 115
  neutrophil and, 685
  phagocytosis and, 704-705, *705*
15Nitrogen, 547
Nitrogen mustard, 898, 900
  neutropenia and, 695
Nitrous oxide, 142
NK cell(s). *See* Natural killer cell(s)
N:L ratio. *See* Neutrophil:lymphocyte ratio
NMB. *See* New methylene blue
Noninfectious hemolytic anemia, 627-654
  copper poisoning and, 627-628
  Heinz body formation and, 632-640
  immune-mediated, 647-650, 649t
  lead poisoning and, 628-632
  metabolic diseases and, 642-647
  poisonous plants and, 640-642
  water toxicosis and, 650-651
Nonspecific collagenase, 714
Nonspecific esterase, 910t, 911t, 912t, 915-919
  technique for, 930
  monocytes and, 776
Nonspecific opsonin, 707
Nonsplenic pool of platelet(s), 442
Noradrenaline, canine platelet and, 121
Normal internal fluidity, 550
Normal macrophage(s), 774
Normal value(s) in blood. *See* Blood value(s)
Normoblast(s), 12
Normochromatic metarubricyte(s), XIX
Normochromic anemia(s)
  macrocytic, 565-566
  normocytic. *See* Normocytic normochromic anemia(s)
Normochromic rubricyte(s), 12
Normocytic normochromic anemia(s), 566, 585
  erythroid hypoplasia and, 668
  liver disease and, 670
  neoplasia and, 671
  riboflavin deficiency and, 660
  vitamin deficiency and, 660
NRA. *See* Neutrophil releasing activity
NRF. *See* Neutrophil releasing factor
5'NT. *See* 5'-Nucleotidase
Nuclear chromatin, 16
  cat, 133, 134
  cattle, 196
  dog, 113-117, 119
  elephant, 338
  goat, 236, 238
  guinea pig, 287
  hamster, 310
  horse, 158
  hyena, 341, *342*
  llama, 337
  lymphocytes and, 791
  mink, 317
  monkey, 314
  mouse, 306, 307
  muskrat, 319
  pig, 252
  rabbit, 281

sheep, 218, 220
water buffalo, 328
Nuclear membrane(s)
  dog neutrophil and, 113-115, 119
  lymphocytes and, 791
Nuclear pocket in lymphocyte(s), 791-792
Nuclear segmentation, neutrophils and, 7, 676
Nucleated erythrocyte(s), 6, 47
  anemia and, 569
  bird, 256, 257, 259
  cat, 130
  pig, 247-248
  reticulocytes and, 499
Nucleated thrombocyte(s), birds and, 256, 257-258, 259
Nucleolus(i),
  blast cell, 15
  lymphocyte, 791, *793*, *794*
  plasma cell, 812
Nucleopore filter(s), 81
Nucleoprotein synthesis, 659
5'-Nucleotidase, 912t, 922
Nucleus(ei)
  asynchronous maturation of cytoplasm and, 16
  cattle neutrophil, 195
  dog neutrophil, 113-115, 119
  double, 16, 115
  doughnut-shaped, 115
  horse neutrophil, 158
  leukocyte, 7
  lymphocyte, 791
  monocyte, 119, 771
  old blood sample and, 5
  plasma cell, 812
  prorubricyte, 492
Null cell(s), 798
Numerical aperture(s), 22
NuRBC. *See* Nucleated erythrocyte(s)
Nurse cell(s), 488. *See also* Reticulum cell(s)
Nutritional deficiency(ies)
  anemia and, 655-656
  erythrocyte survival time and, 548
  niacin and, 659-660
  pantothenic acid and, 660
  riboflavin and, 660
  vitamin B₁₂ and, 656-657
  vitamin B₆ and, 660
  vitamin C and, 660
  vitamin E and, 660-661
Nylon fiber(s), neutrophil migration and, 692
NZW rabbit(s). *See* New Zealand White rabbit(s)

O antigen, 991, 992, 995-996
Ocelot, 334t
Ocular lens(es), 21, 22
Odocoileus virginianus, 321
Oesophagostomiasis, 745, 973
OF. *See* Osmotic fragility
Oil immersion, 22
Okapi, 333t, 341
OLA. *See* Ovine lymphocyte antigen
Oligemia, 87
Oligocythemia, 87
Oligopotential stem cell(s), 365-366
Onchocerca volvulus, 744
Oncornavirus, C-type
  leukemia complex of cattle and, 884
  ovine lymphoma and, 895-896
Oncovin. *See* Vincristine
Onion poisoning
  Heinz bodies and, 634
  hemolytic anemia and, 641-642
Opsonin, 707-708
Optical density(ies)
  avian blood and, 261

Optical density(ies) *(Continued)*
  plasma and, 92
Orangutan, 334t
Orbital sinus blood, 25t, 26, *27*
Organelle(s)
  cytoplasmic, in basophils, 760
  platelet, 452
Organophosphorus inhibitor, 700
Orthochromic leptocyte(s), 542
Oryx, 329, 330t
-osis suffix, 823
Osmotic fragility. *See* Erythrocyte osmotic fragility
Osteoclast(s), 14
  bone marrow and, 15
  mononuclear phagocyte system and, 768
Osteopetrosis, 266
Ostertagia, 585
  plasma proteins and, 973
Ovalocyte(s), *530*, 541
  etymology of, 534t
Ovine lymphoctye antigen, 1002. *See also* Sheep
Ovine plumbism, 631
Owl, 267
Oxidative denaturation of hemoglobin, 644
Oxygen
  cat hemoglobin and, 130
  eggshell and, 258
  inflammatory response and, 713
  monocytes and macrophages and, 780, 784
  neutrophils and, 709-712
  polycythemia and, 572
Oxygen transport, 258
Oxygen-hemoglobin dissociation curve, 258
Oxyhemoglobin method for hemoglobin study, 44, 645
Oxytetracycline, 707, 719

^{32}P. *See* Radiophosphate
P5N. *See* Erythrocyte pyrimidine-specific 5'nucleotidase
Packed cell volume(s), 2, 3, 36-41, *37*, 320. *See also* Hematocrit
  anemia and, 566-567
  cat, 127-129
  cattle, 188
  clinical condition and, 58t
  deer, 321, 322
  determination of, 92-93
  dog, 104, 107-108
  donkey, 339
  error in, 53
  feline infectious anemia and, 604
  haemobartonellosis and, 605
  goat, 225-226, 229t, 230t
  guinea pig, 282
  hamster, 308
  hemorrhage and, 98
  horse. *See* Packed cell volume(s), horse
  microhematocrit and, 41
  monkey, 313
  mouse, 299
  muskrat, 318-319
  pig, 241, 244, 245
  rabbit, 280
  rat, 289, 296
  sheep, 209-212
  Wintrobe hematocrit and, 37
Packed cell volume(s), horse, 140, 141t
  excitation and, 142, 144t
  foal and, 146
  hot-blooded horse and, 151, 154, 156, 157t
  muscular activity and, 168t
  pigment intake of, 160
Pancytopenia
  aplastic anemia and, 665
  tropical canine, 480-481, 976

Panleukopenia, 830
  case report of, 1150
  cat, 130t, 133, 135, 1071-1074, 1150
  hemogram and, 1073t
  immune deficiency and, 981
  leukocyte count in, 1074t
Panthera, 334t, 340-341
Pantothenic acid, 660
Papain
  erythrocytes treated with, 75
  immunoglobulins and, 951
Papio sp., 333t
Pappenheimer body(ies), 6, 570, XII
Parachromatin, 16
  goat blood cell and, 238
Parahaemoproteus, 269
Parakeet, 267, 270
Paralysis
  of jaw of dog, 878, *878*
  Marek's disease and, 264
Paranaplasma, 590
  ultrastructural studies of, 594-595, *594*
Paraprotein(s), 965
Paraproteinemia(s), 965
Parasite(s), blood. *See* Blood parasite(s)
Parrot(s), 267
Partial thromboplastin time, activated, 419-420, 421-422
Parturition
  cattle hemogram and, 191, 192t, *193*
  hemoglobinuria and, 642-643
  pig, 245-247, 246t, 247t
Parvovirus
  Aleutian disease of mink and, 971
  canine, 830
  feline, 1071
PAS. *See* Periodic acid-Schiff reaction
Passer domesticus, 270
Passeriformes, 267
Passerine, 270
Passive transfer of maternal immunoglobulin(s), 979-981
Pasteurella, 780
PBI. *See* Protein-bound iodine
PCV. *See* Packed cell volume(s)
Peanut agglutinin(s), 796
Peccary, 333t, 341-342
Pelger-Huët anomaly, *116*, 117, 117t, 716
  dog and, 734
-penia suffix, 823
Penicillamine, 970
Penicillin(s)
  albumin and, 947
  thrombocytopenia and, 478
Pentobarbital, sodium, 94, 283
Pepsin, 915
Peptide chain(s), globin synthesis and, 516-517
Perching bird(s), 267
Perforation of rectum, 1158-1160
Pericarditis, traumatic, 1076t
Periodic acid-Schiff reaction, 911t, 912t, 919-920,
  neutrophils and, 685
  technique for, 931-932
Peripheral blood, 1-11
  acute blood loss and, 577-581, 577t, 579t
  basophils and, 764
  B-lymphocytes in, 796-797
  collection of, 1-2
  haemobartonellosis and, 604
  handling of sample of, 2
  hemogram development and, 2-5
  lymphocytes in, 796-797, 811-812
  microfilariae and, 82
  normal values and, 7-11, 8t, 9t, 10t. *See also* Blood value(s)

old blood and, 5
physiology and, 7
reticulocytes and, 499-500, 567t
species variation and, 5-7
T-lymphocytes in, 796-797
Peripheral lymphoid organ(s), 798, 801-802
Peripheral zone(s), platelet and, 450-451
Peritoneum. *See also* Peritonitis
monocytes and, 771
mouse macrophage and, 784
Peritonitis
feline infectious. *See* Feline infectious peritonitis
granulocytosis and, 689
leukemoid reaction in, 1105-1106
lymphopenia and anemia in, 1138
Pernicious anemia, 381, 657
Peromyscus maniculatus bairdii, 310-311
Peromyscus maniculatus borealis, 310-311
Peroxidase, 910t, 911t, 920-921, 932-933
basophils and, 760
in canine granulocytic leukemia, 879, *879*
eosinophils and, 737-738, 747
macrophages and, 775-776
technique for, 932-933
Persistent lymphocytosis, bovine, 884
Pertussis, 811
Petechia(iae), 476, 1019. *See also* Thrombocytopenia; Thrombocytopenic purpura
Peyer's patch(es), 798, 799, 801
PF. *See* Platelet factor(s)
PF-3 test. *See* Platelet factor 3 test
PG. *See* Prostaglandin(s)
PGA. *See* Pteroylglutamic acid
PGI$_2$. *See* Prostacyclin
Ph^1. *See* Philadelphia chromosome
PHA. *See* Phytohemagglutinin
Phagocyte(s). *See also* Mononuclear phagocyte system; Phagocytosis
neutrophils and, 719
number of active, 704
Phagocyte system, mononuclear. *See* Mononuclear phagocyte system
Phagocytic index, 704
Phagocytic vacuole(s), 702, *704*
Phagocytin, 711
Phagocytosis, 779-781
anaplasmosis and, 592
coliform mastitis and, *1079*
energy source and, 684
eosinophils and, 739, 743, 744
erythrocytes and, 554-556, 781, *859*
feline myeloproliferative disorder and, *859*
immunoglobulin G and, 1014
microbial resistance to, 709t
neutrophils and, 701-707
platelets and, 459
scanning electron photomicrographs of, *703*
Phagocytosis stimulating factor, 708
Phagolysosome(s), 702, *704*, 780
Phagosome(s), 702
Phase contrast microscopy, anaplasmosis and, 593, *594*
Pheasant(s), 270
Phenothiazine, 633-634, 1152-1153
Phenylbutazone, 462
Phenylepinephrine, 750
Phenylhydrazine, 634
Philadelphia chromosome, 367
-philia suffix, 823
Phlebotomus sand fly, 1068
Phloxine, 261, 262
Phorbol myristate acetate, 703, 706
Phosphasome(s), 679, 683, 914
Phosphatase, alkaline. *See* Alkaline phosphatase
Phosphate buffer(s), 32

Phosphoenol pyruvate, 645
Phospholipase
lymphocyte migration and, 806
microbicidal mechanism of, 712
Phospholipid(s). *See also* Cholesterol-to-phospholipid ratio
acanthocyte and, 540
coagulation and, 396
cholesterol and, 531-532
erythrocyte membrane and, 544
platelet, 76
Phosphonate ester(s), 700
Phosphorus
iron absorption and, 582
postparturient hemoglobinuria and, 643
Phylloquinone, 408
Physiologic leukocytosis, 825-826
cat, 126, 132, 133t
dog, 111-113, 113t
young horse, 166-169, *167*, 168t
Physiologic saturation with iron, 382
Physiologic solution(s), 46, 48
Physiologic thrombocytosis, 469
Physiology in blood value interpretation, 7
Phytohemagglutinin, 798, 896
PIE. *See* Pulmonary infiltrate(s) with eosinophilia
Pig(s)
blood collection from, 25t, 26, 27
blood volume and, 90t, 94, 95
chemotaxis and, 718
copper and, 628, 664
endotoxemia and, 832
eosinophils and, 248, *251*, 252, 737
eperythrozoonosis in, 609-610
erythrocytes and. *See* Pig erythrocyte(s)
fetus of, 240-241
hematology and, 244-250
hemoglobin and, 243-244, 518t
iron requirement of suckling, 243-244
lead poisoning and, 631-632
leptospirosis and, 616
leukemia in, 896-897
leukocyte number and, 9t
leukocytes and, 241, 243, 245-249, 246t
lymphocyte antigen and, 1002
lymphocytes and, 248-249, *251*, 252, 805-806
morphology of blood cells, 8t, 250-252
myeloid:erythroid ratio of, 18t, 250
neonatal, 241-244, 650, 1006
neonatal isoerythrolysis and, 650
neonatal thrombocytopenic purpura in, 1006
normal blood values for, 10t, 240
nutritional deficiency anemia and, 655-656, 656t
platelet number in, 469t
riboflavin deficiency in, 660
soil contact and, 243
thrombocytopenia and, 479, 483
trypanosomiasis and, 612
venous hematocrit and, 94
vitamin deficiency anemia and, 656
Pig erythrocyte(s), 250-252, 528
metabolism in, 545
neonatal pig and, 241, 242t, 243
pregnancy and lactation and, 245-247, 246t
Pigeon(s), 267, 270
Piggyback phagocytosis, 701
Pink tooth, 646, 1167-1168
Pinocytosis, 701, 779-781
Pipette(s)
care of, 22
filling of, 45-46, *46*
Piromen
marrow reserve assessment and, 688
neutropenia and, 693

Piroplasma, 596, 610. *See also* Babesiosis; Theileriasis
Piroplasmosis, 596-601, *597*, 610
PL. *See* Persistent lymphocytosis
Pl^A antigens, 1005
Placenta(s), retained, 191
Plant(s)
  poisonous, 640-642
  lectin of, 806
Plasma, 3
  bilirubin and, 523
  blood volume and, 87
  bovine viral diarrhea and, 356t, 357t
  cat, 136-137
  copper in, 664
  disseminated intravascular coagulopathy and, 415
  dog, 11, 122-123
  fibrinogen in. *See* Plasma fibrinogen
  erythropoietin in, 504
  goat, 225, 229t, 232
  guinea pig, 284t, 288
  hamster, 310
  hemoglobinemia and, 521
  horse, 149, 159-161, 161t
  in vitro alteration and, 92
  lactescence of, 11
  monkey, 314
  mouse, 300t, 303t, 307
  optical density and, 92
  pig, 250
  polycythemia and, 575
  protein in. *See* Plasma protein(s)
  rabbit, 277t, 282
  rat, 290t, 293t, 297-298
  separation of cells and, 28
  sheep, 216-218
  transfusion of, 408, 996
  trapped, 92, 188, 225, 229t
  turbid, 40-41
  viscosity of, 156
  vitamin B$_{12}$ and, 657
  volume of. *See* Plasma volume(s)
  Wintrobe hematocrit and, 39-41
Plasma cell(s), 14, 790, 812-814. *See also* Plasma cell
    dyscrasia(s); Plasma cell myeloma(s)
  bone marrow and, 15, 16
  equine multiple myeloma and, 893, *895*
  sheep, *221*
  ultrastructure of, 812, *813*
Plasma cell dyscrasia(s)
  diagnosis of, 924
  in dog, *966*, 968-969
Plasma cell myeloma(s), 16, 812, 971
  case report of, 1130-1132, *1134*, *1135*
Plasma fibrinogen. *See* Fibrinogen
Plasma inhibitor of fibrinolysis, 400-401
Plasma protein(s), 2, 5, 57-58, 58t, 940-989, 961t
  albumin in, 947
  blood loss and, 578
  cat, 136
  cattle, 187-188, 961t
  ceruloplasmin in, 949
  concentration of, 57t, 942-945, 955-957
  C-reactive protein in, 949-950
  disease and, 57-58, 58t
  dog, 122, 961t
  dysproteinemias in, 957-976. *See also*
    Dysproteinemia(s)
  erythrocyte sedimentation rate and, 55
  factors governing, 942-945
  α-fetoprotein in, 950
  fibrinogen and, 59, 188, 947-948, 960-962, 961t, 962t,
    963t
  fox, 320
  functions of, 940, 941t

  glycoproteins in, 948
  goat, 232
  guinea pig, 288
  half-life of, 942t
  haptoglobin in, 948-949
  hemopexin in, 948-949
  horse, 142, 144, 145t, 160-161, 172t, 961t
  immune deficiency disorders in, 976-982
  immunoglobulins in, 951-955
  lipoproteins in, 950-951
  methodology in, 955-957
  pig, 241-243, 250
  prealbumin in, 945-947
  rabbit, 282
  rat, 297, 298
  refractive index and, 56-57
  refractometer and total, 2-5, 56-58
  sheep, 216-218
  transferrin in, 948
Plasma protein:fibrinogen ratio, 59, 188, 960-962, 961t,
    962t, 963t
Plasma transfusion(s), 408, 996
Plasma turbidity, 11
Plasma viscosity, 156
Plasma volume(s)
  acute blood loss and, 577
  measurement and, 87-93
  neonate and, 94-95
  polycythemia and, 575
  pregnancy and, 95
Plasmablast(s), 813
Plasmacytosis, 812
Plasmapheresis, 944, 970
Plasminogen, 399
Plasminogen activator, 399
  macrophages and, 785
  mast cells and basophils and, 761t
Plasminogen proactivator, 399
Plasmodium sp., 268-269
Plastic(s), embedding of marrow in, 19
Platelet(s), 14
  aggregation and, 6, 457-458, 460-461
  antibodies and. *See* Antiplatelet antibody(ies)
  arachidonic acid metabolism and, 452t, 455-456
  autoimmune thrombocytopenia and, 1018, 1020
  biochemistry of, 454-455
  bird, 6, 256, 257-258, 259, 262
  blood collection and, 1, 2
  blood film and, 62
  buffy coat and, 38
  cat, 136, 447, *449*, 469t
  cattle, 197, 447, *449*, 469t
  cell counting error and, 52
  chinchilla, 319
  coagulation and, 391-392, 397, 407, 411
  count of, 2, 3, 52, 65-66
  disseminated intravascular coagulopathy and, 411
  distribution and removal of, 441-442
  dog, 119-122, *120*, 447, *449*, 469t
  donkey, 339
  elephant, 339
  fish, 6
  functions of, 456-460
  goat, 231, 238, 447, *449*, 469t
  guinea pig, 286t, 288
  hamster, 310
  hemostasis and, 389-390
  horse, 6, 159, 447, *449*, 469t
  kinetics, 441-442
  laboratory animal, 275
  life span of, 121, 441
  mammalian, 6
  megakaryocytes and, 437-438
  megakaryocytopoiesis and, 438-441

mink, 317
monkey, 314
morphology of, 446-454
mouse, 302t, 305t, 307
nucleated, 256, 257-258, 259
pig, 249-250, 252
platelet factor 3 test and, 75-77
qualitative or functional defects of, 466-468
quantitative disorder of, 469-483, 469t, 470t
rabbit, 279t, 282
raccoon, 318
rat, 297
release reaction and, 461-462
satellitism and, 446
severance of vessel and, 389
sheep, 216, 222, 447, *449*, 469t
spiny anteater, 275
spleen and, 377, 1022
thrombocythemia and, 471-472
thrombocytopenia; *See also* Thrombocytopenia
thrombocytosis and, 469-471, 470t, *471*
thrombus and, 416
transfusions of, 994
von Willebrand's disease and, 468-469
water buffalo and, 328
Platelet activating factor, 761t, 763
Platelet aggregating factor, eosinophil and, 746
Platelet antibody(ies), 1005-1006, 1021. *See also*
Antiplatelet antibody(ies)
Platelet antigen(s), 1005-1006
autoantibody against, 1021
Platelet contractile protein, 455
Platelet count(s), 2, 3, 52, 65-66
Platelet factor(s) 1 through 4, 391-392, 458
Platelet factor 3 test, 75-77
Platelet phospholipid(s), 76
Platelet poor plasma, 76
Platelet rich plasma, 65, 76
Platelet survival, 121, 441
Platelet transfusion(s), 994
Pl^E antigens, 1005
Pleokaryocyte(s), 716
Pleomorphic granule(s), 679, *682*
Pleural effusion fluid, equine, 892
Plumbism. *See* Lead poisoning
Pluripotent stem cell(s), 365-367, 798
cell line from, 853, *853*
megakaryocytopoiesis and, 431
regulation of, 339-370
PNA. *See* Peanut agglutinin(s)
Pneumococcus (pneumococci)
phagocytosis and, 707, 711
susceptibility to, 701
PNP. *See* Purine nucleoside phosphorylase
PO. *See* Peroxidase
PO$_2$50, 258
Poietin(s), 368
Poikilocyte(s), *536, 539*, 542, 583, *583. See also*
Poikilocytosis
anemia and, 570
etymology of, 534t
goat, *232*, 234, 235
Poikilocytosis, 6, 247
erythrocyte and, 528
mink, 317
Poisoning
amporolium, 483
bracken fern, 481, 483
copper, 509, 627-628, 949
dicumarol, 1111-1113
hemolytic anemia and, 640-642
lead. *See* Lead poisoning
warfarin, 408-409, 1020, 1111-1113
Pokeweed mitogen(s), 799

Polar bear(s), 335t, 342
Polyacrylamide gel electrophoresis, 532
Polycarbonate filter(s), 81
Polychromasia
cat, 131, 856
guinea pig, 283
mouse, 306
rat, 296
Polychromatic erythrocyte(s), 6
horse bone marrow and, 163
poodle macrocytosis and, 661
Polychromatic rubricyte(s), 12, 16, 490, IV, VI
plasma cell and, 16
Polychrome methylene blue, 31
Polyclonal gammopathy(ies), 965, *965*
Polycythemia(s), 87, 572-575, 572t, *574. See also*
Polycythemia vera
erythropoietin and, 506-507
familial, 574
primary, 572, 573-575
relative, 572, 575
secondary, 572, 575, 1108-1109
Polycythemia vera, 573. *See also* Polycythemia(s)
blood volume and, 95
dog, 1107-1108
erythrocyte survival time and, 550
Polyglutamate, 657
Polymerization of hemoglobin, 234, *234, 235, 236*
Polymorphonuclear leukocyte(s), 7. *See also*
Neutrophil(s)
Polymyxin B sulfate, 702
Polyp(s), stomach, 972
Polypeptide band(s), 532
Polypeptide chain(s), 516, 519-520
Polyploidy, 115, 826
Polyribosome(s)
lymphocytes and, 794
reticulocytes and, 496, *497, 499*
Pongo pygmaeus, 334t
Poodle(s)
babesiosis and, 600-601
macrocytosis and, 571, 661-662, 663t
normal blood values and, 107
Pool(s)
leukocyte migration and, 692
neutrophil, 687-690
Porcine entries. *See* Pig(s)
Porphyria, congenital, 646-647, 1167-1168
Postnatal period
hematopoiesis and, 350-359, 361-262
morphology and, 355-359, *355*, 356t, *358, 359*
Postparturient hemoglobinuria, 642-643. *See also*
Parturition
Postprandial lipemia(s), 11, 1089-1090
Posttransfusion purpura, 1006
Potassium, erythrocyte destruction and, 551
Potassium dichromate
icterus index and, 3, 40
pipette and, 22
Potos flavus, 335t
PP:F. *See* Plasma protein:fibrinogen ratio
PPP. *See* Platelet poor plasma
Prealbumin, 945-947
Pre-B cell(s), 794, 798
Prednisolone
cat leukocyte and, 134, *134*
cattle response to, 200, 201
dog leukocyte and, 111, *111*, 112t
feline eosinophilic leukemia and, 863, 865
marrow reserve assessment and, 688
Waldenström's macroglobulinemia and, 968
water buffalo and, 329
Prednisone, 898, 899
autoimmune hemolytic anemia and, 1016

Prednisone *(Continued)*
  autoimmune thrombocytopenic purpura and, 1024
  plasma cell myeloma and, 968
Pregnancy(ies)
  blood volume and, 95
  cat, 128
  cattle hemogram and, 191
  α-fetoprotein and, 950
  goat erythrocyte and, 229
  haemobartonellosis and, 605
  mature hot-blooded horse and, 151
  neutrophil activity and, 719
  pig, 245-247, 246t, 247t
  plasma proteins and, 944-945
  plasma volume and, 95
  total blood volume and, 95
Prekallikrein, 394
Preleukemia, 839
  feline, 867-869, *868*
Prenatal erythrocyte(s), 355-359, *355*, 356t, *358*, *359*
Prenatal hematopoiesis, 350-359. *See also* Fetal blood
      value(s)
  cat, 351-352
  cow, 352, 354-355
  dog, 350-351
Pre-T cell(s), 794, 798
Primary granule(s), 679, 683
Primary hemostasis, 389-391. *See also* Coagulation
Primary immune deficiency(ies), 976-982
Primary lymphoid organ(s), 798
Primary pathologic fibrinolysis, 410
Primary polycythemia, 572, 573-575
Primate(s), blood collection from, 25t, 27-28, *28*
Primitive cell(s), 854, *854*, *855*
Proactivator(s), plasminogen, 399
Procarbazine, 899
Procoagulant factor(s), 779
Proerythroblast(s). *See* Rubriblast(s)
Progenitor cell(s)
  committed, 367-368, 370-373, 501-502. *See also* Colony
      forming unit erythrocyte(s)
  erythroid, 370, 488-490, *488*, 488t
  granulocytic, migration of, 367
  megakaryocyte and, 431
  pluripotential stem cells and, 369-370
  regulation of, 369-373
Progranulocyte(s). *See* Promyelocyte(s)
Prolymphocyte(s), 850-851, *850*
Promazine hydrochloride, 142
Promegakaryocyte(s), 14, 15, 432-433, *434*
  ultrastructure and cytochemistry of, 434-435
Promonocyte(s), 772
Promyelocyte(s), 13, 16, 677
  cat, 135, *135*, 861
  electron microscopy and, 679
  eosinophilic, 736
Promyelocytic leukemia(s), 918
Pronormoblast(s). *See* Rubriblast(s)
Proplatelet(s), 437-438, *437*
Propranolol hydrochloride
  eosinopenia and, 750
  neutrophil migration and, 692
Proptoporphyrin III, 515
Propylene glycol, 64
Prorubricyte(s), 12, 490, 658
  ultrastructure of, 491-492, *492*, *493*
Prosimian, blood collection and, 27-28
Prostacyclin. *See also* Prostaglandin(s)
  action of, 456
  hemostasis and, 389
  platelets and, 455-456
Prostaglandin(s). *See also* Prostacyclin
  degranulation and, 703
  eosinophils and, 746
  erythropoiesis and, 370

  granulopoiesis and, 697
  progenitor cell regulation and, 371
Protamine sulfate test, 425
Protease
  inflammatory response and, 713
  microbicidal mechanism of, 712
Protein(s). *See also* Plasma protein(s)
  bacterial permeability increasing, 712
  band 3, 532
  cationic, 711, 713, 738
  C-reactive, 949-950
  electrophoresis of. *See* Electrophoresis
  enteropathy and loss of, 971-972
  eosinophils and, 738
  erythrocyte membrane and, 531, 532
  erythrocyte production and, 508-509
  inflammatory response and, 713
  microbicidal mechanisms of, 711
  half-life of, 942t
  monocytes and macrophages and, 780, 784
  platelet contractile, 455
  serum. *See* Protein(s), serum
  sulfhydryl groups of membrane, 628
Protein C, 398
Protein(s), serum
  electrophoresis of, 967. *See also* Electrophoresis
  foal, 149
  guinea pig, 288
  horse, 160-161, 172t
  infection and, 975
  mink, 317
  monkey, 314
  mule, 340
  pig, 250
  sheep, 216
  total, concentrations of, 955-957
Proteinase, 784
Protein-bound iodine, 1063
Protein-losing gastroenteropathy(ies), 971-972
Proteolytic enzyme(s), 784
Prothrombin
  coagulation and, 395-396
  coagulopathy and, 419-420
  hemostasis and, 390
Prothrombin time
  coagulopathy and, 419-420
  hemostasis and, 422-423
Protoporphyrin production, 271
Protozoon(a)
  babesiosis and, 596
  flagellated, 612
  leukocyte response and, 827
  phagocytosis and, 707
Prozone phenomenon(ena), 74
PRP. *See* Platelet rich plasma
Pseudo-eosinophil(s), 276
  chinchilla, 319
  guinea pig, *287*
  rabbit, 281
Pseudo-LE cell(s), 79
Pseudo-left shift(s), 117
Pseudo-neutrophilia, 692, 825
Pseudomonas aeruginosa
  bovine mastitis and, 1076
  marrow reserve assessment and, 688
  neutropenia and, 693
Pseudo-Pelger-Huët anomaly, 117, 716, 826
  interpretation of, 829
Pseudopod(s), 453, 702
Psittaciformes, 267
Psittacosis-lymphogranuloma group, 830
Psychologic factor(s), cattle hemogram and, 189
PT. *See* Prothrombin time
PTT. *See* Partial thromboplastin time, activated

Pteroylglutamic acid(s), 659
Puffin(s), 270
Pulmonary infiltrate(s) with eosinophilia, 749
Pulmonary megakaryocyte(s), 438
Pulp, splenic, 375
Punctate reticulocyte(s), 63
  cat, 578
Purine metabolism, 922
Purine nucleoside phosphorylase, 912t, 922
Purpura
  isoimmune neonatal, 1004, 1005
  posttransfusion, 1006
  thrombocytopenic. *See* Thrombocytopenia;
    Thrombocytopenic purpura
Pus, leukocyte response and, 827
PWM. *See* Pokeweed mitogen(s)
Pyelonephritis, 1158, 1159
Pyknocyte(s), 534t
Pyometra
  cat, 1140-1142
  dog. *See* Pyometra, canine
Pyometra, canine, 1051-1054
  degenerative left shift in, 1102-1104
  hemogram and, 1052t
  leukocyte response and, 827
  regenerative left shift in, 1102, 1103
Pyridoxine(s), 509
Pyrogen(s), bacterial, 688
Pyronin, 919. *See also* Methyl green-pyronin reaction
Pyroninophilia, 266
Pyropoikilocyte(s), 534t
Pyropoikilocytosis, 543-544
Pyruvate kinase, 546
  deficiency of, 645-646, 646t

Quarter horse(s), 149-163. *See also* Horse(s)
  corticosteroids and, 163
  foals of, 144-149
  normal values for, 149, 150t
Quick stain(s), 34
Quick's one stage prothrombin time, 422
Quinidine, 1023
Quinine, 1023
Quinoline, 598

R antigen(s), 991, 992, 995-996
Rabbit(s), 276-282, 283t
  antiplatelet antibody and, 77
  blood collection from, 25t, 26
  blood volume and, 91t, 94
  hemoglobin and, 518t
  leukocytes of, 278t, 279t, 280-282
Rabbit anticanine globulin, 77
Raccoon(s), 16t, 318
Radial immunodiffusion technique, 957
Radiation
  antilymphocyte serum and, 1005
  aplastic anemia and, 666-668, *667*
  canine hematopoietic neoplasia induced by, 882-884
  cyclic hematopoiesis and, 118
  leukemias and, 844, 899-900
  thrombocytopenia and, 483
  whole body gamma, 483
Radiation syndrome, 666-668, *667*
Radiation-induced neoplasia, 882-884
Radioactive diisopropyl fluorophosphate
  erythrocytes and, 155, 306, 313, 547
  granulokinetics and, 686-687, 689, 690t
Radioactive sulfate, 686-687
Radiocarbon. *See* Carbon 14
Radiochromate, 547-548
  albumin labeled with, 972

erythrocytes and. *See* Radiochromate, erythrocytes
  labeled with
  granulokinetics and, 686-687, 689, 690t
  lymphokinetics and, 802, 803
Radiochromate, erythrocytes labeled with, 87, 93, 547-
  548
  horse, 155
  monkey, 313
  pig, 247
Radioimmunoassay, 957
Radioiodine, 87, 93
Radioiron, 547
Radiophosphate
  bacteria labeled with, 704
  erythrocytes and, 547-548
  granulokinetics and, 686-687
  lymphokinetics and, 802
Rat(s), 288-298
  blood collection from, 25t, 26
  blood volume and, 91t, 94
  erythropoietin and, 383
  hemoglobin and, 518t
  leukocytes of, 291t, 292t, 294t, 295t, 296-297
RBC. *See* Erythrocyte(s)
RCF. *See* Relative centrifugal force
RE nucleus(ei), 15
Reactive monocyte(s), 778
Reactive thrombocytosis, 469
Rebuck skin window technique, 690, 698-699
Receptor(s)
  for C3b and C3d, 797
  for Fc portion of immunoglobulin, 797
  surface, 741-742, 776-777
Recipient and donor blood compatibility, 71
Red blood cell(s). *See* Erythrocyte(s)
Red blood cell mass, 3
  neonate and, 94-95
  strenuous exercise and, 141-142, 141t
Red blood count(s), 3, 45-52
  erythropoiesis and, 507
  prenatal and early postnatal hematopoiesis in cat
    and, 352
Red cell antigen(s), 991-993
Red cell aplasia, 665-666
Red deer, 337
Red granule(s), avian leukocyte and, 262-263
Red maple(s), hemolytic anemia and, 642
Red splenic pulp, 375
Red thrombus(i), 416
Red water disease, 617
Reed-Sternberg cell(s), 852, 876
Refractometer(s)
  plasma fibrinogen by, 58-59
  total plasma protein by, 56-58, 955
Regenerative left shift(s), 823, 824
  in pyometra, 1102, 1103
Reindeer, 337
Rejection of graft(s), 1005, 1007
Relative centrifugal force, 37, *38*
Relative leukocyte count(s), 824. *See also* Leukocyte
  count(s)
Relative polycythemia, 572
Renal disease or failure
  in dog, 669-670, 1040-1043, 1041t
  erythrpoietin and, 505
  platelet disorder and, 467
Renal granulopoiesis factor, 696
Renal hypoxia, 505
Reptile(s), 275
RER. *See* Rough endoplasmic reticulum
RES. *See* Reticuloendothelial system
Resident macrophage(s), 774
Resolving power, 21
Respiration(s) in bird(s), 258-259

Respiratory burst, 706
Restoration, blood, 96-99. *See also* Transfusion(s)
Retained fetal membrane(s), 191, 192t, *193*
Retained placenta(s), 191
Reticulated reticulocyte(s), 62-63
Reticulitis, traumatic, 1076t, 1163-1165
Reticulocyte(s), 6, 13, 490-491. *See also* Reticulocytosis
  aggregate, 129
  bird, 257
  cat, 128-130, 500, 567, IV
  cattle, 194, 499-500
  cell transit and, 364
  chinchilla, 319
  counts of, 3, 62-63, 567-568, 567t
  development of, 495-501, *497, 498*
  dog, 108, 500, 567t, 568
  erythrocytes and, 495, *497, 498,* 500-501
  fox, 320
  generation time of, 502
  goat, 229
  guinea pig, 283
  hamster, 308
  horse, 156-158, 163, 499
  liver disease anemia and, 670
  mink, 317
  monkey, 313
  mouse, 299
  pig, 245, 247-248
  punctate, 129
  rabbit, 280
  rat, 296
  sheep, 214
  spleen and, 378
  staining and counting of, 62-63
  types of, 62-63
Reticulocyte count(s), 3, 62-63, 501, 567-568, 567t
Reticulocyte production index, 63, 108
Reticulocytosis
  acute blood loss and, 578
  anemia and, 567-569
  cat, 129
  cow, 499-500
  horse, 499
Reticuloendothelial system, 380, 768. *See also*
    Mononuclear phagocyte system
Reticuloendotheliosis, 267
  feline, 853, 854-856
Reticulosis, histiocytic medullary, XIII
Reticulum cell(s), erythropoiesis and, 488
Reticulum cell sarcoma, *851*
Retinol-binding protein, 947
Retraction, clot, 456, 458
Retrovirus
  RNA, birds and, 264, 265t, 266
  type D, acquired immune deficiency syndrome and,
    982
Reverse transcriptase activity, 844
RGF. *See* Renal granulopoiesis factor
Rh antigen, 650, 996
Rhesus monkey, 311-315, 312t
  acquired immunodeficiency syndrome and, 982
Rheumatoid arthritis
  antinuclear antibody and, 77
  erythropoietin and, 507
Rhino(s), white, 275
Rhipicephalus sanguineus, 1066
Rhopheocytosis, 495
Rib(s), marrow aspiration and, 66, 67
Ribavirin, 481
Riboflavin, 509
Ribonucleic acid
  inhibition of, 812
  lympholysis and, 812
  messenger. *See also* Ribonucleic acid, messenger

  pyroninophilia and, 919
  prorubricyte and, 492, 495
Ribonucleic acid, messenger
  globin synthesis and, 516
  prorubricyte and, 492, 495
Ribonucleic acid virus, 843, 844
  bird, 264, 265t, 266
Ribosome(s)
  lead poisoning and, 629
  lymphocytes and, 792, *793,* 794
  reticulocytes and, 496, *497,* 499
Rickettsia canis, 1066
Rickettsial infection, 830-831
  dog, 1066, 1129-1130
  leukocyte response and, 827
  leukopenias and, 830-831
  plasma proteins and, 975-976
Rieder cell(s), 196
Rift Valley fever, 830
Right shift(s), 115, *116,* 823
Rinderpest virus, 830
Ring-tailed lemur(s), 334t
  heterophils of, 276
Ristocetin, 121
RNA. *See* Ribonucleic acid
Rocket immunoelectrophoresis, 957
Rocky mountain spotted fever, 481
Rodenticide(s)
  intoxication from, in dog, 1113
  vitamin K antagonism and, 408
Romanowsky stain(s), 31-35
Ropheocytosis, 582
Rosenthal needle(s), 67
Rosette(s)
  LE test and, 1027
  lymphocytes and, 796, *797*
  neutrophils and, 79
Rough endoplasmic reticulum, 812, *813,* 814
Rouleau formation, 6, 11
  cat, 132
  erythrocyte sedimentation rate and, 54
  giraffe, 341
  goat, 229
  horse, 155
  pig, 250
  sheep, 214, 218
  water buffalo, 327
  wet-film method and, 59, *60*
Roundworm, filarial, 270
Rous sarcoma(s), 843
RPI. *See* Reticulocyte production index
Rubriblast(s), 12, 489-490, 491, *491*
  development of, *488*
Rubricyte(s)
  basophilic, 490, V, VI
  cell transit and, 364
  iron deficiency anemia and, 583, XVII
  plasma cells and, 16
  polychromatic, 16, 490, IV, VI
Ruminant(s)
  acute blood loss and, 578
  copper and, 628
  nitrate poisoning and, 642
  theileriasis and, 610
  vitamin B_{12} and, 657
Runt disease, 374
Russell's viper venom time, 423
RVVT. *See* Russell's viper venom time

[35]S. *See* Radioactive sulfate
Salmon poisoning, 1129-1130
Salmonella choleraesuis, 249
Salmonella typhosa endotoxin, 688

Salmonellosis
  calf, 202
  experimental hog cholera and, 249
  horse, 169, 1160-1162
  marrow leukocyte reserve and, 688
  phagocytosis and, 709
Sand fly(ies), 1068
Saphenous vein(s), 25t, 26
Sarcocytosis, 616
Sarcoma(s)
  avian, 266
  reticulum cell, of cat, *851*
Satellitism, 446
Saturated solution of iron sulfate, 244
Scavenger(s), 781-782
Schistocyte(s), 6, *536, 539,* 542
  anemia and, 570
  entymology of, 534t
Schistosoma mansoni
  eosinophils and, 744, 745
  neutrophils and, 714
Schistosomiasis
  eosinophils and, 744, 745
  neutrophils and, 714
  sheep, 586
Schizocyte(s). *See* Schistocyte(s)
Schizont(s), 268, 269
Schumauch body, 131
SD antigen(s). *See* Serologically defined antigen(s)
Sea-blue histiocyte(s), 1022
  macrophages and, 782
Seasonal variation(s) in blood values
  cattle, 189-190
  goat, 229
  horse, 151-154
  sheep, 212
Secondary granule(s), 679
Secondary immune deficiency(ies), 976-982
Secondary lymphoid organ(s), 798
Secondary polycythemia, 572, 1108-1109
Secretory code, 706
Secretory role of monocytes and macrophages and, 779, 779t, 784-785
Sedimentation rate, erythrocyte. *See* Erythrocyte sedimentation rate
Sedormid, 1023
Segmented neutrophil(s), 13, 676, VII. *See also* Neutrophil(s), hypersegmentation of
Selective immunoglobulin deficiency(ies), 981-982
Selenium
  anemia and, 665
  bactericidal activity and, 719
  pig, 244
  water buffalo, 329
Selenocyte, *535,* 542
  etymology of, 534t
[75]Selenomethionine, 155
Sensitivity(ies). *See also* Allergy(ies); Hypersensitivity(ies)
  drug, in dog, 1113-1114
  transfusions and, 995
Sensitization,
  platelet, 1022
Septicemia, 836
  cattle, 201-204
  degenerative left shift and, 824
  leukocyte response and, 826-827
  leukopenias and, 836
Serine proesterase, 700
Serologically defined antigen, 999
Serology. *See also* Serum(a) .
  babesiosis and, 601
  bovine leukemia virus and, 885
  feline leukemia virus and, 844

leptospirosis and, 617
Seromucoid, 948
Serotonin, 712
  canine platelet and, 121
  eosinophils and, 746
  horse platelet and, 159
  mast cells and basophils and, 761t
Serum(a). *See also* Serology
  antilymphocyte, 1004-1005
  bilirubin in, 188, 339
  collection of, 1
  electrophoresis and, 956
  feline lymphoma and, 852
  guinea pig, 284t, 288
  immunoglobulins in, 952t. *See also* Immunoglobulin(s)
  iron deficiency and, 583-584
  microfilariae and, 82
  mink, 317
  monkey, 314
  proteins in. *See* Protein(s), serum
  radioiodine labeled albumin in, 87, 93
Serum albumin labeled with radioiodine, human, 87, 93
Serum bilirubin
  cattle, 188
  donkey, 339
Serum complement, 852
Serum ferritin, 583-584
Serum immunoglobulin level(s), 952t
Serum protein. *See* Protein(s), serum
Serval cat(s), 335t
Sessile nodule(s), 115, *116*
Sex chromatin
  female dog, 115-117
  goat, 236
  guinea pig leukocyte and, 287
  hyena, 341, *342*
Sex difference(s) in blood values, 7
  cat, 128, 602
  cattle, 191-193
  dog, 107
  goat, 229
  horse, 151
  laboratory animal, 276
  pig, 247
Sex hormone(s), lymphopoiesis and, 811-812
Sex lobe, neutrophil and, 115-117
Sheep, 208-224
  age and, 208-215, 210t, 211t, 213t
  anaplasmosis, 590-596, 591t, 592t, *593, 594*
  anemia and, 209, 215, 585, 586, 627-628, 671
  bacillary hemoglobinuria in, 617-618, 618t
  bilirubin and, 524-525
  blood volume and, 89t, 94, 95
  bone marrow and, 222
  collection of blood from, 25t
  copper and, 627-628, 662, 664-665
  2,3-diphosphoglycerate and, 547
  eperythrozoonosis in, 609
  erythrocytes and. *See* Sheep erythrocyte(s)
  fascioliasis of, 549, 586
  fetal blood and, 208, 212t
  globulin concentration in pregnancy and, 945
  glutathione deficiency and, 640
  Haemonchus and, 585
  hemoglobin and, 212, 215, 518t
  hypoproteinemia and, 585
  kale and, 634
  leukemia complex in, 895-896
  leukocyte count and, 9t, 11
  leukocytes and, 209, 210t, 215-216, 217t
  lymphocytes and, 216, *219,* 220-222, *221,* 804
  molybdenosis of, 548

Sheep *(Continued)*
  morphology and, 8t, 218-222, 447, *449*
  myeloid:erythroid ratio of, 18t, 222
  normal blood values and, 10t, 208-218, 210t, 211t, 213t
  platelets and, 216, 222, 447, *449*, 469t
  plumbism and, 631
  schistosomiasis in, 586
  theileriasis and, 610
  thrombocytopenia and, 483
Sheep erythrocyte(s), 528
  age and, 208-215, 210t, 211t
  central pallor to, 218, 219
  erythropoiesis and, 508
  fascioliasis and, 549
  life span of, 214
  membrane permeability and, 552
  metabolism and, 545, 546
  morphology and, 360t
Shetland pony(ies), 159
Shift
  to left. *See* Left shift(s)
  to right, 115, *116*, 823
Shift neutrophilia, 692
Shift reticulocyte(s), 501
Shock, 97
  thrombocytopenia and, 483
Sialic acid
  erythrocytes and, 531
  reticulocytes and, 364
Sialoprotein(s), 532
Sickle cell(s), 6, 519-520
  deer erythrocyte and, 275, 321, *321, 322*
  goat, 234
  species variation and, 528
Sickle cell anemia, 519-520. *See also* Sickle cell(s)
Sideroblast(s), 64, 542, XV
  anemia and, 571
  cat with myeloproliferative disorder and, 860
  erythroid precursor and, 495
Siderocyte(s), 64, 495, 542, XII
  cat with myeloproliferative disorder and, 860
  etymology of, 534t
Sideroleukocyte(s), 63-64
Siderosome(s), 582
Silver black fox, 320
Simulium sp., 269
Sinus(es), venous, 25t, 26, *27, 353*, 362
Sinusoid(s), megakaryocytes and, 437
Site(s) of blood collection, 24-26, 25t
Skin window technique of Rebuck, 690, 698-699
SLA. *See* Swine lymphocyte antigen
SLE. *See* Systemic lupus erythematosus
Slide(s), 29, *30*
  care of, 22
Sloth bear(s), 335t, 342
Slow reacting substance of anaphylaxis
  basophils and, 760, 761t
  eosinophils and, 746
SMAF. *See* Specific macrophage arming factor
Smear(s). *See* Blood film(s)
Smoldering leukemia, feline, 867-869, *868*
Snake venom(s), 121
Snow leopard(s), 335t
Sodium, erythrocyte destruction and, 551
Sodium acid phosphate, 643
Sodium chloride solution
  osmotic fragility test and, 70, 70t
  physiologic, 46, 48
Sodium citrate, 1, 2, 24
  avian blood and, 260
Sodium dodecyl sulfate, 532
Sodium pentobarbital
  blood values and, 283
  venous hematocrit and, 94

Sodium pertechnetate, 87
Sodium radiochromate. *See* Radiochromate
Soil contact, pig and, 243
Sol-gel zone(s), platelets and, 451-452
Sorghum vulgare var sudanensis, 642
Sow(s). *See* Pig(s)
Species variation, 5-7
  erythrocytes and, 527-546, *529, 530, 533*, 534t, *535-539. See also* Erythrocyte(s)
Specific collagenase, 714
Specific gravity, babesiosis and, 598
Specific macrophage arming factor, 783
Spectacled bear(s), 342
Spectrin, 532
Spectrophotometry for hemoglobin, 44-45
Sphering in platelet(s), 453
Spherocyte(s), *530, 535, 538*, 543
  anemia and, 570, 648-649, 1010, 1014, *1015*
  autoimmune hemolytic anemia and, 648-649, 1010, 1014, *1015*
  etymology of, 534t
Spherocytosis, autoimmune hemolytic anemia and, 648-649. *See also* Spherocyte(s)
Spheroechinocyte(s), canine, 104
Sphingomyelin, 544-545
Spiculated erythrocyte(s), *536*, 543
  acanthocyte as, 532, 540
Spider monkey(s), 334t
Spiny anteater(s), 275
Spiny mouse(mice), 310-311
Spirochetosis, 270
Spleen(s). *See also* Splenomegaly
  circulating red cell mass and, 94
  contraction of, 7, 97, 189, 575
  cross section of, *376*
  erythrocyte destruction and, 555
  feline mast cell leukemia and, 866
  Heinz body and, 633
  hematopoiesis and, 307-308, 375-379
  horse, 140-142
  leukocyte migration and, 691
  lymphocyte recirculation and, 806
  lymphopoiesis and, 801
  platelets and, 438, 441, 1022
  prenatal and early postnatal hematopoiesis and, 350, 352, 354
  sheep, 214
  splenectomy and. *See* Splenectomy
  splenitis and, 1163-1165
Splenectomy, 6. *See also* Spleen(s)
  Anaplasma ovis and, 596
  anaplasmosis and, 595
  autoimmune hemolytic anemia and, 1017
  autoimmune thrombocytopenic purpura and, 1025
  haemobartonellosis and, 607
  horse, 142-144, 145t
  Howell Jolly bodies and, 6
  infection and, 378
  sheep erythrocyte and, 214
  thrombocytopenia and, 479-480
  thrombocytosis and, 469
Splenic contraction(s), 7
  blood loss and, 97
  fear or excitement and, 189
  polycythemia and, 575
Splenic pool of platelets, 442
Splenitis, 1163-1164
Splenomegaly. *See also* Spleen(s)
  case report of, 1114-1116
  platelets and, 441-442
  thrombocytopenia and, 475, 479-480
Spotted hyena, 335t, 341
Sprague-Dawley rat(s), 293t, 294t, 295t
Springbok, 329, 330t

erythrocyte survival and, 548
Sprue, 972
Spur cell(s), 534, 540, 544-545. *See also* Acanthocyte(s)
   liver disease anemia and, 670
Spur-cell anemia, 544-545
SRA-A. *See* Slow reacting substance of anaphylaxis
Stain(s), 34-36
   avian blood and, 262
   Azure dye, 31
   babesiosis and, 598
   basic principles of, 31
   blood film. *See* Blood film(s)
   brilliant cresyl blue, 62
   determination of overall degree of staining in, 926
   Giemsa, 31-32, 33
   Heinz body and, 63
   haemobartonellosis and, 602
   iron, 64
   methylene blue. *See* Methylene blue
   microfilariae and, 80
   monocytes and, 775-776
   neutral, 32
   neutrophils and, 676-677
   new methylene blue. *See* New methylene blue
   poor staining of, causes and correction of, 34-35
   quick, 34
   reticulocytes and, 62-63
   Romanowsky, 31-35
   sideroleukocytes and, 63-64
   Wright, 31, 32-33
   Wright-Leishman, 33-34
Standardbred horse(s), 149-163. *See also* Horse(s)
   normal values for, 149, 150t
   total plasma proteins and, 160
Staphylococcus (staphylococci). *See also Staphylococcus
     aureus*
   microbicidal activity and, 712
   phagocytosis and, 708, 719
Staphylococcus aureus, 780
   bovine mastitis and, 1076
   heat-labile chemotactic factor and, 699
   superoxide anion and, 710
Starch-gel electrophoresis, 941
Starry sky effect, 876, 882
Steatorrhea, 972
Steer(s). *See* Cattle
Stem cell(s)
   basophils and, 756
   differentiation of, 369t
   hematopoiesis and, 118, 350, 365-368
   monocytes and, 769
   pluripotent. *See* Pluripotent stem cell(s)
Steroid(s). *See* Corticosteroid(s) or steroids
Sticktight flea(s), 584
Stigiformes, 267
Stimulated reticulocyte(s), 501
Stippling
   basophilic, 131, 629
   cat reticulocyte and, 129, 131
   erythrocyte, 630
Stomach
   hematopoiesis and, 381-382
   polyps of, protein loss and, 972
Stomatocyte(s), *535, 537, 539,* 543
Stomatocytic erythrocyte(s), canine, 104
Storage cell(s), 967
Storage pool(s) of leukocytes, 687-689
Streptococcus (streptococci), 707, 1076
Streptococcus agalactiae, 1076
Streptokinase
   fibrinolysis and, 401
   thrombosis and, 418-419, 418t
Streptolysin O, 719
Streptomycin, 478

Stress(es)
   cat, 126, 132, 133t
   eosinopenia and, 750-751
   erythrocytes and, 556
   haemobartonellosis and, 602, 604
   horse, 163, 166-169
   leukocytes and, 11
   neutrophilia and, 692
   pig, 244
   plasma proteins and, 943-944
   sheep, 214
Stress hormone(s), 11
Striped hyena(s), 335t, 341
Strongylus vulgaris, 973
[90]Strontium
   canine hematopoietic disorder and, 883
   swine lymphoma and, 897
Stuart-Prower factor, 395
Subleukemic leukemia, 838, 862, 862t
Substage mirror(s), 22
Suckling pig(s), iron needs of, 243-244
Sudan black B stain. *See also* Sudanophilia
   basophils and, 760
   neutrophils and, 685
   technique for, 933-934
Sudan grass(es), 642
Sudanophilia, 910t, 911t, 921, 933-934. *See also* Sudan
     black B stain
Sulfa drug(s), 719
Sulfhydryl group(s) of membrane proteins, 628
Sulfinpyrazone, 418, 418t
   platelet release reaction and, 462
Superoxide anion(s)
   macrophages and, 780-781
   methemoglobinemia and, 644
   phagocytosis and, 710
Superoxide dismutase
   macrophages and, 780-781
   methemoglobinemia and, 644
   phagocytosis and, 710
Suppressor T cell(s), 798
Surface antigen(s), 796, 797
Surface immunoglobulin(s), 796, 797
Surface phagocytosis, 701
Surface receptor(s), 707, 741-742
   eosinophils and, 741-742
   monocytes and macrophages and, 776-777
   neutrophils and, 707
Surgery, blood loss and, 97
Surra, 612
Swamp buffalo, 329
Swine. *See* Pig(s)
Swine fever, 483
Swine lungworm, 287
Swine lymphocyte antigen, 1002
Syndrome(s)
   Bernard-Soulier, 453
   black-tongue, 659
   Chédiak-Higashi, 197, 317, 318, 453, 717, 719
   Cushing's. *See* Canine Cushing's syndrome
   gray collie, 719
   gray platelet, 453
   Hermansky-Pudlak, 453
   Hurler's, 716, 782
   hyperviscosity, 969-971
   lazy leukocyte, 718
   Loeffler's, 750
   Maroteaux-Lamy, 716
   nephrotic, 974-975
   Wiscott-Aldrich, 453
Systemic lupus erythematosus, 77-79, 1026
   canine, 1027-1029, 1121-1123

T₃. *See* Triiodothyronine
T₄. *See* Thyroxine
T-1824, 92
T cell(s), 790-791
    antibody production and, 807-808
    bird, 259
    characterization of, 795-798
    eosinophilopoiesis and, 740-741
    immune deficiencies and, 978
    immunogenesis and, 374-375
    immunoregulatory influence and, 808
    killer function of, 809
    Kurloff cells and, 288
    lymphokines and, 809
    macrophages and, 782
    migration of, 804
    nonspecific esterase and, 918
    preferential recirculation of, 804
    proliferative response of, 799-800
    thymus and, 264, 801
    viral immunity and, 714
T helper cell(s), 807-808
T suppressor cell(s), 807-808
Tabanus, 595
Taenia hydatigena, 232
Tamarin, 27-28
Target cell(s)
    anemia and, 570
    lipid content and, 544
Tart cell(s), 79
Tayassu sp., 333t
Tayassuidae, 341-342
⁹⁹ᵐTc. *See* Technetium 99m
TdT. *See* Terminal deoxynucleotidyl transferase
Technetium 99m, 87
Temperature(s),
    environmental, hemogram and, 189-190
    erythrocytes and, 543-544
Terminal deoxynucleotidyl transferase, 912t, 921
Terrier(s), Bedlington, 628
Tertiary granule(s), 679
Tetracycline(s)
    anaplasmosis and, 595
    neutrophils and, 719
Tetrahydrofolate, 657-658, *658*
Tetralogy of Fallot
    blood volume and, 95
    polycythemia and, 575, 1108-1109
Texas fever, 596
TG. *See* 6-Thioguanine
Thalarctos maritimus, 335t
Theileria annulata, 610
Theileria mutans, 610, 611
Theileria parva, 610
Theileriasis, 610-612
Thesaurocyte(s), 967
THF. *See* Tetrahydrofolate
Thiamine, 509
Thiamylal sodium, 67
6-Thioguanine, 898, 900
Thoracic duct lymphocyte(s), 805
Thorn test, 64
Thoroughbred horse(s), 149-163. *See also* Horse(s)
    corticosteroids and, 163
    foals of, 144-149
    hematology of, 152t
    normal values for, 149, 150t
    platelet counts and, 159
    serum bilirubin and, 159
    total plasma proteins and, 160
Threshold setting for Coulter Counter, 50
Thrombasthenia, Glanzmann's, 453, 468
Thrombin
    canine platelet and, 121

coagulation and, 395-396
    hemostasis and, 390, 391, 423
    platelets and, 121, 458
Thrombin time, 423
Thrombocyte(s). *See* Platelet(s)
Thrombocythemia, 471-472
Thrombocytopenia, 472-483, 472t, 473t, 474t, *475*, 480.
        See also Thrombocytopenic purpura
    amyloidosis with, 1119-1121
    autoimmune. *See* Autoimmune thrombocytopenia
    bleeding tendency and, 475-476
    disease and, 480-483
    disseminated intravascular coagulation and, 480
    dog, 473t, 474t, *475*, 476-478, 480-481
    drug sensitivity and, 478
    estrogen and, 476-478, 478t, 1100-1102
    hypersplenism and, 479-480
    immune-mediated, 478-479
    induction of, 694
    isoimmune or neonatal, 479, 1004, 1005, 1006
    leptospirosis and, 616
    pig, 250
    platelet transfusion and, 459
    radiation and, 667
Thrombocytopenic purpura. *See also* Thrombocytopenia
    drug sensitivity and, 1113-1114
    idiopathic, 442, 472, 1114-1116
    neonatal pig, 1006
Thrombocytosin, 440
Thrombocytosis, 469-471, 470t, *471*
    iron deficiency and, 583
Thrombocytosis-stimulating factor, 439
Thrombopathia, hereditary, 468
Thromboplastic tissue, 396
Thromboplastin, 421-422, 458
Thromboplastin time, activated partial, 419-420, 421-422
Thrombopoiesis. *See also* Platelet(s)
    acute blood loss and, 580-581
    bird, 364
    factors influencing, 369t
    inhibitors of, 440
    regulation of, 438-441
Thrombopoietin, 439
    inhibitor of, 440
Thrombosis, 415-419
    diffuse intravascular, 410. *See also* Disseminated
        intravascular coagulation
    eosinophils and, 747
    platelets and, 459
Thrombosthenin, 391
Thromboxane
    neutrophil migration and, 692
    platelets and, 455, 461
Thrombus(i), 415. *See also* Thrombosis
Thymectomy, 373-374, 802
Thymic corpuscle(s), 373
Thymic hypoplasia, 979
Thymosin injection, 979
Thymus, 264
    hematopoiesis and, 372, 373-375
    lymphocytes and, 801
    lymphoma and, 848
    prenatal development of dog and, 351
    structure and function of, 373-375
Thymus-dependent and thymus-independent
        lymphocyte, 790. *See also* T cell(s)
Thyroid, dog, 1063-1066
Thyroid hormone(s)
    anemia and, 671
    dog, 1063-1066
    erythropoiesis and, 370
    plasma proteins and, 943
Thyroid-stimulating hormone(s), 1063
Thyroxine, 1063

folate metabolism and, 657
prealbumin and, 947
Tick(s), 270
anaplasmosis and, 595
babesiosis and, 596, 599, 601
ehrlichiosis and, 1066
ixodid, 596
theileriasis and, 610-611
Tiger(s), Bengal, 334t
Tissue culture(s), feline leukemia virus and, 844
Tissue hypoxia
erythropoietin and, 503
sheep hemoglobin and, 215
Tissue injury(ies)
neutrophils and, 712-714
nitrogen loss and, 943
platelets and, 458-459
Tissue macrophage(s), 770-771
Tissue mast cell(s), 757
Titriplex IV, 24
Toluidine blue, 262
Torocyte(s), *535*, *537*, *543*
etymology of, 534t
Total leukocyte count(s). *See* Leukocyte count(s)
Total plasma protein(s). *See* Plasma protein(s)
Total Solids meter, 56, *56. See also* Refractometer(s)
Toxemia(s)
bacterial, 836
cattle, 195
granulopoiesis in, 1133, 1136
leukopenias and, 836
pyometra and, 1140-1142
Toxic granule(s), 16, 679
cattle, 195
horse, 158, 169
neutrophils and, 715
Toxic monocyte(s), 778
Toxic neutrophil(s), 715, 836
cattle, 195
dog, 115, VIII
horse, 1158-1160
in perforation of rectum, 1158-1160
Toxicity. *See also* Toxemia(s)
chloramphenicol, 137-138
drug. *See* Drug(s)
lead. *See* Lead poisoning
nitrate, 642
phenothiazine, 633-634, 1152-1153
water, 185, 650-651
Toxin(s). *See* Endotoxin(s)
Toxoplasma gondii, 62, XIV
Toxoplasmosis, 62, XIV
case report of, 1137-1138
TPNH. *See* Triphosphopyridine nucleotide, reduced
Tr antigen, 991, 992, 995-996
Tranquilizing drug(s)
toxicity of, 633-634, 1152-1153
venous hematocrit and, 94
Transcobalamin, 657
Transfer of maternal immunoglobulin, 979-981
Transfer factor, 810
Transferrin, 948
iron transportation and, 582
mucosal, 582
reticulocytes and, 364
Transfusion(s), 993-996
anemia and, 572, 649t, 650, 1010, *1011*, 1017
cross-matching blood for, 71-72, 951
plasma, 408, 996
haemobartonellosis and, 606
hemolytic reactions and, 74, 994-995
horse blood and, 71-72
leukocyte antibodies and, 1003
nitroblue tetrazolium reduction and, 115

platelet, thrombocytopenia and, 459
precautions for, 995-996
reactions to, 74, 994-995
Transfusion reaction(s), 74, 994-995
Transient hypogammaglobulinemia, 982
Transient microcytosis in cat, 127
Transit, cell
bone marrow and, 362-364
granulopoiesis and, 686-687, 687t
neutrophil, 433, *435*
Transitional macrophage(s), 774
Transmigration of neutrophils, 433, *435*
Transmission of infection in transfusions, 995
Transplantation, bone marrow, 1006-1007
cyclic hematopoiesis and, 118
histocompatibility antigens and, 1003
Transplantation antigen(s), 998, 1003-1004
Trapped plasma, 92
cattle hematocrit and, 188
goat erythrocyte and, 225, 229t
Trauma
erythrocyte sedimentation rate and, 56
tissue, 943
Traumatic pericarditis, 1076t
Traumatic reticulitis in cattle
hemogram and, 1076t
dehydration and, 1164-1165
neutrophilia and lymphocytosis in, 1163-1164
Trichinella spiralis, 740-741, 744, 749
Trichinosis, 740-741, 743-746, 749
Trichlorethylene poisoning, 481, 483
Trichostrongyloidosis, 585,
anemia and, 671
cattle, 585, 1165, 1167
plasma proteins and, 973
Trichostrongylus, 585, 973
Triglyceride metabolism, 764
Triiodothyronine, 1063
prealbumin and, 947
Triphosphopyridine nucleotide, reduced, 546
Tritiated thymidine
granulocytes and, 686-687, 689, 690t
lymphocytes and, 799, 802, 803
Trophozoite(s), 597
Tropical canine pancytopenia. *See also* Ehrlichiosis
plasma proteins and, 976
thrombocytopenia and, 480-481
Trypanosoma congolense, 483
Trypanosoma cruzi
eosinophils and, 744
neutrophils and, 714
Trypanosoma theileri
eosinophils and, 744
immune deficiency and, 981
neutrophils and, 714
Trypanosoma vivax, 483
Trypanosomiasis, 612-615, *613*
eosinophils and, 744
immune deficiency and, 981
neutrophils and, 714
plasma proteins and, 973
thrombocytopenia and, 483
Trypsin, 806
Tryptophan, 659
TS meter. *See* Total Solids meter
TSF. *See* Thrombocytosis-stimulating factor, 439
TSH. *See* Thyroid-stimulating hormone
TT. *See* Thrombin time
Tuftsin, 708
Tumor(s). *See also* Malignancy(es); Neoplasia(s)
armed macrophages and, 783-784
iron deficiency anemia and, 581
metastasis and, 460
new methylene blue stain and, 62

Turbidity, plasma, 11
Turkey(s), 267, 270
TxA₂, 461
Type D retrovirus, 982
Type I hypersensitivity reaction, 954
Typing reagent(s) for blood, 993

Ulcerative colitis
    erythrogenesis and, 123
    protein loss and, 972
Ultrastructure
    Babesia bovis, 597
    erythrocytes and, 491-495, *491-494*
    Haemobartonella canis, 606
    neutrophils and, 677-682
    Paranaplasma and, 594-595, *594*
Uncia, 340-341
Unclassified cell(s), 15
Uncompensated hemolytic anemia, 589
Uniconcavity, 528, *529*
Unicytopenia, 665
Unipotential progenitor cell(s), committed, 367-368
Unipotential stem cell(s), 365-366
Unit(s) of measurement value, 2, 3
Unopette method
    avian leukocytes and, 261-262
    for blood dilution, 48, *49*
    for cell counting, 48-49, *49*
    platelet and, 65
Uremia
    dog, 669-670, 1090, 1091, 1092-1093
    neutrophils and, 719
    platelet disorder and, 467
Urinary antiseptic(s)
    cat hemolytic anemia and, 131
    Heinz bodies and, 638
Urine
    bacillary hemoglobinuria and, 617-618, 618t
    erythropoietin in, 504
    leptospirosis and, 617
Urobilinogen, 571
Urokase, 401. *See also* Urokinase
Urokinase
    fibrinolysis and, 401
    thrombosis and, 418-419, 418t
Uroporphyrin, 516
Uroporphyrinogen III, 514
Ursidae, 342

V antigen, 992
Vaccine(s)
    leukemia complex and, 899
    for Marek's disease, 267
Vacuole(s)
    monocyte cytoplasm and, 119
    neutrophils and, 715
Vacutainer(s), 1, 2, 23, 26
Vaginal smear(s), 62
Van den Bergh test, 160, 523
Vascular endothelium
    arachidonic acid metabolism and, 455
    lymphocytes and, 804-805
    neutrophil adherence to, 700-701
    platelet aggregation and, 460
Vascular sinus(es), 25t, 26, 27, *353*, 362
Vascular sinusoid(s), 437
Vasoactive substance release, 763
Vector(s), tick. *See* Tick(s)
Velban. *See* Vinblastine
Venipuncture(s), 26
Venoject tube(s), 23
Venom, 121, 423

Venous hematocrit, 94
Venous sinus(es), 25t, 26, 27, *353*, 362
Very low-density lipoprotein(s), 950-951
Vesper mouse(mice), 310-311
Vessel(s)
    severing of, 389
    wall injury of, *390, 391*
Vicuna(s), 336-337
Vinblastine, 898
    leukocyte movement and, 700
    platelets loaded with, 1025
Vinca alkaloid(s),
    neutrophils and, 719
Vincristine, 898, 899, 900
    autoimmune thrombocytopenic purpura and, 1024-1025
    leukocyte movement and, 700
    platelets loaded with, 1025
    systemic lupus erythematosus and, 1029
    thrombocytosis and, 440
Viral arteritis, 830
Viral diarrhea, bovine. *See* Bovine viral diarrhea
Viral diseases. *See* Virus(es)
Virus(es), 829-830
    bird neoplasias and, 264-268, 265t
    bovine diarrhea. *See* Bovine viral diarrhea
    bovine leukemia, 884-886
    canine lymphoproliferative disorders and, 869
    feline infectious peritonitis. *See* Feline infectious
        peritonitis
    feline leukemia. *See* Feline leukemia virus
    feline panleukopenia and, 1071
    hemolytic anemia and, 618-619
    leukemia, 843-844
    leukocyte response and, 827
    leukopenias and, 829-830
    lymphopenia and, 812
    monocytes and macrophages and, 779-780
    neutrophils and, 714, 719
    Newcastle disease, 215
    ovine lymphoma and, 895-896
    panleukopenia, 981, 1071
    phagocytosis and, 707
    pig, 483, 897
    plasma proteins and, 975-976
    thrombocytopenia and, 473, 475, 481
Virus particle(s), 844, *845*
Visceral organ(s) in myeloproliferative disorders of cat,
    855t
Viscosity test, DNA, 67-69, *68*, 69t
Vitamin(s), erythrocyte production and, 509. *See also*
        specific vitamin
Vitamin A, 509
Vitamin B₂, 509
Vitamin B₆, 509
Vitamin B₁₂, 658
    deficiency of, 16-17, 716
    erythropoiesis and, 509
    hematopoiesis and, 381
    neutrophils and, 716
Vitamin C
    folate metabolism and, 657
    vitamin deficiency anemia and, 660
Vitamin D, 407-408
Vitamin E
    erythropoiesis and, 509
    neutrophils and, 719
    pig, 244
    vitamin deficiency anemia and, 660-661
Vitamin K
    coagulation factor synthesis and, 397-398
    thrombus and, 417
Volume(s), blood. *See* Blood volume(s)
von Willebrand's disease, 402-403, 403t, 405-406, 406t